High Risk Pregnancy

Management Options

High Risk Pregnancy

Management Options

Edited by

D.K. JAMES, MA, MD, FRCOG, DCH
P.J. STEER BSc, MD, FRCOG
C.P. WEINER MD, FACOG
B. GONIK MD, FACOG

W. B. SAUNDERS COMPANY LTD
London · Philadelphia · Toronto · Sydney · Tokyo

W. B. Saunders Company Ltd 24–28 Oval Road
London NW1 7DX, England

The Curtis Center
Independence Square West
Philadelphia, PA 19106–3399, USA

Harcourt Brace & Company
55 Horner Avenue
Toronto, Ontario M8Z 4X6, Canada

Harcourt Brace Jovanovich & Company Australia
30–52 Smidmore St
Marrickville, NSW 2204, Australia

Harcourt Brace & Company Japan Inc.
Ichibancho Central Building, 22–1 Ichibancho
Chiyoda-ku, Tokyo, 102, Japan

A catalogue record for this book is available from the British Library.

ISBN 0 7020 1575 X

Editorial and Production Services by Fisher Duncan
10 Barley Mow Passage, London W4 4PH

Typeset by Photo·graphics, Honiton, Devon
Printed and bound in Great Britain by The Bath Press, Avon

Contents

Contributors

L. D. Allan MD
Professor of Fetal Cardiology,
Department of Paediatrics,
Columbia Presbyterian Medical School,
630 West 168th Street,
New York,
NY10032, USA

H. Albar MD
Maternal and Fetal Medicine Division,
735 Notre Dame Avenue,
Women's Hospital, WR-120,
Winnipeg, Manitoba,
Canada R3E 0LR

S. Arulkumaran MD
Associate Professor,
Department of Obstetrics and Gynaecology,
National University Hospital,
Lower Kent Ridge Road,
Singapore 0511

T. Asrat MD
Staff Perinatologist,
Long Beach Memorial Women's Hospital,
2801 Atlantic Avenue,
Long Beach, CA 90801,
USA

D. Ware Branch MD
Department of Obstetrics/Gynecology,
University of Utah Medical Center,
50 North Medical Drive,
Room 2B200,
Salt Lake City,
UT 84132, USA

J. P. Brettes MD
Centre Hospitalier Regional et Universitaire de
Brest,
Hôpital Augustin Morvan,
Service de Gynecologie Obstetrique,
29609 Brest Cedex,
France

F. A. Chervenak MD
Director of Obstetrics and Maternal Fetal Medicine,
Department of Obstetrics and Gynecology, M-036
New York Hospital/Cornell Medical Center,
525 East 68th Street,
New York, NY 10021, USA

W. H. Clewell MD
Director, Fetal Medicine and Surgery,
Division of Perinatology,
Phoenix Perinatal Associates,
and Good Samaritan Hospital,
1111 E McDowell Road,
Phoenix,
AZ 85006, USA

D. B. Cotton MD
Department of Obstetrics and Gynecology,
Hutzel Hospital,
4707 St Antoine Boulevard,
Detroit, MI 48201,
USA

T. A. Cowles MD
Department of Obstetrics and Gynecology,
University of Kansas Medical Center,
3901 Rainbow Blvd,
Kansas City, KS 66160, USA

C. A. Crowther MD
Department of Obstetrics and Gynaecology,
The University of Adelaide,
Adelaide,
South Australia 5000

P. J. Danielian MD
Department of Obstetrics and Gynaecology,
West London Hospital,
Hammersmith Road,
London W6 7DQ, UK

P. C. Dennen MD
60 Westwood Avenue,
Waterbury,
CT 06708,
USA

J. E. Dickinson MB BS FRACOG
King Edward Memorial Hospital for Women,
374 Bagot Road,
Subiaco WA 6008,
Australia

M. I. Evans MD
Center for Fetal Diagnosis and Therapy,
Department of Obstetrics,
Gynecology & Molecular Biology & Genetics,
Wayne State University/Hutzel Hospital,
4707 St Antoine,
Detroit, MI 48201, USA

N. M. Fisk PhD FRACOG MRCOG DDU
Royal Postgraduate Medical School,
Institute of Obstetrics and Gynaecology,
Queen Charlotte's and Chelsea Hospital,
Goldhawk Road,
London W6 0XG, UK

S. G. Gabbe MD
Professor,
Department of Obstetrics and Gynecology,
Ohio State University College of Medicine,
Fifth Floor, Means Hall,
1634 Upham Drive,
Columbus, OH 43210-1228, USA

L. C. Gilstrap III MD
Professor of Obstetrics and Gynecology,
Division of Maternal–Fetal Medicine,
The University of Texas, Southwestern Medical
Center at Dallas,
5323 Harry Hines Blvd,
Dallas TX 75235, USA

Y. Giovangrandi MD
Centre Hospitalier Regional et Universitaire de
Brest,
Hôpital Augustin Morvan,
Service de Gynecologie Obstetrique,
29609 Brest Cedex,
France

B. Gonik MD
Professor and Director of Maternal-Fetal Medicine,
Department of Obstetrics/Gynecology, and
Reproductive Sciences
University of Texas Health Science Center,
The Medical School at Houston,
6431 Fannin, Suite 3·204,
Houston, TX 77030, USA

M. G. Gravett MD
Emanuel Hospital and Health Center,
Department of Obstetrics and Gynecology,
2801 N Gantenbein Avenue,
Portland OR 97227, USA

D. R. Griffin MRCOG
Consultant in Obstetrics and Gynaecology,
Watford General Hospital,
Vicarage Road,
Watford,
Herts WD1 8HB, UK

C. Harman MD
Director, Fetal Assessment Unit,
Maternal and Fetal Medicine Division,
735 Notre Dame Avenue,
Women's Hospital, WR-120,
Winnipeg, Manitoba,
Canada R3E 0LR

E. P. Hoffman PhD
University of Pittsburgh School of Medicine,
Department of Molecular Genetics and Biochemistry,
Biomedical Science Tower,
Pittsburgh, PA, USA

R. H. Hayashi MD
Women's Hospital,
Room L 3228,
1500 East Medical Center Dr,
Ann Arbor ME 48109-0264, USA

W. Holzgreve MD
Zentrum für Frauenheilkunde,
Westfälische Wilhelms-Universität,
Albert-Schweitzer-Strasse 33,
D48129 Münster,
Germany

J. Hutton MD
Professor of Obstetrics and Gynaecology,
Department of Obstetrics and Gynaecology,
PO Box 7343,
Wellington South,
New Zealand

G. Isaacson MD
Department of Obstetrics and Gynecology,
M-036, New York Hospital/Cornell Medical Center,
525 East 68th Street,
New York, NY 10021, USA

N. B. Isada MD
Center for Fetal Diagnosis and Therapy,
Department of Obstetrics and Gynecology &
Molecular Biology & Genetics,
Wayne State University/Hutzel Hospital,
4707 St Antoine,
Detroit, MI 48201, USA

D. James MA MD FRCOG DCH
Professor of Feto-Maternal Medicine,
University Department of Obstetrics and
Gynaecology,
C Floor East,
Queen's Medical Centre,
Nottingham NG7 2UH, UK

R. D. Jelsema MD
Department of Maternal-Fetal Medicine,
Butterworth Hospital,
100 Michigan Street,
NE Grand Rapids MI 49503-2560, USA

M. P. Johnson MD
Center for Fetal Diagnosis and Therapy,
Department of Obstetrics & Gynecology &
Molecular Biology and Genetics,
Wayne State University/Hutzel Hospital,
4707 St Antoine,
Detroit, MI 48201, USA

C. T. C. Kennedy MA FRCP
Consultant Dermatologist,
Department of Dermatology,
Bristol Royal Infirmary,
Bristol BS2 8HW, UK

J. C. Konje MD
Lecturer/Registrar,
University Department of Obstetrics and
Gynaecology,
St Michael's Hospital,
Southwell Street,
Bristol BS2 8EG, UK

M. B. Landon MD
Assistant Professor,
Department of Obstetrics and Gynecology,
Division of Maternal-Fetal Medicine,
Ohio State University College of Medicine,
1654 Upham Drive,
Columbus, OH 43210, USA

E. A. Letsky MB BS FRC Path
Consultant Haematologist,
Queen Charlotte's Hospital for Women,
Goldhawk Road,
London W6 0XG, UK

B. B. Little MA PhD
Associate Professor of Obstetrics and Gynecology,
Division of Prenatal Diagnosis and Clinical
Genetics,
University of Texas,
Southwestern Medical Centre,
5322 Harry Hines Road,
Dallas TX 75235, USA

L. Littmann RDMS
Center for Fetal Diagnosis and Therapy,
Department of Obstetrics and Gynecology &
Molecular Biology & Genetics,
Wayne State University/Hutzel Hospital,
4707 St Antoine,
Detroit, MI 48201, USA

I. Z. Mackenzie MA MD FRCOG
Consultant Obstetrician and Gynaecologist,
Nuffield Department of Obstetrics and Gynaecology,
John Radcliffe Maternity Hospital,
Headington,
Oxford OX3 9DU, UK

C. A. Major MD
Assistant Professor
Department of Obstetrics and Gynecology,
University of California at Irvine,
101 City Drive So,
Orange, CA 92668, USA

F. Manning MD
Maternal and Fetal Medicine Division,
735 Notre Dame Avenue,
Women's Hospital, WR-120,
Winnipeg, Manitoba,
Canada R3E 0LR

M. Maresh MD
Consultant Obstetrician,
St Mary's Hospital for Women and Children,
Whitworth Park,
Manchester,
M13 0JH, UK

S. E. Meagher BSc, MB MRCOG, MRCPI
Fellow in Fetal Medicine,
Maternal-Fetal Medicine Unit,
Monash Medical Centre,
Clayton Campus,
246 Clayton Road,
Clayton 3168,
Victoria, Australia

S. Menticoglou MD
Maternal and Fetal Medicine Division,
735 Notre Dame Avenue,
Women's Hospital, WR-120,
Winnipeg, Manitoba,
Canada R3E 0LR

P. Miny MD
Institut für Humangenetik der Westfälischen
Wilhelms,
University of Münster,
D-4400 Münster,
Germany

B. Morgan MB ChB FCAnaes
Department of Anaesthesia,
Institute of Obstetrics and Gynaecology,
Queen Charlotte's and Chelsea Hospital,
Goldhawk Road,
London W6 0XG, UK

I. Morrison MD
Maternal and Fetal Medicine Division,
735 Notre Dame Avenue,
Women's Hospital, WR-120,
Winnipeg, Manitoba,
Canada R3E 0LR

M. P. Nageotte MD
Medical Director,
Women's Hospital,
Memorial Medical Center,
2801 Atlantic Avenue,
Long Beach CA 90801, USA

K. Neales MD
St Mary's Hospital for Women and Children,
Whitworth Park,
Manchester M13 0JH, UK

J. G. Pastorek II, MD FACOG, FACS
Department of Obstetrics and Gynecology,
Louisiana State University,
1542 Tulane Avenue,
New Orleans, LA 70112-2822, USA

Z. J. Penn MB MRCOG
Academic Department of Obstetrics and
Gynaecology,
Charing Cross and Westminster Medical School,
Chelsea and Westminster Hospital,
369 Fulham Road,
London SW10 9NH, UK

M. Pillai MD
Consultant Obstetrician,
Directorate of Obstetrics,
Gynaecology and ENT,
St Michael's Hospital,
Southwell Street,
Bristol BS2 8EG, UK

M. Ramsay MA MD MRCOG
Fetomaternal Medicine Fellow,
Department of Obstetrics and Gynaecology,
Queen's Medical Centre,
Nottingham NG7 2UH, UK

P. A. Ramsay MRACOG
Registrar,
Department of Fetal Medicine,
King George V and Royal Prince Alfred Hospitals,
Missenden Road,
Camperdown,
Sydney, NSW 2050, Australia

J. S. Robinson MD
Professor of Obstetrics and Gynaecology,
Department of Obstetrics and Gynaecology,
The Queen Victoria Hospital,
160 Fullarton Road,
Rose Park,
South Australia 5067

S. K. Rosevear MD
Lecturer/Senior Registrar,
University Department of Obstetrics and
Gynaecology,
St Michael's Hospital,
Bristol BS2 8EG, UK

A. Saleh MD
Department of Obstetrics and Gynecology,
Wayne State University,
4707 St Antoine Blvd,
Detroit, MI 48201, USA

J. E. Sampson MD
Department of Obstetrics and Gynecology,
Brigham and Women's Hospital,
75 Francis St,
Boston, MA 02115, USA

B. Savage MD
Clinical Instructor,
Department of Obstetrics and Gynecology,
Ohio State University College of Medicine,
Fifth Floor, Means Hall,
1654 Upham Drive,
Columbus, OH 43210-1228, USA

P. J. Schubert MD
Fellow in Maternofetal Medicine,
Assistant Professor,
Department of Obstetrics and Gynecology,
Ohio State University College of Medicine,
Fifth Floor, Means Hall,
1654 Upham Drive,
Columbus, OH 43210-1228, USA

C. O. Slocumb MD FACOG
Active Candidate in the American Board of
Obstetrics and Gynecology and the Division of
Maternal-Fetal Medicine of the American Board;
Director Perinatology Center,
Summit Medical Center,
350 Hawthorne Avenue,
Oakland, CA 94609, USA

J. Smoleniec MD
RCOG Fetal Medicine Fellow,
University Department of Obstetrics and
Gynaecology,
St Michael's Hospital,
Bristol BS2 8EG, UK

P. W. Soothill MD
Senior Lecturer/Consultant,
Fetal Medicine Unit,
Department of Obstetrics and Gynaecology,
University College London Medical School,
86 Chenies Mews,
London WC1E 6HX;
and Institute of Child Health,
30 Guilford Street,
London WC1E, UK

P. J. Steer BSc MD FRCOG
Academic Department of Obstetrics and
Gynaecology,
Charing Cross and Westminster Medical School,
Chelsea and Westminster Hospital,
Fulham Road,
London SW10 9NH, UK

D. K. Still MD
Associate Professor,
Department of Obstetrics and Gynecology,
1D1 Walter C. Mackenzie Health Sciences Centre,
University of Alberta,
Edmonton, Canada T6G 2R7

G. Stirrat MD
Professor of Obstetrics and Gynaecology,
University Department of Obstetrics and
Gynaecology,
St Michael's Hospital,
Southwell Street,
Bristol BS2 8EG, UK

P. Stone MD
Senior Lecturer,
Department of Obstetrics and Gynaecology,
Wellington School of Medicine,
PO Box 7343,
Wellington,
New Zealand

J. Streltzoff MD
Department of Obstetrics and Gynecology,
M-036, New York Hospital/Cornell Medical Center,
525 East 68th Street,
New York, NY 10021, USA

J. M. Svigos MB BS FRCOG FRCAG
124 Sturt Street,
Adelaide 5000,
South Australia

M. de Swiet MD
Consultant Physician,
Royal Postgraduate Medical School,
Institute of Obstetrics and Gynaecology,
Queen Charlotte and Chelsea Hospital,
Goldhawk Road,London W6 0XG, UK

G. Turner FRCOG
Professor of Obstetrics and Gynecology,
National Women's Hospital,
Claude Road,
Epsom, Auckland,
New Zealand

R. Vigneswaran MD
124 Sturt Street,
Adelaide 5000,
South Australia

R. J. Walley MD
Professor of Maternal and Child Health,
St Clare's Mercy Hospital,
St John's,
Newfoundland,
Canada A1C 5B8

B. N. J. Walters MD
Clinical Senior Lecturer in Obstetric Medicine,
King Edward Memorial Hospital for Women,
Bagot Road,
Subiaco,
Western Australia 6008, Australia

R. Warwick MD
Queen Charlotte's Hospital for Women,
Goldhawk Road,
London W6 0XG, UK

C. P. Weiner MD
Professor of Obstetrics and Gynecology,
Department of Obstetrics and Gynecology,
Director, Maternal Fetal Medicine,
University of Iowa College of Medicine,
200 Hawkins Drive,
Iowa City IA 52242-1080, USA

M. J. Whittle MD FRCOG FRCP (Glas)
Professor of Fetal Medicine,
Birmingham Maternity Hospital,
Edgbaston,
Birmingham B15 2TG, UK

H. I. J. Wildschut PhD
Academic Medical Centre,
Department of Obstetrics and Gynaecology,
9 Meibergdreef,
1105 AZ Amsterdam,
The Netherlands

R. A. Williamson MD
Department of Obstetrics and Gynecology,
University of Iowa Hospitals and Clinics,
Iowa City,
IA 52242-1080, USA

Preface

This new international textbook in obstetrics will, we believe, be of major value to all practising clinicians, be they trainees or established in practice.

It aims to assist with the questions: How do I manage this patient? or How do I perform this procedure?

It presents a wide range of reputable management options. Unlike many traditional texts, based on a single individual's experience and view, all the contributors to each section were asked to give their preferred management in all areas of their section. Each resulting chapter reflects that wide range of acceptable practice. This means you will have a *choice* about which option or combination of options suits you and your patient.

This book is designated to be practical. It addresses those difficult questions which arise in practice, which often stem not only from the medical facts, but from the constraints of time, facilities, finance, and patient acceptability. Moreover, we have standardized the presentation of each topic as far as possible (while still allowing the personality of the original authors to shine through!) to enable the reader to become familiar with the format.

We have deliberately chosen a panel of contributors who are both leaders in their field and who can represent practice in the USA, Europe and Australasia and this we feel gives the text a unique universality.

Finally it is our intention that the book is comprehensive. We hope that we will have something to say on all the important problems you come across. If you find any exceptions, please let us know, with your comments, in time for the next edition.

D. K. James
P. J. Steer
C. P. Weiner
B. Gonik

1

Prepregnancy Education

GILLIAN TURNER

INTRODUCTION

In Utopia, preparation for conception, pregnancy, parturition and parenthood would be part of general education from childhood, so that every pregnancy would be planned and the parents would be at the peak of health, both mentally and physically. Indeed, in Newfoundland, Canada, School Boards in the province have 'family life programs' in elementary and high schools which emphasize the importance of a healthy lifestyle, and develop awareness of reproductive responsibility and health. General health education is sadly fragmented, underfunded and unsuccessful in many countries and frequently it is not until a woman is actually pregnant that the opportunity arises for further education.

Pregnancy provides the opportunity to impart information of all sorts, the audience is captive and the majority motivated. It is also an opportunity to screen. But is it the appropriate time? It is certainly an opportunistic time, but any individual can only retain a small part of the information given, and do changes in lifestyle have any real impact on the current pregnancy? The major improvement in pregnancy outcome has resulted from improvements in the socioeconomic and nutritional status of the previous generation.

Life skills and healthy living habits need to be inculcated from childhood to have an effect and not rushed into in pregnancy or just prepregnancy, although some good may result. The socioeconomically deprived, poorly educated, smoking, 'junk food consuming' population at greatest risk of poor pregnancy performance is the very group least likely to seek advice prepregnancy, to attend regularly when pregnant, to heed advice or change habits. Financial inducements may be what is needed here.

Healthy living habits encompass not only nutrition and exercise, but also stress management and work patterns. More and more women are in paid employment for their own survival and that of their family unit, their income being an essential contribution. Governments vary in their provision of maternity benefits and increasingly women find themselves continuing to work through much if not all of their pregnancy. Is this harmful? Does harm depend on the type of occupation, level of stress, degree of mental or physical exhaustion? And what harm may result? These questions have received scant attention and advice is usually given empirically by physicians, midwives and carers using common sense and experience as their guides.

With regard to high risk pregnancy, prepregnancy education assumes particular importance, since interventions may provide the opportunity to influence and decrease the risk.

Doctors are not renowned as educators and often criticized as poor communicators so the question of who is the most effective educator needs to be addressed. Initially parents and teachers can be very effective, then information sources are legion with the media playing a major role. A pre-pregnancy counselor needs to be informed, enthusiastic, dedicated and skilful but not necessarily medically qualified.

Smoking, alcohol and drug dependence are the subject of Chapter 5 and will not be detailed here except to say that advice to abstain during pregnancy if the dependence is not going to be eradicated totally is vital for all pregnancies, not just those at high risk.

NUTRITIONAL PREPARATION FOR PREGNANCY

Risks

General

History-taking in the antenatal clinic usually includes a question such as 'do you eat a normal diet?' The reply 'yes' is duly recorded, yet exactly what the respondent means by a normal diet may be very different from what is regarded as a diet suitable for normal pregnancy.

The main nutritional disorder in the affluent industrialized world is obesity, whereas in the developing world malnutrition is the major life hazard for mother, fetus and infant. The main risks to the obese mother relate to impaired glucose tolerance and gestational diabetes and the difficulties inherent in monitoring the progress of pregnancy and labor in the very obese, with the attendant anesthetic and operative complications. The fetus is also at risk because of difficulties in assessing fetal well-being because of maternal obesity.

Malnutrition is a cause of anemia in the mother with its associated problems, and intrauterine growth deficiency as sequela for the fetus; though this problem is rarely seen in developed countries. Hytten[1] analysed the components of weight gain in pregnancy and estimated that the pregnant woman should consume an extra 350 kcal per day and if the diet is well balanced it will contain more than the 8.5 g of extra protein, carbohydrate and fat that is necessary. Undernutrition in pregnany in women of low socioeconomic status is associated with the delivery of low birthweight (<2500 g) infants.[2]

Vitamins

Hytten[3] draws attention to vulnerable groups such as Asian women who spend much time indoors and whose calcium absorption may be impaired by an excess of wholemeal cereals in the diet and who therefore should have vitamin D supplements.

Vitamin deficiency is associated with fetal abnormalities, and that there is strong evidence for an association between maternal vitamin status and pregnancy outcome is generally accepted.[4] Neural tube defects comprise a significant proportion of severe congenital malformations, but there are problems demonstrating exactly the deficiency of which vitamin or vitamins are implicated. Pregnative Forte F® (Bencard), a preparation containing folic acid, ascorbic acid and riboflavin, together with vitamins A and D, thiamine, pyridoxine and nicotinamide, has been given periconceptually to women who have previously delivered an infant with a neural tube defect. These women have a significant risk of an affected child in a subsequent pregnancy. Smithells et al.[5,6] and Sheppard et al.[7] found a significant effect of vitamin supplementation, although the study designs are criticized and the results reviewed with scepticism by others.[8] Current advice for women who have had an affected infant is to take folic acid or Pregnavite Forte F® periconceptually and for the first trimester. This advice has been extended in some prepregnancy clinics to those at greater risk of congenital abnormalities, e.g. diabetic women. Many women have decided, in view of the paucity of side-effects and possible benefits, to take periconceptual folic acid and or multivitamins.

Minerals

The extra requirement for calcium in pregnancy is about 30 g, a minute proportion of the mother's skeletal calcium and easily obtained from a normal diet without extra milk or dairy products.[3] Routine iron supplementation, although apparently 'correcting' the physiological hematological changes of pregnancy, may in fact do harm, increasing red cell size and blood viscosity, reducing uteroplacental blood flow. This has been proposed as the mechanisms for the observed increase in low birthweight babies when the mother has been supplemented.[9] There is no good evidence that most pregnant women are deficient in zinc ('the new cult metal'[3]) and universal supplementation may do harm.[10]

Management Options

Prepregnancy advice, if given at all, is usually:

- avoid alcohol

- stop smoking

- eat a healthy diet.

In pregnancy, the same advice applies. Dietary improvement in the form of financial support is available in some countries to mothers on social assistance. In many countries, vitamin supplements are either bought over the counter or physician prescribed, but in most cases these are unnecessary. The patient with known diabetes or impaired glucose tolerance or previous gestational diabetes should be seen for specific prepregnancy counseling and this is the subject of Chapter 19.

Improved nutrition for all would probably make little impact on pregnancy outcome in affluent countries, but improved nutrition in the developing world if sustained for two generations would have major beneficial effects on reproductive performance.

More precise enquiry is required to ascertain just how often fruit and fresh vegetables are eaten (and how the latter are cooked), how much fibre is eaten, the source and amount of protein and how much fat is eaten. This sort of information could be obtained in the form of a questionnaire, but the population at greatest risk of malnutrition is also the one to respond poorly to a questionnaire.

The general advice for the pregnant woman is very similar to that for the non-pregnant woman:

- eat a well-balanced diet

- low in salt and saturated fats

- high in fibre, fruit and fresh vegetables

- with more white meat and fish than red meat

- dairy products in moderation

- little alcohol and caffeine.

Pregnant women should beware undercooked meats and eggs, avoid patés and soft cheeses, wash all produce thoroughly and pay attention to kitchen hygiene.[11] Vitamin and mineral supplements are not substitutes for healthy eating and are unnecessary if a well-balanced diet is taken. True deficiences and anemia must be identified, proven and corrected by appropriate supplementation. Periconceptual folic acid may be taken empirically, or prescribed specifically for those who have delivered infants with neural tube defects.

Healthy eating is not necessarily expensive and dieticians should be urged to devise low-cost, budget-conscious healthy eating plans presented in attractive leaf-

---

PREPREGNANCY EDUCATION: NUTRITION
Summary of Management Options

Risks

Malnutrition

For obesity the risks include:

- Gestational diabetes

- Hypertension

- Monitoring difficulties

For the undernourished the risks include:

- Fetal growth retardation

- Anemia

Vitamin deficiency

For folic acid deficiency there is a risk of:

- Neural tube defects

Management options

Take a detailed dietary history

Supplementation if a high-risk group:

- Vegan (iron and vitamin supplementation)

- Inappropriate diets (e.g. no fruit or vegetables) (improve intake of specific deficiency)

- Ethnic groups lacking sunlight (vitamin D)

- Highly parous (general) improvement in nutritional status

- Previous infant with a neural tube defect (folic acid, 5 mg daily; or Pregnavite Forte F®, one tablet daily)

Healthy balanced diet for all

lets for distribution at prepregnancy and pregnancy clinics, since the socioeconomically deprived are those at greatest risk. Some countries produce nutritional guidelines.[11,12]

Identification of specific groups at risk (vegans, Asians, the malnourished, the highly parous, those who have had an infant with a neural tube defect) for targeted supplementation is important.

EXERCISE AND STRESS

Risks

Regular exercise is urged as part of healthy living but little if any enquiry about exercise levels is made during routine history-taking at the antenatal clinic. It is usually the pregnant woman who initiates the enquiry, asking if she can continue with her particular physical activity.

There is a wealth of experimental animal data[13,14] relating to exercise and pregnancy which is not directly applicable to humans, since there are species differences in the physiological mechanisms concerned among other things. Human studies on exercise during pregnancy are currently limited. Severe physiological adaptations due to pregnancy are similar to those occurring in non-pregnant women due to strenuous exercise. For instance, a regular exercise program expands blood volume, as does pregnancy. Clapp[15] suggests that several of the physiological adaptations to pregnancy and to exercise actually complement one another and in turn modify the thermal, hemodynamic and metabolic changes induced by exercise; modifications which ultimately protect the conceptus.

The potential risks of exercise to the mother depend on several factors.[16] Her general physical condition, her expertise at the particular exercise, the type of exercise, environment and time spent exercising all have to be considered. Certain anatomical changes such as the increased laxity of ligaments, particularly of the pelvic and sacroiliac joints, the increased lumbar lordosis and weight gain may make exercise more difficult and perhaps dangerous.[17]

There is an increased risk of back strain and musculoskeletal injury, especially if there is a prior history of such problems. Joints loosened by the effects of relaxin in pregnancy[18] may be subjected to increased stress from weight-bearing activities such as jogging. It is apparent from several studies[19–21] that in most women pregnancy modifies exercise performance so that the amount of physiological and anatomical stress is reduced as the pregnancy advances. The pregnancy itself regulates the exercise level as women find exercise of many forms uncomfortable and tiring and their performance is reduced.

Potential risks to the fetus include hyperthermia, hypoxia, intrauterine growth deficiency and increased uterine activity associated with preterm labor. There are, in addition, potential problems for the fetus associated with barometric pressure changes experienced at high altitudes or under water. Sky diving and scuba diving are to be avoided in pregnancy.

A rise in the mother's core body temperature, as would occur in a sauna, could raise maternal lactate levels, which in turn could increase fetal lactate levels,[22] but there is no empirical evidence to support this theoretical concern. However, maternal hyperthermia has been shown to increase the risk of fetal abnormalities in animals and in human studies.[23,24] In very early gestation when the tissue mass is small, a rise in temperature is likely to have the most significant effect, whereas in later pregnancy substrate delivery and changes in the hormonal milieu caused by altered blood flow are most important to fetal growth and maturation.[15] Physiological adaptations such as the decreased peripheral resistance, increased skin temperature and increased heat loss, and the 40% increase in maternal blood volume which transfers heat from the fetus protect against hyperthermia.

Artal et al.[25] found an association between increased uterine activity and exercise during pregnancy, and Clapp and Dickstein[26] an association between exercise in pregnancy and prematurity and low birthweight. But a more detailed study[27] cast doubt on these findings and refuted any such direct relationship. Pommerance et al.,[28] Hauth et al.[29] and Collings et al.[30] all carried out various studies looking at measures of obstetric outcome and none found any detrimental effects of exercise.

Indeed, there are positive benefits to the mother who exercises. She has better cardiorespiratory function and therefore less breathlessness and lower blood pressure. Also labors are shorter and deliveries are easier. These findings are coupled with higher self-esteem and confidence.[31] Clapp,[15] in a more recent review, found that fit women who continue regular running or aerobics throughout pregnancy have a significant reduction in fetal distress as evidenced by meconium staining, abnormal fetal heart rate, cord entanglement and an Apgar score of less than 7 at 1 min. Also the women delivered 7 days earlier on average than those who did not exercise and their offspring had less body fat than control offspring of the non-athletes, and this accounted for 70% of the observed 300 g reduction in birthweight in the exercisers' offspring.

Management Options

Exercise prescriptions should ideally be individualized.[32] The pregnant woman should continue the physical activity to which she is accustomed and at the level at which her body response is comfortable. She

PREPREGNANCY EDUCATION   5

PREPREGNANCY EDUCATION: EXERCISE
Summary of Management Options

Risks   **Benefits**

Maternal   *Maternal*

- Injury   • Improved cardiovascular function

- Tiredness   • Lower blood pressure

- (due to lax joints, altered posture   • Improved self-esteem and confidence
  Increased weight)
                                              • Easier labor and delivery

Fetal   **Management options**

- Hyperthermia   • Moderation

- Dehydration   • Non-aerobic

- Growth retardation   • Non-weightbearing

- Hypoxia   • Supervised

- Preterm labor   • Comfortable and enjoyable

                                              • Avoid
                                                · hyperthermia
                                                · dehydration
                                                · high altitude
                                                · hyperbaric pressures

---

should not 'go for the burn', become dehydrated, overheated or exhausted. She must remember the relative laxity of her joints, her altered posture, sense of balance and centre of gravity. If she 'listens to her body', she will be aware of these changes.

Moderate non-aerobic exercises are safe and will improve health during pregnancy; indeed, they are to be encouraged. Moderate aerobic exercises are likewise of benefit to the experienced but should probably be avoided if there are complications such as hypertension, multiple pregnancy, cardiorespiratory compromise, antepartum hemorrhage or preterm labor. Non weightbearing exercise such as swimming is preferable to weightbearing exercise like jogging and any exercise in the supine position is to be avoided.[16] Exercise at high altitude, sky diving and underwater diving should be avoided, as should water skiing.[33]

Supervision of exercise before and during pregnancy by qualified, nationally certified fitness instructors is to be encouraged and opportunities for such should ideally be provided by prepregnancy and antenatal clinics. At least clinic staff and family practitioners should know where such supervised activities are available and offer advice accordingly.

WORK AND PREGNANCY
Risks

In answer to the question 'What work do you do?', many housewives will reply 'I don't work', assuming paid employment is meant. In its guidelines on work in pregnancy, the American College of Obstetricians and Gynecologists (1977) made no mention of housework and child care, although toddlers are heavy weights to lift and many household chemicals are toxic. Hours are long and there is no time off. The effects of work depend on the physical requirements of the job, the general environment in which the job is done and in certain instances on specific exposures related to the job. As Lumley and Astbury[34] point out, much confusion arises from regarding paid employment as a single category; most women in paid employment carry out housework as well, and what is regarded as housework varies vastly from culture to culture.

There has been concern that work will lead to growth-deficient infants and preterm labor, but studies in the UK and Europe have failed to confirm this. In 1976, a national survey was carried out in France involving 3218 women who delivered in that year, 61% of whom worked during pregnancy. Saurel and Kaminski,[35] reviewing these data, found there was no relationship between employment and growth deficiency or mean birthweight. Indeed, intrauterine growth retardation and preterm delivery appeared to be less common in those who worked. Similarly, analyzing data from the 1958 British Perinatal Mortality Survey, Peters et al.[36] found that the hours worked even in pregnancy have no influence on growth deficiency at term or on the incidence of preterm delivery. Likewise, Murphy et al.,[37] studying data from the Cardiff Births Survey 1964–1979 relating to the effect of work in 20 613 married primigravidae, found that the non-employed group had a greater number of preterm deliveries, low birthweight babies and higher perinatal mortality.

In his review, Jewell[38] emphasizes that paid work for women is a very heterogeneous entity and that for many the housework they do in addition will be more physically demanding than their paid employment. He also urges care in the interpretation of studies relating to work, since the 'healthy worker effect' must be considered – that is, that employment selects a group of women who are already at low risk because of their health.

In contrast, Tafari et al.[39] studied 130 women attending antenatal clinics in Addis Ababa. Housework in this culture, including grinding grain and carrying heavy loads of water long distances, was deemed light if domestic help was available. Heavy work included housework with no help and physical labor outside the home. They found that those carrying out light work delivered babies with a mean weight of 3270 g, compared with 3068 g for those born to women involved in heavy work. However, another factor in this study was that overall food intake was below World Health Organization recommendations and the women delib-erately further restricted their intake in the last trimester to ensure smaller babies.

Specific work hazards

There are recognized specific work hazards related to certain occupations about which advice should be given, although identification of specific industrial hazards is a difficult epidemiological problem. Leck[40] expands on this problem and reviews the criteria for determining a teratogen.

Concern has been expressed about emissions from visual display units (VDUs), but Blackwell and Chang[41] have concluded that there is no evidence that working with VDUs is associated with increased pregnancy loss. Peters et al.[36] found that there was an increase in anencephaly and spina bifida in those working with glazes in the pottery and glass industry, and an increase in perinatal mortality in those working in the dry cleaning and laundry industry. Attention to the increased miscarriage rate among anesthetists and those working in operating theaters was first drawn by Tomlin.[42] Subsequently, Vessey and Nunn[43] reviewed the subject and advised that women wishing to become pregnant should avoid contaminated environments even though the introduction of scavenging systems in operating theaters has probably removed the hazard.

Management Options

It would appear that in general there are no detrimental effects of paid employment on pregnancy, a conclusion reached by Garcia and Elbourne[44] and Chamberlain.[45] Advice, however, has to be individualized and the adviser in the prepregnancy clinic needs to ascertain precisely the details of the woman's activities in the home, at work and the journey between before suggestions are made.

There are benefits from working that must not be forgotten – job satisfaction, self-esteem and confidence not least among these. Also, the income helping toward financial peace of mind will in most instances be greatly missed and not compensated for by maternity benefit and child care allowance when work stops. The advice to stop work should not be given lightly and not without ascertaining the financial problems this might cause, which might subsequently be reflected in the type of food purchased.

Specifically, chemical hazards are of increasing concern in the home and workplace but the number of chemicals proven to be teratogenetic is low. Women may be advised to discuss their worries with their Health and Safety Officer or seek advice from the central office of the Health and Safety Executive.

General advice given before and during pregnancy

should include: avoiding the smoking canteen and greasy food at lunchtime and taking a walk in the park with a wholemeal sandwich and fruit instead; altering hours to avoid peak travel times; changing duties to avoid heavy lifting if possible; and ensuring at least 8 h rest at night. Employment at home and in the workplace may continue for as long as the woman wishes, provided she and her baby remain well.

PREPREGNANCY EDUCATION: WORK
Summary of Management Options

Risks

- Specific

- Chemicals (rare)

- Gases (should be minimized with scavenging systems)

- Radiation

  Note: No proof that work in general has an effect on fetal growth or preterm labor

  VDUs appear to be free from radiation risk, though adverse effects on posture, etc., still possible

Benefits

- Financial

- Satisfaction, confidence and self-esteem

Management options

- Detailed history
  - avoid adverse factors, e.g. smoke-filled environment, rare specific risks
  - avoid excess lifting/exercise

- Continue with work if woman wishes this and is not unduly tired.

CONCLUSION

A healthy lifestyle does not guarantee a successful outcome to pregnancy, but it is ideally a goal to be set for all from childhood. Advice in prepregnancy clinics for the healthy woman and those at risk on the subjects of nutrition, exercise and work needs to be individualized. It is most likely to be effective when it is given in knowledge of the woman's current situation, attitudes, wishes and understanding of these matters.

In general, the pregnant woman should eat a healthy balanced diet which will provide all the nutrients, vitamins and minerals required for pregnancy; supplementation is reserved for identified groups at particular risk. She should be encouraged to continue moderate exercise in whatever form she enjoys, is competent at and is comfortable doing while pregnant. She may continue to work for as long as she wishes and is comfortable.

REFERENCES

1 Hytten F (1980) Nutrition. In Hytten F, Chamberlain G (eds) *Clinical Physiology in Obstetrics*, pp. 163–192. Oxford: Blackwell Scientific.
2 Crawford MA, Doyle W, Craft IL *et al.* (1986) A comparison of food intakes during pregnancy and birthweight in high and low socioeconomic groups. *Progress in Lipid Research* **25**:249–254.
3 Hytten F (1990) *Midwifery* **6**:93–98.
4 Cockcroft DL (1991) Vitamin deficiences and neural tube defects: Human and animal studies. *Human Reproduction* **6**:148–157.
5 Smithells RW, Sheppard S, Schorah CJ, Seller MJ, Nevin NC, Harris R, Read AP, Fielding DW (1981) Apparent prevention of neural tube defects by periconceptional vitamin supplementation *Archives of Diseases of Childhood* **56**:911–918.
6 Smithells RW, Nevin NC, Sellar MJ, Sheppard S, Harris R, Read AP, Fielding DW, Walker S, Schorah CJ, Wild J (1983) Further experience of vitamin supplementation for prevention of neural tube defect recurrences. *Lancet* **i**:1027–1031.
7 Sheppard S, Nevin NC, Sellar MJ, Wild J, Smithells RW, Read AP, Harris R, Fielding DW, Schorah CJ (1989) Neural tube defect recurrence after 'partial' vitamin supplementation. *Journal of Medical Genetics* **26**:326–329.
8 Wald NJ, Polani PE (1984) Neural tube defects and vitamins: The need for a randomised clinical trial. *British Journal of Obstetrics and Gynaecology* **91**:516–523.
9 Mahomed K, Hytten FE (1989) Iron and folate supplementation. In Chalmers I, Enkin M, Keirse M (eds) *Effective Care in Pregnancy and Childbirth*, pp. 301–307. Oxford: Oxford University Press.
10 Hytten FE (1985) Do pregnant women need zinc supplements? *British Journal of Obstetrics and Gynaecology* **92**:873–874.
11 Department of Health (1991) *While You are Pregnant:*

Safe Eating and How to Avoid Infection from Food and Animals. London: HMSO.

12 *Canadian Food Guide* (1988) Department of National Health and Welfare. Ottawa: Federal Government of Canada publication.

13 McMurray RG, Katz VL (1989) Thermoregulation in pregnancy. Implications for exercise. *Sports Medicine* **10**(3):146–158.

14 Lotgering FK, Gilbert RD, Longo LD (1985) Maternal and fetal responses to exercise during pregnancy. *Physiological Reviews* **65**:1–36.

15 Clapp JF (1991) Exercise and fetal health. *Journal of Developmental Physiology* **15**:9–14.

16 Wolfe LA, Hall P, Webb KA, Goodman L, Monga M, McGrath MJ (1989) Prescription of aerobic exercise during pregnancy. *Sports Medicine* **8**(5):273–301.

17 Joseph J (1991) The bones, joints and ligaments of the female pelvis. In Philipp E, Setchell M, Ginsburg J (eds) *Scientific Foundations of Obstetrics and Gynaecology,* Vol. 7, pp. 74–83. Oxford: Butterworth-Heinemann.

18 Calguneri M, Bird HA, Wright V (1982) Changes in joint laxity occurring during pregnancy. *Annals of Rheumatic Disease* **41**:126–128.

19 Clapp JF, Wesley M, Sleamaker RH (1987) Thermoregulatory and metabolic responses to jogging prior to and during pregnancy. *Medicine and Science in Sports and Exercise* **19**:124–130.

20 Cohen GC, Prior JC, Vigna Y, Pride SM (1989) Intense exercise during the first two trimesters of unapparent pregnancy. *The Physician and Sportsmedicine* **17**:87–94.

21 Clapp JF, Capeless EL (1990) Neonatal morphometrics following endurance exercise during pregnancy. *American Journal of Obstetrics and Gynecology* **163**:1805–1811.

22 Hytten FE (1984) The effect of work on placental function and fetal growth. In Chamberlain G (ed.) *Pregnant Women at Work*, pp. 15–25. London: Royal Society of Medicine.

23 Smith DW, Clarren SK, Harvey MA (1978) Hyperthermia as a possible teratogenic agent. *Journal of Pediatrics* **92**:878–883.

24 Miller P, Smith DW, Shephard TH (1978) Maternal hyperthermia as a possible cause of anencephaly. *Lancet* **i**:519–521.

25 Artal R, Platt LD, Sperling M, Kammula RK, Jilek J, Nakamura R (1981) Exercise in pregnancy: Maternal cardiovascular and metabolic responses in normal pregnancy. *American Journal of Obstetrics and Gynecology* **140**:123–127.

26 Clapp JF, Dickstein S (1983) Maternal exercise performance and pregnancy outcome. In *Abstracts of the Thirteenth Annual Meeting of the Society for Gynecological Investigation*, Washington, 195, p. 104.

27 Veille JC, Hohimer AR, Burry K, Speroff L (1985) The effect of exercise on uterine activity in the last eight weeks of pregnancy. *American Journal of Obstetrics and Gynecology* **151**:727–730.

28 Pommerance JJ, Gluck L, Lynch VA (1974) Physical fitness in pregnancy: Its effect on pregnancy outcome. *American Journal of Obstetrics and Gynecology* **119**:867–876.

29 Hauth JC, Gilstrap LC, Widmern K (1982) Fetal heart rate reactivity before and after maternal jogging during the third trimester. *American Journal of Obstetrics and Gynecology* **142**:545–547.

30 Collings CA, Curet LB, Mullin JP (1983) Maternal and fetal responses to a maternal aerobic exercise program. *American Journal of Obstetrics and Gynecology* **145**:702–707.

31 Wallace AM, Boyer DB, Dan A *et al.* (1986) Aerobic exercise, maternal self esteem and physical discomforts during pregnancy. *Journal Nurse Midwife* **31**:255–262.

32 Jarski RW, Trippett DL (1990) The risks and benefits of exercise during pregnancy. *Journal of Family Practice* **30**(2):185–189.

33 Tweedale PG (1973) Gynecological hazards of water-skiing. *Canadian Medical Association Journal* **108**:20–22.

34 Lumley J, Astbury J (1989) Advice for pregnancy. In Chalmers I, Enkin M, Keirse KJNC (eds) *Effective Care in Pregnancy and Childbirth*, pp. 237–254. Oxford: Oxford University Press.

35 Saurel MJ, Kaminski M (1983) Pregnant women at work. *Lancet* **i**:475.

36 Peters TJ, Adelstein P, Golding J, Butler NR (1984) The effects of work in pregnancy: Short- and long-term associations. In Chamberlain G (ed.) *Pregnant Women at Work*, pp. 87–104. London: Royal Society of Medicine.

37 Murphy JF, Dauncey M, Newcombe R, Garcia J, Elbourne D (1984) Employment in pregnancy: Prevalence, maternal characteristics, perinatal outcome. *Lancet* **i**:1163–1166.

38 Jewell D (1990) Prepregnancy and early pregnancy care. In *Ballière's Clinical Obstetrics and Gynaecology,* **4**(1):1–23. London: Ballière Tindall.

39 Tafari N, Naeye RL, Gobezie A (1980) Effects of maternal undernutrition and heavy physical work during pregnancy on birth weight. *British Journal of Obstetrics and Gynaecology* **87**:222–226.

40 Leck I (1983) Fetal malformation. In Baron SL, Thomson AM (eds) *Obstetrical Epidemiology*, pp. 263–318. London: Academic Press.

41 Blackwell R, Chang A (1988) Video display terminals and pregnancy: A review. *British Journal of Obstetrics and Gynaecology* **95**:446–453.

42 Tomlin PJ (1979) Health problems of anaesthetists and thier families in the West Midlands. *British Medical Journal* **i**:779–784.

43 Vessey MP, Nunn JF (1980) Occupational hazards of anaesthesia. *British Medical Journal* **281**:696–698.

44 Garcia J, Elbourne D (1984) Future research on work in pregnancy. In Chamberlain G (ed.) *Pregnant Women at Work*, pp. 273–287. London: Royal Society of Medicine.

45 Chamberlain G (1992) Work in pregnancy. In *ABC of Antenatal Care*, pp. 27–30. London: British Medical Journal.

2

Genetic Counseling

DAVID JAMES

DEFINITION OF GENETIC COUNSELING

Genetic counseling is the process whereby patients or relatives at risk of a disorder that may be hereditary are advised of the consequences of the disorder, the probability of developing and transmitting it and of the ways in which this may be prevented or ameliorated.

PROVISION OF GENETIC COUNSELING SERVICES

The range of professionals who provide genetic counseling is varied. While all developed countries have clinical geneticists, often supported by a team of nurse counselors, these experts are relatively small in numbers. They may only be found in tertiary referral centers. It is clear that in practice, therefore, for many women requiring genetic counseling, this service is provided by other professionals including obstetricians, pediatricians, family doctors, perinatal pathologists, radiologists, nurses, midwives, cytogeneticists and social workers.

The confidence and degree to which an obstetrician will provide genetic counseling will vary with training, experience, special interests and local availability of counseling resources. However, most obstetricians feel able to and do provide counseling on chromosomal abnormalities and many of the more common Mendelian conditions. They generally feel less able to provide more than superficial information about syndromes and organ/system anomalies, preferring to refer the case to a clinical geneticist.

GENETIC COUNSELING: GENERAL

It is important that in providing counseling for genetic disorders, adequate time is allowed and also that the setting for the consultation is quiet and free of disturbance. Depending on the nature of the problem, it may be advisable for the obstetrician to arrange a separate consultation away from the routine prenatal clinic.

Obtaining Information

The first requirement in providing genetic counseling is to obtain accurate and complete information. The aim is to construct a family tree for the specific condition. The agreed notation for this exercise is shown in **Figure 1**. In obtaining this information, the following points are important.

- Ensure that miscarriages, stillbirths and neonatal deaths are not omitted and that any postmortem information available is documented.

- Directly ask whether consanguinity exists (especially important for autosomal recessive conditions).

- Illegitimacy may explain discrepancies in what otherwise is a logical explanation for a family pedigree.

- Take detailed information about both sides of the family and not just the apparently affected side.

- Administrative issues such as recording dates of birth, maiden names and addresses should not be forgotten.

- Affected individual(s) should always be examined by an expert and, if necessary, investigated to confirm the diagnosis.

- Apparently unaffected individuals should also be assessed to exclude mild or early disease.

- All documented information about the condition should be obtained (specialists' letters, results of laboratory or necropsy investigations, treatments, etc.).

Calculating Risks

Once the comprehensive information has been obtained, the clinician is then in a position to estimate and convey to the individual or family the risks for the development of a particular disorder. However, the method of obtaining a risk estimate is not the same for every condition and the reliability of such a derived figure varies. The four main types of risk estimate are summarized in **Table 1**.

Counseling About Risks

It is important to judge the best way in which the information should be presented to the individual(s). Some

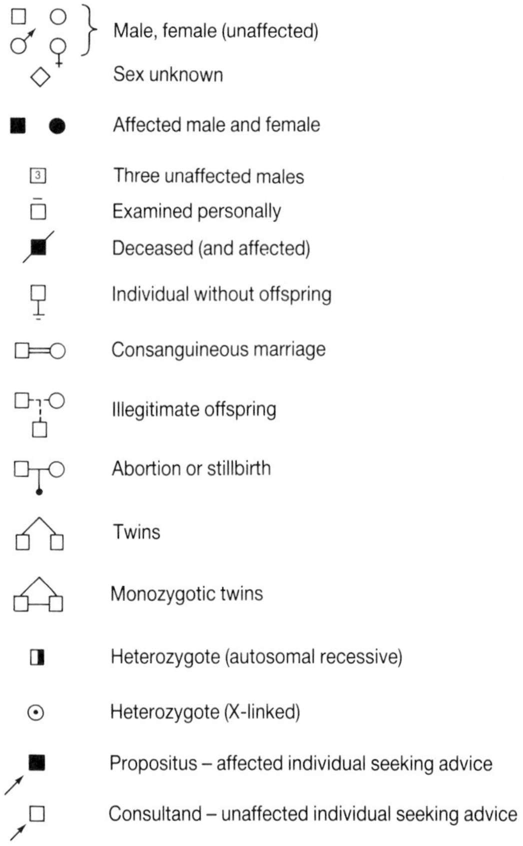

Figure 1. Symbols conventionally used for constructing a family pedigree.

are unable to grasp anything more complex than 'high' or 'low' risk, while others require a precise risk figure and even a detailed discussion about mode of inheritance and mechanisms of genetic disease. Giving risk information in the form of probabilities or odds has the advantage that it is less likely to lead to confusion – the perception of what constitutes 'high' or 'low' risk

Table 1
Types of risk estimation

Risk type	Characteristics	Examples
Empiric	Risk based on observed data; reliable provided population studied and data collection unbiased	Most non-Mendelian or chromosomal disorders
Mendelian	Only applicable to disorders with Mendelian inheritance; clear risk predictions	Mendelian disorders
Modified	Underlying/background risk is modified by additional clinical or laboratory-based information	1. Huntingdon's disease and a man's age 2. Down's syndrome and maternal AFP and HCG
Composite	Where a genetic condition is inherited in different ways and pattern not clear in an individual, an intermediate risk is given as a 'compromise'	Osteogenesis imperfecta

varies with the individual. In conveying risk figures, some clinicians prefer odds, others percentages. It is often necessary to choose the method which seems best for the counselee(s). If a clinician is accustomed to using or has data for a specific condition that is in the form of percentage risk, it is important that he or she makes no mistakes in converting the figure to odds. Thus for a particular disorder:

if percentage risk = x%, then odds risk = 1 in 100/x

The decision as to what constitutes an 'acceptable' risk will vary with the disorder and the individual. However, providing some reference points may be helpful. Some useful examples are given in **Table 2**.

It is important that the counseling should be non-directive. The role of the counselor is to ensure that those whom he or she counsels have fully understood the facts and then to allow them to make their own decisions. It is not easy to be totally non-directive, of course, since one's own views often affect the tone and manner of presentation of the information. Nevertheless, non-directive counseling should be the aim. There is no 'right' or 'wrong' decision in general, rather a couple must make a decision which will be 'right' for their given situation.

COUNSELING FOR CHROMOSOMAL ABNORMALITIES

General

Many chromosomal disorders and their clinical manifestations have been described; however, they gener-

Table 2
Examples of approximate reproductive risks for comparative counseling

Reproductive outcome	Risk	
	Odds	%
Pregnancy ending in spontaneous miscarriage	1:6	16.7
Infertility in a couple	1:10	10.0
Birth of baby with some form of congenital abnormality (major and minor)	1:30	3.3
Perinatal death	1:30 to 1:100	3.3–1.0
Birth of baby with serious physical or mental disability	1:50	2.0
Death of child in first year after the first week	1:150	0.7

These are approximate risks and are for 'developed' countries.

ally have an extremely low risk of recurrence in a family.

Modern cytogenetics techniques can distinguish all 23 pairs of human chromosomes from each other, recognizing fine detail within each chromosome. There is an agreed terminology for the reporting of karyotypes.

- The first figure reports the total number of chromosomes (e.g. 46, 45, 47).

- The next notation is the sex chromosome complement (e.g. XX, XY, XO).

- The final reported information is any abnormalities within chromosomes. In this context, 'p' refers to the short arm of a chromosome, 'q' refers to the long arm of a chromosome, 't( )' refers to a translocation between the chromosomes indicated within the brackets.

Thus '45,XY.t(14q,22q)' denotes a male karyotype with a balanced translocation between the long arms of chromosomes 14 and 22; and '46,XX,5p-' denotes a female karyotype with a deletion of the short arm of chromosome 5. If in any doubt, obstetricians should discuss the report with their cytogenetics laboratory.

Frequency

The frequency of chromosomal abnormalities depends on the source of information. Typical examples which are useful for counseling are given in **Table 3**.

Trisomy 21

Approximately 95–98% of Down's syndrome cases are due to trisomy 21 (the remaining 2–5% are due to translocations involving chromosome 21; see below). It is the most important chromosomal disorder with a population incidence of about 1 in 650 live births. There is a well-known, though often misinterpreted, relationship with maternal age. The great majority of cases arise from non-disjunction in the mother. **Table 4** and **Table 5** give the risks for chromosomal abnormalities according to age. However, when providing information about the risks of trisomy 21, it must be made clear whether the data relate to risks at the start of the second trimester ('at amniocentesis') or at delivery. The risks when providing counseling during the first trimester prior to possible chorion villus sampling are also probably slightly different from the 'amniocentesis' and 'delivery' figures; however, at present, there are no reliable comparable data for use in that situation.

Table 3
Frequency of chromosomal abnormalities[1,2]

Source	Frequency
General population	
All chromosome abnormalities	6.6‰
Autosomal trisomies	1.7‰
trisomy 21	1.5‰ LB
trisomy 18	0.12‰ LB
trisomy 13	0.07‰ LB
Outer autosomal abnormalities	0.4‰
Sex chromosome abnormalities	
in phenotypic males	3.0‰
in phenotypic females	1.8‰
XXY (Klinefelter's syndrome)	2.0‰ LB
45,X (Turner's syndrome)	0.4‰ LB
XYY syndrome	1.5‰ LB
XXX syndrome	0.65‰ LB
Spontaneous miscarriages and stillbirths	
Spontaneous miscarriages	
all chromosomal abnormalities (trisomies 52%, 45X 18%, triploidy 17%)	50%
up to 12 weeks	60%
12–20 weeks	20%
Stillbirths	5%

LB = live births.

When a couple have had prenatal diagnosis which confirms a fetus with trisomy 21 in the current pregnancy, further counseling is necessary. Before undertaking the investigation, the risks of the procedure, the likelihood of finding an abnormality and the response to the diagnosis of an abnormality should have been covered. Nevertheless, it is possible that there may have been a change of heart once a diagnosis is 'real'. For example, a woman may have been expecting a reassuring result and given very little thought to the implications of the alternative, including termination of pregnancy. Thus it is imperative that time is allowed for further counseling, if necessary involving other professional colleagues such as pediatricians, nurse counselors and social workers. Some basic information which might be helpful in this process is provided in **Table 6** (for more detailed texts, see Further Reading).

If a couple have had one child with trisomy 21, their risk of another affected child is increased over the normal population risk. The risk of Down's syndrome recurring (both 'at amniocentesis' and 'at delivery') is approximately 1 in 200 for women under the age of 35 and twice the normal age-specific risk from 35 upwards. The risk for all chromosome abnormalities in such a couple is approximately twice the Down's risk. There is no apparent increased risk for second-degree or more distant relatives. There are very few data concerning the risks related to the rare occurrence of an

Table 4
Risk of Down's syndrome in relation to maternal age (live births)[3]

Maternal age at delivery (years)	Risk
15	1:1578
16	1:1572
17	1:1565
18	1:1556
19	1:1544
20	1:1528
21	1:1507
22	1:1481
23	1:1447
24	1:1404
25	1:1351
26	1:1286
27	1:1208
28	1:1119
29	1:1018
30	1:909
31	1:796
32	1:683
33	1:574
34	1:474
35	1:384
36	1:307
37	1:242
38	1:189
39	1:146
40	1:112
41	1:85
42	1:65
43	1:49
44	1:37
45	1:28
46	1:21
47	1:15
48	1:11
49	1:8
50	1:6

individual with trisomy 21 having a child. Such affected individuals rarely reproduce. An empiric and very approximate risk of 1 in 3 of having a child with trisomy 21 has been quoted for females with the condition themselves.

Other Viable Autosomal Trisomies[13,18]

These are rare as live births in comparison with trisomy 21. There is an increased risk with advancing maternal age (see **Table 5**). When diagnosed prenatally, the same management considerations concerning counseling and discussed above under trisomy 21

Table 5
Risk of chromosomal abnormalities
at amniocentesis[4]

Maternal age (years)	Rate per 1000 cases				
	Trisomy 21	Trisomy 18	Trisomy 13	XXY	All anomalies
35	3.9	0.5	0.2	0.5	8.7
36	5.0	0.7	0.3	0.6	10.1
37	6.4	1.0	0.4	0.8	12.2
38	8.1	1.4	0.5	1.1	14.8
39	10.4	2.0	0.8	1.4	18.4
40	13.3	2.8	1.1	1.8	23.0
41	16.9	3.9	1.5	2.4	29.0
42	21.6	5.5	2.1	3.1	37.0
43	27.4	7.6		4.1	45.0
44	34.8			5.4	50.0
45	44.2			7.0	62.0
46	55.9			9.1	77.0
47	70.4			11.9	96.0

apply (see **Table 6**). There are very few reliable data about recurrence risks, but the figures for the more common Down's syndrome discussed above can be used.

Non-viable autosomal trisomies are very common in spontaneous miscarriages. If such an abnormality is found when karyotyping is undertaken on miscarriage material, there are no data to clarify whether that constitutes an increased risk of recurrence in a future pregnancy and also whether prenatal diagnosis using invasive and potentially dangerous procedures is justified. It may be best to individualize the management by explaining the uncertain implications of the diagnosis and the risks of invasive procedures but to support the

woman's/couple's decision. If the material used was from a late miscarriage or a stillbirth, then the livebirth data are probably more appropriate for use.

Sex Chromosome Abnormalities

The more common features of these conditions are summarized in **Table 7**. Recurrence in a family is exceptional for any of these disorders; however, many women/couples will wish prenatal diagnosis.

Chromosomal Translocations

There are two types of translocations:

- Robertsonian, where a piece or all of one chromosome is transferred on to another;

- non-Robertsonian (reciprocal), where there has been an exchange of chromosome material between two chromosomes but with the total number of chromosomes unchanged.

In either case, if the total amount of chromosome material is normal, then the translocation is 'balanced' and the individual will be phenotypically normal. If, however, there is an excess or a deficiency in the normal amount of chromosome material, then the translocation is 'unbalanced' and this is likely to have an effect either by producing a syndrome, miscarriage, stillbirth or infertility depending on the chromosomes involved.

Table 6
Autosomal trisomies: more common clinical features

	Trisomy 21	Trisomy 18	Trisomy 13
Syndrome	Down's	Edwards'	Patau's
Intelligence	IQ 25–50	Grossly retarded	Grossly retarded
Fertility	Boys, infertile; girls, subfertile	Not relevant	Not relevant
Other problems	Hypotonia, brachycephaly, microcephaly, typical facies and hands; cardiac 40%, emotional 13%	Growth retarded, typical facies, hands and feet; cardiac >50%, renal 10–50%, bowel 10–50%	Holoprosencephaly; seizures; typical hands, feet, facies; neural >50%, cardiac 80%, renal 30%
Prognosis	Tone improves with age; development slows with age; growth-impaired; cardiac defects = main cause of early death	Fetal death common; death after birth: 1 month = 30%, 2 months = 50%; 10% survive 12 months (severe retardation)	Fetal death common; death after birth: 1 month = 44%, 6 months = 69%; 18% survive 12 months (severe retardation)

Table 7
Sex chromosome disorders: more common clinical features

	Chromosome constitution			
	XXY	XYY	45X	XXX
Syndrome	Klinefelter's	XYY	Turner's	Triple X
Phenotypic sex	Male	Male	Female	Female
Gonads	Atrophic testes	Normal	Streak ovaries	Normal (usually)
Fertility	Infertile	Fertile	Infertile	Fertile
Intelligence	Normal or slightly reduced	Normal (usually)	Normal (usually)	Reduced (usually)
Behavioral problems	Sometimes	Sometimes	No	Sometimes
Other problems	Hypogonadism	Tall, acne	Short, web neck, coarctation	

When an unbalanced translocation is identified in association with abnormality, miscarriage or fetal death, the parents' karyotypes should be documented. If the parents have totally normal chromosomes, then the recurrence risk is low. If one of the parents has a balanced translocation, then the risks of recurrence are as summarized in **Table 8**.

Table 8
Risks in a future pregnancy where a parent has a balanced translocation

Balanced translocation in one parent	Risks
D-D group translocation (usually 13/14)	Common translocation; low risks for problems in future pregnancy
Translocation involving chromosome 9	30% risk of unbalanced defect in pregnancy
Other translocations: the risks of other translocations are similar and can be illustrated by the Down's translocations:	
14/21 and 21/22 translocations	2.5–10% risk of Down's offspring; remaining offspring will have either a normal karyotype or a balanced translocation; monosomy 21 is lethal and rarely results in a documented pregnancy
21/21 translocation	100% risk of Down's offspring

Other Chromosomal Abnormalities

Rearrangement of genetic material is recognized by chromosomal banding techniques. When the rearrangement is confined to one arm of a chromosome, there may not be any risk of abnormality in the offspring. However, if the centromere is involved, this will cause problems during meiosis and an unbalanced chromosome complement may be formed. The data available for predicting risk are scanty. If an abnormal child has been born and the inversion is shown to be familial, then the risks are probably comparable with those for translocations (see above). Where it appears to be an incidental finding, prediction of risk is more difficult. Discussion with the cytogenetics laboratory and involvement of a clinical geneticist is advisable. Pericentric inversions of chromosome 9 are common and are probably normal variants.

Chromosomal mosaicism occurs when an individual's tissues/organs contain more than one genetic line of cells. The phenotype will lie somewhere between the full disorder and normal. Accurate figures for the prediction of risk in the offspring of individuals with chromosome mosaicism are not available. Placental mosaicism with a chromosomally normal fetus is a well-recognized phenomenon and is discussed in Chapters 36 and 40.

Loss of part of a chromosome (deletion) can result in a range of abnormalities, some of which are summarized in **Table 9**. Similarly, the new banding techniques and DNA probes have shown minor but consistent chromosome abnormalities in disorders not previously thought to have a cytogenetic defect. Some examples are given in **Table 10**. In these disorders, not all individuals manifest the chromosome abnormality.

Hereditary fragile sites can occur on several chromosomes. On cytogenetic examination, they give the

Table 9
Syndromes associated with chromosome deletions

Chromosome abnormality	Syndrome	Features
4p monosomy	Wolf-Hirschhorn	Characteristic facies, frontal bossing, microcephaly, hypospadias
5p monosomy	Cri-du-chat	Hypertelorism, characteristic cry
Trisomy 8 mosaicism		Craniofacial dysmorphism, everted lower lip, plantar furrows
18p monosomy		Round facies, dental defects, micrognathia
18q monosomy	Depressed mid-face, large fingertips, genital anomalies	
21q monosomy		Small eyes, high forehead, aplastic nasal bridge

Table 10
Genetic disorders associated with minor chromosomal abnormalities

Condition	Chromosome
Prader-Willi syndrome	15q
Angleman syndrome	15q
DiGeorge syndrome	22q
Langer-Giedon syndrome	8q
Retinoblastoma	13q
Wilms' tumor with aniridia	11p
Anorectal atresia with ocular coloboma	22 extra fragment
Miller-Dieker syndrome	17p
Chondrodysplasia punctata (one form)	Xq

appearance of breakage at a specific point. On autosomes they are harmless, occurring only in the heterozygous state. However, on the X chromosome, the occurrence of a fragile site near the end of the long arm is consistently associated in males with a syndrome of X-linked mental retardation and macrorchidism.

COUNSELING FOR CONDITIONS WITH MENDELIAN INHERITANCE

General

An important consideration when assessing a family for a particular condition is whether the disorder is inherited in a Mendelian fashion. This is achieved usually by a combination of the clinical diagnosis and the pedigree. If it is Mendelian inheritance, then precise risks of recurrence can be quoted. If it is not or if the mode of inheritance is not clear, then further information must be ascertained before erroneous predictions are made on premature conclusions.

It is also important to ascertain whether for a given condition there is the possibility of laboratory investigations to permit carrier detection or prenatal diagnosis. It is best to get up-to-date information about these issues from the cytogenetics laboratory or clinical geneticist, since developments in these areas are advancing too rapidly for published literature to keep up to date. Where such tests are available, it is imperative for the obstetrician to be clear about the way in which a particular test will provide information and its limitations. For some investigations, there is an overlap between the abnormal or carrier state and the normal range and the results of such tests are thus not absolute.

Autosomal Dominant Inheritance

Such a disorder is one which is largely or completely expressed in the heterozygote. In general, the homozygous state is very rare or unknown, but when it does occur it tends to be more severe than the hetero zygous form (e.g. familial hypercholesterolemia, achondroplasia). Huntingdon's Disease may be the exception. The risk to the offspring of an affected heterozygote will be 50%. In the pedigree, 'vertical transmission' of the disease can be seen.

Problems arise in counseling, however, where there is late or variable onset of the condition (e.g. Huntingdon's Disease, adult polycystic disease). For such disorders, 'life tables' can be used which give the risks based on the age of the individual. Problems can also arise because of a lack of penetrance of the condition (i.e. failure of individuals known to carry the gene to manifest the condition, e.g. hereditary pancreatitis, retinoblastoma) or variation in clinical expression of the condition (for example achondroplasia, tuberose sclerosis). The maternal intrauterine environment can also influence expression (e.g. myotonic dystrophy, phenylketonuria).

Finally, given these problems of variable onset, penetrance and expression, one must be careful to assume that the occurrence of an autosomal dominant condition in an offspring of apparently normal parents must be a case of a new mutation and thus any future offspring be at low risk of recurrence.

Autosomal Recessive Inheritance

The difficulty with autosomal recessive inheritance is to confirm that this is the mode of inheritance. If this is not possible on the clinical diagnosis, then greater reliance has to be placed on the pedigree and with small family size there may not be enough sibs to be confident.

Once this pattern of inheritance is confirmed, then the main risk is for sibs of an affected individual, for whom the risk is 1:4. Unless the disorder is very common or there is consanguinity, the risks for half-sibs, children of affected individuals and especially children of unaffected sibs is minimally increased over that for the general population. The precise risk will depend on the frequency of the gene in the population and the frequency of the heterozygote in the population.

Once one is confident of autosomal recessive inheritance, then the difficulties of counseling are less than those presented by autosomal dominant disorders. In particular, lack of penetrance and variation in expression are much less common. Genetic heterogeneity in an apparently single clinical entity is arguably the main cause of variation (e.g. different types of recessively inherited polycystic kidney disease, spinal muscle atrophies).

Further points to remember in counseling for recessive conditions are:

- many are amenable to prenatal diagnosis;

- donor insemination might be a therapeutic option to discuss with some couples;

- care must be taken when discussing sterilization with parents of a child with a recessive condition because of the low risk of recurrence if either should remarry.

X-Linked Disease

Over 100 X-linked disorders/traits have been recognized. The majority are X-linked recessive. The terms 'dominant' and 'recessive' must be used with caution in X-linked disease because there can be much greater variability of expression in the heterozygous female than in autosomal disorders. This is largely due to X-chromosome inactivation (the Lyon hypothesis).

The following are general counseling guidelines for an X-linked disorder whether it is recessive, dominant or intermediate in expression:

- male-to-male transmission never occurs (father never passes his X chromosome to son);

- all daughters of an affected male will receive the gene (whether the condition is expressed in that daughter will depend on the dominance of the disorder);

- unaffected males never transmit the disease to their offspring;

- there is a 50% risk of female carriers passing the gene to their sons;

- half the daughters of female carriers will be carriers (and affected if it is a dominant condition);

- affected homozygous females are rare (parents would have to be an affected male and a female carrier).

When an isolated case of an X-linked disorder is identified in a male, it is difficult to determine whether the isolated case represents a new mutation or whether the mother is a carrier. Where the condition has reliable methods for carrier detection (see below) they should be employed. However, even when such tests exist, the variability of gene expression in heterozygotes means that carrier detection in women is difficult. For example, with hemophilia A and Duchenne muscular dystrophy, 20–30% of known carriers have phenotypic carrier tests within the normal range.

Carrier Detection

A carrier is an individual who possesses in heterozygous state the gene determining an inherited disorder and who is essentially healthy at the time of study. The genetic risks for the offspring of an individual with a specific disorder depend on the mode of inheritance of that condition:

- for autosomal recessive conditions the risk to the offspring is very low unless the disorder is extremely common, there is consanguinity or the same disorder is present in the spouse's family;

- for autosomal dominant conditions there is a 50% chance of the condition being acquired by an off-

Table 11
Carrier detection in autosomal recessive conditions

Disorder	Test
Alpha-1-antitrypsin deficiency	Alpha-1-antitrypsin electrophoretic typing; DNA analysis[a]
Combined immunodeficiency (one)	Adenosine deaminase electrophoresis
Congenital adrenal hyperplasia	DNA analysis[a]
Cystic fibrosis	DNA analysis[a]
Galactosemia	Red cell galactose-1-phosphate uridyl transferase
Mucopolysaccharidosis type 1 (Hurler)	White cell alpha-iduronidase
Phenylketonuria	Phenylalanine load; phenylalanine-tyrosine serum ratio; DNA analysis[a]
Pseudocholinesterase deficiency	Pseudocholinesterase level; dibucaine number
Tay-Sachs disease	White cell hexosaminidase A
Thalassemia and other hemoglobinopathies	Red cell morphology; hemoglobin electrophoresis; DNA analysis

[a]DNA analysis only available in family of affected individuals.

Table 12
Carrier detection in variable autosomal dominant conditions

Disorder	Test
Hereditary spherocytosis	Red cell morphology, osmotic fragility
Holt-Oram syndrome	Minor digital abnormalities
Malignant hyperpyrexia	Elevated creatine kinase, muscle biopsy
Multiple epiphyseal dysplasia	Short stature, premature osteoarthritis
Muscular dystrophy (facioscapulohumeral)	Minimal weakness
Myotonic dystrophy	Minimal weakness, lens opacities, electromyography
Neurofibromatosis	Skin lesions, Lisch nodules
Osteogenesis imperfecta	Dental changes, deafness, blue sclerae
Adult polycystic kidney disease	Renal ultrasound, DNA markers
Tuberous sclerosis	Skin lesions (UV light), CT scan, dental pits
Van der Woude syndrome	Lip pits
Von Hippel-Lindau syndrome	Retinal lesions
Waardenburg syndrome	White forelock, hypertelorism

spring of a carrier (the risk of overt disease will vary with the condition);

- for X-linked recessive conditions there is a 50% risk that the offspring of a carrier (female) will acquire the gene; if that offspring is female she will then be a carrier; if male, he will be affected.

The number of genetic conditions where carrier detection is possible is increasing rapidly. Some of the more common examples are given in **Tables 11**, **12** and **13**. These lists are not necessarily comprehensive and the reader is advised to contact the local cytogenetics laboratory and/or clinical geneticist for up-to-date information on a specific condition.

COUNSELING FOR SYNDROMES

General

The study of congenital malformation syndromes is a growing area. In general, the subject concerns those abnormalities that are present at birth. The term 'dys-morphology' has been applied to the study of such birth defects occurring in recognizable combinations as syndromes.

There are many causes for such syndromes, including chromosomal abnormalities, genetic defects and teratogens (e.g. drugs, infections, metabolic causes). For each individual case, it is important to try and establish the cause so that counseling is accurate and complete.

Diagnostic Approach to Dysmorphic Baby/Child

As with all aspects of genetic counseling, accuracy of diagnosis is mandatory before undertaking any counseling. In summary, the important steps are:

- careful and comprehensive examination of the individual with the syndrome;

- photography of the main features as a permanent record;

- radiography may help elucidate the diagnosis;

Table 13
Carrier detection in X-linked conditions

Disorder	Test
Adrenal leucodystrophy[a]	Long chain fatty acid synthesis
Alport's syndrome	Microscopic hematuria
Amelogenesis imperfecta	Patchy enamel hypoplasia
Anhidrotic ectodermal dysplasia[b]	Reduced sweat pores, dental defects
Becker muscular dystrophy[a]	Serum creatine kinase, DNA markers
Lethal centronuclear myopathy[b]	Muscle biopsy
Choroideremia[b]	Pigmentary retinal changes, DNA marker
Chronic granulomatous disease[a]	Partial NADPH oxidase deficiency, discoid lupus-like skin lesions
Duchenne muscular dystrophy[a]	Serum creatine kinase, DNA markers
Fabry's disease[a]	Skin lesions, alpha-galactosidase assay
Glucose-6-phosphate dehydrogenase deficiency[a]	Quantitative enzyme assay and electrophoresis
Hemophilia A[a]	Factor VIII assays
Hemophilia B[a]	Factor IX assays, gene probe
Hunter's syndrome (mucopolysaccharidosis II)	Enzyme assay on hair bulbs and serum
Hypogammaglobulinemia (Bruton type)[b]	Reduced IgG (some individuals only)
Lesch-Nyhan syndrome[a]	HGPRT assay on hair bulbs
Lowe's syndrome	Amnioaciduria, lens opacities
Ocular albinism[b]	Patchy fundal depigmentation
Retinoschisis[b]	Cystic retinal changes
Vitamin D-resistant rickets[b]	Serum phosphate (may be clinical features)
X-linked congenital cataract	Lens opacities
X-linked ichthyosis[a]	Corneal opacities, reduced steroid sulfatase
X-linked mental retardation[b]	Visible fragile site on X chromosome
X-linked retinitis pigmentosa[b]	Pigmentary changes, abnormal electroretinogram, linked DNA marker in some families only

[a]Gene cloned; [b]DNA marker of diagnostic use.

- cytogenetic analysis is usually carried out in most cases if only to exclude chromosomal abnormality;

- other investigations as are suggested by features from the examination;

- obtain a careful obstetric history with especial reference to possible teratogens;

- construct a family pedigree;

- consult a computerized database of malformation syndromes especially for unusual or rare conditions; these databases include information published and presented from all over the world and are especially helpful in rare or atypical disorders.

Syndromes

For many of the more common disorders, empiric risk tables exist and are easy to use and apply (see Further Reading). Those recognizable syndromes with a low risk of recurrence are summarized in **Table 14**. However, the situation commonly occurs where either the diagnosis is not clear or where there is no accurate data upon which to counsel for risk of recurrence. In such circumstances, it is advisable to refer the case to a clinical geneticist for assessment and counseling.

Table 14
Malformation syndromes in which recurrence in sibs is rare

Amniotic bands syndrome
Goldenhar syndrome
Hemifacial microsomia
Klippel-Feil syndrome
Klippel-Trenaunay-Weber syndrome
McCune-Albright (fibrous dysplasia) syndrome
Poland's syndrome
Rubinstein-Taybi syndrome
Russell-Silver syndrome
Sacral agenesis (caudal regression syndrome)
Sturge-Weber syndrome
Weaver's syndrome

COUNSELING FOR ORGAN/SYSTEM ANOMALIES

A large group of disorders exist affecting specific organ systems in which there appears to be a genetic/inherited component but which follows no clear pattern of Mendelian inheritance or identifiable chromosomal abnormality. Some have used the terms 'polygenic' or 'multifactorial' to cover this group. However, this is unsatisfactory. In some cases (e.g. diabetes mellitus), the disorder is not a single entity but a heterogeneous group of disorders, at present indistinguishable, some of which may be inherited in a Mendelian fashion, others where an inherited compo-

GENETIC COUNSELING
Summary of Management Options

GENERAL (see also **Table 2**)

- Allow adequate time in a setting which is free from disturbance

- Obtain accurate and comprehensive information about the condition to make an accurate diagnosis

- Ensure risks quoted are accurate

- If obstetrician cannot fulfill 1, 2 or 3, refer the individual/couple to a clinical geneticist

CHROMOSOME ABNORMALITY (see also **Tables 3, 4, 5, 6, 7, 8, 9, 10**)

- Always check karyotype reports with laboratory if in doubt of meaning

- When providing information, make clear whether data relate to 'at amniocentesis' or 'at delivery'

- Counseling should always be 'non-directive' and supportive

CONDITIONS WITH MENDELIAN INHERITANCE

- Ensure accuracy of diagnosis and mode of inheritance before counseling. Also, where appropriate, check on possibilities for carrier detection and prenatal diagnosis with cytogenetics laboratory or clinical geneticist (see also **Tables 11, 12, 13**)

Autosomal dominant

- 50% risk to offspring with non-lethal conditions

- Life tables for conditions with variable/late onset

- Counseling difficult with variable penetrance and expression

Autosomal recessive

- Risks to sibs of affected child: 25% risk of having the condition and 50% risk of being carriers

- Prenatal diagnosis possible for some

- Careful counseling about donor insemination and sterilization

X-linked

- Male-to-male transmission never occurs

- Daughters of an affected male will be carriers (expression will depend on dominance)

- Unaffected males never transmit the disease

- For female carriers:
  - 50% risk of passing the gene to their sons
  - half the daughters will be carriers (and affected if dominant condition)
- Affected homozygous females are rare

SPECIFIC SYNDROMES

- Establish accurate diagnosis (and cause if possible)

- Provide counseling from empiric risk tables (see Further Reading)

- If doubt about diagnosis or recurrence risks, refer to clinical geneticist

ORGAN/SYSTEM ABNORMALITIES

- Refer to empiric risk tables (see **Table 14** and Further Reading)

- For many conditions, counseling best provided by clinical geneticist

nent and environmental factors interplay and others which are 'acquired' in that environmental factors are largely influential.

Whatever the theoretical basis of these disorders, they represent difficult and specialized counseling problems. For most of these conditions, it is possible to obtain empiric risk data – that is, what the risks to offspring and relatives have been found to be in other individuals with the disorder (see Further Reading). Space does not permit a full discussion of these problems. Furthermore, while it is possible for obstetricians to provide such counseling, it is the author's view that this is best left to a clinical geneticist.

CONCLUSION

The two important principles underpinning genetic counseling are:

- to obtain accurate information

- to impart accurate information.

Individuals or couples seeking counseling about genetic disorders are done a grave disservice if an error is made in the diagnosis of a possible hereditary condition or if the wrong risks are quoted for the correct disorder.

Obstetriciansshould only provide counseling once they are sure of the condition and certain of the risks. When either of these two guidelines are not fulfilled, they should refer the individual/couple to a clinical geneticist.

REFERENCES

1 Jacobs PA, Melville M, Ratcliffe S *et al.* (1974) A cytogenetic survey of 11,680 newborn infants. *Annals of Human Genetics* **37**:359–376.
2 Carr DH, Gedeon M (1977) Population cytogenetics of human abortuses. In Hook EB, Porter IH (eds) *Population Cytogenetics: Studies in Human Reproduction*, pp. 289–326. New York: Academic Press.
3 Cuckle HS, Wald NJ, Thompson SG (1987) Estimating a woman's risk of having a pregnancy associated with Down's Syndrome using her age and serum alpha-feto protein level. *British Journal of Obstetrics and Gynaecology* **94**:387–402.
4 Ferguson-Smith MA (1983) Prenatal chromosome analysis and its impact on the birth incidence of chromosome disorders. *British Medical Bulletin* **39**:355–364.

FURTHER READING

1 Emery AE, Rimoin DL (1983) *Principles and Practice of Medical Genetics*. London: Churchill Livingstone.
2 Fuhrmann WA, Vogel F (1983) *Genetic Counseling: A Guide for the Practicing Physician*, 2nd edn. Berlin: Springer-Verlag.
3 Kelly TE (1986) *Clinical Genetics and Genetic Counseling*. Chicago, IL: Year Book Publishers.
4 Harper PS (1988) *Practical Genetic Counselling*, 3rd edn. Oxford: Butterworth-Heinemann.
5 McKusick VA (1986) *Mendelian Inheritance in Man*, 7th edn. Baltimore, MD: Johns Hopkins University Press.
6 Smith DW (1982) *Recognisable Patterns of Human Malformation*. Philadelphia, PA: W.B. Saunders.

3

Organization of Prenatal Care and Identification of Risk

DAVID JAMES

INTRODUCTION

Definition of Risk

A pregnancy is defined as 'high risk' when there is a likelihood of an adverse outcome to the woman and/or her baby that is greater than the incidence of that outcome in the general pregnant population.[1]

Aims of Prenatal Care

The majority of pregnancies are not 'high risk' by this definition. The aims of care for these 'normal/low-risk' women are:[2]

- To provide advice, reassurance, education and support for the woman and her family.

- To deal with the minor ailments of pregnancy.

- To provide an on-going screening program (clinical and laboratory-based) to confirm that the woman continues to be low risk.

For the minority of pregnant women who are identified as 'high risk' before, during or after pregnancy, these three aims of pregnancy care still apply but, in addition, there is a fourth aim:[2]

- The prevention, detection and management of those problems and factors which adversely affect the health of mother and/or baby.

IS PRENATAL CARE WORTHWHILE: IS IT EFFECTIVE?

Nearly all studies of prenatal care, including the major national surveys, have demonstrated that women who receive no prenatal care have a worse outcome to their pregnancy.[3-7] This leads some to argue erroneously that prenatal care must be beneficial. There are several pitfalls in this argument, which make it unhelpful as a defense of prenatal care.[8] Furthermore, what constitutes 'prenatal care' varies considerably in practice (see below).

A much stronger case for prenatal care can be made by examining whether individual components of care have proven benefit in achieving each of the four aims of prenatal care summarized above.[2,9-12] In general, each suggested strategy of prenatal care can be critically examined and categorized into:[13]

- measures of proven benefit;

- measures where further evidence is needed;

- measures where the available evidence shows no

benefit or even harm (it is reasonable to argue that this group of strategies should no longer be employed in prenatal care).

Space does not allow a detailed discussion of the evidence for classifying a management strategy into one of these three groups and the reader is referred to other texts.[14] Summaries of the available evidence regarding the value of certain management options with respect to the four aims of prenatal care are given in **Tables 1–4**. The evidence for and against specific management options is also discussed at length in individual chapters in this book.

PROVISION OF PRENATAL CARE

There is great variation in the provision and content of prenatal care in developed countries.

Providers

The respective role of obstetricians, family doctors (general practitioners) and midwives in the delivery of prenatal care varies from one country to another.[13] There is no evidence that doctors need to be the medical professionals involved in the prenatal care of every pregnancy.[15]

Within the European Community, Denmark and the Netherlands give a pivotal responsibility to midwives with family doctors playing a supportive role and obstetricians only being involved in problem pregnancies and labor and delivery. In contrast, most of the care is provided by obstetricians in Belgium, Luxembourg and Germany. In France and the UK, the sources of care are more diversified; however, in general, family doctors and midwives share the responsibility for prenatal care with the obstetrician being involved marginally if at all in normal pregnancies. This latter pattern of care also tends to be seen in Australia and New Zealand. In North America, midwives are uncommon, though there are several pilot studies examining an increasing role for such professionals. Most of the prenatal care in the USA and Canada is provided by family doctors and/or obstetricians, though some care is undertaken by nurse practitioners. Traditional birth attendants do not contribute significantly to prenatal care in developed countries.

Education

There is also great variation in the form, content and amount of education and advice that women receive

Table 1

Evidence that advice, reassurance, education and support in preparation for childbirth is effective (aim no. 1 of prenatal care)[14]

Proven strategy	Beneficial effect
1. Improved social and psychological support from caregivers	Better communications, satisfaction with care; less anxieties, postnatal illness and feeding problems
2. Antismoking interventions	Reduced smoking, higher mean birthweight
3. Carbohydrate supplements for malnourished women	Higher mean birthweight
4. Antenatal classes	Less intrapartum analgesia
5. Routine ultrasound with positive feedback	Positive feelings to baby, lower 'postterm' induction rate
Strategy needing more study	Possible beneficial effect
1. Modification of work patterns	Effects on maternal and perinatal morbidity
2. Antenatal classes	Effects of self-esteem and satisfaction with pregnancy
3. Iron, folate, multivitamin and nutritional supplementation for all	Effects of maternal and perinatal morbidity, birthweight, neural tube defects, pre-eclampsia
Strategy of no proven benefit or proven harm	
1. Failure to involve women in decision making	
2. Failure to provide continuity of care	
3. Doctors involved in care of all pregnancies	
4. Prescribing high-density protein supplements	
5. Advising restriction of weight gain	
6. Advising restriction of salt intake	

Table 2
Evidence that minor ailments in pregnancy can be successfully ameliorated
(aim no. 2 of prenatal care)[14]

Proven strategy	Beneficial effect
1. Antiemetics (e.g. antihistamines)	Reduced nausea and vomiting
2. Antacids	Reduced heartburn
3. Increased dietary fibre intake	Reduced constipation
4. Bulking agents and stool softeners	Reduced constipation

Strategy needing more study	Possible beneficial effect
1. Dilute hydrochloric acid	Reduced heartburn
2. Prostigmine	Reduced heartburn
3. Sodium chloride	Reduced leg cramps
4. Calcium	Reduced leg cramps
5. Quinine	Reduced leg cramps
6. Vitamin D	Reduced leg cramps

Strategy of no proven benefit or proven harm

1. Saline cathartics or lubricant oils for constipation

Table 3
Evidence that antenatal screening identifies women at risk
(aim no. 3 of prenatal care)[14]

Proven strategy	Risk identified
1. Selective fetal ultrasound or invasive procedure	Fetal abnormality
2. Maternal serum alpha-fetoprotein testing	Neural tube defect, Down's syndrome
3. Fundal height in high-risk pregnancies	Pathological fetal growth
4. Regular ultrasound measurement of fetal size	Pathological fetal growth
5. Maternal kick-charts	Fetal death
6. Biophysical tests of fetal well-being	Fetal death
7. Doppler ultrasound of fetal circulation	Fetal compromise
8. Rhesus antibody screening	Rhesus hemolytic disease
9. Selective use of ultrasound	Fetal viability, gestational age, placental site, fetal presentation
10. Regular blood pressure measurement and urinalysis	Pre-eclampsia
11. Screening for impaired glucose tolerance	Gestational diabetes
12. Screening for bacteriuria	Asymptomatic bacteriuria and sequelae
13. Screening for syphilis and/or gonorrhea	Maternal and fetal infection

Strategy needing more study	Possible risk identified
1. Fundal height in low-risk pregnancies	Pathological fetal growth
2. Biochemical tests of fetal well-being	Fetal compromise
3. Doppler ultrasound of uteroplacental circulation	Fetal compromise, pre-eclampsia
4. Routine screening for toxoplasmosis, chlamydia, HIV infection	Neonatal infection
5. Regular herpes swabs in women with history of herpes	Neonatal infection
6. Risk scoring, monitoring uterine activity, screening for vaginal sepsis, cervical assessment	Spontaneous preterm labor
7. Maternal/fetal screening	Risk of abruptio placentae
8. Maternal and fetal assessment in post-dates pregnancy	Maternal and fetal risk

Table 4
Evidence that when a specific risk is identified that the subsequent intervention and management improves
the outcome (aim no. 4 of prenatal care)[14]

Proven strategy	Beneficial effect on outcome
1. Multivitamins and folate supplements with previous neural tube fetus	Reduced incidence of neural tube defect in subsequent pregnancies
2. Amniocentesis *vs* chorion villus biopsy	Lower miscarriage rate with amniocentesis
3. Anti-D for Rhesus negative women after delivery of Rhesus positive babies	Reduced subsequent isoimmunization
4. Intravascular fetal blood transfusion for Rhesus hydrops	Improved perinatal mortality
5. 'Routine ultrasound'	Reduced 'post-dates' induction
6. Antihypertensive therapy in women with hypertension	Reduced severe hypertensive pregnancy
7. Tight control of diabetes (rather than moderate)	Reduced urinary infection, preterm delivery, cesarean section, macrosomia, respiratory distress, perinatal mortality
8. Various antifungals	Reduced persistent candidiasis
9. Metronidazole after the first trimester	Reduced *Trichomonas* infestation
10. Intrapartum antibiotics for maternal group B	Reduced neonatal colonization and sepsis
11. Rubella vaccination postpartum	Reduced rubella embryopathy subsequently
12. Cervical cerclage with previous second trimester miscarriage	Reduced delivery before 33 weeks, miscarriage or perinatal death
13. Betamimetics in preterm labor	Reduced delivery within 24 h, 48 h and before 37 weeks
14. Oral betamimetics after inhibition of preterm labor	Reduced recurrence
15. Steroids prior to preterm delivery	Reduced respiratory distress syndrome, periventricular hemorrhage, necrotizing enterocolitis, early neonatal death

Strategy needing more study	Possible beneficial effect
1. Diagnosis of fetal abnormality by ultrasound, biochemical methods and invasive procedures	Reduced incidence of fetal abnormality at birth, and reduced maternal morbidity
2. Identification of pathological fetal growth	Reduced perinatal morbidity and mortality
3. Maternal kick-charts	Reduced perinatal morbidity and mortality
4. Biochemical tests of fetal well-being	Reduced perinatal morbidity and mortality
5. Biophysical tests of fetal well-being	Reduced perinatal morbidity and mortality
6. Doppler ultrasound of fetal circulation	Reduced perinatal morbidity and mortality
7. Plasmapheresis in severe Rhesus disease	Reduced perinatal morbidity and mortality
8. Antiplatelet agents in women at risk of pre-eclampsia and fetal growth deficiency	Reduced recurrence risk
9. Plasma expansion for severe pre-eclampsia	Reduced severe hypertension and renal failure
10. Hospital admission for non-proteinuric hypertension	Reduced development of proteinuria or severe hypertension, maternal and perinatal morbidity
11. Strict bed rest for proteinuric hypertension	Reduced fulminating pre-eclampsia, maternal and perinatal morbidity and mortality
12. Treatment of mycoplasma colonization	Maternal and perinatal morbidity
13. Antiviral agents for active genital herpes	Reduced persistent infection, reduced neonatal infection
14. Cesarean section for herpes with no active disease	Reduced neonatal infection
15. Cervical cerclage with history other than previous second trimester miscarriage	Reduced preterm delivery and perinatal mortality
16. Use of antibiotics with steroids after preterm premature membrane rupture	Reduced infectious morbidity (maternal and fetal)
17. Thyroid-releasing hormone in addition to steroids prior to preterm delivery	Reduced morbidity from respiratory distress syndrome
18. Betamimetics after preterm premature membrane rupture	Reduced maternal and perinatal morbidity

Strategy of no proven benefit or proven harm

1. Prescribing ethanol for inhibition of preterm labor
2. Inducing labor routinely at less than 42 weeks

during pregnancy, not only between but also within countries. Much of the information that a woman acquires about pregnancy is received not from medical professionals, but from relatives and friends.

Frequency of Visits

There is no consensus about what constitutes the 'ideal' number of prenatal visits. For example, the American College of Obstetricians and Gynecologists recommended a visit every 4 weeks until 28 weeks, then every 2 weeks until 36 weeks and weekly until delivery.[16] This amounts to 13 visits if the first visit is at 8 weeks and the last at 40 weeks. In contrast, a recent expert committee suggested a reduction in this number to eight for normal pregnancies.[17] In different European countries, the recommended numbers of prenatal vists vary from 5 to 15.[18] It is likely that the number of prenatal visits could be reduced considerably in normal pregnancies.[19]

Clinical and Laboratory Screening Programs

Despite much variation in other aspects of provision of prenatal care, the clinical and laboratory-based screening that occurs during pregnancy is largely similar in most developed countries. Variations that do exist are often on the basis of the prevalence of problems locally. Factors which are commonly checked during pregnancy are summarized in **Table 5**.

IDENTIFICATION AND MANAGEMENT OF RISK IN PREGNANCY

The third aim of prenatal care stated above is the identification of women at risk. Such identification is made from a woman's history, examination or investigations carried out prior to pregnancy, at first visit or during subsequent antenatal visits. The fourth aim of prenatal care stated above is the management of women at risk. This management is directed at prevention, amelioration or treatment of the adverse outcome.

In practice, identification of risk in pregnancy can be carried out in two ways

- general risk scoring

- specific risk recognition

General Risk Scoring

The main aim of a formal risk scoring system in pregnancy is to permit the classification of women into different categories for which different and appropriate management strategies can be implemented. Other benefits of such general risk scoring methods include aiding teaching and audit, defining populations for epidemiological purposes and for allocation of resources. However, none of these will be considered here.

The main adverse outcome measures for which risk scores have been developed and evaluated with a view to aiding management are:[20,21]

- perinatal death;

- small-for-gestational age or low birthweight fetus;

- preterm labor and delivery;

- perinatal asphyxia;

- or a combination of all four.

There are three ways in which the risk can be calculated:[21]

- by the number of risk factors present;

- by the arithmetic sum of the mathematically weighted risk for each individual factor present in a woman;

- by correcting this weighted risk by a further mathematical process such as Bayes' theorem.

There are theoretical reasons why formal risk scoring may be expected to be less than satisfactory in practice. For example, it tends to lead to a simplistic and inflexible view of pregnancy management, it has the inherent danger of 'ignoring' low risk women, and it requires some form of computerization in the calculation of the score. The fact that such risk scoring systems are not widely used in practice may be partly for these reasons. However, the most likely explanation is that while many of the formal scoring systems proposed do predict the likelihood of an adverse outcome of one form or another, there is little evidence that their use is associated with a reduction in adverse pregnancy outcome.[20] Furthermore, when risk scoring is applied in practice, there is a real danger that a potential yet imprecise risk of an adverse outcome is replaced by the introduction of increased surveillance and possibly

Table 5
Common risk factors sought in prenatal screening

Demographic/general
  maternal age
  ethnicity
  socioeconomic status
  marital status

Past obstetric history
  parity
  ectopics/miscarriages
  mode of delivery
  baby outcome, gestation, size, normality
  other complications of pregnancy

Past medical history
  cigarette smoking
  alcohol abuse
  other drug abuse
  maternal medical disorder
  maternal prescribed medication
  previous surgery
  previous anesthetic problems

Gynecological history
  subfertility
  contraception
  menstrual regularity
  specific problems

Family history
  congenital abnormality
  diabetes
  hypertension
  renal disease

Physical examination
  maternal weight
  maternal height
  general examination
  pelvic examination (not performed by all obstetricians,
    especially if there is no indication and a routine
    pelvis ultrasound is offered)

Factors arising in pregnancy
  multiple pregnancy
  vaginal bleeding
  reduced/abnormal fetal movements
  preterm uterine activity
  hypertension
  abnormal uterine size and/or amniotic fluid volume
  any other problems (weight gain in pregnancy is not
    universally recorded routinely)

Investigations
  urinalysis (glucose, protein, blood, ketones)
  full blood count, group and antibody screen
  serological screening for rubella, syphilis and others
    depending on local prevalence (e.g. hepatitis, HIV)
  serological screening for fetal anomaly (e.g. neural tube
    defect, Down's syndrome)
  routine ultrasound
  cervical smear (depending on local screening policy)

interventions and treatments, many of which may be of unproven value. Examples of such strategies include fetal monitoring and measures claimed to reduce the risks of preterm labor and delivery.[20] Finally, there is the practical limitation that risk scores vary with different populations and for reasons other than just the prevalence of specific adverse outcomes.

It is the author's view that formal risk scoring should not be introduced into routine pregnancy care until the results from a well-designed randomized trial of benefits and dangers are available.

Specific Risk Recognition

In practice, by far the most common way in which risk in pregnancy is identified is by specific risk recognition. A woman is identified to have a risk factor for a specific adverse outcome and as a consequence she receives additional management which may prevent, ameliorate or treat the adverse outcome. This is in addition to the routine prenatal care received by all women in pregnancy. Thus, for example, the woman who weighs over 85 kg is at increased risk for the development of hypertension and gestational diabetes and, accordingly, the clinical and laboratory prenatal screening program must be amended to look specifically for these two complications. In practice, the main problem that besets this approach is that while there may be agreement about what constitutes a risk factor for pregnancy and what the adverse outcome(s) may be, there is less consensus about what the appropriate management strategy should be. For many interventions, the scientific proof of benefit is lacking – an observation that was discussed above (see also **Tables 1–4**).

The way in which this additional care is provided on the basis of identification of risk factors can be empiric or schematic.

Empiric

The obstetrician decides on the specific additional management having identified a given risk factor on a patient-by-patient basis. Thus, faced with the woman (see above example) who weighs over 85 kg and the known increased risk of hypertensive problems and gestational diabetes, the obstetrician may screen for hypertension in several ways:

- no additional measures other than paying strict attention to blood pressure recording at the routine prenatal clinic visits and using a large sphygmomanometer cuff for the measurements;

- increased frequency of clinic attendance for blood pressure readings;

- issuing the woman with a self-assessing sphygmomanometer and giving her guidelines for self-referral.

Similarly, the obstetrician may screen for gestational diabetes by:

- carrying out a random blood glucose on one or more occasions in pregnancy;

- carrying out a fasting blood glucose on one or more occasions in pregnancy;

- carrying out a 'modified' 50 g glucose tolerance test on one or more occasions in pregnancy;

- carrying out a formal 75 g glucose tolerance test on one or more occasions in pregnancy.

Schematic

The obstetrician implements a specific pre-agreed management strategy every time a given risk factor is identified. Examples of such management schemes are given in **Tables 6–11**.[2] There are no studies comparing the schematic approach with the empiric approach with respect to outcome. However, the schematic approach has several theoretical advantages:

- there will be consistency of management for given risk factors;

- it will allow audit of the effectiveness of one management strategy in comparison with another.

One implicit requirement of the schematic approach is that the underlying basic prenatal care program should also be documented. An example is given in **Table 12**.[2]

Table 6
Schematic risk factor management: general factors[2]

Risk factor	Nature of maternal/fetal risk	Principles of management
Age <18 years	Poor antenatal attendance, education and screening	Consider social worker involvement, domiciliary visits
	Hypertensive disease, IUGR	Vigilance for raised BP, Grade I fetal check
Age >35 years	Chromosomal abnormalities	Early consideration for prenatal diagnosis
	Hypertensive disease, IUGR	Vigilance for raised BP, Grade I fetal check
Parity >4	IUGR	Grade I fetal check,
	Anaemia	Iron and folate supplementation
	Further pregnancies	Discuss contraception,
	Malpresentation	Check presentation at 36 weeks
Non-caucasian	Hemoglobinopathy	Hb electrophoresis
	HB-Ag carrier (Far East)	If positive, then clear labeling of notes and implementation of policy guidelines (written)
	HIV (African)	Careful counseling, if positive as for HB-Ag
	Poor English, education and screening	Arrange regular interpreter
Single parent/financial/social	Poor antenatal attendance, education and screening	Domiciliary visits if necessary, discuss plans for labor and delivery, consider social worker
	IUGR	Grade I fetal check

BP, blood pressure; IUGR, intrauterine growth retardation; grade I fetal check, careful check of fetal growth by fundal height measurement and questioning about fetal activity; Hb, hemoglobin; HB-Ag, hepatitis-B antigen.

Table 7
Schematic risk factor management: past obstetric history[2]

Risk factor	Nature of maternal/fetal risk	Principles of management
Previous ectopic	Recurrence, maternal anxiety	Early ultrasound to confirm intrauterine
Previous SB/NND	Risk depends on cause (not all are recurrent)	Try and establish cause, early review and specific management
Baby weight <-2 SD	IUGR	Grade II fetal check
Baby weight $>+2$ SD	Gestational diabetes	Random glucose 28 and 32 weeks
	Further large fetus	Grade II fetal check, vigilance in labor
Congenital anomaly	Possible recurrence	Obtain details/diagnosis, possible prenatal diagnosis
Antibodies	Hemolytic disease	Specific protocol
Proteinuric PET	Recurrence	Assess renal function, Grade II fetal check, carefully check blood pressure
Preterm delivery	Recurrence	Specific plan depending on cause
Uterine scar	Uterine rupture, cesarean section	Review of mode of delivery at 36 weeks
Short labor	Recurrence and neonatal problems (trauma, asphyxia hypothermia)	Specific management plan at 36 weeks
PPH	Recurrence	Specific plan at 36 weeks
Other labor or delivery problems	Recurrence	Specific plan at 36 weeks
Problems with baby	Recurrence, maternal anxiety	Obtain details and make specific plan

SB, stillbirth; NND, neonatal death; <-2 SD, less than 2 standard deviations below mean for gestation; IUGR, intrauterine growth retardation; grade II fetal check, fetal growth by ultrasound every 2–4 weeks and fetal movement chart; $>+2$ SD, more than 2 standard deviations above mean for gestation; PET, pre-eclampsia; PPH, post-partum hemorrhage.

Table 8
Schematic risk factor management: past medical, surgical, gynecological and family history[2]

Risk factor	Nature of maternal/fetal risk	Principles of management
Smoker	IUGR	Advice to reduce/stop, grade I fetal check
Excess alcohol	IUGR	Offer specific help
	Fetal alcohol syndrome	Grade II fetal check, alert pediatricians
Chronic disease and prescribed drugs	Possible adverse effects of disease on pregnancy and pregnancy on disease	Obstetric/physician joint care using pre-agreed specific protocols
Drug abuse	HB-Ag and/or HIV infection	Counseling and serological testing
	IUGR	Grade II fetal check
	Neonatal withdrawal	Alert pediatricians
Hemoglobinopathy	Sickle or thalassemia trait have risk of affected fetus	Test partner, ? offer prenatal diagnosis
	Sickle disease: (1) crisis	Encourage hydration, check renal function, regular MSU
	(2) IUGR	Grade II fetal check
Anesthetic problems	Recurrence	Consultant anesthetist opinion
FH diabetes	Gestational diabetes	Random glucose 28 and 32 weeks
FH congenital anomaly	Possible recurrence	Obtain details/diagnosis
	Maternal anxiety	Obstetrician for possible prenatal diagnosis
Subfertility	Anxiety, multiple pregnancy, hypertension and/or gestational diabetes with PCO	Reassure, vigilance for hypertension and random glucose 28 and 32 weeks if PCO
IUCD in situ	Miscarriage, preterm labor	Remove if threads visible; if not, check at delivery

IUGR, intrauterine growth retardation; grade I fetal check, careful check of fetal growth by fundal-height measurement and questioning about fetal activity; grade II fetal check, fetal growth by ultrasound every 2–4 weeks and fetal movement chart; AN, antenatal; MSU, mid-stream urine; PCO, polycystic ovaries.

Table 9
Schematic risk factor management: factors from examination[2]

Risk factor	Nature of maternal/fetal risk	Principles of management
Weight >85 kg	Hypertension, gestational diabetes	Dietary advice, vigilance for raised BP, random glucose at 28 and 36 weeks
Weight <45 kg	IUGR	Grade I fetal check
Primigravida and height <1.52 m	Cephalopelvic disproportion	Plan for labor if fetal head unengaged at 40 weeks
Cardiac murmur	Asymptomatic heart disease	Consider cardiological opinion

BP, blood pressure; IUGR, intrauterine growth retardation; grade I fetal check, careful check of fetal growth by fundal height measurement and questioning about fetal activity.

Table 10
Schematic risk factor management: factors arising in pregnancy[2]

Risk factor	Nature of maternal/fetal risk	Principles of management
Vaginal bleeding	<20 weeks: miscarriage	Acute referral to hospital, no long-term additional action
	>19 weeks: placenta previa, placental abruption	Acute referral to hospital, long-term grade II fetal check
BP >140/90	Pre-eclampsia, IUGR	(a) If BP >160/100 and/or proteinuria, for hospital admission and care using pre-agreed protocol (b) If BP <160/100 and no proteinuria, for day care using pre-agreed protocol
Multiple pregnancy	Anemia, hypertension, IUGR, preterm delivery, congenital abnormalities	Iron/folate supplements, vigilance for raised BP and preterm uterine activity, grade II fetal check, more frequent visits
SFD	IUGR	Fetal assessment using pre-agreed protocol
LFD	Big baby and complications, gestational diabetes, hydramnios, multiple pregnancy	Fetal assessment using pre-agreed protocol, random glucose
Polyhydramnios	Big baby and complications, abnormal fetus, diabetes	Fetal assessment using pre-agreed protocol, random glucose
Malpresentation after 35 weeks	Delivery problems	Look for causes, make plan for labor
Reduced FM	Poor maternal perception, fetal disease	Immediate NST and fetal assessment
Preterm ROM	Preterm labor, amnionitis	Hospital admission and manage with protocol
UTI	Pyelonephritis, preterm labor	Treat (5 days), monthly MSU

Grade I fetal check, careful check of fetal growth by fundal height measurement and questioning about fetal activity; grade II fetal check, fetal growth by ultrasound every 2–4 weeks and fetal movement chart; BP, blood pressure; IUGR, intrauterine growth retardation; SFD, small for dates; LFD, large for dates; FM, fetal movements; CTG, fetal cardiotocograph; ROM, rupture of membranes; UTI, urinary infection; MSU, mid-stream urine.

Table 11
Schematic risk factor management: factors from investigations[2]

Risk factor	Nature of maternal/fetal risk	Principles of management
Proteinuria	Infection, renal disease, pre-eclampsia	MSU, check BP, investigation if persists
Glycosuria	Lowered renal threshold, gestational diabetes	Random glucose 28 and 36 weeks
Hematuria	Infection, stone, renal disease	MSU, renal investigation if persistent
No rubella antibodies	Susceptible to rubella	Warn mother, offer puerperal vaccination
Rhesus negative	Potential for sensitization	Check antibodies at first visit, 28 and 34 weeks; give anti-D at potential sensitization
Antibodies	Fetal hemolytic disease	Specific protocol of management
Raised AFP	Fetal abnormality	Careful US scan at 18 weeks (amniocentesis)
	If normal, IUGR, placental bleeding, pre-eclampsia	Grade II fetal check, vigilance for raised BP
Low Hb (<10 g/dl)	Pathological anemia	Investigate, treat cause with oral therapy; refer hematologist if uncertain cause, intolerance of therapy, no response to therapy
Raised random glucose (>7 mM)	Gestational diabetes	Formal 75 g oral glucose tolerance test
Abnormal smear	Possible invasive carcinoma	Refer for colposcopy

MSU, mid-stream urine; BP, blood pressure; AFP, α-feto-protein; US, ultrasound; Hb, hemoglobin.

Decision Analysis

In the future, it is possible that some form of decision analysis will be applied to the provision of prenatal care.[22] There are two ways in which this is likely to occur:

- in providing counseling about management options;

- in deciding about the benefits of alternative managements on the basis of the published literature but without the benefit of a randomized trial.

Providing counseling about management options

A simple example is provided by the woman who is 40 years old and is seeking advice about prenatal diagnosis for Down's syndrome. Her likelihood of delivering a baby with the diagnosis is 1:100; her risks of miscarriage are approximately 1:100 for amniocentesis and 1:50 for chorion villus sampling. She is asked to place a relative score on her view of Down's syndrome *vs* miscarriage

- if she fears Down's syndrome three times more than she fears a miscarriage, then she can have either invasive procedure

- if she fears Down's syndrome two times more than she fears a miscarriage, then she should have the amniocentesis

- if she fears a miscarriage to any degree more than she does Down's syndrome, then she should not have an invasive procedure.

Of course, many would argue that currently such decisions are being made 'intuitively' by women and their partners when given all the relevant information in a non-directive way and without the need for complicating the issues with mathematics!

Deciding between alternative managements without a randomized trial

The counsel of excellence is that no management strategy should be implemented without the benefit of a randomized trial. However, some management options would need such large numbers that it is not feasible or likely that they will ever be undertaken. A good

Table 12
Schematic approach to prenatal care: basic care ('for all')[2]

Gestation	Aims and action taken
8–14 weeks	Confirm pregnancy
	Check medical, family and social and past obstetric histories
	General physical examination
	Pelvic examination if there is an indication
	Investigations: urinalysis (glucose/protein/blood)
	mid-stream urine specimen
	full blood count
	ABO/rhesus grouping and antibody screen
	serological tests (rubella, syphilis)
	Discuss pregnancy including the offer of neural tube and Down's screening at 16 weeks and US scan at 18 weeks
	General advice on diet, exercise, breast care, infant feeding, dental health, parentcraft classes, smoking, alcohol, family planning and maternity benefits
	Complete case notes
16 weeks	Serum screening for neural tube defect and Down's syndrome
	Check all booking investigations
18 weeks	Detailed US scan
	Check results from 16 week serum screening
	Confirm/amend estimated date of delivery
22–24 weeks	Routine check (history of any symptoms, especially vaginal bleeding, reduced/absent fetal movements), examination of BP, urinalysis, fundal height with tape measure (charted)
28 weeks	Routine check (as before but includes fetal heart rate and liquor volume), especially BP and fundal height growth
	Full blood count, rhesus antibody screen if rhesus negative
32 weeks	Routine check (as before), especially check BP, fundal height growth and results from 28 week tests
	Discuss labor and parentcraft
36 weeks	Routine check (as before), especially check BP, growth and possible malpresentation
	Full blood count, rhesus antibody screen if rhesus negative
38 weeks	Routine check (as before), especially check BP, growth and possible malpresentation
40 weeks	Routine check (as before), especially check growth and possible malpresentation
	Discuss labor
41 weeks	Review and discuss induction of labor

This is a suggested suitable minimum programme.
At each visit identify risk factors and implement management.

example is provided by the management of breech presentation at term. It is unlikely that a sufficiently large study could be conducted in practice to answer the question of optimum mode of delivery. Nevertheless, it has been argued from decision analysis of the available literature on risks to the mother and baby from cesarean section and the risks from vaginal delivery, that all such breech presentations should be delivered by cesarean section.[23,24]

CONCLUSION

There is great variation in the provision of prenatal care both between and within countries in terms of who sees mothers, when they are seen and what is done. However, there appears to be more consistency in terms of screening programs employed.

Of the four aims of prenatal care, arguably the most important is the prevention, detection and management of those problems and factors which adversely affect the health of the mother and/or her baby. In managing such problems, however, obstetricians should be clear which strategies are of proven benefit and those strategies for which the case remains unproven.

ORGANIZATION OF PRENATAL CARE
Summary of Management Options

Establish what constitutes routine/normal prenatal care for a given population

This is based on available resources

- Personnel

- Buildings/accommodation ('plant')

- Laboratory

    It comprises (see **Table 12** for documented example)

- Who will see the pregnant women

- When they will be seen

- What will be done when they attend

Aims of prenatal care

For the majority of pregnancies ('normal/low-risk')

- Provision of advice, reassurance, education and support

- Manage minor ailments of pregnancy

- On-going screening program (clinical and laboratory) to ensure continuing 'low risk'

For the minority of pregnancies ('high-risk')

- The above three aims *plus*

- Prevention, detection and management of risk factors (*arguably the most important aim*)

Management of risk factors

In practice this will be by specific risk management strategies

- Schematic is arguably more scientific than empiric (see **Tables 6–11** for example)

- Ideally employ strategies for which there is proven benefit (see **Tables 1–4**)

REFERENCES

1 James DK (1988) Risk at the booking visit. In James DK, Stirrat GM (eds) *Pregnancy and Risk*, pp. 45–80. Chichester: John Wiley.

2 James D, Smoleniec J (1992) Identification and management of the at-risk obstetric patient. *Hospital Update* **18**:885–890.

3 Douglas JWB (1948) *Maternity Services in Great Britain*. Oxford: Oxford University Press.

4 Butler NR, Bonham DG (1963) *Perinatal Mortality: The First Report of the British Perinatal Mortality Survey*. Edinburgh: Churchill Livingstone.

5 Butler NR, Alberman ED (1969) *Perinatal Problems: The Second Report of the British Perinatal Mortality Survey*. Edinburgh: Churchill Livingstone.

6 Chamberlain R, Chamberlain G, Howlett B, Claireaux A (1975) *British Births 1970*, Vol. I. London: Heinemann Medical.

7 Chamberlain G (1978) A re-examination of antenatal care. *Journal of the Royal Society of Medicine* **71**:662–668.

8 Hall MH (1989) Critique of antenatal care. In Turnbull A, Chamberlain G (eds) *Obstetrics*, pp. 225–233. Edinburgh: Churchill Livingstone.

9 Parboosingh J, Kerr M (1982) Innovations in the role of obstetric hospitals in prenatal care. In Enkin M, Chalmers I (eds) *Effectiveness and Satisfaction in Antenatal Care*, pp. 254–265. London: Spastics International.

10 Stirrat GM (1989) Late antenatal care. In Turnbull A, Chamberlain G (eds) *Obstetrics*, pp. 247–256. Edinburgh: Churchill Livingstone.

11 Hall MH (1985) The antenatal programme. In Marsh GN (ed.) *Modern Obstetrics in General Practice*, pp. 85–98. Oxford: Oxford University Press.

12 Chamberlain G (1991) Organisation of antenatal care. *British Medical Journal* **302**:647–650.

13 Buekens P (1990) Variations in provision and uptake of antenatal care. *Clinical Obstetrics and Gynaecology* **4**:187–205.

14 Chalmers I, Enkin M, Keirse MJNC (1990) Effective care in pregnancy and childbirth: A synopsis for guiding practice and research. In Chalmers I, Enkin M, Keirse MJNC (eds) *Effective Care in Pregnancy and Childbirth*, pp. 1465–1477. Oxford: Oxford University Press.

15 Keirse MJNC (1990) Interaction between primary and secondary care during pregnancy and childbirth. In Chalmbers I, Edkin M, Keirse MJNC (eds) *Effective Care in Pregnancy and Childbirth*, pp. 197–201. Oxford: Oxford University Press.

16 American College of Obstetricians and Gynecologists (1988) *Guidelines for Perinatal Care*, pp. 54–55. Washington, DC: American Academy of Pediatrics and American College of Obstetricians and Gynecologists.

17 Demographic and Health Surveys (1989) Selected statistics from DHS surveys. *Demographic and Health Surveys Newsletter* **2.2**:10.

18 Blondel B, Pusch D, Schmidt E (1985) Some characteristics of antenatal care in 13 European countries. *British Journal of Obstetrics and Gynaecology* **92**:565–568.

19 Hall MH, Chng PK, McGillivray I (1980) Is routine antenatal care worthwhile? *Lancet* **ii**:78–80.

20 Alexander S, Keirse MJNC (1990) Formal risk scoring during pregnancy. In Chalmers I, Edkin M, Keirse MJNC (eds) *Effective Care in Pregnancy and Childbirth*, pp. 345–365. Oxford: Oxford University Press.

21 Chard T (1991) Obstetric risk scores. *Fetal Medicine Review* **3**:1–10.

22 Lilford RJ (1990) Decision analysis in obstetrics. In Chamberlain G (ed.) *Modern Antenatal Care of the Fetus*, pp. 13–29. Oxford: Blackwell Scientific Publications.

23 Bingham P, Lilford RJ (1987) Management of the selected term breech presentation: Assessment of risks of selective vaginal delivery versus caesarean section for all cases. *Obstetrics and Gynecology* **69**:965–978.

24 Thorpe-Beeston JG, Banfield PJ, Saunders NJStG (1992) Outcome of breech delivery at term. *British Medical Journal* **305**:746–747.

4

Sociodemographic Factors: Age, Parity, Social Class and Ethnicity

HAJO I. J. WILDSCHUT

INTRODUCTION

Maternal age, parity, social class and ethnicity are interrelating and interacting sociodemographic factors that influence maternal health and child-bearing. Despite the fact that numerous investigators have explored this area, problems still arise in the interpretation and practical application of the findings. Investigations of the effects of sociodemographic variables on a wide range of pregnancy outcomes are hampered by two major problems: (1) a lack of consensus regarding appropriate definitions, in particular for social disadvantage and ethnicity, and (2) the scarcity of well-structured multivariate techniques to determine the relative importance of the various sociodemographic factors that have an impact on pregnancy outcomes. In population epidemiology, sociodemographic factors are often considered risk indicators rather than risk factors. Risk factors refer to variables that are involved in the etiology of a disease. Risk indicators refer to those variables that enable identification of high risk groups within the population; they are not necessarily involved in the causation of disease. Risk indicators as such are not amenable to preventive measures, but merely focus on certain high risk groups within the population which could potentially benefit from increased antenatal and intrapartum care.

MATERNAL AGE

Extremes of maternal age are defined inconsistently. The slopes of the upper and lower tails of the fre-

quency distribution for maternal age vary with time and geographical area. According to Golding,[1] there is no consistent evidence to support the view that a particular age is 'ideal' for bearing the first pregnancy, although child-bearing is least hazardous in women aged 20–29 years. Pregnancies in adolescence and pregnancies at advanced maternal age will be considered separately.

PREGNANCY IN ADOLESCENCE

There is no universally agreed definition of 'young maternal age'. Some investigators have advocated the use of the terms 'reproductive age' and 'gynecological age' as measures of physiological maturity.[2–5] 'Reproductive age' refers to the interval from the age of menarche to the chronological age *at conception*, whereas 'gynecological age' relates to the time span from the age of menarche to the chronological age *at delivery*. Conception or delivery within 2 years after the onset of menarche is considered to represent the lower extreme of the distribution of reproductive or gynecological ages, respectively.

Incidence

The incidence of teenage pregnancy shows marked variation between developed countries. The lowest teenage pregnancy rates are found in the Netherlands (14 per 1000 among 15- to 19-year-olds), whereas in Sweden and England and Wales combined they are considerably higher (35 and 44 per 1000, respectively).[6] The highest rates are found in the USA (96 per 1000).[6] In fact, in the USA, approximately one out of every ten girls aged 15–19 years becomes pregnant each year.[7,8] Hence, a woman in the USA has a 20–30% chance of becoming pregnant before her twentieth birthday.[9]

Risks

Teenage pregnancies are associated with social problems rather than physical or medical problems.[1,3,7,10,11] A considerable proportion of teenage mothers originate from working-class families and ethnic minorities. Many are themselves the children of teenage or very young parents.[12] The majority of teenage pregnancies are unplanned and unwanted.[6] Consequently, in Western societies, abortion rates among adolescent women are quite high, ranging from 30 to 60% of all confirmed pregnancies in that age group.[6,8,10,13,14]

Reports on complications of pregnancy in young girls are contradictory and difficult to interpret because of the confounding effects of adverse social circumstances and poor attendance for antenatal care.[10] Typically, cigarette smoking, alcohol consumption and illicit drug use are common among pregnant adolescents.[3,7,15] Adolescents who become pregnant are at particular risk of nutritional deficiencies and sexually transmitted diseases.[3,16] Medical complications associated with adolescent pregnancy include anemia, urinary tract infection, hypertension, preterm labor and low birthweight, a higher analgesia requirement, operative assistance during labor, short interval to next pregnancy and the sudden infant death syndrome.[3,17] It has been suggested that competition for nutrients between the fetus and the mother could affect pregnancy outcome in young pregnant girls by interrupting the normal growth process.[18] Contrary to common belief, biological 'immaturity' does not affect appreciably the reproductive performance of young teenagers in terms length of labor and route of delivery.[3,10,19]

Management Options

Prevention and prepregnancy management

Primary prevention focuses on preventing pregnancy through sexual education in schools with an emphasis on the importance of family planning and related matters.[6,13,14,20] In this respect, teenagers should be encouraged to discuss openly with their friends and classmates the realities of pregnancy and parenthood.[11] The media could, in this respect, play an important role. Education should also include information about

values, responsibilities and the right to say 'no'.[8] Secondary prevention is directed at sexually active women through a flexible approach toward the use and provision of contraceptives for both males and females. Tertiary prevention involves adolescents who become pregnant. Women are encouraged to seek early adequate antenatal care and discuss the options for the resolution of pregnancy.[13]

Prenatal

Compliance with antenatal care tends to be poor,[3,6,21] especially among teenagers in their second pregnancy.[22] Obviously, the provision and utilization of health care services is beneficial to both mother and child, although it is not clear to what extent antenatal care *per se* exerts a positive effect on pregnancy outcome. Routine ultrasonography during early pregnancy is advisable to confirm gestational age. Furthermore, timely identification of risk factors is important. Strategies for intervention should be focused on individual medical and social risk factors, in particular poor nutritional status, adverse health habits and perceived isolation. It is often difficult to determine the real needs of the pregnant teenager and her family. Nevertheless, they should be offered social support where feasible, preferably in close cooperation with the family doctor, an empathetic midwife and/or a social worker.[23] Also, information on pregnancy, delivery and child-rearing should be made available.

Labor/delivery

There are usually no specific programs for the intrapartum management of teenage pregnancies. It is important that the well-being of mother and child is monitored effectively. In this respect, continuous active support during labor by the mother's partner and/or a member of the family should be promoted. Confinement may take place in a non-specialist unit if no risk factors other than age are present. In the exceptionally young adolescents, however, confinement in a specialist unit is recommended because of an increased likelihood of obstructive labor due to the small size of the immature pelvis.[18]

Postnatal

Infant feeding practices, infant growth and infant safety should be reviewed.[13] Symptoms of medical problems in the infant need to be considered. Social and financial concerns should be discussed. Teenage girls should be encouraged to continue secondary education.[6,8,11] Effective contraception should be implemented. In

PREGNANCY IN ADOLESCENCE
Summary of Management Options

Prepregnancy

- Education and advertising directed toward sexual behaviour and family planning. Emphasize self-referral for care when pregnant

Prenatal

- Encouragement of early referral for prenatal care and regular attendance

- Confirm gestation with early ultrasound

- Stress advice about diet and adverse habits (e.g. smoking)

- Mobilize social support

- Extra advice and education about pregnancy and child-rearing

Labor/delivery

- Ensure adequate psychological support

- Delivery in a specialist unit if dystocia is an anticipated problem

Postnatal

- Advice and support for infant feeding and care

- General social and financial support, especially if secondary education is to be continued

- Discussion about contraception

fact, a large percentage of teenagers who give birth before the age of 17 years will have a repeat pregnancy before they are 19 years old.[8]

Conclusion

Pregnancy has a tremendous impact on the adolescent woman and her family. Detrimental effects of age can be largely explained by poor social circumstances. Available data indicate that most pregnant adolescents are biologically mature when they conceive. Teenagers tend to book late for pregnancy and on the whole do not make proper use of the facilities for antenatal care. Attention should be focused on individual risk factors. Overall, clinicians have an important role in providing guidance for pregnant teenagers and their families.

ADVANCED MATERNAL AGE AND PREGNANCY

Definitions

In 1958, the Council of the International Federation of Gynecology and Obstetrics recommended that the age of 35 years should be accepted as the international standard for the 'elderly' nullipara.[24]

Incidence

Whereas in the late 1960s and early 1970s, there was a fall in the number of live births generally and a drop in the proportion of mothers aged 35 and over,[25-27] in the last decade, there has been a trend toward deferred child-bearing, especially among healthy well-educated women with career opportunities.[28-30] The proportion of pregnant women aged 35 and over varies from country to country. It should be noted that both socio-economic circumstances and the nature of the population of elderly women have changed with time. In former days, pregnant women aged 35 and over tended to have several, unplanned children, whereas today there is a growing proportion of first births to elderly pregnant women.

Risks

Advanced maternal age is a risk indicator rather than a risk factor.[31,32] It is associated with a number of pregnancy complications including miscarriage, chromosomal abnormalities, twins, uterine fibroids, hypertensive disorders, gestational diabetes, prolonged labor, cephalopelvic disproportion necessitating operative delivery, bleeding disorders including placenta previa, low birthweight, preterm delivery, ante- and intra-partum fetal loss and neonatal mortality.[28,29,33–35] However, most reports of pregnancy outcome in 'elderly' primiparous women have not taken into account influences other than age, such as details of general health, smoking habits and past reproductive history, including a history of previous miscarriage or infertility and its treatment.[24,28] Information as to whether there was a deliberate postponement of the first pregnancy is often lacking. Recently, Berkowitz *et al.* reported that although pregnancy complications are more common in primiparous women aged 35 and over, the risk of poor neonatal outcome was not appreciably increased.[30] The women in their study represented a highly select group of private patients who were predominantly White, married, college educated and non-smoking and who were delivered of a single infant in a tertiary center. Hence, their study population was not representative of the population at large. The findings of this study should be interpreted with caution, since they may not be applicable to other populations.

Advanced maternal age is associated with an increased risk of miscarriage. It is assumed that the increased risk of miscarriage among elderly women is a function of the age-related risk of chromosomal abnormalities, since approximately 40–60% of conceptions that abort are chromosomally abnormal.[28,36] The relative frequency of chromosomally normal miscarriages also rises with age, possibly resulting in a decline of uterine function with age.[28] Maternal age has no effect on the incidence of birth defects of unknown etiology.[37]

Maternal Age and Chromosomal Abnormalities

The risk of fetal chromosomal abnormalities, in particular trisomy 21 or Down's syndrome, rises sharply with maternal age.[27,38–40] Estimates of the magnitude of age-related risk of chromosomal abnormalities are often based on information related to maternal age at birth. In **Table 1**, the estimates of maternal age-specific rates of chromosomal abnormalities are based on findings among live births.[39] However, rates derived from studies of chorionic villus samples in early pregnancy[41] and amniotic fluid samples in mid-pregnancy[40] are usually higher (**Table 2**). In fact, the prevalence of Down's syndrome and other autosomal trisomies in live births does not represent the actual incidence of these conditions. There are several reasons for this discrepancy. Apart from the selective termination of abnormal fetuses, the incongruity in rates may be explained by the relatively high rates of miscarriage and intrauterine death of fetuses with Down's syndrome or other chromosomal abnormalities. It has been suggested that the risk of spontaneous death of fetuses with Down's syn-

Table 1

Estimated maternal age-specific rates per 1000 live births for chromosomal aneuploidy (i.e. trisomy 21, 18, 13; XXY and XYY genotypes)[a]

Maternal age years[b]	Rate per 1000 live births	Ratio	Ratio range (2 SD)
35	5.6	1:179	156–213
36	6.7	1:150	128–182
37	8.1	1:123	105–152
38	9.5	1:105	85–123
39	12.4	1:81	68–100
40	15.8	1:63	53–80
41	20.5	1:49	41–65
42	25.5	1:39	32–52
43	32.6	1:31	25–41
44	41.8	1:24	19–32
45	53.7	1:19	15–26
46	68.9	1:14	11–20

[a]These estimates are derived from studies of data available in the 1960s and early 1970s before the widespread use of prenatal diagnosis.[39]
[b]Maternal age at birth.

Table 2

Predicted maternal age-specific rates for chromosomal abnormalities (i.e. the autosomal trisomies 21, 18 and 13; XXY, XYY, XO genotypes and unbalanced translocations) based on data available at the time of amniocentesis[40]

Maternal age years[a]	Rate per 1000 pregnancies	Ratio	Ratio range (2 SD)
35	7.3	1:137	101–213
36	8.6	1:116	88–172
37	10.5	1:95	78–123
38	13.0	1:77	63–98
39	16.4	1:61	52–75
40	20.7	1:48	41–58
41	26.5	1:38	32–45
42	34.1	1:29	25–36
43	41.6	1:24	20–30
44	48.0	1:21	18–25
45	59.3	1:17	14–21
46	73.6	1:14	11–17

[a]Maternal age at amniocentesis.

drome detected at second trimester amniocentesis is approximately 26% (range 18–34%).[42,43] Furthermore, underreporting of affected live births and selection bias may also explain differences in age-specific prevalence rates of Down's syndrome.[40]

Maternal age-specific chromosomal abnormalities arise mostly from maternal non-disjunction during the first meiotic division.[40,43,44] In contrast, translocation trisomy (inherited or arising *de novo*) is not associated with maternal age, while Turner's syndrome (45, X pregnancies) shows an inverse relationship with maternal age.[40,45]

Paternal Age

Several investigators have shown that advanced paternal age has little or no independent effect on the risk of autosomal trisomies when the influence of maternal age is taken into account.[28,38,40,46]

Management Options

Prenatal

In clinical practice, maternal age normally refers to the age of the pregnant woman at the time she consults the doctor or midwife for the initial prenatal evaluation. This is particularly important for genetic counseling. Counseling should carefully distinguish the risk of an abnormality in a live birth from the risk of an abnormality detectable in early pregnancy or in mid-pregnancy.[39,40,41,45,47] Screening for detection of fetal chromosomal abnormalities can be performed by means of chorionic villus sampling (CVS) or amniotic fluid sampling (amniocentesis). The timing of CVS should take account of the higher baseline rate of spontaneous first-trimester miscarriages at advanced maternal age.[41,48–50]

Throughout Europe, prenatal diagnosis programs are mainly intended for women who are above a particular age limit at the time of invasive procedure. However, different centers use different limits. For instance, in the Netherlands, chromosomal analysis is offered to pregnant women aged 36 and over, in the UK to women aged 35 and over and in France to those aged 38 years and over. Recently, the 'triple test' was intro-

---

ADVANCED MATERNAL AGE AND PREGNANCY
Summary of Management Options

Prepregnancy

- Discussion of risks: miscarriage, chromosomal abnormalities, twins, fibroids, hypertension, gestational diabetes, labor problems, perinatal mortality and mortality. However, the main aim is to put these risks into perspective. In practice, management in pregnancy is not altered in the woman of advanced age apart from discussion about prenatal diagnosis of chromosomal abnormalities. Thus the other risks are considered to be of relatively low importance

Prenatal

- Discussion of prenatal diagnosis of chromosomal abnormalities and the offer of CVS or amniocentesis if requested

Labor/delivery

- Optional: delivery in a specialist unit because of the theoretical risk of dystocia and other labor problems

Postnatal

- Discussion of long-term contraception

duced as a prenatal screening device for Down's syndrome.[51,52] This test, which is based on maternal serum levels of alpha-fetoprotein, unconjugated estriol and human chorionic gonadotrophin at approximately 15–20 weeks gestation, could be offered to produce a modified risk assessment for consideration for amniocentesis or CVS thereby taking into account maternal age.[53]

While other complications are statistically more common in women aged 35 years and over[54] (see above), in practice normal antenatal care is usually not modified unless some other risk factor or complication is identified.

Labor/delivery

Elderly women are usually advised to be delivered in a specialist unit because of the risk of dystocia during labor. However, the impression is often gained that the woman's age in itself contributes strongly to the decision to intervene.[29] Close monitoring of fetal condition (intermittent monoaural auscultation or CTG) and progress in the second stage of labor are warranted. In fact, intrapartum care will not be modified substantially because of 'the extremes of maternal age'.

Postnatal

Discussion of long-term contraception is recommended.

Conclusion

It is widely held clinically that advanced maternal age is associated with poor reproductive outcome. Apart from the risk of chromosomal abnormalities, in particular trisomy 21 which rises exponentially with age, evidence about adverse effects of maternal age *per se* on pregnancy outcome is inconclusive.

MATERNAL PARITY

Incidence

In Western societies, nulliparous women constitute almost half of all pregnant women.

Definitions

Definitions of parity tend to differ from country to country.[1] In obstetrics, parity usually refers to the number of times a woman has given birth to an infant,

dead or alive, after 28 weeks gestation. A nullipara is a woman who has never borne a 'viable' child; a primipara is a woman who has had one pregnancy which resulted in a 'viable' child, irrespective of the mode of delivery. A multipara is a woman who has had two or more pregnancies which resulted in a 'viable' child. Plural pregnancies are counted as 'one'. Any previous abortions or ectopic pregnancies are not counted. The Netherlands and the Scandinavian countries use 16 weeks as the cut-off point. From the social perspective, it is perhaps more appropriate to obtain information on the number of children the mother already has to look after, including stepchildren and adopted children.[1] The term 'grande multipara' is applied to the woman who has given birth to four or five children of at least 28 weeks gestation.

Risks

Differences in mortality risk between the offspring of primiparous and multiparous women is accounted for by birthweight.[55] Parity is closely associated with maternal age and, to a certain extent, with social class. It is often difficult to establish precisely how these factors are implicated in the etiology of adverse pregnancy outcome. On the whole, the risk of adverse outcome with parity does not show a consistent pattern.[1,22,56] Mean birthweight for infants born to nulliparous women is consistently lower than for infants born to multiparous women.[1] Some investigators have suggested that differences in the mean birthweight of women of different parity could be explained by differences in maternal weight.[55,57] It is well known that nulliparity is associated with an increased risk of pregnancy-induced hypertension, which in itself is strongly related to low birthweight.[32] Furthermore, in nulliparous women, there is an increased risk of perineal trauma, either by episiotomy or spontaneous tear, compared with multiparous women.

Women of high parity tend to receive inadequate obstetric care as exemplified by late booking and poor attendance for antenatal care.[21] High parity is associated with an increased likelihood of abnormal fetal presentation and obstetric hemorrhage. It has been shown that parity does not have a significant effect on the incidence of Down's syndrome when the influence of maternal age is taken into account.[38]

Management Options

Prenatal

Nulliparity is a non-specific risk factor. In this respect, no specific precautions need to be taken, provided the course of pregnancy is uneventful. In fact, there is no need to be under specialist care on the grounds of nulliparity alone.[58]

In parous women, it is of fundamental importance to obtain all clinically relevant details of previous obstetric performance. Reproductive history is a very informative predictor of pregnancy outcome. Consequently, information of this kind has its implications for the management of subsequent pregnancies. In order to facilitate the provision of antenatal care to parous women, it would be useful to provide space, and manpower, to accommodate accompanying children.

Labor/delivery

On empirical grounds, it is known that there is a difference in normal labor patterns of nulliparous and multiparous women. In fact, median duration of the second stage of labor (i.e. from full dilatation of the cervix to delivery) is approximately 45 min in nulliparous women *vs* approximately 20 min in multiparous women, who, at least, have experienced a vaginal delivery previously. Clinically, however, the duration of the second stage of labor is highly variable. In both nulliparous and multiparous women, policies for imposing limits on the length of the second stage tend to be rather subjective, and are usually based on uncontrolled observational data. If the maternal and fetal condition is satisfactory, and there is evidence that progress is occurring with descent of the presenting part, 'therapeutic' intervention is not warranted. Cephalopelvic disproportion must be considered when progress in labor is slow.

PREGNANCIES IN WOMEN AT THE EXTREMES OF PARITY
Summary of Management Options

Prepregnancy

- Discussion of the risks with an emphasis on the effects of parity alone (as opposed to age and socioeconomic status)

Nulliparity

- Pregnancy-induced hypertension

- Perineal trauma

'Grande multiparity'

- Abnormal fetal presentation

- Obstetric hemorrhage

- Poor attendance

Prenatal

- Encourage regular attendance for care in those of high parity

- Vigilance for pregnancy-induced hypertension in those of nulliparity

- Vigilance for abnormal presentation from 36 weeks in those of high parity

- Consideration of iron and folate prophylaxis with high parity

- Plan for care of existing children for labor/delivery

Labor/delivery

- Nothing specific on the grounds of parity alone; however, a careful review of the past delivery details is necessary in those of high parity for specific risk factors which may modify management (e.g. postpartum hemorrhage, rapid labor and delivery)

Postnatal

- Discussion of long-term contraception in those of high parity

Postnatal

Discussion of long-term contraception is recommended.

Conclusion

First births have an increased risk over second births, although the pattern of risk varies with age.[1] In fact, parity, age and socioeconomic status are all intercorrelated and they all exert an influence on birthweight and pregnancy outcome in terms of perinatal mortality. In some women, the effects tend to act in the same direction to produce high rates of adverse pregnancy outcome. Overall, the relative importance of parity is limited where fetal outcome is concerned. Nulliparity is associated with an increased risk of pregnancy-induced hypertension, while 'grande multiparity' is associated with abnormal fetal presentation and obstetric hemorrhage. Empirically, the duration of 'normal' labor in multiparous women is shorter than in nulliparous women.

MATERNAL SOCIAL FACTORS

The importance of maternal social factors on the health and well-being of the offspring has been recognized for a long time. Infant mortality, for example, is closely associated with social class and large differences still exist. For several reasons, caution should be exercised in interpreting studies concerning the impact of the social class on pregnancy outcome. These include variations in definitions and practices with time and geographical area, availability of reliable data, and interpretation of the findings.[59–61]

Variations in Definitions

The concept of 'social class index' is not simple. Various measures of social status exist. Some of these tend to be rather vague and meaningless. In England and Wales, for example, the maternal social class index is traditionally derived from the Registrar General's Classification, which is based on the occupation of the father of the child (see **Table 3**). Although there is a

Table 3
Social class by occupation of father

I	Higher professionals
II	Other professionals, including those in managerial positions
IIIa	Skilled workers, non-manual
IIIb	Skilled workers, manual
IV	Semi-skilled workers
V	Unskilled workers

strong association between social class thus derived and infant mortality, this observation does not explain why some babies die. Other methods of categorization of social class include those based on ranking of educational attainment, income, type of health care coverage, employment profile, legitimacy, family affluence and household characteristics.[61] Accurate information of this kind is usually not readily available.

Interpretation Difficulties

It should be emphasized that social risk factors, however defined, are descriptive rather than explanatory. Social disadvantage in itself is unlikely to have a direct causal effect on the outcome of pregnancy.[62] Social class should merely be regarded as a risk indicator, identifying high-risk groups within the population.[31] Social adversity probably represents a wide range of behavioral, environmental, medical and psychological factors that are causally related to pregnancy outcome, some of these being more amenable to intervention than others.[63–66] In this context, it is assumed that women of high social class have better financial, educational and medical resources when compared with women of low social class. Many social risk factors are interrelated. In the absence of logically structured multivariate analyses, the independence of their effects cannot be established.[55] In scientific research, social class correlations should be the impetus for further investigation, rather than the end-point of an analysis.[54]

Risks

Substantial differences in pregnancy outcome persist between socioeconomic groups.[67] Smoking has been suggested as the key factor underlying socioeconomic differences in infant mortality.[68–71]

Management Options

Prenatal

Socially disadvantaged women are less prone to seek prenatal care and also have more pregnancy complications. Some claim that apart from recognizing the increased risk associated with socioeconomic disadvantage, there is little to do in terms of prevention. Social support, however, does benefit women psychologically, although the effect of social interventions on mean birthweight, low birthweight and preterm delivery is limited.[23,72,73] From a public health point of view, the greatest reduction in adverse pregnancy outcome may be anticipated from prenatal services which are directed at socially disadvantaged women.[74] In this respect, widespread health education and serious anti-smoking measures are needed.[55,67,68,75,76]

Labor/delivery

Intrapartum management need not be substantially modified if no risk factors other than social class are present.

PREGNANCIES IN WOMEN WITH POOR SOCIOECONOMIC BACKGROUND
Summary of Management Options

Prepregnancy

- Health education measures especially directed at antismoking and family planning

Prenatal

- Extra specific and directed social support

- Plan for care of existing children for labor/delivery

- Vigilance for clinical evidence of poor fetal growth

Labor/delivery

- No additional measures on the basis of adverse socioeconomic factors alone

Postnatal

- Extra specific and directed social support

- Discussion of contraception

Conclusion

There seems little doubt from many studies around the world that the maternal environment exerts a pronounced effect on birthweight and pregnancy outcome. The environmental index, usually expressed as 'social class', does not provide direct information about the circumstances in which the pregnant woman lives. Social class differences may reflect differences in material conditions in life and differences in behavior (e.g. smoking habits). Caution must be exercised in the extrapolation of associations between social class, however defined, and pregnancy outcome, since mechanisms underlying these associations are often unclear. Clinically, it is difficult to alleviate the effects of social deprivation. Social support may have a beneficial effect on emotional well-being, but is unlikely to override the cumulative effects and problems of social disadvantage.[72]

ETHNICITY

Race and ethnicity are complex and controversial sociological issues which are difficult to measure accurately. Race and ethnicity are often regarded as surrogate measures for standard of living and lifestyle.[55,77] However, not only between but also within ethnic populations there are marked variations in cultural beliefs and practices, language, household structure, sexual behavior, contraceptive patterns, general health, perception of illness and disease, childbirth and child-rearing policies, customs related to the postnatal period, dietary habits, housing, education, employment status, economic situation, level of assimilation, stress and access to health care services.[78–81] Some of these attributes have little to do with health or disease, others may be important. In clinical research, the terms 'race' and 'ethnicity' are often inadequately defined, if at all. Epidemiological associations with health problems should, therefore, be interpreted with caution. From the public health point of view, information on 'race' or 'ethnicity' could be relevant for the identification of specific health problems and medical needs.[81]

Risks

Ethnicity is one of the factors most strongly associated with low birthweight.[66,79,82–84] Low birthweight in itself is closely related to infant mortality and childhood morbidity.[82] In the USA, preterm birth rather than growth retardation is implicated as the most important cause of low birthweight in women labeled as Black.[84,85] Given the high rates of preterm delivery, crude survival rates for Black infants are less favourable than for White infants.[84,86,87] Evidence to date is inconclusive about the precise biological explanation for the high preterm delivery rate among Black women.

Apart from preterm delivery, it has also been suggested that newborns designated as White and Black differ in their patterns of intrauterine growth.[55,88] At term, for example, Black infants are on average smaller than White infants.[88,89] Moreover, average duration of gestation in Black women is slightly shorter than in White women.[88] It has been argued that birthweight distribution is an intrinsic genetic feature of ethnicity, just like the sex of the infant.[89] Hence, for each ethnic group, different norms for gestational age and birthweight distributions should be applied.[90] Others, however, have refuted this assumption by claiming that ethnic disparities in birthweight distribution are most likely the result of disparities in maternal health and socioeconomic circumstances.[55,66,86,91]

It has been suggested that, in the preterm category, birthweight-specific mortality in Black infants is lower than in White infants. Wilcox and Russell postulated that this finding has been built on an artefact.[89,90] They stated that over the whole spectrum of adjusted birthweight, Black infants are less likely to survive the perinatal period than White infants.[89,90] The excess birthweight-specific mortality in Black infants may be compounded by a failure to seek and/or receive optimal medical care.[92,93]

Many diseases and problems during pregnancy have both ethnic and geographical distributions. The risks are summarized in **Table 4**. They include:

- *Genetic disorders*: such as Tay Sachs disease with high gene frequencies in Ashkenasi Jews, hereditary hemoglobinopathies including sickle cell disease which is highly prevalent among couples of African descent, and alpha- and beta-thalassemias which occur frequently among women from the Mediterranean, X-linked disorders such as glucose-6-phosphate dehydrogenase deficiency (Mediterranean, American Blacks), and genetic disorders resulting from consanguinity.

- *Viral infections*: including HTLV-I with high prevalences in Jamaica and Japan,[94] human immunodeficiency viruses, HIV-1 (previously called HTLV-III) and HIV-2 (Caribbean and African countries), cytomegalovirus and herpes virus.[95]

- *Specific medical disorders in women originating from endemic areas in developing countries*: such as rheumatic fever, acquired immunodeficiency syndrome (AIDS) and AIDS-related complex (ARC), tuberculosis, yaws, malaria, hepatitis and parasitic infections such as hookworm disease (uncinariasis) among others.

- *Other maternal conditions resulting from diseases and/or deprivation in infancy or childhood*: Female circumcision is still practiced in some parts of Africa, in particular the Horn of Africa, and may affect childbirth.[96]

- *Miscellaneous conditions affecting pregnant women*: Systemic lupus erythematosus appears to occur more frequently in women of African descent residing in North America or the Caribbean.[97] Uterine fibroids occur more often in Black women than in White women.[98,99] Non-engagement of the fetal head late in pregnancy is not uncommon in Black primigravidas.[100] The available date on ethnic differences in the frequency of dysfunctional labor are inconclusive, since differences in duration of labor may be attributed to a wide range of confounding variables including maternal age, stature, birthweight of the infant, poor communication and unfavorable sociocultural circumstances among others.[98,99,101,102]

Management Options

Information, screening and appropriate counseling services should be made available for communities regarded as being at risk for specific diseases (see **Table 4**).

Prenatal

Communication is often a problem due to language barriers. Video displays and informative pamphlets or brochures written in several languages should be made available. Standard information should be centered on guidelines for lifestyle and nutrition and on preparation for parturition and parenthood, preferably in keeping with sociocultural features of the relevant ethnic communities. Use of interpreters either in person or by telephone is advisable for dealing with specific problems.

Once prenatal care has been initiated, women at risk for specific diseases, such as sickle cell disease, may be selected for further testing and/or treatment. In parous women, it is of importance to try to get all necessary information on both course and outcome of previous pregnancies. Immunization status should be checked. Fetal growth should be monitored.

Labor/delivery

Continuous emotional support during labor by the husband or any other family member will probably benefit

Table 4
Risks in pregnancy associated with certain ethnic groups

Ethnic group	Risks
Mediterranean islands, parts of Italy and Greece, Middle East, South-East Asia, and parts of the Indian Subcontinent	Beta-thalassemias: (a) *Minor*: anemia in pregnancy, treated with oral iron and folate but not parenteral iron. (b) *Major*: rare to survive to reproductive age but those that do often have pelvic bony deformities and problems with labor/delivery; also iron overload with subsequent hepatic, endocrinological and myocardial damage (c) *Major/minor*: possible risks of inheriting the disease requiring prenatal counseling and diagnosis Alpha-thalassemias (a) *Minor*: usually asymptomatic (b) *Major*: rare but a spectrum of presentation: in adult life usually manifests as a hemolytic anemia of variable severity (c) *Major/minor*: possible risks of inheriting the disease requiring prenatal counseling and diagnosis; homozygous alpha-thalassemias in the fetus can manifest as hydrops fetalis and associated severe pre-eclampsia in the mother
Afro-Caribbean, Mediterranean, Middle East, India	Sickling disorders (especially HbSS, HbSC): (a) *Maternal*: infection, sickling crises, pre-eclampsia, renal compromise, jaundice. Though HbSC tends to be a milder disease (Hb levels usually within normal limits), can present with massive sickling crisis if diagnosis has not been made. HbAS (carrier state) mothers are only rarely at risk of sickling crises with, for example, anoxia, dehydration, acidosis (b) *Fetus*: possible risks of inheriting the disease requiring prenatal counseling and diagnosis; growth retardation a risk with HbSS and HbSC
Mediterranean, American Blacks	Glucose-6-phosphate dehydrogenase deficiency: (a) *Mother*: hemolytic anemia (b) *Fetus*: risks of inheriting the disease requiring prenatal counseling and diagnosis; fetal hydrops
Far East	Hepatitis B (chronic carriers): risks of transmission to fetus/neonate and health care workers
Africa, Caribbean, Hawaii	HIV infection: risks to the mother of developing symptomatic infections to the fetus and to health care workers of acquiring the infection
Africa (especially Horn of Africa)	Female circumcision: problems with vaginal delivery (dystocia, trauma, hemorrhage)
Developing countries	Varied effects of endemic infection on mother and/or fetus

maternal well-being and will also facilitate the assessment of fetal well-being. It is unlikely that ethnicity in itself affects the duration of labor and delivery.

Postnatal

Contraceptive advice should take account of individual sociocultural norms and values.

PREGNANCIES IN WOMEN FROM DIFFERENT ETHNIC BACKGROUNDS
Summary of Management Options

Prepregnancy

- Education, screening and counseling for communities at specific risk (see **Table 4**)

Prenatal (see Table 4)

- Overcoming language and cultural barriers (e.g. regular interpreter, 'routine' pregnancy literature in appropriate language)

- Screening and counseling where specific risk

- Offering prenatal diagnosis if appropriate

- Maternal surveillance appropriate to any specific risk

- Fetal surveillance appropriate to any specific risk

Labor/delivery

- Interpreter who can be present for the whole of labor and delivery

- Consideration of cultural norms in provision of care

Postnatal

- Contraceptive advice taking account of individual sociocultural norms and values

Conclusion

Variations in health care coverage and reproductive outcome among racial and ethnic groups are still large.[77,103,104] Reasons for differences in pregnancy outcome between ethnic groups are not entirely clear, although social environment, age, parity and genetic and constitutional factors may play an important part. A number of diseases show clear ethnic differences among pregnant women. These include genetic defects, such as the hereditary hemoglobinopathies, and specific conditions acquired in endemic areas, such as malaria, AIDS and tuberculosis.

REFERENCES

1 Golding J (1990) Maternal age and parity. In Golding J (ed.) *Social and Biological Effects on Perinatal Mortality. Vol. III: Perinatal Analyses*. Report on an international comparative study sponsored by the World Health Organization, pp. 183–218. Bristol: University of Bristol Printing Unit.
2 Sandler DP, Wilcox AJ, Horney LF (1984) Age at menarche and subsequent reproductive events. *American Journal of Epidemiology* **119**:765–774.
3 McAnarney ER (1987) Young maternal age and adverse neonatal outcome. *American Journal of Diseases of Children* **141**:1053–1059.
4 Scholl TO, Hediger ML, Salmon RW, Belsky DH, Ances IG (1989) Association between low gynaecological age and preterm birth. *Paediatric and Perinatal Epidemiology* **3**:361–370.
5 Mitchell LE, Bracken MB (1990) Reproductive and chronologic age as a predictor of low birth weight, preterm delivery and intrauterine growth retardation in primiparous women. *Annals of Human Biology* **17**:377–386.
6 Bury JK (1985) Teenage pregnancy. *British Journal of Obstetrics and Gynaecology* **92**:1081–1083.
7 Hamburg DA, Nightingale EO, Takanishi R (1987) Facilitating the transitions of adolescence: Council on Adolescent Development. *Journal of the American Medical Association* **257**:3405–3406.
8 McGrew MC, Shore WB (1991) The problem of teenage pregnancy. *Journal of Family Practice* **32**:17–21.
9 Bader M (1987) Adolescent pregnancy: Incidence and cost. *Journal of the American Medical Association* **258**:1890.
10 Barron SL (1986) Sexual activity in girls under 16 years of age. *British Journal of Obstetrics and Gynaecology* **93**:787–793.
11 Hollingsworth DR, Felice M (1986) Teenage pregnancy: A multiracial sociologic problem. *American Journal of Obstetrics and Gynecology* **155**:741–746.
12 Anonymous (1989) Adolescent pregnancy. *Lancet* **2**:1308–1309.
13 Van Winter JT, Simmons PS (1990) A proposal for obstetric and pediatric management of adolescent pregnancy. *Mayo Clinics Proceedings* **65**:1061–1066.
14 Fielding JE, Williams CA (1991) Adolescent pregnancy

in the United States: A review and recommendations for clinicians and research needs. *American Journal of Preventive Medicine* **7**:47–52

15 Davis RL, Tollestrup K, Milham S (1990) Trends in teenage smoking during pregnancy. Washington State: 1984 through 1988. *American Journal of Diseases of Children* **144**:1297–1301.

16 Hardy PH, Hardy JB, Nell EE, Graham DA, Spence MR, Rosenbaum RC (1984) Prevalence of six sexually transmitted disease agents among pregnant inner-city adolescents and pregnancy outcome. *Lancet* **2**:333–337.

17 Babson SG, Clarke NG (1983) Relationship between infant death and maternal age: Comparison of sudden infant death incidence with other causes of infant mortality. *Journal of Pediatrics* **103**:391–393.

18 Moerman ML (1982) Growth of the birth canal in adolescent girls. *American Journal of Obstetrics and Gynecology* **143**:528–532.

19 Sukanich AC, Rogers KD, McDonald NM (1986) Physical maturity and outcome of pregnancy in primiparous women younger than 16 years of age. *Pediatrics* **78**:31–36.

20 Pearson JF (1991) Preventing unwanted pregnancies. *British Medical Journal* **303**:598.

21 Blondel B, Kaminsky M, Breart G (1980) Antenatal care and maternal demographic and social characteristics: Evolution in France between 1972 and 1976. *Journal of Epidemiology and Community Health* **34**:157–163.

22 Sweeney PJ (1989) A comparison of low birth weight, perinatal mortality, and infant mortality between first and second births to women 17 years old and younger. *American Journal of Obstetrics and Gynecology* **160**:1361–1370.

23 Oakley A (1988) Is social support good for the health of mothers and babies? *Journal of Reproduction and Infant Psychology* **6**:3–21.

24 Barkan SE, Bracken MB (1987) Delayed childbearing: No evidence for increased risk of low birth weight and preterm delivery. *American Journal of Epidemiology* **125**:101–109.

25 Jones DC, Lowry RB (1975) Falling maternal age and incidence of Down syndrome. *Lancet* **1**:753–754.

26 Mikkelsen M (1979) Epidemiology of trisomy 21: Population, peri- and antenatal data. In Burgio GR, Fraccaro M, Tiepolo L, Wolf U (eds) *Trisomy 21*, pp. 211–226. Berlin: Springer-Verlag.

27 Holloway S, Brock DJH (1988) Changes in maternal age distribution and their possible impact on the demand for prenatal diagnostic services. *British Medical Journal* **296**:978–981.

28 Stein ZA (1985) A woman's age: Childbearing and child rearing. *American Journal of Epidemiology* **121**:327–342.

29 Tuck SM, Yudkin PL, Turnbull AC (1988) Pregnancy outcome in elderly primigravida with and without a history of infertility. *British Journal of Obstetrics and Gynaecology* **95**:230–237.

30 Berkowitz GS, Skovron ML, Lapinski RH, Berkowitz RL (1990) Delayed childbearing and the outcome of pregnancy. *New England Journal of Medicine* **322**:659–664.

31 Gunning-Schepers L (1989) The health benefits of prevention: A similation approach. In Blanpain J, Davis K, Gunji A (eds) *Health Policy*, Vol. 12. Amsterdam: Elsevier.

32 James WH (1976) Birth order, maternal age and birth interval in epidemiology. *International Journal of Epidemiology* **5**:131–132.

33 MacGillivray I (1983) *Pre-eclampsia: The Hypertensive Disease of Pregnancy*. London: W.B. Saunders.

34 MacGillivray I, Samphier M, Little J (1988) Factors affecting twinning. In MacGillivray I, Campbell DM, Thompson B (eds) *Twinning and Twins*, pp. 67–97. Chichester: John Wiley.

35 Spiekerman JCM, Treffers PE, Van Enk A (1986) Specialistische begeleiding bij de bevalling van de oudere nullipara gewenst? *Nederlands Tijdschrift voor Geneeskunde* **130**:213–217.

36 Hassold T, Warburton D, Kline J, Stein Z (1984) The relationship of maternal age and trisomy among trisomic spontaneous abortions. *American Journal of Human Genetics* **36**:1349–1356.

37 Baird PA, Sadovnick AD, Yee IML (1991) Maternal age and birth defects. *Lancet* **337**:527–530.

38 Smith GF, Berg JM (1976) *Down's Anomaly*, 2nd ed. Edinburgh: Churchill Livingstone.

39 Hook EB (1981) Rates of chromosome abnormalities at different maternal ages. *Obstetrics and Gynecology* **58**:282–285.

40 Ferguson-Smith MA, Yates JRW (1984) Maternal age specific rates for chromosome aberrations and factors influencing them: Report of a collaborative European study on 52 965 amniocenteses. *Prenatal Diagnosis* **4**:5–44 (suppl.).

41 Hook EB (1990) Chromosome abnormalities in older women by maternal age: Evaluation of regression-derived rates in chorionic villus biopsy specimens. *American Journal of Medical Genetics* **35**:184–187.

42 Creasy MR, Polani PE (1978) High risk of Down's syndrome at advanced maternal age. *Lancet* **1**:716–717.

43 Hook EB, Topol BB, Cross PK (1989) The natural history of cytogenetically abnormal fetuses detected at midtrimester amniocentesis which are not terminated electively: New data and estimates of excess and relative risk of late fetal death associated with 47, +21, and some other abnormal karyotypes. *American Journal of Human Genetics* **45**:855–861.

44 Giraud F, Ayne S, Mattei JF, Mattei MG (1979) Maternal age and trisomy 21. In Burgio GR, Fraccaro M, Tiepolo L, Wolf U (eds) *Trisomie 21*, pp. 239–240. Berlin: Springer-Verlag.

45 Stein Z, Stein W, Susser M (1986) Attrition of trisomies as a maternal screening device: An explanation of the association of trisomy 21 with maternal age. *Lancet* **1**:944–947.

46 Hook EB (1987) Issues in analysis of data on paternal age and 47, +21: Implications for genetic counselling for Down syndrome. *Human Genetics* **77**:303–306.

47 Hook EB (1976) Risk of Down syndrome in relation to maternal age. *Lancet* **2**:465–466.

48 Cohen-Overbeek TE, Hop WCJ, Den Ouden M, Pijpers L, Jahoda MGJ, Wladimiroff JW (1990) Spontaneous

abortion rate and advanced maternal age: Consequences for prenatal diagnosis. *Lancet* **336**:27–29.

49 MRC Working Party on the Evaluation of Chrion Villus Sampling (1991) Medical Research Council European Trial of chorion villus sampling. *Lancet* **337**:1491–1499.

50 Canadian Collaborative CVS–Amniocentesis Clinical Trial Group (1989) Multicentre Randomised clinical trial of chorion villus sampling and amniocentesis. *Lancet* **1**:1–6.

51 Wald NJ, Cuckle HS, Densen JW, Nanchahal K, Royston P, Chard T, Haddow JE, Knight GJ, Palomaki GE, Canick JA (1988) Maternal serum screening for Down's syndrome in early pregnancy. *British Medical Journal* **297**:883–887.

52 Wald N, Cuckle H, Wu T, George L (1991) Maternal serum unconjugated oestriol and human chorionic gonadotrophin levels in twin pregnancies: Implications for screening for Down's syndrome. *British Journal of Obstetrics and Gynaecology* **98**:905–908.

53 Sheldon TA, Simpson J (1991) Appraisal of a new scheme for prenatal screening for Down's syndrome. *British Medical Journal* **302**:1133–1136.

54 Golding J, Tejeiro A, Rojas Ochoa F (1990) The uses and abuses of national statistics. In Golding J (ed.) *Social and Biological Effects on Perinatal Mortality. Vol. III: Perinatal Analyses.* Report on an international comparative study sponsored by the World Health Organization, pp. 355–384. Bristol: Bristol University Printing Unit.

55 Kline J, Stein Z, Susser M (1989) Ch 12: Preterm delivery—II. Risk factors; Ch 13: Fetal growth and birthweight—I. Indices, patterns and risk factors. In Kline J, Stein Z, Susser M (eds) *Conception to Birth: Epidemiology of Prenatal Development*, pp. 191–230. New York: Oxford University Press.

56 Forman MR, Meirik O, Berendes HW (1984) Delayed childbearing in Sweden. *Journal of the American Medical Association* **252**:3135–3139.

57 Naeye RL, Tafari N (1983) Fetal growth. In Naeye RL, Tafari N (eds) *Risk Factors in Pregnancy and Diseases of the Fetus and Newborn*, pp. 19–75. Baltimore, MD: Williams and Wilkins.

58 Hall MH (1990) Antenatal care. *Clinical Obstetrics and Gynaecology* **4**:65–76.

59 Jones IG, Cameron D (1984) Social class analysis: An embarrassment to epidemiology. *Community Medicine* **6**:37–46.

60 Oakley A, Rajan L, Robertson P (1990) A comparison of different sources of information about pregnancy and childbirth. *Journal of Biosocial Science* **22**:477–487.

61 Krieger N (1991) Women and social class: A methodological study comparing individual, household, and census measures as predictors of black/white differences in reproductive history. *Journal of Epidemiology and Community Health* **45**:35–42.

62 Antonovsky A, Bernstein J (1977) Social class and infant mortality. *Social Science and Medicine* **11**:453–470.

63 Chalmers I (1985) Short, Black, Himsworth and social class differences in fetal and neonatal mortality rates. *British Medical Journal* **2**:231–233.

64 Chalmers B (1986) Psychological aspects of pregnancy: Some thoughts for the eighties. *Social Science and Medicine* **16**:323–331.

65 Elbourne D, Pritchard C, Dauncey M (1986) Perinatal outcomes and related factors: Social class differences within and between geographical areas. *Journal of Epidemiology and Community Health* **40**:301–308.

66 Kleinman JC, Kessel SS (1987) Racial differences in low birth weight: Trends and risk factors. *New England Journal of Medicine* **317**:749–753.

67 Haggerty RJ (1985) The limits of medical care. *New England Journal of Medicine* **313**:383–384.

68 Kramer MS (1987) Intrauterine growth and gestational duration determinants. *Pediatrics* **80**:502–511.

69 Anonymous (1989) Obstetrics and social change. *Lancet* **2**:657–658.

70 Brooke OG, Anderson HR, Bland JM, Peacock JL, Stewart CM (1989) Effects on birth weight of smoking, alcohol, caffeine, socioeconomic factors and psychosocial stress. *British Medical Journal* **289**:795–801.

71 Leon DA (1991) Influence of birthweight on differences in infant mortality by social class and legitimacy. *British Medical Journal* **303**:964–967.

72 Oakley A, Rajan L, Grant A (1990) Social support and pregnancy outcome. *British Journal of Obstetrics and Gynaecology* **97**:155–162.

73 Bryce RL, Stanley FJ, Garner JB (1991) Randomized controlled trial of antenatal social support to prevent preterm birth. *British Journal of Obstetrics and Gynaecology* **98**:1001–1008.

74 Greenberg RS (1983) The impact of prenatal care in different social groups. *American Journal of Obstetrics and Gynecology* **145**:797–801.

75 Macarthur C, Knox EG (1988) Smoking in pregnancy: Effects of stopping at different stages. *British Journal of Obstetrics and Gynaecology* **95**:551–555.

76 Ershoff DH, Quinn VP, Mullen PD, Lairson DR (1990) Pregnancy and medical cost outcomes of a self-help prenatal smoking cessation program in HMO. *Public Health Reports* **105**:340–347.

77 Terry PB, Condie RG, Settatree RS (1980) Analysis of ethnic differences in perinatal statistics. *British Medical Journal* **281**:1307–1308.

78 Houdek Jimenez M, Newton N (1979) Activity and work during pregnancy and the postpartum period: A cross-cultural study of 202 societies. *American Journal of Obstetrics and Gynecology* **135**:171–176.

79 Barron SL (1983) Birthweight and ethnicity. *British Journal of Obstetrics and Gynaecology* **90**:289–290.

80 Helman C (1986) Culture factors in epidemiology. In Helman C (ed.) *Culture, Health and Illness*, pp. 181–193. Bristol: John Wright.

81 Cruickshank JK, Beevers DG (1989) Migration, ethnicity, health and disease. In Cruickshank JK, Beevers DG (eds) *Ethnic Factors in Health and Disease*, pp. 3–6. London: Butterworth.

82 McCormick MC (1985) The contribution of low birth weight to infant mortality and childhood morbidity. *New England Journal of Medicine* **312**:82–90.

83 Shiono PH, Klebanoff MA, Graubard BI, Berendes HW, Rhoads GG (1986) Birth weight among women of dif-

ferent ethnic groups. *Journal of the American Medical Association* **255**:48–52.

84 Lieberman E, Ryan KJ, Monson RR, Schoenbaum SC (1987) Risk factors accounting for racial differences in the rate of premature birth. *New England Journal of Medicine* **317**:743–748.

85 Shiono PH, Klebanoff MA (1986) Ethnic differences in preterm and very preterm delivery. *American Journal of Public Health* **76**:1317–1321.

86 Paneth N, Wallenstein S, Kiely JL, Susser M (1982) Social class indicators and mortality in low birth weight infants. *American Journal of Epidemiology* **116**:364–375.

87 Behrman RE (1987) Premature births among black women. *New England Journal of Medicine* **317**:763–765.

88 Alexander GR, Tompkins ME, Altekruse JM, Hornung CA (1985) Racial differences in the relation of birth weight and gestational age to neonatal mortality. *Public Health Reports* **100**:539–547.

89 Wilcox AJ, Russell IT (1986) Birthweight and perinatal mortality: III. Towards a new method of analysis. *International Journal of Epidemiology* **15**:188–196.

90 Wilcox A, Russell I (1990) Why shall small black infants have a lower mortality rate than small white infants: The case for population specific standard of birthweight. *Journal of Pediatrics* **116**:7–10.

91 Rahbar F, Momeni J, Fomufod A, Westney L (1985) Prenatal care and perinatal mortality in a black population. *Obstetrics and Gynecology* **65**:327–329.

92 Hendricks CH (1967) Delivery patterns and reproductive efficiency among groups of differing socioeconomic status and ethnic origins. *American Journal of Obstetrics and Gynecology* **97**:608–624.

93 Wildschut HIJ, Wiedijk V, Oosting J, Voorn W, Huber J, Treffers PE (1989) Predictors of foetal and neonatal mortality in Curacao. *Social Science and Medicine* **28**:837–842.

94 Dalgleish AG, Richardson JH, Cruickshank JK (1989) Human retroviruses: Human T-cell leukaemia lymphoma virus (HTLV-I) and disease. In Cruickshank JK, Beevers DG (eds) *Ethnic Factors in Health and Disease*, pp. 155–162. London: Butterworth.

95 Nicoll A, Logan S (1989) Viral infections of pregnancy and childhood. In Cruickshank JK, Beevers DG (eds) *Ethnic Factors in Health and Disease*, pp. 95–102. London: Butterworth.

96 De Silva S (1989) Obstetric sequelae of female circumcision. *European Journal of Obstetrics, Gynecology and Reproductive Biology* **32**:233–240.

97 Fessel WJ (1974) Systemic lupus erythematosus in the community: Incidence, prevalence, outcome and first symptoms; the high prevalence in black women. *Archives of Internal Medicine* **134**:1027–1035.

98 Barron SL, Vessey MP (1966) Immigration: A new social factor in obstetrics. *British Medical Journal* **1**:1189–1194.

99 Tuck SM, Cadozo LD, Studd JWW, Gibb DMF (1983) Obstetric characteristics in different racial groups. *British Journal of Obstetrics and Gynaecology* **90**:892–897.

100 Briggs ND (1981) Engagement of the fetal head in the negro primigravida. *British Journal of Obstetrics and Gynaecology* **88**:1086–1089.

101 Thom MH, Chan KK, Studd JWW (1979) Outcome of normal and dysfunctional labour in different racial groups. *American Journal of Obstetrics and Gynecology* **135**:495–498.

102 Doornbos JPR, Nordbeck HJ (1985) Perinatal mortality: Obstetric risk factors in a community of mixed ethnic origin in Amsterdam. PhD thesis, University of Amsterdam.

103 Robinson MJ, Palmer SR, Avery A, James CE, Beynon JL, Taylor RW (1982) Ethnic differences in perinatal mortality: A challenge. *Journal of Epidemiology and Community Health* **36**:22–26.

104 Mason JO (1991) Reducing infant mortality in the United States through 'Healthy Start'. *Public Health Reports* **106**:479–483.

5

Smoking, Alcohol and Drug Abuse

PHILLIP J. SHUBERT, BEVERLY SAVAGE

INTRODUCTION

The problem of substance abuse in pregnancy transcends racial, social and cultural borders. The exact incidence of substance abuse among pregnant women varies by the population being studied. In a telephone survey of 35 perinatal centers, Chasnoff[1] found the prevalence of substance abuse in a pregnant population to be approximately 11% (range 0.4–27%). The true incidence of illicit drug use during pregnancy is probably much higher if one includes the occasional user or those who abstain later in pregnancy.

In general, substance abuse has been associated with poor perinatal outcomes. However, relating the perinatal outcome to specific substances of abuse is difficult given the concurrent use of multiple substances among drug abusers. But the increased incidence of birth defects, spontaneous miscarriages, preterm labor, intrauterine growth deficiency (IUGD), abruption and maternal morbidity among substance abusers has been well described.[2] Thus the obstetrician must have a clear understanding of the complex management issues these patients present.

ALCOHOL

The incidence of alcohol abuse during pregnancy varies but ranges between 1 and 2% of all pregnant women in the USA.[3] The incidence of fetal alcohol syndrome (FAS) ranges between 1:300 and 1:2000.[4] It is now the leading documented cause of mental retardation.[5] Alcohol abuse has been one of the most widely studied areas of substance abuse, and its effects have been well-documented in the medical literature.

Maternal Risks

Neurological

Coma due to acute alcoholic intoxication is a medical emergency. The main concern is maintenance of a good airway. Unless the patient has a blood alcohol level of greater than 500 mg/dl, supportive care is all that is required. If the blood alcohol level is greater than 500 mg/dl, hemodialysis should be instituted.

Tremors and seizures may occur with alcohol withdrawal in the chronic user. Tremors reach their peak approximately 24–36 h after complete cessation of drinking. Tremors are frequently associated with anorexia, flushed facies and tachycardia, all of which usually resolve within a few days. Ideally, the patient should remain hospitalized until the above symptoms have subsided.

Seizures are typically of the grand mal type, either singular or in clusters of two or more over several hours. Almost 30% of patients with generalized seizure activity go on to develop delirium tremors.[6]

The most severe form of alcohol withdrawal is termed delirium tremens. Approximately 5% of delirium tremens end fatally.[6] It is characterized by confusion, hallucinations, tremors, agitation, sleeplessness and increased activity of the autonomic nervous system.

Cardiac

Alcohol appears to have a direct effect on the excitability and contractility of the heart muscle. It is now generally accepted that prolonged intoxication has a damaging effect on cardiac muscle. There is also some evidence that excessive drinking may predispose to cardiac arrhythmias, especially atrial fibrillation.

Gastrointestinal

Alcohol can have significant effects on the liver, including hypertriglyceridemia, fatty liver, impaired gluconeogenesis and hypoglycemia. The latter can invalidate diabetes screening in both the pregnant and non-pregnant state. Alcoholics are also predisposed to gastritis and pancreatitis.

Nutritional

The Wernicke-Korsakoff syndrome, secondary to the poor nutritional status of the alcoholic, is a life-threatening complication. This syndrome results from depletion of the B vitamins in the alcoholic. In addition to the above-mentioned effects of alcohol abuse, the following lesser known entities have also been described.

- *Central nervous system (CNS)*: a central positive myelinosis – seen in severely malnourished alcoholics.

- *Marchiafava-Bignami disease*: primary degeneration of the corpus callosum with cerebral atrophy.

Fetal Risks

Fetal alcohol syndrome (FAS) is diagnosed when a child whose mother is known to have abused alcohol or a sibling with FAS is found to have the following characteristics:

- intrauterine or postnatal growth retardation – defined as weight, length and/or head circumference below the tenth percentile

- central nervous system abnormalities, such as neurological abnormalities (i.e. irritability in infancy and hyperactivity in childhood), developmental delay or impaired intellect

- two of the characteristic facial abnormalities in FAS: microcephaly, microopthalmia or shortened palpebral fissures, poorly developed philtrum with a thin upper lip and a flattened maxillary area.

Intrauterine growth deficiency is the most consistent manifestation of FAS and may occur in the absence of the full-blown syndrome. Microcephaly is a relatively common finding, and fetal length appears to be more profoundly affected than fetal weight.[7]

A woman is supposed to be at increased risk of FAS when her daily alcohol intake exceeds 80 g alcohol/day (10 g alcohol = 1 unit is equivalent to one glass of wine, a half pint of beer/lager/cider or one measure of a 'short'). Fetal growth can be compromised with as little as 40 g (4 units) alcohol/day.

It is thought that high blood concentrations of alcohol exert a deleterious effect on the developing CNS of the fetus. The gestational age at which the fetus is exposed to alcohol also determines its effect. During the first trimester, alcohol probably acts as a teratogen altering the embryonic organization of tissue. During the third trimester, when the fetus is undergoing rapid growth and neurological development, alcohol probably causes the intellectual impairment seen in children with FAS.[8] Thus, it is believed that cessation of alcohol abuse, at any time during pregnancy, can have a positive effect on fetal development.[9] Aside from CNS involvement, abnormalities of almost every other organ system have been noted to occur with increased frequency in the offspring of alcoholic mothers. Of note are cardiac defects – ventricular septal defect (VSD) being the most common – atrial septal defect and great vessel anomalies (tetralogy of Fallot). The skeletal abnormalities include pectus excavatum, nail hypoplasia, scoliosis and radiolunar synostosis, an anomaly which is rarely seen in the general population. Finally, although an association cannot be proven, case reports have described an increased incidence of neural tube defects, clubbed foot, gastroschisis and an isochromosome with a long arm of number 9.

Management Options

Prenatal

The health care professional needs to address pertinent questions regarding alcohol use in all patients. Attention must be given to the issue of alcohol consumption while taking a general history in the obstetric-gynecologic patient. Almost all the adverse effects of alcohol show a threshold phenomenon. There is no evidence of adverse fetal effects at intake levels of less than 40 g of absolute alcohol per day. However, there is a clear relationship between heavy alcohol intake and adverse fetal outcome.[10] Indentification of at-risk pregnancies and alcohol counseling must be the first step in establishing a means to stop women from drinking during pregnancy.

Once problem drinkers have been identified, immediate attention should be made to withdraw them from alcohol. At Boston City Hospital,[11] in-patient withdrawal was performed over periods of 3–4 days. No adverse effects to the mother or fetus were described.

If medications are required for withdrawal, a short-acting barbiturate (i.e. pentobarbital) can be used. Benzodiazepines should be avoided, if possible, given the concerns about possible teratogenicity in pregnancy and sedative effects in the newborn.[12] Also, disulfiram (Antabuse®) is a potential teratogen, with possible limb defects described,[13] and should be avoided in pregnancy.

In addition to the detoxification of the patient, emphasis should be placed on adequate dietary intake, supplementary prenatal vitamins, screening for additional substance abuse, and referral to support groups such as 'Alcoholics Anonymous' and 'Women for Sobriety'.

As with other antepartum patients, routine prenatal laboratory work should include CBC, urine for culture and sensitivity, serology, rubella screen, Pap smear, and type and rhesus. In addition, these patients should be offered HIV testing as well as urine toxicology screening throughout their pregnancy. Standard serum MSAFP screening should be obtained at 15–16 weeks. In addition, a targeted ultrasound and fetal echo cardiography should be offered at 18 weeks and approximately 22 weeks, respectively. The mother should be screened with an electrocardiogram, liver function tests and a hepatitis profile screen. Even though no formal genetic counseling is indicated, some time should be spent on the genetic or familial aspects of alcoholism. Most family studies show an alcoholism risk of 5–10% for first-degree female relatives.[14]

Poor nutrition can have a significant impact on the mother and fetus. Screening for nutritional deficiencies is advised, including a total protein and serum albumin. Studies in mice have suggested that zinc deficiency may potentiate the teratogenicity of alcohol.[15] As discussed previously, decreased thiamine levels predispose to a Wernicke's encephalopathy. Thus, patients with a history of alcohol abuse should be given liberal thiamine replacement and prenatal vitamins early in pregnancy.

In addition to obtaining a targeted ultrasound at 18 weeks, patients should have serial ultrasounds approximately every 4–6 weeks to assess fetal growth. At approximately 30 weeks, consideration can be given to non-stress testing given the increased risks of growth

retardation in these patients. Bi-weekly ultrasound fluid evaluation may be instituted. Lastly, heavy drinkers should receive care in a high risk center. These patients can experience alcoholic ketoacidosis, characterized by ketoacidosis and dehydration in the presence of normal glucose levels. This may occur with increased frequency during pregnancy as heavy drinkers alter alcohol and food intake.[16] In addition to alcoholic ketoacidosis, the clinical manifestations of alcohol withdrawal must be recognized.

Labor/delivery

The management of the pregnant alcoholic during labor and delivery must reflect an understanding of the disease process of alcoholism. Alcoholics often abuse other substances, and consequently may have a high tolerance for sedation and analgesics in labor. The high doses of opiates required can have a respiratory depressant effect in the neonate. Attention should be given to this possibility in the immediate postpartum period, both on the part of the obstetrician and the pediatrician. Administration of thiamine (100 mg b.i.d.) and vitamin replacement therapy is important throughout the course of pregnancy and should be continued during labor and delivery.

The biggest risks to the patient result from the manifestations of alcohol withdrawal. As described previously, the tremors can begin approximately 48 h after termination of drinking and usually subside within a few days. If the patient shows signs of increased sympathomimetic activity, consideration should be given to sedation with either hydroxyzine or benzodiazepine. It should be noted that if benzodiazepine is used, it may have a prolonged effect on the fetus and can delay the initial response to pediatric resuscitation. It must be noted that up to 15% of patients with delirium tremens die; thus one should have a low threshold for instituting medical therapy in this setting.

Alcohol withdrawal seizures or 'rum-fits' begin within 12–48 h after cessation of drinking.[6] These are usually of the grand mal type. Anticonvulsant medications are required if they persist. In the event that multiple seizures persist, attempts must be made to evaluate the patient for a possible CNS abnormality. Also transfer to an intensive care facility/ward should be considered.

Postnatal

Treatment of the pregnant alcoholic does not end with delivery of the fetus. In the event that medications are required for withdrawal, the patient should be maintained on these medications for approximately 1 week postpartum. The effects of maternal drinking during breast-feeding are not known. Alcohol does cross freely into the breast milk, reaching levels that approximate those in the maternal serum.[17] Ethanol has also been shown to block the secretion of oxytocin, thereby preventing milk ejection.[18] It may be necessary for the continuing abuser to stop breast-feeding while using alcohol or during the withdrawal period if there are problems with the newborn (especially feeding difficulties).

Clearly, the most important aspect of the postpartum period is one of continuing counseling and self-help programs. Instituting good dietary intake, vitamin supplementation and intensive counseling would also be indicated.

OPIATES

Natural opiates, such as codeine and morphine, are harvested from the opium-producing poppy, *Papaver somniferum*.[19] Semi-synthetic narcotics derived from opium include hydromorphone and oxycodone. Meperidine fentanyl, propoxyhphene and methadone are all synthetic drugs. Synthetic and semi-synthetic narcotics are termed opioids; opiates are durgs derived naturally from opium.[19] Heroin (diacetyl-morphine) and methadone are the two narcotics most commonly used – heroin (illegally) and methadone (usually under medical supervision).[12] Heroin is the drug of choice among addicts because of its greater solubility and possibly because it enters the CNS more rapidly than

---

ALCOHOL ABUSE
Summary of Management Options

Prenatal

- Careful enquiry about alcohol intake to identify the at-risk pregnancy

- Implementation of a withdrawal program

- Consider support groups

- Consider vitamin supplementation (especially thiamine)

- Avoid benzodiazepines

- Avoid disulfiram (Antabuse®)

- Offer hepatitis B and HIV screening

- Offer urine toxicology screening

- Check liver function

- Check cardiac function

- Screen for protein deficiency

- Screen for fetal anomaly

- Screen for fetal growth

- Vigilance for ketoacidosis

- Vigilance for withdrawal syndrome

Labor/delivery

- Vigilance with increased analgesia requirement leading to neonatal sedation

- Vigilance for withdrawal syndrome

- If 'DTs', consider
  - sedation
  - anticonvulsants
  - intensive care

Postnatal

- Continue sedation, etc., if necessary

- Consider bottle-feeding if breast-feeding difficult

- Continued counseling and support in liaison with the appropriate group.

morphine. Methadone is a synthetic opiate that is chemically different than morphine but produces similar effects.

It is currently estimated that there are 9000 births per year to narcotic-addicted women in the USA, with over 300 000 children perinatally exposed to either heroin or methadone.[20] Moreover, studies have shown that narcotic use spans all socioeconomic strata.[19] Therefore, the obstetrician must be alert and informed when caring for his or her patients.

Maternal Risks

Acute opiate overdose can be a life-threatening complication to the mother. It is characterized by varying degrees of unresponsiveness, myosis, respiratory depression, bradycardia and hypothermia. In the most advanced stage, the pupils dilate, the skin and mucous membranes become cyanotic, and the circulation fails.[21]

Addiction

The opiate withdrawal or abstinence syndrome depends mainly on the dose of the drug and the duration of the addiction. After the first 8–16 h of abstinence, the patient will exhibit symptoms of anxiety, restlessness, yawning, nausea, diarrhea, lacrimation and abdominal cramping. These symptoms increase in intensity over a 1–3 day period. During this period, the patient develops severe anxiety, tremors, vomiting, diarrhea, fever, chills, hypertension and muscle spasms. After approximately 7 days, all clinical signs of the abstinency syndrome are gone. The withdrawal from opiates is earely fatal.

There is an increased risk of sexually transmitted diseases in this population. Screening for gonorrhea, chlamydia and syphilis must be done. Documenting HIV status is of critical importance in the narcotic addict. This will be discussed more fully later.

Fetal Risks

Opioids have been clearly associated with fetal loss and growth retardation.[22,23] In addition, there appears to be a propensity toward prematurity and low birthweight infants in heroin-addicted mothers.[24]

Neonatal abstinence syndrome (NAS) or withdrawal occurs in approximately 30–90% of infants exposed to either heroin or methadone *in utero*.[24,25] Signs of NAS include tremors, hypertonia, seizures, sneezing, fever, sweating, diarrhea, vomiting and poor feeding. These findings are usually evident within 3–5 days of delivery when the mother has been taking heroin, but can take longer (up to 14 days) with methadone due to its longer half-life.

There does not appear to be an increased risk of teratogenicity due to opiate use.[19] However, additional teratogenetic risk may be due to the contaminants of the street drugs (e.g. strychnine, quinine, coumadin).

Management Options

Prepregnancy

In the unlikely event that an addict presents for prepregnancy care, attempts should be made to enter the patient into an interdisciplinary withdrawal program.

Prenatal, labor/delivery

Up to 50% of pregnant street addicts first present at the time of labor. If a patient presents with no prenatal care and any physical stigmata of opioid use (i.e. cellulitis, sking tracts), a drug screen should be performed.

Screening

The workup of the pregnant addict should include the following laboratory data:

- CBC with differential
- blood group and rhesus
- urine culture
- TB skin test (possibly chest x-ray)
- hemoglobin electrophoresis
- serum creatinine and urea
- total protein serum albumin
- liver functions
- rubella titer
- serology – VDRL, FTA
- HIV titer
- gonorrhea and *Chlamydia* cultures
- hepatitis B screen
- cervical smear
- early ultrasound and serial scans for growth every 4–6 weeks.

Treatment

Once the diagnosis of opioid addiction is established, attempts should be made to alter the patient's drug dependence as soon as possible in the pregnancy. One of the approaches to treatment of the opioid-dependent pregnant woman is to place her on an alternative drug that is hoped will reduce the street drug use. This approach was established because of the reports of intrauterine demise associated with withdrawal from opioids in the early 1970s. The only drug available to treat opioid-addicted women at the present time is methadone. The advantage of methadone is that it can be taken orally, is long acting and allows for relatively constant blood levels in the patient.

Determining the dose of methadone required to block withdrawal and craving, without producing intoxication, is difficult. Whereas pregnant opioid addicts can be converted to methadone as out-patients, the simplest way to determine methadone dosage is to admit pregnant addicts to an in-patient substance abuse unit for drug regulation. The aim is to make the mother comfortable by avoiding further drug craving, and titrating her to the lowest acceptable dose in the pregnancy. A target goal of 20 mg/day of methadone should be attempted in the pregnancy. It has been shown that when the methadone dose, at delivery, was no greater than 20 mg/day, only 18% of newborns developed withdrawal symptoms.[26]

However, disagreement exists whether opiate-abusing pregnant women are best managed by methadone detoxification or maintenance. If methadone detoxification is to be performed, this should be done only during the second trimester and then at a pace of approximately 2–5 mg reduction per week. During the period of detoxification, special concern must be given to fetal movement counts. It would appear that excessive movement is a potential sign of fetal compromise *not* well-being, as the increased fetal movement is an indication of fetal withdrawal.

If a woman is already stabilized on methadone at her first prenatal visit, continuation of a daily methadone dose is recommended in most circumstances.[19] Signs of overdosage or withdrawal would be an indication for further dose adjustment. Once the patient is established on a dose of methadone, this may remain fixed or may be adjusted for the duration of the pregnancy, depending upon the position of maintenance or detoxification.

If methadone detoxification is not desirable, clonidine may be used as an alternative modality.[27] Clonidine is an alpha-adernegic agonist that suppresses opiate withdrawal.[28] Patients undergoing withdrawal may be given 0.1–0.2 mg sublingually every hour up to 0.8 mg if signs of withdrawal persist. The maintenance dose is 0.8–1.2 mg/day in divided doses for the first 7 days, with tapering for the following 3 days.

Treatment of acute opiate overdose consists of gastric lavage after oral ingestion. If the patient is unresponsive, an endotracheal tube should be placed. Administration of naloxone hydrochloride (Narcan®), an opiate antagonist, is both diagnostic as well as a treatment of choice. Typically, the dose of naloxone is 0.7 mg /70 kg body weight given intravenously, and repeated once or twice if necessary, at 5 min intervals for an adequate respiratory response.[21] Once stable, usually after approximately 8 h, the patient may suffer from sneezing, pruritus and urinary retention.

In labor, women on methadone maintenance should be given their oral dose on the day of delivery. If patients show signs of withdrawal in labor, prompt treatment is required. Moreover, narcotics with significant mixed agonist–antagonist properties (e.g. pentazocine) are contraindicated and may precipitate acute withdrawal.[19] During the course of labor, narcotics for pain management are not contraindicated and should be given as to anyone else in labor; however, larger doses than normal may be necessary.

Postnatal

After pregnancy, attention must be directed toward further withdrawal or maintenance of the addict. Once the patient has been withdrawn, she must be encouraged to continue follow-up in substance abuse treatment programs. Additionally, because relapse is a feature of all addictions, the opioid addict may further benefit from behaviour modification programs. Clearly, the emphasis must be placed on education and self-help if inroads are to be made in changing the patient's lifestyle.

The approach to a woman who wishes to breast-feed is controversial. Some feel that continued addiction to any drug contraindicates breast-feeding; others argue that drugs such as methadone, codeine and morphine are not contraindications to breast-feeding. However, most agree that if the mother remains addicted to heroin, breast-feeding is contraindicated. Methadone is felt by some to be compatible with breast-feeding if the mother receives no more than 20 mg in any 24 h period.[29] In fact, breast-feeding by a methadone-maintained woman may reduce the severity of the neonatal abstinence syndrome. Clearly, if she wishes to breast-feed, establishing her HIV status prior to making the recommendation is of utmost importance.

OPIATE ABUSE
Summary of Management Options

Prepregnancy

- Education

- Interdisciplinary withdrawal program

Prenatal

- Screening program (checklist in text)

- Options for management of dependency
  - withdrawal (with clonidine)
  - methadone maintenance program

- Vigilance and prompt treatment (intubation and naloxone) for acute opiate overdose

Labor/delivery

- Continue methadone on day of delivery

- Avoid narcotics with mixed agonist–antagonist properties (e.g. pentazocine)

- May need larger doses of narcotics for analgesia

Postnatal

- Neonatal surveillance for withdrawal (up to 5 days with heroin; up to 14 days with methadone)

- Advice about breast-feeding is controversial

COCAINE

Cocaine abuse by both pregnant and non-pregnant individuals has increased markedly in the USA over the past 5 years.[1,5,30,31] The incidence of infants testing positive for cocaine at birth ranges from 6 to 11%[32–34] in both urban and suburban hospitals. However, populations with an incidence as high as 27% have been identified.[32] Cocaine has detrimental effects on both the mother and fetus.

Cocaine is an alkaloid derived from the *Erythroxylum* coca plant. It is available in a water-soluble salt form, cocaine hydrochloride, which can be absorbed from any mucosal surface (e.g. 'snorting').[31] Alkalinization of the salt and subsequent extraction in a solvent forms free cocaine base, a relatively pure form of cocaine, which is smoked.[35] Cocaine works via several mechanisms resulting in stimulation of the CNS. It inhibits uptake of neuronal catecholamines, stimulates release of dopamine and releases or blocks serotonin. It also inhibits sodium channels in neural tissue causing local anesthetic effects.[36] It is a drug of abuse because of the euphoria and mental stimulation it produces.

Cocaine is lipophilic and readily crosses biologic membranes,[31] including the placenta. It is detectable in urine or blood for 6–12 h after exposure.[31] However, its metabolites (benzoylecgonine, ecgonine methylester and norecgonine) can be present for up to 6 days. In general, cocaine testing is based on identification of these metabolites, which can be detected in urine for approximately 72 h after administration.

Maternal Risks

Acute intoxication

Cocaine produces feelings of stimulation and euphoria; however, higher doses with excessive CNS stimulation, result in agitation, paranoia, sleeplessness or frank psychosis.[36] Dysphoric agitation may be the first sign of intoxication, and this can be fatal.[37] Hypertension, tachycardia, hyperthermia or seizures in association with the above psychiatric abnormalities are sign of cocaine intoxication.[36]

Withdrawal

Cocaine cause depletion of dopamine reserves in the 'pleasure' centers of the brain. Thus without cocaine, the addict is unable to fill basic needs such as eating, drinking or sexual desires.[36]

Signs of cocaine withdrawal include depression, irritability, appetite and sleep dysfunction, and an intense desire for cocaine. It is the latter than can force female cocaine addicts into high-risk sexual behaviors (e.g. prostitution) to obtain cocaine with resultant risks of abuse, sexually transmitted diseases (STDs) and HIV infection. Addicts are also likely to be nutritionally impaired.

Cardiovascular

Cocaine, secondary to the increase in available catecholamines, causes increases in heart rate, blood pressure and myocardial oxygen demand. It has been associated with myocardial infarction in young, otherwise healthy individuals.[38] Anyone with underlying cardiovascular diseases would be at increased risk of cardiovascular compromise with the use of cocaine. Hypertension can also result in aortic dissection and pulmonary edema.[36]

Cocaine has been associated with cardiac arrhythmias; either secondary to the effect on catecholamines or as a direct effect of the drug.[38] Sinus tachycardia, ventricular premature beats and ventricular tachycardia progressing to fibrillation and asystole have been reported.[38] Myocardial infarction and hyperpyrexia will also predispose to arrhythmias.

Central nervous system

Apart from the psychiatric effects of cocaine mentioned above, the drug can cause permanent CNS damage. Subarachnoid hemorrhage, ruptured aneurysms and strokes have been reported. All are probably related to transient hypertension secondary to cocaine use.[38] Increases in sympathomimetic neurotransmitters may cause cerebral vasoconstriction and/or vasospasm.[37]

Cocaine lowers the seizure threshold and thus seizure activity can be first uncovered during ingestion of cocaine.[36] The hyperpyrexia induced by cocaine also contributes to a lowering of the seizure threshold. Seizures usually occur soon after taking the drug.[37]

Placental abruption

Placental abruption associated with cocaine use was first reported by Acker et al.[39] Other reports of abruption associated with cocaine use have since been reported in the literature.[33,34,40,41] Abruption is thought to be secondary to the acute hypertension and vasoconstriction induced by cocaine. Obviously, this complication can be fatal to both mother and fetus.

Fetal Risks

Many adverse effects of cocaine on pregnancy have been reported and include placental abruption, preterm labor, premature rupture of the membranes and IUGD.[33,34,38,40,42,43]

The incidence of positive toxicology screens in patients with preterm labor is higher than in control patients; the most common drug identified is cocaine.[34,42] Often, it is difficult to separate the effects of cocaine from other drug use, environmental or socioeconomic factors, and poor prenatal care,[31,44] all of which have been associated with preterm labor, IUGD and premature rupture. It is prudent to screen all women with these conditions for cocaine abuse and warn pregnant women who abuse cocaine of the signs of preterm labor, premature rupture and abruption.

Cocaine has been implicated as a teratogenic agent; however, as with many other potential teratogens, a direct casual link has been difficult to prove. A recent review summarized the probable effects of cocaine on neurological and developmental outcome in the neonate.[43] Vasospasms of both fetal and placental vessels are thought to be the responsible mechanisms. Animal studies have also implicated an effect of cocaine on neuronal differentiation, possibly secondary to altered ratios of neurotransmitters in the CNS. Cerebral infarction may result in destructive brain lesions in the fetus. These may be ischemic or hemorrhagic lesions and result in motor and intellectual impairment. Microcephaly appears to be the most common measurable brain abnormality. Sudden infant death syndrome appears to be more common in cocaine-exposed infants. A neurological syndrome consisting of tremors, sleeplessness, poor feeding, irritability and seizures has been reported; however, this is self-limited. Long-term developmental delays are thought to be associated with cocaine abuse; however, these have been difficult to prove with conventional tests and will require more sophisticated tests and longer follow-up than is currently available. Again, study of cocaine's effect on development is confounded by socioeconomic and environmental factors.

Management Options

Prenatal

As with all substance abuse, treatment is dependent on the identification of substance abusers. Cocaine is abused by all segments of society and all pregnant women should be asked about drug use. Not all women who abuse cocaine will report it, even on anonymous questionnaires.[32] The use of routine toxicology screens has been advocated. Routine prenatal testing as described in the alcohol section should be performed. Cocaine abuse should be suspected in cases of IUGD, preterm labor or placental abruption.

Once identified, pregnant women should be encouraged to stop using the drug and be enrolled in an in-patient or out-patient treatment center. Outcome can be improved by comprehensive prenatal care.[43] They should be screened for STDs, hepatitis B and HIV infection, and other drug use. Education on the features of premature membrane rupture, preterm labor and abruption should be given and encouragement to report early if identified. The use of regular cervical examinations is controversial. Serial ultrasound scans should be used to detect pathological fetal growth. Toxicology screens can be used to monitor continued cocaine abuse and/or as a positive reinforcement for the abstaining addict.

Acute intoxication with cocaine can be life-threatening at any point in gestation. Usually this is self-limiting and prolonged intoxication should raise suspicions of continued ingestion (e.g. body packing). Agitation and psychosis can be managed with haloperidol if needed. Hypertension may resolve with sedation (e.g. benzodiazepines alone). Hypertensive crises may be life-threatening and can be treated with labetalol[37] or nitrites,[45] although consideration to decreasing uteroplacental perfusion with resultant fetal distress must be given. Any antihypertensive used must be titratable and short acting. Hyperthermia is aggressively treated with cold water and fans.

Seizures may be self-limited or require aggressive management with benzodiazepines. If seizures are refractory, consideration to paralysis and further antiseizure medication must be given. Seizures, hyperthermia and rhabdomyolysis are responsible for many of the deaths attributable to cocaine.

Evidence of cardiac arrhythmias or infarctions are treated in the usual manner and require admission to an intensive care setting. Attention to fetal monitoring and adequate maternal oxygenation should be part of any therapeutic measures. Obstetrical complications of cocaine abuse are treated in the usual manner. Placental abruption is treated aggressively with large bore intravenous access, fetal monitoring, availability of blood and DIC screens as described in Chapter 9. Delivery may be indicated with evidence of maternal or fetal compromise. Preterm labor is arrested with magnesium sulfate tocolysis. B-Mimetics (ritodrine, terbutaline) should also be avoided when cocaine intoxication is suspected.

After acute intoxication has resolved, the patient should be referred to a treatment program. Hospitalization until a referral can be made should be considered.

Labor/delivery

As with women addicted to opiates, larger doses of narcotics may be necessary to achieve analgesia.

COCAINE ABUSE
Summary of Management Options

Prepregnancy

- General counseling about risks

- Interdisciplinary withdrawal program

- Screen for STDs, hepatitis B, HIV

Prenatal

- Screen for identification of abusers (history, toxicology)

- General counseling about risks

- Detoxification programs

- Screen for STDs, hepatitis B, HIV

- Screen for abuse of other drugs

- Check fetal growth

- Warn about early referral with premature membrane rupture, preterm labor, antepartum hemorrhage

- Vigilance and prompt treatment for complications:
  - hypertension
  - hypothermia
  - seizures
  - arrhythmias

Labor/delivery

- May need larger doses of narcotics for analgesia

Postnatal

- Neonatal surveillance for withdrawal

- Advice about breast-feeding is controversial

Postnatal

The same issues relating to management of the newborn with respect to

- vigilance for and treatment of signs of withdrawal

- advice about breast-feeding

discussed above in the opiate section apply to those patients who are addicted to cocaine.

TOBACCO SMOKING

Smoking is the number one preventable cause of low birthweight (LBW) babies, yet many women continue to smoke throughout their pregnancy. Although the prevalence of smoking has declined in recent years and some women stop smoking when they become pregnant, at least 25% of pregnant American women continue to smoke throughout pregnancy.[46] Of the 4000 compounds in tobacco smoke, nicotine, carbon monoxide and cyanide are thought to have the greatest adverse effect on the mother and fetus.

Maternal Risks

Cardiovascular disease

Premature coronary heart disease is one of the most important consequences of cigarette smoking. Women who use contraceptives prior to pregnancy increase their risk of suffering an aucte myocardial infarction by more than five-fold.[47] Cigarette smoking produces an imbalance between myocardial oxygen supply and demand and an increase in platelet aggregation.

Neoplastic

The number of women dying from lung cancer has steadily risen over the past decade. Cigarette consumption by women increased in the USA during this period, and lung cancer mortality is currently increasing at a faster rate in women than in men. In fact, lung cancer has now replaced breast cancer as the number one killer in women. Five-year survival rates for lung cancer remains approximately 10%. Roughly 80% of lung cancer deaths are attributable to cigarette smoking.[48] Squamous cell and oat cell carcinoma are the histologic types most commonly associated with cigarette smoking.

Respiratory disease

Cigarette smoking contributes to the development of chronic bronchitis and emphysema. Cigarette smoking has also been associated with an increased incidence of respiratory infections and death from pneumonia and influenza.

Gastrointestinal

There is an increased prevalence of gastric and duodenal ulcers in smokers. Moreover, smoking impairs ulcer healing.

Fetal Risks

Cigarette smoking is associated is associated with low birthweight babies. Studies report an average reduction of 200 g in the birthweight of babies of mothers who smoke. Nieburg et al.[49] described the fetal tobacco syndrome (FTS) in discussing the major effect cigarette smoking has on birthweight. Fetal tobacco syndrome has been defined in terms of the following

- mother smoking five or more cigarettes per day

- no maternal history of hypertension in pregnancy

- fetal growth retardation at term (greater than 37 weeks, less than 2500 g)

- no other causes for IUGD.

A likely cause of growth retardation in fetuses of smoking mothers is induction of fetal hypoxemia and/or ischemia, which could be produced by both carbon monoxide and nicotine. Nicotine could impart effects secondary to its vasoconstrictive properties. Carbon monoxide binds to fetal hemoglobin, thereby reducing oxygen availability to the fetus.[50] Naeye[51] found increased placental masses in smoking women with microscopic lesions characteristic of periodic interrruptions of placental perfusion.

Long-term follow-up of children born to smoking mothers has also demonstrated impaired intellectual and emotional development.[52–54] Again, fetal hypoxemia has been considered to be a contributory cause of these abnormalities (i.e. hyperactivity, short attention span, lower scores on spelling and reading tests).

Smoking does not appear to increase the risk of teratogenicity. To date, there is no good scientific evidence for an association between congenital anomalies and maternal tobacco use.

Maternal use of tobacco has been associated with an increased risk of early second trimester miscarriages, placental abruption, preterm premature rupture of the membranes, preterm labor, intrauterine fetal demise, neonatal mortality and sudden infant death syndrome.[55] Kline et al.[56] noted an 80% excess of spontaneous miscarriages in smokers vs non-smokers. The increased incidence of placental abruption is not surprising given the vasoconstrictive properties of nicotine. Nicotine causes arteriolar constriction, which then leads to uterine decidual ischemia. Numerous studies have substantiated the increased risks of smoking with preterm premature rupture of the membranes. In particular, Meyer and Tonascia[57] described a three times greater risk of preterm premature rupture of the membranes in smokers vs non-smokers before 34 weeks. Several retrospective studies have noted a relationship between maternal smoking and sudden infant death syndrome (SIDS).[55,58] SIDS mothers are more likely to have smoked during pregnancy than non-SIDS mothers. It is unclear whether prenatal or postnatal exposure is more important for this relationship.

Management Options

Prenatal, labor/delivery

Once a smoking history has been elicited, it is important to quantitate maternal smoking consumption because the effects of cigarette smoking appear to be dose-related and there is good evidence that cessation of smoking over the second half of pregnancy reduces the maternal and fetal complications.

Directing attempts at smoking cessation or reduction should be performed at each visit. Providing the patient with educational materials on smoking cessation should be done early in her prenatal care. Directing patients to self-help smoking cessation materials has been shown to be helpful in assisting them to stop smoking.[46] A 9–40% reduction in smoking has been described using these programs. Self-help materials instruct patients on how to give up smoking and the use of pregnancy's specific behavioral strategies.

Unfortunately, it is unclear exactly what information is useful in assisting pregnant smokers to cease. Some authors have[59] sampled maternal cotinine levels (a smoking by-product) as an adjunct to smoking cessation and Bauman et al.[60] sampled maternal carbon monoxide levels. However, neither study showed that maternal blood sampling helped to reduce maternal smoking. Also, instructing patients regarding a reduction in birthweight may not be persuasive in helping them to give up smoking. Sexton and Habel[61] confronted the myth about small babies and easy labors as an intrinsic component of their smoking reduction trial.

Nicotine replacement therapy is clearly benefical as an adjunct to smoking cessation therapy, particularly in more highly dependent smokers.[46] Nicotine replacement therapy poses less risk to the mother and fetus, since cigarettes contain a significant amount of carbon monoxide in addition to nicotine. Someone who smokes 20 cigarettes a day consumes an average of 20 mg of nicotine and 200–300 ng of carbon monoxide per day.[46] Also, nicotine levels are significantly higher in smokers vs those patients using replacement therapy (20–35 vs 10–15 ng/ml transdermal nicotine). In addition, cigarette smoking delivers nicotine more rapidly, through pulmonary absorption, producing higher concentrations in the brain and other organs.

TOBACCO SMOKING
Summary of Management Options

Prepregnancy

- Explanation of risks

- Advise to reduce

- Specific programs for cessation

Prenatal

- Advise to reduce

- Specific programs for cessation

- Vigilance for small-for-dates, premature membrane rupture, preterm labor and antepartum hemorrhage

Labor/delivery

- Advise cessation of smoking for 48 h prior to elective delivery

Postnatal

- Continued support if cessation has taken place in pregnancy

A criticism of transdermal nicotine replacement is that nicotine levels remain sustained over a 24 h period with no overnight nadirs as seen in cigarette smokers. What effect, if any, this has on the maternal–fetal environment remains to be established.

In addition to helping the patient stop smoking, it is important for the obstetrician to develop a management strategy for the persistent smoker. As described, smoking significantly increases the risks of IUGD, premature rupture of the membranes, preterm labor, abruption and IUFD. The site of insult clearly appears to be at the placenta. Thus performing serial ultrasounds for growth and fluid volume is indicated. Performing cervical cultures and vaginal pH may be useful in screening for the likelihood of premature rupture of the membranes. Cervical ultrasound may benefit those patients who complain of preterm labor symptoms. However, the value of these predictive programs in reducing the incidence of premature rupture of the membranes and preterm labor needs to be established in large randomized trials.

Postnatal

Nicotine has been found in breast milk of smoking mothers and the concentrations of nicotine parallel the number of cigarettes smoked.[62] The impact on the baby of nicotine in breast milk is currently not well-demonstrated. Pneumonia and bronchitis requiring hospitalization have been reported as being more common in the offspring of smoking mothers.

Relapse of the smoking mother usually occurs during the 3-month interval immediately after quitting. Successful programs emphasize maintenance of the non-smoking state during this critical time.

BARBITURATES

There continues to be a high incidence of barbiturate abuse in both therapeutic and non-therapeutic settings. More than 15 000 deaths secondary to barbiturate poisoning have been reported annually in the USA. Therefore, the improper use of barbiturates should be a matter of concern to all in the medical profession.

Maternal/Fetal Risks

The greatest risks of barbiturate ingestion involve either acute intoxication or chronic addiction. The main risk to the fetus is of addiction and withdrawal *in utero* and in the newborn phase.

Management Options

Prenatal

If acute intoxication is suspected, blood levels of barbiturates should be measured to confirm the diagnosis. Clinically, it can be useful to recognize three degrees of acute intoxication: mild, moderate and severe.[63] Mild intoxication results in drowsiness similar to alcohol intoxication. Moderate intoxication results in a more depressed state of consciousness with depressed or absent deep reflexes and shallow respirations. Severe intoxication can evolve into pulmonary edema, cyanosis and slow, shallow, irregular respirations. The temperature may be subnormal and blood pressure may drop to shock levels.

The management of acute intoxication is clearly dependent on its severity. In mild or moderate intoxication, close observation and supportive care is all that is frequently required. In cases of severe respiratory depression or unresponsiveness, prompt intervention must be instituted. Clearly, maintaining a potent airway by means of endotracheal tube must be done immediately. In an unresponsive intubated patient, gastric lavage may be performed. Adequate intravenous fluid volume should be assured to promote renal clearance of the drug. If the patient is in shock, use of norepinephrine and fluid resuscitation may be necessary. Hemodialysis should be used in all patients in a profound coma. Hemodialysis is especially effective in cases of coma due to long acting barbiturates and if anuria develops.

Prolonged maternal consumption of barbiturates may result in tolerance and dependence in both the mother and fetus.[12] Tolerance to barbiturates does not develop as rapidly as to opiates.[63] Abrupt withdrawal before delivery may be accompanied by intrauterine fetal withdrawal, not unlike that seen in narcotic addicts. However, when the pregnant barbiturate addict is identified, she can be withdrawn with controlled decremental doses of pentobarbital without risk of serious neonatal withdrawal. Typically, 0.2 g pentobarbital given orally every 6 h is sufficient.

Labor/delivery, postnatal

As stated previously, substance-abusing patients frequently present with little or no prenatal care. Therefore, identifying the patient during labor and delivery can be difficult. Clearly, a high index of suspicion must be maintained when caring for patients with a blunted sensorium, cerebellar incoordination or emotional lability.

One of the major risks for the chronically intoxicated barbiturate addict is the advent of the abstinence or withdrawal syndrome. With phenobarbital, the onset of withdrawal symptoms may not occur until 48–72 h after the final dose. In its most severe form, seizures and delirium can occur. Death has been reported under these circumstances.[63] Therefore, maintaining close observation of these patients throughout their hospital course is of utmost importance.

AMPHETAMINES

Amphetamine and its D-isomer, dextroamphetamine, are sympathomimetic drugs that are used to stimulate the central nervous system. These drugs are useful for the treatment of narcolepsy and appetite suppression. The major abuse potential has focused on their illicit use as stimulants. Recently, 'ice', a smokable type of methamphetamine, similar to 'crack' cocaine, has become popular.[64]

Maternal Risks

The toxic signs of amphetamine use are generally characterized by restlessness, excessive speech, increased motor activity, tremors and insomnia. Amphetamine use has further been associated with hypertension, tachycardia and hyperthermia. It follows, then, that in patients with underlying pathology, there

may also be an increased incidence of cerebrovascular accidents, myocardial infarction and cardiac arrythmia.

Fetal Risks

The frequency of congenital anomalies does not appear to be increased among amphetamine-abusing women.[65] To date, no consistent abnormalities have been conclusively shown to be associated with amphetamine use.

Management Options

The principles of management are very similar to other drugs of abuse. Attempts should be made to try and stop the consumption of the drug during pregnancy. Vigilance and prompt treatment are needed for the complications of hypertension, tachycardia and hyperthermia.

SUMMARY

The management of the prenant substance abuser involves treating the medical, social and psychological aspects of the illness. Moreover, the obstetrician has the well-being of both mother and fetus at stake. Recognizing that substance abuse is a multidimensional illness is a necessary first step toward instituting adequate patient care.

It is important to develop a three-part approach to these patients. Addressing issues that are unique to the mother, fetus and maternal–fetal unit assures that in the antepartum, intrapartum and postpartum periods, optimal patient care will be given.

BARBITURATES
Summary of Management Options

Prenatal

- Acute intoxication
  - close observation and supportive care if mild/moderate
  - maintain potent airway
  - i.v. diuresis or even dialysis if severe

- Chronic addiction
  - avoid abrupt withdrawal of drug

Labor/delivery, postnatal

- Vigilance for withdrawal syndrome

REFERENCES

1 Chasnoff IJ (1989) Drug use and women: Establishing a standard case. *Annals of the New York Academy of Sciences* 562:208.
2 Evans AT, Gillogley K (1991) Drug use in pregnancy: Obstetric perspectives. *Clinics in Perinatology* 18(1).
3 Little BB, Snell LM, Gilstrap LC III *et al.* (1989) Alcohol abuse during pregnancy: Changes in frequency in a large urban hospital. *Obstetrics and Gynecology* 74:547–550.
4 Council on Scientific Affairs, American Medical Association (1983) Fetal effects of maternal alcohol use. *Journal of the American Medical Association* 249:2517–2521.
5 Pietrantoni M, Knuppel R (1991) Alcohol use in pregnancy. *Clinics in Perinatology* 18(1):93–111.
6 Victor M, Adams RD (1980) Alcohol. In Isselbacher KJ, Adams RD, Braunswald E, Petersdorf RG, Wilson

JD (eds) *Principles of Internal Medicine* 9th edn, pp. 969–977. New York: McGraw-Hill.

7   Abel EL (1989) *Fetal Alcohol Syndrome: Fetal Alcohol Effects*. New York: Plenum Press.

8   Kosch HL, Weiner L (1985) Alcohol and pregnancy: A clinical perspective. *Annual Review of Medicine* **36**:73–80.

9   Rosett HL, Weiner L, Austin L *et al.* (1983) Patterns of alcohol consumption and fetal development. *Obstetrics and Gynecology* **61**(5):539–546.

10 Ernhart L, Sokol R, Martier S *et al.* (1987) Alcohol teratogenicity in the human: A detailed assessment of specificity, critical period and threshold. *American Journal of Obstetrics and Gynecology* **156**:33–39.

11 Rosett HL, Weiner L (1984) *Alcohol and the Fetus: A Clinical Perspective*. New York: Oxford University Press.

12 Rogers BD, Lee RV (1988) Drug abuse. In Burrow GN, Ferris TF (eds) *Medical Complications During Pregnancy*, 3rd edn, pp. 570–581. Philadelphia, PA: W.B. Saunders.

13 Nora AH, Nora JI, Blue J (1977) Limb reduction anomalies in infants born to disulfiram-treated alcoholic mothers. *Lancet* **2**:644.

14 Berini RY, Kahn E (1978) *Psychiatric Disorders: Alcoholism. Clinical Genetics Handbook*, Vol. 43, p. 268. Ordell, NJ: Medical Economics Books.

15 Keppen DL, Pysher T, Rennert M (1985) Zinc deficiency acts as a co-teratogen with alcohol in fetal alcohol syndrome. *Pediatric Research* **19**:944.

16 Jenkins DW, Eckle RE, Craig JW (1971) Alcoholic ketoacidosis. *Journal of the American Medical Association* **217**:177.

17 Anonymous (1983) Alcohol and the fetus – is zero the only option? *Lancet* **1**:682.

18 Kiessling KH, Pilstrom L (1967) Effects of ethanol on rat liver: The influence of vitamin electrolytes and amino acids on the structure and function of mitochondria from rats receiving ethanol. *British Journal of Nutrition* **21**:547.

19 Haegerman G, Schnoll S (1991) Narcotic use in pregnancy. *Clinics in Perinatology* **18**(1):51–76.

20 Zagon IS, McLaughlin PJ, Weaver DJ *et al.* (1982) Opiates, endorphins and the developing organism: A comprehensive bibiliography. *Neuroscience and Behavioural Reviews* **6**:439–479.

21 Victor M, Adams RD (1980) Opiates and synthetic analgesics. In Isselbacher KJ, Adams RD, Braunwald R, Petersdorf RG, Wilson JD (eds) *Principles of Internal Medicine*, 9th edn, pp. 978–990. New York: McGraw-Hill.

22 Chasnoff I, Burns KA, Burns WJ *et al.* (1986) Prenatal drug exposure: Effects on neonatal and infant growth and development. *Neurobehavioral Toxicology and Teratology* **8**:357–362.

23 Naeye RL, Blanc W, LeBlanc W *et al.* (1973) Fetal complications of maternal heroin addiction: Abnormal growth, infections and episodes of stress. *Journal of Pediatrics* **83**:1055–1061.

24 Stone ML, Salerno LJ, Green M *et al.* (1971) Narcotic addiction in pregnancy. *American Journal of Obstetrics and Gynecology* **109**:716–723.

25 Zelson M, Lee SJ, Casalino M (1973) Neonatal narcotic addiction. *New England Journal of Medicine* **289**:1216–1220.

26 Zuspan FP (1992) Detoxification and medical management of the pregnant drug abuser. Presented at the *First National Conference of the OSAP National Resource Center for the Prevention of Perinatal Abuse of Alcohol and Other Drugs*, July.

27 Gold MS, Pottash AC, Sweeney DR *et al.* (1980) Opiate withdrawal using clonidine – a safe, effective and rapid neoopiate treatment. *Journal of the American Medical Association* **243**:343–346.

28 Washton AM, Resnick RB, Rawson RA (1980) Clonidine for outpatient detoxification (Letter). *Lancet* **1**:1078–1079.

29 Committee on Drugs, American Academy of Pediatrics (1989) Transfer of drugs and other chemicals into human milk. *Pediatrics* **84**:924–936.

30 Chavkin W, Kendall S (1990) Between a 'rock' and a hard place: Perinatal drug abuse. *Pediatrics* **85**(2):223–225.

31 Farrar M, Kearns G (1989) Cocaine clinical pharmacology and toxicology. *Journal of Pediatrics* **115**(5):665–675.

32 Schutzman D, Frankfield-Chernicoff M, Clatterbaugh M, Singer J (1991) Incidence of intrauterine cocaine exposure in a suburban setting. *Pediatrics* **88**(4):825–827.

33 Neerhof M, MacGregor S, Retzity S, Sullivan T (1989) Cocaine abuse during pregnancy: Peripartum prevalence and perinatal outcome. *American Journal of Obstetrics and Gynecology* **161**(3):633–638.

34 Matera C, Warner W, Moomjy M, Fink D, Fox M (1990) Prevalence of use of cocaine and other substances in an obstetric population. *American Journal of Obstetrics and Gynecology* **163**(3):797–801.

35 Chasnoff I (1991) Cocaine and pregnancy: Clinical and methodologic issues. *Clinics in Perinatology* **18**(1):113–123.

36 Mueller P, Benowitz N, Olsen K (1990) Cocaine. *Emergency Medicine Clinics of North America* **8**(3):481–492.

37 Cocaine in substance abuse and withdrawal: Alcohol, cocaine and opioids: In Civetta JM, Taylor RW, Kirby RR (eds) (1988) *Critical Care*, pp. 721–725. Philadelphia, PA: J.B. Lippincott.

38 Cregler L, Mark M (1986) Medical complications of cocaine abuse. *New England Journal of Medicine* **315**(23):1495–1500.

39 Acker D, Sachs B, Tracey K, Wise W (1983) Abruptio placentae associated with cocaine use. *American Journal of Obstetrics and Gynecology* **146**(2):220–221.

40 Chasnoff I, Barns W, Schnoll S, Burns K (1985) Cocaine use in pregnancy. *New England Journal of Medicine* **313**(11):666–669.

41 Macgregor S, Keith L, Chasnoff I, Rosner M, Chisom G, Shaw P, Minogue J (1987) Cocaine use during pregnancy: Adverse perinatal outcome. *American Journal of Obstetrics and Gynecology* **157**:686–690.

42 New J, Dooley S, Keith L, Bachicha J, Chasnoff I, Socol M (1990) The prevalence of substance abuse in

patients with suspected preterm labor. *American Journal of Obstetrics and Gynecology* **162**:1562–1567.

43 Macgregor S, Keith L, Bachicha J, Chasnoff I (1989) Cocaine abuse during pregnancy: Correlation between prenatal care and perinatal outcome. *Obstetrics and Gynecology* **74**:882–885.

44 Chasnoff I (1991) Drugs, alcohol, pregnancy, and the neonate – pay now or pay later. *Journal of the American Medical Association* **266**(11):1567–1568.

45 Renzi F (1991) Cocaine. In Rippe JM, Irwin RS, Alpert JS, Fink MP (eds) *Intensive Care Medicine* 2nd edn, pp. 1126–1130. Boston, MA: Little, Brown.

46 Benowitz NL (1991) Nicotine replacement therapy during pregnancy. *Journal of the American Medical Association* **266**:3174–3177.

47 Holbrook JH (1980) Tobacco smoking. In Isselbacher KJ, Adams RD, Braunswald E, Petersdorf RG, Wilson JD (eds) *Principles of Internal Medicine*, 9th edn, pp. 938–941. New York: McGraw-Hill.

48 Huddleston J (1992) Tobacco abuse: Perinatal effects and prevention. *Perinatal Outlook* **IV**:5.

49 Nieburg O, Marks JS, McLaren NM, Remington PL (1985) The fetal tobacco syndrome. *Journal of the American Medical Association* **253**:2998–2999.

50 Longo LD (1976) Carbon monoxide: Effects on oxygenation of the fetus *in utero. Science* **194**:523–525.

51 Naeye RL (1978) Effects of maternal cigarette smoking on the fetus and placenta. *British Journal of Obstetrics and Gynaecology* **85**:732.

52 United States Department of Health and Human Services (1983) *The Health Consequences of Smoking for Women: A Report of the Surgeon General*, p. 191. Pub. 410-889/1284. Bethesda MD, DHHS.

53 Butter MR, Goldstein H (1973) Smoking in pregnancy and subsequent child development. *British Medical Journal* **4**:573.

54 Naeye RL, Peters EL (1984) Mental development of children whose mothers smoked during pregnancy. *Obstetrics and Gynecology* **64**:601.

55 Bergman AB, Wiesner LA (1976) Relationship of passive cigarette smoking to sudden infant death syndrome. *Pediatrics* **58**:665.

56 Kline J, Stein ZA, Susser M, Warburton D (1977) Smoking: A risk factor for spontaneous abortion. *New England Journal of Medicine* **297**:793.

57 Meyer M, Tonascia J (1977) Maternal smoking, pregnancy complications and perinatal mortality. Am J Obstet Gynecol. *American Journal of Obstetrics and Gynecology* **128**:494.

58 Naeye RL, Ladis B, Droge JS (1976) Sudden infant death syndrome. A prospective study. *American Journal of Diseases of Children* **130**:1207.

59 Haddow JE, Knight GJ, Kloza EM, Palomaki GE, Weld NJ (1991) Cotinine assisted intervention in pregnancy to reduce smoking and low birth weight delivery. *British Journal of Obstetrics and Gynaecology* **98**:859–865.

60 Bauman KE, Bryan ES, Dent CW, Koch GG (1983) The influence of observing carbon monoxide levels on cigarette smoking by public prenatal patients. *American Journal of Public Health* **73**:1089–1091.

61 Sexton M, Hebel JR (1984) A clinical trial of changes in maternal smoking and its effect on birth weight. *Journal of the American Medical Association* **251**:911–915.

62 Perlman HH, Donnenberg AM, Sokoloff N (1942) The excretion of nicotine in breast milk and urine from cigarette smoking: Its effect on lactation and nursing. *Journal of the American Medical Association* **120**:1003.

63 Victor M, Adams RD (1980) Barbiturates. In Isselbacher KG, Adams RD, Braunswald E, Petersdorf RG, Wilson JD (eds) *Principles of Internal Medicine*, 9th edn, pp. 982–985. New York: McGraw-Hill.

64 McGregor SN, Keith LG, (1992) Drug abuse during pregnancy. In Rayburn RF, Zuspan FP, (eds) *Drug Therapy in Obstetrics and Gynecology*, 3rd edn, pp. 164–189. St Louis, MO, Mosby Year Book.

65 Kolter H, Workany J (1983) Congenital malformations: Part two *New England Journal of Medicine* **308**:491–497.

6

Maternal Weight and Weight Gain

HAJO I. J. WILDSCHUT

INTRODUCTION

Despite the fact that routine weighing of pregnant women has become an important feature of prenatal care, surprisingly little is known about the effectiveness of weighing as a screening procedure for predicting fetal demise or about the clinical and practical implications of 'abnormal' weight changes in pregnancy. From the epidemiological point of view, prepregnancy weight may be regarded as a risk indicator, identifying women who are at increased risk of pregnancy complications and poor reproductive outcome. In fact, prepregnancy weight is a gross reflection of nutritional status, which is largely determined by maternal genotype and environmental factors including the mother's own obstetric history and her nutrition during childhood. Consequently, prepregnancy weight itself is, by and large, not amenable to intervention. By contrast, weight gain can be considered a risk factor, as it is potentially amenable to intervention.[1] Moreover, weight gain is arguably directly related to birth weight and the subsequent health of the child.

PREPREGNANCY WEIGHT

Definitions

There are no uniform definitions for abnormal maternal weight and constitution. Perhaps the best way to assess the abnormalities of nutritional status, namely undernutrition and obesity, is to refer to the weight for height standard tables, using information on prepregnancy weight and maternal height.[2] Quetelet's index (weight (kg)/height (m²)) is commonly used for this purpose. Naeye, for instance, classified pregnant women into four categories according to arbitrary levels of the Quetelet index: <20 thin; 20–24 normal; 25–30 mildly overweight; >30 obese.[3] In clinical practice, however, these standard definitions of body mass index are difficult to apply, since information on prepregnancy weight is usually unavailable. A considerable number of investigators, therefore, have limited the definitions for abnormal nutritional status to information on body weight. In this regard, subjective criteria for 'initial' body weight have been propagated; values of less than 45 kg (99 lb) have been used to describe 'underweight' women, and 85 kg (187 lb) and over to describe 'overweight' women.[4,5] Alternatively, skinfold thickness measurements are used to define maternal constitution in terms of body fat content. For this purpose, various parameters have been published.[2] Estimates of skinfold measurements, however, are effected by alterations in maternal body composition during pregnancy.[6,7] Since one can not fully rely on the accuracy of these measurements during pregnancy, any results should be interpreted carefully.

Incidence

Since no uniform definitions for abnormalities of maternal constitution exist, it is difficult to elaborate on prevalence rates for 'undernutrition' and 'obesity' in pregnancy. Apart from the diagnostic criteria used, prevalence rates depend on the characteristics of population studied, since body weight is correlated with factors such as age, parity, social class and ethnicity.[2,8]

UNDERNUTRITION

Nutritional deprivation may arise due to starvation, dieting or chronic eating disorders, such as anorexia nervosa and bulimia. The latter conditions are of great public health concern in affluent societies.[9]

Anorexia nervosa is a syndrome characterized by severe weight loss, a distorted body image and an intense fear of becoming obese.[9] Anorexia nervosa is not synonymous with bulimia, although bulimic symptoms can be encountered in women with anorexia nervosa. Bulimia is characterized by recurrent episodes of secretive binge eating followed by self-induced vomiting, fasting or the use of laxatives or diuretics.[9] Depression, alcohol and drug abuse are also prominent features of this disorder.[10] Bulimics exhibit frequent weight fluctuations but are not likely to suffer significant weight loss as seen in women suffering from anorexia nervosa. Both syndromes, which primarily afflict adolescents and young adults from middle-class and upper middle-class families, are often associated with oligo- and amenorrhea.[9] Despite menstrual irregularities, women with chronic eating disorders may become pregnant.[11] Recently Stewart et al.[12] reviewed the outcome of pregnancies in women who suffered from anorexia and bulimia.

Risks

Nutritional deprivation has a negative effect on birthweight, albeit of small magnitude.[13,14] Underweight women are more likely than women of normal weight to give birth to infants who are small for gestational age.[4,15,16] Intrauterine growth deficiency may result in prenatal and postnatal asphyxia and neonatal complications such as hypoglycemia and hypothermia. There is evidence that underweight women are more prone to anemia and preterm delivery.[15] Perinatal mortality rates in 'thin' women (Quetelet's index <20) are increased.[3]

The outcome of pregnancy in women suffering from anorexia and bulimia varies. If the eating disorder is in remission, then an uneventful pregnancy and a favorable pregnancy outcome can be anticipated. However, expectant women with active anorexia nervosa or bulimia at the time of conception may experience a number of severe health problems, including electrolyte imbalances, dehydration, depression, social problems and poor fetal growth. Appropriate psychiatric treatment is then warranted.[12]

Management Options

Prepregnancy

Anorexic and bulimic women who wish to become pregnant are advised to wait until the eating disorder is in remission.[12] It has been suggested that the treatment of underweight women with anovulatory infertility should be focused on restoration of weight by an integrated multidisciplinary approach rather than on ovulation induction.[9,16]

PREGNANCY IN UNDERWEIGHT WOMEN
Summary of Management Options

Prepregnancy

- Improve calorie intake for those who are undernourished

- Appropriate multidisciplinary treatment for those women with eating disorders

Prenatal

- Screening for intrauterine growth retardation with early confirmation of gestational age with ultrasound

- Appropriate multidisciplinary treatment for those women whose eating disorders are not in remission

Labor/delivery

- Continuous electronic fetal heart rate monitoring of fetus if small

Postnatal

- Nil specific

Prenatal

In view of the increased risk of low birthweight, prenatal care should focus on the early detection of intrauterine growth retardation. Careful dating of gestation is important. Adequate weight gain should be ensured (see below). However, beneficial effects of dietary advice with or without specific food supplements are controversial.[9,17]

Labor/delivery

If fetal growth deficiency is suspected, confinement should take place in a specialist unit and continuous electronic fetal monitoring is advised. Emergency neonatal services should be readily available.

Postnatal care

There are no additional specific management strategies which need to be considered.

OBESITY

Risks

Hypertensive disorders, including pre-existent hypertension and pregnancy-induced hypertension, are more common in overweight women, though the prevalence rates in different reports vary widely (7–46%).[18] Gestational diabetes is also more frequent, affecting 7–17% of obese women.[18] Other problems associated with obese women include urinary tract infections, postnatal hemorrhage, uncertain fetal presentation and, possible, thrombophlebitis.[2,18] Obese women are more prone to give birth to large for gestational age infants. In fact, intrauterine growth deficiency is infrequently observed in obese women.[2] Despite the higher mean birthweight of the infant, there is no clear evidence that obese women without prenatal complications are at increased risk of labor/delivery complications, such as dysfunctional labor, shoulder dystocia and birth asphyxia.[2] Moreover, obese women without prenatal complications do not appear to be more prone to either augmentation with oxytocin for poorly progressing labor or cesarean section for dystocia when compared with matched non-obese controls.[2,19]

There is conflicting evidence about the effect of obesity on perinatal mortality. Based on the findings of the Collaborative Perinatal Study in the USA, Naeye concluded that perinatal mortality rates are directly related to Quetelet index values, even when the effects of demographic factors, smoking and the presence or absence of prenatal complications were taken into account.[3] He showed that nearly half the increase in perinatal mortality among obese women could be ascribed to preterm birth. Increased rate of twins may also partly explain the relatively high rates of preterm birth and subsequent increased perinatal mortality rates among obese women.[3] Other investigators could not establish an association between perinatal mortality and obesity. Such a lack of association could be the effect of prenatal care through early recognition and appropriate management of prenatal complications arising in the obese woman.[18] Various studies have suggested that the cesarean section rate for obese women is slightly higher than for women of normal weight.[19] In fact, the increased need for abdominal delivery in obese women can mainly be attributed to the relatively high rates of prenatal complications and factors such as advanced age and high parity. When an operative delivery is required, obese women are more prone to wound infection when compared with non-obese women.[18]

Management Options

Prepregnancy

If an obese woman wishes to reduce her weight, she should be encouraged to lose weight before or after pregnancy. Dietary manipulation should not be advocated during pregnancy as this is possibly detrimental to the birthweight, and subsequent health, of the child and of no benefit to the mother.[13,20] Apart from a balanced diet, daily exercise programs should be promoted. Given that the woman insists on severe caloric restriction for weight reduction, the problem of maintaining reduced weight for prolonged periods should be addressed. In fact, the recurrence rate of obesity after weight reduction is high.[21] Massively obese women failing dietary control sometimes opt for surgical treatment of obesity. Pregnancies following intestinal bypass surgery are often complicated by fetal growth deficiency.[21] In contrast, most pregnancies occurring after gastric bypass surgery appear to have a generally benign course, since the latter procedure is seldom associated with nutritional and metabolic abnormalities.[22] Pregnancy should be avoided if electrolyte imbalance is present.

Prenatal

Prepregnancy weight and maternal height should be documented routinely in the prenatal health records and/or medical records. It is common practice to record weight at each prenatal visit, using calibrated weighing scales. Blood pressure should also be monitored with an appropriate sized cuff, since obese women tend to show artificially high readings when the standard cuff is used.[23]

In grossly obese women, it could be difficult to assess fetal growth and well-being. Ultrasonic measurements of fetal size may be untrustworthy if adipose tissue frustrates proper visualization of the fetus. Ascertainment of fundal height in overweight women by either palpation or measurement could also present problems in terms of accurate estimation of fetal size. There is no simple solution. Moreover, in massively obese women, it may be difficult to ascertain fetal presentation. Ultrasonography becomes particularly important in sorting out problems of presentation. Prior to delivery, anesthesia consultation is needed if medical problems arise, such as hypertension, diabetes mellitus or pulmonary dysfunction.

It is recommended to screen obese women for gestational diabetes at the first prenatal visit and have it repeated in the second and/or third trimester if the previous findings were normal.[19] Women should be screened for asymptomatic bacteriuria by culture and colony count of clean catch voided urine.[8,24] Screening for asymptomatic bacteriuria reduces the risk of pyelonephritis and its consequences.[24]

Labor/delivery

Potential problems in labor include poor progress due to cephalopelvic disproportion, shoulder dystocia and birth asphyxia. Attempts to derive a prediction score to identify large for gestational age infants have failed due to the occurrence of unacceptably high false positive rates.[25]

Procedure: Cesarean Section

Preoperative considerations

Anesthesia

In view of the advances of modern technology, there should no longer be a hesitancy to perform a cesarean section in morbidly obese women. In the case of non-emergent deliveries, epidural anesthesia warrants serious consideration. Even in the massively obese woman, epidural anesthesia is technically possible and is to be preferred over general anesthesia, at least in experienced hands.[2]

Prophylactic measures

Prophylactic antibiotics during both elective and emergency cesarean section are clearly indicated.[26] Additionally, prophylactic administration of low-dose heparin is recommended, beginning preoperatively and continuing until the patient is fully ambulatory.[5]

Type of incision

In obese women, the type of incision for abdominal delivery, midline vertical vs low transverse (Pfannenstiel), is often subject to debate. Gross reviewed the benefits and risks of the two operative approaches in obese women.[5] He concluded that the favorable aspects of the Pfannenstiel incision are: (1) less postoperative pain and early ambulation, thus avoiding atelectasis and embolism; (2) a more secure closure; and (3) less adipose tissue to incise. Morover, the Pfannenstiel incision gives a better cosmetic result than the midline incision. The potential adverse effects of the Pfannenstiel incision are: (1) the incision is more prone to infection as it is located in a warm and moist area; (2) access to the infant may be restricted; and (3) exposure of the upper abdomen is more difficult.

In theory, prolongation of the operation increases risk of wound infection. The extent to which the type of incision affects the duration of operation in overweight women is unknown. It is the author's clinical impression that the total duration of the operation in obese women appears to be only marginally affected by the type of incision used. The time interval from incision to delivery using the Pfannenstiel technique may be somewhat longer, since extraction of the baby may be more difficult, particularly when the baby is large. Incision closure may be more difficult when the midline incision is used.

Use of a 'full-thickness' or 'one-layer' closure technique (incorporating peritoneum together with rectus sheath) with non-absorbable suture material could avoid the problem of wound dehiscence (see Chapter 67).[5] Placing surgical drains at the time of closure of the abdomen in obese women is a matter of debate.

Postnatal

Specific complications following abdominal delivery in obese women include wound infection, wound dehiscence, atelectasis and pulmonary emboli. Prophylactic administration of anticoagulants should be continued until the patient is fully mobilized. Early mobilization appears to improve maternal outcome.

In newborn infants born to grossly obese women, postnatal blood sugars should be monitored during the first hours of life, in particular when the baby is large for gestational age.

Conclusion

Obese women are more likely to have prenatal complications, such as hypertensive disorders of pregnancy, gestational diabetes and urinary tract infection. Consequently, the need for cesarean section is slightly increased. In general, obese women are more likely to give birth to large for gestational age infants and, as a result, more prone to intrapartum complications. Overweight women appear to be more likely to develop postnatal complications such as thrombophlebitis and thromboembolism. Furthermore, the likelihood of postoperative wound infection following cesarean section in obese women is increased. Maintaining awareness of the specific medical and obstetric problems associated with obesity will enable the clinician to maximize efforts to improve maternal health and fetal outcome.

PREGNANCY IN OVERWEIGHT WOMEN
Summary of Management Options

Prepregnancy

- Reduce weight with a program of diet and modest exercise which also addresses maintenance of normal weight once achieved. Consider other methods (e.g. surgery) if this is unsuccessful

- Explain risks of hypertension, diabetes, urinary infections, large fetal size and postpartum hemorrhage

Prenatal

- Avoid obsessive attempts to manipulate diet *during* pregnancy

- Screen for hypertension (using appropriately sized cuff), diabetes and bacteriuria

- Monitor fetal growth (excessive and reduced) using ultrasound, though this may be technically difficult. Vigilance for growth deficiency, especially if history of intestinal bypass surgery

- Anesthetic opinion of abdominal delivery is anticipated

Labor/delivery

- Vigilance for cephalopelvic disproportion and shoulder dystocia which are difficult to predict in obese women

- If cesarean section:
  - consider regional rather than general anesthesia
  - prophylactic antibodies
  - prophylactic low-dose subcutaneous heparin (until fully ambulatory)
  - no agreement over which incision is best
  - value of wound drains is debated

Postnatal

- Subcutaneous heparin until fully ambulatory

- Early mobilization

- Continue with measures to reduce weight

MATERNAL WEIGHT GAIN IN PREGNANCY

Physiology

Weight gain

The total weight gain of a healthy nulliparous woman eating without restriction is about 12.5 kg (27.5 lb).[7] However, large variations in weight gain are seen in women with normal outcome.[7,27] In Western societies, average total weight gain ranges from 10 to 16 kg (22 to 35 lb).[28] This variation is a function of prepregnancy weight, age, parity and dietary habit during pregnancy. In healthy, well-nourished women with uncomplicated pregnancies, the proportional weight gain (i.e. total weight gain at term expressed as a proportion of the weight before pregnancy) is 17–20%.[6] The increase is mostly accounted for by an increase in total body water [averaging about 7.5 kg (16.4 lb) when no edema is present] and body fat mass [about 2.2–3.5 kg (5.0–7.7 lb)].[7,29,30] The remainder, approximating 0.9 kg (2 lb), is due to a rise in protein content, half of which is fetal.[7] Mean weight gain in pregnancy from conception to birth does not show a linear trend. The normal lean nulliparous woman, who eats to appetite, gains only a little weight during the first trimester [0.65–1.1 kg (1.4–2.4 lb) by 10 weeks].[7,30] In the second trimester, the average weekly weight gain is approximately 0.45 kg (1 lb) and thereafter about 0.36 kg (0.8 lb).[2] Weight loss or a failure to gain weight over a 2-week interval in the third trimester is not uncommon in both nulliparous and parous women. There is some evidence that the average weight gain in parous women is slightly less than in nulliparous women. The maximum rate of weight gain is found to occur between 17 and 24 weeks of pregnancy.[17,27] Subcutaneous fat is laid down over the abdomen, back and upper thighs mainly in the first and second trimesters.[18]

Postpartum weight

Recently, a study from the Netherlands showed that in a highly selective group of healthy women, postpartum weight was 2.9 kg (6.4 lb) above weight before pregnancy.[30] Following delivery, the most rapid weight loss occurs between 4 and 10 days postpartum, which is mainly due to loss of fluid. In the following weeks, weight loss is much more gradual – about 0.25 kg (0.55 lb) per week – consistent with a gradual mobilization of fat stores.[31] Eventually, the average woman will lose most of the weight she gains during pregnancy, taking into account the effects of age and weight gain over time.[7,32] In fact, pregnancy in itself does not have a lasting effect on body fat mass. Breast-feeding in excess of 60 days has a favorable effect on the rate of weight loss postpartum, because it is assumed that maternal caloric consumption is generally insufficient to meet the increased needs of lactation.[33]

Risks

There is a positive correlation between maternal weight gain and birthweight, regardless of maternal age and parity.[1,27,33] Women who gain little weight in pregnancy are at increased risk of having babies of low birthweight. The magnitude of the association between inadequate maternal weight gain and low birthweight depends on prepregnancy weight: women of low prepregnancy weight experiencing little weight gain during pregnancy are more likely to give birth to an infant of low birthweight than overweight women having a similar net weight gain during pregnancy. In fact, net weight gain in underweight women is strongly related to birthweight, while in overweight women net weight gain is only marginally related to birthweight.[17,34] It has been suggested that the optimum weight gain in terms of minimum perinatal mortality is 7.3 kg (16 lb) for overweight women, 9.1 kg (20 lb) for women of normal weight and 13.6 kg (30 lb) for underweight women.[7]

The possibility of an eating disorder should be considered in women who fail to gain appropriate weight or who present with intractable vomiting.[12]

Management Options

Prenatal

Over the last several decades, there have been significant changes in the recommendations made to women about weight gain during pregnancy. Until the 1970s, it was common practice to advise women to restrict food intake. These recommendations were aimed at curtailing weight gain to approximately 6.8 kg (15 lb) or 11.3 kg (25 lb) at most.[2,34] The main objectives for dietary restriction were three-fold: (1) the reduction of the incidence of pre-eclampsia, (2) the promotion of easier labor and (3) the preservation of the woman's figure after birth.[34] Later, when the association of low birthweight and inadequate weight gain became obvious, and in view of the fact that dietary restriction could not avert the problem of pre-eclampsia, medical attitudes toward weight gain in pregnancy were relaxed.[20] At present, there is no evidence to support the view that imposing caloric restriction during pregnancy is beneficial to women of average prepregnancy weight in terms of maternal and fetal health.[35] By increasing energy intake, however, the expectant woman could promote excessive fat accretion.[31]

Hence, a modest reduction in nutrient intake may avert the problem of retaining undesirable amounts of fat postpartum.[31]

Despite the fact that the rational for dietary management of pregnant women with 'inappropriate' weight gain is rather obscure, dietary policies vary markedly from hospital to hospital, with some clinicians advocating the strict control of maternal caloric intake during pregnancy and others encouraging women to 'eat to appetite'. Recommendations for minimal weight gain in pregnancy should take account of the weight before pregnancy: underweight women need to gain more than overweight women.[18,34] However, there is little evidence that perinatal mortality can be improved by dietary measures aimed at increasing birthweight.[18] It has been suggested that attention should be focused on dietary quality rather than quantity.[2] The dietician could be called in to attune a healthy and well-balanced diet to the needs of the pregnant woman, in terms of energy expenditure, thereby taking account of her background, assets and life style.

ABNORMAL WEIGHT GAIN IN PREGNANCY
Summary of Management Options

Prenatal

- Check for abnormal fetal growth, with ultrasound if clinically suspected

- Consider physical or psychological pathology in women who fail to gain appropriate weight, especially if associated with other clinical features

- Encourage those women with poor weight gain (especially if also underweight prepregnancy) to improve diet (quality rather than quantity)

- Other prenatal measures:
  - for poor weight gain, as for women who are underweight (p. 68)
  - for excessive weight gain, as for women who are overweight (p. 69)

Labor/delivery

- For poor weight gain, as for women who are underweight (p. 69)

- For excessive weight gain, as for women who are overweight (p. 70)

Postnatal

- Management options for weight gain as for women who are overweight (p. 70)

Labor/delivery

This is discussed in the previous section.

Conclusion

Mean infant birthweight is a function of maternal weight before pregnancy and weight gain in pregnancy. However, independent effects of weight gain over and above those of prepregnancy weight on the infant's birthweight are not always seen. In fact, weight gain in pregnancy seems to have a far greater impact on birthweight of infants born to underweight women than of those born to overweight women.

REFERENCES

1 Brown JE, Abrams BF, Lederman SA, Naeye RL, Rees JM, Taffel S, Worthington-Roberts BS, Tharp TM (1990) Report of a Special Panel on Desired Prenatal Weight Gains for Underweight and Normal Weight Women. *Public Health Reports* **105**:24–28.

2 Kliegman RM, Gross T (1985) Perinatal problems of the obese mother and her infant. *Obstetrics and Gynecology* **66**:299–305.

3 Naeye RL (1990) Maternal body weight and pregnancy outcome. *American Journal of Clinical Nutrition* **52**:273–279.

4 Dawes MG, Grudzinskas JG (1991) Repeated measurement of maternal weight during pregnancy. Is this a useful practice? *British Journal of Obstetrics and Gynaecology* **98**:189–194.

5 Gross TL (1983) Operative considerations in the obese pregnant patient. *Clinics in Perinatology* **10**:411–421.

6 Durnin JVGA (1987) Energy requirements of pregnancy: An integration of the longitudinal data from the five-country study. *Lancet* **ii**:1131–1133.

7 Hytten FE (1991) Weight gain in pregnancy. In Hytten FE, Chamberlain G (eds) *Clinical Physiology in Obstetrics*, 2nd edn, pp. 173–203. Oxford: Blackwell Scientific Publications.

8   Heliövaara M, Aromaa A (1981) Parity and obesity. *Journal of Epidemiology and Community Health* **35**:197–199.

9   Herzog DB, Copeland PM (1985) Eating disorders. *New England Journal of Medicine* **313**:295–302.

10 Feingold M, Kaminer Y, Lyons K, Chaudhury AK, Costigan K, Cetrulo C (1988) Bulimia nervosa in pregnancy. *Obstetrics and Gynecology* **71**:1025–1027.

11 Treasure JL, Russell GFM (1988) Intrauterine growth and neonatal weight gain in babies of women with anorexia nervosa. *British Medical Journal* **296**:1038.

12 Stewart DE, Raskin J, Garfinkel PE, MacDonald OL, Robinson E (1987) Anorexia nervosa, bulimia, and pregnancy. *American Journal of Obstetrics and Gynecology* **157**:1194–1198.

13 Lind T (1984) Nutrition: The changing scene. Would more calories per day keep low birthweight at bay? *Lancet* **i**:501–502.

14 Lumey LH (1988) Obstetric performance of women exposed after *in utero* exposure to the Dutch famine (1944–1945). PhD thesis 8827610, Ann Arbor, Michigan: Columbia University.

15 Kramer MS (1987) Intrauterine growth retardation and gestational duration determinants. *Pediatrics* **80**:502–511.

16 Spuy ZM van der, Steer PJ, McCusker M, Steele SJ, Jacobs HS (1988) Outcome of pregnancy in underweight women after spontaneous and induced ovulation. *British Medical Journal* **296**:962–965.

17 Hytten FE (1979) Restriction of weight gain in pregnancy: Is it justified? *Journal of Human Nutrition* **33**:461–463.

18 Drife JO (1986) Weight gain in pregnancy: Eating for two or just getting fat? *British Medical Journal* **293**:903–904.

19 Garbaciak JA, Richter M, Miller S, Barton JJ (1985) Maternal weight and pregnancy complications. *American Journal of Obstetrics and Gynecology* **152**:238–245.

20 Campbell DM (1982) Dietary restriction in obesity and its effect on neonatal outcome. In Campbell DM, Gillmer MDG (eds) *Nutrition in Pregnancy*, pp. 243–254. Proceedings of the Tenth Study Group of the Royal College of Obstetricians and Gynaecologists. London: Royal College of Obstetricians and Gynaecologists.

21 Friedman CI, Kim MH (1985) Obesity and its effect on reproductive function. *Clinical Obstetrics and Gynecology* **28**:645–663.

22 Richards DS, Miller DK, Goodman GN (1987) Pregnancy after gastric bypass for morbid obesity. *Journal of Reproductive Medicine* **32**:172–176.

23 Swiet M de (1991) Blood pressure measurement in pregnancy. *British Journal of Obstetrics and Gynaecology* **98**:239–240.

24 Wang E, Smaill F (1989) Infection in pregnancy. In Chalmers I, Enkin M, Keirse MJNC (eds) *Effective Care in Pregnancy and Childbirth*, Vol. 1, pp. 534–564. Oxford: Oxford University Press.

25 Scott A, Moar V, Ounsted M (1982) The relative contribution of different maternal factors in large-for-gestational-age pregnancies. *European Journal of Obstetrics, Gynecology and Reproductive Biology* **13**:269–277.

26 Enkin M, Enkin E, Chalmers I, Hemminki E (1989) Prophylactic antibiotics in association with caesarean section. In Chalmers I, Enkin M, Keirse MJNC (eds) *Effective Care in Pregnancy and Childbirth*, Vol. 2, pp. 1246–1269. Oxford: Oxford University Press.

27 Dawes MG, Grudzinskas JG (1991) Patterns of maternal weight gain in pregnancy. *British Journal of Obstetrics and Gynaecology* **98**:195–201.

28 Anonymous (1991) Maternal weight gain in pregnancy. *Lancet* **338**:415.

29 Durnin JVGA, McKillop FM, Grant S, Fitzgerald (1987) Energy requirements of pregnancy in Scotland. *Lancet* **ii**:897–900.

30 Raaij JMA van, Vermaat-Miedema SH, Schonk CM, Peek MEM, Hautvast JGAJ (1987) Energy requirements of pregnancy in the Netherlands. *Lancet* **ii**:953–955.

31 Lawrence M, McKillop FM, Durnin JVGA (1991) Women who gain more fat during pregnancy may not have bigger babies: Implications for recommended weight gain during pregnancy. *British Journal of Obstetrics and Gynaecology* **98**:254–259.

32 Greene GW, Smiciklas-Wright H, Scholl TO, Karp RJ (1988) Post partum weight change: How much of the weight gained will be lost after delivery? *Obstetrics and Gynecology* **71**:701–707.

33 McAnarney ER (1987) Young maternal age and adverse neonatal outcome. *American Journal of Diseases of Children* **141**:1053–1059.

34 Abrams BF, Laros RK (1986) Prepregnancy weight, weight gain, and birth weight. *American Journal of Obstetrics and Gynecology* **15**:503–509.

35 Green J (1989) Diet and the prevention of pre-eclampsia. In Chalmers I, Enkin M, Keirse MJNC (eds) *Effective Care in Pregnancy and Childbirth*, Vol. 1, pp. 281–300. Oxford: Oxford University Press.

7

Bleeding in Early Pregnancy

SYLVIA ROSEVEAR

INTRODUCTION

Irregular vaginal bleeding in a woman of reproductive age must be viewed as a complication of pregnancy until the diagnosis of pregnancy is excluded. Failure to make an accurate diagnosis may cause unnecessary pain and distress and may compromise a woman's reproductive future. Occasionally, it may lead to significant morbidity and even mortality. The differential diagnosis of bleeding in the woman of reproductive age includes dysfunctional uterine bleeding, miscarriage (spontaneous, threatened, missed, incomplete, complete, septic), ectopic pregnancy, hydatidiform mole and gestational trophoblastic disease. Vaginal bleeding occurs in about a quarter of pregnancies. Half of all pregnancies complicated by bleeding will miscarry spontaneously.[1] In Stabile and coworkers' series of 466 patients with bleeding in pregnancy,[1] only 48.7% progressed normally beyond 20 weeks gestation; 12.8% had an ectopic pregnancy, 0.2% had a hydatidiform mole and 32.7% miscarried. Termination of pregnancy was elected in the remaining 5.6%.

INITIAL MANAGEMENT (see **Figure 1**)

Assess Blood Loss and Need for Resuscitation

It is mandatory to identify the patient who requires resuscitation by estimating the blood loss and the rap-

idity of the loss. While the signs of shock are pallor, generalized sweating, cool peripheries, pulse greater than 100 beats/min and blood pressure less than 100/70 mmHg, young fit women compensate by maintaining their arterial blood pressure until very late when it may be difficult to reverse the shock. Early pregnancy hemorrhage may be catastrophic and yet it may be intraperitoneal and hidden. Regular recordings of pulse and blood pressure (approximately every 5 min) should be made in a potentially shocked patient. Irrespective of the amount of revealed bleeding, the patient that is shocked should be managed as though there has been a large loss of blood.

Where severe blood loss has occurred or is suspected, i.v. access should be established. Blood should be taken for hemoglobin concentration, clotting screening and to cross-match blood (4 units would be a minimum with a shocked patient). Subsequent management of the resuscitation is discussed in Chapter 71).

Make the Diagnosis

History

A detailed menstrual history should be taken. Special attention should be paid to the date of the last menstrual period and how the woman recalls it. It can be inaccurate if she recalls it from memory. What is the patient's usual menstrual cycle? What irregularity has there been in vaginal bleeding? Specific questions must be asked about the symptoms of early pregnancy (early morning nausea and vomiting, breast tenderness, uri-

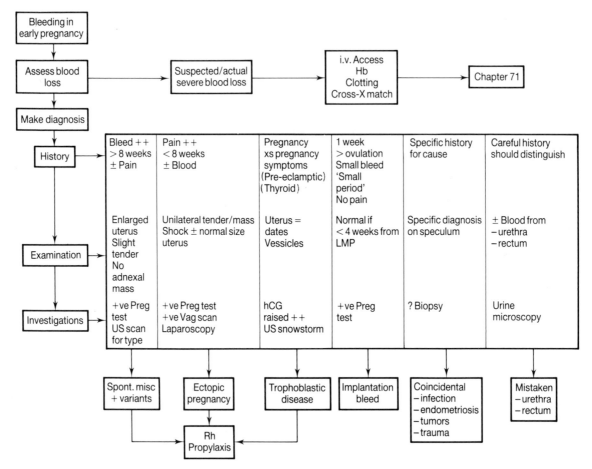

Figure 1. Bleeding in early pregnancy: Initial assessment and management.

nary frequency and generalized fatigue) and to determine whether these symptoms are still present. If they are no longer present, it should be noted when they diminished in intensity or disappeared.

The timing and degree of vaginal bleeding in relation to the menstrual cycle should be established and whether there is any associated low back pain or abdominal pain. Is the pain unilateral, central or generalized? Is it cramping in nature? Shoulder tip pain suggests diaphragmatic irritation from intra-abdominal bleeding. The details and the reliability of contraceptive use should be documented. The presence of an IUCD does not exclude the possibility of an ectopic pregnancy.

Examination of the bleeding patient

Recording the pulse and blood pressure are critical. Vital signs identify the effects of blood loss, both observed and concealed. Findings on abdominal examination of intraperitoneal bleeding are rebound tenderness and guarding. The shape of the abdomen may be convex. Pelvic examination should begin with inspection. The external genitalia and vagina may show evidence of trauma as the cause for bleeding. Bleeding from the cervix may be a possible pathological cause of the bleeding. Whether the cervical os is open or closed should be determined. A cervical os that is open implies either an incomplete or inevitable miscarriage. If there is dilatation of the cervix without bleeding in the second trimester and the fetus is viable, the diagnosis is cervical incompetence (see below for the technique of cervical cerclage in such instances).

Bimanual examination includes moving the cervix laterally to assess the presence or absence of 'cervical excitation', that is, pain thought to be caused by stretching of the broad ligament and indicative of an ectopic pregnancy. A bimanual examination assesses the size, shape, consistency and location of the uterus and the clinical diagnosis of an intrauterine pregnancy. Palpation of the adnexae may identify a mass which may be an ectopic pregnancy. Other signs of pregnancy on vaginal examination are: Chadwick's sign (a blue color of the cervix and vagina) and Hegar's sign (the softening of the isthmic portion of the uterus which gives the impression that the upper and lower portions of the uterus are separate).

Special investigations

Pregnancy test/human chorionic gonadotrophin (hCG)

A pregnancy test is essential in a woman of reproductive age presenting with irregular vaginal bleeding with or without pain. The pregnancy test is based on assaying for human chorionic gonadotrophin (hCG). Human chorionic gonadotrophin is a glycoprotein consisting of an alpha and beta subunit secreted by the trophoblast. The usefulness of the pregnancy test chosen depends on the sensitivity of the test to detect lower concentrations of hCG. The beta subunit of hCG cross-reacts with luteinizing hormone and follicle-stimulating hormone. Thus, some pregnancy tests can be falsely positive, for example when a luteinizing hormone peak occurs at ovulation or when pituitary gonadotrophins are increased in later reproductive life to stimulate an aging ovary to ovulate.[2]

Human chorionic gonadotrophin concentrations are generally reported as IU/l (less commonly as mIU/ml) using the International Reference Preparation (IRP). There is a Second International Standard (2IS) and this gives results which are about half that of the IRP. For the remainder of this chapter, the results will be given as IU/l using IRP.

Human chorionic gonadotrophin is secreted by the syncytiotrophoblast as early as 8 days after the luteinizing hormone peak, which is about the time when uteroplacental circulation begins to be established. By 11 days after the luteinizing hormone peak, hCG can be detected in all normal pregnancies if a suitable assay system is used. The concentration at the time of the first missed period is 100 IU/l. It then rises to a peak of about 100 000 IU/l between 8 and 10 weeks of gestation (dated from the last menstrual period), thereafter falling to a stable low point of 10 000 IU/l at 20 weeks, usually for the rest of pregnancy.

These features of the secretion of hCG have been exploited by the different types of commercially available pregnancy tests:

- *Slide or tube agglutination inhibition tests* were developed by Wide and Gemzell[3] in the 1960s and performed on urine but not serum. The urine specimen is mixed with a solution of hCG antibody, which will bind any hCG present in the test specimen. A suspension of hCG-coated latex beads or

erythrocytes is then added. If hCG is present in the test specimen, the binding of hCG-coated latex particles or erythrocytes to the antibody will be blocked, and the agglutination reaction is inhibited. Therefore, with the agglutination inhibition test, pregnancy is indicated if there is no agglutination, whereas if the specimen agglutinates (presence of fine flocular precipitant), the patient is not pregnant. Latex particles are used in the slide pregnancy tests. They are very simple, taking only 2–3 min to perform, but they lack sensitivity. The minimal concentration of hCG required to give a positive result is at least 1000 IU/l, which has been reduced to 500 IU/l with the use of monoclonal antibodies. There is a direct correlation between hCG levels and the mass of viable cyto-synctiotrophoblast cells present. The hCG level in a normal pregnancy at the time of a missed menstrual period 13–14 days after ovulation is 100–600 IU/l.[4] Pregnancy tests on hemagglutination take 1–2 hours and are more sensitive. With the use of subunit-specific monoclonal antibodies, the sensitivity of this assay is 75–150 IU/l.

- *Radioimmunoassays* which are rapid and highly specific for hCG have a sensitivity of 40 IU/l. However, they require specially trained laboratory staff and a coulter counter.

- *ELISA tests* are a two-site, enzyme-linked immunosorbent assay as sensitive as rapid radioimmunoassays *in vitro*, and can be readily performed by attending staff. The blue color change on a dipstick (testing urine) is only observed if the woman is pregnant. ELISA tests are sensitive to 25–50 IU/l and therefore can give a positive result as early as 8–10 days after fertilization. The false-negative rates are less than 2% for most ELISAs. Also, most ectopic pregnancies associated with a negative hCG assay are likely to resorb, making serious hemorrhagic complications very unlikely. Genuine negative hCGs with ectopic pregnancies may be because there is a genuine defect in beta-hCG synthesis, and hCG is simply not produced.

Quantitative estimations of beta-hCG can provide useful information on the viability or abnormality of a gestation. During the first and second trimesters of pregnancy, abnormally low levels may indicate the likelihood of impending miscarriage or an ectopic gestation. Abnormally high levels may be found in gestational trophoblastic disease and multiple pregnancy. In early pregnancy, the hCG concentration increases exponentially until 6 weeks. This means that the time taken for the hCG concentration to double is constant. Similarly, the amount by which the serum hCG concentration increases (expressed as a proportion or percentage of the initial value) over any fixed time interval is also constant.

If it is uncertain whether the pregnancy is intrauterine or an ectopic pregnancy, then before proceeding to laparoscopy, serial hCG estimations and an ultrasound scan should be carried out.

HCG levels do not always distinguish between normal and abnormal pregnancies. On average, hCG levels at a given gestational age are lower in ectopic than in normal pregnancies, but the overlap is so large that the two conditions cannot be separated on the basis of a low-for-date hCG value. Knowledge of the urinary hCG does allow determination of whether the serum hCG is above or below the discriminatory hCG zone.

Using transvaginal ultrasonography, an intrauterine gestational sac should be imaged in normal pregnancies when the quantitative hCG is greater than 1500 IU/l. In patients in whom an intrauterine gestation sac is not identified during a transvaginal ultrasonography, there is no adnexal mass, and the quantitative hCG is less than 1500 IU/l, a repeat quantitative hCG should be done.

The doubling time of hCG is of diagnostic value if an ectopic pregnancy is present and the ultrasound findings are non-diagnostic. In total, 87% of patients in a prospective study with ectopic pregnancies had an hCG doubling time of more than 2.7 days.[5] Serum measurements for hCG were made 48 h apart. If the increase in the serum hCG was <66% or the doubling time was >2.7 days, then an ectopic pregnancy was excluded. The sensitivity of the test was 85% on average, and its false-positive rate was 15%, which means that the likelihood ratio (sensitivity/false positive rate) is 5.6. No normal intrauterine pregnancies were associated with a doubling time of hCG of > 7days.[6]

Falling hCG values identify a pregnancy as abnormal. The traditional approach of performing a curettage and proceeding to a laparoscopy only if villi are not recovered is only applicable if the half-life of hCG is between 1.4 and 7 days. More rapidly clearing hCG values (i.e. half-life of < 1.4 days) signify that residual trophoblastic activity has almost certainly ceased and the pregnancy will resolve without any intervention and that villi will usually not be recovered by curettage even if the pregnancy is intrauterine. Therefore, these patients will require only expectant management. If the half-life of hCG is > 7 days, the woman is most likely to have an ectopic pregnancy.

The serial estimations of hCG and the introduction of abdominal and more recently transvaginal ultrasound have become invaluable in the differentiation between normal, ectopic and molar pregnancies. In general, patients with an ectopic pregnancy have a positive but low level of hCG. In normal pregnancies and in early ectopic pregnancies, the hCG titers may be normal but increase at different rates. In the normal intrauterine pregnancy, the titer doubles every 2–3 days with a titer of 6000 IU/l usually being associated with a normal intrauterine pregnancy visible on ultrasound.

If the hCG titer is below 6000 IU/l but doubles every 2 days, expectant management is indicated. Should the titer not double, then a laparoscopy should be performed. With transvaginal ultrasound, an intrauterine pregnancy may be indentified with hCG titers of 1000–1500 IU/l, usually around 5–6 weeks after the last menstrual period, but failure of the titer to double in the absence of an intrauterine pregnancy would again indicate the need for a laparoscopy.

Ultrasound scan

Ultrasound scanning identifies fetal viability, growth parameters and the early features of pregnancy. It has become an accurate means of diagnosing the etiology of early pregnancy bleeding problems. At 5 weeks from the last menstrual period, a pregnancy in the uterine cavity is characterized by a gestation sac with decidual reaction. The intrauterine gestational sac may have an eccentric, asymmetrical trophoblast ring which may have a double-sac appearance (amniotic and yolk sac). This double decidual sign is suggestive of a normal intrauterine pregnancy. It consists of two concentric rings surrounding the gestational sac. The inner ring represents decidua capsularis, chorionic villi and chorion surrounding an anechoic area representing the gestational sac; the outer ring represents the decidua parietalis. The anechoic ring between these two layers is the remnant of the obliterated uterine cavity.

With conventional abdominal real-time ultrasound, the gestational sac of a normal intrauterine pregnancy becomes visible at 6 weeks of amenorrhea. By 6–7 weeks a fetal pole may be identified, at 7 weeks a fetal heart and at 9 weeks morphological features of the fetus. The features of a normal intrauterine pregnancy on vaginal ultrasound scan at 6.4 weeks gestation (CRL = 5 mm) are illustrated in **Figure 2**.

Abdominal ultrasound can only reliably diagnose an ectopic pregnancy when a live fetus is demonstrated outside of the uterus, which only occurs in 5–19% of cases (**Figure 3**). A pseudogestational intrauterine sac is seen in 10–20% of cases of ectopic pregnancy. Therefore, a definitive diagnosis of a viable intrauterine pregnancy must include the demonstration of fetal heart activity within the uterine cavity. A pseudogestational sac is due to a collection of blood within the hyperplastic endometrium, i.e. a decidual cast. This is always concentrated in the center of the uterine cavity and may be distinguished from an early (< 6 weeks) gestational sac which is often eccentrically located.

Other ultrasonic features of an ectopic gestation

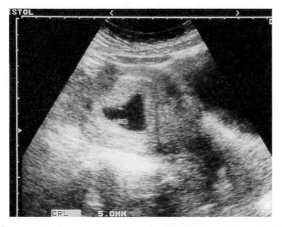

Figure 2. Normal pregnancy, 6/40 gestation. Yolk sacs to right of fetus.

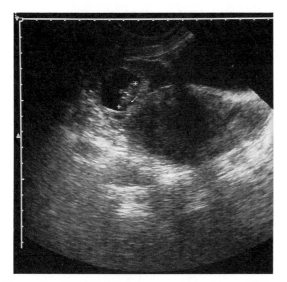

Figure 3. Ectopic pregnancy with fetus (CRL = 19 mm) and fetal heart visualized.

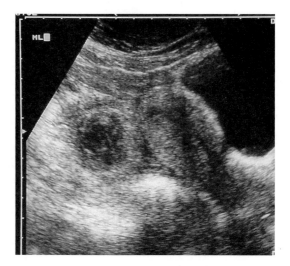

Figure 4. Complex cystic adenexal mass and free fluid in the pouch of Douglas.

include visualization of complex cystic adnexal masses and free fluid in the peritoneal cavity (**Figure 4**). Cystic or complex masses with ectopic pregnancy have been reported in 60–90% of cases. However, this does not take account of other complex cystic masses (such as ovarian tumors, abscesses, endometriosis), which it does not discriminate between.

Transabdominal ultrasonography for fetal diagnostic imaging uses transducers with frequencies of between 1.6 and 3.5 MHz and requires a full bladder. However, imaging smaller structures such as the ovary, endometrium and uterus, pregnant or otherwise, with lower frequency transducers is less than optimal. Axial resolution, that is the ability to distinguish two separate points in the direct line of the ultrasound beam, is a function of the transducer's frequency. Axial resolution improves with increased frequency. Unfortunately, the higher the frequency of sound, the greater the attenuation or loss of sound intensity as it passes through tissue. This rapid attenuation limits the depths at which structures can be imaged with higher frequency sound. The development of the transvaginal probe has allowed the use of higher frequencies, since the pelvic structures are closer to the ultrasound probe. The vaginal probe operates at a higher frequency (5 or 7.5 MHz) and allows greater accuracy of definition. With vaginal scanning, the structures being imaged are closer to the transducer and therefore the problem of tissue attenuation is not as critical, resulting in much better resolution of pelvic structures. A vaginal ultrasound examination is carried out with an empty bladder with the pelvis tilted at a 30° angle.

A last menstrual period that is in agreement with the ultrasound estimate of gestational age and hCG levels is reassuring and gives added confidence to gestational dating. A last menstrual period not in agreement with these other markers warrants close follow-up with serial evaluation until the gestational age and normal or abnormal status of the pregnancy is evident.

It is possible to image a 1 mm gestational sac at 4.2 weeks from the last menstrual period with vaginal ultrasound.[7] Dating a pregnancy from the last menstrual period has an inherent risk of error because it is based on a 28-day cycle with ovulation occurring on day 14. Deviation from a 28-day menstrual cycle implies a variation in timing of ovulation which must be taken into account when imaging a pregnancy. In addition, there may be inherent biological variation in early embryonic development which also causes discrepancies. Therefore, imaging of a 1 mm sac may not be possible until the fifth week or even longer from the last menstrual period. In general, early gestational structures are seen about 1 week earlier using transvaginal ultrasound compared with the transabdominal technique.

The gestational sac diameter increases in size from 2 to 4 mm by 5.0 weeks and is 5 mm by 5.2 weeks. A gestational sac of 2, 5, 10, 20 and 25 mm diameter roughly corresponds to a pregnancy of about 4, 5, 6, 7 and 8 weeks from the last monthly period (LMP), respectively.[4,7] The gestational sac volume increases from 1 ml at 6 weeks to 31 ml at 10 weeks and 100 ml at 13 weeks.[8] However, since the gestational sac is frequently irregular in shape and the method of evaluation of the volume is complex, the use of gestational sac volumes is of less value than measurements of crown rump length (CRL). Furthermore, the sac is not always round, and therefore a single maximal diameter is preferable for measurement.

In normal pregnancy, the sac diameter increases by 1.2 mm/day. No growth, or growth of less than 0.7 mm/day, is a poor prognostic sign. Failure of a gestational sac of 25 mm diameter to increase in size by 75% in 1 week is highly suggestive of a blighted ovum.[9] Gestational age by sac size in the first 50–60 days of pregnancy can be calculated by the formula: [age (day from last monthly period) = mean sac diameter (mm) + 30].[10]

The yolk sac is a bright rounded structure with an internal anechoic area and well-circumscribed edge. It is visualized by week 5 or 6 of pregnancy and disappears at week 10. Its greatest diameter is 5 mm at week 7. The yolk sac is the first structure that can be accurately identified within the gestational sac. Initially, it is much larger than the embryo. A diagnosis of a blighted ovum that will inevitably miscarry is suggested when there is a gestational sac larger than 20 mm in diameter with no yolk sac or greater than 25 mm without a fetus. A large yolk sac (> 10 mm) diameter is also associated with poor outcome.[11]

Fetal cardiac activity may be seen almost as soon as the fetus is identified as a separate entity. Fetal cardiac activity can generally be noted using a 3.5 MHz transabdominal sector transducer by 5.6 weeks to 6.1 weeks of gestation (41–43 days since the LMP). The gestational sac should measure 8–16 mm and the CRL 2–4 mm. A fetal heart should always be present in a normally developing embryo of 5–6 mm or about 6.5 weeks from the LMP.[12] Fetal cardiac activity should be present in all cases when the sac diameter is greater than 30 mm. It should be visualized by the end of the 7th week of amenorrhea. When fetal cardiac activity is noted in a pregnant patient with vaginal bleeding, the woman can be reassured that the prognosis is good; 97% of embryos with cardiac activity present have a normal outcome. The risk of spontaneous miscarriage is reduced from about 40–50% to 1.3–2.6%, depending

on the gestational age when the fetal heart is first imaged and the age of the woman.[1] The fetal heart rate is also a prognostic sign in early ultrasound scanning. Fetal bradycardia is associated with a poor prognosis. At 5–6 weeks, the fetal heart rate is 100 beats/min, which increases to 140 beats/min by 8–9 weeks gestation. A pregnancy with a heart beat of less than 85 beats/min usually results in spontaneous miscarriage.[13]

Other causes of bleeding in early pregnancy diagnosed by ultrasound scan include:

- a second empty gestational sac, and

- subchorional hemorrhage

A second gestational sac occurred in 3.9% of cases in the study quoted above.[1] When an ultrasound diagnosis of a twin pregnancy was made before a gestational age of 10 weeks, 71.4% of the twins vanished. At 10–15 weeks, 62.5% vanished. After week 15, no second twin vanished.[14] In this study, an intrauterine hematoma or retroplacental clot 0.7–16 ml in size was noted in 5.4% of cases. An intrauterine or subchorionic hematoma does not necessarily predict a poor prognosis when less than 50 ml in size and in the presence of a viable fetus.

Background data for interpreting the history: Expected outcome of any pregnancy (see also Chapter 8)

The outcome of previous pregnancies is relevant to a woman's overall risk of successful outcome of any pregnancy. In a prospective study,[15] the overall incidence of clinically recognizable spontaneous miscarriage before 20 weeks gestation was 12% (50/407 pregnancies). In primigravidas and women with a history of consistently successful pregnancies, the incidence of miscarriage is low (5 and 4% respectively). Women with histories only of unsuccessful pregnancy outcome have a much greater risk of miscarrying (24%). The outcome of the last pregnancy also influences outcome – 5% of women miscarried when their previous pregnancy was successful, compared with 19% when the outcome of the last pregnancy was miscarriage. For women with two successive miscarriages, the probability of a third is between 17 and 35%; for those who have had three or more, the probability of another is between 25 and 46%.[16] It is important to realize that even after three or more consecutive losses, the chance of a successful pregnancy is still at best 75% and at worst 54%, compared with the 85% expected by chance.

SPONTANEOUS ABORTION/MISCARRIAGE

Spontaneous abortion or miscarriage used to be defined as the spontaneous termination of a pregnancy prior to 28 completed weeks (196 days) of pregnancy (UK Infant Life (Preservation) Act 1929). The complexity of the legal situation arising from this act was worsened by the lack of any adequate definition of 'capable of being born alive' or the increasing downward trend for fetal viability. This UK definition was changed to 24 weeks (168 days) on 1 October 1992. The World Health Organization (WHO) recommendation is that a record should be kept of all babies born alive or dead of 22 weeks (154 days) gestational age or weighing 500 g or more if born earlier. The incidence of spontaneous miscarriage is between 15 and 20% of all clinically diagnosed pregnancies.[17] However, the actual loss may be as high as 60% of 'chemical' pregnancies diagnosed before the first missed period by estimation of the beta-hCG.

Maternal and Fetal Risks

Miscarriage may be associated with increased maternal mortality and morbidity from hemorrhage and infection, especially in neglected cases. An important part of the management of miscarriage is the psychological trauma and grief reaction resulting from the loss of a wanted pregnancy.[18]

Management Options (Figure 5)

Miscarriage may be classified as threatened, inevitable, incomplete, complete, missed, septic or recurrent and the management depends on the type. The diagnosis may be made from the history, physical examination, special laboratory and ultrasound scan investigations.

Threatened miscarriage

The patient presents characteristically with a history of vaginal spotting or mild vaginal bleeding but with minimal low back or pelvic pain and without the passage of tissue. Approximately 15% of all pregnancies are complicated by threatened miscarriage and of these 16–18% progress to miscarriage depending on the amount of bleeding.[19] Pregnancy is rarely successful if vaginal bleeding in the first 12 weeks of pregnancy is as heavy as the patient's normal menstrual blood loss.[20] When bleeding is slight and resolves, pregnancy may continue satisfactorily, but the threatened miscarriage tends to adversely affect subsequent perinatal out-

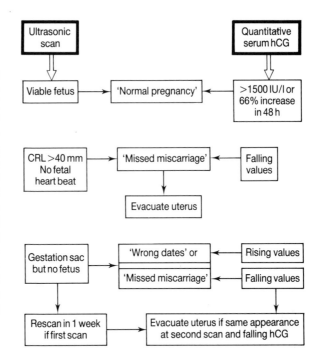

Figure 5. Amenorrhea, positive pregnancy test and vaginal bleeding: Summary of management options.

come.[21] On pelvic examination, bleeding from the cervix may be seen but the os is closed.

Ultrasound examination is an essential investigation which should be performed and interpreted completely in the light of the gestation of pregnancy. Should the ultrasound scan indicate a normal pregnancy, the patient should be managed expectantly with reassurance and should be advised to avoid strenuous activity. However, it is probably of no value to the outcome of the pregnancy to restrict normal daily activity.

If there is no further bleeding, the patient should be re-examined by ultrasound scan in 7 days. Failure of the gestational sac to increase in size, or failure to observe a fetal pole or heart activity would indicate failure of the pregnancy. If the uterine cavity is empty, it is important to consider the possibilities of a complete miscarriage, an ectopic pregnancy or that the pregnancy is not sufficiently advanced to observe an intrauterine pregnancy.

In approximately 50% of patients with first trimester bleeding, the pregnancy proceeds normally, although there is some evidence of an increased incidence of problems later in pregnancy, which include prematurity, small for gestational age, placental abnormalities, breech presentation, perinatal asphyxia, as well as increased incidence of perinatal death.[21–23]

Inevitable miscarriage

A miscarriage becomes inevitable when the internal cervical os dilates. In the majority of cases, this is preceded by crampy low abdominal pain and increased vaginal bleeding. In the first trimester pregnancy, the uterus requires evacuation using either suction or sharp curettage. In the late second trimester miscarriage, complete evacuation may be accomplished using an intravenous oxytocin drip. After 16 weeks when the cervix dilates due to incompetence, and when the membranes are intact, insertion of a cervical suture may salvage the pregnancy. Results from emergency cerclage may be very good if the complications of membrane rupture during the procedure and infection are avoided (see below).

Complete and incomplete miscarriage

In cases of complete miscarriage, the fetus, placenta and membranes may be passed intact with minimal bleeding or pain. On examination, the uterus is well contracted and the cervix is closed. These patients often do not require further treatment.

Incomplete miscarriage presents with a history of the passage of some of the products of conception, of crampy low abdominal pain associated with increased vaginal bleeding. On vaginal examination in many circumstances, tissue may be seen coming through the dilated cervix. The tissue should be removed to prevent uterine bleeding and cervical shock. An intravenous oxytocin drip of 20 units of oxytocin in 1000 ml of N-saline, 5% dextrose or Hartman's solution should be commenced and run at 10–12 mIU/min. Evacuation of the uterus should be carried out promptly to reduce blood loss and the possibility of infection. If blood loss has been significant, transfusion is indicated. Alternatively, the os may be closed and the blood loss either minimal or settling, and an ultrasound scan may reveal retained products of conception (**Figure 6**). Once again, evacuation of the uterus is indicated.

Missed miscarriage

A missed miscarriage is the failure to expel the products of conception following fetal death, recognized by failure of the pregnancy to have developed to the expected uterine size for gestation. The condition is commonly recognized in patients who present with a small amount of dark red or brown vaginal loss with a closed cervical os but with some uterine cramps. The symptoms of pregnancy have frequently disappeared or there have not been any perceived fetal movements where the length of amenorrhea suggests the pregnancy should be second trimester. No fetal heart beat is detectable and the uterine size is less than expected.

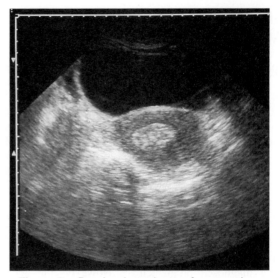

Figure 6.   Retained products of conception.

The definitive diagnosis is made by ultrasound scan when no fetal heart activity or movements are noted and other signs of fetal death are seen, such as a loss of the circular shape to the gestation sac (crenation), a decrease in the sac volume for the gestational age and failure of the conceptus to measure appropriately for gestational age based on the length of amenorrhea (**Figure 7**). In addition, the serial estimation of hCG will show a declining trend. Once the diagnosis is confirmed, evacuation of the uterus should be carried out.

A vaginal pessary containing PGE_2 (10 mg) may be given to facilitate the curettage, if the os is closed. If a missed miscarriage is diagnosed later in pregnancy (14 weeks onwards), it may be appropriate to induce

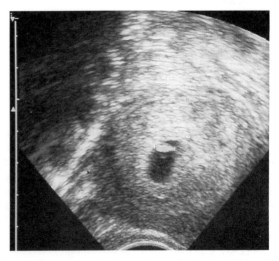

Figure 7.   Missed miscarriage CRL; inappropriate for gestation. No fetal heart activity visualized with CRL = 7 mm.

spontaneous miscarriage by vaginal, intra- or extra-amniotic administration of prostaglandins. A suggested regimen is 40 mg of prostaglandin $PGF_{2-alpha}$ or 16, 16-dimethyl-prostaglandin E_1 intra-amniotically under ultrasound guidance.[24] Alternatively, gemeprost is given vaginally every 3 h in a dose of 1 mg[25] or prostaglandin E_2 1.5–2 mg extra-amniotically as a slow release gel.[26]

Late second trimester missed miscarriage may be complicated by disseminated intravascular coagulation (DIC) with severe generalized hemorrhage. The risk of DIC increases with gestational age and with the duration of the missed miscarriage with retained products, but it does not usually arise until at least 4 weeks. In such cases, a coagulation profile should include platelet count, prothrombin time, partial thromboplastin time and fibrin degradation products. Should DIC occur, blood, fresh frozen plasma, cryoprecipitate or platelets should be transfused before evacuation of the uterus (see also Chapter 71).

Blood should be available at the time of evacuation of the uterus in second trimester evacuations only, as bleeding is often moderate to profuse. Rarely, hysterectomy may be necessary when there is heavy bleeding and the placenta is very adherent to the uterus.[27]

Septic miscarriage

Spontaneous miscarriage may be associated with infection. Historically, septic abortion commonly resulted from illegal termination of pregnancy. Before the legislation liberalizing the abortion laws in the UK in 1967, septic abortion was responsible for 0.7% of maternal deaths.[28] Between 1982 and 1984, according to the Confidential Enquiry into Maternal Mortality in England and Wales, for the first time there were no deaths from criminal abortion.

The clinical signs of a septic miscarriage are that the patient is febrile and usually has significant tenderness over the uterus and lower abdomen. There may be offensive as well as bloodstained vaginal discharge. Initially, infection is confined to the uterus, but it tends to spread through the uterine wall into the connective tissues of the broad ligament and lateral pelvic wall, leading to pelvic cellulitis and possibly septicemia. In severe cases, endotoxic shock can develop, sometimes with DIC. Such patients are at risk of acute renal failure.

Blood should be taken for full blood count and blood grouping and cross-matching. Urine analysis should be performed. Swabs should be taken for culture from the endocervix and lower uterine cavity, and peripheral blood sent for culture. Ultrasound scan of the pelvis and, if there is peritonitis, an abdominal x-ray should be obtained to detect any intra-abdominal or intrauterine gas (suggesting clostridial infection or uterine perforation). An x-ray or ultrasound should also demonstrate an intrauterine foreign body.

A septic miscarriage should be evacuated after the patient has been stabilized and antibiotic therapy instituted within 6 h.

Procedure: Evacuation of the Uterus

Indications

Surgical evacuation of the uterus is indicated when there are retained products of conception as with inevitable, incomplete, missed or septic miscarriages. If the cervical os is not dilated as in a missed miscarriage, particularly in a primagravida, gemeprost 1 mg should be administered intravaginally to facilitate dilatation of the cervix. PGE$_2$ 10 mg is an acceptable alternative.[29]

Description

Evacuation of the uterus is normally performed under general anaesthesia. The patient should be starved for 6 h. Premedication may be given (e.g. temazepam 20 mg or diazepam 10 mg with metachlopramide 10 mg). Ketamine is an effective alternative when inhalational general anesthesia is not available. Ketamine is given 2 mg/kg i.v. or 8 mg/kg i.m., which provides dissociative anesthesia for approximately 20 min. An alternative to ketamine is a benzodiazepine (e.g. midazolam 0.3 mg/kg) in a fit unpremedicated patient. Benzodiazepines are less predictable in their anesthetic effect than many of the more traditional regimens. A newer alternative is total intravenous anesthesia (TIA) which may be given as follows: Propofol 2–3 mg/kg for induction followed by boluses to maintain anesthesia. Infusion pumps are now available with programmed software to maintain anesthesia. Regional anesthesia by subarachnoid block (spinal anesthesia), paracervical block or intracervical block is an effective alternative when general anesthesia is unavailable.

The patient is placed in the lithotomy position. An Ovard's or Sim's speculum is inserted into the vagina for access. The vagina and cervix are cleaned with an antiseptic solution and any blood clot removed. It is common practice for the anesthetist to administer 5–10 units of

Syntocinon® at some stage during the procedure.

The evacuation is done using suction curettage preferably. Vosellum forceps, concave side upwards, are applied to the anterior lip of the cervix for traction while dilating. The cervix is dilated up to size 8–10 Hegar using metal dilators. It is not necessary to sound the uterine cavity, but clinical examination prior to cervical dilation under anesthesia should confirm the size of the uterus and whether there are any adenexal masses.

After cervical dilatation, usually a size 8 Karmen curette is introduced through the cervix. If the gestation is advanced, then a larger suction curette may be necessary, such as a 10 or rarely a 12. The Karmen curette is connected through clear tubing to a suction apparatus. The suction apparatus should supply a vacuum pressure of up to 70 cmHg. A pressure of at least 50 cmHg is required but not more than 70 cmHg (76 cmHg = 1.04 kg/cm^2).

The Karmen catheter is inserted and operated in a vacuuming fashion. Sometimes, it gets blocked with the placental tissue and it is necessary to remove this separately from the uterus with polyp forceps. Suction curettage is continued until there is a characteristic 'grating' feel when curetting the walls of the uterus. In the case of a missed miscarriage, it is often possible to identify characteristic amniotic fluid and white tissue. Occasionally, it is possible to glide over the products of conception. If an ultrasound scan has clearly demonstrated products of conception, then more than 50 ml should be obtained. Failure to do so may indicate that a false passage has been made and the products therefore not evacuated. Alternatively, failure to obtain products of conception suggest an ectopic pregnancy. A sharp curette may be introduced gently with a fingertip action to the fundus of the uterus and then it is depressed and gently stroked along the uterine wall to check the cavity for any remaining products of conception.

Complications

In a study of evacuation of the uterus in first trimester miscarriages using prostaglandin priming of the cervix,[29] uterine perforation occurred at a rate of 8/1000,

three of which required laparotomy. Other complications included a need for re-evacuation (1%) and hemorrhage in excess of 500 ml (0.1%) but no blood transfusions.

Products of conception

At the time of evacuation of the uterus, the products of conception should be sent for:

1. histology if the diagnosis of an intrauterine pregnancy is in doubt

2. karyotype if it is a recurrent miscarriage

3. culture if the diagnosis is uncertain

Histology

The presence of chorionic villi or trophoblastic tissue among products of conception are essential in confirming that a pregnancy has occurred.

In about 40–50% of placentae of spontaneous miscarriages, the chorionic villi correspond with the length of the gestational period. In 20–30% of cases, there are changes that occur after fetal death, i.e. sclerosis and obliteration of fetal vessels, stromal fibrosis, and an increased number of syncytial knots. In 20–40% of cases, the villi are swollen, edematous and hypovascular or avascular (termed hydropic degeneration). Uterine curettings from a patient with an unsuspected ectopic pregnancy will vary depending on whether the fetus is alive or dead, and if dead the time-lapse. If the ectopic pregnancy is viable, there will be the usual signs of pregnancy in the endometrium, i.e. decidualization of the stroma and hypersecretory changes in the glands. A focal Arias-Stella change is present in 60–70% of cases,[30] though this does not always specifically indicate an extrauterine pregnancy. An endometrium with an ectopic pregnancy present has a characteristically 'clean' appearance, without any of the decidual necrosis and inflammatory cell infiltration that characterizes an intrauterine gestation.[31] There is an absence of placental villi, extraplacental fetal membranes or fetal tissues, with no evidence of a placental site reaction. Trophoblastic infiltration of the decidua will be absent, with no trophoblastic migration into the spiral arteries and no transformation of spiral arteries into uteroplacental vessels.

Confusion may arise, because folowing the death of an ectopically sited fetus, the entire uterine lining may be sloughed off as a decidual cast, this showing the typical 'clean' appearance as previously described. If the decidua disintegrates and is irregularly shed, the tissue may show a crumbling decidua with areas of hemorrhage, necrosis and inflammation. Similar appearances are often found after miscarriage of an intrauterine pregnancy. For confirmation of an intrauterine pregnancy, it is therefore necessary to identify placental villi, or a placental site reaction. A similar picture may be obtained from an intrauterine pregnancy that has miscarried if the biopsy has been taken away from the placental site.

Karyotype (see also Chapter 8)

The frequency of karyotype abnormalities in spontaneous miscarriages has been quoted as between 2 and 64%.[32] Types of karyotype abnormalities include autosomal trisomy (45%), 45XO monosomy (20–30%), triploidy (15–20%) and tetraploidy (5%).

It is difficult to grow fetal cells adequately from retained products of conception. This is optimized if the tissue is transported in transport media for tissue culture samples which usually contains 100 ml hams F10 with 2 ml glutamine (200 mm and 40 μl penicillin/streptomycin mix (5000 units penicillin; 5000 μg streptomycin/ml with 5% fetal calf serum).

Tissue must be sent in a sterile container, such as a plastic universal with tissue culture medium as above preferably, or in sterile normal saline. There should be no delay in despatching the sample. Large products of conception may be sent dry, but excessive blood clots should be avoided.

Culture

Products of conception may be sent for culture and sensitivity in a sterile container.

Complications of Miscarriage

The immediate complications of spontaneous miscarriage are a failure to remove all products of conception resulting in retained products of conception with hemorrhage; perforation of the uterus; failure to empty the uterus; intractable bleeding (indication for a laparoscopy) and infection. Very occasionally, a hysterectomy needs to be done for uncontrollable bleeding after alternative methods have been exhausted, such as intramyometrial injection of $PGF_{2\text{-alpha}}$ or ligation of the internal iliac artery. A long-term complication of vigorous curettage is the development of uterine synechiae (Asherman's syndrome) with resulting amenorrhea and infertility.

Septic miscarriage occurs because bacteria in the vagina gain access to the uterus and infect its contents. This may occasionally arise before the miscarriage or more commonly when the membranes are ruptured (often after the first trimester). When the cervix is dilated, bacteria gain entry to the uterus and then infection may spread to the parametrium and thence to the peritoneal cavity. Death may occur from septic shock, hemorrhage due to DIC, or renal failure. Peritonitis, pelvic thrombophlebitis and abscess formation will often lead to long-term morbidity and secondary infertility. Antibiotic treatment is directed toward organisms responsible for septic miscarriage. They are pathogenic organisms of the bowel and vaginal flora. Anerobic organisms are common and include anaerobic streptococci, bacteroides and clostridia; aerobic organisms include *Escherichia coli* and group B beta-hemolytic streptococci. Co-amoxiclav 1.2 mg i.v. every 8 h is appropriate as an ideal single agent for anaerobic and aerobic organisms. It is a potent beta-lactamase inhibitor. It may be given orally at a dose of one tablet every 8 h (one tablet contains 500 mg amoxycillin/100 mg clavulanic acid). A contraindication to its use is penicillin allergy. Alternative antibiotics include penicillin as a crystalline penicilln G (10 million units i.v. every 4 h); ampicillin 2 gm every 4 h; ofloxacin 400 mg as a once daily dose because of the long elimination half-life. For anaerobic organisms: metronidazole 500 mg i.v. every 8 h; clindamycin 600 mg i.v. every 8 h; chloramphenicol 1 gm in 100 ml of saline every 6 h.[33] **Table 1** lists alternative antibiotics that may be used and their sensitivities to particular organisms. If endotoxic shock develops, such patients are at risk of renal failure.

The pathogenesis of sepsis

Sepsis and septic shock is caused by Gram-negative organisms in 30–80% of cases and is due to Gram-positive organisms in 6–24% of cases.[34] Septic syndrome is defined by the criteria given in **Table 2**.

Table 1
Bacteria – antibiotic sensitivity

	Co-amoxiclav	Cefuroxime	Metroni-dazole	Ampicillin/amoxycillin	Gentamicin	Cefotaxime	Flucloxacillin
Steph. aureus (pen. sensitive)	S	S	R	S	S	S	S
Steph. areus (pen. resistant)	S	S	R	R	S	S	S
Strep. pyogenes and *Strep. pneumoniae*	S	S	R	S	R	S	S
Strep. faecalis	S	R	R	S	R	R	R
N. gonorrhoeae	S	S	R	r	—	S	—
N. meningitidis	—	—	R	S	—	S	—
H. influenzae	S	S	R	r	—	S	R
E. coli	S	S	R	r	S	S	R
Klebsiella spp.	S	S	R	R	S	S	R
Proteus mirabilis	S	S	R	S	S	S	R
Serratia spp.	R	R	R	R	S	S	R
Pseudomonas aeruginosa	R	R	R	R	S	r	R
Bacteroides fragilis	S	r	S	R	R	r	R
Bacterioides spp./other anaerobes	S	S	S	S	R	r	R

S, sensitive; R, resistant; r, some strains resistant; — sensitive but not appropriate; pen, pencillin.

Table 2
Clinical evidence of infection

Bacteremia
Positive blood cultures

Sepsis
Tachypnea (>20 breaths/min)
Tachycardia (>90 beats/min)
Hyperthermia (>38.3°C)
Hypothermia (<35°C)
Evidence of inadequate organ perfusion
Hypoxemia
Elevated plasma lactate
Oliguria (<0.5 ml/kg body weight for at least 1 h in patients with a catheter)

Early septic shock

Sepsis syndrome is associated with hypotension (sustained decrease in systolic blood pressure <90 mmHg, or drop >40 mmHg for at least 1 h) when volume replacement is adequate and the patient is taking no antihypertensive medication, and occurs in the absence of other causes of shock such as hypovolemia, myocardial infarction and pulmonary embolism.[35] Early sepsis is responsive to conventional therapy such as intravenous fluid administration and antibiotic intervention. Refractory septic shock is treated with the above plus vasopressors such as dopamine (>6 μg/kg/h). Septic shock associated with sepsis can have a poor prognosis. Bone[36] reported that sepsis

without shock had a mortality of 13%, sepsis syndrome presenting with shock had a mortality of 28% and shock developing after the sepsis syndrome had a mortality of 43%.

Recently, it has been suggested that Gram-negative bacteremia and septic shock may be treated with HA-1A human monoclonal antibody against endotoxin (Centroxin®). HA-1A is a human monoclonal IgM antibody that binds specifically to the lipid A domain of endotoxin and prevents death in laboratory animals with Gram-negative bacteremia and endotoxemia. A randomized controlled trial of its use[37] using a single 100 mg i.v. dose of HA-1A (in 3.5 g of albumin) showed a reduction in mortality in those presenting with Gram-negative septicemia and shock.

Second Trimester Miscarriage

Cervical incompetence is an important yet potentially treatable cause of second trimester miscarriage.[38] Restoration of the internal cervical os is achieved surgically be cervical cerclage. (For details see **Figures 3, 4, 5**, Chapter 8.) A non-absorbable suture such as mersilene tape or nylon is inserted in a purse string fashion at the level of the internal cervical os. The knot is tied anteriorly. Even with cervical dilatation up to 10 cm, a successful outcome has been reported.[39] A survival rate of 63% (12/19) was achieved where gestation was prolonged from 1 to 12 weeks and gestational age at delivery ranged from 25 to 41 weeks.[39] Infection is suggested by the presence of contractions despite tocolysis, a persistent pyrexia or a C-reactive protein greater than 30 mg/l (normal, < 120 mg/l). There is between a 40–90% chance of a successful outcome.[38,40] Beta-sympathomimetic drugs (ritrodine hydrochloride given as a dose titrated to maternal side-effect: 50–100 µg/min and increased up to 20 min; maximum dosage 350 µg; half-life of ritrodine is 6–9 min) are often given intravenously for 1–2 days after the operation and then orally until pregnancy is clearly seen to be progressing satisfactorily. Patients undergoing cervical cerclage with the cervix dilated more than 2 cm and more than 18 weeks gestation should receive prophylactic antibiotics. Co-amoxiclav, ampicillin or cefoxitin can be given intravenously 30 min preoperatively and repeated at 6 h. A combination of gentamicin and clindamycin may be used in the patient allergic to penicillin or cephalosporins.

Differential diagnosis of a second trimester miscarriage includes those diagnoses in **Table 3**.

Table 3
Differential diagnosis of second trimester miscarriage

Uterine fibroids undergoing necrobiosis
Torsion of an ovarian cyst
Appendicitis
Cholecystitis
Intestinal obstruction
Previous uterine surgery: ruptured uterus, TOPs, etc.
Advanced extrauterine pregnancy
Pregnancy in a rudimentary horn of a double uterus

ECTOPIC PREGNANCY
(see **Figure 8**)

Approximately 2% of pregnancies are tubal and the incidence is increasing, especially among young women. The peak age specific incidence rate is found in women aged 25–34 years. This increase is due to a rise in prevalence of infertility, endometriosis, sexually transmitted diseases, tubal sterilization and reconstruction, and the association with intrauterine contraceptive devices which preclude a pregnancy in the uterus but not in the tubes. The rate in Scotland between 1970 and 1985 rose by 50% to 6/1000 pregnancies. In the USA, the increase was four-fold to 20/1000 pregnancies.[41]

A history of infertility gives a four-fold increased risk of an ectopic pregnancy compared with normal patients.[42] The diagnosis should be suspected in any women of reproductive age who present with irregular vaginal bleeding. The presentation may not be classical. The risks of an undiagnosed ectopic pregnancy are catastrophic hemorrhage with tubal rupture and compromise of future fertility.

The management of bleeding in a woman of reproductive age includes the exclusion of an ectopic pregnancy. Clinically, an ectopic pregnancy is most likely with a history of amenorrhea, irregular vaginal bleeding and abdominal pain. The irregular vaginal bleeding occurs often because the pregnancy dies and the loss of hormonal stimulation causes endometrial instability.

Maternal Risks

Ectopic pregnancy is a leading cause of maternal mortality, though in recent years there has been a dramatic fall in incidence from 3.5 deaths/1000 ectopic pregnancies in 1970 to 0.5/1000 ectopic pregnancies in 1983.[41] Deaths occur from delay, inadequate surgical treatment and inadequate therapy of profound hemorrhagic shock.

Diagnosis

Clinical

The diagnosis is often made on clinical suspicion. Rupture of the ectopic gestation with resulting intrauterine bleeding is the classic but infrequent presentation. It can be made from the history and physical examination. More commonly, the diagnosis is less easy and the history and physical findings not typical. The history of amenorrhea may not be obtained. It is important to ask about the last period, its timing, duration and amount of bleeding, as well as details of the previous menstrual period. The vaginal bleeding may have been light and prolonged. Subjective signs of pregnancy may not be present or may have disappeared due to the non-viability of the conceptus. The history of pain may also be mild, intermittent and prolonged. Physical examination may produce minimal, poorly localized tenderness in the abdomen, without peritonism and no pelvic mass may be found. The uterus may feel soft and enlarged.

The vague history and inconclusive physical signs can be shared by other conditions. The differential diagnosis includes a normal pregnancy with a ruptured corpus luteum of pregnancy, torsion of an ovarian cyst or pedunculated fibroid, appendicitis and renal colic; other causes of early pregnancy bleeding already discussed; and gynecological conditions such as pelvic inflammatory disease and endometriosis. Ectopic pregnancy has been nicknamed 'the great masquerade'. It is therefore of paramount importance to be aware of the possibility of an ectopic pregnancy in any woman who presents with abnormal vaginal bleeding and mild abdominal or pelvic pain.

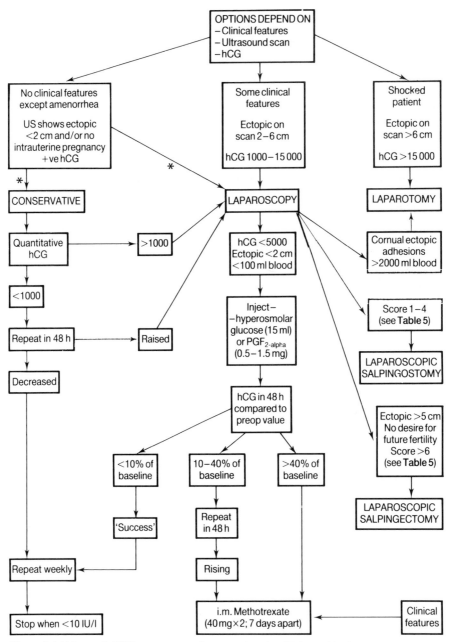

Figure 8. Ectopic pregnancy: Summary of management options.

* Some obstetricians prefer NOT to use a conservative approach and would always at least perform a laparoscopy

Special investigations

In the clinical situation where an ectopic pregnancy is suspected and a urine test for hCG is positive, serial quantitative estimations of the serum level of beta-hCG are helpful diagnostically. The concept of a 'discriminatory zone' for hCG has been introduced because of inconsistencies with the calibration of hCG assays and because of variation in ultrasonographers' abilities with transabdominal and transvaginal ultrasound scanning. This zone was first defined as between 6000 and 6500 IU/l above which a normal intrauterine pregnancy could be visualized by a transabdominal ultrasound scan in 94% of cases and below which an intrauterine gestational sac could not be visualized. A level above the discriminatory zone in the absence of an intrauterine sac is diagnostic of an ectopic pregnancy in 86% of cases. However, over 75% of ectopic pregnancies will have an hCG concentration of less than 6000 IU/l at the initial evaluation.[5]

The pattern of hCG production in ectopic gestation has been studied to provide a means of detection at an early stage. In the normal pregnancy, the hCG doubling time is 1.5 days in early pregnancy and 3 days at 7 weeks gestation. If at around 6 weeks gestation there is less than a 66% increase in hCG levels in 48 h, then an ectopic gestation is present or a pregnancy is present that is about to be aborted.[5]

Progesterone secretion has been studied and compared in ectopic and normal gestations to provide a predictor of abnormal gestations. The progesterone level is found to be lower in ectopic pregnancies than normal pregnancies. The normal pattern of progesterone secretion is a rise during the luteal phase and then a plateau during the first 8 weeks. Thus a single serum level which is below normal may indicate an abnormal pregnancy even when the hCG levels are below the discriminatory zone for ultrasound scan examination. A progesterone level of 25 ng/ml or above indicates a normal intrauterine pregnancy and a level below 15 ng/ml strongly suggests an abnormal pregnancy. However, serum progesterone estimations cannot discriminate between an abnormal intrauterine pregnancy and an ectopic pregnancy.

Culdocentesis, the needle aspiration of the cul-de-sac in search of blood in the peritoneal cavity, was formerly advocated to determine whether laparotomy was indicated. However, this examination could be misleading, especially when an ectopic pregnancy has not ruptured and consequently there is no intraperitoneal bleeding; yet with other disorders mimicking an ectopic gestation blood may be found.

Laparoscopy

The definitive diagnosis is made by laparoscopy, but there have been reports of an ectopic gestation missed at early stages of amenorrhea. The decision as to whether to do a laparoscopy or not is often confounded by an ultrasound report of an intrauterine sac, but it is important to be aware of the possibility of a pseudogestational sac caused by the presence of blood clot in the uterus. If there is doubt or the intrauterine findings are not consistent with expected hCG levels and the length of amenorrhea, and the woman presents with pain, then a laparoscopy is indicated.

Laparoscopy definitively confirms or excludes an ectopic pregnancy. Most ectopic pregnancies (95%) are found in the fallopian tube, most frequently in the isthmic or ampullary portion. Those occurring in the interstitial (cornual) portion of the tube, while much less common are of significance as they may rupture early with life-threatening hemorrhage. Ovarian pregnancies account for 1% of all ectopic gestations and are often only diagnosed at laparotomy because their presentation is similar to tubal pregnancy, or at pathological examination as they may appear grossly as a hemorrhagic ovarian cyst. Cervical pregnancies are very rare, and abdominal pregnancies which may continue to viability probably start out as tubal pregnancies which are 'aborted' into the peritoneal cavity. Others may result from rupture of a previous cesarean section scar. Fertilization of an ovum that is released on to the abdominal peritoneum has also been documented in rare circumstances.

Laparoscopy has greatly improved diagnosis as it allows for the direct visualization of the fallopian tubes and thus confirmation or exclusion of an ectopic pregnancy. Laparoscopy should be performed when there is both a real possibility of an ectopic pregnancy and doubt about the diagnosis. It gives a certain diagnosis for the problem of abdominal pain, with minimal risk (procedure-related risks also include problems of the condition; the risk of laparoscopy in a patient without an ectopic pregnancy is not the same as a patient with an ectopic pregnancy) and enables definitive investigation of the patient within 24 h. It eliminates the prolonged, expensive, anxiety-creating observation period and the need for unnecessary laparotomy when other conditions in the differential diagnosis not requiring surgical treatment are thought to be present from the symptoms and signs.

Management Options

Earlier diagnosis of ectopic pregnancy as a result of beta-hCG and ultrasound scanning and laparoscopy probably decreases the incidence of ruptured tubal pregnancy. Surgical management, in the absence of hemodynamic instability, should aim to preserve tubal function and avoid decreasing fertility.

Medical management of the ectopic pregnancy

Medical management options for ectopic pregnancies include systemic injection of methotrexate and intrasac injection of the ectopic with methotrexate, $PGF_{2-alpha}$, hyperosmolar glucose and other substances. These methods are possible largely because the presentation is so much earlier than previously.

Methotrexate

The cytotoxic drug methotrexate has been used for both systemic and localized injection. It may be used systemically as a 5 day course of treatment with a daily i.v. dose of 20–25 mg or, alternatively, 50 mg (1.0 mg/kg body weight) every other day combined with folinic acid (0.1 mg/kg body weight). The cytotoxic side-effects include nausea, stomatitis and fatigue. The blood cell count and liver enzymes are moderately affected but the risk of serious, acute side-effects appears minimal.

In a review of the non-surgical management of ectopic pregnancies, Pansky et al.[43] found 118 cases treated with systemic methotrexate with a failure rate of 5.9%. They defined the criteria for systemic treatment as the following: (1) pregnancy diameter of < 3 cm; (2) unruptured tube; (3) non-active bleeding; (4) beta-hCG serum level <1500 IU/l; (5) no fetal cardiac activity during ultrasonography; and (6) less than 100 ml of blood in the pouch of Douglas.

Methotrexate is also used as a second-line therapy, in cases with persistent trophoblast after conservative surgery or prostaglandin injection. It is given as two 40 mg i.m. doses 1 week apart. Methotrexate has been used by transvaginal directed ultrasonography for direct injection into the tubal gestation sac: 10 mg of methotrexate is used.[44] The theoretical objection to this is the possible effects of an anti-metabolite injected so close to the oocytes, though there are insufficient data to know if this is relevant in practice.

Potassium chloride

There have been isolated reports[45,46] of transvaginal ultrasonically directed injection of potassium chloride into the ectopic gestation. The advantage of potassium chloride as opposed to methotrexate is its lack of systemic side-effects. However, it acts mainly on the fetal heart and causes asystole and fetal death. It has no effect on the trophoblastic tissue, which may continue to proliferate and cause tubal rupture.

Prostaglandins

Ribic-Paucelj et al.[47] advocated the local injection of PGE_2. However, Feichtinger and Kemeter[48] reported less success with this substance.

$PGF_{2\text{-alpha}}$ affects tubal function by causing an increase in tubal peristalsis and vasospasm of arteries in the mesosalpinx. It is also a luteolytic agent that induces a decrease in progesterone production of the corpus luteum. Linblom et al.[49,50] injected $PGF_{2\text{-alpha}}$ 0.5–1.5 mg locally into the tubal pregnancy laparoscopically. Egarter et al.[51] used a combination of a local injection of both the tube and the corpus luteum in the ovary. They reported severe hemodynamic and cardiac side-effects in 3 out of 18 patients. One had massive pulmonary edema as a result of malignant hypertension

and complete artrioventricular block and another severe cardiac arrhythmia. These complications were explained by the massive absorption of the drug through the ovarian vasculature to the circulation. They then recommended a change in the protocol of treatment to an injection of estrogen (E_2) into the corpus luteum to induce luteolysis.

Hyperosmolar glucose

Lang et al.[52] performed a randomized study with laparoscopic local injection of hyperosmolar glucose in nine patients who had unruptured tubal pregnancies. They used local injection of $PGF_{2\text{-alpha}}$ combined with systemic PGE_2 in another nine patients. Better results were obtained with the hyperosmolar glucose, with no need for subsequent surgery.

Comments on medical management

The chief risk of injection is failure of resorption of the conceptus necessitating further treatment. This occurs in 5% of cases. Success is dependent on appropriate selection. It has been suggested that the following criteria are used for injection of ectopic pregnancies: hCG < 1000 IU/l; < 100 ml of blood in the pouch of Douglas; absence of fetal heart on ultrasonography; minimal clinical symptoms; size of hematosalpinx < 3 cm. Fernandez et al.[53] have proposed a scoring system for delineating which ectopics should be treated by non-surgical management (**Table 4**) and which should be treated by laparoscopy. A score of greater than 6 should be treated laparoscopically.

However, it should be noted that ectopics, particularly those diagnosed early, may resolve of their own accord. Treatment (medical or surgical) may be decided on the basis of whether the hCG is rising or

Table 4
Non-surgical treatment of ectopic pregnancies

Score	1	2	3
Gestational age (weeks of amenorrhea)	> 8	7–8	6
HCG level (IU/l)	< 1000	1000–5000	> 5000
Progesterone level	< 5	5–10	> 10
Abdominal pain	Absent	Induced	Spontaneous
Hematosalpinx	< 1	1–3	> 3
Hematoperitoneum	0	1–100	> 100

Source: Fernandez et al.[53]

not and whether it is less than 1000 IU/l. The difficulty of using criteria obtained at laparoscopy is that not giving definitive treatment at the same time may seem negligent. It has been suggested that ectopics with the following criteria may be managed expectantly and that they will resolve spontaneously: hCG level < 1000 IU/l; less than 50 ml of blood in the pouch of Douglas; and a hemosalpinx less than 2 cm in diameter.

Surgical treatment of ectopic pregnancy

Laparoscopy

Laparoscopy is essentially a safe surgical procedure. However, the morbidity and mortality associated with laparoscopy have largely been determined from laparoscopies related to sterilization and diagnostic laparoscopies. In 1978, the Royal College Confidential Enquiry into Gynaecological Laparoscopy in the UK found an overall complication rate of 34/1000 with a mortality rate of 0.8/1000.[54]

In order to identify those ectopics suitable for salpingostomy compared with salpingectomy, a scoring system has been developed, as shown in **Table 5**.[55] If the score is between 1 and 4, a laparoscopic conservative procedure is suitable; if 6 or above, a radical (salpingectomy) procedure is advisable. Using this criteria, between January 1988 and August 1991 in Clermont-Ferrand, there were 270 salpingectomies performed laparoscopically, 71 salpingostomies and 34 salpingectomies using laparotomy. The complications from 10 years experience from 467 salpingectomies by laparoscopy were 0.6%. There was one deep vein thrombosis, one delayed retroperitoneal hematoma requiring laparotomy and one epigastric vein injury.

Table 5
Predictive score for success of laparoscopic salpingostomy (1–4) or laparoscopic salpingectomy score (> 6)

History of infertility	2
Previous ectopic pregnancy	2
Tuboplasty	2
Tubal occlusion	2
Localization	
isthmic	1
ampullary	0
fimbria	−1
Tubal rupture	1

Source: Pouly et al.[55]

Laparoscopic Treatment of Ectopic Pregnancy

Laparoscopic salpingostomy

Conservative surgical treatment for an ectopic pregnancy is laparoscopic linear salpingostomy, i.e. the tube with the ectopic is conserved by surgical techniques. Various kinds of techniques may be used. An incision is made over the antimesenteric border of the tube along two-thirds of the length of the hematosalpinx. The incision may be made with a needle electrode (on 15 W coagulation and 30 W cutting, blend 1; Valley Lab force 2 diathermy). Unipolar current is generally thought to be a potentially hazardous technique, because of the potential for surrounding tissue damage to a radius of 5 cm. Bipolar coagulation limits tissue damage to 2–5 mm. Alternatively, a laser may be used: a carbon dioxide (CO_2 laser) potassium titanyl phosphate (KTP laser), neodymium-yttium aluminium garnet (Nd-Yag laser) or argon laser. The CO_2 laser operates by vaporization and limitation of tissue damage to 0.1–0.2 mm. A power density of 4000 W/cm^2 and beam diameter of 5 mm is required. Power densities greater than 4800 W/cm^2 in the continuous mode and greater than 2375 W/cm^2 in the pulse mode are needed to limit circumferential tissue damage.[56] The argon laser has a depth of penetration of 0.4–0.8 mm.

A three puncture laparoscopy technique is used with two suprapubic operative trocars placed one to the left and one to the right of an imaginary Pfannenstiel incision line. A 7 mm trocar is inserted in the midline. Any hematoperitoneum is aspirated.

Argipressin (10 units in 0.5 ml diluted in 20 ml Hartman's solution) is injected into the mesosalpinx through a 20 gauge spinal needle. Blanching of the fallopian tube and transient ischemia will be seen and provide a bloodless operating field.

A 10–15 mm incision is made in the antimesenteric portion of the hematosalpinx with the needle electrode (Figure 9), coagulation and scissors, or with the laser, as chosen. A suction/irrigation unit is used for evacuation of the clot and tro-

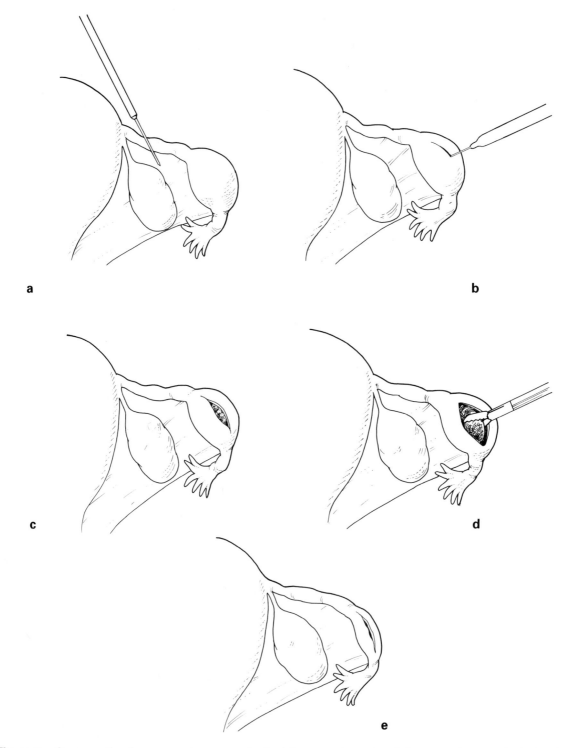

Figure 9. Conservative laparoscopic surgery by incision over hematosalpinx on antemesenteric border of the tube. (**a**) Injection into mesosalpinx of Argipressin for hemostasis. (**b**) Incision of tube. (**c**) Linear salpingostomy exposing trophoblast in tube. (**d**) Removal of tube contents. (**e**) Tube left open to heal by secondary intention

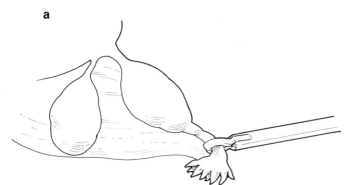

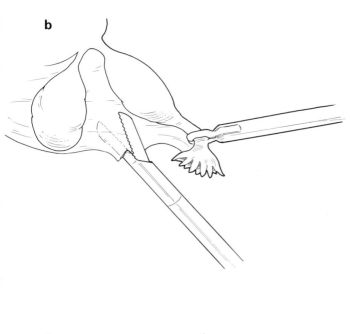

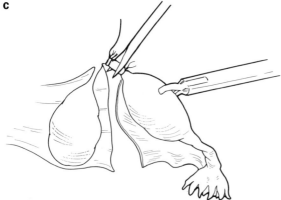

Figure 10. (a) Coagulation of mesosalpinx using bipolar diathermy forceps. (b) Scissors are used to cut diathermed mesosalpinx. (c) Removal of tube (salpingectomy) using a clip for occlusion of tube.

phoblast. If the clot is too organized making suction difficult, then 10 mm spoon-shaped grasping forceps (Semm forceps) may be introduced through a 10 mm portal to remove all the tissue. Alternatively, a combined instrument (the triton) is efficient for opening the tube and removing the ectopic. The salpingostomy site is left open for healing, since this decreases the risk of obstruction and allows better healing of the circumferential mucosal folds.[57]

Laparoscopic salpingectomy

Salpingectomy is performed laparoscopically, either by using a suture loop or by coagulation with bipolar diathermy forceps (3 mm) before cutting the tube (**Figure 10**). The excised tube is removed through a 10 mm portal.

The results from the largest reported series (321 cases) of conservative laparoscopic treatment for ectopic pregnancies are very favorable in terms of tubal patency, subsequent intrauterine pregnancy and acceptable numbers who sustain a repeat ectopic pregnancy.[55] Previous fertility history influences subsequent outcome. In that series, in those without a history of infertility the postoperative intrauterine pregnancy rate was 85.5% (n=62), compared with 41.1% (n=56) in those with a history of infertility or previous ectopic. The subsequent ectopic rates were 16.1 and 28.6%, respectively. Fifteen cases (4.8%) required a subsequent laparotomy or second laparoscopic procedure because of persistent trophoblastic tissue. Of 118 patients desiring a further pregnancy, 76 (64.4%) had an intrauterine pregnancy and 26 (22%) had a second ectopic pregnancy; 45.8% (11/24 patients) attempted conception following surgery to their only remaining fallopian tube and had an intrauterine pregnancy. Of this group, 29.9% had a second ectopic pregnancy. It is difficult to know whether conservative laparoscopic surgery should be advocated where the patient has had two previous ectopic pregnancies. It depends on the availability of *in vitro* fertilization services and the risk the operator and patient are prepared to take for a repeat ectopic pregnancy.

Vermeesh *et al.*[58] found that in a series of 10 patients, only 20% had a subsequent term pregnancy, with a 66.7% repeat ectopic pregnancy rate. This is in accordance with Hallatt's study[59] of 27 patients, where there were three (11.1%) intrauterine pregnancies and four repeat ectopic gestations (57% of conceptions).

DeCherney et al.[60] reported four (30.8%) intrauterine pregnancies and one repeat ectopic pregnancy (20%) in a group of 13 patients. Thus they came to the conclusion that those with two ectopic pregnancies could be treated conservatively.

Vermeesh and Presser[61] analysed the results from a randomized trial of laparoscopic salpingostomy vs laparotomy for the treatement of ectopic pregnancy. At the end of 1 year of study, 56 and 58% of patients had conceived after laparoscopy and laparotomy, respectively, at the end of 3 years, 74 and 86%, respectively. The differences were not statistically significantly different. A life table analysis showed that pregnancy occurred sooner after laparoscopy than after laparotomy, with 75% of all conceptions after laparoscopy occurring within 16 months, whereas only 54% of conceptions after laparotomy occurred within this same time period. There was a higher rate of recurrence of ectopic pregnancy after laparotomy. One explanation may be the extent of tubal and peritubal damage which is increased in laparotomy.

Laparotomy

Abdominal procedures are performed where there is not the laparoscopic expertise to deal effectively with ectopic pregnancies or for specific indications. Approximately 10% of cases will require a laparotomy for definitive treatment of the ectopic pregnancy. These patients are identified because:

- they are hemodynamically unstable, i.e. in shock;

- the serum HCG level is > 15 000;

- extensive intra-abdominal adhesions are present.

Tubal pregnancy was first treated by salpingectomy as a life-preserving procedure by Lawson Tait in 1884.[62] Since then, the objectives of management have changed. Stromme[63] described the first successful salpingostomy in 1953. Conservation procedures are indicated when fertility preservation is important and the patient is hemodynamically stable. A simple procedure – in particular, for an ampullary ectopic pregnancy – is to 'milk' the unruptured ectopic gestation through the end of the fallopian tube. This should not be done, however, as the anatomical site of the ectopic pregnancy is in the muscularis mucosa. Thus it is outside the mucosa. Excessive handling of the tube can only cause further damage to the mucosa.

Procedure

Laparotomy – salpingostomy

Salpingostomy with laser or cautery is possible when the ectopic pregnancy is unruptured. It is particularly indicated when the other tube has been previously removed. A small linear incision is made over the site of the ectopic (usually the antemesenteric border of the tube) and the products of conception are evacuated. Careful attention to securing hemostasis with cautery is important. The incision is left open to heal by secondary intention. Alternatively, bleeding points may be secured with fine nylon sutures or 4/0 absorbable vicryl. Resection of a small portion of an isthmic portion of a fallopian tube with an early ectopic pregnancy may be possible, leaving sufficient proximal and distal portions for immediate end-to-end anastomosis if the patient's condition will allow, or at a later date when because of less vascularity this procedure will be easier.

Laparotomy–salpingectomy

Most procedures may be performed through a minilaparotomy incision. Salpingectomy to remove the ectopic pregnancy will be the treatment of choice in the presence of severe bleeding, gross tubal damage or where the ectopic pregnancy is large (greater than 10–15 cm diameter). A salpingectomy is performed as follows: the fimbrial end of the tube is elevated and the base of the mesosalpinx is clamped with a mosquito forceps at its free edge. The tissue is then divided with cautery, scissors or a scalpel. The entire mesosalpinx is transected by taking identical 'bites' successively until the cornual end of the fallopian tube is reached. The pedicles are stitched with 4/0 vicryl. The tube is then clamped at its cornual end, transected and sutured with 2-0 or 3-0 vicryl. The abdomen is closed after irrigation with Hartman's solution.

In assessing success of a surgical technique where infertility is involved, it is necessary to take account of the cumulative pregnancy rates in the normal population and the etiological conditions of infertility (see **Figure 11**).[64]

Evaluating the literature on the surgical treatment of ectopic pregnancy is difficult because of the limited numbers of randomized controlled trials evaluating medical or surgical procedures. It seems axiomatic that one should adopt a surgical procedure resulting in the least disturbance to reproduce anatomy. Thus the techniques of a laparoscopic approach would seem justifiable. However, there is some recent evidence which disputes this assumption and argues that the prognosis for future pregnancies is reliant on the underlying pathology evident in the history or otherwise of infertility.[42] Sultana *et al.* concluded that there is no difference in pregnancy rates after treatment for an ectopic pregnancy by either laparoscopic salpingostomy or laparotomy. Fewer patients conceived in the group with a history of infertility (*n*=59) and 10.4% of these delivered, compared to 21 (35.6%) who did not have a history of infertility. This means that with a history of normal fertility after a surgical treatment for an ectopic pregnancy, the chances of conception are four times more likely than those with a history of infertility. The chance of a repeat ectopic is about 12%.[42]

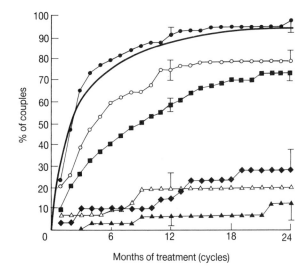

Figure 11. Cumulative rates of conception in couples with single cause of infertility managed as appropriate, excluding use of donor insemination or *in vitro* fertilization, compared with normal rates (highest rates reported in couples of proved fertility). Rates for couples with each cause shown as: — normal; ●—● amenorrhea; ○—○ oligomenorrhea; ■—■ unexplained infertility; △—△ tubal damage (moderate/severe); ◆—◆ failure of sperm penetration of mucus (normal semen); ◇—◇ oligospermia and failure to penetrate mucus. Standard error of proportions are given at 12 and 24 months.

GESTATIONAL TROPHOBLASTIC DISEASE (GTD) (see **Figure 12**)

There is a wide variation in the incidence of hydatidiform moles from 1:1000 to 1:1500 pregnancies in Western countries to 15 times that number in Asian countries. The explanation is thought to be racial and perhaps dietary. It is more common in the extremes of the reproductive age groups when defective ova may be a factor. In 7.5% of cases, chemotherapy is required for invasive mole or choriocarcinoma.[65]

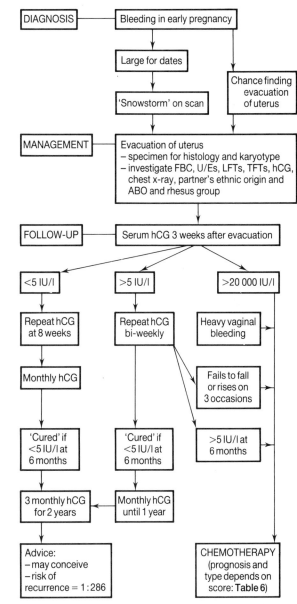

Figure 12. Hydatidiform mole: Summary of management options.

Maternal Risks

The risk to the mother from benign trophoblastic disease is from hemorrhage with spontaneous miscarriage usually without a fetus, but in the case of a partial mole, infection, anemia, severe prolonged vomiting in early pregnancy, early pregnancy-induced hypertension and rarely hyperthyroidism. Malignant gestational trophoblastic disease is fatal in 0.2% of cases.[65] In subsequent pregnancies, the risk of a second hydatidiform mole is 1:76 and that of a third 1:6.5.

Management Options

Diagnosis

With complete moles, patients will present with a uterus that is not compatible with dates. Approximately 50% will have a uterus larger than dates. Over 90% will have vaginal bleeding as early as the fourth week as the most common presentation. Spontaneous passage of grape-like material (the hydropic vesicles) is frequent by 6–8 weeks, with complete miscarriage by 16 weeks. Approximately 20% of patients will present with large, benign theca-lutein cysts because of the stimulation of the ovaries by hCG. Other clinical presentations may result from the complications. There is absence of a fetal heart.

The signs and symptoms of a partial mole may be delayed and the patient may present as a missed miscarriage or as a spontaneous miscarriage with the passage in addition of a fetus. The uterus is more often small for dates and hCG levels are lower.

An ultrasound examination shows a characteristic 'snowstorm' appearance of mixed echogenic appearance, indicating hydropic villi and intrauterine hemorrhage. The serum hCG level is markedly raised, usually in excess of 20 000 IU/l.

Investigation

Laboratory investigations should include a complete blood count, liver, renal and thyroid function tests and a baseline estimation of hCG. A baseline chest x-ray should be performed to rule out metastases and a pelvic ultrasound scan should be performed to determine uterine size and presence or absence of theca-lutein cysts of the ovary. Other investigations relevant to a prognosis of hydatidiform mole are ethnic group, ABO and Rh blood group, including those of the partner, and the use of oral contraceptives.

Evacuation procedures

Evacuation of the uterus is safest using suction curettage followed by sharp curettage. Some advocate oxytocin stimulation to ensure hemostasis. Major complications of the evacuation may include hemorrhage, infection, fluid retention due to the antidiuretic effect of oxytocin when used in large amounts with hypotonic intravenous and rarely trophoblastic emboli. Therefore, all patients should have close hemodynamic monitoring.

Total abdominal hysterectomy is indicated in older patients and for those who do not wish to have further pregnancies. Evacuation of the uterus via induction of labor or hysterotomy are not recommended, as there is an increased risk of hemorrhage due to incomplete evacuation of the uterus.

Oophorectomy or ovarian cystectomy of the thecalutein cysts is not indicated simply on the basis of size, and is only indicated in the presence of torsion or hemorrhage.

Postevacuation

Follow-up 3 weeks after evacuation of the uterus is necessary to check on whether the mole has been successfully treated or not. If the serum hCG falls to normal after 8 weeks (< 5 IU/l, then follow-up is by monthly serum hCG samples for 6 months. If these are normal at 6 months, then samples should be done monthly for 1 year and then every 3 months for up to 2 years after evacuation. If serum hCG values are normal for 6 months, then the risks of malignant gestational trophoblastic disease are very small (1:286), and a subsequent pregnancy could be embarked upon.

Chemotherapy for treatment of a molar pregnancy postevacuation is instigated (approximately 10% of cases) in any of the following situations: (1) if 4 weeks after evacuation the serum beta-hCG level is > 20 000 IU/l; (2) the hCG rises on more than three occasions or fails to fall; (3) there is heavy uncontrolled vaginal bleeding and the hCG is raised; (4) there is evidence of metastases in the brain, liver or gastrointestinal tract, or radiological opacities greater than 2 cm on chest x-ray.[66]

In the UK, the Charing Cross prognostic score identifies the chemotherapeutic regimen that should be adopted (see **Table 6**). A low risk is indicated by a score of less than 50, a medium risk by a score of 55–95 and a high risk by a score greater than 95 (see **Table 7**). Chemotherapy should only be undertaken in collaboration with an experienced oncological team. The following are guidelines for treatment.

For a low score, a single agent is used – methotrexate 35 mg/m² i.m. for 4 days alternating with folinic acid 6 mg i.m. or 15 mg orally. For a medium risk, a

Table 6
Categorization of patients with gestational trophoblastic tumours[a]

Risk factors	0	10	20	40
Age	< 39	> 39		
Parity	1,2,>4	3 or 4		
Antecedent pregnancy	Mole	Abortion	Term	
Interval (AP-chemotherapy)				
in months	< 4	4–7	7–12	> 12
hCG (plasma mIU/ml or urine IU/day)	10^3–10^4	10^4	10^4–10^5	10^5
ABO	A × A	O × O	Bx	
	× B	A × O	ABx	
	× AB	–	–	
No. of metastases	Nil	1–4		> 8
Site of metastases	Not detected	Spleen	4–8	Brain
	Lungs	Kidney	GI tract	
	Vagina	–	Liver	
Largest tumor mass	< 3 cm	3–5 cm	> 5 cm	
Lymphocytic infiltration		Moderate,		
	Marked	unknown	Slight	
Immune status	Reactive		Unreactive	Two drugs or
Previous chemotherapy	Nil		Single drug	more

Source: Newlands.[66]
[a]Scores for individual risk factors are added and risk group determined by the total score as follows: low risk 50 or less, medium risk 55–95, high risk >95.

Table 7
Survival of patients by their prognostic score on admission (analysis up to 1973)

	0–40	40–80	90–120	130–180	> 180
Total	94	99	68	45	15
Deaths	0	2	16	24	15
% Alive	100	98	76	47	0

Source: Modified from Bagshawe.[67]

sequence of viniplastin (VP 16-213) in a dose of 100 mg/m^2 in 200 ml of saline is given i.v. for 5 days, with hydroxyurea and 6-mercaptopurine (6MP), methotrexate and folinic acid for 8 days. High-risk patients have a schedule of two courses consisting of actinomycin-D, VP-16-213, hydroxyurea, methotrexate, vincristine and cyclophosphamide. The sequence is repeated until the patient is in complete remission. Cranial prophylaxis is given as methotrexate 12.5 mg intrathecally on each alternate course.

Prognosis is related to both the score and the interval from the antecedent pregnancy to commencing chemotherapy. If the interval from the antecedent pregnancy to starting chemotherapy is less than 4 months, the survival rate is 97%, in contrast to 48% when the interval is 13–24 months (see Table 7).[67] In some cases of persistent vaginal hemorrhage, hysterectomy is indicated.

Hysterectomy at the time of starting chemotherapy may reduce the duration of treatment, but hCG follow-up is essential.

Oral contraception should be avoided because there is evidence that the recurrence rate is higher when taking the combined oral contraceptive.[68]

RHESUS PROPHYLAXIS

All pregnant women need to have a blood group test to establish whether they are rhesus negative and therefore at risk of rhesus sensitization with pregnancy loss, either at miscarriage or with an ectopic pregnancy. In order to prevent antibody formation and the subsequent risk of rhesus disease in a future pregnancy, passive immunization is given at times of recognized risk of feto-maternal transfusion which includes threatened, inevitable and missed miscarriages and ectopic pregnancy. All Rh negative patients without Rh anti-D antibodies should recieve anti-D gammaglobulin. An intramuscular injection of 250 IU (50 µg) of anti-D is given within 72 h. After 20 weeks gestation, the dose is 500 IU (100 µg). A Kleihauer test[69] determines whether the dose of anti-D is effective in removing all fetal red blood cells from the maternal circulation. Altogether 250 IU (50 µg) neutralizes 2 ml of fetal blood. The blood volume of the fetus is 70 ml/kg, but the placental circulation is much greater. Current prophylaxis still fails to prevent 600–700 RhD negative women being immunized per year in the UK. The operative factors in this are: failure to give anti-D immunoglobulin when indicated, failure of protection by passive anti-D immunoglobulin and intrapartum immunization. Altogether, 25% of the failures of administration of anti-D occur after miscarriage.

IMPLANTATION HEMORRHAGE

Implantation hemorrhage may occur on day 21 following the last menstrual period in women with a regular 28 day cycle, as the blastocyst implants in the endometrium. Bleeding after normal implantation of pregnancy can result from the decidua parietalis, the lining of the pregnancy uterus away from the implantation site. Clinically, the blood loss is minimal and may resemble a menstrual period, but it is not associated with crampy abdominal pain. It has no effect on the continuation of the pregnancy or on the health of the mother and she should be reassured. The bleeding may, however, be confused by the patient as a menstrual period, especially if ovulation is delayed, which in turn can lead to inaccurate calculation of the expected date of confinement.

BLEEDING IN EARLY PREGNANCY
Summary of Management Options

Initial general assessment and management (see **Figure 1**)

Subsequent specific management

- Spontaneous abortion or miscarriage (see **Figure 5**)

- Ectopic pregnancy (see **Figure 9**)

- Gestational trophoblastic disease (see **Figure 12**)

- Implantation bleed—reassure

CONCLUSION

The management of bleeding in early pregnancy is complex in terms of accurate assessment and may require quick intervention to maintain hemodynamic equilibrium, to avoid morbidity and mortality. The objective in management of bleeding in early pregnancy is to diagnose accurately a normal viable intrauterine pregnancy. If this is not established, then alternative differential diagnoses must be considered and accurately managed. These include the complications of intrauterine pregnancy: (miscarriage – incomplete, complete, inevitable and septic) ectopic pregnancy; and hydatidiform mole. It is important to manage the bleeding in terms of the acute situation and the woman's reproductive career. Adequate management may require cross-specialty cooperation.

REFERENCES

1   Stabile I, Campbell S, Grudinskas JG (1987) Ultrasonic assessment of complications during first trimester of pregnancy. *Lancet* **2**:1237–1240.
2   Lind T (1988) How positive is a positive pregnancy test? *British Medical Journal* **296**:730–731.
3   Wide L, Gemzell CA (1960) An immunological pregnancy test. *Acta Endocrinologica* **35**:261–267.
4   Bernaschek G, Rudelstrofer R, Csaicsich P (1988) Vaginal sonography versus serum human chorionic gonadotropin in early detection of pregnancy. *American Journal of Obstetrics and Gynecology* **158**:608–612.
5   Kadar N, Freedman M, Zacher M (1990) Further observations on the doubling time of human chorionic gonadotropin in early asymptomatic pregnancies. *Fertility and Sterility* **54**:783–787.
6   Kadar N, De Vore G, Romero R (1981) Discriminatory hCG zone: Its use in the sonographic evaluation for ectopic pregnancy. *Obstetrics and Gynecology* **58**:156–161.
7   de Crespigny LC, Cooper D, McKenna M (1988) Early detection of intrauterine pregnancy with ultrasound. *Journal of Ultrasound in Medicine* **7**:7–10.
8   Robinson HP (1975) 'Gestation sac' volumes as determined by sonar in the first trimester of pregnancy. *British Journal of Obstetrics and Gynaecology* **82**:100–107.
9   Robinson HP (1975) The diagnosis of early pregnancy failure by sonar. *British Journal of Obstetrics and Gynaecology* **82**:849–857.
10 Nyberg DA, Filly RA, Mahony BS *et al.* (1985) Early gestation: Correlation of hCG levels and sonographic identification. *American Journal of Roentgenology* **144**:951–954.
11 Nyberg DA, Mack LA, Harvey D, Wang K (1988) Value of the yolk sac in evaluating early pregnancies. *Journal of Ultrasound in Medicine* **7**:129–135.
12 Batzer FR, Weiner S, Corson SL *et al.* (1983) Land-

marks during the first forty-two days of gestation demonstrated by the beta-subunit of human chorionic gonadotropin and ultrasound. *American Journal of Obstetrics and Gynecology* **146**:973–979.

13 Robinson HP (1973) Fetal heart rates as determined by sonar in early pregnancy. *Journal of Obstetrics and Gynaecology of the British Commonwealth* **80**:805–809.

14 Levi S (1976) Ultrasonic assessment of the high rate of human multiple pregnancy in the first trimester. *Journal of Clinical Ultrasound* **4**:3.

15 Reagan L, Braude PR, Trembath PL (1989) Influence of past reproductive performance on risk of spontaneous abortion. *British Medical Journal* **299**:541–545.

16 Stirrat GM (1990) Recurrent miscarriage 1: Definition and epidemiology. *Lancet* **336**:673–675.

17 WHO (1970) *Spontaneous and Induced Abortions.* WHO Technical Report Series no. 41, Geneva.

18 Leppert PC, Pahlika BS (1984) Grieving characteristics after spontaneous abortions: A management approach. *Obstetrics and Gynecology* **64**:119–122.

19 Evans JH, Beischer NA (1970) The prognosis of threatened abortion. *Medical Journal of Australia* **2**:165–168.

20 Peckham CH (1970) Uterine bleeding during pregnancy. *Obstetrics and Gynecology* **35**:937–941.

21 Thompson JF, Lein JN (1961) Fetal survival following threatened abortion. *Obstetrics and Gynecology* **18**:40–43.

22 Turnbull EPN, Walker J (1956) The outcome of pregnancy complicated by threatened abortion. *Journal of Obstetrics and Gynaecology of the British Empire* **63**:553–559.

23 South J, Naldrett J (1973) The effect of vaginal bleeding in early pregnancy on the infant born after the 28th week of pregnancy. *Journal of Obstetrics and Gynaecology of the British Commonwealth* **80**:236–241.

24 Hill NCW, MacKenzie IZ (1989) 2308 second trimester terminations using extra-amniotic or intra-amniotic prostaglandin E_2: An analysis of efficacy and complications. *British Journal of Obstetrics and Gynaecology* **96**:1424–1431.

25 Cameron IT, Baird DT (1984) The use of 16,16-dimethyl trans Δ^2 prostaglandin E_1 methyl ester (gemeprost) vaginal pessaries for termination of pregnancy in the early second trimester: A comparison with extra-amniotic prostaglandin E_2. *British Journal of Obstetrics and Gynaecology* **91**:1136–1140.

26 Mackenzie IZ, Embrey MP (1976) Single extra-amniotic injection of prostaglandins to induce abortion. *British Journal of Obstetrics and Gynaecology* **83**:505.

27 Medical Protection Society (1969) *The Abortion Act 1967.* Proceedings of a symposium held by the Medical Protection Society in collaboration with the Royal College of General Practitioners, London, February. London: Pitman Medical.

28 Tietze C, Lewitt S (1972) Joint programme for the study of abortion (JPSA): Early medical complications of legal abortion. *Studies in Family Planning* **3**:97.

29 McKenzie IZ, Jackson C, McKinlay E, Millar J (1990) Cervical priming before first trimester aspiration abortion: A single blind study comparing gemeprost 1 mg and Prostaglandin E_2 10 mg pessaries. *Journal of Obstetrics and Gynaecology* **10**:513–517.

30 Bernhardt RN, Bruns PD, Druse VE (1966) Atypical endometrium associated with ectopic pregnancies. *Obstetrics and Gynecology* **28**:849–853.

31 Robertson WB, Khong TY, Brosens I, DeWolf F, Sheppard BL, Bonnar J (1986) Placental bed biopsy: A review from three European centres. *American Journal of Obstetrics and Gynecology* **155**:401–412.

32 Hamerton JL (1971) *Human Cytogenetics*, Vol. 2: *Clinical Cytogenetics.* New York: Academic Press.

33 Cavanagh D, Knuppel A, Shepherd JH *et al.* (1982) Septic shock and the obstetrician/gynecologist. *Southern Medical Journal* **75**:809–813.

34 Kreger BE, Craven DE, McCabe WR (1980) Gram-negative bacteremia IV. Re-evaluation of clinical features and treatment in 612 patients. *American Journal of Medicine* **68**:344–355.

35 Bone RC (1991) Sepsis, the sepsis syndrome, multiorgan failure: A plea for comparable definitions. *Annals of Internal Medicine* **114**:332–333.

36 Bone RC (1991) The pathognesis of sepsis. *Annals of Internal Medicine* **115**:457–469.

37 Ziegler EJ, Fisher CJ, Sprung CL *et al.* (1991) Treatment of gram-negative bacteremia and septic shock with HA-1A human monoclonal antibody against endotoxin. *New England Journal of Medicine* **324**:429–436.

38 Stray-Pederson B, Stray-Pederson S (1984) Etiologic factors and subsequent reproductive performance in 195 couples with prior history of habitual abortion. *American Journal of Obstetrics and Gynecology* **148**:140–146.

39 MacDougall J, Siddle N (1991) Emergency cervical cerclage. *British Journal of Obstetrics and Gynaecology* **98**:1234–1238.

40 Beischer NA, Mackay EV (1986) Bleeding in early pregnancy. In Beischer NA, Mackay EV (eds) *Obstetrics and the Newborn*, p. 140. London: Ballière Tindall.

41 American College of Obstetricians and Gynaecologists (1990) *Ectopic Pregnancy* **150**:1–8.

42 Sultana CJ, Easley K, Collins R (1992) Outcome of laparoscopic versus traditional surgery for ectopic pregnancies. *Fertility and Sterility* **57**:285–289.

43 Pansky M, Golan A, Bukovsky I, Caspi E (1991) Non-surgical management of tubal pregnancy. *American Journal of Obstetrics and Gynecology* **164**:888–895.

44 Feichtinger W, Kemeter P (1987) Conservative treatment of ectopic pregnancy by transvaginal aspiration under sonographic control and injection of methotrexate. *Lancet* **i**:381–382.

45 Robertson DE, Smith W, Craft I (1987) Reduction of ectopic pregnancy by injection by ultrasound control. *Lancet* **i**:974–5(Letter).

46 Timor-Tritch I, Baxi L, Peisner DB (1988) Transvaginal salpingocentesis: A new technique for treating ectopic pregnancy. *American Journal of Obstetrics and Gynecology* **160**:459–461.

47 Ribic-Paucelj M, Novak-Antolic Z, Urhovec I (1989) Treatment of ectopic pregnancy with prostaglandin E_2. *Clinical and Experimental Obstetrics and Gynecology* **16**:106–109.

48 Feichtinger W, Kemeter P (1989) Treatment of unruptured ectopic pregnancy by needling of sac and injection

of methotrexate or PGE$_2$ under transvaginal sonography control: Report of 10 cases. *Archives of Gynecology and Obstetrics* **246**:85–89.

49   Lindblom B, Hahlin M, Kallfelt B, Hamberger (1987) Local prostaglandin F$_{2alpha}$ injection for termination of ectopic pregnancy. *Lancet* **i**:776–777.

50   Lindblom B (1989) Management of ectopic pregnancy: What does the future hold? *Human Reproduction* **4**:855–857.

51   Egarter C, Husslein P (1988) Treatment of tubal pregnancy by prostaglandins. *Lancet* **i**:1104–1105.

52   Lang PF, Weiss PAM, Mayer HO *et al.* (1990) Conservative treatment of ectopic pregnancy with local injection of hyperosmolar glucose solution or prostaglandin - F$_2$ $_{alpha}$: A prospective randomised study. *Lancet* **336**:78–81.

53   Fernandez H, Lelaidier C, Thouvenez V, Frydman R (1991) The use of a pretherapeutic, predictive score to determine inclusion criteria for the non-surgical treatment of ectopic pregnancy. *Human Reproduction* **6**:995–998.

54   Chamberlain G, Brown JC (1978) *Gynaecological Laparoscopy*. London: Royal College of Obstetricians and Gynaecologists.

55   Pouly JL, Mahnes H, Mage G, Canis M, Bruhart MA (1986) Conservative laparoscopic treatment of 321 ectopic pregnancies. *Fertility and Sterility* **46**:1093–1097.

56   Taylor, MV, Martin DC, Poston W *et al.* (1986) Effect of power density and carbonization of residual tissue coagulation using the continuous wave carbon dioxide laser. *Colposcopy and Gynecologic Laser Surgery* **2**:169–175.

57   Stock R (1990) Histopathology of fallopian tubes with recurrent tubal pregnancy. *Obstetrics and Gynecology* **75**:9–14.

58   Vermeesh M, Silva PD, Rosen GF *et al.* (1989) Management of unruptured ectopic gestation by linear salpingostomy: A prospective randomized clinical trial of laparoscopy versus laparotomy. *Obstetrics and Gynecology* **73**:400–404.

59   Hallat JG (1986) Tubal conservation in ectopic pregnancy: A study of 200 cases. *American Journal of Obstetrics and Gynecology* **154**:1216–1221.

60   de Cherney A, Kase N (1979) The conservative surgical management of unruptured ectopic pregnancy. *Obstetrics and Gynecology* **54**:451–455.

61   Vermeesh M, Presser (1992) Reproductive outcome after linear salpingostomy for ectopic gestation: A prospective 3-year follow up. *Fertility and Sterility* **57**:682–684.

62   Tait L (1884) Five cases of extra-uterine pregnancy operated upon at the time of rupture. *British Medical Journal* 1250–1251.

63   Stromme WB (1973) Conservative surgery for ectopic pregnancy. *Obstetrics and Gynecology* **41**:215–223.

64   Hull MGR, Glazener CMA, Kelly NJ *et al.* (1985) Population study of causes, treatment and outcome of infertility. *British Medical Journal* **291**:1693–1697.

65   Bagshawe KD, Dent J, Webb J (1986) Hydatidiform mole in England and Wales 1973–83. *Lancet* **2**:673–677.

66   Newlands ES (1983) Treatment of trophoblastic disease. In Studd J (ed.) *Progress in Obstetrics and Gynaecology*, Vol. 3, pp. 158–173. Edinburgh: Churchill Livingstone.

67   Bagshawe KD (1976) Risk and prognostic factors in trophoblastic neoplasia. *Cancer* **38**:1373–1385.

68   Stone M, Bagshawe KD (1979) An analysis of the influences of maternal age, gestational age, contraceptive method and the primary mode of treatment of patients with hydatidiform moles on the incidence of subsequent chemotherapy. *British Journal of Obstetrics and Gynaecology* **86**:782–792.

69   Kleihauer E, Braun H, Betke K (1957) Demonstration von fetaleim haemoglobin in den erythrocyten eines blutanssstrichs. *Klinische Wisschenschaft* **35**:637.

8

Recurrent Miscarriage

G. STIRRAT

INTRODUCTION

The biological definition of miscarriage is the expulsion of the conceptus before viability has been achieved. An alternative epidemiological definition is the expulsion or extraction from its mother of an embryo or fetus weighing 500 g or less. The overall conception loss rate is thought to be about 50%.[1] At least 15% of fertilized ova are lost before implantation and the early loss rate among clinically recognized pregnancies is also reckoned to be 12–15%.[2–4] However, only about 3% of pregnancies which are healthy at 8 weeks gestation subsequently result in miscarriage and virtually all of these occur by 14–16 weeks.[5] If a woman has had one or two miscarriages, the likelihood of a successful subsequent pregnancy is still about 80%.

Furthermore, even if she has had three consecutive miscarriages, there is still a 55–75% chance of a successful pregnancy.[5]

The most rigorous definition of recurrent miscarriage, particularly necessary for data collection and further research, is three or more consecutive spontaneous abortions. The definition can be further subdivided into primary (all pregnancies lost) and secondary (one, usually the first, successful pregnancy followed by losses) recurrent miscarriage.

In clinical practice, a less rigorous working definition of two or more consecutive losses may be justified if, for example, the woman is 35 years of age or above or has previously suffered from infertility. In this situation, one is responding appropriately to the concern of the couple. However, little is gained from extensive investigation of otherwise healthy women and their partners who have suffered from only two consecutive miscarriages. This is because the spontaneous chance of the next pregnancy being successful is greater than 80% (see below) and the likelihood of extensive and expensive investigation finding any relevant 'cause' is less than 1 : 10.

A clear and consistent definition of three consecutive losses is necessary to:

- allow sensible and cost-effective questions to be asked about causation

- provide a prognosis

- suggest possible remedies

- guide further research

Therefore, unless patients have suffered from three consecutive losses, they should not be classified as suffering from recurrent miscarriage.

RISK FACTORS FOR RECURRENT MISCARRIAGE

In considering risk factors for recurrent miscarriage, it is important to distinguish between those that are causal and those that are merely associations. This section contains information which will be of value in counseling couples presenting with recurrent miscarriage.

Epidemiological Factors

Gravidity

The risk of miscarriage tends to increase with gravidity whatever the outcome of the previous pregnancy. This is particularly, but not solely, evident when all previous pregnancies have been lost.[7]

Reproductive compensatory factor

Much of the apparent risk may be explained by the wish of the couple to compensate for a previous reproductive loss.[6] They therefore continue to try to produce a healthy child until the desired family size is achieved. In a society where this is a small number, it follows that the greater the gravidity of the woman, the more likely she is to have had several miscarriages which may be consecutive.

Outcome of the last pregnancy

The risk of miscarriage varies between 4 and 20%, depending on whether the last pregnancy was successful or unsuccessful, respectively.[5]

Maternal age

Teenage may be a risk factor. The miscarriage rate for chromosomally normal as well as abnormal pregnancies rises with maternal age above 35 years, but the direct effects of maternal age are confounded by the reproductive compensation effect discussed above.[6]

Genetic Factors

Chromosome abnormality

The incidence of chromosome imbalance in spontaneous aborted conceptuses is at least 50% in the first trimester and 20% in the second trimester.[8]

Parental chromosomal rearrangements

These may occur in up to 10% of couples with two or more miscarriages. These are mainly translocations (4–5%) or mosaicisms (4–5%).[9] Of the translocations, most are balanced (i.e. reciprocal) with some Robert-

sonian. These are illustrated in **Figure 1**. The incidence of balanced translocations in the general population is about 0.4%. The mosaicism usually occurs in the female. Maternal X chromosome mosaicism is by far the most common and results in miscarriage in up to 50% of affected women, probably due to fetal monosomy X. The remaining 1% are due to chromosomal deletions or inversions. The latter result when a chromosome breaks and the fragment is re-inserted in an inverted position. The most common form is the pericentric inversion in which the long and short arms of the chromosome each have a break with reorientation of the fragment around the centromere. This is found in about 0.1% of both partners in couples experiencing recurrent miscarriage. If chromosomal imbalance occurs in the conceptus as a result of parental inversion, there is an increased risk of miscarriage or fetal anomaly.

Aneuploidy

Autosomal trisomies are the most common chromosomal defects found in first trimester miscarriages. Particular trisomies do not tend to be recurrent, only trisomies in general. The recurrence risk is mainly, and possibly solely, a function of increasing maternal age.

Previous chromosome abnormality

If the chromosome complement of a first aborted conceptus is abnormal and the woman miscarries a second time, the likelihood of the second also being abnormal is about 80%. Conversely, if the chromosomal complement of the first was normal, it will be normal again in about 70% of second miscarriages.[8]

Chance

Even if there is no pre-existing parental chromosomal abnormality, the frequency of aneuploidy and polyploidy among sporadic miscarriages still makes them significant contributors to recurrent losses as a matter of mere chance.

Molecular mutations

These may cause recurrent losses even though the conceptus has a normal karyotype[10] as a result of:

- mutations in genes which code for products critical for normal development

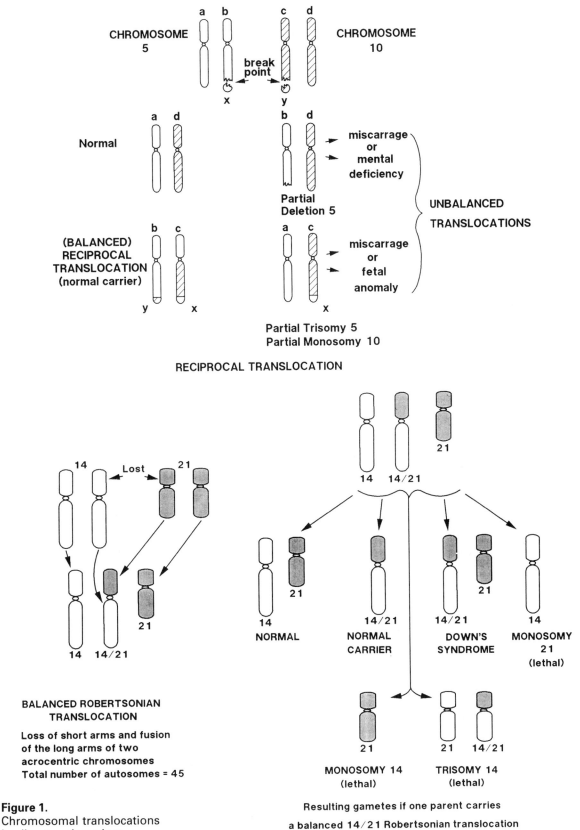

Figure 1.
Chromosomal translocations leading to miscarriage.

- mutations in homeobox genes which control groups of genes by transcriptional regulation

- mutations which lead to fatal metabolic errors in the fetus

- lethal single point mutations possibly linked to Major Histocompatibility Complex (MHC) genes

- disorders of proto-oncogenes and oncogenes.

Anatomical Disorders

Congenital uterine malformations

Figure 2 illustrates the typical anomalies which can result from failure of proper fusion of the Mullerian ducts. They occur to a significant degree in only about 0.1% of the female population, but have been reported to be present in between 15 and 30% of women suffering from recurrent pregnancy loss, which classically occurs in the second trimester.[11] However, there is still controversy regarding their incidence and classification, the extent of reproductive failure associated with them and their optimal treatment.[12]

Cervical incompetence

This is defined as an inherent or acquired inability of the uterine cervix to maintain an intrauterine pregnancy and is another frequently quoted cause for pregnancy loss, particularly in the mid-trimester. Characteristically, painless effacement and dilatation of the cervix, perhaps manifested by asymptomatic membrane rupture, precedes the loss.

Intrauterine adhesions (Ascherman's syndrome)

These result from too vigorous or repeated endometrial curettage or evacuation of retained products of conception, and are said to be associated with recurrent miscarriage.

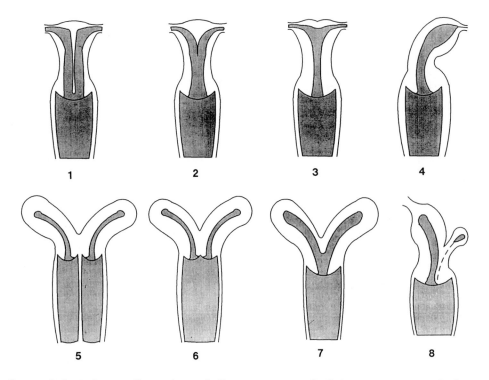

Figure 2. Congenital uterine malformations; 1. Septate uterus. 2. Subseptate uterus. 3. Arcuate uterus. 4. Unicornuate uterus. 5. Double uterine horns, cervix and vagina. 6. Double uterine horns and cervix. 7. Double uterine horns, single cervix. 8. Double uterine horns (one rudimentary), single cervix.

Fibroleiomyomas (fibroids)

The role of these benign tumors in causing recurrent miscarriage is open to question.

Endocrine Causes

Luteal phase defects

These result in progesterone deficiency and may be associated with recurrent miscarriage,[13] but in most cases it is far more likely that the fall in progesterone is an inevitable secondary effect of a pregnancy failing for other reasons. The reported incidence of luteal phase inadequacy varies between 20 and 60%, but there is no reliable way of recognizing inadequate luteal function in the already pregnant patient.[13] The evaluation of corpus luteum function in non-fertile cycles cannot be extrapolated to the pregnant woman because the corpus luteum of pregnancy is, by definition, different from that of the non-fertile cycle. Basal body temperature recordings do not reflect the adequacy of the luteal phase, short-term fluctuations in serum progesterone levels make them unreliable measures, and endometrial biopsy is invasive and open to sampling and interpretative errors.[14]

Prepregnancy hypersecretion of luteinizing hormone (LH)

This is frequently but not necessarily associated with polycystic ovary syndrome and may be associated with infertility, miscarriage and, by inference, recurrent losses.[15,16]

Diabetes mellitus

Diabetic women with elevated blood glucose and glycosylated hemoglobin levels in the first trimester are at a significantly increased risk of miscarriage, whereas diabetic women with good metabolic control are not.[17] However, the incidence of subclinical diabetes is no higher in women who miscarry recurrently than in the general population.

Subclinical thyroid dysfunction

There is no evidence that this contributes to recurrent pregnancy losses.

Reproductive Tract Infections

Although sporadic pregnancy loss has been associated with such organisms as *Ureaplasma urealyticum*, *Mycoplasma hominis*, *Chlamydia trachomatis* and *Toxoplasma gondii*, there is no convincing association with repeated miscarriage.[18] The mere presence of an organism at the time of the loss cannot be assumed to be proof of cause. For an organism to cause such a recurrent outcome, it would have to:

- persist for long periods of time without producing significant maternal symptoms to allow it to escape diagnosis and treatment

- gain access to the intrauterine environment to infect fetal tissue and/or stimulate an inflammatory response.

Anti-Cardiolipin Antibody (ACA) Syndrome

An increasing number of women with poor reproductive histories are found to carry an anti-cardiolipin IgG or IgM antibody which acts on the clotting cascade.[19] This 'lupus anticoagulant' or 'inhibitor' causes all phospholipid-dependent coagulation tests, such as the activated partial thromboplastin time (APTT) or kaolin clotting time (KCT), to be prolonged and to remain so after the addition of normal plasma. The successful pregnancy rate is 10–15% in untreated women carrying anti-cardiolipin antibodies.[20] Fetal losses are often the initial manifestation.

The pregnancy loss, which may follow an initial successful pregnancy, characteristically occurs in the second trimester. This is different from women who have antinuclear antibodies (either first or second trimester losses) or those with no detectable antibodies (predominantly first trimester miscarriages). Other pregnancy complications (e.g. fetal growth deficiency and pre-eclampsia) are common if the pregnancy progresses into the third trimester. The association with systemic lupus erythematosus (SLE) is highly variable and often relatively weak at the time of initial presentation. However, women with established SLE are often positive for ACA and are at risk of recurrent miscarriage. Finally, about one-third of women who have ACA syndrome during pregnancy may develop a variety of serious health problems within the following decade.

Disorders of Materno–Fetal Allo-immune Relationships

One of the most popular hypotheses for an immunological cause for recurrent pregnancy loss invokes classical T-cell dependent, major histocompatibility complex (MHC) related immune mechanisms which must be blocked by specific antibodies for pregnancy to be successful. The available evidence is, at best, confusing and conflicting.[21] For example, the lack of classical Class I or Class II MHC antigens on syncytiotrophoblast, the major population of trophoblast exposed to maternal blood, suggests that neither T- nor B-cell responses are possible against that tissue. In addition, although cellular immunity may be changed in some women who recurrently miscarry, circulating blocking factors are not necessary for pregnancy to be successful.[22]

Another hypothesis implicates so-called trophoblast–lymphocyte cross-reactive TLX antigens.[23,24] It is suggested that maternal recognition of TLX antigens and production of anti-TLX antibodies is the key to fetal survival and that failure of the mother to produce these antibodies can lead to loss of the pregnancy. The immunological, biochemical and functional basis for this hypothesis remains to be elucidated and, at best, its current status must remain unproven.

A third hypothesis arises from the observation that couples suffering from recurrent miscarriages may tend to share HLA haplotypes more often than can be ascribed to chance.[25] The immunological arm of this proposal suggests that a facilitating maternal recognition of the fetus is impaired because they share some polymorphic genes, the products of which the mother sees as 'self' and to which, therefore, she would not respond. A protective blocking antibody response would not occur, allowing a rejection reaction to set it. The second arm of this hypothesis suggests that the unfortunate embryo shares not only HLA antigens with the parents but also a recessive lethal gene linked to HLA.[26] However, the balance of evidence suggests that excessive sharing of HLA haplotypes between partners neither precludes successful pregnancy nor is a strong enough association to be a satisfactory explanation for recurrent losses.[27,28]

Environmental Effects

Maternal smoking and alcohol

The relatively high frequency of these exposures in modern society means that, despite a small adverse effect on the outcome in an individual pregnancy, they could play a significant role in recurrent losses.

Video display terminals

Claims that women working with these are at increased risk of miscarriage have not been confirmed.[29,30]

Environmental pollutants

Low-level exposure to, for example, anesthetic gases, formaldehyde, lead and ethylene oxide have all been implicated as associated with sporadic miscarriage.[31] The evidence is not yet convincing and fails to address the question of recurrent loss.

Psychological Causes

Without denying the deep hurt suffered by couples experiencing recurrent miscarriage, there is no good evidence that psychological stress contributes significantly to recurrent pregnancy loss.

MANAGEMENT OPTIONS

Most published studies on management contain important confounding variables which either weaken or totally invalidate their conclusions. Among the defects are inconsistent definitions (common); different investigative protocols (universal); lack of normal controls (difficult to achieve); and time over which the study population was gathered (inevitable). There is also considerable psychological pressure to find a 'cause' so that 'something can be done about it'. This should be resisted. However, one of the most important aspects of care in these couples is constant reassurance and alleviation of anxiety.

'Prepregnancy' at the third miscarriage

When a woman presents with what appears to be her third consecutive miscarriage, it is important that the opportunity is taken to provide additional management which may subsequently be helpful in caring for her later.

Thus, if a surgical evacuation of retained products is performed, it is important to document any suspected uterine abnormalities such as bicornuate/septate uterus or fibroids. With a first trimester miscarriage, products of conception (not decidua) should be sent for histology to confirm the diagnosis and for karyotyping (see **Table 1**). In the event of a mid-trimester loss, check the fetal karyotype and encourage the couple to agree to a full autopsy examination. Too much reliance cannot be placed on the karyotype of the trophoblast, because mosaicism or unusual aneuploidies are not necessarily reflected in the fetus.

Finally, the patient should be offered subsequent follow-up assessment and counseling.

Table 1
Tissue collection for chromosome analysis from conceptus

	Technique	Comment
Handling tissue	Sterile technique. Send all fetal tissue collected	Tissue from curettage will be contaminated by maternal cells. Trophoblast may contain mosaicisms or aneuploidy not present in fetus
Container	Sterile Universal container with secure cap placed inside plastic Ziplock bag	Label clearly with patient's name, birth date and number. Give clear clinical history on request form
Medium	Either use sterile culture medium supplied by cytogenetics lab or sterile normal saline	Formaline must not be added. Culture medium must be regularly renewed.
Transport	Get to lab as quickly as possible in a padded container. Keep at room temperature if being transported within a few hours. Refrigerate at 4°C if not being sent until following day	Discuss the case with the lab and notify them of impending arrival of specimen

Adapted from Olsen and Magenis.[8]

Prepregnancy assessment and counseling

In couples complaining of recurrent miscarriage, as for subfertility, it is best to deal with both partners together. The following principles should be followed:

- The couple must be dealt with sympathetically and compassionately; a 'recurrent miscarriage' clinic may be better at providing this than busy gynecology or antenatal clinics.

- Recognize the pressure to 'find a cause' and 'do something about it'.

- The provision of accurate information to the couple is a primary responsibility (see 'Risk Factors for Recurrent Miscarriage'). They should, in general, be allowed to make their own decision in the light of this information.

- As much of the preliminary investigation and counseling as possible should take place in the primary health care setting.

- Subsequent management of particular risk factors must only be carried out by those with the appropriate expertise, for example, clinical genetics, endoscopic surgery, immunology or reproductive endocrinology.

History and examination

The first prerequisite is the taking of a comprehensive history. As much information as possible should be gained about the circumstances surrounding the losses such as:

- At what gestations did they occur?

- Was pregnancy confirmed biochemically, by ultrasound and/or histologically on each occasion?

- Was a live embryo or fetus observed by ultrasound at any stage?

During this history-taking, it is important to try and confirm the diagnosis of 'recurrent miscarriage' by documenting the validity of the previous pregnancy losses as accurately as possible. To do this, communication with other doctors and hospitals may be necessary. The importance of taking a comprehensive history cannot be over-emphasized, because it can direct appropriate investigations and the subsequent management.

Physical examination has the dual purpose of opportunistic screening (e.g. blood pressure, cervical cytology, breast palpation), and as a check on some risk factors raised by history (for example, cervical competence). The rubella antibody status of the woman should be checked and immunization offered if it is negative.

Routine investigation of recurrent miscarriage

This should include:

- Karyotyping of both partners to check for translocations and mosaicism.

- Hysterosalpingography or, if the expertise is available, pelvic imaging by vaginal ultrasound and/or hysteroscopy to check for uterine malformation, cervical incompetence, intrauterine adhesions or submucous fibroids.

- Activated partial thromboplastin time (APTT) or kaolin clotting time (KCT) to screen for lupus inhibitor and ACA. If the history is of secondary recurrent miscarriage, screen for SLE.

- Mid-follicular LH concentration. The author seriously doubts the value of measuring luteal phase progesterone concentrations.

- It may be justifiable to measure antipaternal complement fixing antibody levels in discussion with a clinical immunologist.

Other investigations will be determined by positive findings in the history and examination.

Epidemiological factors

The woman's age, gravidity and the outcome of previous pregnancies are immediately apparent from the history. Frank discussion about the effect of these factors and the potential importance of the reproductory compensatory mechanism[6] noted above can be very reassuring if described in the correct manner. If not done sympathetically, it can seem that one is merely dismissing the problem.

One of the most important messages to impart in prepregnancy counseling is the chance of a subsequent successful pregnancy without active intervention. It has already been noted that, after two miscarriages, the spontaneous chance of the next pregnancy being successful is greater than 80%. Indeed, even when three or more consecutive losses have occurred, the chance of a successful pregnancy has been estimated at between 55 and 75%.[5] It is also important that the results of any interventions be interpreted in that knowledge.

Genetic factors

Screening for parental chromosomal rearrangements by karyotyping may be carried out on both partners.[9] The significance of any abnormality should be discussed with a clinical geneticist. For couples with a balanced translocation, the outlook for subsequent pregnancy is good. Many of the fertilized ova with unbalanced translocations fail to implant and they are present in no more than 4% of established pregnancies. If the chance of a subsequent successful pregnancy is low, the possibility of gamete donation can be raised. As in all prepregnancy counseling, it is for the couple to make their own decision in light of this information. Prenatal diagnosis may be offered in subsequent pregnancies. The couple must then make their decision in light of the predicted risk of an abnormal result, the reassurance given by a normal result and the procedure-related risk of miscarriage.[32]

If there is a history of recurrent aneuploidy, prenatal diagnosis can be offered in a subsequent pregnancy. The relative risk of a recurrent trisomy must be set against that of the diagnostic procedure in a possibly older couple who have already suffered several pregnancy losses.[32] No amount of counseling can lessen the acuteness of that dilemma for the couple.

In any event, should the woman miscarry in a fourth or subsequent pregnancy, an attempt should be made to carry out chromosome analysis of the products of conception. **Table 1** shows the recommended method of tissue collection.[8] Curettings are unsuitable for culture because they are likely to contain maternal tissue.

There is, as yet, no way to detect molecular mutations in euploidic pregnancies, but DNA analysis is likely to become available for at least some mutations in the future.

Anatomical disorders

The shape of the uterine cavity should be checked in all women suffering from three or more consecutive pregnancy losses to include congenital uterine malformations, particularly if they have occurred in the second trimester. The traditional method of investigation is hysterosalpingography but, in expert hands, vaginal ultrasound and or hysteroscopy may be as informative, if not more so (see Further Reading).[11]

Minor defects do not warrant surgical correction. Abdominal metroplasty is the traditional corrective procedure for uterina septa, but it has never been properly evaluated prospectively and is associated with a significant degree of postoperative subfertility (see Further Reading).[12] The results of the more recent transcervical hysteroscopic resection of septae look encouraging, but this procedure must also be evaluated prospectively in a proper controlled trial before a clear judgment can be made. It must only be performed by those who have proper training and experience in hysteroscopic surgery (see Further Reading).

There is an increased risk of preterm labor in women with congenital uterine anomalies. Prophylactic oral tocolytic therapy is not warranted, but regular evaluation of cervical effacement and dilatation should be carried out at each prenatal visit. Cervical incompetence may be associated with uterine anomalies and should be dealt with as discussed below.

Cervical incompetence is difficult to diagnose objectively and, although the diagnosis is often postulated in cases of recurrent second trimester loss, the actual risk of abortion without treatment and the effectiveness of treatment remain open to question.

Prepregnancy investigation involves hysterosalpingography (without using a Spackman cannula, which artificially dilates the internal os) or, more recently, transvaginal ultrasound. The internal diameter of the internal os should not exceed 8–9 mm in a nulliparous woman. Too easy passage of an 8 or 9 mm Hegar dilator in non-pregnant women is indicative but not diagnostic. Grant[33] has reviewed the evidence for the benefits and hazards of treatment by cervical cerclage to prolong pregnancy. He suggests that cervical cerclage in women with a previous second trimester miscarriage (or preterm delivery) may help to prevent one delivery before 33 weeks for every 20 sutures inserted. However, the surgical procedure can also *cause* early delivery, and be associated with puerperal pyrexia. It should, therefore, be used only in cases with a high likelihood of benefit such as recurrent second trimester miscarriage. The technique used is probably of less importance than the skill of the surgeon. Cerclage is usually carried out at 12–14 weeks gestation and can be removed at 37–38 weeks. The details of the various techniques are given at the end of the chapter.

Intrauterine adhesions (Ascherman's syndrome) are diagnosed by HSG and/or hysteroscopy. These adhesions can be divided hysteroscopically and an intrauterine device inserted for 6 weeks to inhibit their re-formation. A broad-spectrum antibiotic should be prescribed for 1 week postoperation. Fetal growth should be observed carefully in any subsequent pregnancy because the implantation site may be less than ideal. There may be an increased risk of placenta accreta.

Fibroleiomyomas (fibroids) are diagnosed by HSG or vaginal ultrasound followed by hysteroscopy. Abdominal (or possibly hysteroscopic) myomectomy (see Further Reading) may occasionally be warranted for women with significant submucous fibroids who are experiencing repeated second trimester losses. A temporary reduction in size by GnRH analogs is a more recent alternative which has not yet been fully evaluated (see Chapter 35).

Residual fibroids tend to increase in size during pregnancy and the larger they are the more likely it is that they will become painful due to hemorrhage within their substance ('red degeneration'). Treatment is conservative with adequate analgesia and reassurance. If delivery by cesarean section is required for other obstetric reasons, no attempt must be made to remove intramural or submucous fibroids because of the risk of hemorrhage.

Endocrine causes

The difficulties in making a valid diagnosis of luteal phase defects have been discussed above.[14] Despite them, the most common criteria used are a luteal phase consistently lasting less than 10 days suggested by basal temperature recordings and/or serum progesterone levels at less than 15 nmol/litre in five consecutive cycles. Goldstein *et al.*[34] have reviewed the evidence for claims of improved pregnancy outcomes after hormone treatment and conclude that:

- There is no evidence that progestogens reduce the risk of sporadic miscarriage, stillbirth or neonatal death.

- The data are suggestive of some protective effect of progesterone in idiopathic recurrent miscarriage, but not strongly enough to justify its use except within larger better trials with adequate follow-up.

- A small trial suggests the possibility of some benefit from human chorionic gonadotrophin therapy[35] but more evidence is necessary.

None of the evidence has, therefore, stilled the controversy over preferred treatment options which range from:

- 'Do nothing'.

- No routine therapy but twice weekly measurement of progesterone levels to suggest whether pregnancy support with progestogens is or is not necessary. The lower cut-off level is usually taken to be about 30 nmol/l. Therapy can be continued to about 16 weeks gestation.

- Routine pharmacological 'support' of the pregnancy. This is frequently advocated empirically in all pregnancies following recurrent losses because 'it can do no harm'. In the author's view, this is an unacceptable argument which has no place in ethical treatment regimens.

- Treat only within properly designed prospective trials (with adequate follow-up). This is the author's preferred option.

A variety of progestogen regimens have been advocated (e.g. 17 alpha-hydroxy progesterone caproate

125 or 250 mg i.m. twice weekly from recognition of pregnancy to 14–16 weeks gestation). Therapy with 19-norsteroid progestogens should be avoided because of the risk of masculinization of the female fetus.

In contrast to the controversy about diagnosis and management of possible luteal phase defects, prepregnancy hypersecretion of luteinizing hormone with or without polycystic ovary syndrome represents a more likely potential correctable cause of recurrent miscarriage. Although more work needs to be done on this to provide greater certainty, it could offer a possibility of a predictive test before pregnancy in women at particular risk. Ultrasonic imaging of the ovaries to look for multiple follicular cysts and serial blood sampling can be carried out to determine whether LH concentrations are elevated (10 IU/l or more) in the mid-follicular phase of the menstrual cycle.[16] If levels in one cycle are normal, do no more; if elevated, the test should be repeated in subsequent cycles. If confirmed, the hypersecretion may then be treated with GnRH analogs or, perhaps, ovarian electrodiathermy[16] in a Reproductive Medicine subspecialty unit.

Routine testing of women with no history suggestive of diabetes for diabetes mellitus is unnecessary. Optimal control of known diabetics before pregnancy maximizes their chances of success. Similarly, routine investigation of thyroid function is not necessary and empirical therapy unjustifiable.

Reproductive tract infections

No routine screening for such infections (save for rubella to determine the need for immunization) is indicated on current evidence. Better studies are badly needed. The empirical use of antimicrobial drugs in the treatment of women with recurrent losses is not justified.

Anti-cardiolipin antibody (ACA) syndrome

An auto-immune screen and a phospholipid dependent test of coagulation (such as the APTT or KCT) should be carried out on all women with recurrent pregnancy loss. More specific tests of autoimmune status, and for lupus inhibitor and antinuclear antibodies are indicated in those with abnormal screening tests, a history of thrombotic episodes or auto-immune disorders. If there is a history suggestive of auto-immune disorders but the ACA screening test is negative before pregnancy, it may be worthwhile to repeat it in the second trimester of a subsequent pregnancy.

Successful pregnancies have been reported in women with the ACA syndrome[36] after treatment with prednisone (40–60 mg per day in divided doses) and aspirin (75 mg per day) throughout pregnancy, but this regime needs to be the subject of a randomized controlled trial before its value can be assumed.

All pregnancies must be intensively and carefully monitored in the presence of anti-cardiolipin or anti-DNA antibodies, particularly if therapy is needed. The predominant risks are of placental dysfunction leading to fetal growth retardation or an increased risk of abruption and of pre-eclampsia. For a more detailed discussion of the management of these conditions and of women with SLE, see Chapter 27.

Disorders of materno–fetal allo-immune relationships

It has already been stressed that the scientific basis for routine investigation or therapy is not strong. The most frequently advocated regimen involves a series of injections of paternal lymphocytes before and during the first half of pregnancy.[37,38] It may produce some benefit for women suffering first trimester losses who do not carry antipaternal complement dependent antibodies (APCA); but probably not for those who have APCA or a history of secondary recurrent miscarriage.[39] The uncontrolled therapeutic use of potent immune stimuli is to be deprecated and further evidence relating to the efficacy of immunotherapy is badly needed. Thus, if its use is justified at all, this treatment should only be offered to women who do not carry APCA in the context of properly designed controlled trials in a few designated centers.

Other regimens such as donor (allogeneic) lymphocytes,[40] intravenous immunoglobulin[41,42] or trophoblast membrane preparations[43] from pooled placenta are not recommended either because no properly designed studies have been carried out or, in the case of trophoblast, initial successes have not been confirmed.

Couples with less than three consecutive losses

Couples with several non-consecutive first trimester miscarriages but who also have had successful pregnancies should be reassured that no investigation or treatment is necessary. A history of second or third trimester losses should be considered more carefully, especially if the 'successful' pregnancies resulted in delivery of growth-retarded infants and/or were complicated by pre-eclampsia. The postmortem findings in the failed pregnancies should be reviewed carefully for evidence of fetal dysmorphology, genetic disorders and placental dysfunction, and any risk factors managed accordingly (see Chapters 18, 27 and 42).

In couples with only two consecutive losses, the only routine investigations which can be justified in the absence of specific risk factors is parental karyotyping, and, possibly, a full auto-immune screen (including for lupus inhibitor).

Prepregnancy/treatment options

In considering any possible treatments for recurrent miscarriage before or during a subsequent pregnancy, unproven therapy should not be justified merely because 'it can do no harm'. New interventions should only be initiated within properly controlled trials. Specific conditions for which prepregnancy treatment may be considered were discussed in the previous section. The prepregnancy treatment options for these conditions are summarized in **Table 2**.

Table 2
Management options for recurrent miscarriage before pregnancy[a]

Condition	Management option
Parental chromosome rearrangement	Gamete donation
Uterine septa	Hysteroscopic resection or abdominal metoplasty
Presumed cervical incompetence with failed cerclage in pregnancy	Cervical cerclage before conception
Ascherman's syndrome	Hysteroscopic division of adhesions and intrauterine device
Fibroids	GnRH analogs or myomectomy
LH hypersecretion	GnRH analogs or ovarian electrodiathermy or wedge resection
ACA syndrome/SLE	Aspirin and prednisolone
APCA negative patients	Immunotherapy

[a] See text for discussion.

Management during subsequent pregnancy, delivery and puerperium

The couple will understandably be very anxious about the outcome. They need reassurance that, in general, their chances of success are high. The intensity of prenatal care should be determined by an early assessment of the degree of risk to the pregnancy by an obstetrician and the wishes of the couple. Frequent ultrasonic scans of the viable fetus can be reassuring in the first trimester. Even more effort than usual should be made to provide continuity of care throughout. Where routine alpha-feto protein screening and/or fetal anomaly ultra-

sound scan are offered, particular care must be taken to counsel the couple so that they can make the decisions they feel to be appropriate.

Management of the subsequent pregnancy should be on the basis of recognized risk factors. Intervention merely on the basis of a history of recurrent miscarriage is not justified. Specific management options for specific conditions have been discussed above and are summarized in **Table 3**. Maternal age is a factor which influences pregnancy management, but all that is required is careful surveillance.

Table 3
Management options for recurrent miscarriage during subsequent pregnancy, delivery and puerperium[a]

Conditions	Management option
General	Reassurance (? frequent early scans) Careful discussion about prenatal diagnosis, especially if chromosome rearrangements
Cervical incompetence	Cervical cerclage at 14 weeks
Fibroids	See Chapter 34
Proven progesterone deficiency	Progesterone support (oral, rectal or depot) until 16 weeks
Diabetes	Continue tight blood glucose control
ACA syndrome/SLE	Aspirin and prednisolone, possibly subcutaneous heparin. Careful screening for pre-eclampsia and/or pathological fetal growth
APCA negative patients	Immunotherapy during first half of pregnancy

[a] See text for discussion.

CONCLUSION

The responsibility for the care of couples suffering from recurrent miscarriage can be demanding. It is frequently rewarding but, regrettably, not always so. Equally, one must guard against taking the credit for spontaneous success and the blame for unexplained failure. Those caring for the couple must at all times be open and truthful; aware of the danger of confusing 'causes' with 'association'; unwilling to intervene merely to be seen 'to do something'; and committed to the pursuit of new knowledge about this stressful condition.

Procedure: Cervical Cerclage

General

The incidence of cervical incompetence has been reported as between 2.7 and 18.4 per 1000 live births. This variation probably reflects the lack of a universally agreed definition.[44]

Indications

The most common indication for the insertion of a cervical suture is a previous mid-trimester miscarriage. Approximately 95% of women receiving such sutures are parous, nearly 95% have had a previous mid-trimester loss, and the great majority have a history of some preceding cervical trauma such as dilatation and curettage, termination of pregnancy or cervical surgery such as cone biopsy.[44] The multicenter randomized trial of cervical cerclage[45] demonstrated that the use of cervical cerclage where the indication was just 'previous spontaneous mid-trimester loss' (irrespective of the clinical details of that loss) was associated with a significantly greater likelihood of a successful outcome in the pregnancy. However, it should be stressed that there are other causes of second trimester pregnancy loss and it is likely that cervical incompetence is over-diagnosed. Nevertheless, until there is a better means of diagnosing the condition, it is difficult to reduce this problem and resolve the dilemma.

Operations

Once a decision has been taken that there is an indication to insert a cervical suture, there are then two further decisions to be made:

● **When to insert the suture – during or before pregnancy?**

The majority of obstetricians insert sutures at 14 weeks. The arguments to support this view are that the time of risk for 'normal' miscarriage has passed and that insertion before pregnancy may impair conception. Insertion before conception is only indicated after one or more unsuccessful attempts at insertion during pregnancy. There is no guidance available from randomized controlled trials to resolve this issue.[44]

● **Which procedure to use?**

Many techniques have been described but those most commonly used in practice are:

1. Vaginal techniques
McDonald suture
Shirodkar suture

2. Abdominal techniques
These are commonly reserved for cases where there has been one or more unsuccessful vaginal sutures previously

There are no data to indicate which technique is best or in which circumstances.

Vaginal – McDonald suture (**Figure 3**)

This is the simplest and least traumatic of the suture techniques. It involves insertion of a purse string of a non-absorbable suture material such as 'Mersilene' tape around the cervix at the cervico-vaginal junction.[46]

Vaginal – Shirodkar suture (**Figure 4**)

The essential features of this operation and its variants are that an incision is made in the supravaginal portion of the cervix to expose and then reflect the bladder so that a non-absorbable suture can be placed around the cervix at the level of the internal os. Once the suture is in place, the cervical skin is covered over the operative field and sutured with absorbable material.[47]

Abdominal (**Figure 5**)

Through a low transverse abdominal incision, the peritoneum at the vesico-cervical fold is incised transversely and the bladder reflected downwards. Long fine curved forceps are insinuated around the uterus above the level of the internal os, through the uterosacral ligaments posteriorly and keeping close to the uterine wall to stay inside and avoid the uterine

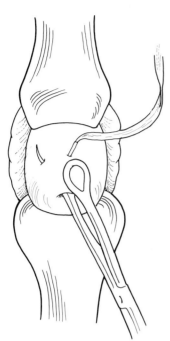

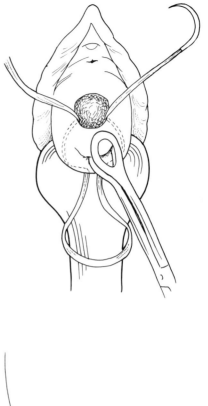

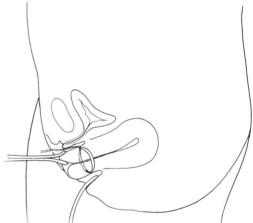

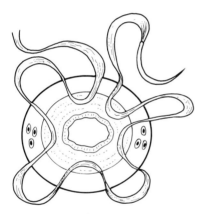

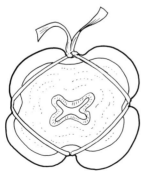

Figure 3. Technique for insertion of McDonald suture. The aim is to place the suture at the level of internal os.

Figure 4. Technique for insertion of Shirodkar suture. The aim is to place the suture at the level of internal os.

blood vessels. A non-absorbable suture is pulled through and tied anteriorly. The peritoneum is repaired and the abdominal wall closed.[48]

Postoperative care

The use of tocolytics and antibiotics following the procedure varies. There is no consensus view or evidence to resolve whether their use is justified. Similarly,

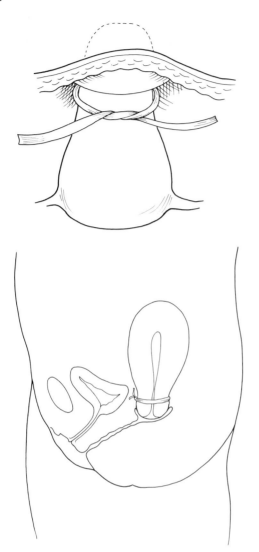

Figure 5. Technique for insertion of cervical suture by abdominal route. The aim is to place the suture at the level of internal os.

while many advocate regular checks that vaginal sutures are in place, there is no evidence that this is of benefit.

Removal of a vaginal suture is routinely undertaken at 37–38 weeks or sooner if the patient threatens to miscarry or go into preterm labor. Removal of the McDonald suture is usually easy, often accomplished without any analgesia or sedation. However, removal of the Shirodkar suture can be more difficult with general anesthesia being occasionally necessary.

Delivery with an abdominal suture in place has to be by elective lower segment cesarean section. If the patient wishes more pregnancies, the suture may be left in place and only removed after her family is complete. If the patient threatens to miscarry before viability with an abdominal suture in place, the obstetrician is faced with the dilemma either of carrying out a hysterotomy with the potential for leaving the suture in place for future pregnancies or of removing it abdominally and allowing a vaginal delivery without opening the uterus.

Complications

These include bleeding, urinary and other trauma, urinary and vaginal infection and membrane rupture. Failure of the operation resulting in spontaneous miscarriage or preterm delivery is arguably the most common complication. Rare but serious problems reported are vesicovaginal fistulae and uterine rupture when the suture has not been removed in a laboring patient.[44]

REFERENCES

1 Little AB (1988) There's many a slip twixt implantation and the crib. *New England Journal of Medicine* **319**:241–242.

2 Miller JF, Williamson E, Glue J *et al.* (1980) Fetal loss after implantation. *Lancet* **ii**:554–556.

3 Edmonds DK, Lindsay KS, Miller JF *et al.* (1982) Early embryonic mortality in women. *Fertility and Sterility* **38**:447–453.

4 Hertz-Piccioto I, Samuels SJ (1988) Incidence of early loss of pregnancy. *New England Journal of Medicine* **319**:1483–1484.

5 Regan L (1988) A prospective study of spontaneous abortion. In Beard RW, Sharp F (eds) *Early Pregnancy Loss: Mechanisms and Treatment*, pp. 23–27. London: Royal College of Gynaecologists.

6 Alberman E (1987) Maternal age and spontaneous abortion. In Bennett MJ, Edmonds DK (eds) *Spontaneous and Recurrent Abortion*, pp. 77–89. Oxford: Blackwell Scientific.

7 Regan L, Braude PR, Trembath PL (1989) Influence of past reproductive performance on risk of spontaneous abortion. *British Medical Journal* **299**:541–545.

8 Olsen SB, Magenis RE (1988) Cytogenetic aspects of recurrent pregnancy loss. *Seminars in Reproductive Endocrinology* **6**:191–202.

RECURRENT MISCARRIAGE
Summary of Management Options

'Prepregnancy' at the third miscarriage

- Carefully document any suspected uterine abnormality at surgical evacuation

- Send products of conception for histology or autopsy and karyotype

- Offer follow-up assessment and counseling

Prepregnancy assessment and counseling

- General approach is important (e.g. see couple together, sympathy, etc.)

- History and examination for causative and associated factors

- Investigations:

  - karyotype both partners
  - hysterosalpingography, transvaginal ultrasound, hysteroscopy
  - APTT, KCT, lupus inhibitor, ACA
  - mid-follicular LH
  - ? antipaternal complement fixing antibody
  - others determined by positive features in history/examination

- Counseling with the following key principles/guidelines:
  - the true rate of recurrent miscarriage is affected by a reproductive compensation effect

- even after three consecutive losses and intensive investigation, a probable cause is determined in only about 12% of couples
- the most important cause is probably repeated but sporadic chromosome abnormalities occurring consecutively by chance
- anatomical defects of the uterine fundus and cervix, parental chromosomal rearrangements, gene mutations, anti-cardiolipin antibodies and, possibly, hypersecretion of luteinizing hormone also play a role
- a causative role for progesterone deficiency, infective agents, and immune rejection is uncertain
- psychological stress and subclinical thyroid disorders or diabetes mellitus are probably not relevant
- even after three consecutive losses, the chance of success without treatment is probably more than 60%

Prepregnancy treatment options

- Do not advocate 'unproven' treatments

- Specific options for specific conditions (see **Table 2**)

Management during subsequent pregnancy, delivery and puerperium

- Psychological support, reassurance, etc.

- Specific options for specific conditions (see **Table 3**)

---

9 Sachs ES, Jahoda MGJ, Van Hemel JO *et al.* (1985) Chromosome studies of 500 couples with two or more abortions. *Obstetrics and Gynecology* **65**:375–378.

10 McDonough PG (1988) The role of molecular mutation in recurrent euploidic abortion. *Seminars in Reproductive Endocrinology* **6**:155–161.

11 Patton PE, Novy MJ (1988) Reproductive potential of the anomalous uterus. *Seminars in Reproductive Endocrinology* **6**:217–233.

12 Bennett MJ (1987) Congenital abnormalities of the fundus. In Bennett MJ, Edmonds DK (eds) *Spontaneous and Recurrent Abortion*, pp. 109–129. Oxford: Blackwell Scientific.

13 Daya S, Ward S, Burrows E (1988) Progesterone pro-

files in luteal phase defect cycles and outcome of progesterone treatment in patients with recurrent spontaneous abortion. *American Journal of Obstetrics and Gynecology* **158**:225–232.

14 Fritz MA (1988) Inadequate luteal function and recurrent abortion. *Seminars in Reproductive Endocrinology* **6**:129–143.

15 Sagle M, Bishop K, Ridley N *et al.* (1988) Recurrent early miscarriage and polycystic ovaries. *British Medical Journal* **297**:1027–1028.

16 Regan L, Owen EJ, Jacobs HS (1990) Hypersecretion of luteinising hormone, infertility and miscarriage. *Lancet* **336**:1141–1144.

17 Mills JL, Simpson JL, Driscoll SG *et al.* (1988) Incidence of spontaneous abortion among normal women and insulin dependent diabetic women whose pregnancies were identified within 21 days of conception. *New England Journal of Medicine* **319**:1617–1623.

18 Watts DH, Eschenback DA (1988) Reproductive tract infections as cause of abortion and pre-term birth. *Seminars in Reproductive Endocrinology* **6**:203–215.

19 Lubbe WF, Liggins GC (1988) Role of lupus anticoagulant and autoimmunity in recurrent pregnancy loss. *Seminars in Reproductive Endocrinology* **6**:181–190.

20 Branch DW, Scott JR, Kochenow NK, Hershgold E (1985) Obstetric complications associated with the lupus anticoagulant. *New England Journal of Medicine* **313**:1322–1326.

21 Sargent IL, Redman CWG, Stirrat GM (1982) Maternal CMSI in normal and pre-eclamptic pregnancy. *Clinical and Experimental Immunology* **50**:601–609.

22 Sargent IL, Wilkins T, Redman CWG (1988) Maternal immune responses to the fetus in early pregnancy and recurrent miscarriage. *Lancet* **ii**:1099–1103.

23 Faulk WP, Temple A, Loviun RE, Smith N (1978) Antigens of trophoblast: A working hypothesis for their role in normal and abnormal pregnancies. *Proceedings of the National Academy of Sciences* **75**:1947–1951.

24 McIntyre JA (1988) In search of trophoblast–lymphocyte cross reactive antigens. *American Journal of Reproductive Immunology and Microbiology* **17**:100–110.

25 Hong-Nerng H, Gill TJ, Rhong-Phong N *et al.* (1990) Sharing of human leukocyte antigens in primary and secondary recurrent abortions. *American Journal of Obstetrics and Gynecology* **163**:178–188.

26 Gill TJ, Ho H-N, Kanbour A *et al.* (1988) Immunogenetic factors influencing the survival of the fetal allograft. In Beard RW, Sharp F (eds) *Early Pregnancy Loss: Mechanisms and Treatment*, pp. 277–286. London: Royal College of Gynaecologists.

27 Christiansen OB, Riisom K, Lauritsen JG, Grunnet N (1989) No increased histocompatibility antigen-sharing in couples with idiopathic habitual abortion. *Human Reproduction* **4**:160–162.

28 Ober CL, Hanck WW, Kostyn DD *et al.* (1985) Adverse effects of human leukocyte antigen-DR sharing on fertility: A cohort study in a human isolate. *Fertility and Sterility* **44**:227–332.

29 Bryant HE, Love EJ (1989) Video display terminal use and spontaneous abortion risk. *International Journal of Epidemiology* **18**:132–138.

30 Schnorr TM, Grajewski BA, Hornung RW *et al.* (1991) Video display terminals and the risk of spontaneous abortion. *New England Journal of Medicine* **324**:727–733.

31 Hemminki K, Mutanen P, Saloneimi I (1982) Spontaneous abortions in hospital staff engaged in sterilising instruments with chemical agents. *British Medical Journal* **285**:1461–1463.

32 Cohen-Overbeck TE, Hop WCJ, Den Ouden M *et al.* (1990) Spontaneous abortion rate and advanced maternal age: Consequences for prenatal diagnosis. *Lancet* **336**:27–29.

33 Grant A (1989) Cervical cerclage to prolong pregnancy. In Chalmers I, Enkin M, Keirse MJNC (eds) *Effective Care in Pregnancy and Childbirth*, pp. 633–646. Oxford: Oxford University Press.

34 Goldstein PA, Sacks HS, Chalmers TC (1989) Hormone administration for the maintenance of pregnancy. In Chalmers I, Enkin M, Keirse MJNC (eds) *Effective Care in Pregnancy and Childbirth*, pp. 612–623. Oxford: Oxford University Press.

35 Harrison RF (1988) Early recurrent pregnancy failure: Treatment with hCG. In Beard RW, Sharp F (eds) *Early Pregnancy Loss: Mechanisms and Treatment*, pp. 421–428. London: Royal College of Gynaecologists.

36 Lubbe WF, Butler WS, Palmer SJ (1983) Fetal survival after prednisone suppression of maternal lupus anticoagulant. *Lancet* **1**:1361–1363.

37 Mowbray JF, Gibbings C, Liddell H *et al.* (1985) Controlled trial of treatment of recurrent spontaneous abortion by immunisation with paternal cells. *Lancet* **i**:941–943.

38 Beer AE (1988) Pregnancy outcome in couples with recurrent abortions following immunological evaluation and therapy. In Beard RW, Sharp F (eds) *Early Pregnancy Loss: Mechanisms and Treatment*, pp. 337–349. London: Royal College of Gynaecologists.

39 Carp HJ, Ben-Shlomo I, Maschiach S (1990) Recurrent miscarriage. *Lancet* **336**:1191.

40 Taylor CG, Maclachlan NA, Wilson JK *et al.* (1988) In Beard RW, Sharp F (eds) *Early Pregnancy Loss: Mechanisms and Treatment*, pp. 369–372. London: Royal College of Gynaecologists.

41 Scott JR, Ware Branch D, Kochenour NK, Ward K (1988) Intravenous immunoglobulin treatment of pregnant patients with recurrent pregnancy loss caused by antiphospholipid antibodies and Rh immunisation. *American Journal of Obstetrics and Gynecology* **159**:1055–1056.

42 Mueller-Eckhardt G, Heine O, Nespert J *et al.* (1989) Prevention of recurrent spontaneous abortion by intravenous immunoglobulin. *Vox Sanguinis* **56**:151–154.

43 Johnson PM, Chia KV, Hart CA *et al.* (1988) Trophoblast membrane infusion for unexplained recurrent miscarriage. *British Journal of Obstetrics and Gynaecology* **95**:342–347.

44 McDonald IA (1980) Cervical cerclage. *Clinical Obstetrics and Gynaecology* **7**:461–679.

45 Medical Research Council/Royal College of Obstetricians and Gynaecologists' Multicentre Randomized Trial of Cervical Cerclage (1988) Interim Report. *British Journal of Obstetrics and Gynaecology* **95**:437–445.

46 McDonald IA (1957) Suture of the cervix for inevitable miscarriage. *Journal of Obstetrics and Gynaecology of the British Empire* **64**:346–350.

47 Shirodkar VN (1960) Habitual abortion in the second trimester. In Shirodkar VN (ed) *Contribution to obstetrics and gynaecology*. Edinburgh: Livingstone.

48 Herron MA, Parer JT (1988) Transabdominal cervical cerclage for fetal wastage due to cervical incompetence. *Obstetrics and Gynecology* **71**:865–868.

FURTHER READING

1 Friedman EA (ed.) (1985) *Atlas of Gynecological Surgery*, 2nd edn. New York: Thierne-Stratton.

2 Gomel V, Taylor PJ, Yuzpe AA, Rioux JE (1986) *Laparoscopy and Hysteroscopy in Gynecologic Practice*. Chicago, IL: Year Book Medical.

3 Hawkins J, Hudson CN (1983) *Shaw's Textbook of Operative Gynaecology*, 5th edn. Edinburgh: Churchill Livingstone.

4 Karasick S, Karasick D (1987) *Atlas of Hysterosalpingography*. Springfield, IL: Charles C. Thomas.

5 Mattingly RF, Thompson JD (eds) (1985) *Te Linde's Operative Gynecology*, 6th edn. Philadelphia, PA: J. B. Lippincott.

6 Monaghan JM (ed.) (1986) *Bonney's Gynaecological Surgery*, 9th edn. London: Baillière Tindall.

7 Siegler AM, Lindemann HJ (eds) (1984) *Hysteroscopy: Principles and Practice*. Philadelphia, PA: J. B. Lippincott.

8 Whitehouse GH (1981) *Gynaecological Radiology*. Oxford: Blackwell Scientific Publications.

9

Bleeding in Late Pregnancy

JUSTIN C. KONJE, ROBERT J. WALLEY

DEFINITION AND INCIDENCE

Any bleeding from the genital tract after the 22nd week of pregnancy should be regarded as 'late bleeding'. In the past, 28 weeks was the cut-off point, but because of improved neonatal intensive care facilities, fetal survival can now occur as early as 22 weeks. For this reason, the World Health Organization redefined any perinatal death as that of any fetus born after 22 weeks or weighing 500 g or more. 'Antepartum hemorrhage', which will be used interchangeably with 'late bleeding' in this chapter, is regarded as bleeding after 22 weeks gestation. It complicates 2–5% of all pregnancies.[1-3] **Table 1** shows the various causes of bleeding in late pregnancy.

RISKS OF BLEEDING IN LATE PREGNANCY

Placenta Previa: Maternal Risks

The main risks or associations of placenta previa are:

- *Maternal mortality*: This has dropped from 5% to less than 0.1% with the introduction of conservative management.[4]

- *Postpartum hemorrhage*: This is due to inefficient occlusion of the venous sinuses in the lower segment following delivery.

Table 1
Causes of bleeding in late pregnancy

Cause	Incidence (%)
Placenta previa	31
Abruptio placenta	22
'Other bleeding'	47
marginal	(60.0)
'show'	(20.0)
cervicitis	(8.0)
trauma	(5.0)
vulvovaginal varicosities	(2.0)
genital tumors	(0.5)
genital infections	(0.5)
hematuria	(0.5)
vasa previa	(0.5)
others	(0.5)

- *Anesthetic and surgical complications*: These occur especially in those with major previa delivered by emergency cesarean section where preparation for surgery is suboptimal.

- *Air embolism*: It occurs when the sinuses in the placental bed are torn.[4]

- *Postpartum sepsis*: This is secondary to ascending infection of the raw placental bed.

- *Placenta accreta*: This occurs in up to 15% of women with placenta previa.

- *Recurrence*: The risk of recurrence is about 4–8% after one previous previa.

Placenta Previa: Fetal Risks

The main fetal risks or associations of placental previa include

- *Prematurity*: Cotton et al.[5] reported a perinatal mortality of 100% at less than 27 weeks, 19.7% between 27 and 32 weeks, 6.4% between 33 and 36 weeks and 2.6% after 36 weeks. The overall perinatal mortality has dropped from 126 per 1000[5] to 42–81 per 1000[6] with conservative management.

- *Intrauterine growth retardation*: This may occur in up to 16% of cases. The incidence is higher in those with multiple episodes of antepartum hemorrhage.[7]

- *Congenital malformations*: The incidence of serious malformations is doubled in women with placenta previa. The most common are those of the central nervous, cardiovascular, respiratory and gastrointestinal systems.[3]

- *Other risks* to the fetus include umbilical cord complications such as prolapse and compression,[4] malpresentations, fetal anemia and unexpected intrauterine death (where vasa previa ruptures or from severe maternal hypovolemic shock).

Abruptio Placenta: Maternal Risks

These include

- *Recurrence*: This is generally reported as 5–17% after one episode, but rises to 25% after two. About 7% of women with abruption so severe to kill the fetus will have the same outcome in subsequent pregnancy[8] and 30% of all future pregnancies of women who have abruptio placenta fail to produce a living child.[1]

- *Hypovolemic shock*: There is a tendency to underestimate blood loss in abruptio placenta. This is because concealed bleeding into the myometrium may be difficult to estimate.

- *Acute renal failure*: This is often a complication of hypovolemia, although it can also result from disseminated intravascular coagulation.

- *Disseminated intravascular coagulation*: This follows the 'consumption' of most clotting factors due to either thromboplastin release or excessive blood loss and presents with coagulation failure.

- *Postpartum hemorrhage*: This results from coagulation failure or from a 'couvelaire uterus', where severe bleeding has occurred into the myometrium.

- *Maternal mortality*: This is thought to be in the order of 1%. In the last confidential enquiry (1985–1987) into maternal deaths in England, Scotland, Northern Ireland and Wales,[9] 4 of the 174 maternal deaths were due to placental abruption. Maternal mortality has fallen from 8% in 1919 to under 1%.[10] While severe hemorrhage is usually the major cause of other complications leading to mortality, disseminated intravascular coagulation itself may cause severe hemorrhage, renal failure and death.

- *Feto-maternal hemorrhage*: This leads to severe rhesus sensitization in rhesus negative patients. All rhesus negative patients must therefore have a Kleihauer test and anti-D immunoglobulin given to neutralize fetal cells in maternal circulation.

Abruptio Placenta: Fetal Risks

These are

- *Intrauterine growth retardation*: This is said to occur in about 80% of infants born before 36 weeks gestation.[1]

Table 2
Reported perinatal mortalities in various studies in patients with abruptio placenta

Reference	Period of study	PNMR/1000
Page et al. (1954)[69]	1930–50	448
Paintin (1962)[55]	1949–58	510
Hibbard and Hibbard (1963)[56]	1952–58	252
Chamberlain et al. (1978)[2]	1970	44
Knab (1978)[57]	1963–77	317
Paterson (1979)[15]	1968–75	144
Hurd et al. (1983)[67]	1979–81	300
Abdella et al. (1984)[14]	1970–80	335
Okonofua and Olatubosun (1985)[13]	1982–83	673

PNMR, perinatal mortality rate.

- *Congenital malformations*: These may be as high as 4.4% (twice that in the population[11]). The rate of major malformations is increased three-fold[3] and most of them involve the central nervous system and could be as high as five times the normal incidence.[10]

- *Abnormal neonatal hematology*: Anemia results from significant fetal bleeding.[12] In addition, Green[3] reported transient coagulopathies in newborns of women with abruptio placenta.

- *Perinatal mortality*: It varies from 14.4%[2] to 67.3%[13] **Table 2** shows various reported perinatal mortality rates. Over 50% of the perinatal deaths are stillborns.[4] Of those delivered alive, Abdella et al.[14] reported 16% mortality within 4 weeks and most weighed less than 2500 g. Perinatal mortality is closely related to gestational age. Paterson[15] reported survival rates varying from 23% at 28–32 weeks to 87.6% at 37–40 weeks. The higher incidence of fetal malformations[10,11] and intrauterine growth retardation[1] contribute to the high perinatal mortality. For babies weighing more than 2500 g, the reported survival rate is 98%.[16] In the presence of associated complications such as hypertension, fetal mortality increases three-fold.[14]

'Other Bleeding'

The risks of 'other bleeding' depend on the cause. The more serious ones are dealt with in Chapters 28, 29, 30, 32 and 35. This type of bleeding can be associated with a higher perinatal mortality which has been reported to vary between 3.5 and 15.7%.[17–19] This is higher than that from placenta previa (4.2–8.1%), suggesting that some degree of placental compromise occurs in these patients. Preterm delivery, which is more common in such patients, is a major contributor to the associated higher perinatal mortality.

In cases of vasa previa, fetal exanguination following rupture or compromise of placental circulation due to compression of the abnormal vessels may cause fetal death. Seventy-five per cent of deaths in vasa previa are due to exanguination. Other fetal risks include an increased incidence of intrauterine growth retardation and congenital malformations. The main risk to the mother is that of bleeding, but often maternal blood loss is mild and not life-threatening.

MANAGEMENT OF BLEEDING IN LATE PREGNANCY

Antepartum hemorrhage is unpredictable and any time

before, during or after presentation, the patient's condition may deteriorate abruptly. The management must therefore aim to treat or prevent such a deterioration. It is only after this has been achieved that specific measures can be instituted. The general measures discussed below will apply to all cases of antepartum hemorrhage, although modifications will have to be made depending on the severity of the bleeding. Specific measures implemented once a diagnosis is made will be discussed under the various causes of bleeding in late pregnancy.

Initial Assessment and General Measures (see **Figure 1**)

Management of any patient with bleeding in late pregnancy should be in the hospital with adequate facilities for transfusion, delivery by cesarean section and neonatal resuscitation and intensive care. Immediate transfer to the hospital via ambulance or the fastest means available is recommended when at home. Initial management must include a brief history, evaluation of the patient's general condition and initiation of various laboratory tests and treatment.

History

This must ascertain any initiating factors such as trauma or coitus, the amount and character of bleeding, association of abdominal pain or regular uterine contractions, a history of ruptured membranes or previous vaginal bleeds, known gestational age either by previous ultrasound scan or by last menstrual period, information about placenta sites from previous scans and fetal movements.

Physical examination

This is aimed at assessing both maternal and fetal conditions and should include:

- Measuring maternal pulse, blood pressure and respiratory rate.

- Looking for clinical evidence of shock (restlessness, pallor, cold and clammy extremities).

- Abdominal examination to ascertain whether the uterine fundus is compatible with the estimated gestational age, the presence of tenderness, the number of fetuses and viability, the presence of uterine contractions.

- Vaginal examination. Unless placenta previa has been excluded, this is usually confined to inspection only in order to assess quickly the amount of blood loss and to determine whether bleeding has stopped or is continuing. Where placenta previa has been excluded, a speculum examination may be performed and, if the bleeding is suspected to be fetal, the Apt test can be performed.

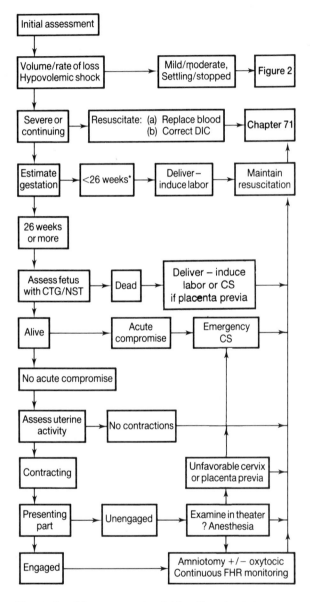

Figure 1. Management of bleeding in late pregnancy: Initial assessment and management of severe bleed. *The gestation after which survival rates are considered sufficiently significant so as to influence mode of delivery of the preterm fetus varies in different centers between 24 and 28 weeks.

Procedure: The Apt Test

This test is based on the principle that fetal hemoglobin is alkaline stable, whereas adult hemoglobin is not. It is designed to distinguish fetal from maternal blood passed per vaginam.

1. A sample of blood is collected vaginally.

2. 5 ml of water is added to each of two 10 ml test tubes.

3. To one test tube, add two drops of adult blood (from patient or volunteer).

4. To the second test tube, enough vaginal blood is added to match the color of the tube containing the adult blood.

5. Add 1 ml of 1% sodium hydroxide to each test tube.

6. The tube containing adult blood will change from pink to yellow brown in 2 min (as the adult hemoglobin is denatured by the alkali).

7. If the second tube contains fetal blood, it will remain pink for much longer (fetal hemoglobin is relatively resistant to denaturization).

Investigations and immediate management

As a general rule, all patients presenting with antepartum hemorrhage should initially be investigated and managed as outlined below, but subsequent management should be determined by the severity and type of bleeding and the gestational age of the pregnancy. The initial management should include the following:

- An intravenous line with a wide bore cannula (preferably size 14–16 French gauge) must be established.

- Blood must be obtained for immediate hemoglobin or hematocrit estimation, full blood count and grouping and reserving of serum. If the bleeding is continuing or is heavy, then at least 4 units of blood must be crossmatched. Where abruptio placenta is suspected, a coagulation profile, urea and electrolytes and liver function tests should also be performed. Other tests that may be performed are the Kleihauer test on maternal blood and the Apt test on vaginal blood.

- Intravenous fluids should be given if bleeding is continuing or is severe while crossmatched blood is being awaited. Colloids are the most suitable fluids in such situations.

- Ultrasound scan to exclude placenta previa if this has not been done or to exclude a major abruption with placental separation if it is suspected. However, this should only be performed if and when maternal and fetal conditions are stable.

After this initial management, the patient may fall into one of the following categories where:

- the bleeding has stopped

- the bleeding is continuing but remains mild or moderate and non-life-threatening

- the bleeding is continuing and is severe and life-threatening

- the fetus is in distress irrespective of the bleeding pattern

- the fetus is dead.

Subsequent management will therefore be determined by the above circumstances. It can be divided into (a) immediate delivery or (b) expectant management. These will be discussed under the various types of antepartum hemorrhage. The flow charts in **Figures 1** and **2** outline the general and specific managements.

Specific Measures: Placenta Previa

This is a placenta inserted partially or wholly in the lower uterine segment. With the advent of ultrasound, up to 45% of cases may be diagnosed early in the second trimester.[20] Four grades have been defined (**Table 3**). **Figure 3** shows grades of placenta previa.

The exact etiology of placenta previa is unknown, but various risk factors have been identified. These include age, parity and previous cesarean section.[6,21-23]

A single cesarean section scar increases the risk by 0.65%, three scars by 2.2% and four or more scars by 10%.[23] Other risk factors include smoking[24] and previous placenta previa. The recurrence risk is 4–8% after one placenta previa.[25]

Clinical presentation

Placenta previa characteristically presents with unprovoked painless vaginal bleeding. Occasionally, however, it may be provoked by sexual intercourse. Threatened miscarriage in the second trimester may precede placenta previa,[26] though such bleeding may have been minor and in some cases unreported. The initial episode of bleeding has a peak incidence at about 34 weeks[3] and occurs in over 50% of cases before 36 weeks and in only 2% after 40 weeks.[4]

The absence of pain is often regarded as a significant distinguishing factor between placenta previa and abruptio placenta, but 10% of women with placenta previa will have a co-existing abruption.[4] Such patients and those presenting for the first time in labor (25%)[27] may present a diagnostic problem.

Since routine early pregnancy ultrasound scanning is performed in most centers, some cases of placenta previa may be asymptomatic. However, diagnosis based on a single scan in the early mid-trimester should be regarded with caution.

Abdominal findings in cases of placenta previa are malpresentation, which in 35% of cases is either breech or transverse,[5] slight but consistent deviation of the presenting part from the midline and difficulties with palpating the presenting part.

Diagnosis

Various approaches have been used to diagnose placenta previa.

Vaginal examination

There is no place for routine vaginal examination in the diagnosis of placenta previa. This is because such examination may cause a torrential hemorrhage. Those who used to advocate this practice justified it because it excluded local causes of vaginal bleeding. However, since local causes are likely to be benign, vaginal examination, even by speculum, is probably wisely deferred until after an ultrasound scan has excluded the diagnosis. Vaginal examination is only indicated during examination in the theater with full preparation for cesarean section (see below).

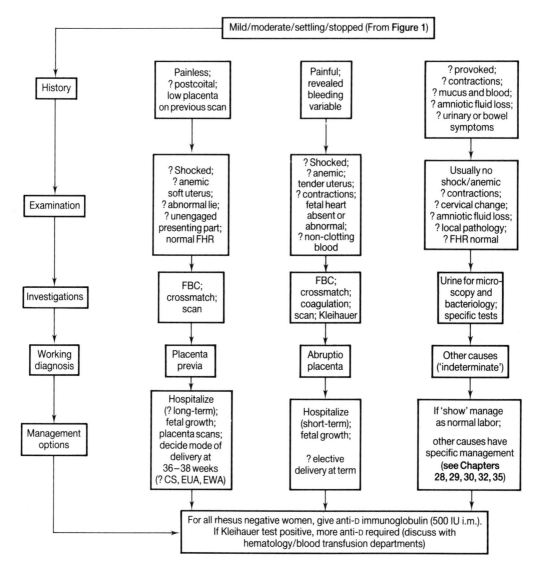

Figure 2. Management of bleeding in late pregnancy: Subsequent assessment and specific management of mild bleed. FHR, fetal heart rate, FBC, full blood count; CS, cesarean section; EUA/EWA, examination in theater with and without anesthetic, respectively.

Table 3
Grading of placenta previa

Grade	Description
I	The placenta is in the lower segment but the lower edge does not reach the internal os
II	The lower edge of the low-lying placenta reaches but does not cover the internal os
III	The placenta covers the internal os asymmetrically
IV	The placenta covers the internal os symmetrically

Placental localization

Various methods have been used for placentography. Some, such as soft tissue placentography (using x-rays), radioisotope radiography, pelvic angiography and thermography are no longer used. Magnetic resonance imaging may be a technique of the future but at present high cost limits availability.[28,29] Thus the mainstay for diagnosis in developed countries is ultrasonography.

Figure 4 shows grade III placenta previa.

Ultrasound is safe, fairly accurate and convenient. It is common practice in many obstetric units in developed countries to scan all pregnancies before 20 weeks gestation. However, the earlier the scan is performed, the more likely is over-diagnosis of placenta

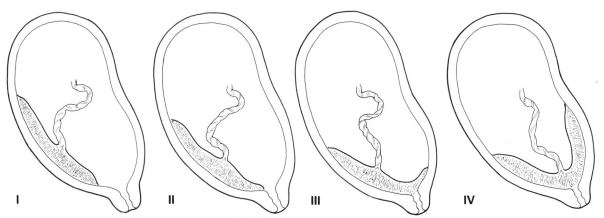

Figure 3. Grades of placenta previa. **I** Encroaching on lower segment. **II** Reaching internal os. **III** Asymmetrically covering internal os. **IV** Symmetrically covering internal os.

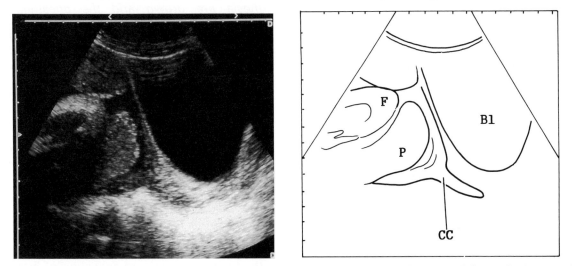

Figure 4. Ultrasound illustration of placenta previa, with tracing for clarification. (F fetus, P placenta, Bl bladder, CC cervical canal)

previa. For example, about 28% of placentas of women scanned before 24 weeks are found to be low-lying, but by 24 weeks this drops to 18% and only 3% are low-lying by term.[4,5,30] Conversely, false negative scan results are found in as many as 7% of cases.[5,31] Such results are more common when the placenta is posterior, the bladder is overfilled, the fetal head obscures the margin of the placenta or the operator fails to scan the lateral uterine wall.[32]

A low-lying placenta is more common in early pregnancy because the lower segment does not exist. This apparent change in placental position is due to enlargement of the upper segment and formation of the lower segment with many apparently low placentas being found to be above the lower segment. Comeau *et al.*[33] and Ruparelia and Chapman[34] have shown that the more advanced the pregnancy is, the more likely a diagnosis of placental previa on scan will be correct. Some obstetricians advocate that all women with a low placenta on an early scan should be rescanned at 32–34

weeks. Because of the fairly low incidence of placenta previa at term, the rationale for this practice has been questioned. Routine rescanning not only increases the workload of ultrasound departments but generates enormous patient anxiety. While some units are continuing with such a practice, others only rescan if there is an indication such as abnormal presentation, vaginal bleeding or the placenta was covering the os on the first scan.

Management Options: Placenta Previa (see **Figure 2**)

General management options have already been discussed (**Figure 1**). Specific measures will be either:

- immediate delivery, or

- expectant management

Immediate delivery

If bleeding continues but is neither profuse nor life-threatening and fetal maturity is more than 36 weeks, delivery would be preferred after commencing resuscitation. In such patients, the mode of delivery will depend on the degree of placenta previa and the state of the cervix. Placental localization occasionally fails to grade placenta previa accurately. In addition, some units do not have facilities for placental localization. The options available in this situation are immediate cesarean section or examination in the theater with or without anesthesia – the so-called 'double set-up'. Where the bleeding is profuse and life-threatening, cesarean section is the only option.

Procedure: Examination in Theater (Double Set-up)

Indications

This provides the most accurate assessment of the relationship of the lower edge of the placenta to the cervical os.[35] It should be done only when delivery is going to be undertaken. It is contraindicated in the presence of active profuse hemorrhage mandating immediate delivery, fetal malposition precluding vaginal delivery, fetal distress or clear ultrasonographic evidence of complete placenta previa.[3] It may be considered when ultrasonographic evidence of placenta previa is inconclusive or grade I or II anterior previa is suspected in patients with ongoing but not life-threatening uterine bleeding in active labor.

Preparation

Before this procedure is undertaken, crossmatched blood must be available. An anesthestist must be present, a midwife or theater nurse must be scrubbed and gowned and a cesarean section trolley laid. Ideally, a second obstetrician should be scrubbed and ready to operate. The procedure must be performed by an experienced obstetrician and a pediatrician must be present.

Opinions vary as to whether the procedure should be carried out under general anesthesia or not. The advantages of general anesthesia include proper relaxation of the patient, thereby making examination easier, and a quicker progression to cesarean section should the need arise. The main disadvantage is that of waking the patient up from anasthesia before inducing labor if vaginal delivery is considered to be possible. In addition, if cesarean section eventually becomes necessary, a second anesthetic will increase the risks. Performing such a procedure under epidural is an alternative, but this causes peripheral vasodilatation and may therefore make hypovolemia worse in the case of severe hemorrhage. A compromise aappears to be one where the drugs for induction of general anesthesia are drawn and the anesthetic machines and instruments all well-prepared. With such precautions, the interval between the examination and delivering the fetus can be short.

Procedure

The patient should be placed in the lithotomy position and draped with sterile towels after cleaning the vulva but not the vagina. The bladder is catheterized and two fingers introduced into the vagina, care being taken to avoid the cervical os. Each vaginal fornix is palpated in turn, the objective being to feel whether there is placenta between the presenting part and the finger. If there is, a sensation of 'bogginess' will be felt. If the four fornices are empty, the index finger is gently introduced into the cervical os and the surroundings felt for the placental edge. Where the cervix is closed, it should not be forced and cesarean section should be performed.[36] If no placental tissue is felt, the fetal membranes should be ruptured. A blood clot in the cervix, however, may be confused for placental tissue. Persistent bright red bleeding following membrane rupture should be an indication for cesarean section. If the placental edge is felt anteriorly but not extending to the os and no bleeding is provoked, some obstetricians advocate rupturing of fetal membranes and anticipating a vaginal delivery.[36] If at any stage during the procedure there is brisk vaginal bleeding, the procedure should be abandoned immediately and cesarean section performed.

Expectant management

Perinatal mortality in placenta previa is directly related to gestational age at delivery.[5,37–39] The introduction of expectant management by Macafee[37] and Johnson et al.[40] in the management of placenta previa was aimed at achieving maximum fetal maturity while minimizing the risks to both mother and fetus, the overall objective being to reduce perinatal mortality while at the same time reducing maternal mortality. The basis of this approach is that most episodes of bleeding are usually self-limited and not fatal to either fetus or mother in the absence of provoking trauma (e.g. intercourse, vaginal examination) or labor. Another major advantage of expectant management is that a proportion of cases, particularly those presenting early with lesser degrees of previa, may resolve to permit vaginal delivery.

In his regime, Macafee[37] advocated that the patient should remain in a fully equipped and fully staffed maternity hospital from the time of initial diagnosis to delivery. Various workers have, however, advocated a policy of permitting selected women to return home as part of expectant management.[5,41,42] This remains controversial, as reports from some units have been conflicting. Cotton et al.[5] reported no difference in their perinatal and maternal mortality rates in those sent home and those managed in hospitals, while D'Angelo and Irwin[43] suggested that retention of the mother in the hospital until delivery was justified on the grounds that neonatal mortality and morbidity and cost of treatment were reduced. However, in a review of 355 maternities managed at home, Kaunitz et al.[44] reported one intrapartum death from placenta previa.

Severe hemorrhage (heavy vaginal bleeding producing maternal hypovolemia) in the past was considered a contraindication to expectant management.[37] Some obstetricians now pursue an alternative expectant approach in such women with some success. In one study, where approximately 20% of the women lost over 500 ml of blood, half of them were managed expectantly with a mean gain of 16.8 days.[5] While only 43–46% of patients were managed successfully without an aggressive expectant approach by Hibbard[41] and Crenshaw et al.,[39] Cotton et al.[5] successfully managed 66% of women expectantly using an aggressive approach.

During expectant management, preterm labor remains a problem. Brenner et al.[45] found that 40% of women with placenta previa had rupture of the membranes, spontaneous labor or other problems that resulted in delivery before 37 weeks gestation. Inhibiting contractions in those with preterm labor would seem logical, but some physicians regard antepartum hemorrhage as a contraindication to the use of tocolytics.[46] This is because with vaginal bleeding and uterine contractions, placental abruption which is widely regarded as a contraindication cannot be excluded. In addition, abruptio placenta is said to coexist with placenta previa in 10% of cases and tocolytics cause maternal tachycardia and palpitations – features that could be confused with hypovolemia. Sampson et al.[47] and Silver et al.[42] advocate the use of tocolytics in cases of placenta previa and uterine contractions after 21 weeks and have claimed a reduction in perinatal mortality to 41 per 1000.

Perinatal mortality is directly related to the total amount of blood lost antepartum.[41] Liberal use of blood transfusion, however, will nullify this effect.[5] There is no limit to the number of blood transfusions a patient can have and, in order to optimize oxygen supply to the fetus and protect the mother against anticipated future blood loss, the aim of transfusion should be to maintain a hemoglobin of at least 10 g/dl or a hematocrit of 30%.

Despite the aggressive approach of expectant management, 20% of women with placenta previa are still delivered earlier than 32 weeks. These cases account for 73% of perinatal deaths.[5] They remain a major problem, and though the use of cervical cerclage has been advocated,[3] this is generally not used. Perinatal mortality and morbidity can be reduced in this group by the use of steroids and thyroid-releasing hormone.[48]

The main disadvantage of continuous hospitalization are cost and the psychological effect on families. For many families, this means prolonged separation and, in some extreme cases, the break-up of marriages. However, the advantages include easy access to resuscitation and delivery and ensuring bed rest and limitation of activities. With improvement in transportation facilities and ambulance services, highly motivated women who clearly understand the necessity of restriction of activity and are within, for example, 15–30 min of the hospital, perhaps may be monitored at home. This will only apply to cases of grade I–III placenta previa and or asymptomatic grade IV. In all cases of expectant management, cross-matched blood (2 units) must be ready at all times.

Procedure: Method of Delivery

In general, the diagnosis of placenta previa means delivery by cesarean section. Where the degree of placenta previa is minor (grade I or II anterior) and the fetal head is engaged, pregnancy may be allowed to continue beyond 37–38 weeks and vaginal delivery anticipated. In such patients, amniotomy followed by syntocinon can be considered. In those with more major grades of placenta previa, delivery is usually by cesarean section. This can be as an emergency or electively. Elective delivery is ideal; since emergency delivery exerts a negative effect on perinatal mortality and morbidity, independent of gestational age.[3] Cotton et al.[5] found that 27.7% of babies born as emergencies had anemia, compared with 2.9% delivered electively. Cesarean section for placenta previa poses several problems. It should therefore never be left to an inexperienced obstetrician.

Although epidurals are increasingly being advocated for cesarean section, Moir[49] considers placenta previa an absolute contraindication to epidural anesthesia. This is because epidurals, by lowering the blood pressure, may critically reduce uterine and placental perfusion. Crawford,[50] however, feels that in experienced hands, an epidural is safe. Where the patient is stable and there is no active bleeding, epidural or spinal anesthesia should not be regarded as contraindicated provided an experienced anesthetist is available. The severe anxiety generated in the couple by the sight of profuse bleeding during cesarean section is a reason for careful consideration before allowing partners in the theater.

The incision on the uterus is commonly a transverse lower segment incision provided there is a lower segment. Where the lower segment is non-existent or is very vascular, some obstetricians advocate a classical or a De Lee's incision. Scott,[51] however, believes that such incisions are rarely justified because of their consequences and long-term disadvantages. When difficulties are encountered with transverse lower segment incisions, these may be converted to inverted T-, J- or U-shaped incisions.

If the incision on the uterus is transverse and the placenta is anterior, two approaches are available: going through the placenta or defining its edge and going through the membranes above or below the placenta. The former approach requires speed and may result in significant fetal blood loss.[52] The latter, however, may be associated with undue delay in the delivery of the fetus, more troublesome bleeding from a partially separated placenta and therefore fetal blood loss and anoxia. Although Myerscough[52] does advise against cutting or tearing

through the placenta, some obstetricians have found it easier and quicker than defining and going through the membranes at the edge.

Because the lower segment is less muscular, contraction and retraction, which result in the occlusion of the sinuses of the placental bed, are inadequate and intraoperative hemorrhage is therefore not uncommon.[53] Where hemostasis is difficult to achieve, bleeding sinuses could be oversewn with atraumatic sutures.[51] If this is unsuccessful, packing the uterus is possible, but the major disadvantages are that the pack may be stitched during closure of the uterus and the bleeding may continue but remain concealed for some time as the pack is soaking through. The intramyometrial injection of prostaglandin F2-alpha has been shown to be useful in such cases.[3,54] When the bleeding remains uncontrollable, ligation of the internal iliac artery or even hysterectomy may be the last resort.

Specific Measures: Abruptio Placenta

This is bleeding following premature separation of a normally situated placenta. The incidence varies from 0.49 to 1.8%.[2,8,55–57] The wide variation in reported incidences is thought to be due to diagnostic difficulties. Fox[58] found evidence of abruption in 4.5% of placentas examined routinely, suggesting that small episodes of abruptio placenta are more common than is realized. Abruptio placenta is concealed in 20–35% and revealed in 65–80% of cases.[29,35] The concealed type is the most dangerous with more severe complications. Four grades of abruptio placenta have been described (**Table 4**). The most severe (grade III) occurs in 0.2% of pregnancies.[35]

The etiology of abruptio placenta is unknown in the majority of cases. In a few, however, it is obvious, such as in direct trauma to the uterus. Various risk factors have been reported to be associated with abruptio placenta. The risk of recurrence varies from 8.3%[59] to 16.7%.[15,36] It occurs more frequently in older women, but this increase has been attributed to parity, and is independent of age.[1] Cigarette smoking increases the incidence of abruptio placenta. Naeye[24] reported an incidence of 1.69% in non-smokers, 2.46% in smokers and 1.87% in smokers who had given up. In the smokers, evidence of decidual necrosis at the edge of the placenta was found. This may represent the effect of smoking on uteroplacental blood flow.[60]

Table 4
Grading of abruptio placenta

Grade	Description
0	Asymptomatic: diagnosed when a small retroplacental clot is discovered
I	There is vaginal bleeding. Uterine tetany and tenderness may be present. There are no signs of maternal shock or fetal distress
II	External vaginal bleeding may or may not be present. There are no signs of maternal shock. Signs of fetal distress are present
III	External bleeding may or may not be present. There is marked uterine tetany, yielding a board-like consistency on palpation. Persistent abdominal pain, maternal shock and fetal demise are present. Coagulopathy may become evident in 30% of cases

Other etiological factors include sudden decompression of the uterus after membrane rupture in patients with hydramnios and multiple pregnancy, external cephalic version,[61] placental abnormalities – especially circumvallate placenta[62,63] – and abdominal trauma.[64] Although in general maternal hypertension is regarded as a risk factor, there is no consensus on whether hypertension precedes the abruption or vice versa. While Paintin,[55] Hibbard and Hibbard[56] and Naeye et al.[65] found no evidence of placental abruption with hypertension, Abdella et al.[14] observed in their series that the incidence of abruptio placenta in those with pre-eclampsia was twice that in those without. The suggestion that folic acid deficiency may have an etiological role in abruptio placenta[1] has not been confirmed. Large prospective studies[12,66] have failed to show any association between abruptio placenta and folate supplementation. Although inferior vena caval compression and lupus anticoagulant have been suggested as possible etiological factors, there has been no convincing evidence.[36]

Clinical presentation

Abruptio placenta classically presents with vaginal bleeding, abdominal pain, uterine contractions and tenderness. Vaginal bleeding, however, is a symptom in only 70–80% of cases.[3,35] This bleeding is characteristically dark and non-clotting. It occurs after the 36th week of gestation in about 50% of cases.[35] In a study of 193 cases, Paterson[15] found that 18% presented before 32 weeks, 40% between 34 and 37 weeks and 42% after 37 weeks. Because labor is the most common factor precipitating placental separation,[4] nearly 50% of patients (with abruptio placenta) are in established labor. The presence of uterine contractions may, however, be difficult to distinguish from the abdominal pain of abruption. Where this distinction is possible, the contractions are characteristically of high frequency[67] – more than five in 10 min.

Though abdominal pain is common, it is not invariable. This is evidenced by the so-called 'unsuspected or silent abruption' referred to by Notelovitz et al.[68] and the higher pathological incidence of abruptio placenta found by Fox.[58] The presence of pain probably indicates extravasation of blood into the myometrium. In severe cases (grade III), the pain is sharp, severe and sudden in onset.[3] Some patients may, in addition, present with nausea, anxiety, thirst, restlessness and a feeling of faintness, while others may complain of absent or reduced fetal movements.

If blood loss is significant, there may be signs of shock (tachycardia with a weak and thready pulse, pallor or cyanosis, cold clammy skin). The presence of hypertension may mask true hypovolemia, but an increasing abdominal girth or a rising fundal height must raise the suspicion of significant hemorrhage. The uterus is typically described as 'woody hard' in severe abruptio placenta. In such cases, the fetus is difficult to palpate and a sonicaid or fetal monitor may have to be used to identify the fetal heart beat. The fetus may be distressed or dead. The former occurs in grades I and II, but in grade III the latter is an almost invariable occurrence.[36,69] In severe cases complicated by disseminated intravascular coagulation, there may be absence of clotting in the vaginal blood loss which is dark-colored. The incidence of coagulopathy is approximately 35%[59,70] and occurs mainly in the severe forms.

Typically, there will be blood clots in the vagina, but if the blood is non-clotting there will be none. Serous fluid from a retroplacental clot may be confused with amniotic fluid. The cervix may be dilating as 50% of cases are in labor. If the membranes are ruptured, blood-stained amniotic fluid may be seen.

Diagnosis

This is usually made on clinical grounds, but ultrasonography may be helpful in certain cases. The symptoms and signs presented above will be diagnostic in moderate to severe cases. In the mild variety, the diagnosis may not be quite obvious until after delivery when a retroplacental clot is identified.

Ultrasonography is not a sensitive method of diagnosing abruptio placenta,[3] but it is useful in excluding coincident placenta previa, which is present in 10% of cases. Where the retroplacental clot is large, ultrasonography identifies it as hyperechogenic or isoechogenic when compared with the placenta. Such echogenicity may therefore be misinterpreted as a thick placenta.[71] Resolving retroplacental clots appear hyperechogenic within 1 week and sonoluscent within 2 weeks.[3] Though ultrasonography is not an accurate diagnostic tool, it is useful in monitoring cases managed expectantly, and Rivera-Alzima et al.[72] used it to determine the time of delivery. The size of the hematoma, location and change in size over time and fetal growth are all parameters monitored by ultrasound scan. The Kleihauer test may be useful in making the diagnosis when a patient presents with abdominal pain but without vaginal bleeding or even in cases of 'unsuspected or silent abruption'.

The differential diagnosis of abruptio placenta can broadly be classified into two groups: these are other causes of vaginal bleeding and causes of abdominal pain in the late second and third trimesters. The former group are discussed elsewhere in this chapter. The latter group includes acute appendicitis (ruptured or unruptured), pyelonephritis, red degeneration of uterine fibroids, retroperitoneal hemorrhage, hematoma of the rectus sheath, chorioamnionitis and orthopedic problems such as lumbar or sacral stain (see Chapter 34).

Management Options: Abruptio Placenta (see Figure 2)

Once the diagnosis of abruptio placenta has been made, the management will depend on the severity, associated complications, the state of the patient and the fetus and gestational age. This is divided into general and specific measures. For the purpose of management, Sher and Statland[73] divided abruptio placenta into three grades of severity. These are: grade I, not recognized clinically before delivery and usually diagnosed by the presence of a retorplacental clot; grade II, intermediate, the classical signs of abruption are present but the fetus is still alive; and grade III, the fetus is dead and coagulopathy may be present.

The general management options have already been discussed (see Figure 1). Specific measures will be divided into:

- immediate delivery

- expectant management

- management of complications.

Immediate delivery

This will depend on the severity of abruption and whether the fetus is alive or dead. Where the fetus is dead, vaginal delivery should be the goal. Emphasis must, however, be placed on resuscitation, since fetal death occurs commonly in the severe variety of abruptio placenta, often with coagulopathy. In such patients, once resuscitation has been initiated, the fetal membranes should be ruptured to hasten the onset of labor. This is effective in most cases, but in a few augmentation with Syntocinon® may be needed. This must be administered cautiously, as uterine rupture could occur from an overstimulated uterus. Barron[36] believes that membrane rupture should be reserved for dead fetuses or those in advanced labor.

When the fetus is alive, the decision on how best to achieve delivery is not always easy. This is compounded by the fact that the outlook for the fetus is poor, not only in terms of immediate survival but also because studies have shown that as many as 15.4% of live-born infants do not survive.[14] However, when the perinatal mortality of vaginal delivery is compared to that of cesarean section – 52 vs 16% (Okonofua and Olatubosun,[13]), 20 vs 15% (Hurd et al.[67]) – it is clear that delivery by cesarean section is associated with better figures. Hibbard[4] has even gone further and stated that many of the poor results from cesarean section are due largely to indecision and delay in cases occurring in the last quarter of pregnancy. He states that cesarean section must be considered in all cases where the fetus is alive, particularly if there is evidence, transiently, of fetal distress. However, the presence of coagulopathy adds considerable risk to the mother and morbidity and mortality could be increased by surgery. Furthermore, some of the better figures associated with cesarean section may reflect selection bias rather than an inherent benefit of that mode of delivery.

If the decision is to deliver and the fetus is alive, the degree of abruption and the state of the fetus will be important determining factors. Where the abruption is severe, cesarean section must be performed once resuscitation is commenced. Such delivery should be performed promptly. Knab[57] noted that most postadmission fetal deaths occurred in fetuses delivered more than 2 h after admission. Once again, however, selection bias may distort these figures.

In mild to moderate cases of abruption, the mode of delivery will be determined by the state of baby, its presentation and the state of the cervix. Fetal distress will be an indication for immediate delivery by cesarean section. However, if the decision is to deliver vaginally, continuous fetal monitoring must be available in order to identify early fetal distress. Golditch and Boyce,[12] Luncan,[16] Knab[57] and Okonofua and Olatubosun[13] have all shown that perinatal mortality is higher with vaginal delivery in the absence of electronic fetal monitoring. There is a place for the use of prostaglandins in the ripening of the cervix of women with mild abruption, but the danger of inducing tetanic contractions must always be borne in mind. Where artificial rupture of fetal membranes is feasible, this often hastens delivery, but where it is not possible, prostaglandins can be used, though once again maintaining vigilance for hyperstimulation.

Expectant management

This expectant management is aimed at prolonging pregnancy with the hope of improving fetal maturity and therefore survival. It should be considered in cases of mild abruptio placenta occurring before 37 weeks gestation. In such patients, vaginal bleeding is slight, abdominal pain is mild and usually localized and they are cardiovascularly stable. Once a decision has been made on conservative management, the fetal condition must be monitored closely. Intrauterine growth retardation is common in placenta abruption. Timing of delivery will depend on further vaginal bleeding, the fetal condition, gestation and neonatal care facilities. If the bleeding episodes are recurrent, induction at 36–38 weeks is advised provided fetal indices (e.g. biophysical parameters and growth: (see also Chapters 39, 42 and 43) are satisfactory. It is our practice to see such patients once or twice weekly for cardiotocography, umbilical artery Doppler recordings and biophysical profiles. If the initial ultrasound scan showed a retroplacental clot, such clots may be monitored by serial ultrasound scans. With deterioration in fetal condition, delivery is effected.

Some cases of mild abruption may be complicated by labor. In such cases, it is difficult to establish which came first. The use of tocolytics in the presence of abruptio placenta is regarded to be contraindicated by many obstetricians because they may worsen the process of abruption.[46] Sholl,[74] however, stated that a trial of tocolytics in mild abruptio placenta and labor may successfully prolong pregnancy without jeopardizing the mother and fetus. There have as yet been no large trials to confirm Sholl's statement.

Management of complications of abruptio placenta

The major complications of abruptio placenta are hemorrhagic shock, disseminated intravascular coagulation, ischemic necrosis of distal organs (especially the kidneys and pituitary) and postpartum hemorrhage.

Hemorrhagic shock (see also Chapter 71)

This usually occurs when blood loss is in excess of 1000 ml. Because bleeding is often concealed, there is a tendency to underestimate blood loss. During shock,

there is tissue hypoperfusion. The objective of treatment should be to restore effective perfusion by restoring blood volume. Estimating external blood loss could be difficult but as a rule of thumb, trebling the volume of blood clot provides a rough estimate.

In hemorrhagic shock, plasma expanders or uncrossmatched O-negative blood could be commenced pending the availability of blood. Coagulation disorders must be excluded as the presence of such a complication may worsen the hemorrhage and additional appropriate corrective measures must be taken.

At least 4 units of whole blood should be crossmatched. Whole blood is preferred to packed cells as it contains some plasma constituents. Fresh whole blood is ideal but this is unlikely to be available because of the requirements for infection screening.

Because massive hemorrhages are often associated with a shift of fluid from the intravascular to the intracellular compartment, the initial hemoglobin (hematocrit) may be deceptively high. Initial replacement must therefore be of large volumes of fluid. The fluids preferentially used are colloids such as plasma expanders, human albumin and other blood susbstitutes, even uncrossmatched blood (O-negative blood or the patient's type). Dextran has the major disadvantage of interfering with clotting and blood crossmatching.

Fluid replacement in patients with hemorrhagic shock must be monitored closely to avoid overloading the circulatory system. Clinically, this can be done by measuring changes in blood pressure, pulse rate and assessing the patient's general state. Since kidney perfusion is closely reflected in urinary output, the degree of perfusion could be monitored by hourly urinary output. An indwelling urethral catheter must therefore be passed and urinary output should be at least 30 ml/h. Where the hemorrhage is massive or there is superimposed pre-eclampsia, a central venous pressure (CVP) should be employed. Pulmonary capillary wedge pressure via a Swan-Ganz catheter is thought to better reflect circulatory adequacy than the CVP, but should only be employed by units experienced in its use.

In the treatment of hemorrhagic shock, problems of massive transfusion (defined as transfusion in excess of $1–1\frac{1}{2}$ times the patient's blood volume or the administration of 10 or more units of blood) must be considered and precautions taken to correct them. These problems are more frequent with stored blood. They include clotting disorders (which may be confused with DIC), thrombocytopenia, hyperkalemia and hypocalcemia. Platelet counts, fibrinogen levels and serun potassium and calcium therefore need to be monitored. Green[3] advocates platelet transfusion if the platelet count is less than $50\,000/mm^3$ and fibrinogen replacement if levels fall below 100 mg/ml. Because of the risk of hyperkalemia, the maternal ECG should be monitored.

Disseminated intravascular coagulation (DIC) (see also Chapter 71)

This occurs in approximately 10% of cases of abruptio placenta but is more common in severe abruption marked by fetal death or massive hemorrhage.[3] The reported incidence of DIC in placental abruption varies widely. Fraser and Watson[29] suggested two reasons for this variation. First, the defect may be less common in recent years because of improved care, particularly resuscitation and, secondly, the criteria on which the diagnosis is made varies. Letsky[75] has classified the severity of DIC into three stages based on laboratory measurements. In stage I (low-grade compensated) there are raised fibrinogen degradation products and increased soluble fibrin complexes; in stage II (uncomplicated, but no hemostatic failure) there are, in addition, a fall in fibrinogen levels, platelet counts and Factors V and VII; while in stage III (rampant, with hemostatic failure) there are very low platelet counts and fibrinogen levels and high fibrinogen degradation products. The incidence of DIC in severe abruptio placenta (grade III) varies from 35%[70] to 38%[59]. Letsky's stage I and II occur in mild to moderate abruption, while stage III occurs in severe abruption.

Investigations that should be performed in patients with suspected DIC include whole blood clotting time, bleeding time, fibrinogen levels, fibrinogen degradation products (FDP), platelet count, euglobulin clot lysis time, prothrombin time (PT), partial thromboplastin time (PTT) and thrombin time. In DIC, the bleeding time is normal, clot retraction is abnormal, there is thrombocytopenia, elevated FDP and fibrinogen split products, normal to prolonged PT and PTT, low fibrinogen levels and a short thrombin time. Tissue thromboplatin released from the site of placental injury initiates widespread coagulation with consumption of the various clotting factors. Fibrinolysis of the clots is responsible for the raised FDPs, which themselves act as anticoagulants.

The ultimate treatment of DIC complicating abruptio placenta is delivering the fetus and placenta. This removes the source of tissue thromboplastin and arrests the process of widespread coagulation and fibrinolysis. Pritchard and Brekken[59] have shown that spontaneous resolution can occur after delivery. While the platelet count may be slower to rise after delivery, fibrinogen levels rise faster. Although delivering the fetus and placenta is the perceived end-point, the initial management must be geared toward replacing lost blood volume and replacing 'lost' or consumed clotting factors. Fibrinogen and platelet replacement is believed to 'fuel the fire'[3,29,75] because these factors encourage further DIC and fibrinolysis with resultant increases in FDPs and fibrinogen split products. Nevertheless, it is the authors' view that such replacement of clotting factors is necessary until the uterus is emptied.

The ideal fluid for replacement is fresh blood, but as this is rarely available (due to the requirements to screen blood for infections), stored banked blood or red cell concentrates with fresh frozen plasma are the best alternatives. Fresh plasma is preferred to freeze-dried as the latter is deficient in Factors V and VII. Cryoprecipitate, which is rich in Factors VII, XII and fibrinogen, may also be used with stored blood. The fibrinogen concentration of fresh frozen plasma (1 g/unit) is four times that in cryoprecipitate (0.25 g/unit). Although platelets and fibrinogen are said to worsen the process of DIC, if the patient is to be taken to theater, platelets should be given if the count is less than 50 000/mm^3. Once the treatment process has been initiated, delivery must be effected. This is by artificial rupture of membranes when the baby is dead or cesarean section if the fetus is alive (see above). Severe hemorrhage during and after cesarean section is a major risk.

The use of heparin in DIC is controversial. Although heparin may stop the process of disseminated coagulation, its use is considered inappropriate where the circulation is not intact.[29] Green[3] states that the use of heparin is now nearly universally condemned. However, it has a place in cases where microvascular plugging of distal organs such as kidneys occurs. Antifibrinolytic agents such as epsilon-aminocaproic acid (EACA) must be used with extreme caution, as they may cause unchecked intravascular coagulation in vessels of organs like the kidneys and brain.[75] It is the authors' view that the mainstays of treatment for DIC complicating abruptio placenta are emptying the uterus and replacement of blood products. Heparinization and the use of other agents are rarely if ever needed. If they are considered, then they should be used in close collaboration with a hematologist. During treatment of DIC, serial frequent measurements of the various parameters discussed above must be undertaken.

If the patient needs delivering by cesarean section (for fetal distress or because vaginal delivery is not possible), general anesthesia is preferred. Spinal and epidural anesthesia are regarded by most authorities as contradicted in severe abruption and DIC. This is because of the risk of hemorrhage in the dural and epidural spaces and the effect of sympathetic outflow block on blood pressure and venous return. In a hypovolemic patient, this may be made worse.

Renal failure (see also Chapters 28 and 71)

This occurs either because of hemorrhagic shock (prerenal) or in DIC with microvascular clotting in the kidneys (renal). Treatment of renal failure should be in collaboration with renal physicians. Barron,[36] states that oliguria during the first 12 h following abruption is common and does not necessarily imply renal damage. If this is associated with renal tubular necrosis, recovery is usually complete, but if there is cortical necrosis, the prognosis will depend on the extent of cortical necrosis. Fluid replacement in these patients must be monitored closely and it is in them that the CVP is important. Renal function must be monitored by urea and electrolytes, serum creatinine and creatinine clearance once or twice daily. Diuretics should be used with caution.[73]

Postpartum hemorrhage
(see also Chapters 68 and 71)

The causes include poor myometrial contractility following infiltration with blood as in Couvelaire uterus, and the inhibitory effect of FDPs on myometrial contractility in DIC.[76] Postpartum hemorrhage occurs in 25% of cases of abruptio placenta. Rapid blood transfusion, the use of ergot derivatives (Syntometrine®, ergometrine and Syntocinon®) and prostaglandins (PG2-alpha) injected intramyometrially have been used at various times. When all these fail, internal iliac artery ligation or hysterectomy may be performed.

Rhesus sensitization

Feto-maternal hemorrhages during abruption tend to be extensive.[77] All rhesus negative women with abruption must have a Kleihauer test and an appropriate dose of anti-D immunoglobulin given to destroy fetal cells. Large doses may be necessary. This must be given within 72 h of the onset of the process of abruption. Where management is expectant and intermittent recurrent bleeding occurs, we perform weekly Kleihauer testing and assays of anti-D immunoglobulin levels can be performed to provide guidelines for further anti-D administration. Collaboration with the hematologist and blood bank is advisable to determine the correct dose where the Kleihauer test is positive.

'Other Bleeding'

The exact cause of bleeding in late pregnancy is unknown in 47% (reported incidence 38–74%) of patients.[1,2,17–19,55,78,79] The cause of bleeding may later become apparent, but in the majority of cases no cause can be demonstrated.[29] Where causes have been identified, they include marginal sinus rupture (60%), 'show' (20%), cervicitis (18%), trauma (5%), vulvovaricosities (2%), genital tumors, hematuria, genital infections and vasa praevia (0.5% each). Although this group is referred to as 'other bleeding', it will invariably include unrecognized cases of minor abrup-

tion or placenta previa. Marginal sinus rupture is the most common source of bleeding in antepartum hemorrhage of unknown cause.[51,62]

Clinical presentation

The patients present with painless vaginal bleeding of unknown origin. There are usually no signs and symptoms diagnostic of either placenta previa or abruption. In the majority of cases, the bleeding is mild and settles spontaneously.[51] About 60% of cases present after 37 weeks and, of these, 15% will deliver within 10 days of the initial hemorrhage.[19] Where there is marginal bleeding with clot formation, serum separated from the clot may be confused with amniotic fluid following spontaneous rupture of fetal membranes.[80]

Diagnosis

This is often made after excluding abruptio placenta and placenta previa. An ultrasound scan is therefore necessary to exclude placenta previa as minor grades may present in a similar manner.

Vaginal examination is routinely performed in patients with 'other bleeding'. The timing of this examination varies. Some believe that it should be delayed until bleeding has stopped, whereas others advocate immediate examination once placenta previa has been excluded. Those who advocate immediate examination do so because they want to exclude advanced labor and local causes of bleeding. On the other hand, those who advocate delayed examination believe that this does not affect management and that other local causes of bleeding are usually benign and therefore need no immediate action. There are no controlled trials to compare these different forms of management. A vaginal examination is indicated, however, if there is the need to exclude fetal bleeding as the cause of antepartum hemorrhage. The test performed for this diagnosis is the Apt test (see Procedure above). If this test is not to be performed, a speculum examination may be delayed until the postnatal visit when appropriate treatment for local causes can be offered. If there are associated contractions, a vaginal examination should then be performed.

Management Options: Other Bleeding

If placenta previa and abruption have been excluded, further management will depend on gestational age, nature of bleeding (persistent or recurrent and severity), the state of the fetus (absence or presence of fetal distress) and the presumed cause.

Further management will either be expectant or

delivery. Where the pregnancy is 37 weeks or more and the bleeding is recurrent, significant or there are associated fetal factors such as growth retardation or distress, delivery is the management of choice. There is no contraindication to vaginal delivery provided there is no fetal compromise. In those presenting before 37 weeks, if episodes of bleeding are recurrent and significant, there may be need for immediate delivery. The mode of delivery will be determined by the state of the fetus, its lie and other associated factors like the state of the cervix.

If the decision is to manage expectantly, then the patient may either be monitored at home or in the hospital. Presently, most units tend to monitor the patients in the hospital until bleeding has stopped for at least 24 h before discharging them. In a retrospective review, Watson[19] showed no significant advantage in managing patients in the hosptial. There is need to conduct a randomized control trial comparing in-patient vs out-patient care in these cases. This is even more important now that emphasis is being placed on community care. Irrespective of where the patient is being managed, fetal surveillance must be provided. Although it is generally recommended that induction should be performed at 38 weeks, the real danger to the fetus is that of prematurity.[18,79] Where awaiting spontaneous onset of labor is the practice,[18] the perinatal mortality is not increased. Those advocating induction at 38 weeks do so based on the fact that placental function is damaged by bleeding.[51,81] In our unit, the practice is to await the spontaneous onset of labor if fetal growth and welfare are satisfactory.

One of the potential hazards of vaginal bleeding in late pregnancy is fetal exanguination from vasa previa. Classically, profuse vaginal bleeding follows amniotomy with subsequent fetal bradycardia. The diagnosis of this condition before these events is difficult, but the experienced observer may be able to feel vessels coursing over the membranes. A speculum examination may also show the vessels. In some cases, where there is mild bleeding after amniotomy but a normal fetal heart rate, this diagnosis cannot be excluded. An Apt test (see above)[82] will therefore have to be performed. If fetal blood is documented, the baby should be delivered immediately by cesarean section.

CONCLUSION

Bleeding in late pregnancy is an important cause of fetal and maternal morbidity and mortality. The etiology of the various types is poorly understood. Various management options are, however, available. Initial assessment of patients and subsequent planned management aimed at resuscitation and prolongation of pregnancy if possible, or immediate delivery either for

---

**BLEEDING IN LATE PREGNANCY
Summary of Management Options**

Initial assessment of severity –

If severe and continuing bleeding

- resuscitate

- deliver/empty uterus
  (see **Figure 1**)

If mild/moderate and settling or stopped

- establish cause

- specific management of the cause
  (see **Figure 2**).

---

fetal or maternal indications, is associated with a better outcome.

REFERENCES

1   Hibbard BM, Jeffcoate TNA (1966) Abruptio placentae. *Obstetrics and Gynecology* **27**:155–167.
2   Chamberlain GVP, Philipp E, Howlett B, Masters K (1978) *British Births, 1970.* London: Heinemann.
3   Green JR (1989) Placenta abnormalities: Placenta praevia and abruptio placentae. In Creasy RK, Resnik R (eds) *Maternal–Fetal Medicine: Principles and Practice.* Philadelphia, PA: W.B. Saunders.
4   Hibbard BM (1988) Bleeding in late pregnancy. In Hibbard BM (ed.) *Principles of Obstetrics.* London: Butterworth.
5   Cotton DB, Read JA, Paul RH, Quilligan EJ (1980) The conservative aggressive management of placenta praevia. *American Journal of Obstetrics and Gynecology* **137**:687–695.
6   McShane PM, Heye PS, Epstein MF (1985) Maternal and perinatal mortality resulting from placenta praevia. *Obstetrics and Gynecology* **65**:176–182.
7   Varma TR (1973) Fetal growth and placental function in patients with placenta praevia. *Journal of Obstetrics and Gynaecology of the British Commonwealth* **80**:311–315.

8 Pritchard JA (1970) Genesis of severe abruption. *American Journal of Obstetrics and Gynecology* **108**:22–27.

9 Department of Health (1991) *Report on Confidential Enquiries into Maternal Deaths in the United Kingdom 1985–87*. London: HMSO.

10 Egley C, Cefalo RC (1985) Abruptio placenta. In Studd J (ed.) *Progress in Obstetrics and Gynaecology*, Vol. 5. Edinburgh: Churchill Livingstone.

11 Niswander KR, Friedman EA, Hoover DB, Petrowski H, Westphal MC (1966) Fetal morbidity following potentially anoxigenic obstetric conditions. 1 Abruptio placentae. *American Journal of Obstetrics and Gynecology* **95**:838–845.

12 Golditch IA, Boyce NE (1970) Management of abruptio placenta. *Journal of the American Medical Association* **212**:288–293.

13 Okonofua FE, Olatubosun OA (1985) Caesarean versus vaginal delivery in abruptio placentae associated with live fetuses. *International Journal of Gynaecology and Obstetrics* **23**:471–474.

14 Abdella TN, Sibai BM, Hays JM, Anderson GD (1984) Relationship of hypertensive diseases to abruptio placentae. *Obstetrics and Gynecology* **63**:365–370.

15 Paterson MEL (1979) The aetiology and outcome of abruptio placentae. *Acta Obstetrica et Gynecologica Scandinavica* **58**:31–35.

16 Lunan CB (1973) The management of abruptio placentae. *Journal of Obstetrics and Gynaecology of the British Commonwealth* **80**:120–124.

17 Macafee CHG, Harley JMG (1963) Antepartum haemorrhage. In Claye A (ed.) *British Obstetric Practice: Obstetrics*, 3rd edn. London: Heinemann.

18 Willocks J (1971) Antepartum haemorrhage of uncertain origin. *Journal of Obstetrics and Gynecology of the British Commonwealth* **78**:987–991.

19 Watson R (1982) Antepartum haemorrhage of uncertain origin. *British Journal of Clinical Practice* **36**:222–226.

20 Wexler P, Gottersfeld KR (1977) Second trimester placenta praevia: An apparently normal presentation. *Obstetrics and Gynecology* **50**:706–709.

21 Naeye RL (1978) Placenta praevia: Predisposing factors and effects on the fetus and the surviving infants. *Obstetrics and Gynecology* **52**:521–525.

22 Newton ER, Barss V, Cetrulo CL (1984) The epidemiology and clinical history of asymptomatic mid-trimester placenta praevia. *American Journal of Obstetrics and Gynecology* **148**:743–748.

23 Clark SL, Koonings PP, Phelan JP (1985) Placenta praevia, accreta and prior caesarean section. *Obstetrics and Gynecology* **66**:89–92.

24 Naeye RL (1980) Abruptio placenta and placenta praevia: Frequency, perinatal mortality and cigarette smoking. *Obstetrics and Gynecology* **55**:701–704.

25 Kelly JV, Iffy L (1981) Placenta praevia. In Iffy L, Kaminetzky HA (eds) *Principles and Practice of Obstetrics and Perinatology*, Vol. 2. New York: John Wiley.

26 Konje JC, Ewings PD, Adewunmi OA, Adelusi B, Ladipo OA (1992) The effect of threatened abortion on pregnancy outcome. *Journal of Obstetrics and Gynaecology* **12**:150–155.

27 Hibbard LT (1981) Placenta praevia. In Sciarra JJ (ed.) *Gynecology and Obstetrics*, Vol. 2. New York: Harper and Row.

28 Powell MC, Buckley J, Price H, Worthington BS, Symonds EM (1986) Magnetic resonance imaging and placenta praevia. *American Journal of Obstetrics and Gynecology* **154**:565–569.

29 Fraser R, Watson R (1989) Bleeding during the latter half of pregnancy. In Chalmers I (ed.) *Effective Care in Pregnancy and Childbirth*. Oxford: Oxford University Press.

30 Chapman MG, Furness ET, Jones WR, Sheat JH (1989) Significance of the location of placenta site in early pregnancy. *British Journal of Obstetrics and Gynaecology* **86**:846–848.

31 McClure N, Dornan JC (1990) Early identification of placenta praevia. *British Journal of Obstetrics and Gynaecology* **97**:959–961.

32 Laing FC (1981) Placena praevia: Avoiding false-negative diagnosis. *Journal of Clinical Ultrasound* **9**:109–113.

33 Comeau J, Shaw L, Marcell CC, Lavery JP (1983) Early placenta praevia and delivery outcome. *Obstetrics and Gynecology* **61**:577–580.

34 Ruparelia BA, Chapman MG (1985) Early low-lying placenta-ultrasonic assessment, progress and outcome. *European Journal of Obstetrics and Gynecology and Reproductive Biology* **20**:209–213.

35 Knuppel AR, Drukker JE (1986) Bleeding in late pregnancy: Antepartum bleeding. In Hayashi RH, Castillo MS (eds) *High Risk Pregnancy: A Team Approach*. Philadelphia, PA: W. B. Saunders.

36 Barron SL (1989) Antepartum haemorrhage. In Chamberlain G, Turnbull A (eds) *Obstetrics*. London: Churchill Livingstone.

37 Macafee CHG (1945) Placenta praevia: A study of 174 cases. *Journal of Obstetrics and Gynaecology of the British Empire* **52**:313–324.

38 Macafee CHG, Millar WG, Harley G (1962) Maternal and fetal mortality in placenta praevia. *Journal of Obstetrics and Gynaecology of the British Commonwealth* **69**:293–212.

39 Crenshaw C, Jones DED, Parker RT (1973) Placenta praevia: A survey of 20 years experience with improved perinatal survival by expectant therapy and caesarean delivery. *Obstetrical and Gynecological Survey* **28**:461–470.

40 Johnson HW, Williamson JC, Greeley AV (1945) The conservative management of some varieties of placenta praevia. *American Journal of Obstetrics and Gynecology* **398**:406.

41 Hibbard LT (1969) Placenta praevia. *American Journal of Obstetrics and Gynecology* **104**:172–184.

42 Silver R, Depp R, Sabbagha RE, Dooley SL, Socol ML, Tamura RK (1984) Placenta praevia: Aggressive expectant management. *American Journal of Obstetrics and Gynecology* **150**:15–22.

43 D'Angelo LJ, Irwin LF (1984) Conservative management of placenta praevia: A cost benefit analysis. *American Journal of Obstetrics and Gynecology* **149**:320–323.

44 Kaunitz AM, Spence C, Danielson TS, Rochat RW, Grimes DA (1984) Perinatal and maternal mortality in a religious group avoiding obstetric care. *American Journal of Obstetrics and Gynecology* **150**:826–831.

45 Brenner WE, Edelman DA, Hendricks CH (1978) Characteristics of patients with placenta praevia and results of 'expectant management'. *American Journal of Obstetrics and Gynecology* **132**:180–189.

46 Besinger RE, Niebyl JR (1990) The safety and efficacy of tocolytic agents for the treatment of preterm labour. *Obstetrical and Gynecological Survey* **45**:415–440.

47 Sampson MB, Lastres O, Thomasi AM, Thomason JL, Work BA (1984) Tocolysis with terbutaline sulphate in patients with placenta praevia complicated by premature labour. *Journal of Reproductive Medicine* **29**:248–250.

48 Ballard RA, Ballard PL, Creasy RK, Padbury J, Polk DH, Bracken M, Moya FR, Gross I (1992) Respiratory disease in very-low-birthweight infants after prenatal thyrotropin-releasing hormone and glucocorticoid. *Lancet* **339**:510–515.

49 Moir DD (1980) *Obstetric Anaesthesia and Analgesia*, 2nd edn. London: Baillière Tindall.

50 Crawford JS (1985) *Principles and Practices of Obstetric Anaesthesia*, 15th edn. Oxford: Blackwell Scientific.

51 Scott (1986) Antepartum haemorrhage. In Whitfield CR (ed.) *Dewhurst's Textbood of Obstetrics and Gynaecology for Postgraduates*, 4th edn. Oxford: Blackwell Scientific.

52 Myerscough PR (1982) *Munro Kerr's Operative Obstetrics*, 10th edn. London: Baillière Tindall.

53 Williamson HC, Greeley AV (1945) Management of placenta praevia: 12 year study. *American Journal of Obstetrics and Gynecology* **50**:987–991.

54 Bigrigg A, Chui D, Chissell S, Read MD (1991) Use of intramyometrial 15-methyl prostaglandin F2α to control atonic postpartum haemorrhage following vaginal delivery and failure of conventional therapy. *British Journal of Obstetrics and Gynaecology* **98**:734–739.

55 Paintin DB (1962) The epidemiology of antepartum haemorrhage: A study of all births in a community. *Journal of Obstetrics and Gynaecology of the British Commonwealth* **69**:614–623.

56 Hibbard BM, Hibbard ED (1963) Aetiological factors in abruptio placentae. *British Medical Journal* **2**:1439–1436.

57 Knab DR (1978) Abruptio placentae: An assessment of the time and method delivery. *Obstetrics and Gynecology* **52**:625–629.

58 Fox H (1978) *Pathology of the Placenta*. London: W.B. Saunders.

59 Pritchard JA, Brekken AL (1967) Clinical and laboratory studies on severe abruptio placentae. *American Journal of Obstetrics and Gynecology* **97**:681–700.

60 Lehtovirta P, Forss M (1978) The acute effect of smoking on intervillous blood flow of the placenta. *British Journal of Obstetrics and Gynaecology* **85**:729–737.

61 Savona-Ventura C (1986) The role of external cephalic version in modern obstetrics. *Obstetrical and Gynecological Survey* **41**:393–400.

62 Scott JS (1960) Placenta extrachoralis (placenta marginata and placenta circumvallata). *Journal of Obstetrics and Gynaecology of the British Empire* **67**:904–918.

63 Wilson D, Paalman RJ (1967) Clinical significance of circumvallate placenta. *Obstetrics and Gynecology* **29**:774–778.

64 Crosby WM, Costila JP (1971) Safety of lap-belt restrain for pregnant victims of automobile collisions. *New England Journal of Medicine* **284**:632–635.

65 Naeye RL, Harkness WL, Utts J (1977) Abruptio placenta and perinatal death: A prospective study. *American Journal of Obstetrics and Gynecology* **128**:740–746.

66 de Valera E (1986) Abruptio placentae. *American Journal of Obstetrics and Gynecology* **100**:599–606.

67 Hurd WW, Miodovnik M, Lavin JP (1983) Selective management of abruptio placentae: A prospective study. *Obstetrics and Gynecology* **61**:467–473.

68 Notelovitz M, Bottoms SF, Dase DF, Leichter PJ (1979) Painless abruptio placentae. *Obstetrics and Gynecology* **53**:270–272.

69 Page EW, King EB, Merril JA (1954) Abruptio placentae: Dangers of delay delivery. *Obstetrics and Gynecology* **3**:385–393.

70 Green-Thompson RW (1982) Antepartum haemorrhage. *Clinical Obstetrics and Gynaecology* **9**:479–515.

71 Nyberg DA, Cyr DR, Mack LA et al. (1987) Sonographic spectrum of placental abruption. *American Journal of Radiology* **148**:161–167.

72 Rivera-Alzima ME, Saldana LR, Maklad N, Korp S (1983) The use of ultrasound in the expectant management of abruptio placentae. *American Journal of Obstetrics and Gynecology* **146**:924–927.

73 Sher G, Statland BE (1985) Abruptio placentae with coagulopathy: A rational basis for management. *Clinical Obstetrics and Gynaecology* **28**:15–23.

74 Scholl JS (1987) Abruptio placentae: Clinical management in nonacute cases. *American Journal of Obstetrics and Gynecology* **156**:40–51.

75 Letsky EA (1985) *Coagulation Problems During Pregnancy*. Edinburgh: Churchill Livingstone.

76 Basu HK (1969) Fibrinolysis and abruptio placentae. *Journal of Obstetrics and Gynaecology of the British Commonwealth* **76**:481–496.

77 Pritchard JA, MacDonald PC, Gant NF (1985) Obstetric hemorrhage. In *William's Obstetrics*, pp. 389–423. New York: Appleton-Century-Crofts.

78 Butler NR, Bromham DG (1963) *The First Report of the 1958 British Perinatal Mortality Survey*. Edinburgh: E. Livingstone.

79 Roberts G (1970) Unclassified antepartum haemorrhage: Incidence and perinatal mortality in a community. *Journal of Obstetrics and Gynaecology of the British Commonwealth* **77**:492–495.

80 Naftolin F, Khudr G, Benirschke K, Hutchinson DL (1973) The syndrome of chronic abruptio placentae, hydrorrhoea and circumvallate placenta. *American Journal of Obstetrics and Gynecology* **116**:347–350.

81 Walker J, MacGillivray I, MacNaughton MC (1976) *Combined Textbook of Obstetrics and Gynaecology*, 9th edn. Edinburgh: Churchill Livingstone.

82 Apt L, Downey WS (1955) Melena neonatorum, the swallowed blood syndrome. *Journal of Pediatrics* **47**:6–16.

10

Multiple Pregnancy Including Delivery

CAROLINE ANN CROWTHER

INCIDENCE

Multiple pregnancy rates vary worldwide. The lowest prevalence for twin births is in Japan (6.7 per 1000 deliveries), with an intermediate prevalence in North America and Europe (11 per 1000 deliveries) and the highest prevalence in Africa, particularly Nigeria (40 per 1000 deliveries). The frequency of twin births in tertiary centers ranges from 1:25 to 1:100, the higher rate reflecting the hospital referral population rather than the true population.

The incidence of monozygous twinning is relatively constant worldwide at 3.5 per 1000 births.[1] Dizygous twinning rates vary widely and are affected by age, parity, racial background and the use of assisted reproductive techniques.

RISKS

Multiple pregnancy is associated with greater risks for both mother and fetuses compared with a singleton pregnancy. These are also discussed in Chapter 55.

Maternal Risks

Multiple pregnancy poses particular risks to the mother (**Table 1**).

Table 1
Maternal risks associated with multiple pregnancy

Increased symptoms of early pregnancy
Increased risk of miscarriage
The vanishing twin syndrome
Anemia
Preterm labor/delivery
Hypertension
Antepartum hemorrhage
Hydramnios
Possible need for prenatal hospitalization
Antepartum fetal death
Minor disorders of pregnancy
Risk of an operative delivery
Increased likelihood of cesarean delivery
Postpartum hemorrhage
Postnatal problems

Increased symptoms of early pregnancy

Nausea and vomiting are common and may arouse the suspicion of a multiple pregnancy. Higher levels of pregnancy hormones are implicated.[2]

Increased risk of miscarriage

Miscarriage occurs more frequently in multiple pregnancy than singleton pregnancy.

Vanishing twin syndrome

Twins and higher order multiple pregnancies are more often conceived than born. During the first trimester of pregnancy, arrest of development and subsequent reabsorption of one or more of the fetuses may occur. This can be seen ultrasonically and is known as the 'vanishing twin' phenomenon.[3] Vaginal bleeding in the first trimester may be related to the vanishing twin syndrome, but the prognosis for the remaining fetus is good.

Anemia

Anemia is often reported as being more frequent in multiple than singleton pregnancies. The greater increase in blood volume compared with the red cell mass lowers the hemoglobin concentration. Mean corpuscular hemoglobin concentrations, used as a measure of anemia are, however, not different in multiple or singleton pregnancies. Fetal demands in a multiple pregnancy are greater, particularly for folate, and megaloblastic anemias have been reported.

Preterm labor/delivery

Preterm delivery (before 37 weeks gestation) occurred in 43.6% of all twin pregnancies compared with 5.6% of singleton pregnancies in a recent Scottish twin study.[4] The mean duration of pregnancy decreases as the number of fetuses in utero increases. The risks to the mother of a preterm delivery relate to the need for hospitalization and possible use of tocolytic therapy, such as beta mimetics. There is an increased risk of pulmonary edema with such tocolysis in twin pregnancies. Premature rupture of membranes occurs more frequently in multiple gestation and preterm labor and delivery are frequent sequelae.

Hypertension

The incidence of pregnancy-induced hypertension, pre-eclampsia and eclampsia are all increased in multiple pregnancy. Primigravid women with a twin pregnancy have a five times greater risk of severe pre-eclampsia than with a singleton pregnancy: and for multigravid women the risk is 10 times greater.[5] The risk of hypertension is reported to be greater in monozygotic twins.[6]

Antepartum hemorrhage

Given the greater surface area of the placental bed in multiple pregnancy, antepartum hemorrhage from placenta previa and placental abruption would have been expected to be increased. However, the available evidence does not support this view.

Hydramnios

Hydramnios may be suspected clinically in up to 12% of multiple pregnancies[7] and is associated with an increased risk of preterm labor. Acute hydramnios may occur, particularly with monoamniotic twins. Apart from preterm labor, hydramnios may cause significant abdominal discomfort for the mother. Hydramnios may be associated with the twin–twin transfusion syndrome discussed later under fetal risks.

Possible need for prenatal hospitalization

With the increased risk of threatened preterm labor, hypertension, fetal growth restriction and the so-called minor disorders of pregnancy, multiple pregnancy often requires admission to hospital, sometimes for prolonged periods during the prenatal period. For the mother, prolonged separation from her family is often a disruptive and stressful experience.[8]

Antepartum death of one fetus

The mother who has a fetal death of one twin during the antepartum period has to adjust to a future without one of the twins while developing a bonding to the surviving twin. In such cases, it is important that parents are encouraged to grieve for the loss of the one twin.[9] The mother also has to adjust to the additional risks to the surviving twin of death and morbidity from cerebral and renal lesions.[10] Physically, the mother is at risk of disseminated intramuscular coagulopathy with a reported 25% incidence.[11]

Minor disorders of pregnancy

The extra weight carried with a multiple pregnancy exaggerates all the minor symptoms of pregnancy. Backache, breathlessness, difficulty with walking – especially towards the end of pregnancy – and pressure problems such as varicose veins are all more frequent with multiple pregnancy.

Risk of an operative delivery

Compared with a vaginal singleton birth, there is an increased likelihood of an operative delivery of one or both twins with the associated risks of trauma, infection and hemorrhage to the mother.

Increased likelihood of cesarean delivery

Twins are more frequently delivered by cesarean section compared with singletons, either as an elective procedure or an emergency before or after the delivery of the first twin. The higher the order of multiple birth, the higher the likelihood of cesarean delivery.[12]

Postpartum hemorrhage

There is a significant risk of postpartum hemorrhage in multiple pregnancy due to the increased placental site, uterine overdistension and the greater tendency to uterine atony.

Postnatal problems

Learning to cope with the demand of two or more babies is often stressful. A higher percentage of depression is reported in mothers of twins.[13] Given the increased perinatal mortality among multiple pregnancies, the problems of coping with the loss of one or more babies may be an added burden in the postnatal period.

Fetal Risks

Multiple pregnancy is associated with many risks to the fetuses, as summarized in **Table 2**. A more detailed discussion of fetal problems in multiple pregnancy is dealt with in Chapter 55.

Stillbirth and neonatal death

In recent reports from Australia, the UK, the USA, Scandinavia and Zimbabwe, multiple pregnancy was associated with up to 10% of all perinatal mortality.[4,14-18] Not only is the perinatal mortality rate of twins up to 10 times that of singletons,[4,7,14,19] but if a broader concept of loss is used, including late abortion, late neonatal death and related infant death,[20] the increased risk is further doubled. Cause-specific mortality among twins is considerably higher for every major cause of death.[21]

Preterm labor and delivery

Preterm delivery (before 37 completed weeks gestation) is the main reason for the poor perinatal outcome in multiple pregnancy. All the studies in perinatal mortality in multiple pregnancy agree that being born preterm is the greatest single threat to the infants. The preterm delivery rate in multiple pregnancy varies between populations from 30%[22] to 50%.[23] Triplets have a higher risk of preterm delivery than twins.[24]

Intrauterine growth restriction

The incidence of light-for-dates babies (defined as less than the 10th percentile on birthweight for gestational age standards in pregnancy) is very common in multiple pregnancy. Rates between populations vary from 25%[23] to 33%.[25] Light-for-dates babies experience increased perinatal mortality and morbidity.

Congenital abnormality

Major congenital abnormalities are twice as common in multiple pregnancies compared with singletons. Abnormalities found exclusively in multiple pregnancy are conjoined twins (rate 1:200 monozygotic twins)[26] and acardia (rate of 1:100 monozygotic twins).[27] Triplet pregnancy is associated with an increased risk of acardia and conjoined twins. Specifically, neural tube defects,[28] bowel atresia[29] and cardiac anomalies[30] have all been reported to be increased in twin pregnancies.

It has recently been suggested that the risk of chromosomal abnormalities in one or both twins may be greater for a given maternal age than with a singleton pregnancy.[31]

Twin–twin transfusion syndrome

Placental vascular anastomosis, usually arteriovenous, can result in the twin–twin transfusion syndrome and is a serious complication usually of monozygotic monochorionic twins. The incidence of the twin–twin transfusion syndrome ranges from 5 to 15% of all twin pregnancies with a continuation of dysfunction after birth.[32] Acute, severe twin–twin transfusion syndrome occurs in about 1% of monochorionic gestations.[33]

Table 2
Fetal risks associated with multiple pregnancy

Stillbirth or neonatal death
Preterm labor and delivery
Intrauterine growth restriction
Congenital abnormalities
Twin–twin transfusion
The 'stuck' twin phenomenon
Hydramnios
Cord accident
Risk of asphyxia
Operative vaginal delivery, especially for the second twin
Death of co-twin
Twin entrapment

Once the unequal vascular anastomosis is established, the donor twin becomes anemic, hypovolemic, oligohydramniotic and poorly grown. In contrast, the recipient twin becomes polycythemic, hypervolemic, polyuric and hydramnios develops. Ascites, pleural and pericardia effusions may be evident. The mortality for twins with the acute syndrome presenting at 18–26 weeks is high, ranging from 79%[34] to 100%.[35–37] The resultant acute hydramnios predisposes to preterm labor or preterm rupture of the membranes, thus the high mortality.

Single fetal death may cause significant increased morbidity in the surviving twin. The appearance of multiple cystic lesions in the brain and kidneys, possibly caused by thrombi secondary to disseminated intravascular coagulation (DIC) initiated by the dead twin, have been described.[37] Alternatively, acute hemodynamic and ischemic changes at the time of the intrauterine death have been suggested to account for the cerebral and renal lesions seen.[38]

The 'stuck' twin phenomenon

This complicates 8% of twin pregnancies. Although common in monochorionic diamniotic gestations (about 35% of cases), the phenomenon has also been described in dichorionic and dizygotic pregnancies.[36,39] In the 'stuck twin' phenomenon, one fetus in a diamniotic pregnancy lies against the uterine wall in a severely oligohydramniotic sac while the co-twin lies in a severely polyhydramniotic sac.[40] Most but not all cases of the 'stuck twin' syndrome result from the twin–twin transfusion syndrome. Mortality rates for both twins are high at over 80%.[39,40] Premature labor from uterine overdistension is common.

Hydramnios

Hydramnios may occur in one gestational sac in both the twin–twin transfusion syndrome and the 'stuck twin' phenomenon as described previously. It may also be caused by fetal anomalies, such as upper gestational tract atresias and hydrops fetalis, possibly secondary to congenital heart anomalies. In some cases of gross hydramnios in both sacs, no causal factor is evident.[41] Hydramnios is a major cause of preterm labor because of the increased intrauterine volume. The associated perinatal mortality is high.

Cord accident

Preterm labor, premature rupture of the membranes, hydramnios, malpositions and malpresentations all predispose to an increased risk of cord prolapse in multiple pregnancies compared with singleton pregnancies. Monoamniotic monochorionic twins accounting for less than 2% of all monozygotic pregnancies are at risk of cord entanglement and knotting.[42] Cord accidents carry a very high perinatal mortality of up to 50%.[43]

Risk of asphyxia

The risk of mortality from asphyxia for a twin is 4–5 times that of a singleton.[21] Increased risk factors of intrauterine growth restriction, cord prolapse and hydramnios are considered to be of importance.

Operative vaginal delivery, especially for the second twin

The likelihood of an operative delivery is increased, especially for the second twin for whom internal podalic version is more common. Operative delivery is associated with an increased risk of birth trauma, low Apgar scores and hyperbilirubinemia compared with a normal vaginal delivery.

Death of a co-twin

Fetal demise of one twin has been reported to occur in 0.5 – 6.8% of twin pregnancies after the first trimester.[44,45] After the death of one twin, the risks of death for the surviving twin is reported as 20%, usually due to preterm delivery. The morbidity of the co-twin is highest for monochorionic twins with a higher frequency of neurological damage.[10] By contrast, the prognosis for a surviving dichorionic twin is relatively good.[46]

Twin entrapment

Twin entrapment is rare and reported to occur in 1:817 twin pregnancies.[47] The risk of fetal death of the first twin is high, as is the risk of fetal hypoxia to both twins. Twin entrapment is typically found with monoamniotic twins.

Management Options
(see also Chapter 55)

Prepregnancy

The risk of multiple pregnancy for women undergoing ovulation induction is increased to 20–40%. After clomiphene, the twinning rate ranges from 5 to 10%. Appropriate counseling of this increased risk should be given. The risk of a multiple pregnancy following the

IVF and GIFT reproductive techniques correlates directly with the number of embryos, zygotes or oocytes returned. When three are transferred, the multiple pregnancy rate (at 20 weeks) following *in vitro* fertilization-embryo transfer (IVF-ETs) is 32%, for zygote intrafallopian transfers (ZIFT) 27% and for gamete intrafallopian transfers (GIFT) 16%.[49] The risk of triplet pregnancy after IVF-ETs is reported as 4.1% and after GIFT 4.3%.[50] When deciding how many embryos, zygotes or oocytes to transfer, a compromise between a wanted high conception rate and an acceptable multiple pregnancy risk is necessary. The best way of reducing the risk of multiple pregnancy is to reduce the number of embryos, zygotes or oocytes transferred after full discussion with the couple.

Prenatal

Regular prenatal attendance for pregnancy care is accepted practice. Most clinicians increase the number of times women with a multiple pregnancy are seen during the prenatal period. A wide range of forms of care is practised, ranging from modified shared care with the general practitioner seeing the woman at the hospital for alternate prenatal visits, to seeing her weekly at the hospital prenatal clinic from the 20th week of gestation. No evidence is available to suggest that one form of care is better than another, nor which style of care women prefer.

Frequent prenatal visits permit extra vigilance in the early detection of pregnancy-induced hypertension if this develops. Gestational diabetes should be screened for as a routine. Antepartum hemorrhage can be neither predicted nor prevented by additional prenatal visits or any other strategy. Iron and folate supplementation is frequently advised from the beginning of the second trimester for women with a multiple pregnancy.

Given the increased risk of congenital abnormalities, an anomaly scan of each fetus is suggested between 18 and 20 weeks gestation. In centers offering routine ultrasound at this stage of pregnancy, any as yet undetected multiple pregnancy should be diagnosed. Early diagnosis enables appropriate counseling and planning of future care, and has been claimed to reduce the perinatal loss related to twin pregnancy.[51] Conjoined twins, if present, can be diagnosed if an ultrasound is done at this stage.

In a recent review, prenatal ultrasonography with cardiac screening limited to the four chamber view resulted in detection of 39% of all major congenital anomalies in twins. However, none of the cardiac lesions were detected. Of the non-cardiac major anomalies, 55% were detected, as were 69% of the major anomalies which could alter prenatal management.[52]

The prediction of amnionicity and chorionicity by ultrasound is possible, though its accuracy remains to be determined on a large sample.[53] The hazards for monochorionic and monoamniotic twins include twin–twin transfusion syndrome, 'stuck twin' phenomenon and cord entanglement. In theory, knowledge of the amnionicity and chorionicity may be useful to differentiate the twin–twin transfusion syndrome from a twin pregnancy complicated by growth restriction. Similarly, this knowledge may be useful in the management of twins where one has a major congenital malformation and selective termination is considered, or in the management of a pregnancy after a single fetal death.[54] However, at present, screening for amnionicity and chorionicity is not normal practice for most obstetricians.

Preterm labor and subsequent delivery presents the greatest risk for fetal morbidity and mortality. Counseling as to the signs and symptoms of preterm labor may be of value, together with a written patient information sheet. If uterine activity is noted, prompt presentation to the hospital is encouraged.

Prediction of who will go into preterm labor is difficult. Cervical assessment has been suggested as a useful way of evaluating preterm delivery risk, either by digital examination,[55–57] or by ultrasound assessment.[58] How frequently such an assessment should be made (e.g. weekly/fortnightly/monthly) is uncertain, and whether such assessments are more harmful than beneficial is not known. Cervical assessment allows calculation of the cervical score (cervical length in centimeters minus cervical dilatation in centimeters). In one study, a cervical score of 2 or less at or before 34 weeks is reported to have a positive predictive value of 75% for preterm delivery.[56] In another recent study, a cervical score of 0 or less also had a positive predictive value of 75% for preterm delivery.[57]

If there is cervical change, admission to hospital is the most generally accepted management. Routine hospital admission and subsequent rest, however, seems of little benefit in delaying labor.[59] It is unknown whether prophylactic tocolysis is of value to this identifiable group at high risk of preterm delivery.

Several prenatal interventions have been tried to reduce the risk of preterm delivery in multiple pregnancies, including prophylactic cervical cerclage,[60,61] prophylactic beta-mimetic agents,[62,63] bed rest in hospital[64] and home uterine activity monitoring.[65] To date, however, none of these has proven to be of value in reducing the incidence of preterm delivery and the associated high perinatal mortality in multiple pregnancy.

Prophylactic cervical cerclage in twin pregnancy fails to show any benefit when the results of randomized trials are reviewed.[66] It seems prudent to reserve the insertion of a cervical suture to cases where there is evidence of cervical incompetence. Prophylactic tocolytic agents are occasionally used in multiple pregnancy. The meta-analysis of the trials of betamimetics fails to show a benefit in the incidence of preterm labor,[67] so their use cannot be recommended.

The admission of women with an uncomplicated twin pregnancy to hospital for rest does not reduce the risk of preterm delivery as previously widely believed. A meta-analysis of randomized trials of routine hospitalization for rest actually showed an increased likelihood of preterm delivery in women who were admitted, compared with a control group who continued normal activity at home.[68] Admission to hospital for rest in an uncomplicated twin pregnancy should only be considered if the woman requests admission. This may be due to discomfort or the fact that she cannot cope at home, or she may live a significant distance from the hospital.

The value of admission to hospital for rest in triplet or higher order multiple pregnancy is unproven. In the only small randomized study to date of 19 triplet pregnancies, hospitalization for rest suggested a beneficial trend in reducing the incidence of preterm delivery and of increased birthweight in the hospitalized group.[69] All of these beneficial results are also compatible with chance variation. There is a need for a multicenter trial to evaluate further the effects of admission to hospital for rest in triplet pregnancy.

Home uterine activity monitoring has been suggested to permit diagnosis of preterm labor at an early stage, enabling successful tocolysis and fewer preterm births. In one small randomized trial of 45 women, such benefits were reported.[65] Uterine activity monitoring may be of value in multiple pregnancies, but much larger studies are necessary to prove the benefits and exclude the harmful effects of this intensive and expensive prenatal procedure.

Fetal assessment during pregnancy includes regular ultrasound for fetal growth and well-being. The range of frequency for scanning varies from every 2 weeks from the 24th week to every 3–4 weeks from the 20th week of gestation. Biophysical profiles have been suggested from the 30th week of gestation.

If the death of one fetus occurs during pregnancy before the delivery of the survivor(s), extra vigilance of the well-being of the survivor(s) and screening for the early features of disseminated intravascular coagulation by regular maternal platelet counts is advised.

If hydramnios develops, therapeutic amniocentesis (see Chapter 48) may be considered if the mother is experiencing great discomfort. If the twin–twin transfusion is suspected, therapeutic options that have been advocated include: non-steroidal anti-inflammatory agents, repeated therapeutic amniocentesis and various methods of interrupting the pathological placental circulation. There is no convincing evidence to suggest that any of these improves fetal outcome.

During the prenatal period, discussion with the couple as to the most likely mode of delivery, conduct of labor and use of analgesia, especially epidural, is necessary. Many countries have multiple pregnancy support groups. The opportunity to contact such local groups during the prenatal period, to attend their meetings and make personal links with other families who have had a multiple pregnancy is recommmended.

Labor/delivery

Delivery in a hospital should be planned with many advising delivery in a tertiary unit. Induction of labor may be indicated for complications such as pregnancy-induced hypertension or growth restriction. There is controversy as to whether elective delivery at 38 weeks to reduce the risk of antepartum stillbirth secondary to intrauterine growth restriction is necessary.

Intrapartum blood loss is greater in multiple pregnancy, as is the risk of postpartum hemorrhage. An intravenous access line should be inserted early in labor and blood taken to estimate the maternal hematocrit and to hold serum for crossmatching if needed later.

For a vaginal delivery, it is recommended that both twins are continuously monitored. Initially, only external fetal monitoring will be possible. Whenever feasible, a scalp electrode should be placed on the first twin with continuation of external monitoring for the second twin. Recently, twin fetal heart rate monitors have become available, allowing the simultaneous print-out of the two fetal heart rate traces. If it is impossible to reliably record the second twin continuously, some recommend a cesarean section because of the higher risk of fetal asphyxia in twins, which may go undetected without adequate monitoring.

Epidural analgesia is widely used and provides adequate pain relief for the mother and minimizes the risk of her pushing prior to full dilatation. In addition, adequate analgesia is provided should there be a need for an operative delivery, internal podalic version or progression to cesarean section. The widespread use of epidural anesthesia often negates the need for emergency general anesthesia with the above complications, although this may still be necessary for an emergency cesarean section for fetal distress.

The most frequent mode of delivery for triplets and higher order multiple births is by cesarean section,[70–72] although no randomized studies are available to support this method of delivery over vaginal delivery. Reports suggest the risk of lower Apgar scores for higher birth order neonates is less when delivered by cesarean section[73,74] and there are fewer perinatal deaths.[73]

The optimal mode of delivery in multiple pregnancies remains controversial. The literature on twin pregnancy offers insight to permit some recommendations to be made. The mode of delivery is often influenced by the presentations of the twins, which may be divided into three groups:

- first twin vertex, second twin vertex

- first twin vertex, second twin non-vertex

- first twin non-vertex.[75]

First twin vertex, second twin vertex

The most common presentation of twins at delivery is vertex–vertex and most obstetricians would recommend a vaginal delivery.[75–78] The recent literature now supports the vaginal delivery of very low birthweight infants under 1500 g for the vertex–vertex twin gestation.[75,78,79]

First twin vertex, second twin non-vertex

For twins presenting as first twin vertex/second twin non-vertex, opinion is divided as to the optimal mode of delivery. Some recommend elective cesarean delivery,[77,80] suggesting reduced neonatal mortality and morbidity. Others suggest there is no increase in neonatal risk by vaginal delivery of the second twin weighing ≥1500 g, either as a breech after internal podalic version if not a longitudinal lie, or as a cephalic after external cephalic version.[81–85] The only randomized study to date found no difference in neonatal outcome in 60 non-vertex second twins at 35 weeks gestation or more, who were randomly allocated to either vaginal delivery or cesarean section.[86] Assessment as to whether vaginal breech delivery is appropriate is necessary using the standard criteria as for a singleton delivery. These include exclusion of cephalopelvic disproportion, an estimated fetal weight of <3500 g and a flexed fetal head on ultrasound.

For a non-vertex, second twin of very low birthweight (<1500 g), mode of delivery is controversial. Some recent reports recommend cesarean delivery to minimize birth trauma to the preterm infant,[75,81,83,84] whereas others fail to show any neonatal benefit and stress that vaginal delivery entails reduced risks for the mother.[87] No randomized studies exist which compare vaginal and cesarean delivery in such infants.

First twin non-vertex

When the first twin is non-vertex, delivery by cesarean section is often advised,[75] although there is no series which suggests vaginal delivery is inappropriate. By following such a policy, the risk of twin entrapment by interlocking chins or heads can be avoided.

Procedure: Twin Delivery

For delivery of twins, at least one experienced obstetrican, anesthetist, pediatrician and neonatal nurse should be in attendance. Depending on gestational age (e.g. if preterm) and circumstances (operative delivery, abnormal CTG), a double pediatric team (two pediatricians and two neonatal nurses) may be appropriate. For higher order multiple births, one pediatric team should be present for each baby delivered. Some would recommend a nurse scrubbed and ready for emergency cesarean section.

For a vaginal birth, the delivery of the first twin should be as for a singleton. After delivery, an experienced obstetrician assesses the lie and presentation of the second twin. This can be done by vaginal examination, abdominal palpation or transabdominal ultrasound assessment. The lie should then be corrected to longitudinal either by external version or internal podalic version.

*External version (**Figure 1**) gently turns the fetus so that the vertex lies above the pelvic brim. Amniotomy can then be performed provided that there are uterine contractions (see below) and delivery is completed. Version is more likely to be successful with epidural anesthesia and when the twins are of similar weights*

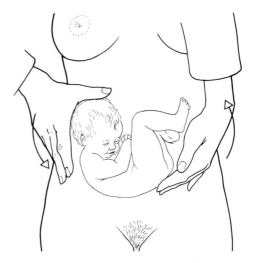

Figure 1. Modified external version for delivery of second twin.

(< 500 g difference).[82] In two reported series, external version was less likely than breech extraction to result in a vaginal delivery.[84,88] Emergency cesarean section and complications such as cord prolapse and fetal distress were more frequent in the external version group. Although these were not randomized studies, in view of the findings, internal podalic version if necessary and delivery as a breech is recommended by some obstetricians if the lie is non-longitudinal or the breech is presenting. However, others prefer to use external cephalic versions and only perform an amniotomy once the lie is longitudinal and there are regular uterine contractions. They advocate a cesarean section if the lie remains non-longitudinal.

A Syntocinon® infusion is mandatory if there is uterine inertia. Once there are contractions and the lie is longitudinal, an amniotomy is performed and with maternal effort during contractions, delivery is effected. A scalp electrode can be applied after amniotomy to permit continuous fetal heart rate monitoring, or an external monitor can be used. Most advise continuous monitoring of the second twin throughout the second stage of labor, given this twin's increased risk of intrapartum asphyxia.

If fetal distress develops and delivery cannot be safely achieved or if the second twin fails to descend into the pelvis, emergency cesarean section is necessary.

After delivery of the second infant, active management of the third stage is recommended with an oxytocic agent. As a prophylactic against uterine atony, some recommend that an infusion of Syntocinon® is continued for 3–4 h.

Internal podalic version (**Figure 2**)

For delivery of the second twin when a non-longitudinal lie and the membranes are intact.

1. Under adequate analgesia, usually epidural but possibly general anesthetic.

2. Lithotomy position.

3. Continuous fetal heart rate monitoring.

4. Aseptic technique; catheterize patient.

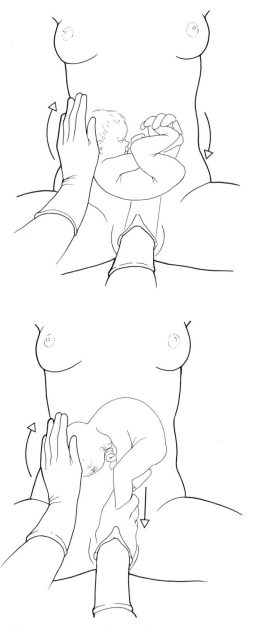

Figure 2.   Internal podalic version.

5. Pediatrician present.

6. Determine the lie of the second twin by abdominal palpation, internal examination or transabdominal ultrasound. Perform an amniotomy.

7. Locate a fetal foot. Confirm definitely a foot by palpating fetal heel and so exclude a fetal wrist.

8. Grasp foot and pull down into vagina. Grasp both feet if possible.

9. With maternal effort during contractions, deliver fetus as an assisted breech delivery.

Complications

1. Risk of fetal trauma secondary to breech delivery, e.g. dislocated hips.

2. Fetal anoxia.

3. Maternal trauma, e.g. ruptured uterus.

4. Endometritis.

5. Cord accident.

6. Placental abruption.

7. Difficulty with delivery of the after-coming head of breech.

8. Inadvertent delivery of a hand–shoulder presentation.

Twin entrapment

Twin entrapment may occur if the first twin is delivering as a breech and the second twin is cephalic and the head of the second twin enters the pelvis before the head of the leading twin.

Some maintain the risk of twin entrapment can be avoided by performing a cesarean section if the first twin is breech and the second twin is cephalic.

In the emergency situation, an attempt may be made to separate the locked twins by passing a hand vaginally between the chins of the fetuses and pushing the second twin upwards. If this fails, emergency cesarean section is necessary. Alternatively, an attempt may be made to push back the first twin presenting as a breech and then allow the 'second' twin presenting cephalically to deliver first. Again if this fails, emergency cesarean section is necessary.

At cesarean section, the head of the first twin is maneuvered upwards, enabling delivery of the second twin's head and body. The 'first' twin may then be delivered. Some recommend that a second obstetrician should be available to manipulate the babies vaginally if necessary.

If the first twin is already dead, rather than a cesarean delivery there is the option of decapitation, delivery of the second twin vaginally, followed by delivery of the head of the first twin. It is recommended that such a destructive operation should be performed under general anesthesia so that the mother is protected from seeing the procedure. Many would advocate that this option should not be used in modern obstetrics. They would argue an abdominal delivery might be expected to be associated with a lower incidence of perinatal asphyxia for the second twin.

Complications

The risk of fetal death of the first twin in twin entrapment is high, as is the risk of fetal hypoxia for both twins. Maternal risks relate to the need for emergency cesarean section, endometritis and possible general anesthesia.

Conjoined twins

Conjoined twins are usually diagnosed antenatally. This identifies the conjoined site and permits discussion prior to delivery of the prognosis and the possibility of surgical correction with the parents. If the diagnosis is made prior to viability, some parents might opt for termination of the pregnancy. Unless delivery is necessary for other reasons, preterm cesarean section is recommended. The use of steroids to stimulate surfactant production is advisable. Some would test for fetal lung maturity before delivery. Many obstetricians favor elective cesarean delivery at 38 weeks; however, this can be difficult technically. Some recommend a classical incision, but this would seem to offer little fetal benefit over a lower segment incision and does increase the maternal risks, particularly of uterine scar rupture in any subsequent pregnancy.

At delivery, two neonatal teams should be available, with the neonatal surgical team and operating theater on standby.

Postnatal

A prolonged in-hospital stay is often required for a mother with twins and should be offered. Breast-feeding needs to be encouraged and additional midwifery help is important. The provision of adequate contraception is necessary and needs to be discussed.

Prior to discharge, if extra help is not available at home, the provision of additional community support may need to be arranged. Maintaining the links made with the local multiple births support group during the puerperium is of importance.

REFERENCES

1   Little J, Thompson B (1988) Descriptive epidemiology. In MacGillivray I, Campbell DM, Thomson B (eds) *Twinning and Twins*, pp. 37–66. Chichester: John Wiley.

2   Vandekerckhove F, Dhont M, Thiery M, Derom R (1984) Screening for multiple pregnancy. *Acta Geneticae Medicae et Gemellologiae* **33**(4):571–574.

3   Landy HJ, Weiner S, Corson SL, Batzer FR, Bolognese RJ (1986) The 'vanishing twin': Ultrasonographic assessment of fetal disappearance in the first trimester.

MULTIPLE PREGNANCY
Summary of Management Options (see also Chapter 55)

Prepregnancy

- The risks of multiple pregnancy need to be appreciated by women undergoing ovulation induction and other assisted reproduction techniques (GIFT, IVF, ET, ZIFT)

Prenatal

- Regular antenatal care with routine anomaly ultrasound scan at 18–20 weeks gestation

- Iron and folate supplementation from the second trimester

- Vigilance for the early signs and symptoms of preterm labor; prompt self-referral if suspected

- Screening for hypertension and gestational diabetes

- Possible assessment of cervical change

- Regular fetal growth assessment by ultrasound

- Hospitalization at patient's request or if complications detected

- Prenatal education about pregnancy, possible modes of delivery, analgesia and conduct of labor

- Introduction to multiple pregnancy self-help support groups

- Consider therapeutic amniocentesis (repeating if necessary) if extreme maternal distress

- If death of one fetus, monitor the well-being of the survivor(s) and maternal platelet count

Labor/delivery

- Hospital delivery

- Experienced obstetrician

- Await spontaneous labor or induce at term

- Aim for vaginal delivery unless leading twin has non-longitudinal lie. Some would suggest elective cesarean if the first twin is not cephalic

- Pediatrician, neonatal nurse and anesthetist to be available at delivery. Two pediatricians if preterm, operative delivery planned or fetal problems anticipated with twins

- Continuous monitoring of all fetuses during labor

- Epidural analgesia recommended

- Vaginal delivery of the first twin, if appropriate

- If longitudinal lie of the second twin, amniotomy if regular contractions and delivery

- If non-longitudinal lie, convert to longitudinal lie by external version, or, if this fails internal podalic version

- May need Syntocinon® infusion for uterine inertia

- Consider prophylactic Syntocinon® infusion after delivery to reduce risk of postpartum hemorrhage

Postnatal

- Extra support while in hospital to assist with care of babies

- Offer longer in-patient stay

- Arrange support at home

- Link with multiple pregnancy support groups

- Adequate contraceptive advice

American Journal of Obstetrics and Gynecology **155**:14–19.

4 Patel N, Barrie W, Campbell D, Howat R, Melrose E, Redford D, McIlwaine G, Smalls (1983) *Scottish Twin Study 1983: Preliminary Report*, pp. 12–13. Glasgow: Greater Glasgow Health Board.

5 MacGillivray I, Campbell DM (1988) Management of twin pregnancies. In MacGillivray I, Campbell DM, Thompson B (eds) *Twinning and Twins*, pp. 111–139. Chichester: John Wiley.

6 McMullan PF, Norman RJ, Marivate M (1984) Pregnancy-induced hypertension in twin pregnancy. *British Journal of Obstetrics and Gynaecology* **91**:240–243.

7 Keith L, Ellis R, Berger GS, Depp R, Filstead W, Hatcher W, Keith DM (1980) The North West University multi-hospital twin study. *American Journal of Obstetrics and Gynecology* **138**:781–789.

8 White M, Ritchie J (1984) Psychological stressors in antepartum hospitalisation: Reports of pregnant women. *Maternal Child Nursing Journal* **13**:47–56.

9 Theroux R (1989) Multiple birth: A unique parenting experience. *Journal of Perinatal and Neonatal News* **3**(1):35–45.

10 Fusi C, Gordon H (1990) Twin pregnancy complicated by single intra-uterine death: Problems and outcome with conservative management. *British Journal of Obstetrics and Gynaecology* **97**:511–516.

11 Landy HJ, Weingold AB (1989) Management of a multiple gestation complicated by an antepartum fetal demise. *Obstetrical and Gynaecological Survey* **44**(3):171–176.

12 Lipitz (1990) High order multifetal gestation: Management and outcome. *Obstetrics and Gynecology* **76**:215–218.

13 Thorpe K, Golding J, MacGillivray I, Greenwood R (1991) Comparison of prevalence of depression in mothers of twins and mothers of singletons. *British Medical Journal* **302**:875–878.

14 Hawrylyshyn PA, Barkin M, Bernstein A, Papsin FR (1982) Twin pregnancies – a continuing perinatal challenge. *Obstetrics and Gynecology* **59**:463–466.

15 Hartikainen-Sorri A, Kauppila A, Tuimala R, Keivisto M (1983) Factors related to improved outcome for twins. *Acta Obstetrica et Gynecologica Scandinavica* **62**:23–25.

16 Chervenak FA, Youcha S, Johnson RE, Berkowitz RL, Hobbins JC (1984) Twin gestation: Antenatal diangosis and perinatal outcome in 385 consecutive pregnancies. *Journal of Reproductive Medicine* **29**:727–730.

17 Crowther CA (1987) Perinatal mortality in twin pregnancy: A review of 799 twin pregnancies. *South African Medical Journal* **71**:73–74.

18 Doherty J (1988) Perinatal mortality in twins, Australia 1973–1980. *Acta Geneticae Medicae et Gemellologiae* **37**:313–319.

19 Fowler MG, Kleinman JC, Kiely JL, Kessel SS (1991) Double jeopardy: Twin infant mortality in the United States 1983 and 1984. *American Journal of Obstetrics and Gynecology* **165**:15–22.

20 Whitfield CR, Smith MC, Cockburn F, Gibson A (1986) Perinatally related wastage – a proposed classification of primary obstetric factors. *British Journal of Obstetrics and Gynaecology* **93**:694–703.

21 Kleinman JC, Fowler MC, Kessel SS (1991) Comparison of infant mortality among twins and singletons: United States 1960–1983. *American Journal of Epidemiology* **133**:133–143.

22 Kauppila A, Jouppila A, Koivisto M, Moilaneu I, Ylikorkala O (1975) Twin pregnancy: A clinical study of 335 cases. *Acta Obstetrica et Gynecologica Scandinavica* **44**:5–8 (suppl.).

23 Houlton MCC, Marivate M, Philpott RHP (1981) The prediction of fetal growth retardation in twin pregnancy. *British Journal of Obstetrics and Gynaecology* **188**:264–273.

24 Sassoon DA, Castro LC, Davis JL, Hobel CJ (1990) Perinatal outcome in triplet versus twin gestations. *Obstetrics and Gynecology* **75**:817–820.

25 Jeffrey RL, Watson A, Bowes JR, Delaney JJ (1974) Role of bed rest in twin gestation. *Obstetrics and Gynecology* **43**:822–826.

26 Hanson JW (1975) Incidence of conjoined twinning. *Lancet* **ii**:1257.

27 Little J, Bryan E (1988) Congenital anomalies. In MacGillivray I, Campbell DM, Thompson B (eds) *Twinning and Twins* pp. 207–240. Chichester: John Wiley.

28 Kallen B (1986) Congenital malformations in twins: A population study. *Acta Geneticae Medicae et Gemellologiae* **35**:167–178.

29 Little J, Bryan E (1986) Congenital anomalies in twins. *Seminars in Perinatology* **10**(1):50–64.

30 Burn J, Corney G (1984) Congenital heart defects and twinning. *Acta Geneticae Medicae et Gemellologiae* **33**:61–69.

31 Rodis JF, Egan JF, Craffey A, Ciareglio L, Greenstein R, Scorza W (1990) Calculated risk of chromosomal abnormalities in twin gestations. *Obstetrics and Gynecology* **76**:1037–1041.

32 Tan KL, Tan R, Tan SH, Tan AM (1979) The twin tranfusion syndrome: Clinical observations on 35 affected pairs. *Clinics in Pediatrics* **18**:111–114.

33 Elliott JP, Urig MA, Clewell WH (1991) Aggressive therapeutic amniocentesis for treatment of twin–twin transfusion syndrome. *Obstetrics and Gynecology* **77**:537–540.

34 Gonsoulin W, Moise KJ, Kirshon B, Cotton DB, Wheeler JM, Carpenter RJ (1990) Outcome of twin–twin transfusion diagnosed before 28 weeks of gestation. *Obstetrics and Gynecology* **75**:214–216.

35 Weir PE, Raten E, Beischer N (1979) Acute polyhydramnios – a complication of monozygous twin pregnancy. *British Journal of Obstetrics and Gynaecology* **86**:849–853.

36 Chescheir NC, Seeds JW (1987) Polyhydramnios and oligo-hydramnios in twin gestations. *Obstetrics and Gynecology* **71**:882–884.

37 Urig MA, Clewell WH, Elliott JP (1990) Twin–twin transfusion syndrome. *American Journal of Obstetrics and Gynecology* **163**:1582–1526.

38 Fusi L, McParland P, Fisk N, Nicolini U, Wigglesworth J (1991) Acute twin–twin transfusion: A possible mechanism for brain-damaged survivors after intrauterine death of a monochorionic twin. *Obstetrics and Gynecology* **78**:517–520.

39 Patten RM, Mack LA, Harvey D, Cyr DR, Pretorius DH

(1989) Disparity of amniotic fluid volume and fetal size: Problem of the stuck twin – US studies. *Radiology* **172**:153–157.

40 Mahoney BS, Filly RA, Callen PW (1985) Amnionicity and chorionicity in twin pregnancies: Predictions using ultrasound. *Radiology* **155**:205–209.

41 Lange I, Harman CR (1990) Hydramnios in twin pregnancy – a reply. *American Journal of Obstetrics and Gynecology* **161**:1626.

42 Nyberg DA, Filly RA, Golbus MS (1984) Entangled umbilical cords: A sign of monoamniotic twins. *Journal of Ultrasound in Medicine* **3**:29.

43 Benirschke K, Kim CK (1973) Multiple pregnancy. *New England Journal of Medicine* **288**:1276–1284.

44 Benirschke K (1961) Twin placenta in perinatal mortality. *New York State Journal of Medicine* **61**:1499–1508.

45 Litschgi M, Stucki D (1980) Course of twin pregnancy after fetal death *in utero*. *Geburtschilfe Perinatol* **184**:227.

46 Bejar R, Vigliocco G, Gramajo H, Solana C, Benirschke K, Berry C, Coen R, Resnik R (1990) Antenatal origin of neurologic damage in newborn infants: Multiple gestations. *American Journal of Obstetrics and Gynaecology* **162**:1230–1236.

47 Cohen M, Kohl SG, Rosenthal AH (1965) Fetal interlocking complicating twin gestation. *American Journal of Obstetrics and Gynecology* **91**:407–411.

48 Pritchard JA, MacDonald PC, Grant NF (1985) Multifetal pregnancy. In *Williams' Obstetrics* 17th edn, p. 503. Norwalk, CT: Appleton-Century-Crofts.

49 Bollen N, Tournaye H, Camus M, DeVroey P, Staessen C, Van Steirteghem A (1991) The incidence of multiple pregnancy after *in vitro* fertilization and embryo transfer, gamete or zygote intra fallopian transfer. *Fertility and Sterility* **55**:314–318.

50 National Perinatal Statistics Unit, Fertility Society of Australia (1987) *IVF and GIFT Pregnancies, Australia and New Zealand 1986.* Sydney, November.

51 Persson P, Grennert L, Gennser G, Kullander S (1979) On improved outcome in twin pregnancies. *Acta Obstetrica et Gynecologica Scandinavica* **58**:3–7.

52 Allen SR, Gray LJ, Frentzen BH, Cruz AC (1991) Ultrasonographic diagnosis of congenital anomalies in twins. *American Journal of Obstetrics and Gynecology* **165**:1056–1060.

53 Mahoney BS, Filly RA, Callen P (1985) Amniocity and chorionicity in twin pregnancies: Prediction using ultrasound. *Radiology* **155**:205–209.

54 D'Alton ME, Mercer BM (1990) Antepartum management of twin gestation: Ultrasound. *Clinical Obstetrics and Gynecology* **33**(1):42–51.

55 Houlton MCC, Marivate M, Philpott RHP (1982) Factors associated with preterm labour and changes in the cervix before labour in twin pregnancy. *British Journal of Obstetrics and Gynaecology* **89**:190–194.

56 Neilson JP, Verkuyl DAA, Crowther CA, Bannerman C (1988) Preterm labour in twin pregnancies: Prediction by cervical assessment. *Obstetrics and Gynaecology* **72**:719–723.

57 Newman RB, Godsey RK, Ellings JM, Campbell BA, Eller DP, Miller MC (1991) Quantification of cervical change: Relationship to preterm delivery in the multifetal gestation. *American Journal of Obstetrics and Gynecology* **165**:264–271.

58 Michaels WH, Schreiber FR, Padgitt RJ, Ager J, Pieper D (1991) Ultrasound surveillance of the cervix in twin gestations: Management of cervical incompetency. *Obstetrics and Gynecology* **78**:739–744.

59 Crowther CA, Neilson JP, Verkuyl DAA, Bannerman C, Ashurst H (1989) Preterm labour in twin pregnancies: Can it be prevented by hospital admission? *British Journal of Obstetrics and Gynaecology* **96**:850–854.

60 Weekes ARL, Menzies DN, De Boer CH (1977) The relative efficacy of bed rest, cervical suture and no treatment in the management of twin pregnancy. *British Journal of Obstetrics and Gynaecology* **84**:161–164.

61 Sinha DP, Nandakumar VC, Brough AK, Beebeejaun MS (1979) Relative cervical incompetence in twin pregnancy: Assessment and efficacy of cervical suture. *Acta Geneticae Medicae et Gemellologiae* **78**:322–331.

62 TambyRaja RL, Atputharajah V, Salmvu V (1978) Prevention of prematurity in twins. *Australia and New Zealand Journal of Obstetrics and Gynaecology* **18**:179–181.

63 Ashworth MF, Spooner SF, Verkuyl DAA, Waterman R, Ashurst HM (1990) Failure to prevent preterm labour and delivery in twin pregnancy using prophylactic oral salbutamol. *British Journal of Obstetrics and Gynaecology* **97**:878–882.

64 Crowther CA, Chalmers I (1989) Bed rest and hospitalisation during pregnancy. In Chalmers I, Enkin M, Keirse MJNC (eds) *Effective Care in Pregnancy and Childbirth*, pp. 624–632. Oxford: Oxford University Press.

65 Knuppel RA, Lake MF, Watson DL, Welch RA, Hill WC, Fleming A, Martin RW, Bentley DL, Moenning RK, Morrison JC (1990) Preventing preterm birth in twin gestation: Home uterine activity monitoring and prenatal nursing support. *Obstetrics and Gynecology* **76**:245–275.

66 Grant A (1989) Cervical cerclage to prolong pregnancy. In Chalmers I, Enkin M, Keirse MJNC (eds) *Effective Care in Pregnancy and Childbirth*, pp. 633–645. Oxford: Oxford University Press.

67 Keirse MJNC, Grant A, King JF (1989) Preterm labour In Chalmers T, Enkin M, Keirse MJNC (eds) *Effective Care in Pregnancy and Childbirth*, pp. 694–749. Oxford: Oxford University Press.

68 Crowther CA (1991) Hospitalisation for bed rest in twin pregnancy: Editorial overview. In Chalmers I (ed.) *Oxford Database of Perinatal Trials.*

69 Crowther CA, Verkuyl DAA, Ashworth MF, Bannerman C, Ashurst HM (1991) The effects of hosptialisation for bed rest on duration of gestation, fetal growth and neonatal morbidity in triplet pregnancy. *Acta Geneticae Medicae et Gemellologiae* **40**:63–68.

70 Newman RB, Hamer C, Millar MC (1989) Outpatient triplet management: A contemporary review. *American Journal of Obstetrics and Gynecology* **161**:547–555.

71 Lipitz S, Reichman B, Paret G, Modan M, Shaler J, Serr D, Mashiach S, Frenkel Y (1989) The improving out-

come of triplet pregnancies. *American Journal of Obstetrics and Gynecology* **161**:1279–1284.

72 Collins MS, Bleyl JA (1990) Seventy one quadruplet pregnancies: Management and outcome. *American Journal of Obstetrics and Gynecology* **162**:1384–1392.

73 Crowther CA, Hamilton RA (1989) Triplet pregnancy: A 10 year review of 105 cases at Harare Maternity Hospital, Zimbabwe. *Acta Geneticae Medicae et Gemellologicae* **38**:1–8.

74 Petrikovsky BM, Vintzilees AM (1989) Management and outcome of multiple pregnancy of high fetal order: Literature review. *Obstetrical and Gynecological Survey* **44**:578–584.

75 Chervenak FA, Johnson RE, Youcha S, Hobbins JC, Berkowitz RL (1985) Intrapartum management of twin gestation. *Obstetrics and Gynecology* **65**:119–124.

76 Rayburn WF, Lavin JP, Miodovnik M, Varner MW (1984) Multiple gestation: Twin interval between delivery of the first and second twins. *Obstetrics and Gynecology* **63**:502–506.

77 Cetrulo CL (1986) The controversy of mode of delivery in twins: The intrapartum management of twin gestation. *Seminars in Perinatology* (Part One) **10**:39–40.

78 Morales WJ, O'Brien WF, Knuppel RA, Gaylord S, Hayes P (1989) The effect of mode of delivery on the risk of intraventricular haemorrhage in non-discordant twin gestations under 1500 g. *Obstetrics and Gynecology* **73**:107–110.

79 Hays PM, Smeltzer JS (1986) Multiple gestation. *Clinical Obstetrics and Gynecology* **29**:269–285.

80 Barrett JM, Staggs SM, Hooydonk JE, Growdon JH, Killam AP, Boehm FM (1982) The effect of type of delivery upon neonatal outcome in premature twins. *American Journal of Obstetrics and Gynecology* **143**:360–365.

81 Acker D, Lieberman M, Holbrook H, James O, Phillippe E, Edelin K (1984) Delivery of the second twin. *Obstetrics and Gynecology* **59**:710–711.

82 Chervenak FA, Johnson RE, Berkowitz RL, Hobbins JC (1983) Intrapartum external version of the second twin. *Obstetrics and Gynecology* **62**:160–164.

83 Blickstein I, Swartz-Shoram Z, Lautz M, Borenstein R (1987) Vaginal delivery of the second twin in breech presentation. *Obstetrics and Gynecology* **69**:774–776.

84 Gocke SE, Nageotte MP, Garite T, Towers CV, Dorcester W (1989) Management of the non-vertex second twin: Primary caesarean section, external cephalic version or primary breech extraction. *American Journal of Obstetrics and Gynecology* **161**:111–114.

85 Adam C, Alexander CA, Baskett TF (1991) Twin delivery: Influence of the presentation and method of delivery on the second twin. *American Journal of Obstetrics and Gynaecology* **165**:23–27.

86 Rabinovici J, Barhai G, Reichman B, Serr DM, Mashiach S (1988) Internal podalic version with unruptured membranes for the second twin in transverse lie. *Obstetrics and Gynaecology* **71**:428–430.

87 Doyle LW, Hughes CD, Guaran RL, Quinn MA, Kitchen WH (1988) Mode of delivery of preterm twins. *Australia and New Zealand Journal of Obstetrics and Gynaecology* **28**:25–28.

88 Wells SR, Thorp JM, Bowes WA (1991) Management of the nonvertex second twin. *Surgery* **172**:383–385.

11

Threatened and Actual Preterm Labour Including Mode of Delivery

JOHN M. SVIGOS, JEFFREY S. ROBINSON, RASIAH VIGNESWARAN

DEFINITIONS AND INCIDENCE

Preterm labor refers to the onset of labor after the gestation of viability (20–28 weeks, depending on definition) and before 37 completed weeks of pregnancy. The onset of labor may be determined by documented uterine contractions (at least one every 10 min) and reptured fetal membranes or documented cervical change with an estimated length of less than 1 cm and/or a cervical dilation of more than 2 cm. Threatened preterm labor may be diagnosed when there are documented uterine contractions but no evidence of cervical change. Despite these apparently clearly defined entities, because of the need for early management of suspected preterm labor, the diagnosis is commonly made in clinical practice before the above criteria are met, and hence the reported incidence of threatened and actual preterm labor may be open to question.

O'Driscoll[1] suggested that the pregnant woman's diagnosis of preterm labor based on the perception of uterine contractions may be incorrect in as many as 80% of instances, while Kragt and Keirse[2] demonstrated that 33% of women presenting with contractions could be safely discharged home in 48 h without treatment. Amon and Petrie[3] believe that 50% of women presenting with uterine contractions do not need tocolytics, whereas Gonik and Creasy[4] in their review found that only 18–20% of women presenting with possible preterm labor were candidates for long-term tocolytic agents. Even more sobering was Gonik and Creasy's assessment of a 20–45% efficacy rate of placebo treatment for suspected preterm labor.

In South Australia in 1990, the overall preterm delivery rate was 6.7%, of which one-third or 2% was due to preterm labor (PTL) without preterm premature rupture of the membranes (PPROM) as the initiating event.[5] If treatment is only 50% effective, then it is likely that the actual PTL rate without PPROM is 4%; however, if 20–30% can be successfully treated with placebo, then it is likely that there is a 5–6% incidence overall of threatened and actual PTL without PPROM, presenting for management. Tertiary referral centers providing maternal and neonatal intensive care will obviously attract a greater number of women with threatened and actual PTL, which will give workers in those units an exaggerated impression of the true overall incidence. As an illustration, in 1990 the Queen Victoria Hospital – the major perinatal center in South Australia – had a 17.8% preterm birth rate for its obstetric population compared with the 6.7% incidence overall for the state.[6]

Maternal Risks

In considering preterm birth, it is clear that many of its causes have their origins in maternal pathology, which carries a risk for the mother as well as the fetus. Excluding PPROM and 'idiopathic' PTL, which constitute approximately 66% of causes, the two most common maternal conditions associated with preterm birth are pregnancy-induced hypertension and antepartum hemorrhage.[4] These two conditions may either precipitate PTL spontaneously, or prompt the deliberate induction of PTL as a way to resolve the maternal problem or to deliver the fetus from an adverse environment. Induction of labor may of itself carry risks for the mother. Additionally, if 'idiopathic' PTL is studied in detail[7] the following associations have been recognized, viz. intrauterine infection (47%), placental abruption or previa (40%), uterine factors (anomalies, hydramnios, 20%), cervical incompetence (17%), immunological factors (33%), maternal factors (systemic infection, pre-eclampsia, 10%), fetal anomalies (7%), trauma (surgical, others, 3%) and 'idiopathic' (1%). Often more than one factor may be present and will contribute to the maternal risks associated with PTL.

Another area of significant risk to pregnant women with threatened or actual PTL is the risk from the treatment regimens currently employed.

Although beta-sympathomimetic agents have been studied in randomized controlled trials to determine their efficacy in the treatment of PTL, unfortunately the total number of women studied is not able to provide meaningful information regarding the incidence of serious maternal hazards associated with such therapy.[8] Observational studies document subjective maternal symptoms associated with beta-sympathomimetic use and these include palpitations, tremor, nausea, vomiting, headaches, vague uneasiness, thirst, nervousness, restlessness, chest discomfort and shortness of breath, which are all reversible with cessation of the therapy. Pulmonary edema has become increasingly recognized as a serious maternal hazard, with many but not all cases probably being due to fluid overload.[8] The actual incidence of this condition is difficult to estimate from the literature, but varies from 5% of treated women[9] to 'a few cases'.[10] Women receiving associated corticosteroid therapy for fetal lung maturity enhancement, combinations of tocolytic agents (viz, beta-sympathomimetics and magnesium sulfate) and those with multiple pregnancies are reported to be at increased risk of pulmonary edema.[8] Myocardial ischemia, possibly as a result of diffuse myocardial micronecrosis, has been reported in women receiving beta-sympathomimetic tocolytic therapy and constitutes an infrequent but serious maternal hazard.[8,9] A number of maternal biochemical effects occur with these agents, but they rarely cause serious problems unless there are underlying maternal diseases such as diabetes, thyrotoxicosis and cardiac disease. Blood sugar levels increase in approximately 40% of women receiving beta-sympathomimetic agents, particularly if combined with corticosteroid administration, which may occasionally result in severe ketoacidosis in pregnant diabetic women.[8] Serum potassium levels generally fall due to a net influx of potassium from the maternal extracellular into the intracellular fluid compartments as a result of the changes in carbohydrate metabolism. The resulting hypokalemia is usually transient and unlikely to be of serious concern.[8]

Although beta-sympathomimetic tocolytic agents remain the mainstay of contemporary regimens for the treatment of PTL, other agents have been used either solely or in combination and these have the potential to contribute to maternal hazards associated with PTL. Perhaps the most widely used agent in this regard is the prostaglandin synthesis inhibitor, indomethacin. The most likely maternal side-effects of treatment include peptic ulceration, gastrointestinal bleeding, thrombocytopenia and allergic reactions irrespective of the mode of administration and these must be considered when determining the management regimen for PTL.[11-13]

Magnesium sulfate infusions have been used for tocolysis in a number of perinatal centers and an adult respiratory distress-like syndrome has been reported. Additionally, hypermagnesemia may lead to maternal respiratory depression, cardiac arrest and death on rare occasions.[14] Calcium antagonists have been used for tocolysis intermittently following the initial favorable report of Read and Wellby,[15] but insufficient data have so far been collected to make meaningful comments regarding maternal safety. Ethanol, diazoxide and relaxin are no longer used for tocolysis, while progesterone and oxytocin analogs are still undergoing evaluation at this time.[8]

Cesarean section as the preferred mode of delivery for the very preterm infant is a practice which did not receive adequate evaluation before it came into common use, and with it came significant maternal morbidity related to a poorly formed lower uterine segment resulting in an increase in operative hemorrhage, infection and compromised uterine function – all this without documented improvement in perinatal mortality or morbidity.[16,17,18]

A survey of members of the Society of Perinatal Obstetricians (SPO) conducted by Amon et al.[16] regarding the use of elective cesarean section for extreme prematurity demonstrated a doubling of the rate for infants born between 24 and 28 weeks gestation over a 5-year period. Sanchez-Ramos et al.[17] however, were able to demonstrate that a significant decrease in the cesarean section rate over the same 5-year period for very low birthweight infants did not alter the neonatal mortality, the incidence of low Apgar scores, cord blood gas values, intraventricular hemorrhage and the median length of stay in the neonatal intensive care unit.

There is currently no way of accurately assessing the psychosocial trauma experienced by the patient, her partner and her family in relation to the management of threatened or actual PTL. The physical limitations imposed by the medical management, the impersonality of the multidisciplinary approach, the geographical dislocations which are commonly necessary, the uncertainty of the perinatal outcome and delayed maternal–infant bonding are probably the major conflicts experienced and these need to be addressed in order to reduce the maternal risk associated with threatened and actual PTL.

Fetal/Neonatal Risks

Compromised fetal well-being may be the precipitating factor in threatened or actual PTL. Hence the association of intrauterine fetal death, intrauterine growth retardation, major congenital anomalies, unrecognized intrauterine infection and complicated multiple pregnancy will contribute to the perinatal mortality and morbidity associated with PTL.

The fetal gestation at which threatened or actual PTL presents influences both management and outcome. In women presenting between 20 and 25 weeks gestation, the management decision after discussion with the parents may be to allow delivery to occur because of the maternal risks of treatment, and the likely poor prognosis for the baby if, as is often the case, delivery can only be postponed for a few hours or days.

Fetal intrapartum hypoxia and birth trauma associated with PTL involving the very low birthweight infant, whether birth is by the vaginal or abdominal route, will contribute to the perinatal risk. The risks in the neonatal period are those of congenital malformation, the sequelae of intrauterine growth retardation, respiratory distress syndrome, intracranial hemorrhage, convulsions and septicemia.

The fetal and neonatal risks associated with the medical management of preterm labor have not been accurately quantified but certainly require consideration in the overall management of PTL. Beta-sympathomimetic tocolytic agents cross the placenta and may cause fetal tachycardia and occasionally other adverse fetal cardiac effects which may be significant in an already compromised fetus.[8,19] The often associated maternal hyperglycemia with these agents may result in troublesome neonatal hypoglycemia. There is a suggestion that neonatal intraventricular hemorrhage may be associated with oral beta-sympathomimetic drug use, although the data are preliminary.[20] No long-term ill-effects for the neonate otherwise have been observed but the study groups are numerically small.[8]

Prostaglandin synthesis inhibitors cross from the mother to the fetus potentially resulting in prolonged bleeding time, cardiopulmonary effects – predominantly premature closure or constriction of the ductus arteriosis – persistent fetal circulation, renal dysfunction and reduced urinary output.[21] Necrotizing enterocolitis and neonatal intraventricular hemorrhage have also been recorded in association with the use of these agents.[21-23] Consequently, the use of prostaglandin synthesis inhibitors has been limited to short-term therapy (72 h) before 32 weeks gestation.[8]

Magnesium sulfate also readily crosses the placenta and may compromise fetal cardiac activity, with reduced baseline variability of the fetal heart rate demonstrated by cardiotocography being a common association, which in turn may lead to unnecessary intervention, while the neonate may exhibit hypotonia and hypocalcemia as a consequence of hypermagnesemia.[24] Calcium antagonists have not been adequately evaluated with regard to fetal or neonatal effects, but some animal studies have demonstrated profound metabolic alterations in the fetus.[4]

Maternal corticosteroid administration to enhance fetal lung maturity may have a number of possible risks for the neonate, but the available data are inconclusive at this time, particularly with regard to infection, and must be balanced against the proven potential beneficial effect on neonatal pulmonary function.[25] The higher risk of fetal death *in utero* in the preliminary work of Liggins and Howie[26] has not been supported by other studies. The Dutch trial[27] which looked at the effects of maternal prenatal corticosteroid administration suggested a long-term increase in the incidence of pharyngeal and ear infections in treated infants, but also reported no clear evidence of significant fetal or neonatal infection in PTL associated with intact membranes.

Other agents used to enhance fetal or neonatal lung maturity such as antenatal thyrotropin releasing hormone (TRH) and artificial surfactant have not been adequately evaluated for comments to be made at this time.

Management Options

Prepregnancy

The prevention and treatment of preterm birth has been the subject of extensive study. Risk scoring strategies have been devised to assess individual potential for preterm birth based on socioeconomic status, clinical history, lifestyle, and past obstetric and current prenatal complications. Unfortunately, there is insufficient evidence from randomized trials of preterm preventive programs based on prospective risk scoring, whether they be hospital based or requiring local social intervention, to suggest that there has been an overall reduction in the incidence of preterm delivery.[28] This failure is due both to the poor predictive value and specificity of risk factors, and the lack of effective treatments. Hewitt and Newnham's study[29] of very low birthweight infants (weighing less than 1500 g) illustrated the limitations of preterm preventive programs. For infants born without major congenital anomalies, only 24% of the mothers overall had a history of a previous preterm birth. Forty-eight percent of the women were in their first pregnancy, and therefore by definition had no risk factors related to past obstetric history; and of the multiparous women, 38% had no factors in their previous pregnancies indicating high risk. Another important feature revealed by this study was that uncomplicated PTL, the subject of the present chapter, was not the major factor in delivery at early gestations, occurring in only 17% of the women studied, while PPROM occurred in 30% of cases, hypertension in 19%, prenatal hemorrhage in 17%, major anomalies in 8% and fetal death *in utero* in 5%.

Thus blanket preventive programs aimed indiscriminately at preterm delivery would not appear logical other than as part of a scientific trial. However, in counseling individual women with a previous preterm birth, the contribution of a perinatal pathologist[30] can be important in some cases by identifying the likely precipitating etological factor. This can help determine the specific management of further pregnancies.

In the situation of preterm birth without known causation, it is useful in prepregnancy counseling to estimate the likely recurrence risk. In their prospective study of preterm deliveries without uterine anomalies or medical problems, Ashmead *et al.*[31] determined that women with one previous preterm delivery had a 15% chance of another preterm delivery and those with two previous preterm births had a 41% incidence of preterm delivery in a subsequent pregnancy. These statistics may be useful in counseling patients who live in an area remote from tertiary perinatal care, as it can be suggested that they move to temporary accommodation near to an intensive care neonatal unit during the critical period of a subsequent pregnancy. This will at least maximize the availability of skilled perinatal care should they have another preterm birth, and is likely to enhance the chances of the infant's survival.

More general advice with regard to daily work activity (avoidance of heavy manual labor or mental stress, where family economics permit) and specific habits such as smoking, alcohol and drug abuse should be given, as there is some evidence that these factors may play a role in preterm birth.[32]

In summary, therefore, at the present time specific prepregnancy preventative measures for PTL might be considered for multiparous patients; however, for nulliparous patients, apart from those with a known genital tract anomaly where surgical intervention might be possible, there do not appear to be any proven strategies to prevent PTL.[28,29,31]

Prenatal

Assessment of risk

At the first prenatal visit, a risk score for preterm delivery based on the history and examination may be useful as an initial screen to identify women at particularly high risk. The score can be updated during the preg-

nancy if complications develop. An adaptation of the score devised by Creasy *et al.*[33] which combines socioeconomic factors, previous medical history, daily habits and aspects of the current pregnancy, is probably the most acceptable system, but its predictive value overall is not great due to the multifactorial nature of PTL.

In all women, but particulary those at risk of PTL, it is preferable that gestational age be confirmed by an early ultrasound scan.

Women with previous preterm labor delivery

If cervical incompetence is suspected on the basis of previous mid-trimester miscarriage, or known physical damage to the cervix (e.g. following surgery), then cervical cerclage (ideally as a planned procedure) can be performed at 12–14 weeks gestation. This is usually a vaginal procedure, but on rare occasions it may have to be performed by the abdominal route. Late cervical cerclage in the face of cervical dilation is a less successful procedure and should only be considered under exceptional circumstances.[34]

In acknowledgement of the increasing emphasis on the role of subclinical infection in PTL,[35] particularly if an infective etiology is suspected from a previous preterm birth, it seems reasonable to take vaginal and cervical microbiological swabs electively in high-risk women at 20–24 weeks gestation. Even if the patient is not subjected to prophylactic antibiotic therapy (see later), a knowledge of the potential microbiological milieu at the time of PTL will assist both the obstetrician in the management of maternal pyrexia and the neonatologist in the management of suspected infection in the perterm infant.

Education of the patient with a previous preterm birth of the signs and symptoms of PTL is a useful option to consider. The perception of contractions, menstrual-like cramps, pelvic pressure sensation, low dull backache, abdominal cramping with or without diarrhea, an increase or change in vaginal discharge and a 'show' may all prove to be significant, but are not particularly predictive individually for determining the onset of PTL.[36] Nonetheless, if they occur in any women at risk of PTL, careful cervical assessment should be performed.

In those women suspected of being at an increased risk of PTL, more frequent prenatal assessment – particularly in the latter half of pregnancy – is a common option employed. The rationale for this form of management is based on indirect evidence that absent or delayed onset of prenatal care is associated with an increased rate of preterm birth and low birthweight infants. Of course, it is possible that those patients who are sufficiently motivated to seek more regular prenatal care are intrinsically healthier and better motivated than those who do not seek early prenatal care, but this is only one aspect to consider. Not only is the frequency of care related to outcome, but also the type of care. Beuscher and Ward[37] have shown that a greater use of non-medical support services in addition to traditional prenatal care improves the outcome when comparing care given by general practitioners as distinct from hospital-based care with its greater capacity to provide support services. Bowes[38] perhaps best summarized the contributions of prenatal care in preterm birth management by suggesting that success is related to continuity of care, time available for patients to talk about their problems, ready access to ancillary services when needed, and a prenatal record that provides failsafe reminders of critical procedures and screening tests.

Out-patient and home monitoring of uterine contractility have been used either solely or in conjunction with cervical examination[4,39,40] to identify women at high risk of preterm delivery in the index pregnancy. Although the devices currently used are able to detect uterine activity, there is substantial overlap between those women experiencing Braxton-Hicks contractions and those experiencing the contractions of early labor, which must cast some doubt on tocography as a screening test. However, those women who go on to deliver preterm appear to have more than average uterine activity.[39,40] There is some evidence that twice daily uterine activity monitoring of very high-risk women in conjunction with daily nursing support and immediately available obstetric care may prevent preterm births, but it is not clear if tocography is the major contributor to this success.[4,39,40] An analysis of the relevant randomized trials conducted to date reveals that they are of limited size, and their randomization procedures have also been questioned. At the present time, prenatal tocography cannot be recommended as part of the routine management of women at risk of PTL.[39]

Regular cervical assessment on a weekly basis from 24 weeks gestation as a predictor of PTL has had varying support for many years. A sensitivity of at least 60% and specificity of 75% makes cervical assessment the most reliable clinical method available at present for predicting PTL.[4,40,41] Early concerns regarding the possibility of precipitating PTL, PPROM or ascending uterine infection by digital cervical assessment[42] have not been confirmed by subsequent studies.[43,44] Additionally, cervical assessment has been shown to be an even more sensitive predictor of PTL in multiple pregnancy than in singleton pregnancy.[44] Cervical dilation has been shown to be a better predictor than cervical effacement of PTL and this casts doubt on the studies of ultrasound assessment of cervical length as a predictor of PTL,[45,46] although Stock and Haines[47] have shown that the measurement of cervical dilatation by ultrasound is more promising.

A number of strategies using prophylactic oral tocolytics, antibiotics and corticosteroids have been employed in the prenatal management of women at high risk of PTL and deserve further discussion. Several controlled trials of the prophylactic administration of beta-sympathomimetic drugs for the prevention of PTL have been reported in the literature.[8] They give no indication that these agents decrease the incidence of preterm delivery or low birthweight in multiple or singleton pregnancies, with the odds ratios being 1.17 and 1.02, respectively.[8] Consideration of the three available prospectively randomized trials of prophylactic antibiotic therapy in the prevention of PTL[35] suggests that there is no significant difference in the incidence of preterm birth and low birthweight between the treated and the placebo groups, although there may be a possible reduction in the incidence of PPROM. The outcome of further studies is awaited with interest.

The use of prophylactic maternal corticosteroids to enhance fetal lung maturity in women at very high risk of PTL, particularly those women with higher-order multifetal pregnancies, has not been examined in detail, although this is a common practice. The Collaborative Group on Antenatal Steroid Therapy[48] raised questions regarding the dosage and frequency of administration of corticosteroids in this situation but to date these questions remain unanswered.

Women presenting with threatened or actual preterm labor

Once the diagnosis of threatened or actual PTL is established, parenteral tocolytic therapy should be considered. After a careful clinical appraisal of the maternal and fetal condition, the following preliminary investigations should be performed. Ultrasound will determine fetal well-being, fetal number, estimated fetal weight, fetal morphology and presentation, volume of amniotic fluid and the placental site. Fetal breathing movements may also be assessed during this evaluation and have been used to predict the likelihood of PTL.[49]

Testing for an infective etiology is important in the initial assessment and includes vaginal and cervical microbiological cultures, midstream specimen of urine culture, complete blood picture and C-reactive protein. Amniocentesis may be considered if infection is suspected and at the same time fetal lung maturity and possibly fetal karyotype can also be evaluated, though not all obstetricians would perform this procedure because of the possibility of inducing uterine activity. Determination of the presence or absence of PPROM by clinical and if necessary additional investigations is essential to the management.

Once fetal gestation is established, the universally poor fetal outcome of infants born between 20 and 25 weeks gestation[16,50] requires considerable discussion between the parents, the obstetrician and the neonatologist either before or shortly after the initiation of tocolytic therapy. The parents may choose to allow delivery to occur in the face of extreme fetal immaturity, but caution must be exercised because fetal weight and gestational estimates are subject to great variation between 20 and 25 weeks. Perhaps a more pragmatic method of dealing with this dilemma is to transfer the patient to a tertiary center and allow her to deliver vaginally without intervention but with a neonatologist present at delivery to assess the delivered neonate with regard to the potential of further neonatal support. Whether continuous fetal monitoring should be carried out during such a labor is a matter of dispute. Some argue that recording a potentially abnormal fetal heart rate while prescribing non-intervention is distressing for parents and staff, while others argue that the normality or otherwise of the fetal heart rate may be important for the pediatrician when he decides whether or not to resuscitate/support the neonate.

The use of tocolytic therapy between 25 and 34 weeks gestation is not only to facilitate the *in utero* transfer of the fetus to a tertiary referral centre,[51] but also to enable sufficient time to enhance fetal lung maturity by the concomitant use of maternal corticosteroid therapy. Overall, the data of the 15 studies considered by Keirse *et al.*[8] demonstrate that beta-sympathomimetic drug therapy results in a lower incidence of preterm birth than observed without such treatment. Although the low birthweight incidence was reduced by beta-sympathomimetic therapy, the relationship to an observed lengthening of gestation did not reach statistical significance. This negative relationship and a lack of a detectable decrease in perinatal mortality and morbidity may have been due to the use of tocolysis after 34 weeks gestation when any beneficial effect was unlikely, and there may have been direct adverse effects (previously discussed) and indirect adverse effects, including the prolongation of the pregnancy contrary to the best interests of the baby, i.e. in the presence of abruptio placenta, hypertension and intrauterine growth retardation.[8] Contraindications to parenteral tocolysis, particularly beta-sympathomimetic agents, include fetal death, fetal distress, fetal abnormality incompatible with survival, fetal lung maturity demonstrated by an L/S ratio >2, chorioamnionitis, antepartum hemorrhage, maternal disease (cardiac, hyperthyroidism), obstetric indications for delivery (severe pre-eclampsia) and possibly PPROM.

With all tocolytics but particularly beta-sympathomimetics, the danger of pulmonary edema must be counteracted by careful attention to the patient's fluid balance and the known side-effects of these agents. Magnesium sulfate, although of unproven benefit, can be given intravenously as an alternative tocolytic and therapeutic levels must be monitored every 8 h by magnesium blood levels and careful clinical assessment. Calcium gluconate should be available to reverse any toxic effects of magnesium sulfate.

Tocolytic therapy should be continued if possible for 48 h to try to maximize the fetal lung enhancement effect of maternally administered corticosteroids. Data from 12 controlled trials reviewed by Crowley *et al.*[52] and a more recent meta-analysis by R. J. Lilford (personal communication) demonstrated that corticosteroids reduce the occurrence of respiratory distress syndrome overall, and this reduction in respiratory morbidity was also associated with reductions in the risk of intraventricular hemorrhage, necrotizing enterocolitis and neonatal death.

The Queen Victoria Hospital is the coordinating center for a randomized controlled trial of the concomitant use of maternally administered thyrotropin-releasing hormone (TRH), which has been shown in preliminary studies to enhance lung maturity (C. Crowther, personal communication). The results of this trial have yet to be evaluated and at the present time TRH cannot be recommended as an option in the routine management of PTL.

If the initially selected tocolytic agent is unsuccessful, or is not tolerated in the suppression of PTL, then an alternative agent may be considered. This can be given alone or in combination with the initial agent. Any such strategy should only be instituted after careful re-evaluation of maternal and fetal well-being.

After the initial 48 h of labor suppression, some workers have used oral tocolytic agents until 34–37 weeks gestation in an effort to prolong gestation. Although this option has shown some benefit,[8] it has not been commonly employed by many perinatal centers.

Treatment of PTL after 34 weeks gestation has received considerable attention in the literature and it would appear that the neonatal morbidity following delivery between 34 and 37 weeks is unchanged whether or not attempts to arrest labor are successful.[53] The additional expense and the maternal risks of tocolytics do not appear justified in the treatment of PTL after 34 weeks gestation.

Labor/delivery

When preterm delivery seems inevitable, then clearly the mode of delivery and the neonatal outcome should be discussed with the parents. Not only should the parents discuss the management with an obstetrician and a neonatologist, but an experienced obstetric anesthetist[54] is essential in establishing management guidelines acceptable to all parties. In those cases where labor is usually attended by midwives, they should also be included in all discussions concerning management.

In general, before 26 weeks gestation, vaginal delivery should be the accepted mode with expert neonatal evaluation at delivery to determine if further supportive neonatal care is warranted. Between 26 and 34 weeks gestation, the management of labor should not differ from that past 34 weeks gestation,[17,18] with perhaps the preterm breech presentation having special consideration (see Chapter 13).[55] Continuous electronic fetal monitoring and a preference for epidural analgesia are unproven but are commonly employed options in the contemporary management of established preterm labor.

Evaluation of the randomized trials available would suggest that 'prophylactic' outlet forceps or 'elective' episiotomy do not contribute favorably to the neonatal outcome and hence should only be performed for standard obstetric indications.[55] Early cord clamping has not been proven to confer an advantage to the fetus and so cannot be recommended in the routine management of a preterm birth.[56] Standard management of the third stage is recommended in preterm delivery.[55]

From the neonatal aspect, the significantly higher risk of mortality and morbidity when extremely premature infants are delivered outside a tertiary care center makes a compelling argument for maternal–fetal transport to a perinatal center with neonatal intensive care facilities,[57] providing such transport does not jeopardize the safety of the mother. However, it is estimated that maternal–fetal transport is not possible in up to 50% of high-risk pregnancies. In these situations, a specifically trained neonatal retrieval team with nursing and medical personnel should be present at the delivery in order to stabilize the premature infant prior to transfer to the tertiary perinatal center if this seems necessary.[57]

Postnatal

Maternal considerations

Encouragement of parent–infant bonding is a major consideration in postnatal management. Continuous access of the parents to the neonatal nursery should be encouraged to facilitate the bonding process. Breastfeeding should be encouraged in a compassionate and pragmatic manner.

Continuing psychosocial support utilizing the services of a domiciliary midwife, a social worker and if indicated a psychiatrist are essential factors in the management, particularly if there is neonatal death.

An early postnatal evaluation of possible etiological factors related to the PTL should be considered by the perinatal team, which should include an obstetrician, a neonatologist and a perinatal pathologist, with input from other professionals such as an obstetric physician, pediatric surgeon, a geneticist and an ultrasonologist where indicated in order to construct a rational plan of management for further pregnancies.

Neonatal considerations
(see also Chapter 72)

Premature birth requires adaptation to extrauterine life while the different organ systems undergo continued structural and functional development and maturation. Thus premature infants can be expected to have a variety of problems in the neonatal period with the risk of complications being proportional to the degree of prematurity.

Premature infants are likely to have difficulties in maintaining body temperature and in oral feeding. They are also at greater risk of infection. Lung maturity of premature infants is proportional to their gestation, and immaturity is the major cause of respiratory distress syndrome in these infants. Poorly developed respiratory control may lead to recurrent apnea in premature infants.

Congestive cardiac failure may occur as a result of a patent ductus arteriosus associated with prematurity. Due to liver immaturity, neonatal jaundice is likely to be more severe and the baby is more vulnerable to the neurotoxic effects of unconjugated bilirubin. There is an increased risk of intracranial hemorrhage and necrotizing enterocolitis in these infants, while in the extremely premature infant chronic lung disease, retinopathy of prematurity and developmental delay are all more likely.[58]

Lung maturity is the key factor determining the ultimate prognosis of the premature infant. Minimizing the incidence and severity of respiratory distress has been the major factor in the substantial improvement in neonatal morbidity and mortality over the past two decades. Previously mentioned strategies of regionalization of high-risk maternal and neonatal care, effective use of tocolytic agents and antenatal administration of corticosteroids to enhance fetal lung maturity have all been positive contributing factors. Evaluation of the 'prophylactic use' of exogenous surfactant has demonstrated a favorable outcome with a reduction in the incidence of respiratory distress syndrome,[59,60] while the course of established respiratory distress can be significantly modified by the administration of surfactant therapy in association with mechanical respiratory support.[61]

A summary of three separate reports based on a careful assessment of gestational age has shown a significant increase in survival rates at 26–27 weeks of gestation over the past decade.[62] However, it appears that prematurity per se has a deleterious effect on neonatal growth and development, consequently contributing to a poor outcome (E. Q. Goldson, unpublished). This aspect must be taken into account particularly when assessing survival rates in premature infants in the less than 26 weeks gestational age group (so-called 'previable group').[63]

Despite substantial medical advances in neonatal

THREATENED AND ACTUAL PRETERM LABOR/DELIVERY
Summary of Management Options

Prepregnancy (previous preterm delivery)

- Establish cause/precipitating factors
- Estimate risk of recurrence
- Honesty about value of preventitive measures
- General non-specific strategies (advice about diet, smoking, alcohol and drug abuse)

Prenatal

Assessment of risk

- Formal scoring system
- Establish gestational age early and accurately

Previous preterm labor/delivery

- General non-specific strategies (advice about diet, smoking, alcohol and drug abuse)
- If cervical incompetence, suture at 12–14 weeks
- Patient education about clinical features
- ? Value of bacteriological vaginal screening
- ? Value of increased attendance
- Other strategies which need more research work but of no current proven value in reducing incidence of preterm labor delivery:
  - monitoring uterine activity
  - regular cervical assessments
  - prophylactic beta-sympathomimetics
  - prophylactic antibiotics
  - steroids (though these are sensible to reduce risks of RDS in women at risk)

Presenting with threatened or actual preterm labor

Initial assessment to determine whether genuine preterm labor

- Uterine activity, bleeding, membrane rupture, presentation, engagement of head, cervical status, fetal breathing
- Gestational age

Search for a cause/precipitating factor, e.g.

- Fetal abnormality
- Placental bleeding
- Infection
- Multiple pregnancy

- Membrane rupture

Consider specific management strategies

- Transfer to tertiary center
- i.v. tocolytic therapy (influenced by factors including gestation, cause, contraindications)
- Beta-sympathomimetics most widely used (alternatives are magnesium sulfate, indomethacin, nifedipine). Justified for at least 48 h to administer steroids; probably not justified beyond 34 weeks
- Consider oral therapy after successful i.v. treatment
- BEWARE PULMONARY EDEMA AND HYPERGLYCEMIA
- Steroids (? plus TRH)

Labor/delivery

Before 26 weeks

- Careful discussion with parents
- Aim for vaginal delivery; experienced pediatrician in attendance

After 26 weeks

- If cephalic presentation, aim for vaginal delivery with cesarean for normal obstetric indications
- If breech presentation, see Chapter 13
- Continuous fetal heart rate monitoring
- Many use regional analgesia
- Instrumental vaginal delivery only for standard obstetric indications
- Experienced pediatrician in attendance (see also Chapters 71 and 72)

Postnatal

Maternal

- Encourage breast-feeding
- Psychological support
- Give adequate information about baby
- Allow continuous access to neonatal care unit
- Look for causes/precipitating factors and establish plan for future pregnancies

Neonatal

- See Chapter 72

intensive care, it must be emphasized that every premature newborn infant cannot be salvaged and on occasions survival will be accompanied with severe handicap – physical and/or mental. Prolonging life in these circumstances may not be beneficial to the infant and may be unacceptably burdensome to the parents. Consideration of withdrawing life support in such tragic situations should be undertaken after detailed and extensive consultation and counseling of the parents.[64]

The final measure of the quality of a neonatal intensive care unit is its long-term follow-up program. All tertiary care centers should be prepared to maintain this essential service in order to practice early intervention for physical and mental handicaps in premature infants and also to provide advice, support, reassurance and counseling for the parents who bear the brunt of the care of the infant who is born prematurely.

FUTURE DEVELOPMENTS

The placebo-controlled trials of tocolytic agents in active PTL have demonstrated that many women are treated unnecessarily while in other women the treatment is ineffective in significantly delaying delivery.

It seems likely that the etiology of PTL will take a long time to unravel because of its multi-factorial nature, and thus specific preventive measures are unlikely to make significant headway in reducing preterm birth in the near future. Consequently, future developments should perhaps focus on distinguishing which women in threatened preterm labor will actually go on to deliver and those who will not, in order that women need not be exposed to treatments from which they will not benefit. To this end, the presence of an elusive biochemical marker has been sought for some time and the recent preliminary studies of onco-fetal fibronectin[65,66] appear to show some promise for the future.

REFERENCES

1   O'Driscoll M (1977) Preterm labour. In Anderson A, Beard R, Brudenall JM, Dunn PM (eds) *Proceedings of the Fifth Study Group of the Royal College of Obstetricians and Gynaecologists*, pp. 369–370. London: Royal College of Obstetricians and Gynaecologists

2   Kragt H, Keirse MJNC (1989) How accurate is a women's diagnosis of threatened preterm delivery. In Chalmers I, Enkin M, Keirse MJNS (eds) *Preterm Labour: Effective Care in Pregnancy and Childbirth*, Vol. 1, pp. 694–745. Oxford: Oxford University Press.

3   Amon E, Petrie RH (1988) Tocolytic Agents. In Charles D, Glover DD (eds) *Current Therapy in Obstetrics*, pp. 267–270. Toronto: Decker.

4   Gonik B, Creasy RK (1986) Preterm labor: Its diagnosis and management. *American Journal of Obstetrics and Gynecology* **154**:3–9.

5   Chan A, Scott J, McCaul K (1992) *Pregnancy Outcome in South Australia 1990*. Annual Report of the Pregnancy Outcome Unit, Epidemiology Branch, South Australian Health Commission.

6   *Pregnancy and Neonatal Care Bulletin* (1990) Obstetric profile, Queen Victoria Hospital. Pregnancy Outcome Unit, Epidemiology Branch, South Australian Health Commission.

7   Lettieri L, Vintzileos A, Albini M, Martins M, Salafia C, Mead J (1992) Does 'idiopathic' preterm labor exist? 12th Anuual SPO Meeting No. 313. *American Journal of Obstetrics and Gynecology* **166**:363.

8   Keirse MJNC, Grant A, King JF (1989) Preterm labour. In Chalmers I, Erkin M, Keirse MJNC (eds) *Preterm Labour: Effective Care in Pregnancy and Childbirth*, Vol. 1, pp. 694–745. Oxford: Oxford University Press.

9   Katz M, Robertson PA, Creasy RK (1981) Cardiovascular complications associated with terbutaline treatment for preterm labor. *American Journal of Obstetrics and Gynecology* **25**:182–183.

10   Ingemarsson I, Azulkumaran S, Kottegoda SR (1985) Complications of betamimetic therapy in preterm labor. *Australia and New Zealand Journal of Obstetrics and Gynaecology* **25**:182–185.

11   Zuckerman J, Reiss U, Rubinstein I (1974) Inhibition of human premature labor by indomethacin. *Obstetrics and Gynecology* **44**:787–790.

12   Zuckerman H, Shalev E, Gilad G, Katzuni E (1984) Further study of the inhibition of premature labor by indomethacin. Part II: Double-blind study. *Journal of Perinatal Medicine* **12**:25–28.

13   Gamissans O, Balasch J (1984) Prostaglandin synthetase inhibitors in the treatment of preterm labor. In Fuchs F, Stubblefield PG (eds) *Preterm Birth: Causes, Prevention and Management*, pp. 223–248. New York: Macmillan.

14   Ferguson JE, Hensleigh P, Kredenster D (1984) Adjunctive use of magnesium sulphate with ritodrine for preterm labor tocolytics. *American Journal of Obstetrics and Gynecology* **148**:166–171.

15   Read MD, Wellby DE (1986) The use of a calcium antagonist (nifedipine) to suppress preterm labour. *Births Journal of Obstetrics and Gynaecology* **93**:933–937.

16   Amon E, Moyn S (1992) Caesarean section for fetal indications at the limits of fetal viability (1986–1991). 12th Annual SPO Meeting No. 4. *American Journal of Obstetrics and Gynecology* **166**:274.

17   Sanchez-Ramos L, Walker C, Briones D, Cullen MT (1992) Decreasing caesarean section rates in very low birthweight infants: Effective on perinatal outcome. *American Journal of Obstetrics and Gynecology* **166**:444–446.

18   Todd AL, Trudinger BJ, Cole MJ, Cooney GH (1992) Antenatal tests of fetal welfare and development at age 2 years. *American Journal of Obstetrics and Gynecology* **167**:66–69.

19   Friedman DM, Blackstone J, Hoskins I (1992) Adverse fetal cardiac effects of oral ritodrine tocolysis. 12th

Anuual SPO Meeting No. 17. *American Journal of Obstetrics and Gynecology* **166**:326.

20 Groome LJ, Goldenberg RL, Cliver SP, Davis RD, Copper RL (1992) Neonatal intraventricular haemorrhage (IVH) following maternal betasympathomimetic tocolysis. 12th Anuual SPO Meeting No. 5. *American Journal of Obstetrics and Gynecology* **166**:275.

21 Gersony WM, Peckham GJ, Ellison RC, Miettinen OS, Nadas AS (1983) Effects of indomethacin in premature infants with patent ductus arteriosus: Results of a national collaborative study. *Journal of Pediatrics* **102**:895–896.

22 Gleason CA (1987) Prostaglandins and the developing kidney. *Seminars in Perinatology* **11**:12–21.

23 Hennessy MD, Livinston EC, Papagianos J, Killam AP (1992) The incidence of ductal contriction and oligohydramnios during tocolytic therapy with ibuprofen. 12th Annual SPO Meeting No. 163. *American Journal of Obstetrics and Gynecology* **166**:324.

24 Wright JW, Wright BD, Ridgeway LE, Covington DI, Bobitt JR (1992) Effects of magnesium sulphate on fetal heart rate monitoring in the preterm fetus. 12th Annual SPO Meeting No. 138. *American Journal of Obstetrics and Gynecology* **166**:317.

25 Taeusch HW (1975) Glucocorticoid prophylaxis for respiratory distress syndrome: A review of potential toxicity. *Journal of Pediatrics* **87**:617–619.

26 Liggins GC, Howie RN (1972) A controlled trial of antepartum glucocorticoid treatment for prevention of the respiratory distress syndrome in premature infants. *Pediatrics* **50**:515–517.

27 Smolders de Haas H, Neuvel J, Schmard B, Treffers PE, Koppe J, Hocks J (1990) Physical development and medical history of children who were treated antenatally with corticosteroids to prevent respiratory distress syndrome: A 10–12 year follow-up. *Pediatrics* **74**:132–138.

28 Connon AF (1992) An assessment of key aetiological factors associated with preterm birth and perinatal mortality. *Australia and New Zealand Journal of Obstetrics and Gynaecology* **32**:200–202.

29 Hewitt BG, Newnham JP (1988) A review of the obstetric and medical complications leading to the delivery of very low birth weight infants? *Medical Journal of Australia* **1**:149:234–237.

30 Chambers H (1990) The perinatal autopsy. *Medical Journal of Australia* **1**:153:578–579.

31 Ashmead G, Burrows W, Krew M, Ashmead J, Mann L (1990) Predicting preterm labour and birth. 12th Annual SPO Meeting No. 486. *American Journal of Obstetrics and Gynecology* **164**:379.

32 Fox SH, Brown C, Koontz AM, Kessel SS (1990) NHIS findings. *Public Health Reports* **102**:73–75.

33 Creasy RK, Gummer BA, Liggins GC (1980) A system for predicting spontaneous preterm birth. *Obstetrics and Gynecology* **55**:692–698.

34 Balucci J, Drews M, Rawlinson K, Fenton AN (1991) Cervical cerclage: Risks versus benefits. *American Journal of Obstetrics and Gynecology* **165**:380.

35 Gibbs RS, Romero R, Hillier SL, Eschenbach DA, Sweet RL (1992) A review of premature birth and subclinical infection. *American Journal of Obstetrics and Gynecology* **166**:1515–1528.

36 Iams JD, Parker M, Johnson FF (1992) Prospective evaluation of symptoms preceding preterm labor. 12th Annual SPO Meeting No. 324. *American Journal of Obstetrics and Gynecology* **166**:366.

37 Beuscher PA, Ward NI (1992) Preterm birth and low birth weight incidence with comprehensive prenatal care. *Public Health Reports* **107**:54–57.

38 Bowes WA (1992) Editorial. *Obstetrical and Gynecological Survey* **47**:474.

39 Rhoads GG, McNellis DC, Kessel SS (1991) Home monitoring of uterine contractility. Am. J. Obstet. *American Journal of Obstetrics and Gynecology* **165**:2–7.

40 Catalano PM, Ashinkaga T, Mann LI (1989) Cervical change and uterine activity as predictors of preterm delivery. *American Journal of Perinatology* **6**:185–187.

41 Smeltzer J, Lewis J, Van Dorsten P, Cruikshank D (1992) Cervical dilation is the best predictor of risk for preterm birth. *American Journal of Obstetrics and Gynecology* **166**:364–366.

42 Lenihan JP (1984) Relationship of antepartum pelvic examinations to premature rupture of the membranes. *Obstetrics and Gynecology* **83**:33–35.

43 Holbrook RH, Lirette M, Creasy RK (1985) Weekly examination in the patient as high risk for preterm delivery. *Proceeding of the Society of Perinatal Obstetrics* **1**:27.

44 Dyson DC (1990) Preterm birth prevention in twin gestations. 10th Annual SPO Meeting. *American Journal of Obstetrics and Gynecology* **164**:324.

45 Paraskos J, Waxman M, Johnson F, Teteris J, Iams JD (1992) Ultrasound assessment of cervical length in preterm labor. *American Journal of Obstetrics and Gynecology* **166**:364–365.

46 Mulla WR, Eife S, Jackson GM, Ludmir J (1992) Observer variability in sonographic assessment of cervical length. *American Journal of Obstetrics and Gynecology* **166**:332.

47 Stock A, Haines CJ (1992) Transabdominal ultrasound assessment of cervical dilation in preterm labour. *Australia and New Zealand Journal of Obstetrics and Gynaecology* **32**:280–281.

48 Collaborative Group on Antenatal Steroid Therapy (1981) Effect of antenatal dexamethasone therapy on prevention of respiratory distress syndrome. *American Journal of Obstetrics and Gynecology* **141**:276–279.

49 Boddy K, Dawes GD, Robinson J (1974) Intrauterine fetal breathing movement. In Gluck L (ed.) *Modern Perinatal Medicine*, pp. 381–392. Chicago, IL: Year Book Publishers.

50 Robertson PA, Sniderman SH, Laros RK, Cowan R, Heilbron D, Goldenberg RL, Iams JD, Creasy RK (1992) Neonatal morbidity according to gestational age and birthweight from five tertiary care centres in the United States 1983 through 1986. *American Journal of Obstetrics and Gynecology* **166**:1629–1635.

51 Tsokos N, Newnham J, Langford SA (1988) Intravenous tocolytic therapy for long distance aeromedical transport of women in preterm labour in Western Australia. *Asia-Oceania Journal of Obstetrics and Gynaecology* **14**:21–22.

52 Crowley P, Chalmers I, Keirse MJNC (1990) The effects of corticosteroid administration before preterm

delivery: An overview of the evidence from controlled trials. *British Journal of Obstetrics and Gynaecology* **97**:11–17.

53 Fox JF, McCaul RW, Martin WE, Roberts WE, McLaughlin B, Morrison JC (1992) Neonatal morbidity between 34–37 weeks gestation. *American Journal of Obstetrics and Gynecology* **166**:360–363.

54 Crowhurst JA (1992) Epidural blockade in obstetrics – how safe? *Medical Journal of Australia* **157**:220–222.

55 Weiner C, Estle E, (1992) Vaginal breech delivery in the 1980s – preterm gestation. *American Journal of Obstetrics and Gynecology* **166**:396.

56 Keirse MJNC (1989) In Chalmers I, Enkin M, Keirse MJNC (eds) *Preterm Labour: Effective Care in Pregnancy and Childbirth*, Vol. 2, pp. 695–745. Oxford: Oxford University Press.

57 Paneth N (1987) The effect of the choice of place of delivery and hospital level on mortality in all singleton births in New York City. *American Journal of Diseases of Children* **141**:60–66.

58 Kitchen W, Yu VYH, Orgill AA (1982) Infants born before 29 weeks gestation: Survival and morbidity at 2 years of age. *British Journal of Obstetrics and Gynaecology* **89**:887–889.

59 Corbett A, Bucciarelli R, Goldman S (1991) Decreased mortality rate in small premature infants treated at birth with a single dose of synthetic surfactant: A multicentre controlled trial. *Journal of Pediatrics* **118**:277–280.

60 Long, W, Stevenson D, Pauly T (1991) Effects of a single prophylactic dose of Exosurf Neonatal in 215, 500–700 gram infants. *Pediatric Research* **29**:223A.

61 Gitlin JD, Soll RF, Parar RB (1987) A randomised controlled trial of exogenous surfactant for the treatment of hyaline membrane disease. *Pediatrics* **79**:31–33.

62 Creasy RD (1990) Assessment and care of the fetus. In Eden RD, Buehm FK (eds) *Preterm Labor* pp. 617–633. New York: Oxford University Press.

63 Nwaesi CG, Young DC, Byrne JM (1987) Preterm birth at 23–26 weeks gestation: Is active management justified? *American Journal of Obstetrics and Gynecology* **157**:890.

64 Young ENT, Stevenson DK (1990) Limiting treatment for extremely premature low birth weight infants (500–700 grams). *American Journal of Diseases of Children* **144**:549–552.

65 Garite TJ (1991) Oncofetal fibronectin in cervico-vaginal secretions is highly predictive of preterm delivery. *American Journal of Obstetrics and Gynecology* **164**:259–260.

66 Nageotte MP, Hollenback KA, Vanderwahl BA, Hutch KM (1992) Circulating cellular fibronectin in the prediction of preterm labor. *American Journal of Obstetrics and Gynecology* **166**:270–273.

12

Premature Rupture of the Membranes

JOHN M. SVIGOS, JEFFREY S. ROBINSON, RASIAH VIGNESWARAN

DEFINITIONS AND INCIDENCE

Premature rupture of the membranes (PROM) is an obstetric conundrum; poorly defined with an obscure etiology, difficulties in diagnosis, associated significant maternal, fetal and neonatal risks, and management strategies which are often diverse and controversial. It may be defined as rupture of the fetal membranes with a latent period before the onset of spontaneous uterine activity. The length of this latent period varies in different definitions from not being specified to up to 8 h.

It is generally accepted that PROM occurs in 10% of all pregnancies,[1] with the majority of cases occurring after 37 completed weeks of gestation. If PROM occurs before 37 completed weeks of gestation, then the condition is referred to as preterm premature rupture of the membranes (PPROM). This occurs in approximately 2% of all pregnancies.[2-4] These statistics refer to the general obstetric population, but clearly the incidence of PROM recorded for any particular hospital will be determined by the level of perinatal care provided, and hence in a hospital accepting fetal–maternal transfers the incidence of PPROM may be recorded as 5% of all pregnancies delivering there.[5]

Maternal Risks

There are significant maternal risks associated with PROM, more particularly with PPROM, and these can occur antepartum, intrapartum and postpartum. Although the incidence of subclinical chorioamnionitis may be as high as 30% with PROM,[6] serious maternal systemic infection is rare if treatment is initiated promptly.[7]

The use of a number of therapeutic agents such as corticosteroids, antibiotics and tocolytic agents, particularly with PPROM, may pose some maternal risk and these must be considered in the overall management. Abruptio placenta is evident in 4–7% of women with PPROM, and hence vaginal bleeding in the presence of premature rupture of the membranes must be regarded seriously and managed accordingly.[8-10]

The undoubted psychosocial sequelae particularly related to PPROM, with the disruption created by maternal hospitalization and continued observation associated with the uncertain fetal/neonatal prognosis, should never be underestimated and should be addressed on an individual basis in the overall management.

The maternal intrapartum consequences of PROM are predominantly related to the induction of labor. The latent phase of labor under these circumstances may be as long as 16–20 h, and thus unrealistic limits must not be set regarding the duration of labor when counseling the patient and attendant staff. The increased likelihood of operative delivery associated with induction of labor will increase the chance of maternal complications.[11]

Pathological examination of placentas associated with PROM demonstrates an increased incidence of marginal cord insertion and battledore placentas, which may account for the increased incidence of retained placentas in this condition.[12] This in turn may be associated with the known increase in the incidence of primary and secondary postpartum hemorrhage. The latter complication is also probably associated with the 10% incidence of endomyometritis which occurs with premature rupture of the membranes.

The complications described above account for a significant proportion of puerperal maternal morbidity, while the impaired maternal–infant bonding particularly seen with PPROM, and which results in maternal psychological and lactation problems, will contribute to the remainder.

Neonatal Risks

Prematurity is the most significant factor in the increased perinatal morbidity and mortality associated with premature rupture of the membranes, because delivery occurs within 7 days of PPROM in over 80% of cases.[13,14]

Although the incidence of chorioamnionitis is 30%, the reported incidence of neonatal sepsis is only 2–4%.[15–17] Gestational age at the time of rupture of the membranes will have some influence on the incidence of neonatal sepsis (the earlier the gestation the greater the chance of infection), as will the length of the latent period (the longer the latent period the less the chance of infection).

Oligohydramnios, particularly if there is prolonged PPROM, may result in the neonatal 'oligohydramnios tetrad' of facial anomalies, limb position defects, pulmonary hypoplasia and impaired fetal growth, all of which will add to the neonatal morbidity.[13]

Fetal distress is also more likely to be due to the greater possibility of cord prolapse, cord compression and abruptio placenta associated with premature rupture of the membranes, particularly with PPROM. Neonatal morbidity will also be increased because of the mechanical difficulties encountered with delivery, either by the vaginal or abdominal route, as a result of the increased incidence of malpresentations and reduced volume of amniotic fluid.

Management Options

Prepregnancy

Prepregnancy counseling has only a limited role in the management of premature rupture of the membranes, particularly in relation to PPROM. The recurrence rate for PPROM has not yet been examined in depth, but Naeye's observations in 1982 suggested a 21% recurrence rate,[18] while in a smaller but more recent study Asrat *et al.*[19] have suggested that the recurrence rate may be of the order of 32%.

In considering the known etiological associations of PPROM examined in detail by Harger *et al.*,[20] the only independent risk factor which might be amenable to

prepregnancy interventional strategies was cigarette smoking.

Increasing emphasis has been placed on the association of premature rupture of the membranes with maternal vaginal colonization of potentially pathogenic microorganisms. Hence prepregnancy vaginal cultures and antimicrobial treatment may offer some potential benefit, although this has not been proven.[21] Antimicrobial treatment of the sexual partner is even more controversial, while the restriction of coital activity during the course of further pregnancies would appear to be unnecessarily restrictive given the evidence available at present.

Prenatal

Diagnosis and further assessment

The diagnosis of premature rupture of the membranes requires a judicious assessment of the history, clinical findings and specialized testing. Whenever the history is suggestive of PROM, a sterile vaginal speculum examination should be performed. Visualization of amniotic fluid draining through the cervix provides the most reliable diagnosis. In cases of doubt, demonstration that vaginal fluid has an alkaline pH on nitrazine yellow testing (the pH indicator turning black) is suggestive, but not conclusive evidence, of PROM. The normal vaginal pH is acid, and becomes neutral or alkaline due to the presence of amniotic fluid; however, such loss of acidity can also be due to vaginal infections, urine or even bathwater. Ferning on microscopy is also a useful sign that the fluid is of amniotic origin, although this is not a convenient test to perform and is not widely used.

When the diagnosis is in doubt, then further investigations, including the ultrasound evaluation of amniotic fluid volume and intra-amniotic dye injections, may be required. However, ultrasound diagnosis of oligohydramnios is often only possible with a large fluid loss that is clinically obvious. Furthermore, intra-amniotic injection of dyes is not without risk and is not widely practiced. Alternatively, if conservative management is deemed appropriate, a 'wait and see' policy may be adopted. Repeatedly dry pads and a normal amniotic fluid volume on scan make the diagnosis less likely, while the converse is also true.

In the future, other tests such as fluid prolactin or alpha-fetoprotein and fetal fibronectin estimations, may have a role in the more precise diagnosis of premature rupture of the membranes.

The initial clinical assessment of the patient with premature rupture of the membranes will determine the further management. All efforts must be directed initially to the exclusion of overt chorioamnionitis with attention to the detection of maternal tachycardia, pyrexia, uterine tenderness, purulent vaginal discharge and fetal tachycardia. Thereafter, there should be an evaluation of the fetal gestational age (from the history, clinical examination and ultrasound assessement), the immediate fetal well-being (clinical examination and fetal cardiotocography), and the exclusion of abruptio placenta and preterm labor.

The subsequent management of the patient will depend very heavily on the particular combination of the above features. The management alternatives which can be considered include:

Expectant management

This consists of hospitalization and continued clinical observation of the mother and fetus. The role of bedrest is controversial but may aid diagnosis by allowing a pool of amniotic fluid to collect in the posterior fornix. Maternal activity also seems sometimes to increase the rate of fluid leakage, perhaps by dislodging the presenting part. Specialized assessment of continued fetal well-being using cardiotocography (NST) and/or biophysical profiles[22,23] have been advocated, while bi-weekly obstetric ultrasound evaluation of fetal growth would usually be performed.

The detection of covert chorioamnionitis using serial white cell differential counts and C-reactive protein estimations in association with an initial and then weekly vaginal microbiological cultures, has been advocated. The use of amniocentesis in clarifying the possibility of covert chorioamnionitis is more controversial, and has yet to be tested adequately.[24]

Of recent interest are the observations that early intrauterine infection appears to be associated with disturbances in fetal behavioral physiology. Abnormalities of the fetal heart rate (NST) and the biophysical profile score (BPS) correlate closely with proven intrauterine sepsis. These non-invasive tests have obvious advantages over amniocentesis. However, at present, it is not known whether the use of these tests will be helpful in determining the appropriate management and improving fetal outcome.

Active management

This may be defined as the above management, plus the use of one or more of the following pharmacological agents, viz. maternal corticosteroids, tocolytics and prophylactic antibiotic administration.

The use of corticosteroids in PPROM to enhance fetal lung maturity cannot be strongly supported from the available literature, despite a weak inference of efficacy from Ohlsson's meta-analysis, in which the author acknowledged that one study of marginal quality biased the conclusions of the analysis.[25] Contrary to the use of corticosteroids is the reported increase in the risk of maternal endometritis from earlier studies,[26–28] but the more recent study by Cunningham and Evans[29] demonstrating that both specific and non-specific maternal and neonatal immune function remain unaltered by maternal corticosteroid administration, should offer some reassurance to those who wish to use these agents. Hence at this time we believe that corticosteroids should only be administered to women with PPROM under the conditions of a clinical trial, which will ultimately provide conclusive evidence as to its efficacy [*Editor's note*: despite these caveats, the use of corticosteroids with PPROM has now become the norm in many centers.]

With regard to the use of tocolytic agents in pregnancies complicated with PPROM, the results of the available studies are even more inconclusive, with no study being able to show an improved neonatal outcome from the reported prolongation of gestation allegedly associated with their use. There is, however, some support for the limited use of these agents in the facilitation of maternal–fetal transfer to an appropriate tertiary care center.[30] It would seem unwise to give tocolytics if there is any evidence of overt chorioamnionitis, as prompt delivery is likely to minimize maternal risk from sepsis. At certain critical gestations (e.g. 24–28 weeks), however, simultaneous administration of tocolytics and antibiotics may improve the chances for a successful neonatal outcome by prolonging the gestation, although the significant maternal risks from such a strategy must be discussed fully with the parents before it is implemented.

From the very limited available studies, routine prophylactic antibiotic therapy does not appear to alter the overall fetal outcome as measured by perinatal mortality.[31–33] There are a number of potential disadvantages to consider, including a possible inability to deliver therapeutic concentrations to the amniotic cavity and the fetus, the masking of perinatal infection, the potential of drug resistance and an interference with neonatal microbiological cultures.

Further studies are urgently required in this area as the demonstrated microbiological association with PPROM continues to escalate,[34] but other than the treatment of women colonized with streptococci there is no strong support for the use of prophylactic antibiotics, unless once again it is under the conditions of a clinical trail.

Aggressive management

This is employed where delivery is deemed necessary as a result of obstetric indications, such as fetal distress, maternal sepsis or abruptio placenta, or is requested by the parents in the face of marked fetal immaturity (<26 weeks) or of demonstrated fetal maturity (after 34 weeks). This form of management implies an increased incidence of induction and augmentation of labor, and operative delivery and the associated maternal and fetal morbidity. Comparison of expectant, active and aggressive management in well-designed prospective randomized trails should be a major goal for the 1990s. Division of these studies into prelabor PROM at term and PPROM at different gestational age groups will be essential.

Management strategies

Generally, the recommended management of premature rupture of the membranes is expectant, with accurate assessment of fetal gestational age being crucial to the decision-making process. It is useful to consider prenatal management strategies in relation to five gestational periods.

• PPROM at less than 26 weeks gestation

The most appropriate management at this gestation is not clear, and must be individualized, with the wishes of the parents being paramount. Aggressive management is almost always indicated if active labor, abruptio placenta or clinical evidence of maternal–fetal infection are present. It may also be requested by the parents if they fear delivery at a subsequent gestation at which there is the possibility of survival but also a high likelihood of serious neonatal complications and long-term handicap (e.g. 26–27 weeks).

Expectant management is being increasingly considered, but with reported neonatal survival rates of less than 60% at gestations <26 weeks, even in the very latest and most optimistic studies,[35,36] and with 'normal' neonatal development in only 40–70% after a 12-month follow-up period, care must be taken to ensure that parental counseling is thorough and cautious when there is PPROM at less than 26 weeks gestation. The parents must be helped to understand that the neonatal prognosis is at best guarded, and the likelihood of neonatal death and morbidity is significant.

In view of the uncertainty of the outcome, an alternative management strategy has evolved for women who experience PPROM at less than 26 weeks gestation. After initial hospitalization for 72 h, the patient can be managed at home restricting her physical activity, taking her own temperature and reporting weekly for prenatal evaluation and microbiological/hematological surveillance. This management alternative has yet to be tested scientifically, but would clearly have merit with regard to hospital bed cost implications.

• PPROM at 26–31 weeks gestation

At this gestation, the greatest risk to the fetus is still prematurity, and this currently outweighs any potential advantage in delivering a patient with occult intrauterine infection. Consequently, expectant management is the most favored option at this gestation.

The use of amniocentesis to detect the possibility of occult amniotic infection remains controversial at this gestation, particularly as fetal lung maturity is unlikely. It may be specifically indicated in certain circumstances, for example if there are some signs (mild pyrexia, raised white cell count or CRP) of chorioamnionitis but the parents request expectant management rather than prompt delivery.

A randomized study by Carlan et al.,[37] which assessed hospital *vs* home management after 72 h of PPROM at 26–31 weeks gestation, suggested that home management was a safe protocol to adopt in terms of neonatal and maternal outcome with significant savings in maternal hospital bed days. Hoffmann et al.[38] suggested that this form of management may be more appropriate for a subset of patients with PPROM, characterized by the absence of labor or evidence of infection for 1 week, with adequate amniotic fluid volume demonstrated by ultrasound assessment. We await the outcome of similar larger randomized studies to determine the appropriate management of PPROM at this gestation.

Included in the prenatal management of PPROM at 26–31 weeks gestation must be a discussion with the parents regarding the likely mode of delivery should expectant management not be appropriate. In this regard, some interesting trends in clinical practice have evolved. A survey of members of the Society of Perinatal Obstetricians conducted by Amon et al.,[39] regarding the use of cesarean section for fetal indications, particularly at the limits of fetal viability in women delivering between the years 1986 and 1992, showed a doubling of the cesarean section rate for infants delivered between 24 and 28 weeks gestation. Sanchez-Ramos et al.,[40] however, were able to demonstrate that a significant decrease in the cesarean section rate from 55% to 40% (*P*<0.05) for very low birthweight infants/delivering between the years 1986 and 1990, did not alter the neonatal mortality, the incidence of low Apgar scores, cord blood gas values, the incidence of intraventricular hemorrhage or the median length of stay in the neonatal intensive care unit. Weiner and Estle[41] specifically studied breech presentation before 32 weeks gestation, and they concluded that cesarean section reduced the perinatal mortality by a reduction in the incidence of intraventricular hemorrhage, confirming the study of Olofsson et al.[42]

On balance, it would appear that aiming for vaginal delivery of the very low birthweight infant would be a reasonable management option to put before the parents during counseling, with resort to cesarean section for standard obstetric indications, save perhaps for those infants presenting by the breech before 32 weeks gestation (for a fuller description of the mode of delivery of the preterm breech, see Chapter 13).

● *PPROM at 31–33 weeks*

In our institution, neonatal survival at this gestation exceeds 95%, and thus the risk from prematurity is similar to the risk to the neonate from sepsis. While the use of amniocentesis would appear to be an attractive refinement in the management of patients with PPROM at this gestation, its value has never been adequately evaluated.[44] Success rates in obtaining amniotic fluid at amniocentesis in women with PPROM have varied from 45 to 97%.[10,43–45] If fluid is obtained successfully, then the lack of a 'gold standard' for the diagnosis of occult intrauterine infection *vs* colonization, makes interpretation of the results of Gram stain, fluid microbiological culture, leucocyte esterase testing and gas liquid chromatography studies particularly difficult. Fisk's review[46] of six studies using culture or Gram staining to diagnose infection of the amniotic fluid revealed sensitivities of between 55 and 100%, and specificities of 76–100%. The outcome studied is important in interpreting the sensitivity and specificity of tests designed to diagnose occult infection; for example, if the presence of pathogenic organisms is regarded as diagnostic of infection, then sensitivity of demonstrating such organisms on Gram staining and culture of the amniotic fluid is by definition 100%, whereas if neonatal death from sepsis is used as the end-point, sensitivity will be much lower and significant morbidity will be ignored. Fisk used histopathological evidence of chorioamnionitis as definitive evidence of infection, but this has been disputed by Ohlsson and Wang[47] who accepted clinical chorioamnionitis and all its shortcomings, Dudley *et al.*[24] who used neonatal sepsis (proven or suspected) and Vintzileos[23] who used both clinical chorioamnionitis and neonatal sepsis (proven or possible).

With regard to fetal lung maturity, Dudley and coworkers[24] demonstrated its presence in 58% of specimens obtained at amniocentesis at this gestation. This result was consistent with other studies,[45,48] which showed a 50–60% incidence of fetal lung maturity. With regard to outcomes, pulmonary maturity testing (L/S ratio) had a positive predictive value of 68%, and a negative predictive value of 79% with regard to neonatal respiratory distress with PPROM.[24] The specific situations of occult amniotic fluid infection but fetal lung immaturity, and fetal lung maturity but absent fluid infection, have not been adequately evaluated to determine the correct management option.

If amniocentesis is unsuccessful in obtaining an adequate amniotic fluid sample, then the management must be on a clinical basis with its inherent limitations, in association with the less precise hematological parameters of serial C-reactive protein estimations and complete blood pictures[49] to assess the presence of infection. Although Yeast *et al.*[50] found no evidence that amniocentesis induces labor, the procedure is not entirely complication-free and this must be considered when counseling the parents. It would appear that further evaluation of the role of amniocentesis in the management of PPROM, particularly at this gestation, requires a large prospective randomized trial before it can take its place as a legitimate management option.

● *PPROM at 34–36 weeks*

Although an expectant management policy is commonly employed at this gestation, this is by no means the standard approach, with many favoring induction of labor as outlined by Olofsson *et al.*[42] in their review of the practice of Swedish obstetricians with regard to PPROM. The possibility of failed induction is more likely at this gestation than at term, but this has not been adequately evaluated to date. Clearly, aggressive management is indicated if there is evidence of possible intrauterine infection, abruptio placenta or fetal distress.

● *PROM after 36 weeks*

In women with premature rupture of the membranes after 36 weeks gestation, an expectant management policy may be justified initially because 75–85% of these women are likely to labor within 24 h. Indeed, Naeye in 1982 reported that efforts to accomplish delivery by induction of labor resulted in increased morbidity and cesarean section rates.[18] However, there is still considerable debate whether this is the most appropriate option, because of Johnson and coworkers' large study,[51] which suggested greater neonatal and maternal infectious morbidity after 48 h of ruptured membranes.

There have been eight randomized controlled trials to date which have addressed the question of active *vs* conservative management of PROM at term.[52–59] All of these studies are of insufficient power, with potential biases in the method of randomization of treatment and detection of neonatal infection, to be able to give a clear management option. The meta-analysis of relevant clinical trials in this area, published in the Oxford Data Base of Perinatal Trials,[30] suggests that a routine policy of induction of labor results in an increased cesarean section rate and possibly a higher maternal infection rate, but there is a possible decreased risk of serious neonatal infection.

The favorability of the cervix (Bishop score > 4) has been proposed as a factor which might influence the choice of induction of labor, rather than the adoption of the conservative management option. This argument suggests that induction should be employed if the cervix is favorable and the likelihood of failed induction small, while conservative management should be reserved for women in whom the cervix is unripe.

Additionally, a number of trials[60,61] have attempted

to demonstrate an advantage with the use of prostaglandin E_2 preparations, compared with the use of oxytocin in inducing labor with ruptured membranes. There does not appear to be a clear advantage, although the Oxford Data Base meta-analysis[30] showed a tendency for a reduced cesarean section rate, and a reduction in infectious morbidity. However, these differences did not reach statistical significance.

In answer to the question of the most appropriate management option for women with PROM after 36 weeks, we await the results of a multicentre randomized trial currently being coordinated by the Women's College Hosptial, Toronto.[60]

Special circumstances

The 'hindwater' leak

This poorly defined clinical entity is of unknown frequency, and is often a diagnosis of exclusion. The natural history of this phenomenon is unknown and awaits further evaluation.

'Resealed' PPROM

Once again, this is a poorly defined clinical entity, which may encompass a number of women with a 'hindwater' leak. Carlan et al.[63] examined 349 women with PPROM, of whom 14 (4%) apparently resealed after initial confirmation of PPROM. An analysis of these 14 women suggested that they were of a younger age group, had PPROM at an earlier gestation, and had larger pockets of residual amniotic fluid at the initial ultrasound than the women with PPROM who did not reseal. After resealing, the pregnancies proceeded normally without any increased likelihood of re-rupture.

Multiple pregnancy and PPROM

Currently, there is little information regarding the latency period and perinatal outcome after PPROM in multiple gestations. Additionally, the relative risks of morbidity and mortality between presenting and non-presenting infants have not been addressed. Mercer and coworkers' study[64] has shown only a brief latency period, regardless of gestational age, with no difference in infant survival between twins but with a significant increase in respiratory morbidity in the non-presenting infant. In their case controlled study, Montgomery et al.[65] have suggested that the natural history of PPROM in the twin gestation parallels that in the singleton pregnancy, and that similar antepartum management strategies are appropriate for both groups.

Labor/delivery

If labor occurs in the presence of premature rupture of the membranes, then it should be monitored closely and augmented promptly if there is any delay, because of the increased risk of infection. The only exception to this rule is to allow transfer to a tertiary care center if labor is preterm and begins in a hospital without appropriate neonatal care facilities. Vaginal delivery should generally be the objective, with decisions regarding the mode of delivery and the need for cesarean section not differing substantially from other preterm deliveries.

Once labor is established, maternal antibiotic therapy is often commenced, particularly if signs of intrauterine infection are present. Although this policy has not been addressed specifically by controlled studies, earlier reservations regarding the possibility of inducing superinfection with resistant bacteria and complicating the diagnosis of infection in the neonate, have not been borne out in clinical practice. This has been demonstrated in particular by the controlled trials of antibiotic use in maternal group B hemolytic streptococcal colonization.[30] A documented reduction in anticipated maternal puerperal infectious complications has been confirmed in most studies advocating this approach.[66,67]

Labors following PROM carry an increased risk of fetal distress, often as a result of umbilical cord compression due to the associated oligohydramnios. The use of amnio-infusion to counter this complication has shown some promise in the controlled trial of Nageotte et al.[68] and in the more recent prospective randomized study conducted by Schrimmer et al.[69]

At the time of delivery, the presence of a neonatologist, with the back-up of an appropriate neonatal support team, is essential to the perinatal outcome.

Postnatal

With regard to the woman delivering after premature rupture of the membranes, an awareness of the risks associated with endometritis, not only postpartum genital sepsis/septicemia but also postpartum hemorrhage and venous thrombosis, is essential for effective management. Active promotion of maternal–infant bonding, particularly with PPROM, deserves special consideration.

All infants born after premature rupture of the membranes should be thoroughly screened for sepsis, irrespective of the antepartum or intrapartum use of maternal antibiotic therapy. Screening investigations usually include neonatal blood culture, endotracheal aspirate culture, urinary latex particle agglutination testing and a complete blood picture. Lumbar puncture and cerebrospinal fluid examination should be reserved

PREMATURE RUPTURE OF THE MEMBRANES
Summary of Management Options

Prepregnancy (previous PPROM)

- Counsel about recurrence risks

- Search for causes/precipitating factors

- Advise against cigarette smoking

- Vaginal bacteriological screening and antimicrobial treatment not proven

Prenatal

Diagnosis

- Careful history and examination (especially sterile speculum)

- Repeated pad checks to confirm diagnosis

- Additional tests ('ferning', alkaline pH turning nitrazine blue/black, presence of vernix or meconium) all have limitations, especially being unreliable/inappropriate at preterm gestations

- Intra-amniotic injection of dyes is not without risk and is not widely practiced

- Ultrasound diagnosis of oligohydramnios only detectable with large fluid loss (usually clinically obvious)

- Future tests might include:
  - monoclonal antibody detection of AFP
  - fluid prolactin
  - fetal fibronectin

Management

- Vigilance for chorioamnionitis:
  - clinical (maternal fever, tachycardia uterine pain/tenderness, purulent vaginal discharge, fetal tachycardia)
  - laboratory investigations (unreliable)
    - white cell count (band count)
    - C-reactive protein
    - amniotic fluid Gram stain, white cells and culture
    - gas chromatography
  - biophysical testing (NST and/or BPS)

- Delivery is indicated if:
  - chorioamnionitis is diagnosed
  - fetal 'distress' occurs (NST/BPS)
- If no chorioamnionitis:
  - Before 26 weeks
    - Careful counseling of parents
    - If decision is to continue with pregnancy, then implement surveillance for sepsis (see above) (? domiciliary)
  - 26–33 weeks
    The upper gestational age chosen will vary with different institutions depending on survival rates:
    - conservative rather than aggressive approach tends to be followed
    - sepsis surveillance (see above)
    - use of steroids, tocolytics and antibiotics is controversial (many obstetricians use steroids but not tocolytics or antibiotics)
    - assessment of fetal pulmonary maturity is erratic
  - 34–36 weeks
    Options used in practice are:
    - conservative (as in 26–33 weeks above)
    - aggressive (delivery)
    - combination (conservative for 24 h, then delivery)
  - 37 weeks or more
    Options used in practice are:
    - conservative (wait for 24 h and if then not in labor opt for induction)
    - aggressive (induce labor at presentation)

Labor/delivery

- Maintain vigilance and screening for infection

- Use of maternal antibiotics prophylactically once in labor remains controversial

- Continuous fetal heart rate monitoring

- Pediatrician for delivery

Postnatal

- Maintain vigilance and screening for infection

- Neonatal screen for sepsis (see Chapter 72)

for clinically septic neonates, and those with positive blood cultures. Initial antibiotic therapy using a combination of intravenous penicillin and gentamicin may be employed while awaiting the results of the screening investigations (see also Chapter 72). Often the results are inconclusive or equivocal, and discontinuation of the antibiotic therapy may then have to be based on clinical judgement.

Prematurity remains the greatest hazard encountered with premature rupture of the membranes, and hence hyaline membrane disease requiring mechanical ventilation is common. This can be aggravated by pulmonary hypoplasia, which is usually only significant if PPROM occurs before 25 weeks gestation, with a latent period of more than 5 weeks before delivery.[70] The outcome of PPROM at later gestations is more optimistic than is reported for other causes of oligohydramnios.[46]

The other complications associated with prematurity and its management, including intracranial hemorrhage, jaundice and feeding difficulties, must be attended to in the usual fashion, while there should be provision made for long-term neonatal follow-up (see Chapter 72).

CONCLUSIONS

The controversy surrounding premature rupture of the membranes, and preterm premature rupture of the membranes, appears to be on-going, but with continued research into the etiology of this condition we may be able to offer appropriate management options based on an understanding of the pathophysiology. However, until this is achieved, we must be willing to revise our management options on the basis of quality clinical trials.

REFERENCES

1   Mead PB (1980) Management of the patient with premature rupture of the fetal membranes: A review. *Clinics in Perinatology* 7:243–260.
2   Gibbs RS, Blanco JD (1982) Premature rupture of the membranes. *Obstetrics and Gynecology* 60:671–673.
3   Graham L, Gilstrap LC, Hauth JC, Kodeck-Garza S (1982) Conservative management of patients with premture rupture of fetal membranes. *Obstetrics and Gynecology* 59:607–610.
4   Cox S, Williams L, Leveno K (1988) The natural history of preterm ruptured membranes: What to expect of expectant management. *Obstetrics and Gynecology* 71:558–561.
5   Queen Victoria Hospital (1991) *Perinatal Statistics Annual Report.* Queen Victoria Hospital, Adelaide.
6   Levy DL, Arquembourg PC (1981) Maternal and cord blood complement activity: Relationship to premature rupture of the membranes. *American Journal of Obstetrics and Gynecology* 139:38–39.
7   Garite TJ, Freeman RK (1982) Chorioamnionitis in the preterm gestation. *Obstetrics and Gynecology* 59:539–543.
8   Breese MW (1961) Spontaneous premature rupture of the membranes. *American Journal of Obstetrics and Gynecology* 81:1086–1088.
9   Nelson DM, Stempel LE, Zuspan FP (1986) Association of prolonged preterm premature rupture of the membranes and abruptio placentae. *Journal of Reproductive Medicine* 31:429–431.
10 Vintzileos AM, Campbell WA, Nochimson DJ, Weinbaum PJ (1987) Premature rupture of the membranes: A risk factor for the development of abruptio placentae. *American Journal of Obstetrics and Gynecology* 156:1235–1236.
11 Asrat T, Garite TJ (1991) Management of preterm premature rupture of membranes. *Clinical Obstetrics and Gynecology* 34:730–738.
12 Allen SR (1991) Epidemiology of premature rupture of the fetal membranes. *Clinical Obstetrics and Gynecology* 34:685–687.
13 Taylor J, Garite TJ (1984) Premature rupture of the membranes before fetal viability. *Obstetrics and Gynecology* 140:34–38.
14 Beydoun SN, Yasin SY (1986) Premature rupture of the membranes before 28 weeks: Conservative management. *American Journal of Obstetrics and Gynecology* 155:471–473.
15 Knudsen FU, Steinrud J (1976) Septicaemia of the newborn associated with ruptured fetal membranes, discoloured amniotic fluid or maternal fever. *Acta Paediatrica Scandinavica* 65:725–726.
16 Cederquist LL, Zervoudaikas IA, Ewool LC (1979) The relationship between prematurely ruptured membranes and fetal immunoglobulin production. *American Journal of Obstetrics and Gynecology* 134:784–787.
17 Siegel JD, McCracken GH Jr (1981) Sepsis neonatorum. *New England Journal of Medicine* 304:642–644.
18 Naeye RI (1982) Factors that predispose to premature rupture of the fetal membranes. *Obstetrics and Gynecology* 60:93–98.
19 Asrat T, Lewis DF, Garite TJ, Major CA, Nageotte MP, Towers CV, Montgomery DM, Dorchester WA (1991) Rate of recurrence of preterm premature rupture of membranes in consecutive pregnancies. *American Journal of Obstetrics and Gynecology* 165:1111–1115.
20 Harger JH, Hsing AW, Toomala RE, Gibbs RS, Mead PB, Eschenbach DA, Knox GE, Polk BF (1990) Risk factors for preterm premature rupture of fetal membranes: A multicenter case-control study. *American Journal of Obstetrics and Gynecology* 163:130–138.
21 Seo K, McGregor JA, French JI (1990) Infection and premature rupture of the membranes. *Fetal Medicine Review* 2:1–15.
22 Roussis P, Rosemond RL, Glass C, Boehm FH (1991) Preterm premature rupture of membranes: Detection of infection. *American Journal of Obstetrics and Gynecology* 165:1099.
23 Vintzileos AM, Campbell WA, Rodis JF (1991) Ante-

partum surveillance in patients with preterm PROM. *Clinical Obstetrics and Gynecology* **34**:779–783.

24 Dudley J, Malcolm G, Ellwood D (1991) Amniocentesis in the management of preterm premature rupture of the membranes. *Australia and New Zealand Journal of Obstetrics and Gynaecology* **31**:331–334.

25 Ohlsson A (1989) Treatments of preterm premature rupture of the membranes: A meta-analysis. *American Journal of Obstetrics and Gynecology* **160**:890–898.

26 Taeusch HW, Frigoletto F, Kitzmiller J (1979) Risk of respiratory distress syndrome after prenatal dexamethasone treatment. *Paediatrics* **63**:64–66.

27 Garite TJ, Freeman RK, Linzey EM, Braly PS, Dorchester WL (1981) Prospective randomised study of corticosteroids in the management of premature rupture of the membranes and the premature gestation. *American Journal of Obstetrics and Gynecology* **141**:508–512.

28 Iams JD, Talbert ML, Barrows H, Sachs L (1985) Management of preterm prematurely ruptured membranes: A prospective randomised comparison of observations versus use of steroids and timed delivery. *American Journal of Obstetrics and Gynecology* **151**:32–37.

29 Cunningham DS, Evans EE (1991) The effects of betamethasone on maternal cellular resistance to infection. *American Journal of Obstetrics and Gynecology* **165**:610–613.

30 Keirse MJNC, Ohlsson A, Treffers PE, Kanhai HHH (1989) Pre-labour rupture of the membranes preterm. In Chalmers I, Enkin M, Keirse MJNC (eds) *Effective Care in Pregnancy and Childbirth*, Vol. 1, pp. 666–692. Oxford: Oxford University Press.

31 Harlass FE (1991) The use of tocolytics in patients with preterm premature rupture of the membranes. *Clinical Obstetrics and Gynecology* **34**:751–753.

32 Veille JC (1988) Management of preterm premature rupture of membranes. *Clinics in Perinatology* **15**:851–853.

33 Greenberg RT, Hankins GDV (1991) Antibiotic therapy in preterm premature rupture of membranes. *Clinical Obstetrics and Gynecology* **34**:742–744.

34 Romero R, Quintero R, Oyarzun E (1988) Intra-amniotic infection and the onset of labor in preterm premature rupture of the membranes. *American Journal of Obstetrics and Gynecology* **159**:661–664.

35 Majors CA, Kitzmiller JL (1990) The healthy neonate – expectant management of midtrimester rupture of membranes. Soc Perinat Obstet Abstract No. 104. *American Journal of Obstetrics and Gynecology* **163**:14.

36 Morales W, Talley T (1991) Premature rupture of membranes < 24 weeks – a management dilemma. Soc Perinat Obstet Abstract No. 228. *American Journal of Obstetrics and Gynecology* **164**:310.

37 Carlan SJ, Parsons M, O'Brien WF, Lense JJ (1991) Preterm PROM: Safety and cost of home *vs* hospital management. Soc Perinat Obstet Abstract No. 234. *American Journal of Obstetrics and Gynecology* **164**:311.

38 Hoffmann D, Hansen G, Ingardia C, Philipson E (1992) Preterm premature rupture of membranes: Is outpatient management appropriate? Soc Perinat Obstet Abstract No. 467. *American Journal of Obstetrics and Gynecology* **166**:403.

39 Amon E (1992) Caesarean section for fetal indications at the limits of fetal viability (1986 to 1991). Soc Perinat Obstet Abstract No. 4. *American Journal of Obstetrics and Gynecology* **166**:274.

40 Sanchez-Ramos L, Walker C, Briones D, Cullen MT (1992) Decreasing caesarean section rates in very low-birthweight infants: Effect on perinatal outcome. Soc Perinat Obstet Abstract No. 655. *American Journal of Obstetrics and Gynecology* **166**:444.

41 Weiner C, Estle E (1992) Vaginal breech delivery in the 1980s: Preterm gestation. Soc Perinat Obstet Abstracts No. 438. *American Journal of Obstetrics and Gynecology* **166**:396.

42 Olofsson P, Rydhstrom H, Sjoberg NO (1988) How Swedish obstetricians manage premature rupture of the membranes in preterm gestations. *American Journal of Obstetrics and Gynecology* **159**:1028–1031.

43 Brockhuizen FF, Gilman M, Hamilton PR (1985) Amniocentesis for Gram stain and culture in preterm premature rupture of the membranes. *Obstetrics and Gynecology* **66**:316–318.

44 Burke M, Porreco RP (1986) Use of amniotic fluid analysis in the management of preterm premature rupture of the membranes. *Journal of Reproductive Medicine* **31**:31–32.

45 Garite TJ, Freeman RK, Linzey EM, Braly P (1979) The use of amniocentesis in patients with premature rupture of the membranes. *Obstetrics and Gynecology* **54**:1266–1269.

46 Fisk NM (1988) Modifications to selective conservative management in preterm premature rupture of the membranes. *Obstetrical and Gynaecological Survey* **43**:328–338.

47 Ohlsson A, Wang E (1990) An analysis of antenatal tests to detect infections in preterm premature rupture of the membranes. *Journal of Obstetrics and Gynecology* **162**: 809–811.

48 Cotton DB, Hill LM, Strassner HT, Platt LD, Ledger WJ (1984) Use of amniocentesis in preterm gestation with ruptured membranes. *Obstetrics and Gynecology* **63**:38–40.

49 Norman K, Louw JP (1991) C-Reactive protein in premature rupture of membranes. *Contemporary Reviews of Obstetrics and Gynaecology* **3**:148–151.

50 Yeast JD, Garite TJ, Dorchester W (1984) The risks of amniocentesis in the management of premature rupture of the membranes. *American Journal of Obstetrics and Gynecology* **149**:505–507.

51 Johnson JWC, Daikoku NH, Niebyl JR, Johnson TRB, Khouzami VA, Witter FR (1981) Premature rupture of the membranes and prolonged latency. *Obstetrics and Gynecology* **57**:547–550.

52 Duff P, Huff RW, Gibbs RS (1984) Management of premature rupture of the membranes and unfavourable cervix in term pregnancy. *Obstetrics and Gynecology* **63**:697–701.

53 Fayez JA, Hasan AA, Jones HS, Miller GL (1978) Management of premature rupture of the membranes. *Obstetrics and Gynecology* **52**:17–25.

54 Morales WJ, Lazar AJ (1986) Expectant management of rupture of membranes at term. *Southern Medical Journal* **79**:955–957.

55 Van der Walt D, Venter PF (1989) Management of term pregnancy with premature rupture of the membranes and unfavourable cervix. *South African Medical Journal* **75**:54–59.

56 Wagner MV, Chin VP, Peters CJ, Drexler B, Newman LA (1989) A comparison of early and delayed induction of labor with spontaneous rupture of membranes at term. *Obstetrics and Gynecology* **74**:93–97.

57 Mahmood TA, Dick MJW, Smith NC (1989) Management of spontaneous rupture of the membranes and no uterine activity in health primigravidae after 34 weeks gestation. *Lancet* **2**:721–723.

58 Tamsen L, Lyrenas S, Cnattingius S (1990) Premature rupture of the membranes: Intervention or not. *Gynecological and Obstetrical Investigations* **29**:128–130.

59 Ray DA, Garite TJ (1990) Prostaglandin E$_2$ induction in term patients with premature rupture of membranes. In *Proceedings of the 10th Annual Meeting of the Society of Perinatal Obstetrics Houston, Texas No. 80.*

60 Noah ML, DeCoster JM, Fraser TJ, Orr JD (1987) Pre-induction cervical softening with endocervical PGE$_2$ gel: A multicentre trial. *Acta Obstetrica et Gynecologica Scandinavica* **66**:3–9.

61 Ekman G, Gronstram L, Ulmsten U (1986) Induction of labour with intravenous oxytocin or vaginal PGE$_2$ suppositories: A randomised study. *Acta Obstetrica et Gynecologica Scandinavica* **65**:857–860.

62 Hannah ME (1991) Personal communication.

63 Carlan SJ, O'Brien WF, Glock JL (1992) Clinical characteristics and outcome of patients with resealed, preterm, premature rupture of membranes. Soc Perinat Obstet Abstract No. 657. *American Journal of Obstetrics and Gynecology* **166**:445.

64 Mercer B, Crocker L, Dahmus M, Pierce F, Sibai B (1992) Outcome of multiple gestation complicated by preterm PROM. Soc Perinat Obstet Abstract No. 297. *American Journal of Obstetrics and Gynecology* **166**:359.

65 Montgomery DM, Perlow JH, Asrat T, Morgan MA, Bahado-Singh RO, Garite TJ (1992) Preterm premature ruptured membranes in the twin gestation: A case control study. Soc Perinat. Obstet. Abstract No. 301. *American Journal of Obstetrics and Gynecology* **166**:360.

66 Sperling RS, Ramamurthy RS, Gibbs RS (1987) A comparison of intrapartum versus immediate postpartum treatment of intra-amniotic infection. *Obstetrics and Gynecology* **70**:861–863.

67 Gilstrap LC, Leveno KJ, Cox SM, Burris JS, Mashburn M, Rosenfeld CR (1988) Intrapartum treatment of acute chorioamnionitis: Impact on neonatal sepsis. *American Journal of Obstetrics and Gynecology* **159**:579–582.

68 Nageotte MP, Freeman RK, Garite TJ, Dorchester W (1985) Prophylactic intrapartum amnio-infusion in patients with preterm premature rupture of the membranes. *American Journal of Obstetrics and Gynecology* **153**:557–561.

69 Schrimmer DB, Macri CJ, Paul RH (1991) Prophylactic amnio-infusion as a treatment for oligohydramnios in laboring patients: A prospective, randomised trial. *American Journal of Obstetrics and Gynecology* **165**:972–974.

70 Nimrod MB, Varela-Gittings F, Machin G, Campbell D, Wesenberg R (1984) The effect of very prolonged membrane rupture on fetal development. *American Journal of Obstetrics and Gynecology* **148**:540–543.

13

Breech Presentation

ZOE J. PENN, PHILIP J. STEER

INTRODUCTION

The management of breech presentation is an area of intense controversy. A variety of committed opinions have been expressed on every aspect of management from the mode of delivery ('Once a breech always a caesarean section'[1]) to the place of external cephalic version in modern management of the breech ('there are those who express . . . a rather elegant distaste for it'[2]).

However, the most fundamental shift in opinion over the last 10–15 years has been the realization that breech presentation may well be a bad prognostic variable of itself.[3] Any studies, clinical trials or proposed clinical management must take account of this.

Breech presentation has been recognized for centuries. At one time, it was regarded as advantageous, probably because the midwife could pull on the legs to expedite delivery.[4] Mauriceau described a maneuver for the gentle delivery of the aftercoming head in the sixteenth century and the mode of delivery of the breech remained essentially unchanged until the late 1950s, when cesarean section was first recommended on a routine basis. It was thought that this might minimize the perinatal morbidity and mortality of the breech presenting fetus.

INCIDENCE

The incidence of breech presentation overall is said to be of the order of 3–4%,[5] and in those of birthweight greater than 2.5 kg the incidence is 2.6–3%. The incidence of breech presentation in the preterm pregnancy is higher and at 29–32 weeks gestation the incidence is 14%.[6]

ETIOLOGY

Breech presentation may be a benign error of orientation, or it may be associated with maternal or fetal abnormality. One of the most common causes of breech presentation is prematurity. In this case, it is usually the chance lie of a highly mobile fetus in relatively copious amniotic fluid.

However, there is a well-recognized association with fetal abnormality for both the term and the preterm fetus. Lamont et al.,[7] in a series of preterm breech infants, found that 18% were congenitally abnormal. Collea et al.[8] quoted a 5% incidence of congenital abnormality in term breech fetuses, two to three times higher than in their vertex counterparts (2.1%). Approximately 50% of all cases of hydrocephalus, myelomeningocele, Prader-Willi syndrome and trisomy are born in breech presentation.[9] It has also been noted that 90% of all abnormalities in breeches occurred in fetuses weighing greater than 2000 g.[10] Central nervous system abnormalities are the most commonly noted.[10] Presumably, this reflects the fact that preterm breeches are in breech presentation primarily because of their gestational age, which will affect normal and abnormal fetuses more or less equally, whereas at term, fetal abnormality of itself plays a part in determining the presentation.

Term breech presentations are associated with relatively short cords,[11] reduced fetal growth[12] and abnormalities in amniotic fluid volume (either oligo- or hydramnios). Breech fetuses tend to have reduced feto-placental ratios, to be small for dates and have an increased head circumference regardless of the mode of delivery. This difference in weight remains until 18 months of age, but disappears after the age of 4 years.[13] Breech presentation appears to be associated with a shorter mean gestation,[13] but at present it is not clear whether this is purely due to the increased likelihood of breech presentation at preterm gestations or whether breech presentation *per se* predisposes to preterm labor.

Uterine size or shape may also influence presentation. It seems that the narrower cephalic pole of the fetus will normally occupy the narrower lower segment, especially if the legs of the fetus are flexed at the knee. This configuration of uterus and fetus will produce the usual cephalic presentation. But if the knees are extended, the hips flexed and uterine space is limited, the head and feet may lie alongside each other, making the cephalic pole of the fetus larger and encouraging a breech presentation. Uterine space is often limited in the nullipara and breech presentation is reported to be more common in nulliparous women.[12]

Other less benign conditions may alter the uterine capacity or the intrauterine shape. Uterine anomaly, such as bicornuate uterus, is associated with breech presentation.[14] Placenta previa is well recognized in association with breech presentation as this changes the intrauterine shape.[15] By contrast, cornual implantation of the placenta, a completely benign condition, is strongly associated with breech presentation; only 5% of vertex presenting fetuses have a cornual placenta in comparison with 73% of those presenting by the breech.[16] A contracted pelvis is also associated with breech presentation, probably by limiting uterine space in the lower segment.[14]

Women who have had a previous breech presentation at term are significantly more likely to have one in a subsequent pregnancy. This is usually associated with extended fetal legs. Multiple pregnancy is strongly associated with breech presentation, but aside from the choice of mode of delivery, we refer the reader to the Chapter 10 on multiple pregnancy. Medication with anticonvulsants in pregnancy also seems to be associated with breech presentation,[17] as does maternal alcohol abuse: both are substances which have a profound influence on intrauterine fetal neurological function.

RISKS AND SIGNIFICANCE

It is almost impossible to distinguish the risks of breech presentation *per se* and the risks of breech delivery and there is a paucity of published data in this area. It is clear from the data reported above that the fetus presenting by the breech has a higher rate of congenital anomaly. Manzke[18] also reported a higher incidence of breech presentation in fetal alcohol syndrome and trisomy-21 syndrome. Antepartum stillbirth and neonatal death rate are both higher with breech presentation, regardless of mode of delivery.[19] Schutte *et al.*[20] report that even after correction for gestational age, congenital defects and birthweight, the perinatal mortality rate is higher in breech than in vertex infants, again regardless of the mode of delivery.

As enumerated above, the breech fetus tends to be smaller at any given gestation than its cephalic presenting counterpart[21] and have a lower feto-placental ratio and a smaller head circumference.[22] Many retrospective reviews of breech presentation and trials of antepartum and intrapartum management compare the vertex presenting infant with the breech presenting infant and in any comparison of this sort the breech presenting infant will compare unfavourably, regardless of the mode of delivery.[23] This reflects inherent differences between the vertex and breech presenting infant. Westgren and Ingemarsson[9] report that in prospective follow-up studies and matched control studies, breech infants will score less favourably neurologically, regardless of the mode of delivery. They felt that this reflected prenatal factors rather than birth injuries.

Nelson and Ellenberg[24] looked at all the obstetric factors that could be associated with the development of cerebral palsy using a multiple-regression technique. They found that breech presentation was a predictor for cerebral palsy but that breech delivery *per se* was not.

Bearing in mind the inherent link between breech presentation and fetal abnormality, the risks to the breech fetus of vaginal delivery are difficult to ascertain. Estimates of the risk of perinatal mortality vary from zero to 35 per 1000 births.[5] Rovinsky *et al.*[25] calculated the fetal risk of breech delivery, corrected for the abnormality that may have caused the breech presentation, to be of the order of four times that of a cephalic presentation. The inherent difficulty with this approach is that detected abnormalities may not include all the features that confer this increased risk.

The risks to the mother are rather easier to quantify. Breech presentation confers an increased likelihood of cesarean section with its attendant morbidity and mortality.[8,26,27] The rate of cesarean section for breech presentation has risen in recent years.[28–30] It has been calculated by some that the risk of maternal mortality in cesarean section is up to 38 times that of a vaginal delivery.[31] However, others have suggested a relative risk as low as seven-fold, decreasing to five-fold after exclusion of women with medical or life-threatening complications.[32] In the latter study, most of the surplus risk occurred in emergency cesareans, when the relative risk was eleven-fold, compared with elective cesareans when the risk was only four-fold. This excess risk for emergency cesareans has led one set of authors to use decision analysis to recommend routine elective cesarean section for the delivery of the term breech presentation.[33]

DIAGNOSIS

Three clinical types of breech presentation are recognized. These types are useful in that they may predict the cause of the presentation and indicate the complications to be anticipated. As with any clinical classification, there may be overlap between the groups.

- The frank (or extended) breech indicates that the legs of the fetus are flexed at the hip and extended at the knee. This type accounts for 60–70% of all breech presentations at term. The risk of feto-pelvic disproportion and of cord prolapse are lowest in this group.

- The complete (or flexed) breech indicates that the hips and knees are flexed so that the feet are presenting in the pelvis.

- The incomplete (or footling) breech indicates that one leg is flexed and the other extended.

The woman with a breech presentation, especially toward term, may complain of subcostal discomfort and of feeling the baby kick in the lower part of the uterus. On palpation, the hard round ballotable head is found at the fundus and the softer breech at the lower pole. The fetal heart sounds are more commonly heard above the umbilicus. One diagnostic pitfall is the confusion of the deeply engaged head and the breech presentation. The examiner thinks that the shoulders are above the pelvic brim, when in fact the breech is over the pelvis.

At vaginal examination, if the cervix is sufficiently dilated, the fetal ischial tuberosities and the sacrum provide the bony landmarks. The anus and the genitalia may also be felt but are less useful in diagnosis due to their softness and compressibility. If the membranes are ruptured, the examining finger in the anus may produce meconium staining. The main diagnostic confusion is face presentation. Face presentation produces the characteristic bony landmarks of the malar eminences, mouth and mentum that produce a bony triangle, whereas the ischial tuberosities and the sacrum are in line.[8,34] The mouth, in contrast to the anus, has a firm unyielding margin of bone.

Engagement of the breech implies that the bitrochanteric diameter has passed the pelvic brim.

MANAGEMENT OPTIONS FOR BREECH PRESENTATION

These are best considered under two headings:

- Breech presentation at term

- Preterm breech presentation

Management Options for Breech Presentation at Term

Version of the breech

Spontaneous version of the breech

The fact that breech presentation is so common at early gestations and relatively uncommon at term implies that spontaneous version does occur. It becomes less frequent as the third trimester progresses. However, the incidence of spontaneous version after 32 weeks may be as high as 57% and after 36 weeks gestation may still be as high as 25%.[35] Spontaneous version is more likely in multiparas without a previous breech birth and less likely in the nulliparous woman and in the breech with extended legs. It follows from this that if the woman is to be delivered by cesarean section at term simply because of breech presentation, the presentation should be re-checked immediately prior to cesarean section (preferably by ultrasound scanning), as the chances of spontaneous version even at this late stage are not insignificant.[35]

Promotion of spontaneous version

There is a growing interest in techniques to promote spontaneous version. Hofmeyr et al.[36] noted that in a proportion of women in whom a ultrasound scan was performed prior to enrolment in a randomized controlled trial of external cephalic version (ECV), spontaneous version of the breech to cephalic had occurred in the short period of time between the scan and the attempted ECV. This led him to postulate that the full bladder required for a successful scan had disengaged the breech and promoted version as the woman rolled off the examination couch. The combination of disengagement and postural change at the same time he judged worthy of further investigation. A variety of midwifery techniques are in use and claim a measure of success.[31]

One technique is for the woman to assume the knee–chest position, with the buttocks higher than the torso and the chest lying on a flat surface, for 10 min every day. Although it appears to be common for this advice to be given, there has been no randomized controlled trial to determine the value of this technique. Bung *et al.*[37] reported another technique which was to elevate the pelvis and abduct the thighs and breathe in a relaxed fashion for a prescribed period of time throughout the day. The results were inconclusive. It seems likely that these techniques are harmless in themselves and may be worth trying, but cannot be recommended in the absence of objective supporting data.

External cephalic version

"There are those who enthusiastically recommend it and those who violently oppose it, and still others who express a rather elegant distaste for it".[2] External cephalic version fell from favour in the mid-1970s. Prior to this time, it was performed without medication (except occasionally sedation), without tocolysis and usually prior to 36 weeks gestation. It was thought that as ECV was easier to perform prior to 36 weeks, it must therefore be safer.[14] Without tocolysis it was usually unsuccessful after 36 weeks. In 1975, Bradley-Watson reported a 1% fetal mortality rate for external cephalic version done prior to 36 weeks without tocolysis which was considered an unacceptably high complication rate.[38] In 1978, Lyons and Papsain reported increasing use of cesarean section for the delivery of the breech.[39] As a result, the use of ECV declined and was almost abandoned in most institutions as cesarean section was seen as a safer alternative.

Another significant disadvantage of preterm ECV in contrast with term ECV is that fetal bradycardia immediately after ECV may require immediate delivery by cesarean section, following which respiratory distress syndrome poses a significant threat to the preterm infant. To avoid this, it was traditional to manage acute bradycardia by reversion of the fetus to breech, which did not always work and in any case defeated the objective of the ECV. In addition, more spontaneous reversion to breech occurred prior to delivery. Thus its effectiveness was controversial, especially as the fetal mortality was reported to be higher in the preterm than the term breech.[40] Three randomized controlled trials have now shown no effect of early version on the incidence of breech birth, cesarean section rates or perinatal outcome.[41–43] There are no published data on the use of ECV in the management of the preterm breech in labor. The antecedents of the preterm breech in labor are often abnormal and ECV is therefore less relevant as a management strategy.

Any consideration of the efficacy and safety of the technique of external cephalic version should include a likelihood of spontaneous version, the effectiveness of ECV of producing a cephalic presentation at the time of birth, the risks to the mother and the baby, and the utility of cephalic presentation at birth to the mother and the baby (i.e. if some pre-existing abnormality or fetal compromise determines the mode of delivery rather than the presentation itself and also if the prognosis of the baby is determined by its condition rather than the mode of delivery, correction of the breech presentation will then not alter the outcome for the fetus).

In recent years, a spate of randomized controlled trials on the use of ECV with tocolysis after 37 weeks has increased its use. The advantages of the use of ECV at term are that it allows time for spontaneous version to occur, and the clarification of conditions which may require delivery by cesarean section of themselves, e.g. antepartum hemorrhage and growth deficiency. This results in fewer unnecessary attempts being made. Also, any complications of ECV itself may be managed by prompt cesarean delivery of a mature infant. It is also clear that ECV performed after 36 weeks gestation has a lower incidence of complications.[40]

There are now five randomized controlled trials on the use of ECV in the management of the term breech presentation.[36,44–47] A meta-analysis of these data performed by Hofmeyr[48] showed that the typical odds ratio for the reduction in breech births was 0.13 and for reduction in cesarean section 0.36. The three European and North American trials showed a reduction in the rate of breech birth from 78 to 44% and of cesarean section from 29 to 15%.[44,45,47] The implications of these data are that every 100 ECV attempts should prevent 34 breech births and 14 cesarean sections. A conservative estimate of the impact of performing ECV on 2% of the 750 000 pregnancies in the UK every year would be a reduction in the number of breech births of 5100 and a reduction in the number of cesarean sections of 2100.[48]

Two of the above trials were performed in Africa on Black African women.[36,49] The success rates quoted in these trials are higher than in the European and North America trials. This is probably due to the tendency for late engagement of the presenting part in the pelvis in the Black African woman.

Although most of these trials have either used tocolysis routinely or have advocated its use routinely, as originally proposed by Saling and Muller-Holve,[40] it may be that it is unnecessary in many pregnancies.[49,50] On the one hand, Van Vellen *et al.*[44] did not use tocolysis or any other medication, but none the less reported a 25% success rate at one attempt of ECV and achieved cephalic presentation at delivery in 48% after repeated attempts. On the other hand, Van Dorsten *et al.*[45] used tocolysis and achieved a 68% successful version rate and all patients presented in labor with a cephalic presentation. The value of tocolysis remains unconfirmed by a randomized controlled trial and thus requires further investigation before it can be recommended unequivocally.

• Benefits to the fetus of ECV

It is clear that ECV reduces the incidence of breech presentation at term and of breech delivery, whether vaginal or by cesarean section. It should be remembered, however, that although cesarean section is often seen as eliminating the risks of fetal trauma attendant upon vaginal delivery, this is not always the case.[51,52] Cesarean section may also increase the risks of pulmonary hypertension in the newborn.[53] It will, however, decrease the incidence of cord prolapse and unattended precipitate breech birth. Unattended or precipitate breech birth has been shown to have an eightfold increase in the risk of poor condition at birth in comparison to women expertly attended and assessed for vaginal delivery antepartum.[51,54]

• Risks of ECV to the fetus

The risk to the fetus is difficult to quantify because there is at present no randomized controlled trial large enough to clarify this issue. However, in a review of 979 reported cases of ECV at term with neither inhalational analgesia nor general anesthesia, there were no fetal losses.[31] An 8% incidence of bradycardias has been reported in association with ECV.[55] In 1983, Hofmeyr reported and published the fetal heart rate changes associated with the procedure of ECV itself.[36] These were transient and returned quickly to normal. He ascribed them to transient fetal hypoxia rather than direct pressure on the fetus or cord, or placental abruption, by interpretation of the characteristics of the fetal heart rate trace. Kouam[56] followed up 116 children born after ECV. Developmental screening at 2–5 years showed no developmental delay. Although the short-term neonatal outcomes reported in these randomized controlled trials are essentially normal and compare favorably with controls, they are only surrogates for definitive follow-up studies of the effects of this procedure.

Feto–maternal hemorrhage has been reported in association with ECV.[57] The risk has been quoted at approximately 5% using tocolysis, whereas the risk without tocolysis has been reported to be as high as 28%.[58] The experience of ECV prior to 36–37 weeks demonstrates that the risks to the fetus are related to gestational age and the use of general anesthesia.[31] It may be that anterior placenta also represents a risk. However, the risks of ECV, set in the overall context of the risks of breech presentation in itself or of the risks of breech delivery vaginally or abdominally, are small.

• Benefits to the mother of ECV

There will be a decrease in the number of vaginal breech deliveries, which often entails episiotomy and forceps delivery, and of the number of cesarean sections performed. Maternal morbidity is usually higher after cesarean section than after vaginal delivery.[59] Tatum et al.[51] quoted a rate of significant maternal complications of 42% after cesarean section compared with 1.1% in the group delivered vaginally (excluding episiotomy). Cesarean section may compromise future reproductive function[60] and there may be adverse emotional sequelae on the mother and the maternal–infant pair.[61] All these aspects are aside from the higher maternal death rate associated with cesarean section quoted above.

Procedure: External Cephalic Version (ECV)

Indications/Contraindications

The contraindications for the performance of ECV are outlined in **Table 1**. The absolute contraindications are uncontroversial. However, the relative contradindications are more debatable. Fortunato et al.[62] also add uterine anomaly to this list. These authors also noted that a body weight 20% above ideal was associated with decreased success of ECV; however, Ferguson[63] noted no effect of maternal weight on success rates. Some authors emphasize the performance of a contraction stress test prior to commencement of ECV. Others claim that the presence of an engaged breech or previous uterine surgery is a contraindication to ECV.[45] An amniotic fluid volume less than 2 cm in any pocket, an engaged breech and the presence of the fetal back lying anteriorly are also thought to decrease the chance of success.[62] The chances of success are increased with increasing parity and a breech lying more in the iliac fossae than in the midline.[63] Fetal abdominal circumference is related to the chances of success, whereas the biparietal diameter is not. Gestational age and estimated weight, provided the attempt was after 37 weeks, had no relationship to the chances of success, as success rates were found to be the same at 37, 38 and 40 weeks.

Table 1
Indications and contraindications for ECV

Indications

Any breech presentation after 36–37 weeks gestation
Suspected feto-pelvic disproportion
Unengaged breech

Contraindications to ECV

Absolute
Multiple pregnancy
Antepartum hemorrhage
Placenta previa
Ruptured membranes
Significant fetal abnormality
Need for cesarean section for other indications

Relative
Previous cesarean section
Intra-uterine growth deficiency
Severe proteinuric hypertension
Obesity
Red cell iso-immunization
Evidence of macrosomia
(Grand multiparity)
(Anterior placenta)
('Previous baby')
(Previous APH)

Any suspected fetal compromise: unreactive
   cardiotocogram
If tocolysis is to be used, exclude women with congenital
   or acquired heart disease, diabetes or thyroid disease
   because of possible adverse reactions

Prerequisites for the performance of ECV

These are:

1. Recent ultrasound to confirm a normal fetus and an adequate volume of amniotic fluid.

2. Reactive CTG.

3. Informed consent: the mother should be specifically advised of the risks of premature labor, ruptured membranes, and cord and placental accidents.

4. Facilities for the performance of a cesarean section.

Procedure for ECV
(see **Figure 1**, Chapter 10)

External cephalic version may be performed in the labor room or the clinic room if there is rapid access to delivery facilities. The woman is positioned either in steep or slight lateral tilt or in Trendelenberg. It is sometimes recommended that a Kleihauer test be performed before and after the procedure. Some also recommend the placement of an intravenous line and the crossmatching of blood for a possible cesarean section. If tocolysis is to be used, some practitioners perform an electrolyte and glucose estimation as well. A clinical pelvimetry should be judged as adequate. An ultrasound scan should be performed in order to assess the volume of amniotic fluid, fetal attitude and position of fetal legs. The CTG should be reactive prior to commencement. Some authorities also recommend that a contraction stress test be performed prior to version. It has even been suggested that the maternal blood pressure should be taken every 5 min throughout the procedure[45] and that the maternal heart rate should be monitored electronically. This is probably unnecessary if the mother appears well throughout, but could be important if tocolysis is used.

If tocolysis is employed, this can be given in a variety of ways:

10 μg hexaprenaline i.v. over 1 min
0.25 mg terbutaline s.c.
0.25 mg terbutaline in 5 ml of normal
   saline i.v. over 5 min
0.5 μg/min terbutaline i.v.
0.5 μg/min terbutaline i.v. over 15–20 min
0.2 mg/min ritodrine i.v. for 20 min

Some authors give the chosen tocolytic as a stat dose and commence the ECV almost immediately. Others increase the dose steadily or wait until adequate uterine relaxation is achieved, all contractions have ceased or there is softening of the uterus and easy palpation of fetal parts.

The ECV should be performed in one sitting by one operator and continuous pressure on the uterus should be limited to 5 min. The uterine manipulation should only continue for 10 min. Mohamed et al.[49] report that 55% are successful after 1 min and only 15% require up to 5 min continuous pressure on the abdomen. The increased incidence of fetal heart rate abnormalities with failed ECV suggests that persistence in an attempt beyond these suggested times may be counter-

productive. Van Dorsten et al.[45] report the incidence of fetal heart rate abnormalities among ECV failures to be 63% compared with 29% when the ECV is successful. Mohamed et al.[49] also report that 73% were deemed by the obstetricians to be easy conversions with 90% of women reporting little or no discomfort.

A variety of techniques of ECV are also employed. A forward or backward somersault can be performed: the forward somersault is the classically described maneuver. Hofmeyr et al.[64] describe a technique which involves placing the woman in a steep lateral tilt with her back against the wall behind the examination couch. They recommend performing a forward somersault if the fetal back is downward and a backward somersault if the fetal back is upward. If the breech is engaged, the breech must first be pushed out of the pelvis with the operator's right hand prior to correction of the presentation. There is a general consensus that vaginal disengagement should not be performed if the breech will not easily come out of the pelvis with abdominal pressure. Occasionally, the fetal head is caught under the costal margin and this prevents the disengagement of the breech. In such a case, the fetal head should be manipulated down and sideways prior to the disengagement of the breech and forward somersault. The actual version is accomplished using flexion of the fetal head and encouragement of a forward somersault by pressure on the uterus. Some practitioners pause as the breech is about to negotiate the transverse diameter of the uterus and apply acoustic stimulation. This may cause fetal kicking, which assists the version. Ferguson et al.[63] suggest that as the frank breech is more difficult to convert to a cephalic presentation due to the extension of the fetal legs, the legs should be converted to a flexed position prior to ECV. How this feat is to be accomplished is not, however, made clear.

After successful version the attitude of the fetus should be maintained manually for a few minutes.[45]

The fetal heart can be monitored continuously through the procedure or every 2 min. A repeat CTG should be performed immediately after the ECV. If this is normal, the woman may go home. She should return within a few days so that the position of the fetus can be rechecked. Some practitioners perform a cesarean section if the breech presentation recurs, whereas others follow their protocol for selection for vaginal breech delivery. Others continue to correct the presentation repeatedly. There is some evidence that the latter approach does result in more vertex presentations at delivery.

Current evidence indicates that ECV performed at term and particularly with tocolysis is a safe procedure for carefully selected women. The short-term complications are negligible and, although the long-term complications are harder to determine overall, it seems likely that the benefits will outweigh the risks. A randomized controlled trial is awaited that will more properly quantify these risks and benefits, particularly in the long term.

Assessment of the fetus

The presentation of the fetus should be checked using ultrasound scanning. This should be possible in most cases even if the woman presents in labor. The fallibility of conventional abdominal palpation as a screening test for malpresentation has been demonstrated many times including personally by the authors! Thorp et al.[65] showed that palpation only had a sensitivity of 28% and a specificity of 94% in the detection of breech presentation, using ultrasound scanning as the 'gold standard'.

X-ray examination of the fetus is being supplanted by CT scanning which reduces the radiation dosage.[66] X-ray examination has been customary during the investigation of erect lateral pelvimetry (see below) to investigate pelvic capacity and the presentation of the fetus can be confirmed at the same time. The attitude of the fetus can also be assessed, determining not only the attitude of the fetal legs but also the presence of extension of the neck. Radiological exclusion of a nuchal arm, with an estimated incidence of 4%, has also been suggested,[67] since this complication can produce delay and trauma during the second stage of labor.

Increasingly with the abandonment of erect lateral pelvimetry in the management of breech presentation, the attitude of the fetus is assessed with ultrasound.[4] Ultrasound examination will also provide an estimate of fetal weight that is so crucial to the management of breech delivery. However, it should always be remembered that estimation of fetal weight has at best an error of ± 15%, which is ± 600 g in the 4 kg fetus. Assessment of the volume of amniotic fluid is also possible and many congenital abnormalities can be detected. Placenta previa should also be excluded, as far as possible, prior to any decision about ECV or the mode of delivery.

The validity of ultrasound measurement of fetal parameters, especially the biparietal diameter, have long been debated. Bader et al.[68] performed ultrasound measurements in 450 fetuses in breech presentation and compared them with 1880 fetuses in cephalic presentation between 15 and 40 weeks gestation. They found no difference between the biparietal diameter (BPD), head circumference and the cephalic index (CI = BPD/occipital frontal distance × 100) in the two groups in uncomplicated pregnancy. However, in complicated breech pregnancies, the CI was found to be lower in breech presenting fetuses, indicating the dolichocephalic head shape that is commonly noted (the complications included premature rupture of the membranes, premature labor, intrauterine growth deficiency, fetal anomaly, hydramnios, drug and alcohol abuse, maternal diabetes and hypertension).

Neck hyperextension (the star gazing fetus) is an important condition that can cause spinal cord and brain injuries at delivery. Proposed etiologies are cord around the neck, fundal placenta, spasm of the fetal musculature and fetal and uterine anomalies. It is of interest that most mammals other than the human deliver their young with the neck of the fetus in a hyperextended position. Flexion of the neck in the human fetus is probably an adaptation to the necessity of delivering a large brain in a large fetal skull through a relatively small human pelvis. Although the incidence of neck extension in the fetus has been quoted as 7.4%,[35] its significance is hard to ascertain. Ophir et al.[69] looked specifically for hyperextension of the fetal head, using X-ray examination as part of their selection protocol. They found hyperextension requiring elective cesarean section delivery to be present in only one of 71 women screened. It is regarded as an unfavorable prognostic sign with regard to successful vaginal breech delivery, but few authors indicate how it is to be diagnosed antepartum. Erect lateral pelvimetry limits the X-ray field of view so as to limit radiological exposure and often the fetal head is not on the film. With the gradual abandonment of erect lateral pelvimetry in many centers, information about the fetal neck is no longer available from this source. There is no validation of the success of determination of the attitude of the fetal head by ultrasonography, especially in the term fetus. Ballas and Toaff[70] examined the radiological diagnosis of hyperextension of the fetal head. They found that of 58 cases in the literature where the angle of extension of the neck could be measured, 20 had an angle of extension greater than 90°. Of these, 11 were delivered vaginally and included 8

cases of damage to the cervical cord. On the basis of this, they recommend that elective cesarean section be performed when the angle of extension exceeds 90°.

Other adverse features if ECV or vaginal breech delivery are contemplated include intrauterine growth deficiency and rhesus iso-immunization.

Choice of mode of delivery

Estimates of the risk to the fetus of vaginal breech delivery have been estimated at 0–35 per 1000 deliveries.[5] It was not until the late 1950s with the increasing safety of the cesarean section that it started to become the preferred mode of delivery and was recommended on a routine basis to minimize morbidity and mortality.

Risks of vaginal breech delivery for the fetus

The risks and benefits of vaginal breech delivery are shown in **Table 2**.

Short-term effects

Many of the studies performed to assess the mortality and morbidity of the fetus undergoing vaginal breech delivery are poor. They are mostly retrospective reviews of practice and often simply compare babies delivered vaginally by the breech and by the head.[4] This is not comparing like with like and is therefore invalid. Increasingly of recent years, vaginal breech delivery is only performed when the woman presents in advanced labor. The birth of the baby is therefore unattended and often the pregnancy has not been assessed for its suitability for vaginal breech delivery.

Table 2
Risks and benefits for the fetus of vaginal breech delivery

Risks
Poor condition at birth
Intracranial hemorrhage
Medullary coning
Severance of the spinal cord
Brachial plexus injury
Occipital diastasis
Fracture of the long bones
Epiphyseal separation
Rupture of internal organs
Long-term neurological damage
Genital damage in the male[71]
Hypopituitarism[72]
Damage to the mouth and pharynx[73]

Benefits
Reduction in idiopathic pulmonary hypertension

These women are a high-risk group. Many of the long- and short-term follow-up studies of vaginally delivered breech babies were performed on populations born in the 1950s and 1960s and reflect the standards of care being offered at that time.

More recent studies reporting careful selection criteria for vaginal breech delivery and a cesarean section rate of 20–60% have reported no difference in short-term outcome for the fetus.[9,20,51,54,69,74–76,78–82] Croughan-Minihane[76] reviewed 1240 fetuses presenting by the breech with regard to birth injury, asphyxia, head trauma and neonatal seizures and found no difference between those delivered vaginally and those delivered by cesarean section after multiple-regression techniques had controlled for excess of low birthweight and premature infants in the vaginally delivered group. They also noted no difference in perinatal mortality once the antepartum stillbirths and babies with abnormalities incompatible with life had been excluded. This hospital had a cesarean section rate for breech presentation of 65% and a vaginal delivery rate of 35%. Schutte et al.[20] reviewed 57 819 singleton deliveries in the Netherlands. Altogether, 8% of these were breech. They reported an excess perinatal mortality rate with breech presentation even after correction for gestational age and birthweight. Cesarean section was more often performed for breech presentation (25%) than the vertex (6.8%), but did not appear to improve the outcome, either in relation to babies in cephalic presentation delivered by cesarean section or in relation to the vaginally delivered breech baby. Green et al.[75] noted a cesarean section rate for breech presentation that had increased from 22 to 94% during the 1970s with no decrease in the rate of birth asphyxia.

Mecke et al.[80] demonstrated a higher 1-min Apgar score in breech neonates delivered by cesarean section compared with those delivered vaginally. Babies delivered by cesarean section also had higher pH values at delivery. Similar differences were observed when babies in cephalic presentation were compared by mode of delivery. That the breech delivered vaginally has a lower pH than the cephalic infant or the breech infant delivered vaginally is not in doubt,[83] it is what this difference means clinically that is difficult to ascertain.

Certain conditions in the breech seem to increase the chances of trauma during delivery. Ballas and Toaff[70] emphasize the importance of excluding the breech with a greater than 90° neck extension. The risks of cord prolapse depend on the attitude of the fetal legs. The rate of cord prolapse appears to be of the order of 1.4–6%,[21,84] but if there is an incomplete breech the risk may be as high as 15%.[51] This compares with the risk of cord prolapse in the non-breech of 0.24–0.5%. The risks of brachial plexus injury is of the order of 8.5% at term, but 70% of these have fully resolved at 3 months of age. Brachial plexus injury is more common if the arms are caught across the back of the neck at delivery (nuchal arm). A proportion of cases with this complication are due to injudicious manipulation during delivery.

Long-term effects

Long-term follow-up studies fall into two main groups: those that review the infants delivered prior to 1970 and those after 1970. The standards of obstetric and neonatal care have changed so dramatically over this period that studies prior to this time demonstrate more about other factors than the mode of delivery.

Epidemiological studies of the link between cerebral palsy and spastic hemiplegia reveal an excess of breech infants, as might be expected. Dale and Stanley[85] reported that 11.5% of children with cerebral palsy were born in breech presentation compared with 2.9% of controls. Lagergren[86] found a 9.4% incidence of vaginal breech deliveries when reviewing all motor handicapped children aged 4–16 years in a Swedish county in 1976. Neither study evaluated breech presentation as a single variable.

Minimal brain damage and learning difficulties are subtle and have a complex relationship to perinatal events. In a recent review of the link between birth asphyxia and cerebral palsy. Hall[87] noted that only 8% of cases of cerebral palsy could be related to perinatal events.

Follow-up studies are difficult to interpret. They are largely retrospective and uncontrolled reviews of small numbers of subjects with variable lengths of follow-up and completeness of examination.[18]

Neligan[88] followed up all breech delivered infants born between 1960 and 1970 in Newcastle-upon-Tyne and found more mild neurological abnormality at 4 years in those breech infants delivered vaginally compared with those delivered by cesarean section. These differences had disappeared by the age of 10 years on more sophisticated examination. Nilssen and Bergsjo[89] followed up a series of breech infants delivered between 1960 and 1963 at 18 years of age and found no differences in mortality, morbidity or intelligence. Westgren and Ingemarsson[9] summarized the condition of the breech born infants born in this period as showing an increasing incidence of neurological abnormality in pre-school and school-age infants, but these differences disappeared on later testing in adulthood.

Those studies reviewing later born (1970–80) children reflect the impact of rising cesarean section rates and more modern obstetric care. They are still mostly retrospective reviews of practice.[19,20]

Faber-Nijolt et al.[19] performed a case-controlled study of breech delivered infants compared with cephalic delivered infants. They were matched for sex, birthweight, gestational age, maternal age, parity and year of delivery, and matching was successful in 60%

of cases (the breech delivered infants showed an excess of premature deliveries and growth-deficient babies, which made matching difficult). The group where matching was possible were evaluated at 4–10 years of age. A slight excess of minor neurological dysfunction was found, but it was not statistically significant.

A variety of other prospective evaluations of long-term outcome showed no difference in neurological outcome, psychomotor problems or cerebral palsy.[13,91,92] Long-term follow-up of infants born by the breech either spontaneously or using the Bracht maneuver for delivery of the head showed that psychometric and intellectual development were superior in those infants delivered spontaneously.[93]

Maternal risks

The relative risks of vaginal *vs* cesarean section delivery for the mother are summarized in **Table 3**.

Choice of mode of delivery: Conclusions

There has been a small randomized controlled trial of the mode of delivery of the breech. Collea *et al.*[74] randomized 208 women at term in labor to receive a cesarean section or a vaginal delivery. Altogether, 55% of the latter delivered vaginally and 45% delivered by cesarean section. Despite some difficulties with methodology, they showed no statistically significant differences in short-term neonatal outcome between those delivered vaginally and those delivered by cesarean section. By contrast, they showed 'striking and concerning differences in maternal outcome'.

Songane *et al.*[33] used decision analysis to demonstrate that a trial of vaginal delivery, by exposing the mother to the dangers of emergency cesarean section with its higher morbidity and mortality, is riskier than performing an elective cesarean section in all cases of term breech presentation. Although they conclude that

Table 3
Risks for the mother of vaginal vs cesarean section

Risks of vaginal breach
Perineal discomfort and morbidity
Difficult birth experience

Risks of cesarean section
Short-term morbidity: increased pospartum pyrexia, increased need for blood transfusion
Increased maternal mortality
Reduction in future fertility[60]
Difficult birth experience
Entering the subsequent pregnancy with a scar on the uterus

vaginal delivery is more dangerous to the fetus, they also comment that in the latter years of their review of breech delivery their elective cesarean section rate had risen to 33% from 14% (over 10 years) and that in the latter years of the review no intrapartum or neonatal deaths had occurred.

The optimum mode of delivery of the breech in order to minimize the risks to both mother and baby is a matter of great concern both to professionals and parents. Despite the fact that many studies are of dubious quality, they are remarkably consistent in reporting minimal risk of long-term neurological damage after careful selection for vaginal delivery – handicap rates will not be higher than for infants born head first or by cesarean section. The 'ideal' cesarean section rate with regard to the fetus is not known, but it seems likely to be in the range of 30–65%.

Vaginal delivery still carries the risk of cord prolapse and extended arms at delivery as well as difficult delivery of the head. This risk may be approximately 1–2%.[54,74] Therefore, obstetric expertise should be retained for dealing with these situations and for the late presenting breech in labor in whom cesarean section is logistically impossible; this may account for 11% or more of all breech deliveries.[51,54]

Assessment for vaginal breech delivery (Table 4)

All the available literature stresses the importance of utilizing a protocol for the assessment of women for vaginal breech delivery. These protocols have produced elective cesarean section rates of 25–65% with no significant differences in the outcome for the fetus whether delivered by cesarean section or vaginally. It is impossible to say, with the current evidence, what is the ideal cesarean section rate. This will be partly determined by the ethnic group of the population and whether external cephalic version is employed as well as a number of other population variables.

Assessment of pelvic capacity

Clinical pelvimetry

Clinical pelvimetry is a low-technology screening investigation probably only of benefit if there is gross contraction of the pelvis. It will make a subjective assessment of the bony features of the pelvic cavity, including the sacral promontory, the curvature of the sacrum, whether the side walls are convergent, or the ischial spines prominent, whether the sacrospinous ligaments will accommodate two fingers and whether the intertuberous diameter will accommodate the clenched fist and whether the pubic arch is greater than 90°.[34]

Table 4
Assessment for vaginal breech delivery

1. Assessment of the cause of the breech presentation
   exclude placenta previa
   exclude multiple pregnancy
   exclude fibroids/pelvic tumors
   exclude hydramnios
   exclude hydrocephalus/anencephaly
   exclude other congenital abnormalities

2. Assessment of the fetal condition
   exclude intrauterine growth retardation
   exclude rhesus disease
   exclude fetal abnormalities
   exclude others

3. Assessment of the fetal weight and attitude

4. Assessment of the maternal pelvis
   clinical pelvimetry
   X-ray erect lateral pelvimetry
   CT scanning pelvimetry

5. Assessment of the maternal condition
   exclude significant maternal disease: diabetes
   exclude proteinuric hypertension
   exclude cardiac or renal disease

6. Assessment of maternal and parental wishes
   Close consultation with the mother and partner and
   counseling about the implications of the choice of
   vaginal breech delivery *vs* elective cesarean section is
   important

The success or otherwise of clinical pelvimetry is hard to assess and most discussions about the assessment of pelvic capacity now center on X-ray pelvimetry. With regard to a clinical assessment of the size of the pelvis, a consideration of the woman's height alone is useful.[94]

X-ray and CT pelvimetry

No trials have ever been performed to assess the value of pelvimetry in the pelvis with borderline or reduced dimensions in relation to cephalic presentation. The value of pelvimetry in the assessment for vaginal breech delivery is even more controversial.[95–97] Mahamood[97] reported that there was no absolute level of pelvic contraction as assessed by X-ray pelvimetry below which vaginal delivery was impossible and that prenatal assessment of fetal weight was a more important determinant of the success of attempted vaginal delivery.

The value of CT scanning for pelvimetry is clear – it will reduce the radiation dosage and is more accurate;[66] however, there is no evidence that it will predict the outcome of a trial of vaginal breech delivery. Normal measurements do not guarantee vaginal delivery and many authorities now recommend the abandonment of X-ray pelvimetry for breech presentation.[5,25]

Criteria for selection for vaginal breech delivery

A variety of criteria are proposed. Broadly, the fetus should be neither too small nor too big and should have a well-flexed head, the mother should have at least an average capacity pelvis, judged clinically, and the mother and the baby should be in 'good' condition. An estimated fetal weight of 1500–3900 g is appropriate (for further discussion of the delivery of the preterm breech, see below). Other favorable features are frank or complete breech (not a footling) and absence of detectable congenital abnormalities.

X-ray pelvimetry may be omitted and a clinical assessment made instead. The limits of fetal weight and gestation are also contentious, with many different limits being suggested. Estimation of fetal weight is unreliable,[33] even when ultrasound is used, with a margin of error ± 15%. Some authors would exclude the primigravid woman with a breech from consideration of vaginal delivery and others consider the multiparous patient to be at higher risk.[21,25,98]

Procedure

Practical considerations in the conduct of assisted vaginal breech delivery

The essence of the assisted vaginal breech delivery is allowing as much spontaneous delivery by uterine action and maternal effort as possible. Operator intervention should be minimized and limited except for the maneuvers described below or to correct any deviation from the normal mechanism of spontaneous delivery. The operator may make the delivery more complicated by injudicious traction that encourages displacement of the fetal limbs from their normal flexed position across the fetal body or by promoting hyperextension of the fetal head. Injudicious traction will also cause the fetal body to be subjected to compression and traction forces which will predispose to further injury of soft tissue and bony parts. The fetal body should, at all times, be treated with the utmost care and grasped, if at all, by the bony parts. There are many described procedures for the vaginal delivery of the breech.[99–101]

First stage

Many authors recommend that labor should be spontaneous, as this increases the chance of successful vaginal delivery. If delivery is required before the onset of spontaneous labor, elective cesarean section is recommended by many authors.

Labor should be conducted in a labor ward with all facilities to perform a cesarean section, with a full anesthetic service and senior obstetric staff available. The woman should be instructed to arrive early in labor so that her progress and the condition of the fetus may be monitored. Similarly, should the membranes rupture, she should attend the hospital because of the risks of cord prolapse. Rupture of the membranes at any point during the labor should prompt immediate vaginal examination.

On presentation in labor, an intravenous line should be sited and blood taken for group and crossmatch. Because of the relatively high risk of cesarean section, oral intake should be avoided for the duration of the labor. After the usual assessment of the woman in labor, she should be told that continuous electronic fetal monitoring is advisable and that an epidural anesthetic may be advisable. It will make any manipulation in the second stage more comfortable and make any urge to push prior to full dilatation easier to resist. Bearing down prior to full dilatation may push the relatively smaller breech through the incompletely dilated cervix and entrap the aftercoming head behind the cervix. Epidural anesthesia is not essential, and some obstetricians suggest that there is a higher chance of spontaneous vaginal delivery without one. There is little doubt that epidural anesthesia obtunds the urge to bear down. However, the counterargument is that if a baby does not deliver easily with an epidural in situ, then it is better delivered by cesarean as there is likely to be mild relative disproportion. Because there is no clear scientific evidence to resolve this issue, it seems appropriate at the present time to allow the woman a major degree

of personal choice in this respect. Whatever she chooses, however, an anesthetist should be in attendance during the second stage of labor in case rapid anesthesia should be required for an unexpectedly difficult delivery. Although on first principles the labor should be unstimulated if possible, if the labor progress is slow there is no evidence that the careful use of oxytocin is dangerous. Oxytocin is particularly appropriate if there is a primary dysfunctional labor (slow progress in the active phase, less than 1 cm cervical dilatation every 2 h). The use of an intrauterine pressure transducer may reassure the obstetrician that excessive uterine activity is not being generated. The fear with oxytocin is that it will produce descent of the breech in the presence of feto-pelvic disproportion, hence the disproportion will only be detected when the head is entrapped above the pelvic brim and the body is already delivered. The bitrochanteric diameter is usually smaller than the biparietal, and if the former does not easily traverse the pelvis neither will the latter.[10] Collea et al.[74] demonstrated that the use of oxytocin in selected patients does not produce an excessive rate of maternal or neonatal complications.

Failure to progress in the first stage of labor over a 4-h period suggests that cesarean section is necessary. Failure to make expected progress in cervical dilatation or for the breech to descend appropriately in the first 4 h of labor or the appearance of cardiotocographic abnormalities should prompt careful consideration of whether cesarean section is advisable. Total labor duration should be similar to that in cephalic presentation, although descent of the breech may be slow. The progress of the labor should therefore be plotted on a partogram in the usual way.[101]

Meconium staining of the amniotic fluid is common in breech labor and its predictive value for asphyxia is poor. In early labor, it is often found on the glove at the end of a vaginal examination. Its passage when the breech is still high in the birth canal in the first stage may indicate 'fetal distress' and careful evaluation of the fetal heart rate pattern at this stage will be necessary. Cardiotocographic fetal heart rate abnormalities should be further investigated using fetal blood sampling, *obtaining the blood from the fetal breech, avoiding the genitalia. The region around the ischial tuberosity is the best site for blood sampling. The blade may have to be pressed more firmly onto the buttock in order to ensure a good flow of capillary blood.[99] The passage of meconium in the second stage is almost universal and is of no prognostic value.*

Second stage (*see* **Figure 1**)

The second stage should be attended and supervised by a senior obstetrician. An active second stage with vaginal breech delivery does not start until the cervix is fully dilated and the fetal anus is just seen on the perineum. The woman is then placed in the lithotomy position with her buttocks just over the end of the delivery couch and is cleaned and draped as for ventouse or forceps delivery. Care should be taken to avoid the completely supine position to avoid hypotension due to caval compression, and lateral tilt using a wedge is probably advisable. The bladder and the bowel should preferably be empty and elective bladder catheterization is probably advisable, with an 'in and out' catheter. If effective regional anesthesia is not in place, a pudendal block with perineal infiltration should be used. An episiotomy is generally advised and should be performed at this point. Episiotomy will always be required if forceps are to be used to achieve delivery of the head, if extensive manipulation of the fetus is anticipated and in all nulliparas. The breech, legs and abdomen should be allowed to deliver spontaneously to the level of the umbilicus. The breech should be encouraged to deliver in a sacro-anterior position if it is not already in this position. At this point, the obstetrician is permitted to deliver the legs, if they are extended, by abduction of the thigh and flexion of the fetal knee (using finger pressure in the popliteal fossa), allowing the fetal thigh to pass lateral to the fetal body. A loop of umbilical cord should be brought down at this point to minimize traction and possible tearing with consequent loss of fetal blood. The prognostic significance of the absence of cord pulsation is controversial. Fetal condition may be assessed at this point by noting

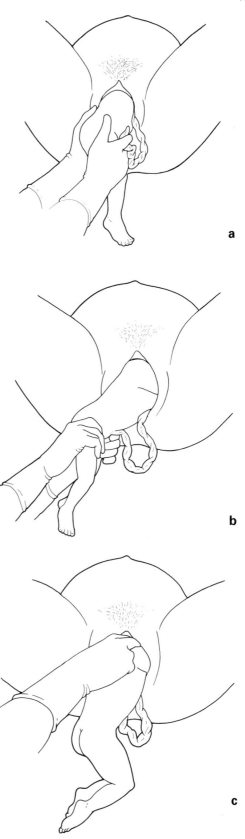

a

b

c

Figure 1.

the tone and color of the fetus at the vulva.

Delivery to this point should be achieved in one contraction and one maternal expulsive effort. Delivery of the rest of the body, to delivery of the mouth, should be achieved over the next one or two contractions. The duration of time that should be allowed to elapse between delivery to just below the umbilicus to delivery of the mouth is 5–10 min. Arulkumaran et al.[102] examined two different ways of delivering the breech. They allowed spontaneous delivery to the hip with one contraction and maternal effort followed by an assisted delivery of the rest of the body and head in the next contraction in one group of women, and in another group they assisted delivery to the shoulders with one contraction and then an assisted delivery of the head was performed with the next contraction. The former method produced babies with a smaller reduction in the fetal blood pH and in better condition at delivery, judged by the Apgar score and need for ventilation. They hypothesized that this was due to exposure, stretching and compression of the umbilical cord over a longer period of time during the delivery of the latter group, or possibly due to premature separation of the placenta.

Once the legs and abdomen have emerged, the fetus should be allowed to hang from the vulva until the wing of the posterior scapula is seen. The arms are often found folded over the fetal chest, flexed at the shoulder and elbow and in this case no particular maneuver is required to effect their delivery. If injudicious traction is exerted in order to deliver the breech, the arms may become extended over the fetal head. In this case, the Lovsett's maneuver may be used to free the arm. This involves wrapping the fetus in a warm, dry towel and grasping the body over the bony pelvis with the thumbs along the sacrum. The fetal back should then be turned through 180°, until the posterior arm comes to lie anteriorly. The elbow will appear below the symphysis pubis and that arm and hand can be delivered by sweeping it across the fetal body. This maneuver is repeated in reverse to deliver the other arm. If these maneuvers fail, it is the traditional last resort to induce deep anesthesia and push the body of the fetus well up, pass the hand along its ventral aspect and bring down the most accessible arm. Having pushed the fetus up successfully, it may well be safer to proceed with cesarean section.[103] The nuchal arm, where the arm is flexed at the elbow and extended at the shoulder coming to lie behind the fetal head, may be dealt with by a modified Lovsett's maneuver: rotating the fetal back through 180° in the direction of the trapped arm may draw the elbow forward toward the face and over the fetal head by friction on the birth canal and render it amenable to a traditional Lovsett's to deliver the arm. If this technique does not suffice to release the nuchal arm, it may be forcibly extracted by hooking the finger over it, in which case a fracture almost always follows.[100]

The fetus should be allowed to hang from the vulva for a few seconds again until the nape of the neck is visible at the anterior vulva. This allows descent of the head into the pelvis and at this point the head may be delivered. Clinch[101] advises that this technique combined with downward traction may result in hyperextension of the fetal head rather than flexion and descent, so again operator interference may cause complications in the delivery. If the head negotiates the inlet of the pelvis easily, there is little danger that the progress of the head will be arrested in mid-cavity. If there is difficulty with the head in the mid-cavity or the outlet, a properly performed Mauriceau-Smellie-Veit maneuver will overcome this (see below for a full description). Should the head fail to descend into the pelvis after the shoulders have delivered, the body of the fetus should be turned sideways and suprapubic pressure used to flex the head and push it into the pelvis in the occipitotransverse position. A vaginal finger in the mouth of the fetus may also tend to flex the head and help it to descend into the pelvis prior to delivery.[101] Continued failure of the head to descend into the pelvis is the only indication for symphysiotomy.[104] The causes of this feared complication may be hydrocephalus, in which case the head should be perforated and the cerebrospinal fluid drained. Alternatively, the cervix may not be fully dilated, in which case the cervix must be incised. If there are locked twins, there is no choice but to do a cesarean section. If none of these causes is present, then the operator must assume that cephalo-pelvic disproportion is present and there is a strong case for the performance of a sym-physiotomy.[103] With proper predelivery assessment and conduct of labor, this situation should not arise.

The techniques for delivery of the head are various (see **Figure 2**). Some authorities advise that the body should be supported on the right forearm of the operator and not be raised above the horizontal in order to minimize the chance of hyperextension of the fetal head. Others advise that the operator's assistant should grasp the ankles of the fetus and raise the body vertically above the mother's abdomen prior to any attempt to deliver the fetal head, as this will promote flexion of the fetal head and place it in the antero-posterior diameter of the pelvis. The latter technique is called the Burns-Marshall technique. The Burns-Marshall technique may flex the head and deliver it over the perineum without further intervention. It is therefore advisable to cover the perineum with the hand to prevent precipitate delivery of the head as the body is swung upward. The operator's hand can then be opened slowly in order to allow the rest of the head to deliver slowly.[101] Often, however, further assistance is required to deliver the head. The head may be delivered from this position using forceps applied below the fetal body and in the usual fashion. The operator should remember that the smallest part of the head is lowest in the vagina and that the tip of the forceps blade must accommodate the occiput; therefore, premature straightening of the forceps blade during application will cause undue pressure on the side of the fetal head.[101]

The forceps should be of a type with a long enough shank to permit the operator to visualize the maneuver, as often the fetal arms obstruct the view and if the fetal body is in the horizontal position access is further reduced. The head should be delivered over 1 min to reduce the compression–decompression forces on the fetal skull that may cause tentorial tears and intracranial bleeding.

The other often described technique of delivering the fetal head is the Mauriceau-Smellie-Veit maneuver. This is actually a variety of techniques. The principle is that of traction down the axis of the birth canal and encouraging flexion of the fetal head to present the most favorable diameters to the pelvis. With the fetus supported on the right forearm, the middle finger of the right hand is passed into the fetal throat and the forefinger and the ring finger are placed either on the fetal shoulders or the malar eminences. Traction is applied to flex and deliver the head. The middle finger should not be just inside the fetal mouth, as traction can produce dislocation or fracture of the mandible.[99] If the finger is inserted too far down the throat, creation of a pseudo-diverticulum of the pharynx has been described. The left hand is used to exert pressure upward and posteriorly on the fetal occiput to encourage flexion. Alternatively, suprapubic pressure can be applied to encourage head flexion and descent. All these maneuvers can be performed with the operator's assistant elevating the fetal body above the horizontal. Clinch[101] notes that the traction downward of the fetal shoulders tends to stretch the cervical spine, and in combination with flexion of the fetal head will draw the base of the skull away from the vault thus causing a tentorial tear. He therefore recommends that traction on the trunk should not be used. All these permutations have been described by various authors as the Mauriceau-Smellie-Veit maneuver.

A pediatrician should be present at delivery and the breech should have the mouth and pharynx sucked out on the perineum prior to complete delivery of the head.

Practical considerations in the performance of breech extraction (see **Figure 3**)

This is rarely performed nowadays because of the risks of fetal and maternal trauma and because of the effects of injudicious traction on the fetal body. It is occasionally indicated for the delivery of a second twin after internal podalic version or if cord prolapse complicates the late second stage. It may also be appropriate if the fetus is dead. In breech extraction, the traction is exerted on the body of the fetus to expedite delivery. Groin traction is performed to draw the breech over

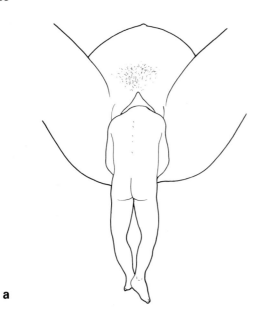

a

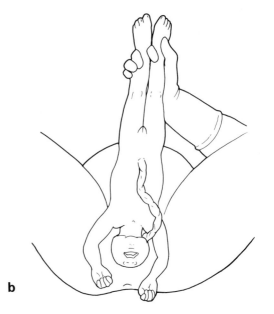

b

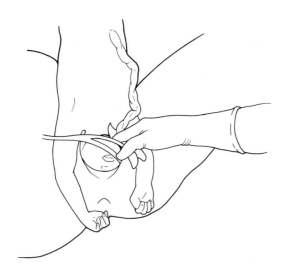

c

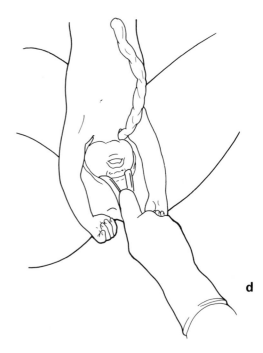

d

Figure 2.

the perineum, Lovsett's maneuver is employed routinely and downward traction is exerted to bring the head into the pelvis. All the above stages of assisted breech delivery are achieved actively by the obstetrician.[99]

Practical considerations in the performance of cesarean section for the delivery of the term breech

The orthodox obstetric practice of considering any woman with a breech pres-

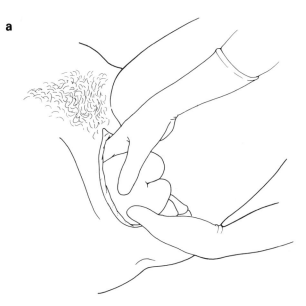

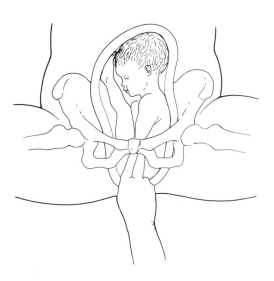

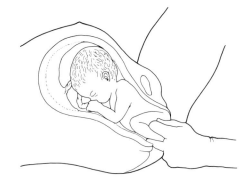

Figure 3.

entation and any other medical or obstetric complication for an elective cesarean section has much to recommend it. Elective and even emergency cesarean section for the term breech should present few technical problems. It should be remembered that the performance of a cesarean section does not prevent the possibility of birth injury and many of the above considerations about the careful delivery of the aftercoming head and the dangers of traction on the fetal spine still apply. The lower segment will be the site of choice for the incision with a term breech presentation. Schutterman and Grimes[105] reviewed 416 breeches of all gestations allocated randomly to transverse or low vertical incisions in the uterus and found no advantages for low vertical incisions. An elective cesarean section when adequate amniotic fluid is still present and the uterus is less likely to contract rapidly before completion of delivery of the breech will present less of a problem to the operator. Forceps may be employed for delivery of the aftercoming head. Delivery at full dilatation in the absence of amniotic fluid may be difficult, as an arm may prolapse through the uterine incision and should be immediately pushed back. Instead, a leg should be grasped and brought through the incision. Traction will then effect the rest of the delivery. The head can be trapped in a well-contracted lower segment and the incision will then need to be enlarged in a J-shaped fashion to increase the access. In general, the mode of effecting delivery through the uterine incision is the same as for the vaginal breech delivery and many of the same complications may arise.

'Active breech delivery'

With increasing consumer pressure over the last few years toward less interventionist obstetrics, a demand for an active method of delivering the breech has appeared. This demand has been satisfied in the UK by a group of mainly midwife practitioners who have started to perform the so-called 'active breech delivery'. This encourages women to be active during labor and while encouraging the woman to adopt the most comfortable birthing position, they favor a standing *position for the delivery itself. They emphasize non-pharmacological analgesia, and encourage maternal participation in the birth. The breech is usually allowed to deliver spontaneously without any interference from the birth attendants. There is no evidence to suggest that this method is better than an assisted breech delivery.*

Management Options for Preterm Breech Presentation

The search for methods of preventing or suppressing preterm labor has proved disappointing[106] and obstetricians have been forced to look at other techniques for optimizing the condition of preterm infants at birth to minimize neonatal complications. This has focused predominantly on the mode of delivery and has led to an increase in the cesarean section rate. At a time of popular concern in many countries about escalating cesarean section rates, the controversy about mode of delivery, and the balance between fetal/neonatal and maternal risk, has been particularly fierce in relation to the preterm baby in breech presentation.

Risks

Approximately 15% of all babies delivered between 26 and 32 weeks gestation are in breech presentation, and the proportion of babies delivered between these gestations has been remarkably constant over the years at 7%. However, the mortality and morbidity of babies delivered between 33 and 36 weeks inclusive is now very low, and not significantly influenced by mode of delivery provided cesarean section is undertaken for the usual clinical indications. Discussion is focused here on the gestation range of 26–32 weeks, when approximately 2% of all pregnant women with viable fetuses will deliver. Most breech presentations at these gestations are due to the chance lie of a very mobile fetus in the relatively copious amniotic fluid. Thus at 26–32 weeks, about 25% of all presentations will be by the breech giving an overall incidence of 0.5%.

The premature breech presentation shares many of the characteristics of the mature breech. The premature breech also has a higher rate of congenital abnormality than its vertex presenting counterpart; Lamont et al.[107] have shown that up to 18% of preterm breech infants are congenitally abnormal. The correlation of abnormal

premature presentation and congenital abnormality is well documented.[108] The preterm breech has a higher antepartum stillbirth and neonatal death rate than babies presenting by the head, regardless of mode of delivery.[9,19] It is probably even more true of the preterm breech than the term infant that poor outcome in survivors, such as mild neurological dysfunction, cannot safely be attributed solely to the fact of vaginal breech delivery, but also to the abnormalities associated with breech presentation. The premature breech shows other striking differences from the premature cephalic presenting infant; it is more commonly small for gestational age and has a lower feto-placental ratio.[21] It also tends to have a larger head circumference for a given birthweight than babies delivered in vertex presentation, probably due to the lack of the compressive effect of the lower segment.[22] It seems likely that in many cases, presentation at delivery, prematurity and poor fetal outcome are all determined by the same prenatal influence.

At delivery

Experienced obstetricians have recognized that cesarean section is not always an atraumatic option for the fetus and the preterm breech infant faces some formidable difficulties whichever route of delivery is employed. Wigglesworth and Husemeyer[109] have emphasized the vulnerability of the occipital bone to damage during vaginal breech delivery, due to its impact on the maternal pubis during descent of the fetal head into the pelvis during the second stage. These forces tend to separate the squamous part of the occipital bone from the lateral part (occipital diastasis). This produces a ridge in the posterior fossa and hence bruising or laceration of the cerebellum. The squamous part of the occipital bone is forced anteriorly to distort the foramen magnum and produce pressure on the spinal cord. Cerebellar bruising can be present in the absence of occipital diastasis and although the fracture may be easily diagnosable post-delivery with a lateral skull X-ray, the cerebellar bruising alone will not be diagnosable unless the cerebellum is scanned routinely by the neonatologist using ultrasound. The injury is commonly not discovered at postmortem examination if traditional dissection techniques have been used. The damage to the brain may not be clinically apparent until the stage of approximately 2 years, when the child will manifest signs of clumsiness and poor coordination consequent upon its cerebellar damage (ataxic cerebral palsy).[88]

In addition, the preterm infant is vulnerable to the intraventricular and periventricular damage secondary to hemorrhage or ischemia, which can be due to hypoxic or acidotic insults in the antepartum, intrapartum and neonatal periods. The premature breech may be still more susceptible to these as a consequence of the peculiar circumstances surrounding delivery. However, avoiding vaginal delivery will not necessarily prevent intracranial bleeding. Tejani *et al.*[110] have shown that premature labor of itself can produce intracranial hemorrhage even if delivery is delayed or by cesarean section.[110]

A traumatic breech delivery in which there is widespread limb and body bruising can produce gross skeletal muscle damage that results in large quantities of hemoglobin and myoglobin being liberated. This can lead to severe jaundice and damage to the kidneys in a premature infant whose hepatic capacity to deal with bilirubin is limited and whose renal excretory capacity is poor. This can produce a form of 'shock lung' in the neonate, manifesting as severe respiratory distress syndrome.

The premature breech infant is also susceptible to damage to the internal organs, transection of the spinal cord and other nerve palsies consequent on traction, especially the brachial plexus, and fractures of long bones[52] similar to its more mature counterpart. Because the widest diameter of the fetus is the biparietal diameter and the discrepancy between the diameters of the head and the body are most pronounced in the premature fetus, it is possible for the body and limbs of the premature breech to slip through a cervix that is still incompletely dilated and the head will be unable to follow. This 'entrapment' of the head is more likely in the mother who commences active pushing prior to the second stage, with a footling presentation, especially with the preterm fetus where the subcutaneous fat has not yet been laid down and the liver is not of the large size reached in the mature fetus; hence the abdominal circumference is relatively smaller. Recommended management is usually to incise the cervix with scissors at 4 and 8 o'clock, but inevitably there is delay in delivery and therefore an increase in the hypoxic stress to the fetus, together with an increase in traumatic morbidity to both mother and child.

However, injuries are not confined to babies delivered vaginally in breech presentation. Any very low birthweight baby is susceptible to trauma from a difficult delivery through a poorly formed lower segment. If the presentation is breech, then a limited uterine incision can impede the delivery of the head to the same degree as can a difficult vaginal delivery and is analogous in every way to the entrapment of the head that is such a feared complication of the premature breech delivered vaginally. To some extent, this can be avoided by performing an anterior vertical uterine incision (ideally De Lee's incision, but often in a very small uterus it becomes a classical). However, this carries increased risks for the mother, particularly in respect of a rupture in a future pregnancy or labor, but occasionally also in terms of poor healing and postpartum hemorrhage.

Management of the preterm breech in labor

Most elective deliveries of the preterm breech where the woman is not in labor are for fetal or maternal indications where elective cesarean section is the preferred method of delivery. Most of the controversy about management centers on the preterm breech presentaiton in labor.

Management of the premature breech in labor rests on the accurate diagnosis of premature labor, the confirmation of presentation and the exclusion of fetal abnormality. It is evident that in up to 80% of cases where the mother thinks she is in premature labor, contractions cease spontaneously and the pregnancy continues. The definitive diagnosis of labor, therefore, rests on demonstrating progressive dilatation of the cervix. Careful cervical assessment of all women in suspected premature labor is imperative to confirm or refute the diagnosis. In the presence of ruptured membranes, this should be done using the full aseptic technique and the number of examinations limited to minimize the risk of introducing infection, causing chorioamnionitis. Vaginal examination can confirm the presentation and can even reveal the presence of fetal abnormality (e.g. anal atresia!).

In view of the recognized association of fetal abnormality with premature breech presentation, all previous ultrasound examinations should be carefully reviewed. A further detailed ultrasound scan should be performed if possible to confirm the normality of the fetus and check on placental position at the same time. An estimate of fetal weight may allow a more rational decision to be made about the optimum place and mode of delivery. Ultrasound fetal weight estimation is possible to ± 15% in skilled hands, although when performed by junior residents out of normal hours, errors greater than 15% have been reported in over 40% of cases.[111] This has led some workers to suggest that the outcome for the infant is best predicted by accurate knowledge of gestational age.[106]

Administration of tocolytics may be appropriate in an effort to delay delivery for long enough to administer steroids to promote surfactant production in the fetal lung prior to preterm delivery, or to arrange delivery in a site with appropriate neonatal intensive care facilities. It is now clear that tocolytic therapy is ineffective in preventing premature delivery in the longer term and that its use beyond 48–72 h is probably inappropriate.[106]

Optimum mode of delivery of the preterm breech

The preterm breech on the labor ward presents the obstetrician with rather a heterogeneous group of clinical problems. Some will present not in labor but with spontaneous rupture of the membranes only; others will present at 7 cm dilatation in strong labor and deliver after only a short interval. As with all premature deliveries, premature vaginal breech delivery may well be precipitate and in many cases unattended by skilled medical attendants. It is important to realize that, also in common with all preterm labors, the antecedents are often clearly pathological and therefore a decision about the mode of delivery is uncontentious. If there has been a placental abruption or cord prolapse, then clearly cesarean section is indicated.

However, if the clinical situation is one of 'the uncomplicated preterm breech in labor' (i.e. if fetal and maternal condition are good, and labor is progressing at a normal rate), it is necessary to decide whether a vaginal delivery is to be allowed, or a cesarean section undertaken.

One of the first suggestions that cesarean section should be undertaken routinely for the delivery of the preterm breech was in 1977 when Goldenberg and Nelson reviewed the outcome of 224 babies less than 1500 g delivered between 1975 and 1979.[112] They compared babies delivered vaginally in breech presentation with babies delivered vaginally in vertex presentation, and all those delivered by cesarean section. For reasons enumerated earlier (in particular, the differing incidence of congenital anomaly), their comparisons were not valid. The other problem highlighted by these authors was the non-comparability of the study groups in other respects. The authors report that many fetuses below 1000 g were not monitored as they were thought to be non-viable, or, if they were monitored, when signs of fetal distress supervened surgical intervention was often not performed as the fetus was thought to be 'too small to live'. This approach resulted in infants being delivered vaginally who happened to survive despite non-intervention, being compared with infants who were thought to be viable and not 'too small to live' and who were therefore delivered electively by cesarean section, attended by senior and experienced members of staff. Such a comparison is inherently likely to show a better outcome for the latter group and therefore lead to the (potentially) erroneous conclusion that cesarean section improves the outcome for the preterm breech infant. The outcomes for the babies were also assessed in 500 g weight intervals as the number of infants involved was so small. This can lead to substantial differences in mean weights between the groups within individual bands. The optimum size of weight band is probably 100 g, which allows the very real differences between the survival rates at 28 and 32 weeks to become apparent.[114] These very small weight bands require much larger numbers of infants before comparisons can be held to be valid.

Further retrospective reviews of clinical practice

were published over the next few years: some correctly comparing vaginally delivered breech with the breech delivered by cesarean section, but then only stratifying by birthweight below and above 2500 g[39] or in other similarly wide weight bands.[115] Some advocated cesarean section[39,115] and some advised that selected preterm breeches should be allowed to deliver vaginally.[116–119] Most of these latter authors felt that outcome was more related to obstetric variables rather than the mode of delivery. Other authors advised that all premature infants are best delivered by classical cesarean section.[120]

Further evidence of the non-comparability of groups of vaginally delivered and cesarean delivered infants is shown in a paper by Woods.[117] He noted that in his group (1000–1500 g birthweight) there was a marked difference in the average weight, with the babies delivering vaginally being significantly lighter than those delivered by cesarean section – a difference likely to account for any differences in survival. These discrepancies in weight or gestational age are also found in other papers reporting improved outcomes for preterm breeches after cesarean section.[121] A further series of retrospective and uncontrolled studies were then reported to show a better outcome after cesarean section for babies weighing 1000–1500 g, but no advantage to babies weighing less than this.[107,122] In 1986, Bodmer et al. concluded the opposite: that babies <1000 g or from 25–28 weeks gestation were most likely to benefit, although it was in this group that cesarean section was least often used.[123]

Even more recently, Weissman et al. reported that in the weight bands 500–999 g, 1000–1499 g and 1500–1999 g, there was no statistically significant difference in survival rates or the rates of intraventricular hemorrhage by mode of delivery, but that those preterm breech babies delivered by cesarean section had statistically significant lower long-term morbidity.[124]

In order to overcome the non-comparability of groups in these retrospective reviews of practice, there has been a series of attempts at using statistical techniques to determine the contribution that mode of delivery makes to outcome for the preterm breech.[125,126] Only Kitchen et al.[126] found that mode of delivery was a significant factor in the likelihood of survival for the preterm breech. Others have found that variables such as gestational age or administration of steroids prenatally are more significantly associated with outcome.

Thus the current evidence has major methodological flaws that makes it unreliable as a guide to clinical decision making and has led to a number of calls for a randomized controlled trial to settle the question of optimum mode of delivery. Despite this, there has only been one such randomized trial that has actually been completed.[127] Viegas et al. randomized 23 women but unfortunately their analysis of the results was fundamentally flawed by inappropriate withdrawals and no conclusions can be drawn from their results. Two other randomized trials of the optimum mode of delivery of the preterm infant (both vertex and breech presenting) have been initiated, but both were terminated prematurely and produced no interpretable results.[128,129] Lumley et al.[128] randomized just 4 subjects of a possible 33 who were eligible over a 5-month period and terminated the trial after drawing the conclusion that clinicians were unwilling to randomize their management. Wallace et al.[129] aborted their randomized trial of the optimum mode of delivery of the preterm infant because they found that an unacceptably high number of the babies (63%) were above the 1500 g upper weight limit for the trial. They concluded that a more accurate way of estimating fetal weight prior to delivery was needed before a further attempt was feasible. The subjects they did randomize were analysed according to the eventual mode of delivery, not according to the randomized mode of delivery, thereby invalidating the randomizing process.

A prospective randomized multicenter trial recruiting subjects to determine the best mode of delivery for the preterm breech (26–32 weeks) has just been abandoned in the UK. This was funded by Birthright and coordinated from the West London Hospital. The recruitment rate was disappointing, with only 10% of eligible subjects being randomized, despite high numbers of women consenting to take part in the trial and sufficient numbers of premature breeches available for randomization. No definitive conclusion was reached. This appears to reflect obstetricians' reluctance to abandon individualized decisions about management even in the presence of a high degree of scientific uncertainty about the basis on which their decisions are being made, and despite the fact that preliminary data show that 30% of preterm breeches not entered in the trial were allowed to deliver vaginally. It therefore appears likely that the optimum mode of delivery of the preterm breech will remain uncertain for the foreseeable future. At gestations above 32 weeks and when the fetus weighs 1500 g or more, current evidence does not suggest any advantage to routine cesarean section. Under this gestation and weight but at more than 26 weeks gestation, the best mode of delivery remains uncertain in the absence of any clinical feature specifically indicating cesarean section. The advantage, if any, that routine section confers on the fetus is likely to be small, otherwise it would already be obvious in the multiplicity of published data already available. What is certain is that if a policy of routine cesarean section for the preterm breech fetus is followed, a number of cesarean sections will be performed unnecessarily – for the fetus that is congenitally abnormal, for the fetus that is >1500 g and therefore unlikely to benefit, for babies mistakenly thought to be in breech presentation (of which there were two in the Birthright study) and for some that will not actually be in established premature labor and were destined to deliver at a later gestation. A policy of routine cesarean section will also expose the mother to an established risk of maternal mortality[27] consequent on emergency cesarean section, and morbidity already discussed with relation to the term breech fetus above.

Procedure: Conduct of Delivery

Vaginal delivery of the preterm breech should be supervised by an experienced obstetrician. An effective epidural anesthetic is preferable to prevent the woman from pushing prior to full dilatation, to allow manipulation of the breech, or painless operative intervention either with forceps or rapid recourse to cesarean section. The anesthetist and pediatrician should be in attendance for the second stage. There is no clear evidence to favor the use of obstetric forceps to the head; the pelvis will be relatively capacious for the premature neonate and it will not be subject to the rapid compression–decompression forces applied to the head of the mature infant in breech presentation. There is some evidence that delivery with intact membranes is an advantage.[112] Should the cervix clamp down over the head or the body be delivered through an incompletely dilated cervix, the head should be flexed abdominally and the finger of the vaginal hand should be inserted in the mouth of the fetus to flex the head and facilitate delivery. If this is not possible, then scissors with the intracervical blade guarded by a finger should be introduced at 4 and 8 o'clock and the cervix should be incised. The carefully flexed head should now deliver easily. The cervix is usually repaired easily provided analgesia is adequate.

If cesarean section is indicated, the abdominal incision used should be considered carefully. Although a Pfannenstiel will give good access for a lower segment uterine incision, if this needs to be extended in an emergency (e.g. if the head becomes entrapped), then a vertical midline incision will be an advantage (it can be extended upward as far as is necessary). The advent of mass closure with nylon has reduced the morbidity of the midline approach so that it is now on a par with the Pfannenstiel, apart from the obvious cosmetic drawback. As well as providing improved access, it is also quicker. If a transverse uterine incision needs extending, then a J-shape is to be preferred to an inverted T, as the latter leaves a point of marked scar weakness at its center, which may rupture in a future pregnancy. The De Lee or classical uterine incision appears to confer little benefit on the fetus in terms of reduced trauma, from 28 weeks onwards (Patterson, Stacey and Steer, unpublished data). On the other hand, neonatal mortality below 28 weeks can be up to 50%.[113] *Because of the maternal morbidity involved, it is probably unwise to use the classical approach to try to salvage the preterm baby if its viability seems doubtful.*

CONCLUSIONS

The management of the preterm breech in labor is a paradigm of the difficult obstetric problem. Priorities in management include the exclusion as far as possible of congenital abnormality and placenta previa and accurate determination of presentation (preferably with ultrasound), accurate diagnosis of premature labor by careful vaginal examination, careful observation of fetal and maternal condition, epidural anesthesia, and the participation of an experienced obstetrician. Clear-cut recommendations about the optimum mode of delivery will have to await the performance of a properly conducted trial, which in the light of current experience seems unlikely ever to be performed. In the absence of such evidence, the decision about the mode of delivery should be reached after close consultation with the laboring woman and her partner.

The presence of breech presentation in both the term and the preterm pregnancy confers an increased risk on the fetus regardless of the mode of delivery. This increased risk is only partly due to an increased rate of congenital malformations. The use of external cephalic version in the appropriately assessed woman after 37 weeks gestation shows a clear benefit in the reduced numbers of cesarean sections and an increased rate of vaginal delivery in the cephalic position.

There is no definitive evidence to show that elective cesarean section for the term or the preterm breech presentation confers any benefit on the fetus either in the short or the long term.

Women should be selected for vaginal breech delivery using a protocol which should consider fetal morphology, weight, attitude and well-being, placental location, an assessment of the maternal pelvis, and any

maternal conditions which would preclude vaginal delivery. The current paucity of evidence offers few clues as to what the ideal elective cesarean section rate should be, nor what emergency cesarean section rate might be expected using the different vaginal breech delivery protocols. Currently, the mode of delivery should be decided taking all the above factors into consideration and in close consultation with the pregnant woman and her family.

BREECH PRESENTATION
Summary of Management Options

Breech presentation at term

- Consider external cephalic version (? with tocolysis)

- Fetal assessment
  - confirm diagnosis and determine placental site
  - normality
  - attitude
  - fetal size

- Choice of mode of delivery
  - no clear evidence for elective cesarean section or trial of vaginal delivery being the better method
  - if vaginal breech delivery is to be considered, a written procol is advisable (see **Table 4**) and critical review of labor is mandatory

Preterm breech presentation

- Elective delivery
  - usually by cesarean section for fetal and/or maternal reasons

- Preterm breech in labor
  - confirm in labor (including vaginal examination)
  - confirm normality (if time)
  - no clear indication of which method is better (a protocol is to be encouraged also)

REFERENCES

1 O'Leary JA, Pasley WW (1983) Once a breech, always a caesarean section. In Zuspan FP, Christiann CD (eds) *Reid's Controversies in Obstetrics and Gynaecology*, Vol. III, pp. 235–239. Philadelphia, PA: W.B. Saunders.

2 MacArthur JL (1964) Reduction of the hazards of breech presentation by external cephalic version. *American Journal of Obstetrics and Gynecology* **88**:302–306.

3 Hytten F (1982) Breech presentation: Is it a bad omen? *British Journal of Obstetrics and Gynaecology* **60**:417–420.

4 Confino E, Gleicher N, Elrad H, Ismajovich B, David MP (1985) The breech dilemma: A review. *Obstetrical and Gynecological Survey* **40**:330–337.

5 Kauppila O (1975) The perinatal mortality in breech deliveries and observations on affecting factors: A retrospective study of 2227 cases. *Acta Obstetrica et Gynecologica Scandinavica* **39**:1–79 (suppl.).

6 Haughey MJ (1985) Fetal position during pregnancy. *American Journal of Obstetrics and Gynecology* **153**:885–886.

7 Lamont RF, Dunlop PDM, Crowley P *et al.* (1983) Spontaneous preterm labour and delivery at under 34 weeks gestation. *British Medical Journal* **286**:454–457.

8 Collea JV, Rabin SC, Weghorst GR *et al.* (1978) The randomised management of term frank breech presentation: Vaginal delivery versus caesarean section. *American Journal of Obstetrics and Gynecology* **134**:186.

9 Westgren LM, Ingemarsson I (1988) Breech delivery and mental handicap. *Baillières Clinical Obstetrics & Gynecology* **2**:187–194.

10 Mazor M, Hagay ZJ, Leiberman J, Biale Y, Insler V (1985) Fetal abnormalities associated with breech delivery. *Journal of Reproductive Medicine* **30**:884–886.

11 Soernes T, Bakke T (1986) The length of the human umbilical cord in vertex and breech presentations. *American Journal of Obstetrics and Gynecology* **154**:1086–1087.

12 Westgren LMR, Songsetr G, Paul RH (1985) Preterm delivery: Another retrospective study. *Obstetrics and Gynecology* **66**:481–484.

13 Luterkort M, Polberger S, Persson PH, Bjerre I (1987) Role of asphyxia and slow intrauterine growth among breech delivered infants. *Early Human Development* **14**:19–31.

14 Ranney B (1973) The gentle art of external cephalic version. *American Journal of Obstetrics and Gynecology* **116**:239–248.

15 Stevenson CS (1950) The principal cause of breech presentation in single term pregnancies. *American Journal of Obstetrics and Gynecology* **60**:41–53.

16 Fianu S, Vaclavinkova V (1978) The site of placental attachment as a factor in the aetiology of breech presentation. *Acta Obstetrica et Gynaecologica Scandinavica* **58**:209–210.

17 Robertson IS (1984) Breech presentation associated with anticonvulsant drugs. *Journal of Obstetrics and Gynecology* **4**:174–177.

18 Manzke H (1987) Morbidity among infants born in breech presentation. *Journal of Perinatal Medicine* **6**:127–138.

19 Faber-Nijolt R, Huisjes HJ, Touwen BCL, Fidler VJ (1983) Neurological follow-up of 281 children born in breech presentation: A controlled study. *British Medical Journal* **286**:9–12.

20 Schutte MF, Van Hemel DJS, van de Berg C, Van de Pol A (1985) Perinatal mortality in breech presentation as compared vertex presentation in singleton pregnancy: An analysis based upon 57819 computer registered pregnancies in the Netherlands. *European Journal of Obstetrics, Gynecology and Reproductive Biology* **19**:391.

21 Brenner WF, Bruce RD, Hendricks CH (1974) The characteristics and perils of breech presentation. *American Journal of Obstetrics and Gynecology* **118**:700–712.

22 Duignan NM (1982) Management of breech presentation. In Studd J (ed.) *Progress in Obstetrics and Gynaecology*, Vol. 2, pp. 73–84. Edinburgh: Churchill Livingstone.

23 O'Connell P, Keane A (1985) The term breech: Subsequent growth and development. In Clinch J, Matthews T (eds) *Perinatal Medicine*, pp. 217–235. Lancaster: MTP Press.

24 Nelson KB, Ellenberg JH (1986) Antecedents of cerebral palsy: Multivariate analysis of risks. *New England Journal of Medicine* **315**:81–86.

25 Rovinsky JJ, Miller JA, Kaplan S (1973) Management of breech presentation at term. *American Journal of Obstetrics and Gynecology* **115**:497–513.

27 Hall MH (1990) Commentary: Confidential enquiry into maternal death. *British Journal of Obstetrics and Gynaecology* **97**:752–753.

28 Notzon FG, Placek PJ, Taffel SM (1987) Comparisons of national caesarean section rates. *New England Journal of Medicine* **316**:386–389.

29 Taffel SM, Placek PJ, Liss T (1987) Trends for the United States: Cesarean section rates and reasons for the 1980–1985 rise. *American Journal of Public Health* **77**:955–959.

30 Anderson GM, Lomas J (1984) Determinants of the increasing caesarean section rates: Patients, facilities or policies? *Canadian Medical Association Journal* **132**:253–259.

31 Hofmeyr GJ (1989) Breech presentation and abnormal lie in late pregnancy. In Chalmers I, Enkin M, Kierse MJNC (eds) *Effective Care in Pregnancy and Childbirth*, pp. 653–665. Oxford: Oxford University Press.

32 Lilford RJ, Van Coeverden De Groot HA, Moore PJ, Bingham P (1990) The relative risks of caesarean section (intrapartum and elective) and vaginal delivery: A detailed analysis to exclude the effects of medical disorders and other acute pre-existing physiological disturbances. *British Journal of Obstetrics and Gynaecology* **97**:883–892.

33 Songane FF, Thobani S, Malik H, Bingham P, Lilford RJ (1987) Balancing the risks of planned caesarean section and trial of vaginal delivery for the mature selected singleton breech presentation. *Journal of Perinatal Medicine* **15**:531–543.

34 Llewelyn-Jones D (1983) Antenatal care. In *Fundamentals of Obstetrics and Gynaecology*, Vol. 1, *Obstetrics*, pp. 70–71. London: Faber and Faber.

35 Westgren M, Edvall H, Nordstrom E, Svalenius E
(1985) Spontaneous cephalic version of breech presentation in the last trimester. *British Journal of Obstetrics
and Gynaecology* **92**:19–22.

36 Hofmeyr GJ (1983) Effect of external cephalic version
in late pregnancy on breech presentation and caesarean
section rate: A controlled trial. *British Journal of
Obstetrics and Gynaecology* **90**:392–399.

37 Bung P, Huch R, Huch A (1987) Ist die undische
avendung der Beckenendelage frequenz. *Geburtsh
Frauenheilk* **47**:202–205.

38 Bradley-Watson PJ (1975) The decreasing value of
external cephalic version in modern obstetrics. *American Journal of Obstetrics and Gynecology* **13**:237–241.

39 Lyons ER, Papsain FR (1978) Caesarean section in the
management of breech presentation. *American Journal
of Obstetrics and Gynecology* **130**:558–561.

40 Saling E, Muller-Holve W (1975) External cephalic version under tocolysis. *Journal of Perinatal Medicine*
3:115–121.

41 Mensinck WFA, Huisjes HJ (1980) Is external version
useful in breech presentation? (English abstract). *Nederlands Tijdschrift voor Geneeskunde* **124**:1828–1831.

42 Kasule J, Chimbira THK, Brown IMcL (1985) Controlled trial of external cephalic version. *British Journal
of Obstetrics and Gynaecology* **92**:14–18.

43 Brosset A (1956) The value of prophylactic external
version in cases of breech presentation. *Acta Obstetrica
et Gynecologica Scandinavica* **35**:555–562.

44 Van Vellen AF, Van Cappellan AW, Flu PK, Straub
MJPF, Wallenberg HCS (1989) Effect of external
cephalic version in late pregnancy on presentation at
delivery: A randomised controlled trial. *British Journal
of Obstetrics and Gynaecology* **96**:916–921.

45 Van Dorsten JP, Schifrin BS, Wallace RL (1981) Randomised controlled trial of external cephalic version
with tocolysis in late pregnancy. *American Journal of
Obstetrics and Gynecology* **141**:417–424.

46 Mahomed K (1988) Breech delivery: A critical evaluation of the mode of delivery and the outcome of labour.
International Journal of Gynecology and Obstetrics
27:17–20.

47 Brocks V, Philipsen T, Secher NJ (1984) A randomised
controlled trial of external cephalic version with tocolysis in late pregnancy. *British Journal of Obstetrics and
Gynaecology* **91**:653–656.

48 Hofmeyr GJ (1991) ECV at term: How high the stakes?
British Journal of Obstetrics and Gynaecology **98**:1–3.

49 Mohamed K, Seeras R, Coulson R (1991) External
cephalic version at term: A randomised controlled trial
using tocolysis. *British Journal of Obstetrics and
Gynaecology* **98**:8–13.

50 Robertson AW, Kopelman JN, Read JA, Duff P, Mag-
elssen DJ, Dashow EE (1987) External cephalic version
at term: Is a tocolytic necessary? *Obstetrics and Gynecology* **70**:896–898.

51 Tatum RK, Orr JW, Soong S, Huddleston JF (1985)
Vaginal breech delivery of selected infants weighing
more than 2000 g: A retrospective analysis of 7 years
experience. *American Journal of Obstetrics and Gynecology* **152**:145–155.

52 Ilagan NB, Key-Chyang Liang, Piligan J, Poland R

(1987) Thoracic spinal cord transection in a breech presenting caesarean section delivered preterm infant.
American Journal of Perinatology **4**:232–233.

53 Heritage CK, Cunningham MD (1985) Association of
elective repeat caesarean section and persistent pulmonary hypertension of the newborn. *American Journal of
Obstetrics and Gynecology* **152**:627–629.

54 Gimovsky ML, Petrie RH (1989) The intrapartum management of the breech presentation. *Clinics in Perinatology* **16**:976–986.

55 Phelan JP, Stine LE, Mueller E, McCart D, Yeh S
(1984) Observations of fetal heart rate characteristics
related to external cephalic version and tocolysis. *American Journal of Obstetrics and Gynecology* **149**:658–
661.

56 Kouam L (1985) Child development after abdominal
version of the fetus from breech presentation near term
(English Abstract). *Geburtsh Frauenheilk* **45**:83–90).

57 Alexander L, Newton J (1969) Acute renal failure after
attempted external cephalic version. *Journal of Obstetrics and Gynaecology of the British Commonwealth*
76:711–712.

58 Gjode P, Rassmussen TB, Jorgensen J (1980) Feto-
maternal bleeding during attempts at external version.
British Journal of Obstetrics and Gynaecology **87**:571.

59 Miller JM (1988) Maternal and neonatal morbidity in
caesarean section. *Obstetrics and Gynecology Clinics of
North America* **15**: 629–638.

60 Hemminki E (1987) Pregnancy and birth after caesarean
section: A survey based on the Swedish Birth Register.
Birth **14**:12–17.

61 Garel M, Lelong N, Marchand A, Kaminski M (1990)
Psychological consequences of caesarean childbirth: A
4 year follow-up study. *Early Human Development*
21:105–114.

62 Fortunato SJ, Mercer LJ, Guzick DS (1988) External
cephalic version with tocolysis: Factors associated with
success. *Obstetrics and Gynecology* **72**:59–62.

63 Ferguson JE, Armstrong MA, Dyson DC (1987)
Maternal and fetal factors affecting success of antepartum external cephalic version. *Obstetrics and Gynecology* **70**:722–726.

64 Hofmeyr GJ (1983) Effect of external cephalic version
in late pregnancy on breech presentation and caesarean
section rate: A controlled trial. *British Journal of
Obstetrics and Gynaecology* **90**:393–399.

65 Thorp JM, Jenkins T, Watson W (1991) Utility of Leopold manoeuvres in screening for malpresentation.
Obstetrics and Gynecology **78**:394–396.

66 Kopelman JN, Duff P, Karl RT, Schipul AH, Read JA
(1986) Computed tomograpic pelvimetry in the evaluation of breech presentation. *Obstetrics and Gynecology* **68**:455.

67 Sherer DM, Menashe M, Palti Z, Aviad I, Ron M (1989)
Radiologic evidence of a nuchal arm in the breech presenting fetus at the onset of labor: An indication for
abdominal delivery. *American Journal of Perinatology*
6:353–355.

68 Bader B, Graham D, Stinson S (1987) Significance of
ultrasound measurements of the head of the breech
fetus. *Journal of Ultrasound Medicine* **6**:437–439.

69 Ophir E, Oettinger M, Yagoda A, Markovits Y, Rojan-

sky N, Shapiro H (1989) Breech presentation after a caesarean section: Always a section? *American Journal of Obstetrics and Gynecology* **161**:25–28.

70 Ballas S, Toaff R (1976) Hyperextension of the fetal head in breech presentation: Radiological evaluation and significance. *British Journal of Obstetrics and Gynaecology* **83**:201–204.

71 Tiwary CM (1989) Testicular injury in breech delivery: Possible implications. *Urology* **34**:210–212.

72 Van den Broek J, Vandershueren-Lodeweyckx M, Malvaux P, Craen M, Van Vleit G, Dooms L, Eggermont E (1987) Growth hormone deficiency: A hidden obstetric trauma? *European Journal of Obstetrics Gynecology and Reproductive Biology* **26**:329–334.

73 Tank ES, Davis R, Holt JF, Morley GW (1971) Mechanism of trauma during breech delivery. *Obstetrics and Gynecology* **38**:761.

74 Collea JV, Chien C, Quilligan EJ (1980) The randomised management of term frank breech presentation: A study of 208 cases. *American Journal of Obstetrics and Gynecology* **137**:253–239.

75 Green JE, McLean F, Smith LP, Usher R (1982) Has an increased caesarean section rate for term breech delivery reduced the incidence of birth asphyxia, trauma and death? *American Journal of Obstetrics and Gynecology* **142**:643–648.

76 Croughan-Minihane MS, Pettiti DB, Gordis L, Golditch I (1990) Morbidity amongst breech infants according to method of delivery. *Obstetrics and Gynecology* **75**:821–825.

77 Davidson S, Cohen WR (1990) Influence of presentation on neonatal outcome of vaginally delivered low birth weight infants: A matched pair analysis. *Journal of Perinatology* **10**:38–42.

78 Sarno AP Jr, Phelan JP, Ahn MO, Strong TH Jr (1989) Vaginal birth after caesarean delivery: Trial of labour in women with breech presentation. *Journal of Reproductive Medicine* **34**:831–833.

79 Myers SA, Gleicher N (1987) Breech delivery: Why the dilemma? *American Journal of Obstetrics and Gynecology* **156**:6–10.

80 Mecke H, Weisner D, Freys I, Semm K (1989) Delivery of breech presentation infants at term: An analysis of 304 breech deliveries. *Journal of Perinatal Medicine* **17**:121–126.

81 Otamiri G, Berg G, Ledin T, Leijon I, Nilsson B (1990) Influence of elective caesarean section and breech delivery on neonatal neurological condition. *Early Human Development*, **23**:53–66.

82 Roumen FJ, Luyben AG (1991) Safety of term vaginal breech delivery. *European Journal of Obstetrics Gynecology and Reproductive Biology* **40**:171–177.

83 Christian SS, Brady K (1991) Cord blood acid–base levels in breech presenting infants born vaginally. *Obstetrics and Gynecology* **78**:778–789.

84 Hall JE, Kohl SG, O'Brien F *et al.* (1965) Breech presentation and perinatal mortality. *American Journal of Obstetrics and Gynecology* **91**:665–683.

85 Dale A, Stanley PJ (1980) An epidemiological study of cerebral palsy in Western Australia 1956–1975. II: Spastic cerebral palsy and perinatal factors. *Developmental Medicine and Child Neurology* **22**:13–25.

86 Lagergren J (1981) Children with motor handicaps. *Acta Paediatrica Scandinavica* **289** (suppl.) 255–259.

87 Hall DMB (1989) Birth asphyxia and cerebral palsy. *British Medical Journal* **299**:279–282.

88 Neligan GA, Prudham D, Steiner H (eds) (1974) *The Formative Years: Birth, Family and Development in Newcastle-upon-Tyne.* Oxford: Oxford University Press.

89 Nilssen ST, Bergsjo P (1985) Males born in breech presentation 18 years after birth. *Acta Obstetrica et Gynecologica Scandinavica* **64**:323–325.

90 Rosen MG, Debanne S, Thompson K, Bilenker RM (1985) Longterm neurological morbidity in breech and vertex births. *American Journal of Obstetrics and Gynecology* **157**:718–723.

91 Hutchcroft SA, Wearing MP, Buck CW (1981) Late results of caesarean section and vaginal delivery in cases of breech presentation. *Canadian Medical Association Journal* **125**:726–730.

92 Hochuli E (1980) Der Versuch einer Kosten-und nutzenanalyse im Perinatalbereich. *Zeiteschrift für Gerburtshilfe und Perinatologie* **184**:383–394.

93 Krause W, Voigt C, Donzik J, Michels W, Gstottner H (1991) Assisted spontaneous delivery veresus Bracht manual aid within the scope of vaginal delivery in breech presentation: Late morbidity in children 5–7 years of age. *Zeiteschrift für Gerburtshilfe und Perinatologie* **195**:76–81.

94 Todd WD, Steer CM (1963) Term breech: Review of 1006 term breech deliveries. *Obstetrics and Gynecology* **22**:583–595.

95 Dunn LJ, Van Voorhis L, Napier J (1965) Term breech presentations: A report of 499 consecutive cases. *Obstetrics and Gynecology* **25**:170–176.

96 Beischer NA (1966) Pelvic contraction in breech presentation. *Journal of Obstetrics and Gynaecology of the British Commonwealth* **73**:421–427.

97 Mahamood TA (1990) The influence of maternal height, obstetrical conjugate and fetal birthweight in the management of patients with breech presentation. *Australia and New Zealand Journal of Obstetrics and Gynaecology* **30**:10–14.

98 Fischer-Rasmussen W, Trolle D (1967) Abdominal versus vaginal delivery in breech presentation. *Acta Obstetrica et Gynecologica Scandinavica* **46**:69.

99 Liu DTY, Fairweather DVI (1985) *Labour Ward Manual*, pp. 101–105. London: Butterworths.

100 Cunningham FG, MacDonald PC, Gant NF (1989) Techniques for breech delivery. In *Williams' Obstetrics*, 18th edn, pp. 393–404. New York: Appleton and Lange.

101 Clinch J (1989) Breech presentation. In Turnbull A, Chamberlain G (eds) *Obstetrics*, pp. 802–808. Edinburgh: Churchill Livingstone.

102 Arulkumaran S, Thavarasah AS, Ingemarsson I, Ratnam SS (1989) An alternative approach to assisted vaginal breech delivery. *Asia and Oceania Journal of Obstetrics and Gynecology* **15**:47–51.

103 Menticoglou SM (1990) Symphysiotomy for the trapped aftercoming parts of the breech: A review of the literature and a plea for its use. *Australia and New*

Zealand Journal of Obstetrics and Gynaecology **30**:1–9.

104 Gebbe D (1982) Symphysiotomy. *Clinics in Obstetrics and Gynaecology* **9**:663–683.

105 Schutterman EB, Grimes DA (1985) Comparative safety of the low transverse versus the low vertical uterine incision for the delivery of breech infants. *Obstetrics and Gynecology* **61**:593–597.

106 Kierse MJNC (1989) Preterm delivery. In Chalmers I, Enkin M, Kierse MJNC (eds) *Effective Care in Pregnancy and Childbirth*, pp. 666–693. Oxford: Oxford University Press.

107 Lamont RF, Dunlop PDM, Crowley P *et al.* (1983) Spontaneous preterm labour and delivery at under 34 weeks gestation. *British Medical Journal* **286**:454–457.

108 Karp LE, Doney JR, McCarthy T *et al.* (1979) The premature breech: Trial of labour or caesarean section? *Obstetrics and Gynecolgoy* **53**:88–92.

109 Wigglesworth JS, Husemeyer RP (1977) Intracranial birth trauma in vaginal breech delivery. *British Journal of Obstetrics and Gynaecology* **84**:684–691.

110 Tejani N, Rebold B, Tuck S *et al.* (1984) Obstetric factors in the causation of early periventricular–intraventricular haemorrhage. *Obstetrics and Gynecology* **64**:510–515.

111 Tahilrameny MP, Platt LD, Sze-Ya Yeh, DeVore GR, Sipos L, Paul RH (1985) Ultrasonic examination of weight in very low-birth weight fetus: A resident versus staff physician comparison. *American Journal of Obstetrics and Gynecology* **151**:90–91.

112 Goldenberg RL, Nelson KG (1977) The premature breech. *American Journal of Obstetrics and Gynecology* **27**:240–244.

113 Haddad NG, Irvine DS (1988) Classical versus lower segment caesarean section in very preterm deliveries (Letter). *Lancet* **i**:762.

114 Miller EC, Kouam S, Schweintek S (1980) The problem of the increased perinatal mortality rate in premature breech deliveries, compared to premature vertex deliveries. *Geburtsh Frauenheilk* **40**:1013–1021.

115 Nissel H, Bistoletti, Palme C (1979) Preterm breech delivery. *Acta Obstetrica et Gynecologica* **133**:503–508.

116 Paul RH, Koh KS, Monfared AH (1979) Obstetric factors influencing outcome in infants weighing from 1001 to 1500 grams. *American Journal of Obstetrics and Gynecology* **133**:503–508.

117 Woods JR (1979) Effects of low birthweight breech delivery on neonatal morbidity. *Obstetrics and Gynecology* **53**:735–740.

118 Cox C, Kendall AC, Hommes H (1982) Changed prognosis for breech presenting low birth weight infants. *British Journal of Obstetrics and Gynaecology* **89**:881–886.

119 Effer SB, Saigal S, Rand C *et al.* (1983) Effect of delivery mode on outcome in the very low birth weight breech infant: Is the improved survival rate related to caesarean section or other perinatal manoeuvres? *American Journal of Obstetrics and Gynaecology* **145**:123–128.

120 Haesslin HC, Goodlin RC (1979) Delivery of the tiny newborn. *American Journal of Obstetrics and Gynecology* **134**:192–200.

121 Greisen G, Jacobsen JC, Ulrichsen H *et al.* (1983) Method of delivery of low birth weight infants: A retrospective analysis. *Journal of Perinatal Medicine* **11**:162–168.

122 Yu VYH, Bajuk B, Cutting D *et al.* (1984) Effect of mode of delivery on the outcome of very low birth weight infants. *British Journal of Obstetrics and Gynaecology* **91**:633–639.

123 Bodmer B, Benjamin A, McLean FH, Usher RH (1986) Has the use of caesarean section reduced the risks of delivery in the preterm breech presentation? *American Journal of Obstetrics and Gynaecology* **154**:244–250.

124 Weissman A, Blazer S, Zimmer EZ, Jakobi P, Paldi E (1988) Low birth weight breech infants: Short term and long term outcome by method of delivery. *American Journal of Perinatology* **5**:289–292.

125 Rosen MG, Chik L (1984) The effect route of delivery on outcome in breech presentation. *American Journal of Obstetrics and Gynaecology* **148**:909–914.

126 Kitchen W, Ford GW, Doyle LW, Rickards AL, Lissenden JV, Pepperell RJ, Duke JE (1985) Caesarean section or vaginal delivery at 24–28 weeks gestation: Comparison of survival and neonatal and two year morbidity. *Obstetrics and Gynecology* **66**:149–157.

127 Viegas OAC, Ingemarsson I, Low PS, Singh K, Cheng M, Ratnam SS, Chow KK, Ho TH, Vengadasalam D (1985) Collaborative study on preterm breeches: Vaginal delivery versus caesarean section. *Asia and Oceania Journal of Obstetrics and Gynecology* **11**:359–365.

128 Lumley J, Lester A, Renon P, Wood C (1985) A failed RCT to determine the best mode of delivery for the very lowbirth weight infant. *Controlled Clinical Trials* **6**:120–127.

129 Wallace RL, Schifrin BS, Paul RH (1984) The delivery route for very-low-birth-weight infants. *Journal of Reproductive Medicine* **29**:736–740.

14

Unstable Lie

IAN Z. MACKENZIE

DEFINITION

An unstable lie is generally a description used beyond 37 weeks gestation when the fetal lie and presentation repeatedly change, the lie varying between longitudinal, transverse and oblique. By 36 weeks, the fetus usually adopts a 'stable' lie and presentation which will be unchanging until labor and delivery; the fetal position, describing the relationship of the fetal back to the maternal side may, however, change.

ETIOLOGY

Unstable lie is much more common in multiparas than nulliparas, but may be caused by or associated with a number of factors as illustrated in **Figure 1**.

- *High parity*: Increasing laxity in the maternal anterior abdominal wall musculature; which thereby fails to act as a brace to encourage and maintain a fetal longitudinal lie, is probably the most frequent associated factor. In addition, there is a commonly held view that the highly parous uterus has reduced myometrial tone discouraging a stable lie; this has not been proven and is of doubtful relevance.

- *Hydramnios*: Excessive volumes of amniotic fluid may produce marked uterine distension enabling the fetus to move around more freely. This prob-

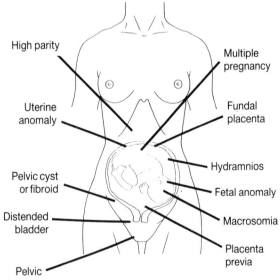

Figure 1. Etiological factors and conditions associated with an unstable lie in late pregnancy.

ably represents the most common 'pathological' cause for an unstable lie and also potentially the most hazardous for mother and fetus (see Chapter 48).

- *Multiple pregnancy*: When the lie of one or both fetuses repeatedly changes, this usually indicates the presence of hydramnios. The discovery of an abnormal lie during the last 3 weeks of pregnancy should arouse suspicion of a multiple pregnancy, particularly if a previous ultrasound examination has not been performed.

- *Placenta praevia*: A repeatedly changing fetal lie may be the only clinical feature leading to the diagnosis of placenta previa. In addition, a placenta situated in the fundus may predispose to an unstable lie.[1]

- *Pelvic tumors*: Ovarian cysts and low-lying fibroids, occupying the pelvic cavity and preventing the entry of the fetal head or breech, may result in an unstable lie.

- *Pelvic inlet contracture and/or fetal macrosomia*: As with pelvic tumors, a fetal pole is unable to enter the pelvic brim, leading to instability of the lie.

- *Fetal anomaly*: Significant hydrocephaly, tumors of the neck or sacrum, fetal abdominal distension, and fetal neuromuscular dysfunction may impede or discourage engagement of a fetal pole in the maternal pelvis.

- *Uterine anomaly*: Uterus cordiformis, subseptus or septus may predispose to a fetal transverse lie, discouraging but not preventing one or other pole from engaging in the maternal pelvis. More severe forms of uterine anomaly, including uterus bicornuus and uterus didelphus, virtually prevent an unstable lie in late pregnancy due to the restricted uterine capacity; these anomalites may predispose to a fetal breech presentation.

- *Distended maternal urinary bladder*: Maternal urinary retention with a distended bladder can cause a changing fetal lie. This is usually only temporary, resolution being achieved by urinary voiding or catheterization of the bladder.

INCIDENCE

Figures are not generally available for the incidence of unstable lie. It is likely to be influenced mainly by the proportion of multiparas and particularly the numbers of grand-multiparas in the population. Similarly, in societies where malnutrition is prominent and maternal and/or fetal skeletal deformities are common, the incidence will be higher. In a well-nourished and developed population where high parity (greater than four) is relatively uncommon, the incidence will be in

the range 0.1–1.0%. The rate of transverse lie in labor is in the region of 0.4%.[2]

Risks

There are no major hazards to mother or fetus during the prenatal period from an unstable lie *per se*. It is possible that cord entanglement is a small risk, although this has never been scientifically demonstrated. During the latter weeks of pregnancy, spontaneous resolution to a longitudinal lie before labor starts occurs in about 85% of cases.[3–5] There are, however, serious risks to mother and fetus if the lie is not longitudinal at the onset of labor. Once the membranes rupture, with or without accompanying uterine contractions, there is a risk of cord presentation and prolapse if the fetal lie is oblique or transverse, or the presenting part is high above the pelvic inlet (see Chapter 62). If labor starts when the lie is not longitudinal, a compound presentation may result or the pelvis may remain empty. If left unattended, fetal distress will eventually supervene, resulting ultimately in fetal death. In addition, uterine rupture is a possible outcome, especially in multiparas, with serious consequences for mother and fetus (see Chapter 61).

Management Options

Assessment

Once an unstable lie or persistent transverse lie has been identified, investigations should be performed to try to establish the cause. This will be easier before the onset of labor. Findings from such investigations may influence subsequent pregnancy and delivery management.

Clinical history and examination

The prenatal history should be checked carefully to ensure reliability of gestational assessment. Any relevant family or previous obstetric history (such as diabetes, macrosomia or fetal anomaly) should be highlighted. Abdominal examination should identify significant hydramnios and, if present, further specific investigations should be arranged to identify any associated fetal anomaly. A pelvic examination by an experienced clinician should enable an assessment to be made of pelvic shape and capacity. This examination will also identify any tumor in the pelvis, obstructing the entry of a fetal pole. Such an examination should not be performed if there is a history of antepartum hemorrhage of uncertain origin, or if placenta previa has been diagnosed or suspected.

Ultrasound examination

The key investigation in cases of unstable lie is real-time ultrasound. It can be used to identify significant fetal malformations or pelvic tumors, and localize the placenta. It is of less value for demonstrating congenital uterine anomalies, particularly as most are of a minor degree.

Radiology

There is virtually no place for a radiological examination of the abdomen if ultrasound equipment and competent experienced sonographers are available. In their absence, x-rays can be used to identify gross fetal skeletal anomalies, although soft tissue tumors are often missed. Radiological views of the maternal pelvis can be obtained to assess pelvic size and shape. These are largely of academic interest, since gross distortions to pelvic shape and reductions in pelvic capacity should be diagnosed by experienced clinical examination, and lesser deviations from 'normal', which may escape clinical notice, should not alter clinical management.

Prenatal

During the prenatal period, management can be non-interventionist or interventionist, expectant or active, while delivery can either await spontaneous labor onset or be arranged as a planned event. An algorithm of the various options is illustrated in **Figure 2**.

Non-intervention

Once an unstable lie is identified, no specific action is taken in anticipation that the lie will become longitudinal before the membranes rupture or labor starts: this is likely to occur in more than 80%.[3–5] Manipulation to a longitudinal lie at a prenatal examination can be performed. Exclusion of an obvious mechanical cause for the unstable lie should be made, since if such a cause is discovered, obstructed labor can be predicted and elective cesarean section should therefore be performed, if possible before the onset of labor. The pregnant woman should be advised of the risks associated with an unstable lie and the need for urgent attention should labor start or the membranes rupture.

A number of physical exercises, frequently associated with the woman adopting the knee–elbow position for short periods on a number of occasions each day, have been advocated to promote spontaneous version, generally from a breech to cephalic presentation.[6–9] Such maneuvers possibly increase the incidence of a longitudinal lie by 5–10%, but this has not been scientifically proven.

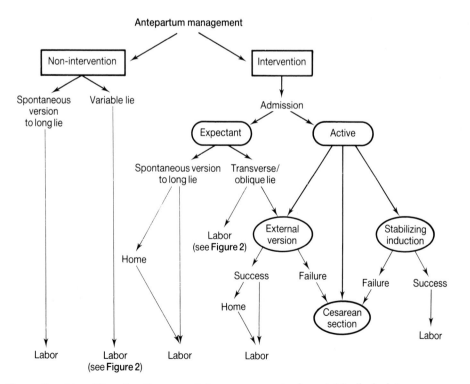

Figure 2. Algorithm for the prenatal management of unstable lie in late pregnancy.

Intervention

Admission may be advised from 37 weeks gestation onward. This enables daily observations of fetal lie and presentation, the opportunity for active treatment to correct the lie if necessary and the possibility of immediate clinical assistance being given upon membrane rupture or labor onset if the lie is not longitudinal, fetal distress occurs, or the cord is presenting or prolapsed.

Expectant daily observation

This involves awaiting spontaneous resolution to a longitudinal lie. Once a cephalic or breech presentation has been established and maintained for 48 h, the patient may be discharged home to await spontaneous labor.

Active

There are three options:

- *External cephalic version*: Once admitted, external cephalic version (see Chapter 13) is attempted where facilities permit immediate delivery in the event of acute fetal distress being caused.[10,11] If a longitudinal lie is established and maintained, the patient may be allowed home to await spontaneous labor onset. Rhesus immunoprophylaxis should be given to at-risk women either before or soon after the version attempt and a Kleihauer test may be checked about 20 min after the attempt, to determine whether additional prophylaxis is necessary. If a longitudinal lie is not maintained, the version can be repeated as often as necessary and if not successful the patient kept in hospital until labor supervenes. The success of version prenatally in unstable lie is unclear, but in cases of breech presentation it is 40–65%.[12–14] Tocolysis can be used, such as intravenous infusions of ritodrine 50 μg/min for 15 min[14] or terbutaline sulfate 25 μg i.v. over 1–2 min,[15] but is often unnecessary with a transverse or oblique lie.

- *Stabilizing induction*: A stabilizing induction may be performed either immediately following admission or when convenient during the following days or weeks. Following transfer to the labor ward, an external cephalic version is performed converting the fetal lie to longitudinal. Once in position, regular abdominal palpations are performed to confirm the longitudinal lie is maintained and a titrated intravenous infusion of oxytocin is commenced to stimulate uterine contractility.[16] As soon as contractions are occurring at 10-min inter-

vals or more freqeuntly, a low amniotomy is performed having ensured the lie is still longitudinal and the presentation is not compound and in particular that the cord is not presenting. If the cord presents, an emergency cesarean section is then necessary. Once low amniotomy is performed, a reasonable volume of amniotic fluid should be released, again confirming the cord is not presenting and the presenting part is fixed in the pelvic brim. Thereafter, once labor is established, management continues as for an uncomplicated labor.

An alternative approach is to perform an external cephalic or podalic version and, having established a longitudinal lie, to stimulate uterine contractility with a titrated intravenous oxytocin infusion. Having confirmed the lie is longitudinal, a Drew Smythe catheter[17] is passed through the cervix, behind the presenting part between the uterine wall and the fetal membranes, avoiding trauma to the fetus and a posteriorly situated placenta. The stylet within the catheter is advanced to puncture the membranes and allow a controlled release of amniotic fluid. This procedure should reduce the chances of cord prolapse occurring. Uterine contractility can also be stimulated with local (vaginal) or oral prostaglandins, but this is probably less advisable, since the response to prostaglandins is occasionally unpredictable and hyperstimulation can occur which would require acute tocolytic management or emergency cesarean section, especially if the lie reverted to oblique or transverse.

- *Elective cesarean section*: Following admission, an elective cesarean section may be performed at a convenient time, often at 38–39 weeks gestation;[5] ideally converting the lie to longitudinal at laparotomy and then performing the lower segment operation rather than the classical operation. This approach is particularly appropriate if there is a contraindication to external version, external version fails, or there is a mechanical obstruction to vaginal delivery.

Intrapartum

When the membranes rupture or labor starts, the options for management illustrated in the algorithm in **Figure 3** are as follows:

Longitudinal lie

If the lie is longitudinal, check that the fetal heart rate pattern is healthy. Then perform a vaginal examination

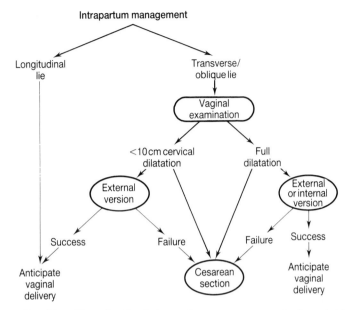

Figure 3. Algorithm for the intrapartum management of unstable lie.

to identify which pole is presenting, exclude gross pelvic contracture and pelvic tumors, exclude cord presentation and prolapse, and assess the degree of cervical dilatation. Allow labor to establish and progress or augment with an oxytocic such as titrated intravenous oxytocin, ensuring the lie remains longitudinal and the fetal heart rate pattern remains healthy. Management of the labor then continues as normal.

Non-longitudinal lie

If the lie is not longitudinal, confirm that the fetal heart rate pattern is healthy. Then perform a vaginal examination, exclude any mechanical obstruction to a vaginal delivery, exclude cord presentation or prolapse, and exclude full dilatation of the cervix.

Version

If the uterus is contracting, either attempt an external version between contractions or infuse a tocolytic such as ritodrine 100 μg/min for 10–15 min prior to attempting the version; if necessary, the infusion rate can be increased at 50 μg/min increments to a maximum of 350 μg/min in the absence of distressing maternal side-effects.[18] If version is successful, repeat the vaginal examination to exclude cord presentation or prolapse and allow labor to establish and progress or augment with an oxytocic. Continue management as for normal labor. If the version is unsuccessful, arrange delivery by cesarean section (see later).

If cord presentation or prolapse is found on vaginal examination, or significant fetal heart rate abnormalities occur, immediate delivery by cesarean section should be arranged (see later).

If full dilatation of the cervix is found, the lie is not longitudinal and vaginal delivery is considered mechanically safe, attempt an external cephalic version. If this is not successful, an internal podalic version may be considered (see Chapter 13). This requires that there be adequate anesthesia (a general anesthetic or epidural anesthetic suitable for cesarean section) and intact membranes with at least a normal amniotic fluid volume. If this is also unsuccessful, proceed to delivery by cesarean section (see below).

Cesarean section

If the lie is not longitudinal and all observations are satisfactory, delivery by cesarean section can be performed without any attempt at securing a vaginal delivery. An external cephalic version may be attempted prior to the start of the cesarean section or immediately before making the incision in the uterus; if the lie can be corrected to longitudinal, the lower segment operation should be used. If the lie is transverse, the classical incision may be advisable, particularly if the fetal back is downward. This is because it may prove difficult to bring a fetal pole down into the incision for delivery, particularly if the lower segment is poorly formed. In such an event, an inverted T or U-shaped incision may become necessary to secure delivery, with compromised scar integrity in a subsequent pregnancy.

Postnatal

No specific management is required following delivery, whether achieved vaginally or by cesarean section, compared with delivery following a stable lie in late pregnancy. If a classical cesarean section is performed, this should be taken into account both in relation to the slightly higher postoperative morbidity rates and when considering advice for future pregnancy management.

Conclusions

The recognition that the fetal lie is repeatedly changing at 37 weeks gestation and later should alert the attendants to the risks to mother and fetus if the membranes rupture or labor starts. Investigations to determine the possible cause for the unstable lie should be organized as the results can influence subsequent management.

Prenatally, a non-interventionist approach may be followed, but the risks should be explained to the woman and advice given for early referral to a major obstetric unit once the membranes rupture or labor starts. Alternatively, admission can be advised and with the woman remaining in hospital until the lie becomes longitudinal spontaneously or active treatment has corrected the lie, with maintenance of the longitudinal lie for several days. Alternatively, delivery can be planned by a stabilizing labor induction or cesarean section.

If labor commences or the membranes rupture and the lie is not longitudinal, version with or without tocolytic assistance can be attempted if the conditions are favorable, or delivery arranged by lower or upper segment cesarean section as appropriate either as a primary decision or if a version attempt fails.

UNSTABLE LIE
Summary of Management Options

Prenatal

Assessment: Establish cause

- History/examination

- Real-time ultrasound

*Management options (see **Figure 2**)*

- Non-intervention

  - if still unstable when in spontaneous labor, see opposite **(Intrapartum)**

- Intervention

  - expectant: await onset of spontaneous labor in hospital; then as opposite **(Intrapartum)**

  - active
    — external version
    — stabilizing induction
    — elective cesarean

Intrapartum

Assessment: Establish cause

- History/examination

- Real-time ultrasound

*Management options (see **Figure 3**): Assess lie*

- Longitudinal lie: allow normal labor and delivery

- Non-longitudinal lie: assess cervix
  - not full dilatation:
    — external version
    — cesarean section

  - full dilatation:
    — external version
    — internal podalic version
    — cesarean section

REFERENCES

1   Steven CS (1949) Transverse or oblique presentation of the fetus in the last ten weeks of pregnancy: Its causes, general nature and treatment. *American Journal of Obstetrics and Gynecology* **58**:432–446.

2   Pritchard JA, MacDonald PC (eds) (1980) *Williams' Obstetrics*, 16th edn, pp. 813–817. New York: Appleton-Century-Crofts.

3   Fried AW, Cloutier M, Woodring JH, Shier RW (1984) Sonography on the transverse fetal lie. *American Journal of Radiology* **142**:421–423.

4   Hughey MJ (1985) Fetal position during pregnancy. *American Journal of Obstetrics and Gynecology* **153**:885–886.

5   Phelan JP, Boucher M, Mueller E, McCart D, Horenstein J, Clark SL (1986) The nonlabouring transverse lie: A management dilemma. *Journal of Reproductive Medicine* **31**:184–186.

6   Elkins VH (1980) quoted in Enkins M, Chalmers I (eds) *Effectiveness and Satisfaction in Antenatal Care*, p. 216. London: Spastics International Medical Publishers.

7   Hofmeyr GJ (1983) Effect of external cephalic version in late pregnancy on breech presentation and caesarean section rate: A controlled trial. *British Journal of Obstetrics and Gynaecology* **90**:392–399.

8   Bung P, Huch R, Huch A (1987) Ist die indische wendung eine erfolgreiche methode zur senking der beckenendlage-frequenz? *Geburtsch Frauenheilk* **47**:202–205.

9   Chenia F, Crowther C (1987) Does advice to assume the knee–chest position reduce the incidence of breech presentation at delivery? A randomised clinical trial. *Birth* **14**:75–78.

10 Ranney B (1973) The gentle art of external cephalic version. *American Journal of Obstetrics and Gynecology* **116**:239–245.

11 Hibbard LT, Schumann WR (1973) Prophylactic external cephalic version in an obstetric practice. *American Journal of Obstetrics and Gynecology* **116**:511–516.

12 Saling E, Muller-Holve W (1975) External cephalic version under tocolysis. *Journal of Perinatal Medicine* **3**:115–122.

13 Fall O, Nilsson BA (1979) External cephalic version in breech presentation under tocolysis. *Obstetrics and Gynecology* **53**:712–715.

14 Brocks V, Philipsen T, Secher NJ (1984) A randomised trial of external cephalic version with tocolysis in late pregnancy. *British Journal of Obstetrics and Gynaecology* **91**:653–656.

15 Dyson DC, Ferguson JE, Hensleigh P (1986) Antepartum external cephalic version under tocolysis. *Obstetrics and Gynecology* **67**:63–68.

16 Edwards RL, Nicholson HO (1969) The management of the unstable lie in late pregnancy: *Journal of Obstetrics and Gynaecology of the British Commonwealth* **76**:713–718.

17 Drew Smythe HG (1931) Indications for the induction of premature labour. *British Medical Journal* **1**:1018–1020.

18 Phelan JP, Stine LE, Edwards NB, Clark SL, Horenstein J (1985) The role of external version in the intrapartum management of the transverse lie presentation. *American Journal of Obstetrics and Gynecology* **151**:724–726.

15

Previous Cesarean Section

JAN E. DICKINSON

INTRODUCTION

The medical pendulum has swung in both directions during the 20th century in the management of pregnancy following cesarean section. In the first half of the century, a cesarean section meant that all subsequent pregnancies were very likely to be delivered the same way. This policy resulted from the fear of uterine scar rupture. This fear was well-founded when the original procedure was still likely to be a classical cesarean section. When the lower uterine segment operation largely replaced classical cesarean section, the fear of catastrophic uterine rupture was retained without the same basis in fact. With time, it became apparent that a vaginal delivery could occur both successfully and safely following a previous lower uterine segment cesarean section. This observation was made initially by chance when women went into labor before their scheduled repeat cesarean section and delivered vaginally before the operation could take place. In 1957, a review of the obstetric literature by Dewhurst[1] showed that the feared event of catastrophic uterine rupture occurred almost exclusively in those women who had previously undergone a classical cesarean section. When uterine rupture occurred with a previous lower uterine segment cesarean section, it was not the disastrous event associated with the vertical upper segment incision. This observation heralded the era of the 'trial of scar' or 'Vaginal Birth After Cesarean' (VBAC).

Over the past 10 years, the pendulum reached and passed the midpoint of its arc. The 1980s were remarkable for the multitude of articles supporting vaginal birth after cesarean section, particularly from the hitherto conservative North American medical fraternity. In the absence of a recurring indication, one previous lower uterine segment cesarean section no longer dictated an elective repeat cesarean section. The American College of Obstetricians and Gynecologists formally endorsed a policy of trial of labor under most circumstances.[2] This change in attitude was probably ignited by a drive to halt the ever-increasing cesarean section rate, postulated to reach 30% in the early 1990s in the USA. In the USA, the most common indication for cesarean section in multiparous women is previous cesarean section. However, current medical evidence indicates that upwards of 70% of women can achieve a vaginal delivery following a previous cesarean delivery. Hence, the opportunity to decrease the number of procedures performed, and therefore patient risk and health care cost, is large.

The contemporary medical literature has also begun to question the validity of other obstetric dogmas, and now suggests that a trial of labor be allowed after more than one cesarean section,[3–6] and after previous cesarean section despite the presence of a breech presentation or twins in the subsequent pregnancy.[7,8]

The pendulum has threatened potentially to swing too far to the left. The early 1990s have marked some call to restraint with several articles appearing in the literature reporting catastrophic complications during trial of labor after cesarean section.[9–11] These publications are timely in that they serve to remind us that while there is no doubt that a trial of labor is a relatively safe procedure, it is not risk-free and should not be undertaken in a casual fashion. It is to be hoped that the 1990s will provide a level, educated perspective on the management of labor following previous cesarean section, based on the results of well-conducted clinical trials and conducted in a manner to provide the optimal outcome for mother and infant.

SCOPE OF THE ISSUE

There has been a dramatic rise in the cesarean birth rate over the past 20 years, particularly in the USA, where 25% of live births are delivered abdominally.[12] In Europe, cesarean delivery rates have also risen but are approximately half those in the USA.[13] This increase in abdominal delivery has created an expanding obstetric subpopulation: women with a previous cesarean section scar. Parallelling the increase in the cesarean section rate has been an increase in information on management of the subsequent pregnancies of these women.

When evaluating any two alternative methods of patient management, several issues are raised: medical, social and ethical. Management of the patient following a previous cesarean section is an object lesson in medical decision-making processes. Some issues are straightforward, for example management of the patient with a prior classical cesarean section. Although a vaginal delivery is certainly possible, and most clinicians have had the experience of delivering a patient vaginally only to find later she has had a previous classical cesarean section, the risk of catastrophic uterine rupture is too high to warrant this as a management protocol. Other issues are now accepted as standard obstetric practice: one previous low transverse cesarean section in a patient with no adverse risk factors is an indication for a trial of labor in subsequent pregnancies. The data are solid on this issue and really do not warrant further extensive discussion. The interested reader can investigate more in some excellent review articles,[14,15] but this issue is no longer a dilemma. The more controversial areas now are management of labor after more than one lower uterine segment cesarean section, management of the multifetal gestation after a previous cesarean section, the use of oxytocin and prostaglandins, and the use of regional analgesia.

Risks of Vaginal Birth After Cesarean Section

As cesarean section became a viable obstetric option in the first two decades of this century, the performance of elective repeat cesarean section became an established practice. In 1981, only 9% of women with a previous cesarean section received a trial of labor in the USA.[16] The obstetric literature in the UK has been more positive toward the option of a trial of labor, and

hence the procedure has been more prevalent in that country over the past 30 years. During the 1980s, there was an abundance of literature published in the USA supporting the concept of a trial of labor following a lower uterine segment procedure. The American College of Obstetrics and Gynecology (ACOG) has formally supported the management plan of trial of vaginal delivery after a low uterine segment cesarean section and it is to be hoped that the repeat cesarean section rate in the USA will soon reflect the ACOG stance.

In the face of the available clinical data, one is left to ponder the reluctance of obstetricians to allow a trial of labor following one lower segment cesarean section. Several reasons appear to have produced this mindset. First, the fear of uterine rupture in labor with the threat of risk to mother and/or fetus. Second, the belief by many obstetricians and patients that cesarean section is a simple, convenient procedure essentially free of hazard. Why accept a risk of uterine rupture or failed vaginal delivery when a planned procedure at a mutually convenient time can be performed? It is these two concepts that appear to have led to the rapid rise in elective repeat cesarean section over the past 20 years.

If a trial of labor is undertaken, what percentage of women can realistically expect a vaginal delivery following a previous transverse lower uterine segment cesarean section? As Enkin[14] has commented in his erudite dissertation, there are no randomized controlled trials comparing the results of elective repeat cesarean section with a trial of labor for women with a previous cesarean section, nor in view of the proven low risk of VBAC are there ever likely to be. However there are a number of published prospective cohort studies. In seven series[17-23] involving 8899 women, analyzed by Enkin, 6097 women (68.5%) were permitted a trial of labor, of whom 79.9% (4874) delivered vaginally and 20.1% (1223) by cesarean.[14] This results in an overall vaginal delivery rate for all women with a previous cesarean section in these seven series of 54.8% (4874/8899).

What are the risks of a trial of labor following a prior transverse lower uterine segment cesarean section? How often do these adverse outcomes occur? Again, assessment of the published prospective trials provides a guide. Enkin[14] analyzed six eligible studies[17-21,24] and reported on their maternal morbidity statistics (see **Table 1**). These data reveal a uterine dehiscence/rupture rate of 1.5% for elective repeat cesarean section cases and 1.7% for all women undergoing a trial of labor (irrespective of eventual delivery mode), i.e. no significant difference. It is notable that the majority of the scar separations were minor (dehiscences rather than ruptures) with no maternal mortality or significant difference between the groups in terms of hysterectomy. Not permitting a trial of labor in an eligible candidate is simply not justified on the basis of fear of uterine rupture.

Maternal morbidity is not measured solely in terms of scar separation. Assessment of other morbidity parameters shows a 19.7% incidence of febrile/infectious morbidity in women undergoing elective repeat cesarean section compared with 11.7% in women having a trial of labor. In fairness, further analysis of the trial of labor group shows the greatest risk for febrile morbidity to be in the subgroup who failed a trial of labor (39.3%). This figure is offset, however, by the 3.3% incidence of febrile morbidity in women who successfully achieved a vaginal delivery, and who form the majority of those attempting a trial of labor. Indeed, all measured parameters of maternal morbidity were lower in the trial of labor groups compared with the elective cesarean section group (e.g. thromboembolic phenomena, pneumonia, anesthetic complications).

What of the infants? It is impossible from the nature of the available trials to make valid direct comparisons between perinatal outcomes in women undergoing elective repeat cesarean section and those undergoing a trial of labor, for they are not randomized controlled trials and thus, by their very nature, the groups are different. A clinician may permit a trial of labor in certain circumstances, such as a dead or severely anomalous fetus, but if the fetus was normal, perform an elective repeat cesarean section. However, analysis of the available evidence does not support an association between increased perinatal mortality and trials of labor.[25]

Risks of Elective Repeat Cesarean Section

Although there are several confounding variables, the available data suggest the maternal mortality rate associated with elective cesarean section is approximately 2–4 times that of vaginal delivery. In 1982, Petitti et al.[26] reported that the maternal mortality rate associated with all forms of cesarean section to be 40.9/100 000 births, some four-fold greater than that associated with vaginal deliveries (9.8/100 000 births).

However, the maternal mortality rate associated with elective repeat cesarean section was much lower at 17.9/100 000 births (see **Table 2**).

Maternal morbidity is probably a more useful statistic when comparing the two modes of delivery than maternal mortality, as either delivery route has a low mortality rate. The overwhelming trend from the available studies is that related maternal morbidity is greater with cesarean section than vaginal delivery. Operating time is longer in women with multiple cesarean sections.[27] Kirkinen[27] reported a 13% incidence of cesarean hysterectomy in a cohort of 64 women with multiple cesarean sections. In addition to the inherent risks in any surgical procedure (e.g. anesthesia, operative trauma), there are several reports which discuss the negative impact of cesarean section on subsequent fertility[28,29] and psychological status.[30]

For an individual patient, the incidence of placenta previa increases with increasing numbers of cesarean deliveries.[31] The presence of placenta previa in a woman with a previous cesarean section is a recognized risk factor for placenta accreta. There is an increased tendency for placental implantation in the vicinity of the uterine scar with secondary trophoblast invasion of the myometrium.[32] With the increased cesarean delivery rate, the incidence of placenta accreta is increasing. Clark et al.[33] reported a 24% incidence of

Table 2
Maternal mortality via delivery mode

Delivery mode	Maternal mortality
Cesarean section (overall)	40.9/100 000 births
Vaginal delivery (overall)	9.8/100 000 births
Elective repeat cesarean section	17.9/100 000 births
Uncomplicated vaginal delivery	4.9/100 000 births

Adapted from Petitti et al.[26]

Table 1
Previous cesarean section: maternal morbidity

	Dehiscence	Fever/infection	Other
Elective cesarean section (n = 2027)	31 (1.5%)	399 (19.7%)	129 (6.4%)
Trial of labor overall (n = 4153)	69 (1.7%)	491 (11.8%)	88 (2.1%)
vaginal delivery (n = 3142)	40 (1.3%)	104 (3.3%)	32 (1.0%)
cesarean section (n = 1011)	29 (2.9%)	397 (39.3%)	51 (5.0%)

Adapted from Enkin.[14]

placenta accreta in women with one previous cesarean section and placenta previa. The incidence rose to 67% with four previous cesarean sections. Cesarean hysterectomy is the usual management for such patients, increasing the potential maternal morbidity for repeat cesarean section.

The effect of cesarean section on the infant centers around iatrogenic preterm birth and respiratory distress. With careful and meticulous dating criteria, the incidence of iatrogenic preterm birth can be reduced.[34] There are differences in respiratory function when infants born by cesarean section are compared with those delivered vaginally. Reduced lung gas volumes, elevated mid-volume total pulmonary resistance,[35] and lower pharyngeal aspirate lecithin/sphingomyelin ratios[36] have been reported.

Although most recent data are overwhelmingly in support of a trial of labor after one lower uterine segment cesarean section, there have been several recent papers reporting complications from trial of labor and warning against complacency.[9–11] These are timely, not in that they imply trial of labor after cesarean is too dangerous to contemplate, but in that they remind the obstetrician that no generalized management plan for a disorder should supersede individualization of patient care and constant attention during pregnancy and labor.

There are certain basic requirements expected of any institution managing the labor of a woman with a previous cesarean section. These are well-outlined in the recommendations of the panel of the Canadian Consensus Conference on Aspects of Caesarean Birth (1986). This panel states: 'Hospitals providing obstetric care should ensure the availability of blood, operating rooms, neonatal resuscitation, and nursing, anaesthetic and surgical personnel so that a cesarean section can be started within approximately 30 minutes for any woman in labor, including a woman undergoing a trial of labor.'

Management Options

Eligibility for a trial of labor

The policy of trial of labor following a previous cesarean section is one of assessing the available options and selecting the appropriate choice for the individual patient. There is a subset of women who are not candidates for a trial of labor, another subset who are eligible for a trial of labor but in whom the chances of success are low, and a final subset who have a high chance of achieving a vaginal delivery. The risk of uterine rupture is not significantly greater in a trial of labor and the overall maternal morbidity is significantly lower.

Based on the published data, it is appropriate to offer a trial of labor to any woman with a low uterine seg-

ment cesarean section and no other adverse obstetric feature. This is now a common approach in many obstetric institutions throughout the world.

The factors affecting the success or lack thereof in a trial of labor following previous cesarean section are listed in **Table 3**. The highest success rates are found among women in whom the original cesarean was performed for a breech presentation, and those in whom a subsequent vaginal delivery has already occurred. A meta-analysis of indicators for success of vaginal birth after cesarean section by Rosen et al.[37] reported an odds ratios of 2.1 (95% CI 1.8–2.3) for a successful vaginal delivery if the prior cesarean was performed for a breech presentation. A vaginal delivery subsequent to the cesarean section provided an odds ratio of 2.1 (95% CI 1.7–2.5). Adverse predictors of a successful trial of labor were a history of more than one cesarean section (odds ratio 0.7) and a requirement for oxytocin during the trial of labor (odds ratio 0.3). A woman with a history of cesarean delivery for cephalo-pelvic disproportion has the lowest success rate for vaginal birth after cesarean section. However, she still has more than a 50% chance of a successful vaginal delivery if permitted a trial of labor (**Table 3**), indicating that a prior diagnosis of cephalo-pelvic disproportion should not limit a trial of labor.

Patient preference cannot be ignored in the delivery equation. Patients with a prior diagnosis of dystocia, cephalo-pelvic disproportion or failure to progress have the lowest acceptance of a trial of labor.[18] This is not difficult to understand, as these women usually have recollections of a long, augmented and often unpleasant previous labor, and if they cannot be assured a successful vaginal delivery in the current pregnancy (which is always the case), may be reluctant to face another labor which may go the same way. However, an agreement to restrict the length of a trial of labor to a mutually agreed length, or allowing the

Table 3
Factors affecting outcome of a trial of labor after cesarean section

Reason for the primary cesarean section	
	Success rate
dystocia	66%
malpresentation	84%
fetal distress	75%
other	78%

Previous vaginal delivery
Uterine incision type
Gestational age at previous cesarean section
Scar integrity
Oxytocin usage
Number of prior cesarean deliveries
Fetal macrosomia

woman to 'blow the whistle' and ask for cesarean section if she finds the labor unacceptable at any time, may sometimes reassure them sufficiently to go ahead with a trial.

Multiple cesarean sections

The obstetrics world, having accepted the concept of trial of labor after one previous cesarean section, is now turning its attention to the delivery mode of the woman with more than one cesarean section. Several papers have appeared over the past 30 years supporting the feasibility and safety of the vaginal delivery route after more than one cesarean section.[3–6,19,20,38–40] These data consistently demonstrate the frequent success of a trial of labor in this subpopulation. Of the studies with sufficient data available for analysis (**Table 4**), 68% of women permitted a trial of labor successfully achieved a vaginal delivery. Of note was the absence of increased risk of maternal or fetal mortality or morbidity in these labors. Phelan et al.,[4] in the largest series published to date with 1088 women with two or more prior cesarean sections, reported an overall uterine dehiscence rate of 3%, which is higher than that commonly reported for one previous cesarean section. However, the dehiscence rate in women attempting a vaginal delivery was 1.8% vs 4.6% in those who underwent an elective repeat cesarean section. Therefore, the relatively high overall dehiscence rate he reports is most likely to be due to the ease of diagnosis of scar dehiscence at laparotomy.

Twin gestation

As attempts are made to broaden the indications for vaginal birth after cesarean section, previously contraindicated areas are being re-evaluated. The management of the woman with a previous low segment cesarean section and a twin gestation has received some study in the recent literature.[41,42] In 1989, Strong et al.[41] presented a non-randomized cohort study of 56 women with a twin gestation and a prior cesarean section. An elective repeat cesarean section was performed in 31 (55%) and 25 (45%) attempted a vaginal

Table 4
Published series of outcomes with more than one previous cesarean section, 1961–89

Total	Elective cesarean section	Trial of labor	Vaginal delivery	Repeat cesarean section
1975	1147 (58.1%)	828 (41.9%)	563 (68%)	265 (32%)

From References 3–6, 19, 20, 38–40.

delivery. A successful vaginal delivery of both twins occurred in 18 out of 25 (72%). A dehiscence rate of 4% (1/25) was reported for the trial of labor group compared with 2% for singleton trial of labor pregnancies in that same time period. There were no significant differences in maternal or neonatal morbidity and mortality rates in women having a trial of labor vs women not having a trial of labor. As long ago as 1959, concern was expressed that uterine overdistension would increase the risk of uterine rupture.[43] This concern has not been borne out in other studies.[42,44,45] The published data suggest that vaginal birth after cesarean in twin gestation is not associated with an increased risk of perinatal or maternal morbidity or mortality and that it is a reasonable consideration in the properly selected patient. Guidelines for selection include a vertex presentation in the leading twin and the availability of continuous electronic fetal heart rate monitoring. Intrauterine manipulation of the second twin, although the published experience is limited, does not appear an unreasonable maneuver if indicated by malpresentation of the second twin, especially if the alternative is a 'crash' cesarean section.

Breech presentation

The current weight of obstetric opinion supports repeat cesarean section in the patient with a breech presentation and previous cesarean section.[46] There has recently been some evidence to challenge this belief, although it is preliminary and the numbers are small. Ophir et al.[7] have presented a retrospective review of 71 breech deliveries following previous cesarean section. A trial of labor was conducted in 47 (66%), with 37 out of 47 (79%) achieving a vaginal delivery. However, in an era when vaginal breech delivery is rapidly becoming a lost obstetric technique, it is unlikely that repeat cesarean section will be displaced as the standard delivery mode in this subpopulation.

Suspected fetal macrosomia

Five series describing outcomes for women with previous cesarean section delivering macrosomic infants have been published.[22,45,47–49] An overall success rate of 69% (556/807) was achieved, which compares favorably with published outcomes for non-macrosomic infants. In the largest series, a retrospective cohort study by Flamm et al.,[48] 55% (165/301) of women with at least one previous cesarean section delivered vaginally. When compared to a similar number of control patients with no previous uterine surgery, the rate of vaginal birth was significantly lower in the study group (79 vs 55%), but there was no significant difference in maternal or perinatal morbidity.

The caution that has been shown toward a trial of labor in a woman with a previous cesarean section and a fetus with suspected macrosomia appears to be based on concern about a potential increase in the risk of uterine rupture. The literature does not support this contention. It would seem prudent, however, not to be cavalier in continuing a trial of labor when progress is abnormal. This attitude is reflected in the lower success rates for vaginal delivery in Flamm and co-workers' series, presumably secondary to a low threshold for surgical intervention in the scar cohort.

A major confounding variable in any discussion of the management of a pregnancy with suspected fetal macrosomia is our poor prospective ability to diagnose such infants. Prenatal clinical assessment of fetal weight is approximately correct in only 35% of cases.[50] The predictive accuracy of ultrasound decreases as fetal weight approaches 4000 g[51] and the specificity with which macrosomia can be identified before birth is not currently acceptable.

The evidence at present – diabetic pregnancies excluded – does not support elective cesarean section for suspected fetal macrosomia in women with previous cesarean section.

Unknown uterine scar

As a classical uterine incision is associated with an increased likelihood of uterine rupture, documentation of the type of prior uterine incision is an important prerequisite to a trial of labor. Several authors have reported series in which the type of prior uterine incision was unknown, and this did not significantly alter the incidence of subsequent vaginal birth.[52,53] However, in Pruett's series,[52] the only full-thickness uterine rupture was in the undocumented scar group, and was subsequently found to be associated with a previous vertical incision. Although the incidence of classical cesarean section is low, and 90–95% of undocumented scars will be transverse lower segment scars, it would seem prudent to document the nature of a previous uterine incision in the prenatal period whenever possible.

Intrapartum issues

As the number of women eligible for a trial of labor following a previous cesarean section increases, several intrapartum management issues are raised. Can oxytocin be used safely? What is the role of prostaglandins for cervical ripening? Is regional analgesia safe? Should the scar be palpated after delivery?

Prostaglandins

The use of prostaglandins prior to induction of labor is accepted management in the woman with an unfavorable cervix. Concern has been expressed regarding the safety of these agents in the scarred uterus for fear of increased risk of uterine rupture. There are few published data to make a decision either way. MacKenzie[54] published a series in 1984 using prostaglandin gel to ripen the cervix in 143 patients with a prior cesarean delivery who desired a trial of labor. This was followed by oxytocin induction or augmentation of labor. A 76% vaginal delivery rate was reported and there were no uterine dehiscences or ruptures.

Oxytocin

Although many clinicians believe oxytocin to be contraindicated in the presence of a previous cesarean section, the obstetric literature does not support this view. Current obstetric opinion is that a previous cesarean section is not a contraindication to the use of oxytocin for the induction or augmentation of labor. Oxytocin can be used safely without increased maternal or fetal risk if standard management guidelines are adhered to.

The published series indicate high vaginal delivery rates and low scar dehiscence rates in association with oxytocin usage. Flamm et al.[55] reported a series of 1776 patients with previous cesarean section and permitted trial of labor, of whom 27% (485) received oxytocin for either induction or augmentation of labor. There was no significant difference in maternal or perinatal morbidity when the obstetric outcomes of those who received oxytocin was compared with those who did not. In particular, there was no difference in the incidence of uterine rupture between the two groups, although the rate of full-thickness uterine rupture was higher in the oxytocin group (4/1000 vs 1/1000). Interestingly, there was a significant difference in the vaginal delivery rate between the two groups. Successful vaginal delivery occurred in 64% of cases when oxytocin was used and 78% when it was not. This tendency to a lower vaginal delivery rate when oxytocin is required in patients with a previous cesarean section has been noted in similar series.[56,57] Sakala et al.[58] attempted to determine why oxytocin use was associated with a lower successful vaginal delivery rate in patients with previous cesarean section. They suggested the difference in success was a function of initial cervical dilatation rather than the use of oxytocin.

Chazotte and Cohen[9] recently reported two cases of uterine rupture during labor associated with the use of oxytocin for correction of prolonged arrest disorders. They suggest a trial of labor should be discontinued if a prompt response to uterine stimulation does not occur. This approach is sensible, given the increase in full-thickness uterine rupture reported by Flamm et al. in their oxytocin cohort.[55]

Regional analgesia

Regional analgesia, particularly epidural analgesia, is commonly used in labor to provide effective pain relief. It was believed that the use of epidural analgesia might mask the perception of pain which could herald uterine scar rupture.[59] Despite the presence of one case report supporting this viewpoint,[60] the majority of published reports provide no evidence of complications with regional analgesia and the interpretation of clinical signs of scar rupture.[19,23,61,62] As signs of impending uterine scar rupture, pain and tenderness are neither sensitive nor specific. Scar dehiscences are usually asymptomatic and even overt rupture may not be associated with any of the classic signs irrespective of whether regional analgesia is being used.[21] Indeed, studies report emergency cesarean sections performed for uterine tenderness in which no scar separation was found.[63,64] There is no evidence to support an increased risk of or from uterine rupture associated with epidural analgesia. Needless to say, standard protocols of maternal and fetal monitoring must be used in the presence of an epidural catheter. To deny adequate pain relief based on the presence of a uterine scar is not justified and should not be a deterrent for women desiring a trial of labor.

Postpartum scar palpation

In an attempt to discern uterine scar integrity following a vaginal delivery after cesarean section, the practice of postpartum scar palpation has been advocated.[21,65] Apart from the inherent technical difficulties in this procedure,[66,67] no study has ever demonstrated any benefit from routine manual exploration of the scarred uterus. The procedure may in fact do more harm than good, with the potential for infection, converting a dehiscence into a larger rupture, or even falsely identifying a separation in the thin soft anterior wall of the lower uterine segment.

Michaels et al.[68] prospectively evaluated ultrasound as a means to determine the integrity of the lower uterine segment prior to the onset of labor. There was a false positive rate of 7.1%. No report of the function of the uterine scar during labor was provided and at present this is an interesting but purely investigational tool. Hysterography has been used intermittently to assess the uterine scar with little predictive ability. Most defects found radiologically are benign and not predictive of uterine rupture.

In the asymptomatic patient, the therapy for a dehiscence discovered fortuitously is uncertain, as most reports indicate these patients do well without

---

PREVIOUS CESAREAN SECTION
Summary of Management Options

Eligibility for trial of labor

- One previous lower uterine segment section with no other adverse features

- Twins, breech, non-diabetic macrosomia are probably not adverse features

- More than one previous cesarean section is more controversial as an adverse feature

- Generally accepted contraindications include:
  - previous classical cesarean section
  - diabetic macrosomic fetus

- Patient preference may influence choice of method (e.g. prolonged labor, dystocia, problems with baby)

Conduct of trial of labor

- Critical review of progress of labor

- Continuous fetal heart rate monitoring

- The issues of intravenous access and crossmatching blood are more controversial

- Prostaglandins can be used

- Caution should be exercised with i.v. oxytocin (also lower success rate)

- Regional analgesia not contraindicated

- Digital palpation/examination of scar only necessary with persistent postpartum bleeding

intervention. As previously stated, manual exploration of the lower segment cannot be advocated as a routine procedure, but may be indicated in women when persistent postpartum bleeding suggests a possible rupture which needs surgery.

CONCLUSION

The 1980s have witnessed a change in attitude toward management of the labor of the woman with a previous cesarean delivery, particularly in the USA. The stimulus for the interest in vaginal birth after cesarean section is probably the progressive increase in the cesarean section rate which has had a profound medical and social impact. The weight of the published clinical evidence indicates that vaginal birth after a lower uterine segment cesarean section is advantageous to the mother and has no adverse impact on the fetus. There has not been – and it is doubtful if there ever will be – a prospective randomized trial comparing elective repeat cesarean section with a trial of labor to demonstrate superior maternal and neonatal outcome definitively with either approach. Each delivery method has its advantages and disadvantages. It is ultimately the responsibility of the obstetrician to ensure the delivery plan is appropriate for the individual patient.

REFERENCES

1 Dewhurst CJ (1957) The ruptured caesarean section scar. *Journal of Obstetrics and Gynaecology of the British Empire* **64**:113–118.
2 Committee on Obstetrics (1988) *Maternal and Fetal Medicine: Guidelines for Vaginal Delivery after a Previous Cesarean Section.* ACOG Committee Opinion No. 64. Washington, DC: American College of Obstetricians and Gynecologists.
3 Farmakides G, Duvivier R, Schulman H et al. (1987) Vaginal birth after two or more cesarean sections. *American Journal of Obstetrics and Gynecology* **156**:565–566.
4 Phelan JP, Ahn MO, Diaz F et al. (1989) Twice a cesarean, always a cesarean? *Obstetrics and Gynecology* **73**:161–165.
5 Pruett KM, Kirshon B, Cotton DB et al. (1988) Is vaginal birth after two or more cesarean sections safe? *Obstetrics and Gynecology* **72**:163–165.
6 Novas J, Myers SA, Gleicher N (1989) Obstetric outcome of patients with more than one previous cesarean section. *American Journal of Obstetrics and Gynecology* **160**:364–367.
7 Ophir E, Oettinger M, Yagoda A et al. (1989) Breech presentation after cesarean section: Always a section? *American Journal of Obstetrics and Gynecology* **161**:25–28.
8 Strong TH, Phelan JP, Ahn MO et al. (1989) Vaginal birth after cesarean delivery in the twin gestation. *American Journal of Obstetrics and Gynecology* **161**:29–32.
9 Chazotte C, Cohen WR (1990) Catastrophic complications of previous cesarean section. *American Journal of Obstetrics and Gynecology* **163**:738–742.
10 Scott JR (1991) Mandatory trial of labor after cesarean delivery: An alternative viewpoint. *Obstetrics and Gynecology* **77**:811–814.
11 Jones RO, Nagashima AW, Hartnett-Goodman MM et al. (1991) Rupture of low transverse cesarean scars during trial of labor. *Obstetrics and Gynecology* **77**:815–817.
12 Taffel SM, Placek PJ, Liss T (1987) Trends in the United States cesarean section rate and reasons for the 1980–85 rise. *American Journal of Public Health* **77**:955–959.
13 Notzon FC, Placek PJ, Taffel SM (1987) Comparisons of national cesarean section rates. *New England Journal of Medicine* **316**:386–389.
14 Enkin M (1989) Labour and delivery following previous caesarean section. In: Chalmers I, Enkin M, Kierse MJNC (eds) *Effective Care in Pregnancy and Childbirth*, pp. 1196–1215. Oxford: Oxford University Press.
15 Porreco RP (1988) Once a cesarean, always a cesarean? In Phelan JP, Clark SL (eds) *Cesarean Delivery*, pp. 467–475. New York: Elsevier.
16 National Institutes of Health Consensus Development Task Force (1981) Statement on cesarean childbirth. *American Journal of Obstetrics and Gynecology* **139**:902–909.
17 Gibbs CE (1980) Planned vaginal delivery following cesarean section. *Clinics in Obstetrics and Gynecology* **23**:507–515.
18 Meier PR, Porreco RP (1982) Trial of labor following cesarean section: A two year experience. *American Journal of Obstetrics and Gynecology* **144**:671–678.
19 Martin JN, Harris BA, Huddleston JF et al. (1983) Vaginal delivery following previous cesarean birth. *American Journal of Obstetrics and Gynecology* **146**:255–263.
20 Paul RH, Phelan JP, Yen S-Y (1985) Trial of labor in the patient with a prior cesarean birth. *American Journal of Obstetrics and Gynecology* **151**:297–304.
21 Phelan JP, Clark SL, Diaz F et al. (1987) Vaginal birth after cesarean. *American Journal of Obstetrics and Gynecology* **157**:1510–1515.
22 Molloy BG, Sheil O, Duignan NM (1987) Delivery after cesarean section: Review of 2176 consecutive cases. *British Medical Journal* **294**:1645–1647.
23 Duff P, Southmayd K, Read JA (1988) Outcome of trial of labor in patients with a single previous low transverse cesarean section for dystocia. *Obstetrics and Gynecology* **71**:380–384.
24 Beneditti TJ, Platt L. Druzen M (1982) Vaginal delivery after cesarean section for a non-recurrent cause. *American Journal of Obstetrics and Gynecology* **142**:358–359.
25 Rosen MG, Dickinson JC, Westhoff CL (1991) Vaginal birth after cesarean section: A meta-analysis of morbidity and mortality. *Obstetrics and Gynecology* **77**:465–470.
26 Petitti DB, Cefalo RC, Shapiro S et al. (1982) In-hospital maternal mortality in the United States: Time trends

and relation to method of delivery. *Obstetrics and Gynecology* **59**:6–11.

27 Kirkinen P (1987) Multiple cesarean sections: Outcomes and complications. *British Journal of Obstetrics and Gynaecology* **95**:778–782.

28 Hurry DJ, Larsen B, Charles D (1984) Effects of postcesarean section febrile morbidity on subsequent fertility. *Obstetrics and Gynecology* **64**:256–260.

29 Hemminki E, Graubard BI, Hoffman HJ *et al.* (1985) Cesarean section and subsequent fertility: Results from the 1982 national survey of family growth. *Fertility and Sterility* **43**:520–528.

30 Garel M, Lelong N, Kaminski M (1987) Psychological consequences of caesarean childbirth in primiparas. *Journal of Psychosomatic Obstetrics and Gynecology* **6**:197–209.

31 Weckstein LN, Masserman JSH, Garite TJ (1987) Placenta accreta: A problem of increasing clinical significance. *Obstetrics and Gynecology* **69**:480–482.

32 Read JA, Cotton DB, Miller FC (1980) Placenta accreta: Changing clinical aspects and outcome. *Obstetrics and Gynecology* **56**:31–34.

33 Clark SL, Koonings PP, Phelan JP (1985) Placenta previa-accreta and previous cesarean section. *Obstetrics and Gynecology* **66**:89–92.

34 Frigoletto FD, Phillippe M, Davies IJ *et al.* (1980) Avoiding iatrogenic prematurity with elective repeat cesarean section without the routine use of amniocentesis. *American Journal of Obstetrics and Gynecology* **137**:521–524.

35 Boon AW, Milner AD, Hopkins IE (1981) Lung volumes and lung mechanics in babies born vaginally and by elective and emergency lower segmental cesarean section. *Journal of Pediatrics* **98**:812–814.

36 Callen P, Goldsworthy S, Graves L *et al.* (1979) Mode of delivery and the lecithin/sphingomyelin ratio. *British Journal of Obstetrics and Gynaecology* **86**:965–968.

37 Rosen MG, Dickinson JC (1990) Vaginal birth after cesarean: A meta-analysis of indicators for success. *Obstetrics and Gynecology* **76**:865–869.

38 Porreco RP, Meier PR (1983) Trials of labor in patients with multiple cesarean sections. *Journal of Reproductive Medicine* **28**:770–772.

39 Riva HL, Teich JC (1961) Vaginal delivery after cesarean section. *American Journal of Obstetrics and Gynecology* **81**:501–510.

40 Saldana LR, Schulman H, Reuss L (1979) Management of pregnancy after cesarean section. *American Journal of Obstetrics and Gynecology* **135**:555–561.

41 Strong THE, Phelan JP, Ahn MO *et al.* (1989) Vaginal birth after cesarean delivery in the twin gestation. *American Journal of Obstetrics and Gynecology* **161**:29–32.

42 Brady K, Read JA (1988) Vaginal delivery of twins after previous cesarean section. *New England Journal of Medicine* **319**:118–119.

43 Kaltreider D, Krone W (1959) Delivery following cesarean section. *Clinics in Obstetrics and Gynecology* **2**:1029–1042.

44 Pedowitz P, Schwartz RM (1957) The true incidence of silent rupture of cesarean section scars. *American Journal of Obstetrics and Gynecology* **74**:1071–1080.

45 Phelan JP, Eglinton GS, Horenstein JM *et al.* (1984) Previous cesarean birth: Trial of labor in women with macrosomic infants. *Journal of Reproductive Medicine* **29**:36–40.

46 Cruikshank DP (1986) Breech presentation. *Clinics in Obstetrics and Gynecology* **29**:258–263.

47 Graham RA (1984) Trial labor following previous cesarean section. *American Journal of Obstetrics and Gynecology* **149**:35–45.

48 Flamm BL, Goings JR (1989) Vaginal birth after cesarean section: Is suspected fetal macrosomia a contraindication? *Obstetrics and Gynecology* **74**:694–697.

49 Ollendorf DA, Goldberg JM, Minogue JP *et al.* (1988) Vaginal birth after cesarean section for arrest of labor: Is success determined by maximum cervical dilatation during the prior labor? *American Journal of Obstetrics and Gynecology* **159**:636–639.

50 Ong HC, Sen DK (1972) Clinical estimation of fetal weight. *American Journal of Obstetrics and Gynecology* **112**:877–880.

51 Simon NV, Levisky JS, Shearer DM *et al.* (1987) Influence of fetal growth patterns on sonographic estimation of fetal weight. *Journal of Clinical Ultrasound* **15**:376–383.

52 Pruett KM, Kirshon B, Cotton DB (1988) Unknown uterine scar and trial of labor. *American Journal of Obstetrics and Gynecology* **159**:807–810.

53 Beall M, Eglinton GS, Clark S *et al.* (1984) Vaginal delivery after cesarean section in women with unknown types of uterine scar. *Journal of Reproductive Medicine* **29**:31–35 (suppl.).

54 MacKenzie IZ, Bradley S, Embrey MP (1984) Vaginal prostaglandins and labour induction for patients previously delivered by caesarean section. *British Journal of Obstetrics and Gynaecology* **91**:7–10.

55 Flamm BL, Goings JR, Fuelberth N-J *et al.* (1987) Oxytocin during labor after previous cesarean section: Results of a multicenter study. *Obstetrics and Gynecology* **70**:709–712.

56 Horenstein JM, Phelan JP (1984) Previous cesarean section: The risks and benefits of oxytocin usage in trial of labor. *American Journal of Obstetrics and Gynecology* **151**:564–569.

57 Flamm BL, Dunnett C, Fischerman E (1984) Vaginal delivery following cesarean section: Use of oxytocin augmentation and epidural anesthesia. *American Journal of Obstetrics and Gynecology* **148**:759–763.

58 Sakala EP, Kaye S, Murray RD *et al.* (1990) Oxytocin use after previous cesarean section: Why a higher rate of failed labor trial? *Obstetrics and Gynecology* **75**:356–359.

59 Plauche WC, Von Almen W, Muller R (1984) Catastrophic uterine rupture. *Obstetrics and Gynecology* **64**:792–797.

60 Pearce J, Ravi P (1976) Rupture of uterine scar in a patient given epidural analgesia. *Lancet* **i**:1177–1178.

61 Flamm BL, Dunnett C, Fischermann E *et al.* (1984) Vaginal delivery following cesarean section: Use of oxytocin augmentation and epidural analgesia with internal tocodynamic and internal fetal monitoring. *American Journal of Obstetrics and Gynecology* **148**:759–763.

62 Hadley CB, Mennuti MT, Gabbe SG (1986) An evalu-

ation of the relative risks of a trial of labor versus elective repeat cesarean section. *American Journal of Perinatology* **3**:107–114.

63 Case B, Corcoran R, Jeffcoate N (1971) Caesarean section and its place in modern obstetric practice. *Journal of Obstetrics and Gynaecology of the British Commonwealth* **78**:203–214.

64 Cosgrove RA (1951) Management of pregnancy and delivery following cesarean section. *Journal of the American Medical Association* **145**:884–886.

65 Greenhill JP (1970) Editorial. *Year Book of Obstetrics and Gynecology*, pp. 202–203. Chicago, IL: Year Book Publishers.

66 Poidevin LO, Bockner VY (1958) A hysterographic study of uteri after caesarean section. *Journal of Obstetrics and Gynaecology of the British Empire* **65**:278–283.

67 Baxter J (1958) Vaginal delivery after caesarean section: Rupture of the lower segment scar. *Journal of Obstetrics and Gynaecology of the British Empire* **65**:87–88.

68 Michaels WH, Thompson HO, Boutt A *et al.* (1988) Ultrasound diagnosis of defects in the scarred uterine segment during pregnancy. *Obstetrics and Gynecology* **71**:112–120.

16

Prolonged Pregnancy

SABARATNAM ARULKUMARAN

INTRODUCTION

Management of prolonged pregnancy is a subject of concern because of its known association with increased fetal morbidity and mortality.[1-4] Women worry when they have not delivered by the expected date of delivery (EDD) because they think post-EDD is the same as prolonged pregnancy, and they have heard that prolonged pregnancy carries a risk to the fetus. Such anxiety should not arise if women are counseled at their first visit that they are likely to deliver between 38 and 42 weeks but not necessarily on the EDD, and that prolonged pregnancy refers to gestations longer than 42 weeks. Even doctors become anxious when a woman does not deliver by 41 weeks, because unexpected morbidity and mortality can occur between 41 and 42 weeks even though it is rare. Hence prenatal tests of fetal well-being are commonly instituted after 41 weeks,[5] even though they are probably not justified in low-risk pregnancies until week 43. One should be aware that trials of induction *vs* conservative management in prolonged pregnancy have been on selected populations in which the fetus was thought to have 'minimal risk' (there is no such thing as a 'no-risk' population) based on tests of fetal well-being at the end of 42 completed weeks. There is a wide variation in the availability of tests for fetal well-being and therefore in the ability to manage pregnancies after 42 weeks conservatively while minimizing the risk of unexpected intrauterine death. The availability of appropriate medication for successful induction of labor (usually prostaglandins, if the cervix is unfavorable) may also determine the timing of induc-

tion. Based on these factors, it is difficult to derive a policy for the management of prolonged pregnancy which will suit all obstetric units. The management has to be tailored to suit the facilities available in each centre. Any management policy should weigh the risk–benefit ratio of intervention vs non-intervention and should also take into consideration the patient's wishes after having counseled her with the relevant information.

DEFINITION

Prolonged pregnancy, postdate pregnancy, postterm, postdatism and postmaturity are all expressions which have been used to denote a pregnancy which has gone beyond 42 weeks or 294 days from the date of the first day of the last menstrual period.[6] These expressions are used with the idea of conveying a risk situation; however, to aid communication, it is useful to keep to a single definition. Prolonged pregnancy conveys its meaning most accurately and is defined by the International Federation of Gynaecologists and Obstetricians (FIGO) as any pregnancy which exceeds 294 days from the first day of the last menstrual period.[7] The expressions 'postdates' and 'postdatism' appear to convey different meanings to patients and doctors, some considering it to refer to a pregnancy which has gone past the EDD. To avoid confusion, it is preferable to describe the duration of pregnancy as 'so many days post the EDD' or as '41 weeks and 4 days', unless it is more than 294 days when it can be labeled as prolonged pregnancy.

Postmaturity syndrome refers to the description of a newborn who is coated with meconium, has dry peeling skin, overgrown nails, well-developed creases on the palm and soles, abundance of scalp hair, little vernix or lanugo hair, a scaphoid abdomen, minimal subcutaneous fat and an attentive apprehensive look.[1] Though such a picture is associated with infants born after 42 weeks, infants from prolonged pregnancies constitute only a small proportion of the babies with this appearance. Infants with such features may be born even at 39 and 40 weeks and hence the features described are not always characteristic of prolonged pregnancy. Therefore, the term 'prolonged pregnancy' should be preferred to 'postmaturity' for pregnancies beyond 42 weeks.

INCIDENCE

The incidence of prolonged pregnancy varies from 3 to 10% or more depending on whether it is calculated in a prospective or retrospective manner. It will also vary depending on whether the calculation is based on the history and clinical examination alone or whether early ultrasound examination (in the first half of pregnancy) is used to calculate the gestation.[8–11] The definition of prolonged pregnancy adopted and the consideration of factors such as cycle length when calculating the period of gestation will also influence the incidence. The incidence is bound to be uncertain if the population contains a high proportion of women who are not sure of the date of their last menstrual period, or the period occurred immediately after discontinuing hormonal contraceptives or breast-feeding. The literature suggests that about 20–40% of women in most populations cannot remember the date of their last menstrual period (LMP) and are unsure of their date of conception.[12] One should be aware that perinatal mortality is increased in women with unknown dates[13] and some of these deaths may be associated with unrecognized cases of prolonged pregnancy.

Some women have a normal menstrual period followed a few weeks later by a short episode of bleeding and then no further menstruation. It is sometimes construed that the woman conceived after the last normal period and that the short episode of bleeding was a threatened miscarriage in early pregnancy. But more often than not, the short episode of bleeding or 'spotting' was the actual LMP.[14] In places where women book in the first trimester and/or in centers where a dating scan is done in the first half of pregnancy, the incidence of prolonged pregnancy is less than 5%.[10,11] A high incidence of induction for whatever reasons will also reduce the true incidence of prolonged pregnancy.[9,15]

Maternal Risks

The main risk for the mother in prolonged pregnancy is that of operative delivery, whether associated with spontaneous or induced labor. Induction of labor is performed as a routine by week 42 in some centers, while in others it is done when abnormalities of fetal function on antepartum testing prompt delivery. The incidence of operative delivery in prolonged pregnancy of spontaneous onset has been reported in some series as being lower than that in induced labor,[16] while others have found no difference[17] and some have even reported an increase in operative delivery in those managed conservatively with the help of antepartum testing compared with those induced.[18] The risks of induction are largely those of operative delivery such as cesarean section. Other morbidity such as postpartum hemorrhage and infection usually only occur if labor is prolonged.

The success of induction will depend mainly on the parity of the woman and the state of her cervix (Bishop score). The influence of the period of gestation largely acts through the favorability or otherwise of the cervix, the Bishop score usually improving with advancing gestation. In order to counsel the patient properly, the risk of cesarean section when labor is induced should be known according to parity, cervical score and method of induction, for the unit in which she will have her baby. **Table 1** summarizes typical risks of cesarean section for failed induction of labor, classified by parity and cervical score, when labor was induced for various indications by amniotomy and oxytocin infusion in our own unit in Singapore.[19] For this study, the cervix was assessed by giving a score of 0–2 for each of the cervical characteristics of position, consistency, length, dilatation, and the station of the fetal head in relation to the maternal ischial spines. The rate of cesarean section (CS) in multiparas, and nulliparas with a good cervical score, was not high. However, nulliparas with a score of 3 or less had a CS rate of 65% for all indications and 45% for failed induction. In this study, the diagnosis of failed induction was made when a CS was done for reasons other than fetal distress, cephalo-pelvic disproportion or failure to pro-

Table 1
Cesarean section rate for failed induction of labor according to parity and cervical score

Cervical score	Para 0		Para 1 or more	
	n	*(%)*	*n*	*(%)*
0–3	27/59	(45.8)	2/26	(7.7)
4–6	30/292	(10.3)	10/257	(3.9)
7–10	3/208	(1.4)	2/215	(0.9)

gress due to malposition. Those who had CS for failed induction did not have a maximum cervical dilatation of more than 4 cm and thus did not enter the active phase of labor despite intravenous infusion of oxytocin for a period of 10–12 h.

The incidence of failed induction in nulliparas with poor cervical score can be reduced by pretreating the cervix with porstaglandins or lamicel prior to the use of oxytocin and artificial rupture of membranes.[20,21] Alternatively, labor can be induced by prostaglandin vaginal pessaries or gel.[22,23] Nulliparas with a cervical score of ≤ 6 induced with oxytocin and artificial rupture of the membranes have a significantly higher CS rate than when induction is carried out with prostaglandin E_2 vaginal pessaries (3 mg); each pessary being inserted 4 h apart, followed if necessary by oxytocin and artificial rupture of membranes 24 h later (**Table 2**).[24] Even so, the CS rates after induction with prostaglandins are much higher than the CS rates in nulliparas admitted in spontaneous labor.[25] A particular advantage of the use of prostaglandins is that they allow postponement of the induction if the woman does not become established in labor and the fetal heart rate pattern is normal, because the amniotic membranes are left intact.

In prolonged pregnancy, the need for prostaglandins will be confined to a relatively small number of nulliparas with a poor score, as appreciable numbers of women will be multiparous or nulliparous with a good cervical score. In an appropriately selected population with a favorable Bishop score, the overall CS rate in induced labor is likely to be insignificantly different from a similar group managed conservatively. Whenever induction is contemplated for uncomplicated prolonged pregnancy, the likelihood of CS based on par-

ity, cervical score and treatment modality should be estimated and explained to the pregnant woman when counseling her for induction or conservative management.

Fetal/Neonatal Risks

Though small, there is an increased risk of perinatal mortality after 42 weeks.[26,27] The incidence of antepartum stillbirths, intrapartum stillbirths and neonatal deaths are all approximately equal in prolonged pregnancy, whereas between 37 and 42 weeks antepartum deaths contribute about two-thirds of the total perinatal mortality.[26] There is also an increased morbidity in prolonged pregnancy due to hypoxia, shoulder dystocia and birth injuries, even when delivery is spontaneous rather than instrumental.

Management Options

Prepregnancy

The occurrence of prolonged pregnancy cannot be predicted. There is some evidence to suggest that it is more likely to occur in first pregnancies. Those women who have had one previous prolonged pregnancy and those who have had two prolonged pregnancies have a 30% and 40% chance of another prolonged pregnancy, respectively.[27] There is conflicting evidence in relation to the effect of maternal age. Accurate diagnosis of prolonged pregnancy relies upon either accurate menstrual data or routine second trimester scanning. In communities where routine scanning is not available for logistical or economic reasons, improved education aimed at increasing the proportion of women recording accurately the date of their last menstrual period might have a favorable impact on the increased rate of obstetric interference and perinatal mortality associated with prolonged pregnancy, by allowing timely intervention.[28]

Prenatal

Assessment of EDD

Unless routine second trimester scanning is available, clinical assessment of gestational age is most reliably performed in the first trimester. Once the patient misses her period, an early pregnancy test helps to define the limits of probability of gestational age. If a pregnancy test is positive 5 weeks after the last menstrual period, a women is unlikely to be more than 5 weeks gestation (unless her last period was in fact a threatened miscarriage) and cannot be less or the level of

Table 2
The indication for cesarean section in nulliparas with a cervical score <6, according to the method of induction

Treatment regimen	Oxytocin 2nd amniotomy $n = 230$	(%)	Prostaglandins $n = 152$	(%)
Fetal distress	27	(11.7)	13	(8.6)
CPD or malposition	10	(4.4)	8	(5.3)
Failed induction	55	(23.9)	14	(9.2)
Others	8	(3.5)	1	(0.7)
Total	100	(43.5)[a]	36	(23.7)

[a]$P < 0.001$.
CPD, cephalo-pelvic disproportion.

beta-hCG would be insufficient to provide a positive test (although this does of course assume that the test was not a false positive). This compares with a pregnancy test which is done at 7 weeks amenorrhea, when she could be 5, 6 or 7 weeks pregnant and which is therefore of less value for defining gestational age. A vaginal examination in the first trimester of pregnancy can also be useful in the estimation of gestational age; the assessment of uterine size in the second trimester is not so valuable.

An ultrasonic examination in the first or second trimester is now the preferred method of establishing gestational age in many maternity units. A crown rump length (CRL) at 7–10 weeks or a biparietal diameter at 18–22 weeks can estimate true gestational age within ±5 days, as validated, for example, in artificially conceived pregnancies when the times of fertilization and implantation are known with great accuracy. This relative precision is due to the consistency of fetal growth rates in the first half of pregnancy when maternal constraints are usually least important; later in pregnancy, growth rates diverge and hence measures of size become less closely related to gestational age. Assessment of gestational age by early ultrasound examination has reduced the apparent incidence of prolonged pregnancy by one-half to two-thirds in many centres.[10,11] This is because at least half of all apparently prolonged pregnancies occur in women who cannot remember their LMP accurately or who have long or irregular cycles; in these women, the presumption of prolonged pregnancy is erroneous.

Evaluation at 41 weeks

• Presence of risk factors

Once pregnancy proceeds beyond 41 weeks, it should be carefully reassessed, in case there are potential risk factors which have been overlooked. There is epidemiological evidence that women who have had pregnancy complications such as antepartum hemorrhage of unknown origin, or who have a history of stillbirth or neonatal death, are at increased risk of perinatal mortality.[29] These women are probably best delivered by 40 weeks. There is a slightly increased incidence of hypertension when pregnancy advances into the late third trimester. In the majority of cases, mild hypertension has no major consequence for the mother or fetus. However, they should be checked for signs of intrauterine growth deficiency, and induction offered if there is evidence of poor fetal growth.

• Counseling for induction of labor or conservative management

Obstetrics is a fine art built on facts gathered by scientific research. The same situation can often be managed differently with but equal effectiveness. The option chosen will usually depend on the knowledge and experience base of the obstetrician and the facilities available. When tests of fetal well-being are readily available for the conservative management of prolonged pregnancy, one can argue that it is appropriate to inform the pregnant woman of the options open to her, and involve her in the decision making. She will need to be told about the tests available, and their reliability or otherwise, should she wish to wait a few more days until the onset of spontaneous labor. On the other hand, the alternative – induction of labor – should also be explained, including the likelihood of vaginal delivery based on her parity, cervical score and method of induction. Her choice of option is likely to be based on her own knowledge and experience (for example, whether she knows someone who had a postmature stillbirth, or alternatively someone who had a difficult or painful induction of labor), her social life and other personal considerations. A recent prospective study[62] looked at the attitude of 500 pregnant women at 37 weeks gestation to a proposal of conservative management of prolonged pregnancy. Most women were unwilling to accept the conservative management of prolonged pregnancy and the proportion increased if still undelivered at 41 weeks. The reasons for such an attitude varied from 'could not stand the thought of being pregnant for more than 42 weeks' to concern regarding fetal size or the feeling that 'there is no benefit in waiting'.

Conservative management

• Maternal weight gain

The use of regular weight measurements in pregnancy is controversial. Some centres no longer recommend routine weighing as this practice has never been shown to produce lower perinatal morbidity or mortality. Sudden excessive weight gain might suggest the possible onset of pre-eclampsia or even diabetes, while static weight or weight loss over a few weeks has been considered to indicate failing placental function with resulting intrauterine growth deficiency. Static weight or weight loss at term has been used as an indication for induction in many centers,[19] but this view has changed as confidence has grown in the newer methods of fetal surveillance. Reduction in amniotic fluid volume signifies possible fetal compromise but is difficult to quantify clinically especially in obese women. The use of ultrasound is helpful and will be discussed later.

• Symphysial fundal height

The assessment of fetal size by measurement of symphysial fundal height can be influenced by obesity, the amount of amniotic fluid, the level of the presenting part, the fetal lie and abdominal wall tension. Although serial measurements are useful in following the progress of pregnancy, single measurements are of limited value in prolonged pregnancy. They may help to identify an association case of growth retardation or a macrosomic baby which has been missed in earlier examinations.

• *Tests of fetal well-being*

The occurrence of prolonged pregnancy is unpredictable. Hence the mainstay of prenatal management lies first in the correct diagnosis of prolonged pregnancy. Once diagnosed, the pregnancy can be terminated by induction of labor or managed conservatively until spontaneous onset of labor. If the option of awaiting spontaneous onset of labor is chosen, fetal well-being should be monitored by appropriate available tests.

1. Biochemical methods: Only a few centers now use biochemical methods to monitor fetal well-being. For a correct interpretation of the results, the period of gestation must be known. Further, serial measurements are needed to draw meaningful conclusions because of the wide range of normal values.[30] The results obtained represent fetal status over the previous few days and do not prognosticate fetal health except very indirectly. Results are usually not available until many hours after dispatching the test samples. In prolonged pregnancy, the value of such tests is limited as the patient might deliver prior to the results becoming known. Low estriol values in an otherwise healthy fetus should suggest the rare condition of placental sulfatase deficiency (which occurs in 1:5000 pregnancies). These women may be carrying a fetus with the autosomal recessive disorder of congenital icthyosis.[31]

2. Fetal movement chart: Fetal activity, measured as fetal movements, has been found to be correlated with other indices of fetal health.[32] A monitoring technique which has been widely promoted is that of the 'count to 10' fetal movement chart where 10 episodes of fetal activity are expected within a period of 12 h.[33] Most mothers feel 10 episodes of fetal movements within a few hours; however, anxious mothers commonly over-report slightly less than optimal movements, which can lead to unnecessary intervention. Busy or less intelligent gravidas sometimes fail to seek attention or come late even with no fetal movements, thus preventing any action which might be taken to lessen the risk of a poor fetal outcome. Yet other pregnant women are unable to perceive fetal movements at all, and for them the method is clearly not suitable. Although inexpensive, the value of fetal movement counting in monitoring the fetus in prolonged pregnancy has not been validated. A randomized study involving 68 000 women showed no benefit in providing fetal movement charts as a routine compared with selective use when indicated.[34] Based on current data, a fetal movement chart alone is probably not sufficient to monitor fetal health in prolonged pregnancy.

3. Maternal perception of sound-provoked fetal movements: The normal fetus exhibits flexion–extension limb movements or a startle reflex in response to a vibroacoustic stimulus, indicating an intact central nervous system and a somatomotor sensory pathway.[35,36] Maternal perception of sound-provoked fetal movement (mp SPFM) correlates well with a reactive non-stress test (NST)[37,38] and may be of value in centers where facilities for performing a NST are limited. The correlation of mp SPFM with the NST is reported in **Table 3**.

The sensitivity of mp SPFM in the prediction of a positive NST was 92.8%, the specificity 76.9%, positive predictive value 99.7% and negative predictive value 11.9%. The three women who had a positive mp SPFM but a non-reactive NST were less than 33 weeks of gestation and were on multiple antihypertensive therapy for severe pre-eclampsia, which may have accounted for the decreased variability and lack of accelerations of fetal heart rate (FHR).[39] The incidence of prolonged pregnancy in this population was 12.8% and none had an adverse outcome. It may be possible to use mp SPFM to assess fetal well-being in prolonged pregnancy in centers where facilities for NST are not regularly available; however, this approach needs further investigation before it can be recommended.

4. Non-stress test: Antepartum recording of the FHR continuously on a cardiotocograph for a period of 20–40 min to evaluate fetal well-being has been called the 'non-stress test' (NST). In recent years, it has become one of the most popular methods of prenatal fetal surveillance, particularly in relation to prolonged pregnancy.[40] Definitions of normal, suspicious and abnormal FHR patterns have been described by the FIGO.[41] A normal reactive FHR trace is one which over a period of 10 min has a baseline rate of between 110 and 150 beats/min, baseline variability of 10–25

Table 3
Correlation of the results of the mp SPFM

mp SPFM	FM present ($n = 1009$)	(%)	FM absent ($n = 88$)	(%)	Total ($n = 1097$)	(%)
NST reactive	1006	(99.7)	78	(88.6)	1084	(98.8)
NST non-reactive	3	(00.3)	10	(11.4)	13	(1.2)

beats/min, no decelerations and two FHR accelerations of 15 beats or more above the baseline for >15 s. If accelerations do not occur within the first 10 min, the trace should be continued for at least 40 min prior to confirming it as a non-reactive trace. The fetal acoustic stimulation test (FAST), where a vibroacoustic stimulus is used to elicit acelerations of the FHR, is a useful way to reduce the number of non-reactive traces and to shorten the testing time.[42] The reliability of the NST in the prediction of continuing fetal well-being for 1 week after testing has been studied by amalgamating the results from four studies which together included 10 169 tests.[43-46] The number of falsely reassuring tests was 7:1000 cases. Some of those fetuses who died within a week of a reassuring trace had lethal malformations. In other studies where fetuses died, a reactive trace (with accelerations) was coupled with decelerations indicating possible oligohydramnius.[47-49] Compromise to the fetus in prolonged pregnancy is often due to oligohydramnios and will be discussed later. In a reactive trace with good baseline variability, isolated decelerations which are <15 beats from the baseline rate lasting <15 s or <30 s following an acceleration do not signify fetal compromise. However, if the trace is not reactive despite stimulating the fetus or if it shows decelerations >15 beats/min, then it indicates possible compromise and this is usually an indication for terminating the pregnancy.

5.   Contraction stress test/Fetal acoustic stimulation test: A good outcome has been reported following a contraction stress test (CST) used as the primary means of assessing fetal well-being in prolonged pregnancy.[50] Though reliable, it is invasive, requires the patient to be restricted to bed and necessitates a short stay in hospital. However, similarly valid information can be obtained by more convenient out-patient techniques. It may be of particular value when a non-reactive NST is encountered. However, in current practice, this latter problem is probably more conveniently investigated by the use of a fetal acoustic stimulation test (FAST). Not only does FAST produce a reactive trace, it also reduces the testing time.[42] It may not represent the stress of uterine contractions and thus not reveal a situation of potential compromise in labor, but produces a reactive trace comparable to the NST and the perinatal outcome is similar whether the trace was reactive spontaneously or as a result of the FAST.[51] In fact, there is some evidence to suggest that the use of FAST in such a situation is more discriminatory in selecting fetuses in good health.[52]

6.   Assessment of amniotic fluid volume: Fetal urine contributes significantly to the volume of amniotic fluid. Severe oligohydramnios is a common finding in bilateral renal agenesis. With diminished placental function, maintained perfusion of the brain and heart is associated with reduced perfusion of other organ systems including the kidneys. This leads to a reduction of fetal urine formation and thus oligohydramnios commonly complicates severe intrauterine growth retardation. Thus fetal compromise due to a gradual decline in placental function can be monitored by assessing the amniotic fluid volume. In prolonged pregnancy, a common mechanism of fetal compromise appears to be cord compression[53] and in this context evaluation of amniotic fluid volume is even more useful.[54] Evaluation of amniotic fluid volume by palpatation may be deceptive and measurement using ultrasound is more objective. Compared with the assessment of the vertical depth of the largest pool (after excluding loops of cord), adding the vertical pockets in the four quadrants of the uterus (the amniotic fluid index: AFI) correlates better with perinatal outcome.[55] In prolonged pregnancy, an amniotic fluid index <5 cm or <2 cm depth of the largest pocket is suggestive of reduced placental function. In these situations, there is a possibility of fetal compromise either prenatally or in labor because of cord compression. Delivery by induction and continuous electronic fetal monitoring during labor is desirable in such cases. In prolonged pregnancy, the AFI can decline at a surprisingly fast rate in some cases and it is therefore wise to determine the AFI twice weekly.

7.   Biophysical profile: Biophysical profile measurement consists of an ultrasound examination to evaluate fetal movements, fetal tone, fetal breathing movements, and the vertical depth of the largest amniotic fluid pocket, coupled with a non-stress test. Each of these variables is scored 0 or 2, there being no intermediate score of 1. A score of 8 or 10 indicates a fetus in good condition. Retesting should be performed at intervals depending on the level of obstetric risk. In prolonged pregnancy, it is best performed twice weekly. If the score is 6, then the score has to be re-evaluated 4–6 h later and a decision made based on the new score. A score of 4 or less is an indication for delivery.[56] Good perinatal outcome has been reported with biophysical profile scoring both in high-risk pregnancy[57] and as a primary modality of testing in prolonged pregnancy.[58]

A modified biophysical profile where only the ultrasound parameters are evaluated (without NST) has been found to be equally reliable.[59] Due to the time and expertise needed to perform a biophysical profile, many centers perform an NST, if needed with FAST (when NST is not reactive) and an AFI. Excellent perinatal outcome in high-risk pregnancies has been reported with this approach.[60] A simple plan for fetal surveillance is given in **Figure 1**. The cycle of investigation should be carried out twice weekly in prolonged pregnancy. Indications for terminating the pregnancy are an AFI <6, a non-reactive NST despite FAST and

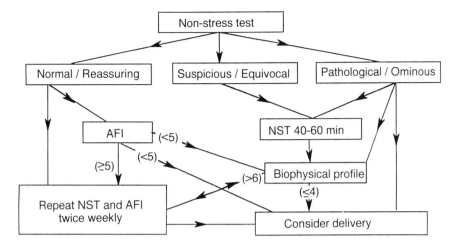

Figure 1. Suggestion for prenatal fetal monitoring of prolonged pregnancy.

retesting, decelerations >15 beats last >15 s or >30 s if following an acceleration. There was a higher incidence of meconium-stained amniotic fluid, cesarean section for fetal distress and babies with poor Apgar scores in cases of prolonged pregnancy when the pregnancy was terminated based on an abnormal result in the above scheme compared with a control group of patients with prolonged pregnancy but normal test results.[61]

Labour/delivery

Fetal surveillance in labor

- *Admission test*

The fetus undergoing a prolonged pregnancy appears to be more at risk of hypoxia during labor and in the postnatal period than a fetus at term.[27,61] Those fetuses who maintain just enough oxygenation in the prenatal period may show evidence of compromise with the contractions of early labor. An admission cardiotocgram or 'admission test' should pick up such cases.[63] In some cases, delay in intervention on admission might result in a severely asphyxiated neonate or a stillbirth. The absence of the normal accelerations and baseline variability which are the hallmark of fetal health should alert the clinician to possible fetal hypoxia. In such a case, the baseline rate may be normal (110–150 beats/min) but shallow decelerations of <15 beats are ominous when the baseline variability is <5 beats/min (**Figure 2**). Often the significance of such a trace is missed, confidence being falsely generated by the baseline rate which is in the normal range. It is unusual for a fetus in labor to be hypoxic without any decelerations, but they may be very shallow when

the baseline variability is <5 beats/min, as shown in **Figure 2**. In addition, the absence of accelerations in any part of the trace should always be considered ominous.

In order to screen those at risk, it is useful to advise women after 41 weeks to come early when in labor and to have an admission test on arrival. Precious time should not be wasted with administrative admission procedures prior to the admission test. Electronic fetal monitoring at least for a brief period is necessary to pick up any subtle changes in the fetal heart rate pattern prior to reliance on intermittent auscultation. When there are no accelerations and the trace is suspicious, fetal acoustic stimulation can be employed to reduce the number of non-reactive traces.[64] This combined approach helps in selecting those fetuses who are already compromised or likely to be compromised in labor. An ominous trace in early labor in the presence of thickly meconium-stained and scanty amniotic fluid warrants immediate delivery and not procrastination to await further cervical dilatation so as to perform a fetal scalp blood sampling. A suspicious or an abnormal admission test trace is an indication for subsequent continuous electronic fetal monitoring.

- *Continuous electronic fetal monitoring*

Prolonged pregnancy is a high-risk situation and continuous electronic fetal monitoring is preferable if equipment is available and there is no objection from the woman. When there is limitation of equipment or reluctance by the patient for continuous monitoring, a normal admission test followed by meticulous intermittent auscultation may suffice in the presence of clear amniotic fluid. However, a 20–30 min cardiotocogram every 2–3 h gives more information and may be useful. Added risk factors such as thick meconium-stained fluid or no fluid at membrane rupture, induction or

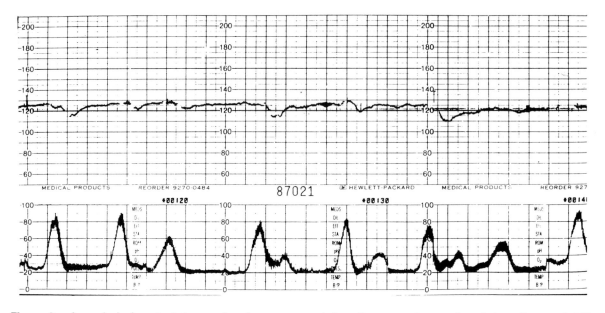

Figure 2. An admission test trace showing a normal baseline rate but reduced baseline variability (<5 beats/min) with shallow decelerations which are ominous in a non-reactive trace.

augmentation with oxytocin or prostaglandin, use of epidural analgesia and cases suspected of intrauterine infection following a prolonged period of membrane rupture dictate the use of continuous monitoring as the fetal heart rate can become abnormal within a short time.

● *Color and quantity of amniotic fluid*

Meconium passage *in utero* is largely a function of fetal maturity and the incidence of meconium-stained fluid is higher in prolonged pregnancy.[66] However, fresh thick meconium staining of scanty amniotic fluid should prompt the initiation of cardiotocograph monitoring because of the increased risk associated with intrapartum hypoxia if an abnormal fetal heart rate pattern occurs in conjunction with meconium staining.[65–67] Abnormal fetal heart rate patterns suggestive of hypxoia are more common with thick meconium-stained amniotic fluid. On the other hand, the risk associated with thin or moderate meconium staining of the amniotic fluid appears not to be substantially increased.[68,69] The incidence of low Apgar scores is doubled when an abnormal FHR pattern occurs in the presence of thickly meconium-stained fluid when compared with a similar tracing in the presence of clear amniotic fluid.[66] A similar increase in low Apgar scores with meconium staining of the fluid may not be seen if the FHR pattern is normal.[66] Neither does the umbilical cord arterial blood pH differ according to whether the amniotic fluid is meconium stained or not, so long as the FHR pattern is normal. However, if the FHR trace is abnormal, cord arterial pH values are sig-

nificantly lower in those with meconium-stained fluid compared with those with clear fluid.[70]

Since hypoxia and acidosis are particularly undesirable in the presence of meconium-stained amniotic fluid, particular care should be taken to avoid hypotension if an epidural anesthetic is administered, and hyperstimulation with oxytoxics should be avoided at all costs. Prompt action should be taken in the presence of meconium staining of the fluid if the FHR pattern becomes abnormal. Meconium aspiration leading to pneumonitis is the major threat with thick meconium, and there is some correlation between asphyxia and meconium aspiration.[71,72] The meconium-stained fluid in prolonged pregnancy tends to be more particulate with the presence of exfoliated skin, hair and vernix and this may block the airways causing more problems than non-particulate meconium-stained fluid found in pregnancies of earlier gestation. Post-term fetuses may be more prone to hypoxia due to reduced amniotic fluid volume leading to the greater possibility of cord compression with uterine contractions.[53] The appearance of meconium, the degree of staining based on the quantity of amniotic fluid and the FHR pattern have to be kept in mind in monitoring a patient with prolonged pregnancy.

● *Amnioinfusion in labor*

Since a major problem with labors in prolonged pregnancy is oligohydramnios and cord compression, and since these often co-exist with meconium staining of the amniotic fluid, it may be posible to use amnioinfusion of warm saline to reduce the likelihood of fetal hypoxia and/or meconium aspiration. Preliminary studies[73-75] where amnioinfusion has been used in such situations are encouraging. The catheters used for such a purpose have an amnioinfusion port at the base of the catheter through which fluid is infused. Intrauterine pressure recordings can be obtained simultaneously through a separate channel of the catheter connected to a pressure transducer.[76] The results of further large-scale randomized studies which are in progress should reveal whether amnioinfusion in labor will reduce the morbidity to the mother and fetus in prolonged pregnancy.

Monitoring progress of labor

There has been some debate about whether the progress of labor is usually normal in prolonged pregnancy, some claiming an increase in dysfunctional labour, whereas others have found no such increase. In cases of poor progress, the problem should be either poor uterine contractions or disproportion in the fetopelvic relationship, or a combination of both. The rate of fetal weight gain is maximal at 270 days and subsequent weight gain is not marked,[77] although inevitably there is a higher proportion of heavy babies associated with prolonged pregnancy.[78] Despite popular belief, there is no evidence to suggest that the skull bones are significantly more ossified and that there is therefore less molding, contributing to disproportion. Poor progress of labor in prolonged pregnancy can therefore be managed in the same way as in term pregnancy.

In prolonged pregnancy, increased perinatal morbidity and mortality have been attributed to birth trauma.[27] The only reasonable approach to this is careful monitoring of labor progress and appropriate intervention. At the onset of labor, one should estimate the birthweight as around 2, 3, 4 or more kg. This estimation should be made early and not after 16–18 h of labor at the time of cesarean section or after traumatic instrumental vaginal delivery. A prolonged first stage, especially secondary arrest late in the first stage of labor, when the cervix is loosely applied to the presenting part, followed by a prolonged second stage with marked caput and molding and difficulty in palpating the fetal ear, are all indicators of the possibility of a difficult and traumatic instrumental vaginal deilvery. In addition, the presence of meconium and/or an abnormal fetal heart rate pattern signifies the possibility of meconium aspiration and/or hypoxia. Shoulder dystocia should always be considered a possibility with abnormal labor patterns in prolonged pregnancy and each labor ward should have a protocol for a definitive plan of action should it occur. The delivery should be conducted in a stepwise fashion in the form of a drill – 'shoulder dystocia drill'.[79]

Care of the neonate at and after delivery

If the amniotic fluid is meconium-stained, the neonate deserves particular care at delivery. The oropharynx and nasopharynx should be sucked out when the head is delivered but with the trunk still in the maternal pelvis. Once the shoulders are delivered, the oropharynx should be sucked out again. It is advisable to have a pediatrician in attendance to visualize the vocal cords using the laryngoscope and to observe if there is any meconium below them. If meconium is present below the vocal cords a bronchial lavage has been advocated by some.[80] To prevent subsequent vomiting and aspiration of the stomach contents, a gastric lavage can be undertaken to clear the thick particulate meconium from the stomach. The baby should be checked carefully so as to detect any birth injury. Hypoglycemia can be a problem in a large neonate and regular checks of its blood sugar are advisable. Early feeding is likely to be beneficial. In infants followed up for 2 years after prolonged pregnancy no adverse mental or physical delay in milestones has been identified.[81]

CONCLUSION

Prolonged pregnancy cannot be predicted, but when uncomplicated carries little risk to the fetus or the mother. Attempts to prevent prolonged pregnancy have taken the form of induction by medication or by alternative means such as breast stimulation.[82] These attempts are undertaken because of anxiety about declining placental function postterm and the associated fetal morbidity and mortality. Current biophysical methods of fetal health assessment are probably fairly reliable and a combination of NST and AFI starting from the end of week 41 appears to be adequate. Such testing is most reassuring when performed twice weekly. The patient's wishes regarding induction or conservative management and the facilities available for antepartum testing should be taken into consideration when management is planned. Simple tests like the mp SPFM may be useful in centers with limited facilities for other forms of testing. The method of induction should be tailored according to the parity and cervical score to minimize the risk of failed induction and the cesarean section rate. When managed conservatively, about 40–50% of nulliparas and multiparas deliver within 4 or 5 days after 42 weeks.[11] An admission test, continuous cardiotocography and knowledge of the quantity and color of amniotic fluid are essential to provide optimal care to the fetus in labor. Amnioinfusion when warranted and a combined obstetric–pediatric approach to reduce the incidence of meconium aspiration may help us to reduce the morbidity and mortality associated with prolonged pregnancy to a minimum.

PROLONGED PREGNANCY
Summary of Management Options

Prepregnancy

- Counsel about risks of recurrence (30% with one and 40% with two previous prolonged pregnancies)

Prenatal

- Establish estimated date of delivery as accurately as possible in first half of pregnancy

- At 41 weeks:
  - re-evaluation for possible risk factors (APH, poor fetal growth, hypertension, etc.)
  - in normal pregnancy, counsel for relative risks and benefits of induction *vs* conservative management

- If conservative management:
  - fetal monitoring (methods will be determined by local availability and experience)

Labor/delivery

- Admission test

- Continuous fetal heart rate monitoring

- Critical review of progress of labor

- Vigilance and precautions for potential difficult delivery

- Normal management if meconium staining of amniotic fluid (see Chapters 62 and 71)

REFERENCES

1 Clifford SH (1954) Postmaturity with placental dysfunction. *Journal of Pediatrics* 44:1–13.
2 Nesbitt REL Jr (1955) Prolongation of pregnancy: A review. *Obstetrical and Gynecological Survey* 10:311.
3 Evans TN, Koeff ST, Morely GW (1963) Fetal effects of prolonged pregnancy. *American Journal of Obstetrics and Gynecology* 85:701–702.
4 Naeye RL (1978) Causes of perinatal mortality excess in prolonged gestation. *American Journal of Epidemiology* 108:429.
5 Guidetti DA, Divon MY, Langer O (1989) Postdate fetal surveillance: Is 41 weeks too early? *American Journal of Obstetrics and Gynecology* 161:91–93.
6 Gibb D (1984) Prolonged pregnancy. In Studd JWW (ed.) *The Management of Labour*, pp. 108–122. Oxford: Blackwell Scientific Publications.
7 FIGO (1980) International classification of diseases: Update. *International Journal of Obstetrics and Gynecology* 17:634–640.
8 Bierman J, Siegel E, French FE, Simonian K (1965) Analysis of the outcome of all pregnancies in a community Kauai pregnancy study. *American Journal of Obstetrics and Gynecology* 91:37–45.
9 Lindell A (1956) Prolonged pregnancy. *Acta Obstetrica et Gynecologica Scandinavica* 35:136–163.
10 Eik-Nes SH, Okland O, Aure JC, Ulstein M (1984) Ultrasound screening in pregnancy: A randomised controlled trial. *Lancet* i:1347.
11 Ingemarsson I, Heden L (1989) Cervical score and onset of spontaneous labor in prolonged pregnancy dated by second-trimester ultrasonic scan. *Obstetrics and Gynecology* 74:102–105.
12 Hall MH, Carr-Hill RA, Fraser C, Campbell D, Samphier MI (1985) The extent and antecedents of uncertain gestation. *British Journal of Obstetrics and Gynaecology* 92:445–451.
13 Dewhurst CJ, Beazley JM, Campbell S (1972) Assessment of fetal maturity and dysmaturity. *American Journal of Obstetrics and Gynecology* 118:141.
14 McCarthy TG (1975) Relationship of a short period to conception. *British Journal of Obstetrics and Gynaecology* 82:158.
15 Chamberlain G, Philip E, Howlett B, Masters K (1970) *British Births 1970*: Vol. 2. *Obstetric Care*. London: Heinemann Medical.
16 Gibb DMF, Cardozo LD, Studd JWW, Cooper DJ (1982) Prolonged pregnancy: Is induction of labour indicated? A prospective study. *British Journal of Obstetrics and Gynaecology* 89:292–295.
17 Cardozo L, Fysh J, Pearce JM (1986) Prolonged pregnancy: The management debate. *British Medical Journal* 293:1059–1063.
18 Dyson DC, Miller PD, Armstrong MA (1987) Management of prolonged pregnancy: Induction of labor versus antepartum fetal testing. *American Journal of Obstetrics and Gynecology* 156:928–934.
19 Arulkumaran S, Gibb DMF, Tamby Raja RL, Heng SH, Ratnam SS (1985) Failed induction of labour. *Australia and New Zealand Journal of Obstetrics and Gynaecology* 25:190–193.
20 Tromans PM, Beazley JM, Shenouda PI (1981) Comparative study of oestradiol and prostaglandin E$_2$ gel upon subsequent labour. *British Medical Journal* 282:679–681.
21 Sorensen SS, Brocks V, Lenstrup C (1985) Induction of

labour and cervical ripening by intracervical prostaglandin E_2. *Obstetrics and Gynecology* **65**:110–114.

22 Pearce MF, Shepherd JH, Sims CD (1979) Prostaglandin E_2 pessaries for induction of labour. *Lancet* **1**:572–575.

23 Arulkumaran S, Adaikan G, Anandakumar C, Viegas OAC, Piara Singh S, Ratnam SS (1989) Comparative study of a two dose schedule of PGE 3 mg pessary and 1700 µg film for induction of labour in nulliparae with poor cervical score. *Prostaglandins, Leukotrienes and Essential Fatty Acids*. **38**:37–41.

24 Kurup A, Chua S, Arulkumaran S, Tham KF, Tay D, Ratnam SS (1991) Induction of labour in nulliparas with poor cervical score: Oxytocin or prostaglandin vaginal pessaries? *Australia and New Zealand Journal of Obstetrics and Gynaecology* **31**:223–226.

25 Arulkumaran S, Gibb DMF, TambyRaja RL, Heng SH, Ratnam SS (1985) Rising caesarean section rates in Singapore. *Singapore Journal of Obstetrics and Gynaecology* **16**:6–15.

26 Crowley P (1989) Post-term pregnancy: Induction or surveillance? In Chalmers I, Enkin M, Keirse MJNC (eds) *Effective Care in Pregnancy and Childbirth*, Vol. 1, pp. 776–791. Oxford: Oxford University Press.

27 Bakketeig L, Bergsjo P (1989) Post-term pregnancy: Magnitude of the problem. In Chalmers I, Enkin M, Keirse MJNC (eds) *Effective Care in Pregnancy and Childbirth*, Vol. I, pp. 765–775. Oxford: Oxford University Press.

28 Hall MH, Carr-Hill RA (1985) The significance of uncertain gestation for obstetric outcome. *British Journal of Obstetrics and Gynaecology* **92**:452–460.

29 Butler NR, Bonham DG (1963) *Perinatal Mortality: The First Report of the 1958 British Perinatal Mortality Survey under the Auspices of the National Birthday Trust Fund*. Edinburgh: E.&S. Livingstone.

30 Arulkumaran S (1989) Antenatal monitoring of the high risk fetus. *Singapore Medical Journal* **30**:202–204.

31 Harkness RA, Taylor NF, Crawford MA, Rose FA (1983) Recognising placental steroid sulphatase deficiency. *British Medical Journal* **287**:2.

32 Sadovsky E, Yaffe H, Polishuk WZ (1974) Fetal movements in pregnancy and urinary oestriol in prediction of impending fetal death in utero. *Israel Journal of Medical Science* **10**:1096–1099.

33 Pearson JF (1982) Monitoring high risk pregnancy. In Bonnar J (ed.) *Recent Advances in Obstetrics and Gynaecology*, Vol. 14, pp. 3–34. Edinburgh: Churchill Livinstone.

34 Grant A, Elbourne D, Valentin L, Alexander S (1989) Routine formal fetal movement counting and risk of antepartum late death in normally formed singletons. *Lancet* **i**:345–349.

35 Gelman SR, Wood S, Spellacy WN, Abrams RM (1982) Fetal movements in response to sound stimulation. *American Journal of Obstetrics and Gynecology* **143**:484–485.

36 Divon MY, Platt LD, Cautrell CJ, Smith CV, Yeh SY, Paul RH (1985) Evoked fetal startle response: A possible intrauterine neurological examination. *American Journal of Obstetrics and Gynecology* **153**:454–456.

37 Westgren M, Almstrom H, Nyman M, Ulmsten U (1987) Maternal perception of sound provoked fetal movements as a measure of fetal wellbeing. *British Journal of Obstetrics and Gynaecology* **94**:523–527.

38 Arulkumaran S, Anandakumar C, Wong YC, Ratnam SS (1989) Evaluation of maternal perception of sound provoked fetal movements as a test of antenatal fetal health. *Obstetrics and Gynecology* **73**:182–186.

39 Montan S, Solum T, Sjoberg NO (1984) Influence of beta-andrenoceptor blocker atenolol on antenatal cardiotocography. *Acta Obstetrica et Gynecologica Scandinavica* **118**:99–102 (suppl.).

40 Cario GM (1984) Conservative management of prolonged pregnancy using fetal heart rate monitoring only: A prospective study. *British Journal of Obstetrics and Gynaecology* **91**:23–30.

41 FIGO Subcommittee on Perinatal Medicine (1987) Guidelines for the use of fetal monitoring. *International Journal of Obstetrics and Gynecology* **25**:159–167.

42 Smith CV, Phelan JP, Paul RH, Broussard P (1985) Fetal acoustic stimulation testing: A retrospective experience with the fetal acoustic stimulation test. *American Journal of Obstetrics and Gynecology* **153**:567–568.

43 Kubli F, Boos R, Ruttgers H, Van Hagen SC, Vanselow H (1977) Antepartum fetal heart rate monitoring and ultrasound in obstetrics. In Beard RW, Campbell S (eds) *Proceedings of a Scientific Meeting of the Royal College of Obstetricians and Gynaecologists*, pp. 28–47. London: Royal College of Obstetricians and Gynaecologists.

44 Schifrin BS, Foye G, Amato J, Kates R, Mackenna J (1979) Routine fetal heart rate monitoring in the anteparum period. *Obstetrics and Gynecology* **54**:21–25.

45 Keagan KA, Paul RH (1980) Antepartum fetal heart rate monitoring: Non-stress test as a primary approach. *American Journal of Obstetrics and Gynecology* **136**:75–80.

46 Flynn Am, Kelly J, Mansfield H, Needham P, O'Connor M, Viegas OAC (1982) A randomised controlled trial of non-stress antepartum cardiotocography. *British Journal of Obstetrics and Gynaecology* **89**:427–433.

47 Barss VA, Frigoletto FD, Diamond F (1985) Stillbirth after nonstress testing. *Obstetrics and Gynecology* **65**:541–544.

48 Smith CV, Nguyen HN, Kovacs B, McCart D, Phelan JP, Paul RH (1987) Fetal death following antepartum fetal heart rate testing: A review of 65 cases. *Obstetrics and Gynecology* **70**:18–20.

49 Garite TJ, Linzey EM, Freeman RK *et al.* (1979) Fetal heart rate patterns and fetal distress in fetuses with congenital anomalies. *Obstetrics and Gynecology* **53**:716–719.

50 Freeman RK, Garite TJ, Modanlou H, Dorchester W, Rommal C, Devaney M (1981) Postdate pregnancy: Utilization of contract stress testing for primary fetal surveillance. *American Journal of Obstetrics and Gynecology* **140**:128–135.

51 Smith CV, Phelan JP, Platt LD (1986) Fetal acoustic stimulation testing II: A randomized clinical comparison with the nonstress test. *American Journal of Obstetrics and Gynecology* **155**:131–134.

52 Trudinger BJ, Boylan P (1980) Antepartum fetal heart

rate monitoring: Value of sound stimulation. *Obstetrics and Gynecology* **55**:265–268.

53 Leveno KJ, Quirk JG, Cunningham FG, Nelson SD, Santos-Ramos R, Toofanian A, De Palma RT (1984) Prolonged pregnancy. I. Observations concerning the causes of fetal distress. *American Journal of Obstetrics and Gynecology* **150**:465–473.

54 Crowly P (1980) Non-quantitative estimation of amniotic fluid volume in suspected prolonged pregnancy. *Journal of Perinatal Medicine* **8**:249–251.

55 Moore RT (1990) Superiority of the four-quadrant sum over the single-deepest pocket technique in ultrasonic identification of abnormal amniotic fluid volumes. *American Journal of Obstetrics and Gynecology* **163**:762–767.

56 Manning FA, Platt LD, Sipos L (1980) Antepartum fetal evaluation: Development of a biophysical profile. *American Journal of Obstetrics and Gynecology* **136**:787–790.

57 Manning FA, Morrison I, Harman CR, Lange IR, Menticoglou S (1987) Fetal assessment based on fetal biophysical profile scoring: Experience in 19,221 referred high-risk pregnancies. *American Journal of Obstetrics and Gynecology* **157**:880–884.

58 Johnson JM, Hareman CR, Lange IR, Manning FA (1986) Biophysical profile scoring in the management of posterm pregnancy: An analysis of 307 patients. *American Journal of Obstetrics and Gynecology* **154**:269–273.

59 Eden RD, Seifert LS, Kodack LD, Trofatter KF, Killam AP, Gall SA (1988) A modified biophysical profile for antenatal fetal surveillance. *Obstetrics and Gynecology* **71**:365–369.

60 Clark SL, Sabey P, Jolley K (1989) Nonstress testing with acoustic stimulation and amniotic fluid volume assessment: 5973 tests without unexpected fetal death. *American Journal of Obstetrics and Gynecology* **160**:694–697.

61 Rutherford SE, Phelan JP, Smith CV, Jacobs N (1987) The four-quadrant assessment of amniotic fluid volume: An adjunct to antepartum fetal heart testing. *Obstetrics and Gynecology* **70**:353–356.

62 Roberts LJ, Young KR (1991) The management of prolonged pregnancy – an analysis of women's attitudes before and after term. *British Journal of Obstetrics and Gynaecology* **98**:1102–1106.

63 Ingemarsson I, Arulkumaran S, Ingemarsson E, Tamby Raja RL, Ratnam SS (1986) Admission test: a screening test for fetal distress in labor. *Obstetrics and Gynecology* **68**:800–806.

64 Ingemarsson I, Arulkumaran S, Paul RH, Ingemarsson E, Tamby Raja RL, Ratnam SS (1988) Fetal acoustic stimulation in early labor in patients screened with the admission test. *American Journal of Obstetrics and Gynecology* **158**:70–74.

65 Miller FC, Sacks DA, Yeh SY *et al.* (1975) The significance of meconium during labor. *American Journal of Obstetrics and Gynecology* **122**:573–580.

66 Steer PJ (1985) Fetal distress. In Crawford J (ed.) *Risks of Labour*, pp. 11–31. Chichester: John Wiley.

67 Wong WS, Wong KS, Chang A (1985) Epidemiology of meconium staining of amniotic fluid in Hong Kong. *Australia and New Zealand Journal of Obstetrics and Gynaecology* **25**:90–93.

68 Meis PJ, Hall M, Marshall JR *et al.* (1978) Meconium passage: A new classification for risk assessment during labor. *American Journal of Obstetrics and Gynecology* **131**:509–513.

69 Arulkumaran S, Yeoh SC, Gibb DMF, Ingemarsson I, Ratnam SS (1985) Obstetric outcome of meconium stained liquor in labour. *Singapore Medical Journal* **26**:523–526.

70 Starks GC (1980) Correlation of meconium stained amniotic fluid, early intrapartum fetal pH, and Apgar scores as predictors of perinatal outcome. *Obstetrics and Gynecology* **56**:604–609.

71 Bowes WA (1982) Steps to prevent meconium aspiration syndrome. *Contemporary Obstetrics and Gynecology* **19**:135–138.

72 Mitchell J, Schulman H, Fleischer A *et al.* (1985) Meconium aspiration and fetal acidosis. *Obstetrics and Gynecology* **65**:352–355.

73 Wenstrom KD, Parsons MT (1989) The prevention of meconium aspiration in labor using aminoinfusion. *Obstetrics and Gynecology* **73**:647–651.

74 Sadovsky Y, Among E, Bade ME, Petrie RH (1989) Prophylactic amnioinfusion during labor complicated by meconium: A preliminary report. *American Journal of Obstetrics and Gynecology* **161**:613–617.

75 Owen J, Henson BV, Hauth JC (1990) A prospective randomized study of saline solution amnioinfusion. *American Journal of Obstetrics and Gynecology* **162**:1146–1149.

76 Arulkumaran S, Ynag M, Chia YT, Ratnam SS (1991) Reliability of intrauterine pressure measurements. *Obstetrics and Gynecology* **78**:896–899.

77 Gruenwald P (1967) Growth of human fetus. In McLaren A (ed.) *Advances in Reproductive Physiology, Vol. 2*, pp. 279–309. London: Logos Press.

78 Boyd ME, Usher RH, McLean FH (1983) Fetal macrosomia: Prediction, risks, proposed management. *Obstetrics and Gynecology* **61**:715–722.

79 Arulkumaran S, Montan S (1991) The fetus at risk in labour: Identification and management. In Ratnam SS, Ng SC, Sen DK, Arulkumaran S (eds) *Contributions to Obstetrics and Gynaecology, Vol. I*, pp. 179–190. Singapore: Churchill Livingstone.

80 Carsons BS, Losey RW, Bowes WA, Simmons MA (1976) Combined obstetric and paediatric approach to prevent meconium aspiration syndrome. *American Journal of Obstetrics and Gynecology* **126**:712–715.

81 Shime J, Librach CL, Gare DJ, Cook CJ (1986) The influence of prolonged pregnancy on infant development at one and two years of age: A prospective study. *American Journal of Obstetrics and Gynecology* **154**:341–345.

82 Elliot JP, Flaherty JF (1984) The use of breast stimulation to prevent postdate pregnancy. *American Journal of Obstetrics and Gynecology* **149**:628–632.

17

Medication During Pregnancy: Maternal and Embryofetal Considerations

LARRY C. GILSTRAP, BERTIS B. LITTLE

INTRODUCTION

Scientific data regarding the maternal and embryofetal effects of most therapeutic agents is alarmingly sparse, but it seems that the majority of pregnant women (40–90%) are exposed to medications during pregnancy. These medicines include a variety of agents such as vitamins, minerals, antibiotics, laxatives, antiemetics, sedatives, antacids, diuretics and antihistamines (**Table 1**).[1,2] Many women take medications without their physician's advice or prior to recognition of the pregnancy. Importantly, treatment of pregnant women with medications is sometimes essential as therapy for serious or life-threatening medication conditions.

INCIDENCE

In one survey of over 1000 pregnant women, approximately 97% took medications prescribed by a physician, and two-thirds took non-prescription medications without medical advice.[3] Similarly, in a 1987 survey of nearly 500 pregnant women, approximately 10% reported that they took neither prescription nor over-the-counter drugs.[4] The incidence of medication use during pregnancy seems considerably lower in the UK compared with the USA. In one report, fewer than 10% of pregnant women in the UK took medications other than prenatal vitamins and iron supplements during the first trimester.[5]

DRUGS KNOWN TO BE POTENTIALLY HARMFUL TO THE EMBRYO AND/OR FETUS

Medications may cause harm to the unborn child via either

- 'teratogenic effects' or

- 'fetal effects'

Teratogenic effects are those which occur during the period of organogenesis (embryonic period), with vulnerability encompassing the second through the eighth

Table 1
Medications frequently utilized by pregnant women[1,2]

Vitamins
Iron
Analgesics
Diuretics
Antiemetics
Antimicrobials
Antihistamines
Hypnotics and sedatives
Laxatives

weeks postconception. It is important to differentiate embryonic age from menstrual age in this discussion. Menstrual age is approximately 2 weeks greater than embryonic age because the former is calculated from the first day of the last menstrual period and the latter is an estimate of the day of conception. A medication which is a teratogen will cause a malformation in the unborn child when given during the period of the embryo.[2]

A drug's fetal effects are those that cause alterations in structure or function of organ systems normally formed during organogenesis.[2] The medications strongly suspected or proven to have adverse fetal or teratogenic effects are summarized in **Table 2**.

Thalidomide

This hypnotic/sedative is the best known of all human teratogens. Maternal ingestion between days 27 and 42 days postconception has resulted in the teratogenic effect known as phocomelia,[6,7] and involved absence

Table 2
Medications known or suspected of being human teratogens or having adverse fetal effects[2]

Retinoids
Isotretinoin
Etretinate

Hormones
Androgens
Diethylstilbestrol
Danazol

Anticoagulants
Warfarin

Antineoplastics
Aminopterin
Methotrexate
Busulfan
Cyclophosphamide

Anticonvulsants
Phenytoin and other hydantoins
Trimethadione and paramethadione
Valproic acid
Carbamazepine

Antibiotics
Tetracycline

Others
Lithium
Penicillamine
Thalidomide

of the long bones of the upper and/or lower limbs, among other defects. This agent is no longer commercially available for use as a sedative, but is used in the therapy for tuberculosis. Accordingly, alternative antituberculoric drug regimens are indicated for treatment of women of reproductive age (see Chapter 24).

Retinoids (see also Chapter 31)

Both isotretinoin and etretinate are derivatives of retinoic acid (vitamin A). Isotretinoin (Accutane®) is utilized primarily for the treatment of intractable cystic acne, a relatively common dermatologic disorder among women of reproductive age. Clinicians providing health care for pregnant women are likely to encounter use of this medication during early pregnancy, despite the stern warning in the manufacturer's package insert that using this drug during pregnancy is a known cause of devastatingly severe congenital anomalies of the ears, brain, heart and thymus. Scientific studies have supported the manufacturer's warning that isotretinoin is a significant teratogen and is associated with serious congenital anomalies, summarized in **Table 3**.[2,6–12]

In one review of approximately 60 pregnancies exposed to isotretinoin during early pregnancy, one-third were associated with a bad outcome: 16% had miscarriages and 19% had malformation.[12,13] Because of isotretinoin's relatively short terminal half-life (96 h; personal communication from the manufacturer), the risk of malformed offspring does not appear to be increased if the medication is discontinued prior to conception.[2,14]

Etretinate (Tegison®) is used primarily for the treatment of psoriasis and has been reported to be associated with central nervous system, craniofacial and skeletal anomalies in the progeny of pregnant women who received this medication during or prior to pregnancy.[2,8,15] Unlike isotretinoin, this agent has an unusually long half-life and there are reports of newborns with central nervous system and craniofacial

Table 3
Fetal anomalies reported to be associated with maternal isotretinoin (Accutane®) use[2,6–12]

Microtia
Anotia
Micrognathia
Cleft palate
Heart defects
Eye anomalies
Brain anomalies
Hydrocephalus
Thymic agenesis

abnormalities born to mothers who had discontinued etretinate up to 18 months prior to conception.[16,17] The manufacturer reports that serum etretinate levels are persistently in the therapeutic range for more than 5 years following cessation of therapy (personal communication from the manufacturer). Fortunately, psoriasis is relatively uncommon during pregnancy and when it does occur it generally does not require extensive therapy. If therapy is necessary, topical agents should be used because they will primarily be metabolized in the skin, resulting in negligible serum concentration.

Antineoplastics (see also Chapters 23 and 32)

Most antineoplastics have been reported to be teratogenic in humans (**Table 2**). In particular, folate antagonists (e.g. aminopterin and methotrexate) are very well-known human teratogens. Aminopterin has also been utilized as an abortifacient. Congenital anomalies reported to be associated with the fetal aminopterin syndrome are summarized in **Table 4**.[2,18–20] Methotrexate was associated with similar anomalies when used during the first trimester in two uncontrolled reports.[21,22]

Busulfan (Myleran®), alkylating agent used to treat some forms of leukemia, was associated with fetal growth retardation, cleft palate and eye defects in an infant whose mother received this antineoplastic in early pregnancy.[22] Similar defects were reported in animal teratology studies.[2] Cyclophosphamide (Cytoxan®) is another alkylating agent utilized to treat certain forms of leukemia as well as other forms of cancer (ovarian, cervical, endometrial and breast carcinomas). Reports of congenital anomalies associated with cyclophosphamide use during pregnancy include cleft palate, absence of digits, imperforate anus and fetal growth deficiency.[2,23,24] Craniofacial anomalies occurred in non-human primates whose mothers were given this drug during organogenesis.[25]

It is impossible to quantitate the teratogenic risk of the alkylating agents to the human fetus from available anecdotal data. In one review of maternal exposure to alkylating agents in the first trimester, 14% of the offspring had major congenital anomalies,[26] with the remainder apparently 'normal'.

Anticonvulsants (see also Chapter 26)

An increased risk of congenital anomalies has been reproted to be associated with a variety of anticonvulsant agents (phenytoin, trimethadione, carbamazepine and valproic acid).[2] The hydantoin agents, phenytoin (Dilantin®, Diphenylan®), ethotoin (Peganone®) and mephenytoin (Mesantoin®), are well known for their association with a constellation of congenital anomalies called the fetal hydantoin syndrome (see **Table 5**).[27] A review of several studies that included over 450 infants born to women who received hydantoin anticonvulsants during pregnancy suggest that approximately one-third of the infants exposed to phenytoin during gestation had minor anomalies (craniofacial and digital) and 10% had major congenital anomalies (cardiac defects, cleft lip/palate).[28]

The dione anticonvulsants, paramethadione (Paradione®) and trimethadione (Tridione®), are primarily used to treat petil mal seizures. A fetal dione syndrome has been described that consisted of abnormalities strikingly similar to the fetal hydantoin syndrome.[29]

For many years, carbamazepine (Tegretol®) was thought to be relatively safe for use during pregnancy, and was the drug of choice to treat pregnant women with seizure disorders.[30] In one report of almost 100 infants of mothers who received this agent during early pregnancy, the frequency of malformations was not increased over that expected for the general population.[31] However, it was recently reported that carbamazepine use during early pregnancy may be associated with a pattern of malformations very similar to that caused by phenytoin (i.e. craniofacial abnormalities, minor limb defects, growth retardation, mental retardation and neural tube defects).[32] According to a 1991 report from the Federal Drug Administration

---

Table 4
Features of the fetal aminopterin syndrome[2,18–20]

Short stature
Craniosynostosis
Calvarial ossification delay
Hydrocephalus
Hypertelorism
Micrognathia
Cleft palate

Table 5
Features of the fetal hydantoin syndrome[a]

Craniofacial abnormalities
  cleft lip/palate
  hypertelorism
  broad nasal bridge
Hypoplasia of distal phalanges and nails
Growth deficiency
Mental deficiency

[a]Adapted from Hansen and Smith.[27]

(FDA), the risk for neural tube defects seems to be 1–2% among carbamazepine-exposed offspring.

It is presently unclear whether it is the epilepsy *per se*, the anticonvulsant medication, or a combination of both or other factors that is responsible for the embryopathy.[30] Interestingly, it has been shown recently that cultured amniocytes obtained from pregnancies that resulted in fetuses with features of the fetal hydantoin syndrome were deficient in epoxide hydrolase enzyme activity.[33] This enzyme is essential for the elimination of a toxic phenytoin epoxide metabolite, and it was postulated that this epoxide metabolite may be responsible for the teratogenicity of the various anticonvulsant medications that have this metabolic pathway in common.[33,34] Thus, there may be a pharmacogenetic component to the etiology of the anticonvulsant embryopathies.

Valproic acid (Depakene®) is one of the most commonly utilized agents for petit mal seizures. It is reported to be associated with an increased risk of neural tube defects, estimated to be in the range 1–2%.[35,36] In addition, a constellation of anomalies of the face and digits – called the fetal valproate syndrome – has been described.[37–39]

If anticonvulsants do produce a direct effect on embryogenesis, this may be due in part to their effects on folate metabolism (especially phenytoin). Thus it is reasonable to administer folate supplements prepregnancy and prenatally in such patients.

Anticoagulants (see also Chapter 20)

The coumarin anticoagulant, warfarin, is a relatively small molecule and readily crosses the placenta.[30] A distinct pattern of anomalies called the warfarin embryopathy occurred in 15–25% in offspring whose mothers used this agent during the first trimester of pregnancy.[40,41] The two most common features are nasal hypoplasia and stippling of epiphyses. Other characteristic features of this syndrome are summarized in **Table 6**.[40] This anticoagulant may also result in adverse fetal effects such as intracerebral hemorrhage, microcephaly, cataracts, blindness and mental retardation when utilized during the second or third trimester of pregnancy.[40]

Hormones

Maternal androgen therapy (i.e. testosterone) may result in virilization of the external genitalia of the female fetus, including clitoral enlargement and labioscrotal fusion.[42] Most of these genital tract abnormalities can be surgically corrected and normal female development can be anticipated at puberty.[2]

The anti-endometriosis drug, danazol, is a testosterone derivative that has weak androgenic activity and may result in clitoromegaly and labial fusion with female fetal exposure.[43–46] The exact risk of this complication is unknown. Apparently this agent has no adverse effects in male fetuses exposed *in utero*.

Diethylstilbestrol (DES) is a non-steroidal synthetic estrogen, and is associated with clear-cell adenocarcinoma of the vagina in the progeny of women exposed to it during late embryogenesis.[47] The exact risk of this serious complication is unknown because the number of pregnant women actually exposed to this hormone during gestation is unknown. A variety of other non-malignant anomalies has also been reported among the female and male offspring of mothers exposed to this agent during pregnancy (see **Table 7**).[2,47–57] Importantly, increased frequencies of preterm labor, miscarriages and ectopic pregnancy have been reported among women whose mothers used diethylstilbestrol during pregnancy.[52]

Antibiotics

Tetracyclines are the only antibacterial agents known to have teratogenic effects. Fortunately, the adverse effects caused by this antibiotic, yellowish-to-brown

Table 6
Characteristic features of the fetal warfarin syndrome[a]

Nasal hypoplasia
Stippled bone epiphyses
Hydrocephaly
Microcephaly
Growth deficiency
Ophthalmologic anomalies
Postnatal development delay

[a]Adapted from Hall *et al.*[40]

Table 7
Abnormalities in the offspring of pregnant women exposed to diethylstilbestrol[2,47–57]

Female offspring
Clear-cell adenocarcinoma of the vagina or cervix
Vaginal adenosis
T-shaped uterus
Uterine hypoplasia
Paraovarian cyst
Incompetent cervix

Male offspring
Epididymal cyst
Hypoplastic testes
Cryptorchidism

discoloration of the deciduous teeth, is purely cosmetic and does not affect the permanent teeth, the frequency of dental caries or bone growth.[58-60] Importantly, the use of tetracyclines during pregnancy does not appear to be associated with an increased frequency of structural congenital anomalies.[61-63] Tetracyclines are not recommended for use during pregnancy because of the adverse effects on the deciduous teeth, except for the treatment of life-threatening infections in penicillin-allergic patients (e.g. syphilis).

Psychotropics

Lithium is utilized primarily for the treatment of affective mental disorders.[30] The use of this agent by pregnant women during early gestation is reportedly associated with an increased risk of cardiovascular anomalies in exposed offspring. In one review of over 200 infants born to mothers who took this medication during early pregnancy, 8% had serious congenital heart defects, and almost 3% had the very rare and unusually lethal cardiovascular malformation, Ebstein's anomaly.[64] The usual frequency of Ebstein's anomaly is less than 1:20 000 live births. The precise risk of cardiovascular anomalies due to maternal exposure to this agent during embryogenesis is unknown.[30] The risk of non-cardiovascular abnormalities does not appear to be increased substantially above background rises.[64]

Others

Penicillamine is used to treat rheumatoid arthritis and cystinuria.[2] It can also be used as a chelating agent for heavy metal poisoning (e.g. lead). This agent has been reported to be associated with connective tissue disorders in the offspring of exposed mothers,[65] although the risk is quantitatively unknown.[66] It is, therefore, contraindicated for use during pregnancy.

USE OF OTHER MEDICATIONS DURING PREGNANCY

The majority of medications currently available are 'not proven' to be human teratogens, although fewer than 40% have been adequately studied for use in human pregnancy. A clinically useful discussion of the use of medications during pregnancy is given below in the context of the medical indications for their use.

Dermatologic Medications (see also Chapter 31)

Retinoic acid analog, tretinoin (Retin-A, StieVAA®), is a topical agent utilized for the treatment of acne. It seems unlikely that a significant amount is absorbed systemically because this is a topical agent that is largely metabolized in the skin. Thus, this agent has little, if any, access to the fetus and would not be expected to be associated with a significant teratogenic risk. Although there are no studies with this agent in pregnant women, it has not been shown to be teratogenic in animal studies.[2] Other dermatologic agents are discussed under antimicrobials.

Seizure Disorders (see also Chapter 26)

Anticonvulsants known to be associated with teratogenic effects (i.e. phenytoin, carbamazepine, valproic acid, trimethadione) have already been discussed. Although these agents are associated with such adverse effects as birth defects, their benefits often outweigh the risks. Importantly, seizure activity in the untreated gravid epileptic may itself be teratogenic (i.e. from fetal hypoxia). Accordingly, it is usually recommended that anticonvulsant therapy be continued in pregnant epileptics, if necessary to control seizures.

Some anticonvulsant agents (i.e. phenytoin and barbiturates) may be associated with hemorrhage secondary to vitamin K deficiency. It seems reasonable to supplement pregnant women on these medications with vitamin K and possibly their newborns. Two anticonvulsants which have not been discussed are phenobarbital and ethosuximide.

Phenobarbital

There are no convincing scientific data to support the speculation of this agent as being teratogenic.[30] In one large study of over 1000 mother–infant pairs in which phenobarbital was used during the first trimester of pregnancy, the frequency of infant malformations detected at birth was not increased compared with controls.[62] In addition, this agent was not associated with congenital anomalies when prescribed for other (non-seizure) indications during pregnancy.

Ethosuximide

This agent is a succinimide anticonvulsant utilized primarily for treatment of petit mal seizures. There are no reports of congenital anomalies attributed to the use of this agent.[30] While phenobarbital appears to be 'relatively' safe for use during pregnancy, ethosuximide (Zarontin®) has not been studied sufficiently to make such an assessment.

Antimicrobials (see also Chapters 29 and 30)

A variety of infections occur commonly during pregnancy. Thus, clinicians providing care for pregnant women may need to prescribe antimicrobial agents, including antibacterial, antifungal, antiviral and antiparasitic agents.

Antibacterial agents

Antibacterial agents are among the most commonly prescribed medications during pregnancy, and it appears as though most of these drugs are safe for use during pregnancy. The antibiotics that may be associated with adverse fetal effects are summarized in **Table 8**. All the penicillins are apparently safe for use during pregnancy in patients not allergic to these drugs. The use of amoxicillin, penicillin and ampicillin has been studied, and congenital anomalies as well as other adverse effects were not increased in frequency. Other more recently developed broad-spectrum penicillins (e.g. piperacillin, mezlocillin), and those combined with the beta-lactamase inhibitors such as clavulanic acid (Timentin®, Augmentin®) and sulbactam (Unasyn®), have not been adequately studied during pregnancy. However, a significant risk for adverse effects seems unlikely, although small risks cannot be ruled out. It is important to note that the maternal serum levels of all the penicillins may be significantly lower in pregnant women compared with non-pregnant patients because blood volume is increased as much as 40% during pregnancy, and increased renal clearance is associated with the gravid state.[67] All the penicillins cross the placenta and may result in significant fetal levels as summarized in **Table 9**.[68,69] For this reason, the penicillins are the drugs of choice for treating syphilis during pregnancy, and prevention of congenital syphilis.

There are three major classes of cephalosporins: first-, second- and third-generation derivatives. All cephalosporins probably cross the placenta to a similar degree, resulting in significant fetal levels similar to those in the mother.[67–69] These drugs have been given to numerous pregnant women to treat serious conditions, although there are no controlled scientific studies regarding cephalosporin use during pregnancy. It should be noted that second- and third-generation cephalosporins containing the N-methylthiotetrazole (MTT) side chain have been reported to be associated with testicular hypoplasia in newborn animals,[70] but this adverse effect has not been described in the human. One of the most commonly used second-generation cephalosporins, cefoxitin, does not contain the MTT side chain. Thus, cefoxitin would appear to be the rational choice when therapy with broad-spectrum cephalosporins is indicated during pregnancy or in nursing mothers.

Erythromycin belongs to the macrolide group of

Table 9
Ratio of cord blood to maternal blood for some of the penicillins and cephalosporins[a]

	Ratio
Ampicillin	0.7
Mezlocillin	0.4
Ticarcillin plus clavulanic acid	0.8
Ampicillin plus sulbactam	1.0

[a]Adapted in part from Gilstrap et al.[30]

Table 8
Antibiotics with potentially adverse fetal effects[a]

Antibiotic	Potential adverse effect(s)
Tetracyclines	Yellow-brown discoloration of the deciduous teeth
Aminoglycosides	Ototoxicity (VIIIth cranial nerve damage)
Sulfonamides	Hyperbilirubinemia, transient
Nitrofurantoin	Hemolytic anemia, transient
Fluoroquinolones	Irreversible arthropathy
MTT-containing cephalosporins	Testicular hypoplasia[b]

[a]Adapted from Gilstrap et al.[30]
[b]Adverse effect only described in animals (see text).

antibiotics and has not been reported to be associated with adverse fetal effects. Apparently, this agent does not cross the placenta in appreciable quantity. Importantly, congenital syphilis has been reported among the offspring of penicillin-allergic mothers who received erythromycin for syphilis during pregnancy.[71] The most prudent approach to treating penicillin-allergic gravidas seems to be to desensitize pregnant women infected with syphilis and treat the disease in the mother and fetus with penicillin. Alternatively, the pregnant woman with syphilis may be treated with tetracycline, although this would not be the choice of many clinicians because of the risk of discoloration of the deciduous teeth.[72,73]

All the aminoglycosides cross the placenta to some degree[68,74,75] and result in significant fetal levels. A related compound, streptomycin, has been reported to be associated with eighth cranial nerve damage (sensorineural deafness) in fetuses whose mothers who received it for a significant time during pregnancy.[76,77] The risk of fetal ototoxicity from other aminoglycosides is not known precisely, but appears to be approximately 2%, a 20-fold greater than background risk for sensorineural hearing loss.

Aztreonam (Azactam®) is a recently developed monobactam antibiotic with a spectrum of activity similar to the aminoglycosides. There are no well-controlled studies and little is known about its use in pregnant women. Unlike the aminoglycosides, this group of antibiotics is not known to be associated with either renal or ototoxicity in adults.[30]

Clindamycin is utilized primarily for anaerobic infections and is known to cross the placenta.[74] There are no scientific studies regarding its use during pregnancy. There are few indications for its use in pregnant women, and its effect on the developing coniceptus is virtually unknown.

Chloramphenicol readily crosses the placenta and there is no evidence to suggest that it is a human teratogen,[30] but there may be adverse neonatal effects with high doses of the drug administered to the mother near the time of delivery. It is rarely utilized in current clinical practice because of the risk of maternal aplastic anemia and 'gray baby syndrome' in the newborn.

Sulfonamides and trimethoprim are often used in combination, primarily to treat urinary tract infections. Sulfonamides readily cross the placenta and seem to compete with bilirubin for binding in the fetus. Thus, if utilized during late gestation, it is possible that sulfonamide therapy may result in neonatal hyperbilirubinemia.[67] Trimethoprim is a weak folate antagonist but has not been found to be associated with an increased risk of congenital anomalies.[78]

Nitrofurantoin is another agent used to treat urinary tract infections during pregnancy. This drug was not associated with an increased risk of congenital anomalies in one study, and there are no reports of adverse effects following its use during pregnancy.[30,79]

The fluoroquinolones (ciprofloxacin and norfloxacin) are relatively new antibiotics frequently used to treat urinary tract infections in non-pregnant patients. There are no studies of congenital anomalies in infants whose mothers took these drugs during pregnancy. However, the manufacturer reported that these agents were associated with irreversible arthropathy in dogs whose mothers were given the drug during pregnancy.[30] Accordingly, these agents should not be prescribed for use during pregnancy.

The antituberculosis drugs, rifampin, isoniazid and ethambutol, have not been reported to be associated with an increase in congenital anomalies in one study that summarized case reports.[80] No controlled epidemiological studies are published. As with numerous therapeutic agents, the benefits may outweigh any theoretical risk, depending upon the stage of disease under consideration for treatment (see also Chapter 24).

Antifungals

Antifungals frequently prescribed for use during pregnancy include clotrimazole, miconazole and nystatin. The frequency of malformations among infants whose mothers used these drugs during pregnancy was not increased in two studies.[63,81] There have not been published any epidemiological studies of congenital anomalies in infants whose mothers took butaconazole during pregnancy.

Amphotericin B is used to treat systemic mycotic infections.[30] It was not associated with an increased frequency of malformations among infants who used the drug during pregnancy in one study.[82] Griseofulvin is utilized for the treatment of mycotic infections of the skin and nails. There are no large scientific studies in humans, although there are reports of increased central nervous system and skeletal anomalies in animal studies.[30] Additionally, there is a case report that implicated griseofulvin with conjoined twinning,[83] but a Hungarian study did not confirm this anecdotal finding.[2]

Antiviral agents

Frequently prescribed antiviral agents include zidovudine, acyclovir, amantadine, ramantadine, ribavirin, idoxurdine and vidarabine. Zidovudine (AZT) is currently the primary agent for the treatment of human immunodeficiency virus (HIV) infection. No epidemiological studies regarding its use in pregnant women and congenital anomalies in their progeny are published. However, it is certainly reasonable to conclude that the benefits of its use to treat the fatal disease caused by this virus, AIDS, far outweigh any theoretical risks. Importantly, it is theoretically possible that this drug may prevent congenital HIV infection, since it significantly lowers HIV titer, though this awaits confirmation in practice.[30]

Acyclovir is the drug of choice to treat herpes viruses such as primary genital herpes and varicella. According to the registry maintained by its manufacturer, acyclovir does not appear to be associated with an increase in the frequency of infant malformations or adverse fetal effects in more than 200 pregnancies exposed during the first trimester.[84] Although it is not currently recommended for routine use in pregnant women with genital herpes, it may prove useful in overwhelming varicella infections. Importantly, topical acyclovir resulted in negligible systemic concentrations of the drug, and seems to pose minimal risks of adverse effects in the developing embryo fetus. Given the results of the manufacturer's collaboration with the surveillance by the Centers for Disease Control (CDC) of acyclovir use during pregnancy, inadvertent use of this agent is not grounds for 'therapeutic termination of pregnancy'.

Amantadine was not found to be associated with an increase in the frequency of congenital anomalies in one anecdotal uncontrolled report of 20 patients who used the drug during early pregnancy.[30] There are no reports regarding amantadine use during pregnancy.

Ribavirin is currently administered as an aerosol in the treatment of respiratory syncytial viral infections in infants, although systemic regimens are available. Although there are no human studies, this agent has been found to be teratogenic in animals.[30] It seems to be a potent teratogen because a high frequency of a constellation of malformations was present among the offspring of mothers given the drug at human therapeutic and several times the human therapeutic dose during embryogenesis. Therefore, it should not be prescribed for use during pregnancy, and inadvertent exposure is an indication for prenatal diagnosis.

There are no scientific studies regarding the use of either idoxuridine or vidarabine during human pregnancy.

Antiparasitic agents

One of the more commonly prescribed antiparasitic agents is metronidazole, a nitroimidazole. Metronidazole is prescribed primarily as an antiparasitic agent for the treatment of vaginal trichomoniasis. This was not teratogenic in over 60 offspring of women who took it during the first trimester.[30,85] Although this drug is reported to be carcinogenic in rats and mutagenic in certain bacteria, it is apparently safe for use during pregnancy.

Lindane is a topical agent indicated for treatment of *Pediculosis pubis* and scabies. Although there are no adequate epidemiological studies of its use during human pregnancy, this agent was not teratogenic in experiments involving pregnant animals.[30] The potential for central nervous system toxicity, if this agent is absorbed systemically, motivates some clinicians to recommend a combination of pyrethrins and piperonyl butoxide as an alternative for the initial treatment of *Pediculosis pubis* during pregnancy. However, topical application of lindane over limited surface areas seems to result in minimal systemic absorption.

Chloroquine is a first-line antimalarial agent. It is also used for chemoprophylaxis against malaria in pregnant women who travel to areas where malaria is endemic. Prophylactic low-dose weekly use of chloroquine for malaria appears to pose no teratogenic risk.[30] Quinine is the prototype antimalarial agent and is used to treat chloroquine-resistant *P. falciparum* malaria. There are no large scientific studies regarding the use of this agent during pregnancy. One report suggested an increased risk of congenital anomalies with use of quinine in large doses as an abortifacient, but there is little information regarding its use in therapeutic doses.[86] Anecdotal data suggest that large doses may cause otolithic agenesis, eye defects and vestibular abnormalities among infants born to mothers who took therapeutic, but large doses of this drug during the first trimester.[2]

Pyramethamine is an antiparasitic agent that is effective in the treatment of malaria and toxoplasmosis. In one report of 64 offspring of women who took this drug in early pregnancy, the frequency of malformations was not increased.[87] Two other agents, spiramycin and sulfadiazine, are also used to treat toxoplasmosis, but no scientific studies of the effect of either of these agents on the developing embryo have been published.

Mebendazole is an antiparasitic agent used primarily to treat helminthic infections, including enterobiasis (pinworms), trichuriasis (whipworm), ascariasis (roundworm) and necatoriasis (hookworm). Mebendazole has been reported to be teratogenic in laboratory animals when given during gestation at many times the human therapeutic dose, but it is impossible to extrapolate these results to possible effects in human pregnancy.[30] Thiabendazole is another antihelminth agent. No studies of this agent's use during pregnancy have been published involving animals or humans. Pyrantel pamoate is another antihelminthic agent used to treat ascariasis and enterobiasis. Although the drug was not found to be teratogenic in animal studies, no human studies have been published, and the relevance, if any, of animal teratology studies to the human situation is unknown.

Cardiovascular Diseases (see also Chapters 18, 20 and 33)

Cardiovascular diseases occur among approximately 3–5% of pregnant women. Most gravidas require these medications because they are given to treat life-threatening disorders. With few exceptions, most cardiovascular medications may be given during pregnancy with minimal risks to the unborn child. Cardiovascular agents with potentially adverse embryo or fetal effects are summarized in **Table 10**.[40,88–105]

Anticoagulants

The fetal warfarin syndrome, caused by the use of coumadin anticoagulants during gestation, was discussed previously (see **Table 6**).

Calcium heparin is a very large molecule and does not cross the placenta.[30] Its use during pregnancy is not associated with an increased frequency of congenital anomalies. However, osteoporosis and thrombocytopenia may occur among adults, including pregnant women, with protracted use of this drug. Calcium supplements should be considered in patients who require long-term heparin treatment. Information about the low molecular weight heparins and their use in pregnancy is awaited. Until such information is available, no guidelines on the use of these drugs can be given.

Antihypertensives

Methyldopa (Aldomet®) is used to treat chronic hypertension in pregnant women. There are no large scientific studies of the use of this agent during early pregnancy. Hydralazine (Apresoline®) is another antihypertensive agent used commonly to treat pregnant women, but most clinical experience with this drug has been with it use during the latter half of pregnancy to treat acute severe pregnancy-induced hypertension (PIH). It is usually not prescribed for chronic hypertension. This agent has been used to treat thousands of pregnant women outside the period of embryogenesis without apparent adverse effects on the unborn child.

Numerous beta-adrenergic blocking agents are commercially available for the treatment of hypertension. Beta-blockers commonly prescribed for use during pregnancy include propranolol (Inderal®), labetolol (Normadyne®, Trandate®), metoprolol (Lopressor®), nadolol (Corgard®) and atenolol (Tenormin®). There are no large epidemiological studies of congenital anomalies among infants who took any of these agents during pregnancy. While some investigators have reported an increased frequency of fetal growth deficiency among infants born to women who took some of these agents (e.g. atenalol) chronically during pregnancy,[90,106] others have reported no such association.[107] It is difficult to ascribe the effect to the drug because the disease state being treated, PIH, also causes fetal growth deficiency. Other possible adverse fetal or neonatal effects include transient bradycardia, respiratory depression and hypoglycemia.[90–93]

Clonidine (Catapress®) is an alpha-adrenergic blocker antihypertensive. Although it has been utilized in pregnant women without apparent adverse fetal effects,[108,109] there are no epidemiological studies of the frequency of congenital anomalies among infants whose mothers used the drug during the first trimester.

Table 10
Cardiovascular agents with possible adverse fetal effects[a]

Agent	Potential adverse effect(s)
Warfarin[b]	Fetal warfarin syndrome
Verapamil and other calcium channel blockers	Decrease in uterine blood flow, myocardial depression and fetal cardiac arrest
Propranolol and other beta-adrenergic blockers	Intrauterine growth retardation; bradycardia, respiratory depression and hypoglycemia
Diazoxide	Alopecia and abnormalities of body hair; hyperglycemia
Sodium nitroprusside	Cyanide toxicity in animals
Furosemide	Decrease in uterine blood flow; hyperbilirubinemia
Spironolactone	Feminization of male animal genitalia
Thiazide diuretics	Neonatal thrombocytopenia
Angiotensin-converting enzyme (ACE) inhibitors	Anuria and renal malformations; hypocalvaria

[a]Some of these adverse effects have been described only in animals and are theorized to possibly occur in humans (see text).
[b]See **Table 6**.

Diazoxide (Hyperstat®), a thiazide, has been utilized as both an antihypertensive and a tocolytic agent. No epidemiological studies of congenital anomalies among infants born to women who took this drug during the first trimester are available. Use of this thiazide during pregnancy has been reported to be associated with body hair abnormalities (alopecia) and with transient neonatal hypoglycemia.[94,95]

Sodium nitroprusside (Nipride®, Nitropress®) is a potent antihypertensive utilized for the treatment of serious, life-threatening hypertension. This agent has been reproted to cause cyanide toxicity in fetal animals.[96] However, the human fetus does not appear to be at risk for this complication when therapeutic doses of this agent are utilized.[110] None the less, it seems prudent to avoid the use of this drug during pregnancy unless it is needed to treat a life-threatening condition in which other medications have not proved effective.

Captopril (Capiten®) and enalapril (Vasotex®) are angiotensin-converting enzyme (ACE) inhibitors. There are no large human reproduction studies of the use of these agents during pregnancy. There are case series and case reports that seem to associate neonatal anuria, congenital hypocalvaria, renal anomalies and nephrotoxicity with ACE inhibitor use during the first trimester.[101–105] Thus, ACE inhibitors are contraindicated for use during pregnancy, and are suspected human teratogens.

Diuretics

Diuretics are often used to treat chronic hypertension and pulmonary edema associated with heart disease in pregnant women. There are several major types of diuretics, including thiazides, loop diuretics, potassium-sparing diuretics and carbonic anhydrase inhibitors.

Thiazide diuretics are the ones most commonly prescribed to pregnant women. Neither chlorothiazide (Diuril®) or hydrochlorothiazide (Hydrodiuril®, Esidrix®, Hydro-Chlor®) has been reported to be associated with an increased frequency of congenital anomalies among exposed infants.[30] However, thiazides are known to pose a risk of transient neonatal thrombocytopenia.[100] In the latter half of pregnancy, this group of drugs may also be associated with lowered maternal blood volume and decreased uteroplacental perfusion.

Use of loop diuretics such as ethacrinic acid (Edecrin®) and furosemide (Lasix®, Myrosemide®) during pregnancy is apparently not associated with an increased risk of congenital anomalies. It is important to note that loop diuretics may interfere with the 'normal' pregnancy-associated expansion of the blood volume, and may decrease placental perfusion. Also, maternal use of furosemide seems to displace bilirubin from albumin, possibly causing neonatal hyperbilirubinemia.[98]

Spironolactone (Aldactone®) is a potassium-sparing diuretic which acts as a competitive inhibitor of aldosterone. Although its effect on the developing human conceptus has not been studied, it has mild antiandrogenic effects and was associated with feminization of male rat fetuses born to mothers given large doses of this drug during gestation.[99] For this reason, spironolactone is not recommended for use during pregnancy.

Acetazolamide is a carbonic anhydrase inhibitor diuretic. This agent has not been studied for possible teratogenic effects in the human.[30] However, it has been reported to be associated with characteristic and replicable pattern limb abnormalities in animals born to mothers given the drug during pregnancy.[111] Hence, the use of this diuretic should be avoided during pregnancy.

Anti-arrhythmics

The cardiac glycoside, digoxin, is utilized as both an anti-arrhythmic agent to treat atrial fibrillation, flutter and for congestive heart failure. It has also been successfully used to treat fetal cardiac arrhythmias since it readily crosses the placenta.[112,113]

Quinidine is another agent commonly used to treat arrhythmias (supraventricular tachycardia and ventricular arrhythmia). There are no large epidemiological studies available regarding the use of quinidine during pregnancy. Some clinicians believe it is probably relatively safe for use during pregnancy.[114]

A variety of local anesthetics are employed as anti-arrhythmic agents. The best known are probably lidocaine (Xylocaine®), also known as lignocaine in the UK, and procainamide (Pronestyl®, Rhthmin®, Promine®). Related agents include encainide (Enkaid®), flecainide (Tambocar®), tocainide (Tanocard®) and mexiletine (Mexitil®). All of them probably cross the placenta to some appreciable degree. Although there are no large epidemiological studies for most of these agents, Heinonen and colleagues reported on 293 offspring of mothers who were given lidocaine acutely in early pregnancy and the frequency of malformations among exposed infants was not increased above unexposed controls.[62] However, there is a difference between acute use of the drug as an anesthetic, and chronic administration in the treatment of cardiac arrhythmias. There are no studies reported in which possible association of malformations with any of the other similar agents during pregnancy was analyzed. However, the benefit of their use clearly outweighs any theoretical risk in most instances, because cardiac arrhythmias may be life-threatening.

Disopyramide (Norpace®) is an anti-arrhythmic similar in action to quinidine used to treat supraventricular and ventricular arrhythmias.[115] Although there are no studies of its use during human pregnancy and the frequency of congenital anomalies, it was reported to cause uterine contractions.[113,114,116] Therefore, alternative treatment regimens with similar action should be employed.

Bretylium (Bretylol®) is used to treat ventricular tachycardia and fibrillation. There are no adequate studies of the potential risk of congenital anomalies following its use in human pregnancy. However, if this agent is clearly indicated for treatment of life-threatening arrhythmias where other agents have failed, it should be used, regardless of the stage of pregnancy.

Amiodarone (Cardarone®) is another agent used to treat life-threatening arrhythmias, ventricular tachycardia and fibrillation. There is one case report of a possible association of fetal cretinism with the use of this agent,[117] but there are no published epidemiological studies of the use of amiodarone during pregnancy. As with bretylium, it would seem reasonable to utilize this agent during pregnancy if indicated for treatment of serious ventricular arrhythmias where other agents have not proved effective.

Anti-anginal agents

The organic nitrites are the most commonly utilized anti-anginal agents and include nitroglycerin, amyl nitrate, erythrityl tetranitrate (Cardilate®), isorbide dinitrate (Isodil®, Sorbitrate®) and pentaerythritol tetranitrate (Pentritol®, Peritrate®). Nitroglycerin has also been utilized acutely to 'blunt' the hypertensive effect of intubation during general anesthesia in the hypertensive or cardiac patient who is pregnant. No epidemiological studies of the use of organic nitrites during human pregnancy are published but it is prudent to utilize them in life-threatening conditions.

A variety of calcium channel blocking agents have anti-anginal effects. Some of these agents are also used to treat supraventricular tachycardia and hypertension. Verapamil (Clan®, Isoptin®) is probably the best known of this group of drugs. Although it has been utilized in many pregnant women without apparent adverse fetal effects, verapamil has been reported to be associated with a decrease in uterine blood flow in animals[88] and may cause cardiac depression or even arrest in neonates whose mothers received it peripartum for supraventricular tachycardia associated with heart failure.[89] Other calcium antagonists could theoretically be associated with similar adverse effects. Thus, these agents as a group are indicated for use during pregnancy only when life-threatening conditions exist and other therapeutic agents have not proven effective.

Dipyramidole (Persantine®) is a selective coronary vasodilator and inhibits platelet aggregation. It is utilized as an adjunct in the prevention of thromboembolism, myocardial infarction and transient ischemic events. No epidemiological studies of the use of this agent in human pregnancy have been published. According to the manufacturer, dipyramidole was not teratogenic in animal studies, but the relevance of this to the human situation is unknown.

Asthma (see also Chapter 24)

Asthma is encountered among 1–3% of gravidas.[30] The two major classes of medications utilized for the treatment of asthma – bronchodilators and immunosuppressants – seem to be relatively safe for use during pregnancy.

Bronchodilators

Theophylline salts are the most commonly utilized bronchodilators for treating both the pregnant and nonpregnant patient with asthma. Aminophylline is the parenteral form and there are numerous oral forms of theophylline. This agent has been utilized extensively in pregnant women without apparent adverse effects.

Epinephrine is another bronchodilator which is reserved for acute asthmatic attacks and is usually given in a dose of 0.3–0.5 ml s.c. in a 1:1000 dilution.[30] An increased frequency of malformations was reported in the Collaborative Perinatal Project,[62] but it is unclear as to whether the effects may have been related to the maternal illness for which it was given or to the drug itself. In the authors' opinion, it seems very unlikely that epinephrine is a human teratogen. However, its use should be reserved for treatment of acute asthma attacks, and not be given chronically. Another agent, terbutaline (Brethaire®, Brethine®, Bricanyl®), has significant bronchodilating activity. There are no reports of an association of the use of this agent during early pregnancy and congenital anomalies. In one study of protracted maternal use of terbutaline during pregnancy but outside the first trimester, no adverse effects were noted among the offspring.[118]

Albuterol (Proventil®, Ventolin®) and metaproterenol (Alupert®, Metaprel®) are beta-adrenergic blocking bronchodilators that are self-administered inhalation aerosols. Systemic concentrations resulting from inhalation should be small. There are no epidemiological studies of their use during pregnancy. They are commonly used to treat asthma among pregnant patients. However, potential adverse effects on the developing conceptus have yet to be published.

Immunosuppressants

Cromolyn sodium (Nasalcrom®, Rynacrom®) is an agent that inhibits mast-cell histamine release and is given via nasal insufflation. It has little benefit during an acute asthmatic attack and is utilized primarily for prophylaxis in chronic asthma.[30] No studies of its use during human pregnancy are published, but according to the manufacturer it was not teratogenic in several animal species given several times the usual human dose during gestation.

A number of glucocorticoids are used to treat pregnant women with asthma. The most commonly used agents are beclamethasone, betamethasone, cortisone and prednisone. Beclamethasone (Vanceril®, Beclovent®) is utilized primarily as an inhalational aerosol or nasally. Dexamethasone (Decadron®, Respihaler®, Turbinaire®) is also utilized in this fashion. In some pregnant asthmatics, it is occasionally necessary to use large doses of parenterally administered corticosteroids to treat a life-threatening acute asthmatic attack. Among some gravidas, it may also be necessary to prescribe chronic steroid maintenance therapy as prophylaxis to prevent exacerbation of respiratory symptoms.

Acute asthmatic attack may be life-threatening. Therefore, these agents should be utilized because any potential risks are clearly outweighed by the potential benefit of saving the mother's life.

Psychotropics

Psychiatric illness occurs among approximately 1–2% of gravidas. Treatment of most psychiatric disorders should continue during pregnancy for the benefit of the patient. Abrupt discontinuation of psychotropic therapy may have adverse effects, including suicide gestures.

Sedatives, hypnotics and tranquilizers

Numerous sedatives, hypnotics and tranquilizers are commercially available and belong to several different pharmacological categories. The most commonly encountered agents include phenobarbital, secobarbital, butalbital, diazepam, chlordiazepoxide, chloral hydrate and meprobamate.

Phenobarbital has often been implicated in causing congenital anomalies when used with other anticonvulsant agents.[30] As previously discussed under anticonvulsants, it is unclear whether it is the anticonvulsant medication *per se*, the seizure disorder or a combination of both that is associated with an increased risk of congenital anomalies. Phenobarbital is often prescribed to pregnant women as a sedative and there is no evidence that it is teratogenic when utilized for this indication. Importantly, among more than 1000 offspring exposed to this agent during the first trimester, the frequency of malformations was not increased.[62] The major risk of the barbiturates as a group is maternal drug dependence and possible transient neonatal withdrawal.

Secobarbital (Seconal®, Novosecobarb®) is a short-acting barbiturate given primarily as a sleep medication. There is no scientific evidence that this agent is teratogenic in humans and it seems to be relatively safe for use during pregnancy, especially if utilized over a short period of time.

Butalbital is a short-acting barbiturate that is found in combination with a variety of other medications such as aspirin (Fiorinol®, Axotal®, etc.), acetaminophen (Fioricet®, Rogesic®, etc.) and codeine. Among more than 100 pregnant women exposed to this agent during the first trimester, the frequency of malformations among exposed offspring was not statistically increased compared with controls.[62]

Diazepam (Valium®, Vazepam®, Meval®) and chlordiazepoxide (Librium®, Librax®, Lipoxide®, Medilium®, Novopoxide®) are benzodiazepines commonly used as minor tranquilizers and sedatives. Diazepam is also utilized as an amnestic and as an anticonvulsant. Initially, diazepam was thought to be associated with an increased risk of facial clefts,[119–121] but this has not been confirmed by several other large studies,[122–124] some of which were a reanalysis of previously reported data. In addition, there have been reports of an association of maternal diazepam and cardiovascular anomalies in the offspring exposed *in utero*,[125,126] but these findings were not confirmed in subsequent studies.[127,128] Cumulatively, available information does not support the notion that diazepam is a human teratogen. However, it is important to remember that this agent may cause transient hypotonia, hypothermia and respiratory depression in the neonate when used chronically by the mother close to delivery. This entity has been termed the floppy infant syndrome, but is not life-threatening when managed medically.

Chlordiazepoxide has been reported to be associated with an increase in congenital anomalies in one study,[129] although such an association was not confirmed in a much larger study that included over 250 offspring whose mothers used the drug during early pregnancy.[62] Similarly, the frequency of malformations was not increased in several other studies of infants whose mothers used the drug in the first trimester.[130–132]

Meprobamate (Equanil®, Miltown®, etc.) is a minor tranquilizer and muscle relaxant. Whether or not it is associated with congenital anomalies is controversial. Some investigators have reported an association of congenital anomalies with the use of this drug during gestation,[63,129] whereas others have failed to demonstrate such an effect.[62] In one study of over 350 offspring, meprobamate exposure during pregnancy was not associated with an increased frequency of malformations.[62] It would seem reasonable to avoid this agent during all stages of pregnancy because of the inconsistencies in the available data.

Chloral hydrate is a minor sedative sometimes prescribed as sleep medication. Although there are no large, well-controlled studies regarding its use during pregnancy, the frequency of congenital anomalies in the offspring of 71 pregnant women who took chloral hydrate during early pregnancy was not increased compared with controls.[62]

Antidepressants

The antidepressants are generally divided into tricyclic and non-tricyclic agents. The former category was the most commonly used until fluoxetine (Prozac®) was introduced recently. These agents are summarized in **Table 11**.

Although limb-reduction defects have been reported with one of the tricyclic agents, amitriptyline,[133,134] during early pregnancy, such an association was not confirmed by other studies.[62,135,136] Such a risk seems very unlikely. There is no information regarding the safety of other tricyclic antidepressants during pregnancy, but several of them are metabolites of amitriptyline. Hence, their risks may be assumed to be similar to those of amitriptyline (i.e. none to negligible).

Tranylcypromine (Parnate®), isocarboxazid (Marplan®) and phenelzine (Nardil®) are monoamine oxidase inhibitors which are utilized as antidepressants. There is no information regarding the safety of these agents for use during pregnancy.

Fluoxetine (Prozac®) is currently one of the most frequently prescribed antidepressants, and has received significant public attention recently because of the possible, yet unproven, potentiation of suicidal tendencies in adults who take this medication. There are few scientific data to date regarding this alleged adverse effect. In one report by the manufacturer of 73 offspring born to mothers who took this antidepressant

Table 11
Commonly utilized tricyclic antidepressants

Imipramine (Tofranil®, Janimine®, Tipramine®)
Amitriptyline (Amitril®, Elavil®, Endep®,
　Emitrip®, Enovil®)
Desipramine (Norpramin®, Pertofrane®)
Doxepin (Adapin®, Sinequan®)
Nortriptyline (Aventyl®, Pamelor®)
Protriptyline (Vivactil®)
Amoxapine (Asendin®)
Clomipramine (Anafranil®)

during pregnancy,[137] the frequency of congenital anomalies was not increased above the expected or background of congenital anomalies in humans (i.e. 2 of 73 or 2.7%).

Antipsychotics

Phenothiazines comprise the largest pharmacologic class of antipsychotics. Several phenothiazines are also prescribed as antiemetics during pregnancy (chlorpromazine, perphenazine, prochlorperazine and triflupromazine).

Chlorpromazine (Thorazine®) has been prescribed for several decades as an antipsychotic to pregnant women. This agent was not associated with an increased risk of congenital anomalies in two studies of over 4000 patients who took the drug during the first trimester for various indications.[62,138] Two of the most common side-effects in the adult are hypotension and extrapyramidal tract symptoms. Similar transient effects were observed among neonates exposed to the drug during late gestation.

Among more than 800 infants born to women who took prochlorperazine (Compazine®) during early pregnancy reported in the Collaborative Perinatal Project,[62] the frequency of congenital anomalies was not increased above background risk. Likewise, no increase in the frequency of malformations was found in the offspring of 63 pregnant women who took perphenazine (Trilafon®) during the first trimester compared with controls.[62]

There are epidemiological studies regarding the safety of the use of thioridazine (Mellaril®) or trifuoperazine (Stelazine®) during pregnancy. Thioridazine has been utilized in many pregnant women without apparent adverse fetal effects such as malformations. However, the lack of such reports is not a reassurance of safety of the drug's use during pregnancy.

Other antipsychotic drugs include haloperidol (Haldol®, Decanoate®), thiothixene (Navane®), loxapine (Loxitane®, Daxolin®), clozapine (Clozaril®), molindone (Moban®, Lidone®) and chlorprothixene (Taractan®). There is no relevant scientific information regarding the safety of using these agents during pregnancy.

Lithium

Lithium is a first line treatment regimen for affective mental disease. Of all the psychotropic agents, it is the one for which the greatest concern exists with regard to teratogenic effects in the human.[32] Use of this agent during early pregnancy has been reported to be associated with an increased risk of cardiovascular anomalies, particularly Ebstein's anomaly.[139] In one report from a registry of over 200 offspring whose mothers used this agent during embryogenesis, 8% of infants exposed during early gestation had cardiovascular anomalies.[139] In addition, hydramnios and fetal diabetes insipidas have been reported as a possible secondary complication of the use of lithium during the second and third trimesters. If possible, exposure to this agent should be avoided during pregnancy during the first trimester. Patients using this drug in the second and third trimesters should be routinely evaluated for increased amniotic fluid volume.

Analgesics

Analgesics are the medications most commonly needed by and prescribed to pregnant women. With few exceptions, most analgesics can be administered to pregnant women with relative safety.

Non-steroidal anti-inflammatory agents (NSAIDs)

A variety of NSAIDs are commercially available for use as analgesics. Frequently prescribed NSAID agents are summarized in **Table 12**. Indomethacin is a commonly used NSAID, which also acts as a tocolytic in perceived premature labor.[140] The frequency of congenital anomalies was not increased in one study of 50 patients who received this agent during the first trimester of pregnancy.[61]

The major concern with NSAIDs as a group is the possible association with premature closure of the ductus arteriosus when given during the latter half of pregnancy. Although there have been reports of fetal and newborn premature ductal arteriosus closure and subsequent pulmonary hypertension due to the maternal use of these agents,[141–143] other investigators have not confirmed such an association.[140,144] These agents have also been reported to be associated with decreased amniotic fluid volume.[145] NSAIDs are generally not recommended for use in pregnant women after 34 weeks gestational age because of the theoreti-

Table 12
Some commonly utilized non-steroidal anti-inflammatory agents

Indomethacin (Indocin®)
Ibuprofen (Advil®, Motrin®, etc.)
Fenaprofen (Fenoproten®, Nalfon®)
Meclofenamate (Meclamen®)
Naproxen (Naprosyn®, Anaprox®)
Tolmentin (Tolectin®)
Diflunisal (Dolobid®)

cal risk for these adverse effects. These agents are probably relatively safe if utilized prior to this gestational age, especially if given acutely.

Salicylates and acetaminophen

Salicylates and acetaminophen are non-narcotic analgesics commonly used by pregnant women. In one report of over 1500 pregnant women, about half utilized aspirin and 41% utilized acetaminophen.[146]

Aspirin is also an NSAID, and has been available for more than a century. Although there are reports of an association with malformations in humans,[147] such an association was not confirmed in other studies.[148,149] Similar to other NSAIDs, aspirin is a prostaglandin synthetase inhibitor and has been reported to be associated with premature closure of the ductus arteriosus and pulmonary hypertension in the newborn[143,150] and oligohydramnios.[150] Large doses of aspirin may also be associated with hemorrhagic disorders in both mother and fetus due to lowered platelet activity. In summary, it is the authors' opinion that the usual adult low-dose aspirin for non-analgesic indications is probably of little risk to the fetus. However, this drug should be avoided for analgesia during pregnancy because safer medications are available (i.e. acetaminophen).

Acetaminophen is the preferred analgesic for use in pregnancy. In one report of over 300 offspring born to mothers who took this agent during pregnancy, the frequency of malformations was not increased.[61] Similar results were reported among more than 200 offspring included in the Collaborative Perinatal Project database.[62] However, this analgesic may result in fetal liver toxicity when used in excessive amounts such as attempted suicide late in pregnancy.[151] Acetaminophen is apparently not associated with premature ductal closure or oligohydramnios.

Narcotic analgesics

A number of narcotic analgesic agents are available. The more frequently prescribed drugs in this class include codeine, meperidine (Demerol®), morphine, pentazocine (Talwin®), butophanol (Stadol®), hydrocodone (Vicodin®, etc.), nalbuphine (Nubain®), hydromorphone (Dilaudid®) and propoxyphene (Darvon®, etc.).

Meperidine and morphine, as with all the opioid-narcotic agents, may cause a transient withdrawal syndrome in the newborn when taken on a chronic basis during pregnancy. However, none of these analgesics was associated with an increased frequency of malformations in the offspring following early pregnancy use by the mother.[62] Acute large doses near the time of delivery, especially morphine, may be associated with newborn respiratory depression, though the effects can be reversed with naloxone. Codeine was not found to be teratogenic in one study of over 500 patients with first trimester exposure.[62] Similarly, the frequency of malformations was not increased compared with unexposed controls among more than 700 newborns whose mothers used propoxyphene during early pregnancy.[62,63] There have been isolated case reports of malformations associated with its use that were probably serendipitous and not causal.[30] Similarly, pentazocine use during early pregnancy was not associated with an increased frequency of congenital anomalies.[30]

There have been no epidemiological studies of congenital anomalies in infants whose mothers used butorphanol, hydrocodone or hydromorphone during pregnancy, although all are potentially associated with neonatal withdrawal if abused or utilized for a protracted period of time during late pregnancy.

Thyroid medications
(see also Chapter 21)

Hypothyroidism infrequently presents during pregnancy, but it is not unusual to encounter pregnant women who were on thyroid replacement therapy before the gravid state was recognized. Hyperthyroidism, on the other hand, is relatively uncommon during pregnancy.[30]

Thyroid replacement

Thyroxine utilized as replacement apparently does not cross the placenta to any great extent, if at all, and was not associated with any known adverse fetal effects in several studies.[30]

Antithyroid medications

Agents utilized to treat hyperthyroidism include propylthiouracil (Propyl-Thyracil®) or PTU, methimazole (Tapazole®), potassium iodide and propranolol. Propranolol use during pregnancy was discussed previously in the section on antihypertensives.

The remaining three antithyroid agents readily cross the placenta. PTU may result in fetal hypothyroidism and goiter formation, although clinically significant effects are relatively uncommon with usual therapeutic regimens of the drug. There is no firm scientific evidence that PTU is related to an increased risk of malformations, although the data are largely inconclusive. Methimazole was reportedly associated with scalp defects in the offspring of mothers receiving this

agent,[152,153] but other investigators have not confirmed such an association.[154,155]

Potassium iodide and sodium iodide block the release of thyroid hormone. The protracted use of these agents may result in fetal hypothyroidism and goiter formation. It is highly unlikely that iodide medication will result in such adverse effects when given acutely for the treatment of thyroid crisis ('thyroid storm') using intravenous sodium iodide or for preoperative prophylaxis prior to thyroid surgery (oral potassium iodide).

Antineoplastics (see also Chapters 23 and 32)

Malignancy occurs among approximately 0.1% of pregnant women.[156] Breast carcinoma, melanoma and Hodgkins' lymphoma are the most common malignancies encountered in pregnant women.[156–159]

Chemotherapeutic agents can be grouped into alkylating, antimetabolite, plant alkaloid, antibiotic and miscellaneous agents. Antineoplastics are often reported to be associated with fetal growth deficiency and congenital anomalies, and causality seems plausible since the majority of chemotherapeutic agents interfere with cell growth and division in some fashion.

From the available information, it seems unlikely that the majority of chemotherapeutic agents are associated with significant fetal risk when utilized after the first trimester except for growth deficiency. Importantly, the potential life-saving benefits of such therapy generally outweigh the risk to the unborn child. Some conditions, such as acute leukemia, mandate chemotherapy as soon as the diagnosis is confirmed, even during the first trimester of pregnancy.

Alkylating agents

Commonly prescribed alkylating agents include busulfan (Myleran®), cyclophosphamide (Cytoxan®), chlorambacil (Leukeran®), melphalan (Alkeran®), trimethylene thiophosphoramide (Thiotepa®) and carmustine (BCNU®). There are no epidemiological studies of congenital anomalies or fetal effects among infants whose mothers used melphalan, trimethylene thiophosphoramide or carmustine during pregnancy.

Busulfan and cyclophosphamide were discussed at the beginning of this chapter and are associated with an increased risk of congenital anomalies. In one report of 44 infants whose mothers received one of several alkylating agent during pregnancy, 6 (14%) had a major congenital anomaly, an apparent increased risk of malformation.[160]

Antimetabolites

Commonly employed antimetabolites in the treatment of neoplasia include methotrexate (Folex®, Mexate®), mercaptopurine (Purinethol®), thioguanine, cytarabine (Cytosan®) and fluorouracil (Efudex®, Fluoroplex®). Methotrexate was discussed in the first section of this chapter and is associated with an increased risk of congenital anomalies, similar to those related to another folate antagonist, aminopterin.[18–22] Although there are only case reports of the possible association of congenital anomalies with the use of other antimetabolites during early pregnancy, common mechanisms of action suggest that the case reports represent a causal relationship. In a review by Doll and associates,[160] 15 (19%) of 77 offspring exposed to antimetabolites *in utero* had major congenital anomalies. Of these 15 malformed infants, 13 were exposed to folate antagonists. Obviously, these agents should be avoided during pregnancy if possible, especially in the first trimester.

Plant alkaloids

The two major plant alkaloids are vinblastine (Velban®, Velsan®) and vinicristine (Oncovin®, Vincasar®, Vincrex®). Although there are reports of a possible association of malformations with first trimester exposure to these agents,[161] there are also reports of normal infants born to women who used this class of drugs during pregnancy.[162] In the review by Doll and associates,[163] only 1 (7%) of 14 infants exposed to this group of agents had a major congenital anomaly. It is important to note that these agents are used to treat life-threatening malignancies (i.e. acute leukemia) and should be given when indicated, even during the first trimester.

Antibiotics

Antineoplastic antibiotics include daunorubicin (Cerabidine®), doxorubicin (Adiramycin®), bleomycin (Blexoxane®) and dactinomycin (Cosmegen®). No epidemiological studies of the use of any of these agents during pregnancy have been published. However, it may be necessary to prescribe anthracycline antibiotics (daunorubicin and doxorubicin) during the first trimester to treat acute leukemia because potentially life-saving therapy should not be withheld.

Miscellaneous antineoplastics

Agents in this category include *cis*-platin (Platinol®), procarbazine and hydroxyurea (Hydrea®). No controlled studies in human pregnancies involving any of these agents have been published. These agents should be avoided during the first trimester if possible, but should not be withheld when clearly needed to treat life-threatening conditions.

Immunosuppressant Agents (see also Chapters 25, 27 and 28)

Immunosuppressants are given primarily for the therapy of autoimmune diseases (rheumatoid arthritis, systemic lupus) and for maintenance therapy in patients with organ transplants. The most frequently prescribed agents in this group include glucocorticoids, azathioprine (Imuran®) and cyclosporine (Sandimmune®). Glucocorticoids are discussed in the section on anti-asthma medications.

Azathioprine

A derivative of 6-mercaptopurine, azathioprine is given as an adjunct in suppression of cell-mediated immunity. There are no controlled studies regarding the use of this agent in pregnant women. However, in two case series involving a total of 154 pregnant women who took azathioprine and prednisone throughout pregnancy,[164,165] malformations were reported among 11 (7.1%) infants. It is impossible to differentiate the effects of monotherapy with this agent from the effects of taking multiple immunosuppressant medications, and from the disease process itself. However, since this medication is usually used to prevent organ rejection in renal transplant patients, it should not be withheld from the pregnant patient because this is a life-threatening condition.

Cyclosporine

Cyclosporine is utilized primarily in the treatment and prevention of allograft rejection. There are no epidemiological studies regarding the maternal or infant effects when used during pregnancy. It should be used when indicated even in pregnant women because it is usually prescribed for potentially life-threatening conditions.

MANAGEMENT OF THE PREGNANT PATIENT WITH MEDICATION EXPOSURE

Management of the pregnant patient who has been exposed to medication during pregnancy, especially during the critical period of organogenesis, presents a unique challenge to the clinician. Several important questions arise. Is the medication or substance a known teratogen? Are there potential adverse fetal or neonatal effects? Additionally, what is the risk to the mother with use of the medication or if it is withheld? Are there other factors that may be as or more important than the medication itself such as the disease being treated? What are the available sources of information regarding the use of the medications during pregnancy? How should the patient be counseled?

Etiology of Malformations

The etiology of the vast majority (65–70%) of congenital malformations is unknown. However, it has been estimated that 20–25% are secondary to genetic abnormalities, 3–5% to intrauterine infection and 4% may be associated with maternal diseases such as diabetes mellitus, phenylkeonuria or epilepsy.[166] Although less than 1% seem to be due to prescribed medications, many patients, their physicians and lawyers often suspect that a particular medication caused a malformation in the exposed infant.[167]

Evaluating the Risk

As stated earlier, few medications are known human teratogens. However, for the vast majority of medications – perhaps more than 60% – available information is inadequate to assess risks for congenital anomalies or adverse fetal effects.

Sources of information

Where can one go to find such information? There are several major textbooks written on the subject which can serve as a starting point. In addition, there are computerized databases such as TERIS or TOXLINE[2] that provide useful information to assess potential risks (Table 13). Ultimately, referral to a tertiary care center with a clinical teratologist on the maternal–fetal medicine staff is the preferred scenario. In the UK, the Regional Drug Information Centres fulfil the same function.

Federal Drug Administration fetal risk categories

In 1979, the FDA established a risk category system for medications intended to classify drugs with regard to potential adverse effects on the fetus.[1,2,168] Category A medications are those which are felt to be relatively safe for use during pregnancy; category B agents are those in which there are no known risks but controlled human studies are lacking; and category C agents are those for which there is little or no information available and most new drugs are placed in this category. Agents for which there is a definite risk but such medications may be deemed necessary for use during pregnancy based upon a risk–benefit assessment (i.e. anticonvulsants) are category D. Category X are drugs whose use during pregnancy is a definite risk for which potential risks outweigh benefits and are thus contraindicated. Few medications are listed as category A drugs (an example would be some of the prenatal vitamins). An example of a category B medication is ampicillin (i.e. no controlled human studies). An example of a category X drug is isotretinoin (Accutane®). Unfortunately, the FDA pregnancy categories most often do not reflect current scientific information regarding the potential teratogenic risk of a specific medication[169] and these categories should not be con-

Table 13
Sources of information on drugs and medications during pregnancy[a]

Databases
TERIS: Department of Pediatrics, University of Washington, Seattle, WA (Tel.: 206/543-4365)
TOXLINE: National Library of Medicine, Bethesda, MD (Tel.: 800/638-8480)

Textbooks
Berkowitz RL, Coustan DR, Mochizuki TK (1982) *Handbook for Prescribing During Pregnancy*, 2nd edn. Boston, MA: Little, Brown and Co.
Briggs GG, Freeman RK, Yaffe SJ (1990) *Drugs in Pregnancy and Lactation*. Baltimore, MD: Williams and Wilkins.
Gilstrap LC, Little BB (1992) *Drugs and Pregnancy*. New York: Elsevier.
Niebyl JR (1988) *Drug Use in Pregnancy*. Philadelphia, PA: Lea and Febiger.
Rubin PC (1987) *Prescribing in Pregnancy*. London: British Medical Journal.
Schardein JL (1985) *Chemically Induced Birth Defects*. New York: Marcel Dekker.
Shepard TH (1989) *Catalog of Teratogenic Agents*, 6th edn. Baltimore, MD: Johns Hopkins University Press.

[a]Adapted in part from Little *et al.*[2]

sidered primary directives for prescribing medication during pregnancy.

Counseling the Patient

Prior to counseling the patient and her family, it is important to take a detailed medical history and do a physical examination. The history should include gestational dating criteria such as last menstrual period, and detailed information regarding the drug exposure (class, dose, route of administration, timing, disease being treated) should be obtained. Information on other concomitant medication use, ionizing radiation exposure, a detailed family history and genetic pedigree, and a review of any other medical conditions that may affect the risk of malformations should also be taken.[2]

Establishing gestational age and the timing of exposure is of paramount importance and ultrasound evaluation should be carried out if gestational age is questionable or not confirmed by physical examination. If it can be determined that a medication was taken prior to conception or after the period of organogenesis, counseling for most medications may consist of simply reassuring the patient. It is necessary to differentiate between embryonic age and menstrual age because menstrual age includes 2 weeks when the patient was not actually pregnant. It is also important to ascertain whether or not a particular agent is absorbed from the maternal gastrointestinal tract, resulting in significant serum levels. Some agents such as stool softeners have a local effect with little or no systemic absorption. Such agents would be expected to result in none or minimal embryo or fetal exposure.

Similarly, it is necessary to determine whether or not significant amounts of a specific agent have access to the embryo fetal compartment (i.e. cross the placenta). For example, heparin crosses the placenta poorly, if at all, and has no known direct adverse fetal effects. Most drugs (99%), however, do cross the placenta.

For known teratogens (such as isotretinoin) with reasonably established risk figures, the patient can be counseled that there are definite risks for exposure during a given gestational time period. Therapeutic options in such a case should include pregnancy termination. All counseling should begin with an explanation of the 'background' risk of congenital anomalies in the general population (i.e. 3–5%).

There are few scientific studies regarding the use of more than half of the currently available agents during pregnancy. Although a small risk cannot be ruled out, the risk of spontaneous anomalies (i.e. 3–5%) is probably greater than any risk that can be estimated from available information for most medications that have been studied.[167] For certain medical illnesses (e.g. diabetes, seizure disorders), the risk of the condition itself,

---

MEDICATION IN PREGNANCY
Summary of Management Options

Inadvertent exposure to medication

- Obtain accurate details of exposure, especially gestational age

- Check for confounding family or medical history

- Get up-to-date information regarding published risks of the specific drug in humans

- Emphasize 'background' risks in counseling

- Be clear about what is known, but do not assume absence of data means no risk

Consideration of commencing/continuing medication

- Medication should be used only if expected benefits (usually to mother) are greater than risks (usually to fetus)

- Try and avoid first trimester

- Use drugs which have been extensively used in pregnancy rather than new/untried drugs

- Use minimum dose for desired effect

- Absence of data does not imply safety

---

especially if untreated, generally far outweighs any known or theoretical risk of medications to the conceptus. Such medications should not be withheld from a woman because she is pregnant. For obvious reasons, preconceptional counseling is preferred in such patients, but the opportunity for this is rare.

Finally, when medications are being considered for the woman who is already pregnant, it is important to consider whether the initiation of therapy can be delayed until after the completion of the first trimester (i.e. embryogenesis). If it is unsafe to do so, the medication should be initiated when needed, even if risk is involved. An exaggerated example is chemotherapy for acute leukemia which should be begun as soon as the diagnosis is confirmed, regardless of gestational age.

REFERENCES

1   Gilstrap LC, Cunningham FG (1987) Drugs and medications during pregnancy. In *Williams' Obstetrics*, 17th edn. Supplement 13. Norwalk, CT: Appleton & Lange.

2   Little BB, Gilstrap LC, Cunningham FG (1991) Medication use during pregnancy. Part. 1. Concepts of human teratology. *Williams' Obstetrics*, 18th edn. Supplement 10. Norwalk, CT: Appleton & Lange.

3   Nelson MM, Forfar JO (1971) Association between drugs administered during pregnancy and congenital abnormalities of the fetus. *British Medical Journal* 1:523–527.

4   Centers for Disease Control (1987) Use of supplements containing high-dose vitamin A – New York. *Morbidity and Mortality Weekly Report* 336:80.

5   Rubin PC (1986) Prescribing in pregnancy. *British Medical Journal* 293:1415–1417.

6   Centers for Disease Control (1984) Isotretinoin – A new recognized human teratogen. *Morbidity and Mortality Weekly Report* 33:171–173.

7   Medical Letter (1983) Update on isotretinoin (Accutane) for acne. *Medical Letter: Drugs and Therapy* 25:105–106.

8   Ross FW, Wilk AL, Kelsey FO (1986) Teratogen update: Vitamin A congeners. *Teratology* 33:355–364.

9   Rosa FW (1983) Teratogenicity of isotretinoin. *Lancet* 2:513.

10 Strauss JS, Cunningham WJ, Leyden JJ, Pochi PE, Shalita AR (1988) Isotretinoin and teratogenicity. *Journal of the American Academy of Dermatology* 19:353–354.

11 Thomson EJ, Cordero JF (1989) The new teratogens: Accutane and other vitamin-A analogs. *American Journal of Maternal–Child Nursing* 14:244–248.

12 Lammer EJ, Chen DT, Hoar RM, Agnish ND, Benke PJ, Braun JT (1985) Retinoic acid embryopathy. *New England Journal of Medicine* 313:837–841.

13 Lammer EJ, Hayes AM, Schunior A, Holmes LB (1987) Risk for major malformation among human fetuses exposed to isotretinoin (13-*cis*-retinoic acid). *Teratology* 35:68.

14 Dai WS, Hsu MA, Itri LM (1989) Safety of pregnancy after discontinuation of isotretinoin. *Archives of Dermatology* 125:362–365.

15 Happle R, Traupe H, Bounameaux Y, Fisch T (1984) Teratogenicity of etretinate in humans. *Deutsche Medizinische Wochenschrift* 109:1476–1480.

16 DiGiovanna JJ, Zech LA, Ruddel ME, Gantt, G, McClean SW, Gross EG, Peck GL (1984) Etretinate: Persistent serum levels of a potent teratogen. *Clinical Research* 32:579.

17 Lammer EJ (1988) Embryopathy in infant conceived one year after termination of maternal etretinate. *Lancet* 2:1080–1081.

18 Char F (1979) Denoument and discussion: Aminopterin embryopathy syndrome. *American Journal of Diseases of Children* 133:1189–1190.

19 Reich EW, Cox RP, Becker MH, Genieser NB, McCarthy JG, Converse JM (1977) Recognition in adult patients of malformations induced by folic-acid antagonists. *Birth Defects* 14:139–160.

20 Warkany J (1978) Aminopterin and methotrexate: Folic acid deficiency. *Teratology* 17:353–358.

21 Milunsky A, Graef JW, Gaynor MF (1968) Methotrexate-induced congenital malformations. *Journal of Pediatrics* 72:790–795.

22 Diamond I, Anderson, MM, McCreadie SR (1960) Transplacental transmission of busulfan (Myleran) in a mother with leukemia: Production of fetal malformations and cytomegaly. *Pediatrics* 25:85–90.

23 Kirshon B, Wasserstrum N, Willis R, Herman GE, McCabe ERB (1988) Teratogenic effects of first trimester cyclophosphamide therapy. *Obstetrics and Gynecology* 72:462–464.

24 Murray CL, Reichert JA, Anderson J, Twiggs LB (1984) Multimodal cancer therapy for breast cancer in first trimester of pregnancy. *Journal of the American Medical Association* 252:2607–2608.

25 McClure HM, Wilk AL, Horigan EA, Pratt RM (1979) Induction of craniofacial malformations in rhesus monkeys (*Macaca mulatta*) with cyclophosphamide. *Cleft Palate Journal* 16:248–256.

26 Doll DC, Ringenberg S, Yarbro JW (1988) Management of cancer during pregnancy. *Archives of Internal Medicine* 148:2058–2064.

27 Hanson JW, Smith DW (1975) The fetal hydantoin syndrome. *Journal of Pediatrics* 87:285–290.

28 Kelly TE (1984) Teratogenicity of anticonvulsant drugs. I. Review of the literature. *American Journal of Medical Genetics* 19:413–434.

29 Zackai EH, Mellman WJ, Neiderer B, Hanson JW (1975) The fetal trimethadione syndrome. *Journal of Pediatrics* 87:280–284.

30 Gilstrap LC, Little BB, Cunningham FG (1991) Medication use during pregnancy. Part 2. Special considerations. *Williams' Obstetrics*, 18th edn. Supplement 11. Norwalk, CT: Appleton & Lange.

31 Niebyl JR, Blake DA, Freeman JM, Luft RD (1979) Carbamazepine levels in pregnancy and lactation. *Obstetrics and Gynecology* 53:139–140.

32 Jones KL, Lacro RV, Johnson KA, Adams J (1989) Pattern of malformations in the children of women treated with carbamazepine during pregnancy. *New England Journal of Medicine* 320:1661–1666.

33 Buehler BA, Delimont D, van Waes M, Finnell RH (1990) Prenatal prediction of risk of the fetal hydantoin syndrome. *New England Journal of Medicine* 322:1567–1572.

34 Strickler SM, Dansky LV, Miller MA, Seni MH, Andermann E, Spielberg SP (1985) Genetic predisposition to phenytoin-induced birth defects. *Lancet* 2:746–749.

35 Centers for Disease Control (1983) Valproate: A new cause of birth defects – Report from Italy and follow-

up from France. *Morbidity and Mortality Weekly Report* **32**:348.

36 Robert E, Robert JM, Lapras C (1983) Is valproic acid teratogenic? *Revue Neurologique* **139**:445–447.

37 Dalens B, Raynaud EJ, Gaulme J (1980) Teratogenicity of valproic acid. *Journal of Pediatrics* **97**:332–333.

38 DiLiberti JH, Farndon PA, Dennis NR, Curry CJR (1984) The fetal valproate syndrome. *American Journal of Medical Genetics* **19**:473–481.

39 Jager-Roman E, Deichl A, Jakob S, Hartmann AM, Koch S, Raging D, Steldinger R, Nau H, Helge H (1986) Fetal growth, major malformations, and minor anomalies in infants born to women receiving valproic acid. *Journal of Pediatrics* **108**:997–1004.

40 Hall JG, Pauli RM, Wilson K (1980) Maternal and fetal sequelae of anticoagulation during pregnancy. *American Journal of Medicine* **68**:122–140.

41 Stevenson RE, Burton M, Ferlauto GJ, Taylor HA (1980) Hazards of oral anticoagulants during pregnancy. *Journal of the American Medical Association* **243**:1549–1551.

42 Schardein JL (1985) *Chemically Induced Birth Defects*. New York: Marcel Dekker.

43 Kingsbury AC (1985) Danazol and fetal masculinization: A warning. *Medical Journal of Australia* **143**:410–411.

44 Quagliarello J, Greco MA (1985) Danazol and urogenital sinus formation in pregnancy. *Fertility and Sterility* **43**:939–942.

45 Rosa FW (1984) Virilization of the female fetus with maternal danazol exposure. *American Journal of Obstetrics and Gynecology* **149**:99–100.

46 Shaw RW, Farquhar JW (1984) Female pseudohermaphroditism associated with danazol exposure in utero: Case report. *British Journal of Obstetrics and Gynaecology* **91**:386–389.

47 Herbst AL, Hubby MM, Azizi F, Makii MM (1981) Reproductive and gynecologic surgical experience in diethylstilbestrol-exposed daughters. *American Journal of Obstetrics and Gynecology* **141**:1019–1028.

48 Herbst AL, Poskanzer DC, Robboy SJ, Friedlander L, Scully RE (1975) Prenatal exposure to stilbestrol: A prospective comparison of exposed female offspring with unexposed controls. *New England Journal of Medicine* **292**:334–339.

49 Bibbo M (1979) Transplacental effects of diethylstilbestrol. In Grundman E (ed.) *Perinatal Pathology* pp. 191–211. New York: Springer-Verlag.

50 Robboy SJ, Szyfelbein WM, Goellner JR, Kaufman RH, Taft PD, Richard RM, Gaffey TA, Prat J, Virata R, Hatab PA, McGorray SP, Noller KL, Townsend D, Labarthe D, Barnes AB (1981) Dysplasia and cytologic findings in 4589 young women enrolled in Diethylstilbestrol-Adenosis (DESAD) project. *American Journal of Obstetrics and Gynecology* **140**:579–586.

51 Robboy SJ, Noller KL, O'Brien P, Kaufman RH, Townsend D, Barnes AB, Gunderson J, Lawrence WD, Berstrahl E, McGarray S (1984) Increased incidence of cervical and vaginal dysplasia in 3980 diethylstilbestrol-exposed young women: Experience of the National Collaborative Diethylstilbestrol Adenosis Project. *Journal of the American Medical Association* **252**:2979–2983.

52 Stillman RJ (1982) *In utero* exposure to diethylstilbestrol: Adverse effects on the reproductive tract performance in male and female offspring. *American Journal of Obstetrics and Gynecology* **142**:905–921.

53 Kaufman RH, Noller K, Adam E, Irwin J, Gray M, Jeffries JA, Hilton J (1984) Upper genital tract abnormalities and pregnancy outcome in diethylstilbestrol-exposed progeny. *American Journal of Obstetrics and Gynecology* **148**:973–984.

54 Barnes AB, Colton T, Gunderson J, Noller KL, Tilley BC, Strama T, Townsend DE, Hatab P, O'Brien PC (1980) Fertility and outcome of pregnancy in women exposed *in utero* to diethylstilbestrol. *New England Journal of Medicine* **302**:609–613.

55 Herbst AL (1981) Clear cell adenocarcinoma and the current status of DES-exposed females. *Cancer* **48**:484–488.

56 Herbst AL, Hubby MM, Blough RR, Azizi F (1980) A comparison of pregnancy experience in DES-exposed and DES-unexposed daughters. *Journal of Reproductive Medicine* **24**:62–69.

57 Sandberg EC, Riffle NL, Higdon JV, Getman CE (1981) Pregnancy outcome in women exposed to diethylstilbestrol *in utero*. *American Journal of Obstetrics and Gynecology* **140**:194–205.

58 Rendle-Short TJ (1962) Tetracycline in teeth and bone. *Lancet* **1**:1188.

59 Kutscher AH, Zegarelli EV, Tovell HM, Hocberg B, Hauptman J (1966) Discoloration of deciduous teeth induced by administration of tetracycline antepartum. *American Journal of Obstetrics and Gynecology* **96**:291–292.

60 Genot MG, Golan HP, Porter PJ, Kass EH (1970) Effect of administration of tetracycline in pregnancy on the primary definition of the offspring. *Journal of Oral Medicine* **25**:75–79.

61 Aselton P, Jick H, Milunsky A, Hunter JR, Stergachis A (1985) First-trimester drug use and congenital disorders. *Obstetrics and Gynecology* **65**:451–455.

62 Heinonen OP, Slone D, Shapiro S (1977) *Birth Defects and Drugs in Pregnancy*. Littleton, MA: Publishing Sciences Group.

63 Jick H, Holmes LB, Hunter JR, Madsen S, Stergachis A (1981) First trimester drug use and congenital disorders. *Journal of the American Medical Association* **246**:343–346.

64 Weinstein MR (1980) Lithium treatment of women during pregnancy and in the post-delivery period. In Johnson FN (ed.) *Handbook of Lithium Therapy*, p. 421. Baltimore, MD: University Park Press.

65 Harpey J-P, Jaudon M-C, Clavel J-P, Galli A, Darbois Y (1983) *Cutis laxa* and low serum zinc after antenatal exposure to penicillamine. *Lancet* **2**:858.

66 Rosa FW (1986) Teratogen update: Penicillamine. *Teratology* **33**:127–131.

67 Landers DV, Green JR, Sweet RL (1983) Antibiotic use during pregnancy and the postpartum period. *Clinics in Obstetrics and Gynecology* **26**:391–406.

68 Gilstrap LC, Bawdon RE, Burris JS (1988) Antibiotic concentration in maternal blood, cord blood and placental membranes in chorioamnionitis. *Obstetrics and Gynecology* **72**:124–125.

69 Maberry M, Trimmer K, Bawdon R, Sobhi S, Dax J, Gilstrap LC (1990) *Antibiotic Concentrations in Maternal Blood, Cord Blood and Placental Membranes in Women with Chorioamnionitis.* St. Louis, MO: Society for Gynecologic Investigation, March, A-543.

70 Martens MG (1989) Cephalosporins. *Obstetrics and Gynecology Clinics of North America* **16**:291–304.

71 Fenton LG, Light LJ (1976) Congenital syphilis after maternal treatment with erythromycin. *Obstetrics and Gynecology* **47**:492–494.

72 Kline AH, Blattner RJ, Lunin M (1964) Transplacental effects of tetracyclines on teeth. *Journal of the American Medical Association* **188**:178–180.

73 Rendle-Short TJ (1962) Tetracycline and teeth and bone. *Lancet* **1**:1188.

74 Weinstein AJ, Gibbs RS, Gallasher M (1976) Placental transfer of clindamycin and gentamicin in term pregnancy. *Obstetrics and Gynecology* **124**:688–691.

75 Yoshioka H, Monma T, Matsuda S (1972) Placental transfer of gentamicin. *Journal of Pediatrics* **80**:121–123.

76 Conway N, Birt DN (1965) Streptomycin in pregnancy: Effect on the foetal ear. *British Medical Journal* **2**:260–263.

77 Donald PR, Sellars SL (1981) Streptomycin ototoxicity in the unborn child. *South African Medical Journal* **60**:316–318.

78 Brumfitt W, Pursell R (1973) Trimethoprim/ sulfamethoxazole in the treatment of bacteriuria in women. *Journal of Infectious Diseases* **128**:657–665.

79 Lenke RR, VanDorsten JP, Schifrin BS (1983) Pyelonephritis in pregnancy: A prospective randomized trial to prevent recurrent disease evaluating suppressive therapy with nitrofurantoin and close surveillance. *American Journal of Obstetrics and Gynecology* **146**:953–957.

80 Snyder DE Jr, Layde PM, Johnson MW, Lyle MA (1980) Treatment of tuberculosis during pregnancy. *American Review of Respiratory Diseases* **122**:65–79.

81 Rosa FW, Baum C, Shaw M (1987) Pregnancy outcomes after first trimester vaginitis drug therapy. *Obstetrics and Gynecology* **69**:751–755.

82 Ismail MA, Lerner SA (1982) Disseminated blastomycosis in a pregnant woman: Review of amphotericin B usage during pregnancy. *American Review of Respiratory Diseases* **126**:350–353.

83 Rosa FW, Hernandez C, Carlo WA (1987) Griseofulvin teratology, including two thorapagus conjoined twins. *Lancet* **1**:171.

84 Andrews EB, Yankaskas BC, Cordero JF, Schoeffler, K, Hampps S (1992) Acyclovir in pregnancy registry: Six years experience. *Obstetrics and Gynecology* **79**:7–13.

85 Hammill HA (1989) Metronidazole, clindamycin, and quinolones. *Obstetrics and Gynecology Clinics of North America* **16**:317–328.

86 Nishimura H, Tanimura T (1976) *Clinical Aspects of the Teratogenicity of Drugs.* Amsterdam: Excerpta Medica.

87 Hengst P (1972) Investigations of the teratogenicity of daraprim (pyrimethamine) in humans. *Zentralblatt für Gynakologie* **94**:551–555.

88 Murad SH, Tabsh KM, Shilyanski G, Kapur PA, Ma C, Lee C, Conklin KA (1985) Effects of verapamil on uter-ine blood flow and maternal cardiovascular function in the awake pregnant ewe. *Anesthesia and Analgesia* **64**:7–10.

89 Kleinman CS, Copel JA (1991) Electrophysiological principles and fetal antiarrhythmic therapy. *Ultrasound in Obstetrics and Gynceology* **1**:286–297.

90 Pruyn SC, Phelan JP, Buchanan GC (1979) Long-term propranolol therapy in pregnancy: Maternal and fetal outcome. *American Journal of Obstetrics and Gynecology* **135**:485–489.

91 Tunstall ME (1969) The effect of propranolol on the onset of breathing at birth. *British Journal of Anaesthesia* **41**:792.

92 Habib A, McCarthy JS (1977) Effects on the neonate of propranolol administered during pregnancy. *Journal of Pediatrics* **91**:808–811.

93 Rubin PC (1981) Current concepts: Beta-blockers in pregnancy. *New England Journal of Medicine* **305**:1323–1326.

94 Milner RD (1972) Neonatal hypoglycaemia – a critical reappraisal. *Archives of Diseases of Childhood* **255**:679–682.

95 Milsap RL, Auld PAM (1980) Neonatal hyperglycemia following maternal diazoxide administration. *Journal of the American Medical Association* **243**:144–145.

96 Lewis PE, Cefalo RC, Naulty JS, Rodkey FL (1977) Placental transfer and fetal toxicity of sodium nitroprusside. *Gynecologic Investigations* **8**:46.

97 Gant NF (1986) Lupus erythematosus, the lupus anticoagulant, and the anticardiolipin antibody. *Williams' Obstetrics*, Supplement 6. Norwalk, CT: Appleton & Lange.

98 Turmen T, Thom P, Louridas AT, LeMourvan P, Aranda JV (1982) Protein binding and bilirubin displacing properties of bumetanide and furosemide. *Journal of Clinical Pharmacology* **22**:551–556.

99 Hecker A, Hasan SH, Neumann F (1980) Disturbances in sexual differentiation of rat foetuses following spironolactone treatment. *Acta Endocrinologica* **95**:540–545.

100 Rodriguez SU, Leikin SL, Hiller MC (1964) Neonatal thrombocytopenia associated with antepartum administration of thiazide drugs. *New England Journal of Medicine* **270**:881–884.

101 Boutroy MJ, Vert P, Hurault de Ligny BH, Miton A (1984) Captopril administration in pregnancy impairs fetal angiotensin converting enzyme activity and neonatal adaptation. *Lancet* **2**:935–936.

102 Boutroy MJ (1989) Fetal effects of maternally administered clonidine and angiotensin-converting enzyme inhibitors. *Developmental Pharmacology and Therapeutics* **13**:199–204.

103 Rothberg AD, Lorenz R (1984) Can captopril cause fetal and neonatal renal failure? *Pediatric Pharmacology* **4**:189–192.

104 Barr M, Cohen MM (1991) ACE inhibitor fetopathy and hypocalvaria: The kidney–skull connection. *Teratology* **44**:485–495.

105 Rosa F, Bosco L (1991) Infant renal failure with maternal ACE inhibitors. *American Journal of Obstetrics and Gynecology* **164**:273.

106 Sibai BM, Gonzales AR, Mabie WD, Moretti M

(1987) A comparison of labetalol plus hospitalization versus hospitalization alone in the management of preeclampsia remote from term. *Obstetrics and Gynecology* **70**:323–327.

107 Rotmensch HH, Elkayam U, Frishman W (1983) Antiarrhythmic drug therapy during pregnancy. *Annals of Internal Medicine* **98**:487–497.

108 Horvath JS, Phippard A, Korda A, Henderson-Smart DS, Child A, Tiller DJ (1985) Clonidine hydrochloride – a safe and effective antihypertensive agent in pregnancy. *Obstetrics and Gynecology* **66**:634–638.

109 Raftos J, Bauer GE, Lewis RG, Stokes GS, Mitchell AS, Young AA, Maclachlan I (1973) Clonidine in the treatment of severe hypertension. *Medical Journal of Australia* **1**:786–793.

110 Shoemaker CT, Meyers M (1984) Sodium nitroprusside for control of severe hypertensive disease of pregnancy: A case report and discussion of potential toxicity. *American Journal of Obstetrics and Gynecology* **149**:171–173.

111 Hirsch KS, Wilson JG, Scott WJ, O'Flaherty EJ (1983) Acetazolamide teratology and its association with carbonic anhydrase inhibition in the mouse. *Teratogenesis Carcinogenesis and Mutagenesis* **3**:133–144.

112 Lingman G, Ohrlander S, Ohlin P (1980) Intrauterine digoxin treatment of fetal paroxysmal tachycardia: Case report. *British Journal of Obstetrics and Gynaecology* **87**:340–342.

113 Harrigan JT, Kangos JJ, Sikka A, Spisso KR, Natarajan N, Rosenfeld D, Leiman S, Korn D (1981) Successful treatment of fetal congestive failure secondary to tachycardia. *New England Journal of Medicine* **304**:1527–1529.

114 Rotmensch HH, Rotmensch S, Elkayam U (1987) Management of cardiac arrhythmias during pregnancy: Current concepts. *Drugs* **33**:623–633.

115 Rotmensch HH, Elkayam U, Frishman W (1983) Antiarrhythmic drug therapy during pregnancy. *Annals of Internal Medicine* **98**:487–497.

116 Leonard RF, Braun TE, Levy AM (1978) Initiation of uterine contractions by disopyramide during pregnancy. *New England Journal of Medicine* **299**:84–85.

117 Pinsky WW, Rayburn WF, Evans MI (1991) Pharmacologic therapy for fetal arrhythmias. *Clinics in Obstetrics and Gynecology* **34**:304–309.

118 Wallace RL, Caldwell D, Ansbacher R, Otterson W (1978) Inhibition of premature labor by terbutaline. *Obstetrics and Gynecology* **51**:387–392.

119 Aarskog D (1975) Association between maternal intake of diazepam and oral clefts. *Lancet* **2**:921.

120 Safra MJ, Oakley BP Jr (1975) An association of cleft lip with or without cleft palate and prenatal exposure to diazepam. *Lancet* **2**:478–480.

121 Saxen I, Saxen L (1975) Association between maternal intake of diazepam and oral clefts. *Lancet* **2**:498.

122 Czeizel A (1988) Lack of evidence of teratogenicity of benzodiazepine drugs in Hungary. *Reproductive Toxicology* **1**:183–188.

123 Rosenberg L, Mitchell A, Parsells JL, Pashayan H, Louik C, Shapiro S (1983) Lack of correlation of oral clefts to diazepam use during pregnancy. *New England Journal of Medicine* **309**:1982–1985.

124 Shiono PH, Mills JL (1984) Oral clefts and diazepam use during pregnancy. *New England Journal of Medicine* **311**:919–920.

125 Rothman KJ, Fyler DC, Goldblatt A, Kreidberg MB (1979) Exogenous hormones and other drug exposures of children with congenital heart disease. *American Journal of Epidemiology* **109**:433–439.

126 Bracken MB, Holford TR (1981) Exposure to prescribed drugs in pregnancy and association with congenital malformations. *Obstetrics and Gynecology* **58**:336–344.

127 Bracken MB (1986) Drug use in pregnancy and congenital heart disease in offspring. *New England Journal of Medicine* **314**:1120.

128 Zierler S, Rothman KJ (1985) Congenital heart disease in relation to maternal use of bendectin and other drugs in early pregnancy. *New England Journal of Medicine* **313**:347–352.

129 Milkovich L, van den Berg BJ (1976) An evaluation of the teratogenicity of certain antinauseant drugs. *American Journal of Obstetrics and Gynecology* **125**:244–248.

130 Crombie DL, Pinsent RJ, Fleming DM, Rumeau-Rouquette C, Goujard J, Huel G (1975) Fetal effects of tranquilizers in pregnancy. *New England Journal of Medicine* **293**:198–199.

131 Kullander S, Kallen B (1976) A prospective study of drugs and pregnancy. *Acta Obstetrica et Gynecologica Scandinavica* **55**:25–33.

132 Hartz SC, Heinonen OP, Shapiro S, Siskind V, Slone D (1975) Antenatal exposure to meprobamate and chlordiazepoxide in relation to malformations, mental development and childhood. *New England Journal of Medicine* **292**:726–728.

133 McBride WG (1972) Limb deformities associated with iminodibenzyl hydrochloride. *Medical Journal of Australia* **1**:492.

134 Morrow AW (1972) Imipramine and congenital abnormalities. *New Zealand Medical Journal* **75**:228–229.

135 Crombie DL, Pinsent R, Fleming D (1972) Imipramine in pregnancy. *British Medical Journal* **1**:745.

136 Scanlon FJ (1969) Use of antidepressant drugs during the first trimester. *Medical Journal of Australia* **2**:1077.

137 Goldstein DJ (1990) Outcome of fluoxetine exposed pregnancies. *American Journal of Human Genetics* **47**:A136 (suppl.).

138 Farkas G, Farkas G Jr (1971) Teratogenic effects of hyperemesis gravidarum and of the customary drugs used in its therapy. *Zentralblatt für Gynakologie* **10**:325–330.

139 Weinstein MR (1980) Lithium treatment of women during pregnancy and in the post-delivery period. In Johnson FN (ed.) *Handbook of Lithium Therapy* pp. 421–429. Baltimore, MD: University Park Press.

140 Niebyl J, Blake D, White R, Kumor KM, Dubin NH, Robinson JC, Egnor PG (1980) The inhibition of premature labor with indomethacin. *American Journal of Obstetrics and Gynecology* **136**:1014–1019.

141 Manchester D, Margolis HS, Sheldon RE (1976) Possible association between maternal indomethacin therapy and primary pulmonary hypertension in the new-

born. *American Journal of Obstetrics and Gynecology* **126**:467–469.

142 Csaba I, Sulyok FE, Ertl T (1978) Relationship of maternal treatment with indomethacin to persistence of fetal circulation syndrome. *Journal of Pediatrics* **92**:484.

143 Levin DL, Fixler DE, Morriss FC, Tyson J (1978) Morphologic analysis of the pulmonary vascular bed in infants exposed *in utero* to prostaglandin synthetase inhibitors. *Journal of Pediatrics* **92**:478–483.

144 Dudley DKL, Hardie MJ (1985) Fetal and neonatal effects of indomethacin used as a tocolytic agent. *American Journal of Obstetrics and Gynecology* **151**:181–184.

145 Hickok DE, Hollenbach KA, Reilley SD, Nyberg DA (1989) The association between decreased amniotic fluid volume and treatment with nonsteroidal anti-inflammatory agents for preterm labor. *American Journal of Obstetrics and Gynecology* **160**:1525–1531.

146 Streissguth AP, Treder RP, Barr HM, Shepard TH, Bleyer WA, Sampson PD, Martin DC (1987) Aspirin and acetaminophen use by pregnant women and subsequent child IQ and attention decrements. *Teratology* **35**:211–219.

147 Agapitos M, Georgiou-Theodoropoulou M, Koutselinis A, Papacharalampus N (1986) Cyclopia and maternal ingestion of salicylates. *Pediatric Pathology* **6**:309–310.

148 Slone D, Siskind V, Heinonen OP, Monson RR, Kaufman DW, Shapiro S (1976) Aspirin and congenital malformations. *Lancet* **1**:1373–1375.

149 Turner G, Collins E (1975) Fetal effects of regular salicylate ingestion in pregnancy. *Lancet* **2**:338–339.

150 Sibai B, Amon EA (1988) How safe is aspirin use during pregnancy? *Contemporary Obstetrics and Gynecology* **32**:73–79.

151 Haibach H, Akhter JE, Muscato MS, Cary PL, Hoffmann MF (1984) Acetaminophen overdose with fetal demise. *American Journal of Clinical Pathology* **82**:240–246.

152 Milham S, Elledge W (1972) Maternal methimazole and congenital defects in children (Letter). *Teratology* **5**:125.

153 Mujtaba Q, Burrow GN (1975) Treatment of hyperthyroidism in pregnancy with propylthiouracil and methimazole. *Obstetrics and Gynecology* **46**:282–286.

154 Momotani N, Ito K, Hamada N, Ban Y, Nishikawa Y, Mimura T (1984) Maternal hyperthyroidism and congenital malformations in the offspring. *Clinical Endocrinology* **20**:695–700.

155 Van Dijke CP, Heydendael RJ, De Kleine MJ (1987) Methimazole, carbimazole, and congenital skin defects. *Annals of Internal Medicine* **106**:60–61.

156 Donegan WL (1983) Cancer and pregnancy. *A Cancer Journal for Clinicians* **33**:194–197.

157 Donegan WL (1986) The influence of pregnancy on the management of cancer. *The Cancer Bulletin* **38**:278–284.

158 Parente JT, Amsel M, Lerner R, Chinea F (1988) Breast cancer associated with pregnancy. *Obstetrics and Gynecology* **71**:861–864.

159 Yazigi R, Cunningham FG (1990) Cancer and pregnancy. *Williams' Obstetrics*, Supplement 4. Norwalk, CT: Appleton & Lange.

160 Doll DC, Ringenberg S, Yarbro JW (1988) Management of cancer during pregnancy. *Archives of Internal Medicine* **148**:2058–2064.

161 Metz SA, Day TG, Pursell SH (1989) Adjuvant chemotherapy in a pregnant patient with endodermal sinus tumor of the ovary. *Gynecologic Oncology* **32**:371–374.

162 Caliguri MA, Mayer RJ (1989) Pregnancy and leukemia. *Seminars in Oncology* **16**:388–396.

163 Witter FR, Niebyl JR (1986) Inhibition of arachidonic acid metabolism in the perinatal period: Pharmacology, clinical application, and potential adverse effects. *Seminars in Perinatology* **20**:316–333.

164 Penn I, Makowski EL, Harris P (1980) Parenthood following renal transplantation. *Kidney International* **18**:221–233.

165 Registration Committee of the European Dialysis and Transplant Association (1980) Successful pregnancies in women treated by dialysis and kidney transplantation. *British Journal of Obstetrics and Gynaecology* **87**:839–845.

166 Beckman DA, Brent RL (1984) Mechanism of teratogenesis. *Annual Review of Pharmacology and Toxicology* **24**:483–500.

167 Brent RL (1982) Drugs and pregnancy: Are the insert warnings too dire? *Contemporary Obstetrics and Gynecology* **20**:42–49.

168 Federal Drug Administration (1979) Pregnancy labeling. *FDA Drug Bulletin* **9**(4):23–24.

169 Friedman JM, Little BB, Brent RL, Cordero JF, Hanson JW, Shepard TH (1990) Potential human teratogenicity of frequently prescribed drugs. *Obstetrics and Gynecology* **75**:594–599.

18

Hypertensive Disorders of Pregnancy

TRACY COWLES, ABDELAZIZ SALEH, DAVID B. COTTON

INTRODUCTION

Hypertension associated with pregnancy is a relatively frequent occurrence, affecting 5–7% of all pregnancies. On a superficial basis, hypertension is easily diagnosed (e.g. by serial blood pressure measurements). However, the underlying pathophysiology of this heterogeneous complex of diseases has alluded our understanding in many respects, making this still one of the major reasons for maternal mortality in the world today. Complicating the issue is the fact that across continental boundaries, even basic definitions differ, thereby further confusing our understanding of this complication of pregnancy.

Definitions and Classification

The following definitions are consistent with those adopted by the American College of Obstetricians and Gynecologists:[1]

Pre-eclampsia

The triad of pre-eclampsia consists of proteinuria, edema and hypertension. Other terms such as 'pregnancy-induced hypertension' and 'toxemia' have been used interchangeably, although this remains inconsistent in the literature.

Hypertension

This is defined as either:

- diastolic pressure of at least 90 mmHg, or

- systolic pressure of at least 140 mmHg, or

- a rise in diastolic pressure of at least 15 mmHg, or

- a rise in systolic pressure of 30 mmHg.

These blood pressure elevations should be documented on at least two occasions 6 h or more apart.

Proteinuria

This is defined as 300 mg/l or more of protein in a 24-h urine collection or a protein concentration of 1 g/l or more on at least two random urine samples collected 6 h or more apart.

Edema

This is defined as generalized accumulation of fluid, represented by greater than 1+ pitting edema after 12 h of bed rest or weight gain of 5 lb or more in 1 week.

In general, pre-eclampsia occurs after 20 weeks of gestation. Earlier onset pre-eclampsia may be the earliest presentation of a hydatidiform mole. Pre-eclampsia is classified as either mild or severe. The criteria for severe pre-eclampsia can be found in **Table 1**.

Eclampsia

This is defined as pre-eclampsia plus the development of generalized tonic–clonic seizures *not* caused by coincidental neurologic disorders.

Chronic hypertension

This definition refers to pre-existing elevations in blood pressure according to the following criteria:

- persistent hypertension of at least 140/90 mmHg or greater, before 20 weeks gestation in the absence of hydatidiform mole or extensive molar changes of the placenta, or

- persistent hypertension beyond 6 weeks postpartum.

Superimposed pre-eclampsia or eclampsia

This is defined as the development of pre-eclampsia or eclampsia in women with chronic hypertensive vascular or renal disease.

Transient hypertension

This is defined as the development of isolated hypertension later in pregnancy or early in the puerperium.

Table 1
Criteria for severe pre-eclampsia

Blood pressure ≥ 180 mmHg systolic or ≥ 110 mmHg diastolic, recorded on at least two occasions at least 6 h apart with patient at bed rest

Proteinuria ≥ 5 g in 24 h (3+ or 4+ on qualitative examination)

Oliguria (< 400 ml in 24 h)

Cerebral or visual disturbances

Epigastric pain

Pulmonary edema or cyanosis

Impaired liver function of unclear etiology

Thrombocytopenia

Alternative definitions and classifications adopted by FIGO (International Federation of Gynaecologists and Obstetricians) and the International Society for the Study of Hypertension in Pregnancy are given in Appendices 1–5.[98]

PRE-ECLAMPSIA/ECLAMPSIA

General

The conditions associated with an increased incidence of pre-eclampsia include:

- multiparity

- increased trophoblastic mass

- pregnancies with a different partner

- previous use of barrier contraceptives

- pregnancies after oocyte donation.

The conditions associated with a decreased incidence of pre-eclampsia include:

- previous miscarriage

- frequent exposure to seminal fluid

- pregnancies with a previous blood transfusion and leucocyte immunization

- pregnancies from consanguineous marriages[2]

The patheogenesis of pre-eclampsia remains incompletely understood despite years of research. Although hypertension is a hallmark feature of pre-eclampsia, it is neither the cause of pre-eclampsia nor the earliest symptom. Pre-eclampsia is clearly a complex clinical syndrome potentially involving all of the organ systems.

The physiologic changes of normal pregnancy allow the gravida to accommodate the growing products of conception. Maternal blood volume increases by approximately 50% over non-pregnant levels; cardiac output increases by 40–50% by midterm and remains elevated throughout pregnancy. Despite these increases, there is a concomitant decrease in blood pressure early in pregnancy, reaching a nadir in the mid-trimester and returning to prepregnant levels near term. This decrease in pressure is secondary to a reduction in peripheral vascular resistance.[3]

Patients with pre-eclampsia fail to demonstrate the physical changes characteristic of normal pregnancy. Blood pressure is, by definition, elevated. There is little if any increase in blood volume. Studies using invasive monitoring, prior to treatment, often reveal a hyperdynamic cardiac state in which output and systemic vascular resistance (SVR) are elevated.[4] Pre-eclamptics lose the resistance to the pressor effects of angiotensin II seen in normal pregnancy.[5]

The vasospastic process accounts for many of the pathologic findings of pre-eclampsia. Intense vasospasm may cause injury to the vascular endothelium, resulting in platelet adherence and fibrin deposition. These fibrin plugs cause red cell fragmentation, thrombocytopenia, decrease fibrinogen and increase fibrin-degradation products. Although the bleeding time may be prolonged secondary to these hematologic changes, overt disseminated intravascular coagulation (DIC) is uncommon in pre-eclamptics.

Other organ systems are affected by the pathologic changes of pre-eclampsia. The characteristic renal finding in pre-eclampsia has been designated 'glomerular capillary endotheliosis'.[6] Enlarged glomeruli show evidence of endothelial damage with partial or complete obstruction of the capillary lumen. This leads to the proteinuria characteristic of pre-eclampsia, a decrease in uric acid clearance and, in severe cases, a reduction in creatinine clearance and oliguria.

In the liver, subendothelial fibrin deposition, similar to that seen in the kidney, suggests endothelial damage. Hepatic manifestations may include elevated liver enzymes and hyperbilirubinemia. The underlying mechanism again appears to be vasospasm with fibrin deposition in the hepatic sinusoids.[7]

There has been no consensus regarding the pathophysiology of eclamptic seizures; vasospasm, ischemic hemorrhage and cerebral edema have all been proposed.[8] Clearly, hypertensive encephalopathy, alone, cannot account for the central nervous system (CNS) complications seen in some patients. Retinal hemorrhages, exudates and papilledema are the hallmarks of hypertensive encephalopathy, and are rarely seen in eclamptics. In addition, at least 20% of eclamptics will never demonstrate a systolic blood pressure ≥ 140 mmHg or a diastolic blood pressure ≥ 90 mmHg. Most likely, the etiology of eclampsia depends on an interplay between vasospasm, microinfarctions and edema, with vasospasm being an early and prominent feature.

The underlying etiology of the vasospasm and increased sensitivity to circulating pressors seen in pre-eclamptics has received a great deal of attention. It has been proposed that an imbalance in two of the vasoactive ecosanoids, prostacyclin (PGI_2) and thromboxane A_2(TXA_2), explains the vasospasm seen in pre-eclampsia.[9-16] PGI_2, synthesized in the endothelium, is a potent vasodilator and an inhibitor of platelet aggregation. TXA_2, produced primarily by platelets, stimulates platelet aggregation and causes vasoconstriction. Both substances are increased in pregnancy. However, Walsh et al. reported that the placentas of women with pre-eclampsia produced seven times more TXA_2 than PGI_2.[11] This imbalance in the TXA_2/PGI_2 ratio has also been demonstrated in maternal blood,[16] urine [17] and amniotic fluid.[18]

Friedman and Roberts[19] proposed that this imbalance is not a primary defect but a phenomenon secondary to endothelial cell damage. They noted that failure of the spiral arterioles to properly invade the myometrium between weeks 16 and 22 of gestation caused a decrease in uteroplacental blood flow in pre-eclamptics. Thus, the placental vasculature failed to become a high-volume, low-pressure system, which is the earliest difference that can be detected between pre-eclamptic and normal pregnancies. These investigators speculated that the decrease in placental profusion led to the release of some yet-to-be-identified toxin which induced the endothelial cell damage. This in turn led to an imbalance in the TXA_2/PGI_2 ratio, vasospasm and the subsequent pathology of pre-eclampsia.

Maternal/Fetal Risks

Maternal mortality

Pregnancy-induced hypertension (PIH) is the third leading cause of maternal mortality, comprising 18% of all maternal deaths in the USA.[20] In all likelihood, this percentage underestimates the impact of this disease on maternal mortality. Other assigned 'causes of death' (e.g. abruptio placenta, CNS complications, DIC, etc.) may well have, as an underlying unrecognized etiology, hypertension associated with pregnancy. Of interest, maternal deaths are equally divided between those presenting with pre-eclampsia and those with eclampsia. In both groups, when a precipitating etiology could be identified, cerebrovascular insults or other neurologic complications were responsible for the majority of deaths. No data are currently available to assess newer critical care management approaches to these types of patients; nor is accurate information available to determine if the cause of death preceded health care provider contact. Therefore, it is unclear whether mortality for PIH can be significantly reduced in the future. Empirically, improved overall health care should impact positively on this condition.

Central nervous system complications

Eclamptic seizures, intracranial hemorrhage, cerebral edema, amaurosis and headache are separate but related neurologic conditions that may occur in pre-eclampsia. The precise cause of seizures in pre-eclampsia remains unknown. Hypertensive encephalopathy, as well as vasospasm, hemorrhage, ischemia and edema of the cerebral hemispheres have been proposed as etiologic factors.[8] Intracranial hemorrhage is thought to result from the combination of severe hypertension and hemostatic compromise.[21] It occurs most often in the older parturient and is not specifically correlated with seizure activity. When small intracranial hemorrhages occur, the patient may complain initially of only drowsiness or seeing flashes of light. With progression, focal neurological deficits worsen; hemiplegia or rapidly progressive coma may ensue with massive bleeds. Cerebral edema is most likely due to a combination of factors influencing local hydrostatic changes and reduced oncotic pressure. The cerebral edema associated with pre-eclampsia is thought to occur secondary to generalized anoxia or loss of local cerebral vascular autoregulation.[22] Cerebral edema may present insidiously with a variety of neurologic findings, and should be considered in the patient who has a rapidly deteriorating mental status. Amaurosis (temporary blindness) may occur in 1–3% of pre-eclamptics.[23] Although the precise etiology of this latter event is speculative, both retinal vascular and occipital lobe injuries have been implicated. Headache is one of the symptoms which defines severe pre-eclampsia – it can occur in 40% of pre-eclamptics and up to 80% of eclamptics.[24] The headache is usually a severe, throbbing, frontal headache unresponsive to common analgesics. It may be associated with nausea, excitability, apprehension and visual disturbances.[25]

Renal complications

A hallmark finding in the pre-eclamptic patient is that of renal vascular spasm. Therefore, it is not surprising that renal blood flow and glomerular filtration rate are decreased in these patients. Clinically, renal dysfunction typically presents as a reduction in urine output. Although oliguria (defined as less than 20–30 ml of urine production per hour over two consecutive hours) is a common event in the pre-eclamptic, its progression to renal failure is rare. Pritchard and associates[26] have shown that in 245 cases of eclampsia, none required dialysis for renal failure. In those rare cases of renal failure associated with pre-eclampsia, the predominant insult is acute tubular necrosis, a rapidly reversible disorder. Abruptio placenta, DIC and hypovolemia usually precede this complication. Permanent renal failure can occur as the result of renal cortical necrosis.

HELLP syndrome

The HELLP syndrome, characterized by hemolysis, elevated liver enzymes and low platelets, occurs in 4–12% of patients with pre-eclampsia.[27,28] This potentially severe complication is identified twice as often in the multigravid patient as in primigravidas. Because the HELLP syndrome can present with rather atypical features, it sometimes is confused with other medical conditions, such as thrombotic thrombocytopenia purpura and hemolytic uremic syndrome. Patients present with non-specific findings including nausea, vomiting and epigastric pain. Hypertension, characteristic of pre-eclampsia, is not always seen on initial presentation. The laboratory features associated with this syndrome are listed in **Table 2**. Other findings which frequently accompany this condition include DIC, abruptio placenta, fetal demise, ascites and hepatic rupture.

Hematologic complications

Isolated hematologic abnormalities have been described in association with pre-eclampsia. The most frequent abnormality is thrombocytopenia, which is thought to result from peripheral platelet destruction secondary to vascular spasm. This has been noted in up to 50% of pre-eclamptic patients studied in this regard.[29] Vascular spasm and injury can also result in microangiopathic hemolytic anemia in these patients. Of interest, neonates of pre-eclamptic mothers have been shown to demonstrate neutropenia and thrombocytopenia, although the exact pathophysiology of this finding remains unidentified.

Hepatic complications

Hepatic failure is not a direct consequence of pre-eclampsia. However, abnormalities in liver function

Table 2
Laboratory values used to diagnose the HELLP syndrome

Hemolysis
Abnormal peripheral smear
Increased bilirubin
Increased lactic dehydrogenase

Elevated liver enzymes
Increased serum oxaloacetic transaminase (SGOT)
Increased serum glutamic pyruvic transaminase (SGPT)
Increased lactic dehydrogenase (LDH)

Low platelets
Platelet count less than 100×10^9/l

can be seen in pre-eclampsia and may relate to alternations in liver perfusion or hepatic congestion. The most life-threatening of these complications is rupture of the hepatic capsule, which carries with it a 60% maternal mortality rate.[30] Initial symptomatology includes constant right upper quadrant or epigastric pain and vomiting. Subsequently, hypovolemic shock develops from intra-abdominal hemorrhage. Laboratory studies may demonstrate liver function abnormalities, although few warning signs typically precede this catastrophic complication.

Pulmonary complications

Pulmonary edema complicates the course of pre-eclampsia in as much as 2% of cases.[31] The etiology of this condition appears to be multifactorial and may be iatrogenically induced.[32] Altogether, 80% of patients who develop pulmonary edema do so in the postpartum period. The etiology of pulmonary edema involves various degrees of capillary leakage, increases in hydrostatic pressure and alterations in colloid osmotic pressure (COP).

Capillary leakage is a consequence of both local vascular spasm and endothelial cell injury. Increases in hydrostatic pressure can result from depressed myocardial function and increases in SVR. COP is lower in pre-eclamptic patients than in normal pregnant patients,[33] and these changes disrupt the normal COP to pulmonary capillary wedge pressure (PCWP) gradient. A decreased COP–PCWP gradient has long been correlated with the development of pulmonary edema.[34] COP decreases further postpartum secondary to fluid redistribution with supine positioning, blood loss at delivery and injudicious use of crystalloid solutions.[35] These postpartum changes, along with the persistent hemodynamic alterations associated with pre-eclampsia, make the postpartum period a time of particular risk.

Cardiovascular complications

Although profound cardiovascular alterations are found in pre-eclamptic patients, these do not directly lead to an increase in maternal morbidity. Based on a limited number of studies utilizing invasive hemodynamic monitoring, pre-eclampsia is typically associated with hyperdynamic cardiac function and an increase in SVR.[36] While earlier studies suggested that the pre-eclamptic patient routinely maintains a hypovolemic state, recent data support a more variable picture of differing hemodynamic subsets in pre-eclamptic patients.[37] The clinical impact of this latter observation centers on the occurrence of oliguria, which should not be automatically tested with fluid challenges in these patients.

The issue of chronic hypertension as a sequela of pre-eclampsia is controversial. Most authorities would agree that 'pure' pre-eclampsia is a self-limiting condition, without the subsequent risk of future hypertension. However, the development of pre-eclampsia during pregnancy may unmask the presence of previously undetected hypertension, thus confusing our understanding of the natural history.

Fetal mortality

Perinatal mortality is increased in the presence of pre-eclampsia. The majority of these cases are in patients whose pregnancies are complicated by severe pre-eclampsia. Individual factors contributing to this increase in mortality, and associated morbidity, include preterm delivery, uteroplacental insufficiency, abruptio placenta and unexplained fetal demise.

Preterm delivery is often necessitated by the fact that definitive treatment of pre-eclampsia mandates termination of pregnancy, regardless of the gestational age of the fetus. The uteroplacental bed is not spared the vasoconstrictive effects of pre-eclampsia. It is, therefore, understandable that this decrease in perfusion can result in fetal growth restriction, reduction in amniotic fluid volume and an inability to tolerate the *in utero* environment. Abruptio placenta is not an infrequent consequence of these factors as well. Data demonstrate this complication to occur more frequently in pregnancies complicated by severe pre-eclampsia, the HELLP syndrome and superimposed pre-eclampsia (**Table 3**).[38]

Management Options (see also Chapter 73)

Prepregnancy

Because pre-eclampsia is primarily a disorder of primigravid women, prepregnancy counseling in the otherwise healthy patient is not applicable. On the other hand, well-established risk factors such as low socioe-

Table 3
Incidence of abruptio placenta

Patients	Incidence (%)
Normotensive	1
Mild pre-eclampsia	1
Severe pre-eclampsia	10
Eclampsia	11
Superimposed pre-eclampsia	15
HELLP syndrome	20

conomic status, race and pre-existing medical diseases allow for the identification of a subpopulation who may benefit from counseling. Basic recommendations for early prenatal care, prepregnancy diabetes and hypertension control, and adequate nutrition should be discussed.

In those patients with a history of pre-eclampsia, prepregnancy counseling may be of benefit. The recurrence risk of pre-eclampsia is influenced by the certainty of the original diagnosis. 'Pure' pre-eclampsia is unlikely to recur unless new medical conditions are identified subsequent to the index pregnancy. Although limited data are available, Chesley[39] found that when the pregnancy of multiparas is complicated by eclampsia, approximately 50% of them experience hypertension in subsequent pregnancies, while only 33% of primigravidas with eclampsia have recurrent hypertension.

Prenatal

Prediction of pre-eclampsia

Many clinical and laboratory parameters have been used in an attempt to predict pre-eclampsia with varying degrees of success. The 'roll over test' was introduced 20 years ago as a means of predicting the development of pre-eclampsia as early as 28–32 weeks, but did not have high specificity.[40] Increased vascular reactivity to intravenous infusion of angiotensin II, as demonstrated by an increased pressure response, has been reported to be predictive as early as 26 weeks of gestation.[5] In the 1980s, high plasma cellular fibronectin showed some promise, but has not developed into a useful clinical tool.[41,42] An increase in platelet intracellular calcium when exposed to arginine vasopressin,[43] a decrease in urinary calcium excretion[44] and higher fasting insulin levels[45] have all been used in attempts to predict the development of pre-eclampsia. Campbell *et al.*[46] reported that Doppler velocimetry of the uterine and umbilical vessels can predict pre-eclampsia as early as 18 weeks of gestation. In those patients who developed pre-eclampsia, there was a characteristic notching of the diastolic waveform suggesting increased peripheral vascular resistance. None of these predictive tests is currently used in clinical practice, primarily because of their lack of sensitivity and specificity.

Prevention

Our lack of understanding of the underlying pathophysiology in pre-eclampsia has impeded our attempts at preventing this disorder. Regardless, several empiric approaches have been investigated with varying degrees of success. These include dietary supplementa-tion, the use of diuretics, antihypertensives and low-dose aspirin.

Manipulation of sodium, magnesium and calcium intake have received interest. However, prospective trials have failed to produce consistent results. Calcium supplementation, the best studied agent, seems to show the most promise in this regard. Epidemiologic data have demonstrated an inverse relationship between calcium intake and the development of eclampsia.[47] Both animal and human data suggest that calcium supplementation can significantly reduce blood pressure. Studies in pregnant women are much more limited, but have suggested calcium can lower blood pressure and reduce the incidence of pre-eclampsia.[48] Additional confirmatory data are needed before one can recommend calcium as an agent to prevent pre-eclampsia.

The prophylactic administration of diuretics or antihypertensive medications has not been shown to prevent the development of pre-eclampsia.[49] However, one report has shown a decreased incidence of proteinuria in hypertensive gravidas treated with atenolol.[50] This preliminary finding requires additional study.

Aspirin inhibits the enzyme cyclooxygenase which is essential for the synthesis of prostaglandins such as thromboxane (TXA_2) and prostacyclin (PGI_2).[9] Low-dose aspirin (60–80 mg/day) selectively inhibits platelet TXA_2 release but does not effect endothelial cell production of PGI_2. It is on this basis that recent clinical trials have focused on the use of low-dose aspirin as a preventative agent.

Wallenburg *et al.*[51] studied 207 primigravidas who were screened for pre-eclampsia at 28 weeks with angiotensin II infusions. The 46 patients who had a positive screen were randomized to receive either aspirin 60 mg/day or placebo. None of the aspirin-treated group developed pre-eclampsia, while three in the control group developed severe pre-eclampsia and one eclampsia. Intrauterine growth deficiency occurred in 19% of the aspirin-treated group and in 39% of the control group. Benigni *et al.*[52] studied 33 patients at risk for pre-eclampsia. These patients were similarly randomized. The aspirin-treated group had longer gestations and higher neonatal birth weights. Schiff *et al.*[53] screened 791 women at risk for pre-eclampsia utilizing the roll over test at 28–29 weeks. Sixty-five patients had positive screening and were randomized to receive either aspirin 100 mg/day or placebo. The incidence of PIH was significantly lower in those treated with aspirin compared with the placebo group (2.9 *vs* 22.6%). It is important to note that the above-mentioned studies included small numbers of patients at risk for the development of pre-eclampsia. The use of low-dose aspirin for preventing pre-eclampsia is awaiting the results of multicenter clinical trials to evaluate the safety and effectiveness of its use.

Diagnosis

The diagnostic criteria for pre-eclampsia are well established, and in the usual circumstances this diagnosis can be easily made. Difficulties can arise when the patient presents with atypical features or when other medical conditions confound the clinical picture. The diagnosis of pre-eclampsia is made when hypertension (as previously defined) and either proteinuria or edema are present. Two forms of pre-eclampsia are traditionally discussed, mild and severe. Reasons for this distinction relate to increasing maternal and perinatal risks and therefore the need for more aggressive management. The criteria for the diagnosis of severe pre-eclampsia are listed in **Table 1**. Some of the confusion in the international literature centers on the fact that, in the absence of proteinuria, some clinicians do not feel justified in establishing the diagnosis of pre-eclampsia. As a result, data from different trials are not always comparable.

Chronic hypertension is a known risk factor for the development of pre-eclampsia. Distinguishing between these two entities may be difficult. Chronic hypertensive patients have a tendency to show a more pronounced drop in mean arterial blood pressure in the second trimester, followed by a rebound elevation of blood pressure early in the third trimester.[54] This rebound may be misinterpreted as the development of superimposed pre-eclampsia. Patients with pheochromocytoma may also have episodes of acute elevation in blood pressure during pregnancy. Patients with chronic renal disease can develop acute hypertensive crises, but usually have concomitant manifestations of long-standing disease (e.g. elevated serum creatinine). Exacerbations of systemic lupus erythromatosus – or other autoimmune conditions – during the third trimester of pregnancy can also be difficult to differentiate from pre-eclampsia. Thyrotoxicosis can cause an acute elevation in blood pressure, but this is usually in association with tachycardia, hyperthermia, goiter and abnormal thyroid function tests. Provided there is no underlying renal disease, an elevated serum uric acid may help distinguish pre-eclampsia from some of these conditions.

Treatment

Pre-eclampsia, when firmly diagnosed at term, mandates delivery. In pregnancies remote from term, expectant management in an appropriate level hospital setting can be instituted. It is important to recognize that all therapeutic modalities currently in use are palliative, and that the disease continues to be progressive until delivery has been accomplished.

The mainstays of therapy include bed rest, serial blood pressure determinations, monitoring for evidence of disease progression and fetal surveillance. There is no evidence that fluid or sodium restriction improves pregnancy outcome. Similarly, diuretic therapy is of little value in the management of these patients. The use of low-dose aspirin once the diagnosis of pre-eclampsia has been established is of no proven benefit. Antihypertensive therapy can reduce blood pressure and thus some of the maternal risk, but does not improve the disease process and theoretically may mask disease progression.

It should be anticipated that with the above conservative measures, most non-severe pre-eclamptics will respond favorably. The markers of improvement include a reduction in blood pressure, decreased edema, weight loss and a decrease in the degree of proteinuria. These improvements in clinical status are temporary in nature. Routine laboratory tests should include a 24-h urine collection for creatinine clearance and total protein, platelet count and serum fibrinogen. Evidence of disease progression will dictate the need for additional laboratory studies. Fetal surveillance during expectant management is mandatory. A variety of recommended surveillance schemes has been proposed. Regardless of the scheme employed, tests should include both amniotic fluid assessment and fetal heart rate monitoring. Since fetal growth restriction can be a complication of pre-eclampsia, serial ultrasound measurement is recommended. Recently, Doppler velocimetry has been used in assessing fetal well-being; the value of this tool remains unclear.[55]

The timing of delivery in pregnancies complicated by pre-eclampsia can represent a dilemma. Where there is obvious placental involvement with compromised fetal growth (and usually abnormal umbilical artery Doppler recordings), to deliver before the biophysical parameters (such as NST, amniotic fluid volume or biophysical profile score) become abnormal may result in the baby suffering the consequences of preterm delivery. However, to wait until the tests become abnormal may increase the likelihood of asphyxial injury while lessening the effects of prematurity. There are no controlled studies of short- or long-term outcome to help resolve this issue. If preterm delivery is contemplated, administration of steroids to enhance fetal surfactant production is advisable.

Intrapartum

The intrapartum management of pre-eclampsia has the following goals:

- prevention of eclamptic seizures
- delivery of the patient within a reasonable time
- recognition and treatment of associated complications
- minimize maternal and fetal morbidity.

To accomplish these goals, general guidelines should include care in an appropriate facility, adequate support personnel and the availability of consultative services. Because the fetus is at substantial risk of intrapartum distress, continuous electronic fetal heart rate monitoring should be employed. The maternal condition should be carefully assessed on a frequent basis to include the following parameters: hourly vital signs, accurate intake and output assessments, and evaluation of pulmonary and neurologic status. Further evaluation should be dictated by the clinical condition of the individual patient.

Fluid therapy

The injudicious use of intravenous fluids during the intrapartum period can precipitate iatrogenic complications in the pre-eclamptic patient. Therefore, the clinician must limit fluid administration to no more than 150 ml/h. Some suggest an even more cautious approach of 1 ml/kg/h. Not infrequently, the laboring patient is noted to have a reduction in urine output; unless this is clearly due to hypovolemia, empiric fluid boluses should not be utilized. Similarly, fluid boluses for 'fetal distress' should be avoided. If, however, conduction anesthesia is initiated, an additional 1000–1500 ml of fluid beyond the maintenance rate is usually necessary to avoid hypotension and subsequent fetal distress.

Crystalloid solutions are the mainstay of fluid therapy in the pre-eclamptic patient, despite the lower COP found in most pre-eclamptics. Administration of colloid solutions can transiently elevate oncotic pressure, although there is no evidence to suggest this improves the clinical picture. Close monitoring of fluid intake and output must be undertaken in order to prevent an imbalance of hydrostatic and oncotic forces that can potentiate the occurrence of pulmonary edema.

Anticonvulsant medication

Magnesium sulfate has been used for more than 60 years to prevent and treat eclamptic convulsions.[26,56,57] Despite the success of magnesium sulfate in obstetrics, other medical disciplines have generally decried its use. The objection had been that no central inhibitory action could be identified and that magnesium sulfate merely masked seizures via peripheral neuromuscular blockage. However, Cotton *et al.*[58] recently demonstrated magnesium sulfate to have central anticonvulsant activity in an animal model via suppression of the *N*-methyl-D-aspartate receptor in the hippocampus. These objective data, as well as a vast amount of clinical experience, support the use of magnesium sulfate for seizure prophylaxis.

A 6 g loading dose over 20 min, followed by 2–3 g/h continuous intravenous infusion, should provide therapeutic magnesium levels within a reasonable period of time. Plasma magnesium levels maintained at 4–7 meq/l are felt to be therapeutic in preventing eclamptic seizures. Patellar reflexes are usually lost at 8–10 meq/l and respiratory arrest may occur at 12–14 meq/l. Clinical signs of toxicity should be utilized to alert the clinician to check magnesium sulfate levels and adjust the maintenance infusion (**Table 4**). Calcium gluconate or calcium chloride, oxygen therapy and the equipment for endotracheal intubation should be available in the event of magnesium toxicity. Since magnesium sulfate is excreted primarily through the kidneys, urine output should be closely monitored; in patients with renal dysfunction, the magnesium sulfate infusion will need to be decreased.

Table 4
Magnesium toxicity

Sign	Magnesium level (mg/dl)
Loss of patellar reflex	8–12
Feeling of warmth, flushing	9–12
Somnolence	10–12
Slurred speech	10–12
Muscular paralysis	15–17
Respiratory difficulty	15–17
Cardiac arrest	30–35

Although seizure prophylaxis with magnesium sulfate is standard of care in the USA, less than 20% of obstetricians in European communities utilize this agent. Alternative therapies include the use of other anticonvulsants such as dilantin and phenobarbital, the use of sedatives such as valium and chlormethiazole,[59] or the use of antihypertensives with no specific seizure prophylaxis.[60] Details of some these agents are given in Chapter 73 together with a discussion of the management options regarding the choice of an anticonvulsant.

Antihypertensive therapy

Although magnesium sulfate prevents and treats eclamptic seizures, it is not an antihypertensive agent. Careful control of hypertension must be achieved in order to prevent complications such as maternal cerebral vascular accidents and placental abruption. Pharmacologic intervention is usually undertaken when systolic blood pressure exceeds 160–180 mmHg, or the diastolic blood pressure exceeds 100–110 mmHg.[61,62] Although many different antihypertensive agents are available, this discussion will center on those agents most commonly used for acute hypertensive crises in pregnancy. Oral agents which can be used in pre-eclampsia for more long-term control of maternal blood pressure are discussed later under 'Chronic Hypertension'.

Hydralazine hydrochloride has long been the agent of choice for the management of acute hypertension in pre-eclamptics. Hydralazine reduces vascular resistance via direct relaxation of arteriolar smooth muscle, affecting the precapillary resistance vessels more than the postcapillary capacitance vessels.[63] Assali[64] noted the hypotensive effect to be marked and prolonged in pre-eclamptic patients, moderate in patients with essential hypertension and slight in normotensive subjects. An initial intravenous dose of 5 mg should be followed by 15–20 min observation for hemodynamic effects. If an appropriate change in blood pressure is not achieved, additional 5–10 mg doses may be administered intravenously at 20-min intervals to a total dose of 30–40 mg. Hypertension refractory to hydralazine therapy warrants central hemodynamic monitoring and the use of more potent antihypertensive agents.[65,66]

Labetalol is a combined alpha- and beta-adrenoceptor antagonist that may be used to induce a controlled, rapid decrease in blood pressure via decreased SVR in patients with severe hypertension. Reports on the efficacy and safety of labetalol in the treatment of hypertension during pregnancy have been favorable.[67–74] Mabie and coworkers[72] compared bolus intravenous labetalol with intravenous hydralazine in the acute treatment of severe hypertension and found that labetalol had a quicker onset of action and did not result in reflex tachycardia. Labetalol may exert a positive effect on early fetal lung maturation in patients with severe hypertension who are remote from term.[70,71] Lunell et al.[74] studied the effects of labetalol on uteroplacental perfusion in hypertensive pregnant women and noted increased uteroplacental perfusion and decreased uterine vascular resistance.

Labetolol can be parenterally administered by either repeated intravenous injection or by slow continuous infusion. An initial dose of 20 mg should be administered, followed by additional doses of 40 or 80 mg at 10-min intervals until the desired effect is achieved or a total of 300 mg has been given. If a continuous infusion is used, labetolol should be initiated at a dose of 2 mg/min. Maximum effect should be seen in approximately 5 min after intravenous administration.[62] Oral dosage of labetolol should begin at 100 mg twice daily and can be increased to a maximum of 2400 mg per day.

Sodium nitroprusside is another potent antihypertensive agent that may be used to control severe hypertension. A dilute solution may be started at 0.25 µg/kg/min and titrated to the desired effect by increasing the dose by 0.25 µg/kg/min every 5 min. The solution is light-sensitive and so should be covered in foil and changed every 24 h. Arterial blood gases should be monitored to watch for developing metabolic acidosis, which may be an early sign of cyanide toxicity. Treatment time should be limited because of the potential for fetal cyanide toxicity.[75] Correction of hypovolemia prior to initiation of nitroprusside infusion is essential in order to avoid abrupt and often profound decreases in blood pressure.

Nifedipine is administered at an initial oral dose of 10 mg, which may be repeated after 30 min if necessary for the acute management of severe hypertension; 10–20 mg may then be administered orally every 6–8 h as needed.[62] Care must be taken when nifedipine is administered to patients receiving concomitant magnesium sulfate because of the possibility of an exaggerated hypotensive response.[76] Although nifedipine appears safe for the treatment of hypertensive crises in pregnancy, further controlled clinical trials are needed prior to general clinical use.

Nitroglycerin relaxes predominantly venous, but also arterial, vascular smooth muscle. It decreases preload at low doses and afterload in high doses. It is a rapidly acting potent antihypertensive agent with a very short hemodynamic half-life. Using invasive hemodynamic monitoring, Cotton and associates[66] noted that the ability to control blood pressure precisely was dependent on volume status. Nitroglycerin is administered via an infusion pump at an initial rate of 10 µg/min, and titrated to the desired pressures by doubling the dose every 5 min. Methemoglobinemia may result from high-dose (>7 µg/kg/min) intravenous infusion. Patients with normal arterial oxygen saturation who appear cyanotic should be evaluated for toxicity, defined as a methemoglobin level greater than 3%.[77]

Management of renal complications

Oliguria is a relatively frequent finding during the intrapartum period. It may be due to some combination of hypovolemia, renal artery vasospasm or renal injury. Using invasive hemodynamic monitoring, Clark and associates[37] have described three different hemodynamic subsets of oliguria. The first group had low PCWP with a mild to moderate increase in SVR. Those patients responded to volume replacement. The second group had normal or increased PCWP, normal SVR and were best managed with pharmacologic pre- and/or afterload reduction. The last group had elevated PCWP, elevated SVR with depressed ventricular function. Volume restriction and afterload reduction were helpful in correcting oliguria in this last group.

Close monitoring of fluid intake and output is of paramount importance in all patients diagnosed with pre-eclampsia and decreased urine output. In most cases, aggressive management is not necessary, since a timely delivery should reverse the adverse effects of pre-eclampsia on renal function. When confronted with oliguria, it is reasonable to consider a single fluid challenge of 500–1000 ml of normal saline or lactated Ringer solution over 30 min. If the urine output does not respond to this empiric fluid challenge, pulmonary artery catheterization is indicated if further hemodynamic manipulation is contemplated in an effort to resolve the oliguria. Repetitive fluid challenges are to be avoided in the absence of invasive monitoring, as pulmonary edema can evolve very quickly in this setting.

Management of pulmonary edema

Patients with pre-eclampsia can present with pulmonary edema, or develop this complication during the intrapartum or postpartum periods. Dyspnea and chest discomfort are the usual complaints. Tachypnea, tachycardia and pulmonary rales are noted on examination. Chest x-ray, pulse oximetry and arterial blood gases help to confirm the diagnosis. Other life-threatening conditions such as thromboembolism should be included in the differential diagnosis, and excluded by appropriate diagnostic studies.

Initial management includes oxygen administration and fluid restriction. A pulse oximeter should be placed so that oxygen saturation may be monitored continuously. Use of a pulmonary artery catheter may be important in severe pre-eclamptic patients who develop pulmonary edema during the antepartum period. This invasive tool can help distinguish between fluid overload, left ventricular dysfunction and pulmonary edema associated with vascular bed injury.

Furosemide administered in a 10–40 mg dose intravenously over 1–2 min is the first line of conventional therapy. If adequate diuresis does not commence within 1 h, up to an 80 mg dose can be slowly administered to achieve diuresis. In severe cases, a diuresis of 2–3 l may need to be achieved before oxygenation begins to improve. An alternative approach involves attempts at 'preload reduction', using agents such as intravenous nitroglycerin. While hydrostatic derangements can be quickly corrected with these agents, rapid improvement in arterial oxygenation has not been seen.[66,77] 'Afterload reduction' with arterial vasodilators such as hydralazine or sodium nitroprusside may be necessary for the treatment of pulmonary edema secondary to left ventricular failure.[78]

If hypoxemia persists despite initial treatment, mechanical ventilation may be required for respiratory support pending correction of the underlying problem. In all cases, close monitoring of the patient's respiratory status with frequent arterial blood gases should be performed. Fluid balance is maintained by careful monitoring of intake and output. An indwelling catheter with urometer should be placed to follow hourly urine output. Serum electrolytes should also be closely monitored especially in patients receiving diuretics. Pulmonary edema, left unattended, can progress to adult respiratory distress syndrome (ARDS), which carries with it a significant increase in maternal mortality.

Management of hematologic abnormalities

It is unusual for the clinician to be required to actively manage many of the hematologic derangements associated with pre-eclampsia. These tend to resolve spontaneously following delivery of the fetus. Thrombocytopenia is the most common hematologic aberration noted among pre-eclamptic patients, particularly in those with severe pre-eclampsia or the HELLP syndrome. Neiger *et al.*[79] found most pre-eclamptic patients with thrombocytopenia reached nadir levels 27 h following delivery. The mean time required for the platelet count to return to greater than 100×10^9/l was 60 h; this recovery time was inversely related to the severity of the thrombocytopenia. Leduc and associates[80] followed 100 pre-eclamptic women and noted that the platelet count was an excellent screening marker by which to gauge the occurrence of other hematologic abnormalities. None of their study subjects had an abnormal fibrinogen level, or a prolonged prothrombin (PT) or partial thromboplastin time (PTT), in the absence of thrombocytopenia.

In the patient who is not actively bleeding, platelet transfusion is not usually necessary until the platelet count falls below 20×10^9/l. At this point, there is a high likelihood of spontaneous pulmonary hemorrhage if the platelet count is not expeditiously corrected. If cesarean delivery is contemplated, a platelet count of at least 50×10^9/l is recommended. One way to manage such patients is to prepare 10 units of platelet concentrate and to infuse 5 units in the operating room just prior to making the incision. The remaining 5 units are infused as uterine closure is begun. The transfused platelets tend to have a relatively short functional half-life (~12 h). Complications of platelet transfusion include allergic reactions and the development of platelet-associated antibodies.

Red cell hemolysis and other clotting disorders are most often seen with the HELLP syndrome or in the pre-eclamptic patient with abruptio placenta. Again, these rarely require direct therapy because of their tendency for spontaneous resolution following delivery. There are no absolute laboratory cut-off values which dictate the need for blood transfusion or the replacement of specific blood components. These should be managed according to the clinical status of the individual patient. Somewhat arbitrarily, some clinicians suggest the use of either fresh frozen plasma or cryoprecipitate in order to maintain a fibrinogen level above 100 mg/dl and to correct for a prolonged PT or PTT.

Plasmapheresis has been used in the recent past to remove 'toxic substances' within the pre-eclamptic's systemic circulation.[81] Anecdotal reports are available describing the use of plasmapheresis in patients with the HELLP syndrome, and in those with delayed recovery following delivery. Although it currently seems inappropriate to suggest the use of this method to attempt prolongation of the pregnancy, some reports suggest that there may be a role for plasmapheresis in the management of the postpartum pre-eclamptic with severe hematologic abnormalities, resistant to more conservative therapies.

Management of central nervous system complications

Eclampsia is a life-threatening condition for mother and baby. After securing the patient's airway, intravenous access is established and a slow bolus of 6 g of magnesium sulfate is administered. Convulsions not responding to magnesium sulfate administration should be treated with the slow intravenous administration of 100 mg of thiopental sodium or 1–10 mg of intravenous diazepam. Sodium amobarbital, up to 250 mg i.v., may also be administered. Computed tomographic (CT) evaluation is indicated if the patient has repetitive seizures despite a therapeutic magnesium level, late postpartum eclampsia and/or focal neurological deficits. The timing of delivery in eclamptic patients is controversial. Pritchard[26] has advocated delivery of the patient as soon as convulsions are controlled, the patient is conscious, and certainly within 48 h of the seizures. Recently, some investigators have advocated more conservative management attempts to achieve fetal lung maturity before delivery.[82] This latter approach, if confirmed to be safe, would only apply to the rare eclamptic patient. There are no specific contraindications to labor induction associated with eclampsia. Indications for cesarean delivery should be based on obstetrical issues, provided the patient's condition is not rapidly deteriorating. The rate of cesarean delivery in eclamptic patients ranges between 11 and 57%.[83]

General therapeutic principles in the treatment of cerebral edema include correction of hypoxemia and hypercarbia, avoidance of volatile anesthetic agents, control of body temperature and control of blood pressure. Assisted hyperventilation reduces intracranial hypertension and the formation of cerebral edema. The administration of hypertonic solutions such as mannitol increases serum osmolality and draws water from the brain into the vascular compartment, thus reducing brain tissue water and volume. Steroid therapy is thought to be most effective in the treatment of focal chronic cerebral edema which may occur in association with a tumor or abscess and is less beneficial in cases of diffuse or acute cerebral edema.[84] Other pharmacologic agents that have been used to reduce intracranial

pressure and cerebral edema include acetazolamide, furosemide, spironolactone and ethacrynic acid.

Cerebral hemorrhage complicating pre-eclampsia tends to be a morbid event, in which the only available management option is supportive care. Acute surgical intervention (e.g. to remove a large intracerebral hematoma) is rarely beneficial. Control of subsequent seizure activity and severe hypertension are critical. Monitoring for the development of DIC, which may aggravate the condition, should be done. Ventilatory support for respiratory failure may be needed as progressive function is lost. Obviously, neurosurgical consultation should be obtained, and the patient should be managed in an appropriate critical care setting.

Anesthesia

The use of conduction anesthesia in pre-eclampsia for either labor management or cesarean delivery is controversial. Epidural anesthesia leads to peripheral vasodilation, which in turn can reduce SVR and arterial blood pressure in a patient with an already compromised blood volume.[85] These hemodynamic changes can lead to a reduction in uteroplacental perfusion and fetal compromise. Alternatively, general endotracheal anesthesia for cesarean delivery has been shown to result in a significant rise in the systemic arterial blood pressure and PCWP at the time of induction.[86] These features of general anesthesia in the pre-eclamptic patient can precipitate acute hypertensive crisis, abruptio placenta, cerebral hemorrhage and pulmonary edema.

During labor, pain relief can be accomplished with the use of intermittent doses of narcotic analgesia. In the hands of a skilled anesthesiologist, cautious use of epidural anesthesia is reasonable for both control of labor pain and for non-emergent cesarean delivery.[87] To avoid excessive hypotension, the patient should be placed on the left side (preventing vena caval compression) and preloaded with crystalloid solution to compensate for the anticipated peripheral vasodilation. Ephedrine is the drug of choice to correct hypotension unresponsive to volume replacement.

Invasive monitoring

There is a large body of literature available describing the use of the pulmonary artery catheter (Swan-Ganz catheter) in patients with severe pre-eclampsia. Although these studies have broadened our understanding of the hemodynamic characteristics of this disease, they have also confused the issue of when this invasive tool is needed *clinically*. As a basic guide, the pulmonary artery catheter should be placed when specific hemodynamic data are needed to alter the management plan of the individual patient. Suggested indications for placement are:

PRE-ECLAMPSIA
Summary of Management Options

Prepregnancy

- Advise early prenatal care, prepregnancy diabetic and hypertensive control, good nutrition for those at risk

Prenatal

- Diagnosis at term mandates delivery

- Mild pre-eclampsia remote from term can be managed conservatively with bed rest, fetal surveillance and monitoring for disease progression

- Severe pre-eclampsia requires delivery of the fetus if:
  - the patient is at term or at a stage where fetal viability is not a concern
  - at any stage of pregnancy if there is evidence of serious maternal or fetal complications:
    — renal failure
    — hepatocellular damage/failure
    — falling platelets or DIC
    — HELLP syndrome
    — imminent or actual eclampsia
    — uncontrollable hypertension
    — acute or chronic fetal compromise

- Laboratory studies utilized during expectant management include 24-h urine collections for quantitative protein and creatinine clearance, platelet counts, liver function tests, serum fibrinogen, PT and PTT

Labor/delivery

- The judicious use of fluid therapy and careful, frequent assessment of maternal vital signs is critical

- Continuous electronic fetal monitoring is necessary to evaluate fetal status

- Magnesium sulfate is the most common drug used in the USA for seizure prophylaxis; alternative antiseizure agents are acceptable (see Chapter 73)

- Antihypertensive medications are employed to maintain blood pressures below 160 mmHg systolic and 100 mmHg diastolic

- Potential complications include oliguria, pulmonary edema, the HELLP syndrome and seizures

- Invasive hemodynamic monitoring is infrequently needed. It should be employed to provide specific hemodynamic data to effect management decisions in patients who are unstable or in whom the volume status is uncertain

Postnatal

- Continue seizure prophylaxis in pre-eclamptics approximately 24-h postpartum

- In patients who have severe disease in the mid-trimester, eclampsia or the HELLP syndrome, slow resolution of the disease process may dictate close monioring and continuation of seizure prophylaxis for 2–4 days

- Patients who still require antihypertensive medication on discharge from the hospital should be evaluated weekly. A full work-up should be initiated for those persistently hypertensive and/or proteinuric more than 6 weeks postpartum

- Complications related to central volume status (e.g. pulmonary edema or persistent oliguria) arise and require intervention.

- Intractable severe hypertension, unresponsive to first line agents, requires continuous infusion of vasodilators such as nitroglycerin or nitroprusside.

- Conduction anesthesia is needed in a patient who is hemodynamically unstable or has an uncertain intravascular volume status.[91]

Pulmonary edema can be due to elevated hydrostatic forces (as measured by elevated PCWP), reduced oncotic forces (as measured by COP) or an increase in pulmonary capillary permeability. When COP values are 'normal' (i.e. 22–26 mmHg), PCWP levels around 18 mmHg are associated with pulmonary congestion and frank pulmonary edema is seen when the PCWP exceeds 25 mmHg.[88] In pre-eclampsia, baseline COP values are known to be reduced, and further decline postpartum to levels which range between 12 and 14 mmHg on average.[33] This implies the pre-eclamptic is at risk for pulmonary edema when even modest elevations in PCWP occur. The management of this clinical complication, therefore, first depends on differentiating the above mechanisms causing the pulmonary edema. Most of the time, simple fluid restriction and diuretic therapy will be sufficient. However, when these measures fail, pulmonary artery catheterization (with COP determinations to determine the PWCP:COP gradient) can help to better define the management plan. High PCWP values mandate aggressive diuresis and afterload reduction; normal or low values (with the PCWP:COP difference greater than 4) support the diagnosis of pulmonary capillary injury and increased permeability. These latter patients require supportive care without specific hemodynamic manipulations.

Postnatal

Magnesium sulfate (or other selected agent) for seizure prophylaxis should be continued for 24 h after delivery. During this time, close monitoring of the patient (vital signs, reflexes, intake and output) must be maintained. Approximately 25% of eclamptic seizures occur in the puerperium.[83] Although most patients begin to show resolution of the disease process during the initial 24 h after delivery, those with severe disease in the mid-trimester, eclampsia or the HELLP syndrome may require intensive monitoring for 2–4 days. Until signs of improvement are seen in these patients, magnesium sulfate infusion should be continued. These patients are also at particular risk for pulmonary edema.

Most patients will be normotensive on discharge from hospital and they may take oral contraceptive pills without increased risks. A minority of pre-eclamptic patients will continue to need antihypertensive medication to control their blood pressure. These patients should be evaluated weekly until they no longer require medication. If they are still hypertensive 6 weeks postpartum and/or have proteinuria, a complete work-up to assess the hypertension and identify the underlying causes is necessary so that appropriate long-term management can be instituted (**Table 5**).

Table 5
Investigation of persistent hypertension and/or proteinuria at 6 weeks postnatal

Urea and electrolytes
24-h urine collection for protein
Creatinine clearance
Renal ultrasound and i.v. urogram

If any of these abnormal, refer to renal physicians for further assessment and management

CHRONIC HYPERTENSION

General

Chronic hypertension is defined as a persistent elevation in blood pressure of 140/90 mmHg or greater before 20 weeks gestation, or persistent hypertension beyond 6 weeks postpartum. Because of the physiologic decrease in blood pressure seen in mid-pregnancy, chronic hypertensive patients may actually have pressures in the normotensive range for a good portion of their pregnancy. This will make the diagnosis difficult in those with scant prenatal care.

The literature on chronic hypertension during pregnancy is clouded by inconsistencies in criteria used to select study patients. Americans tend to use the above definition, whereas Europeans and Australasians tend to include patients with all forms of hypertension. Classification schemes also vary. In this chapter, patients with mild chronic hypertension will be those with systolic blood pressures between 140 and 159 mmHg and diastolic pressures between 90 and 109 mmHg, while those with a systolic blood pressure ≥ 160 mmHg or a diastolic blood pressure ≥ 110 mmHg will be classified as severe. However, in practice, antihypertensive therapy is started often when the systolic exceeds 160 mmHg and/or the diastolic exceeds 100 mmHg, suggesting that many obstetricians consider ≥ 100 mmHg to be a more practical definition of 'severe' hypertension.

Depending on the population studied and the criteria used, the incidence of chronic hypertension in pregnancy ranges from 0.5 to 3%. Essential hypertension is responsible for 90% of the chronic hypertension associated with pregnancy. Causes of secondary hypertension can include renal disease (glomerulonephritis, nephropathy or renovascular disease), endocrinologic disorders (diabetes with vasular involvement, thyrotoxicosis, pheochromocytoma) or collagen vascular disease (lupus erythematosus, scleroderma).

Maternal/Fetal Risks

Maternal and perinatal morbidity and mortality are not generally increased for patients with uncomplicated, mild chronic hypertension. However, risks to both mother and fetus increase dramatically when the pregnancy is complicated by severe disease, superimposed pre-eclampsia or the risk factors listed in **Table 6**.

Maternal risks include exacerbation of hypertension, superimposed pre-eclampsia, congestive heart failure, intracerebral hemorrhage, acute renal failure, abruptio placenta with DIC or death as a result of any of these. Of these, superimposed pre-eclampsia and abruptio placenta are the two most common complications. Superimposed pre-eclampsia complicates approximately 5–50% of the pregnancies of chronic hypertensives, depending on whether the diagnosis of pre-eclampsia was made simply on the basis of exacerbation of the hypertension or if significant proteinuria was part of the definition. In patients with risk factors, the incidence of superimposed pre-eclampsia is 25–50%. The incidence of abruptio placenta ranges from 0.5 to 2% in mild, uncomplicated hypertensives and from 3 to 10% in those with severe hypertension. Of interest, neither the incidence of superimposed pre-eclampsia or abruption is influenced by the use of antihypertensive medications.[89]

Fetal morbidity and mortality are directly related to the severity of the hypertension and are particularly high in the presence of superimposed pre-eclampsia and abruptio placenta. Decreased uteroplacental perfusion can lead to fetal growth restriction. Spontaneous or intentional interruption of the pregnancy adds the compounding complications of prematurity. Mid-trimester death *in utero* is higher in chronic hypertensives, especially in those not receiving prenatal care. Again, perinatal complications are not particularly increased for those with mild, uncomplicated hypertension.

Management Options

Prepregnancy

In the past, women with severe chronic hypertension were advised not to get pregnant and many terminated an early pregnancy out of concern over maternal risks. Today, those women with severe disease who desire pregnancy should be encouraged to receive prepregnancy care. The cause of the chronic hypertension should be established if possible, along with the severity of the disease.

The patient should be taken off antihypertensives with potential adverse effects on the fetus, such as angiotensin-converting enzyme inhibitors and diuretics. This should be done, however, under strict physician supervision. At times, these medications are continued into pregnancy, despite their potential for fetal risks, because of difficulties controlling hypertension otherwise. Adequate time must be allowed preconceptionally to gauge the patient's response to any new medications utilized for control of the hypertension. Renal function should be assessed in more severe cases by measuring serum creatinine and a 24-h urine collection for creatinine clearance. Once conception occurs, early prenatal care within an appropriate setting is important.

Prenatal

Early and frequent prenatal care is essential to optimize perinatal outcome in hypertensive patients. During the initial visits, a detailed evaluation of the etiology and severity of the chronic hypertension should be made, and careful attention given to the history of cardiac or renal disease, diabetes, thyroid disease and the outcome of previous pregnancies. Baseline laboratory studies evaluating organ systems likely to be affected include: urine analysis and culture, electrolytes, uric acid, blood sugar and a 24-h urine for creatinine clearance and protein. Patients with severe hypertension or proteinuria in the first trimester should also have a chest x-ray, electrocardiogram, antinuclear antibody testing and, when indicated, serum complement studies. In those with severe, long-standing hypertension, an echocardiogram should be performed to evaluate cardiac function. Those with recurrent pregnancy loss or recent thromboembolic disease should be evaluated

Table 6
Characteristics of high risk chronic hypertension patients

Maternal age > 40 years
Duration of hypertension > 15 years
Blood pressure > 160/110 mmHg early in pregnancy
Diabetes (class B–F)
Renal disease (all causes)
Cardiomyopathy
Connective tissue disease
Coarctation of the aorta

Reproduced with permission from Sibai.[89]

for the presence of lupus anticoagulant and anticardiolipin antibodies.

Women classified as low-risk (having mild chronic hypertension and none of the above listed risk factors) should be seen every 2–4 weeks in the first two trimesters and then weekly after that. Sibai recommends the discontinuation of all antihypertension medication at the first prenatal visit in women that fall into this category.[90] Only half will require subsequent medication; the treatment of those needing antihypertensive agents can be tailored to their individual needs at that time. Fetal evaluation should include serial ultrasound examinations to document adequate fetal growth and weekly antepartum fetal non-stress testing beginning at about 34 weeks gestation. In the absence of superimposed pre-eclampsia or the inability to document fetal wellbeing, routine induction of labor prior to 41 weeks gestation is probably not warranted.

Pregnancies in hypertensive women with additional risk factors are associated with increased maternal and perinatal complications. These pregnancies should be managed in consultation with appropriate specialists (e.g. maternal–fetal medicine, nephrology). Very close monitoring is essential and multiple hospitalizations may be necessary to control maternal hypertension and associated medical complications. Severe hypertension mandates an aggressive pharmacologic approach to the patient. Carefully selected antihypertensive medications may also be beneficial to those with mild hypertension, but with additional complicating factors such as diabetes, renal disease or cardiac dysfunction. Intensive fetal surveillance is critical to optimize fetal outcome. Serial ultrasonagraphy for fetal growth and weekly (or more frequently depending on the fetal condition) antepartum fetal non-stress testing beginning as early as 26 weeks should be employed. The pregnancy may be continued until term, until the onset of superimposed pre-eclampsia or until the development of fetal growth restriction or distress. The development of severe, superimposed pre-eclampsia places the patient at highest risk for maternal and perinatal complications. This development after 28 weeks is an indication for delivery; prior to 28 weeks, the pregnancy may be followed conservatively in a tertiary center with daily evaluation of maternal and fetal condition, although this latter approach remains quite controversial.[91]

Antihypertensive therapy

Although the maternal and fetal benefits of antihypertensive medications are well documented in the treatment of pregnancies complicated by severe hypertension, the benefits of these medications in those pregnancies with mild uncomplicated hypertension is much less clear. There are no randomized trials in the treatment of severe hypertension. In practice, obstetricians vary in when they start therapy. In general, however, they treat when the diastolic blood pressure reaches 100–110 mmHg. This is to prevent cerebral vascular accident, the largest cause of maternal death in hypertensive patients.

In the USA, methyldopa and hydralazine are the first-line agents because of extensive experience in their use and lack of known fetal effects. Labetalol, first popularized in European studies, is a reasonable second-line antihypertensive for use in these pregnant women. Nifedipine is also gaining in popularity. There are no studies to indicate which oral agent is best for controlling chronic hypertension during pregnancy.

The treatment of gravidas with mild to moderate chronic hypertension is more controversial. The many reports of antihypertensive use in this group of patients are difficult to evaluate because of differences in definitions, populations and treatments. The trials are more limited by sample size, selection bias and frequent initiation of therapy late in the second or third trimesters. Nevertheless, a few generalizations can be made from these reports.[60,90,92] The use of methyldopa or labetolol in women with mild, uncomplicated hypertension does not significantly improve gestational age at delivery, birthweight, rates of intrauterine growth deficiency or the perinatal death rate over those women who were untreated or received placebo. Trials comparing the efficacy of methyldopa with a beta-blocker in mild hypertension showed little significant differences.[93–95] The use of these agents does not lower the incidence of superimposed pre-eclampsia or abruptio placenta, the conditions responsible for the majority of adverse perinatal outcomes in mild chronic hypertensive patients.

Labor/delivery

Intrapartum management is directed at the avoidance of acute maternal and fetal complications. Maternal blood pressure can be controlled with oral or intravenous hydralazine or labetolol (see Pre-eclampsia: Antihypertensive medications and Chapter 73). Judicious use of intravenous fluids and close attention to non-invasive hemodynamic parameters (e.g. blood pressure, pulse, oximetry) are crucial. Fetuses may be compromised by long-standing growth restriction and hypoxemia prior to the onset of labor. Therefore, continuous electronic fetal monitoring and intermittent fetal scalp pH sampling, as needed, are important to assess the ability of the fetus to tolerate labor.

Postnatal

High-risk chronic hypertensive patients should be monitored closely for at least 48 h after delivery because they are at risk for the development of hyper-

CHRONIC HYPERTENSION
Summary of Management Options

Prepregnancy

- Establish the etiology, if possible, and the severity of the hypertension. Evaluate renal function

- The patient with mild to moderate disease should be taken off antihypertensive medication or switched to medication known to have few fetal side-effects. Patients difficult to control with severe diseases may need to remain on prepregnancy medications, regardless of potential fetal risks

- Encourage early prenatal care in an appropriate setting

Prenatal

- Early and frequent prenatal care is crucial to optimize maternal and fetal outcome

- Antihypertensive medication can be discontinued unless the maternal diastolic pressure exceeds 100–110 mmHg. Oral medications (methyldopa, hydralazine or labetolol) are used in severe hypertensives and in those with mild hypertension complicated by known risk factors

- Laboratory studies include 24-h urine collection for creatinine clearance and quantitative protein, uric acid, blood sugar, electrolytes and, where appropriate, antinuclear antibody, serum complement studies and antiphospholipid antibodies

- Fetal surveillance should include serial ultrasound evaluations for fetal growth, and antepartum testing beginning about 26 weeks in women with severe hypertension and/or risk factors, and about 34 weeks in women with mild, uncomplicated hypertension. Both fetal heart rate monitoring and amniotic fluid volume should be assessed

- Watch for superimposed pre-eclampsia

Labor/delivery

- Continuous electronic fetal monitoring is necessary to evaluate the fetus which may be compromised by long-standing growth restriction and hypoxemia

- Antihypertensive medications are employed to maintain blood pressures below 160 mmHg systolic and 100–110 mmHg diastolic

- Monitor for potential complications, including superimposed pre-eclampsia and abruptio placenta

Postnatal

- Close monitoring in the first 48 h postpartum is needed to anticipate the development of hypertensive encephalopathy, pulmonary edema or renal failure

- Oral or intravenous medication (methyldopa, hydralazine or labetolol) is used to control hypertension

- Evaluation should occur in the postpartum period for deterioration in cardiac or renal status

- Although detectable in breast milk in minute amounts, most antihypertensives are not contraindicated in breast-feeding mothers. Thiazide diuretics should be avoided in this group.

tensive encephalopathy, pulmonary edema and renal failure. Either oral or intravenous hydralazine, methyldopa or labetalol can be used to control severe hypertension. Diuretic therapy should be used in those with evidence of circulatory congestion or pulmonary edema. These women should be evaluated after the postpartum period for deterioration in cardiac or renal function and to adjust antihypertensive medication.

After delivery, oral antihypertensive medications usually need to be continued to control hypertension. Minute amounts of all antihypertensives are found in breast milk. Limited data suggest no short-term effects on the breast-feeding infant exposed to methyldopa, hydralazine or beta-blockers.[96] However, thiazide diuretics have been reported to inhibit adequate breast milk production.[97]

APPENDICES
CLASSIFICATION AND DEFINITION OF THE HYPERTENSIVE DISORDERS OF PREGNANCY

(from Davey and MacGillivray[98])

Appendix 1
CLINICAL CLASSIFICATION OF HYPERTENSIVE DISORDERS OF PREGNANCY

A. Gestational hypertension and/or proteinuria
Hypertension and/or proteinuria developing during pregnancy, labor or the puerperium in a previously normotensive non-proteinuric woman and subdivided into:

1. Gestational hypertension (without proteinuria)
   (a) developing during pregnancy (prenatal)
   (b) developing for first time in labor
   (c) developing for first time in the puerperium

2. Gestational proteinuria (without hypertension)
   (a) developing during pregnancy (prenatal)
   (b) developing for first time in labor
   (c) developing for first time in puerperium

3. Gestational proteinuric hypertension (pre-eclampsia)
   (a) developing during pregnancy (prenatal)
   (b) developing for first time in labor
   (c) developing for first time in puerperium

B. Chronic hypertension and chronic renal disease
Hypertension and/or proteinuria in pregnancy in a woman with chronic hypertension or chronic renal disease diagnosed either before or during or persisting after pregnancy and subdivided into:
1. Chronic hypertension (without proteinuria)
2. Chronic renal disease (proteinuria and hypertension)
3. Chronic hypertension with superimposed pre-eclampsia
   (Proteinuria developing for the first time during pregnancy in a woman with known chronic hypertension)

C. Unclassified hypertension and/or proteinuria
Hypertension and/or proteinuria found either
   (a) **at first 'booking' examination after the 20th week** of pregnancy (140 days) in a woman without known chronic hypertension or chronic renal disease, or
   (b) **during pregnancy, labor, or the puerperium where information is insufficient to permit classification** is provisionally regarded as unclassified and subdivided into:

1. Unclassified hypertension (without proteinuria)
2. Unclassified proteinuria (wihtout hypertension)
3. Unclassified proteinuric hypertension (pre-eclampsia)

D. Eclampsia, is regarded as one of the complications of the hypertensive disorders of pregnancy and should be included in a separate classification of complications.

NOTES ON CLASSIFICATION
1. Women found to have hypertension and/or proteinuria at the first visit before the 20th week of pregnancy are presumed (in the absence of trophoblastic disease) to have either:
 (i) **chronic hypertension** (if they have hypertension only), or
(ii) **chronic renal disease** (if they have proteinuria with or without hypertension)

2. Women with unclassified hypertension and/or proteinuria may be reclassified after delivery:

A. If the hypertension and/or proteinuria disappears into:
 (i) **Gestational hypertension** (without proteinuria), or
 (ii) **Gestational proteinuria** (without hypertension), or
(iii) **Gestational proteinuric hypertension (pre-eclampsia)**

B. If the hypertension and/or proteinuria persist after delivery or other tests confirm the diagnosis into:

(i) **Chronic hypertension** (usually without proteinuria), or
(ii) **Chronic renal disease** (usually proteinuria with or without hypertension), or
(iii) **Chronic hypertension with superimposed pre-eclampsia**

Appendix 2
DEFINITIONS

Hypertension in pregnancy
Hypertension is diagnosed on the basis of the diastolic blood pressure (DBP) as measured by sphygmomanometry using the 'point of muffling' (Phase IV Korotkoff sounds) in women lying on their side at 15–30% to the horizontal. Blood pressure may be taken with the patient sitting but if raised must be confirmed with the patient lying after 2–3 min rest.
Hypertension is defined as either:
A. One measurement of DBP of 110 mmHg or more, or
B. Two consecutive measurements of DBP of 90 mmHg or more 4 h or more apart

Proteinuria in pregnancy
The definition of proteinuria in pregnancy is based on either the quantitative measurement of the total protein in one 24-h urine collection or the detection of 'significant' proteinuria in two random urine specimens tested by reagent strip (Multistix SG), or sulfosalicylic acid 'cold' test.
'Significant' proteinuria is defined as either:
A. One 24-h urine collection with a total excretion of 300 mg or more/day, or
B. Two random clean-catch or catheter specimens of urine collected 4 h or more apart, with

(i) **2+(1 g albumin/l) or more** on reagent strip or sulfosalicylic acid 'cold' test, or
(ii) **1+(0.3 g albumin/l) if SG less than 1030,** or
(iii) **A protein/creatinine index of 300 or more**

The volume and concentration of the urine greatly affects the protein concentration and may give rise to both false positive and false negative results in tests on random urine specimens. If the SG is less than 1030 tests may give false negative results and if 1030 or more false postitive results and unreliable specimens should be discarded. If the close correlation between the protein/creatinine index and the 24-h total protein excretion found in non-pregnant subjects is confirmed in pregnancy, this index may provide the best method of measuring and confirming significant proteinuria.

Appendix 3
RECOMMENDED STANDARD METHOD FOR THE MEASUREMENT OF BLOOD PRESSURE BY SPHYGMOMANOMETRY

1. Preparation
(a) **Preparation.** Remove any tight clothing so that the right upper arm is fully exposed and the sphygmomanometer cuff can be easily applied.
(b) **Position.** Arrange that the patient rests comfortably on a couch or bed on her right side with 15–30° tilt and that the right upper arm is well supported at the same level as the heart.
(c) **Sphygmomanometer.** Position the sphygmomanometer so that the 90 mmHg mark is at eye-level when the blood pressure is taken with the stethoscope fixed in the ears and the bell applied to the antecubital fossa.

2. Application of cuff
(a) **Position.** Place the center of the bladder in the sphygmomanometer cuff directly over the brachial artery on the inner side of the right upper arm with the cuff at the same level as the sternum at the 4th intercostal space.
(b) **Application.** Apply the cuff evenly and firmly but not tightly around the arm with the connecting tubes pointing upward (toward the head) and the antecubital fossa free.
(c) **Size of cuff.** If possible use a cuff with the acceptable range of arm circumference marked on the sleeve. If arm circumference is too large, use a large cuff. If no large cuff is available, note that the blood pressure reading is unsatisfactory and may be erroneous.

3. Taking the blood pressure

(a) **Position of stethoscope.** Palpate the brachial artery in the antecubital fossa and place the stethoscope directly over the artery and hold in place without undue pressure.

(b) **Initial cuff pressure.** Rapidly pump up the pressure in the sphygmomanometer cuff to 20–30 mmHg above the point at which pulsation in the brachial and radial artery cease and the Korotkoff sounds disappear.

(c) **Rate of deflation of cuff.** Let the air out of cuff without delay so that mercury falls steadily at 2–3 mm/s.

(d) **Systolic blood pressure.** Take the systolic blood pressure (SBP) as the point where first clear tapping sound is heard, read top of mercury meniscus, record to nearest 2 or 5 mmHg.

(e) **Diastolic blood pressure.** Take diastolic blood pressure (DBP) in pregnancy as the point where the Korotkoff sounds first become muffled (Phase IV), read top of mercury meniscus to nearest 2 or 5 mmHg. If no clear point of muffling is heard, take point of disappearance of sounds (Phase V) and record which point taken. Ideally, both point of muffling (Phase IV) and of disappearance (Phase V) should be recorded.

(f) **Complete deflation of cuff.** Let down pressure in the cuff completely as soon as blood pressure is taken to minimize patient discomfort and to allow free flow of blood in and out of arm.

4. Choice of arm

(a) **Right arm preference.** The blood pressure should normally be taken in the right arm as most observers stand on the right side of the patient when taking the blood pressure.

(b) **Both arms at first visit.** At first visit take blood pressure in both arms. First take blood pressure in right arm and then turn patient on left side with 30° tilt with left arm well supported at level of heart. Ensure patient rests comfortably for 1–2 min and take blood pressure in left arm in same way as in right arm and record all measurements.

(c) **If BP in left arm higher.** If blood pressure in left arm is 10 mmHg or more higher than in right arm, make special note in records that the left arm should be used for all future measurements.

5. Repeat measurements if blood pressure is uncertain or high

(a) **If BP uncertain.** If the blood pressure reading is uncertain, always repeat measurement. Let cuff down completely and wait 1–2 min before re-inflating cuff and repeating measurement.

(b) **If BP is taken in sitting position and found to be raised.** Arrange that patient lies down on couch on right side with 30° tilt, rests a few minutes and take blood pressure as described above.

(c) **If BP is raised in lying position.** Ensure patient rests comfortably for 1–2 min, repeat blood pressure measurement and if necessary get second experienced observer to check. Record all measurements both initial and repeat and act on lowest DBP (Phase IV) unless it is falsely low measurement.

Appendix 4
RECOMMENDED METHOD FOR TESTING URINE FOR PROTEIN

1. Avoid dilute urine. Patients should not drink large quantities of fluid before passing urine samples – dilute urine may give false negative tests.

2. Obtain clean urine samples. Obtain fresh sample of urine in clean, uncontaminated container without preservative and note any abnormal deposit.

3. Test urine for protein (and if possible pH and SG), with

A. Multiple Reagent Strip ('Dipstick') always test for protein, SG and pH (Multistix – SG Ames).

(i) **Protein;** Trace 0.1 g/l
                1+ 0.3 g/l
                2+ 1.0 g/l
                3+ 3.0 g/l
                4+10.0 g/l

(ii) **SG: if SG less than 1010,** beware of false negative due to dilute urine;
    if SG 1030 or more; beware of false positive due to concentrated urine

(iii) **pH: if pH 8.0 or more,** beware of false positive test with sulfosalicylic acid (very alkaline)

B. Sulfosalicylic acid 'cold' test for protein

(i) Put 4–5 ml urine in clean test tube

(ii) Add 2–3 drops 20% sulfosalicylic acid

(iii) Mix thoroughly and estimate turbidity against a dark background in a good light
    Trace (0.1 g/l) cloudiness only visible against a dark background
    1+ (0.3 g/l) cloud not flocculent or granular

2+ (1.0 g/l) cloud granular but not flocculent
3+ (3.0 g/l) thick flocculent cloud
4+ (10+ g/l) thick deposit to solid mass.

4. Obtain second clean-catch to catheter specimen of urine and repeat test for protein, SG and pH
IF (i) **urine SG less than 1010**
or (ii) **any proteinuria of trace or more**
and (iii) **urine SG 1030 or more** (give 250 ml fluid to drink first)

5. Interpretation of results
IF Negative = **No proteinuria**
IF 2+ or more = **"Significant" proteinuria**
IF 1+ or trace **Arrange for** (in order of preference)
   (i) **24-h urine collection for urinary protein**
IF 300 mg or more/24 h = 'Significant' proteinuria
or (ii) **Repeat urine specimen for protein/creatinine ratio**
IF 10 × protein mg/l = 300 or more equivalent to
      creatinine mmol/l   300 mg protein/24 h
                         = **'Significant' proteinuria**
or (iii) **Repeat urine specimen and check SG and pH**
IF SG 1010 – 1025 trace   = no proteinuria
       and pH 8 1+   = 'Significant' proteinuria

6. Diagnose 'significant' proteinuria on basis of either:
   A. One 24-h urine collection or
   B. Two random clean-catch or catheter urine specimens

A. One 24-h urine collection
The definitive test for proteinuria is the quantitative measurement of the total protein excreted over 24 h. The rate of protein excretion in the urine varies greatly, is increased on exercise and on standing when the urine protein concentration may be increased up to 10-fold. Due to the wide variations in the urine concentration and volume and to the effect of exercise and recumbency random urine specimens may give false negative or false positive results. It is hence recommended that the diagnosis of **'significant' proteinuria** in pregnancy should be based wherever possible on the quantitative measurement of the total protein excreted in a 24-h urine collection.

B. Two random clean-catch or catheter urine specimens
Where a 24-h urine collection is not available or possible, it is recommended that the diagnosis of **'significant' proteinuria** should be based on the finding of proteinuria in at least two **random clean-catch or catheter urine specimens.** This recommendation is made to reduce mistakes in diagnosis resulting from variations in the amount of protein and the urinary concentration and to minimize possible errors in the testing of urine specimens and the recording of results.

Appendix 5
SUGGESTED DEFINITIONS OF SEVERE HYPERTENSION AND SEVERE PROTEINURIA

Severe hypertension is defined as the finding of either:
   A. DBP 120 mmHg or more on one occasion
or **B. DBP 110 mmHg or more on two occasions 4 h or more apart**
These levels usually indicate the need for urgent anithypertensive therapy.

Severe proteinuria is defined as the finding of:
   3 g or more total protein in one 24-h urine collection
It is necessary to ensure that 24-h urine collections are (a) obtained uncontaminated in clean containers with a suitable preservative such as toluene or else kept at 4°C; and (b) complete (the completeness may be checked by estimation of the total 24-h urinary creatinine excretion). It is not considered valid to diagnose 'severe' proteinuria on the basis of tests on random urine specimens.

REFERENCES

1 The American College of Obstetricians and Gynecologists (1986) *Management of Preeclampsia*. ACOG Technical Bulletin No. 91, February.

2 Sibai BM (1991) Immunologic aspects of preeclampsia. *Clinics in Obstetrics and Gynecology* **34**:27–34.

3 Wilson M, Morganti AA, Zervoudakis J *et al.* (1980) Blood pressure, the renin–aldosterone system and sex steroids throughout normal pregnancy. *American Journal of Medicine* **68**:97–102.

4 Clark SL, Cotton DB (1988) Clinical indications for pulmonary artery catheterization in the patient with severe preeclampsia. *American Journal of Obstetrics and Gynecology* **158**:453–458.

5 Gant NF, Daley GL, Chand S *et al.* (1973) A study of angiotensin II pressor response throughout primigravid pregnancy. *Journal of Clinical Investigation* **52**:2682–2689.

6 Spargo B, McCartney CP, Winemiller R (1959) Glomerular capillary endotheliosis in toxemia of pregnancy. *Archives of Pathology* **68**:593–599.

7 Arias F, Mancilla-Jiminez R (1976). Hepatic fibrinogen deposits in preeclampsia. *New England Journal of Medicine* **295**:578–582.

8 Sibai B (1988) Eclampsia. In Rubin PC (ed.) *Handbook of Hypertension*, Vol. 10, pp. 320–340. Amsterdam: Elsevier.

9 Walsh SW (1985) Preeclampsia: An imbalance in placental prostacyclin and thromboxane production. *American Journal of Obstetrics and Gynecology* **152**:335–340.

10 Goodman RP, Killam P, Brash AR *et al.* (1982) Prostacyclin production during pregnancy: Comparison of production during normal pregnancy and pregnancy complicated by hypertension. *American Journal of Obstetrics and Gynecology* **142**:817–822.

11 Walsh SW, Behr, MJ, Allen NH (1985) Placental prostacyclin production in normal and toxemic pregnancies. *American Journal of Obstetrics and Gynecology* **151**:110–115.

12 Makila UM, Jouppila P, Kirkinen P *et al.* (1986) Placental thromboxane and prostacyclin in the regulation of placental blood flow. *Obstetrics and Gynecology* **68**:537–540.

13 FitzGerald GA, Brash AR, Falardeau P *et al.* (1981) Estimated rate of prostacyclin secretion into the circulation in normal man. *Journal of Clinical Investigation* **68**:1272–1276.

14 Remuzzi G, Marchesi D, Mecca G *et al.* (1980) Reduction of fetal vascular prostacyclin activity in preeclampsia. *Lancet* **2**:310.

15 Makila UM; Viinikka L, Ylikorkala O (1984) Evidence that prostacyclin deficiency is a specific feature in preeclampsia. *American Journal of Obstetrics and Gynecology* **148**:772–774.

16 Koullapis EN, Nicolaides KH, Collins WP *et al.* (1982) Plasma prostanoids in pregnancy-induced hypertension. *British Journal of Obstetrics and Gynaecology* **89**:617–621.

17 Ylikorkala O, Pekonen F, Viinikka L (1986) Renal prostacyclin and thromboxane in normotensive and pre-eclamptic pregnant women and their infants. *Journal of Clinical Endocrinology and Metabolism* **63**:1307–1312.

18 Ylikorkala O, Makila UM, Viinikka L (1981) Amniotic fluid prostacyclin and thromboxane in normal, preeclamptic and some other complicated pregnancies. *American Journal of Obstetrics and Gynecology* **141**:487–490.

19 Friedman SA, Taylor RN, Roberts JM (1991) Pathophysiology of preeclampsia. *Clinics in Perinatology* **18**:661–682.

20 Atrash HK, Koonin L, Lawson HW *et al.* (1990) Maternal mortality in the United States, 1979–1986. *Obstetrics and Gynecology* **76**:1055–1060.

21 Romero R, Lockwood C, Oyarzun E, Hobbins JC (1988) Toxemia: New concepts in an old disease. *Seminars in Perinatology* **12**:302–323.

22 Benedetti TJ, Quilligan EJ (1980) Cerebral edema in severe pregnancy-induced hypertension. *American Journal of Obstetrics and Gynecology* **137**:860–862.

23 Seidman DS, Sen DM, Ben-Rafael Z (1991) Renal and ocular manifestations of hypertensive diseases of pregnancy. *Obstetrical and Gynaecological Survey* **46**:71–78.

24 Sibai BM, McCubbin JH, Anderson G *et al.* (1981) Eclampsia I. Observation from 67 recent cases. *Obstetrics and Gynecology* **58**:609–613.

25 Royburt M, Seidman DS, Serr DM, Mashiachi S (1991) Neurologic involvement in hypertensive disease of pregnancy. *Obstetrical and Gynaecological Survey* **46**:656–664.

26 Pritchard JA, Cunningham G, Pritchard SA (1984) The Parkland Memorial Hospital protocol for treatment of eclampsia: Evaluation of 245 cases. *American Journal of Obstetrics and Gynecology* **148**:951–963.

27 Pritchard JA, Weisman R, Ratnoff OD, Vosburgh GJ (1954) Intravascular hemolysis, thrombocytopenia, and other hematologic abnormalities associated with severe toxemia of pregnancy. *New England Journal of Medicine* **150**:89–98.

28 Sibai BM, Taslimi MM, El-Nazer A *et al.* (1986) Maternal–perinatal outcome associated with the syndrome of hemolysis, elevated liver enzymes and low platelets in severe preeclampsia–eclampsia. *American Journal of Obstetrics and Gynecology* **155**:501–509.

29 Burrows RF, Hunter DJS, Andrew M, Kelton JG (1987) A prospective study investigating the mechanism of thrombocytopenia in preeclampsia. *Obstetrics and Gynecology* **70**:334–338.

30 Bis KA, Waxman B (1976) Rupture of the liver associated with pregnancy: A review of the literature and report of 2 cases. *Obstetrical and Gynecological Survey* **31**:763–773.

31 Sibai BM, Mabie BC, Harvey CJ, Gonzalez AR (1987) Pulmonary edema in severe preeclampsia–eclampsia: Analysis of 37 consecutive cases. *American Journal of Obstetrics and Gynecology* **156**:1174–1179.

32 Benedetti TJ, Kates R, Williams V (1985) Hemodynamic observations in severe preeclampsia complicated by pulmonary edema. *American Journal of Obstetrics and Gynecology* **152**:330–334.

33 Benedetti TJ, Carlson RW (1979) Studies of colloid osmotic pressure in pregnancy-induced hypertension.

American Journal of Obstetrics and Gynecology **135**:308–311.

34 Fein A, Grossman RF, Jones JG *et al.* (1979) The value of edema fluid protein measurement in patients with pulmonary edema. *American Journal of Medicine* **67**:32–38.

35 Weil MN, Henning RJ, Puri VK (1979) Colloid osmotic pressure: Clinical significance. *Critical Care Medicine* **7**:113–116.

36 Cotton DB, Lee W, Huhta JC, Dorman KF (1988) Hemodynamic profile of severe pregnancy-induced hypertension. *American Journal of Obstetrics and Gynecology* **158**:523–528.

37 Clark SL, Greenspoon JS, Aldahl D, Phelan JP (1986) Severe preeclampsia with persistent oliguria: Management of hemodynamic subsets. *American Journal of Obstetrics and Gynecology* **154**:490–494.

38 Abdella TN, Sibai BM, Hays JM, Anderson GD (1984) Relationship of hypertensive disease to abruptio placentae. *Obstetrics and Gynecology* **63**:365–370.

39 Chesley LC (1980) Hypertension in pregnancy: Definitions, familial factors and remote prognosis. *Kidney International* **18**:234–240.

40 Gant NF, Chand S, Worley RJ *et al.* (1971) A clinical test useful for predicting the development of acute hypertension of pregnancy. *American Journal of Obstetrics and Gynecology* **120**:1–7.

41 Lazarchick J, Stubbs TM, Remein L et al. (1986) Predictive value of fibronectin levels in normotensive gravid women destined to become preeclamptic. *American Journal of Obstetrics and Gynecology* **154**:1050–1052.

42 Lockwood CJ, Peters JH (1990) Increased levels of ED1+ cellular fibronectin precede the clinical signs of preeclampsia. *American Journal of Obstetrics and Gynecology* **162**:358–362.

43 Zemel MB, Zemel PC, Berry S *et al.* (1990) Altered platelet calcium metabolism as an early predictor of increased peripheral vascular resistance and preeclampsia in urban black women. *New England Journal of Medicine* **323**:434–438.

44 Sanchez-Ramos L, Jones DC, Cullen MT (1991) Urinary calcium as an early marker for preeclampsia. *Obstetrics and Gynecology* **77**:685–688.

45 Sowers JR, Saleh AA, Niyogi T *et al.* (1992) Midgestational hyperinsulinemia and development of preeclampsia. *American Journal of Obstetrics and Gynecology* **166**:294.

46 Campbell S, Pearce JMF, Hackett G *et al.* (1986) Quantitative assessment of uteroplacental blood flow: Early screening test for high risk pregnancies. *Obstetrics and Gynecology* **68**:649–653.

47 Belizan JM, Villar J (1980) The relationship between calcium intake and edema-, proteinuria- and hypertension-gestosis: An hypothesis. *American Journal of Clinical Nutrition* **32**:2202–2210.

48 Villar J, Repke JT (1990) Calcium supplementation during pregnancy may reduce preterm delivery in high risk populations. *American Journal of Obstetrics and Gynecology* **163**:1124–1131.

49 Collins R, Yusuf S, Peto R (1985) Overview of randomized trials of diuretics in pregnancy. *British Medical Journal* **290**:17–23.

50 Rubin PC, Butters L, Clark DM *et al.* (1983) Placebo-controlled trial of atenolol in treatment of pregnancy-associated hypertension. *Lancet* **1**:431–434.

51 Wallenburg HLS, Dekker GA, Makowitz JW (1986) Low-dose aspirin prevents pregnancy-induced hypertension and preeclampsia in angiotensin-sensitive primigravidae. *Lancet* **1**:1–3.

52 Benigni A, Gregorini G, Frusca T *et al.* (1989) Effect of low-dose aspirin on fetal and maternal generation of thromboxane by platelets in women at risk for pregnancy-induced hypertension. *New England Journal of Medicine* **321**:357–362.

53 Schiff E, Peleg E, Goldenberg M *et al.* (1989) The use of aspirin to prevent pregnancy-induced hypertension and lower the ratio of thromboxane A_2 to prostacyclin in relatively high risk pregnancies. *New England Journal of Medicine* **321**:351–356.

54 Chesley LC, Annitto JE (1947) Pregnancy in the patient with hypertensive disease. *American Journal of Obstetrics and Gynecology* **53**:372.

55 Fairlie, FM (1991) Doppler flow velocimetry in hypertension in pregnancy. *Clinics in Perinatology* **18**:749–778.

56 Lazard EM (1925) A preliminary report on the intravenous use of magnesium sulphate in puerperal eclampsia. *American Journal of Obstetrics and Gynecology* **9**:178–188.

57 Pritchard JA (1955) The use of the magnesium ion in the management of eclamptogenic toxemias. *Surgery Gynecology and Obstetrics* **100**:131–140.

58 Cotton DB, Janusz CA, Berman RF (1992) Anticonvulsant effects of magnesium sulfate on hippocampal seizures: Therapeutic implications in preeclampsia–eclampsia. *American Journal of Obstetrics and Gynecology* **166**:1127–1136.

59 Chamberlain GVP, Lewis PJ, Swiet M De, Bulpitt CJ (1978) How obstetricians manage hypertension in pregnancy. *British Medical Journal* **1**:626–629.

60 Walker JJ (1991) Hypertensive drugs in pregnancy: Antihypertension therapy in pregnancy, preeclampsia, and eclampsia. *Clinics in Perinatology* **18**:845–873.

61 Lubbe WF (1987) Hypertension in pregnancy: Whom and how to treat. *British Journal of Clinical Pharmacology* **24**:15–20 (suppl).

62 Naden RP, Redman CWG (1985) Antihypertensive drugs in pregnancy. *Clinics in Perinatology* **12**:521–538.

63 Koch-Weser J (1976) Hydralazine. *New England Journal of Medicine* **295**:320–322.

64 Assali NS, Kaplan S, Oighenstein S, Suyemoto R (1953) Hemodynamic effects of 1-hydrazinophthalazine (Apresoline) in human pregnancy: Results of intravenous administration. *Journal of Clinical Investigation* **32**:922–930.

65 Clark SL, Cotton DB (1988) Clinical indications for pulmonary artery catheterization in the patient with severe preeclampsia. *American Journal of Obstetrics and Gynecology* **158**:453–458.

66 Cotton DB, Longmire S, Jones MM *et al.* (1986) Cardiovascular alterations in severe pregnancy-induced hypertension: Effects of intravenous nitroglycerin

coupled with blood volume expansion. *American Journal of Obstetrics and Gynecology* **154**:1053–1059.

67 Riley AJ (1981) Clinical pharmacology of labetalol in pregnancy. *Journal of Cardiovascular Pharmacology* **3**:53–S59 (suppl).

68 Lunnell NO, Hjemdahl P, Fredholm BB *et al.* (1981) Circulatory and metabolic effects of a combined and β-adrenoceptor blocker (labetalol) in hypertension of pregnancy. *British Journal of Clinical Pharmacology* **12**:345–348.

69 Coevoet B, Leuliet J, Comoy E *et al.* (1980) Labetalol in the treatment of hypertension of pregnancy: Clinical effects and interactions with plasma renin and dopamine betahydroxylase activities, and with plasma concentrations of catecholamine. *Kidney International* **17**:701.

70 Michael CA (1979) Use of labetalol in the treatment of severe hypertension during pregnancy. *British Journal of Clinical Pharmacology* **8**:211–215.

71 Michael CA (1982) The evaluation of labetalol in the treatment of hypertension complicating pregnancy. *British Journal of Clinical Pharmacology* **13**:127–131 (suppl).

72 Mabie WC, Gonzalez AR, Sibai BM, Amon E (1987) A comparative trial of labetalol and hydralazine in the acute management of severe hypertension complicating pregnancy. *Obstetrics and Gynecology* **70**:328–333.

73 Pickles CJ, Symonds EM, Pipkin FB (1989) The fetal outcome in a randomized double-blind controlled trial of labetalol versus placebo in pregnancy-induced hypertension. *British Journal of Obstetrics and Gynaecology* **96**:38–43.

74 Lunell NO, Lewander R, Mamoun I *et al.* (1984) Utero-placental blood flow in pregnancy-induced hypertension. *Scandinavian Journal of Clinical and Laboratory Investigation* **169**:28–35.

75 Pasch T, Schulz V, Hoppelshauser G (1983) Nitroprusside-induced formation of cyanide and its detoxification with thiosulfate during deliberate hypotension. *Journal of Cardiovascular Pharmacology* **5**:77–85.

76 Waisman GD, Mayorga LM, Cámera MI *et al.* (1988) Magnesium plus nifedipine: Potentiation of hypotensive effect in preeclampsia? *American Journal of Obstetrics and Gynecology* **159**:308–309.

77 Herling IM (1984) Intravenous nitroglycerin: Clinical pharmacology and therapeutic considerations. *American Heart Journal* **108**:141–149.

78 Strauss RG, Keefer JR, Burke T, Civetta JM (1980) Hemodynamic monitoring of cardiogenic pulmonary edema complicating toxemia of pregnancy. *Obstetrics and Gynecology* **55**:170–174.

79 Neiger R, Contag SA, Coustan DR (1991) The resolution of preeclampsia-related thrombocytopenia. *Obstetrics and Gynecology* **77**:692–699.

80 Leduc L, Wheeler JM, Kirshon B *et al.* (1992) Coagulation profile in severe preeclampsia. *Obstetrics and Gynecology* **79**:14–18.

81 Watson WJ, Katz VL, Bowes WA (1990) Plasmapheresis during pregnancy. *Obstetrics and Gynecology* **76**:451–457.

82 Anderson WA, Harbert GM Jr (1977) Conservative management of preeclamptic and eclamptic patients: A re-evaluation. *American Journal of Obstetrics and Gynecology* **129**:260–267.

83 Dildy GA, Cotton DB, Phelan JP (1991) Complications of pregnancy induced hypertension. In Clark SL, Cotton DB, Hankins GDV, Phelan JP (eds) *Critical Care Obstetrics*, 2nd edn, Vol. 3, pp. 251–288. Oxford: Blackwell Scientific.

84 Miller JD (1979) The management of cerebral edema. *British Journal of Hospital Medicine* **21**:152–166.

85 Lindheimer MD, Katz AL (1985) Current concepts: Hypertension in pregnancy. *New England Journal of Medicine* **313**:675–680.

86 Connell H, Dalgleish JG, Downing JW (1987) General anesthesia in mothers with severe preeclampsia/eclampsia. *British Journal of Anaesthesia* **59**:1375–1380.

87 Gutsche B (1986) The experts opine: Is epidural block for labor and delivery and for cesarean section a safe form of analgesia in severe preeclampsia or eclampsia? *Survey of Anesthesiology* **30**:304–311.

88 Cotton DB, Benedetti TJ (1980) Use of the Swan-Ganz catheter in obstetrics and gynecology. *Obstetrics and Gynecology* **56**:641–645.

89 Sibai BM (1991) Chronic hypertension in pregnancy. *Clinics in Perinatology* **18**:833–844.

90 Sibai BM (1991) Diagnosis and management of chronic hypertension in pregnancy. *Obstetrics and Gynecology* **78**:451–461.

91 Sibai BM, Akl S, Fairlie F, Moretti M (1990) A protocol for managing severe preeclampsia in the seond trimester. *American Journal of Obstetrics and Gynecology* **163**:733–738.

92 Weitzc C, Khouzami V, Maxwell K *et al.* (1987) Treatment of hypertension in pregnancy with methyldopa: A randomized double-blind study. *International Journal of Gynaecology and Obstetrics* **25**:35–40.

93 Sibai BM, Mabie WC, Shamsa F *et al.* (1990) A comparison of no medication versus methyldopa or labetalol in chronic hypertension during pregnancy. *American Journal of Obstetrics and Gynecology* **162**:960–967.

94 Mabie WC, Gonzalez AR, Sibai BM *et al.* (1987) A comparative trial of labetalol and hydralazine in the acute management of severe hypertension complicating pregnancy. *Obstetrics and Gynecology* **70**:328–333.

95 Plouin PF, Breart G, Mallard F *et al.* (1988) Comparison of antihypertensive efficacy and perinatal safety of labetalol and methyldopa in the treatment of hypertension in pregnancy: A randomized controlled trial. *British Journal of Obstetrics and Gynaecology* **95**:868–876.

96 Committee on Drugs, American Academy of Pediatrics (1989) Transfer of drugs and other chemicals in human milk. *Pediatrics* **84**:924–936.

97 Healy M (1961) Suppressing lactation with oral diuretics. *Lancet* **1**:1353.

98 Davey DA, MacGillivray I (1986) The classification and definition of the hypertensive disorders of pregnancy. *Clinics of Experimental Hypertension – Hypertension in Pregnancy* **B5(1)**: 97–133.

19

Diabetes Mellitus

MARK B. LANDON, STEVEN G. GABBE

INTRODUCTION

Prior to the discovery of insulin in 1921, pregnancy in the diabetic woman was uncommon and was accompanied by high maternal and fetal mortality rates. Through improved understanding of the pathophysiology of diabetes in pregnancy, as well as the implementation of care programs emphasizing normalization of maternal glucose levels, fetal and neonatal mortality have been reduced from approximately 65% before the discovery of insulin to 2–5% at the present time (**Figure 1**). If optimal care is delivered to the diabetic woman, the perinatal mortality rate, excluding major congenital malformations, is nearly equivalent to that observed in normal pregnancies.

Controversy still exists regarding the management of pregnancy complicated by diabetes. While the benefit of careful regulation of maternal glycemia is well accepted, questions remain regarding those factors which contribute to intrauterine deaths and congenital malformations, as well as the significant neonatal morbidity observed in the infant of the diabetic mother (IDM). There is also debate concerning the timing of and need for obstetric intervention including the assessment of fetal well-being and maturity. Finally, the significance of lesser degrees of carbohydrate intolerance during pregnancy such as the diagnosis of gestational diabetes (GDM) has been the subject of debate.

During normal pregnancy, maternal metabolism adjusts to provide adequate nutrition for both the mother and the growing feto-placental unit. Early in pregnancy, glucose homeostasis is affected by increases in estrogen and progesterone which lead to

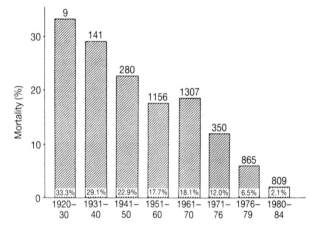

Figure 1. Perinatal mortality in pregnancies complicated by insulin-dependent diabetes mellitus, classes B through R. The number at the top of each column indicates the number of cases in each time period. Adapted from Gabbe.[13]

beta-cell hyperplasia and increased insulin secretion.[1] Increased peripheral utilization of glucose result in lower maternal fasting glucose levels. Glycogen deposition increases in peripheral tissues, accompanied by a decrease in hepatic glucose production. Insulin-dependent diabetics therefore commonly experience periods of hypoglycemia in the first trimester. Additionally, maternal circulating levels of amino acids are reduced, whereas levels of fatty acids, triglycerides and ketones are increased. Maternal mechanisms to offset this state of 'accelerated starvation' include increased protein catabolism and accelerated renal gluconeogenesis.[2]

Lipids become an important maternal fuel as pregnancy advances. Early in pregnancy, fat storage increases. With the rise of human placental lactogen (hPL), a polypeptide hormone produced by the syncytiotrophoblast, lipolysis is stimulated in adipose tissue.[3] The release of glycerol and fatty acids reduces both maternal glucose and amino acid utilization, and in doing so spares these fuels for the fetus. The actions of hPL are responsible, in part, for the 'diabetogenic state' of pregnancy. In the normal pregnant woman, glucose homeostasis is maintained by an exaggerated rate and amount of insulin release which accompanies decreased sensitivity to insulin.[4] Other hormones which appear to modify this response include elevated levels of free cortisol, estrogen and progesterone.

Glucagon, which has both glycogenolytic and gluconeogenic actions, appears to contribute little to the 'diabetogenic stress' of pregnancy. Levels of this hormone show a modest increase over non-pregnant values as pregnancy advances.[5] In normal pregnant women, glucagon levels appear to be suppressed in response to glucose administration. This results in 'facilitated anabolism', periods after meals marked by more prolonged hyperglycemia which counterbalance the 'accelerated starvation' of the fasting state.

With placental growth, larger amounts of contrainsulin factors are synthesized. A woman with overt diabetes cannot respond to this stress and requires additional insulin therapy as pregnancy progresses. Her increased insulin requirement, approximately 30% over the prepregnancy dose, is roughly equivalent to the endogenous increase seen in a normal gestation. If the pregnant woman has borderline pancreatic reserve, or if she is obese and therefore insulin-resistant, it is possible that her endogenous insulin production will be inadequate. Diabetes will then be revealed for the first time, particularly in late gestation. Unlike known insulin-requiring patients, obese GDM with beta-cell reserve, but presumed peripheral insulin resistance, may experience large increases in both their insulin secretion and requirement during pregnancy. In these women, postprandial insulin response is sluggish, and peak insulin levels occur 1 h after a meal, in contrast to 30 min in normal individuals.[6] In addition to decreased first-phase insulin response, impaired suppression of hepatic glucose production is observed in GDM in late gestation.[7] With weight loss following pregnancy, most GDM women will exhibit normal glucose homeostasis and will no longer require insulin.

Maternal glucose appears to pass to the fetus by carrier-mediated facilitated diffusion. Fetal blood glucose levels usually remain 20–30 mg/dl lower than those of the mother. There is a close correlation between fetal glucose uptake and maternal blood levels.[8] The fetal level is normally maintained within narrow limits because maternal glucose homeostasis is well regulated. Protein hormones such as insulin, glucagon, growth hormone and hPL do not cross the placenta. Ketoacids appear to diffuse freely across the placenta and may serve as a fetal fuel during periods of maternal starvation.[9]

During pregnancy in the insulin-dependent diabetic woman, periods of hyperglycemia result in fetal hyperglycemia. Persistently elevated levels of glucose will stimulate the fetal pancreas, resulting in beta-cell hyperplasia and fetal hyperinsulinemia (**Figure 2**).[10] Other potent insulin secretagogues, such as amino acids, may be elevated in the sera of diabetic women and may be transferred in increased quantity to the fetus. These nutrients appear to play the major role in inducing excessive fetal growth. Metzger and colleagues have demonstrated that birthweight can be correlated with fasting concentrations of several maternal plasma amino acids.[11] In studies of GDM women, Kalkoff has confirmed this relationship for the amino acids serine, prolene and ornithine.[12] Hyperinsulinism also contributes to the increased risk of intrauterine death, respiratory distress syndrome, hypoglycemia, and other morbidity seen in the IDM.

Maternal/Fetal Risks

Perinatal morbidity and mortality

In the past, sudden and unexplained stillbirth occurred in 10–30% pregnancies complicated by insulin-depen-

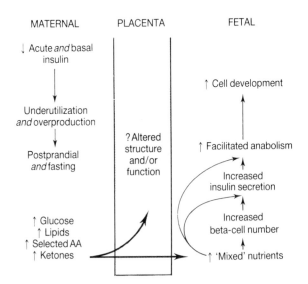

Figure 2. The modified Pedersen hypothesis as described by Freinkel et al.[26] Glucose and other substrates stimulate fetal insulin release resulting in macrosomia and other morbidity observed in the infant of the diabetic mother.

dent diabetes mellitus (IDDM).[13] Although relatively uncommon today, such losses still plague the pregnancies of patients who do not receive optimal care. Stillbirths have been observed most often after the 36th week of pregnancy in patients with vascular disease and pre-eclampsia, or in patients with poor glycemic control exhibiting fetal macrosomia and hydramnios. The precise cause of the excessive stillbirth rate in pregnancies complicated by diabetes remains unknown. Because extramedullary hematopoiesis is frequently observed in stillborn IDMs, chronic intrauterine hypoxia has been cited as a likely cause of these intrauterine fetal deaths.

Maternal diabetes may produce alterations in red blood cell oxygen release and placental blood flow.[14] Reduced uterine blood flow is thought to contribute to the increased incidence of intrauterine growth retardation (IUGR) observed in pregnancies complicated by diabetic vasculopathy. Investigations using radioactive tracers have also suggested a relationhip between poor maternal metabolic control and reduced uteroplacental blood flow.[15] Ketoacidosis and pre-eclampsia – two factors known to be associated with an increased incidence of intrauterine deaths – may further decrease uterine blood flow. In diabetic ketoacidosis, hypovolemia and hypotension caused by dehydration may reduce flow through the intervillous space, while in pre-eclampsia, narrowing and vasospasm of spiral arterioles may result.

Alterations in fetal carbohydrate metabolism may also contribute to intrauterine asphyxia.[16–18] There is considerable evidence linking hyperinsulinemia and fetal hypoxemia: Hyperinsulinemia induced in fetal lambs by an infusion of exogenous insulin produces an increase in oxygen consumption and a decrease in arterial oxygen content.[19] Thus, hyperinsulinemia in the fetus of the diabetic mother may increase fetal metabolic rate and oxygen requirements in the face of several factors such as hyperglycemia, ketoacidosis, pre-eclampsia and maternal vasculopathy, which can reduce placental blood flow and fetal oxygenation.

Congenital malformations

With the reduction in stillbirths and a marked decrease in neonatal mortality related to hyaline membrane disease, congenital malformations have emerged as the most important cause of perinatal loss in pregnancies complicated by IDDM. In the past, these anomalies were responsible for approximately 10% of all perinatal deaths. At present, however, malformations account for 30–50% of perinatal mortality.[20] Neonatal deaths now exceed stillbirths in pregnancies complicated by IDDM, and fatal congenital malformations account for this changing pattern.

Most studies have documented a two to four-fold increase in major malformations in infants of IDDM mothers. Kucera, in reviewing 47 articles, reported an incidence of anomalies in offspring of diabetic mothers of 4.8% (**Figure 3**).[21] In a prospective analysis, Simpson observed an 8.5% incidence of major anomalies in the IDDM population, while the malformation rate in a small group of concurrently gathered control subjects was 2.4%.[20] Similar figures were obtained in the Diabetes in Early Pregnancy Study in the USA.[22] The incidence of major anomalies was 2.1% in 389 control patients and 9.0% in 279 IDDM women. In general, the incidence of major malformations in worldwide studies of offspring of IDDM mothers has ranged from 5 to 10%.

The insult that causes malformations in IDM impacts on most organ systems and must act before the 7th week of gestation (**Table 1**).[23] Central nervous system malformations, particularly anencephaly, open

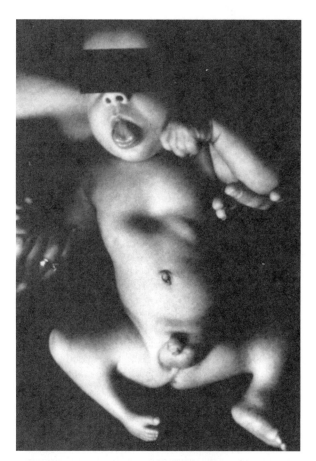

Figure 3. Infant of a diabetic mother with caudal regression syndrome. The mother of this infant presented with class F diabetes at 26 weeks, in poor glycemic control. Ultrasound examination revealed absent lower lumbar spine and sacrum and hypoplastic lower extremities.

Table 1
Congenital malformations in infants of diabetic mothers

Cardiovascular
Transposition of the great vessels
Ventricular septal defect
Atrial septal defect
Hypoplastic left ventricle
Situs inversus
Anomalies of the aorta

Central nervous system
Anencephaly
Encephalocele
Meningomyelocele
Holoprosencephaly
Microcephaly

Skeletal
Caudal regression syndrome
Spina bifida

Genitourinary
Absent kidney (Potter syndrome)
Polycystic kidneys
Double ureter

Gastrointestinal
Tracheoesophageal fistula
Bowel atresia
Imperforate anus

spina bifida and, possibly, holoprosencephaly, are increased several fold. Cardiac anomalies, which are the most common malformations, consist primarily of ventricular septal defects and complex lesions such as transposition of the great vessels. The congenital defect thought to be most characteristic of diabetic embryopathy is sacral agenesis or caudal dysplasia, an anomaly found 200–400 times more often in the offspring of diabetic women.[21]

It appears that a derangement in maternal metabolism, possibly in association with a greater genetic susceptibility, contributes to abnormal embryogenesis.[24] The Diabetes in Early Pregnancy Study demonstrated an association between certain maternal HLA haplotypes and malformations in the offspring of diabetic women.[24]

Several mechanisms have been proposed by which the above teratogenic factors produce malformations. Maternal hyperglycemia has been proposed by most investigators as the primary factor, but hyperketonemia and hypoglycemia also have been suggested.[25] Freinkel suggested that anomalies might arise from inhibition of glycolysis, the key energy-producing process during embryogenesis. He found that D-mannose added to the culture medium of rat embryos inhibited glycolysis and produced growth deficiency and derangements of neural tube closure.[26] Freinkel stressed the sensitivity of normal embryogenesis to alterations in these key energy-producing pathways, a process he labeled 'fuel-mediated' teratogenesis. Goldman and Baker have suggested that the mechanism responsible for the increased incidence of neural tube defects in embryos cultured in a hyperglycemic medium may involve a functional deficiency of arachidonic acid, because supplementation with arachidonic acid or myo-inositol will reduce the frequency of neural tube defects in this experimental model.[27] Pinter and colleagues have reported that supplemental arachidonic acid reverses gross as well as ultrastructural abnormalities produced by the in vitro culture of rat embryos in a hyperglycemic medium.[28] Finally, somatomedin inhibitors may act synergistically with hyperglycemia and elevated ketone levels to produce structural defects.[29]

Studies using a variety of animal models suggest a role for hypoglycemia in the pathogenesis of malformations, yet human data conflict with these observations.[30] Data from both the Diabetes in Early Pregnancy Study and the California Diabetes and Pregnancy Program results have failed to show a relationship between maternal hypoglycemia and congenital anomalies.[22,31]

Macrosomia

Excessive growth may predispose the IDM to shoulder dystocia, traumatic birth injury and asphyxia. Newborn adiposity in offspring of GDM women may be associated with a significant risk for obesity and carbohydrate intolerance in later life.[32]

Some have defined macrosomia as a birthweight in excess of 4000–4500 g, but others prefer categorizing infants as large for gestational age (LGA: a birthweight above the 90th percentile) using population-specific growth curves. According to these definitions, macrosomia has been observed in as many as 50% of pregnancies complicated by gestational diabetes mellitus (GDM) and 40% of IDDM pregnancies. Delivery of an infant weighing greater than 4500 g occurs *ten times* more often in diabetic women than in a non-diabetic control population (**Figure 4**).[33]

Fetal macrosomia in the IDM is reflected by increased adiposity and muscle mass and organomegaly. Because brain growth is not increased, the head circumference usually remains in the normal range.[34] This disproportionate increase in the size of the trunk and shoulders when compared with the head may contribute to the likelihood of a difficult vaginal delivery.[35] The most eloquent descriptions of the characteristic appearance of the macrosomic IDM have been given by Farquhar.[36] In noting that these infants closely resemble each other, he stated the 'fat confers anon-

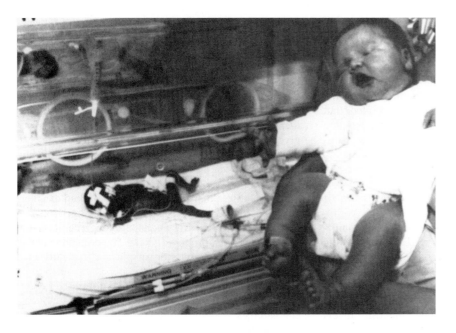

Figure 4. Two extremes of growth abnormalities in infants of diabetic mothers. The small growth-deficient infant on the left weighed 470 g and is the offspring of a woman with nephropathy and hypertension, delivered at 28 weeks gestation. The neonate on the right is the 5100 g baby of a woman with suboptimally controlled class C diabetes.

ymity and a brotherhood of identicality in IDMs'. An increase in total body fat in the IDM has been supported by direct measurements as well as by assessment of subcutaneous stores using skinfold thickness measurements. Brans and colleagues performed anthropometric measurements in a large series of IDMs and noted that 67% had increased skinfold thickness when compared with non-diabetic controls.[37] Skinfold thickness can also be correlated with birthweight.[35,38] Enzi and coworkers found that skinfold thickness, body fat mass and fat-cell weight in full-term newborns of GDM women and insulin-dependent diabetes women were greater than in infants of non-diabetic mothers.[39] These authors analyzed gluteal fat biopsies in 8 infants of IDDM women and 17 of GDM women as well as 17 controls. Fat-cell number was similar in the diabetic and control groups, but fat-cell hypertrophy was observed in the IDM, probably secondary to an increase in triglyceride content of the adipocytes. The amount of subcutaneous fat present in the IDM may be an indication of the quality of diabetic control achieved during gestation. In Enzi and coworkers' study, maternal blood glucose levels as well as neonatal immunoreactive insulin levels measured in cord blood were significantly correlated with fat-cell weight.

Farquhar also suggested that the plethoric appearance of these newborns was not a result of edema, but actually reflected excess adipose tissue. Several investigations have confirmed that total body water is actually decreased in the IDM when compared with controls of similar birthweights.[38,40] The reduction in total body water is even more pronounced in LGA IDMs, since less intracellular water may be found in cells which have increased fat content.[38]

Several autopsy studies have confirmed the existence of pancreatic islet hyperplasia in the IDM.[34,40] Milner and colleagues, using cytochemical techniques, have demonstrated a specific increase in beta-cell mass in the pancreatic islets of IDMs when compared with control infants.[41] This finding was observed in approximately 40% of the IDMs. Increased beta-cell mass may be identified as early as the second trimester.[42]

Using a rhesus monkey model, Susa and coworkers have confirmed the central role of excess insulin in disordered fetal growth and development.[43] Subcutaneous minipumps were implanted in the monkeys to provide a constant insulin infusion for 2 weeks during the third trimester. In order to observe the independent effect of fetal hyperinsulinemia, maternal and fetal glucose levels were kept within the normal range. The findings of increased body weight, as well as organomegaly of the liver, placenta and heart, in the infused rhesus fetuses mimic the features characteristic of the human macrosomic IDM.

Futher evidence supporting the Pedersen hypothesis has come from studies of amniotic fluid and cord-blood insulin and C-peptide levels. Both are increased in the amniotic fluid of insulin-treated diabetic women at term.[44] Elevated amniotic fluid insulin levels are observed in LGA infants of insulin-dependent diabetic mothers, as well as those of women with GDM.[44,45] Lin *et al.* found that C-peptide levels in amniotic fluid could be correlated with both maternal glucose control and birthweight.[46] These authors noted that 78% of macrosomic infants had elevated amniotic fluid C-peptide levels compared with a 48% rate overall in 33 diabetic subjects. Persson and colleagues have also confirmed a positive relationship between maternal blood glucose and amniotic fluid C-peptide in pregnancies complicated by IDDM and GDM.[47]

Cord-blood levels of C-peptide are also increased in the IDM.[48] IDMs exhibit a more brisk insulin response to a glucose load than infants of non-diabetic women. This response appears to be greater in the macrosomic IDM.[49] Interestingly, Sosenko's study revealed that only macrosomic infants who developed hypoglycemia had elevated C-peptide levels at birth. These data suggest that fetal hyperinsulinism cannot completely explain the high incidence of macrosomia found in the IDM.

Over the past two decades, well-organized plans of care emphasizing control of blood glucose within physiological ranges have eliminated much of the morbidity and mortality suffered by the IDM. The results of several clinical series have validated the Pedersen hypothesis inasmuch as good maternal glycemic control has been associated with a decline in the incidence of macrosomia. In a series of 260 insulin-dependent women achieving fasting plasma glucose levels between 109 and 140 mg/dl, Gabbe observed 58 (22%) macrosomic infants.[50] Kitzmiller and Cloherty reported that 11% of 134 women achieving fasting levels between 105 and 121 mg/dl were delivered of an infant with a birthweight in excess of 4000 g.[51] Several reports have demonstrated a reduction in the rate of macrosomia when more physiological control is achieved. Roversi instituted a program of 'maximally tolerated' insulin administration and observed macrosomia in only 6% of cases, while Jovanovic and coworkers eliminated macrosomia in 52 women who achieved a mean glucose level of 80–87 mg/dl throughout gestation.[52,53] On the other hand, it has been reported that the incidence of macrosomia in pregnancies complicated by diabetes mellitus does not increase significantly until mean glucose values approach 130 mg/dl.[54] Most recently, Jovanovic and colleagues have suggested that non-fasting blood glucose levels obtained during the third trimester best correlate with birthweight.[55] Differences in methodology employed in the assessment of glycemic control may in part explain some of the disparate findings cited above. In a study using daily capillary glucose values obtained during the second and third trimesters in insulin-dependent patients, only 9% of infants of women with mean capillary glucose values less than 110 mg/dl were found to be LGA compared with 34% of infants of women with less optimal control.[56] Thus, it appears that the frequency of excessive fetal growth may be reduced by maintaining excellent glucose control in women with IDDM.

Hypoglycemia

Neonatal hypoglycemia, a blood glucose below 40 mg/dl during the first 12 h of life, results from a rapid drop in plasma glucose concentrations following clamping of the umbilical cord. The degree of hypoglycemia may be influenced by at least two factors: (1) maternal glucose control during the latter half of pregnancy and (2) maternal glycemic control during labor and delivery. Maternal blood glucose levels greater than 90 mg/dl during delivery have been found to increase significantly the frequency of neonatal hypoglycemia.[57] Presumably, prior poor maternal glucose control can result in fetal beta-cell hyperplasia, leading to exaggerated insulin release following delivery. IDMs exhibiting hypoglycemia have elevated cord C-peptide and free insulin levels at birth and an exaggerated pancreatic response to glucose loading.[58]

Other mechanisms for neonatal hypoglycemia in the IDM have been proposed. Fetal hyperinsulinemia is associated with suppression of plasma free fatty acid levels and diminished glycogenolysis. Limited data also suggest that the IDM may have diminished counter-regulatory responses of both glycagon and catecholamines.[59]

Neonatal hypoglycemia is commonly observed in the IDM. In reported series, the frequency of this complication has ranged from 18 to 49%.[51,60] Gabbe observed that 99 of 257 IDMs (39%) became hypoglycemic after delivery, while Kitzmiller and Cloherty reported that 65 of 113 IDMs (49%) developed hypoglycemia despite mean maternal fasting blood glucose levels of 105–121 mg/dl.[50,51] Although Karlsson and Kjellmer were unable to correlate maternal blood glucose control with the incidence of hypoglycemia, a few cases of neonatal hypoglycemia have been noted in several recent series in which physiological maternal glucose levels were maintained.[61] Jovanovic et al. reported only one case of hypoglycemia in the offspring of diabetic women whose mean blood glucose was less than 87 mg/dl.[53] Similarly, Roversi et al. found that only 35 of 240 (15%) infants became hypoglycemic after birth. In this study, the mean fasting plasma glucose was 70 mg/dl.[52] Ylinen and colleagues have also demonstrated that maternal glucose control during late pregnancy may influence the development of neonatal hypoglycemia.[62] In their series of 104 diabetic women, mean HbA1c levels were higher in women whose offspring became hypoglycemic after delivery.

Respiratory distress syndrome

The precise mechanism by which maternal diabetes affects pulmonary development remains unknown. Experimental animal studies have focused primarily on the effects of hyperglycemia and hyperinsulinemia on pulmonary surfactant biosynthesis. An extensive review of the literature confirms that both of these factors are involved in delayed pulmonary maturation in the IDM.[63]

In vitro studies have documented that insulin can interfere with substrate availability for surfactant biosynthesis. Smith and colleagues, using monolayers of cultured cells from fetal lungs, demonstrated that insulin stimulates H^3 choline incorporation into phosphatidylcholine (lecithin).[64] More significantly, these investigators noted that when insulin was added to cultures with cortisol present, steroid-enhanced lecithin synthesis was abolished. The incorporation of substrates into lecithin may be in part dependent on the concentration of insulin present. Engle found that low concentrations of insulin could increase glucose incorporation into lecithin, while higher levels resulted in diminished glucose and choline uptake by fetal rate type II alveolar cells.[65] Hyperglycemia *per se* did not alter *de novo* lecithin synthesis, suggesting that hyperinsulinism is primarily responsible for inhibition of surfactant formulation.

Smith has postulated that insulin interferes with the normal timing of glucocorticoid-induced pulmonary maturation in the fetus.[66] Apparently, cortisol acts on pulmonary fibroblasts to induce synthesis of fibroblast-pneumocyte factor, which then acts on type II cells to stimulate phospholipid synthesis.[67] Carlson and coworkers have shown than insulin blocks cortisol action at the level of the fibroblast by reducing the production of fibroblast-pneumocyte factor.[68] An alternative explanation for insulin's antagonism of cortisol-induced lung lecithin synthesis has been proposed by Rooney and Ingleson.[69] In their study of cultures of fetal rat lung cells, dexamethasone-induced stimulation of choline phosphate cytidyltransferase was prevented by insulin administration. This important enzyme is involved in the pathway which eventually converts phosphatidic acid to phosphatidylglycerol (PG).

Clinical studies investigating the effect of maternal diabetes on fetal lung maturation have produced conflicting data. In a series of 805 infants of diabetic mothers delivered over a 10-year period, Robert and coworkers found that corrected risk for respiratory distress syndrome (RDS) to be nearly six times that of mothers without diabetes mellitus.[70] With the introduction of protocols which have emphasized glucose control and antepartum surveillance until lung maturity has been established, RDS has become a less common occurrence in the IDM. Several studies agree that in well-controlled diabetic women delivered at term, the risk of RDS is no higher than that observed in the general population.[71,72] In studies which have emphasized glycemic control, RDS has virtually been eliminated.[53,60]

Calcium and magnesium metabolism

Neonatal hypocalcemia, serum levels below 7 mg/dl, occurs at an increased rate in the IDM when one con-

trosl for predisposing factors such as prematurity and birth asphyxia.[73] Hypocalcemia in the IDM has been associated with a failure to increase parathyroid hormone synthesis normally following birth.[73] Decreased serum magnesium levels have also been documented in pregnant diabetic women as well as their infants. Mimouni has described reduced amniotic fluid magnesium concentrations in women with IDDM.[74] These findings may be explained by a drop in fetal urinary magnesium excretion, which would accompany a relative magnesium-deficient state. Paradoxically, then, magnesium deficiency may inhibit fetal parathyroid hormone secretion.

Maternal classification and risk assessment

Priscilla White first noted that the patient's age at onset of diabetes, the duration of the disease and the presence of vasculopathy significantly influenced perinatal outcome. Her pioneering work led to a classification system which has been widely applied to pregnant women with diabetes.[75] A modification of this scheme is presented in **Table 2**. Some clinicians prefer to categorize IDDM women into two groups – those with and without vascular complications. Thus, the White classification is of greatest value when comparing series of patients between institutions. Counseling a patient and formulating a plan of management requires assessment of both maternal and fetal risk. The identification of vascular complications facilitates this evaluation.

Class A_1 diabetes mellitus includes those patients who have demonstrated carbohydrate intolerance during a 100-g 3-h glucose tolerance test (GTT); however,

Table 2
Modified White classification of pregnant diabetic women

Class	Diabetes onset age (years)		Duration (years)	Vascular disease	Insulin need
Gestational diabetes					
A_1	any		any	0	0
A_2	any		any	0	+
Pregestational diabetes					
B	> 20		< 10	0	+
C	10–19	or	10–19	0	+
D	< 10	or	> 20	+	+
F	any		any	+	+
R	any		any	+	+
T	any		any	+	+
H	any		any	+	+

Modified from White.[75]

their fasting and 2-h postprandial glucose levels are less than 105 mg/dl and 120 mg/dl, respectively. These patients are generally managed by dietary regulation alone. If fasting or postprandial hyperglycemia requires insulin, patients are designated class A_2.

The Third International Workshop Conference on Gestational Diabetes, sponsored by the American Diabetes Association in cooperation with the American College of Obstetricians and Gynecologists, has recommended the continued use of the term 'gestational diabetes', rather than class A diabetes, to describe women with carbohydrate intolerance of variable severity with onset or recognition during pregnancy.[76] The term 'gestational diabetes' fails to specify whether the patient requires dietary adjustment alone or treatment with diet and insulin. This distinction is important because those patients who are normoglycemic while fasting have a significantly lower perinatal mortality rate.[77] They do not appear to experience an increased incidence of intrauterine deaths in late pregnancy. Gestational diabetics who require insulin are at greater risk for a poor perinatal outcome than those controlled by diet alone. This observation probably relfects more marked maternal hyperglycemia and, in some cases, a delay in the institution of insulin therapy.

Patients requiring insulin are designated by the letters B, C, D, R, F and T. Class B patients are those whose onset of disease occurs after age 20. They have had diabetes less than 10 years and have no vascular complications. Included in this subgroup of patients are those who have been previously treated with oral hypoglycemic agents. Oral hypoglycemics are not used during pregnancy in the USA. Class C diabetes includes patients who have the onset of their disease between the ages of 10 and 19 or have had the disease for 10–19 years. Vasular disease is not present. Class D represents women whose disease is of 20 years duration or more, or whose onset occurred before age 10, or who have hypertension or benign retinopathy. The latter includes microaneurysms, exudate and venous dilation.

Nephropathy

Class F diabetes describes the 5–10% of patients with underlying renal disease. This includes those with reduced creatinine clearance and/or proteinuria of at least 300 mg in 24 h measured during the first trimester. Patients with nephropathy are at increased risk for pre-eclampsia, fetal growth deficiency and premature delivery. Women with subnephrotic range proteinuria and normal creatinine clearance usually progress well into the third trimester before requiring delivery. However, several factors present prior to 20 weeks gestation appear to be predictive of poor perinatal outcome in class F women (e.g. perinatal death or birthweight less than 1100 g). These include:

- proteinura >3.0 g/24 h

- serum creatinine >1.5 mg/dl

- anemia with hematocrit <25%

- hypertension (mean arterial pressure >107 mmHg).

In a series of 27 class F women, if any one of the above factors was present early in gestation, over half of the pregnancies resulted in perinatal deaths or infants weighing less than 1100 g.[78] In contrast, when no risk factors were present, over 90% experienced a successful perinatal outcome.

Several studies have failed to demonstrate a permanent worsening of diabetic renal disease as a result of pregnancy.[79,80] Kitzmiller and colleagues reviewed 35 pregnancies complicated by diabetic nephropathy.[79] Proteinuria increased in 69%, including one patient with an excretion of 2 g in the first trimester which increased to 20 g by the end of gestation. Hypertension developed in 73% of women. Following delivery, proteinuria declined in 65% of cases. In only two patients did protein excretion increase after gestation. Changes in creatinine clearance during pregnancy are variable in class F patients. Kitzmiller, in reviewing 44 patients from the literature, noted that about one-third had an expected rise in creatinine clearance during gestation, compared with one-third who had a decline of more than 15% by the third trimester.[81] Of interest, most patients with a severe reduction in creatinine clearance (<50 ml/min) measured during the first trimester did not demonstrate a further reduction in clearance during pregnancy.[81] However, a decline in renal function was evident in 20–30% of cases. Hayslett and Reece have confirmed that any deterioration of renal function after pregnancy is consistent with the natural course of diabetic nephropathy and is not related to pregnancy *per se*.[82]

With improved survival of diabetic patients following renal transplantation, a small group of kidney recipients has now achieved pregnancy (class T). Nine cases of pregnancy complicated by diabetes and prior renal transplantation have been described.[83] In this series, there were no episodes of renal allograft rejection. Prednisone and azathioprine were administered throughout gestation without any significant effects. A single maternal death and two fetal deaths did occur in patients with pre-existing peripheral vascular disease. Superimposed pre-eclampsia was observed in six patients. All seven surviving infants were delivered prior to term, with fetal distress documented in six of these cases.

Retinopathy

Class R diabetes designates patients with proliferative retinopathy. Retinopathy is observed with a similar frequency in women who have or have not experienced pregnancy. Klein and colleagues prospectively evaluated 171 pregnant diabetic women, comparing them with 298 non-pregnant controls. They found that pregnancy conveyed greater than a two-fold independent risk for progression of retinopathy.[84] Retinopathy may worsen significantly during pregnancy despite the major advances that have been made in diagnosis and treatment. Laser photocoagulation therapy during pregnancy with careful follow-up has helped maintain many pregnancies which in the past may have been terminated prior to a gestational age at which neonatal survival would be possible. Fortunately, most patients who require laser photocoagulation respond to this therapy and should therefore be promptly treated. However, those women who demonstrate severe florid disc neovascularization which is unresponsive to laser therapy during early pregnancy may be at great risk for deterioration of their vision. Termination of pregnancy should be considered in this group of patients. All insulin-dependent patients should undergo ophthalmologic examination in early pregnancy. Patients with minimal disease are followed each trimester, whereas patients with significant fundoscopic changes are examined more frequently.

In a large series of 172 patients, including 40 cases with background retinopathy and 11 with proliferative changes, only one patient developed new onset proliferative retinopathy during pregnancy.[85] Progression to proliferative retinopathy during pregnancy rarely occurs in women with background retinopathy or those without any eye ground changes. In Kitzmiller's review, of 561 women in these two categories, only 17 (3.0%) developed neovascularization during gestation.[86] In contrast, 23 of 26 (88.5%) with untreated proliferative disease experienced worsening retinopathy during pregnancy.

Moloney and Drury have reported that pregnancy may increase the prevalence of some background changes.[87] These authors noted a characteristic increase in streak-blob hemorrhages and soft exudates which often resolved between examinations.[87] Retinopathy progressed despite strict metabolic control. Phelps and colleagues have related worsening retinal disease to plasma glucose at the first prenatal visit as well as the magnitude of improvement in glycemia during early pregnancy.[88] Chang and colleagues have also reported the development of proliferative changes with rapid normalization of glucose control.[89] Whether improved control contributes to a deterioration of background retinopathy remains uncertain.

In addition to background and proliferative eye disease, Sinclair and colleagues have described vaso-occlusive lesions associated with the development of macular edema during pregnancy.[90] Cystic macular edema is most often found in patients with proteinuric nephropathy and hypertensive disease leading to retinal edema. Macular capillary permeability is a feature of this process. The degree of macular edema is directly related to the fall in plasma oncotic pressure present in these women. In Sinclair's series, seven women with minimal or no retinopathy before becoming pregnant developed severe macular edema associated with pre-proliferative or proliferative retinopathy during the course of the pregnancies. Although proliferation was controlled with photocoagulation, the macular edema worsened until delivery in all cases and was often aggravated by photocoagulation.[90] While both macular edema and retinopathy regressed after delivery in some patients, in others these pathologic processes persisted, resulting in significant visual loss.

Coronary artery disease

Class H diabetes refers to the presence of diabetes of any duration associated with ischemic myocardial disease are at an increased risk for mortality during gestation.[91] This is especially true of women with a previous myocardial infarction or an infarction during pregnancy. For these cases, maternal mortality rates exceed 50%.[92] While there are a few reports of successful pregnancies following myocardial infarction in diabetic women, cardiac status should be assessed carefully early in gestation or preferably prior to pregnancy. If electrocardiogram (ECG) abnormalities are encountered, echocardiography may be employed to assess ventricular function or modified stress testing may be undertaken. Based on these findings, a decision must then be made whether to continue the pregnancy.

Management Options

Prepregnancy

Anomalies of the cardiac, renal and central nervous systems arise during the first weeks of gestation, a time when it is most unusual for patients to seek prenatal care. Therefore, the management and counseling of women with diabetes in the reproductive age group should begin prior to conception (**Table 3**). Unfortunately, few diabetic women seek prepregnancy care.[93]

Fuhrmann has reported that intensive treatment begun prior to conception in 307 diabetic women reduced the malformation rate to 1%.[94] Nearly 90% of women in this study maintained mean glucose levels less than 100 mg/dl. In contrast, the incidence of anomalies in the offspring of 593 diabetic women who registered for care after 8 weeks gestation was 8.0%

Table 3
Congenital malformation rates (percentages in parentheses) in offspring of diabetic women according to timing of prenatal care

Author	Pre- or periconceptional enrolment	Late enrolment
Fuhrmann[94]	2/185 (1.1)	31/473 (6.6)
Steel[137]	2/114 (1.8)	9/86 (10.5)
Mills[22]	17/347 (4.9)	25/279 (9.0)
Kitzmiller[31]	1/84 (1.2)	12/110 (10.9)

(47/593), only 20% of whom had mean daily glucose levels of less than 100 mg/dl. Mills has reported that diabetic women registered prior to pregnancy had fewer infants with anomalies when compared with late registrants (4.9 *vs* 9.0%).[22] While the incidence of 4.9% remains higher than that in a normal control population (2%), normalization of glycemia was not established in the early entry group. Most recently, Kitzmiller has reported normalization of the major malformation rate in diabetic women who were well controlled before conception.[31]

Glycosylated hemoglobin levels obtained prior to or during the first trimester may be used to counsel diabetic women regarding the risk for an anomalous infant. Overall, the risk of a major fetal anomaly may be as high as 1:4 or 1:5 when the glycosylated hemoglobin level is several percent above normal values.[95,96] Regardless of the glycosylated hemoglobin value obtained, all patients require a careful program of surveillance as outlined earlier to detect fetal malformations. It is unclear whether the risk of miscarriage is elevated in diabetic women.[97] It does appear to be increased with marked elevations in glycosylated hemoglobin. However, for diabetic women in good control, there appears to be no greater likelihood for miscarriage.[98]

With the increasing evidence that poor control is responsible for the congenital malformations seen in pregnancies complicated by diabetes, it is apparent that preconception counseling involving the patient and her family should be instituted. Physicians who care for young women with diabetes must be aware of the importance of such counseling. At this time, the nonpregnant patient may learn techniques for self-glucose monitoring as well as the need for proper dietary management. Questions may be answered regarding risk factors for complications and the plan for general manatement of diabetes in pregnancy. A thorough evaluation for vascular complications can also be accomplished. Planning for pregnancy should optimally be accomplished over several months. Glycosylated hemoglobin measurements are performed to aid in the timing of conception. The patient should attempt to achieve a glycosylated hemoglobin level within two standard deviations of the mean for the reference laboratory.[99] Finally, because recent evidence suggests that folic acid supplementation may decrease the risk of fetal spina bifida, diabetic women attempting to conceive may be started on 4 mg of folate daily to be continued through the first 12 weeks of pregnancy.[100]

Prenatal

Detection of diabetes in pregnancy

Altogether, 90% of the cases of diabetes which complicate pregnancy are gestational diabetes (GDM).[101] The detection of GDM is, therefore, an important diagnostic challenge. Patients with GDM represent a group with significant risk for developing glucose intolerance later in life. It has been reported that 50% of these patients will become diabetic in the 15 years following pregnancy.[102]

The normal values for the diagnostic glucose tolerance test (GTT), according to the National Diabetes Data Group, Carpenter's and the World Health Organization (WHO) are listed in **Table 4**. The WHO criteria are not different from non-pregnant thresholds, thus representing a more stringent approach to diagnosis. Carpenter's plasma modification of O'Sullivan's data may actually represent a more valid transformation of the original whole blood cut-off points.[103,104] The patient must have two abnormal postprandial glucose determinations to be designated a gestational diabetic. Women who demonstrate one abnormal value on the diagnositc 3-h GTT are apparently at increased risk for fetal macrosomia.[105] While Langer and colleagues prefer to recognize and treat such patients as GDM, further confirmation is necessary to insure that these patients are at a risk for adverse perinatal outcomes equal to that of women who meet the present diagnostic criteria for GDM.[105] Recent data from a collaborative European study suggests that these lesser degrees of carbohydrate intolerance do not pose an increased risk for fetal complications such as macrosomia.[106] Since O'Sullivan's original data were based on the subsequent maternal development of diabetes and not perinatal outcome, debate continues as to the true significance of GDM. Until a large prospective study of untreated women with varying degrees of carbohydrate tolerance is performed, to ascertain what level of glycemia poses a risk to the fetus, practitioners will have to rely on the present criteria for diagnosis and treatment.

As noted above, GDM is a state restricted to pregnant women whose impaired glucose tolerance is discovered during pregnancy. Because, in most cases, patients with GDM have normal fasting glucose levels, some challenge of glucose tolerance must be under-

Table 4

Detection of diabetes during pregnancy (glucose mg/dl)

Authors	Load	Fasting	Hours 1	Hours 2	Hours 3	Specimen
NDDG	100 g	105	190	165	145	Plasma
Carpenter[103]	100 g	95	180	155	140	Plasma
O'Sullivan[76]	100 g	90	165	145	125	Whole blood
WHO	75 mg	≤ 140		≤ 200		Plasma

NDDG, National Diabetes Data Group; WHO, World Heath Organization.

taken. Traditionally, obstetricians have relied upon historical and clinical risk factors to select those patients most likely to develop GDM. This group included patients with a family history of diabetes, or those whose past pregnancies were marked by an unexplained stillbirth, or the delivery of a malformed or macrosomic infant. Obesity, hypertension, glycosuria and maternal age over 30 years were other indications for screening. Interestingly, over half of all patients who exhibit an abnormal GTT lack the risk factors mentioned above. Coustan and colleagues have reported that, in a series of 6214 women, using historical risk factors and an arbitrary age cut-off of 30 years for screening, would miss 35% of all cases of GDM.[107]

It is therefore recommended that *all* pregnant women be screened for gestational diabetes. A number of methods have been proposed.[103] The technique we employ is a 50-g oral glucose load followed by a glucose determination 1 h later.[76] The patient need not be fasting when this test is performed. However, sensitivity is improved if the test is performed in the fasting state.[108] The sensitivity of this screening technique is approximately 80%, and its specificity approaches 90%. The test is generally performed at 24–28 weeks gestation. Patients whose plasma glucose level equals or exceeds 130–140 mg/dl should be evaluated with a 3-h GTT. A lower threshold will enhance sensitivity while diminishing specificity, thus requiring more diagnostic 3-h GTTs to be performed. A normal glucose screen in early pregnancy does not necessarily rule out later development of GDM. We reserve screening in early pregnancy for women with a previous history of GDM, marked obesity, a strong family history of diabetes, or those receiving glucocorticoid therapy for another disease. One can expect approximately 15% of patients with an abnormal screening value to have an abnormal 3-h GTT. However, most patients whose 1-h screening value exceeds 190 mg/dl will exhibit abnormal glucose tolerance.[103] In these women, it is preferable to check a fasting glucose level before administering a 100-g carbohydrate load.

Treatment of the insulin-dependent patient

Fetal glucose levels reflect those of the mother. Therefore, the benefits of careful regulation of maternal glucose homeostasis will be apparent in improved perinatal outcomes. Self blood glucose monitoring combined with aggressive insulin therapy has made the maintenance of maternal normoglycemia (levels of 60–120 mg/dl) a therapeutic reality (**Table 5**). In most institutions, patients are taught to monitor their glucose control using glucose-oxidase impregnated reagent strips and glucose reflectance meter.[109] Glucose determinations are made in the fasting state and before breakfast, lunch, dinner and bedtime. Postprandial and nocturnal values are also helpful.

During pregnancy, most insulin-dependent patients will require multiple insulin injections. A combination of intermediate-acting and regular insulin before breakfast and at dinner time is employed in 70% of our patients.[110] As a general rule, the amount of intermediate-acting insulin taken in the morning will exceed that of regular by a 2:1 ratio.[111] Patients usually receive two-thirds of their total insulin dose at breakfast and the remaining third at suppertime. An alternative regimen is to administer separate injections of regular insulin at dinner time and intermediate-acting insulin at bedtime to reduce the frequency of nocturnal hypoglycemia and pre-breakfast hyperglycemia.[111] The latter may occur when the mother is in a relative fasting state,

Table 5

Target plasma glucose levels in pregnancy

Time	mg/dl
Before breakfast	69–90
Before lunch, supper, bedtime snack	60–105
After meals	≤ 120
02.00–0.600 h	> 60

while placental and fetal glucose consumption continue. Insulin requirements vary greatly among pregnant women, although an increased requirement is generally not observed until after the second trimester. On average, we have observed a 30% increase in insulin requirement by the end of gestation. This increase is likely to be several fold greater in obese women with adult-onset diabetes. All patients and their families should be instructed in the use of glucagon for the treatment of serious hypoglycemia. Patients who have achieved good glycemic control during early pregnancy can be managed as out-patients. Early hospitalization is necessary for those pregnant women who are poorly controlled or unfamiliar with self-monitoring techniques.

The presence of maternal vasculopathy should be thoroughly assessed early in pregnancy. The patient should be evaluated by an ophthalmologist familiar with diabetic retinopathy. Baseline renal function is established by assaying a 24-h urine collection for creatinine clearance and protein. An electrocardiogram and urine culture are also obtained.

Diet therapy is critical to successful regulation of maternal diabetes. A program consisting of three meals and several snacks is employed for most patients. The goal of diet planning is to minimize hyperglycemia and hypoglycemia while providing adequate nutrition for mother and fetus during the entire day. Dietary composition should be 50–60% carbohydrate, 20% protein and 25–30% fat, with less than 10% saturated fats, up to 10% polyunsaturated fatty acids and the remainder derived from monosaturated sources.[112] Caloric intake is established based on prepregnancy weight and weight gain during gestation. Weight reduction is not advised. Patients should consume approximately 30 kcal/kg ideal body weight. Obese women may be managed with an intake as low as 1600 calories per day, although if ketonuria develops, this allowance may be increased.

Patients who fail to maintain adequate control despite multiple insulin injections and dietary adjustment may be candidates for continuous subcutaneous insulin infusion (CSII) pump therapy. The initiation of this treatment almost always requires hospitalization. A basal infusion rate is established which is approximately 1 unit/h. Bolus infusions are then given with meals and snacks. Multiple blood glucose determinations are made to prevent periods of hyper- and hypoglycemia. Many groups have now treated pregnant patients for varying periods of time with CSII. Glucose values may become normalized, with large fluctuations in glucose levels eliminated in a select group of pregnant diabetics. Episodes of hypoglycemia are usually secondary to errors in dose selection or failure to adhere to the required diet.[113] The risk of nocturnal hypoglycemia, which is markedly increased in the pregnant state, necessitates that great care be made in

selecting candidates for CSII. Patients who fail to exhibit normal counter-regulatory responses to hypoglycemia should probably be discouraged from using an insulin pump. While this technique may be valuable for a small group of pregnant women with diabetes mellitus, it has not been demonstrated to be superior to multiple injection regimens. Coustan and colleagues randomized 22 pregnant women to intensive conventional therapy with multiple injections *vs* pump therapy.[114] There were no differences between the two treatment groups with respect to out-patient mean glucose levels, glycosylated hemoglobin levels or glycemic excursions.[114] In our experience with hundreds of IDDM pregnancies, we have found it necessary to institute pump therapy to achieve good glycemic control in only one patient. However, we have chosen to maintain women who have demonstrated good control using continuous infusion devices prior to pregnancy on this therapy throughout gestation.

After the initial visit, patients are followed closely with frequent telephone contact to arrive at a stable insulin regimen. Following careful review of the patient's daily glucose values, adjustments in insulin dosage are made. The patient is instructed to contact her physician should periods of hypoglycemia or hyperglycemia occur. Fetal growth is evaluated by serial ultrasound examinations at 4- to 6-week intervals. In the third trimester, pregnancy-induced hypertension may become evident, necessitating hospitalization (see also Chapter 18).

Fetal surveillance

During the past 15 years, the understanding of the importance of maternal glycemic control in relation to fetal outcome has played a major role in reducing perinatal mortality in pregnancies complicated by diabetes. Some have therefore questioned the value of rigorous antepartum fetal testing schemes in well-controlled patients.[115] Despite these considerations, programs of fetal surveillance are often initiated in the third trimester when the risk of sudden intrauterine death appears to be greatest. Well-controlled patients, as well as those without vasculopathy or significant hypertension, rarely have abnormal tests of fetal condition. Most importantly, the presence of reassuring antepartum testing allows the obstetrician to await further fetal maturation and avoid unnecessary premature intervention.

Maternal monitoring of fetal activity is recommended for all patients during the third trimester. Several methods of counting fetal movements are available which compare favorably with heart rate testing.The contraction stress test (CST) was the first biophysical test introduced, and remains an important tool in the assessment of fetal well-being in pregnancies complicated by diabetes.[50] It has been repeatedly demonstrated that in a well-controlled patient, a negative CST predicts fetal survival for 1 week.[116] Positive CSTs, observed in approximately 10% of insulin-dependent diabetic patients, have been associated with an increased perinatal mortality rate, late decelerations during labor, low Apgar scores, respiratory distress syndrome and growth retardation. The CST does have a significant false positive rate of up to 60%.

The non-stress test (NST) appears to be the preferred antepartum heart rate screening test in the management of patients with diabetes mellitus.[93] An NST which is non-reactive requires that a CST or a biophysical profile (BPP) be performed. In most cases, heart rate monitoring is begun at approximately 32–34 weeks gestation and should be performed twice weekly.[116,117] In patients with vascular disease or poor control, in whom the incidence of abnormal tests and intrauterine deaths is greater, testing is performed earlier in gestation and more frequently.

Most recently, the BPP, rather than the CST, has been used to evaluate the significance of a non-reactive NST result. Golde and colleagues observed that 430 of 434 BPPs performed after a reactive NST were associated with reassuring scores of 8 or greater.[118] Of 25 BPPs performed after a non-reactive NST result, 21 had scores of 8 and four had lower scores. In this series, even patients with low scores had good perinatal outcomes. The BPP did not appear to add more information about fetal condition if the NST result was reactive, but a score of 8 based on ultrasound parameters was as reliable in predicting good fetal outcome as was a reactive NST.

Johnson and associates have also described their experience with the BPP in diabetic women.[119] These authors performed twice-weekly tests in 50 women with insulin-dependent diabetes and weekly exams in 188 women with GDM. There were no stillbirths in this series. The incidence of abnormal BPPs was low – only 8 of 238 tests (3.3%). The 230 fetuses with a normal score before delivery experienced minimal morbidity. In contrast, of eight patients with an abnormal score, 37.5% suffered significant neonatal morbidity. Although this study did not demonstrate the superiority of the BPP over the NST alone, it did establish that the BPP may also be used for fetal surveillance with few unnecessary interventions, thereby allowing prolongation of pregnancy beyond 37 weeks in most of the patients studied.

Ultrasound has been shown to be an extremely valuable tool in evaluating fetal growth, estimating fetal weight, and detecting hydramnios and malformations. A determination of maternal serum alpha-fetoprotein at week 16 of gestation should be used in association with a detailed ultrasound study at weeks 18–20 to detect neural tube defects and other anomalies. Care must be used in interpreting alpha-fetoprotein results,

since the values may be lower in diabetic pregnancies. Fetal echocardiography is performed at 20–22 weeks gestation for the investigation of possible cardiac defects. Using such an approach to screen for anomalies, Greene and Benaceraff detected 18 of 32 malformations in a series of 432 diabetic women. The specificity was 99.5%, and the negative predictive value was 97%.[120] Spina bifida was identified in all cases; however, ventricular septal defects, limb abnormalities and facial clefts were commonly missed.

Ultrasound examinations are repeated at 4- to 6-week intervals to assess fetal growth. Prenatal detection of the macrosomic or growth-deficient fetus will facilitate selection of the optimal time and route of delivery in pregnancies complicated by diabetes. An increased rate of cephalopelvic disproportion and shoulder dystocia accompanied by significant risk of traumatic birth injury and asphyxia have been consistently associated with the vaginal delivery of large infants. The risk of such complications rises exponentially when fetal weight exceeds 4 kg and is greater for the fetus of a diabetic mother when compared with a fetus of similar birthweight whose mother does not have diabetes.[121]

The macrosomic IDM is characterized by selective organomegaly, with increases in insulin-sensitive tissues including fat, muscle mass and hepatomegaly. A disproportionate increase in the size of the trunk and shoulders is common in large-for-gestational (LGA) IDMs. Thus, sonographic measurements of the fetal abdominal circumference (AC) have proven most helpful in predicting fetal macrosomia. Using an AC>90th percentile obtained within 2 weeks of delivery, Tamura correctly identified 78% of macrosomic fetuses.[122]

We have found serial ultrasonography to be most useful in detecting growth abnormalities in diabetic pregnancies.[123] In our study of 79 diabetic women examined on at least three occasions during the third trimester, growth curves were similar for femoral length and head circumference for both normally grown and LGA fetuses. In contrast, growth of the AC was accelerated as early as week 32 in the LGA group. An AC growth velocity ≤1.2 cm/week detected LGA fetuses with 84% sensitivity and 85% specificity. More recently, we have described the use of soft tissue measurements of the upper humerus to identify LGA fetuses of GDM women.[124] This technique compares favorably with AC measurements and may identify disproportionately large fetuses.

Doppler umbilical artery velocimetry has been proposed as a clinical tool for antepartum fetal surveillance in pregnancies at risk for placental vascular disease. As women with insulin-dependent diabetes are at increased risk for the development of pre-eclampsia and fetal growth deficiency, Doppler ultrasonography could be helpful in this population. In a serial study of 35 patients, umbilical artery waveforms were abnormal in 50% of fetuses of women with vascular disease compared with 12% of those without hypertension or nephropathy.[125] In women with vascular disease, increased placental resistance was correlated with fetal growth deficiency. Two studies have demonstrated that umbilical artery waveform measurements appear to be independent of lycemic control.[125,126] Although still somewhat investigational, umbilical and uterine artery Doppler studies may be helpful in the early identification of pregnancies complicated by vasculopathy which are at increased risk for fetal growth deficiency.

Management of gestational diabetes

Women with GDM generally do not need hospitalization for dietary instruction and management. Once the diagnosis is established, patients are begun on a dietary program of 2000–2500 calories daily with the exclusion of simple carbohydrates.[127] Obese women with GDM may be managed on as little as 1200–1800 kcal/day with less weight gain and no apparent reduction in fetal size.[128,129]

The single most important therapeutic intervention in pregnancy complicated by GDM is the careful monitoring of maternal glucose levels throughout the third trimester. Fasting and 2-h postprandial glucose levels are monitored at least weekly.We prefer daily self-glucose monitoring to better ascertain the level of glycemic control achieved by diet therapy.[130] If the fasting plasma glucose level exceeds 105 mg/dl, and/or 2-h postprandial values are greater than 120 mg/dl on several occasions, therapy with human insulin is begun.

Langer and colleagues have proposed that a repetitive fasting blood glucose ≤95 mg/dl justifies insulin therapy to reduce the frequency of macrosomia.[131] However, the level of glycemia necessary to reduce fetal and neonatal complications in GDM pregnancies is debatable. 'Prophylactic' insulin given to patients who would normally be treated by diet alone may also reduce the frequency of macrosomia, cesarean section and birth trauma. It has been suggested that insulin may reduce subtle degrees of postprandial hyperglycemia which can promote excessive fetal growth.[132] Alternatively, insulin may regulate maternal levels of other fetal insulin secretagogues such as branched-chain amino acids. In contrast, Persson and coworkers performed a prospective randomized investigation of 'prophylactic insulin' therapy. These authors noted similar rates of macrosomia and no differences in skinfold thickness in the offspring of diet *vs* diet and insulin-treated GDM women.[133] Until large prospective randomized studies indicate the benefit of prophylactic insulin, insulin should be reserved for women who demonstrate significant fasting or postprandial hyperglycemia not controlled by diet.

Patients with GDM who are well controlled are at low risk for intrauterine death. However, gestational diabetics requring insulin undergo fetal testing in a manner similar to uncomplicated insulin-dependent patients.[134] Prenatal fetal heart rate testing prior to term has been recommended in three groups of patients with GDM: (1) those who require insulin; (2) those with hypertension; and (3) those who have a history of a prior stillbirth. Maternal assessment of fetal activity is begun at 28 weeks. Gestational diabetics may be safely followed until 40 weeks as long as fasting and postprandial glucose values remain normal. At 40 weeks, fetal surveillance is begun with non-stress testing. As with pregestational diabetic patients, ultrasound is employed to identify macrosomia and help select the safest route of delivery.

Labor/delivery

Timing of delivery

In the past, elective preterm delivery of the insulin-dependent patient to avoid an unexpected intrauterine fetal death was commonplace. Such empiric scheduled preterm delivery often resulted in a high incidence of neonatal morbidity and mortality. With improved glycemic control and better methods of prenatal fetal surveillance, most patients are now delivered at term.[115] Nevertheless, the rate of elective intervention still remains high in pregnancies complicated by diabetes. In most centers, elective delivery will be planned at 38–39 weeks gestation. It is important to use not only the results of prenatal testing, but to recognize all the clinical features involving mother and fetus before a decision is made to intervene. This includes evaluation of the degree of glycemic control, hypertension, nephropathy and the patient's ophthalmologic status.

Unless accurate gestational dating has been established in a well-controlled patient who has reached 39 weeks gestation, an amniocentesis should be considered prior to elective delivery to document fetal pulmonary maturity. The value of the lecithin/ sphingomyelin ratio (L/S) has been questioned in diabetic pregnancies. Most series, however, report a low incidence of respiratory distress syndrome (RDS) with a mature L/S ratio.[135] The presence of the acidic phospholipid phosphatidylglycerol (PG) is a final marker of fetal pulmonary maturation. Several studies have suggested that fetal hyperinsulinemia may be associated with delayed appearance of PG and an increased incidence of RDS. In one series, four infants who developed RDS at delivery had L/S ratios between 2.0 and 3.0, but absent PG.[136] These authors noted reduced amounts of PG compared with phosphatidyinositol (Pl) in amniotic fluid from gestations complicated by diabetes. Caution must therefore be used in planning the delivery of patients with a mature L/S and absent PG.

If prenatal assessment remains reassuring, delivery may be delayed for another week. In addition, the clinician must be familiar with the laboratory analysis of amniotic fluid in his or her institution and the neonatal outcome at various L/S ratios in the presence or absence of PG.

When prenatal testing suggests fetal compromise, delivery must be considered (**Figure 5**). If amniotic fluid analysis yields a mature L/S ratio, delivery should be executed promptly. When the L/S ratio is immature, the decision to proceed with delivery should be based on confirmation of deteriorating fetal condition by several positive test results. For example, if the results of both the NST and the CST or BPP indicate fetal compromise, delivery is indicated.

Route of delivery

The route of delivery for the diabetic patient remains controversial. Delivery by cesarean section is usually favored when fetal distress has been suggested by prenatal heart rate monitoring. An elective delivery is scheduled if, at 37–38 weeks of gestation, the fetus has a mature lung profile and is at significant risk for intrauterine demise because of the mother's poor metabolic control or a history of stillbirth. We now reserve elective cesarean section for cases in which the cervix cannot be ripened with prostaglandin gel or when fetal macrosomia is suspected. Although there are clear limitations to the accuracy of sonographic estimation of fetal weight, we favor cesarean delivery if the fetus is believed to weigh greater than 4000 g. In well-controlled patients without vascular disease and an unfavorable cervix, we often delay intervention until week 40. Despite this approach, the cesarean section rate for women with classes B–R diabetes remains as high as 50%.

Glucose control

Because neonatal hypoglycemia is related directly to maternal glucose levels during labor as well as to the degree of prenatal metabolic control, it is important to maintain maternal plasma glucose levels at approximately 100 mg/dl during labor. Neonatal hypoglycemia may result from beta-cell stimulation *in utero* as a result of elevated blood glucose levels during labor. A continuous infusion of both insulin and glucose has proven most valuable to control maternal glycemia during labor and delivery.

In well-controlled patients, the usual dose of NPH insulin is given at bedtime, and the morning insulin dose is withheld. Once active labor begins or the glucose levels fall to <70 mg/dl, the infusion is changed from saline to 50% dextrose at a rate of 2.5 mg/kg/min.[111] Glucose levels are monitored and the infusion rate is adjusted accordingly. Regular insulin is administered if glucose values exceed 140 mg/dl. It is important to use a flow sheet that summarizes glucose values, insulin dosage and other metabolic parameters during labor.

When cesarean section is to be performed, it should be scheduled for early morning. This simplifies intrapartum glucose control and allows the neonatal team to prepare for the care of the newborn. The patient should not eat or drink after midnight, and her usual morning insulin dose is withheld. Epidural anesthesia is preferred because it allows the anesthesiologist to detect early signs of hypoglycemia and also permits the mother to interact with her newborn infant.

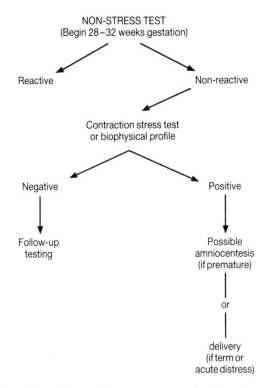

NON-STRESS TEST
(Begin 28–32 weeks gestation)

Reactive   Non-reactive

Contraction stress test
or biophysical profile

Negative   Positive

Follow-up   Possible
testing   amniocentesis
                   (if premature)

                   or

                   delivery
                   (if term or
                   acute distress)

Figure 5. Scheme for antepartum fetal testing in pregnancy complicated by diabetes mellitus.

Postnatal

Insulin requirements are usually significantly lower postnatally than prepregnancy. The objective of 'tight control' used in the prenatal period is relaxed for several days, and glucose values of 150–200 mg/dl are acceptable. Patients who deliver vaginally and are able to eat a regular diet are given one-third to one-half of their end-pregnancy dose of NPH insulin the morning after delivery. An occasional patient may require little or no insulin during the first 24–48 h postnatally. Frequent glucose determinations are used to guide the insulin dose. If the patient has been given supplemental regular insulin in addition to the morning NPH dose, the amount of NPH insulin on the following morning is increased to an amount equal to two-thirds of the additional regular insulin. Most patients are stabilized on this regimen within a few days after delivery.

Women with diabetes are encouraged to breast-feed. Dietary adjustments for breast-feeding are made as they are in non-diabetic patients. The insulin dose may be somewhat lower in lactating women because of the caloric expenditure associated with nursing.

DIABETES MELLITUS AND PREGNANCY
Summary of Management Options

Prepregnancy

- Explanation of general risks and management of diabetes in pregnancy

- Evaluate any additional risks with appropriate specialist referral (e.g. renal, ophthalmologic)

- Optimize blood glucose control

- Discuss effective contraception until good glucose control (?avoid estrogen containing preparations with vascular disease)

- Folate supplementation (4–5 mg daily) for at least 2 months before and during first trimester.

Prenatal

- Screen for gestational diabetes ideally in all pregnancies (controversy over which test and whether just at 24–28 weeks)

- Regular capillary glucose series

- Avoid oral hypoglycemic agents

- Appropriate diet

- Amend insulin regimen to keep capillary glucose values as normal as possible (see **Table 5**)

- Instruct partners/relatives in glucagon use for hypoglycemic attacks

- Baseline renal and possibly cardiac function

- Regular ophthalmologic review

- Monitor for hypertensive disease

- Fetal surveillance
  - normality
  - growth
  - well-being (NST, BPP)

- Gestational diabetics: initially try to control with diet rather than insulin; otherwise, as for established diabetics

Labor/delivery

- Timing: can be delayed until term if diabetes is well-controlled and pregnancy uncomplicated

- Method: will depend on complications in mother (e.g. hypertension, opthalmic) and/or fetus (e.g. macrosomia, acute fetal compromise) when cesarean section more likely

- Maintain good perinatal glucose control

Postnatal

- Reduced insulin requirements

- Continue capillary glucose monitoring

- Encourage breast-feeding

- Give contraceptive advice

REFERENCES

1 Kalkhoff RK, Kissebah AH, Kim HJ (1979) Carbohydrate and lipid metabolism during normal pregnancy: Relationship to gestational hormone action. In Merkatz IR, Adam PAJ (eds) *The Diabetic Pregnancy: A Perinatal Perspective.* New York: Grune and Stratton.

2 Freinkel N, Metzger BE, Mitzan M *et al.* (1972) Accelerated starvation and mechanisms for the conservation of maternal nitrogen during pregnancy. *Israel Journal of Medical Science.* **8**:426.

3 Kaplan SL (1974) Human chorionic somatomammotropin secretion, biologic effects and physiological significance. In Jaffe RB (ed.) *The Endocrine Milieu of Pregnancy, Puerperium and Childhood.* Columbus, OH: Ross Laboratories.

4 Yen SSC (1973) Endocrine regulation of metabolic homeostasis during pregnancy. *Clinics in Obstetrics and Gynecology* **16**:130.

5 Spellacy WN (1975) Maternal and fetal metabolic interrelationships. In Sutherland HW, Stowers JM (eds) *Carbohydrate Metabolism in Pregnancy and the Newborn.* New York: Churchill Livingstone.

6 Hollingsworth DR, Grundy SM (1981) Pregnancy-associated hypertriglyceridemia in normal and diabetic women: Differences in insulin-dependent, non-insulin-dependent, and gestational diabetes. *Diabetes* **31**:1092.

7 Catalano P, Tyzbier ED, Wolfe RR *et al.* (1992) Longitudinal changes in carbohydrate metabolism in pregnant control subjects and women with gestational diabetes. *Society for Gynecological Investigation*, Abstract 458, San Antonio, TX.

8 Beard RW, Turner RC, Oakley N (1971) Fetal response to glucose loading. *Postgraduate Medical Journal* **47**:68.

9 Felig P (1973) Maternal and fetal fuel homeostasis in human pregnancy. *American Journal of Clinical Nutrition* **26**:998.

10 Pedersen J *The Pregnant Diabetic and Her Newborn*, 2nd edn. Baltimore, MD: Williams and Wilkins.

11 Metzger BE, Phelps RL, Freinkel N *et al.* (1980) Effects of gestational diabetes on diurnal profiles of glucose, lipids, and individual amino-acids. *Diabetes Care* **3**:402–409.

12 Kalkoff R (1991) Impact of maternal fuels and nutritional state of fetal growth. *Diabetes* **40**:61–65 (suppl. 2).

13 Gabbe SG (1980) Management of diabetes in pregnancy: Six decades of experience. In Pitkin RM, Zlatnik F (eds) *The Yearbook of Obstetrics and Gynecology.* Chicago, IL: Year Book Medical Publishers.

14 Madsen H (1986) Fetal oxygenation in diabetic pregnancy. *Danish Medical Bulletin* **33**:64.

15 Nyland L, Lunell NO, Lewander R *et al.* (1982) Uteroplacental blood flow in diabetic pregnancy: Measurements with indium 113m and a computer linked gamma camera. *American Journal of Obstetrics and Gynecology* **144**:298.

16 Kitzmiller JL, Phillippe M, von Oeyen P *et al.* (1981) Hyperglycemia, hypoxia, and fetal acidosis in rhesus monkeys. Presented at the *28th Annual Meeting of the Society for Gynecologic Investigation*, St. Louis, MO, March.

17 Phillips AF, Dubin JW, Matty PJ *et al.* (1982) Arterial hypoxemia and hyperinsulinemia in the chronically hyperglycemic fetal lamb. *Pediatrics Research* **16**:653.

18 Shelley JH, Bassett JM, Milner RDG (1975) Control of carbohydrate metabolism in the fetus and newborn. *British Medical Bulletin* **31**:37.

19 Carson BS, Phillips AF, Simmons MA *et al.* (1980) Effects of a sustained insulin infusion upon glucose uptake and oxygenation of the ovine fetus. *Pediatrics Research* **14**:147.

20 Simpson JL, Elias S, Martin AO *et al.* (1983) Diabetes in pregnancy, Northwestern University Series (1977–1981). I. Prospective study of anomalies in offspring of mothers with diabetes mellitus. *American Journal of Obstetrics and Gynecology* **146**:263.

21 Kucera J (1971) Rate and type of congenital anomalies among offspring of diabetic women. *Journal of Reproductive Medicine* **7**:61–70.

22 Mills JL, Knopp RH, Simpson JP *et al.* (1988) Lack of relations of increased malformation rates in infants of diabetic mothers to glycemic control during organogenesis., *New England Journal of Medicine* **318**:671.

23 Mills JL, Baker L, Goldman A (1979) Malformations in infants of diabetic mothers occur before the seventh gestational week: Implications for treatment. *Diabetes* **28**:292.

24 Simpson JL, Mills JL, Ober C *et al.* (1990) DR3+ and DR4+ diabetic women have increased risk for anomalies: Evidence for genetic susceptibility in diabetic embryopathy. Presented at the *37th Annual Meeting of the Society for Gynecologic Investigation*, Abstract 391, St Louis. MO.

25 Sadler TW, Horton WE Jr (1986) Mechanisms of diabetes induced congenital malformations as studied in mammalian embryo culture. In Jovanovic L, Peterson CM, Fuhrmann K (eds) *Diabetes in pregnancy: Teratology, Toxicity and Treatment.* New York: Praeger.

26 Freinkel N, Lewis NJ, Akazama S *et al.* (1984) The honeybee syndrome: Implication of the teratogenecity of mannose in rat-embryo culture. *New England Journal of Medicine* **310**:223.

27 Goldman AS, Baker L, Piddington R *et al.* (1985) Hyperglycemia-induced teratogenesis is mediated by a functional deficiency of arachidonic acid. *Proceedings of the National Academy of Sciences USA* **82**:8227.

28 Pinter E, Reece EA, Leranth CZ *et al.* (1986) Yolk sac failure in embryopathy due to hyperglycemia ultrastructural analysis of yolk sac differentation associated with embryopathy in rat conceptuses under hyperglycemic conditions. *Teratology* **33**:73.

29 Sadler TW, Phillips LS, Balkan W *et al.* (1986) Somatomedin inhibitors from diabetic rat serum alter growth and development of mouse embryos in culture. *Diabetes* **35**:861.

30 Buchanan TA, Schemmer JK, Freinkel N (1986) Embryotoxic effects of brief maternal-induced hypoglycemia during organogenesis in the rat. *Journal of Clinical Investigation* **78**:643.

31 Kitzmiller JL, Gavin LA, Gin GD *et al.* (1991) Preconception management of diabetes continued through

early pregnancy prevents the excess frequency of major congenital anomalies in infants of diabetic mothers. *Journal of the American Medical Association* **265**:731.

32 Pettit DJ, Bennett PH, Knowler WC *et al.* (1985) Gestational diabetes mellitus and impaired glucose tolerance during pregnancy: Long term effects on obesity and glucose tolerance in the offspring. *Diabetes* **34**:119 (suppl. 2).

33 Spellacy WN, Miller S. Winegar A *et al.* (1985) Macrosomia – maternal characteristics and infant complications. *Obstetrics and Gynecology* **66**:158.

34 Naeye RL (1965) Infants of diabetic mothers: A quantitative morphologic study. *Pediatrics* **35**:980–988.

35 Modanlou HD, Komatsu G *et al.* (1982). Large-for-gestational age neonates: Anthropometric reason for shoulder dystocia. *Obstetrics and Gynecology* **60**:417–423.

36 Farquhar JW (1959) The child of the diabetic woman. *Archives of Disease in Childhood* **34**:76–82.

37 Brans YW, Shannon DL (1983) Maternal diabetes and neonatal macrosomia. II. Neonatal anthropometric measurements. *Early Human Development* **8**:297–305.

38 Brans YW, Shannon DL (1983) Maternal diabetes and neonatal macrosomia. III. Neonatal body water estimates. *Early Human Development* **8**:307–316.

39 Enzi G, Inelman EM (1980) Development of adipose tissue in newborn of gestational diabetic and insulin-dependent diabetic mothers. *Diabetes* **29**:100–104.

40 Driscoll SG, Ernirschke K (1960) Neonatal deaths among infants of diabetic mothers. *American Journal of Diseases of Children* **100**:818–830.

41 Milner RDG, Wirdnam PK (1981) Quantitative morphology of B, A, D and PP cells in infants of diabetic mothers. *Diabetes* **30**:271–274.

42 Reiher H, Fuhrmann K. (1983) Age dependent insulin secretion of the endocrine pancreas *in vitro* from fetuses of diabetic and nondiabetic patients. *Diabetes Care* **6**:446–451.

43 Susa JB, McCormick KL (1979) Chronic hypertension in the fetal Rhesus monkey. *Diabetes* **28**:1058–1068.

44 Falluca F, Gargiulo P (1985) Amniotic fluid insulin, C peptide concentrations, and fetal morbidity in infants of diabetic mothers. *American Journal of Obstetrics and Gynecology* **153**:534–540.

45 Weiss PAM, Hofinan H (1984) Gestational diabetes and screening during pregnancy. *Obstetrics and Gynecology* **63**:776–780.

46 Lin CC, River P (1981) Prenatal assessment of fetal outcome by amniotic fluid C-peptide levels in pregnant diabetic women. *American Journal of Obstetrics and Gynecology* **141**:671–676.

47 Persson B, Pschera H (1986) Amino acid concentrations in maternal plasma and amniotic fluid in relation to fetal insulin secretion during the last trimester of pregnancy in gestational and type I diabetic women and women with small-for-gestational age infants. *American Journal of Perinatology* **3**:98–103.

48 Sosenko IR, Kitzmiller JL (1979) The infant of the diabetic mother: Correlation of increased cord C-peptide levels with macrosomia and hypoglycemia. *New England Journal of Medicine* **301**:859–862.

49 Phelps RL, Freinkel N (1978) Carbohydrate metabolism in pregnancy. XV. Plasma C-peptide during intravenous glucose tolerance in neonates from normal and insulin-treated diabetic mothers. *Journal of Clinical Endocrinology and Metabolism* **46**:61–68.

50 Gabbe SG, Mestman JH, Freeman RK *et al.* (1977) Management and outcome of pregnancy in diabetes mellitus, Classes B–R. *American Journal of Obstetrics and Gynecology* **129**:723–732.

51 Kitzmiller JL, Cloherty JP (1978) Diabetic pregnancy and perinatal morbidity. *American Journal of Obstetrics and Gynecology* **131**:560–580.

52 Roversi GD, Gargiulo M (1979) A new approach to the treatment of diabetic pregnant women. *American Journal of Obstetrics and Gynecology* **135**:567–576.

53 Jovanovic L, Druzin M, Peterson CM (1981) Effect of euglycemia on the outcome of pregnancy in insulin-dependent diabetic women as compared with normal control subjects. *American Journal of Medicine* **72**:921–927.

54 Willman SP, Leveno KJ, Whalley P (1986) Glucose threshold for macrosomia in pregnancy complicated by diabetes. *American Journal of Obstetrics and Gynecology* **154**:470–475.

55 Jovanovic-Peterson L, Peterson CM, Reed GF *et al.* (1991) Maternal postpartum glucose levels and infant birthweight: The Diabetes in Early Pregnancy Study. *Journal of Obstetrics and Gynecology* **164**:103–110.

56 Landon MB, Gabbe SG, Piana R *et al.* (1987) Neonatal morbidity in pregnancy complicated by diabetes mellitus: Predictive value of maternal glycemic profile. *American Journal of Obstetrics and Gyncecology* **156**:1089–1095.

57 Soler NG, Soler SM, Malins JM (1978) Neonatal morbidity among infants of diabetic mothers. *Diabetes Care* **1**:340.

58 Kuhl C, Anderson GE, Hartil J *et al.* (1982) Metabolic events in infants of diabetic mothers during first 24 hours after birth. *Acta Paediatrica Scandinavica* **71**:19.

59 Bloom SR, Johnson DI (1972) Failure of glucagon in infants of diabetic mothers. *British Medical Journal* **4**:453.

60 Coustan DR, Berkowitz RL, Hobbins C (1980) Tight metabolic control of overt diabetes in pregnancy. *American Journal of Medicine* **68**:845–852.

61 Karlsson K, Kjellmer (1972) The outcome of diabetic pregnancies in relation to the mother's blood sugar level. *American Journal of Obstetrics and Gynecology* **112**:213–220.

62 Ylinen K, Raivio K (1981) Hemoglobin A1c predicts the perinatal outcome in insulin-dependent diabetic pregnancies. *British Journal of Obstetrics and Gynaecology* **88**:961–967.

63 Bourbon JR, Farrell PM (1985) Fetal lung development in the diabetic pregnancy. *Pediatrics Research* **19**:253–267.

64 Smith BT, Giroud CJP *et al.* (1975) Insulin antagonism of cortisol action on lecithin synthesis by cultured fetal lung cells. *Journal of Pediatrics* **87**:953–955.

65 Engle M, Langan SM *et al.* (1983) The effects of insulin and hyperglycemia on surfactant phospholipid biosynthesis in organotypic cultures on type II pheumocytes. *Biochemica Biophysica Acta* **753**:6–13.

66 Smith BT (1984) Pulmonary surfactant during fetal development and neonatal adaptation: Hormonal control. In Robertson B, Van Golde LMG, Batenburg JJ (eds) *Pulmonary Surfactants*, pp. 357–381. Amsterdam: Elsevier.

67 Post M, Barsoumian A *et al*. (1986) The cellular mechanisms of glucocorticoid acceleration of fetal lung maturation. *Journal of Biochemical Chemistry* **261**:2179–2184.

68 Carlson KS, Smith *et al*. (1984) Insulin acts on the fibroblast to inhibit glucocorticoid stimulation of lung maturity. *Journal of Applied Physiology* **57**:1577–1579.

69 Rooney SA, Ingleson LD (1980) Insulin antagonism of dexamethasone induced stimulation of cholineophosphate cytidyltransferase in fetal rat lung in organ culture. *Lung* **158**:151–155.

70 Robert MF, Neff RK *et al*. (1976) Association between maternal diabetes and the respiratory distress syndrome in the newborn. *New England Journal of Medicine* **294**:357–360.

71 Gabbe SG, Lowenshon RI, Wu PK *et al*. (1978) Current patterns of neonatal morbidity and mortality in infants of diabetic mothers. *Diabetes Care* **1**:335–339.

72 Dudley DKL, Black DM (1988) Reliability of lecithin/sphingomyelin ratios in diabetic pregnancy. *Obstetrics and Gynecology* **66**:521–524.

73 Tsang RC, Chen I-W, Friedman MA *et al*. (1975) Parathyroid function in infants of diabetic mothers. *Journal of Pediatrics* **86**:399.

74 Mimouni F, Miodovnik M, Tsang RC *et al*. (1987) Decreased amniotic fluid magnesium concentration in diabetic pregnancy. *Obstetrics and Gynecology* **69**:12.

75 White P (1949) Pregnancy complicating diabetes. *American Journal of Medicine* **7**:609.

76 O'Sullivan Summary and Recommendations of the Third International Workshop (1991) Conference on gestational diabetes. *Diabetes* **40**:197 (suppl. 2).

77 Gabbe SG, Mestman JH, Freeman RK *et al*. (1977) Management and outcome of class A diabetes mellitus. *American Journal of Obstetrics and Gynecology* **127**:465.

78 Main EK, Main DM, Landon MB, Gabbe SG (1986) Factors predicting perinatal outcome in pregnancies complicated by diabetic nephropathy (class F). *Sixth Annual Meeting of the Society of Perinatal Obstetricians*, San Antonio, February.

79 Kitzmiller JL, Brown ER, Phillippe M *et al*. (1981) Diabetic nephropathy and perinatal outcome. *American Journal of Obstetrics and Gynecology* **141**:741.

80 Reece EA, Coustan DR, Hayslett JP *et al*. (1988). Diabetic nephropathy: Pregnancy performance and fetomaternal outcome. *American Journal of Obstetrics and Gynecology* **159**:56.

81 Kitzmiller JL (1988) Diabetic nephropathy In Reece EA, Coustan DR (eds) *Diabetes Mellitus in Pregnancy: Principles and Practice*. New York: Churchill Livingstone.

82 Hayslett JP, Reece EA (1987) Effects of diabetic nephropathy on pregnancy. *American Journal of Kidney Diseases* **9**:344.

83 Ogburn PL Jr, Kitzmiller JL, Hare JW *et al*. (1986) Pregnancy following renal transplantation in class T diabetes mellitus. *Journal of the American Medical Association* **255**:911.

84 Klein BEK, Moss SE, Klein R (1990) Effect of pregnancy on the progression of diabetic retinopathy. *Diabetes Care* **13**:34.

85 Horvat M, Maclear H, Goldberg L, Crock CW (1980) Diabetic retinopathy in pregnancy: A 12 year prospective study. *British Journal of Ophthalmology* **64**:398.

86 Kitzmiller JL, Gavin LA, Gin GD *et al*. (1988) Managing diabetes and pregnancy. *Current Problems in Obstetrics, Gynecology and Fertility* **11**:113.

87 Moloney JBM, Drury Ml (1982) The effect of pregnancy on the natural course of diabetic retinopathy. *American Journal of Ophthalmology* **93**:745.

88 Phelps RL, Sakol P, Metzger BE *et al*. (1986) Changes in diabetic retinopathy during pregnancy: Correlations with regulation of hyperglycemia. *Archives of Ophthalmology* **104**:1806.

89 Chang S, Fuhrmann M, and the Diabetes in Early Pregnancy Study Group (1985) Pregnancy, retinopathy, normoglycemia: A preliminary analysis: *Diabetes* **34**:3A (suppl.).

90 Sinclair SH, Nesler C, Foxman B *et al*. (1984) Macular edema and pregnancy in insulin dependent diabetes. *American Journal of Ophthalmology* **97**:154.

91 Silfen SL, Wapner RJ, Gabbe SG (1980) Maternal outcome in class H diabetes mellitus. *Obstetrics and Gynecology* **55**:749.

92 Hare JW (1989) Maternal complications. In Hare JW (ed.) *Diabetes Complicating Pregnancy: The Joslin Clinic Method*. New York: Alan R. Liss.

93 Landon MB, Gabbe SG, Sachs L (1990) Management of diabetes mellitus and pregnancy: A survey of obstetricians and maternal–fetal specialists. *Obstetrics and Gynecology* **75**:635.

94 Fuhrmann K, Reiher H, Semmler K *et al*. (1983) Prevention of congenital malformation in infants of insulin-dependent diabetic mothers. *Diabetes Care* **6**:219.

95 Miller E, Hare JW, Cloherty JP *et al*. (1981) Elevated maternal HbA$_1$ in early pregnancy and major congenital anomalies in infants of diabetic mothers. *New England Journal of Medicine* **304**:1331.

96 Ylinen K, Aula P, Stenman UH *et al*. (1984) Risk of minor and major fetal malformations in diabetics with high haemoglobin A$_{1c}$ values in early pregnancy. *British Medical Journal* **289**:345.

97 Kalter H (1987) Diabetes and spontaneous abortion: An historical review. *American Journal of Obstetrics and Gynecology* **156**:1243–1253.

98 Mills J, Simpson JL, Driscoll SG *et al*. (1988) Incidence of spontaneous abortion among normal and insulin-dependent diabetic women whose pregnancies were identified within 21 days of conception. *New England Journal of Medicine* **319**:1617.

99 Freinkel N. (1988) Diabetic embryopathy and fuel-mediated organ teratogenesis: Lessons from animal models. *Hormones, Metabolism Research* **20**:463.

100 MRC Vitamin Study Research Group (1991) Prevention of neural tube defects: Results of the Medical Research Council Vitamin Study. *Lancet* **338**:131.

101 Freinkel N (1980) Gestational diabetes 1979: Philo-

sophical and practical aspects of a major health problem. *Diabets Care* **3**:399.

102   O'Sullivan JB (1982) Body weight and subsequent diabetes mellitus. *Journal of the American Medical Association* **248**:949.

103   Carpenter MW, Coustan DR (1982) Criteria for screening tests of gestational diabetes. *American Journal of Obstetrics and Gynecology* **144**:768.

104   Sacks DA, Abu-Fadil S, Greenspoon J *et al.* (1989) Do the current standards for glucose tolerance testing in pregnancy represent a valid conversion of O'Sullivan's original criteria? *American Journal of Obstetrics and Gynecology* **161**:638.

105   Langer O, Anyaegbunam A, Brustman L *et al.* (1989) Management of women with one abnormal oral glucose tolerance test value reduces adverse outcome in pregnancy. *American Journal of Obstetrics and Gynecology* **161**:593.

106   Lind T, Phillips PR *et al.* (1991) Influence of pregnancy on the 75-g OGTT: A prospective multicenter study. *Diabetes* **40**:8–13. (suppl. 2).

107   Coustan Dr, Nelson C, Carpenter NW *et al.* (1989) Maternal age and screening for gestational diabetes: A population based study. *Obstetrics and Gynecology* **73**:557.

108   Coustan DR, Widness JA, Carpenter MW *et al.* (1986) Should the fifty-gram one-hour plasma glucose screening test be administered in the fasting or fed state? *American Journal of Obstetrics and Gynecology* **154**:1031.

109   Landon MB, Gabbe SG (1985) Glucose monitoring and insulin administration in the pregnant diabetic patient. *Clinics in Obstetrics and Gynecology* **28**:496.

110   Landon MB, Marger R, Gabbe SG *et al.* (1992) Are current guidelines for insulin therapy in women with pregestational diabetes mellitus appropriate? *Society for Gynecologic Investigation*, March.

111   Jovanovic L, Peterson CM (1980) Management of the pregnant, insulin-dependent diabetic woman. *Diabetes Care* **3**:63.

112   American Diabetes Association (1979) Principles of nutrition and dietary recommendations for individuals with diabetes mellitus. *Diabetes* **28**:1027.

113   Rudolf MCJ, Coustan DR, Sherwin RS *et al.* (1981) Efficacy of insulin pump in the home treatment of pregnancy diabetics. *Diabetes* **30**:891.

114   Coustan DR, Reece EA, Sherwin RS *et al.* (1986) A randomized clinical trial of the insulin pumps *vs* intensive conventional therapy in diabetic pregnancies. *Journal of the American Medical Association* **255**:631.

115   Landon MB, Langer O, Gabbe SG *et al* (1992) Fetal surveillance in pregnancies complicated by insulin dependent diabetes mellitus. *American Journal of Obstetrics and Gynecology* **167**:617–621.

116   Barret JM, Salyer SL, Boehm FH (1981) The nonstress test: An evaluation of 1000 patients. *American Journal of Obstetrics and Gynecology* **141**:153.

117   Miller JM, Horger EO (1985) Antepartum heart rate testing in diabetic pregnancy. *Journal of Reproductive Medicine* **30**:515.

118   Golde SH, Montoro M, Good-Anderson B *et al.* (1984) The role of non-stress tests, fetal biophysical profile,

and CTSs in the outpatient management of insulin-requiring diabetic pregnancies. *American Journal of Obstetrics and Gynecology* **148**:269.

119   Johnson JM, Lange IR, Harman CR *et al.* (1988) Biophysical profile scoring in the management of the diabetic pregnancy. *Obstetrics and Gynecology* **72**:841.

120   Greene MF, Benacerraf B (1991) Prenatal diagnosis in diabetic gravidas: Utility of ultrasound and MSAFP screening. *Obstetrics and Gynecology* **77**:420.

121   Acker DB, Sachs BP, Friedman EA (1985) Risk factors for shoulder dystocia. *Obstetrics and Gynecology* **66**:762.

122   Tamura RK, Sabbagha RE, Depp R *et al.* (1986) Diabetic macrosomia: Accuracy of third trimester ultrasound. *Obstetrics and Gynecology* **67**:828.

123   Landon MB, Mintz MG, Gabbe SG (1989) Sonographic evaluation of fetal abdominal growth: Predictor of the large-for-gestational age infant in pregnancies complicated by diabetes mellitus. *American Journal of Obstetrics and Gynecology* **160**:115.

124   Landon MB, Sonek J, Foy P *et al.* (1991) Sonographic measurement of fetal humeral soft tissue thickness in pregnancy complicated by GDM. *Diabetes* **40**:66 (suppl. 2).

125   Landon MB, Gabbe SG, Bruner JP, Ludmir J (1989) Doppler umbilical artery velocimetry in pregnancy complicated by insulin dependent diabetes mellitus. *Obstetrics and Gynecology* **73**:961.

126   Johnstone FD, Steel JM, Haddad NG *et al.* (1992) Doppler umbilical artery flow velocity waveforms in diabetic pregnancy. *British Journal of Obstetrics and Gynaecology* **99**:135–140.

127   Hollingsworth DR, Ney DM (1988) Dietary management of diabetes during pregnancy. In Reece EA, Coustan DR (eds) *Diabetes Mellitus in Pregnancy: Principles and Practice.* New York: Churchill Livingstone.

128   Algert S, Shragg P, Hollingsworth DR (1985) Moderate caloric restriction in obese women with gestational diabetes. *Obstetrics and Gynecology* **65**:489.

129   Dornhorst A, Nicholls JSD, Probst F, *et al.* (1991) Calorie restriction for treatment of gestational diabetes. *Diabetes* **40**:161–164 (suppl. 2).

130   Goldberg J, Franklin B, Lasser L *et al.* (1986) Gestational diabetes: Impact of home glucose monitoring on neonatal birth weight. *American Journal of Obstetrics and Gynecology* **154**:546.

131   Langer O, Berkus M, Brustman L *et al.* (1991) Rational for insulin management in gestational diabetes mellitus. *Diabetes* **40**:186–190 (suppl. 2).

132   Coustan DR, Imarah J (1984) Prophylactic insulin treatment of gestational diabetes reduces the incidence of macrosomia, operative delivery, and birth trauma. *American Journal of Obstetrics and Gynecology* **150**:836.

133   Persson B, Stangenberg M, Hasson U, Nordlander E (1985) Gestational diabetes mellitus: Comparative evaluation of two treatment regimens, diet versus insulin and diet. *Diabetes* **34**:101 (suppl. 2).

134   Landon MB, Gabbe SG (1985) Antepartum fetal sur-

veillance in gestational diabetes mellitus. *Diabetes* **34**:50 (suppl. 2).

135   Kjos SL, Walther FJ, Montoro M *et al.* (1990) Prevalence and etiology of respiratory distress in infants of diabetic mothers: Predictive value of fetal lung maturation tests. *American Journal of Obstetrics and Gynecology* **163**:898.

136   Gabbe SG, Lowenshon RI, Mestman JH *et al.* (1977) The lecithin/sphingomyelin ratio in pregnancies complicated by diabetes mellitus: *American Journal of Obstetrics and Gynecology* **128**:757.

137   Steel JM, Johnstone FD, Smith AF, Duncan LJP (1982) Five years experience of a 'prepregnancy' clinic for insulin-dependent diabetics. *British Medical Journal* **285**:353–356.

20

Cardiac Disease

RUSSEL D. JELSEMA, DAVID B. COTTON

GENERAL

Maternal/Fetal Risks

Cardiac disease in pregnancy represents a condition in which a pregnancy is complicated by impaired heart function. This condition may increase either maternal or fetal morbidity and mortality. Cardiac disease may be pre-existent, or it may be induced by the pregnant condition. The incidence of significant cardiac disease in pregnancy is <2%.[1] If mitral valve prolapse is included, the incidence approaches 10–15%.[2]

The main maternal risks associated with pregnancies complicated by cardiac disease include infection, worsening of the pre-existing condition, cardiac arrhythmia and the development of cardiomyopathy. Infective endocarditis occurs in approximately 0.005–1.0% of cases. Mortality from this complication has been reported at 20%.[3] Recurrent rheumatic fever is also a recognized risk. Maternal mortality occurs in less than 1% of cases for many of the common cardiac problems, including mitral valve prolapse, atrial and ventricular septal defects. With the more rare entities such as primary pulmonary hypertension and Eisenmenger's syndrome, it approaches 50%.

The risk of fetal development of congenital heart disease is reported to be between 10 and 24% if maternal or paternal congenital heart disease is present; the highest risk occurring in the presence of maternal disease.[4–6] The risk of prematurity and intrauterine growth retardation are also increased in the gravida with any form of cardiac disease.[7]

Management Options: General

Prepregnancy

Prepregnancy management for individuals with recognized cardiac disease should include discussion of the maternal and fetal risks (see below), as well as effective contraception. Consultation with a cardiologist should be obtained to determine the current status of the disease as well as to provide information on long-term outcome. Medical management should be optimized preconceptually and surgically correctable lesions ideally should be repaired before pregnancy to reduce maternal risks.[8]

Prenatal

In established cardiac disease complicating pregnancy, the principles of management include determining the functional class of the gravida based upon the New York Heart Association classification system (**Table 1**)[9] and determining her mortality risk associated with pregnancy (**Table 2**).[10] Approximately 90% of gravidas with cardiac disease are either class I or II, and with appropriate medical care usually tolerate pregnancy without significant problem. Pregnant women with class III or IV cardiac disease account for only 10% of heart disease in pregnancy, but contribute 85% of cardiac deaths.[11]

Factors that aggravate pre-existing disease, such as anemia, anxiety, arrhythmias, rigorous exercise and thromboembolic disease, should be minimized. Weight

Table 1
New York Heart Association heart functional classification[7]

Class I: Patients have no limitation of physical activity. Ordinary physical activity does not cause undue fatigue, palpitation, dyspnea or anginal pain

Class II: Patients have slight limitation of physical activity. Ordinary physical activity results in fatigue, palpitation, dyspnea or anginal pain

Class III: Patients have marked limitation of physical activity. Less-than-ordinary activity causes fatigue, palpitation, dyspnea or anginal pain

Class IV: Patients have an inability to carry on any physical activity without discomfort. Symptoms of cardiac insufficiency or of anginal syndrome may be present, even at rest. If any physical activity is undertaken, discomfort is increased

Table 2
Mortality risk associated with pregnancy[8]

Group I: Mortality < 1%
Atrial septal defect[a]
Ventricular septal defect[a]
Patent ductus arteriosus[a]
Pulmonic/tricuspid disease
Corrected tetralogy of Fallot
Porcine valve
Mitral stenosis, NYHA class I and II

Group II: Mortality 5–15%
Mitral stenosis with atrial fibrillation
Artificial valve
Mitral stenosis, NYHA class III and IV
Aortic stenosis
Coarctation of aorta, uncomplicated
Uncorrected tetralogy of Fallot
Previous myocardial infarction
Marfan's syndrome with normal aorta

Group III: Mortality 25–50%
Pulmonary hypertension
Coarctation of aorta, complicated
Marfan's syndrome with aortic involvement

[a]Uncomplicated.

gain should be monitored closely in an effort to detect incipient congestive heart failure. Elastic support hose should be worn to prevent venous blood pooling and assist venous return to the heart. Diagnostic tests that include radiation exposure are usually avoided unless they will affect management. Endocarditis prophylaxis should be given according to the American Heart Association recommendations (**Table 3**).[12] Prophylactic antibiotics are recommended for gravidas at risk for developing endocarditis who are undergoing those procedures most likely to produce bacteremia with organisms that commonly cause endocarditis (**Table 4**).

Labor/delivery

Laboring in the left lateral position is preferred to minimize the hemodynamic fluctuations associated with

Table 3
American Heart Association recommendations for endocarditis prophylaxis

CARDIAC CONDITIONS

Endocarditis prophylaxis recommended
Prosthetic cardiac valves, including bioprosthetic and homograft valves
Previous bacterial endocarditis, even in the absence of heart disease
Most congenital malformations
Rheumatic and other acquired valvular dysfunction, even after valvular surgery
Hypertrophic cardiomyopathy
Mitral valve prolapse with valvular regurgitation

Endocarditis prophylaxis not recommended
Isolated secundum atrial septal defect
Surgical repair without residua beyond 6 months of secundum atrial septal defect, ventricular septal defect, or patent ductus arteriosus defect
Previous coronary artery bypass graft surgery
Mitral valve prolapse without valvular regurgitation (mitral valve prolapse associated with thickening and/or redundancy of the valve leaflets may be at increased risk for endocarditis)
Physiologic, functional or innocent heart murmurs
Previous Kawasaki disease without valvular dysfunction
Previous rheumatic fever without valvular dysfunction
Cardiac pacemakers and implantable defibrillators

SURGICAL PROCEDURES

Endocarditis prophylaxis recommended
Urinary catheterization if urinary tract infection is present
Vaginal delivery in the presence of infection

Endocarditis prophylaxis not recommended
Cesarean section
In the absence of infection for urethral catheterization, dilatation and curettage, uncomplicated vaginal delivery, therapeutic delivery, sterilization procedures, or insertion or removal of intrauterine devices
(In patients who have prosthetic heart valves, a previous history of endocarditis, or surgically constructed systemic-pulmonary shunts or conduit, physicians may wish to administer prophylactic antibiotics even for low-risk procedures that involve the genital tract)

Table 4
Recommended drug regimens for genito-urinary procedures

Standard regimen
Intravenous or intramuscular administration of ampicillin 2.0 g, plus gentamicin 1.5 mg/kg (not to exceed 80 mg), 30 min before procedure: followed by amoxicillin 1.5 g orally 6 h after initial dose. Alternatively, the parenteral regimen may be repeated once 8 h after initial dose

Ampicillin/amoxicillin/penicillin-allergic patient regimen
Intravenous administration of vancomycin 1.0 g over 1 h plus intravenous or intramuscular administration of gentamicin 1.5 mg/kg (not to exceed 80 mg) 1 h before procedure; may be repeated once 8 h after initial dose

Alternate low-risk patient regimen
Amoxicillin 3.0 g orally 1 h before procedure, then 1.5 g at 6 h after the initial dose

labor and delivery. Continuous electrocardiographic monitoring is utilized to detect arrhythmias. Invasive monitoring should be employed in severe cases, and includes measurement of systemic arterial and pulmonary artery pressures. Monitoring of the fetus is also necessary as a higher incidence of growth retardation exists in the gravida with severe cardiac disease, predisposing the fetus to abnormal heart rate patterns. Cesarean delivery should be reserved for obstetrical indications.

Postnatal

Postnatal management for the first 48–72 h should include continued use of invasive monitoring as significant intravascular fluid shifts usually occur during this time period. These changes predispose the patient to cardiopulmonary complications. Ideally, contraception should be discussed and implemented as soon as possible.

ATRIAL SEPTAL DEFECT

Maternal/Fetal Risks

Uncorrected atrial septal defect (ASD) is not only the most frequent congenital heart disease seen in pregnancy, but it is commonly first diagnosed during pregnancy.[13] The most common etiology of ASD is an ostium secundum defect, resulting from the absence of tissue in the fossa ovalis. Although the mortality of an uncorrected ASD approaches 75% by age 50, maternal mortality with uncomplicated ASD is rare but reported (1 in 219 pregnancies).[14,15]

The major risks associated with an ASD include paradoxical emboli from leg veins to systemic circulation, infective endocarditis and pulmonary hypertension.[16] The risk of an ASD occurring in the fetus of a mother with an ASD is 3–11%.[17]

Management Options

Prepregnancy

Prepregnancy management should be directed toward determining the presence of secondary problems such as recurrent supraventricular tachycardia or pulmonary hypertension. The presence of pulmonary hypertension usually contraindicates pregnancy.

Prenatal

Prenatal management of pregnancies complicated by an ASD differs only slightly from normal prenatal care, excluding the use of support hose and heparin to prevent paradoxical emboli.

Labor/delivery

Intrapartum management includes electrocardiographic monitoring for arrhythmias, systemic arterial blood pressure monitoring and fluid restriction. Although associated with increased pulmonary blood flow, ASD is uncommonly complicated by pulmonary hypertension. In the absence of pulmonary hypertension, pulmonary artery catheterization is unnecessary. Anesthetic management should include lumbar epidural for both vaginal and cesarean delivery because of its negative effect upon systemic vascular resistance. The use of bacterial endocarditis prophylaxis with ASD has been controversial,[8,9] but current recommendations are that it is not necessary (**Table 3**).[12]

Postnatal

Postnatal management is directed primarily toward the prevention of emboli.

PATENT DUCTUS ARTERIOSUS

Maternal/Fetal Risks

An uncorrected patent ductus arteriosus (PDA) is not commonly seen in women of child-bearing age. It can occur as a result of premature birth, maternal rubella syndrome and living at high altitude.[17] Maternal risks with PDA depend upon the its size. Small, asymptomatic lesions represent minimal risk except for infective endocarditis, whereas large PDAs with left-to-right shunt and pulmonary hypertension have been associated with significant maternal mortality.[18] However, a recent series has reported no maternal deaths.[19] The risk of PDA in a fetus with a mother with PDA is 4–11%.

Management Options

Prepregnancy

Prepregnancy management should be directed toward determination of the severity of the PDA as well as the presence of secondary pulmonary hypertension.

Prenatal

Prenatal management is dependent upon the presence or absence of pulmonary hypertension. All pregnancies complicated by PDA should have echocardiography for evidence suggestive of pulmonary hypertension. In the absence of pulmonary hypertension, patients with uncomplicated PDA should be at bed rest, with the use of supplemental oxygen considered.

Labor/delivery

Intrapartum care includes cardiac monitoring and fluid restriction. Systematic hypotension must be avoided to prevent reversal of blood flow across the shunt. Pulmonary artery catheterization may be indicated if pulmonary hypertension is present. Endocarditis prophylaxis should be used routinely.

Postnatal

Postnatal management consists of careful attention to volume status and thromboemboli prevention.

COARCTATION OF THE AORTA

Maternal/Fetal Risks

Coarctation of the aorta is uncommon, and is often associated with a bicuspid aortic valve. It is usually located immediately distal to the origin of the left subclavian artery and the ligamentum arteriosum. Most patients with uncomplicated coarctation are asymptomatic for the first two decades of life, and are diagnosed following a workup for hypertension. Maternal risks

include aortic dissection, endocarditis, intracranial hemorrhage and death (3.5%).[20,21] The risk of a fetus developing coarctation in a mother with coarctation is 2–10%.[3]

Management Options

Prepregnancy

Preconceptual management should be directed toward surgical repair.

Prenatal

Prenatal management in the patient with coarctation includes determining the presence of associated disease such as aortic valvular disease or systemic vascular aneurysm, which significantly increase the risk of death to 15%.[10] For this subset of patients, therapeutic abortion should be considered.

Labor/delivery

Intrapartum care is directed toward preventing hypertension. Anesthetic management should include epidural anesthesia. For the gravida with a history of repaired coarctation, the continued presence of a bicuspid aortic valve or intracranial aneurysms, this substantially increases maternal risk for morbidity.[22]

Postnatal

The management goals oulined prior to delivery should be continued into the postpartum period. Hypertension should be controlled, and the parturient should be monitored for evidence of aortic dissection or intracranial hemorrhage.

AORTIC VALVULAR DISEASE (NON-RHEUMATIC)

Maternal/Fetal Risks

A functionally normal bicuspid aortic valve is very common, is often associated with mild aortic regurgitation, and is well tolerated in pregnancy. Bicuspid aortic valvular stenosis is uncommon, and like stenosis secondary to rheumatic disease, if severe, not well tolerated in pregnancy. Maternal risks with both aortic stenoses (AS) and aortic regurgitation (AR) are primarily related to infective endocarditis, although death has been reported secondarily to these conditions. The risk of fetal AS and AR in a mother with AS or AR is unknown, but probably approximates that of other congenital heart disease, i.e. 2–8%.[5]

Management Options

Prepregnancy

Patients with an aortic valve area <1.0 cm² should be advised against pregnancy, and if pregnancy occurs, abortion should be considered.[13]

Prenatal, labor/delivery and postnatal

The prenatal, labor/delivery and postnatal management of AS and AR are discussed under rheumatic heart disease.

VENTRICULAR SEPTAL DEFECTS

Maternal/Fetal Risks

A ventricular septal defect (VSD), whether isolated or part of a syndrome, often closes spontaneously after birth (50%) or is recognized and corrected in childhood.[23] Uncorrected isolated VSD is rare, with the prognosis being directly related to the size of the lesion. In larger defects, the size of the shunting that occurs is determined by the relative vascular resistance in the pulmonic and systemic systems. Pregnancy following repair of an uncomplicated VSD should be relatively uncomplicated.

In the pregnant woman with unrepaired VSD, maternal risks include congestive heart failure (5%), arrhythmias (5%) and hypertension (5%).[4] Maternal mortality (1 in 278 pregnancies) is uncommon.[14] The fetal risks of congenital heart disease in a mother with VSD are 19–23%, and 50% of these lesions are an isolated VSD.[4]

Management Options

Prepregnancy

Preconceptual management of unrepaired isolated VSD includes consideration for repair. The risk of fetal recurrence of VSD as well as other congenital heart disease should be thoroughly discussed.

Prenatal

Prenatal management requires echocardiography or pulmonary artery catheterization to determine the degree of left-to-right shunting and the presence of pulmonary hypertension. If pulmonic blood flow exceeds systemic blood flow by 1.5 times, surgery is recommended.[15] Termination of pregnancy is also an option for severe cases. As with ASD, the potential for paradoxical emboli exists, and efforts to prevent this with elastic stockings and heparin are indicated.

Labor/delivery

Intrapartum care is directed toward bacterial endocarditis prophylaxis (**Table 3**) and avoidance of systemic hypotension which may precipitate shunt reversal and circulatory collapse. Circulatory collapse has also been associated with difficult forceps delivery.[24]

Postnatal

With small VSDs, the postnatal risks are minimal. In the case of large defects, diligence should be maintained to avoid large fluid shifts. Early evidence of congestive heart failure should be treated aggressively. Continuous monitoring for cardiac arrhythmias should be undertaken during the first 24 h after delivery.

EISENMENGER'S COMPLEX AND EISENMENGER'S SYNDROME

Maternal/Fetal Risks

Eisenmenger's complex (EC) is a non-restrictive ventricular septal defect (VSD) with pulmonary vascular obstruction resulting in pulmonary hypertension. This complex usually develops in infancy. Eisenmenger's syndrome (ES) is pulmonary hypertension secondary to an uncorrected left-to-right shunt from VSD, an atrial septal defect (ASD) or patent ductus arteriosus (PDA). Both EC and ES produce the same result, right-to-left shunting across the VSD, ASD or PDA. For the remainder of this discussion, EC will be discussed as ES. Pulmonary vascular resistance determines the amount of right-to-left shunt, and the risk of mortality with pregnancy. The risk of maternal mortality with ES is 30–70%, and occurs primarily during the labor/delivery.[25] The fetal risk of developing ES with a mother with ES is unknown, but intrauterine growth retardation complicates 30% of pregnancies and fetal wastage approaches 75%.

Management Options

Prepregnancy

Preconceptual counseling of patients with ES should strongly advise against pregnancy.

Prenatal

For those patients with ES who do become pregnant, contrast echocardiography should be performed to detect the presence of right-to-left shunting. If right ventricular hypertrophy or right-to-left shunting is suspected, cardiac catheterization should be performed to determine the degree of pulmonary vascular resistance. If significant pulmonary hypertension is present, termination of pregnancy should be offered. Preferred methods of termination as well as prenatal, labor/delivery and postnatal management of ES/EC are discussed below under pulmonary hypertension management.

Labor/delivery

Vaginal delivery is associated with a 35% maternal mortality, compared with a 75% mortality for cesarean delivery in one series.[26] This is thought to be secondary to sudden changes in systemic vascular resistance, producing changes in the degree of right-to-left shunting, resulting in fatal syncope.[15]

Postnatal

Subacute bacterial endocarditis prophylaxis and heparin therapy should be used during the labor/delivery. Despite intensive peripartum monitoring, delayed sudden death has been reported in the distant (4–6 week) postnatal period. Permanent sterilization should be considered because of the high mortality of this condition.

TETRALOGY OF FALLOT

Maternal/Fetal Risks

Tetralogy of Fallot is the complex of ventricular septal defect (VSD), overriding aorta, right ventricular hypertrophy and pulmonary stenosis. Most tetralogy of Fallot lesions are corrected in infancy or early childhood. A woman with a corrected tetralogy will usually have an excellent pregnancy outcome. In a series of 309 patients, 18 women had 40 pregnancies without morbidity.[15] Because of the relative lack of morbidity in patients with corrected tetralogy, the remainder of this discussion will be limited to pregnancies complicated by uncorrected tetralogy of Fallot.

Uncorrected tetralogy of Fallot is associated with a 50% mortality by the age of 25 years.[27] For the surviving patient with unrepaired tetralogy, fertility is uncommon (1:20 in one series), and of 26 reported cases of pregnancy with unrepaired tetralogy, three

mothers died.[28,29] Although this mortality risk is less than that associated with pulmonary hypertension, the morbidity rates including congestive heart failure approach 40%.[28] The prognosis is especially poor when right ventricular pressure exceeds 120 mmHg, hematocrit exceeds 60%, or in the presence of repeated syncopal attacks.[30]

The fetal risk of development of tetralogy of Fallot in a mother with uncorrected tetralogy is 15% and less than 2% with corrected maternal tetralogy.[4,14] Uncorrected tetralogy is also associated with an increased risk of intrauterine growth retardation and perinatal mortality.[31] Corrected tetralogy is not associated with intrauterine growth retardation or increased perinatal mortality.[4]

Management Options

Prepregnancy

The management of patients with uncorrected tetralogy should include preconceptual counseling that advises surgical correction.

Prenatal

Prenatal care should include activity restriction and correction of anemia so as to maximize cardiac and pulmonary function. Polycythemia should be corrected by venisection only if there is evidence of thromboembolic disease or intrauterine growth retardation.[11] Aggressive treatment of arrhythmias is mandatory as are antibiotics for endocarditis prophylaxis. Use of supplemental oxygen at low flow rates during the night may be helpful.[32]

Labor/delivery

Care of the patient with uncorrected tetralogy during labor/delivery must focus upon maintaining stable maternal blood pressure. The required attention to maternal volume status may necessitate central monitoring of pressures. Although recommended for use with pregnancies complicated by pulmonary hypertension, the routine use of the pulmonary artery catheter is controversial, with several maternal deaths being attributed directly to it from pulmonary artery rupture and fatal arrhythmia.[33,34] Preload should be maximized to avoid hypotension. Although over-hydration may predispose to pulmonary edema, it is preferable to hypovolemia. Diuresis should be reserved for frank pulmonary edema. Pain and bearing down, both of which increase pulmonary artery resistance and decrease venous return, should be minimized by adequate anesthesia.

Intrapartum anesthesia for uncorrected tetralogy is controversial. Regional anesthesia associated hypotension must be avoided to prevent increasing right-to-left shunt. Because of this, some have recommended general endotracheal anesthesia only.[35] Intrathecal narcotics, which have minimal effect on systemic blood pressure as well as preventing paralysis of the lower masculature, may represent an alternative approach.[36] We have successfully used this method ourselves in a patient with atrial septal defect and pulmonary hypertension, without the use of a pulmonary artery catheter.

Postnatal

Close observation must be continued for 48–72 h postnatally. Even with successful pregnancy outcome in cases of unrepaired tetralogy, permanent sterilization should be considered.

PRIMARY PULMONARY HYPERTENSION

Maternal/Fetal Risks

Primary pulmonary hypertension, like Eisenmenger's syndrome, is associated with sudden death. The exact etiology of this sudden death phenomenon is unknown, but it has been hypothesized that a decreased venous return in the presence of a fixed pulmonic vascular resistance results in decreased biventricular output. This reduced cardiac output leads to a reduction in cardiac and brain perfusion, as well as arrhythmias.[15] With the increased cardiac output and decreased systematic vascular resistance of normal pregnancy, the risk of sudden death increases to 50%.[26]

Current medical treatment for patients with heart failure includes continuous oxygen, digoxin, diuretics and anticoagulation. Vasodilators such as hydralazine, with its side-effect of systemic hypotension, and prostacyclin, which requires continuous intravenous infusion, have not been particularly effective.[37] Surgical treatment is limited to heart–lung transplantation. The risk of development of primary pulmonary hypertension in the fetus of a mother with primary pulmonary hypertension is 3–10%.

Management Options

Prepregnancy

Preconceptual counseling should advise against pregnancy.[25]

Prenatal

In the patient who does become pregnant, termination should be recommended. Dilatation and curettage, and dilatation and evacuation, are the recommended methods in the first and second trimesters, respectively. In the continuing pregnancy, consideration should be made for hospitalization, and oxygen administered to maintain a maternal PaO_2 of 70 mmHg. Hyperbaric oxygen has been successfully used in gravidas with primary pulmonary hypertension.[38] Venous return should be encouraged by use of ambulation and support hose. This prevents the cycle leading to sudden death and decreases the risk of thromboembolic phenomena. Because of the risk of thromboembolism, full heparinization in the perinatal period has been recommended. However, Pitts[25] found increased maternal mortality with this therapy. Mini-dose heparinization of 5000 units subcutaneously twice a day may be adequate to prevent thromboemboli. Fetal monitoring should include serial ultrasound examinations to monitor growth. Because of the high risk of fetal loss, third trimester fetal heart rate testing including non-stress and contraction testing is necessary.

Labor/delivery

Attention during labor/delivery must focus primarily upon maintaining stable maternal blood pressure. The required attention to maternal volume status may necessitate central monitoring. Although recommended by many, the routine use of the pulmonary artery catheter has become controversial, with several maternal deaths being attributed directly to it from pulmonary artery rupture and fatal arrhythmia.[33,34] Preload should be maximized to avoid hypotension. Over-hydration is preferable to hypovolemia. Diuresis should be reserved for frank pulmonary edema. Pain and bearing down, both of which increase pulmonary artery resistance, and decrease venous return, should be minimized by adequate anesthesia.

Anesthesia for pulmonary hypertension during labor/delivery is controversial. Because hypotension must be avoided, some have argued for general endotracheal anesthesia.[35] Intrathecal narcotics, which have a minimal effect on systematic blood pressure as well as preventing paralysis of the lower musculature, may represent an alternative approach.[36] As mentioned earlier, we have used this method ourselves, without the use of a pulmonary artery catheter, with excellent results.

Postnatal

Close observation must be continued for 48–72 h postnatally. Despite excellent care during labor/delivery and good results, delayed sudden cardiac death has been reported 4–6 weeks postnatally.[26] This has been attributed to a rebound worsening of pulmonary hypertension secondary to the decreasing concentration of pregnancy hormones. Even with successful pregnancy with pulmonary hypertension, permanent sterilization should be considered.

RHEUMATIC HEART DISEASE: GENERAL

Maternal/Fetal Risks

Over the last five decades, the prevalence and severity of rheumatic heart disease and its sequelae of valvular disease have decreased in the USA and other developed countries.[39] Rheumatic fever affects 0.3% of children with pharyngitis from group A beta-hemolytic streptococcus. The occurrence of rheumatic fever in pregnancy is extremely uncommon, with a reported incidence in an English population in the 1960s of 0.7%.[40] The worst and most common residual effect of rheumatic fever is rheumatic heart disease.

The etiology of cardiac damage in rheumatic fever is probably an immune response to the infection, with some individuals being congenitally susceptible to the infection.[41] The resultant permanent valvular lesions can cause arrhythmias and congestive heart failure.

Although the risk of cardiac decompensation and frank pulmonary edema increases with increasing maternal age and gestational length, it is extremely uncommon, occurring in none of 203 pregnancies complicated by rheumatic valvular heart disease in one report.[33] Although the incidence of life-threatening complications has decreased in the last 30 years, rheumatic heart disease remains one of the leading causes of non-obstetric maternal death in the USA.[42] For patients who survive the pregnancy, there does not appear to be a reduction in their life expectancy.[43] Fetal risks are limited to intrauterine growth retardation, and prematurity.

Management Options

General management principles of pregnant patients with rheumatic heart disease include limitation of activity with bed rest, and continuing antibiotic prophylaxis against recurrent rheumatic fever as well as antibiotic prophylaxis against bacterial endocarditis at delivery. Individual lesions associated with rheumatic heart disease are discussed below.

MITRAL STENOSIS

Maternal/Fetal Risks

Mitral stenosis is the most frequent (90%) rheumatic valvular disorder,[44] and is the leading cause of death from heart disease in young women in most areas of the world.[45] It produces left atrial outflow obstruction, decreased cardiac output, and elevated left atrial, pulmonary venous and pulmonary capillary wedge pressures. When pulmonary capillary wedge pressure exceeds 25 mmHg, pulmonary edema usually develops.[44] Pulmonary capillary hypertension predisposes the patient to reactive pulmonary hypertension, which further limits left atrial filling and cardiac output. The increased atrial pressure also increases left atrial size, which causes atrial fibrillation in a large number of patients with mitral stenosis.[15] The overall result is a fixed cardiac output with limited ability to accommodate the increased intravascular volume and elevated heart rate associated with normal pregnancy.

Management Options

Prepregnancy

Prepregnancy care of the patient with mitral stenosis should include determining the degree of stenosis, cardiac function and reserve by a complete cardiovascular workup including two-dimensional echocardiography with color flow and Doppler. Cardiac catheterization may be necessary to better determine the size of the lesion and the presence of pulmonary hypertension. A severely stenotic valve with an orifice less than 2 cm^2 requires consideration of repair prior to pregnancy, and significantly predisposes the patient to atrial fibrillation or pulmonary edema and death during pregnancy.[15] Because of this, prepregnancy valve surgery is recommended in severe cases. Valve commissurotomy is often preferable to a prosthetic valve.[15] If a prosthesis is necessary, although a tissue valve may require replacement sooner, it is preferable to a mechanical valve because of the latter's requirement for full anticoagulation.[46]

Prenatal

For the pregnant patient with mitral stenosis, symptomatology is often correlated with pregnancy outcome, i.e. the asymptomatic patient often has an uncomplicated pregnancy.[15] Echocardiography should be done routinely in all patients with mitral valvular disease, regardless of symptomatology, with catheterization reserved for the patient with persistent pulmonary edema unresponsive to medical management who may require corrective surgery. Prenatal care should include limitation of physical activity, sodium restriction and endocarditis prophylaxis for procedures.

Atrial fibrillation, if it occurs, should be converted to a sinus rhythm by digitalization or direct current cardioversion if necessary. Recently, beta-blockade using atenolol or propranolol has been used successfully to control heart rate in 25 pregnancies with symptomatic mitral stenosis.[47] Close assessment of the fetus with serial ultrasonographic evaluation of growth and well-being is a necessary part of the prenatal management of patients with cardiac disease.

Labor/delivery

Complications during labor/delivery include pulmonary edema and atrial fibrillation. Attention at this time should be focused upon maternal intravascular volume, heart rate and blood pressure. This requires monitoring of both pulmonary and systematic arterial blood pressures. Because of the fixed valvular area with mitral stenosis, pulmonary capillary wedge pressure will not accurately reflect left ventricular end diastolic pressure. A higher than normal pulmonary capillary wedge pressure may be required to maintain adequate left atrial filling pressures and cardiac output.[10] However, upon delivery, because of the volume increase, pulmonary capillary wedge pressure may increase by up to 16 mmHg over predelivery levels.[42] Since frank pulmonary edema does not occur with pulmonary capillary wedge pressures of less than 30 mmHg, the best predelivery wedge pressure may be less than 14 mmHg. To obtain such a wedge pressure, intravascular volume (preload) reduction must be accomplished cautiously. Because cardiac output is also affected by heart rate, and cardiac output in mitral stenosis is dependent upon diastolic filling time, sinus tachycardia or atrial fibrillation in the peripartum period can lead to rapid hemodynamic decompensation. Control of heart rate should be attained with intravenous beta-blockers, such as rapid acting esmolol or slower acting propranolol.

Anesthetic concerns should be directed toward preventing rapid ventricular rates, which decrease diastolic filling time and decrease cardiac output. Medications such as atropine, ketamine, pancuronium and meperidine should be avoided.[48] Rapid ventricular rates (greater than 110 beats/min) should be treated with beta-blockers such as propranolol, labetolol or esmolol. Medically unresponsive atrial fibrillation or atrial fibrillation in an unstable (angina, hypotension) patient require cardioversion.[3] Pain during labor, hypercarbia and acidosis should be avoided because of their detrimental effect upon heart rate and pulmonary artery function. Drops in systemic vascular resistance which cause reflex tachycardia must also be avoided.

Systematic vascular resistance should be maintained with a vasopressor, e.g. metaraminol. Gradual onset epidural anesthesia is ideal as it limits pain and anxiety-induced tachycardia, and decreases cardiac output fluctuations. Cesarean section is also ideally performed with epidural anesthesia, but general anesthesia may be used with avoidance of the above-mentioned medications. Although mid-forceps have been recommended in the past to limit bearing down and strain on the heart, this may not be necessary.[10] Endocarditis prophylaxis is mandatory as with other rheumatic cardiac structural lesions.

Postnatal

Invasive monitoring should be continued postnatally in order to best manage the changes in intravascular volume that occur in the puerperal period. Clark *et al.* found postnatal elevations over baseline of pulmonary capillary wedge pressure of up to 16 mmHg in mitral stenosis patients, and advocated lowering pulmonary capillary wedge pressure to less than 14 mmHg in the prenatal period to prevent pulmonary edema postnatally.[44] However, such a reduction in preload must not be at the expense of cardiac ouput. Generally, fluid restriction and the fluid losses accompanying labor are often adequate to produce a pulmonary capillary wedge pressure of 14 mmHg or less.

MITRAL REGURGITATION

Maternal/Fetal Risks

Although mitral valve prolapse (discussed later) is the most common cause of mitral regurgitation, rheumatic deformities are the most common cause of hemodynamically significant mitral regurgitation. Mitral regurgitation represents 7% of rheumatic heart disease encountered in pregnancy.[19] It is usually well tolerated in pregnancy, and maternal mortality is rare unless severe ventricular dysfunction is present, when it may reach 5–10%.[49] When greater than 50% of the left ventricular stroke volume is ejected backward into the left atrium, significant decreases in cardiac output occur and left atrial pressure rises.[15] However, if the onset of the increased left atrial pressure is gradual, pulmonary edema is uncommon as the left ventricle is able to adjust to the increased intravascular volume of pregnancy.[15] Patients with mitral regurgitation tolerate the pregnancy's increased heart rate well, but pregnancy does appear to predispose to atrial fibrillation, especially with atrial enlargement. Therefore, some authors have recommended prophylactic digitalization for patients with severe regurgitation.[50]

Management Options

Prepregnancy

Cardiac class status (**Table 1**) should be determined for purposes of prognosis and counseling. Medical therapy should be optimized. On rare occasions, surgical correction is needed, which should ideally be done before pregnancy.

Prenatal

Asymptomatic patients with normal activity do not require treatment during pregnancy. Mildly symptomatic patients require restricted activity and salt restriction. For patients with symptoms at rest, echocardiography or catheterization are helpful. If left heart failure is evident, medical management including digitalis, diuretics and afterload reduction should be utilized. If medical therapy is unsuccessful, surgical repair should be instituted. Rheumatic fever antibiotic prophylaxis should be continued.

Labor/delivery

During the labor/delivery period, increases in systematic vascular resistance should be avoided to prevent increased regurgitation. As discussed with atrial stenosis, atrial fibrillation is not tolerated well and must be treated agressively. The preferred anesthetic technique for both cesarean and vaginal delivery is regional, since it decreases left ventricular afterload. Bacterial endocarditis prophylaxis is necessary with procedures and at delivery. Although uncommon in pregnancy, when present, mitral regurgitation requires close observation to minimize morbidity.

Postnatal

Postnatal care is dictated by prenal and labor/delivery events. The patient should be observed for evidence of cardiac failure and atrial fibrillation.

AORTIC STENOSIS

Maternal/Fetal Risks

Aortic stenosis from rheumatic disease is rare (1% of rheumatic disease) and seldom occurs independently of mitral stenosis. Left ventricular ejection is impaired in aortic stenosis, limiting cardiac output, and reducing both cerebral and coronary blood flow. Left ventricular hypertrophy eventually develops, limiting left ventricu-

lar distension, and increasing left atrial pressure. These changes predispose to tachyarrhythmias that increase myocardial oxygen consumption and decrease cardiac output. Despite these problems, aortic stenosis is remarkably well tolerated, with several series reporting no deaths and one series reporting four deaths in 23 women with 38 pregnancies.[19,51] Two of the four deaths were after therapeutic abortion. Maternal risk is also dependent upon the presence of concurrent mitral valvular disease. Fetal risks are primarily recurrent congenital heart disease and growth retardation. The risk of fetal heart disease is greater in women with uncorrected stenosis than with corrected stenosis, further arguing for correction before conception.[27]

Management Options

Prepregnancy

Prepregnancy management includes establishing a firm diagnosis with a complete echocardiographic evaluation, including two-dimensional echocardiography, with Doppler and color flow imaging as well as catheterization. Severe stenosis should be surgically corrected prior to pregnancy.

Prenatal

Prenatal care emphasizes limitation of activity, avoidance of hypovolemia, and rheumatic disease antibiotic prophylaxis.

Labor/delivery and postnatal

Care during labor/delivery and postnatally may require invasive monitoring, especially if mitral stenosis is coexistent. The primary complications observed with severe stenosis are pulmonary edema secondary to left ventricular failure and low cardiac output from decreased venous return which may result in sudden cardiac standstill. Pulmonary edema should be treated with oxygen, morphine and cardiac inotropes such as dopamine, dobutamine or amrinone.[10] Vigorous diuresis should be avoided because of the negative effect of decreased venous return on cardiac output. Sudden decreases in venous return may be the cause of sudden death in gravidas with aortic stenosis. Venocaval compression by the uterus and hypovolemia must be avoided.

Regional anesthesia can decrease systematic vascular resistance and venous return. Narcotic epidural with local infiltration avoids this problem.[8] Balanced general anesthesia may be the best choice for cesarean delivery. Bacterial endocarditis prophylaxis is necessary.

AORTIC REGURGITATION

Maternal/Fetal Risks

Aortic regurgitation or insufficiency from rheumatic disease is usually associated with mitral stenosis, but may also be seen with Marfan's syndrome or syphilitic aortitis. When aortic regurgitation develops slowly, stroke volume and left ventricular volume increase gradually, producing left ventricular hypertrophy with maintenance of cardiac output. The development of both left ventricular dilatation and hypertrophy, and widened pulse pressure, is extremely uncommon in a woman of child-bearing age.[52] Therefore, aortic regurgitation is extremely uncommon with pregnancy, accounting for 2.5% of rheumatic disease in pregnancy. The increased heart rate of pregnancy, which decreases time for systolic regurgitation, and the decreased systemic vascular resistance with pregnancy, which decreases regurgitation, make aortic regurgitation extremely well tolerated in pregnancy. Szekely reported only one death from pulmonary edema in 19 patients with 38 pregnancies.[18]

Management Options

Prepregnancy

Prepregnancy management includes echocardiography, catheterization and electrocardiography. Symptomatic patients should have medical management including digitalis, diuresis and afterload reduction. If medical management is unsuccessful, surgical replacement of the valve is necessary.

Prenatal

Management is similar to the prepregnancy period, including surgical correction of non-responsive cases. In aortic regurgitation secondary to active endocarditis, maternal mortality is particularly high with medical management, and early surgical repair is preferable.

Labor/delivery and postnatal

Management of labor/delivery and the postnatal period, in the absence of congestive heart failure, can be accomplished without invasive monitoring unless mitral valvular disease is also present. As with mitral regurgitation, lumbar epidural anesthesia is preferred because of afterload reduction. Increased afterload can lead to cardiac failure by increasing regurgitation. Bradycardias, which increase ventricular diastolic time and subsequently regurgitant flow, must also be avoided. If general anesthesia is necessary, myocardial depressants such as halothane and enflurane should be avoided, and atrial fibrillation treated aggressively.[53]

MITRAL VALVE PROLAPSE

Maternal/Fetal Risks

Mitral valve prolapse is caused by a primary connective tissue disease of the mitral valve leaflets, chordae tendineae and annulus producing valvulo-ventricular disproportion and valvular prolapse. The diagnosis may be by auscultation or echocardiography. Mid-systolic click alone is the hallmark of the condition, but a systolic murmur may also be present. Echocardiography should demonstrate inappropriate posterior motion of the mitral valve during systole.[54] Increased left end diastolic volume and lowered systemic vascular resistance decrease the degree of prolapse, making the diagnosis in pregnancy more difficult.[55] The incidence of mitral valve prolapse may approach 17% of otherwise healthy young women of child-bearing age.[2] It is associated with Marfan's syndrome, von Willebrand's disease, autoimmune disorders and hyperthyroidism. Complications are more frequent in patients with systolic murmurs as well as clicks, and include infective endocarditis, spontaneous non-infectious rupture of chordae tendineae, emboli and sustained tachyrhythmia.[18] Sudden death in association with mitral valve prolapse is exceedingly rare. Although no evidence exists for increased pregnancy wastage, the risk of the development of mitral valve prolapse in the child of a mother with mitral valve prolapse is high.[56]

Management Options

Prepregnancy

Prepregnancy management should include two-dimensional echocardiography to document the diagnosis of mitral valve prolapse and to determine the degree of regurgitation.

Prenatal

Prenatal management is directed toward treatment of arrhythmias. Re-entrant supraventricular tachycardia is the most common tachyrhythmia with mitral valve prolapse, and is treated with digitalization.[15] Multiform or repetitive ventricular ectopy may require beta-blockers.

Labor/delivery and postnatal

Management of labor/delivery and the postnatal period should consist of external maternal cardiac monitoring if there is a history of tachyrhythmia or ectopy. The risk of endocarditis is small without concurrent regurgitation, and prophylaxis is recommended for all patients with mitral valve prolapse with regurgitation.[12]

MARFAN'S SYNDROME

Maternal/Fetal Risks

Marfan's syndrome is a generalized connective tissue abnormality that causes mitral valve prolapse and aortic root weakening. Although the mitral valve prolapse of Marfan's syndrome carries the above risks, the aortic root complications of aortic regurgitation and dissection are much more significant. All women with Marfan's syndrome have cardiovascular involvement, and this complication reduces the life expectancy of Marfan's patients to half that of normal.[57] Pregnancy definitely increases the risk of aortic regurgitation and aortic dissection. Aortic dilation accompanied by aortic regurgitation is associated with a 50% mortality in pregnancy.[55] An aortic root diameter of less than 40 mm, a normal valve with no regurgitation, and no dilation is associated with a 5% mortality.[58] Because of the autosomal dominant transmission of Marfan's syndrome, the risk of the fetus developing Marfan's syndrome is 50%.

Management Options

Prepregnancy

Preconceptual counseling should emphasize the high rate of transmission of Marfan's syndrome as well as the significant risk of maternal death. Echocardiographic evaluation of aortic root diameter and post-valvular dilatation must be done to determine risk of mortality. The prophylactic use of propranolol has been recommended to decrease pulsatile pressure on the aortic wall.[59]

Prenatal, labor/delivery and postnatal

Prenatal, labor/delivery and postnatal care should be directed toward recognizing symptoms and signs of aortic dissection, as well as maintaining blood pressure within a small range and especially minimizing systolic hypertension.

CARDIOMYOPATHIES

Maternal/Fetal Risks

Peripartum cardiomyopathy is a dilated cardiomyopathy that develops in the last month of pregnancy (15%) or the first 6 months postpartum (80% occur in the first 2 months) without prior cardiac disease and after the exclusion of other etiologies of cardiac failure.[60] The incidence is 1 in 5000–15 000 pregnancies, depending upon the population. Reported associations include increased parity, age, multiple gestation, malnutrition and hypertension.[15] Multiple gestation, malnutrition and hypertension (both pregnancy-induced and chronic) may aggravate the failure, and not primarily cause it. The majority of patients in the USA are Afro-American.[15] Maternal risks include systemic and pulmonary emboli (50%) and mortality (50%).[61]

Management Options

Prepregnancy

Preconceptual counseling of patients with a history of peripartum cardiomyopathy is controversial. Some authors believe pregnancy is absolutely contraindicated because the reported risk of recurrence and mortality ranges from 10 to 60%.[35] The prognosis is most closely related to the cardiac size 1 year after diagnosis: with a return to normal size, mortality is 11–14%; persistent cardiomegaly is associated with a mortality rate of 15–80%.[58]

Prenatal, labor/ delivery and postnatal

Limited information is available for prenatal labor/delivery and postnatal management of pregnancies complicated by peripartum cardiomyopathy. Therapy should include bed rest, sodium restriction, digoxin, diuretics and afterload reduction with hydralazine or nitrates. Immunosuppressive therapy has been utilized successfully where inflammatory myocarditis has been identified on endomyocardial biopsy. Because of the high risk of thromboemboli, anticoagulation should be routinely used.[15] In view of the high risk of recurrence, counseling regarding contraception and future pregnancies is mandatory.

ARRHYTHMIAS

Maternal/Fetal Risks

Arrhythmias during pregnancy are of two general types: (1) benign dysrhythmias that occur in otherwise uncomplicated pregnancies, and (2) dysrhythmia associated with certain cardiac diseases. Sinus bradycardia, sinus tachycardia, atrial and ventricular premature beats are very common in normal pregnancy. Although bigeminy may occur in normal pregnancy, multiform premature ventricular complexes and ventricular tachycardia are abnormal and require further evaluation including electrocardiography.

Paroxysmal supraventricular tachycardia (PSVT) is the most common sustained tachyrhythmia in pregnancy, and is likely to recur in the third trimester.[62] Atrial fibrillation and flutter are usually associated with organic heart disease such as Wolff-Parkinson-White syndrome. Maternal risks, from arrhythmias are primarily failure and death. Fetal risks are primarily related to cardiac anti-arrhythmic medication effects.

Management Options

Prenatal, labor/delivery and postnatal management should include appropriate anti-arrhythmic medications. For PSVT, emergent treatment may consist of intravenous verapamil or esmolol, followed by maintenance therapy with digoxin. Both quinidine and procainamide may be used in pregnancy, with quinidine the preferred drug because of greater experience with it and the lupus-like syndrome encountered with procainamide. The use of amiodarone, with its long half-life and effect on fetal thyroid function, should be restricted to pregnant patients with Wolff-Parkinson-White syndrome. When medical therapy fails or the patient is unstable (angina, hypotension), cardioversion has been accomplished safely without fetal complication in pregnancy.[3]

ATHEROSCLEROTIC CORONARY HEART DISEASE

Maternal/Fetal Risks

Atherosclerotic coronary heart disease is exceedingly rare in the 17–35 years age group. Coronary disease in pregnancy usually presents as myocardial infarction. Although the increased hemodynamic burden of late pregnancy may cause discovery of unrecognized coronary disease, not all coronary thrombosis is associated with abnormal coronary arteries.[63]

The incidence of atherosclerotic coronary heart disease is 1 in 10 000 deliveries. The overall maternal risk of death is 35%, with increased risk of myocardial infarction later in pregnancy. Women who survive myocardial infarction during pregnancy have an increased risk for miscarriage and stillbirth.[64,65]

Management Options

Preconceptual counseling of women with a history of coronary heart disease must include notification of the increased risk of myocardial infarction with pregnancy as well as the 35% mortality of infarction in pregnancy. Prenatal care must include bed rest to limit myocardial oxygen consumption, control of hypertension, and antianginal medications including nitrates. Myocardial infarction occurring during the prenatal period has been managed medically and surgically by coronary bypass grafting as well as with intra-aortic balloon counterpulsation.[65] Delivery within 2 weeks of infarction is associated with increased mortality.[66] Management of labor/delivery should include external cardiac monitoring for evidence of ischemia, oxygen administration and epidural anesthesia, with invasive pulmonary artery monitoring reserved for those patients with a history of failure. Oral contraception may be contraindicated in these patients.

IDIOPATHIC HYPERTROPHIC SUBAORTIC STENOSIS

Maternal/Fetal Risks

Idiopathic hypertrophic subaortic stenosis (IHSS)is an autosomal dominant condition that may first appear during pregnancy.[15] Septal hypertrophy obstructs left ventricular outflow primarily, and causes mitral regurgitation secondarily. Because of the varied effects of pregnancy, the effect of pregnancy upon IHSS is variable. The increased blood volume of pregnancy improves cardiac output, whereas the fall in systemic vascular resistance with pregnancy decreases it. The increase in maternal heart rate also decreases time for left ventricular filling and increases outflow obstruction. Maternal risks are few, and death has been reported only once.[67] The risk of the fetus developing IHSS in a mother with IHSS is 50%.

Management Options

Preconceptual conseling should discuss the fetal risk of recurrence. Prenatal, labor/delivery and postnatal management should be to limit stress, increase bed rest and avoid tachycardia and hypotension. In cases where maternal bearing down efforts cause hypotension, operative vaginal delivery should be instituted. Cesarean section should be reserved for obstetrical indications. Beta-blockers should be reserved for angina and arrhythmias. Calcium channel blockers have recently been used to improve hemodynamic function.[68] Endocarditis prophylaxis is required in this condition (**Table 3**).

CARDIAC DISEASE
Summary of Management Options

GENERAL: CHECKLIST FOR MANAGEMENT OF PATIENT WITH CARDIAC DISEASE IN PREGNANCY

Prepregnancy

- Discussion of maternal/fetal risks

- Discussion of effective/safe contraception

- Obtain update on cardiac status

- Optimize medical and surgical management

- Advise against pregnancy with certain conditions (see text)

Prenatal

- Assess functional class of heart disease

- Joint management with cardiologist

- Optimize medical management

- Avoid/minimize aggravating factors

- Anticoagulation for certain conditions (? stop warfarin and change to subcutaneous heparin: see Chapter 33)

- Prophylactic antibiotics with certain conditions (see **Tables 3** and **4**)

- Fetal surveillance:
  - growth (especially if left-to-right shunt)
  - detailed fetal cardiac ultrasound if maternal congenital heart disease

Labor/delivery

- Elective induction may be necessary for maternal and/or fetal indications

- Avoid mental and physical stress (? epidural)

- Labor in left lateral or upright position

- Monitor electrocardiogram; more invasive monitoring with certain conditions

- Administer extra oxygen with certain conditions

- Full resuscitation facilities available

- Continuous fetal heart rate monitoring

- Assisted second stage with certain conditions

- Avoid ergometrine for third stage

Postnatal

- Vigilance for cardiac failure

- Continued high-dependency care

- Discuss effective/safe contraception

SPECIFIC: MANAGEMENT OPTIONS FOR THESE CONDITIONS DISCUSSED ON PAGES SHOWN

- Atrial septal defect p. 301

- Patent ductus arteriosus p. 302

- Coarctation of the aorta p. 302

- Aortic valvular disease (non-rheumatic) p. 303

- Ventricular septal defects p. 303

- Eisenmenger's complex/syndrome p. 303

- Tetralogy of Fallot p. 304

- Primary pulmonary hypertension p. 305

- Mitral stenosis p. 306

- Mitral regurgitation p. 308

- Aortic stenosis p. 308

- Aortic regurgitation p. 309

- Mitral valve prolapse p. 309

- Marfan's syndrome p. 310

- Cardiomyopathy p. 310

- Arrhythmias p. 311

- Atherosclerotic coronary heart disease p. 311

- Idiopathic hypertrophic subaortic stenosis p. 311

REFERENCES

1 Sugrue D *et al.* (1981) Pregnancy complicated with maternal heart disease at the national hospital, Dublin, Ireland, 1969–78. *American Journal of Obstetrics and Gynecology* **139**:1–6.

2 Markiewicz W, Stoner J, London E *et al.* (1976) Mitral valve prolapse in one hundred presumably healthy young females. *Circulation* **53**:464–473.

3 Reid CL, Elkayam U, Rhamitoola SH (1992) Infective endocarditis. In Gleicher N (ed.) *Principles and Practice of Medical Therapy in Pregnancy*, pp. 795–801. Norwalk, Conn.: Appleton and Lange.

4 Whittemore R, Hobbins JC, Engle MA (1982) Pregnancy and its outcome in women with and without surgical treatment of congenital heart disease. *American Journal of Cardiology* **50**:641–651.

5 Rose V, Gold RJM, Lindsay G, Allen M (1985) A possible increase in the incidence of congenital heart defects among the offspring of affected parents. *Journal of the American College of Cardiologists* **53**:376–382.

6 Neil CA, Swanson S (1961) Outcome of pregnancy in congenital heart disease (abstract). *Circulation* **24**:1003.

7 Niswander KR, Berendes H, Deutschberger J *et al.* (1967) Fetal morbidity following potentially anoxygenic obstetric conditions. V. Organic heart disease. *American Journal of Obstetrics and Gynecology* **98**:871–876.

8 Mortenson JD, Ellsworth HS (1963) Pregnancy and cardiac surgery. *Circulation* **28**:773.

9 Criteria Committee of the New York Heart Association (1964) *Nomenclature and Criteria for Diagnosis of Disease of the Heart and Great Vessels*, 6th edn. Boston, MA: Little, Brown.

10 Clark SL (1991) Structural cardiac disease in pregnancy. In Clark SL, Cotton DB, Hankins GDV, Phelan JP (eds) *Critical Care Obstetrics*, 2nd edn, pp. 114–135. Oxford: Blackwell Scientific.

11 Ostheimer GW, Alper MA (1975) Intrapartum anesthetic management of the pregnant patient with heart disease. *Clinics in Obstetrics and Gynecology* **18**:81–97.

12 Dajani AS, Bisno AL, Chung KJ *et al.* (1990) Prevention of bacterial endocarditis: Recommendations by the American Heart Association. *Journal of the American Medical Association* **264**:2919–2922.

13 Elkayam U (1992) Pregnancy and cardiovascular disease. In Braunwald E (ed.) *Heart Disease: A Textbook of Cardiovascular Medicine,* 4th edn, pp.1790–1809. Philadelphia: W.B. Saunders.

14 Campbell M (1970) Natural history of atrial septal defect. *British Heart Journal* **32**:820–826.

15 Metcalfe J, McNulty JH, Ueland K (1986) *Heart Disease and Pregnancy: Physiology and Management.* Boston, MA: Little, Brown.

16 Morris CD, Menashe VD (1985) Recurrence of congenital heart disease in offspring of parents with surgical correction *Clinical Research* **33**:68A.

17 Alzamora-Castro V, Battilana G, Abugattas R, Sialer S (1960) Patent ductus arteriosus and high altitude. *American Journal of Cardiology.* **5**:761–763.

18 Szekely P, Snaith L (1974) *Heart Disease and Pregnancy.* Edinburgh: Churchill Livingstone.

19 McFaul PB, Dorman JC, Lamki H *et al.* (1988) Pregnancy complicated by maternal heart disease: A review of 519 women. *British Journal of Obstetrics and Gynecology* **95**:861–867.

20 Deal K, Wooley CF (1973) Coarctation of aorta and pregnancy. *Annals of Internal Medicine* **78**: 706–710.

21 Mortenson JD, Ellsworth HS (1965) Coarctation of the aorta and pregnancy: Obstetric and cardiovascular complications before and after surgical correction. *Journal of the American Medical Association* **191**:596–598.

22 Cobb T, Gleicher N, Elkayam U (1982) Congenital heart disease and pregnancy. In Elkayam U and Gleicher N (eds) *Cardiac Problems in Pregnancy*, pp. 67–69. New York: Alan R. Liss.

23 Alpert BS, Mellits ED, Rowe RD (1973) Spontaneous closure of small ventricular septal defects: Probability rates in the first five years of life. *American Journal of Diseases of Children* **125**:194–196.

24 Hamilton BE, Thomson KH (1941) *The Heart in Pregnancy and the Childbearing Age.* Boston, MA: Little, Brown.

25 Pitts JA, Crosby WM, Basta LL (1977) Eisenmenger's syndrome in pregnancy: Does heparin prophylaxis improve the maternal mortality rate. *American Heart Journal* **93**:321–326.

26 Gleicher N, Midwall J, Hochberger D, Jaffin H (1979) Eisenmenger's syndrome and pregnancy. *Obstetrical and Gynaecological Survey* **34**:721–741.

27 Campbell M (1972) Natural history of cyanotic malformations and comparison of all common cardiac malformations. *British Heart Journal* **34**:3–8.

28 Mendelson CL (1960) Cardiac disease in pregnancy. In Heaton CE (ed.) *Medical Care, Cardiovascular Surgery and Obstetrical Management as Related to Maternal and Fetal Welfare.* Obstetrical and Gynecological Monographs. Philadelphia: Davis.

29 Hamilton BE (1954) Cardiovascular problems in pregnancy. *Circulation* **9**:922–933.

30 Meter EC, Tulsky AS, Sigmann P, Silber EN (1964) Pregnancy in the presence of tetralogy of Fallot: Observation on two patients. *American Journal of Cardiology* **14**:874–879.

31 Jacoby WJ Jr (1964) Pregnancy with tetralogy and pentalogy of Fallot. *American Journal of Cardiology* **14**: 866.

32 Whittemore R (1983) Congenital heart disease: Its impact on pregnancy. *Hospital Practice* **18**:65–74.

33 Barash PG *et al.* (1981) Catheter induced pulmonary artery perforation: Mechanisms, management, and modifications. *Journal of Thoracic and Cardiovascular Surgery* **82**:5–12.

34 Devitt JH, Noble WH, Byrick RJ (1982) A Swan-Ganz catheter related complication in a patient with Eisenmenger's syndrome. *Anesthesiology* **57**:335–337.

35 Sullivan JM, Ramanathan KB (1985) Management of medical problems in pregnancy: Severe cardiac disease. *New England Journal of Medicine* **313**:304–309.

36 Abboud TK, Raya J, Noueihed R, Daniel J (1983) Intrathecal morphine for relief of labor pain in a parturient with severe pulmonary hypertension. *Anesthesiology* **59**:477–479.

37 Palevsky HI, Fishman AP (1991) The management of

primary pulmonary hypertension. *Journal of the American Medical Association* **256**:1014–1020.

38 Slavin AG (1979) Importance of hyperbaric oxygenation for a favourable outcome of labor in primary pulmonary hypertension patients. *Vopr Okhr Materin Det* **24**:64–66.

39 Krause RM (1979) The influence of infection on the geography of heart disease. *Circulation* **60**:972–976.

40 Szekely P, Turner R, Snaith L (1973) Pregnancy and the changing pattern of rheumatic heart disease. *British Heart Journal* **35**:1293–1303.

41 Gray ED, Regelmann EW, Abdin Z, Kholy A *et al.* (1987) Compartmentalization of cells bearing 'rheumatic' cell surface antigens in peripheral blood and tonsils in rheumatic heart disease. *Journal of Infectious Diseases* **155**:247.

42 Hibbard LT (1975) Maternal mortality due to cardiac disease. *Clinics in Obstetrics and Gynecology* **18**:27–36.

43 Chesley LC (1980) Severe rheumatic cardiac disease and pregnancy: The ultimate prognosis. *American Journal of Obstetrics and Gynecology* **136**:552–558.

44 Clark SL, Phelan JP, Greenspoon J *et al.* (1985) Labor and delivery in the presence of mitral stenosis: Central hemodynamic observations. *American Journal of Obstetrics and Gynecology* **152**:984–988.

45 Padmavati S (1978) Rheumatic fever and rheumatic heart disease in developing countries. *Bulletin of the World Health Organization* **56**:543–550.

46 Lakier JB, Khaja F, Magilligan DJ Jr, Goldstein S (1980) Porcine xenograft valves: Long-term (60–89 month) followup. *Circulation* **62**:313–318.

47 Al Kasab SM *et al.* (1990) β-adrenergic receptor blockade in the management of pregnant women with mitral stenosis. *American Journal of Obstetrics and Gynecology* **163**:37–40.

48 Jones MM, Joyce TH (1991) Anesthesia for the patient with pregnancy-induced hypertension and pregnant cardiac patient. In Clark SL, Cotton DB, Hankins GDV, Phelan JP (eds) *Critical Care Obstetrics*, 2nd edn, pp. 559–578. Oxford: Blackwell Scientific Publications.

49 McAnulty JH, Blair N. Walance C, Ueland K (1986) Prosthetic heart valves and pregnancy: Maternal and infant outcome. *Journal of the American College of Cardiologists* **7**:171A.

50 Ueland K (1982) Rheumatic heart disease and pregnancy. In Elkayam U, Gleicher N (eds) *Cardiac Problems in Pregnancy: Diagnosis and Management of Maternal and Fetal Disease*, pp. 79–86. New York: Alan R. Liss.

51 Arias F, Pineda J (1978) Aortic stenosis and pregnancy. *Journal of Reproductive Medicine* **20**:229–232.

52 Spagnuolo M, Kloth H, Taranta A *et al.* (1971) Natural history of rheumatic aortic regurgitation: Criteria predictive of death, congestive heart failure, and angina in young patients. *Circulation* **44**:368–380.

53 Ramanathan J, Sibai BM (1992) Obstetric anesthesia for complicated pregnancies. In Gleicher N (ed.) *Principles and Practice of Medical Therapy in Pregnancy*, pp. 1247–1261. Norwalk, Conn.: Appleton and Lange.

54 DeMaria AN, King JF, Bogren HG *et al.* (1974) The variable spectrum of echocardiographic manifestations of the mitral valve prolapse syndrome. *Circulation* **50**:33–41.

55 Haas JM (1976) The effect of pregnancy on the midsystolic click and murmur of the prolapsing posterior leaflet of the mitral valve. *American Heart Journal* **92**:407–408.

56 Shappell, SD, Marshall CE, Brown RE, Bruce TA (1973) Sudden death and the familial occurrence of mid systolic click, late systolic murmur syndrome. *Circulation* **48**:1128–1134.

57 Murdoch JL, Walker BA, Halpern BL *et al.* (1972) Life expectancy and causes of death in the Marfan syndrome. *New England Journal of Medicine* **286**:804–808.

58 Pyeritz RE (1981) Maternal and fetal complications of pregnancy in the Marfan syndrome. *American Journal of Medicine* **71**:784–790.

59 Slater EE, DeSanctis RW (1979) Dissection of the aorta. *Medical Clinics of North America* **63**:141–154.

60 Demakis JG, Rahimtoola SH, Sutton GC *et al.* (1971) Natural course of peripartum cardiomyopathy. *Circulation* **44**:1053–1061.

61 Homans DC (1985) Peripartum cardiomyopathy. *New England Journal of Medicine* **312**:1432–1437.

62 Schroeder JS, Harrison DC (1971) Repeated cardioversion during pregnancy. *American Journal of Cardiology* **27**:445–446.

63 Henion WA, Hilal A, Matthew PK, Lazarus A, Cohen J (1982) Postpartum myocardial infarction. *New York State Journal of Medicine* **82**:57–62.

64 Reece EA, Assimakopoulos EA (1992) Coronary artery disease. In Gleicher N (ed.) *Principles and Practice of Medical Therapy in Pregnancy*, pp. 817–822. Norwalk, Conn.: Appleton and Lange.

65 Allen JN, Wewers MD (1990) Acute myocardial infarction with cardiogenic shock during pregnancy: Treatment with intra-aortic balloon counterpulsation. *Critical Care Medicine* **18**:888–889.

66 Ueland K (1989) Cardiac diseases. In Creasy RK, Resnik R (eds) *Maternal-Fetal Medicine*, 2nd edn, pp. 746–762. Philadelphia: W.B. Saunders.

67 Oakley GDG, McGarry K, Limb DG, Oakley CM (1979) Management of pregnancy in patients with hypertrophic cardiomyopathy. *British Medical Journal* **1**:1749–1750.

68 Lorell BH, Paulus WJ, Grossman W *et al.* (1982) Modification of abnormal left ventricular diastolic properties of nifedipine in patients with hypertrophic cardiomyopathy. *Circulation* **65**:499–507.

21

Thyroid Disorders

CAROLE A. MAJOR, MICHAEL P. NAGEOTTE

INTRODUCTION

Diseases of the thyroid are common in the female population; therefore, it is not uncommon for obstetricians to care for patients with concomitant thyroid disorders.[1] Pregnancy has a significant impact on the normal maternal thyroid physiology and function. Many of the physiologic changes that occur during pregnancy may mimic thyroid abnormalities. Careful evaluation and correct interpretation of thyroid laboratory values during pregnancy is essential.[2–4]

The thyroid, like most of the other endocrine systems, is regulated by the pituitary gland and hypothalamus. Thyrotropin-releasing hormone (TRH) is synthesized and released from the hypothalamus. This neurotransmitter stimulates the anterior pituitary to both synthesize and release thryoid-stimulating hormone (TSH). In turn, THS, stimulates both the synthesis and release of the thyroid hormones, triiodothyronine (T3) and thyroxine (T4). Both of these thyroid hormones have a classic negative feedback control on TSH; mainly at the level of the pituitary.[5] The steps for thyroid hormone synthesis are outlined in **Table 1**. This is of critical importance; since the therapy of various disorders involves pharmacologic manipulation of different points along this pathway.

Pregnancy causes changes in the structure and function of the thyroid gland which may result in confusion when attempting to diagnose thyroid disfunction (**Table 2**).[6] The overall control of the thyroid gland is not altered in a normal pregnancy. However, the binding of the active thyroid hormone is markedly changed during pregnancy. The amount of thyroid-binding

Table 1
Pathway of thyroid hormone synthesis

1. Trapping:	Accumulation of iodide within the thyroid gland from the plasma by active transport via the iodide pump. This step is stimulated by TSH and iodide deficiency
2. Iodination:	The iodide reacts with a peroxidase and the tyrosyl groups of thyroglobulin to form monoiodotyrosine and diiodotyrosine. This step is inhibited by both propylthiouracil (PTU) and methimozole (TAP)
3. Coupling:	Formed iodotyrosines oxidatively couple to form thyroxine (T4) and triiodothyronine (T3)
4. Release:	The T4 and T3 are released into the circulation by the action of a protease. This step is stimulated by TSH and inhibited by iodine
5. Peripheral conversion:	The circulating T4 is converted to T3 (active) and rT3 (reverse T3-inactive). This step is inhibited by PTU and decreased by propranolol and glucocorticoids

globulin produced by the liver doubles in the first trimester. This change is thought to result from the effects of estrogen increase. This results in an increased amount of total hormone (T4), whereas there is no change in the amount of circulating free hormone

Table 2
Alterations of laboratory tests of thyroid function
during pregnancy

	Non-pregnant	Pregnant	Change in pregnancy
T4 (total)			increased
T3 (total)	5–12.5 µg/dl	6–15 µg/dl	increased
T4 (free)	50–175 ng/dl	125–275 ng/dl	no change
T3 (free)	2.5 ng/dl	2.5 ng/dl	no change
TSH	0.3 ng/dl	0.3 ng/dl	no change
	1.9–5.9 µU/ml	1.9–5.9 µU/ml	
FTI	4.5–12	4.5–12	no change
R3TU	25–35%	15–25%	decreased

(FT4). The renal clearance of iodine increases in pregnancy but more iodine is successfully trapped by the thyroid gland to maintain normal thyroid homeostasis.[7,8]

By the end of the first trimester, the fetal thyroid–pituitary axis is functional. Thyrotropin and thyrotropin releasing hormone can be detected in the fetal pituitary and hypothalamus from about 10 weeks of gestation. Thyrotropin and T4 appear in the circulation from 12 weeks. These levels remain low until the mid-third trimester (30 weeks) when T3 and T4 peak.

HYPERTHYROIDISM

Hyperthroidism in the mother is present in approximately two out of every 1000 pregnancies and 90% of cases of hyperthyroidism are secondary to Graves' disease, which is an autoimmune disorder associated with the presence of circulating thyroid-stimulating antibodies. Not uncommonly, alterations in the immune system during the latter part of pregnancy result in an improvement in Graves' disease. Aggravation of symptoms frequently occur in the postpartum period and need to be followed closely.[9] Other causes of hyperthyroidism include toxic diffuse nodules, toxic multinodular goiter, subacute thyroiditis, Hashimito's thyroiditis and trophoblastic disease.

Diagnosis

Some of the signs and symptoms of hyperthyroidism include tachycardia, weight loss, heat intolerance and systolic flow murmurs. Because of the hyperdynamic state of pregnancy, some of these signs may be overlooked or mistaken as normal physiologic changes in pregnancy.

Infiltrative dermopathy, which is characterized by localized thickening of the skin and opthalmopathy, which is manifested by exopthalmos, are most commonly seen with Graves' disease. However, these signs do not indicate the degree of hyperthyroidism.[10]

Confirmation of the diagnosis can be made by measuring the FT4 and FT3 levels, which are elevated. A less expensive yet reliable test in pregnancy is the free thyroxine index (FT1), which is calculated from total T4 and the T3 resin uptake (FTI-T3RU × TT4/100). The RT3U is the resin uptake test and is an indirect measurement of the thyroid-binding globulin or the amount of thyroid hormone that is protein bound. TSH levels are usually suppressed and are only detected with the new ultrasensitive assays; for many, this represents the best way of diagnosing and monitoring thyroid disorders in pregnancy.

Maternal Risks

Although this disorder causes menstrual irregularities, it appears to have little impact on fertility. In general, pregnancy does not appear to worsen the course and should not alter the management of thyroid disease.[11]

The primary maternal concern related to hyperthyroidism is uncontrolled disease, termed 'thyroid storm'. It is a medical emergency with a mortality rate as high as 25% even with appropriate management. It is most commonly precipitated by infection or stress such as labor, cesarean section or surgery. It is characterized by hyperpyrexia, which invariably begins a few hours after delivery or surgery. The fever can easily exceed 40°C. Tachycardia, which is almost always present, is usually out of proportion to the fever. This tachycardia may even precipitate high output heart failure. Atrial fibrillation with rapid ventricular response may also be present. Other symptoms include diarrhea, vomiting, dehydration, abdominal pains and central nervous system (CNS) abnormalities such as restlessness, seizures, psychosis, stupor and even coma.[12]

Fetal Risks

Very little is known concerning the role of maternal thyroid hormones in fetal development; T3 and TSH do not cross the placenta from the mother to fetus. Although in the hypothyroid fetus some T4 may cross from the mother to the fetus, persistently low T4 levels in the fetus lead to an increase in TSH and thyroid stimulations, as evidenced by the development of goiter in the fetus due to defects in thyroid hormone biosynthesis.[13] Thyroid-stimulating antibodies, TRH, TSH receptor antibodies, PTU, methimozole and iodine all cross the placenta and may subsequently cause alterations in the fetal physiology.[14] The fetal thyroid after 11–12 weeks concentrates iodine at a significantly higher rate than the maternal thyroid; therefore, the use of diagnostic scanning or uptake with radioactive tracers such as iodine 131 or technetium 99 should be avoided after the first trimester due to the risks of exposure to the developing fetus.[15]

Hyperthyroidism has other adverse effects on perinatal outcome.[16] It has been associated with an increased incidence of preterm deliveries (11–25%), stillbirths (8–15%) and an overall decrease in the mean infant birthweight.[2,4] There is also an increased incidence of fetal/neonatal thyrotoxicosis due to the transplacental passage of immunoglobulins associated with Graves' disease. Neonatal thyrotoxicosis occurs in 10% of the offspring of mothers with Graves disease. it is usually transient, lasting only 2–3 months after delivery. The finding of a high titer of thyroid-stimulating immunoglobulins in the blood of an infant is highly predictive of the development of hyperthyroidism, but the absence of such titers does not mean the infant will not develop the disease. Studies have also shown that a high maternal TSH receptor antibody level in the last trimester of pregnancy is helpful in making the presumptive diagnosis of fetal hyperthyroidism. Thyrotoxicosis may also result in the development of craniosynostosis, exopthalmos, heart failure and hepatosplenomegaly. Maternal thioamide therapy may mask the symptoms of neonatal thyrotoxicosis at birth and cause a delay in the onset of its symptoms. The development of neonatal thyrotoxicosis is not dependent on the activity of the maternal thyroid disease.[7]

Management Options

Prepregnancy

Therapy for hyperthyroidism is best begun prior to pregnancy. This will allow for the use of radioactive iodine studies for diagnosis, higher initial doses of pharmacologic agents without fetal concerns, and surgery when needed for unresponsive cases. Counseling should be supportive and reassuring, although absolute guarantees for lack of fetal effects is not possible. Most importantly, patients should be sternly warned against the discontinuation of medications without close supervision. Risks of adverse perinatal outcomes as outlined above should be discussed.[18]

Prenatal

All pregnant patients who have both symptoms and laboratory abnormalities suggestive of hyperthyroidism should be treated. Management for patients who are chemically hyperthyroid and clinically euthyroid is widely debated. Extreme elevations in the thyroid test, despite the lack of symptoms, require immediate treatment. Clinically euthyroid patients with mild labora-

tory abnormalities may be followed closely with clinical evaluations and thyroid studies.[19] The only exceptions to this management are patients with high titers of either TSH receptor antibodies and/or thyroid-stimulating antibodies. In such cases, these patients should be treated to maintain the thyroid tests within the upper limits of normal.[20]

Therapeutic modalities for hyperthyroidism can be divided into five categories (see **Table 3**):

- thioamides
- beta-blockers
- iodides
- radioactive iodine
- surgery

Medical therapy, with the thioamides, is the mainstay of hyperthyroid treatment during pregnancy. Both PTU and tapazole (TAP) are efficacious in treating hyperthyroidism. However, PTU is the preferred agent due to the fact that it not only blocks the incorporation of iodine into tyrosine and thus inhibits thyroxine synthesis, but it also inhibits the peripheral conversion of

Table 3
Pharmacologic agents in hyperthyroidism

Name	Mode of action	Dose	Side-effects
PTU	Inhibits thyroid synthesis and peripheral conversion of T4 to T3	50–150 mg every 8 h	Rash, fever, agranulocytosis
TAP	Inhibits thyroid hormone synthesis	5–20 mg every 8 h	Rash, fever, agranulocytosis
Propranolol	Decreases adrenergic symptoms	10–80 mg every 6–8 h	Bronchospasm, CHF
Iodide	Inhibits thyroid hormone release	see doses for each medication below	Rash
SSKI (potassium iodide)	See above	1–2 drops orally every 8 h	Rash
NaI (sodium iodide)	See above	1 g i.v. every 8 h	Rash

T4 to T3. Side-effects occur in approximately 2–3% of all patients taking these agents and include skin rash, pruritis, agranulocytosis (0.2%), granulocytopenia (5%), nausea, vomiting and diarrhea. A severe complication, agranulocytosis, requires cessation of all thioamide therapy.

The usual starting dose of PTU is 300–450 mg/day and of TAP 30–45 mg/day. Both drugs are given in divided doses orally. Usually, some improvement is seen after 1 week of treatment with thioamides. However, 4–6 weeks may sometimes be needed for a full effect. During therapy, the FT4 and FT1 need to be closely followed to avoid the development of maternal hypothyroidism. As the FT4 and FT1 begin to decrease, the dose of the thioamides needs to be decreased by a quarter to a third over 3–4 week intervals. Lowering of the doses after the first 4–6 weeks of therapy is recommended so that unnecessary fetal

---

HYPERTHYROIDISM
Summary of Management Options

Prepregnancy

- Establish the diagnosis of hyperthyroidism prior to pregnancy so that a complete diagnostic workup can be reformed and therapy instituted
- Counsel regarding the need to continue therapy during pregnancy, potential perinatal risks, and need for serial thyroid function studies

Prenatal

- Continue thioamide therapy to maintain patient clinically euthyroid and laboratory parameters in acceptable ranges for pregnancy (**Table 2**)
- Use beta-blockers for symptomatic complaints (i.e. tachycardia, palpitations)
- Thyroid function studies every 1–3 months
- Serial ultrasonography of the fetus for evidence of growth restriction and/or fetal goiter
- Management of thyroid storm as outlined (**Table 4**)

Labor/delivery

- No specific management needs are associated with the intrapartum process

Postnatal

- Watch for worsening of symptomatology if autoimmune etiology suspected
- Adjust thioamide therapy according to laboratory parameters and symptomatology
- Complete diagnostic evaluation of hyperthyroidism, and when appropriate institute definitive therapy
- Evaluate the neonate for evidence of goiter and transient hypothyroidism

exposure may be reduced. Even doses as low as PTU 100–200 mg/day have been reported to cause mild transient fetal hypothyroidism; therefore, it is important to seek the lowest possible dose to maintain the FT4 and FT1 in the normal range.

Beta-adrenergic receptor blocking drugs are used for symptomatic relief in toxic patients beginning thioamide therapy. This type of medication controls the autonomic (sympathetic) symptoms of hyperthyroidism and also reduces peripheral conversion of T4 to T3.

Iodide treatment is an older mode of therapy and essentially is limited to preoperative use. Otherwise, this therapy results in a high incidence of fetal goiter and hypothyroidism when used chronically and does not result in adequate control of thyrotoxicosis.[35,38]

Surgery is reserved for patients who do not respond to medication or who develop an intolerance to the medication. Surgical excision is not recommended without a complete evaluation with ultrasound and or fine needle aspiration to rule out malignancy (see section: Diagnostic Evaluation of a Fetal Goiter). Thyroid surgery is associated with a high incidence of hypothyroidism post-operatively and therefore surgery has become increasingly less common during pregnancy. Other post-operative complications include hypoparathyroidism (1–2%) and recurrent laryngeal nerve palsy (1–2%). There are also risks of surgical and anesthetic morbidity and mortality. The reported pregnancy loss associated with general anesthesia and surgery of all types in the first trimester is approximately 8%, and decreases in the second trimester. Prior to surgery, patients should be prepared medically with 7–10 days of iodide to decrease gland vascularity and to prevent thyroid storm. Overall, surgery is reserved for failures to the standard medical management.

The use of radioactive iodine ^{131}I is absolutely contraindicated in pregnancy because it destroys the fetal thyroid gland. Radioactive iodine also frequently results in maternal hypothyroidism.[33,34]

Labor/delivery

No specific intrapartum concerns exist, except when the patient presents with an acute exacubation or when a previous diagnosis has not been established. The diagnosis of 'thyroid storm' in a patient with known pre-existing thyroid disease may not be difficult. However, this diagnosis is significantly more difficult in patients without a known history of thyroid disease or obvious findings such as goiter or exophthalmos. Clinical assessment is the only tool available in these cases due to the fact that the results of the diagnostic laboratory tests are not readily available to aid in guiding management. Therefore, if thyroid storm is suspected, thyroid blood tests such as TSH, FT4, FT1 and T3RU should be drawn and sent, but appropriate management should not be delayed while waiting for the test results.

The appropriate therapy of a patient in thyroid storm is outlined in **Table 4**. The therapy involves rapid intervention with supportive measures such as i.v. fluids, electrolyte replacement, vasopressor agents as needed and cooling blankets for the hyperthermia. The medical management includes high doses of PTU (600–1000 mg) or TAP (60–100 mg) orally/rectally initially, followed by subsequent doses of PTU 150–200 mg or TAP 10–20 mg every 8 h for maintenance. Potassium iodide 2–5 drops orally or sodium iodide 0.5–1.0 g i.v. every 8 h should be given approximately 1–2 hours after the initiation of therapy with thioamides. This is done in an attempt to block thyroid hormone release.

Propranolol 40–80 mg orally or 1 mg/min i.v. should be given to reduce adrenergic overactivity. Reserpine or guanethidine have also been used for this purpose in patients in whom beta-blockers are contraindicated.

Dexamethasone 2 mg every 6 h for 24 h may also be given to decrease thyroid hormone release and peripheral conversion of T4 to T3. No data are available to document that continuing steroids for more than 24 h has been found to be beneficial. The use of phenobarbital has also been advocated to aid in decreasing agitation and restlessness.[21,22]

Table 4
Management of 'thyroid storm'

Drug therapy	Supportive therapy
PTU 600–800 mg orally immediately, then 150–200 mg orally every 8 h; or TAP 60–100 mg rectally followed by 10–20 mg rectally every 8 h	i.v. fluids and electrolyte replacement
SSKI 2–5 drops every 8 h orally or NaI 0.5–1.0 g i.v. every 8 h	Antipyretics such as salicylates, acetominophen or cooling blankets
Dexamethasone 2 mg i.v. every 6 h × 4 doses	Calories/glucose
Propranolol 20–80 mg orally or 1–10 mg i.v. every 4 h; if propranolol is contraindicated, then use reserpine or guanethidine	Treat underlying medical illnesses
Phenobarbital 30–60 mg every 6–8 h	Digoxin for treatment of CHF
	Oxygen therapy

Postnatal

Under some circumstances, such as when hyper-thyroidism is caused by an autoimmune event, the disease can worsen following delivery. Conversely, higher doses of the thioamides may have been needed to compensate for the larger volume of distribution in pregnancy, and therefore a decrease in medications may be indicated. If not already completed, a detailed evaluation of the underlying etiology should be initiated after delivery, and when possible definitive treatment instituted.

Thioamides cross the placenta and can affect the fetus as well. These drugs block the fetal thyroid gland and result in fetal goiter in approximately 10% of all cases, with the risks of goiter being dose-related. The incidence of transient neonatal hypothyroidism is 1–5%. With Graves' disease and the presence of antithyroid antibodies, there may be a delayed onset of neonatal thyrotoxicosis resulting from the effects of *in utero* exposure to thioamides. Rarely, TAP can be associated with aplasia cutis. No long-term developmental effects have been found with PTU exposure *in utero*.

HYPOTHYROIDISM

Hypothyroidism most commonly develops secondary to the destruction of the thyroid gland by autoimmune diseases, surgery or radioactive iodine therapy. Rarely, hypothyroidism results from pituitary or hypothalamic disease. The three most common causes of hypothyroidism in adults are idiopathic myxedema, Hashimoto's thyroiditis, and radioactive or surgical ablation of the thyroid gland.[23,24]

Diagnosis

Various historical factors may suggest the diagnosis of hypothyroidism, including a history of previous thyroid surgery, radioiodine treatment or Hashimoto's thyroiditis. The signs and symptoms experienced by patients with hypothyroidism include fatigue, cold intolerance, dry skin, coarse hair, constipation, blunted DTRs, eyelid edema and weight gain. A goiter may or may not be present. The laboratory values reveal a low TT4, low FT1, low FT4 and an elevated TSH. There may also be elevated antimicrosomal antibodies and antithyroglobulin antibodies.

Maternal/Fetal Risks

There is some evidence to suggest that fertility is impaired in patients with hypothyroidism. If pregnancy occurs, the most serious consequence of hypothyroid-ism is myxedema coma. This is extremely rare in pregnancy, but it represents a medical emergency with a 20% mortality rate. The clinical picture of myxedema coma includes hypothermia, bradycardia, decreased DTRs and altered consiousness. Hyponatremia, hypoglycemia, hypoxia and hypercapnia may also be present. Once the diagnosis is made, therapy should begin immediately with supportive care and thyroid hormone replacement. Improvement in symptoms usually occurs after 12–24 h of therapy.[25]

Although documentation in the literature in sparse and conflicting, studies have shown that the fetal effects of maternal hypothyroidism include a theoretical increase in miscarriages, congenital anomalies and stillbirths.[26]

Management Options

Prepregnancy

The patient with hypothyroidism may actually present to their physician with complaints of infertility. Patients should be counseled to delay pregnancy until maintenance drug levels have been achieved. Reassurances should be given for the safety of these agents during pregnancy.

Prenatal

Patients diagnosed as being hypothyroid should receive full thyroid replacement during pregnancy. The therapy is simple, inexpensive and produces dramatic results. Replacement can be accomplished with various different preparations (**Table 5**). However, recommended therapy should be carried out using the following preparation: levothyroxine (Synthroid®) 0.1–0.2 mg/day exclusively. This preparation is a pure T4 preparation, which when used in appropriate doses, results in normal T4 and T3 levels. In fact, thyroid preparations which contain both T4 and T3 (i.e. desiccated thyroid) have resulted in a greater incidence of hypothyroid side-effects when compared with thyroid replacement

Table 5
Thyroid hormone replacement preparations

Name	T3/T4	Dose (mg/day)
Levothyroxine (Synthroid®)	T4	0.10–0.20
Desiccated thyroid	T4/T3	90–180
Liothyronine (Cytomel®)	T3	0.075–0.125
Liotrix (Euthroid®)	T4/T3	0.15/0.0375–0.3/0.75

preparations which have only T4. The effectiveness of replacement should be monitored by following TSH, T4 and FT4 levels. The TSH should be less than 5 mU/ml and the TT4 and FT4 should be within the normal range for pregnancy. Patients who have chronically supplemented hypothyroidism, and become pregnant, do not have to have their doses of medication altered during the pregnancy due to the fact that the rate of turnover of T4 is not altered by pregnancy.[27]

Labor/delivery

In the patient who is adequately controlled, no specific management plans are needed for the labor or delivery process.

HYPOTHYROIDISM
Summary of Management Options

Prepregnancy

- Consider hypothyroidism in differential diagnosis of infertility and/or menstrual disorders

- Delay pregnancy until maintenance drug levels achieved

Prenatal

- Continue full thyroid hormone replacement

- Serial (every trimester) thyroid function studies

- Watch for evidence of myxedema

Labor/delivery

- None specific necessary

Postnatal

- Watch for exacerbation of subclinical thyroid disease, which may present with transient hyperthyroidism

---

Postnatal

Postpartum exacerbations of subclinical thyroid disease have been reported to occur in approximately 5–10% of women. Frequently, these exacerbations are detected by laboratory abnormalities and not clinical findings. The clinical features include transient hyperthyroidism that usually occurs approximately 6–12 weeks postpartum. The hyperthyroidism is followed by a transient hypothyroid phase which is associated with the presence of a goiter and high titers of antithyroid microsomal antibodies. This hypothyroidism resolves spontaneously in approximately 80% of patients in 6–9 months after delivery.

In the 20% of the patients who remain hypothyroid, their course can be predicted by following antimicrosomal antiboy titers. Patients with high titers should be followed for the development of persistent hypothyroidism. Management includes symptomatic treatment with Synthroid® if hypothyroid and with thioamides if hyperthyroid.[28]

FETAL/NEONATAL HYPOTHYROIDISM (see Chapter 55)

Primary neonatal hypothyroidism is most commonly the result of thyroid dysgenesis. Other less common etiologies include inborn errors of thyroid function, pituitary TSH deficiency and drug-induced hypothyroidism. The lack of sufficient thyroid hormone during fetal development and early infancy has a profound effect on the development of the fetal CNS, with the exact mechanisms whereby thyroid hormone deficiency causes abnormal CNS development remaining unclear.

Fetal/Neonatal Risks

Studies have shown that the severity of the neurological abnormalities is directly related to the duration and extent of the lack of thyroid hormone. The majority of infants with congenital hypothyroidism appear normal at birth. The clinical signs and symptoms of congenital hypothyroidism take weeks to months to develop by which time irreversible neurological damage may have occurred.

Diagnosis

It is extremely important that the diagnosis and therapy of neonatal hypothyroidism is made as soon as possible. By law, all newborns in the USA are screened for hypothyroidism with a T4 and a TSH level. In hypothyroidism, the serum T4 if low and the serum TSH is elevated. The clinical signs of neonatal hypothyroidism are macroglossia, large fontanelles, hypotonia, feeding and respiratory difficulties, protracted hyperbilirubinemia, and abdominal distension without vomiting. Less than 30% of all infants with congenital hypothyroidism have one or more of these signs at birth, which as mentioned earlier, take weeks to months to develop.[29]

Management Options

Treatment of congenital hypothyroidism consists of the administration of therapeutic doses of levothyroxine (10 µg/kg). The T4 levels should be used to follow the treatment efficacy. The prognosis of congenital hypothyroidism appears to be good with early therapy. It is not known how the long-term intellectual performance of these treated infants with congenital hypothyroidism compares with infants with temporary thyroid suppression from maternal treatment with thioamides.[30,31]

DIAGNOSTIC EVALUATION OF A MATERNAL THYROID NODULE DURING PREGNANCY

Maternal/Fetal Risks and Management Options

The development of a solitary thyroid nodule in pregnancy is suggestive of a malignancy due to the fact that most goiters which develop during pregnancy are diffuse. Radioactive iodine uptake studies are normally used to evaluate thyroid nodules. However, these studies cannot be used in pregnancy due to their adverse effect on the fetal thyroid. Ultrasound is the preferred mode for evaluating a thyroid nodule in pregnancy. Cystic lesions are usually benign. Fine needle aspiration of a suspicious solitary thyroid nodule is indicated and can be performed safely in pregnancy. This procedure also has high sensitivity and specificity. Pregnancy has a minimal effect on the prognosis of a diagnosed primary thyroid malignancy.[38]

DIAGNOSTIC EVALUATION OF A FETAL GOITER (see Chapter 55)

Fetal Neonatal Risks and Management Options

Occasionally, patients being treated for thyroid disease during pregnancy will develop evidence of fetal goiter demonstrated with ultrasound. Further, women with a history of Graves' disease or familial congenital hypothyroidism may present with fetal growth retardation, tachycardia or fetal goiter. Amniotic fluid thyroid hormone concentrations do not accurately reflect fetal thyroid status in these circumstances. However, utilizing fetal blood sampling techniques, an accurate measure of fetal thyroid status can now be determined. Successful prenatal treatment of fetal hypothyroidism following successful identification of fetal thyroid status in a patient with maternal thyroid-stimulating immunoglobulins receiving propylthiouracil treatment has been reported.[39] When linked with some recent less encouraging reports that suggest not all effects of fetal hypothyroidism are reversed by early neonatal treatment,[40,41] an aggressive approach to *in utero* hypothyroidism might be justified when correctly identified.

REFERENCES

1   Burrow GN (1988) Thyroid diseases. In Burrow GN, Ferris TF (eds) *Medical Complications During Pregnancy*, 3rd edn, pp. 224–253. Philadelphia: W.B. Saunders.

2   Freely J (1979) Physiology of thyroid function in pregnancy. *Postgraduate Medicine* 55:336–339.

3   Barron WM (1991) *Medical Disorders During Pregnancy*, pp. 113–124. Missouri: Mosby-Yearbook.

4   Vander Spuy ZM, Jacobs HS (1984) Management of endocrine disorders in pregnancy. Part 1: Thyroid and parathyroid disease. *Postgraduate Medical Journal* 60:245–252.

5   Aboul-Khair SA, Crooks J, Turnbull AC, Hytten FE (1964) The physiological changes in thyroid function during pregnancy. *Clinical Science* 27:195–207.

6   Brander A, Kivisaari L (1989) Ultrasonography of the thyroid during pregnancy. *Journal of Clinical Ultrasound* 17:403–408.

7   Gibson M, Tulchinsky D (1980) The maternal thyroid. In Tulchinsky D, Ryan (eds) *Maternal-Fetal Endocrinology*, pp. 115–128. Philadelphia: W.B. Saunders.

8   Fisher DA (1985) Control of thyroid hormone production in the fetus. In Malbreecht ED, Pepe GH (eds) *Research in Perinatal Medicine Vol. IV: Perinatal Endocrinology*, pp. 55–62. Ithaca, NT: Perinatology Press.

9   Davis LE, Leveno KJ, Cunningham FG (1988) Hyperthyroidism complicating pregnancy. *American Journal of Obstetrics and Gynecology* 160:63–70.

10 Prout TE (1975) Thyroid diseases in pregnancy. *American Journal of Obstetrics and Gynecology* 122:699–705.

11 Hardisty CA, Munro DS (1983) Serum long acting thyroid stimulating protector in pregnancy complicated by Graves Disease. *British Medical Journal* 286:934–936.

12 Rosenburg IN (1976) Thyroid storm. *Pharmacol Therapy* 423–429.

13 Vulsma T, Gons MH, de Vijlder JJM (1989) Maternal-

fetal transfer of thyroxine in congenital hypothyroidism due to a total organification defect or thyroid agenesis. *New England Journal of Medicine* 321:13–16.

14 Roti E, Gnudi A, Braverman LE (1983) The placental transport, synthesis and metabolism of hormones and drugs which affect thyroid function. *Endocrine Reviews* 4:131–135.

15 Burrow GN (1978) Hyperthyroidism during pregnancy. *New England Journal of Medicine* 298:150–153.

16 Burrow GN (1978) Maternal–fetal consideration in hyperthyroidism. Clin *Endocrinology and Metabolism* 7:115–118.

17 McKenzie JM, Zakarijam M (1978) Pathogenesis of maternal Graves' disease. *Journal of Endocrinology Investigation* 2:182–191.

18 Davis LE, Lucas MJ, Hankins GDV, Mujtaba Q, Burrow GN (1975). Treatment of hyperthyroidism in pregnancy with propyithiouracil and methimazole. *Obstetrics and Gynecology* 46:282–286.

19 Glinoer D, Fernandez M, Bourdoux P *et al.* (1991) Pregnancy in patients with mild thyroid abnormalities: Maternal and neonatal repercussions. *Journal of Clinical Endocrinology and Metabolism* 73:421–427.

20 Mestman J (1991) Hyperthyroidism. *Contemporary Obstetrics and Gynecology* 36–50.

21 Hoffenberg R (1980) Thyroid emergencies in pregnancy. *Clinical Endocrinology and Metabolism* 9:503–509.

22 Lowy C (1980) Endocrine emergencies in pregnancy. Clinical Endocrinology and Metabolism 9:569–574.

23 Kennedy A, Montgomery DL (1978) Hypothyroidism in pregnancy. *British Journal of Obstetrics and Gynecology* 85:225–228.

24 Montoro M, Collea JV, Frasier SD *et al.* (1981) Successful outcome of pregnancy in women with hypothyroidism. *Annals of Internal Medicine* 94:31–34.

25 Nicoloff JT (1985) Thyroid storm and nyxedema coma. *Medical Clinics of North America* 69:1005–1009.

26 Pekonen F, Teramo K, Ikonen E *et al.* (1984) Women on thyroid hormone therapy: Pregnancy course, fetal outcome and amniotic hormone level. *Obstetrics and Gynecology* 63:535–539.

27 Davis LE, Leveno KJ, Cunningham FE (1988) Hypothyroidism complicating pregnancy. *Obstetrics and Gynecology* 72:108–112.

28 Jansson R, Dahlberg PA, Karlsson A (1984) Postpartum thyroid dysfunction. *Scandinavian Journal of Clinical and Laboratory Investigation* 44:371–375.

29 Fischer DA, Dussault JH, Foley TP *et al.* (1979) Screening for congenital hypothyroidism: Results of screening one million North American infants. *Journal of Pediatrics* 94:700–706.

30 Nelson NC, Becker WFL (1969) Thyroid crisis: Diagnosis and treatment. *Annals of Surgery* 9:263–273.

31 Greenman GW, Gabrielson MD, Howard-Flandy J *et al.* (1962) Thyroid dysfunction in pregnancy: Fetal loss and follow up evaluation of surviving infant. *New England Journal of Medicine* 267:426–431.

32 Molitch ME, Beck JR, Dreisner M *et al.* (1984) The cold thyroid nodule: An analysis of diagnostic and therapeutic options. *Endocrine Reviews* 5:185–199.

33 Cooper DS (1984) Antithyroid drugs. *New England Journal of Medicine* 311:1353–1362.

34 Edwards DM (1979) The management of thyroid diseases in pregnancy. *Postgraduate Medical Journal* 55:340–342.

35 Goluboff L, Sission J, Hamburger J (1974) Hyperthyroidism associated with pregnancy. *Obstetrics and Gynecology* 44:107–111.

36 Burrow G (1985) Thyroid diseases: The management of thyrotoxicosis in pregnancy. *New England Journal of Medicine* 313:562–565.

37 Ramsay I (1983) Drug treatment of thyroid and adrenal disease during pregnancy. In Lewis P (ed.) *Clinical Pharmacology in Obstetrics*, pp. 232–250. London: Wright.

38 Cheron R, Kaplan M, Larsen PR *et al.* (1981) Neonatal thyroid function after PTU therapy for maternal Graves disease. *New England Journal of Medicine* 304:525–528.

39 Davidson KM, Richards DS, Schartz DA, Fisher DA (1991) Successful *in utero* treatment of fetal goiter and hypothyroidism. *New England Journal of Medicine* 324:435–439.

40 Heyerdahl S, Kase BF, Lie SO (1991) Intellectual development in children with congenital hypothyroidism in relation to recommended thyroxine treatment. *Journal of Pediatrics* 118:850–857.

41 Fuggle P, Tokar S, Grant DB (1991) Intellectual ability of early treated children with congenital hypothyroidism: Results from the UK National follow up study. *Hormone Research* 35:16–21 (suppl.).

22

Pituitary and Adrenal Disorders

MARK B. LANDON

PITUITARY DISEASE

The anterior lobe of the pituitary gland may significantly enlarge during pregnancy due to lactotroph proliferation. Magnetic resonance imaging has confirmed a more than doubling of the gland size by the end of gestation.[1] Accordingly, prolactin levels increase approximately 10-fold as preparation for lactation occurs.[2]

The levels of other pituitary hormones are also affected by pregnancy. Gonadotropin concentrations decline and exhibit a diminished response to GnRh. Growth hormone response to insulin or arginine stimulation is similarly blunted. Plasma levels of ACTH have been shown to increase throughout pregnancy, but absolute levels remain lower in the pregnant than in the nonpregnant state.[3] The rise in ACTH curiously occurs despite an increase in free and bound cortisol, suggesting an alternate mechanism to the normal negative feedback loop between cortisol and ACTH. The diurnal variation of cortisol, although somewhat blunted, is maintained during pregnancy. Thyrotropin levels are unaffected by pregnancy as free levels of thyroxine and tri-iodo thyronine are unchanged, whereas total levels increase due to estrogen-induced synthesis of throxine-binding globulin.

Posterior pituitary processes are also altered during normal pregnancy. A significant preterm increase in oxytocin is observed, while plasma levels of vasopressin remain similar to those obtained in the nonpregnant state. However, plasma osmolality decreases 5–10 mOsm/kg in pregnant women, indicating that the threshold for vasopressin secretion is lowered for pregnant women. It follows that the plasma osmolality at which thirst is experienced is also lowered during gestation.[4]

PITUITARY DISORDERS: PROLACTIN-PRODUCING ADENOMAS

Maternal/Fetal Risks

With widely available radioimmunoassays for serum prolactin and improved techniques for radiologic diagnosis, an increasing number of prolactin-secreting pituitary adenomas are now being detected in women. Spontaneous ovulation is uncommon when a pituitary tumor is present. Therefore, most patients with this disorder will present with amenorrhea-galactorrhea or anovulatory cycles and infertility. With the use of ovulation induction and suppression of prolactin synthesis by dopaminergic agents such as bromocriptine, pregnancy has become increasingly common in patients with prolactinomas.

As mentioned previously, much of the pituitary gland enlargement is thought to be secondary to hyperplasia of the anterior pituitary lactotrophic cells which are stimulated by estrogen. Although this stimulus may result in the enlargement of adenomas during pregnancy,[5] most patients with a microadenoma – a pituitary tumor less than 1cm in size – have an uneventful pregnancy.[6–8] In those few patients who do become symptomatic, regression usually follows delivery.

Management Options

Prepregnancy

The vast majority of women with prolactin-secreting adenomas will require ovulation induction to conceive. Non-pregnant patients who present with amenorrhea-galactorrhea and hyperprolactinemia (prolactin $\leq$ 20 ng/ml)should be investigated for the presence of a pituitary adenoma. While serum prolactin levels have been correlated with the presence of pituitary adenomas, in a patient considering pregnancy with hyperprolactinemia of any degree, a thorough radiologic investigation is warranted. Debate continues regarding the appropriate sequence of the workup for this disorder, though it appears that computerized axial tomography (CT) and more recently magnetic resonance imaging (MRI) have replaced coned down sella turcica radiographs and polytomography as the procedure of choice to evaluate the size of the pituitary gland.

Once a pituitary tumor is diagnosed, it may be prudent to re-evaluate the gland for growth after several months before attempting ovulation induction. Bromocriptine therapy may be all that is required for therapy of patients with microadenomas. Macroadenomas – tumors measuring 1 cm or more – should be definitively treated with surgery or radiation, as 15–33% of these patients may develop symptoms during pregnancy.[5,8] These patients may require continued bromocriptine therapy following surgery.

Prenatal

Evaluation for possible prolactin-secreting tumors is made difficult during pregnancy by the physiologic rise in serum prolactin which accompanies normal gestation. At term, serum prolactin levels may reach values 20 times normal. Furthermore, prolactin levels do not always rise during pregnancy in women with prolactinomas, nor do they always rise with pregnancy-induced tumor enlargement (**Figure 1**).[9] Therefore, radiologic diagnosis is necessary for the pregnant patient who develops severe headaches or a visual field defect.

Management of the pregnant patient with a previously diagnosed prolactinoma requires careful attention by a team of physicians, including the obstetrician, endocrinologist and ophthalmologist. The development of headaches may reflect tumor enlargement and impingement on the diaphragmatic sella or adjacent dura. Visual disturbances result from optic nerve compression. If the optic chiasm is compressed by superior extension, bitemporal hemianopsia may develop. Visual field and ophthalmologic examinations should, therefore be performed in symptomatic patients.[8] While the limitations of serum prolactin levels have

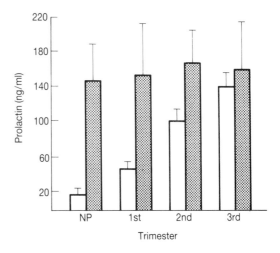

Figure 1. Maternal serum prolactin concentration in microadenoma patients (shaded bars, $n = 237$) and controls (open bars, $n = 215$) while non-pregnant (NP) and during each trimester. Reproduced from Divers and Yen[9] with permission of the American College of Obstetrics and Gynecology.

been discussed, marked elevations outside of the pregnant range for a given gestational age may signal rapid tumor enlargement.

Gemzell and Wang reviewed the course of 85 women during 91 pregnancies with previously untreated microadenomas and reported that only 5% experienced complications.[5] Four of the five pregnancies associated with symptoms of headache and visual disturbance showed resolution following delivery. One patient who had a visual field defect noted early in pregnancy, subsequently underwent a transphenoidal hypophysectomy after a cesarean section for a triplet gestation at 36 weeks. Similarly, Albrecht and Betz have confirmed a low rate of complications in women with untreated microadenomas during gestation.[10] Of 352 such cases, 8 (2.3%) developed visual disturbances and 17 (4.8%) developed headaches.

Maygar and Marshall report that symptoms seem to occur more frequently in the first trimester than in the second or third, noting a median time at onset of 10 weeks gestation.[6] However, the likelihood of developing visual symptoms did not differ in each trimester (**Figure 2**). In their series, symptoms requiring therapy occurred in over 20% of the 91 patients who had untreated tumors, but in only 1% of women with previously treated adenomas.

Molitch has reviewed 16 series of 246 cases of pregnancy and prolactin-secreting pituitary microadenomas.[8] Only 4 of the 246 women (1.6%) had symptoms of tumor enlargement and 11 (4.5%) had asymptomatic enlargement on radiologic examination (**Table 1**). In no case was surgical intervention necessary. Molitch

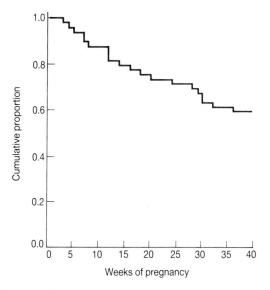

Figure 2. Time from beginning of pregnancy to onset of symptoms (headache or visual disturbances) in 91 pregnancies in women with previously untreated pituitary tumours. Reproduced from Maygar and Marshall[6] with permission.

Table 1
Effect of pregnancy on prolactinomas

Tumor type	Prior therapy	n	Symptomatic enlargement
Microadenomas	none	246	4
Macroadenomas	none	45	7
Macroadenomas	yes	46	2

Adapted from Molitch.[8]

also reviewed 45 cases of women with macroadenomas, of which 7 (15.5%) experienced symptomatic tumor enlargement. Surgery was required in four of these women during pregnancy.[8] The risk of developing symptoms is probably related to the size of the tumor at the onset of pregnancy. Further data will be necessary to define which group of patients with a microadenoma should be treated with bromocriptine for a prolonged period of time prior to conception.

Therapy for complications arising during pregnancy is influenced by both gestational age and the severity of symptoms. If fetal maturity is present, induction of labor or cesarean section should be accomplished. Cesarean section is generally performed for obstetrical indications. Earlier in gestation, if radiologic evidence suggests tumor enlargement, therapy should not be delayed. Treatment employing bromocriptine has been successful in several symptomatic patients, and has become the preferred therapy during pregnancy.[9] This

drug appears to be safe in early pregnancy, as evidenced by its use for induction of ovulation in large groups of hyperprolactinemic women without an increased incidence of congenital malformations.[11,12] Other treatment modalities employed during pregnancy include transphenoidal surgery[6–8] and, in one case, hydrocortisone therapy.[12] The complications of transphenoidal surgery are infection, hypopituitarism, hemorrhage and transient diabetes insipidus. The risk of these complications is probably not increased during pregnancy.

Labor/delivery

The intrapartum care of the patient with a prolactin-producing adenoma does not differ from that of the general obstetric population. On occasion, an undiagnosed case may present with sudden visual impairment, and here the prolactinoma must be differentiated from more common conditions such as pregnancy-induced hypertension, which can produce these same symptoms.

Postnatal

Following delivery, radiologic assessment of tumor size and a serum prolactin assay should be performed at the first postpartum visit. Breast-feeding is not contraindicated in the presence of a prolactin-secreting microadenoma.[7] Since serum prolactin levels may remain elevated while nursing, caution must be used in interpreting these results. However, serum prolactin levels do not appear to be significantly higher than pre-pregnancy levels in women with microadenomas who choose to breast-feed.[13] Counselling patients regarding future pregnancies requires establishing that progression of tumor growth has not not occurred. Gemzell concluded that, in 16 patients with untreated pituitary adenomas, symptoms did not seem to occur with increasing frequency in subsequent pregnancies.[5]

PITUITARY DISORDERS: ACROMEGALY

Maternal/Fetal Risks

Acromegaly results from excessive growth hormone secretion which is most often secondary to an acidophilic or chromophobic pituitary adenoma. Although amenorrhea is common in women with acromegaly, pregnancies do occasionally occur.[14,15] Pregnancy may be accompanied by tumor expansion, necessitating hypophysectomy.[16] Patients with acromegaly are at increased risk for diabetes and hypertension.

Management Options

Lack of suppression of growth hormone levels below 5 mg/ml during a glucose tolerance test can help secure a diagnosis. Measurement of somatomedin C, which mediates the effects of growth hormone, is more useful in establishing the diagnosis of acromegaly in non-pregnant women because levels of this insulin-like growth factor may rise in normal pregnancy. Definitive surgical treatment is recommended prior to conception. Dopaminergic agents may paradoxically decrease growth hormone levels in acromegalic individuals. Case reports have confirmed lack of tumor expansion during pregnancy in women receiving bromocriptine therapy.[17]

PITUITARY DISORDERS: DIABETES INSIPIDUS

Maternal/Fetal Risks

Diabetes insipidus is a rare disorder with fewer than 100 cases complicating pregnancy reported in the literature. The disease results from inadequate or absent antidiuretic hormone (ADV or vasopressin) production by the posterior pituitary gland. The etiology of diabetes insipidus is often unknown, although in most cases it follows pituitary surgery or destruction by tumor of the normal pituitary architecture. It may occur as a primary idiopathic disorder in approximately 30% of cases. Massive polyuria, resulting from failure of the renal tubular concentrating mechanism, and a dilute urine, (specific gravity < 1.005) are characteristic of diabetes insipidus. To combat dehydration and the intense thirst produced by this syndrome, patients consume large quantities of fluid. The diagnosis of diabetes insipidus relies on the demonstration of continued polyuria and relative urinary hyposmolarity when a patient is water restricted. The administration of intramuscular vasopressin to such a patient will result in water retention and an appropriate increase in urine osmolality. This response is not observed in patients with nephrogenic diabetes insipidus, a state in which free water clearance is increased because of renal tubule insensitivity to ADH. Other conditions which cause polyuria such as diabetes mellitus, hyperparathyroidism with hypercalcemia, and chronic renal tubular disease, must also be considered in the differential diagnosis. However, these can usually by distinguished from central diabetes insipidus by appropriate laboratory investigation.

Hime and Richardson[18] reviewed 67 cases of diabetes insipidus complicating pregnancy and noted that 58% of cases seemed to deteriorate during gestation, whereas 20% of cases improved. To explain this phenomenon, it has been suggested that the increased glomerular filtration seen in pregnancy may increase the requirement of ADH.[19] Patients with mild disease may also worsen during pregnancy because of a diminished response of the renal tubule to ADH, possibly as a result of progesterone antagonism.[20] Impaired liver function, including fatty liver of pregnancy, has been observed with diabetes insipidus during pregnancy, suggesting that several factors may explain worsening of this condition.[20]

Management Options

Synthetic vasopressin, in the form of L-deamino-8-D-arginine vasopressin (DDAVP) is the treatment choice. This drug is given intranasally in doses of approximately 0.1 mg up to three times daily. Oxytocic activity is rarely observed. Burrow and colleagues have reported the successful use of DDAVP in pregnancy and the puerperium and suggests that this drug is safe for both mother and fetus as well as during lactation.[21]

Spontaneous labor and lactation seem to occur in most cases of diabetes insipidus. While older reports suggest an increased number of dysfunctional labors in affected patients, oxytocin release appears to be independent of vasopressin secretion.[22]

PITUITARY INSUFFICIENCY

Maternal/Fetal Risks

Fifty-five years ago, Sheehan described postpartum ischemic necrosis of the anterior pituitary.[23] This form of hypopituitarism is usually observed in patients who have experienced severe postpartum hemorrhage with hypotensive shock. Because pituitary necrosis is uncommon with other conditions associated with hypovolemic shock, it has been suggested that the hyperplastic pituitary gland of pregnancy is more susceptible to hypoperfusion. Lymphocytic hypophysitis, an autoimmune form of hypopituitarism, is also more common in women and during the puerperium. It should be considered in cases where hypopituitarism is suspected in the absence of preceding postpartum hemorrhage. Destruction of the gland from tumor invasion, surgery or radiotherapy may also accompany pregnancy, although fertility is often compromised in such patients. Antepartum pituitary infarction has been described as a rare complication of insulin-dependent diabetes mellitus.[24] In these cases, insulin requirements may fall dramatically.

Patients with Sheehan's syndrome may exhibit varying degrees of hypopituitarism, so that specific assays

PITUITARY DISORDERS
Summary of Management Options

PROLACTIN-PRODUCING ADENOMAS

Prepregnancy

- Treatment (bromocriptine/surgery/radiotherapy depending on tumor size)

- Advise against pregnancy until 'cured'

Prenatal

- Bromocriptine is probably safe to fetus

- Screening/monitoring for recurrence or exacerbation is best undertaken by vigilance for clinical features (headaches, visual disturbance) and prompt investigation. Monitoring prolactin not helpful

- Interdisciplinary management

- If enlargement/recurrence, bromocriptine if fetus not mature (possibly surgery in extreme cases); delivery and definitive management if fetus mature

Postnatal

- Can breast-feed

- Monitor symptoms, prolactin, tumor size

ACROMEGALY

Prepregnancy

- Definitive surgical management before conception

- Screen for diabetes and hypertenstion

DIABETES INSIPIDUS

Prenatal

- Continue supplementation with synthetic vasopressin; dose may need increasing

- Monitor disease control with clinical features and specific gravity of urine

Labor/delivery

- Vigilance for dysfunctional labor (minority of cases)

Postnatal

- Vigilance for poor lactation (minority of cases)

PITUITARY INSUFFICIENCY

Prepregnancy and prenatal

- Give appropriate replacement hormones (usually thyroxine and corticosteroids)

- Monitor clinical features and TSH levels

Labor/delivery

- Increase dose of glucocorticiods

Postnatal

- Readjust dose of drugs if necessary

of tropic hormones as well as stimulation and suppression tests may be necessary to establish the diagnosis. During pregnancy, because of normal physiologic changes, adjustments must be made in interpreting both hormone levels and responses to various stimuli. An average delay of 7 years has been observed between the onset and the diagnosis of this disorder. A history of hypovolemic shock and antecedent postpartum hemorrhage has been recorded as a precipitating event in up to 79% of cases.[25] There is no apparent correlation between the degree of hemorrhage and the occurrence of Sheehan's syndrome. The characteristic clinical picture begins with failure to lactate. However, this may not be observed in all cases. Some patients may present with late onset disease and progress to loss of axillary and pubic hair, oligomenorrhea, or amenorrhea with senile vaginal atrophic changes, as well as signs and symptoms of hypothyroidism. Patients with these findings are usually infertile, although the frequency of pregnancy with this disorder is difficult to ascertain. In a review of 19 patients with Sheehan's syndrome documented by endocrinology studies or post-mortem examination, 39 pregnancies occurred after the onset of hypopituitarism.[25] Eleven of these women required hormonal therapy to establish a pregnancy and replacement therapy was used during 15 (38%) of the 39 pregnancies. The treated group had a livebirth rate of 87%, compared with 54% in untreated patients, suggesting that early diagnosis and proper therapy result in a more favorable outcome.

Because pregnancy may occur in women with Sheehan's syndrome, this diagnosis should be considered in all patients with a history of postpartum hemorrhage. Measuring gonadotropins is of little value, since levels decline with normal pregnancy. However, the finding of a low or low normal TSH in conjunction with a low serum T_4 level is consistent with secondary hypothyroidism. Similarly, low cortisol levels with failure to increase with stress as well as diminished ACTH would support the diagnosis.

Management Options

The treatment of pituitary insufficiency involves replacement of those hormones necessary to maintain normal metabolism and respond to stress. Thyroid hormone may be provided as L-thyroxine in doses of 0.1–0.2 mg daily. Corticosteroids are essential for those patients who manifest any degree of adrenal insufficency. The maintenance dosage of cortisone acetate is provided as 25 mg every morning and 12.5 mg every evening, or as prednisone 5 mg and 2.5 mg, respectively. Mineralocorticoid replacement is rarely necessary because adrenal production of aldosterone is not solely dependent on ACTH stimulation. The dose of glucocorticoids should be increased during the stress of labor and delivery.

ADRENAL DISEASE

A two- to three-fold increase in cortisol levels is observed by the end of normal pregnancy.[26] The majority of this increase is due to the estrogen-induced increase in cortisol-binding globulin (CBG) levels; however, the biologically active 'free' levels are also elevated.[27] An elevated urinary free cortisol concentration can thus be measured during gestation.

Increased CBG levels prolong the half-life of cortisol in plasma while cortisol production is also increased. Urinary 17 hydroxycorticosteroid levels are actually lower in pregnancy because excretion of cortisol tetrahydro metabolites is decreased.[28] ACTH levels have been shown to increase throughout pregnancy, but absolute levelas remain lower in the pregnant than non-pregnant states.[29] Both ACTH and cortisol surge during labor. Unlike cortisol, ACTH does not cross the placenta. ACTH is manufactured by the placenta, as is corticotropin-releasing hormone (CRH). The relationship between these placenta hormones and maternal adrenal function remains unknown.

ADRENAL DISEASE: CUSHING'S SYNDROME

Maternal/Fetal Risks

Cushing's syndrome, which is characterized by excess glucocorticoid production, is usually secondary to inappropriate hypersecretion of ACTH by a pituitary adenoma. Primary adrenal disease, usually an adrenal adenoma, has been reported to be more common during pregnancy than in the non-pregnant state. Patients with pituitary disease and secondary adrenal hyperplasia are more likely to demonstrate excess androgen secretion which can inhibit pituitary gonadotropin release. Thus, amenorrhea is common in this setting. In contrast, adrenal adenomas are more likely to be pure cortisol producers and are less likely to impair fertility.[26] Other etiologies for Cushing's syndrome include neoplastic ectopic ACTH production, nodular adrenal hyperplasia, or excessive doses of exogenous corticosteroids.

Because women with Cushing's syndrome are usually infertile, de novo cases are rare in pregnancy. Most occur in patients who have been previously or partially treated. The clinical features of this disorder may be difficult to distinguish from many signs and symptoms which accompany normal pregnancy. Weakness, weight gain, edema, striae, hypertension and impaired glucose tolerance may be observed both during gestation and in Cushing's syndrome. The early onset of hypertension with easy bruising and proximal myopathy should strongly suggest the diagnosis and prompt further evaluation.

Laboratory diagnosis includes the demonstration of elevated serum cortisol levels without diurnal variation, as well as a failure to suppress cortisol secretion with the administration of dexamethasone. Assays for ACTH are of variable accuracy and may confuse the diagnosis. During gestation, there is normally a rise in total and free cortisol. Therefore, laboratory results must be compared with established norms for pregnancy. Diurnal variation in cortisol production is maintained in normal pregnancy, although free plasma cortisol levels at term may be two to three times higher than in non-pregnant women. Furthermore, even in normal pregnant patients, cortisol secretion may not be suppressed with low doses (1 mg) of dexamethasone.[29] Most patients with adrenocortical hyperplasia will demonstrate a reduction in plasma and urinary corticosteroids with an 8 mg dose (2 mg every 6 h for 2 days). If such suppression fails, an adrenal tumor, autonomous adrenal nodule or ectopic ACTH production must be considered.

Several reports have suggested the Cushing's syndrome may be exacerbated by pregnancy with improvement of symptoms following delivery.[26,30,31] In the majority of these cases, Cushing's syndrome was associated with an adrenal adenoma.[26] Keegan[31] has speculated that a latent adrenal tumor may be stimulated by placental ACTH, with falling adrenal cortisol secretion following parturition. That pregnancy may act as a stimulus for the development of Cushing's syndrome is supported by the fact that in virtually all reports of Cushing's syndrome in pregnancy, diagnosis was not established until pregnancy occurred.[26]

Table 2
Cushing's syndrome and perinatal complications in 65 pregnancies

Complication	n (%)	
Miscarriage	2	(3.1)
Perinatal death		
neonatal death	5	(7.7)
stillbirth	5	(7.7)
Premature birth	42	(64.6)
Intrauterine growth deficiency	17	(26.2)

Adapted from Buescher et al.[26]

Pregnancy outcome in Cushing's syndrome is marked by a high rate of preterm delivery (67%) and stillbirths (7%) in cases not electively terminated.[26,27,30–32] It has been suggested that maternal hyperglycemia may be a contributing factor to the intrauterine deaths observed (**Table 2**). Hypertension has been reported in 65% of cases and pre-eclampsia in 9%.[26]

Koerten and colleagues reviewed 33 cases of Cushing's syndrome in pregnancy and concluded that maternal complications are more common with adrenal adenomas than with hyperplasia.[32] In this review, every patient with an adenoma developed hypertension if the pregnancy progressed beyond the first trimester. Seven of 16 (47%) patients developed pulmonary edema and one died. In contrast, only one of the 12 with adrenal hyperplasia demonstrated hypertensive disease. The overall prematurity rate (delivery after 20 weeks) was 20 of 33 cases (61%); stillbirths occurred in four cases.

Management Options

Management of the pregnant patient with cortisol excess includes first identifying the source of the hormone production and then instituting proper therapy. Patients with pituitary disease are most often treated surgically if a tumor can be well-defined. Surgical removal of adrenal adenomas can be accomplished through a posterior incision. Bevan and colleagues have examined maternal and fetal outcomes based on the timing of surgical therapy.[33] Fetal loss occurred in 1 of 11 (9%) patients treated during gestation vs 8 of 26 (31%) in which definitive therapy was delayed. In Buescher's review of 60 cases in which 17 women underwent therapy directed at relieving hypercortisolism, treatment effected a decrease in the prematurity rate from 72 to 47%.[26] Because the incidence of adrenal adenoma and carcinoma appears to be increased in pregnant patients with Cushing's syndrome, prompt investigation employing abdominal CT or MRI is warranted, particularly if failure to suppress excess cortisol production with high levels of dexamethasone is observed. Surgery is indicated if an adrenal tumor is discovered. This treatment may be delayed in the third trimester with early delivery being planned.

ADRENAL DISEASE: PRIMARY ALDOSTERONISM

Maternal/Fetal Risks

Few cases of primary aldosteronism during pregnancy have been reported. The diagnosis is suggested in a patient with hypertension, hypokalemia and metabolic alkalosis. Because aldosterone secretion is increased during pregnancy, the diagnosis can be difficult to establish. Failure to replete serum potassium may also suppress aldosterone secretion, thus obscuring the diagnosis.[34] Amelioration of hypertension and hypokalemia during gestation has been attributed to high levels of progesterone, which may block the action of aldosterone. Despite this, patients often present with severe hypertension and superimposed pre-eclampsia.

Management Options

The management for patients without toxemia is controversial. While prompt surgical excision of underlying adrenal adenomas has been suggested by early case reports, Lotgerring and associates have described successful medical therapy from mid-gestation, consisting of spironolactone, an aldosterone antagonist, as well as other antihypertensive medications.[35]

ADRENAL INSUFFICIENCY

Maternal/Fetal Risks

Adrenal insufficiency is usually primary (Addison's disease) as a result of autoimmune destruction. Pituitary failure or adrenal suppression resulting from steroid replacement may also lead to adrenal insufficiency. Adrenal crisis, an acute life-threatening condition, may accompany stressful conditions such as labor, the puerperium or surgery. Unfortunately, the diagnosis of hypoadrenalism is often made with difficulty, particularly in those patients who possess enough adrenal reserve to sustain normal daily activity. In pregnancy, adrenal crisis during the postpartum period may lead to the diagnosis of adrenal insufficiency for the first time.[36]

The clinical presentation of Addison's disease during gestation is similar to that in non-pregnant state. Fatigue, weakness, anorexia, nausea, hypotension, non-specific abdominal pain, hypoglycemia and increased skin pigmentation are hallmarks for this endocrinopathy. Mineralocorticoid deficiency leads to renal sodium loss with resultant depletion of the intravascular volume. A small cardiac silhouette on chest x-ray is often associated with a state of reduced cardiac output and, eventually, circulatory collapse. Hypoglycemia, which is often common in early pregnancy, may be exacerbated by glucocorticoid deficiency.

Management Options

The diagnosis of adrenal insufficiency is based on specific laboratory findings. Plasma cortisol levels are decreased. However, since cortisol-binding globulin is elevated in pregnancy, even low normal cortisol values may actually reflect a state of adrenal insufficiency.[36]

Stimulation of the adrenal gland by synthetic ACTH may be helpful in establishing a diagnosis.[37] Following the intravenous administration of 0.25 mg of Cortrosyn, plasma cortisol should be increased at least two-fold over baseline values. Failure to respond to this stimulus suggests primary adrenal insufficiency. This test may be used in pregnancy since little ACTH crosses the placenta. Measurement of serum ACTH may also be of benefit in distinguishing primary adrenal insufficiency from hypopituitarism.

Pregnancy usually proceeds normally in treated patients. Maintenance replacement of adrenocortical hormones is provided by cortisone acetate 25 mg orally each morning and 12.5 mg in the evening. As an alternative, prednisone may be substituted in doses of 5 mg and 2.5 mg, respectively. Mineralocorticoid deficiency is treated with fludrocortisone acetate (Florinef®) in a dose of 0.05–0.1 mg per day. The use of a mineralocorticoid requires careful observation for symptoms of fluid overload. The presence of edema, excess weight gain and electrolyte imbalance often requires an adjustment in the dose of mineralocorticoid.

Adrenal crisis is a rare, life-threatening disturbance which demands immediate medical attention. Treatment in an intensive care setting is recommended. As noted, women with undiagnosed Addison's disease may present with a crisis during the puerperium. Symptoms include nausea, vomiting and profound epigastric pain accompanied by hypothermia and hypotension. Treatment initially consists of glucocorticoid and fluid replacement. Intravenous hydrocortisone should be given in a dose of 100 mg, followed by repeat doses every 6 h for a period of up to several days. Mineralocorticoid replacement is indicated in cases of refractory hypotension or hyperkalemia.

All patients with adrenal insufficiency should wear an identifying bracelet. Emergency medical kits have also been prepared to help these patients when they travel. Women with Addison's disease require an increase in steroid replacement during periods of infection or stress, and during labor and delivery.

ADRENAL DISEASE: PHEOCHROMOCYTOMA

Maternal/Fetal Risks

Pheochromocytoma is a rare catecholamine-producing tumor which is uncommonly associated with pregnancy. The tumors arise from chromaffin cells of the adrenal medulla or sympathetic nervous tissue, including remnants of the organs of Zuckerkandl, neural crest tissue which lies along the abdominal aorta. In pregnancy, as in the non-pregnant state, the tumor is located in the adrenal gland in 90% of cases.[38] The incidence of malignancy, which can be diagnosed only when metastases are present, is approximately 10%. Schenker et al. have reported mortality rates of 55% with postpartum diagnosis vs 11% if diagnosed during pregnancy.[38,39] Fetal loss can exceed 50%.

In pregnancy, pheochromocytoma may present as a hypertensive crisis marked by cerebral hemorrhage or severe congestive heart failure. Pheochromocytoma can be easily confused with other medical diseases. The signs and symptoms of pheochromocytoma may mimic those of severe pregnancy-induced hypertension (**Table 3**). Hypertension, headache, abdominal pain and blurring of vision are common to both entities. While not uniformly present, paroxysmal hypertension, particularly before 20 weeks gestation, as well as orthostasis and the absence of significant proteinuria and edema may be helpful in the differential diagnosis. Thyrotoxicosis may also resemble this disease. However, significant diastolic hypertension is rarely observed with hyperthyroidism. An unexplained hypertensive response to anesthesia or circulatory collapse, following delivery, should also warrant evaluation for a possible pheochromocytoma.

Table 3
Symptoms and signs in 89 cases of pheochromocytoma in pregnancy

	%
Paroxysmal or sustained hypertension	82
Headaches	66
Palpitation	36
Sweating	30
Blurred vision	17
Anxiety	15
Convulsion-dyspnea	10

Adapted from Schenker and Chowers.[38]

Management Options

Prepregnancy

If this condition is suspected, a complete diagnostic evaluation should be completed before attempting pregnancy. Definitive therapy should be undertaken, as suggested below.

Prenatal

The definitive diagnosis depends upon the laboratory measurement of catecholamines and their metabolites in a 24 h urine collection. Elevated metanephrine excretion appears to be the most sensitive and specific finding, although isolated elevated vanillylmandelic acid excretion may be present.[38] Because episodic secretion of catecholamines may occur with some tumors, plasma assay of epinephrine or norepinephrine may be helpful during symptomatic episodes.[40] Extraadrenal tumors have characteristic elevations of norepinephrine and not epinephrine.

Pharmacologic testing may establish the diagnosis in the non-pregnant patient. The phentolamine (Rogitiner®) test is based on the observation that marked alpha-adrenergic blockade will produce a fall in blood pressure in many patients with pheochromocytoma. This test is not advised during pregnancy, as it has been associated with both maternal and fetal deaths.[40] Nonetheless, it is of extreme importance that the diagnosis is established. Approximately 90% of maternal deaths due to pheochromocytoma occur in those patients who were undiagnosed prior to delivery.[41] In patients with symptoms suggesting pheochromocytoma and with laboratory findings that support the diagnosis, an effort should be made using radiologic techniques to localize the tumor. CAT of the abdomen or MRI are the procedure of choice. In the non-pregnant state, selective venous catheterization of the adrenals may be performed. The tumor is bilateral in about 10% of cases, including those encountered during gestation.

Prior to surgery, the patient should be stabilized on either oral doses of phenoxybenzamine or intravenous phentolamine in an effort to reduce the catecholamine-medicated effects. Careful evaluation of fluid status with central monitoring is essential when using these preparations. Beta-blockade employing propranolol or similar agents should be reserved for treatment of tachyarrhythmias, and should not be instituted prior to beta-blockade, as hypertensive crisis may ensue.

Schenker and Granat recommend prompt surgical removal of any pheochromocytoma detected prior to 24 weeks gestation.[39] In patients detected during the third trimester, maternal stabilization with medical therapy has been successfully accomplished, thereby allowing further fetal maturation.[41]

Labor/delivery and postnatal

Cesarean section is preferred as it minimizes the potential catecholamine surges associated with labor and vaginal delivery. Adrenal exploration may also be performed at the time of cesarean section. Careful follow-up of these patients is advised, since the tumors may recur and are potentially malignant.

ADRENAL DISEASE
Summary of Management Options

CUSHING'S SYNDROME

Prepregnancy

• Investigate and treat before conception

Prenatal

• If diagnosed in pregnancy, identify and treat cause (usually by surgery); only possible exception is diagnosis in third trimester, where delivery and subsequent definitive management may be an option

PRIMARY ALDOSTERONISM

Prenatal

• If diagnosed in pregnancy, options are medical (antihypertensives and spironolactone) vs surgery

ADRENAL INSUFFICIENCY

Prenatal

• Continue glucocorticoid and mineralocorticoid supplementation

• Vigilance for fluid overload and electrolyte disturbance

• Vigilance for adrenal crisis (treat with i.v. hydrocortisone, i.v. fluids and medical supportive therapy)

Labor/delivery

• Increase glucocorticoid supplementation

PHEOCHROMOCYTOMA

Prepregnancy

• Avoid pregnancy until definitive treatment implemented and 'cured'

Prenatal

• If suspected clinically, establish diagnosis and location of tumor

• Medical stabilization/control of blood pressure prior to and during surgery

Delivery

• Cesarean preferable

• Concomitant surgery debatable

Postnatal

• Monitor for recurrence

REFERENCES

1 Gonzalez JG, Elizondo G, Saldwar D et al. (1988) Pituitary gland growth during normal pregnancy: An in vivo study using magnetic resonance imaging. American Journal of Medicine **85**:217.

2 Tyson JE, Hwang P, Guyden H et al. (1972) Studies of prolactin secretion in human pregnancy. American Journal of Obstetrics and Gynecology **113**:14.

3 Rees LH, Burke SW, Chard T et al. (1975) Possible placental origin of ACTH in normal human pregnancy. Nature **254**:620.

4 Davison JM, Gilmore EA, Durr J et al. (1983) Altered osmotic thresholds for vasopressin secretion and thirst in human pregnancy. American Journal of Physiology **246**:105.

5 Gemzell C, Wang CF (1979) Outcome of pregnancy in women with pituitary adenoma. Fertility and Sterility **31**:363.

6 Maygar DM Marshall JR (1978) Pituitary tumors and pregnancy. American Journal of Obstetric Gynecology **132**:739.

7 Jewelewicz R, VanDeWiele RL (1980) Clinical course and outcome of pregnancy in twenty-five patients with pituitary microadenomas. American Journal of Obstetric Gynecology **136**:339.

8 Molitch ME (1984) Pregnancy and the hyperprolacti-

nemic women. *New England Journal of Medicine* **312**:21.

9 Divers W, Yen SSC (1983) Prolactin producing microadenomas in pregnancy. *Obstetrics and Gynecology* **62**:425.

10 Albrecht BH, Betz G (1986) Prolactin-secreting pituitary tumors and pregnancy. In Olefsky JM, Robbins RJ (eds) *Contemporary Issues in Endocrinology and Metabolism: Prolactinomas*, Vol. 2, pp. 195–218. New York: Churchill Livingstone.

11 Turkalj I, Braun P, Krup P (1982) Surveillance of bromocriptine in pregnancy. *Journal of The American Medical Association* **247**:1589.

12 Jewelewicz R, Zimmerman EA, Carmel PW (1977) Conservative management of a pituitary tumor during pregnancy following induction of ovulation with gonadotropins. *Fertility and Sterility* **28**:35.

13 Zarate A, Canales ES, Alger M (1979) The effect of pregnancy and lactation on pituitary prolactin secreting tumors. *Acta Endocrinologica* **92**:407.

14 Abelove WA, Rupp JJ, Paschkis KE (1954) Acromegaly and pregnancy. *Journal of Clinical Endocrinology and Metabolism* **14**:32.

15 Finkler RS (1954) Acromegaly and pregnancy. Case report. *Journal of Clinical Endocrinology and Metabolism* **14**:1245.

16 Bigazzi M, Ronga R, Lancranjan I et. (1979) A pregnancy in an acromegalic women during bromocriptine treatment: Effects of growth hormone and prolactin in the maternal, fetal, and amniotic compartments. *Journal of Clinical Endocrinology and Metabolism* **48**:9.

17 Luboshitzky R, Dickstein G, Barzilai D (1989) Bromocriptine induced pregnancy in an acromegalic patient. *Journal of the American Medical Association* **244**:584.

18 Hime MC, Richardson JA (1978) Diabetes insipidus and pregnancy. Case report, incidence and review of the literature. *Obstetrical and Gynaecological Survey* **33**:375.

19 Durr JA (1978) Diabetes insipidus in pregnancy. *American Journal of Kidney Disease* **9**:276.

20 Barron WM, Cohen LM, Ulland LA et al. (1984) Transient vasopressin-resistant diabetes insipidus of pregnancy. *New England Journal of Medicine* **310**:442.

21 Burrow GN, Wassenaar W, Robertson GL, Sehl H (1981) DDAVP treatment of diabetes insipidus during pregnancy and the postpartum period. *Acta Endocrinologica* **97**:23.

22 Shangold MM, Freeman R, Kumaresan P et al. (1983) Plasma oxytocin concentrations in a pregnant woman with total vasopressin deficiency. *Obstetrics and Gynecology* **61**:662.

23 Sheehan HL (1937) Postpartum necrosis of the anterior pituitary. *Journal of Pathology and Bacteriology* **45**:189.

24 Dorfman SG, Dillaplain RP, Gambrell RD (1979) Antepartum pituitary infarction. *Obstetrics and Gynecology* **53**:215.

25 Grimes HG, Brooks MH (1980) Pregnancy in Sheehan's syndrome. Report of a case and review. *Obstetrical and Gynaecological Survey* **35**:481.

26 Buescher MA, McClamrock HD, Adashi EY (1992) Cushing syndrome in pregnancy. *Obstetrics and Gynecology* **79**:130.

27 Nolten W, Lindheimer M, Rueckert P et al. (1980) Diurnal patterns and regulation of cortisol secretion in pregnancy. *Journal of Clinical Endocrinology and Metabolism* **51**:466.

28 Migeon CJ, Kenny FM, Taylor FH (1968) Cortisol production rate. VIII. Pregnancy. *Journal of Clinical Endocrinology* **28**:661.

29 Carr BR, Parker CR, Madden JD et al. (1981) Maternal plasma adrenocorticotropsin and cortisol relationships throughout human pregnancy. *American Journal of Obstetric Gynecology* **139**:416.

30 Reschini F, Ciustina G, Crosignani PG et al. (1978) Spontaneous remission of Cushing's syndrome after termination of pregnancy. *Obstetrics and Gynecology* **51**:598.

31 Keegan GT, Gravartis F, Roland AS (1976) Pregnancy complicated by Cushing's syndrome. *Southern Medical Journal* **69**:1207.

32 Koerten JM, Morales WJ, Washington SR, Castaldo TW (1986) Cushing's syndrome in pregnancy. A case report and literature review. *American Journal of Obstetric Gynecology* **154**:626.

33 Bevan JS, Gough MH, Gillmer MDG et al. (1987) Cushing's syndrome in pregnancy. The timing of definitive treatment. *Clinical Endocrinology* **27**:225.

34 Merrill RH, Dombroski RA, MacKenna JM (1984) Primary hyperaldosteronism during pregnancy. *American Journal of Obstetric Gynecology* **160**:785.

35 Lotgerring FK, Derkx FMH, Wallenburg HCS (1986) Primary hyperaldosteronism in pregnancy. *American Journal of Obstetric Gynecology* **155**:986.

36 Brent F (1950) Addison's disease and pregnancy. *American Journal of Surgery* **79**:645.

37 O'Shaughnessy RW, Hackett KJ (1984) Maternal Addison's disease and fetal growth retardation. *Journal of Reproductive Medicine* **29**:752.

38 Schenker JG, Crowers I (1971) Pheochromocytoma and pregnancy: Review of 89 cases. *Obstetrical and Gynaecological Survey* **26**:739.

39 Schenker JG, Granat M (1982) Pheochromocytoma and pregnancy – an update and appraisal. *Australia and New Zealand Journal of Obstetrics and Gynaecology* **22**:1.

40 Shapiro B, Fig LM (1989) Management of pheochromocytoma. *Endocrinology and Metabolism Clinics of North America* **16**:443.

41 Venuto R, Burstein P, Schmeider R (1984) Pheochromocytoma: Antepartum diagnosis and management with tumor resection in the puerperium. *American Journal of Obstetric Gynecology* **150**:431.

23

Hematological Problems

ELIZABETH A. LETSKY, RUTH WARWICK

ANEMIA

There are marked physiological changes in the composition of the blood in healthy pregnancy. The increase in total blood volume and[1] hemostatic changes[2] help to combat the hazard of hemorrhage at delivery. There is a dramatic increase in plasma volume (50%) and an increasing red cell mass (18–25% depending on iron status). These changes cause a dilutional decrease in hemoglobin concentration erroneously called the 'physiologic anemia of pregnancy'. This is maximal at 32 weeks gestation. The World Health Organization[3] recommends that the hemoglobin concentration should not fall below 11.0 g/dl at any time during pregnancy. Anemia of pregnancy due to deficiency of hematinics should not occur with appropriate prophylaxis. In iron-replete women, the hemoglobin returns to normal by the first week postpartum.

Low-grade anemia in a demanding metabolic state such as pregnancy may result in morbidity *per se*. In addition, deficiency of essential hematinics arising from increased requirements and inadequate intake may have far-reaching effects on mother, fetus and neonate which bear no relationship to the impaired oxygen-carrying capacity of the reduced red cell mass.

Pathological anemia of pregnancy is mainly due to iron deficiency[4]. Over 90% of anemia is due to red cell iron deficiency associated with depleted iron stores and deficient intake.[5,6] Occasionally, infection will inhibit the incorporation of iron from the stores into hemoglobin. Folate deficiency is often a minor interacting component and is associated with iron deficiency due to the fact that they are both associated with a poor diet. The effects of folate deficiency are usually masked by iron deficiency.

Vitamin B_{12} deficiency hardly ever causes anemia in pregnancy. Addisonian pernicious anemia does not usually occur in the reproductive years, though if it does it is associated with infertility. Pregnancy only occurs when the B_{12} deficiency is corrected. It is only vegans that may have a vitamin B_{12} deficient diet.

Any miscellaneous disorder or any acquired or chronic genetic disorder with anemia and increased marrow turnover will be exacerbated during pregnancy and will need special treatment.

ANEMIA: IRON DEFICIENCY

Maternal Risks

The female is always in precarious iron balance during the reproductive years. There are increasing demands for iron with advancing pregnancy but the demands of the fetus are maximal in the third trimester. As pregnancy continues, serum iron will fall and serum TIBC will increase due to the increased plasma volume. Plasma and tissue ferritin decreases in pregnancy in any woman whether given hematinics or not. Marrow iron in a woman not given hematinics is not detectable at term whatever her hemoglobin concentration.[4] The main demand for iron arises from the expansion of the red cell mass.

Insensible losses of iron during pregnancy are approximately 1 mg/day. Outside pregnancy, 1–2 mg are absorbed daily from the diet. In pregnancy, the demand is approximately 4 mg daily (2.5 mg in early pregnancy; 6.6 mg in the last trimester). The woman can only meet these demands by a limited increase in absorption and by mobilizing her iron stores;[5,6] if she enters pregnancy with depleted iron stores, then effects of iron deficiency will develop. Vegetarians are at an additional disadvantage because heme iron is more readily absorbed and heme also facilitates absorption of non-heme iron in a mixed diet.

As iron deficiency develops, the ferritin falls first, then the serum iron. A fall in hemoglobin concentration is a late development.[7] The red cell mean cell volume (MCV) also falls and is the first indication in pregnancy of iron deficiency affecting hemoglobin synthesis. There is also an effect on iron-dependent enzymes present in every cell. This causes a profound effect on body functions, e.g. impaired muscle function, neurotransmitter activity, exercise tolerance, epithelial changes and alteration in gastrointestinal function.[8] These abnormalities can be corrected by oral iron.[9,10]

The various effects of iron deficiency on cellular function may be responsible for the reported association between anemia during pregnancy and pre-term birth.[11,12] Overt symptoms of iron deficiency are generally not prominent. Impaired oxygen-carrying capacity due to a gradually reducing hemoglobin concentration is compensated for. However, the impairment of the function of iron-dependent tissue enzymes has profound effects on cellular function as stated on the central nervous system.[13]

It is well known that parenteral treatment of megaloblastic anemia with appropriate hematinics, either vitamin B_{12} or folic acid, results in an immediate subjective feeling of improvement and well-being in the patient long before the hemoglobin rises. This is because of the non-hematological effects of depletion of these vitamins on various tissues. A similar immediate feeling of well-being has been observed in those few patients under our care who have received parenteral iron and in those during the first week of oral iron administration before the hemoglobin level starts to rise, presumably for similar reasons.

Tissue enzyme malfunction undoubtedly occurs even in the very first stages of iron deficiency, and it is obvious that the prevention of nutritional iron deficiency is a desirable objective in this period of maximal stress on the hemopoietic system during pregnancy. Acute blood loss causes dramatic changes in maternal blood volume at both vaginal delivery and cesarean section.

In normal pregnancy, hypervolemia modifies the response to blood loss considerably.[2] The blood volume drops following the acute loss at delivery but remains relatively stable as long as the loss does not exceed 25% of the predelivery volume. There is no

compensatory increase in blood volume and there is a gradual fall in plasma volume due primarily to diuresis. The overall result is that the hematocrit gradually increases and the blood volume returns to non-pregnant levels. ·

The average blood loss which can be tolerated without causing a significant fall in hemoglobin concentration is 1000 ml, but this depends in turn on a healthy increase in blood volume prior to delivery and on iron status. Many studies have shown that women not given iron supplements are profoundly deficient at the end of pregnancy and these studies have been reviewed.[14]

In iron-deficient women, it may take more than a year for the hemoglobin to return to prepregnancy levels. If iron supplements are given, the hemoglobin is in the normal prepregnancy range by 5–7 days after delivery.[9] There is anecdotal evidence that the blood loss at delivery is much greater in those women who are anemic. This is not a surprising association when the effect of iron deficiency on neuromuscular transmission and the vital role myometrial contraction plays on stemming the flow from the placental site is appreciated.

Fetal Risks

The fetus derives its iron from the maternal serum by active transport across the placenta, mainly in the last 4 weeks of pregnancy. The concentration of ferritin in the core blood is substantially higher than that in the mother's circulation at term regardless of whether she is iron-deficient or not.[6,15] All of the cord values obtained are within the normal, predominantly the high normal range, for serum ferritin as defined in the adult. However, the babies born to iron-deficient mothers have significantly decreased cord ferritin levels compared with the others. This reduction in iron accumulated by fetuses of mothers with depleted iron stores may have an important bearing on the iron stores and the development of anemia during the first year of life,[15,16] when oral iron intake is very poor.

Studies have also suggested behavioral abnormalities in children with iron deficiency related to changes in the concentration of chemical mediators in the brain.[13] Iron deficiency in the absence of anemia is also associated with poor performance on the Bayley Mental Development Index and this performance can be improved by the administration of iron.[17]

Even more far-reaching effects of maternal iron deficiency during pregnancy have been suggested in a recent publication from a busy obstetric unit in Oxford, UK.[18] A retrospective study of over 8000 deliveries in a 2-year period between January 1987 and January 1989 showed a correlation between maternal iron deficiency anemia, high placental weight and an increased ratio of placental to birth weight. This suggests that maternal iron deficiency results in poor fetal growth compared with that of the placenta. High blood pressure in adult life has been linked to lower birthweight and with those whose birthweight was lower than would be expected from the weight of the placenta. Prophylaxis of iron deficiency in pregnancy may therefore have important implications for the prevention of adult hypertension, which appears to have its origin in fetal life.[18]

Diagnosis

Hemoglobin concentration

A reduction in concentration of circulating hemoglobin is a relatively late development in iron deficiency, and is preceded first by a depletion in iron stores, then a reduction in serum iron and, finally, detectable decrements in the hemoglobin level. This is the simplest non-invasive practical test available. Hemoglobin values of less than 0.5 g/dl in the second and third trimesters are probably abnormal and require further investigation.

Red cell indices

The appearance of red cells on a stained film is a relatively insensitive gauge of iron status in pregnancy. Useful information relevant to the diagnosis of iron deficiency in pregnancy can be obtained by the examination of red cell indices (**Table 1**). The earliest effect of iron deficiency on the erythrocyte is a reduction in the cell size (MCV), and with the dramatic changes in red cell mass and plasma volume, this appears to be the most sensitive indicator of underlying iron deficiency. Hypochromia and a fall in MCHC only appear with more severe degrees of iron depletion. Of course, some women enter pregnancy with already established anemia due to iron deficiency, or with grossly depleted iron stores, and they will quickly develop florid anemia with reduced MCV, MCH and MCHC. These do not present any problems in diagnosis. It is those who enter pregnancy in precarious iron balance with a normal hemoglobin who present the most difficult diagnostic problems. Recognition of iron deficiency before a fall in hemoglobin or an effect on indices depends on three non-invasive laboratory tests.

Ferritin

This high molecular weight glycoprotein circulates at levels ranging from 15 to 300 μg/l in healthy adult females. A level of 12 μg/l or below indicates iron deficiency. Ferritin is stable and not affected by the recent ingestion of iron, and appears to reflect the iron stores accurately and quantitatively in the absence of inflammation, particularly in the lower range associated with iron deficiency which is so important in pregnancy. In the development of iron deficiency, a low serum ferritin is the first abnormal laboratory test.

Serum iron and total iron-binding capacity (TIBC)

Serum iron together with the TIBC is an estimation of transferrin saturation. Reduced transferrin saturation indicates a deficient iron supply to the tissues and this is the second measurement to be affected in the devel-

Table 1
Red cell indices in iron deficiency and thalassemia[a]

	Normal range	Iron deficiency	Thalassemia
$\dfrac{PCV}{RBC}$ MCH	75–99 fl	Reduced	Markedly reduced
$\dfrac{Hb}{RBC}$ MCH	27–31 pg	Reduced	Markedly reduced
$\dfrac{Hb}{PCV}$ MCHC	32–36 g/dl	Reduced	Normal or slightly reduced

[a]In thalassemia, unlike iron deficiency, there is a disproportionate decrease in MCV and MCH compared with the MCHC, which can be in the normal range.

PCV, packed cell volume; RBC, red cell count; Hb, hemoglobin; MCV, mean corpuscular volume; MCH, mean corpuscular hemoglobin; MCHC, mean corpuscular hemoglobin concentration.

opment of iron deficiency. At this early stage, erythropoiesis is impaired and there is an adverse effect on iron-dependent tissue enzymes.

In health, the serum iron of adult non-pregnant women lies between 13 and 27 μmol/l, but it shows considerable diurnal variation and can fluctuate from hour to hour. The TIBC, which ranges from 45 to 72 μmol/l in the non-pregnant state, rises in association with iron deficiency and decreases in chronic inflammatory states. It is raised in pregnancy because of the increase in plasma volume. In the non-anemic individual, the TIBC is approximately one-third saturated with iron.

In pregnancy, most reports describe a decrease in both serum iron and percentage saturation of the TIBC, which can largely be prevented by iron supplements. Serum iron even in combination with TIBC is not a reliable indicator of iron stores, because it fluctuates so widely and is affected by recent ingestion of iron and other factors not directly involved with iron metabolism such as infection. Nevertheless, a serum iron of less than 12 μmol/l and a TIBC saturation of less than 15% indicate deficiency of iron during pregnancy.

Free erythrocyte protoporphyrin (FEP)

Erythroblast protoporphyrin rises when there is a defective iron supply to the developing red cell but there is a misleading increase in patients with chronic inflammatory disease, malignancy or infection. Although a widely used test in the past, this estimation has largely been dropped from the laboratory investigation of iron status.

Marrow iron

The most rapid and reliable method of assessing iron stores in pregnancy is by examination of an appropriately stained preparation of a bone marrow sample. In the absence of iron supplementation, there is no detectable stainable iron in over 80% of women at term.[4] No stainable iron (hemosiderin) may be visible once the serum ferritin has fallen to below 40 μg/l, but other stigmata of iron deficiency in the developing erythroblasts, particularly the late normoblasts, will confirm that the anemia is indeed due to iron deficiency in the absence of stainable iron. The effects of folate deficiency which often accompanies iron deficiency will also be apparent (see below). A block of incorporation of iron into hemoglobin occurs in the course of acute or chronic inflamation, particularly that arising from urinary tract infection, even if iron stores are replete. This problem will be revealed by examination of the marrow aspirate stained for iron.

Management Options

Prepregnancy

In patients proven to have iron deficiency anemia prior to pregnancy, every attempt should be made to ameliorate this condition before conception. A careful diagnostic evaluation should be undertaken to seek out the cause, and oral iron therapy should be initiated. Patients should be counseled regarding the need to continue therapy throughout gestation, and of the potential risks listed previously. Patients should also be aware of the expected change in stool color secondary to therapy, the potential for gastrointestinal upset, and problems associated with constipation.

Prenatal

The management of iron deficiency in pregnancy has largely become prevention by daily oral supplements. Elemental iron 60–80 mg/day starting in early pregnancy maintains hemoglobin in the recognized normal range for gestation but does not maintain or restore the iron stores. The World Health Organization[3] recommends that supplements of 30–60 mg/day be given to those pregnant women who have adequate iron stores, and 120–240 mg/day to those with none.

Whether all pregnant women need iron is controversial, but if it is accepted that iron is necessary, a bewildering number of preparations of varying expense are available. In those women to whom additional iron cannot be given by the oral route, either because of non-compliance or because of unacceptable side-effects, intramuscular injection of 1000 mg iron more than ensures iron sufficiency for that pregnancy. The injections are painful and can be skin-staining but there is no risk of incurring malignancy at the injection site as once reported.

Side-effects of oral iron administration appear related to the quantity administered.[19] If the daily dose is reduced to 100 mg and introduction is delayed until the 16th week of gestation, they are rare with any preparation. Some women have gastric symptoms but the most common complaint is constipation, usually overcome easily by simple basic measures. Slow-release preparations, which are on the whole more expensive, are said to be relatively free of side-effects. This is only because much of the iron is not released at all, and excreted unchanged. This means that double doses may have to be given to cover requirements, thereby further increasing expense. Since most women tolerate the cheaper preparations with no significant side-effects, these should be tried first.

Virtually all preparations used in pregnancy are combined with an appropriate dose of folic acid (see below). They should be supplied in toddler-proof packaging, preferably blister packs for the mother's benefit, to avoid the hazard of iron overdose in a young child.

Are iron supplements during pregnancy necessary? A review of controlled clinical trials of iron administration during pregnancy in developed western countries concluded that there was no beneficial effect in terms of birthweight, length of gestation, maternal and infant morbidity and mortality in those women receiving iron.[20] Age, economic status and poor nutrition affected the outcome, pregnancy anemia was not related but was simply associated with other risks. However, from the evidence available, it appears that a high proportion of women in their reproductive years do lack storage iron.[4,6] More recent studies have refuted the lack of beneficial effects of iron supplements during pregnancy, especially as far as the fetus and infant is concerned (see above).[13,15,17,18]

It has been suggested that women at risk from iron deficiency anemia can be identified by estimating the serum ferritin concentration in the first trimester.[21] A serum ferritin of less than 50 µg/l in early pregnancy is taken as an indication for daily iron supplements, while women with serum ferritin concentrations of greater than 80 µg/l are unlikely to require iron supplements. Unnecessary supplementation would thus be avoided in women enjoying good nutrition, and any risk to the pregnancy arising from severe maternal anemia would be avoided by prophylaxis and prompt treatment.[21] The management of iron deficiency anemia diagnosed late in pregnancy presents a particular challenge because a satisfactory response has to be obtained in a limited space of time. Poor compliance is the most common cause of failure of oral prophylaxis. Iron sorbitol citrate can be given as a series of intramuscular injections, but it is associated with toxic reactions such as headache, nausea and vomiting if given simultaneously with oral iron.[22,23] Iron dextran (Imferon®), an extensively used preparation, can be administered as a series of intramuscular injections or preferably as a total dose intravenous infusion. Rare anaphylactic reactions do occur in the case of intravenous infusions, but usually during the period when the first few milliliters are being administered.[23] For this reason, the infusion should initially be administered at a slow rate carefully observing the patient during the first few minutes. This preparation does not appear to be associated with toxicity if given simultaneously with oral iron.[19] There is no hematological benefit in prescribing parenteral as opposed to oral iron, but many women fail to take prescribed oral preparations and use of the parenteral route ensures that the patient has received adequate supplementation.

In the absence of any other abnormality, an increase in hemoglobin of 0.8 g/dl/week (1.0 g/dl in the nonpregnant female) can be reasonably expected with adequate treatment. The response is similar whether iron is given orally or parenterally. If there is not enough time to achieve a reasonable hemoglobin for delivery, then transfusion with all its hazards should be considered. If a woman is symptomatic, the decision is easier. However, in the asymptomatic patient, there are no data which provide suitable guidelines for practice.

In summary, negative iron balance throughout pregnancy, particularly in the latter half, may lead to iron deficiency anemia in the third trimester. This hazard, together with the increasing evidence of non-hematological effects of iron deficiency on exercise tolerance, cerebral function and effects on the fetus and its subsequent development, leads to the conclusion that it is safer, more practical and in the long term less expensive in terms of investigation, hospital admission and treatment, to offer all women iron supplements from 16 weeks gestation, especially as this would appear to do no harm.[14,24,25]

Labor/delivery

No specific therapy is indicated for the management of the iron-deficient gravida in labor. If severe blood loss with maternal anemia exists, blood transfusion may be necessary. Thus cross-matching of blood for those who remain anemic early in labor may be prudent.

Postnatal

As the physiologic effects of pregnancy diminish, hemoglobin levels will rise during the puerperium. Patients with clear evidence of iron deficiency anemia should continue oral supplementation, particularly if breastfeeding is being considered.

ANEMIA: FOLATE DEFICIENCY

Maternal Risks

Folic acid, together with iron, has assumed a central role in the nutrition of pregnancy. At a cellular level, folic acid is reduced first to dihydrofolic acid (DHF) and then to tetrahydrofolic acid (THF) which forms the cornerstone of cellular folate metabolism. It is fundamental through linkage with L-carbon fragments both to cell growth and cell division. The more active a tissue is in reproduction and growth, the more dependent it will be on the efficient turnover and supply of folate co-enzymes. Bone marrow and epithelial linings are therefore particularly at risk.

Requirements for folate are increased in pregnancy to meet the needs of the fetus, placenta, uterine hypertrophy and the expanded maternal red cell mass. The placenta transports folate actively to the fetus even in the face of maternal deficiency, but maternal folate metabolism is altered early in pregnancy like many other maternal functions, before fetal demands act directly.

Folic acid, like hemoglobin and iron, must be among the most studied substances in maternal blood, yet there are comparatively few serial data available. It is generally agreed, however, that plasma folate decreases as pregnancy advances, reaching roughly half non-pregnant values by term.[26] Plasma clearance of folate by the kidneys is more than doubled as early as the 8th week of gestation and while some ascribe importance to urinary losses, it is unlikely that increased renal clearance results in a major drain of maternal resources.

The cause of megaloblastic anemia in pregnancy is nearly always folate deficiency. Vitamin B_{12} is only rarely implicated. A survey of reports from the UK over the past two decades suggests an incidence ranging from 0.2 to 5.0%, but a considerably greater number of women have megaloblastic changes in their marrow which are not suspected on examination of the peripheral blood only.[26] The incidence of megaloblastic anemia in other parts of the world is considerably greater and is thought to reflect the nutritional standards of the population. While there is much controversy at the moment about the requirement for folate, particularly during pregnancy, the World Health Organization recommendations for daily intake are as high as 800 µg in the prenatal period and 600 µg during lactation. Food folates are only partially available. The amount of folate supplied in the diet is difficult to quantify. In the UK, folate intake in foodstuffs ranges between 129 and 300 µg, while the content of 24-h food collections in various studies in Sweden and Canada averaged 200 µg (range 70–600 µg). Dietary folate deficiency megaloblastic anemia probably occurs in about one-third of all pregnant women in the world, despite the fact that folate is found in nearly all natural foods. This is because folate is rapidly destroyed by cooking, especially in finely divided foods such as beans and rice,[27] while green vegetables lose up to 90% of their vitamin content during the first few minutes of boiling.

The effects of dietary inadequacy may be further amplified by frequent childbirth, and several reports have shown a markedly increased incidence of megaloblastic anemia in multiple pregnancy.[26]

Fetal Risks

There is an increased risk of megaloblastic anemia occurring in the neonate of a folate-deficient mother, especially if delivery is preterm. There are also data suggesting an association between periconceptional folic acid deficiency and harelip, cleft palate and, most important of all, neural tube defects.[28–30] This subject has been well reviewed in the past,[31] but the association between periconceptional folate deficiency and recurrence of neural tube defects has now been confirmed in a mass multicenter controlled trial of pre-pregnancy folate supplementation.[32] Periconceptional folic acid has been shown to reduce the recurrence of neural tube defects. More recently in Hungary it has also been shown in a large randomized controlled trial[151] that a periconceptional supplement of 800 µg of folic acid in a combined vitamin preparation prevented the first occurrence of neural tube defects.

Diagnosis

Substantial day-to-day variations of plasma folate are possible and postprandial increases have been noted; this will limit its diagnostic value for serum folate estimations when an occasional sample taken at a casual prenatal clinic visit is considered. Estimation of red cell folate does not reflect daily or other short-term variations in plasma folate levels and is thought to give a better indication of overall body tissue levels. However, the turnover of red blood cells is slow and there will be a delay before significant reductions in the folate concentrations of the red cells are evident. In this respect, there is evidence that patients who have a low red cell folate at the beginning of pregnancy develop megaloblastic anemia in the third trimester.[26] Histidine loading leads to increased forminoglutamic acid (FIGLU) excretion in the urine when there is folate deficiency, but this is not a good test in pregnancy. This is because the metabolism of histidine is altered, resulting in increased FIGLU early in normal pregnancy.

The value of the above various investigations in predicting megaloblastic anemia and assessing subclinical folate deficiency has been the subject of numerous reports. Using these various tests, folate 'deficiency' in pregnancy is not invariably accompanied by any significant hematological change. In the absence of any changes, megaloblastic hemopoiesis should be suspected when the expected response to adequate iron therapy is not achieved. No help can be expected from the use of tests of folate status. Usually, abnormal results are obtained with most of the tests, but these are not significantly different from results in healthy pregnant women.

The blood picture is complex and may be difficult to interpret. There is a physiological increase in red cell size in healthy iron-replete pregnancy. The MCV rises on average by 4 fl but may be as much as 20 fl. This increase in red cell size is not prevented by folate supplements.

The physiological macrocytosis may be masked by the effects of iron deficiency which results in the production of small red cells (see above). Outside pregnancy, the hallmark of megaloblastic hemopoiesis is macrocytosis, first identified in routine laboratory investigations by a raised MCV. In pregnancy, macrocytosis by non-pregnant standards is the norm and in any event may be masked by iron deficiency. Examination of the blood film may be more helpful. There may be occasional oval macrocytes in a sea of iron-deficient microcytic cells. Hypersegmentation of the neutrophil polymorph nucleus is significant because in normal pregnancy there is a shift to the left. However, hypersegmentation is observed in pure iron deficiency even if uncomplicated by folate deficiency.

The diagnosis of folate deficiency in pregnancy has to be made ultimately on morphological grounds and usually involves examination of a suitably prepared marrow aspirate.[26]

Management Options

Prepregnancy

As with other anemias, a careful diagnostic evaluation should be undertaken, followed by prompt therapy prior to conception. Risks as outlined should be discussed prior to pregnancy.

Prenatal

Prophylaxis

The case for giving prophylactic folate supplements throughout pregnancy is a strong one,[26,33,34] and the supplement needs to be of the order of 200–300 μg folic acid daily. This should be given in combination with iron supplements (see above) and there are several suitable combined preparations available. The risk of adverse effects from folate supplements in a pregnant woman suffering from B_{12} deficiency is very small (see below). Patients with that degree of B_{12} deficiency are usually infertile and pernicious anemia is generally a disease of older people. More important than this, there is not one report of subacute combined degeneration of the spinal cord occurring among the thousands of women who have received folate supplements during pregnancy: 'It is a hypothetical situation which should not detract from the vast benefit provided by routine use of folate supplements in pregnancy'.[26]

Management of established folate deficiency

Severe megaloblastic anemia is now uncommon in the UK and USA, largely as a result of prophylaxis and prompt treatment. Once megaloblastic hematopoiesis is established, treatment of folic acid deficiency becomes more difficult, presumably due to megaloblastic changes in the gastrointestinal tract resulting in impaired absorption. Treatment initially, if the diagnosis is made in the prenatal period, should be pteroyl-

glutamic acid 5 mg daily, continued for several weeks after delivery. If there is no response to this therapy, parenteral folic acid can be tried. It is far better to intervene before these difficulties arise and give routine prophylaxis throughout pregnancy.

Anticonvulsants and folic acid

Folate status is even further compromised in pregnancy if a woman is on anticonvulsants, in particular phenytoin and phenobarbitone. Although earlier studies suggested that the control of epilepsy became more difficult in pregnancy with folate supplements approaching 5.0 mg daily,[35] more recent studies with supplements between 100 and 1000 μg daily have not substantiated these fears.[36] Anticonvulsant therapy is associated with an increased incidence of congenital abnormality, prematurity and low birthweight, giving extra weight to the argument for folate supplements being given to all epileptic women taking anticonvulsants.

Disorders which may affect folate requirement

Women with hemolytic anemia, particularly hereditary hemolytic conditions such as hemoglobinopathies and hereditary spherocytosis, require extra folate supplements from early pregnancy if the development of megaloblastic anemia is to be avoided. The recommended supplement in this situation is 5–10 mg orally daily. The anemia associated with thalassemia trait is not strictly due to hemolysis but to ineffective erythropoiesis (see below). However, the increased though abortive marrow turnover still results in folate depletion and such women would probably benefit from the routine administration of oral folic acid 5.0 mg daily from early pregnancy.

Folate supplements are of particular importance in the management of sickle cell syndromes during pregnancy if aplastic crises and megaloblastic anemia are to be avoided.

Labor/delivery

There is no specific acute therapy for folate-associated anemia during labor and delivery. This presumes that the patient is hemodynamically stable, and that blood replacement therapy is available if needed.

Postnatal

In the 6 weeks following delivery, there is a tendency for all the parameters discussed to return to non-pregnant values. However, should any deficiency of folate have developed and remained untreated in pregnancy, it may present clinically for the first time in the puerperium and its consequences can be detected for many months after delivery. Lactation provides an added folate stress. A folate content of 5 μg per 100 ml of human milk and a yield of 500 ml daily implies a loss of 25 μg folate daily in breast milk. Red cell folate levels in lactating mothers are significantly lower than that of their infant during the first year of life.

ANEMIA: VITAMIN B$_{12}$ DEFICIENCY

Muscle, red cell and serum vitamin B$_{12}$ concentrations fall during pregnancy. Non-pregnant levels of 205–1025 μg/l decrease to 20–510 μg/l at term, with low levels in multiple pregnancy. Women who smoke tend to have lower serum B$_{12}$ levels, which may account for the positive correlation between birthweight and serum levels in non-deficient mothers.

Maternal/Fetal Risks

Vitamin B$_{12}$ absorption is unaltered in pregnancy but tissue uptake may be increased by the action of estrogens, as oral contraceptives cause a fall in serum vitamin B$_{12}$. Cord blood serum vitamin B$_{12}$ is higher than that of maternal blood. The fall in serum vitamin B$_{12}$ in the mother is related to preferential transfer of absorbed B$_{12}$ to the fetus at the expense of maintaining the maternal serum concentration, but the placenta does not transfer vitamin B$_{12}$ with the same efficiency as it does folate. Low serum vitamin B$_{12}$ levels in early pregnancy in vegetarian Hindus do not fall further, while their infants often have subnormal concentrations. The vitamin B$_{12}$ binding capacity of plasma increases in pregnancy analogous to the rise in transferrin. The rise is confined to the liver-derived transcobalamin II concerned with transport rather than the leucocyte-derived transcobalamin I which is raised in myeloproliferative conditions.

Pregnancy does not make a vast impact on maternal vitamin B$_{12}$ stores. Adult stores are of the order of 3000 μg or more, and vitamin B$_{12}$ stores in the newborn infant are about 50 μg. Addisonian pernicious anemia is very unusual during the reproductive years. Also, vitamin B$_{12}$ deficiency is associated with infertility, and pregnancy is likely only if the deficiency is remedied.

Chronic tropical sprue is another cause of vitamin B$_{12}$ deficiency in pregnancy. The megaloblastic anemia in this case is due to both a long-standing vitamin B$_{12}$ deficiency and folate deficiency. Cord vitamin B$_{12}$ levels remain above the maternal levels in these cases, but the concentration in the breast milk follows the maternal serum levels.

Management Options

Prepregnancy

See iron and folate deficiency.

Prenatal

The recommended intake of vitamin B$_{12}$ is 2.0 μg per day in the non-pregnant and 3.0 μg per day during pregnancy.[3] This will be met by almost any diet which contains animal products. However, in these days of processed foods, certain animal products may lose their B$_{12}$ content in preparation. It has been reported that a surprising number of underprivileged young adults were suffering from B$_{12}$ deficiency in Mexico City.[27] Their sole source of dietary B$_{12}$ was in processed milks which, on investigation, were found to have very little B$_{12}$ content. Strict vegans, who will not eat any animal-derived substances, may have a deficient intake of vitamin B$_{12}$ and their diet should be supplemented during pregnancy.

Labor/delivery

See iron and folate deficiency.

Postnatal

See iron and folate deficiency.

ANEMIA: BONE MARROW APLASIA

Maternal/Fetal Risks and Management Options

There have been sporadic case reports of refractory hypoplastic anemia, sometimes recurrent, developing in pregnancy and appearing to be related in some way to the pregnancy.[37–39] Occasionally, pregnancy occurs when chronic acquired aplastic anemia is present as an underlying disease.[40] It has been generally considered that in both these situations, pregnancy exacerbates the marrow depression, causing rapid deterioration, and the gestation should be terminated. It is true that many cases do remit spontaneously after termination but there is no record of excessive hemorrhage at delivery despite profound thrombocytopenia. Supportive measures in this situation are improving and pregnancy should be maintained as long as the health of the mother is not seriously impaired.[40]

There are a few cases in the literature of pure red cell

COMMON ANEMIAS
Summary of Management Options

Investigate if Hb <10.5 g/dl (opinions vary, 10.0–11.0 g/dl)

- Full blood count

- Blood film

- Red cell indices

- Reticulocyte count

- Assess iron status (e.g. ferritin)

- Red cell folate

- Serum B_{12}

- Other investigations as indicated by clinical findings and laboratory results.

IRON DEFICIENCY

Prepregnancy

- Investigate for cause

- Oral iron therapy

Prenatal

- Prophylaxis is controversial (routine *vs* selective)

- Oral iron and folate for deficiency

- Parenteral iron only if failed oral therapy

- Blood transfusion considered if symptomatic

Labor/delivery

- Cross-match blood if severe anemia

Postnatal

- Continue iron/folate therapy for iron-deficient

FOLATE DEFICIENCY

Prepregnancy

- Public health measures to prevent periconceptional folate deficiency

- Investigate and treat causes

Prenatal

- Strong case for routine prophylaxis

- Prophylaxis with anticonvulsants

- Continue routine oral therapy for hemolytic anemias

- Parenteral therapy if deficiency severe

VITAMIN B_{12} DEFICIENCY

Prenatal

- Deficiency is rare but continue treatment where instituted before conception

- Consider oral supplementation and other components with strict vegans

AUTOIMMUNE HEMOLYTIC ANEMIA

- Monitor carefully

- Use steroids if necessary

- Investigate fetus

aplasia associated with pregnancy, reversible following delivery. One report describes the course of relapsing pure red cell aplasia during three pregnancies.[38] Anemia can be profound and supportive red cell transfusions are necessary, but the outcome is generally good if there are no other interacting complications.

AUTOIMMUNE HEMOLYTIC ANEMIA

Maternal/Fetal Risks and Management Options

The rare combination of autoimmune hemolytic anemia (AIHA) and pregnancy carries great risks to both the woman herself and the fetus. Very careful prenatal supervision and adjustment of steroid therapy is required.[41] There have been a number of reports[42] in which women have been treated with steroids and other immune suppressives throughout pregnancy for a variety of conditions including autoimmune thrombocytopenic purpura (AITP), SLE, AIHA and some forms of malignancy. The problems of their use are essentially the same as those outside pregnancy, but more frequent monitoring and adjustment are required due to the rapidly changing blood volume and changes in the circulating hormones during the prenatal and postnatal periods. There is also concern about the possible effects of azathioprine on the reproductive performance of female offspring (see Chapter 17). The anemia of systemic lupus erythematosis as well as hematologic problems in the newborn due to transplacental passage of IgG antibodies is discussed in Chapter 27.

HEMATOLOGICAL MALIGNANCIES

One in 1000 pregnancies is complicated by malignant disease.[43] Leukemia and lymphoma are the second and fifth leading causes of cancer-related deaths in the 15–35 year age group of women, respectively. The incidence of these diseases in pregnancy may rise as women delay their families and as more children survive malignancies to reach reproductive maturity. The aim of treatment in leukemia and lymphoma is not only to save life but also to cure the patient of their disease. These principles should be no less true in pregnancy. The conditions that will be considered are:

- Leukemias   • Lymphomas
  acute   Hodgkin's disease
  chronic   non-Hodgkin's lymphomas

Most of the papers reporting these conditions give an account of a few cases at best and include a review of the published literature.[44–46,152] Some include a discussion of management considerations.[47,48,153] The management options discussed here are based on these publications. Other malignant conditions are considered in Chapter 32.

ACUTE LEUKEMIAS

Definition and Incidence

Acute leukemia is a malignant proliferation of hemopoietic precursor cells. The marrow is replaced by malignant cells which spill over into the peripheral blood. The incidence in the general population varies from 5 to 10 per 100 000. Patients present with symptoms and signs as a consequence of marrow failure (anemia, neutropenia and thrombocytopenia). Without treatment, death occurs in 2–3 months or less. The incidence of acute leukemia in pregnancy is about 1:75 000.

Maternal/Fetal Risks (General)

The prognosis for the mother and fetus depends on:

- the type of acute leukemia

- the stage of pregnancy

- the management by the obstetrician and hematologist

There are over 300 cases of leukemia reported in the literature predating effective combination chemotherapy. The perinatal mortality in this group approaches 70% and most of the mothers were dead within 3 months. However, there are 70 reported cases which were effectively treated in the last two decades:[47] 14 pregnancies were in patients previously cured of acute lymphoblastic leukemia (ALL), 16 pregnancies were complicated by intercurrent ALL and 40 cases were complicated by intercurrent acute myeloid leukemia (AML). However, caution should be exercised in interpreting these reports since they may not be representative. The gestational distribution is not uniform with very few cases in the first trimester or presenting after 32 weeks gestation. There may be under-reporting of cases resulting in first trimester termination of pregnancy or those where elective delivery was undertaken in the last trimester.

Maternal Risks

There is no evidence that the rate of leukemia is increased in or by pregnancy. One feature of several reports is the delay in diagnosis that can occur because of confusion of symptoms with those of normal pregnancy (fatigue, breathlessness, anemia). However, even a short delay can threaten maternal and fetal survival, since untreated patients have a median survival of only 2 months. Chemotherapy and supportive care (see below) constitute the only chance of survival for the mother and the fetus. There is significant maternal mortality associated with delivery in patients with active uncontrolled disease, especially secondary to hemorrhage and infection. Even if the patient can be brought into remission, infection remains a potential risk at the time of delivery, although it does not affect maternal survival. The prognosis of the mother with acute leukemia in pregnancy is no different from that if she were not pregnant, namely relapse in about 2 years for most with AML, and a 50% survival and hopeful cure at 5 years for those with ALL.

In most cases of AML and ALL, fertility in the mother will be retained and the younger the woman is at the time of diagnosis and treatment, the greater the chance that she will remain fertile. The group of agents with the highest likelihood of inducing infertility are the alkylating agents, but these drugs are not used in the modern treatment of AML and ALL. Patients who are receiving or have recently had chemotherapy may be fertile despite the drug treatment. Thus effective contraception (preferably the oral contraceptive pill) are recommended during chemotherapy.

Patients who have been cured of acute leukemia and who are off maintenance therapy have no additional risks in pregnancy.

There have been some reports of successful pregnancies in women who had prior allogenic bone marrow transplants (BMT) both in those whose conditioning therapy was by use of chemotherapy alone [154] and more recently in women who received total body irradiation.[155]

Fetal Risks

Transmission of maternal malignant cells to the fetus is extremely rare but has been reported in 37 cases since 1866. Only two cases were in infants born to mothers with ALL, both babies dying from the disease in the first year.

Approximately 20% of the babies are small-for-dates. This seems to be primarily not the effect of the drugs, since the incidence is the same in untreated cases. Other suggested explanations include maternal catabolism, chronic maternal anemia, aggregation of leukemic cells in the uteroplacental circulation, recurrent infection and disseminated intravascular coagulation. Preterm delivery is found in 50% of cases and is due to both spontaneous and iatrogenic factors. There are no reported cases of spontaneous labor secondary to chorioamnionitis, which is surprising. The dramatic improvement in medium-term maternal survival with the aggressive use of chemotherapy results in 92% survival when the diagnosis is made after the first trimester (compared to 50% in untreated cases).

There is no evidence of long-term ill-effects in the babies (growth retardation, poor intellectual performance, delayed puberty, loss of fertility, immune deficiency or malignancy) after birth. However, it must be added that the number of children followed for a long period is not large.

There are risks from the chemotherapy, especially if the diagnosis is made in the first trimester. There is undoubtedly increased fetal wastage when the drugs are used in the first trimester, though the degree of this risk is difficult to quantify because of the possibility of under-reporting of such losses. Surprisingly, the fetal abnormality rate is only approximately 10% with first trimester chemotherapy. Since the 1980s, there have been many reports of successful outcomes of pregnancy when treatment was started within the first 12 weeks with daunorubicin, cytosine arabinoside, 6-thioguanine, vincristine and prednisolone.

There appear to be very few problems for the fetus from the chemotherapy started after the first trimester. As already discussed, the 20% small-for-dates rate does not seem to be primarily due to the effects of chemotherapy.

Short-term effects on the fetus noted in the newborn include signs of marrow toxicity (anemia, neutropenia, thrombocytopenia). While there are no reports of long-term adverse effects of chemotherapy given during pregnancy in infancy and later childhood, this is a reflection of the lack of information rather than a proven lack of complications.[49]

Management Options

Prepregnancy

When a woman in her reproductive years is diagnosed to have an acute leukemia and is started on chemotherapy, it is important that she is carefully advised against conception until she is in remission and on no chemotherapy. Even then it is probably wise to give a clear picture of the long-term prognosis for the condition (see above) so that she and her partner can decide whether they wish to consider a pregnancy at all given all the facts. The oral contraceptive pill is a reasonable and effective method for avoiding pregnancy.

Prenatal

When a pregnant woman presents with acute leukemia, the main aim should be to treat with chemotherapy as vigorously as in the non-pregnant state. Untreated or uncontrolled leukemia has an ominous prognosis for both mother and baby. Careful attention to supportive care in terms of blood and blood product transfusions should be maintained and prompt investigation and treatment of infection is mandatory. Further studies are required to determine whether alterations of the non-pregnant regimes are necessary given the alterations in such physiological parameters as glomerular filtration rate and blood volume. If treatment is started in the first trimester there should be careful counseling about the teratogenic risks. The growth and health of the fetus should be monitored through the pregnancy.

Labor/delivery

Delivery should be expedited for the normal obstetric indications. Ideally, delivery should occur when the mother is in remission and the fetus has the optimum chance of survival. The use of steroids to enhance fetal surfactant production should be considered if preterm delivery is contemplated.

Postnatal

It is important that, after delivery, careful counseling about the long-term prognosis is offered. This should include advice about contraception (see above).

CHRONIC LEUKEMIAS

Definition and Incidence

In contrast to the acute leukemias, the chronic leukemias can often run an indolent course and require no treatment for long periods. Chronic myeloid leukemia (CML) has been described in pregnancy and is characterized by splenomegaly, leucocytosis and the presence of the Philadelphia chromosome. The marrow is hypercellular with an excess of granulocytes but there is an apparently normal maturation pattern with no blast cells. In most cases, the disease is controlled with oral alkylating agents such as busulphan. Ultimately, the disease tranforms to an acute form ('blast crisis') within an average of 3 years from the time of diagnosis. While in the stable state, CML can be successfully treated by marrow transplantation. CML accounts for over half the cases of chronic leukemia reported in association with pregnancy, in most cases the diagnosis antedating the pregnancy.

Chronic lymphatic leukemia (CLL) is a relatively benign proliferation of mature lymphocytes found in elderly patients. It is thus extremely unlikely to be encountered in pregnancy. Other myeloproliferative disorders e.g. polycythemia rubra vera and thrombocythemia are seen very occasionally during pregnancy.

Maternal Risks

There is no evidence that pregnancy adversely affects the disease or that in the quiescent form it has any serious effect on the pregnant woman. Blast phase leukemia that is complicating the pregnancy should be managed as AML (see above).

Fetal Risks

As with the acute leukemias, there is an association between CML and both preterm delivery and the delivery of a small-for-dates baby. No other short-term complications have been reported from the disease. Furthermore, extensive follow-up studies of babies born to mothers with CML before the chemotherapeutic era have failed to demonstrate any long-term sequelae in terms of development, growth or handicap.

There have been at least 24 cases in the literature of women receiving busulphan during pregnancy and over half of them received the drug during the first trimester. Two of the 24 gave birth to malformed infants. However, only one of these women received the drug during the first trimester, though she also received 6-mercaptopurine and splenic irradiation in addition; the other was treated with busulphan from 20 weeks.

Management Options

Prepregnancy

The implications and risks for pregnancy (see above) need to be discussed. Giving advice about effective contraception is also mandatory.

Prenatal

Regular hematological review should take place during pregnancy to detect development of the blast phase. If the blast phase should develop, then managment is as for acute leukemia (see above). Busulphan can be given during pregnancy, but it should be avoided during the first trimester if possible. Fetal growth and health should be monitored. Pregnancy has been successful in women who received recombinant interferon alpha$_{2C}$ for management of chronic myeloid leukemia.[156]

HODGKIN'S DISEASE

Definition and Incidence

Hodgkin's disease comprises about 40% of all lymphomas and has a bimodal age distribution at 25 and 70 years. Cure outside of pregnancy with 5-year survival rates as high as 60% has been based on accurate staging followed by the appropriate use of radiotherapy and chemotherapy:

- Stage I: disease in one set of lymph nodes; radiotherapy.

- Stage II: disease in two adjacent sets of lymph nodes; radiotherapy.

- Stage III: disease above and below the diaphragm; chemotherapy.

- Stage IV: disease involving liver, bone marrow and other extralymphatic sites; chemotherapy.

It is by far the most common lymphoma in pregnancy[157] reported to be found in between 1:1000 and 1:6000 pregnancies. As with the acute leukemias, more aggressive management has led to better survival for both the mother and the fetus. However, there are important differences which need to be emphasized.

Maternal Risks

There is no evidence that Hodgkin's disease is adversely affected by pregnancy.[158] The majority of patients who have Hodgkin's disease in pregnancy are asymptomatic and healthy. The dilemma comes when one attempts accurate staging, the necessary prerequisite for successful treatment, since there is the potential for understaging and thus undertreating the mother. Staging may have to be incomplete in pregnancy and the clinician will have to rely more on clinical staging associated with as much as a 30% inaccuracy rate, though the use of CT or MRI scanning is probably justified to improve upon this clinical figure. A staging laparotomy can also be considered in the second trimester (see below). Fortunately, there is good evidence that chemotherapy following inappropriate radiotherapy gives just as good a result as initial chemotherapy.

There is, however, evidence of reduced fertility in women treated for Hodgkin's disease, with a reported incidence as high as 30%, though the majority of such women will successfully conceive. Women who have been successfully treated for Hodgkin's disease are not prone to a higher relapse rate in subsequent pregnancies.

Fetal Risks

These may be divided into risks from:

- the disease itself

- diagnostic techniques (radiation or laparotomy)

- therapeutic radiation

- chemotherapy

There has only been one report of placental involvement with Hodgkin's disease, the infant dying of disseminated Hodgkin's disease at the age of 5 months. Staging involving laparatomy is associated with a greater risk of spontaneous miscarriage and preterm delivery (see also Chapter 34).

Diagnostic radiation carries theoretical risks to the fetus with the following approximate doses:

- chest x-ray   1 mrem

- plain abdominal x-ray   220 mrem

- lymphogram   1100 mrem

- CT scan of abdomen/pelvis   2000 mrem

While the cumulative dose from a series of radiological investigations in a patient with Hodgkin's disease could approach 5 rem, this is not necessarily associated with a high risk (see below).

The effect of diagnostic and/or therapeutic radiation on the fetus depend on both the gestational age and the dose received. When the pelvic radiation dosage exceeds 200 rem, there are well-proven risks:

- high incidence of spontaneous miscarriage with treatment in early pregnancy

- teratogenesis with treatment in the first trimester (approximately one in three)

- increased incidence of microcephaly, mental retardation and growth deficiency with treatment after the first trimester and up to 20 weeks.

In animals, doses as low as 10–15 rem have been shown to carry an increased risk of teratogenesis. However, there is no evidence from human studies of risk when the dosage is less than 100 rem. Unfortunately, the doses of radiation received by the fetus in the first half of pregnancy from radiotherapy to the chest or upper abdomen even without shielding are 50 and 150 rem, respectively, a dosage range for which the human data on fetal risk are not clear. If the dosage of radiation to the fetus can be kept below 10 rem either with diagnostic radiation (see above) or therapeutic radiation with shielding, then this is considered to be relatively safe.

Most of the effects of chemotherapy have been discussed under acute leukemias (see above) with a teratogenic risk of treatment in the first trimester of about 10%.

Management Options

Prepregnancy

Women with the diagnosis should receive counseling about the risks for pregnancy (see above) and contraceptive advice.

Prenatal

Overall, the outlook for patients with Hodgkin's disease in pregnancy is good, though the risks should be discussed with the patient at every stage. Diagnosis is made on clinical grounds and lymph node biopsy in the first instance. However, once a positive lymph node biopsy has been obtained, CT or MRI scanning is probably justified (see above), though a staging laparotomy can be considered early in the second trimester. A careful discussion of the risks (see above) with the mother and her partner is essential.

Stage I and II disease (extra-abdominal) should be treated with radiotherapy, the pelvis and abdomen being shielded to prevent exposure of the fetus. Stage III and IV disease should be treated with chemotherapy from the outset.

For intra-abdominal stage I or II disease, the options are:

- in early pregnancy, either to consider therapeutic abortion and then radiotherapy, or, if the mother wishes to continue with the pregnancy, to use chemotherapy;

- in late pregnancy, either to deliver the fetus once fetal survival can be reasonably assured (and possibly with the use of steroids) and then to use radio-

therapy, or, if the pregnancy is too preterm, to use chemotherapy.

NON-HODGKIN'S LYMPHOMAS

Definition and Incidence

Clinically, non-Hodgkin's lymphomas may be divided into grades:

- *low*: these are usually slow-growing tumours and often require no immediate treatment at presentation but later may need single agent chemotherapy to keep them under control;

- *intermediate*;

- *high*: these require prompt aggressive chemotherapy if the patient is to survive; remission occurs in 70% with a 5-year survival of 40–50%.

These tumors have a peak incidence in the fifth and sixth decades and are, therefore, uncommon in pregnancy. Less than 30 cases have been described in association with pregnancy in the literature; however, most were of the high grade type.

Maternal Risks

The tumors tend to be of the high grade type and about half are widespread with more than one site of involvement at presentation. In approximately 30% of cases, the breast, ovary or uterus is involved. There is a tendency for the clinical course of the disease to be accelerated postpartum. The difficulties of diagnosis and staging are the same as described for Hodgkin's disease.

Fetal Risks

There is no evidence that the disease has a direct effect on the fetus.[159] The neonatal deaths that have occurred were mainly related to preterm delivery necessitated by the severity of the maternal condition. The implications for the fetus with the use of chemotherapy have been discussed above. Radiotherapy is rarely used in this condition, since the disease is often multifocal at presentation.

Management Options

Prenatal

In the majority of cases, the disease is likely to be widespread at diagnosis/presentation and aggressive combination chemotherapy is the only therapeutic option which carries a chance of survival for the mother. If the woman presents in the first trimester, then careful counseling about the risks of that chemotherapy should be undertaken and therapeutic termination of pregnancy is an option that the woman may wish to consider. If the woman presents after the fetus is considered to be viable, then delivery prior to implementation of chemotherapy is also an option for consideration.

HEMATOLOGICAL MALIGNANCIES
Summary of Management Options

ACUTE LEUKEMIAS

Prepregnancy

- Counsel about prognosis
- Advise against conception until in remission and not on chemotherapy

Prenatal

- Start chemotherapy as for non-pregnant
- Supportive therapy (blood, platelets, antibiotics, etc.)
- Careful counseling, especially if treatment commenced in first trimester
- Monitor fetal growth and health

Labor/delivery

- Expedite if normal obstetric indications
- Ideally when mother in remission and fetus mature
- Steroids if preterm delivery contemplated

Postnatal

- Contraceptive advice
- Counseling about long-term prognosis

CHRONIC LEUKAMIAS

Prepregnancy

- Counsel about prognosis both for pregnancy and in long-term
- Give contraceptive advice

Prenatal

- Hematological screening for blast phase

- Manage blast phase as for AML
- Avoid busulphan in first trimester
- Monitor fetal growth and health

HODGKIN'S DISEASE

Prepregnancy

- Counsel about risks
- Give contraceptive advice

Prenatal

- Diagnosis by lymph node biopsy
- Staging by clinical assessment and CT/MRI scanning; laparotomy can be considered early in the second trimester
- Stage I/II
  - extra-abdominal – radiotherapy with shielding
  - intra-abdominal (depends on gestation and mother's wishes)
    — delivery and radiotherapy
    — continue pregnancy and chemotherapy and supportive care
- Stage III/IV
  - chemotherapy with supportive care

NON-HODGKIN'S LYMPHOMA

Prepregnancy

- As for Hodgkin's (above)

Prenatal

- Comments about staging and diagnosis are as for Hodgkin's (above)
- Aggressive combination chemotherapy with supportive care (termination and preterm delivery before chemotherapy are options)

HEMOGLOBINOPATHIES

The hemoglobinopathies are inherited defects of hemoglobin, resulting from:

- impaired globin synthesis (thalassemia syndromes) or

- structural abnormality of globin (hemoglobin variants)

These inherited hemoglobin defects are responsible for significant morbidity and mortality worldwide, and present a vast public health problem concentrated in the populations of the Eastern Mediterranean, Middle East, parts of India, South-East Asia, Africa and the West Indies. Following the influx of immigrants from these parts of the world, obstetricians in the UK, like those in the USA, are now encountering women with genetic defects of hemoglobin seldom seen in the indigenous population.

Under normal circumstances, the carrier states for the most important of these hemoglobinopathies, beta-thalassemia and sickle cell hemoglobin, are symptomless, with no direct effect on the quality of life or life expectancy. Problems which arise during pregnancy include the following:

- With the increased stress on hemopoiesis during the prenatal period, the clinical effects of these hemoglobin defects, even in the heterozygous or carrier state, may complicate obstetric management.

- Prenatal diagnosis of a fetus at risk of a serious hemoglobin defect is now possible and such a fetus has to be identified early enough for the relevant procedures to be planned in advance (see Chapters 36 and 41).[50]

A proper appreciation of these defects requires some understanding of the structure of normal hemoglobin. The hemoglobin molecule consists of four globin chains, each of which is associated with a heme complex. There are three normal hemoglobins in man – HbA, HbA_2 and HbF – each of which contains two pairs of polypeptide globin chains. The synthesis and structure of the four globin chains – alpha, beta, gamma and delta – are under separate control and only conditions affecting the synthesis of Hba ($\alpha_2\beta_2$), which should comprise over 95% of the total circulating hemoglobin in the adult, will be of significance for the

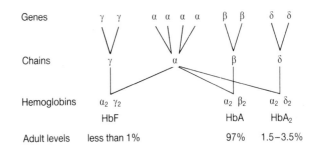

Figure 1. Genetic control of globin synthesis. The adult levels shown are those reached by 6 months of age.

mother during pregnancy. Alpha chain production is under the control of four genes, two inherited from each parent, and the alpha chains are common to all three hemoglobins. Beta chain production, on the other hand, is under the control of only two genes, one inherited from each parent (**Figure 1**).

THE THALASSEMIA SYNDROMES

The thalassemia syndromes, the most common of the genetic blood disorders, constitute a vast public health problem in many parts of the world. The basic defect, a reduced rate of globin chain synthesis, results in red cells being formed with an inadequate hemoglobin content. These syndromes are divided into two main groups, the alpha and beta thalassemias, depending on whether the alpha or beta globin chain synthesis of adult hemoglobin [HbA ($\alpha_2\beta_2$)] is depressed.

BETA-THALASSEMIA

Maternal/Fetal Risks

Thalassemia major, homozygous beta-thalassemia, was the first identified form of the thalassemia syndromes. Since the first cases were described in chldren of Greek and Italian immigrants, the disease was named thalassemia from the Greek thalassa meaning the sea or, in the classical sense, the Mediterranean. We know now that the distribution is virtually worldwide, although the defect is concentrated in a broad band which does include the Mediterranean and the Middle East. If both parents are carriers of beta-thalassemia, the newborn has a 1 in 4 chance of acquiring thalassemia major. The carrier rate in the UK is around 1 in 10 000, compared with 1 in 7 in Cyprus. There are 300–400 patients with thalassemia major in the UK today, most in the Greater London area, but there are over 100 000 babies born worldwide with the condition each year.

Before the days of regular transfusion, a child born with homozygous beta-thalassemia would die in the first few years of life from anemia, congestive cardiac failure and intercurrent infection. Where blood is freely available, survival is prolonged into the teens and early 20s, the greatest management problem being one of iron overload derived mainly from the transfused donor red cells. This results in hepatic and endocrine dysfunction, but most important of all, in myocardial damage. The cause of death is cardiac failure in the vast majority of cases. Puberty is delayed or incomplete and there has only been one case report of successful pregnancy in a truly transfusion-dependent thalassemic girl.[51] It remains to be seen how effective recently instituted intensive iron chelation programmes or future plans to use gene replacement will be. Bone marrow transplantation has been used with success, mainly in cases with histocompatible siblings.

Diagnosis and Management Options

Prepregnancy and prenatal

There are occasions when survival is possible without regular transfusion in thalassemia major, but these patients usually manifest severe bone deformities due to massive expansion of marrow tissue. Although iron loading still occurs from excessive gastrointestinal absorption, stimulated by the accelerated but ineffective marrow turnover, it is much slower than in those who are transfused, and pregnancy may occur in this situation. Extra daily folate supplements should be given but iron in any form is contraindicated. The anemia should be treated by transfusion during the prenatal period.

Perhaps the most common problem associated with the hemoglobinopathies and pregnancy is the anemia developing in the prenatal period in women who have thalassemia minor, heterozygous beta-thalassemia. They can be identified for further examination of the booking blood by observing (as in alpha-thalassemia) small, poorly hemoglobinized cells (low MCV and MCH) (**Table 1**). The level of hemoglobin at the first visit may be normal or slightly below the normal range. The diagnosis will be confirmed by finding a raised concentration of HbA_2 ($\alpha_2\delta_2$) with or without a raised HbF ($\alpha_2\gamma_2$). Excess alpha chains combine with delta and gamma chains because of the relative lack of beta chains (**Figure 1**).

Women with beta-thalassemia minor require the usual oral iron[52] and folate supplements in the prenatal period. Oral iron for a limited period will not result in significant iron loading, even in the presence of replete iron stores, but parenteral iron should never be given. A serum ferritin estimation would be advisable early in pregnancy, and if iron stores are found to be high,

iron supplements can be witheld. Many women with thalassemia minor enter pregnancy with depleted iron stores (as do many women with normal hemoglobin synthesis). To cover the requirements of ineffective erythropoiesis, folic acid 5.0 mg daily is recommended (see above). If the anemia does not respond to oral iron and folate, and intramuscular folic acid has been tried, transfusion is indicated to achieve an adequate hemoglobin for delivery at term.

Labor/delivery and postnatal

No specific management plans are indicated during these periods of pregnancy.

ALPHA-THALASSEMIA

Maternal/Fetal Risks

Alpha-thalassemia, unlike beta-thalassemia, is often but not always a gene deletion defect (**Figure 2**). There are two carrier states: α^+-thalassemia, in which there is deletion of one of the two alpha genes on chromosome 16; and α^0-thalassemia in which both genes are deleted. HbH disease is an intermediate form of alpha-thalassemia in which there is only one functional alpha gene. HbH is the name given to the unstable hemoglobin formed by tetramers of the beta chain (β_4), when there is a relative lack of alpha chains. Alpha-thalassemia major, in which there are no functional alpha genes (both parents having transmitted α^0-thalassemia), is incompatible with life and fetuses inheriting this defect usually develop hydrops and only survive a matter of hours if born alive, often prematurely. The condition is common in South-East Asia. The name HbBarts was given to tetramers of the gamma chain of fetal hemoglobin (γ_4) which forms *in utero* when no alpha chains are made (see **Figure 2**). It was first defined in a Chinese infant born at St Bartholomews Hospital, London.

Managment Options

Prepregnancy

Appropriate counseling should be offered regarding specific fetal risks for acquiring these disorders. Maternal risks, as outlined, should be discussed with the prospective parents.

Prenatal

During pregnancy, with its stress on the hemopoietic system, carriers of alpha-thalassemia, particularly those

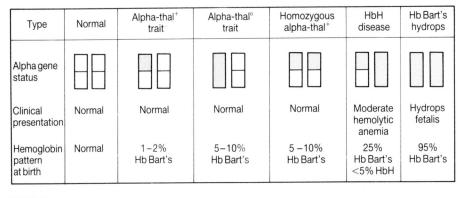

Type	Normal	Alpha-thal+ trait	Alpha-thal° trait	Homozygous alpha-thal+	HbH disease	Hb Bart's hydrops
Alpha gene status						
Clinical presentation	Normal	Normal	Normal	Normal	Moderate hemolytic anemia	Hydrops fetalis
Hemoglobin pattern at birth	Normal	1–2% Hb Bart's	5–10% Hb Bart's	5–10% Hb Bart's	25% Hb Bart's <5% HbH	95% Hb Bart's

☐ Abnormal gene

Figure 2. The alpha-thalassemias: Classification based on genotype, clinical presentation and hemoglobin pattern at birth.

THALASSEMIA SYNDROMES
Summary of Management Options (Prenatal)

BETA-THALASSEMIA

Major (pregnancy rare)

- Avoid iron

- Give folate

- Regular transfusions for anemia

- Screen partner and consider counseling and prenatal diagnosis if trait/minor

Minor/trait

- Give folate

- Oral (not parenteral) iron if low ferritin

- Transfusion for anemia

- Screen partner and consider counseling and prenatal diagnosis if trait/minor

ALPHA-THALASSEMIA

HbH disease

- Give folate

- Transfusion for severe anemia

- Screen partner and consider counseling and prenatal diagnosis if trait/minor

HbBarts hydrops

- No treatment for fetal hydrops (incompatible with life)

Minor/trait

- Iron and folate supplementation

- Screen partner and consider counseling and prenatal diagnosis if trait/minor

with α^0-thalassemia (two defective genes), may become anemic. They can be identified for further tests at their first visit by finding abnormal red cell indices (**Table 1**). They have a reduction in the size of their red cells (MCV) and the individual cell content of hemoglobin (MCH), although the mean cell hemoglobin concentration (MCHC) is usually within the normal range (**Table 1**). These changes are often minimal in α^+-thalassemia (**Figure 1**), but this condition is not so important as α^0-thalassemia in terms of maternal anemia, genetic counseling and prenatal diagnosis. Diagnosis can only be confirmed by globin chain synthesis studies or by DNA analysis of nucleated cells. Hemoglobin electrophoresis does not help make this diagnosis, because there is no abnormal hemoglobin made, nor excess or lack of one or other of the normal hemoglobins (in contrast to beta-thalassemia) (**Figure 1**). These individuals need iron and folate supplements throughout the prenatal period. Sometimes, intramuscular folic acid is helpful but parenteral iron should never be given. If the hemoglobin is not thought to be adequate for delivery at term, transfusion is indicated.

Patients with HbH disease (three defective genes) have a chronic hemolytic anemia and have 5–30% HbH in their peripheral blood. This can be identified by hemoglobin electrophoresis. They have a normal life-expectancy but require daily oral folate supplements to cover the demands of increased marrow turnover. During pregnancy, it is recommended to give women with HbH disease 5.0 mg folate daily. They will transmit either α^0- or α^+-thalassemia to their offspring.

Pregnancy with an alpha-thalassemia hydrops is associated with severe, sometimes life-threatening, pre-eclampsia (cf. severe rhesus hemolytic disease). Vaginal deliveries are associated with obstetric complications, due to the large fetus and very bulky placenta. If routine screening of the parents (see below) indicates that the mother is at risk of carrying such a child (i.e. both parents have the α^0-thalassemia trait), she should be referred, as early as possible in pregnancy, for prenatal diagnosis so that termination of an affected fetus can be carried out before these severe obstetric complications with a non-viable child develop.[53–55] Although at the present time problems arising from α^0-thalassemia are not great in the UK, they may well become more numerous if there is an influx of immigrants from Hong Kong and the Far East, which has already occurred in the USA and Australia.

Labor/delivery and postnatal

There are no specific management schemes established for these types of patients.

HEMOGLOBIN VARIANTS SICKLE CELL SYNDROMES

Over 250 structural variants of the globin chains of normal human hemoglobins have been described but the most important by far, both numerically and clinically, is sickle cell hemoglobin (HbS). This is a variant of the beta globin chain where there is one amino acid substitution at the sixth position, a glutamine replacing a valine residue. HbS has the unique physical property that, despite being a soluble protein in its oxygenated form, in its reduced state the molecules become stacked on one another, forming tactoids, which distort the red cells to the characteristic shape which gives the hemoglobin its name.

Because of their rigid structure, these sickled cells tend to block small blood vessels. The sickling phenomenon occurs particularly in conditions of lowered oxygen tension, but may also be favored by acidosis or dehydration and cooling which cause stasis in small blood vessels.

Maternal/Fetal Risks

The sickling disorders include the heterozygous state for sickle cell hemoglobin, sickle cell trait (HbAS), homozygous sickle cell disease (HbSS), compound heterozygotes of Hb variants, the most important of which is sickle cell/HbC disease (HbSC), and sickle cell/beta-thalassemia. Although these disorders are more commonly seen in Black people of African origin, they can be seen in Saudi Arabians, Indians and Mediterraneans.

The characteristic feature of HbSS is the occurrence of periods of health punctuated by periods of crises. Between 3 and 6 months of age, when normal HbA production usually becomes predominant, a chronic hemolytic anemia develops – the hemoglobin level being between 6 and 9 g/dl. Even if the hemoglobin is in the lower part of the range, symptoms due to anemia are surprisingly few because of the low affinity of HbS for oxygen, which facilitates oxygen delivery to the tissues. The acute episodes due to intravascular sickling are of far greater practical importance, since they cause vascular occlusion resulting in tissue infarction. The affected part is painful and the clinical manifestations are extremely variable, depending on the site at which sickling takes place. Sickling crises are often precipitated by infection and may be exacerbated by any accompanying dehydration. Most deaths are due to massive sickling following an acute infection and to pulmonary embolus which has even been reported with heterozygotes.[56] Renal complications are a constant finding; there is a progressive inability to concentrate urine, subtle protein and potassium secreting defects, and hematuria is common. These deficits result from sickling in the renal medullary circulation. An inability to concentrate the urine adequately makes pregnant women with the sickling disorders unduly prone to dehydration during labor. Also, perhaps due to the anti-aldosterone actions of progesterone, hypercalcemia has been reported in pregnant women with sickle cell disease at levels of renal dysfunction below that observed in non-gravid individuals with SS disease.[57]

The overall prognosis of HbSS depends greatly on the environment: in Africa, a large proportion of children with this disorder die within the first 5 years and probably less than 10% reach adulthood. In the West Indies, however, where prompt treatment and prophylaxis of infection is more easily available, many women with sickle cell disease need management during pregnancy.[58]

Sickle cell hemoglobin C disease (HbSC) is a milder variant of HbSS with normal or near normal levels of hemoglobin. One of the dangers of this condition is that, owing to its mildness, neither the women nor her obstetrician may be aware of its presence. These women are at risk of massive, sometimes fatal, sickling crises during pregnancy and particularly in the puerperium. It is therefore vital that the abnormality is detected, preferably before pregnancy, so that the appropriate precautions can be taken.

Clinical manifestations of the doubly heterozygous condition, sickle cell beta-thalassemia, are usually indistinguishable from HbSS; those who make detectable amounts of HbA are usually less severely affected but still at risk from sickling crises during pregnancy. Sickle cell trait (HbAS) results in no detectable abnormality under normal circumstances, although it is easily diagnosed by specific investigations including hemoglobin electrophoresis (see below). Affected subjects are not anemic even under the additional stress of pregnancy, unless there are additional complications, and sickling crises occur only in situations of extreme anoxia, dehydration and acidosis.

Women with sickle cell disease present special problems in pregnancy.[59,60] Fetal loss is high, which is thought to be due to both impaired oxygen supply and sickling infarcts in the placental circulation.[59] Miscarriage, preterm labor and other complications are more common than in women with normal hemoglobin.[61,62]

Management Options

Prepregnancy

Prepregnancy management can be divided into two basic areas. The first is the optimization of the mother's health status. This relates to the recognized symptomatic complications associated with many of the sickle cell syndromes. In particular, a complete evaluation of renal status is indicated for prognostic as well as therapeutic purposes. The second area relates to counseling for the potential risk of the fetus having a similar condition. This involves both parents and may necessitate several rapid diagnostic screening studies (see below).

Prenatal

At present, there is no effective long-term method of reducing the liability of red cells to sickle *in vivo*. Once a crisis is established, there is no evidence that alkalis, hyperbaric oxygen, vasodilator, plasma expanders, urea or anticoagulants are of any value. Where beneficial effects have been reported, they can usually be attributed to the meticulous care and supportive therapy received by the patient, rather than to the specific measures themselves. Adequate fluid administration alone probably accounts for the benefit. Patients' response to pregnancy varies, and therefore there should not be 'blanket' recommendations for all patients with sickle cell disease.

Many women with sickle cell disease have no complications, although the outcome in any individual case is always in doubt. The only consistently successful way of reducing the incidence of complications due to sickling is by regular blood transfusion at approximately 6-week intervals, to maintain the proportion of HbA at 60–70% of the total. Between 3 and 4 units of blood are given at each transfusion. This regime has two effects: it dilutes the circulating sickle hemoglobin and, by raising the hemoglobin, reduces the stimulus to the bone marrow and therefore the amount of sickle hemoglobin produced. However, the trade-off of such a regime includes alloimmunization[63] and all the other problems of transfusion, including hepatitis and HIV transmission. Sickle cells have a shorter life-span than normal red cells and so the effect of each successive transfusion is more beneficial.

The management of the sickle cell syndromes in pregnancy in the UK is a relatively recent problem and longitudinal data are lacking. It is clear on review of the extensive American literature that although risks remain higher for pregnancy complicated by sickle cell disease, modern obstetric care alone, without transfusion, has reduced the maternal morbidity and mortality dramatically and also improved fetal outcome. Increasing numbers of obstetric centers have adopted prophylactic transfusion regimes, but the real benefit of such regimes remains to be proven by a large trial with contemporary controls.[64] At the time of writing, one such trial is in progress in the UK, while a smaller multicenter trial in the USA suggests that outcome is similar in women transfused prophylactically compared to those transfused only when indications arise.[65]

One of the most worrying complications of transfusion of SS patients has been the development of atypical red cell antibodies, resulting from the fact that the donor population differs in ethnic origin from the recipients and carries different minor red cell antigens. This has resulted in extreme difficulties in finding compatible blood,[63,64] and even in hemolytic disease of the newborn.[60] The general consensus from the USA in 1989, based on the results of one multicenter randomly controlled trial, is that it is wiser to give close obstetric supervision, and deliver women where there are special care baby units available. Transfusion should only be given in preparation for general anesthetic or where there is evidence of maternal distress.[59,60] If the disorder presents late in pregnancy and there is more urgency because, for instance, the woman is profoundly anemic or is suffering a crisis, exchange transfusion can be used.

Standard exchange transfusion regimes for sickle cell disease have been used with success in a large number of pregnant patients. It is obvious that it would be far better to prevent the emergency situation during pregnancy by identification of women before pregnancy and early booking for prenatal care. However, even after preparation with regular transfusion, tissue hypoxia, acidosis and dehydration should be avoided because they will make the patient's own remaining red cells more likely to sickle. Tourniquets should not be used.

The single most important pregnancy precaution is for the woman's partner to be screened, so that the couple can be advised of the risk of a serious hemoglobin defect in their offspring. Screening procedures vary from location to location[66] and often only involve 'high-risk' populations. **Figure 3** shows a scheme used at Queen Charlotte's Maternity Hospital, London, which serves a cosmopolitan population. This involves examination of red cell indices (**Table 1**), hemoglobin electrophoresis and, where indicated, quantitation of HbA_2 and HbF on every sample of blood taken at the first visit (**Figure 1**). If a hemoglobin variant or thalassemia is found, the partner is requested to attend so that his blood can also be examined. By this means, the chances of a serious hemoglobin defect in the fetus will be assessed early in pregnancy, allowing counseling of the parents, and the chance to offer them a prenatal diagnosis by fetal blood sampling or transabdominal chorionicvillis sampling, even though it will result in a later termination of pregnancy, if indicated and desired (see Chapter 60).

Additional regular screening should be implemented for urinary infection, hypertension/pre-eclampsia, abnormal renal or liver function and pathological fetal growth.

Labor/delivery

The worry concerning aspiration pneumonitis, hypoxia and other perioperative pulmonary problems, may be

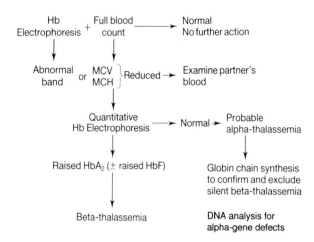

Figure 3. Screening for hemoglobinopathies.

avoided by using regional anesthesia but substitutes the risk of hypotension and venous pooling in the vessels of the lower extremities. These can be reduced by wrapping the legs in elastic bandages and elevation. Although a number of sicklers have been reported in the obstetric literature to have suffered pulmonary emboli,[56,67] there is no good evidence to incriminate regional anesthesia as a significant additional risk factor and indeed there are good physiological data to support it having a protective role. In an emergency, both regional and general anesthesia may have to be undertaken without ideal preparation. Good communication and cooperation between the anesthetist, obstetrician and hematologist, together with meticulous postoperative care, are essential for a successful outcome. Again, as with the controversy over blood transfusion,[68] it is a simple lack of awareness of potential problems and relaxation of vigilance which change the story rather than lack of knowledge or the details of the measures adopted to deal with the many and varied hazards of sickle hemoglobin in pregnancy.[69]

No special preparation with blood transfusion is required in pregnancy for women with sickle cell trait (HbAS). However, as in patients with HbSS, it is essential that hypoxia and dehydration are avoided during anesthesia and labor, particularly in the immediate post-delivery period. In fact, the majority of unexpected deaths associated with HbS have occurred in patients with sickle cell trait in the immediate postoperative or postpartum period.[70]

The main principles of management of labor are to avoid dehydration, sepsis, acidosis, hypoxia or a prolonged labor. Continuous fetal heart rate monitoring is mandatory.

SICKLE CELL SYNDROMES
Summary of Management Options

Prepregnancy

- Counsel against conception until disease status optimized; assess renal and liver function

- Avoid intrauterine contraceptive devices

- Counsel about risks of pregnancy

- Screen partner and if trait or positive counsel regarding prenatal diagnosis

Prenatal

- Hb electrophoresis screening of whole population or high-risk groups (depends on prevalence)

- Screen partner and consider counseling and prenatal diagnosis if trait/disease

- Regular transfusions to keep Hb at 9–12 g/dl with 60–70% HbA but complications exceed benefits

- Prompt treatment of crises (adequate hydration, oxygen, screen for infection) may include exchange transfusion

- Prenatal fetal surveillance and tests for fetal well being

- Screen for
  - urinary infection
  - hypertension/pre-eclampsia
  - renal and liver function
  - pathological fetal growth

Labor/delivery

- Ensure adequate hydration

- Avoid hypoxia (? additional oxygen)

- Continuous cardiotocography (CTG)

Postnatal

- Use of prophylactic antibiotics is controversial

- Maintain good hydration and oxygenation especially for first 24 h

- Contraceptive counseling; avoid IUDs

Postnatal

There is much more longitudinal experience in the USA than there is as yet in the UK. The methods of contraception vary,[71] but problems arise from the assumption that sicklers are at increased risk of thromboembolism if they use oral contraception. The patient's risk is less than that of pregnancy and there are almost no data to suggest that patients with sickle cell disease run a greater risk than any other patients using low-estrogen preparations.[59] The usual contraindications hold true and patients should be monitored meticulously for alterations in blood pressure and liver function.

THROMBOCYTOPENIA

Platelets play an integral part in the homeostasis of thrombosis and coagulation interrelating with the coagulation cascade and the vessel wall. The most common abnormality encountered in platelet pathophysiology is reduction in number, thrombocytopenia, to below 150×10^9 per liter.

With the advent of automatic cell counters in hematology laboratories, it has become apparent that incidental thrombocytopenia during pregnancy is relatively common. In addition to incidental thrombocytopenia, there are a number of clinically significant thrombocytopenic disorders which may have adverse effects on the mother and fetus. It is necessary to distinguish between those conditions which are important clinically and those which will have no bearing on pregnancy outcome. The clinically relevant conditions include those that are specific to pregnancy and those that are coincidental to pregnancy. Both may have relevance to outcome. The management and outcome of the pregnancy for mother and fetus varies with the etiology and it is therefore imperative to distinguish the various types of thrombocytopenia to prevent inappropriate intervention.

In normal pregnancy, the platelet count tends to fall progressively but usually remains within the normal range.[72] This phenomenon is exaggerated in patients developing pre-eclampsia, in whom the count may fall below the lower limit of normal[73] and is discussed in Chapter 18. Similarly, thrombocytopenia may be seen in the HELLP syndrome (Hemolysis, Elevated Liver enzymes and Low Platelets), which is arguably part of the spectrum of pre-eclampisa (see Chapter 8). Low platelets may be seen in pregnant women as a consequence of a severe megaloblastic picture due to folic acid deficiency in association with low white cell counts and macrocytosis.

Disseminated intravascular coagulation (DIC) is another cause of thrombocytopenia seen in pregnancy[74] and is always a secondary phenomenon. It may compli-cate placental abruption, amniotic fluid embolism and prolonged retention of a dead fetus. The widespread precipitation of fibrin through activation of the coagulation cascade leads to depletion of the coagulation factors, platelets and of the fibrinolytic system. This results in a generalized bleeding tendency[75] and sometimes microangiopathic hemolytic anemia. The secondary phenomenon of DIC will be dealt with elsewhere in this volume under the appropriate clinical headings and in Chapter 73.

This section will address incidental thrombocytopenia, immune causes of thrombocytopenia and aspects of other acquired causes of thrombocytopenia.

INCIDENTAL THROMBOCYTOPENIA

Maternal/Fetal Risks

In one study carried out over 1 year, 8.3% of 1357 consecutive normal pregnant women were found to be thrombocytopenic at the time of delivery with platelet counts between $97 - 150 \times 10^9$ per liter.[76] The extension of this study over a 3-year period confirmed that 7.6% of 6715 consecutive women had thrombocytopenia at delivery.[76] Approximately 5% (two-thirds of the total with thrombocytopenia) had no history of immune thrombocytopenia or associated conditions such as pre-eclampsia.

In the first study, there were no adverse effects on any of the mother and infant pairs. In the extended study conducted over 3 years, the rate of neonatal thrombocytopenia in infants born to healthy women with incidental thrombocytopenia was 4%, which was the same frequency as seen in the infants of a control group of mothers who did not have thrombocytopenia. None of the infants born to healthy mothers with thrombocytopenia had a cord platelet count less than 50×10^9 per liter and none had clinical bleeding. Of the 334 women in this group, 17 had platelet counts less than 100×10^9 per liter of which the lowest was 43×10^9 per liter. The infants of all of these women had normal platelet counts (greater than 150×10^9 per liter), except for one who had a count of 136×10^9 per liter. All the maternal platelet counts returned to normal by 7 days postpartum.

Management Options

Prepregnancy

By definition, this is a condition which is identified during pregnancy, making management decisions prior to pregnancy non-applicable. However, in a patient presenting preconceptually with a history of thrombocytopenia during an earlier pregnancy, a careful review should be made of the medical evaluation in that pregnancy. If the patient is currently without significant chemical or laboratory findings and there is no evidence of a pathological cause for the thrombocytopenia, reassurances can be provided for the planned pregnancy.

Prenatal

No specific management recommendations have been established for incidental thrombocytopenia except that an adequate diagnostic evaluation be completed to exclude pathological causes. There appears to be no rationale for the empiric administration of pharmacologic agents in an attempt to increase the platelet count.

Labor/delivery

From the previously cited studies, it was concluded that for healthy women with platelet counts over 80×10^9 per liter, no treatment was required and that the mode of delivery should be determined by obstetric indications only. Many of the patients received epidural anesthesia. Another recent publication suggests that with platelet counts of 80×10^9 per liter and over, there is no increased hazard of bleeding associated with epidural anesthesia.[77] A similar conclusion was reached in a retrospective study carried out over 11 years of 162 women who were found to be thrombocytopenic in pregnancy. Of these, 74 had no preceding history of immune thrombocytopenia and none of their infants had severe thrombocytopenia, i.e. counts below 50×10^9 per liter. However, it must be noted that one group studying incidental thrombocytopenia of pregnancy found that 4 of 31 fetuses were thrombocytopenic at term and one of these had a platelet count of only 35×10^9 per liter.[78]

On the basis of these studies, it has been suggested that vaginal delivery without drug or diagnostic intervention should be standard for pregnant women with non-symptomatic thrombocytopenia based on obstetric criteria.[79,80] This reverses the trend toward aggressive intervention which followed the development of techniques for obtaining fetal blood samples and the concept that all fetuses at risk of thrombocytopenia should be delivered by cesarean section.

Invasive intervention, particularly with fetal blood sampling, seems to have been generally incorporated into management strategies because of the poor fetal outcome in older retrospective analyses (see below) which may have included cases of allo-immune thrombocytopenia. In this condition, which is analogous to anti-rhesus D-allo-immune hemolytic disease, the mother forms antibodies to paternally derived fetal platelet antigens which she lacks. The fetal consequences of allo-immune thrombocytopenia may be devastating. However, it is unusual to see fetal bleeding resulting from auto-immune thrombocytopenia in the mother. Confusion between the consequences of allo-immune *vs* auto-immune thrombocytopenia seems to have had an effect on the management of other types of fetal thrombocytopenia (see also Chapter 46).

Postnatal

Serial assessments of both the maternal and neonatal platelet counts seems appropriate, with the anticipation of a gradual shift toward normalization of these values.

CLINICO-PATHOLOGICAL THROMBOCYTOPENIA

The pathological causes of thrombocytopenia have been well reviewed[160,161] and may be classified as follows:

- Increased comsumption/destruction:
  — removal of platelets by immune processes (e.g. auto-immune thrombocytopenic purpura)
  — activation of coagulation (e.g. DIC: see Chapter 73)
  — formation of platelet thrombi (e.g. thrombotic thrombocytopenic purpura; hemolytic uremic syndrome)
  — mechanical destruction (e.g. hypersplenism)

- Decreased production (e.g. marrow aplasia; malignant infiltration)

AUTO-IMMUNE THROMBOCYTOPENIC PURPURA (see also Chapter 46)

Maternal/Fetal Risks

Auto-immune thrombocytopenic purpura (AITP) occurs in two main forms: the acute, self-limiting type that is most common in children following a prodromal viral ilness and a chronic form usually found in adults. AITP is common in women of child-bearing age and has been found to have an incidence of 1–2 per 10 000 pregnancies.[81] Cases may present with skin bruising, and platelet counts between $30–80 \times 10^9$ per liter, but it is rare to see severe bleeding associated with low platelet counts in the chronic form.

With the screening of pregnant women,[83] very mild thrombocytopenia, as described above, may be discovered as an incidental finding and is not associated with risk to the mother or infant.[83,84] It may be that this incidental thrombocytopenia represents a very mild AITP, but as it is not associated with adverse effects it must be distinguished from cases of AITP in pregnancy resulting in infants affected with severe thrombocytopenia and intracranial hemorrhage.[85–90] There are no serological tests or clinical guidelines which will reliably predict the hazard of thrombocytopenia in any individual fetus and the correlation between maternal and neonatal platelet counts is poor.[85,88] It has been assumed that cesarean section delivery is less traumatic to the fetus than vaginal delivery and while that premise could be debated,[91] recognizing and investigating the minority of pregnancies at risk of significant fetal thrombocytopenia would void many unnecessary fetal blood samples and cesarean sections.

There have been a number of analyses of outcome of cases of maternal AITP from the 1950s onwards. Their findings may not be entirely applicable to current management because some of the documented poor fetal outcomes may have been associated with unrecognized maternal lupus, pre-eclampsia or allo-immune thrombocytopenia. Only symptomatic women and neonates were investigated because there was no general screening of the platelet count in healthy women. This resulted in an exaggerated incidence of both neonatal thrombocytopenia and the morbidity and mortality arising from it.

AITP is a diagnosis of exclusion with peripheral thrombocytopenia and normal or increased megakaryocytes in the bone marrow and the documented absence of other diseases. The red and white cells are essentially normal unless there is secondary anemia. AITP requires the exclusion of SLE, lupus anticoagulant and anti-cardiolipin antibody as they may co-exist with thrombocytopenia. The majority of thrombocytopenic patients are asymptomatic and tests to estimate the bleeding risk in these patients would obviously be helpful.

In chronic platelet consumption disorders, a population of younger larger platelets is established which have enhanced function. Measurement of the mean platelet volume (MPV) or, if this is not available, an examination of the stained blood film, will detect the presence of these large platelets. The risk of bleeding for any given platelet count is less in those patients with younger large platelets. The bleeding time which has recently been severely criticized[90] as a predictor of bleeding at surgery still has a place in this context according to some respected workers.[79] A bleeding time of greater than 15 min indicates a greater risk than in those with a normal bleeding time.

The mechanism of immune destruction of platelets has been shown to be due to auto-antibodies directed against platelet surface antigens. This has special relevance in pregnancy because the placenta has receptors for the constant fragment (Fc) and the IgG immunoglobulin molecule facilitating active transport of immunoglobulin across the placenta to the fetal circulation. The immunoglobulin passage increases with advancing pregnancy[92,93] and may result in fetal thrombocytopenia.

The role of circulating globulin in the pathogenesis of immune thrombocytopenia was first documented in the 1950s.[94,95] However, platelet antibody on the platelet membrane and in the plasma, demonstrated by tests analogous to the direct and indirect Coombs' tests on red cells, have been slow to enter the repertoire of routine hematological laboratories because they have been fraught with technological difficulties, such as the intrinsic reactivity of platelets and the presence of some platelet-associated immunoglobulin in normal individuals.

Antibody from some cases of AITP demonstrates a specificity for the platelet glycoprotein IIb/IIIa[96,97] or for glycoprotein Ib.[98] In one study, the minority of cases of AITP demonstrating this specificity fared less well in their responses to splenectomy.[99] Other specificities of the antibody in chronic AITP have been documented showing variation between patients.[100] While some cases of AITP have normal or increased amounts of immunoglobulin on the platelets or in the plasma,[101–103] 10–35% of patients have no demonstrable platelet-associated IgG (PAIgG). In one study, 57% of patients had raised PAIgG and PAIgM, while 90% had raised PAIgG or PAIgM alone. All patients with PAIgG greater than four times the normal also had raised PAIgM.[104] The presence of IgG rather than IgM antibodies has relevance to the pregnant patient because only IgG antibodies can be transported across the placenta and cause thrombocytopenia in the fetus.

In the study of 162 consecutive pregnant patients with platelet counts of less than 150×10^9 per liter gathered over 11 years, the absence of circulating IgG antiplatelet antibody at term, despite a history of thrombocytopenic purpura, was associated with minimal risk of thrombocytopenia in the fetus.[85] However, no currently available serological test can be used to reliably predict thrombocytopenia in the fetus.[105]

The absence of a history of AITP prior to the index pregnancy is an indicator of low risk for neonatal thrombocytopenia. In contrast, 18 neonates who were born with platelet counts of less than 50×10^9 per liter, out of a total of 178, were all born to mothers with a history of AITP prior to pregnancy. In addition, 40% of mothers with a preceding history delivered infants with platelet counts below 100×10^9 per liter. Of 162 infants delivered in the index pregnancy, ten had bleeding complications, of which five were serious. Intracranial hemorrhage in infants born to women with a prior history of AITP and delivered vaginally numbered two out of 17, while there were no cases of intra-cranial hemorrhage in women with similar histories who were delivered by cesarean section.[85] A more recent review of the literature of AITP in pregnancy[79] shows a neonatal mortality rate of 6 per 1000 AITP patients, about the same or better than the overall per-inatal mortality rate. All the deaths occurred in babies delivered by cesarean section and all events appeared more than 24–48 h after delivery, the time of the plate-let count nadir in the neonate. Thus it is not clear whether cesarean section protects the baby from intra-cranial hemorrhage.[91]

Management Options

The management of pregnancy in AITP is directed at three aspects: prenatal care of the mother, management of the mother and fetus during delivery; and manage-ment of the neonate from the time of delivery.

Prepregnancy

No firm data are available to assist the clinician in counseling AITP patients who desire pregnancy as to prognosis. Given the apparent fluctuations in the nature of this disease process, a poor outcome previously does not always suggest repetitive poor outcomes. Con-versely, a prior successful pregnancy does not imply a no-risk situation. The current state of the disease and prior therapies should be taken into account when assessing pregnancy risk (see below).

Prenatal

The most important decision to make is whether the woman needs any treatment at all. Many patients have significant thrombocytopenia (platelet count less than 100×10^9 per liter), but no evidence of an *in vivo* hemostatic disorder. In general, the platelet count must be less than 50×10^9 per liter for capillary bleeding and purpura to occur.

There is no need to treat any asymptomatic women with mild-to-moderate thrombocytopenia (count above 50×10^9 per liter) and a normal bleeding time. How-ever, the maternal platelet count should be monitored regularly and signs of hemostatic impairment looked for. The platelet count will show a downward trend during pregnancy with a nadir in the third trimester and active treatment may have to be instituted to achieve a safe hemostatic concentration of platelets for delivery at term. The incidence of antepartum hemorrhage is not increased in maternal AITP, but there is a small

increased risk of postpartum hemorrhagic compli-cations not from the placental bed but from surgical incisions such as episiotomy and from soft tissue lacer-ations.

Intervention in the prenatal period is based on clini-cal manifestations of thrombocytopenia. The woman with bruising or petechiae requires measures to raise the platelet count, but the woman with mucous mem-brane bleeding which may be life-threatening requires urgent treatment with platelet transfusions and i.v. IgG, (see below) and occasionally emergency splenectomy.

The real dilemma in the pregnant woman with AITP is that nearly all patients have chronic disease. The long-term effects of treatment which is happily embarked on outside pregnancy have to be considered in the light of the possible complications on the pro-gress of pregnancy in the mother and of any effects on the fetus. The hazard for the mother who is monitored carefully and where appropriate measures have been taken is negligible, but most of her management is ori-ented toward what are thought to be optimal conditions for the delivery of the fetus, who in turn may or may not be thrombocytopenic (see below).

Corticosteroids

Corticosteroids are a satisfactory short-term therapy but are unacceptable as long-term support unless the maintenance dose is very small (e.g. 5–10 mg daily).[106,107] Side-effects for the mother include weight gain, subcutaneous fat redistribution, acne and hyper-tension, which are undesirable during pregnancy. In addition, the prevalence of pre-eclampsia, gestational diabetes, postpartum psychosis and osteoporosis are all increased with the use of corticosteroids. Nevertheless, they are often used, but should be reserved as short-term therapy for patients with obvious risk of bleeding or to raise the platelet count of an asymptomatic woman at term allowing her to have epidural or spinal analgesia for delivery if desired or indicated.

A suggestion in the older literature of an association between steroid administration and cleft lip or palate has been refuted by more recent studies. Suppression of fetal adrenal glands is a theoretical hazard, but approximately 90% of a dose of prednisolone or hydro-cortisone is metabolized in the placenta and never reaches the fetus.[108] This is in contrast to dexame-thasone and betamethasone, which cross the placenta freely. It has been suggested[109] that high doses of corticosteroids given to elevate platelet counts at or near term should be avoided, since they may increase the transplacental passage of IgG antibody and thus expose the fetus to greater risk of severe thrombocyto-penia.[87] In our experience, this is a theoretical hazard not seen in practice.

Intravenous IgG

Intravenous IgG has altered the management options for AITP dramatically. It is known that intravenous administration of monomeric polyvalent human IgG in doses greater than those produced endogenously prolongs the clearance time of immune complexes by the reticulo-endothelial system. It is thought that such a prolongation of clearance of IgG-coated platelets in AITP results in an increase in the number of circulating platelets, but the mechanism is as yet unknown.[110] Used in the original recommended doses of 0.4 g/kg for 5 days by i.v. infusion, a persistent and predictable response was obtained in more than 80% of reported cases. More recently, alternative dosage regimens of this very expensive treatment have been suggested, which are just as effective, but easier to manage and which use less total immunoglobulin.[79] A typical dose is 1 g/kg over 8 h on one day. This dose will raise the platelet count to normal or safe levels in approximately half of the patients. In those in whom the platelet count does not rise, a similar dose can be repeated 2 days later. The advantages of this treatment are that it is safe, has very few side-effects and the response to therapy is more rapid than with corticosteroids. The response usually occurs within 48 h and is maintained for 2–3 weeks. The main disadvantage is that it is very expensive and seldom produces a long-term cure of the AITP.

It has been suggested that IgG given intravenously can cross the placenta and should provoke an identical response in the fetus[111] at risk, but this has never been proved. Indeed, an analysis of the more recent literature indicates that the postulated transplacental effect is unreliable[92,93] and that exogenous IgG may not cross the placenta.[112] The use of IgG has been recommended[109,113] in all pregnant patients with platelet counts of less than 75×10^9 per liter regardless of history or symptoms. There is no doubt about the value of IgG in selected case of severe symptomatic thrombocytopenia where a rapid response is required but its indiscriminate use in all cases with significant thrombocytopenia would have to be shown to improve dramatically both maternal and fetal outcome to justify the high cost.

Splenectomy

Splenectomy will produce a cure or long-term drug-free remission in 60–80% of all patients with AITP. This is because the main site of antibody production is often the spleen and because many of the IgG-coated platelets are sequestered there. All patients should receive pneumovax before splenectomy and twice daily oral penicillin for life following surgery to protect against pneumococcal infection. Reviews of the management of AITP have associated splenectomy during

pregnancy with high fetal loss rates [114] and even an approximate 10% maternal mortality rate in the past,[115] but modern supportive measures and improved surgical practices have reduced the fetal loss rate considerably and the risk of maternal mortality is negligible.[107] In current practice, splenectomy is hardly ever indicated in the pregnant patient and should be avoided given the success of medical management. However, removal of the spleen remains an option if all other attempts to increase the platelet count fail. Splenectomy should be performed in the second trimester because surgery is best tolerated then and the size of the uterus will not make the operation technically difficult. The platelet count should be raised to safe levels for surgery if possible by i.v. IgG. Although transfused platelets will have a short life in the maternal circulation, they may help to achieve hemostasis at surgery. Platelet concentrates should be available but given only if abnormal bleeding occurs.

Other medications

Other medications have been used in AITP but most of them are contraindicated in pregnancy and only have moderate success rates. Danazol, an attenuated anabolic steroid, has been used with moderate success in a few patients. Vincristine has a transient beneficial effect in many patients, but it is not recommended in pregnancy and long-term associated neurotoxicity limits its usefulness.

Very occasionally, immunosuppressives such as azothiaprine and cyclophosphamide have to be used in severe intractable thrombocytopenia which does not respond to any other measures. Cyclophosphamide should be avoided in pregnancy. However, experience with relatively low doses of azothiaprine in the increasing number of transplant patients who have now negotiated a subsequent pregnancy suggests that this drug is not associated with increased fetal or maternal morbidity. The most contentious issue in the management of AITP in pregnancy is the mode of delivery given that the fetus may also be thrombocytopenic and may bleed from trauma during birth.

Assessment of the fetal platelet count

Assessment of the fetal platelet count was suggested by Hegde,[109] who analysed the reported cases in the literature from 1950 to 1983, which suggested an overall incidence of neonatal thrombocytopenia of 52% with significant morbidity in 12% of births. The incidence increased to 70% of deliveries if maternal platelet count was less than 100×10^9 per liter at term. The probability of fetal thrombocytopenia increased with the severity of maternal thrombocytopenia. As a result of this and other analyses, many strategies were developed to predict the fetal platelet count and to determine the optimal mode of delivery, since it was believed that elective cesarean section was the best option for an affected fetus at risk from trauma during a vaginal delivery.

We know now that the incidence in these retrospective analyses was distorted because only symptomatic women were likely to have been investigated and reported (see above). A recent report[85] studied the outcome of 162 consecutive pregnancies in women with presumed AITP presenting in the decade 1979–89. The overall incidence of thrombocytopenia (11.0%) in the offspring of these women was much lower than the earlier reported analyses, but two important factors emerged in predicting neonatal thrombocytopenia. In the absence of a history of AITP before pregnancy or in the absence of circulating platelet IgG antibodies in the index pregnancy in those with a history, the risk of severe thrombocytopenia in the fetus at term was negligible.

These findings are supported by another recent report[116] of 61 infants born to 50 mothers with confirmed AITP. Only three (4.9%) had a cord platelet count $<50 \times 10^9$ per liter. None of the infants had morbidity or mortality as a result of the thrombocytopenia. Two-thirds of the infants had a further fall in platelet count in the first 2–3 days after birth, but in all of them the thrombocytopenia could easily be corrected. Some investigators have suggested that maternal splenectomy increases the probability of neonatal thrombocytopenia.[114,117] Closer scrutiny of published reports[80] shows that this is only in those women with splenectomy and persistent thrombocytopenia (less than 100×10^9 per liter) that the risk of neonatal thrombocytopenia is increased. What has become clear over the years is that analysis of the older literature gives an exaggerated incidence of neonatal thrombocytopenia and of the morbidity and mortality arising from it. However, even with the benefit of accurate automated, easily repeated platelet counts, estimation of IgG platelet antibodies and taking into consideration splenectomy status, it is still impossible to predict the fetal platelet count in any individual case[118] and to plan the mode of delivery based on these maternal parameters is not logical or sensible.

Fetal blood sampling

Fetal blood sampling was thus suggested as the best way of determining fetal risk. A method for direct measurement of the fetal platelet count in scalp blood obtained transcervically prior to or early in labor has been described.[119–121] These authors recommend that cesarean section be performed in all cases where the fetal platelet count is less than 50×10^9 per liter. This approach is more logical than a decision about the mode of delivery made on the basis of maternal platelet count, concentration of IgG or splenectomy status, but

it is not without risk of significant hemorrhage in the truly thrombocytopenic fetus, often gives false positive results[79] and demands urgent action to be taken on the results. Also, the cervix must be sufficiently dilated to allow the fetal scalp to be sampled and the uterine contraction that is needed to achieve this may cause the fetus to descend so far in the birth canal that cesarean section is technically difficult and also traumatic for the fetus.

The only way a reliable fetal platelet count can be obtained so that a decision concerning the optimal mode of delivery can be taken is by a percutaneous transabdominal fetal cord blood sample taken before term.[122–124] This gives time for discussion between the obstetrician, pediatrician, hematologist and anesthetist. It can be performed at 37–38 weeks gestation under ultrasound guidance as the transfer of IgG increases in the last weeks of pregnancy and an earlier sample may give a higher fetal platelet count than one taken nearer term.

The risk of fetal loss associated with the sampling has been claimed to be as low as 1%.[122,123] Sometimes if a free loop of cord is entered, the vessels go into spasm and a cesarean section is precipitated because of fetal distress even if the platelet count proves to be normal. This is another good reason for performing an FBS as late as possible in gestation if it is thought to be justified. There is no point in performing serial fetal platelet counts from earlier in gestation because the fetus is not at risk from spontaneous hemorrhage before labor. Given the low risk of identifying a problem and the risk of associated complications *in utero*, fetal blood sampling cannot be justified in all AITP pregnancies and some would argue that, if there is no convincing evidence to demonstrate that cesarean section is of benefit, then fetal blood sampling with its inherent risks is not justified at all.[91]

Labor/delivery

There is little risk to the mother whatever the mode of delivery. In most cases, the maternal platelet count can be raised to hemostatic levels to cover the event. Even if the mother has to deliver in the face of a low platelet count, she is unlikely to bleed from the placental site once the uterus is empty, but she is at risk of bleeding from any surgical incisions, soft tissue injuries or tears. Platelets should be available but not given prophylactically. It should be remembered that the unnecessary transfusion of platelet concentrates in the absence of hemostatic failure may stimulate more auto-antibody formation synthesis and thus increase maternal thrombocytopenia. Most anesthetists require that the platelet count is at least 80×10^9 per liter and preferably over 100×10^9 per liter before they will administer an epidural anesthetic, but there is no good evidence that counts above 50×10^9 per liter are not sufficient to achieve hemostasis in AITP.[77]

The major risk at delivery is to the fetus with thrombocytopenia who as the result of birth trauma may suffer intracranial hemorrhage. If there is any question that a vaginal delivery will be difficult or traumatic, then elective cesarean section should be carried out.

For many centres the availability of planned or emergency transabdominal fetal blood sampling is severely limited or non-existent and so decisions concerning the mode of delivery will have to be taken without knowing the fetal platelet count. As discussed earlier, maternal platelet count, maternal platelet associated IgG, history and splenectomy status show trends regarding the incidence of fetal and neonatal thrombocytopenia but can never be used to predict fetal thrombocytopenia with absolute confidence in an individual case. It does appear, however, that it is very unlikely for the fetus to have severe thrombocytopenia if the mother has no previous history of AITP before the index pregnancy and if she has no detectable free IgG platelet antibody.[85]

Many of the options proposed in the literature presuppose that cesarean section is less traumatic than an uncomplicated vaginal delivery. There is no objective evidence to support this contention and there are undesirable associated complications of cesarean section *per se* for both mother and fetus.[91] The only advantage is that there is more overall control of the delivery if it is by elective cesarean section and there are usually no unpredictable complications.

Based on an estimate of a 12.7–21% perinatal mortality associated with AITP, it was proposed[125] that all patients should be delivered by cesarean section. The mortality rate quoted is a gross overestimate probably because of the selection of severe symptomatic cases for the analysis. A recent review of the literature of AITP in pregnancy shows a neonatal mortality rate of 6 per 1000 AITP patients,[79] about the same as or better than the overall perinatal mortality rate. All these deaths occurred in babies delivered by cesarean section and all events appeared more than 24–48 h after delivery, the time of the platelet count nadir in the neonate. The incidence of severe thrombocytopenia in the fetus of a woman with proven AITP is no more than 10%. Even if cesarean section is the optimum mode of delivery for the thrombocytopenic fetus, this does not justify this mode of delivery for the nine out of ten fetuses without thrombocytopenia.

Because the risk of severe fetal thrombocytopenia at term (platelet count less than 50×10^9 per liter) is not more than 5% and the maximum neonatal risk period is 2–3 days after delivery, and because the reduction in neonatal morbidity and mortality by prophylactic cesarean section has yet to be established, delivery by cesarean section should be reserved for those cases

with obstetric indications and should not be based on the presence of maternal AITP alone.

It is not now thought to be optimum management to deliver all fetuses with potential or identified thrombocytopenia by cesarean section. If delivery by cesarean section is indicated for obstetric reasons, there is no point in fetal blood sampling to obtain the platelet count and elective cesarean section should be performed. In our hospital, there is considerable expertise in intrauterine fetal blood sampling, but we only recommend this procedure:

- where the women enters pregnancy with a history of AITP together with currently identifiable platelet-associated IgG antibodies, or

- in those women who have to be treated for AITP during the index pregnancy.

Our obstetricians, like many others, prefer to deliver a fetus with significant thrombocytopenia (platelet count $< 50 \times 10^9$ per liter) by cesarean section. However it should be stressed that the above approach is arbitrary and not based on controlled data. Individual units may require different policies, depending on local expertise and practice.

Postnatal

An immediate cord platelet count should be performed following delivery in all neonates of mothers with AITP whenever or however diagnosed. The vast majority of babies will have platelet counts well above 50×10^9 per liter and will be symptom-free. For those with low platelet counts, petechiae and purpura, steroids or preferably i.v. IgG should be administered. If there is mucous membrane bleeding, platelet concentrates should also be administered.

It should be borne in mind that the neonatal platelet count will fall further in the first few days of life and it is at the nadir that most complications occur, rather than at delivery. Measures should be taken to prevent the fall if the cord blood platelet count warrants this, or if clinically there is evidence of skin or mucous membrane bleeding. The platelet count should be repeated daily for the first week in those neonates with thrombocytopenia at delivery.

As previously mentioned, postpartum concerns in the mother relate to bleeding from surgical incisions such as episiotomy and cesarean section sites, or from soft tissue lacerations. These areas should be carefully inspected during the postpartum period.

AITP Associated with HIV Infection

Thrombocytopenia is a well-recognized complication of HIV infection and may be due to drugs and severe infection. The subject has been reviewed.[126,127] However, patients with the immune deficiency syndromes may have thrombocytopenia otherwise indistinguishable from AITP. This may be due to immune platelet destruction resulting from cross-reaction between the human immunodeficiency virus and the platelet glycoproteins IIb/IIIa,[128] which may explain AIDS-free, HIV-associated AITP. It has also been suggested that disturbances in the beta-cell subset, CD5, in HIV-infected patients, may cause immunological changes correlating with the platelet count.[129] It has also been suggested that non-specific deposition of complement and immune complexes on platelets leads to their removal from the circulation.[127]

While most HIV patients have so far been young men, it is possible that this complication will become more common in young pregnant women,[130] although the degree of heterosexual spread of HIV is uncertain.[131] Certainly, young pregnant women in a high-risk group for HIV and thrombocytopenia should be considered for HIV testing.

THROMBOTIC THROMBOCYTOPENIC PURPURA (TTP) AND HEMOLYTIC UREMIC SYNDROME (HUS)

Maternal/Fetal Risks and Management Options

These conditions are both due to the presence of platelet thrombi in the microcirculation, which cause ischemic dysfunction and microangiopathic hemolysis. In HUS, the brunt of the disease process is taken by the kidney. It is most commonly seen in childhood in association with an acute diarrheal illness often due to an *Escherichia coli* verocytotoxin,[132,133] but has also rarely been associated with pregnancy particularly in the postnatal period.[134–136] It has also been seen during pregnancy[136,137] and in association with ectopic pregnancy.[138] It has been postulated that endothelial damage is mediated through neutrophil adhesion in association with infection and leads to the formation of platelet thrombi.[139]

In TTP, the focus shifts to multisystem disease, often with neurological involvement and fever. It has been associated with pregnancy and the postpartum period[140] and with the platelet anti-aggregating agent, ticlopidine.[141] It is associated with abnormal patterns of von Willebrand factor (VWF) multimers in the plasma.[142] Immunohistochemistry has shown the presence of VWF but not fibrinogen in the platelet aggregates in TTP.[143] It has been suggested that a calcium-dependent cysteine protease present in patients' plasma may interact with VWF to render it highly reactive with platelets, thus contributing to the formation of platelet aggregates.[144] The underlying etiology of TTP in pregnancy remains unknown and the various abnormalities which have been described may only be epiphenonema. It is feasible that there is a deficiency of prostacyclin activator or synthesis. The etiology has been reviewed.[145,146]

The pentad of fever, normal coagulation tests with low platelets, hemolytic anemia, neurological disorders and renal dysfunction are virtually pathognomonic of TTP. The thrombocytopenia may range from 5 to 100×10^9 per liter. The clinical picture is severe with a high maternal mortality.

Empirical therapeutic strategies hinge on intensive plasma exchange or replacement. In a random allocation study of 102 non-pregnant patients with HUS, plasma exchange was found to be more effective than plasma infusion, with more than seven exchanges over 9 days.[147] It has been suggested that plasma supplies a factor lacking in patients with TTP that stimulates the release of prostacyclin. Regimens may be supplemented with antiplatelet drugs to prevent relapse,[146] although their use has been contested by some authors.[148] Platelet infusions are contraindicated. Cryosupernatant has been shown to process abnormally large VWF multimers.[149] There is no clear evidence that delivery alters the course of the disease, although it does simplify maternal management.

In one large series of 108 patients with HUS/TTP, of whom 9% were pregnant, steroids alone were judged to be effective in mild cases, while there were 8 deaths and 67 relapses in a group of 78 patients with complicated disease. They were treated with steroids and intensive plasma infusions. The overall survival was 91%. Of the nine pregnant patients, all were in the third trimester and all were delivered of normal infants. Five women went on to further normal pregnancies and deliveries.[148]

In summary, it seems reasonable to treat all TTP patients with steroids. Severe cases will benefit from intensive plasma exchange but, where that is difficult, intensive plasma infusion is indicated. Unresponsive cases may benefit from cryosupernatant infusions. The use of antiplatelet drugs seems non-contributory.[150] Plasma infusion should be tapered but continued until all objective signs have been reversed, in order to prevent recurrence.

THROMBOCYTOPENIA
Summary of Management Options

INCIDENTAL

Prenatal

- Exclude pathological causes

- No specific management indicated if $>100 \times 10^9/l$

AUTO-IMMUNE THROMBOCYTOPENIC PURPURA (see also Chapter 46)

Prenatal

- Check platelet antibodies

- Serial platelet counts

- Steroids if $<50 \times 10^9/l$

- Platelet transfusion if $<50 \times 10^9/l$ and bleeding

- IgG at 36 weeks and delivery within 2–3 weeks if $<50 \times 10^9/l$ and steroids have been unsuccessful

- Splenectomy and platelet transfusion only if ill patient and all else fails

- Fetal blood sampling is controversial

Labor/delivery

- Platelets available if $<50 \times 10^9/l$

- Prompt suturing

- Avoid traumatic delivery

- Case for elective cesarean section not proven

Postnatal

- Check cord blood platelets

- Pediatricians for delivery and ongoing neonatal care

TTP/HUS

Prenatal and postnatal

- Avoid platelet transfusions

- Steroids

- Plasma infusion or exchange in steroid-resistant cases

REFERENCES

1 Hytten F (1985) Blood volume changes in normal pregnancy. In Letsky EA (ed.) *Haematological Disorders in Pregnancy*, pp. 601–612. Clinics in Haematology Vol. 14. London: W.B. Saunders.

2 Letsky EA (1991) The haematological system. In Hytten FE, Chamberlain GVP (eds) *Clinical Physiology in Obstetrics*, 2nd edn, pp. 39–82. Oxford: Blackwell Scientific Publications.

3 World Health Organization (1972) *Nutritional Anaemias*. Technical Report Series No. 503. Geneva: WHO.

4 de Leeuw NKM, Lowenstein L, Hsieh YS (1966) Iron deficiency and hydremia in normal pregnancy. *Medicine* **45**:291–315.

5 Svanberg B (1975) Absorption of iron in pregnancy. *Acta Obstetrica et Gynecologica Scandinavica* **48**:7–108, (suppl.).

6 Fenton V, Cavill I, Fisher J (1977) Iron stores in pregnancy. *British Journal of Haematology* **37**:145–149.

7 Thompson WG (1988) Comparison of tests for diagnosis of iron depletion in pregnancy. *American Journal of Obstetrics and Gynecology* **159**:1132–1134.

8 Finch CA, Cook JD (1984) Iron deficiency. *American Journal of Clinical Nutrition* **39**:471–477.

9 Taylor DJ, Mallen C, McDougall N, Lind T (1982)

Effect of iron supplements on serum ferritin levels during and after pregnancy. *British Journal of Obstetrics and Gynaecology* **89**:1011–1017.

10 Guldholt IS, Trolle BG, Hvidman LE (1991) Iron supplementation during pregnancy. *Acta Obstetrica et Gynecologica Scandinavica* **70**:9–12.

11 Kaltreider DF, Kohl S (1980) Epidemiology of preterm delivery. *Clinics in Obstetrics and Gynecology* **23**:17–31.

12 Klebanoff MA, Shiono PH, Selby JV, Trachtenberg AI, Graubard BI (1991) Anemia and spontaneous preterm birth. *American Journal of Obstetrics and Gynecology* **164**:59–63.

13 Addy DP (1986) Happiness is: Iron. *British Medical Journal* **292**:969–970.

14 Letsky EA (1987) Anaemia in obstetrics. In Studd J (ed.) *Progress in Obstetrics and Gynaecology* **7**:23–58.

15 Krawinkel MB, Bethge M, El Karib AO, Ahmet HM, Mirghani OA (1990) Maternal ferritin values and foetal iron stores (Letter). *Acta Paediatrica Scandinavica* **79**:467.

16 Colomer J, Colomert C, Gutierrez D, Jubert A, Nolasco A, Donat J, Fernandez-Delgado F, Donat F, Alvarez-Dardet C (1990) Anaemia during pregnancy as a risk factor for infant iron deficiency: Report from the Valencia Infant Anaemia Cohort (VIAC) Study. *Paediatric and Perinatal Epidemiology* **4**:196–204.

17 Oski FA (1985) Iron deficiency – facts and fallacies. *Pediatric Clinics of North America* **32**:493–497.

18 Godfrey KM, Redman CWG, Barker DJP, Osmond C (1991) The effect of maternal anaemia and iron deficiency on the ratio of fetal weight to placental weight. *British Journal of Obstetrics and Gynaecology* **98**:886–891.

19 Hallberg I, Ryttinger L, Solvell L (1966) Side effects of oral iron therapy. *Acta Medica Scandinavica* **459**:3–10 (suppl).

20 Hemminki E, Starfield B (1978) Routine administration of iron and vitamins during pregnancy: Review of controlled clinical trials. *British Journal of Obstetrics and Gynaecology* **85**:404–410.

21 Bentely DP (1985) Iron metabolism and anaemia in pregnancy. In Letsky EA (ed.) *Haematological Disorders in Pregnancy*, pp. 613–628. Clinics in Haematology Vol. 14. London: W.B. Saunders.

22 Scott JM (1962) Toxicity of iron sorbiton citrate. *British Medical Journal* **ii**:480–481.

23 Clay B, Rosenburg B, Sampson N, Samuels SI (1965) Reactions to total dose intravenous infusion of iron dextran (Imferon). *British Medical Journal* **i**:29–31.

24 Kullander S, Kallen B (1976) A prospective study of drugs and pregnancy. *Acta Obstetrica et Gynecologica Scandinavica* **55**:287–295.

25 Sheldon WL, Aspillaga MO, Smith PA, Lind T (1985) The effects of oral iron supplementation on zinc and magnesium levels during pregnancy. *British Journal of Obstetrics and Gynaecology* **92**:892–898.

26 Chanarin I (1985) Folate and cobalamin. In Letsky EA (ed.) *Haematological Disorders in Pregnancy*, pp. 629–641. Clinics in Haematology Vol. 14. London: W.B. Saunders.

27 Herbert V (1985) Biology of disease – megaloblastic anaemias. *Laboratory Investigations* **52**:3–19.

28 Smithells RW, Sheppard S, Schorah CJ *et al.* (1980). Possible prevention of neural-tube defects by periconceptional vitamin supplementation. *Lancet* **i**:339–340.

29 Laurence KM, James N, Miller NH, Tennant BG, Campbell H (1981) Double-blind randomised controlled trial of folate treatment before conception to prevent recurrence of neural tube defects. *British Medical Journal* **282**:1509–1511.

30 Smithells RW, Newin NC, Seller MJ *et al.* (1983) Further experience of vitamin supplementation for prevention of neural tube defect recurrences. *Lancet* **i**:1027–1031.

31 Elwood JM (1983) Can vitamins prevent neural tube defects? *Canadian Medical Association Journal* **129**:1088–1092.

32 MRC Vitamin Study Research Group (1991) Prevention of neural tube defects: Results of the Medical Research Council Vitamin Study. *Lancet* **338**:131–137.

33 Baumslag N, Edelstein T, Metz J (1970) Reduction of incidence of prematurity of folic acid supplementation in pregnancy. *British Medical Journal* **1**:16–17.

34 Iyengar L (1971) Folic acid requirements of Indian pregnant women. *American Journal of Obstetrics and Gynecology* **111**:13–16.

35 Reynolds EH (1973) Anticonvulsants, folic acid and epilepsy. *Lancet* **i**:1376–1378.

36 Hiilesmaa VK, Teramo K, Granstrom M-L, Bardy AH (1983) Serum folate concentrations during pregnancy in women with epilepsy: Relation to anti-epileptic drug concentrations, number of seizures and fetal outcome. *British Medical Journal* **287**:577–579.

37 Taylor JJ, Studd JWW, Green ID (1968) Primary refractory anaemia and pregnancy. *Journal of Obstetrics and Gynaecology of the British Commonwealth* **75**:963–968.

38 Picot C, Triadou P, Lacombe C, Casadevall N, Girot R (1984) Relapsing pure red-cell aplasia during pregnancy. *New England Journal of Medicine* **311**:196.

39 Snyder TE, Lee LP, Lynch S (1991) Pregnancy-associated hypoplastic anemia: A review. *Obstetrical and Gynaecological Survey* **46**:264–269.

40 Lewis SM, Gordon Smith EC (1982) Aplastic and dysplastic anaemias. In Hardisty RM, Weatherall DJ (eds) *Blood and its Disorders*, 2nd edn, pp. 1229–1268. Oxford: Blackwell Scientific Publications.

41 Chaplin H, Cohen R, Bloomberg G, Kaplan HJ, Moore JA, Dorner I (1973) Pregnancy and idiopathic auoimmune haemolytic anaemia: A prospective study during 6 months gestation and 3 months post-partum. *British Journal of Haematology* **24**:219–229.

42 Soo-Chin Ng, Wong KK, Raman S, Bosco J (1990) Autoimmune haemolytic anaemia in pregnancy: A case report. *European Journal of Obstetrics and Gynecology and Reproductive Biology* **37**:83–85.

43 Rothman LA, Cohen CJ, Astarloa J (1973) Placental and fetal involvement by maternal malignancy: A report of rectal carcinoma and review of the literature. *American Journal of Obstectrics and Gynecology* **116**:1023–1033.

44 Ewing PA, Whittaker JA (1973) Acute leukaemia in pregnancy. *Obstetrics and Gynecology* **42**:245–251.

45 Gokal R, Durrant J, Baum JD, Bennett MJ (1976) Successful pregnancy in acute monocyte leukaemia. *British Journal of Cancer* **34**:299–302.

46 Nicholson HO. (1968) Leukaemia and pregnancy. *Journal of Obstetrics and Gynaecology of the British Commonwealth* **75**:517–520.

47 Slade R, James DK (1991) Pregnancy and maternal malignant haematological disorders. In Turner TL (ed.) *Perinatal Haematological Problems*, pp. 23–38 Chichester: John Wiley.

48 Lewis BJ, Laros RK (1986) Leukemia and lymphoma. In Laros RK (ed.) *Blood Disorders in Pregnancy*, pp. 85–101. Philadelphia: Lea and Febiger.

49 Blatt J, Mulvihill JJ, Ziegler J *et al.* (1980) Pregnancy outcome following cancer chemotherapy. *American Journal of Medicine* **69**:828.

50 Weatherall DJ (1991) Prenatal diagnosis of haematological disorders. In Letsky EA, Hann IM, Gibson BES (eds) *Fetal and Neonatal Haematology*, pp. 285–314. London: Ballière Tindall.

51 Goldfarb AW, Hochner-Celnikier D, Beller U, Menashe M, Daga I, Palti Z (1982) A successful pregnancy in transfusion dependent homozygous β-thalassaemia: A case report. *International Journal of Gynaecology and Obstetrics* **20**:319–322.

52 Bareford D (1991) Thalassaemia in pregnancy (Letter). *British Medical Journal* **303**:120.

53 Chang JG, Lee LS, Lin CP, Chen PH, Chen CP (1991) Rapid diagnosis of alpha-thalassaemia-1 of southeast Asia type and hydrops fetalis by polymerase chain reaction (Letter). *Blood* **78**:853–854.

54 Ko TM, Tseng LH, Hsieh FJ, Hsu PM, Lee TY (1992) Carrier detection and prenatal diagnosis of alpha-thalassaemia of Southeast Asian deletion by polymerase chain reaction. *Human Genetics* **88**:245–248.

55 Hsia YE (1991) Detection and prevention of important α-thalassemia variants. *Seminars in Perinatology* **15**:35–42 (suppl.1).

56 Van Dinh T, Boor PJ, Garza JR. (1982) Massive pulmonary embolism following delivery of a patient with sickle cell trait. *American Journal of Obstetrics and Gynecology* **143**:722–724.

57 Lindheimer MD, Richardson DA, Ehrlich EN *et al.* (1987) Potassium homeostasis in pregnancy. *Journal of Reproductive Medicine* **32**:517–526.

58 Serjeant GR (1983) Sickle haemoglobin and pregnancy. *British Medical Journal* **287**:628–630.

59 Charache S, Niebyl JR (1985) Pregnancy in sickle cell disease. In Letsky EA (ed.) *Haematological Disorders in Pregnancy*, pp. 720–746. Clinics in Haematology, Vol. 14. London: W.B. Saunders.

60 Tuck SM, Studd JWW, White JM (1983) Pregnancy in sickle cell disease in the United Kingdom. *British Journal of Obstetrics and Gynaecology* **90**:122–117.

61 Aluoch JR, Rogo K, Otieno MB (1990) Maternal and foetal outcome of pregnant patients with sickle cell anaemia at Kenyatta National Hospital Nairobi: A retrospective study. *Trop Geogr Med.* **42**:28–31.

62 Anyaegbunam A, Langer O, Brustman L, Whitty J, Merkatz IR (1991) Third-trimester prediction of small-for-gestational-age infants in pregnant women with sickle cell disease: Development of the ultradop index. *Journal of Reproductive Medicine* **36**:577–580.

63 Rosse WF, Gallagher D, Kinney TR, Castro O, Dosik H, Moohr J, Wang W, Levy PS (1990) Transfusion and alloimmunization in sickle cell disease: The Cooperative Study of Sickle Cell Disease. *Blood* **76**:1431–1437.

64 Tuck SM, James CE, Brewster EM, Pearson TC, Studd JWW (1987) Prophylactic blood transfusion in maternal sickle cell syndromes. *British Journal of Obstetrics and Gynaecology* **94**:121–125.

65 Koshy M, Burd L, Wallace D, Moawad D, Baron J (1988) Prophylactic red cell transfusions in pregnant patients with sickle cell disease. *New England Journal of Medicine* **319**:1447–1452.

66 Perry KG Jr, Morrison JC (1990) The diagnosis and management of hemoglobinopathies during pregnancy. *Seminars in Perinatology* **14**:90–102.

67 Thomas AN, Pattison C, Serjeant GR (1982) Causes of death in sickle cell disease in Jamaica. *British Medical Journal* **285**:633–655.

68 Yeomans E, Lowe TW, Eigenbrodt EH, Cunningham FG (1990) Liver histopathologic findings in women with sickle cell disease given prophylactic transfusion during pregnancy. *American Journal of Obstetrics and Gynecology* **163**:958–964.

69 Koshy M, Burd L (1991) Management of pregnancy in sickle cell syndromes. *Hematol Oncol Clin North Am* **5**:585–596.

70 Pastorek JG II, Saseiler B 91985) Maternal death associated with sickle cell trait. *American Journal of Obstetrics and Gynecology* **151**:295–297.

71 Samuels-Reid JH, Scott RB, Brown WE (1984) Contraceptive practices and reproductive patterns in sickle cell disease. *Journal of the National Medical Association* **76**:879–883.

72 Tygart SG, McRoyan DK, Spinnato JA, McRoyan CJ, Kitay DZ (1986) Longitudinal study of platelet indices during normal pregnancy. *American Journal of Obstetrics and Gynecology* **154**:883–887.

73 Leduc L, Wheeler JM, Kirshon B, Mitchell P, Cotton DB (1992) Coagulation profile in severe preeclampsia. *Obstetrics and Gynecology* **79**:14–18.

74 Letsky EA (1987) Disseminated intravascular coagulation. In Morgan B (ed.) *Problems in Obstetric Anaesthesia*, pp. 69–87. Chichester: John Wiley.

75 Letsky EA (1992) Management of massive haemorrhage – the haematologist's role. In Patel N (ed.) *Maternal Mortality: The Way Forward*, pp. 63–71. London: Royal College of Obstetrics and Gynaecologists.

76 Burrows RF, Kelton JG (1990) Thrombocytopenia at delivery: A prospective survey of 6715 deliveries American Journal of Obstetrics and Gynecology **162**:731–734.

77 Letsky EA (1991) Haemostasis and epidural anaesthesia. *International Journal of Obstetrics and Anesthesia* **1**:51–54.

78 Kaplan C, Daffos F, Forestier F, Tertian G, Catherine N, Pons JC, Tchernia G (1990) Fetal platelet counts in thrombocytopenic pregnancy *Lancet* **336**:979–982.

79 Burrows RF, Kelton JG (1992) Thrombocytopenia during pregnancy. In Greer IA, Turpie AGG, Forbes CD (eds) *Haemostasis and Thrombosis in Obstetrics and Gynaecology*, pp. 407–429. London: Chapman and Hall.

80 Aster RH (1990) 'Gestational' thrombocytopenia: A plea for conservative management. *New England Journal of Medicine* 323:264–266.

81 Kessler I, Lancet M, Borenstein R, Berrebi A, Mogilner BM (1982) The obstetrical management of patients with immunologic thrombocytopenic purpura. *International Journal of Gynecology and Obstetrics* 20:23–28.

82 Weatherall DJ, Letsky EA (1984) Genetic haematological disorders. In Wald NJ (ed.) *Antenatal and Neonatal Screening*, pp. 155–191. Oxford: Oxford University Press.

83 Burrows RF, Kelton JG (1988) Incidentally detected thrombocytopenia in healthy mothers and their infants. *New England Journal of Medicine* 319:532–542.

84 Hart D, Dunetz C, Nardi M, Porges RF, Weiss A, Karpatkin M (1986) An epidemic of maternal thrombocytopenia associated with elevated antiplatelet antibody: Platelet count and antiplatelet antibody in 116 consecutive pregnancies. Relationship to neonatal platelet count. *American Journal of Obstetrics and Gynecology* 154:878–883.

85 Samuels P, Bussel JB, Braitman LE, Tomaski A, Druzin ML, Mennuti MT, Cines BD (1990) Estimation of the risk of thrombocytopenia in the offspring of pregnant women with presumed immune thrombocytopenic purpura. *New England Journal of Medicine* 323:229–235.

86 Martin JN Jr, Morrison JC, Files JC (1984) Autoimmune thrombocytopenic purpura: Current concepts and recommended practices. *American Journal of Obstetrics and Gynecology* 150:86–96.

87 Cines DB, Dusak B, Tomaski A, Mennuti M, Shreiber AD (1982) Immune thrombocytopenic purpura and pregnancy. *New England Journal of Medicine* 306:826–831.

88 Kelton JG (1983) Management of the pregnant patient with idiopathic thrombocytopenic purpura. *Annals of Internal Medicine* 99:796–800.

89 Murray JM, Harris RE (1976) The management of the pregnant patient with idiopathic thrombocytopenic purpura. *American Journal of Obstetrics and Gynecology* 126:449–451.

90 Noriega-Guerra L, Aviles-Miranda A, de la Cadena OA, Espinosa LM, Chavez F, Pizzuto J (1979) Pregnancy in patients with autoimmune thrombocytopenic purpura. *American Journal of Obstetrics and Gynecology* 133:439–448.

91 Browning J, James D (1990) Immune thrombocytopenia in pregnancy. *Fetal Medicine Review* 2:143–157.

92 Tchernia G, Dreyfus M, Laurian Y, Derycke M, Merica C, Kerbrat G (1984) Management of immune thrombocytopenia in pregnancy: Response of infusions of immunoglobulins. *American Journal of Obstetrics and Gynecology* 148:225–226.

93 Nicolini U, Tannirandorn Y, Gonzales P, Fisk NM, Beecham J, Letsky E, Rodeck CH (1990) Continuing

controversy in alloimmune thrombocytopenia: Fetal hypergammaglobulinemia fails to prevent thrombocytopenia. *American Journal of Obstetrics and Gynecology* 163:1144–1146.

94 Harrington WJ, Sprague CC, Minnich V, Moore CV, Aulvin RC, Dubach RC (1953) Immunologic mechanisms in idiopathic and neonatal thrombocytopenic purpura. *Annals of Internal Medicine* 38:433–469.

95 Evans RS, Takahashi K, Duane RT, Payne R, Liu C-K (1951) Primary thrombocytopenic purpura and acquired hemolytic anemia:Evidence for a common etiology. *Archives of Internal Medicine* 87:48–65.

96 Van Leeuwen EF, van der Ven JTM, Englefreit CP, von Dem Borne AEG (1982) Specificity of autoantibodies in autoimmune thrombocytopenia. *Blood* 59:23–26.

97 Woods VL Jr, Kurata Y, Montgomery RR, Tani P, Mason D, Oh EH, McMillan R (1984) Autoantibodies against platelet glycoprotein Ib in patients with chronic immune thrombocytopenic purpura. *Blood* 64:156–160.

98 Woods VL Jr, Oh EH, Mason D, McMillan R (1984) Autoantibodies against the platelet glycoprotein IIb/IIIa complex in patients with chronic ITP. *Blood* 63:368–375.

99 Woods VL Jr, McMillan R (1984) Platelet autoantigens in chronic ITP. *British Journal of Haematology* 57:1–4.

100 Mason D, McMillan R (1984) Platelet antigens in chronic idiopathic thrombocytopenic purpura *British Journal of Haematology* 56:529–534.

101 Cines DB, Schreiber AD (1979) Immune throbocytopenia: Use of a Combe's antiglobulin test to detect IgG and C3 on platelets. *New England Journal of Medicine* 300:106–111.

102 von dem Borne AEG Kr, Helmerhorst FM, van Leeuwen EF, Pegels HG, von Riesz E, Engelfriet CP (1980) Autoimmune thrombocytopenia: Detection of platelet autoantibodies with the suspension of immunofluorescence test. *British Journal of Haematology* 45:319–327.

103 Mueller-Ekhardt C, Kayser W, Mersch-Baumert K, Mueller-Eckhardt G, Breidenbach M, Kugel H-G, Graubner M (1980) The clinical significance of platelet-associated IgG: A study on 298 patients with various disorders. *British Journal of Haematology* 46:123–131.

104 Hegde UM, Ball S, Zuiable A, Roter BLT (1985) Platelet associated immunoglobulins (PAIgG and PAIgM) in autoimmune thrombocytopenia. *British Journal of Haematology* 59:221–226.

105 Harrington WJ (1987) Are platelet antibody tests worthwhile? *New England Journal of Medicine* 316:211–212.

106 McMillan R (1981) Chronic idiopathic thrombocytopenic purpura. *New England Journal of Medicine* 304:1135–1147.

107 Martin JN, Morrison JC, Files JC (1984) Autoimmune thrombocytyopenia purpura: Current concepts and recommended practices. *American Journal of Obstetrics and Gynecology* 150:86–96.

108 Smith BT, Torday JS (1982) Steroid administration in

pregnant women with autoimmune thrombocytopenia. *New England Journal of Medicine* **306**:744–745.

109 Hegde UM (1985) Immune thrombocytopenia in pregnancy and the newborn. *British Journal of Obstetrics and Gynaecology* **92**:657–659.

110 Dwyer JM (1992) Manipulating the immune system with immune globulin *New England Journal of Medicine* **326**:107–116.

111 Morgenstern GR, Measday B, Hegde UM (1983) Auto-immune thrombocytopenia in pregnancy: New approach to management. *British Medical Journal* **287**:584.

112 Pappas C (1986) Placental transfer of immunoglobulins in immune thrombocytopenic purpura. *Lancet* **1**:389.

113 Hegde U (1987) Immune thrombocytopenia in pregnancy and the newborn: A review. *Journal of Infection* **15**:55–58 (suppl.1).

114 Carloss HW, McMillan R, Crosby WH (1980) Management of pregnancy in women with immune thrombocytopenic purpura. *Journal of the American Medical Association* **144**:2756–2758.

115 Bell WR (1977) Hematologic abnormalities in pregnancy. *Medical Clinics of North America* **61**:165–203.

116 Burrows RF, Kelton JG (1990) Low fetal risks in pregnancies associated with idiopathic thrombocytopenic purpura. *American Journal of Obstetrics and Gynecology* **163**:1147–1150.

117 Van Leeuwen EF, Helmerhorst FM, Engelfriet CP, Von Dem Borne AEG (1981) Maternal autoimmune thrombocytopenia and the newborn. *British Medical Journal* **283**:104.

118 Kaplan C, Daffos F, Forestier F, Tertian G, Catherine N, Pons JC, Tchernia G (1990) Fetal platelet counts in thrombocytopenic pregnancy. *Lancet* **336**:979–982.

119 Ayromlooi J (1978) A new approach to the management of immunologic thrombocytopenic purpura in pregnancy. *American Journal of Obstetrics and Gynecology* **130**:235–236.

120 Scott JR, Cruikshank DP, Kochenour NK *et al.* (1980) Fetal platelet counts in the obstetric management of immunologic thrombocytopenic purpura. *American Journal of Obstetrics and Gynecology* **136**:495–499.

121 Tchernia G (1988) Immune thrombocytopenic purpura and pregnancy. *Current Studies in Hematology and Blood Transfusion* **55**:81–89.

122 Moisse KJ, Carpenter RJ, Cotton DB, Wasserstrujm N, Kirshon B, Cano L (1988) Percutaneous umbilical cord sampling in the evaluation of fetal platelet counts in pregnant patients with autoimmune thrombocytopenia purpura. *Obstetrics and Gynecology* **72**:346–350.

123 Scioscia AL, Grannum PAT, Copel JA, Hobbins JC (1988) The use of percutaneous umbilical blood sampling in immune thrombocytopenia purpura. *American Journal of Obstetrics and Gynecology* **159**:1066–1068.

124 Daffos F, Forestier F, Kaplan C, Cox W (1988) Prenatal diagnosis and management of bleeding disorders with fetal blood sampling. *American Journal of Obstetrics and Gynecology* **158**:939–946.

125 Murray JM, Harris RE (1976) The management of the pregnant patient with idiopathic thrombocytopenic purpura. *American Journal of Obstetrics and Gynecology* **126**:449–451.

126 Costello C (1988) Haematological abnormalities in human immunodeficiency virus (HIV) disease. *Journal of Clinical Pathology* **41**:711–715.

127 Walsh CM, Nardi MA, Karpatkin S (1984) On the mechanism of thrombocytopenic purpura in sexually active homosexual men. *New England Journal of Medicine* **311**:635–639.

128 Bettaieb A, Fromont P, Louache F, Oksenhendler E, Vainchencker W, Duedari N, Bierling P (1992) Presence of cross-reactive antibody between human immunodeficiency virus (HIV) and platelet glycoproteins in HIV-related immune thrombocytopenic purpura. *Blood* **80**:162–169.

129 Kouri YH, Basch RS, Karpatkin S (1992) B-cell subsets and platelet counts in HIV-1 seropositive subjects. *Lancet* **339**:1445–1446.

130 Treacy M, Lai L, Costello C, Clark A (1987) Peripheral blood and bone marrow abnormalities in patients with HIV related disease. *British Journal of Haematology* **65**:289–294.

131 Johnson AM (1992) Home grown heterosexually acquired HIV infection: Still difficult to predict. *British Medical Journal* **304**:1125–1126.

132 Karmali MA, Steel BT, Petric M, Lim C (1983) Sporadic cases of HUS associated with faecal cytotoxin and cytotoxin producing *Escherichia coli* in stools. *Lancet* **1**:619.

133 Martin DL *et al.* (1990) The epidemiology and clinical aspects of the HUS in Minnesota. *New England Journal of Medicine* **323**:1161–1167.

134 Robson *et al.* (1968) Irreversible post partum renal failure *Quarterly Journal of Medicine* **37**:423–435.

135 Wagoner *et al.* (1968) Accelerated nephrosclerosis and post-partum acute renal failure in normotensive patients. *Annals of Internal Medicine* **69**:237–284.

136 Hayslett JP (1985) Post-partum renal failure. *New England Journal of Medicine* **24**:1556–1559.

137 Vandewalle, Kanfer A, Kourilsky O (1975) Oliguric thrombotic microangiopathy during the first month of pregnancy *British Medical Journal* **ii**:497.

138 Creasy GW, Morgan J (1987) Haemolytic uremic syndrome after ectopic pregnancy: Post ectopic nephrosclerosis. *Obstetrics and Gynecology* **69**:448–449.

139 Forsyth KD *et al.* (1989) Neutrophil mediated endothelial injury in HUS. *Lancet* **ii**:411–414.

140 Weiner CP (1987) Thrombotic microangiopathy in pregnancy and the postpartum period. *Seminars in Haematology* **2**:119–129.

141 Page Y, Tardy B, Zeni F, Comtet C, Terrana R, Bertrand JC (1991) Thrombotic thrombocytopenic purpura related to ticlopidine. *Lancet* **337**:774–776.

142 Moake JL *et al.* (1982) Unusually large plasma factor VIII: VWF multimers in chronic relapsing TTP. *New England Journal of Medicine* **307**:1432–1435.

143 Asada Y *et al.* (1985) Immunohistochemistry of vascular lesion in TTP with special reference to factor VIII related antigen. *Thrombosis Research* **38**:469–479.

144 Moore JC, Murphy WG, Kelton JG (1990) Calpain proteolysis of VWF enhances its binding to platelet membrane glycoprotein IIb/IIIa: An explanation for

platelet aggregation in TTP. *British Journal of Haematology* **74**:457–464.

145 Aster RH (1985) Plasma therapy for thrombotic thromboeytopenic purpura. *New England Journal of Medicine* **312**: 985–987.

146 Machin SJ (1984) Thrombotic thrombocytopenic purpura *British Journal of Haematology* **56**:191–197.

147 Rock GA, Shumack KH, Buskard NA, Blanchette VS, Kelton JG, Nair RC, Spasoff RA, Canadian Apheresis Study Group (1991) Comparison of plasma exchange with plasma infusion in the treatment of thrombotic thrombocytopenic purpura. *New England Journal of Medicine* **325**:393–397.

148 Bell WR, Braine HG, Ness PM, Kickler TS (1991) Improved survival in thrombotic thrombocytopenic purpura-hemolytic uremic syndrome *New England Journal of Medicine* **325**:398–403.

149 Moake JL, Byrnes JJ, Troll JH, Rudy CK, Hong SL, Weinstein MJ, Colannino NM (1985) Effects of fresh-frozen plasma and its cryosupernatant fraction on von Willebrand factor multimeric forms in chronic relapsing thrombotic thrombocytopenic purpura. *Blood* **65**:1232–1236.

150 Moake JL (1991) TTP: Desperation, empiricism, progress *New England Journal of Medicine* **325**:426–428.

151 Czeizel AE, Dudás, I (1992) Prevention of the first occurrence of neural-tube defects by periconceptional vitamin supplementation. *New England Journal of Medicine* **327**:1832–1835.

152 Caliguiri MA, Mayer RJ (1989) Pregnancy and leukemia. *Seminars in Oncology* **16**:388–396.

153 Zuazu J, Julia A, Sierra J *et al.* (1991) Pregnancy outcome in hematologic malignancies. *Cancer* **67**:703–709.

154 Milliken S, Powles R, Parikh P *et al.* (1990) Successful pregnancy following bone marrow transplantation for leukaemia. *Bone Marrow Transplant* **5**:135–137.

155 Giri N, Vowels MR, Barr AL, Mameghan H (1992) Successful pregnancy after total body irradiation and bone marrow transplantation for acute leukaemia. *Bone Marrow Transplant* **10**:93–95.

156 Reichel RP, Linkesch W, Schetitska D. (1992) Therapy with recombinant interferon alpha-2c during unexpected pregnancy in a patient with chronic myeloid leukaemia. *British Journal of Haematology* **82**:472–473.

157 Ward FT, Weiss RB (1989) Lymphoma and pregnancy. *Seminars in Oncology* **16**:397–409.

158 Lishner M, Zemlickis D, Degendorfer P *et al.* (1992) Maternal and foetal outcome following Hodgkin's disease in pregnancy. *British Journal of Cancer* **65**:114–117.

159 Janov AJ, Anderson J. Cella DF *et al.* (1992) Pregnancy outcome in survivors of advanced Hodgkin disease *Cancer* **70**:688–692.

160 Colvin BT (1985) Thrombocytopenia. *Clinics in Haematology* **14**:661–681.

161 Pillai M (1993) Platelets and pregnancy. *British Journal of Obstetrics and Gynaecology* **100**:201–204.

24

Respiratory Disorders

MICHAEL DE SWIET

INTRODUCTION

All respiratory disorders should be managed in conjunction with a respiratory physician or preferably a physician with particular interests in pregnancy. The help of a respiratory physician is critically important in acute severe asthma, the severity of which may be underestimated by both doctor and patient, in severe pneumonia and in tuberculosis where guidelines for therapy change frequently. A recent review on the topic of respiratory diseases as they relate to pregnancy can also be found in de Swiet.[1]

ASTHMA

Asthma is defined as a reversible airways obstruction. Precipitating factors may be overtly immunological (e.g. allergy to certain animals such as cats), infective or emotional. The condition is more common in atopic individuals. The prevalance of patients with a history of asthma is thought to vary between 0.1 and 2% in pregnancy.[1,2] For useful reviews see Schaefer and Silverman,[3] Greenberger[4] and Barksy.[5]

Maternal/Fetal Risks

Pregnancy does not increase the frequency or severity of asthma[6,7] except in those very few patients who have respiratory failure. In these patients, the increase in oxygen consumption due to pregnancy of about 50 ml/min may be critical.[8] Asthma attacks almost never occur during labor. The usual reasons why asthmatic patients deteriorate in pregnancy is the mistaken belief that treatment for asthma is harmful to the fetus. Medical attendants as well as patients and their relatives are likely to promote this dangerous fallacy. The only risk to the fetus is that of growth deficiency and this only occurs in those very few patients who are permanently hypoxemic.[6] Some authorities cite preterm delivery[9,10] as a risk, but there are no published data to support these opinions.

The risk of the child developing asthma in later life varies between 6 and 30%, depending on whether or not the mother is atopic and whether or not the father also is atopic and has asthma.[11]

Management Options

Prepregnancy

Pregnancy counseling should be given based on the preceding information.

Prenatal

Prenatal care is based on optimizing treatment to prevent asthma attacks with additional rescue therapy, if available, if attacks still occur. Whenever possible, treatment should be by inhalation rather than oral, since this reduces systemic effects. It also reduces any possible effects on the fetus. Patient inhaler techniques should be checked, since even in the long term asthmatic errors can be identified.

The most widely used preventive treatment is inhaled glucocorticoids such as betamethasone. The daily dose of betamethasone can vary from 200 to 2000 μg in divided doses. Relatively little betamethasone is absorbed and there are no consistent reports of adverse effects in the fetus.[12,13] Other inhaled prophylactic agents include disodium cromoglycate and ipratropium, both of which are safe in pregnancy.[14] The new long-acting beta$_2$-agonist salmeterol is also marketed for prophylactic therapy. There are insufficient data to recommend its use in pregnancy at present. Beta$_2$-Agonists such as salbutamol are the standard form of 'rescue therapy' for attacks of asthma.

They should be given by inhalation rather than orally and can be given by nebulizer in severe asthma.

Theophyllines (e.g. aminophylline) are used as both rescue and prophylactic therapy. They may be given intravenously in severe asthma providing the patient has not taken aminophylline within the previous 24 h. The clearance of aminophylline is increased in pregnancy in a rather variable way.[15] Any patient who is taking more than 700 mg of aminophylline per day should have blood measurements made for optimal dosing.

A reasonable strategy would be to use the inhaled betasympathomimetics discussed above as rescue therapy in patients having infrequent attacks. If these occur more than three times a week, start inhaled glucocort-

---

ASTHMA
Summary of Management Options

Prepregnancy

- Adjust maintenance medication to optimize respiratory function

- If possible, minimize precipitating factors by timing of pregnancy (seasonal), avoiding of allergens, and the development of good support systems

- Advise early referral for prenatal care

Prenatal

- Adjust asthma medication as needed to control symptomatology

- On occasion, baseline and serial ventilatory function (especially peak flow) may need to be assessed

- Follow theophylline blood levels, since blood volume expansion in pregnancy may mandate higher doses of drug

- In the stable patient, antepartum non-stress testing is not necessary. If con-

cerns over fetal well-being arise, begin antepartum testing in the late second or early third trimesters

- Seek anesthesiology consultation in preparation for delivery

Labor/delivery

- Maintain adequate maternal oxygenation

- Avoid prostoglandin F$_2$-alpha and ergometrine

- Avoid general anesthesia if possible

- Use parenteral steroids for patients on chronic therapy

Postnatal

- Physiotherapy to maintain adequate pulmonary toilet

- Encourage respiratory therapy to minimize atelectosis

- Restart maintenance drug therapy

icoid therapy, increasing the dose as necessary. The addition of ipratropium, theophylline or oral steroids is a decision for the respiratory physician and can be made independently of pregnancy. This strategy of early and aggressive use of inhaled steroids is relatively new and European. In North America, there is a greater emphasis on treatment with theophylline.

Prednisone and hydrocortisone are not contraindicated in pregnancy. They are not teratrogenic in humans.[9] In doses equivalent to prednisone 25 mg/day, they do not cross the placenta because of placental metabolism[16,17] (the same is not true for betamethasone or dexamethasone). Even in higher doses, the effect of hydrocortisone or prednisone on the fetus in terms of suppression of the hypothalmo-pituitary-adrenal axis is minimal.

Acute severe asthma (status asthmaticus) is a very dangerous condition which should be managed with a respiratory physician in an intensive care environment. The most common mistake is to use insufficient parenteral steroid therapy. Even in the absence of acute severe asthma, there should be a very low threshold for admission, since patients with asthma can deteriorate so suddenly and so fast.[18]

Asthma is not an indication for elective delivery, though if there are other maternal or fetal problems, induction should not be withheld.

Labor/delivery

Asthma is rarely a problem in labor. Prostaglandin F_2-alpha should be avoided for induction because it causes bronchoconstriction.[19] But prostglandin E is used as an induction agent in the majority of delivery suites in any case. In the third stage of labor, oxytocin should be used instead of ergometrine, which has caused severe bronchospasm in asthmatic patients, particularly in association with general anesthsia.

Although pethidine may theoretically cause bronchoconstriction, this is not a problem in practice. Many asthmatic women will have been given pethidine in labor without harm. If anesthsia is required, epidural is preferable to general anesthsia because of the risks of chest infection and atelectasis.

Patients who have taken oral steroids for more than 1 month within a year of delivery should be covered with hydrocordisone 150 mg i.m or i.v every 6 h during labor because of the remote risk of Addisonian collapse due to pituitary suppression.

Postnatal

Breast-feeding is not contraindicated in patients taking any form of asthma treatment including oral prednisone.

SARCOID

Sarcoidosis is a non-caseating granulomatosis condition typically affecting the lung, skin (nodules and erythma nodosum), joints and eyes. Less commonly, the heart, liver and indeed any other organ may be involved. It usually regresses spontaneously, though very occasionally lung disease is progressive (see below).

The incidence and prevalence of diagnosed sarcoid in pregnancy is less than 1%.[20] However, erythma nodosum is not uncommon in pregnancy and some cases may be due to undiagnosed sarcoid; also, mediastinal lymphadenopathy due to sarcoid is often not diagnosed. If pregnant patients were to have routine chest x-rays, it is likely that more cases of undiagnosed sarcoid would be found than of tuberculosis.

Maternal Risks

Pregnancy does not influence the natural history of sarcoid.[21] Very occasionally, patients with sarcoid develop progressive pulmonary fibrosis, hypoxemia, pulmonary hypertension and cor pulmonale. Pulmonary hypertension has a very bad prognosis in pregnancy whatever the cause (see Chapter 20). Such patients would be at risk of dying in pregnancy but they are exceptionally uncommon.

Fetal Risks

There are no specific risks. Sarcoid granulomas have been found in the placenta[22] but not in the fetus.[23]

Management Options

Prepregnancy

Prepregnancy counseling can be given, incorporating the above information.

Prenatal

Even patients who are not developing pulmonary fibrosis can become breathless, whether they are pregnant or not. Patients may also have pain from joints and erythema nodosum. All these symptoms can be improved by steroid therapy, which is not contraindicated in pregnancy (see 'Asthma' above).

Patients with sarcoidosis are very sensitive to vitamin D which causes hypercalcemia whether they are pregnant or not.[24] But patients often take multivitamin

---

SARCOID
Summary of Management Options

Prepregnancy

- Reassure patient of benign nature of sarcoidosis during pregnancy unless there is pre-existing evidence of pulmonary fibrosis, hypoxemia or pulmonary hypertension. Counsel against pregnancy when pulmonary hypertension exists

- Baseline pulmonary function studies may assist in the evaluation of the patient's lung status prior to pregnancy.

Prenatal

- Avoid multivitamins containing vitamin D

- Watch for signs and symptoms of progressive pulmonary disease; institute steroid therapy with evidence of significant disease advancement

Labor/delivery

- With substantial parenchymal disease, avoid inhalation anesthesia

- Recognize that high-block conduction anesthesia may cause significant respiratory compromise

- Obtain early anesthesiology consultation

Postnatal

- No specific disease-related needs

---

preparations in pregnancy. Those containing vitamin D should not be used.

The level of angiotensin-converting enzyme has been used as an index of disease activity in sarcoid. This may be invalid in pregnancy where angiotensin-converting enzyme levels seem to change independently of sarcoid activity.[25]

Labor/delivery

If there is any degree of paraenchymatous lung disease, epidural block would be better than general anesthesia.

Postnatal

No specific recommendations are needed for the post-partum management of the parturient with sarcoid.

TUBERCULOSIS

Tuberculosis is now a rare complication of pregnancy in the developed world. For example, at Queen Charlotte's Hospital in London, the incidence is less than 1 in 5000 deliveries. However, in the developing countries, tuberculosis is still common and patients with HIV infection are also at risk from tuberculosis, particularly from atypical mycobacteria.

Maternal/Fetal Risks

Tuberculosis used to have a sinister reputation in pregnancy,[26] but with the advent of modern chemotherapy, immunocompetent patients should make a complete recovery even if tuberculosis is first diagnosed in pregnancy.[27] Tubercle bacilli very rarely cross the placenta,[28] though granulomata may be found in the placenta. Therefore, there is no risk to the fetus apart from the very questionable teratogenicity of anti-tuberculous drugs (see below). The neonate is only at risk of infection if the mother still has active tuberculosis at the time of delivery. Only under these most unusual circumstances should the mother be separated from her newborn baby. Any remote risks of neonatal infection may be reduced by giving the neonate BCG and prophylactic isoniazid (see below).

Management Options

Prepregnancy

The problem concerning the management of tuberculosis in pregnancy is the possible teratogenicity of some antituberculosis drugs. Prepregnancy counseling may be given, incorporating the information given above. Providing women have had an adequate course of chemotherapy, previous tuberculosis is no contra-indication to pregnancy and tuberculosis is no more likely to be reactivated in pregnancy than at any other time.

Prenatal

For patients who present with tuberculosis in pregnancy, a respiratory physician should always be consulted concerning regimes of anti-tuberculosis therapy. The current recommendation in the UK[29] for uncomplicated tuberculosis is an initial 2-month course of pyrazinamide, rifampicin and isoiazid, followed by a further 4 months of rifampicin and isoniazid, i.e. a total of 6 months treatment.

With regard to teratogenicity, ethambutal and isoniazid should be considered safe.[30] However, there has been concern about rifampicin[31] in the first trimester where 14 of 442 fetuses exposed to the drug were variously and severely affected.[30] Streptomycin has been shown to cause both vestibular and auditory eighth nerve damage[30,32] and should be avoided throughout pregnancy. Pyrazinamide is an extremely potent bactericidal drug and there have not been any major reports of teratogenicity. However, there is sufficient experience with pyrazinamide use in early pregnancy to be completely confident about its safety.

In patients who present after the first trimester, there is no problem. They should be treated according to the UK guidelines. Isoniazid therapy should be supplemented with pyridoxine to reduce the risk of maternal peripheral neuritis, and because of the extra requirement for pyridoxine in pregnancy.[33,34] Treatment in the first trimester must be tailored to the severity of the disease. Patients who are not seriously ill could be treated with isoniazid and ethambutol alone until after the first trimester. They should then start a full 6-month course with pyrazinamide, rifampicin and isoniazid as outlined in the UK guidelines. Patients who are ill and who present in the first trimester should be treated with ethambutal, isoniazid and pyrazinamide, pyrazinamide being used because of its potency, despite the lack of knowledge about teratogenicity.

Labor/delivery

No specific recommendations are needed for labor and delivery except as they relate to infection control issues.

TUBERCULOSIS
Summary of Management Options

Prepregnancy

- It is best to establish this diagnosis, and treat the condition, prior to pregnancy. Therefore, screening at-risk populations is advised

- Counsel regarding the potential teratogenesis of rifampicin and streptomycin

Prenatal

- Outside the first trimester, standard therapy (pyrazinamide, rifampicin and isoniazid) for active tuberculosis should be employed. Within the first trimester, one may withhold rifampicin (and substitute with ethambutol) until later in pregnancy, and pyrazinamide should only be given with severe illness (see text)

Labor/delivery

- No specific recommendations except infection precautions needed with active disease

Postnatal

- Separate mother from baby if open tuberculosis present, until no longer infective (appropriately 10 days into therapy)

- Administer isoniazid and BCG to neonate

Postnatal

After delivery, patients with open tuberculosis (i.e. tubercule bacilli in their sputum) should be separated from their babies until they are no longer overtly infective. Since pyrazinamide renders the sputum sterile in 10 days, this should occur infrequently. In addition, the neonate should be given isoniazid to prevent it acquiring infection from its mother and should be given isoniazid-resistant BCG to boost its immunity.[35]

KYPHOSCOLIOSIS

The prevalence of kyphoscoliosis in pregnancy depends on the criteria used for definition. However, kyphoscoliosis will not affect pregnancy unless there is some degree of respiratory impairment and under these circumstances the prevalence is less than 0.1%. It is remarkable that patients can achieve successful pregnancy despite so much deformity, i.e. the abdominal cavity often appears so contracted that there should be insufficient room for a fetus to develop normally. Nevertheless, babies can and do grow normally in these adverse surroundings.

Maternal/Fetal Risks

The risks to the mother are those of cardiac failure and cor pulmonale in the very few patients with pulmonary hypertension. To develop pulmonary hypertension, the condition has to be severe enough to cause hypoxemia at rest. If vital capacity is less than 1.5 liters, the patient is at risk of respiratory failure, particularly if it is less than 1 liter.[36] The risks to the fetus are intrauterine growth deficiency caused by maternal hypoxemia and preterm delivery,[37] which is often elective because of concern about maternal well-being. Very severe hypoxia in a single patient with kyphoscoliosis (maternal $PaO_2 = 59$ mmHg) has led to brain damage in one fetus.[38]

Management Options

Prepregnancy

Prepregnancy counseling should be given, incorporating the above information. The vital capacity should be measured. If it is greater than 2 liters, there should be no problem; if it is less than 2 liters, then PaO_2 should be estimated. If there is any degree of desaturation, the fetus is at risk of growth deficiency. Also, an estimate of the degree of pulmonary hypertension (if any) should be made. Because of the distortion of the chest, the ECG is particularly poor at estimating

right ventricular hypertrophy in kyphoscoliosis. Therefore, an estimate of the pulmonary circulation should be made by echocardiography, preferably with Doppler ultrasound. Any degree of pulmonary hypertension is a contraindication to pregnancy (see Chapter 20). However, such a drastic recommendation should be based on direct assessment of pulmonary vascular resistance by measurement of pulmonary artery pressure and cardiac output either by formal right-sided cardiac catheterization or using a Swan-Ganz catheter.

Prenatal

Patients who have increased pulmonary vascular resistance, as assessed above, should be offered termination because of the maternal risk. All other patients require optimal medical care directed toward diagnosing and treating respiratory infection and bronchospasm and any cardiac failure. In addition, supplementary domiciliary oxygen therapy to prevent growth deficiency should be considered in those who are hypoxemic. This form of therapy has not been evaluated for this indication; however, it is successful in preventing the development of pulmonary hypertension in non-pregnant patients, and granted the association between growth deficiency and maternal hypoxia, it seems worth pursuing further.

Patients may require admission from about 30 weeks gestation either because of concern about impending respiratory failure or simply because they get so tired.

Obstetric prenatal care relates to detecting intrauterine growth deficiency. Elective preterm delivery may be necessary for maternal reasons, increasing hypoxemia or frank respiratory failure or because of the signs of fetal hypoxia either with or without intrauterine growth deficiency.

Labor/delivery

Many patients with severe kyphoscoliosis are delivered by cesarean section because of associated pelvic deformity. This is better performed with epidural block rather than with general anesthesia. Surprisingly, epidural puncture and catheterization is often possible in these patients. This is because the defect in kyphoscoliosis is often in the upper part of the spine.

Postnatal

No special measures are necessary after delivery apart from a continuation of optimal medical and obstetric care, including early mobilization and physiotherapy.

KYPHOSCOLIOSIS
Summary of Management Options

Prepregnancy

- Counsel regarding risk for increasing pulmonary compromise as pregnancy advances, risks for fetal growth restriction and need for preterm delivery

- Assess pulmonary vital capacity

- Assess for evidence of pulmonary hypertension (unlikely); if present, advise against pregnancy

Prenatal

- Pregnancy termination discussed with pulmonary hypertension

- Early treatment for respiratory infection, bronchospasm and cardiac failure

- Administer supplementary oxygen when hypoxemia present

- In severely compromised patients, begin prenatal surveillance for growth restriction and fetal well-being in early third trimester

- May need early delivery for frank respiratory failure

Labor/delivery

- Supplementary oxygen as needed

- High probability for cesarean section if associated pelvic deformities; attempt conduction anesthesia if possible

Postnatal

- Aggressive pulmonary toilet, especially if cesarean section performed

---

CYSTIC FIBROSIS

This is an autosomal recessive condition. The gene frequency is 1:20, so heterozygotes are common. The incidence is about 1 in 2000 live births. With improved care in childhood, more and more women are surviving to an age at which pregnancy is possible.[39] It is a multisystem disease characterized by impaired cellular secretion. The lungs are most severely affected, and the patient suffers from recurrent pneumonia, bronchitis and bronchospasm. In addition, the pancreas may be affected, leading to malabsorption and diabetes mellitus.

Maternal Risks

If the mother has pulmonary hypertension, she is at risk of heart failure as outlined above under kyphoscoliosis. In addition, women may become emaciated in pregnancy because of the additional nutritional demands of the feto-placental unit. Patients who already have malabsorption are at obvious risk. However, apart from these problems, there is no evidence that pregnancy increases the morbidity or mortality from cystic fibrosis.

Fetal Risks

The fetus is also at risk from intrauterine growth deficiency and iatrogenic preterm delivery, as discussed above under kyphoscoliosis. In addition, the risk of this fetus having cystic fibrosis must be considered. The child will be at least heterozygous and has a considerable risk of being a homozygote in view of the high prevalence of the cystic fibrosis (CF) gene in the community. Unfortunately, because of the polymorphism of the CF gene, reliable tests for the heterozygote are not yet available, nor can prenatal diagnosis exclude cystic fibrosis with complete confidence unless a couple already have an affected child. However, first trimester diagnosis is possible in at least two-thirds of couples presenting with one affected child.[40]

Management Options

Prepregnancy

Prenatal counseling should be given, acting on the above information. As indicated for kyphoscoliosis, the presence of pulmonary vascular disease should be accurately determined if this is to be a reason for precluding or terminating pregnancy. In addition, the couple should be aware that the woman's life-span will be limited and should consider the implications of this for parenting. Although heart and lung transplantation may be possible for some patients with cystic fibrosis, it will not be possible for the majority, if only because of the shortage of donors. Patients who are already significantly malnourished should be warned of the further weakness and emanciation that pregnancy may cause.

Prenatal

The principles of management of patients with cystic fibrosis in pregnancy are also similar to those already discussed under kyphoscolosis: patients with pulmonary hypertension should be offered termination of pregnancy because of the maternal risk.

Patients who are continuing pregnancy require optimal medical care for their respiratory condition. Most patients who survive to become pregnant are giving themselves physiotherapy on a daily basis and they or their partners should be encouraged to continue and increase this treatment. Oral penicillins and cephalosporins should be considered safe in pregnancy, together with inhaled aminoglycoside drugs. Nearly all bronchodilator drugs can be used safely in pregnancy (see 'Asthma' above). There should be no hesitation concerning hospital admission either because of exacerbation of respiratory infection or because of malnutrition. Malnutrition may be the cause of intrauterine growth deficiency, which frequently complicates cystic fibrosis; but this may also be caused by maternal hypoxemia and, as in the case of kyphoscoliosis, there is an unsubstantiated argument for maternal oxygen therapy where the patient has been shown to be hypoxemic.

Intrauterine growth deficiency, decreasing maternal weight and deteriorating respiratory function despite optimal medical treatment in hospital are all indications for preterm delivery, in addition to the usual obstetric reasons.

Labor/delivery

At delivery, the aim should be for a vaginal delivery using epidural rather than opiate analgesia or general anesthesia. Epidural analgesia should also be used electively when there is concern about maternal respiratory function: its efficacy as an analgesic decreases the maternal oxygen requirement. Forceps or vacuum delivery should be considered early in the second stage of labor to avoid or relieve maternal exhaustion.

Postnatal

Most patients with cystic fibrosis should be encouraged to breastfeed, but this is not advisable where maternal nutrition is a problem. Furthermore, if the mother's general health is very poor, bottle-feeding has the advantage that somebody else can do it at night and thus allow the mother to rest. The previous suggestion that breast milk from women with cystic fibrosis has a very high sodium content has not been substantiated.[41,42]

CYSTIC FIBROSIS
Summary of Management Options

Prepregnancy

- Counsel for maternal risks similar to kyphoscoliosis

- Paternal testing for carrier state if available

- Counsel for fetal risks of having cystic fibrosis or being a carrier

Prenatal

- Similar to kyphoscoliosis

Labor/delivery

- Similar to kyphoscoliosis

Postnatal

- Similar to kyphoscoliosis

- Avoid breast-feeding in nutritionally compromised parturient

---

PNEUMONIA

Pneumonia – infection and consolidation of the lung parenchyma – is a rare complication of pregnancy with a general incidence of less than 1%. Indeed, in all but typical cases, the diagnosis should only be made by exclusion since pulmonary infarction due to embolus can mimic pneumonia, and since pulmonary embolism is a leading cause of maternal mortality (see Chapter 33). However, in deprived inner-city areas, the incidence of pneumonia is increasing. At the Sloan Hospital in New York, Berkowitz[43] found that in 1988–89 the incidence was 1:3670 deliveries, compared with 1:2288 deliveries in 1992. The mothers usually had co-existing medical problems including drug abuse, anemia and HIV infection.

Maternal/Fetal Risks

The risks to the fetus are those of miscarriage and pre-term labor; these are non-specific risks associated with any pyrexial illness in pregnancy. In addition, the organism causing pneumonia may present specific risks to the fetus, particularly if it is a virus (e.g. varicella).[44] However, most cases of pneumonia in pregnancy are caused by *Streptococcus pneumoniae* or *Mycoplasma pneumoniae*, which do not affect the fetus. The fetus may also be at risk from maternal conditions which predispose to pneumonia (e.g. HIV infection).

Effective antibiotic therapy has removed the excess maternal risk that pregnancy might have added to bacterial pneumonia. Even though the patients in Berkowitz's series[43] from New York were seriously ill and required aggressive treatment, it is likely that this was because of their other underlying conditions rather than because of pregnancy. However, viral pneumonia is still a worry in pregnancy. Altogether, 10% of maternal varicella infection may be complicated by pneumonia, which can be very severe. In one series, two patients required ventilation and one died.[44] In influenza epidemics, half the cases of maternal mortality have been due to pneumonia,[45] though this has not been a problem recently.

In countries where fungal lung infections are a problem, pregnancy may also be an aggravating factor. In a series of 50 cases of coccidioidmycosis from North America, 22 became disseminated during pregnancy with a maternal mortality of 100% in patients not treated with amphotericin B.[46,47]

Management Options

Prepregnancy

Prepregnancy counseling is not relevant, since pneumonia presents as an acute event without warning.

Prenatal

There should be no hesitation about performing chest radiology in pregnancy for patients who are suspected of having pulmonary disease. The radiation to the fetus is minimal and the likelihood of harm to the fetus from missing a diagnosis such as pneumonia is far greater than the likelihood of harm from radiation.

In patients who present with high fever, purulent sputum, chest pain and clinical and radiological signs of pulmonary consolidation, the diagnosis is not a problem. But patients who only have a modest pyrexia, no sputum and indeterminate physical and radiological signs may well have pulmonary infarction rather than infection. They should be treated for both conditions simultaneously (see Chapter 33) until the diagnosis is

---

PNEUMONIA
Summary of Management Options

Prepregnancy

- None specifically related to pneumonia; in patients with underlying conditions, counsel regarding this possible complication

Prenatal

- Differentiate from other conditions, especially pulmonary embolus

- Use standard techniques for microbiologic assessment

- *Do not avoid* chest x-rays if pulmonary disease suspected

- Begin appropriate antimicrobial therapy based on underlying conditions and presentation; avoid tetracycline therapy in pregnancy

Labor/delivery

- None

Postnatal

- None

best established, usually by radioisotope ventilation perfusion lung scanning.

The treatment of pneumonia in pregnancy is similar to that in non-pregnant patients, except that tetracyclin should not be used in patients suspected of having mycoplasma infection because of its effects on fetal bones and teeth. Patients who present with pneumonia acquired outside hospital should be given penicillin in the first instance. Penicillin-sensitive patients should receive erythromycin, which is also effective in mycoplasma lung infection and Legionnaire's disease. Hospital-acquired infection should be treated with a broad-spectrum antibiotic in the first instance (amoxycillin, cephalosorins, erythromycin) pending the results of microbiological investigations. Ampicillin and amoxycillin dosage should be doubled in pregnancy[15,48] because of increased renal clearance. Patients should receive paracetamol as an antipyretic. Those that are very sick may require assisted ventilation as judged by deteriorating blood gas status.

Because of the high prevalence and morbidity of pneumonia associated with varicella infection in pregnancy, there is a good case for giving parenteral acyclovir to all patients who develop disseminated varicella infection.[49–51] There should be no hesitation in using acyclovir in patients who have varicella pneumonia in pregnancy.[49,52]

REFERENCES

1   de Swiet M (1989) Diseases of the respiratory system. In de Swiet M (ed.) *Medical Disorders in Obstetric Practice*, 2nd edn, Vol. 1, p. 47. Oxford: Blackwell Scientific Publications.

2   Fleming DM, Crombie DL (1987) Prevalence of asthma and hayfever in England and Wales. *British Medical Journal* 294:279–283.

3   Schaefer G, Silverman F (1961) Pregnancy complicated by asthma. *American Journal of Obstetrics and Gynecology* 46:706–715.

4   Greenberger PA (1985) Pregnancy and asthma. *Chest* 87:855–875.

5   Barksy HE (1991) Asthma and pregnancy. *Postgraduate Medicine* 89:125–132.

6   Sims CD, Chamberlain GVP, de Swiet M (1976) Lung function tests in bronchial asthma during and after pregnancy *British Journal of Obstetrics and Gynaecology* 88:434–437.

7   Turner ES, Greenberger PA, Patterson R (1980) Management of the pregnant asthmatic patient. *Annals of Internal Medicine* 6:905–918.

8   Gelber M, Sidid Y, Gassner S, Ovadia Y, Spitzer S, Weinberger A, Pinkhas J (1984) Uncontrollable life-threatening status asthmaticus – an indicator for termination of pregnancy by caesarean section. *Respiration* 46:320–322.

9   Schatz M, Patterson R, Zeitz S (1975) Corticosteroid therapy for the pregnant asthmatic patient. *Journal of the American Medical Association* 233:804–807.

10   Bahna SL, Bjerkedal T (1972) The course and outcome of pregnancy in women with bronchial asthma. *Acta Allergolica* 27:397–400.

11   Sibbald B (1981) A family study approach to the genetic basis of asthma, PhD thesis, University of London.

12   Morrow Brown H, Storey G (1975) Treatment of allergy of the respiratory tract with beclomethasone dipropionate steroid aerosol. *Postgraduate Medical Journal* 51:59–94 (Suppl. 4).

13   Greenberger P, Patterson R (1978) Safety of therapy for allergic symptoms during pregnancy. *Annals of Internal Medicine* 89:234–237.

14   Dykes MHM (1974) Evaluation of an anti asthmatic agent cromolyn sodium (Aarare, Intal). *Journal of the American Medical Association* 277:1061–1062.

15   Rubin PC (1986) Prescribing in pregnancy: General principles. *British Medical Journal of Anaesthesia* 293:1415–1417.

16   Ballard PL, Granberg P, Ballard RA (1975) Glucocorticoid levels in maternal and cord serum after prenatal beclomethasone therapy to prevent respiratory distress. *Journal of Clinical Investigation* 56:1548–1554.

17   Beitins R, Baynoard F, Ances IG, Kowarsk A, Migeon CJ (1972) The transplacental passage of prednisone and prednisolone in pregnancy near term. *Journal of Pediatrics* 81:936–945.

18   Gordon M, Niswander KR, Berendes H, Kantor AG (1970) Fetal morbidity following potentially anoxigenic obstetric conditions. VII. Bronchial asthma. *American Journal of Obstetrics and Gynecology* 106:421–429.

19   Smith AP (1973) The effects of intravenous infusion of graded doses of prostaglandins $F_{2\alpha}$ and E_2 on lung resistance in patients undergoing termination of pregnancy. *Clinical Science* 44:17–25.

20   Grossman JH II, Littner MD (1976) Severe sarcoidosis in pregnancy. *Obstetrics and Gynecology* 50:81–8 (suppl.).

21   Agha FP, Vade A, Amendola MA, Cooper RF (1982) Effects of pregnancy on sarcoidosis. *Surgery, Gynecology and Obstetrics* 155:817–822.

22   Keleman JT, Mandl L (1969) Sarcoidose in der placenta. *Zentralblatt fur Allgemeine Pathologie und Pathologische Anatomie* 281:520–522.

23   Barnes CG (1974) *Medical Disorders in Obstetric Practice*. Oxford: Blackwell Scientific Publications.

24   James DG (1970) Sarcoidosis. *Disease-A-Month* 1:43.

25   Erskine KJ, Taylor KS, Agnew RAL (1985) Serial estimation of serum angiotensin converting enzyme activity during and after pregnancy in a woman with sarcoidosis. *British Medical Journal* 290:269–270.

26   Cohen JD, Patton EA, Badger TL (1952) The tuberculous mother. *American Review of Tuberculosis* 65:1–23.

27   de March P (1975) Tuberculosis and pregnancy: Five-in-ten year review of 215 patients in their fertile age. *Chest* 68:800–804.

28   Kiwanuka A (1984) Carcinoma of the lung complicating pregnancy. *Journal of Obstetrics and Gynecology* 5:103–104.

29   British Medical Association and Royal Pharmaceutical Society of Great Britain (1991) *British National Formulary*, No. 22, p. 210. London: BMA.

30   Snider DE, Layde PM, Johnson MW, Lyle HA (1980)

Treatment of tuberculosis during pregnancy. *American Review of Respiratory Disease* **122**:65–78.

31 Steen JSM, Staintain-Ellis DM (1977) Rifampicin in pregnancy. *Lancet* **ii**:604–605.

32 Conway N, Birt BD (1965) Streptomycin in pregnancy: Effect on the foetal ear. *British Medical Journal* **2**:260–263.

33 Atkins NA (1982) Maternal plasma concentration of pyridoxal phosphate during pregnancy: Adequacy of vitamin B$_6$. Supplementation during isoniazid therapy. *American Review of Respiratory Disease* **126**:714–716.

34 Brummer DL (1972) Letter to the editor. *American Review of Respiratory Disease* **106**:145–185.

35 Gaisford W, Griffiths MI (1961) A freeze-dried vaccine from isoniazid-resistant BCG. *British Medical Journal* **1**:1500–1501.

36 Sawicka EH, Spencer GT, Branthwaite MA (1986) Management of respiratory failure complicating pregnancy in severe kyphoscoliosis: A new use for an old technique? *British Journal of Diseases of the Chest* **80**:191–196.

37 Lao TT, Yeung S, Leung BFH (1986) Kyphoscoliosis and pregnancy. *Journal of Obstetrics and Gynecology* **7**:11–15.

38 Barrett JFR, Dear PRF, Lilford RJ (1991) Brain damage as a result of chronic intrauterine hypoxia in a baby born of a severely kyphoscoliotic mother. *Journal of Obstetrics and Gynecology* **11**:260–261.

39 Matthews LW, Drotar D (1984) Cystic fibrosis – a challenging long term chronic disease. *Pediatric Clinics of North America* **31**:133–152.

40 Super M, Ivinson A, Schwartz M, Giles L, Elles RG, Read AP, Harris R (1987) Clinic experience of prenatal diagnosis of cystic fibrosis by use of linked DNA probes. *Lancet* **ii**:782–784.

41 Whitelaw A, Butterfield A (1977) High breast milk sodium in cystic fibrosis. *Lancet* **ii**:1988.

42 Alpert SE, Cormier AD (1983) Normal electrolyte and protein content in milk from mothers with cystic fibrosis: An explanation for the initial report of elevated milk sodium concentration. *Journal of Pediatrics* **102**:77–80.

43 Berkowitz K, LaSAla A (1990) Risk factors associated with the increasing prevalence of pneumonia during pregnancy. *America Journal of Obstetrics and Gynecology* **163**:981–985.

44 Parayani SG, Arvin AM (1986) Intrauterine infection with varicella-zoster virus after maternal varicella. *New England Journal of Medicine* **314**:1542–1546.

45 Freeman DW, Barno A (1959) Death from Asian influenza associated with pregnancy. *American Journal of Obstetrics and Gynecology* **78**:1172–1175.

46 Harris RE (1966) Coccidiodomycosis complicating pregnancy: Report of three cases and review of the literature. *Obstetrics and Gynecology* **28**:401–405.

47 Moya F, Morishima, HO, Shnider SM, James LS (1975) Influence of maternal hyperventilation on the new born infant. *American Journal of Obstetrics and Gynecology* **91**:76–84.

48 Sangoul F, Fox GS, Houle GL (1975) Effect of regional analgesia on maternal oxygen consumption during the first stage of labor. *American Journal of Obstetrics and Gynecology* **212**:1080.

49 Boyd K, Walker E (1988) Use of acyclovir to treat chickenpox in pregnancy. *British Medical Journal* **296**:393–394.

50 Glaser JB, Loftus J, Ferragamo V, Mootbar H, Castellano M. Varicella-zoster infection in pregnancy. *New England Journal of Medicine* **315**:1416.

51 Haddad J, Simeoni U, Messner J, Willard D (1987) Acyclovir in prophylaxis and perinatal varicella. *Lancet* **i**:161.

52 Cox SM, Cunningham FG, Luby, J (1990) Management of varicella pneumonia complicating pregnancy. *American Journal of Perinatology* **7**: 300–301.

25

Hepatic and Gastrointestinal Disease

BARRY N. J. WALTERS

INTRODUCTION

Disorders of the liver and gastrointestinal tract frequently complicate pregnancy. They may be seen in a maternity hospital or general hospital. There are a number of disorders specific for the gravid individual which are not seen at any other time in life and these are dealt with in this chapter, together with certain pre-existing medical disorders which may complicate the pregnancy. Viral hepatitis is discussed in Chapter 29.

INTRAHEPATIC CHOLESTASIS OF PREGNANCY (See also Chapter 31)

Definition and Incidence

This is an idiopathic condition characterized by cholestasis, which begins in pregnancy and resolves after delivery, and is associated with adverse features for the mother and baby. Pruritus occurring in pregnancy, in the absence of dermatologic abnormalities, is usually due to intrahepatic cholestasis of pregnancy (ICP). The onset of pruritus is usually between 28 and 34 weeks but may be as early as the first trimester.[1,2] Jaundice is not necessary for the diagnosis but follows in more severe cases. Most patients will notice darkening of the urine and often lighter colored stools. The incidence is highly variable,[3] probably reflecting genetic and perhaps geographic or other environmental factors. A prevalence of 1–2 cases per 1000 pregnancies in low-risk populations is exceeded by 10- to 20-fold in others, e.g. the Scandinavian countries, Chile and Poland.

Diagnosis

ICP is suspected at the report of pruritus, usually widespread; severe and distressing for the woman, often pronounced in the palms and soles with hyperhydrosis at those sites (unpublished observation, author). There is bilirubinuria and biochemical analysis shows very high levels (10–100 times normal) of bile acids[4] in all cases, elevated alkaline phosphatase and bilirubin in most, and mild elevations of transaminases in many. The latter (although it may suggest hepatocellular dysfunction) should not detract from the diagnosis of ICP. Hepatitis viral serology, hepatobiliary tract ultrasound and auto-antibody screen (for primary biliary cirrhosis) should be performed in all cases, as these examine valid differential diagnoses.

Maternal/Fetal Risks

For the mother, ICP is not a life-threatening disorder, but it certainly causes considerable suffering through intractable pruritus. It carries a 10–22% risk of obstetric hemorrhage, largely due to hypoprothrombinemia (from vitamin K malabsorption),[1,5,6,7] and of preterm labor.[5] Furthermore, maternal nutritional status may be impaired by steatorrhea.[8] It carries an appreciable risk of present or later cholelithiasis.[6,9,10]

With regard to the fetal prognosis, and given the lack of controlled trials, there is some controversy, views ranging from 'entirely benign'[11] to quite the opposite.[1,5,12] The risks are of stillbirth (up to 15%), fetal distress (up to 25%), preterm delivery (up to 30%)[4,7] and meconium staining of the amniotic fluid (30–40%). The incidence in multiple pregnancy is increased.[4,7] The mechanism of fetal compromise is uncertain, but maternal cholestasis does cause substantial changes in fetal steroid metabolism.[4]

Management Options

Prepregnancy

Preconceptional management is not applicable unless ICP occurred in a previous pregnancy. Then the patient should be counseled about possible recurrence of this condition. Biliary ultrasound should be performed, if not previously done.

Prenatal

The chief aspects of management are monitoring of fetal well-being, timing of delivery, maternal symptom control, vitamin K supplementation and postnatal follow up. It is likely that pruritus alone without biochemical alteration (or with only minimally elevated bile acids) indicates a better prognosis for the fetus than in those cases with frank hepatic enzyme abnormalities.[2,4]

In all but the mildest cases, if pregnancy is to be allowed to progress beyond 37 or 38 weeks, close fetal monitoring is advisable. This should be considered earlier in severe cases, and from 34 to 35 weeks in most, by means of cardiotocography, ultrasound assessment of growth and perhaps Doppler analysis of umbilical artery blood flow. There are those who would deliver electively once fetal lung maturity is demonstrated.[6,13] Estriol levels are likely to be of no value in monitoring as estrogen metabolism is perturbed in ICP.[14]

The pruritus is very resistant to treatment. Cool baths, oatmeal baths and bicarbonate washes often help mild cases. Skin emollients may be useful. Phenol 0.5–1% in aqueous cream with or without menthol 0.5–1% may provide some local relief. Phenobarbitone is traditional but usually ineffective[6] and cholestyramine, while theoretically attractive as a bile acid sequestrant, is similarly disappointing but some have found benefit.[12] Antihistamines may provide slumber and brief respite from the torment.

A recent uncontrolled series of ten cases was treated with oral dexamethasone daily for 10 days. Partial or

---

INTRAHEPATIC CHOLESTASIS OF PREGNANCY
Summary of Management Options

Prepregnancy

- Not applicable, unless diagnosed in previous pregnancy

- Counsel for 40–60% chance of recurrence

Prenatal

- Local antipruritic measures

- Consider cholestyramine

- Vitamin K supplement, both mother and baby

- Monitor fetal well-being

- Consider elective delivery

- Biliary tract ultrasound

Labor/delivery

- Non specific

Postnatal

- Monitor resolution of biochemical parameters

- Use oral contraceptives cautiously

- Consider liver biopsy if diagnosis is suspect, or condition progressive

---

complete relief of pruritus occurred in all cases. At present such treatment remains investigational.[75]

In all cases, particularly after cholestyramine and even when the prothrombin ratio is normal, intramuscular vitamin K 10 mg weekly should be given from 36 weeks. The newborn should also always receive vitamin K.

Postnatal

Prurutis usually subsides within 4–7 days of delivery but may last up to 2 weeks. Biochemical abnormalities may be slower to reverse. In all cases, postnatal biliary tract ultrasound for stones should be performed.

The recurrence rate in future pregnancies is perhaps surprisingly not 100% and is quoted at 40–60%.[4,6] In women who have experienced ICP, the administration of oral contraceptive steroids was often attended by recurrence of liver abnormalities.[15,16] However, these are studies from an epoch when steroid doses were higher than today. Modern combined pills may be considered for women who have had ICP where other contraception is problematic, provided liver enzymes are monitored at reasonable intervals and the medication ceased at the sign of any symptom of pruritus or change in biochemistry. In the occasional case where abnormalities do not resolve after delivery, liver biopsy may need consideration, but this is hardly ever necessary during pregnancy.

ACUTE FATTY LIVER OF PREGNANCY

Definition and Incidence

Acute fatty liver of pregnancy (AFLP) is a rare disorder characterized by microvesicular steatosis on liver histology which is induced by pregnancy, usually appears in the third trimester and may proceed to hepatic failure with maternal and fetal mortality. The incidence is approximately one case in 10 000 pregnancies,[17,18] but may be higher with earlier recognition of the disorder[19] and modern reports of such cases describe a more favorable prognosis.[18–21]

Maternal Risks

The major risk in AFLP is maternal death, which was previously an expected outcome[22] but recently is infrequent.[18–20,23] Death results from hepatic encephalopathy, gastrointestinal or genital tract hemorrhage associated with disseminated intravascular coagulation, and pancreatitis or sepsis.

Early diagnosis is essential for salvage of mother and baby, but because of the severe coagulopathy which is often present, liver biopsy presents unacceptable hazards. Fortunately, the diagnosis may usually be strongly suspected on clinical grounds.[18] Almost all cases present with vomiting in the third trimester. This is accompanied by a systemic illness manifest as malaise, tiredness and abdominal pain for days or weeks followed by jaundice with drowsiness or confusion. With early presentation, most cases will be diagnosed before mental state alteration. Extreme polydipsia or pseudo-diabetes insipidus may be present[18,24,25] and the blood film is often leukemoid[18] or with leukoerythroblastic change.[18,20] Hypoglycemia is frequently present. Biopsy may be performed in the recovery phase. Ultrasound or CT scan may be able to demonstrate fatty infiltration.

Liver enzymes are usually only moderately elevated. There may be renal failure. Hypertension and proteinuria are present in 50%. The uric acid level is often prodigiously elevated.[18]

Fetal Risks

Intrauterine death is the major fetal risk and is frequently observed, although the mortality rate has fallen in recent studies from about 85%[22] to 15–65%.[26] The mechanism of fetal demise is not understood but certainly relates to maternal liver failure, metabolic derangement and probably placental involvement. There may be transient liver abnormalities in the newborn infant and hypoglycemia has been observed.

Management Options

Prepregnancy

This is an acute condition which cannot be predicted prior to pregnancy. The postnatal management section has a discussion of potential recurrence risks.

Prenatal

The first important principle of prenatal management focuses on the diagnosis of this condition. The second overriding principle in the management of this condition is maternal resuscitation and continuous fetal monitoring together with urgent delivery as soon as the diagnosis is made, or even strongly suspected. There is no role for conservative management, but the pathophysiologic derangements must be corrected as rapidly as possible while embarking upon the delivery process.

Labor/delivery

Where possible, more severe cases should be admitted to an intensive care facility during labor, with involvement of a team including a physician, an anesthetist and an obstetrician. Hematologic aspects may also need consultation as vitamin K, fresh frozen plasma, clotting factor replacement, platelet and whole blood transfustion will usually be necessary.[27] The coagulopathy may preclude the use of epidural analgesia and

narcotics may well worsen hepatic encephalopathy, hence pain relief in labor or for cesarean section needs careful consideration. General anesthesia is preferable for cesarean section except in the mildest cases where there is no coagulopathy.

Parenteral glucose will often be necessary, as hypoglycemia is a feature of this disorder.[28] Antacid therapy and histamine receptor blockers will guard against peptic ulceration. Antibiotics should be considered as prophylaxis.

If cesarean delivery is necessary, the wound should be drained in expectation of continued problems with hemostasis after delivery. After vaginal delivery, tears and episiotomy should be sutured by experienced personnel, since vulval hematoma is to be anticipated as is other postpartum hemorrhage.[20] When encephalopathy is present, or worsening jaundice and conscious state, treatment with oral lactulose and neomycin is indicated to clear the bowel and reduce ammonia production by bacteria. Multivitamin supplementation should be given also.

There is no uniformity of opinion concerning the mode of delivery and this will require judgment of the circumstances in each case. Cesarean section may have advantages for the infant but usually the mother is best served by vaginal delivery.

Postnatal

Convalescence may be prolonged after severe disease and postnatal depression is common. Esophageal ulceration may be the precursor of stricture.[18] Liver function steadily returns toward normal and there is no evidence of long-term hepatic compromise as a result of this illness.

Until 1988, there had been only 15 reports of pregnancy following a gestation afflicted by AFLP.[18] In none of these had the disorder recurred. However, there is a single report of death from AFLP in a subsequent pregnancy in a woman who had an undiagnosed hepatic illness in the first pregnancy.[29] There is no evidence that the oral contraceptive pill is contraindicated in these women, but liver function tests should be kept under surveillance.

THE LIVER IN HYPEREMESIS GRAVIDARUM

Definition and Incidence

Nausea and vomiting are such common untoward symptoms of early pregnancy that they have been used as diagnostic features. Nevertheless, vomiting severe enough to require hospital admission afflicts only

---

ACUTE FATTY LIVER OF PREGNANCY
Summary of Management Options

Prepregnancy

- None, except discussion of recurrence risks (see 'Postnatal')

Prenatal

- Establish diagnosis, supportive care and plan delivery

Labor/delivery

- Maternal resuscitation by correction of coagulopathy, hypoglycemia and fluid imbalance
- Treatment of liver failure
- Intense fetal monitoring
- Urgent delivery when maternal condition is stabilized, although vaginal delivery preferable
- Meticulous hemostasis, including adequate wound drainage

Postnatal

- Continue intensive care management
- Watch for postpartum hemorrhage, wound hematoma formation and sepsis
- Recurrence risks difficult to estimate (?1:15–20)

3–10 women per 1000 and this serves as a functional definition of hyperemesis gravidarum.

Maternal Risks

Hyperemesis is often accompanied by dehydration, electrolyte disturbance, protein-calorie malnutrition and vitamin deficiency. In more severe cases, biochemical evidence of liver dysfunction, and even jaundice, are seen in 30–50%.[30,31]

Hyperemesis should be a diagnosis of exclusion. It is mimicked by many intra-abdominal problems, by enteric infections, hepatitis, hypercalcemia, pseudotumor cerebri and, commonly, reflux esophagitis among other medical disorders. The diagnosis should be made only with great circumspection beyond 18 weeks as it is likely to be incorrect. In the third trimester, it is virtually always erroneous and the cause of vomiting may be a serious complication such as acute fatty liver.

Flexible endoscopy is very valuable and carries no excess risk in pregnancy.

Fetal Risks

Other than those that occur as a consequence of maternal compromise, no specific risks to the fetus are identified.

Management Options

Prepregnancy

Given the relatively common nature of this affliction, women contemplating pregnancy should be told of this potential problem. Most can be reassured as to the self limiting nature of hyperemesis gravidarum.

Prenatal

The cause of the liver dysfunction is unknown, though it shares features with the liver changes in kwashiorkor from protein malnutrition. Intravenous fluid and electrolyte replacement is essential. Rest, reassurance (often from an ultrasound examination) and encouragement are combined with a drug regimen including antiemetics such as meclozine, promethazine and metoclopramide. These have no known adverse fetal effects. Transdermal scopolamine may be essayed also.

Attempts at early discharge are doomed, although home visits by medical or nursing staff are valuable. Vitamin supplementation is usually advisable and should always include thiamine, since Wernicke's

encephalopathy is known to complicate severe hyperemesis in some cases.[32]

Gastroesophageal reflux is almost always present, commencing in the first trimester. Antireflux measures including elevation of the bed head, frequent small meals, alginates and metoclopramide should be employed. When severe esophagitis has been revealed by endoscopy, omeprazole should be considered, although information about its safety in pregnancy is still forthcoming.

Unfortunately, vomiting often recurs in subsequent pregnancies. Happily, the prognosis for the fetus is not different from that in normal pregnancy.

THE LIVER IN HYPEREMESIS GRAVIDARIUM
Summary of Management Options

Prepregnancy

- None

Prenatal

- Consider alternative diagnoses

- Intravenous fluid and electrolyte therapy

- Antiemetic regimen

- Vitamin supplementation

- Anti-gastroesophageal reflux measures

Labor/delivery

- None

Postnatal

- None

Labor/delivery and postnatal

Hyperemesis gravidarum has no implications for the labor and delivery process, nor the postnatal period.

THE LIVER IN PRE-ECLAMPSISA
(See also Chapter 18)

Definition and Incidence

In severe pre-eclampsia, the liver is often involved and such cases number 5–20 per 1000 confinements. The hepatic lesion may be clinically silent but biochemically manifest[26] or cliniclally overt, the patient usually presenting with a characteristic symptom of severe epigastric or low substernal pain which has been termed 'pre-eclamptic angina'.[33] This seems to correspond to focal hepatic hemorrhage or infarction.[26] In those instances, hematologic abnormalities are also present, consisting of microangiopathic hemolysis and thrombocytopenia, or the 'HELLP' (Hemolysis, Elevated Liver enzymes, Low Platelets) syndrome.[34,35] This is a varient of pre-eclampsia in which severe hypertension is not always present. It is more often seen in pre-eclampsia of early onset, before 34 weeks, but may be present at any gestation.

Maternal/Fetal Risks

Hepatic involvement marks pre-eclampsia as severe. Jaundice may also be present. The maternal risks are all those accompanying pre-eclampsia (see Chapter 18), in particular, coagulopathy and hepatic hemorrhage or rupture.

For the fetus, intrauterine growth deficiency is often present. Fetal distress in labor is very common and cesarean delivery will usually prove necessary. Placental abruption is to be anticipated in these cases. The remaining fetal risks are those of preterm gestation and low birthweight. In the neonatal period, these babies often show signs of asphyxia and may be born with acidosis.

Management Options

Prepregnancy

Liver disease complicating pre-eclampsia is a condition that is not predictable prior to pregnancy.

Prenatal

It may be difficult to distinguish these cases from AFLP,[36] but the management is very similar. For the fetus, intensive monitoring of well-being is essential. Resuscitation of the mother involves, first, strict control of hypertension and also often includes anticonvulsant therapy (see Chapter 18). Correction of coagulopathy as mentioned above (see 'AFLP') is also necessary. Plasma volume expansion has its advocates,[37] but carries the risk of pulmonary edema. Invasive hemodynamic monitoring may be employed in an intensive care setting but there are no controlled trials to support such aggressive management. However, such measures are palliative and when there is symptomatic liver involvement with pre-eclampsia, the chance of catastrophic maternal or fetal complications is sufficiently great to make prompt termination of the pregnancy by delivery the treatment of choice.

Labor/delivery

The mode of delivery is determined by individual circumstances, but cesarean section will prove necessary in 50–70% of cases. Blood should be available as bleeding complications are frequent.

THE LIVER IN PRE-ECLAMPSIA
Summary of Management Options

Prepregnancy

- None

Prenatal and labor/delivery

- Control of hypertension

- Correct coagulation disturbance

- Consider anticonvulsant prophylaxis

- Close fetal monitoring

- Initiate delivery process

Postnatal

- Anticipate delayed postnatal recovery

Postnatal

Pre-eclampsia will often worsen after delivery for 24–48 h. Full therapy should therefore be maintained during that time. Oliguria is usual and careful fluid management is necessary. Rarely, pre-eclamptic liver disease and coagulopathy will worsen after delivery and there are anecdotal reports of the use of plasmapheresis in this situation, but such therapy is at present experimental.[38] There is no evidence of any lasting hepatic damage from this disorder. Future pregnancies should be closely monitored. Postnatal investigation should include urinalysis, renal ultrasound and autoantibody screen including anti-cardiolipin antibody.

PEPTIC ULCERATION IN PREGNANCY

Incidence

All observers note a remarkable decrease in the frequency of diagnosis of peptic ulceration during pregnancy. The incidence of ulcer complications in those known to harbor or who have been treated for peptic ulceration is also very much reduced. Only six cases of active ulceration were detected in more than 22 000 pregnancies[39] and 90% of 118 women with proven ulceration before pregnancy improved or lost their symptoms during pregnancy.[40] This happy expectation does not, however, imply that *de novo* ulceration and ulcer complications cannot occur in pregnancy.

The reduction in ulcer activity in the pregnant state may be related to increased medical supervision, attention to diet, cessation of cigarette smoking and alcohol intake, or to postulated hormonal or other changes inherent in pregnancy. The other possibility is that ascertainment of the diagnosis is incomplete as there is no doubt that pregnant women are less likely to be investigated for gastrointestinal symptoms. Such symptoms are often attributed to 'morning sickness', uterine contractions or other aberrations of the gravid state.

Maternal Risks

A major risk is the possibility of undiagnosed ulceration. In those with suggestive symptoms, fibre-optic endoscopy of the upper gastrointestinal tract undertaken with due care and consideration of the pregnant state is an invaluable procedure and may be carried out without any added risk in the pregnant woman. Certainly, barium studies are not a valid alternative in pregnancy.

The same risks of peptic ulceration apply as in the non-pregnant individual. Perforation, hemorrhage or obstruction may all occur and have been reported before delivery and in the puerperium.[39,41–43]

There is at least a theoretical expectation of maternal risk accompanying administration of high-dose steroids for fetal lung maturation to the woman with a history of peptic ulceration. While cases confirming this have not been published, the prohibition should be respected as these are potentially life-threatening complications. Either steroid treatment should not be given, or an alternative such as thyrotrophin-releasing hormone can be administered for fetal lung maturation.

Management Options

Prepregnancy

In those with past or active ulceration, advice to cease cigarette and alcohol intake prior to pregnancy is even more pertinent than in the normal woman. It may be necessary to avoid the administration of iron to avert gastric irritation. Also, women with known disease can be offered the expectation of a reduction in symptoms during pregnancy.

Prenatal

During pregnancy, many women with mild symptoms of gastroesophageal reflux respond readily to antireflux measures such as alginates, elevation of the head of the bed, small frequent meals, and avoidance of precipitants. In those with previous ulceration using H_2 receptor antagonists, the therapy should be continued in pregnancy if ulcer recurrence has been a problem in the past. While ranitidine and cimetidine have not been given unconditional approval for pregnancy,[44] there is no evidence so far of danger, particularly in a low nocturnal suppressive dose.

Where ulceration is newly diagnosed in pregnancy, either non-absorbable antacids or H_2 receptor blockers should be used in appropriate dosage as the risks of inadequate treatment outweigh any potential hazards to the fetus, none having thus far been demonstrated. There is a theoretical concern regarding the anti-androgenic effect of cimetidine if administered to a woman bearing a male fetus, but such effects have not been described in this situation. Antacids are still the treatment of choice for proven peptic ulceration in pregnant women. Of course, constipation from aluminum preparations and diarrhea with magnesium-containing agents may need attention in their own right.

Helicobacter pylori is a spiral organism present in 85–100% of cases of duodenal ulcer and up to 80% of cases of gastric ulcer.[45] It has been found that the relapse rate after H_2 blocker treatment is high when such treatment is not combined with eradication of helicobacter.[46,47] Eradication, however, is difficult and requires triple antibiotic therapy combining a bismuth preparation with amoxycillin and metronidazole given concurrently for 2 weeks. The place and safety of such therapy in pregnancy has not been established. Even so, anti-helicobacter therapy should be considered in pregnancy in those with proven duodenal ulcer where the organism has been identified and in whom surgery is being considered, H_2 antagonists have been ineffective, or where bleeding has occurred despite such therapy.

The indications for surgery of peptic ulcer complications in pregnancy are the same as in non-pregnant individuals and there is no increased mortality for the mother.[48] In the third trimester, however, close fetal monitoring is necessary as the state of fetal well-being may well be impaired by the illness leading to surgery or other events surrounding the surgery and anesthetic process.[48]

Labor/delivery

There are no specific management recommendations for peptic ulcer disease at the time of delivery. Maintenance medications should be continued.

Postnatal

There is some suggestion that ulcer symptoms and complications may be exacerbated in the puerperium.[40–42] Therapy should not be discontinued. Cimetidine and ranitidine, as well as crossing the placenta, are both concentrated in breast milk,[48] but the dose received by the suckling infant has not been associated with any adverse effects. The use of gastrointestinal drugs during pregnancy and lactation is reviewed by Lewis and Weingold.[44]

PEPTIC ULCERATION IN PREGNANCY
Summary of Management Options

Prepregnancy

- Discontinue agents which may exacerbate peptic ulcer disease (e.g. alcohol, smoking)

- Anticipate improvement in clinical symptoms with pregnancy

Prenatal

- Adequate endoscopic investigation

  Antacids or histamine receptor blockers

  Consider anti-helicobacter treatment

Labor/delivery

- None

Postnatal

- None

CELIAC DISEASE IN PREGNANCY

Definition and Incidence

In celiac disease, structural damage to the small intestinal mucosa leads to malabsorption of nutrients subsequent to mucosal villous atrophy. This results from sensitivity to dietary gluten, a protein component of wheat and other cereal grains. The disease presents often in childhood with features of malabsorption but may appear at any age. The classic presenting features are malaise, diarrhea and wasting, but less typical presentations are often seen. These include macrocytic anemia due to folate deficiency, other nutritional deficiency states, osteomalacia from vitamin D deficiency or even recurrent miscarriage.[49]

The mainstay of treatment is lifelong rigid adherence to a gluten-free diet without which response will be inadequate. The disease afflicts at least one per 3000 of the population in Western nations.

Maternal/Fetal Risks

The average age at menarche was normal in an early study[50] but delayed by 1–2 years in a recent series,[51] although with good childhood control this should not be the case. Fertility is usually not impaired in adequately treated individuals,[52] but infertility has been reported when the disease was not diagnosed or incompletely controlled,[51,53] and in the latter series 40% of women experienced amenorrhea. Recurrent miscarriage is also considered a possible consequence of this disorder.[51,52] A retrospective review suggested that the miscarriage rate was 4% in 22 pregnancies after treatment, much lower than the 21% rate before treatment[52] in 38 pregnancies of the same women. Others report similar findings.[54]

The risks for the mother and fetus with well-controlled celiac disease in a well-nourished woman are not different from those of the population as a whole. Successful outcome was 86% in a series of 22 treated pregnancies,[52] although with a slight excess of growth-deficient infants (4 of 22 babies). Of two stillbirths, one was anencephalic.

In the undiagnosed parturient, or when malabsorption is not corrected, the risks are of megaloblastic anemia due to folic acid deficiency,[55,56] neural tube defect due to the same deficiency[57] and perhaps zinc deficiency[58] and iron deficiency. Osteomalacia due to an inadequate supply of vitamin D and calcium may result from malabsorption in pregnancy[59] and babies are at risk of neonatal hypocalcemia after such gestations.

Management Options

Prepregnancy

Management ideally commences before conception with close dietary regulation and review by a physician and dietitian in collaboration with an obstetrician. Prepregnancy folic acid supplementation is mandatory in those women who are at great risk of folate deficiency. This recommendation originates in a recent controlled study of folic acid supplementation in women whose previous pregnancy was affected by a fetus with neural tube defect.[60] Together with strict dietary compliance, supplementation with calcium, iron, folic acid, vitamin B_{12} and B complex vitamins is necessary. Blood levels should be estimated before pregnancy and at 4–8 week intervals as the levels of many nutrients will decline as gestation proceeds.

Prenatal

An oral folate dosage of at least 5 mg daily is appropriate, even though the recommended daily allowance for normal pregnant women is only 10% of that. Vitamin D adequacy is assessed by levels of 25-hydroxychole-calciferol. The World Health Organization recommended daily allowance is 400 IU per day of ergocalciferol, but more may be necessary where intestinal absorption is abnormal. Vitamin K malabsorption may lead to coagulation disturbance during or after delivery and the baby may share coagulopathy. The prothrom-

bin ratio should be assessed at 36 weeks and treated, if necessary, with intramuscular or oral vitamin K.

Except for the mildest of cases with no evidence of malabsorption, the administration of B group vitamins by the intramuscular route is advisable at intervals of not greater than 4 weeks during the pregnancy. Iron should be administered to all women and, if not tolerated by mouth, parenteral replacement should be considered. Maternal weight, hemoglobin, ferritin and other nutrient levels should be assessed regularly.

In a small proportion of cases, malabsorption is not corrected by the gluten-free diet. Intercurrent infection, jejunal ulceration and lactase deficiency are possible and steroid therapy may be necessary. All women

---

CELIAC DISEASE IN PREGNANCY
Summary of Management Options

Prepregnancy

- Pre-conception counseling and control

Prenatal

- Careful dietary surveillance

- Folic acid supplement

- Monitor and replace vitamins, minerals and nutritional status

- Give iron

- Monitor fetal growth

Labor/delivery

- None

Postnatal

- Monitor nutritional and vitamin status, in particular if breast-feeding is undertaken

should be offered serum alpha-fetoprotein screening and fetal ultrasound for neural tube defect. Serial ultrasound scanning for fetal growth is advisable in any pregnancy where maternal nutrition is suspect.

Labor/delivery

There are no specific recommendations for the delivery process.

Postnatal

In the puerperium, appropriate diet must be maintained with monitoring. In particular, attention should be given to calcium and vitamin D as lactation presents a challenge to calcium homeostasis. Babies born to mothers with celiac disease may need supplementation with vitamin B_{12}, folic acid or other vitamins, but this should not be necessary if antepartum control has been ideal. Many normal women experience profound weight loss during lactation. The woman with celiac disease is all the more at risk of this and warrants observation during this time with continued nutritional supplements.

INFLAMMATORY BOWEL DISEASE IN PREGNANCY

Definition and Incidence

Inflammatory bowel disease herein refers to Crohn's disease (CD) and ulcerative colitis (UC). The incidence of CD in Western countries is between 1 and 4 per 100 000 population and onset is usually during reproductive life. Fistula formation often leads to malabsorption. UC is more common, its prevalence being approximately 6 per 10 000 population.

Maternal and Fetal Risks

Fertility is dependent on general physical condition; the woman with severe active inflammatory bowel disease who is underweight and malnourished may well be amenorrheic and infertile. In large studies, however, such cases are few and usually do not influence the general conclusions. In particular, fertility was normal in a survey of 256 women with UC over a 20-year period, only 7% reporting unwanted infertility.[61] Earlier suggestions of reduced fertility may be attributed to less adequate control of the disease in those years. However, in CD, several studies concur that fertility is reduced,[62-64] with up to 65% being unable to conceive, particularly those with Crohn's colitis or active dis-

ease.[65] This may relate to poor general health and nutritional factors or to local factors such as tubal adhesions subsequent to inflammation. The matter is reviewed by Gennuso.[66]

The present consensus is that the chance of a full-term normal delivery for women with IBD is the same as that of normal women, with 80–90% generally quoted.[61,67,68] A miscarriage rate of 7–15% is usual with the proviso that active disease at conception nearly doubles the miscarriage rate for both UC[61,68] and CD.[69,70]

The rate of preterm birth was not increased in early studies, but in a recent controlled study,[71] 16% of patients delivered preterm compared with only 6% of controls, supporting previous evidence that prematurity is increased with disease activity during gestation.[65,69]

Numerous studies have failed to identify any adverse effects of systemic or colonic steroid therapy or of sulfasalazine[66,72] in pregnancy or lactation, despite the theoretical consideration that sulfasalazine may interfere with bilirubin metabolism in the newborn.

The risk of a flare of CD is not altered by pregnancy[69,73] and UC behaves in a similar fashion.[61] Notwithstanding this, active disease in early pregnancy is more likely to be followed by a flare later or in the puerperium.[61] Furthermore, severe relapses of UC are not ameliorated by termination of pregnancy[61] and energetic drug or other treatment is required along usual lines.[74] Surgery is rarely necessary during pregnancy and is reserved for major complications of IBD such as toxic megacolon. It is hazardous for the baby and may precipitate preterm labor. The presence of an old or recent stoma does not preclude normal vaginal delivery.[61,67]

Relapses tend to occur in the first trimester and should be investigated, as usual, with flexible colonoscopy.

Management Options

Prepregnancy

Preconception counseling is ideal, giving an opportunity to optimize therapy, nutritional status, and to suggest contraception if the disease is active. Folic acid supplementation should begin with vitamin B_{12} if the terminal ileum is involved. The treatment of malabsorption, considered in this chapter already, is pertinent to patients with fistulas or after resection.

Prenatal

In the prenatal period, usual therapy is continued with reassurance to the mother concerning its safety, otherwise, a number of women will wish to cease their medication. Iron should be administered unless it exacerbates bowel symptoms. The involvement of a gastroenterologist is highly advisable when IBD is active, for example with bloody diarrhea, pain or inadequate weight gain. Bowel sedatives and opiates should be avoided where possible[44,74] and this is often possible as the reduced colonic motility of pregnancy improves diarrhea. Constipation is to be avoided by fluids, a high fiber diet and bulking agents except in those with strictures. Monitoring of fetal growth by ultrasound is advisable.

Labor/delivery

Given the potential for severe perineal disease and scarring, if an operative delivery is necessary, one should anticipate a more complicated procedure. A meticulous surgical approach is needed to avoid additional postoperative complications. Intraoperative consultation with a general surgeon may be needed during cesarian section.

Postnatal

After delivery, continued attention to nutrition, drug therapy and maternal condition is important. Breast-feeding is not contraindicated but should be reviewed where the nursing mother is failing to thrive. Oral contraception may be ineffective when there is diarrhea or malabsorption and, at those times, barrier methods or alternative family planning strategies should be added. Both before and after delivery, hematinics should be given and nutritional status monitored, as for coeliac disease.

INFLAMMATORY BOWEL DISEASE IN PREGNANCY
Summary of Management Options

Prepregnancy

- Preconception counseling and control

Prenatal

- Continue usual drug therapy prenatally

- Attention to nutrition, iron and folate supplementation

- Monitor fetal growth

Labor/delivery

- If operative delivery needed, anticipate adhesional problems

Postnatal

- Oral contraceptives may be ineffective if severe diarrhea and malabosorption is present; consider alternative contraceptives

---

REFERENCES

1 Qiu Z, Wang Q, Liu Y, Miao H (1983) Intrahepatic cholestasis of pregnancy: Clinical analysis and follow-up study of 22 cases. *Chinese Medical Journal* **96**:902–906.

2 Berg B, Helm G, Petersohn L, Tryding N (1986) Cholestasis of pregnancy: Clinical and laboratory studies: *Acta Obstetrica et Gynecologica Scandinavica* **65**:107–113.

3 Reyes H (1982) The enigma of intrahepatic cholestasis of pregnancy: Lessons from Chile. *Hepatology* **2**:87–96.

4 Laatikainen T, Tulenheimo A (1984) Maternal serum bile acid levels and fetal distress in cholestasis of pregnancy. *International Journal of Gynaecology and Obstetrics* **22**:91–94.

5 Reid R, Ivey KJ, Rencoret RH, Storey B (1976) Fetal complications of obstetric cholestasis. *British Medical Journal* **1**:870–872.

6 Shaw D, Frolich J, Wittmann BA, Willms M (1982) A prospective study of 18 patients with cholestasis of pregnancy. *American Journal of Obstetrics and Gynecology* **142**:621–625.

7 Johnston WG, Baskett TF (1979) Obstetric cholestasis: A 14 year review. *American Journal of Obstetrics and Gynecology* **133**:299–301.

8 Roszkowski I, Miedzinska DP (1968) Jaundice in pregnancy II. Clinical course of pregnancy and delivery and condition of the neonate. *American Journal of Obstetrics and Gynecology* **101**:500–503.

9 Furhoff AK (1974) Itching in pregnancy: A 15 year followup study. *Acta Medica Scandinavica* **196**:403–410.

10 Samsioe G, Svendsen P, Johnson P *et al.* (1975) Studies in cholestasis of pregnancy V. *Acta Obstetrica et Gynecologica Scandinavica* **54**:417–423.

11 Haemmerli UP, Wyss HI (1967) Recurrent intrahepatic cholestasis of pregnancy: Report of six cases and review of the literature. *Medicine (Baltimore)* **46**:299–321.

12 Wilson BR, Haverkamp AD (1979) Cholestatic jaundice

of pregnancy: new perspectives. *Obstetrics and Gynecology* **54**:650–652.

13 Fisk NM, Storey GN (1988) Fetal outcome in obstetric cholestasis. *British Journal of Obstetrics and Gynaecology* **95**:1137–1143.

14 Tikkanen MJ, Adlercreutz H (1973) Recurrent jaundice in pregnancy. III. Quantitative determination of urinary estriol conjugates, including studies in pruritus gravidarum. *American Journal of Medicine* **54**:600–604.

15 Orellana-Alcalde JM, Dominguez JP (1966) Jaundice and oral contraceptive drugs. *Lancet* **ii**:1276–1280.

16 Ockner RK, Davidson CS (1967) Hepatic effects of oral contraceptives. *New England Journal of Medicine* **276**:331–334.

17 Kaplan MM (1985) Acute fatty liver of pregnancy. *New England Journal of Medicine* **313**:367–370.

18 Purdie JM, Walters BN (1988) Acute fatty liver of pregnancy: Clinical features and diagnosis: *Australian and New Zealand Journal of Obstetrics and Gynaecology* **28**:62–67.

19 Riely CA, Latham PS, Romero R, Duffy TP (1987) Acute fatty liver of pregnancy: A reassessment based on observations in nine patients. *Annals of Internal Medicine* **106**:703–706.

20 Burroughs AK, Seog NH, Dojcinov DM *et al.* (1982) Acute fatty liver of pregnancy in twelve patients: *Quarterly Journal of Medicine* **204**:481–497.

21 Hague WM, Fenton DW, Duncan SL, Slater DN (1983) Acute fatty liver of pregnancy. *Journal of the Royal Society of Medicine* **76**:652–661.

22 Varner M, Rinderknectht NK (1980) Acute fatty metamorphosis of pregnancy: A maternal mortality and literature review. *Journal of Reproductive Medicine* **24**:177–180.

23 Rolfes DB, Ishak KG (1985) Acute fatty liver of pregnancy: A clinicopathologic study of 35 cases. *Hepatology* **5**:1149–1158.

24 Mizuno O (1987) Transient nephrogenic diabetes insipidus associated with acute hepatic failure in pregnancy. *Endocrinologica Japonica* **34**:449–455.

25 Cammu H, Velkeniers B, Charels K *et al.* (1987) Idiopatic acute fatty liver of pregnancy associated with transient diabetes insipidus: Case report. *British Journal of Obstetrics and Gynaecology* **94**:173–178.

26 Rolfes DB, Ishak KG (1986) Liver disease in pregnancy. *Histopathology* **10**:555–570.

27 Pockros PJ, Peters RL, Reynolds RB (1984) Idiopathic fatty liver of pregnancy: Findings in ten cases. *Medicine (Baltimore)* **63**:1–11.

28 Davies MH, Wilkinson SP, Hanid MA *et al.* (1980) Acute liver disease with encephalopathy and renal failure in late pregnancy and the early puerperium: A study of fourteen patients. *British Journal of Obstetrics and Gynaecology* **87**:1005–1014.

29 Wood EE (1970) A case of acute fatty liver of pregnancy. *Journal of Obstetrics and Gynaecology of the British Commonwealth* **77**:337–342.

30 Adams RH, Gordon J, Combes B *et al.* (1968) Hyperemesis gravidarum: I. Evidence of hepatic dysfunction. *Obstetrics and Gynecology* **31**:659–664.

31 Larrey D, Rueff B, Feldmann G *et al.* (1984) Recurrent jaundice caused by recurrent hyperemesis gravidarium. *Gut* **25**:1414–1415.

32 Wood P, Murray A, Sinha B *et al.* (1983) Wernicke's encephalopathy induced by hyperemesis gravidarium. *British Journal of Obstetrics and Gynaecology* **90**:583–586.

33 Walters BN, Walters T (1991) Pre-eclamptic angina: A characteristic symptom of severe pre-eclampsia. *Clinical and Experimental Hypertension Part B. Hypertension in Pregnancy* **B10**:271.

34 Pitchard JA, Weisman R, Ratnoff OD, Vosburgh GJ (1954) Intravascular hemolysis, thrombocytopenia and other hematologic abnormalities associated with severe toxemia of pregnancy. *New England Journal of Medicine* **250**:89–96.

35 Weinstein L (1982) Syndrome of hemolysis, elevated liver enzymes, and low platelet count: A severe consequence of hypertension in pregnancy. *American Journal of Obstetrics and Gynecology* **142**:159–167.

36 de Swiet M (1985) Some rare medical complications of pregnancy (Editorial). *British Medical Journal* **290**:2–4.

37 Goodlin RC, Holdt D (1981) Impending gestosis. *Obstetrics and Gynecology* **58**:743–745.

38 Schwartz ML (1986) Possible role for exchange plasmapheresis with fresh frozen plasma for maternal indications in selected cases of preeclampsia and eclampsia. *Obstetrics and Gynecology* **67**:136–139.

39 Baird RM (1966) Peptic ulceration in pregnancy: Report of a case with perforation. *Canadian Medical Association Journal* **94**:861–862.

40 Clark DK (1953) Pregnancy and peptic ulcer in women. *British Medical Journal* **1**:1254–1257.

41 Jones PF, McEwen AB, Bernard RM *et al.* (1969) Haemorrhage and perforation complicating peptic ulcer in pregnancy. *Lancet* **ii**:350–351.

42 Parry GK (1974) Perforated duodenal ulcer in the puerperium. *New Zealand Medical Journal* **80**:448–449.

43 Sandweiss DJ, Podolsky HM, Saltzstein HC, Farbman AA (1943) Deaths from perforation and hemorrhage of gastroduodenal ulcer during pregnancy and puerperium. *American Journal of Obstetrics and Gynecology* **45**:131–136.

44 Lewis JH, Weingold AB (1985) The use of gastrointestinal drugs during pregnancy and lactation. *American Journal of Gastroenterology* **80**:912–923.

45 Tytgat GN, Axon AT, Dixon MF *et al.* (1991) *Helicobacter pylori*: Causal agent in peptic ulcer disease? *Journal of Gastroenterology and Hepatology* **6**:102–140.

46 Rauws EA, Titgat GN (1990) Cure of duodenal ulcer associated with eradication of *Helicobacter pylori*. *Lancet* **335**:1233–1235.

47 Blum AL, Armstrong D, Dammann H *et al.* (1991) The effect of *H. pylori* on the healing and relapse of duodenal ulcer. *Gastroenterology* **98**:A22.

48 Becker-Andersen H, Husfeldt V (1971) Peptic ulcer in pregnancy: Report of two cases of surgically treated bleeding duodenal ulcer. *Acta Obstetrica et Gyencologica Scandinavica* **50**:391–395.

49 Joske RA, Martin JD (1971) Coeliac disease presenting as recurrent abortion. *Journal of Obstetrics and Gynaecology of the British Commonwealth* **79**:754–758.

50 Cooke WT, Peeney AL, Hawkins CF (1953) Symptoms, signs, and diagnostic features of idiopathic steatorrhoea. *Quarterly Journal of Medicine* **22**:59–77.

51 Molteni N, Bardella MT, Bianchi PA (1990) Obstetric and gynecological problems in women with untreated celiac sprue. *Journal of Clinical Gastroenterology* **12**:37–39.

52 Ogborn AD (1975) Pregnancy in patients with celiac disease. *British Journal of Obstetrics and and Gynaecology* **82**:293–296.

53 Morris JD, Adjukiewicz AB, Read AE (1970) Coelic infertility: An indication for dietary gluten restriction. *Lancet* **i**:213–214.

54 Green PA, Wollaeger EE (1960) The clinical behavior of sprue in the United States. *Gastroenterology* **38**:399–418.

55 Ek B (1967) On the familial incidence of idiopathic sprue and the significance of pregnancy and partial gastrectomy for the manifestation of the symptoms. *Acta Medica Scandinavica* **181**:125–126.

56 Chanarin I (1979) Megaloblastic anemia in pregnancy. In *The Megaloblastic Anemias*, 2nd edn. Oxford: Blackwell Scientific Publications.

57 Hibbard ED, Smithells RW (1965) Folic acid metabolism and human embryopathy. *Lancet* **i**:1254.

58 Prasad AS (1983) Zinc deficiency in human subjects *Progress in Clinical and Biological Research* **129**:1–33.

59 Walters BN, de Swiet M (1989) Gastrointestinal and hepatic osteomalacia. In de Swiet M (ed.) *Medical Disorders in Obstetric Practice*, pp. 706–707. Oxford: Blackwell Scientific Publications.

60 MRC Vitamin Study Research Group (1991) Prevention of neural tube defects: Results of the Medical Research Council vitamin study. *Lancet* **338**:131–137.

61 Willoughby CP, Truelove SC (1980) Ulcerative colitis and pregnancy. *Gut* **21**:469–474.

62 Fielding JF, Cooke WT (1970) Pregnancy and Crohn's disease. *British Medical Journal* **2**:76–77.

63 De Dombal FT, Burton IL, Goligher JC (1972) Crohn's disease and pregnancy. *British Medical Journal* **3**:550–553.

64 Homan WP, Thorbjarnarson B (1976) Crohn's disease and pregnancy. *Archives of Surgery* **111**:545–547.

65 Korelitz BI (1985) Pregnancy, fertility, and inflammatory bowel disease. *American Journal of Gastroenterology* **80**:365–370.

66 Gennuso R (1985) Crohn's disease and pregnancy: A literature study. *Mount Sinai Journal of Medicine* **52**:398–403.

67 Donaldson RM (1985) Management of medical problems in pregnancy – inflammatory bowel disease. *New England Journal of Medicine* **312**:1616–1619.

68 Nielsen OH, Andreasson B, Bondesen S, Jarnum S (1983) Pregnancy in ulcerative colitis. *Scandinavian Journal of Gastroenterology* **18**:735–742.

69 Nielsen OH, Andreasson B, Bondesen S (1984) Pregnancy in Crohn's disease. *Scandinavian Journal of Gastroenterology* **19**:724–729.

70 Khosla R, Willoughby CP, Jewell DP (1984) Crohn's disease and pregnancy. *Gut* **25**:52–56.

71 Fedorkow DM, Persaud D, Nimrod CA (1989) Inflammatory bowel disease: A controlled study of late pregnancy outcome. *American Journal of Obstetrics and Gynecology* **160**:998–10170.

72 Mogadam M, Dobbins WO, Korelitz BI, Ahmed SW (1981) Pregnancy in inflammatory bowel disease: Effect of sulfasalazine and corticosteroids on fetal outcome. *Gastroenterology* **80**:72–76.

73 Norton RA, Patterson JF (1972) Pregnancy and regional enteritis. *Obstetrics and Gynecology* **40**:711–712.

74 Fagan EA (1989) Disorders of the gastrointestinal tract. In de Swiet M (ed.) *Medical Disorders in Obstetric Practice*, pp. 550–555. Oxford: Blackwell Scientific Publications.

75 Hirvioja ML, Tuimala R, Vuori J (1992) The treatment of intrahepatic cholestasis of pregnancy by dexamethasone. *British Journal of Obstetrics and Gynecology* **99**:109–111.

26

Neurological Diseases

MARY PILLAI, SAVAS MENTICOGLOU

INTRODUCTION

Pregnancy may coincide with a broad range of neurological disorders with the exception of those associated with aging, and which have not therefore been included in this chapter. With the possible exceptions of eclampsia and epilepsy, most obstetricians have too little experience with any particular neurological problem coinciding with pregnancy to be confident in its management without referral to a neurologist and the literature. This chapter has purposely been directed at the obstetric management of neurological problems and disease factors as they relate to pregnancy, rather than an in-depth discussion of the disease as can be found in general neurology texts. Specific questions which concern the patient and physician concern the effect of the patient's disease on the pregnancy, the effect of pregnancy on her disease and how these should influence management of the pregnancy.

The incidence of some neurological diseases are listed in **Table 1**. Certain neurological conditions coincide so infrequently with pregnancy, that the published reviews are based on small numbers, and one must remain objective about their conclusions.

SEIZURES: EPILEPSY

Maternal/Fetal Risks

This is the most common neurological disorder accompanying pregnancy, occurring in 0.15–1.0% of women of child-bearing age. There is no consistent

Table 1
Incidence of neurological disease in child-bearing population

Migraine	1 : 5
Epilepsy	1 : 150
Multiple sclerosis	1 : 1000
Cerebral venous thrombosis[a]	1 : 2500–10 000 deliveries
Ruptured cerebral aneurysm[a]	1 : 10 000 pregnancies
Bleed from cerebral AVM[a]	1 : 10 000 pregnancies
Myasthenia gravis	1 : 25 000
Malignant brain tumor	1 : 50 000
Guillain-Barré syndrome	1.5 : 100 000

AVM: Arterio-venous malformation.
[a] Conditions occurring more commonly in pregnancy.

predictable effect of pregnancy on epilepsy. Several studies have reported an increase in seizure frequency,[1-3] while others find no difference.[4] Prospective studies from Finland,[5] Canada,[6] Germany and Italy[7] found that there was either no change or a reduction in seizure frequency in the majority of pregnancies.

A number of factors lead to decreased serum levels of anticonvulsant drugs in pregnancy, including reduced compliance because of fears of teratogenicity, increased extracellular fluid volume, reduced albumin levels leading to increased clearance of free drug, and failure to prescribe adequate treatment because of pregnancy.[7] However, the reduction in drug level is mostly tolerated without an increase in seizure frequency.[4]

Most complications of pregnancy are increased, especially when epilepsy is poorly controlled.[2,8] An increased incidence of antepartum hemorrhage, post-partum hemorrhage, pre-eclampsia, preterm birth, low birthweight and perinatal mortality have all been reported,[9,10] however, in general, women whose epilepsy is well controlled have few problems from their disease in pregnancy, and seizures increase in those whose disease is poorly controlled at other times.[6,11]

Many studies over the past two decades have demonstrated an increased risk of fetal anomaly. The question of intrinsic association of fetal malformations, maternal epilepsy and the genetics of this disorder remains to be resolved. All anticonvulsant drugs have now been associated with congenital anomalies and specific drug syndromes are recognized for hydantoin,[12,13] valproic acid[14,15] and trimethadone.[16,17] A summary of these is given in **Table 2**. For treated epileptic mothers, the risk of fetal anomaly may be as high as 8–9% (two to three times the general population rate).

Maternal seizures during pregnancy have not specifically been associated with an increased risk of congenital malformations;[18,19] however, fetal hypoxia during seizures may be a further cause of perinatal loss or residual handicap. Congenital anomalies are less likely if good control can be achieved with single rather than multiple drug therapy. Lindhout reported not only an increasing rate of congenital anomalies with increasing number of drugs used, but also anomaly rates which were proportional to the concentration of arene oxide metabolites of anticonvulsants.[20] It is possible that a common metabolite might acount for a specific pattern of anomalies with various different drugs.

Management Options

Prepregnancy

Those considering pregnancy should be adequately counseled about the risks of anticonvulsants, the effects of the disease on pregnancy and of pregnancy on the disease (as above). No increase in the risk of miscarriage or stillbirth has been reported in studies from Finland,[21] Japan[22] and the USA.[23,24] For patients who have been free of seizures for 2 years or more, consideration should be given to discontinuing anticonvulsants prior to conception.

It has been suggested that the original choice of anticonvulsant drugs in girls or young women with epilepsy should avoid sodium valproate, and that those taking phenytoin or valproic acid should consider changing to carbamazepine.[25] This advice has been disputed since the birth defects associated with carbamazepine may be less amenable to prenatal diagnosis than those associated with valproic acid.[26] Peri-conceptional folic acid supplementation is appropriate with phenytoin, phenobarbitone and primidone, since these are

folate antagonists, and since supplementation has now been shown to reduce the incidence of fetal neural tube defects in pregnancies at increased risk for these,[27] without reducing the anticonvulsant efficacy.[28]

It should be emphasized that uncontrolled seizures are more hazardous to the fetus than the risks associated with anticonvulsants in pregnancy. The course of pregnancy on one occasion does not appear to be a reliable guide to the course of subsequent pregnancies in epileptics.[3,29]

A study of family members of epileptics did not find a familial association between epilepsy and congenital malformations, other than an increased risk in the children of women with epilepsy who were taking anticonvulsant medication.[30]

Prenatal

In patients on constant doses of anticonvulsants through pregnancy, a decline in drug concentration will occur in 60–85%.[3,11] The question therefore arises as to whether drug doses should be increased when the concentration falls. In most cases, this fall in drug concentration will not be accompanied by an increase in seizure frequency, and plasma level monitoring–dosage adjustment has not been shown to produce any improvement in overall seizure control in pregnancy.[11] Moreover, consideration of potential adverse effects of the drugs on the fetus mandate use of the lowest possible concentrations of drug in pregnancy. It is therefore the opinion of the author that dosage should not be changed on the basis of concentration data alone, and drug levels are not indicated in those patients who have very infrequent fits but who elect to stay on a low dose of anticonvulsant drug through pregnancy. Drug levels are indicated for those whose frequency of fits is such that convulsions are likely to occur in pregnancy and for those with infrequent fits who experience an increase in pregnancy. Dosages should be adjusted within the therapeutic range to the minimum that controls seizures. Following this protocol, the vast majority of patients do not require any alterations to their anticonvulsant regime.

In view of the suspected teratogenic effects of anticonvulsants, detailed mid-trimester ultrasonography should be offered to all women so exposed in early pregnancy.

Labor/delivery

Essentially, the management is the same as in the non-epileptic obstetric patient. All anticonvulsant drugs except sodium valproate have been shown to be competitive inhibitors of prothrombin precursors resulting in deficiency of vitamin K dependent clotting factors (II, VII, IX, X) in infants of epileptic mothers.

Table 2
Fetal malformations and anticonvulsant drugs[a]

Sodium valproate (Depakene®) (Category D)

Uses: highly effective in most forms of epilepsy
Malformations: 1–3% risk of neural tube defect[14,32,33]
Breast-feeding appears safe. Low concentration in milk

Carbamazepine (Tegretol®) (Category C)

Uses: trigeminal neuralgia, virtually all types of epilepsy,
bipolar depression, excited psychosis, alcohol withdrawal
Malformations: craniofacial defects, fingernail hypoplasia
and developmental delay,[34,35] spina bifida.[36]
Breast-feeding appears safe. No accumulation in infant

Phenytoin (Dilantin®) (Category D)

Uses: A first-line drug in grand mal and focal epilepsy
Malformations: syndrome of microcephaly, mild to
moderate mental retardation, growth deficiency, facial
clefts, limb anomalies, distal phalangeal and nail
hypoplasia, and congenital heart defects[12,13]
Breast-feeding safe if maternal levels in therapeutic range[37]

Trimethadone (Category D)

Uses: petit mal
Malformations: the most potent teratogen among
anticonvulsants, best avoided in women of child-bearing
potential. A syndrome of growth delay, microcephally,
mental retardation, facial dysmorphism, congenital heart
defects, assorted gastrointestinal and genitourinary
anomalies[16,17]
No data on breast-feeding

Phenobarbital (Category D)

Uses: first-line drug for treatment of grand mal and focal
motor epilepsy
Malformations: much less teratogenic than phenytoin, but
non-specific increase in anomalies has been
documented.[38,39]
Neonatal depression and withdrawal more marked than
with other drugs, and may cause vitamin K deficient
hemorrhage
Risk of accumulation in breast-fed infants

**Ethosuximide (Zarontin®) and Clonazepam
(Clonopin®)** (Category C)

Uses: petit mal
Malformations: possibly have low-level teratogenicity but
no specific syndrome descried
Excreted in breast milk but appear safe

---

[a]Categories used by FDA for risk in pregnancy.[40,41]

Maternal clotting studies, however, have been normal. The effect in the neonate can be reversed by giving prophylactic vitamin K at delivery, or to the mother in the last 4 weeks of pregnancy.[31]

Postnatal

Relapse of seizures during the puerperium may result from failure of the patient to receive her daily dose because the obstetrician is unaware of her drug treatment or has forgotten to prescribe the drug in hospital. Loss of sleep further predisposes to fits and is likely to be a factor at this time.[6] Patients who are unable to take their usual oral medication because of complicated labor or delivery should receive the appropriate intravenous alternative until oral medication can be resumed.

If the dose of anticonvulsants has been increased in pregnancy, this should be adjusted back to the prepregnancy dose which gave satisfactory control. Breast-feeding is not contraindicated in women taking anticonvulsants (**Table 2**). For the reasons outlined above, infants of these women should receive prophylactic vitamin K at birth.

SEIZURES: ECLAMPSIA (see also Chapters 18 and 73)

Maternal/Fetal Risks

The occurrence of tonic–clonic seizures or coma distinguishes eclampsia from pre-eclampsia. The advent of seizures is important in several respects. First, if prolonged and uncontrolled, seizures themselves can lead to structural brain damage, enduring neurological deficits, or death. In addition, serious medical complications can result if there are frequent seizures, such as aspiration pneumonia, pulmonary edema or circulatory collapse. Also, seizures may herald the presence of other severe intracranial pathology, such as cerebral infarct or hemorrhage. Seizures are a dramatic manifestation that the patient's disease may have reached a perilous state, and that other severe problems may co-exist, such as acute renal failure, disseminated intravascular coagulation (DIC), subcapsular liver hematoma or abruption. Finally, although the seizure itself may not be detrimental to the fetus, the resultant hypoxemia and hemodynamic alterations can lead to fetal compromise and death.

Management Options

Diagnosis

Not all seizures occurring for the first time in pregnancy or after delivery are due to eclampsia. The diagnosis of eclampsia requires that seizures not be the consequence of some other discernible cause, examples of which are given in **Table 3** and include iatrogenic mishaps such as lidocaine intoxication, or water intoxication from inappropriate fluid and oxytocin use. Nevertheless, one's approach to new onset seizures in the second half of pregnancy or the first 10 days after delivery should be 'eclampsia until proven otherwise'.

The diagnosis of eclampsia is not a problem when a seizure develops in a woman who is being monitored or treated for pre-eclampsia. In other women, seizures develop unexpectedly, even though the preceding prenatal examination has shown no hypertension or proteinuria, but the presence of hypertension with or without proteinuria in the post-seizure period makes eclampsia the likely diagnosis. It is important to note that the blood pressure elevation need not be great; for example, if the woman is known to have low blood pressure at her first visit (e.g. 90/55), then a blood pressure of 135/85, say, is probably enough to justify the diagnosis. A co-existing complication of pre-eclampsia/eclampsia (e.g. concealed blood loss from an abruptio placenta) may lower the blood pressure and muddle the diagnosis. The diagnosis may also be difficult if a woman is found unconscious and no seizures are seen. If she is hypertensive, the initial working diagnosis should be eclampsia; the subsequent 30–60 min observation and management will generally reveal whether she is postictal or whether she has suffered some catastrophic cerebral event. On rare occasions, a pheochromocytoma or cocaine or other ingestion will mimic eclampsia.

In some cases, the diagnosis is not clear-cut at the beginning. Specifically, the diagnosis of eclampsia is difficult to make in the absence of observed hypertension or proteinuria. The approach in such cases is to institute emergency treatment of the presenting problem, namely the seizure or coma, as described in general neurology texts.[42,43] Over the next 1–2 h, careful observation and repeated examination and appropriate consultation will usually clarify the diagnosis. A delay of several hours is not harmful if the diagnosis is eclampsia, as long as the coma and seizures are properly managed, as the patient's condition has to be stabilized in any event before delivery; whereas rushing in

Table 3
Possible causes of prolonged convulsions

Eclampsia
Encephalitis
Meningitis
Cerebral tumor
Drug withdrawal
Toxicity (e.g. heavy metals)
Metabolic disturbance

---

and delivering the mother in ambiguous cases may lead to needless morbidity for mother and fetus as well as divert consideration of the other serious causes of seizure or coma.

Emergency management (see also Chapters 18 and 73)

No matter what the diagnosis or cause of the seizure or coma, certain general principles of management apply to all patients. If, as is usually the case, the seizure begins suddenly, without warning, the first step is to prevent the woman from harming herself by falling on the floor or striking her head. During the tonic phase, when the teeth are tightly clenched shut, efforts to insert an object between the teeth are futile. During the clonic phase, a soft item such as a handkerchief can be inserted between the teeth to prevent injury to the tongue. During a seizure there is prolonged apnea but trying to intubate a patient during the tonic–clonic phase is usually unnecessary and very difficult; in any event, the tonic–clonic phase will usually last only 2–3 min and regular respirations will return postictally. The woman should be placed on her side with her head tilted backward and mouth slightly downward to promote gravity drainage of liquid foreign matter from the mouth. However, if the tonic–clonic phase lasts longer than 3–4 min, or rapidly recurs, the seizure should be stopped promptly with diazepam given at a rate of 5 mg/min until the seizure stops. When the seizure has stopped (almost always by the time 20 mg has been given), maintenance anticonvulsant therapy should be started immediately (see below).

The integrity of the airway must be assured. The combination of the sedative effect of diazepam, the now-relaxed flaccid pharyngeal musculature of the postictal state, and possibly the presence of vomitus or blood in the upper airway can lead to complete or partial airway obstruction and result in asphyxia and cardiac arrest within minutes. It may be necessary to clear the mouth and pharynx of foreign material manually, as well as to extend the head and elevate the jaw to prevent hypopharyngeal obstruction by the base of the tongue. If the woman can breathe adequately on her own, or after airway obstruction is prevented, intubation is not necessary, since the postictal coma is generally brief in duration. However, if the coma is expected to be, or turns out to be, of long duration, or if there is no-one continuously present who has experience in the airway control of the unintubated patient, then intubation by a highly trained person is probably best. This may occasionally prove to be very difficult if there is severe glottic edema. Whether intubated or not, supplemental oxygen should be given. Even the intubated patient has to be observed very closely to ensure that adequate ventilation is occurring.

In an emergency situation, it is easy to forget the most basic things. Supine hypotension must be avoided; it can easily occur in the undelivered comatose patient who is unable to complain of faintness or feeling unwell, and can lead to disaster. If there is any chance that the cause of the seizure or coma is not eclampsia, or if there has been generalized tonic–clonic status eclampticus, then a bolus of glucose should be given intravenously.

As long as the patient is in coma, continuous cardiac monitoring and pulse oximetry are desirable, as well as assessment of the blood pressure. Venous blood should have been drawn for appropriate laboratory tests but arterial blood gases need not be checked routinely. Oxygenation can be assessed with pulse oximetry. The respiratory acidosis caused by the seizure responds to proper airway management and ventilation. The metabolic acidosis will be corrected if seizures are stopped.

The insertion of central venous or pulmonary artery catheters or arterial lines is not usually necessary and is certainly not an immediate priority. They can wait until maintenance anticonvulsant therapy has begun and are usually needed only if there are other complications such as persistent oliguria or pulmonary edema or the need for potent antihypertensives.

It is not useful to monitor the fetus during the immediate seizure episodes. If the fetus is alive, electronic fetal heart rate monitoring may suggest clear-cut fetal distress, probably as a consequence of the combination of maternal hypoxia, acidosis, pyrexia and uterine hypertonus. One may be tempted to do an urgent cesarean section in the expectation of saving the baby, but instead one can end up killing the mother by operating when she is in an unstable condition. Besides, the fetus will recover as the mother's condition improves and her hypoxia and acidosis are corrected.

Anticonvulsant therapy (see also Chapters 18 and 73)

Seizures should be stopped, because repeated seizures of whatever cause can result in brain damage.[42] Repeated and prolonged seizures can also create life-threatening systemic disturbances.[43] If the tonic–clonic phase of the seizure has abated and the patient is postictal, i.v. diazepam is not necessary but maintenance therapy with a long-acting anticonvulsant should start immediately. It will generally take 30 min to set up and administer enough long-acting anticonvulsant, so diazepam should be at hand if the seizures recur in the interim.

The drug most commonly used in North America (and perhaps in South Africa) to stop eclamptic convulsions is magnesium sulfate. Altogether, 4–6 g is given as an i.v. bolus over 15–20 min; giving more

than this amount or giving it too fast can result in lethal respiratory arrest. If seizures recur within the first hour of therapy, additional 2 g i.v. boluses should be given to stop the convulsions up to a maximum of 8 g magnesium sulfate in the first hour. A continuous i.v. infusion is then begun at 2 g/h and usually continued for 24 h postpartum. A therapeutic serum level is said to be 4–8 mg 100/ml but, generally, measuring serum levels is unnecessary, if the seizures do not recur after the first hour, if the serum creatinine and urine output are good (since the kidney is the main source of excretion), if there are normal deep tendon reflexes, and if the respiratory rate is normal. A disadvantage of magnesium sulfate is that when it is being given i.v., the potential for mishap and magnesium intoxication and lethal respiratory arrest is always present. More important than the intermittent measurement of serum levels is the continuous observation of the woman for evidence of toxicity – loss of the deep tendon reflexes and depressed respiratory rate. A perhaps safer method is to replace the continuous i.v. infusion with the i.m. administration of 10 g every 6 h; before each dose, however, the deep tendon reflexes and respiratory rate must still be checked. One virtue of magnesium sulfate is that it does not cause any central nervous system (CNS) depression, leaving the mother awake and alert.

The criticisms against the use of magnesium sulfate are several.[44–46] One is that its use as an anticonvulsant makes no sense in light of what is known about seizure mechanisms and its actions on the brain. Another is that its value has never been proven in a definitive trial with control subjects. Some attribute its empiric success in large series of eclampsia to the accompanying good intensive care and good antihypertensive treatment, arguing that the good results are being achieved despite, and not because of, the magnesium sulfate. Of interest is that two recent randomized studies from Africa compared the use of magnesium sulfate with diazepam in one study,[47] and with dilantin[48] in the other. In each case, magnesium sulfate was more effective in preventing recurrent seizures in patients with eclampsia.

Phenytoin is a credible alternative to magnesium sulfate for maintenance anticonvulsant therapy.[49,50] It has proven effective in non-pregnant status epilepticus. Its central mechanism of action is understood. It is safe to use; serious side-effects such as arrthythmias and hypotension are rarely seen in young women if the infusion rate is not excessive. Like magnesium sulfate, it does not depress consciousness, so the patient is alert. It is simpler to administer than magnesium sulfate. A loading dose of 15–20 mg/kg is given (750–1500 mg). It is diluted in 100 ml normal saline solution and given at a rate of 25 mg/min. In 30–60 min, the infusion is completed and blood levels in the therapeutic range are achieved that will be satisfactory for

12 h or so, making the continuous administration of medication unnecessary. At 12 h, blood levels can be checked and an additional 250–500 mg phenytoin given if necessary. The published experience with phenytoin in cases of eclampsia is limited, but it seems that recurrent convulsions after the initiation of therapy are more frequent with phenytoin than after magnesium sulfate.[48,51–54]

The *infrequent* seizure occurring despite 'therapeutic' levels of magnesium sulfate or phenytoin in a patient under observation is not too serious. On the very rare occasions when frequent or prolonged seizures persist ('status eclampticus') despite the use of adequate dosages of magnesium or phenytoin, there is a real problem. The alternate drug that has not already been given to the woman should be tried, but if this is not successful within 20 min, one may have to resort to a continuous intravenous diazepam drip at 8–10 mg/h, or else to i.v. phenobarbital at 50–100 mg/min until seizures stop or a loading dose of 20 mg/kg has been given.[43,55] By the time this stage is reached, the patient should already have been intubated and the expertise of a neurologist and anesthetist sought.

Usually, once seizures are stopped, the mother will gradually awaken over the next 15–30 min. If there is protracted deep unresponsiveness beyond 30 min, the situation is very serious. Severe permanent brain damage may have occurred because of repetitive seizures or as a result of circulatory or respiratory complications. Another cause might be an intracerebral hemorrhage, in a critical area of the brainstem, or in the supratentorial compartment giving rise to brain herniation. The problem may be diffuse cerebral edema with raised intracranial pressure. The only 'good' possibility is that the enormous cerebral metabolic demands of the seizures, along with the systemic hypoxemia during the attack, have made the postictal coma merely take longer than usual to resolve. In any event, in this serious situation where brain herniation due to increased intracranial pressure is a possibility, the patient should be intubated and hyperventilated to lower the arterial pCO_2 to about 25 mmHg, oxygenation and circulation maintained, urgent help sought from a neurologist, and arrangements made for computed axial tomography (CT scan) of the head. Except for these cases of prolonged coma, and for cases with persistent neurologic deficit, CT scan and magnetic resonance imaging (MRI) are not needed for the evaluation of eclampsia.

Treating the hypertension

It is important to reduce the blood pressure for two reasons: first, to prevent major intracerebral hemorrhage and, second, to reverse the encephalopathy that has led to the convulsions, headache, vomiting or cortical blindness. There are a number of suitable parenteral drugs for the treatment of the hypertension, and the best one is probably the drug with which the physician is most familiar.[45] Continuous infusions are best avoided. Hydralazine in 5–10 mg i.v. boluses, labetalol in 20–40 mg i.v. boluses, diazoxide in 50–60 mg i.v. boluses, or nifedipine in 5 mg sublingual doses, all give a gradual fall in blood pressure. For each drug it may take 15 min or so to observe a blood pressure lowering effect, so it is important to wait this length of time before giving additional boluses. Giving boluses too close together, giving too large boluses or giving a combination of hypotensive agents may cause abrupt and marked falls in blood pressure and the resultant hypoperfusion of the brain or heart may result in a catastrophe.[56] In these cases, the treatment may end up worse than the disease. A reasonable goal of therapy is to lower the diastolic pressure to about 100 mmHg, but the treatment should be individualized.[57] The teenager with a blood pressure of 90/50 at first visit who has had a seizure at a pressure of 150/100 can have her diastolic lowered to 90 or so, whereas the eclamptic woman admitted with a pressure of 200/140 should probably not have the diastolic lowered below 110 in the acute situation.

Delivery

The fundamental step in the care of the woman with eclampsia is delivery. Attempts to prolong the pregnancy in order to improve fetal maturity are unlikely to be of value, unless the gestation is very early, under 26–27 weeks, and at least half a week to a week is gained. For this possible gain, the mother is exposed to the continuing dangers of seizures, hypertension and ongoing multi-organ dysfunction, while the fetus may die *in utero* from a catastrophe such as an abruption. Once eclampsia has occurred, delivery should be effected without regard to the gestation of the pregnancy or the possibility of survival of the baby.

This does not mean that immediate cesarean section is the treatment of choice. To embark on such surgery when the mother's condition is unstable – seizures uncontrolled, hypertension extreme, acidosis, hypoxia, coagulopathy, pulmonary edema untreated – is sometimes to administer the *coup de grace* for the gravely ill mother. Especially to be avoided is the temptation to intervene by urgent cesarean section for presumed fetal distress. It is not commendable to save the baby if it means killing the mother.

Once the seizures are controlled, the mother is awake and alert, the blood pressure reduced to safe levels, and functional derangements of other organ systems attended to, it is time to consider delivery. If labor can easily be induced, vaginal delivery is preferable.

If the gestation is near term but the cervix is unfavorable, an attempt to prime the cervix for a few hours before induction may be considered, but this course of action demands that the mother's condition be very stable and that good labor progress ensues. In the eclamptic woman remote from term with a closed uneffaced cervix and an unengaged presenting part, cesarean section may be best. In the rare woman who is still comatose several hours after admission, despite adequate management, and in whom vaginal delivery cannot be anticipated within several hours, cesarean section should be performed.[56]

STATUS EPILEPTICUS

Maternal/Fetal Risks

This term is appropriate for seizures lasting more than 30 min. The nature of the convulsion should be critically assessed by the physician in order that pseudo-seizures are not misdiagnosed and over-treated. In true seizures, pupillary light reflexes are absent and consciousness is lost. Most commonly, status occurs in the second half of pregnancy, and in known epileptics is associated with subtherapeutic levels of anticonvulsant

---

SEIZURES
Summary of Management Options

EPILEPSY

Prepregnancy

- Counsel about risks (see text)

- Folic acid supplementation

- Control fits with lowest dose of preferably a single agent

Prenatal

- Regular check of clinical control and serum levels of anticonvulsant

- Adjust dose to control fits rather than 'treat' serum levels; avoid toxic doses

- Detailed fetal anomaly scan

Postnatal

- Vitamin K to newborn

- Monitor fit control and serum levels; dose adjustment may be necessary

ECLAMPSIA
(see also Chapters 18 and 73)

- First-aid measures
  - avoid injury
  - semi-prone position
  - maintain airway
  - administer oxygen
  - monitor maternal and fetal conditions

- Control and prevent recurrence of fits

- Treat hypertension

- Avoid fluid overload

- Check renal, liver and coagulation status

- Deliver when stable

STATUS EPILEPTICUS

- First-aid measures (see 'Epilepsy' above)

- Control convulsions
  - anticonvulsant drugs
  - paralyse and ventilate if conservative approach fails

- Search for causes (see **Table 3**)

drugs. When it occurs in women not known to be epileptic, the causes listed in **Table 3** should be considered. Inadvertent intravenous injection of local anesthetic around the time of delivery may also result in prolonged convulsions, as may injudicious use of large quantities (usually greater than 3 liters) of electrolyte-free solutions with syntocinon to augment labor, resulting in hyponatremia.[58]

Without anticonvulsant therapy, status has a high mortality for both mother and fetus.[59] This is not surprising as seizures result in hypertension, hypoglycemia, hypoxia and lactic acidosis, which does not have a chance to resolve spontaneously during status. Cerebral blood flow, oxygen and glucose consumption increase during seizure activity, and the longer seizures last the greater the likelihood of permanent neurological sequelae or death.

Fetal bradycardia usually accompanies seizure activity and may persist for some time following. Stillbirths have been recorded after a single generalized convulsion.[60]

Management Options

The therapeutic aim is to control status as quickly as possible while maintaining the airway and preventing self-injury. Intravenous access is essential and diazepam is the most effective drug, given as a 10 mg i.v. bolus over 2 min, followed by 2 mg/min up to 20 mg. In most cases, less than 20 mg will be effective. Blood should be taken for glucose, electrolytes, calcium and to screen for toxic substances. Face mask oxygen and a bolus of 50 ml 50% dextrose are appropriate as prolonged seizures are likely to cause hypoglycemia.

Next, a loading dose of a long-acting anticonvulsant is appropriate, and phenytoin (Dilantin®) is currently the preferred drug as it does not depress respiration or consciousness. In late pregnancy in conscious patients, a dose of 10 mg/kg initially followed by 5 mg/kg 2 h later has been shown to provide therapeutic-free phenytoin levels for over 24 h without toxic effects.[49] Cardiac monitoring is mandatory during administration of an intravenous bolus, and if signs of toxicity occur infusion should be stopped and then resumed at a slower rate. If seizure activity persists, the assistance of an experienced anesthetist, endotracheal intubation followed by phenobarbital 50 mg/min up to a total dose of 20 mg/kg are appropriate. Failing this, general anesthesia is indicated.

CEREBROVASCULAR DISEASE: 'STROKE'

Although uncommon in this age group, multiple studies attest to the greater risk of cerebral infarction during

Table 4
'Stroke' in pregnancy

Mechanism and causes
Atherosclerosis
Diabetes
Hypertension
Hypercholesterolemia
Increased clotting or blood stasis
Polycythemia
Essential thrombocytosis
Thrombotic thrombocytopenic purpura
Antithrombin III deficiency
Sickle cell crises
Severe dehydration
Embolic
Mitral valve prolapse
Bacterial endocarditis
Paradoxical embolus
Atrial fibrillation
Cardiomyopathy
Vasculitic
Syphilis
Takayusu's disease
Fibromuscular dysplasia
Moyamoya
Autoimmune
SLE
Circulating anticoagulant syndrome
Malignancy
Metastatic choriocarcinoma

and immediately after pregnancy.[61] Wiebers reported a risk 13 times that in the non-pregnant patient of the same age.[62] An incidence of 1:6000 pregnancies was reported between 1984 and 1990 from Dallas,[63] with 40% being hemorrhagic and 60% being due to ischemic causes. Chronic and pregnancy-induced hypertension are well recognized predisposing factors to intracranial hemorrhage.[64,65] Any symptoms suggesting stroke in pregnant women should be investigated promptly because some etiologies of stroke are treatable. Causes to consider are listed in **Table 4**. Management of the pregnancy should be individualized and if pregnancy-induced hypertension plays a causative role, then delivery is indicated. Otherwise, within limits, the pregnancy can be ignored and work up and possible neurosurgical treatment pursued.

CEREBROVASCULAR DISEASE: ARTERIAL OCCLUSIVE DISEASE

Risks and Management Options

Arterial occlusive disease is rare in pregnancy, complicating 1:20 000 live births. Arterial occlusions tend to occur during the second and third trimesters or the first postpartum week, where as venous occlusions are most common 1–4 weeks postpartum.[66–69] Unlike stroke in the elderly, atherosclerosis is a relatively uncommon cause of stroke in this age group, accounting for about one-quarter of cases. Hypertension, diabetes and hypercholesterolemia are predisposing factors. Spontaneous thrombus formation within the heart, extracranial carotid, vertebral or middle cerebral arteries is a more likely etiology, and acute carotid thrombectomy has been reported in the puerperium with good results.[70]

A number of rare vasculitic causes include:

- *Takayasu's disease* characterized by bruits or diminished pulses in a young patient. Hypertension in pregnancy is common and the only treatment is steroids.

- *Fibromuscular dysplasia* affecting cerebral arteries, may be associated with intracranial aneurysms. Treatment has been anticoagulants or antiplatelet regime.

- *Moyamoya disease* is a progressive stenosis of the internal carotid artery with development of a collateral circulation, occurring predominantly in Japanese people. Aneurysmal dilatation may predispose to intracranial hemorrhage, and cases have been reported during pregnancy.[71,72] Optimal therapy of the disease has not been defined, except where hemorrhage occurs there is a consensus of opinion that indications for operation should be the same as in the non-pregnant state.[73–77]

CEREBROVASCULAR DISEASE: CARDIOGENIC EMBOLUS

Maternal Risks

During pregnancy, cardiac disease may produce symptoms of focal cerebral ischemia through various mechanisms, including valve-related embolization, mural thrombus formation and systemic venous thromboembolism through a cardiac defect. Echocardiography is indicated for all young stroke patients, and in some cases a 24 h ECG may be indicated to detect arrhythmias which predispose to emboli.

Cardiac causes include:

- *Infective endocarditis* associated with cerebral embolization in up to 20% of cases. During pregnancy, *Streptococcus viridans* is the most common

agent, particularly in those with pre-existing rheumatic heart disease.[78] Staphylococcal endocarditis should be considered in pregnant drug addicts and carries a high risk of cerebral abscess, lung abscess and mortality.

- *Paradoxical embolus* should be considered in patients with a deep vein thrombosis. Lesions which may be found in association include patent foramen ovale, atrial septal defect or a pulmonary arterio-venous malformation.

- *Cardiomyopathy* may occur coincidentally during the course of pregnancy or may be pregnancy-related, and gives rise to cerebral emboli.

- *Mitral valve prolapse* (MVP) occurrs in approximately 5% of otherwise healthy young women[79,80] and may give rise to stroke by formation of sterile thrombi on abnormal valve leaflets. In the general population, the annual risk of stroke with MVP is around 1:6000; however, no major studies of stroke in pregnancy have been done since widespread availability of echocardiography and recognition of this syndrome. Stroke with MVP generally carries a good prognosis.

- *Prosthetic heart valves*. Such patients may undergo pregnancy and the risk of embolic cerebral complications is high, unless effectively anticoagulated. Because of teratogenic concerns with warfarin, heparin therapy had been advocated in the past. However, heparin is recognized not to prevent thrombosis of cardiac valve prostheses and is associated with greater technical management difficulties than is oral anticoagulation.[81]

Management Options

A dilemma exists regarding anticoagulation even outside pregnancy. Without such treatment, the risk of recurrence of embolization is high, but effective anticoagulation increases the risk of catastrophic hemorrhagic transformation in healthy or infarcted brain tissue. Whatever the source of emboli, if the risk of recurrence is high, then the same principles should apply as in the non-pregnant patient. Guidelines for this have been offered in the absence of prospective trials,[82] and include that anticoagulation should be confined to small defects without evidence of hemorrhagic infarction, large infarcts carrying the greatest risk of hemorrhage. With large infarcts, the CT scan should be repeated in 3–5 days and if negative for hemorrhagic transformation heparin therapy instituted. Acute anticoagulation should always be with heparin, and although warfarin is indicated for long-term therapy, it should not be instituted for at least 6 weeks (to allow growth of a relatively mature neovasculature in the damaged tissue). If by then the woman is into the third trimester, it may be preferable not to change to warfarin until after delivery.

CEREBROVASCULAR DISEASE: VENOUS THROMBOSIS

Maternal Risks

Cerebral venous thrombosis is extremely rare in the developed world, with an estimated incidence of 1:2500 to 1:10 000 deliveries;[67–69] however, in India, reported rates are 10 times higher.[83] When it occurs, it is usually a superior sagittal sinus thrombosis, and usually during the puerperium. Symptoms of headache, vomiting, convulsions, hemiparesis, blurred vision and impaired intellect are typical. Signs of papilloedema, meningism and fever are characteristic. Seizures may be generalized or focal, and the condition may be confused with eclampsia or subarachnoid hemorrhage. Predisposing factors include infection, hyperviscosity syndromes such as sickle hemoglobinopathy and dehydration. The differentiation between venous thrombosis and arterial occlusion can be difficult. However, in addition to a difference in the timing of presentation, focal and generalized seizures, impaired consciousness and increased intracranial pressure are all more common with venous thrombosis. Failure of CT scans to reveal venous thrombosis is well recognized, and digital subtraction angiography has been the gold standard in diagnosis. Where available, MRI scans are noninvasive, present no recognizable risk to the fetus and are superior to CT scans.[84] Although Amias[69] reported a mortality rate of 45% in 1970, anecdotal experiences today suggest most women recover without sequelae.

Management Options

Control of seizures and adequate hydration are fundamental. Some advocate anticoagulation but this is associated with a high risk of death from intracranial hemorrhage.[85,86] The disease may be life-threatening due to increased intracranial pressure, and reduction of intracranial pressure with high-dose steroids may be essential. However, use of mannitol is generally not advised, as it has been associated with fetal vascular depletion and bradycardia.[87] Antihypertensive drugs are also controversial because hypertension is thought to be a major compensating mechanism.

CEREBROVASCULAR DISEASE – 'STROKE'
Summary of Management Options

ARTERIAL OCCLUSIVE DISEASE

- General supportive measures

- Treat any causes/associated factors (see **Table 4**)

- Indications for surgery are as for non-pregnant patient

CARDIOGENIC EMBOLUS

- Consider anticoagulation if no evidence of hemorrhage on CT scan

VENOUS THROMBOSIS

- Control seizures
- Ensure adequate hydration
- Most do not advocate anticoagulation, mannitol or antihypertensive agents

---

CEREBROVASCULAR DISEASE: SUBARACHNOID HEMORRHAGE

Maternal/Fetal Risks

There are relatively few recent data in the obstetric or neurology literature concerning this medical complication of pregnancy. Although the occurrence overall is rare in pregnancy, intracranial hemorrhage (ICH) has increased in importance as other causes of maternal death have declined. A recent review of the English literature documented 157 cases, with an overall maternal mortality of 35% (similar to that of the nongravid population) and a fetal mortality of 17%.[65] Of the various types of non-traumatic ICH, subarachnoid hemorrhage has been the one most commonly associated with pregnancy, with an estimated incidence of 1:10 000 to 5:10 000 pregnancies.[61]

Presentation is the same as in the non-pregnant patient, most often with sudden onset of severe headache, accompanied by signs of meningitic irritation, including neck stiffness, fever, photophobia, nausea and vomiting. There may be acute loss of consciousness at the time of the initial hemorrhage, with the degree of coma and its duration depending on the severity of hemorrhage.

Management Options

Prenatal

A CT scan, if necessary with contrast enhancement, should be performed as soon as possible to confirm the presence of subarachnoid blood, and to detect associated intracerebral and intraventricular hemorrhage. In some, this may also reveal the underlying cause. If the CT scan is not diagnostic, lumbar puncture is indicated. Finding bloody cerebrospinal fluid (CSF) with xanthochromic supernatant is diagnostic. Once ICH has been confirmed, angiography should be performed.[88] In the past, this has been withheld because of perceived risk to the fetus; however, with proper shielding, the radiation exposure to the fetus is minimal. Iodinated contrast agents are physiologically inert and pose little risk to the fetus.[89] Maternal hydration should be maintained during their administration to avoid fetal dehydration.

The majority of bleeds are due to rupture of either an intracranial aneurysm or an arterio-venous malformation (AVM). AVMs account for about 20–50% of subarachnoid hemorrhages during pregnancy, a much higher proportion than in the general population.[65,69,90] They tend to occur in younger women than do aneurysmal hemorrhages, and also are more likely to cause recurrent hemorrhage during pregnancy.[65,91] Bleeding from either source can occur at any time in pregnancy, and the overall risk increases with advancing gestation.[65] Although angiography is the definitive investigation, this procedure may be delayed in patients who have profound alteration in consciousness, because their prognosis is poor (80–90% mortality in the first 2 weeks) and the operative mortality is high (25–35%).[88]

The patient with subarachnoid hemorrhage is at risk for seizures, hyponatremia from inappropriate antidiuretic hormone (ADH) secretion, raised intracranial pressure, hydrocephalus, aneurysmal rebleeding and vasospasm resulting in stroke. The management of all these complications may include anticonvulsants, high-dose steroids and mannitol for lowering intracranial pressure, and nimodipine for reducing posthemorrhagic vasospasm. Detailed discussion of these is beyond the scope of this chapter, though obviously once subarachnoid hemorrhage has been identified, both obstetric and neurologic needs must be addressed.

Surgery is the definitive treatment for both AVM and aneurysms, and should be determined on neurosurgical indications. Such treatment during the course of pregnancy does not appear to adversely affect fetal outcome.[90–94] The major neurosurgical modification imposed by pregnancy is in the choice of anesthetic used to lower intracranial pressure. In comatose patients, supportive treatment only is indicated. Among conscious patients, those with little or no neurological deficit have the best prognosis (10–20% mortality in the first 2 weeks), with most of the deaths in this group resulting from rebleeding in the first 2 weeks. The potential advantages of early operation must be weighed against increased operative mortality during the first week after hemorrhage. In recent years, the tendency has been to utilize early surgery in this group.

Medical treatment with aminocaproic acid to prevent rebleeding has been used in non-pregnant patients, but overall does not seem to improve morbidity and mortality because of increased risk of thrombotic side-effects.[95,96] This treatment has not been tried in pregnancy, as the risk of thrombotic side-effects would be expected to be even higher. Similarly, use of vasopressin to prevent vasospasm would be empirically contraindicated in pregnancy.

Certain groups are at increased risk for aneurysm and include those with a family history and those having a collection of rare disorders (moyamoya disease, fibromuscular dysplasia, polycystic kidneys, coarctation of the aorta, pseudoxanthoma elasticum, Ehlers-Danlos and Marfan's disease). Ideally, asymptomatic aneurysms greater than 7 mm, and particularly those greater than 10 mm, should be treated surgically before pregnancy. Diagnosis of an unruptured aneurysm in pregnancy is rare, and is most likely related to symptoms of mass effect such as cranial nerve palsy. Most aneurysms that produce these symptoms are 10 mm or more in diameter and the likelihood of subsequent rupture is greater than with smaller aneurysms.[97,98] Unruptured aneurysms of this size should be operated on as soon as possible, regardless of pregnancy. Unruptured aneurysms of less than 10 mm warrant further consideration, particularly as the natural history of unruptured aneurysms in pregnancy has not been adequately elucidated. In general, those less than 5 mm should be left alone.

Robinson found that AVMs carried an 87% risk of bleeding and a 27% risk of rebleeding during pregnancy.[91] A more recent review of the natural history of AVMs, found that an unruptured AVM in adults was associated with a 2–3% risk of bleeding per year, with a 1% risk of death per year.[99] There was no correlation between pregnancy and bleeding.[100] Resecting the AVM considerably reduces the risk of bleeding, and new steriotactic radiosurgical techniques suggest that an increasing number of AVMs are treatable. However, the use of methods employing high-dose radiation would be contraindicated by pregnancy. Optimal management must be determined on an individual basis. Both embolization and surgical resection have been attempted during pregnancy.[101]

CEREBROVASCULAR DISEASE-SUBARACHNOID HEMORRHAGE
Summary of Management Options

DIAGNOSIS

- CT Scan

- Lumbar puncture if CT equivocal

MANAGEMENT

Prenatal

- Interdisciplinary care

- Angiograph to identify cause after diagnosis (? defer in those in coma)

- Anticonvulsants, high-dose steroids, mannitol, and nimodipine depending on clinical picture/problems

- Consider surgery for AVMs and aneurysms (see text)

Labor/delivery

- Regional analgesia preferable to narcotic analgesia and general anesthesia

- Minimize pushing in second stage Cesarean section for:
  - normal obstetric indications
  - to save fetus in moribund mother
- Consider life-support machine in patient with brain death to gain fetal maturity

---

Labor/delivery

Dramatic but short-lived hemodynamic changes occur during labor and delivery. The importance of these in promoting intracranial hemorrhage is uncertain. If an intracranial aneurysm has been successfully clipped, then delivery can be managed routinely as in any other pregnant woman. If a ruptured aneurysm cannot be obliterated, the question arises as to whether vaginal delivery increases the risk of aneurysmal bleeding. None of 21 patients reported by Amias bled during labour,[102] and among 142 ruptured aneurysms reviewed from the literature only one occurred during labor and vaginal delivery.[103] It has been proposed that during contractions, intracranial transvessel pressure gradients remain static and therefore labor is not contraindicated. Overall, there is a consensus that the valsalva maneuver should be strictly avoided and delivery effected by forceps. This being the case, regional anesthesia would seem most appropriate,[65,103] and cesarean section reserved for obstetric indications.

AVMs contain fragile vessels which have been considered more liable to bleed during labor than an aneurysm. If the AVM is not operable, elective cesarean section has been recommended.[88,90] Of note, a recent review by Dias[65] found that maternal and fetal outcomes were similar after cesarean section and vaginal delivery with either aneurysmal or angiomatous ICH which had not been surgically treated. They recommend adjunctive measures to decrease the risk of recurrent bleeding during vaginal delivery, including caudal or epidural analgesia, and low forceps.

Cesarean delivery may be appropriate for fetal salvage when the mother is moribund and the fetus is beyond 24 weeks. Equal consideration should be given to maintaining the mother on life-support after confirmation of brain death to achieve further maturity of the fetus.

HEADACHE

Headache is the most common neurological symptom presenting in pregnancy. Most cases do not have severe underlying disease, but it is important to consider this possibility, especially when there are associated focal neurological signs, impairment of intellect or the headaches disturb sleep. Conditions which should be considered include:

- pre-eclampsia

- benign intracranial hypertension

- subarachnoid hemorrhage

- cortical vein thrombosis

- rapid expansion of a brain tumor

- meningitis

These conditions can usually be excluded from the history and a limited neurological examination (which must include ophthalmoscopy, blood pressure, testing for meningism, and an assessment of mental status). In the small minority of patients in whom intracranial disease is suspected, the need for CT scan, EEG and examination of cerebrospinal fluid must be decided on an individual basis. A cerebral CT scan carries minimal risk for the fetus and, if no mass lesion is revealed, pregnancy poses no special contraindication to lumbar puncture.

Most often, headaches which begin in pregnancy are migraine[104] or non-migrainous vascular headaches.

MIGRAINE HEADACHES

Maternal/Fetal Risks

Migraine headaches occur predominantly in women of child-bearing age, and thus the concurrence of migraine and pregnancy is relatively common, occurring in up to 20% of pregnancies.[104–106] In the largest study of 703 women, 116 (16.5%) fulfilled migraine criteria of the International Headache Society.[106] Overall, studies suggest that 60–70% of women with migraine will improve during pregnancy (**Table 5**).[104,106,107] However, migraine may also have its onset during the course of pregnancy.[104,105,108–110]

Wainscott reviewed the reproductive histories of 77 women with migraine and compared them with 182 non-migrainous controls.[111] There was no excess of

miscarriage, toxemia, congenital anomalies or stillbirth in migraine sufferers. Migraine is sometimes subdivided into common migraine (without aura), classical migraine (with aura), focal migraine (with neurological symptoms) and status migrainous, where the headache lasts for more than 72 h. Neurological deficit temporarily accompanying focal migraine may create great anxiety, making awareness of this condition and its benign course important.[108]

Hormonal factors appear to play a role in triggering migraine.[112] Girls are more frequently affected than boys after the menarche.[113] Two-thirds of women implicate the menstrual cycle as a factor in their attacks.[114] The oral contraceptive pill may precipitate migraine during withdrawal intervals.[115] Women with 'menstrual migraine' typically experience exacerbations before and during menstruation, are improved during pregnancy, but are very prone to postpartum headache.[116]

Management Options

The treatment for an acute attack of migraine is now well documented as comprising rest, an antiemetic and analgesics. The benefit of aspirin has been known for many years. Gastric stasis is one of the major problems in the treatment of an acute attack and a significant advance in treatment followed assessment of the effect of metoclopramide on the absorption of aspirin during the acute attack.[117] The antiemetic used should increase gastric motility and be taken at the onset of attack. Domperidone (Motilium®) in a dose of 30 mg has also been shown to be beneficial in preventing an attack when taken at the very first appearance of warning signals,[118,119] but as yet there are few data on its safety in pregnancy. Patients should be warned of the possibility of extrapyramidal side-effects with these antiemetics. Antiemetics should be followed by 900 mg soluble aspirin or 1 g paracetamol (Acetaminophen®)

Table 5
Studies of migraine in pregnancy[104–107]

	No. of women studied	No. with migraine	No. pregnancies with migraine	Improved	Same/worse	Onset in pregnancy
Lance (1966)	NS	120	252	145	107	NS
Callaghan (1968)	200	41	41	4	4	33
Somerville (1972)	200	38	38	24	7	7
Ratinahirana (1990)	703	116	147	102	21	16
Totals	1103	195/1103	478	275/422	139/422	56/1103
%		17.8%		65.2%	32.9%	5.1%

NS: not stated.

preferably 10–15 min later, and these drugs can be repeated in 4–6 h.[120] Although aspirin is the analgesic of choice for migraine,[121] it readily crosses the placenta, and may be associated with undesirable fetal and maternal effects when taken at this dose at certain times in pregnancy. In early pregnancy, there is uncertainty about teratogenicity.[122] In late pregnancy, the theoretical risk of closure of the fetal ductus arteriosus seems small in practice; however, this dose would be expected to affect platelet function for the platelet lifespan (7 days in late pregnancy). Thus should labor occur within 1 week of the dose, many maintain that epidural analgesia is contraindicated. Similarly, should operative delivery be necessary, there may be a theoretical adverse influence on blood loss. Of importance, this dose has also been associated with a hemorrhagic tendency in the newborn.[123,124] Paracetamol may, therefore, be preferable to aspirin in the first and last trimesters, and particularly in the last few weeks of pregnancy. Ergotamine-containing compounds are beneficial in patients who do not respond to antiemetic analgesic regimes; however, they are strictly contraindicated in pregnancy.

The importance of rest, particularly sleep if this can be achieved, should not be forgotten and non-pharmacological treatment including biofeedback, relaxation and psychotherapy can be helpful. This may be particularly appropriate in pregnancy to minimize the use of medications.[125]

Avoidance of precipitating factors is fundamental. If attacks are frequent, disabling and not adequately controlled by moderate doses of analgesics, then prophylaxis may be warranted in pregnancy. Of drugs used for this there is greatest experience with beta-blockers in pregnancy (predominantly in the management of hypertensive disease). A meta-analysis of studies evaluating propranolol in the management of recurrent migraine revealed substantial support for its short-term effectiveness.[126] Propranolol readily crosses the placenta, and may be associated with fetal bradycardia and loss of reactivity of non-stress tests.[127] However, a 1988 review of beta-blockers, including propranolol, during pregnancy and lactation concluded that they were relatively safe.[128] Newborn infants of women consuming propranolol near delivery should be observed for bradycardia and hypoglycemia over the first 24–48 h.

POSTPARTUM HEADACHE

Risks and Management Options

Headache is a frequent symptom of the puerperium, with a reported incidence of 30–40%,[116,129,130] and a peak incidence on days 4–6.[116] Women with a previous or family history of migraine were particularly suscep-

tible;[116,130] however, the severity of the headaches is rarely equivalent to migraine. Rest and simple analgesics are usually sufficient.

SPINAL HEADACHE

Maternal Risks

Another etiology of headache for which pregnant women are at risk is that associated with accidental dural puncture during attempted insertion of an epidural. Postpartum headache complicates 85% of such punctures.[131] Factors which predispose to this complication are the patient's inability to be still during painful contractions, the large size of needle diameter, and involuntary expulsive efforts later on in labor. The mechanism of headache is thought to be CSF hypotension (possibly by producing traction on pain-sensitive structures) as a result of leakage of spinal fluid into the epidural space.

Management Options

Relief, at least transiently, may be obtained by epidural injection of physiological saline,[132] which can be done at the time of puncture. The most effective treatment is epidural blood patch, involving injection of 2–3 ml of autologous blood near the dural perforation. This procedure is best reserved for those with persistent headache more than 24 h after dural puncture. When it is performed in the first 24 h, the failure rate is 71%, compared with only 4% thereafter.[133] During the initial 24 h, conservative treatment with analgesia, adequate hydration and lying flat are recommended. In the small percentage that fail to be cured by blood patch, a repeat procedure may be effective.[134]

Factors proposed to explain the beneficial effects of blood patch include that it seals the dural perforation impeding the flow of CSF through it, and that compression of the dura results in an immediate augmentation of subarachnoid pressure.[133,135] Contraindications to epidural blood patch are the same as those to epidural, namely hemorrhagic tendency, anticoagulant therapy and cutaneous lumbar lesions.

BENIGN INTRACRANIAL HYPERTENSION (BIH)/PSEUDOMOTOR CEREBREI

Maternal Risks

This syndrome of prolonged increased intracranial pressure (ICP) not associated with a space occupying lesion rarely accompanies pregnancy, and the incidence may be lower than expected during pregnancy.[136] Other causes of high ICP are listed in **Table 6**. Presentation is with symptoms due to raised ICP, namely, headache (95%) and visual disturbance (15%) without localizing signs or any impairment of intellect. The only signs are bilateral papilloedema (100%) and, occasionally, a VIth cranial nerve palsy. Eighty percent of cases occur in women of child-bearing age, and over 90% of these women are obese. In pregnancy, BIH is most commonly reported between the second and fifth months[136,138] and appears not to affect the outcome. Recurrence during subsequent pregnancies has been described.[137,147]

Management Options

Prenatal

The diagnosis is essentially one of exclusion with a normal CT scan, and on lumbar puncture the cerebrospinal fluid (CSF) pressure is high (often pressure > 200 mm H$_2$O).[137] Lumbar puncture is obviously unsafe in patients with raised intracranial pressure due to a space occupying lesion, which must therefore first be excluded.

The natural history of BIH is spontaneous resolution, usually within a few months of onset. However, the term 'benign' may be misleading, as prolonged high ICP may cause optic atrophy. Treatment is aimed at preserving vision, and to this end monitoring the size of the blind spot, acuity and color discrimination are appropriate. Visual deterioration is an absolute indication for treatment. Outside pregnancy, acetazolamide

Table 6
Causes of raised intracranial pressure

Benign intracranial hypertension
Cerebral edema
  Hyptertensive encephalopthy
  Lead poisoning
  Viral encephalitis
Impaired reabsorption CSF
  Venous sinus thrombosis
  High CSF protein
    Guillain-Barré syndrome
    spinal cord tumor
  Post-meningitis
Drugs
  Hypervitaminosis A
  Tetracycline
  Indomethacin
  Nitrofurantoin
Space occupying lesion

(Diamox®), steroids, glycerol and serial lumbar puncture are used. On theoretical grounds, osmotic diuretics, like glycerol, may reduce circulating volume and uteroplacental blood flow, and are probably best avoided in pregnancy. Acetazolamide is a carbonic anhydrase inhibitor that reduces CSF production, and has been used in pregnancy without any apparent adverse effects,[136] although there are few data on possible teratogenicity. Serial lumbar punctures are the mainstay of treatment, and may be more effective if combined with acetazolamide. Generally, up to 30 ml of fluid are removed to lower ICP to normal,[139] at 10–14 day intervals. The rate of CSF production is such that this quantity would be expected to be reproduced in 90 min;[140] however, symptomatic improvement is generally maintained for several days, possibly reflecting a continuing CSF leak.

Weight reduction has been associated with a dramatic reduction in ICP in obese women[141] and, provided the dietary regime is sensible, will not adversely affect the pregnancy.

In patients whose symptoms do not respond to medical therapy, or who continue to have progressive visual loss, surgical intervention in the form of either shunting or a decompression procedure is appropriate. Because the ventricles are normal or small in BIH, shunting is best achieved by lumbar subarachnoid peritoneal shunt. This has been successfully utilized in pregnancy.[136,137] The procedure is safe and can prevent or improve deteriorating vision in most patients.[142,143] Shunt malfunction may be a problem and, as with ventriculoperitoneal shunts, the risk may be increased during the last trimester due to increasing uterine size. Unlike ventriculoperitoneal shunts, these do not contain a reservoir, so if malfunction occurs, assessment of fetal lung maturity and consideration of early delivery (versus serial lumbar punctures) may be appropriate.

Labor/delivery

Vaginal delivery is not contraindicated.[144] As lumbar puncture is safe in the treatment of the condition, its use for analgesia in labor is obviously not contraindicated. The usual objection posed by post-lumbar puncture headache is not relevant in patients with BIH. In anecdotal case reports, the spread of local anesthetic in BIH patients undergoing spinal[137] and epidural[145] anesthesia was not different from that in normal patients. As pethidine (Meperidine®) increases cerebral blood flow and general anesthesia increases ICP, regional anesthesia is the method of choice. Where the condition was present at the time of labor, its resrolution within 72 h of delivery occurred in seven cases reported by Koontz.[146]

HEADACHE
Summary of Management Options

INDICATIONS FOR INVESTIGATION (e.g. CT scan, EEG)

- Focal/abnormal neurological signs

- Impaired intellect

- Intractible pain

- Pain which disturbs sleep

MIGRAINE

- Avoid precipitating factors

- Bed rest, antiemetics, simple analgesics for acute attacks (avoid aspirin in pregnancy)

- Ergotamine-containing preparations are contraindicated

- Consider propranolol or sumatriptan succinate in refractory cases

POSTPARTUM HEADACHES

- Bed rest

- Simple analgesics

SPINAL HEADACHES

- Injection of physiological saline at time of dural tap/puncture

- Analgesia, adequate hydration, lying flat

- Autologous blood patch if this fails after 24 hours

BENIGN INTRACRANIAL HYPERTENSION

Prenatal

- Monitor visual function

- If evidence of deterioration of visual function consider:
  - serial lumbar puncture or acetazolamide
  - ? weight reduction
  - shunting for decompression if fail to respond to conservative measures

Labor/delivery

- Regional analgesia preferred

PRIMARY CEREBRAL TUMOURS

Maternal/Fetal Risks

Brain tumors in pregnancy have been extensively reviewed in the published literature;[148–152] however, the total numbers reported are relatively small and interest in the subject appears to have declined with a dearth of publications over the past two decades. Simon[153] estimated the incidence of pregnancy coinciding with brain tumor at 89 women per year in the USA (2.3 per 100 000 births), and found approximately 220 cases of brain tumor in the world literature. While it is unclear whether these figures included only malignant brain tumors, undoubtedly they do not include pituitary tumors which are much more common in pregnancy.

Despite the relatively small numbers, every category of tumor has been reported in pregnancy, and with the exception of pituitary tumors, appear no more common than outside pregnancy.[154] Early studies found that 80% of cerebral tumors appear to progress more rapidly in the second half of pregnancy, and then show remission after delivery.[148] Certainly, a long-standing neoplasm may cause symptoms for the first time in pregnancy, which disappear after delivery. This is especially true of pituitary tumors.

Presentation is the same as outside pregnancy with focal neurological defects or insidious onset of raised intracranial pressure. Seizures occurring for the first time in pregnancy, unless accompanied by hypertension and proteinuria, should also be considered as possibly due to a neoplasm. The presence of maternal brain tumor does not seem to pose a risk of later development of brain tumor in the child.[155] However, family members of glioma patients have been found to be at increased risk for development of brain tumors.[156]

Management Options

Prenatal

Minimum investigations would be a CT scan with enhancement, taking appropriate steps to shield the fetus. If seizures are present, an EEG may also be appropriate. The remainder of the diagnostic evaluation must be individualized to each case.

In general, malignant tumors in the early stages of pregnancy hold the worst outlook for the pregnancy, and this led to the recommendation of termination on medical grounds in the 1970s.[157] While therapeutic abortion in early gestation is an option which should be open to women with a malignant brain tumor, more recent techniques of neurosurgery such as stereotaxic decompression under local anesthesia may mean that tumors with a high mortality, such as malignant gliomas, presenting at any time during pregnancy, may be managed with surgery during the 1990s. As yet, there are few data in the literature.

For slow-growing tumors in a favorable location, surgery may reasonably be delayed until after delivery. Some recommend a 2–3 week delay after delivery, as many tumors will tend to involute during this period.

Cerebral edema caused by tumor, whether in pregnancy or not, should be aggressively managed with high-dose steroids. There is insufficient experience with mannitol in human pregnancy to advocate its use in this situation. Hypothermia and hyperventilation have been used to reduce cerebral edema during this type of surgery in pregnancy, without adverse fetal effects.

Termination of pregnancy or preterm delivery is rarely necessary on medical grounds, but would be indicated for a severe uncontrollable rise in intracranial pressure or rapid deterioration in vision not responsive to medical therapy.

Labor/delivery

There is no consensus view in the literature as to mode of delivery in patients with brain tumors. During labor, uterine contractions do not increase intracranial pressure; however, expulsive efforts in the second stage do. Whether this is acceptable may depend on factors such as the nature and location of the tumor and the parity of the woman. Given judicious management of the second stage with forceps delivery if there is concern about increased intracranial pressure, it would seem reasonable to reserve cesarean section for obstetric indications.

METASTATIC TUMORS

Risks and Management Options

Very few malignant brain tumors metastasize outside the CNS. However, non-CNS tumors may metastasize to the brain and in order of frequency they are lung, breast, gastrointestinal, renal, melanoma and thyroid. Maternal cancers which have been identified in the fetus include lymphoproliferative tumors and melanoma.[158] Otherwise, the fetus does not appear at risk of metastatic spread.

Choriocarcinoma during or following normal pregnancy is rare; however, the unique property of trophoblastic tissue to invade the walls of blood vessels results in a high rate of hematogenous spread, including cerebral metastases, in up to 20% of cases.[159] This may manifest as cerebral infarction, hemorrhage or space occupying lesion.[160] Cerebral metastases of choriocarcinoma warrant special consideration. More than 90% of patients with metastatic gestational trophoblastic disease can expect to enter complete and sustained remission with appropriate chemotherapy. Unfortunately, patients who develop brain metastases do not share this favorable prognosis, with survival rates as low as 18% reported.[161] This has been attributed to diagnostic delay, decreased responsiveness of tumor in this location to chemotherapy, and sudden unexpected fatal intracerebral hemorrhage.[162–164] Survival rates for those who present with neurological symptoms as the first sign of gestational trophoblastic disease are significantly higher than those for patients developing brain metastases after resistance to chemotherapy has developed in other metastatic sites.[165,166] Most authorities agree that combination chemotherapy is the treatment of choice in patients with brain metastases. Over the last decade, the combination most often used has been methotrexate, actinomycin D and an alkylating agent. Rustin et al. reported a significant improvement in survival with a weekly schedule alternating etoposide, methotrexate and actinomycin D with vincristine and cyclophosphamide chemotherapy (EMACO).[167]

The role of radiotherapy in the management of brain metastases is controversial. Those recommending radiotherapy contend that irradiation of intracerebral choriocarcinoma not only can prevent intracranial hemorrhage, but may also have a tumoricidal effect. Arguments against center around survival data demonstrating that tumor in this location can be eradicated by chemotherapy alone.

NEUROLOGICAL PROBLEMS OF PROLACTINOMAS IN PREGNANCY

Risks and Management Options
(see also Chapter 22)

Use of bromocryptine has resulted in increasing numbers of pregnant women with prolactinomas. Estrogens stimulate tumor development, so pregnancy in these women can be dangerous.[168,169] Micro-adenomas rarely produce clinically important enlargement in pregnancy,[170] while macro-adenomas have a significant risk of symptomatic tumor enlargement. Without treatment, about 15–35% will develop tumor-related neurological

complications,[170–173] with about 6% being neurological emergencies.[172] Because of this risk, prior to availability of bromocryptine, prepregnancy hypophysectomy or radiation were recommended. However, these procedures frequently resulted in global or partial hypopituitarism with a chronic need for endocrine treatment, and did not abolish the risk of tumor-related complications in pregnancy. Continuous bromocryptine in pregnancy has radically changed all this, having proved very satisfactory in the prevention of tumor-related complications, and has greatly reduced surgery in the management. To date, bromocryptine has not been associated with any adverse effects.[174] Breast-feeding should not be discouraged; however, women with macro-adenomas should be followed closely for possible tumor enlargement throughout lactation.

SPINAL CORD PROBLEMS: PARAPLEGIA

Maternal/Fetal Risks

In women of reproductive age with spinal cord injury fertility, libido and the ability to have intercourse and children are generally not affected. Frequent complications they experience in pregnancy include urinary tract infection, anemia, pressure sores, sepsis, exacerbation of constipation, unattended birth and and autonomic dysreflexia.

Autonomic dysreflexia is a most dangerous complication which occurs during labor in up to two-thirds of women with lesions above the T6 level, and is more severe the higher the level of cord damage. It results from a disordered neurological response to noxious stimuli below the level of cord damage. Such stimulation may occur with bladder, rectal, vaginal or cervical distension, which elicit a spinal reflex of sympathetic and parasympathetic outflow uninhibited by either supraspinal centers below the lesion or elsewhere in the CNS.[175] Acute hypertension is mediated by peripheral and splanchnic vasoconstriction, and commonly reaches levels of 200 systolic and 150 diastolic. Intense vagal stimulation mediates bradycardia and arrhythmias. Characteristic features are sudden onset of headache, marked flushing above the level of the lesion along with pupiliary dilation and nasal stuffiness. Hypertensive crisis with cerebrovascular accident has been described in pregnancy,[176,177] with one maternal death.[176] The incidence of pregnancy-associated hypertension is not increased in paraplegics.[178]

Management Options

Unattended birth results from failure of the woman to perceive labor, and possibly rapid labour.[179] For this

---

CEREBRAL TUMORS
Summary of Management Options

PRIMARY

Prenatal

- Termination of pregnancy *vs* neurosurgery during pregnancy depends on:
    - type of tumor
    - natural history
    - gestation
    - patient's wishes

- High-dose steroids for cerebral edema

Labor/delivery

- Insufficient data to determine whether assisted second stage is of benefit

PROLACTINOMAS

- See Chapter 22 for full discussion

reason, regular cervical assessment in the last trimester and induction at term when the cervix is favorable are appropriate in the management; however, elective hospital admission has been found to confer no benefit until 36 weeks gestation.[180]

Unlike the more common hypertensive complications of pregnancy, the elevation of blood pressure due to autonomic dysreflexia builds rapidly with the contraction, abates markedly between contractions, and disappears rapidly following delivery.[181] Thus blood pressure measurements during labour should be frequent and it should be appreciated that blood pressure measurements between contractions do not reflect the condition or the response to antihypertensives. It has been proposed that the frequency with which this complication leads to cerebrovascular accident may be underestimated owing to misdiagnosis of pregnancy-associated hypertension.[177] It has been suggested that noxious stimuli in labour should be minimized by the use of topical anesthetic prior to procedures such as vaginal examination, bladder catheterization or rectal manipulation, that the bladder should be left on continuous drainage to avoid distension, and fetal heart rate monitoring by means of a scalp clip to avoid abdominal stimulation.[177] Use of a paracervical block to eliminate neurological stimulation during dilatation has not been evaluated.

Regional anesthesia may be optimal for controlling autonomic dysreflexia,[182] and full discussion between the patient, anesthetist and obstetrician with a plan for intrapartum management should be made prior to delivery. If autonomic dysreflexia is not prevented with regional anesthesia, then short-acting antihypertensives should be used, and the second stage expedited with forceps or vacuum extraction. Uterine contractility is not affected by spinal cord damage, and essentially cesarean section is indicated for obstetric reasons only.[181,183]

There is no reason why these women should not breast-feed successfully.

SPINAL CORD TUMORS

Maternal Risks

Spinal cord tumors are uncommon and co-existence with pregnancy is rare. About 75% are in fact arteriovenous malformations (AVM). In general, these AVMs cause progressive neurological symptoms; however, in pregnancy, the course is characteristically intermittent, with exacerbation followed by complete remission after delivery.[184] Mechanisms proposed to explain the intermittent course during pregnancy include the increase in uterine perfusion, a bulky uterus impeding vena caval return resulting in engorgement on the venous side of the AVM, and enlargement of the AVM due to vasodilator effect of hormones on vessels within the shunt.

Management Options

In the presence of cord compression symptoms, investigative studies should be performed regardless of the radiation risk to the fetus. Both plain x-rays and myelography, and examination of CSF are indicated. CSF samples should also be saved for protein electrophoresis and viral studies. Normal results of CSF and myelogram studies suggest a diagnosis of acute or chronic inflammatory demyelinating disease.

SPINAL CORD PROBLEMS
Summary of Management Options

PARAPLEGIA

Prenatal

- Treatment of 'minor problems', e.g.
  - pressure sores
  - urinary infection
  - constipation

Labor/delivery

- Vigilance for unrecognized labor

- Vigilance for spinal dysreflexia syndrome (especially above T6)
  - minimize stimuli (vaginal and rectal examinations, catheterization)
  - ? regional analgesia advisable

- Cesarean section for normal obstetric conditions

SPINAL CORD TUMORS

- Investigate if signs of cord compression

CONGENITAL MALFORMATIONS: NEURAL TUBE DEFECTS

Risks and Management Options

During the last 20 years, significant numbers of children with meningomyelocele and or hydrocephalus have reached reproductive age. The risk of neural tube defect in their offspring appears to be only about 3%.[185] Problems expected in women with spina bifida undergoing pregnancy are a high incidence of urinary tract infection and deterioration in renal function due to increasing hydronephrosis. The author recently experienced a patient who went into renal failure at 25 weeks. Delivery of the infant was associated with a marked improvement in renal function with a return to prepregnancy values within 1 week.

CONGENITAL MALFORMATIONS: CEREBROSPINAL FLUID SHUNTS

Maternal Risks

The prognosis for hydrocephalus has improved dramatically over the past 20 years, with long-term survival in 85% and 60–70% have near normal intelligence.[186,187] In recent years, a number of pregnancies in women with shunted hydrocephalus have been reported.[188–194]

Management Options

Prepregnancy

Patients with well-functioning shunts frequently develop symptoms of raised intracranial pressure (ICP) during pregnancy,[192] which may reflect physiological changes of increased brain water and venous distension. For this reason, a preconception CT or MRI scan has been recommended, and if there is any suspicion of shunt malfunction, additional measurement of ICP and a radioisotope shunt patency study.[192]

Patients on anticonvulsants should have their drugs reviewed and those with hydrocephalus associated with a neural tube defect should be advised of the 2–3% risk of this in her offspring and of the value of folic acid supplementation starting before pregnancy.[27]

Prenatal

During pregnancy it has been found that 58% of women with shunts will develop symptoms and signs of raised intracranial pressure.[192] This may be the result of poor cerebral compliance with limited capacity to respond to the expanded brain volume of pregnancy, exacerbation of pre-existing shunt malfunction by these physiological changes, or blockage of a previously well-functioning shunt. The risk of shunt malfunction appears highest in the third trimester, probably due to an increase in intra-abdominal pressure.[190,195,196] The value of a pregnancy CT or MRI scan becomes apparent in these patients, as the cause of new symptoms may be evaluated by comparison of ventricular size with the baseline value. A radioisotope study of shunt patency may be necessary to reveal a malfunctioning shunt. Conservative treatment with bed rest, fluid restriction, steroids, acetazolamide (Diamox®) and even diuretics may be tried. Shunt aspiration allows measurement of intracranial pressure and periodic aspirations may be used for relief of symptoms. Although this must be weighed against the risk of CNS and or peritoneal infection. Pumping the shunt may be a more benign way of relieving symptoms,[193,194] but is not always effective. Symptoms often resolve spontaneously following delivery, so that for symptomatic women, early delivery as soon as fetal lung maturity has been demonstrated may avoid the need for shunt replacement. If CT or MRI studies demonstrate enlarging ventricles with conservative measures, and delivery is not a reasonable option, then a shunt revision is indicated. Ventriculo-peritoneal shunting is feasible in the first and second trimesters and carries the lowest complication rate.[186,187] In later pregnancy, consideration of a ventriculo-atrial or ventriculo-pleural shunt would be necessary because of the uterine size. Five patients described in the literature had no complications associated with shunt placement prenatally.[192]

Labor/delivery

The mode of delivery advocated depends on the neurological status. For patients with a peritoneal shunt, any abdominal surgery may increase the risk of adhesion formation around the end of the shunt, and also increase the risk of shunt infection. Temporary elevations in CSF pressure are well tolerated by neurologically stable patients, so vaginal delivery with avoidance of a long active second stage is the method of choice.

If the patient is neurologically unstable, elective cesarean section under general anesthesia is advocated,[192] with care not to leave blood in the peritoneal cavity, which may result in shunt blockage by fibrin clot. Because the shunt is a foreign body linking the peritoneal cavity and the brain, and because bacterial contamination of the peritoneal cavity could theoretically result from a retrograde seeding during labor and delivery, antibiotic prophylaxis for these events is recommended.[189,192,194] For analgesia, opiates should be avoided as far as possible as they may cloud consciousness and further increase intracranial pressure. Epidur-

---

CONGENITAL MALFORMATIONS OF THE CENTRAL NERVOUS SYSTEM
Summary of Management Options

NEURAL TUBE DEFECTS

Prenatal

- Serial screening:
  - renal function
  - urinary infection

Labor/delivery

- Mode of delivery depends on pelvic size/shape (often cesarean section)

CEREBROSPINAL FLUID SHUNTS

Prepregnancy

- Check shunt is fully working

- If on anticonvulsants, counseling as for Epilepsy (above)

Prenatal

- Vigilance for raised intracranial pressure (ICP) (confirm with CT scan in comparison with prepregnancy or radiostudy)

- With raised ICP:
  - bed rest
  - fluid restriction
  - steroids
  - acetazolamide
  - shunt pumping or intermittent aspiration
  - delivery *vs* shunt revision if conservative measures fail

Labor/delivery

- Aim for vaginal delivery with short second stage

- Regional analgesia:
  - acceptable if stable
  - contraindicated if raised ICP or NTD

- If cesarean section:
  - avoid leaving blood in abdomen
  - prophylactic antibiotics

---

als may be used with caution in stable patients, but are contraindicated in patients with raised intracranial pressure and those with spina bifida, making general anesthesia the method of choice for surgical delivery.

NEUROMUSCULAR DISEASE: ACUTE DEMYELINATING POLYNEURITIS: GUILLAIN-BARRÉ SYNDROME

Maternal Risks

Sometimes referred to as the Landry Guillain Barré and Strohl syndrome, Guillain-Barré Syndrome (GBS) is now the most common acute paralytic disease encountered. Although it is relatively rare (1.5–1.7 cases per 100 000 population per year[197,198]), it does affect young adults and so may coincide with pregnancy. Pregnancy does not appear to alter the incidence or the course and severity of GBS, and GBS does not appear to adversely affect the pregnancy.[199,200]

Antecedent infection with numerous agents has been reported; however only for campylobacter, cytomegalovirus and Epstein–Barr virus are there supportive controlled data.[201] Essentially, the pathogenesis of the disorder remains unknown.[202]

Clinical features include progressive motor weakness of more than one limb associated with loss of reflexes. Sensory and autonomic involvement are common but are usually mild compared with the degree of motor deficit. The differential diagnosis includes poly-neuritis due to vitamin B_{12} deficiency, acute intermittent porphyria and heavy metal poisoning. Investigations should include a vitamin B_{12} level, heavy metal and porphyrin screens. Normal creatine phosphokinase levels exclude an inflammatory muscle disorder, and lack of fever, a raised protein concentration in CSF without an increase in cell count, and neurophysiological evidence of demyelination are all in keeping with the diagnosis. However, there is no definitive test for the disease.

Management Options

Management is predominantly symptomatic. Serial forced vital capacity measurements should be commenced in the acute phase as respiratory failure is the major complication. Other complications include infection due to an inability to clear secretions, and vascular collapse and arrhythmias from autonomic involvement. These autonomic complications are notoriously difficult to manage and may rarely lead to sudden death. Outside pregnancy, Dyck reported 16% of patients required ventilatory support and a 5% mortality,[198] whereas Winer reported death in 1:8 patients.[203] A review of 32 pregnancies in 29 affected women in the literature suggests that pregnant women with the disease have a slightly increased mortality (13%) and 35% required respiratory support. Fetal survival rate was reported at 96%.[204]

Although the pathophysiology of demyelinating neuropathy is unknown, it is thought to involve a myelinotoxic antibody or substance circulating in the plasma. Randomized controlled trials evaluating the role of plasmapharesis in non-pregnant individuals with the GBS syndrome have demonstrated a marked reduction in both the proportion of patients requiring assisted ventilation, and decreased duration of ventilation in those with respiratory failure.[205,206]

Hurley et al.[207] reported good results with plasmapharesis, with no adverse fetal effects, in three pregnant women. In view of the relatively high mortality in pregnant women requiring ventilation, it is recommended that plasmapharesis should be commenced before ventilation is required. A fluctuating course has been related to plasmapharesis in some patients; however, repeat plasmapharesis is also associated with a favorable response.[208,209] Treatment-related fluctuations are considered to be induced by the temporary effect of plasma exchange on the disease process.

Steroids were popular until a controlled trial in 1978 failed to show evidence of benefit.[210] A trial conducted by the Medical Research Council is in progress to assess the role of methylprednisolone; however, preliminary results suggest that it is ineffective.[211] High-dose intravenous immunoglobulin is the latest treatment option,[212] and analysis of the Dutch Guillain-Barré trial comparing high-dose i.v. immunoglobulin with plasmapharesis is currently in progress. An initial analysis has shown that i.v. immunoglobulin compares favorably with plasmapharesis.[213] It is important that pregnant patients who are unable to move their legs should also receive prophylactic subcutaneous heparin.

The disease is self-limiting and the usual course is complete functional recovery in a median time of 9 months.[203] Relapses may occur in 1–6% of patients, and have been reported in pregnancy.

NEUROMUSCULAR DISEASE: MULTIPLE SCLEROSIS: CHRONIC DEMYELINATING POLYNEUROPATHY

Maternal/Fetal Risks

This chronic demyelinating disorder of white matter typically has its onset in young adults, with an excess among females. Symptoms and signs of visual loss due to optic atrophy, diplopia, spasticity, sensory loss and sphincter disturbance predominate. The diagnosis is one of exclusion, and the natural history of the disease is variable with unpredictable relapses and remissions and cumulative deficits over time.

Infertility, abortion, stillbirth and fetal anomalies do not appear increased in women with multiple sclerosis (MS),[214–216] although the diagnosis may alter a woman's decision about having children, as evidenced by the high rate of unwanted pregnancies reported by Poser and Poser.[216] Children of women with MS have a 3% risk of developing the disease compared with a 0.1% risk in the general population.[217]

A number of retrospective studies have reported reduced exacerbation rates during pregnancy and a tendency to relapse postpartum.[216,218–222] During pregnancy, relapses occur at about half the expected rate outside pregnancy, with the most significant reduction in the last trimester, while during the first 6 months postpartum Birk et al.[223] estimated that the relapse rate was 10 times that observed in the same women during pregnancy. No measures have been shown to reduce the risk of postpartum relapse, including pregnancy termination.

Pregnancy per se does not appear to alter the long-term prognosis of MS.[216,224]

Management Options

Prepregnancy

The risks and complications for pregnancy (see above) should be discussed.

Prenatal

Specific treatments remain disappointing, and thus there is little or no justification for using agents which may be harmful to the fetus. In those with bladder dysfunction, the bladder should be kept free of residual urine by intermittent self-catheterization. Urine should be regularly screened for incipient infection.

Steroids are commonly used to treat acute exacerbations of MS. In animals, high-dose prednisone has been associated with an increased rate of miscarriage, cleft palate and fetal growth deficiency; however, these effects have not been confirmed in humans. Also, it is now recognized that there are maternal conditions where survival of the fetus depends on highly aggressive steroid therapy, and this has alleviated anxiety about its use elsewhere for benefit of the mother.

Immunosuppressives have been used in management and in pregnancy. A recent meta-analysis of published trials of azathiaprine concluded that there was slight benefit in patients treated over 2–3 years, but that it is debatable whether these outweigh the side-effects.[225] In view of this finding, its use cannot be justified during pregnancy for MS.

Labor/delivery

Labor and delivery can be managed routinely and cesarean section is indicated for obstetric reasons only. Anesthesia consists of fewer options for the woman with MS, in that progressive neurological disease with a propensity to relapse in the puerperium relatively contraindicates regional anesthesia. The relative safety of regional compared with general anesthesia in patients requiring cesarean section or complicated vaginal delivery has not been resolved.

Postnatal

Breast-feeding is not contraindicated just because of the propensity to postpartum relapse, or in women receiving steroids or immunosuppressives. Vigilance should be maintained for a relapse in the puerperium.

NEUROMUSCULAR DISEASE: MYASTHENIA GRAVIS (see also Chapter 27)

Maternal/Fetal Risks

This autoimmune disorder presents classically with easy fatiguability, diplopia and difficulty with speaking, swallowing and clearing secretions. All of these result from IgG autoantibodies binding to acetylcholine receptors at the neuromuscular junction, reducing the number of receptors on the post-synaptic membrane and so interfering with neuromuscular transmission.[226] If symptoms of weakness and easy fatiguability of voluntary muscles present for the first time in pregnancy, diagnosis can be made by the electromyogram and response to tensilon. The association of congenital anomalies with myasthenia is very rare, with only seven published reports including 12 infants.[227]

Pregnancy has no consistent effect on myasthenia. A review of 322 pregnancies occurring in 225 myasthenic mothers in the literature reported an exacerbation rate of 41% during pregnancy and 29.8% post partum.[228] Of note, there were nine maternal deaths (40 per 1000), mostly related to exacerbations or treatment complications. Termination for those with exacerbation in the first trimester has not been shown to confer any consistent benefit.[229]

In recent years, the outlook for the disease has improved dramatically;[230] however, the obstetrician should be aware of two particular aspects of the disease – the effects of some commonly used drugs, and the occurrence of neonatal myasthenia in the newborn infants of myasthenic mothers.

Any drugs possessing curare-like properties or neuromuscular blocking properties are contraindicated. These include muscle relaxants, procaine, ether, quinine, quinidine, the aminoglycoside antibiotics (neomycin, streptomycin, kanamycin and gentamicin), and magnesium salts.

Management Options

Prepregnancy

Thymectomy has a well-established role in the management of the disorder. Its introduction was accompanied by a dramatic improvement in mortality and morbidity, particularly in women without a thymoma, and the benefit appears greatest when it is performed early in the course of the disease. A review of the literature supports elective thymectomy prior to pregnancy in the initial treatment of young women, as being associated with a lower incidence of clinical exaceration in pregnancy.[231]

Prenatal

Steroids have an established role, rapidly inducing remission in 80% of patients,[232] probably by protecting acetylcholine receptors from immunological attack. Steroid withdrawal may cause exacerbation, but the dose may be minimized by an alternate day regime.

Concomitant use of immunosuppressives is beneficial in the non-pregnant patient, allowing lower doses of anticholinesterase drugs and steroids to produce a given effect. Azathiaprin has been most extensively used and, although it readily crosses the placenta and is teratogenic in animals, it appears relatively safe in human pregnancy (category B).[41]

Plasmapheresis has also been used successfully for myasthenic crisis during pregnancy.[233]

Labor/delivery

Vaginal delivery is in no way contraindicated by myasthenia, although tiring of voluntary muscles during the second stage may necessitate instrumental delivery. Cesarean section is particularly hazardous because of the effects of muscle relaxants and postoperative difficulties with restricted respiration and clearance of secretions. Narcotic analgesics may worsen myasthenia, making regional anesthesia the method of choice. Magnesium sulfate should not be used for seizure prophylaxis in the event a myasthenic patient presents with concomitant pre-eclampsia.

Postnatal

Transient weakness occurs in a minority (10–20%) of infants of myasthenic mothers.[228,234] This low incidence has been ascribed to an inhibitory effect of alpha-fetoprotein on the binding of antibody to acetylcholine receptors.[235] It usually presents with hypotonia, respiratory and feeding difficulties, occurring in the first 24 h, but may present as late as 3 days. Spontaneous resolution within 1 month is the rule, although antibody may be detected for 3–4 months.[236] Papatestas found that the incidence in infants of mothers who had not undergone thymectomy was twice that in thymectomized women;[237] however, this is contrary to the review by Eden and Gall.[231] These latter authors suggested that the occurrence of neonatal disease could not be predicted by the severity of disease in the mother or the presence or absence of thymectomy. It may even occur when the mother is in remission.[238] The level of maternal antibody also has no predictive value.[239]

Management of the neonate includes careful observation, tube feeding, control of secretions and ventilatory support if needed. Cholinesterase inhibitors can be used but may increase secretions. In severe cases, plasma exchange may be beneficial. The disease is self-limiting within 3–4 weeks. Breast-feeding is not contraindicated in myasthenic mothers, including those using steroids, azathiaprin and anticholinesterase drugs.

NEUROMUSCULAR DISEASE: MYOTONIC DYSTROPHY

Maternal/Fetal Risks

Myotonic dystrophy is an autosomal dominant condition, manifested clinically by a progressive distal myopathy with delayed relaxation, weakness and wasting of affected muscles. Myotonia of the grip detected by shaking a hand of an affected individual is said to be a useful diagnostic aid. Other features may include myopathic facies, cataracts, frontal balding, variable mental retardation and other multi-organ involvement. Diagnosis is confirmed by electromyographic studies.

Pregnancy may be associated with exacerbations of myotonia and weakness, particularly during the third trimester.[240–243] Symptoms of the disease may first be noticed in pregnancy,[244,245] or the mother may be relatively asymptomatic and the disease go unrecognized.[246] Reports reveal a high rate of fetal loss due to early miscarriage,[241,242] premature delivery[241,242,245, 247–249] and neonatal death.[245,247] Cardiac involvement may appear several years after the onset of neuromuscular symptoms, and manifests as conduction defects, arrhythmias and other ECG abnormalities.[250]

Management Options

Prenatal

Continued activity through pregnancy should be encouraged as inactivity is known to cause a deterioration in myotonia.[242] An ECG should be peformed at the first visit and the patient told to report any symptoms suggestive of arrhythmia. Prenatal diagnosis is now possible with either amniotic fluid or chorionic villi sampling, and should be discussed with affected mothers in light of the adverse prognosis for affected fetuses and infants. Originally, the linkage of the gene to the secretor locus was utilized;[251] however, recombinant DNA technology has led to the identification of restriction fragment polymorphic markers close to the gene on chromosome 19,[252,253] allowing prenatal diagnosis with a high degree of certainty.

Hydramnios commonly develops and this together with abnormal myotonic involvement of the uterus are predisposing factors to premature labour.[241,244, 247,254] The presence of hydramnios probably indicates a fetus affected with myotonic dystrophy,[241,248] with a significant risk of stillbirth or neonatal death. For these reasons, clinical and/or ultrasound evaluation of amniotic fluid volume, and some form of fetal surveillance in those fetuses suspected of being affected is indicated in the last trimester. Also, it has been suggested that cervical assessment should be performed at intervals

NEUROMUSCULAR DISEASE
Summary of Management Options

GUILLAIN-BARRÉ SYNDROME

- Monitor respiratory function; ventilation may be necessary

- Nursing and physiotherapy

- Prophylactic heparin

- Consider
  - plasmapheresis
  - immunoglobulin i.v.

MULTIPLE SCLEROSIS

Prepregnancy

- Counsel about risks

Prenatal

- Nursing measures, e.g. intermittent self-catheterization

- Steroids for relapse

Labor/delivery

- Regional analgesia is contraindicated

Postnatal

- Breast-feeding is acceptable

- Vigilance for relapse

MYASTHENIA GRAVIS
(see also Chapter 27)

Prepregnancy

- Counseling about risks

- Review of therapy to improve disease control

- Consider thymectomy

Prenatal

- Continue pre-existing drugs:
  - anticholinesterases
  - steroids
  - (azathiaprine)

- Plasmapheresis for drug-resistant cases

- Fetal surveillance, especially activity (? biophysical profile score)

Labor/delivery

- Minimize stress

- Continue anticholinesterase drugs (parenteral)

- Steroid cover if on steroids

- Regional analgesia preferable to narcotics for pain relief and general anesthesia

- Experienced anesthetist if general anesthesia (advisable to consult in prenatal period)

- Assisted second stage more likely

- Avoid magnesium sulfate in patients with pre-eclampsia

Postnatal

- Review dosage of drugs

- Special care and surveillance of newborn; may need short-term anticholinesterases

MYOTONIC DYSTROPHY

Prenatal

- Offer prenatal diagnosis

- Vigilance for hydramnios, etc. (see Chapter 48 for therapeutic options)

Labor/delivery

- Syntocinon infusion if dystocia in first stage

- May need assisted second stage

- Active third stage

- Regional analgesia preferable to narcotics and general anesthesia

Postnatal

- Careful neuromuscular examination of the newborn

in the last trimester, which will detect those likely to deliver prematurely. Where hydramnios develops, consideration may be given to therapeutic amniocentesis[255] or indomethacin[256] to prolong the gestation (see Chapter 48).

Labor/delivery

Although rapid preterm labor may complicate hydramnios, dysfunction of uterine smooth muscle affected by myotonia may predispose to slow labor. When present, uterine intertia should respond to oxytocin,[241] and maternal weakness may necessitate assisted delivery. There are several reports of postpartum hemorrhage due to uterine inertia,[242,248,257] so the third stage should be actively managed with oxytocic injection.

Muscular wasting may include the diaphragm and accessory muscles, making these patients highly susceptible to apnea with narcotics, halothane and diazepam. Attempts at maintenance or instrumentation of the airway may trigger a myotonic response, preventing successful establishment of the airway and ventilation. Neuromuscular blocking agents used during general anesthesia may also result in a marked generalized contracture of skeletal muscle, preventing airway maintenance.[258,259]

For these reasons, regional anesthesia is the method of choice, and consultation with an anesthetist is appropriate during the prenatal period.

Postnatal

The incidence of the congenital syndrome was reported by Wesstrom et al.[260] to be 1:3500 live births in the Swedish population, and is a condition which is likely to be under-diagnosed when the mother has not complained of any symptoms of the disorder.[246] Once suspected in a baby, it can be confirmed by examination and EMG studies in the mother, as no tests are diagnostic in the newborn.

Congenital myotonic dystrophy is clinically distinct from the adult type,[261] with transmission almost confined to infants of mothers with the disease.[262] This is strong evidence that the intrauterine environment as well as the autosomal dominant gene contribute to the congenital form.[263]

The clinical picture is that of severe generalized hypotonia and weakness, including respiratory and feeding difficulties.[245,254,264] Severely affected babies will fail to establish ventilation and may be misdiagnosed as having perinatal asphyxia. If the baby survives the first few weeks, there is gradual improvement. Although their development is slow, most learn to walk and talk; however, long-term prognosis is poor

with a high incidence of mental retardation and muscle weakness. Dyken and Harper found an average IQ of 56 in 14 patients who had respiratory symptoms in the neonatal period.[265]

MONONEUROPATHIES

A whole variety of peripheral nerve syndromes may be associated with pregnancy or delivery, particularly those involving facial, trigeminal, median and ulnar, lateral cutaneous nerve of the thigh, obturator, peroneal and sciatic nerves. Most resolve spontaneously and require only symptomatic treatment and reassurance.

MONONEUROPATHIES: BELL'S PALSY

Maternal Risks

Idiopathic facial palsy has an incidence of 17 per 100 000 women of child-bearing age, but a well-documented increase in frequency occurs during pregnancy and the first 2 weeks postpartum to 45 per 100 000, with 75% of cases occurring during the last trimester and the early puerperium.[266,267] Diagnosis presents no problem, with the sudden onset of unilateral facial weakness, usually discovered on wakening. Associated loss of taste on the anterior two-thirds of the tongue if the lesion is proximal to the branch of the corda tympani, and hyperacusis if the nerve to stapedius is involved, carry a less favorable prognosis.[268]

The etiology is uncertain; however, in this age group, it may be a viral mononeuropathy, whereas in older age groups, it may be a manifestation of vascular disturbance.

Management Options

A short course of high-dose prednisone dramatically relieves pain associated with Bell's palsy and has become standard treatment. Usually, a 10-day course is sufficient for partial paralysis, while a 3 week course is indicated with total paralysis. However short the course, steroids must not be withdrawn abruptly because rebound inflammation may lead to further denervation. Protection of the eye by use of glasses and eye drops during the day is recommended.[268]

In those with incomplete paralysis, recovery within 3–6 weeks can be expected.

MONONEUROPATHIES: CARPAL TUNNEL SYNDROME

Risks and Management Options

This is the most common nerve compression syndrome in pregnancy, occurring in up to 25% of women during the second half of pregnancy.[269] It is believed to result from edema within the carpal tunnel. The diagnosis is made from the history of pain or paresthesia in the hands, particularly on wakening. In view of the good prognosis, management is symptomatic. Night splints or just reassurance is usually all that is required. Spontaneous resolution occurs in over 80% within 2 months of delivery. For those with residual symptoms, thyroid status should be checked and surgical decompression may be appropriate. Decompression during pregnancy should be considered for those with severe pain and sensory deficit, and can be done under local anesthesia.[269] This provides immediate and lasting relief.

MONONEUROPATHIES: MERALGIA PARESTHETICA

Risks and Management Options

This is a rare mononeuropathy presenting with numbness, tingling and pain over the lateral aspect of the thigh in late pregnancy. Spontaneous resolution is usual after delivery.

REFERENCES

1   Knight AH, Rhind EG (1975) Epilepsy and pregnancy: A study of 153 pregnancies in 59 patients. *Epilepsia* **16**:99–110.
2   Philbert A, Dam M (1982) The epileptic mother and her child. *Epilepsia* **23**:85–99.
3   Zlatkis LS (1966) Effect of pregnancy, childbirth and puerperium on the course of epilepsy. *Sovetskaia Meditsina (Moskva)* **29**:104–108.
4   Gjerde IO, Strandjord RE, Ulstein M (1988) The course of epilepsy during pregnancy: A study of 78 cases. *Acta Neurologia Scandinavica* **78**:198–205.
5   Bardy AH (1982) Seizure frequency in epileptic women during pregnancy and the puerperium: Results of the prospective Helsinki study. In Janz D, Dam M, Richens A, Bossi L, Helge H, Schmidt D (eds) *Epilepsy, Pregnancy and the Child*, pp. 27–31. New York: Raven Press.
6   Remillard G, Dansky L, Andermann E, Andermann F (1982) Seizure frequency during pregnancy and the puerperium. In Janz D, Dam M, Richens A, Bossi L, Helge H, Schmidt D (eds) *Epilepsy, Pregnancy and the Child*, pp. 15–26. New York: Raven Press.
7   Schmidt D, Canger R, Avanzini G, Cusi C, Beck-Mannagetta G, Kock S, Rating D, Janz D (1983) Change of seizure frequency in pregnant epileptic women. *Journal of Neurology, Neurosurgery and Psychiatry* **46**: 751–755.
8   Yerby M, Koepsell, Daling J (1985) Pregnancy complications and outcomes in a cohort of women with epilepsy. *Epilepsia* **26**:631–635.
9   Bjerkedal T, Bahna SL (1973) The course and outcome of pregnancy in women with epilepsy. *Acta Obstetrica et Gynecologica Scandinavica* **52**:245–248.
10   Sonneveld SW, Correy JF (1990) Outcome of pregnancies complicated by epilepsy in Tasmania 1981–1988. *Australia and New Zealand Journal of Obstetrics and Gynaecology* **30**:286–289.
11   Lander CM, Eadie MJ (1991) Plasma antiepileptic drug concentrations during pregnancy. *Epilepsia* **32**:257–266.
12   Hanson JW, Smith DW (1975) Are hydantoins (phenytoins) human teratogens? *Journal of Pediatrics* **87**:285–290.
13   Hanson JW, Myrianthopoulos NC, Harvey MAS, Smith DW (1976) Risks to the offspring of women treated with hydantoin anticonvulsants, with emphasis on the fetal hydantoin syndrome. *Journal of Pediatrics* **89**:662–668.
14   DiLiberti JH, Parndon PA, Dennis, NR, Curry CJ (1984) The fetal valproate syndrome. *American Journal of Medical Genetics* **19**:473–481.
15   Jager-Roman E, Deichl A, Jakob S, Hartmann AM,

MONONEUROPATHIES
Summary of Management Options

BELL'S PALSY

• Protect eye on affected side

• High-dose steroids if severe

CARPAL TUNNEL SYNDROME

• Explanation/reassurance

• Splinting

• ? Diuretics if severe

• ?? Decompression if severe and all else fails

Koch S, Rating D, Steldinger R, Nau H, Helge F (1986) Fetal growth, major malformatoins, and minor anomalies in infants born to women receiving valproic acid. *Journal of Pediatrics* **108**:997–1104.

16 Zackai EH, Mellman WJ, Neiderer B, Hanson JW (1975) The fetal trimethadone syndrome. *Journal of Pediatrics* **87**:280–284.

17 Feldman GL, Weaver DD, Lovrien EW (1977) The fetal trimethadone syndrome. *American Journal of Diseases of Children* **131**:1389–1392.

18 Speidel BD, Meadow SR (1972) Maternal epilepsy and abnormalities of the fetus and newborn. *Lancet* **ii**:839–843.

19 Fedrick J (1973) Epilepsy and pregnancy: A report from the Oxford record linkage study. *British Medical Journal* **ii**:442–448.

20 Lindhout D, Hoppener RJ, Meinardi H (1984) Teratogenicity of antiepileptic drug combinations with special emphasis on epoxidation of carbamazepine. *Epilepsia* **25**:77–83.

21 Hiilesmaa VK, Bardy AH, Teramo K (1985) Obstetric outcome in women with epilepsy. *American Journal of Obstetrics and Gynecology* **152**:499–504.

22 Nakane Y, Okuma T, Takahashi R, Sato Y, Wada T, Sato T *et al.* (1980) Multi-institutional study on the teratogenicity and fetal toxicity of antiepileptic drugs: A report of a collaborative study group in Japan. *Epilepsia* **21**:663–680.

23 Kelly TE, Edwards SP, Rein M, Miller JQ, Dreifruss FE (1984) Teratogenicity of anticonvulsant drugs. II. A prospective study. *American Journal of Medical Genetics* **19**:423–443.

24 Ottman R, Annegers JF, Hauser WA, Kurland LT (1988) Higher risk of seizures in offspring of mothers than of fathers with epilepsy. *American Journal of Human Genetics* **43**:257–264.

25 Saunders M (1989) Epilepsy in women of childbearing age. *British Medical Journal* **299**:581.

26 Firth HV, Lindenbam RH (1989) Epilepsy: Women of child bearing age. *British Medical Journal* **299**:976–977.

27 MRC Vitamin Study Research Group (1991) Prevention of neural tube defects: Results of the Medical Research Council vitamin study. *Lancet* **338**:131–137.

28 Meadow SR (1970) Congenital abnormalities and anticonvulsant drugs. *Proceedings of the Royal Society of Medicine* **63**:48–49.

29 Schmidt D (1982) The effect of pregnancy on the natural history of epilepsy: Review of the literature. In Janz D, Dam M, Richens A, Bossi L, Helge H, Schmidt D (eds) *Epilepsy, Pregnancy and the Child*, pp. 3–14. New York: Raven Press.

30 Annegers JF, Kurland LT, Hauser WA (1983) Teratogenicity of anticonvulsant drugs. In Ward AA Jr, Penry JK, Purpura D (eds) *Epilepsy*, pp. 239–248. New York: Raven Press.

31 Mountain KR, Hirsh J, Gallus AS (1970) Neonatal coagulation defect due to anticonvulsant drug treatment in pregnancy. *Lancet* **i**:265–266.

32 Valproate and malformations. (1982) *Lancet* **ii**:1313–1314.

33 Oakeshoff P, Hunt GM (1989) Valproate and spina bifida. *British Medical Journal* **298**:1300–1301.

34 Jones KL, Lacro RV, Johnson KA, Adams J (1989) Pattern of malformations in the children of women treated with carbamazepine during pregnancy. *New England Journal of Medicine* **320**:1661–1666.

35 Niesen M, Froscher W (1985) Finger and toenail hypoplasia after carbamazepine monotherapy in late pregnancy. *Neuropediatrics* **16**:167–168.

36 Rosa RW (1991) Spina bifida in infants of women treated with carbamazepine during pregnancy. *New England Journal of Medicine* **324**:674–677.

37 Nau H, Cuhnz W, Egger HJ, Rating D, Helge H (1982) Anticonvulsants during pregnancy and lactation. *Clinical Pharmokinetics* **7**:508–543.

38 Smith DW (1977) Teratogenicity of anticonvulsive medications. *American Journal of Diseases of Children* **131**:1337–1339.

39 Greenberg G, Inman WHW, Weatherall JAC *et al.* (1977) Maternal drug histories and congenital abnormalities. *British Medical Journal* **ii**:853–856.

40 US Food and Drug Administration (1980) *Federal Register* **44**:37 434–37 467.

41 Briggs GG, Freeman RK, Yaffe SJ (1990) *Drugs in Pregnancy and Lactation*, 3rd edn. Baltimore, MD: Williams and Wilkins.

42 Plum F, Posner JB (1980) *The Diagnosis of Stupor and Coma*, 3rd edn, pp. 345–364. Philadelphia: F.A. Davis.

43 Engel J (1989) *Seizures and Epilepsy*, pp. 256–280. Philadelphia: FA Davis.

44 Kaplan PW, Lesser RP, Fisher RS, Repke JT, Hanley DF (1988) No, magnesium sulphate should not be used in treating eclamptic seizures. *Archives of Neurology* **45**:1361–1364.

45 Donaldson JO (1988) Eclamptic hypertensive encephalopathy. *Seminars in Neurology* **8**:230–233.

46 Kaplan PW, Lesser RP, Fisher RS, Repke JT, Hanley DF (1990) A continuing controversy: Magnesium sulfate in the treatment of eclamptic seizures. *Archives of Neurology* **47**:1031–1032.

47 Crowther C (1990) Magnesium sulphate versus diazepam in the management of eclampsia: A randomized controlled trial. *British Journal of Obstetrics and Gynaecology* **97**:110–117.

48 Dommisse J (1990) Phenytoin sodium and magnesium sulphate in the management of eclampsia. *British Journal of Obstetrics and Gynaecology* **97**:104–109.

49 Ryan G, Lange I, Nauglen MA (1989) Clinical experience with phenytoin prophylaxis in severe pre-eclampsia. *American Journal of Obstetrics and Gynecology* **161**:1297–1304.

50 Slater RM, Wilcox FL, Smith WD, Donnai P, Patrick J, Richardson T, Mawer GE, D'Souza SW, Anderton JM (1987) Phenytoin infusion in severe pre-eclampsia. *Lancet* **i**:1417–1421.

51 Tuffnell D, O'Donovan P, Lilford RJ, Prys-Davies A, Thornton JG (1989) Phenytoin in pre-eclampsia (Letter). *Lancet* **ii**:273–274.

52 Coyaji KJ, Otiv SR (1990) Single high dose of intravenous phenytoin sodium for the treatment of eclampsia. *Acta Obstetrica et Gynecologica Scandinavica* **69**:15–18.

53 Sibai BM (1990) Eclampsia. VI. Maternal–perinatal outcome in 254 consecutive cases. *American Journal of Obstetrics and Gynecology* **163**:1049–1054.

54 Pritchard JA, Cunningham FG, Pritchard SA (1984) The Parkland Memorial Hospital protocol for treatment of eclampsia: Evaluation of 245 cases. *American Journal of Obstetrics and Gynecology* **148**:951–963.

55 Delgado-Escueta AV, Wasterlain C, Treiman DM, Porter RJ (1982) Current concepts in neurology: Management of status epilepticus. *New England Journal of Medicine* **306**:1337–1340.

56 Richards AM, Moodley J, Bullock MRR, Downing JW (1987) Maternal deaths from neurological complications of hypertensive crises in pregnancy. *South African Medical Journal* **71**:487–490.

57 Richards AM, Moodley J, Graham DI, Bullock MRR (1986) Active management of the unconscious eclamptic patient. *British Journal of Obstetrics and Gynaecology* **93**:554–562.

58 Feeney JG (1982) Water intoxication and oxytocin. *British Medical Journal* **245**:243.

59 Donaldson JO (1989) *Neurology of Pregnancy*, 2nd edn. London: W.B. Saunders.

60 Higgins TA, Commerford JB (1974) Epilepsy and pregnancy. *Journal of the Irish Medical Association* **67**:317–329.

61 Donaldson JO (1978) *Neurology of Pregnancy*, 1st edn. London: W.B. Saunders.

62 Wiebers DO (1985) Ischemic cerebrovascular complications of pregnancy. *Archives of Neurology* **42**:1106–1113.

63 Simolke GA, Cox SM, Cunningham FG (1991) Cerebrovascular accidents complicating pregnancy and the puerperium. *Obstetrics and Gynecology* **78**:37–42.

64 Chopra JS, Prabhakar S (1979) Clinical features and at risk factors in stroke in young. *Acta Neurologia Scandinavica* **60**:289–300.

65 Dias MS, Sekhar LN (1990) Intracranial hemorrhage from aneurysms and arteriovenous malformations during pregnancy and the puerperium. *Neurosurgery* **27**:855–866.

66 Goldman JA, Eckerling B, Gans B (1964) Intracranial venous sinus thrombosis in pregnancy and puerperium: Report of 15 cases. *Journal of Obstetrics and Gynaecology of the British Commonwealth* **71**:791–796.

67 Carroll JD, Leak D, Lee HA (1966) Cerebral thrombophlebitis in pregnancy and the puerperium. *Quarterly Journal of Medicine* **35**:347–368.

68 Cross JN, Castro PO, Jennett WB (1968) Cerebral strokes associated with pregnancy and the puerperium. *British Medical Journal of Clinical Research* **3**:214–218.

69 Amias AG (1970) Cerebral vascular disease in pregnancy: II. Occlusion. *Journal of Obstetrics and Gynaecology of the British Commonwealth* **77**:312–325.

70 Sturm JT, Toro C, Snyder BD (1987) Emergency carotid artery thrombectomy for postpartum hemiplegia. *American Journal of Emergency Medicine* **5**:291–293.

71 Fujita K, Yamasaki S, Tamaki N, Fujita S, Shirakata S, Matsumoto S (1978) Cerebrovascular accident during pregnancy. *Neurologia Medico-Chirurgica (Tokyo)* **6**:989–995.

72 Enomoto H, Goto H (1987) Moyamoya disease presenting as intracerebral hemorrhage during pregnancy: Case report and review of the literature. *Neurosurgery* **20**:33–35.

73 Chen MN, Nakagawa S, Ikeda Y, Tazaki H, Simura T, Yajima K (1982) A case of dural AVM during pregnancy. *Neurologia Medico-Chirurgica (Tokyo)* **10**:549–555.

74 Flieger JRH, Hooper RS, Kloss M (1969) Subarachnoid hemorrhage and pregnancy. *Journal of Obstetrics and Gynaecology of the British Commonwealth* **76**:912–917.

75 Harada H, Fujioka Y, Okamoto H, Shinohara S, Oki S, Uozumi T (1986) Intracranial hemorrhage associated with pregnancy. *Neurologia Medico-Chirurgica (Tokyo)* **14**:221–225.

76 Minielly R, Yuzpe AA, Drake CG (1979) Subarachnoid hemorrhage secondary to ruptured cerebral aneurysm in pregnancy. *Obstetrics and Gynecology* **53**:64–70.

77 Robinson JL, Chir B, Hall CJ, Sedzimir CB (1972) Subarachnoid hemorrhage in pregnancy. *Journal of Neurosurgery* **36**:27–33.

78 Mendelson CL (1948) Pregnancy and subacute bacterial endocarditis. *American Journal of Obstetrics and Gynecology* **56**:645–654.

79 Devereux RB, Perloff JK, Reichek N, Josephson ME (1976) Mitral valve prolapse. *Circulation* **54**:3–24.

80 Procacci PM, Savran SV, Schreiter SL, Bryson AL (1976) Prevalence of clinical mitral valve prolapse in 1,169 young women. *New England Journal of Medicine* **294**:1086–1088.

81 De Sweit M (1989) Heart disease in pregnancy. In De Swiet M (ed.) *Medical Disorders in Obstetric Practice*, 2nd edn, pp. 215–218. Oxford: Blackwell Scientific Publications.

82 Yatsu FM, Hart RG, Mohr JP, Grotta JC (1988) Anticoagulation of embolic strokes of cardiac origin: An update. *Neurology* **38**:314–316.

83 Srinivasan K (1988) Puerperal cereral venous and arterial thrombosis. *Seminars in Neurology* **8**:222–225.

84 Turkewitz LJ, Jacobs AK, Bidwell JK (1991) Atypical MRI findings of venous sinus thrombosis in pregnancy: Clinical significance relating to episodic vascular headache. *Headache* **31**:240–243.

85 Gettelfinger DM, Kokmen E (1977) Superior sagittal sinus thrombosis. *Archives of Neurology* **34**:2–6.

86 Simolke GA, Cox SM, Cunningham FG (1991) Cerebrovascular accidents complicating pregnancy and the puerperium. *Obstetrics and Gynecology* **78**:37–42.

87 Bruns PD, Linder RO, Drose VE, Battaglia F (1963) The placental transfer of water from fetus to mother following intravenous infusion of hypertonic mannitol to the maternal rabbit. *American Journal of Obstetrics and Gynecology* **86**:160–166.

88 Weibers DO (1988) Subarachnoid hemorrhage in pregnancy. *Seminars in Neurology* **8**:226–229.

89 Dalessio DJ (1982) Neurologic diseases. In Burrow GN, Ferris TF (eds) *Medical Complications During Pregnancy*, 2nd edn, pp. 435–447. Philadelphia: W.B. Saunders.

90 Robinson JL, Hall CS, Sedzimir CB (1972) Subarachnoid hemorrhage in pregnancy. *Journal of Neurosurgery* **36**:27–33.

91 Robinson JL, Hall CS, Sedzimir CB (1974) Arterioven-

ous malformations, aneurysms, and pregnancy. *Journal of Neurosurgery* **41**:63–70.

92 Donchin Y, Amirov B, Sahar A, Yarkoni S (1978) Sodium nitroprusside for aneurysm surgery in pregnancy: Report of a case. *British Journal of Anaesthesia* **50**:849–851.

93 Tuttleman RM, Gleicher N (1981) Central nervous system hemorrhage complicating pregnancy. *Obstetrics and Gynecology* **58**:651–656.

94 Lennon RL, Sundt TM, Gronert GA (1984) Combined cesarean section and clipping of intracerebral aneurysm. *Anaesthesiology* **60**:240–242.

95 Adams HP Jr, Nibbelink DW, Torner JC, Sahs AL (1981) Antifibrinolytic therapy in patients with aneurysmal subarachnoid hemorrhage. *Archives of Neurology* **38**:25–29.

96 Kassell NF, Torner JC, Adams HP Jr (1984) Antifibrinolytic therapy in the acute period following aneurysmal subarachnoid hemorrhage. *Journal of Neurosurgery* **61**:225–280.

97 Wiebers DO, Whisnant JP, O'Fallon WM (1981) The natural history of unruptured intracranial aneurysms. *New England Journal of Medicine* **304**:696–698.

98 Wiebers DO, Whisnant JP, Sundt TM Jr, O'Fallon WM (1987) The significance of unruptured intracranial occular aneurysms. *Journal of Neurosurgery* **66**:23–29.

99 Wilkins RH (1985) Natural history of intracranial vascular malformations: A review. *Neurosurgery* **16**:421–430.

100 Itoyama Y, Uemura S, Ushio Y, Kuratsu JI, Nonaka N, Wada H, Sano Y, Fukumura A, Yoshida K, Yano T (1989) Natural course of unoperated intracranial arteriovenous malformations: Study of 50 cases. *Journal of Neurosurgery* **71**:805–809.

101 Stein BM, Wolpert SM (1980) Arteriovenous malformations of the brain. II: Current concepts and treatment. *Archives of Neurology* **37**:69–75.

102 Amias AG (1970) Cerebrovascular disease in pregnancy: I. Hemorrhage. *Journal of Obstetrics and Gynaecology of the British Commonwealth* **77**:100–120.

103 Hunt HB, Schrifrin BS, Suzuki K (1973) Ruptured berry aneurysms and pregnancy. *Obstetrics and Gynecology* **43**:827–837.

104 Callaghan N (1968) The migraine syndrome in pregnancy. *Neurology* **18**:197–201.

105 Somerville BS (1972) A study of migraine in pregnancy. *Neurology* **22**:824–828.

106 Ratinahirana H, Darbois Y, Bousser MG (1990) Migraine and pregnancy: A prospective study in 703 women after delivery. *Neurology* **40**: 437 (suppl.).

107 Lance JW, Anthony M (1966) Some clinical aspects of migraine. *Archives of Neurology* **15**:356–361.

108 Wright GDS, Patel MK (1986) Focal migraine in pregnancy. *British Medical Journal* **293**:1557–1558.

109 Mandel S (1988) Hemiplegic migraine in pregnancy. *Headache* **28**:14–16.

110 Chancellor AM, Wroe SJ, Cull RE (1990) Migraine occurring for the first time in pregnancy. *Headache* **30**:224–227.

111 Wainscott G, Volans GN (1978) The outcome of pregnancy in women suffering from migraine. *Postgraduate Medical Journal* **54**:98–102.

112 Silberstein SD, Merriam GR (1991) Estrogens, progestins and headache. *Neurology* **41**:786–793.

113 Bille B (1981) Migraine in childhood and its prognosis. *Cephalgia* **1**:71–75.

114 Epstein MT, Hockaday JM, Hockaday TDR (1975) Migraine and reproductive hormones throughout the menstrual cycle. *Lancet* **i**:543–548.

115 Magos AL, Zilkha KJ, Studd JWW (1983) Treatment of menstrual migraine by oestradiol implants. *Journal of Neurosurgery and Psychiatry* **46**:1044–1046.

116 Stein G, Morton J, Marsh A, Collins W, Branch C, Desaga U, Ebeling J (1984) Headaches after childbirth. *Acta Neurologia Scandinavica* **69**:74–79.

117 Volgans GN (1978) Migraine and drug absorption. *Clinical Pharmacokinetics* :313–318.

118 Waelkens J (1982) Domperidone in the prevention of complete classical migraine. *British Medical Journal* **ii**:944–945.

119 Amery WK, Waelkens J (1983) Prevention of the last chance: An alternative pharmacologic treatment of migraine. *Headache* **23**:37–38.

120 Wilkinson M (1983) Treatment of the acute migraine attack – current status. *Cephalgia* **3**:61–67.

121 Wilkinson M (1990) Treatment of acute migraine: The British experience. *Headache* **2**:545–549 (suppl.).

122 Collins E (1981) Maternal and fetal effects of acetaminophen and salicylates in pregnancy. *Obstetrics and Gynecology* **58**:57–62 (suppl.).

123 Haslam RR (1975) Neonatal purpura secondary to maternal salicylism. *Journal of Pediatrics* **86**:653.

124 Casteels-Van Daele M, Eggermont E, de Gaetano G, Vermijlen J (1972) More on the effects of antenatally administered aspirin on aggregation of platelets of neonates. *Journal of Pediatrics* **80**:685–686.

125 Hickling EJ, Silverman DJ, Loos W (1990) A non-pharmacological treatment of vascular headache during pregnancy. *Headache* **30**:407–410.

126 Holroyd KA, Penzien DB, Cordingley GE (1991) Propranolol in the management of recurrent migraine: A meta-analytic review. *Headache* **31**:333–340.

127 Marguilis E, Binder D, Cohen AW (1984) The effect of propranolol on the nonstress test. *American Journal of Obstetrics and Gynecology* **148**:340–341.

128 Frishman WH, Chesner M (1988) Beta-adrenergic blockers in pregnancy. *American Heart Journal* **115**:147–152.

129 Pitt B (1973) Maternity blues. *British Journal of Psychiatry* **122**:431–433.

130 Stein GS (1981) Headaches in the first postpartum week and their relationship to migraine. *Headache* **21**:201–205.

131 Brownridge P (1983) The management of headache following accidental dural puncture in obstetric patients. *Anaesthetics and Intensive Care* **11**:4–15.

132 Lee JA, Atkinson RS (1978) *Lumbar Puncture and Spinal Analgesia*, pp. 170–175. New York: Churchill Livingstone.

133 Rosenberg PH, Heavner JE (1985) *In vitro* study of the effect of epidural blood patch on leakage through a dural puncture. *Anesthesia and Analgesia* **65**:501–504.

134 Seebacher J, Ribeiro V, LeGillou JL, Lacomblez L, Henry M, Thorman F, Youl B, Bensimon G, Darbois Y, Bousser MG (1989) Epidural blood patch in the treatment of post dural puncture headache: A double blind study. *Headache* **29**:630–632.

135 Ozdil T, Powell WF (1965) Postlumbar puncture headache: An effective method of prevention. *Anesthesia and Analgesia* **44**:542–545.

136 Kassam SH, Hadi HA, Fadel HE, Sims W, Jay WM (1983) Benign intracranial hypertension in pregnancy: Current diagnostic and therapeutic approach. *Obstetrical and Gynaecological Survey* **38**:314–321.

137 Abouleish E, Ali V, Tang RA (1985) Benign intracranial hypertension and anesthesia for cesarean section. *Anesthesiology* **63**:705–707.

138 Powell JL (1972) Pseudotumor cerebri and pregnancy. *Obstetrics and Gynecology* **40**:713–718.

139 Weisberg LA (1975) Benign intracranial hypertension. *Medicine (Baltimore)* **54**:197–207.

140 Reid AC, Teasdale GM, Matheson MS, Teasdale EM (1981) Serial ventricular volume measurements: Further insight into the etiology and pathogenesis of benign intracranial hypertension. *Journal of Neurology, Neurosurgery and Psychiatry* **44**:636–640.

141 Newborg B, Durham NC (1974) Pseudotumor cerebri treated by rice/reduction diet. *Archives of Internal Medicine* **133**:802–809.

142 Selman WR, Spetzler RF, Wilson CB, Grollmus JW (1980) Percutaneous lumboperitoneal shunt: Review of 130 cases. *Neurosurgery* **6**:255–257.

143 James HE, Tibbs PA (1981) Diverse clinical applications of percutaneous lumboperitoneal shunts. *Neurosurgery* **8**:39–42.

144 Marx GF, Scheinberg L, Romney S (1964) Anesthetic management of the parturient with intracranial tumor. *Obstetrics and Gynecology* **24**:122–126.

145 Palop R, Choed-Amphai E, Miller R (1979) Epidural anesthesia for delivery complicated by benign intracranial hypertension. *Anesthesiology* **50**:159–160.

146 Koontz WL, Herbert WNP, Cefalo RC (1983) Pseudotumor cerebri in pregnancy. *Obstetrics and Gynecology* **62**:324–327.

147 Elian M, Ben-Tovin N, Bechar M, Bornstein B (1968) Recurrent benign intracranial hypertension (pseudotumor cerebri) during pregnancy. *Obstetrics and Gynecology* **31**:685–688.

148 Divry P, Bobow J (1949) Brain tumors in pregnancy. *Acta Neurologia et Psychiatrica Belgica* **49**:59–80.

149 Rand CW, Andler (1950) Tumors of the brain complicating pregnancy. *Archives of Neurology and Psychiatry* **63**:1–41.

150 Kempers RD, Miller RH (1963) Management of pregnancy associated with brain tumors. *American Journal of Obstetrics and Gynecology* **87**:858–864.

151 Toakley G (1965) Brain tumors in pregnancy. *Australia and New Zealand Journal of Surgery* **35**:149–154.

152 Michelsen JJ, New RFJ (1969) Brain tumor and pregnancy. *Journal of Neurology, Neurosurgery and Psychiatry* **32**:305–307.

153 Simon RH (1988) Brain tumors in pregnancy. *Seminars in Neurology* **8**:214–221.

154 Roelvink CA, Kamphorst W, Van Alphen HAM, Rao BR (1987) Pregnancy related primary brain and spinal tumors. *Archives of Neurology* **44**:209–215.

155 Gold E, Gordis L, Tonciscia J, Szklo M (1979) Risk factors for brain tumors in children. *American Journal of Epidemiology* **109**:309–319.

156 Choi NW, Shuman LM, Gullen WH (1970) Epidemiology of primary central nervous system neoplasms. II: Case control study. *American Journal of Epidemiology* **91**:467–484.

157 Carmel PN (1974) Neurologic surgery in pregnancy. In Barber HR, Graber EA (eds) *Surgical Disease in Pregnancy*, pp. 203–224. Philadelphia: W.B. Saunders.

158 Rothman LA, Cohen CJ, Astarloa J (1973) Placental and fetal involvement by maternal malignancy. *American Journal of Obstetrics and Gynecology* **116**:1023–1034.

159 Vaughan HG, Howard RG (1962) Intracranial hemorrhage due to metastatic chorioepithelioma. *Neurology* **12**:771–777.

160 Gurwitt LJ, Long JM, Clark RE (1975) Cerebral metastatic choriocarcinoma. *Obstetrics and Gynecology* **45**:583–588.

161 Jones WB, Wagner-Reiss KM, Lewis JL (1990) Intracerebral choriocarcinoma. *Gynecologic Oncology* **38**:234–243.

162 Song H, Wu B (1979) Brain metastases in choriocarcinoma and malignant mole: An analysis of 98 cases. *Clin Med J* **92**:164–174.

163 Weed JC, Woodward KT, Hammond CB (1982) Choriocarcinoma metastatic to the brain: Therapy and prognosis. *Seminars in Oncology* **9**:208–212.

164 Lui TL, Deppe G, Chang QT, Tan TT (1983) Cerebral metastatic choriocarcinoma in People's Republic of China. *Gynecologic Oncology* **15**:166–170.

165 Bagshawe KD (1976) Risk and prognostic factors in trophoblastic neoplasia. *Cancer* **38**:1373–1385.

166 Gordon AN, Gershenson DM, Copeland LJ, Saul PB, Kavanagh JJ, Edwards CL (1985) High-risk metastatic gestational trophoblastic disease. *Obstetrics and Gynecology* **65**:550–556.

167 Rustin GJS, Newlands EE, Begent RHJ, Dent J, Bagshawe KD (1989) Weekly alternating etoposide, methotrexate, and actinomycin D/vincristine and cyclophosphamide chemotherapy for treatment of CNS metastases of choriocarcinoma. *Journal of Clinical Oncology* **7**:900–903.

168 Child DF, Gordon H, Mashiter K, Joplin GF (1975) Pregnancy, prolactin and pituitary tumors. *British Medical Journal* **4**:87–89.

169 Kitjar T, Tomkin GH (1971) Emergency hypophysectomy in pregnancy after induction of ovulation. *British Medical Journal* **4**:88–90.

170 Molitch ME (1985) Pregnancy and the hyperprolactinemic woman: Current concepts. *New England Journal of Medicine* **312**:1364–1370.

171 Bergh T, Nilliuss J, Wide L (1978) Clinical course and outcome of pregnancies in amenorrhoeic women with hyperprolactinaemia and pituitary tumors. *British Medical Journal* **i**:875–880.

172 Gemzell C, Wang CF (1979) Outcome of pregnancy in

women with pituitary adenoma. *Fertility and Sterility* **31**:363–372.

173   Thorner MO, Edwards CRW, Charlesworth M, Dacie JE, Moult PJA, Rees LH, Jones AE, Besser GM (1979) Pregnancy in patients presenting with hyperprolactinaemia. *British Medical Journal* **ii**:771–774.

174   Konopka P, Raymond RE, Merceron RE, Seneze J (1983) Continuous administration of bromocriptine in the prevention of neurological complications in pregnant women with prolactinomas. *American Journal of Obstetrics and Gynecology* **146**:935–938.

175   Thompson CE, Witham AC (1948) Paroxysmal hypertension and spinal cord injuries. *New England Journal of Medicine* **239**:291–294.

176   Abouleish E (1980) Hypertension in a paraplegic parturient. *Anesthesiology* **53**:348–349.

177   McGregor AJ, Meeuwsen J (1985) Autonomic hyperreflexia: A mortal danger for spinal cord-damaged women in labor. *American Journal of Obstetrics and Gynecology* **151**:330–333.

178   Robertson DN (1972) Pregnancy and labor in the paraplegic. *Paraplegia* **10**:207–210.

179   Young BK, Katz M, Klein S (1983) Pregnancy after spinal cord injury: Altered maternal and foetal response to labour. *Obstetrics and Gynecology* **62**:59–63.

180   Hughes SJ, Short DJ, Usherwood M, Tebbutt H (1991) Management of the pregnant woman with spinal cord injuries. *British Journal of Obstetrics and Gynaecology* **98**:513–518.

181   Comarr AE (1975) Observations on menstruation and pregnancy among female spinal cord injury patients. *Paraplegia* **3**:263–272.

182   Watson DW, Downey GO (1980) Epidural anesthesia for labor and delivery of twins of a paraplegic mother. *Anesthesiology* **52**:259–261.

183   Rossier AB, Ruffieux M, Ziegler WH (1971) Pregnancy and labor in high traumatic cord lesions. *Paraplegia* **7**:210–216.

184   Aminoff MJ, Logue V (1974) Clinical features of spinal vascular malformations. *Brain* **97**:197–210.

185   Carter CO, Evans K (1973) Children of adult survivors with spina bifida cystica. *Lancet* **2**:924–926.

186   Keucher TR, Healey J (1979) Long-term results after ventriculoatrial and ventriculoperitoneal shunting for infantile hydrocephalus. *Journal of Neurosurgery* **50**:179–186.

187   Amacher AL, Wellington J (1984) Infantile hydrocephalus: Long-term results of surgical therapy. *Childs Nervous System (Berlin)* **11**:217–229.

188   Gast MJ, Grubb RL, Strickler RC (1983) Maternal hydrocephalus and pregnancy. *Obstetrics and Gynecology* **62**:290–315.

189   Howard TE, Herrick CN (1981) Pregnancy in patients with ventriculoperitoneal shunts: Report of two cases. *American Journal of Obstetrics and Gynecology* **141**:99–101.

190   Kleinman G, Sutherland W, Martinez M, Khalil T (1983) Malfunction of ventriculoperitoneal shunts during pregnancy. *Obstetrics and Gynecology* **61**:753–754.

191   Nugent P, Hoshek S (1986) Large extra-abdominal

cyst as a postpartum complication of peritoneal shunt. *Journal of Neurosurgery* **64**:151–152.

192   Wisoff JH, Kratzert KJ, Handwerker SM, Young BK, Epstein F (1991) Pregnancy in patients with cerebrospinal fluid shunts: Report of a series and review of the literature. *Neurosurgery* **29**:827–831.

193   Cusimano MD, Meffe FM, Gentili F, Sermer M (1990) Ventriculoperitoneal shunt malfunction during pregnancy. *Neurosurgery* **27**:969–971.

194   Monfared AH, Kee SK, Apuzzo MLJ, Collea JV (1979) Obstetric management of pregnant women with extracranial shunts. *Canadian Medical Association Journal* **120**:562–563.

195   Hanakita J, Suzuki T, Yamamoto Y, Kinuta Y, Nishihara K (1985) Ventriculoperitoneal shunt malfunction during pregnancy. *Journal of Neurosurgery* **63**:459–460.

196   Houston CS, Clein LJ (1989) Ventriculoperitoneal shunt malfunction in a pregnant patient with meningomyelocele. *Canadian Medical Association Journal* **141**:701–702.

197   Kennedy RH, Danielson MA, Mulder DW, Kurland LT (1978) Guillain-Barré syndrome: A 42 year epidemiologic and clinical study. *Mayo Clinic Proceedings* **53**:93–99.

198   Dyck PJ (1984) *Peripheral Neuropathy*, 2nd edn, pp. 2050–2100. Philadelphia: W.B. Saunders.

199   Ravn H (1967) The Landry-Guillain-Barré syndrome: A survey of a clinical report of 127 cases. *Acta Neurologia Scandinavica* **43**:30 (suppl.).

200   Ahlberg G, Ahlmark G (1978) The Landry-Guillain-Barré syndrome and pregnancy. *Acta Obstetrica et Gynecologica Scandinavica* **57**:377–380.

201   Winer JB, Hughes RAC, Anderson MJ, Jones DM, Kangro H, Watkins RPF (1988) A prospective study of acute idiopathic neuropathy. 2. Antecedent events. *Journal of Neurology, Neurosurgery and Psychiatry* **51**:613–618.

202   Winer J (1992) Guillain-Barré syndrome revisited: Pathogenesis still unknown. *British Medical Journal* **304**:65–66.

203   Winer JB, Hughes RAC, Osmond C (1988) A prospective study of acute idiopathic neuropathy. 1. Clinical features and their prognostic value. *Journal of Neurology, Neurosurgery and Psychiatry* **51**:605–612.

204   Nelson LH, McLean WT Jr (1985) Management of Landry-Guillain-Barré syndrome in pregnancy. *Obstetrics and Gynecology* **65**:25–29 (suppl.).

205   Guillain-Barré Syndrome Study Group (1985) Plasmapharesis and acute Guillain-Barré syndrome. *Neurology* **35**:1096–1104.

206   French Cooperative Group on Plasma Exchange in Guillain-Barré Syndrome (1987) Efficiency of plasma exchange in Guillain-Barré syndrome: Role of replacement fluids. *Annals of Neurology* **22**:753–761.

207   Hurley TJ, Brunson AD, Lefler SF, Quirk JG (1991) Landry-Guillain-Barré syndrome in pregnancy: Report of three cases treated with plasmapharesis. *Obstetrics and Gynecology* **78**:482–485.

208   Osterman PO, Fagius J, Safenberg J, Wikstrom B (1988) Early relapse of acute inflammatory polyradicu-

loneuropathy after successful treatment with plasma exchange. *Acta Neurologia Scandinavica* **77**:273–277.

209 Ropper AH, Albers JW, Addison R (1988) Limited relapse in Guillain-Barré syndrome after plasma exchange. *Archives of Neurology* **45**:314–315.

210 Hughes RAC, Davis JMN, Perkin GD, Pierce JM (1978) Controlled trial of prednisolone in acute polyneuropathy. *Lancet* **ii**:750–753.

211 Hughes RAC (1991) Ineffectiveness of high dose intravenous methyl prednisolone in Guillain-Barré syndrome. *Lancet* **338**:1142.

212 Kleyweg RP, van der Meche FGA, Meulstee J (1988) Treatment of Guillain-Barré syndrome with high dose gammaglobulin. *Neurology* **38**:1639–1641.

213 Kleyweg RP, van der Meche FGA (1991) Treatment related fluctuations in Guillain-Barré syndrome after high-dose immunoglobulins or plasma exchange. *Journal of Neurology, Neurosurgery and Psychiatry* **54**:957–960.

214 Sadovnick AD, Baird PA (1985) Reproductive counselling for multiple sclerosis patients. *American Journal of Medical Genetics* **20**:349–354.

215 Poland BJ, Miller JR, Harris M, Livingston J (1981) Spontaneous abortion: A study of 1,961 women and their conceptuses. 102. *Acta Obstetrica et Gynecologica Scandinavica* **102** (suppl.).

216 Poser S, Poser W (1983) Multiple sclerosis and gestation. *Neurology* **33**:1422–1427.

217 Sadovnick AD (1984) Empiric recurrence risks for use in the genetic counselling of multiple sclerosis patients. *American Journal of Medical Genetics* **17**:713–714.

218 Shapira K, Poskanzer DC, Newell DJ, Miller H (1966) Marriage, pregnancy and multiple sclerosis. *Brain* **89**:419–428.

219 Miller JHD, Allison RS, Cheeseman EA, Merrett JD (1959) Pregnancy as a factor influencing relapse in disseminated sclerosis. *Brain* **82**:417–426.

220 Sweeney WJ (1955) Pregnancy and multiple sclerosis. *American Journal of Obstetrics and Gynecology* **66**:124–130.

221 Ghezzi A, Caputo D (1981) Pregnancy: A factor influencing the course of multiple sclerosis? *European Journal of Neurology* **20**:517–519.

222 Leibowitz U, Antonovsky A, Kats R, Alter M (1967) Does pregnancy increase the risk of multiple sclerosis? *Journal of Neurology, Neurosurgery and Psychiatry* **30**:354–357.

223 Birk K, Ford C, Smeltzer S, Ryan D, Miller R, Rudick RA (1990) The clinical course of multiple sclerosis during pregnancy and the puerperium. *Archives of Neurology* **47**:738–742.

224 Thompson DS, Nelson LM, Burns A, Burks JS, Franklin GM (1986) The effects of pregnancy in multiple sclerosis: A retrospective study. *Neurology* **36**:1097–1099.

225 Yudkin PL, Ellison GW, Ghezzi A, Goodkin DE, Hughes RAC, McPherson K, Mertin J, Milanese C (1991) Overview of azathioprine treatment in multiple sclerosis. *Lancet* **338**:1051–1055.

226 Drachman DB, DeSilva S, Ramsay D, Pestronk A (1987) Humoral pathogenesis of myasthenia gravis. *Annals of the New York Academy of Sciences* **505**:90–105.

227 Carr SR, Gilchrist JM, Abuelo DN, Clark D (1991) Treatment of antenatal myasthenia gravis. *Obstetrics and Gynecology* **78**:485–489.

228 Plauche WC (1991) Myasthenia gravis in mothers and their newborns. *Clinics in Obstetrics and Gynecology* **34**:82–98.

229 Hay DM (1969) Myasthenia gravis in pregnancy. *Journal of Obstetrics and Gynaecology of the British Commonwealth* **76**:323–329.

230 Fonseca V, Havard CWH (1990) The natural course of myasthenia gravis: The outlook has improved substantially. *British Medical Journal* **300**:1409–1410.

231 Eden RD, Gall SA (1983) Myasthenia gravis and pregnancy: A reappraisal of thymectomy. *Obstetrics and Gynecology* **62**:328–333.

232 Pascuzzi RM, Coslett HB, Johns TR (1984) Long-term corticosteroid treatment in myasthenia gravis: Report of 116 patients. *Annals of Neurology* **15**:291–298.

233 Levine SE, Keesey JC (1986) Successful plasmapharesis for fulminant myasthenia gravis during pregnancy. *Archives of Neurology* **43**:197–198.

234 Donaldson JO, Penn AS, Lisak RP, Abramsky O, Brenner T, Schotland OL (1981) Anti-acetylcholine receptor antibody in neonatal myasthenia gravis. *American Journal of Diseases of Children* **135**:222–226.

235 Brenner T, Beyth Y, Abramsky O (1977) Inhibitory effect of alpha fetoprotein on the binding of myasthenia gravis antibody to acetylcholine receptor. *Proceedings of the National Academy of Sciences, USA* **77**:3635.

236 Keesey J, Cokley H, Herrmann C Jr (1977) Anti-acetylcholine receptor antibody in neonatal myasthenia gravis. *New England Journal of Medicine* **296**:55.

237 Papatestas AE, Alpert LI, Osserman KE, Osserman RS, Kark AE (1971) Studies in myasthenia gravis: Effects of thymectomy. *American Journal of Medicine* **50**:465–474.

238 Elias SB, Butler I, Appel SH (1979) Neonatal myasthenia gravis in the infant of a myasthenic mother in remission. *Annals of Neurology* **6**:72–75.

239 Gutmann L, Seybold (1980) Acetylcholine receptor antibodies in absence of neonatal myasthenia gravis (Letter). *Archives of Neurology* **37**:738.

240 Hopkins A, Wray S (1967) The effect of pregnancy on dystrophia myotonica. *Neurology* **17**:166–168.

241 Hillard GD, Harris RE, Gilstrap LC, Shoumaker RD (1977) Myotonic muscular dystrophy in pregnancy. *Southern Journal of Medicine* **70**:446–447.

242 Shore RN, MacLachlan TB (1971) Pregnancy with myotonic dystrophy: Course, complications and management. *Obstetrics and Gynecology* **38**:448–454.

243 Jaffe R, Mock M, Abramowicz J, Ben-Aderet N (1986) Myotonic dystrophy and pregnancy: A review. *Obstetrical and Gynaecological Survey* **41**:272–278.

244 Broekhuizen FF, Elejalde M de, Elejalde R, Hamiltin PR (1983) Neonatal myotonic dystrophy as a cause of hydramnios and neonatal death: A case report and literature review. *Journal of Reproductive Medicine* **28**:595–599.

245 Sarnat HB, O'Connor T, Byrne PA (1976) Clinical

effects of myotonic dystrophy on pregnancy and the neonate. *Archives of Neurology* **33**:459–465.

246 Hughes RG, Lyall EGH, Liston WA (1991) Obstetric and neonatal complications of myotonic dystrophy. *Journal of Obstetrics and Gynaecology* **11**:191–193.

247 Dunn LJ, Dierker LJ (1973) Recurrent hydramnios in association with myotonia dystrophica. *Obstetrics and Gynecology* **42**:104–106.

248 Webb D, Muir I, Faulkner J, Johnson G (1978) Myotonia dystrophica: Obstetric complications. *American Journal of Obstetrics and Gynecology* **132**:265–270.

249 Pearse RG, Howeler CJ (1979) Neonatal form of dystrophic myotonia. *Archives of Diseases of Children* **54**:331–338.

250 Moorman J, Coleman R, Packer D *et al.* (1985) Cardiac involvement in myotonic dystrophy. *Medicine* **64**:371–387.

251 Insley J, Bird GWG, Harper PS, Pearce GW (1976) Prenatal prediction of myotonic dystrophy. *Lancet* **i**:806.

252 Brook JD, Shaw DJ, Meredith AL (1985) Myotonic dystrophy and gene mapping on human chromosome 19. *Biotechnology and Genetic Engineering* **3**:311–347.

253 Milunsky A, Skare JC, Milunsky JM, Maher TA, Amos JA (1991) Prenatal diagnosis of myotonic muscular dystrophy with linked deoxyribonucleic acid probes. *American Journal of Obstetrics and Gynecology* **164**:751–755.

254 Harper PS (1975) Congenital myotonic dystrophy in Britain: Clinical aspects. *Archives of Diseases of Children* **50**:505–513.

255 Cabrera-Ramirez L, Harris RE (1976) Controlled removal of amniotic fluid in hydramnios. *Southern Medical Journal* **69**:239–240.

256 Mamopoulos M, Assimakopoulos E, Reece A, Androu A, Zheng X-Z, Mantalenakis S (1990) Maternal indomethacin therapy in the treatment of polyhydramnios.

American Journal of Obstetrics and Gynecology **162**:1225–1229.

257 Cope I (1981) Myotonic dystrophy and pregnancy. *Australia and New Zealand Journal of Obstetrics and Gynaecology* **21**:240–241.

258 Kaufman L (1960) Anesthesia in dystrophia myotonica: A review of the hazards of anaesthesia. *Proceedings of the Royal Society of Medicine* **53**:183–187.

259 Mitchell MM, Ali HH, Savarese JJ (1978) Myotonia and neuromuscular blocking agents. *Anesthesiology* **49**:44–48.

260 Wesstrom G, Bensch J, Schollin J (1986) Congenital myotonic dystrophy: Incidence, clinical aspects and prognosis. *Acta Paediatrica Scandinavica* **75**:849–854.

261 Vanier TM (1960) Dystrophia myotonica in childhood. *British Medical Journal* **2**:1284–1288.

262 Harper PS (1975) Congenital myotonic dystrophy in Britain: Genetic basis. *Archives of Diseases of Children* **50**:514–521.

263 Harper PS, Dyken PR (1972) Early-onset dystrophia myotonica: Evidence supporting a maternal environmental factor. *Lancet* **2**:53–55.

264 Zellweger H, Lonaescu V (1973) Early onset of myotonic dystrophy in infants. *American Journal of Diseases of Children* **125**:601–604.

265 Dyken PR, Harper PS (1973) Congenital dystrophia myotonica. *Neurology* **23**:465–473.

266 Pope TH, Kenan PD (1969) Bells palsy in pregnancy. *Archives of Otolaryngology* **89**:52–56.

267 Hilsinger RL, Adour KK, Doty HE (1975) Idiopathic facial paralysis, pregnancy and the menstrual cycle. *Annals of Otology, Rhinology and Laryngology* **84**:433–442.

268 Adour KK (1982) Diagnosis and management of facial paralysis. *New England Journal of Medicine* **307**:348–351.

269 Voitk AJ, Mueller JC, Farlinger DE, Johnston RU (1983) Carpal tunnel syndrome in pregnancy. *Canadian Medical Association Journal* **128**:277–281.

27

Autoimmune Disease

D. WARE BRANCH

INTRODUCTION

The diagnosis of an *autoimmune disease* is made when a state of *autoimmunity* (i.e. evidence of an immune response to self-constituents) is associated with a recognized pattern of clinical signs and symptoms. The state of autoimmunity is usually confirmed by the detection of characteristic autoantibodies in the patient's circulation. For many conditions, such as autoimmune thyroid disease and myasthenia gravis, there is substantial evidence linking the activity of the autoantibody(ies) or autoimmune effector cells to the disease state. For other conditions, such as systemic lupus erythematosus or multiple sclerosis, there is less evidence that the clinical manifestations of the disease are actually caused by detectable autoantibodies or other effector mechanisms.

Simply put, there are two major theories as to how one might develop a state of autoimmunity. The earliest of these held that autoimmunity resulted from a failure in the normal deletion of lymphocytes that recognized self-antigens. More recently, authorities have suggested that autoimmunity results from a failure of the normal regulation of the immune system (which contains many immune cells that recognize self-antigens but are normally suppressed). Regardless of what fundamental immunological disturbance allows autoimmunity, it appears that a combination of environmental, genetic and host factors must be present for the full expression of an autoimmune disease.

The co-existence of pregnancy and autoimmune disease is far from rare. Some autoimmune diseases can have a profound effect on pregnancy. Others may be influenced by pregnancy, and still others are unique to pregnancy or have unique features associated with pregnancy. For all these reasons, the obstetrician should be familiar with the more common autoimmune diseases, how they influence and are influenced by pregnancy, and what special medical risks may be in store for mother or the conceptus. This chapter details the pertinent aspects of systemic lupus erythematosus, antiphospholipid syndrome, rheumatoid arthritis, systemic sclerosis and myasthenia gravis.

SYSTEMIC LUPUS ERYTHEMATOSUS

Systemic lupus erythematosus (SLE) is an idiopathic chronic inflammatory disease that affects skin, joints, kidneys, lungs, serous membranes, nervous system, liver, and other organs of the body. Like other autoimmune diseases its course is characterized by periods of remission and relapse. Probably the most common complaint among patients with SLE is extreme fatigue (**Table 1**). Fever, weight loss, myalgia and arthralgia are also particularly common symptoms.

The prevalence of SLE is 5–100 per 100 000 individuals, depending upon the population studied. The disease is at least five, and probably closer to ten, times more common among adult women than adult men. Certain populations have higher prevalence rates. For example, the prevalence of SLE is three times greater among Black women than among White women. A genetic predisposition to SLE is strongly implicated by

Table 1
Approximate frequency of clinical symptoms in
SLE

Symptoms	Patients (%)
Fatigue	80–100
Fever	80–100
Arthralgia, arthritis	95
Myalgia	70
Weight loss	> 60
Skin	
butterfly rash	50
photosensitivity	60
mucous membrane lesions	35
Renal involvement	50
Pulmonary	
pleurisy	50
effusion	25
phenumonitis	5–10
Cardiac (pericarditis)	10–50
Lymphadenopathy	50
CNS	
seizures	15–20
psychosis	< 25

several observations. SLE occurs in 5–12% of relatives of patients with SLE, and the concordance rate for SLE among monozygotic twins may be over 50%. A number of genetic markers occur more frequently in SLE patients than in controls. These include HLA-B8, HLA-DR3 and HLA-DR2. Patients with SLE also have a higher frequency of homozygous deficiencies of the early complement proteins C2 and C4.

Diagnosis

The diagnosis of SLE, suspected by the clinical presentation, is confirmed by demonstrating the presence of circulating autoantibodies. A number of categories of autoantibodies are now recognized to be associated with SLE. The best studied are those directed against nuclear antigens, the antinuclear antibodies (ANA). Of these, the first to be described was the serum factor that caused the LE cell phenomenon, an autoantibody now known to be directed against nucleoprotein (DNA-histone). The LE cell phenomenon is no longer necessary for the diagnosis of SLE. It has been replaced by immunofluorescent assays for ANA which now serve as the screening test in the initial diagnostic evaluation of a patient with suspected SLE. A positive ANA can be interpreted to some degree according to the pattern of the binding, even though specific antigen–antibody reactions are much more informative. The four basic patterns of binding are homogeneous, peripheral, speckled and nucleolar. The homogeneous

pattern is found in about 65% of patients with SLE, but the peripheral pattern is the most specific for SLE, even if it is not very sensitive. The speckled and nucleolar patterns are more specific for other autoimmune diseases.

Assays for specific nuclear antigen–antibody reactions offer the most detailed and specific methods of defining the autoantibodies that bind in the ANA assay. Antibodies to double-stranded (native) DNA (dsDNA) are the most specific for SLE and are found in 80–90% of untreated patients at the time of presentation. The presence and titer of anti-dsDNA may be related to the disease activity. Antibodies to single-stranded DNA (ssDNA) are also found in a very high percentage of untreated SLE patients, but anti-ssDNA is less specific for SLE than anti-dsDNA. Patients with SLE may also have antibodies to RNA–protein conjugates, often referred to as soluble or extractable antigens, since they can be separated from tissue extracts. These antigens include the Sm antigen, nuclear ribonucleoprotein (nRNP), the Ro/SSA antigen and the La/SSB antigen. The Sm and nRNP antigens are nuclear in origin and the presence of anti-Sm, found in about 30–40% of patients with SLE, is highly specific for the disease. Anti-Ro/SS-A and La/SS-B, found in the sera of SLE patients and patients with Sjogren's syndrome, are of particular importance to obstetricians, since they are associated with neonatal lupus.

In 1971, the American Rheumatism Association devised criteria for SLE as a framework for comparing studies of patients with SLE. These were revised in 1982,[1] changed by the elimination of Raynaud's phenomenon and alopecia and by the addition of a positive ANA, anti-DNA and anti-Sm (**Table 2**). To be classified as having SLE, an individual must have at least 4 of the 11 criteria at one time or serially. These criteria are very sensitive and specific for SLE, but the

Table 2
Revised ARA classification criteria for SLE (1982)[1]

Malar rash
Discoid rash
Photosensitivity
Oral ulcers
Arthritis (non-deforming polyarthritis)
Serositis (pleuritis and/or pericarditis)
Renal disorder (proteinuria > 0.5 g/day or cellular casts)
Neurological disorder (psychosis and/or seizures)
Hematological disorder (leukopenia or
  lymphopenia/hemolytic anemia/thrombocytopenia)
Immunological disorder (anti-DNA/anti-Sm/LE cell/false-
  positive STS)
Antinuclear antibody

To be classified as having SLE, one must have at least 4 of the 11 criteria at one time or serially.

reader should recognize that they were never intended to form the *sine qua non* for the diagnosis of SLE. Exclusion of patients with an autoimmune diathesis from the diagnosis of SLE by the dogmatic use of strict diagnostic criteria can result in patients being confused and frustrated. Reasonable and sympathetic medical care and counseling are required as much for these patients as for those with clear-cut SLE.

Maternal Risks

General

A number of studies of the relationship between SLE and pregnancy published from the early 1950s through the early 1970s suggested that women with SLE were placing themselves at substantial risk for severe morbidity or mortality during pregnancy. The study of Garenstein *et al.* is representative.[2] The authors studied retrospectively 33 pregnancies in 21 women with SLE and found that the risk of SLE exacerbation was three times greater in the first 20 weeks of pregnancy and six times greater in the first 8 weeks postpartum than in the 32 weeks prior to conception. The mere mention of one maternal mortality in association with pregnancy, even if the investigators felt that the relative risk was not increased,[2] led physicians to the unsubstantiated view that pregnancy might somehow precipitate an SLE-related death in a medically significant proportion of cases. Finally, several early studies suggested that the rate of pregnancy loss among women with SLE was relatively high.[3] Taken together, these concerns led many practitioners to the opinion that SLE patients should not become pregnant. However, the data and conclusions of these early studies should not be applied to clinical decision making today. All studies prior to the 1980s were retrospective and relatively small. There were no generally agreed upon criteria for the classification of SLE, predisposing to the inclusion of a disproportionate number of more severe cases. Also, there were no tested diagnostic criteria for SLE exacerbation. This may have allowed certain events of pregnancy, such as pre-eclampsia or increasing proteinuria, to be incorrectly diagnosed as SLE exacerbation.

The subsequent introduction of classification criteria in 1971 and the development of more sophisticated autoantibody assays allows for a more uniform patient selection and inclusion of less severely affected, typical SLE patients. Additionally, current treatment of SLE and its SLE exacerbations has changed, making it necessary for us to reconsider the risks of this disease in relationship to pregnancy.

Exacerbation of SLE

Patients with SLE and their physicians are understandably concerned about whether pregnancy poses a threat to the course of their autoimmune disease. Perhaps the foremost area of concern is that of an exacerbation or 'flare' of SLE. More recent studies have done much to clarify the relationship of pregnancy to the rate and nature of SLE exacerbations. Overall, about 15–60% of women will have exacerbations during pregnancy or the postpartum period.[4–9] There are several prospective studies that deserve special consideration in regard to this issue. Lockshin *et al.* matched non-pregnant SLE patients with 28 SLE patients undertaking 33 pregnancies.[5] Any SLE exacerbations were defined by a previously published scoring system. There was no difference in the flare score between the cases and controls, and a similar number in either group required a change in their medication. The same investigators have now followed 80 consecutive pregnancies in women with SLE[8] and conclude that exacerbations occur in less than 25% of cases and that most are mild in nature. If only signs or symptoms specific for SLE are included, exacerbations occurred in only 13% of cases. Mintz *et al.* studied prospectively 92 pregnancies in women with SLE and used a 'similar group' of non-pregnant SLE patients on oral contraceptives derived from a previous study as controls.[7] Exacerbations were defined by specific, acceptable criteria, but these were different from those used by Lockshin *et al.* As a matter of policy, all pregnant women were started on 10 mg prednisone daily, even if there was no evidence of SLE activity. The rate of SLE flares per month at risk was similar in both groups. As in Lockshin's studies, most of the exacerbations tended to be easily controlled with low to moderate doses of glucocorticoids, but seven patients (8%) had severe exacerbations requiring more aggressive therapies. Interestingly, the majority (54%) of the exacerbations occurred in the first trimester. Using criteria for SLE flare that differed from either of the other two studies, Petri *et al.* found SLE flares (flares per person years) to be more common among pregnant women than among controls.[9] Fortunately, over three-quarters of the flares were mild to moderate in nature.

In summary, the issue of whether pregnancy predisposes to SLE exacerbation is not yet settled. At most, however, the predisposition to SLE flare during pregnancy is modest. Furthermore, most SLE exacerbations during pregnancy are easily treated with low to moderate doses of glucocorticoids. The routine use of glucocorticoids in all pregnant SLE patients, as suggested by Mintz *et al.*, seems unwarranted in view of the excellent results achieved by Lockshin *et al.* without the routine use of steroids.

A number of investigators feel that serial serological evaluation of complement components of their activation products allows for the time detection of an SLE exacerbation during pregnancy. In two studies, Devoe and colleagues found that SLE exacerbation was 'signaled' by a decline of C3 and C4 into the subnormal range.[10,11] More recently, Buyon et al. found that a lack of the usual rise in C3 and C4 levels during pregnancy was associated with SLE exacerbation.[12] Others have questioned the predictive value of serological determinations in lupus pregnancy. Lockshin and colleagues found the concentration of the C1s–C1 inhibitor complex, which should be increased in the face of classical pathway complement activation, was normal in most pregnant patients with hypocomplementemia.[13] The authors suggested that pregnant SLE patients may actually have relatively poor synthesis (rather than consumption) of some complement components. In a recent prospective study of 19 continuing SLE pregnancies, neither ANA, C3 nor C4 levels predicted which of the nine patients were going to have a flare.[14] Finally, there are several studies which show that hypocomplementemia may occur in pregnant patients without SLE and does not predict a poor pregnancy outcome.[15] Thus, the utility of serial determinations of complement components or their activation products for the timely detection of SLE exacerbations or poor pregnancy outcome remains controversial. None of the studies touting the predictive value of serial serological evaluation has proved that the serological studies are better for the timely diagnosis of SLE exacerbation than relatively frequent, thorough clinical assessment of the patient.

Distinguishing between an exacerbation of SLE involving active nephritis and pre-eclampsia is problematic, since each may present with proteinuria, hypertension and evidence of multi-organ dysfunction. In the typical problem case, the patient develops hypertension and begins to excrete increasing amounts of urinary protein in the latter half of pregnancy. Several laboratory tests may be helpful. Elevated levels of anti-DNA weigh in favor of active SLE. Normal or slightly elevated levels of classical pathway complement components weigh against active SLE, but decreased levels are less helpful since complement activation may be seen in pre-eclampsia.[16] Buyon et al. recently found that frank lupus activity in pregnancy was associated with elevated levels of Ba or Bb, fragments of protein B activation in the alternative pathway of complement activation.[17] The terminal attack complex, Sc5b-9, was also elevated in the patients with active SLE. While elevated concentrations of Ba, Bb and Sc5b-9 were also found in some patients with pre-eclampsia, the combination of these with a decreased CH50 strongly suggested SLE flare. A number of laboratory tests have been put forward as being specific for pre-eclampsia. These include decreased levels of antithrombin-III, increased levels of total plasma or cellular fibronectin,[18] and hypocalciuria. Unfortu-

nately, none of these has been specifically tested as markers for pre-eclampsia in patients with SLE.

In the author's experience, two tests are particularly helpful in distinguishing between active SLE nephritis and pre-eclampsia. An active urinary sediment strongly suggests lupus nephritis. Cellular casts and hematuria are usually present in diffuse proliferative glomerulonephrosis, and often present in focal proliferative glomerulonephrosis, the two conditions most likely to be confused with pre-eclampsia. The second test of immense benefit is the renal biopsy. In severe and confusing cases, the renal biopsy will actually make the correct diagnosis. Of course, there is an understandable reluctance to utilize this invasive procedure in the pregnant patient, and sound clinical judgment is required to decide which patients require a biopsy for optimal management.

As a final point regarding SLE-related hypertension and proteinuria vs pre-eclampsia, it is the author's experience in severe cases that the SLE flare and pre-eclampsia may be indistinguishable as the patient's course advances, rendering the laboratory distinction between the two conditions moot. Concerns about optimizing the mother's SLE management and avoiding serious complications of pre-eclampsia, including fetal hypoxemia, often prompt delivery in a relatively short time.

Renal disease

Clinically obvious renal disease is a rather common complication of SLE, with some renal involvement eventually occurring in about 50% of cases. It is generally held that lupus nephropathy (LN) is due to immune complex deposition, with resultant complement activation and inflammatory tissue damage in the kidney. The most common presentation is proteinuria, which occurs at some time in up to 75% of patients. About 40% of patients will have hematuria or pyuria and about a third will have urinary casts. Renal biopsy findings are very important to prognosis and treatment. In simple terms, renal biopsy findings can be grouped into four basic histologic and clinical categories of LN. Of these, diffuse proliferative glomerulonephritis (DPGN) is the most common, occurring in about 40% of SLE cases with renal involvement. It is also the most severe renal lesion associated with SLE. DPGN typically presents with hypertension, moderate to heavy proteinuria and nephrotic syndrome, hematuria, pyuria, casts, hypocomplementemia and circulating immune complexes. The 10-year survival rate is about 60%. Focal proliferative glomerulonephritis also presents with proteinuria, but the degree of proteinuria is less. Hypertension is less common and less severe, and serious renal insufficiency is uncommon. Membranous GN typically presents with moderate to heavy proteinuria, but lacks the active urinary sediment and does not cause renal insufficiency. Mesangial nephritis appears as the least severe lesion clinically and carries the best long-term prognosis.

The overall prognosis for patients with LN is good, with 80% of patients surviving at least 10 years. Traditionally, the first line of therapy in patients with active LN has been glucocorticoids, usually given as oral prednisone, 40–50 mg/m²/day for several weeks to several months. Thereafter, the dose is tapered while carefully watching the patient for evidence of exacerbation of the LN. Aggressive treatment of hypertension is important for optimal outcome. Severe proliferative lesions, such as seen in moderate to severe DPGN, has been shown to respond best to cytotoxic agents. Cyclophosphamide, in divided monthly dose of 0.5–1.0 g/m², is now generally used.

A woman with LN who becomes pregnant faces several special problems. The underlying renal disease probably presages an increased risk for maternal and fetal morbidity and mortality. In addition, those with chronic renal disease resulting in proteinuria are likely to have worsening proteinuria during gestation as the renal blood flow increases. This inevitably poses the question as to whether the increased proteinuria represents an exacerbation of underlying renal disease, pre-eclampsia or both.

Early reports suggested that LN was a major contributor to serious maternal morbidity or death.[2,3,19] For example, Estes et al. noted progression of renal disease in all 10 pregnant patients with LN, with two of these dying within a year after delivery.[3] Bear et al. noted worsening of renal disease in five of six patients with LN, and three suffered permanent deterioration.[19] Such

reports were interpreted by many practitioners to strongly recommend against pregnancy in woman with LN. However, larger, more recent stories suggest that the course of renal disease in pregnant women with LN is not so serious.[10,20–24] All the studies were retrospective and patient selection doubtlessly varied from one study to the next; however, the summary shown in **Table 3** may be useful in counseling patients with LN. The median rate of SLE exacerbation was 34%, probably no different from that observed in unselected SLE patients. Deterioration of renal status occurred in about a quarter of the patients undertaking pregnancy. Altogether, 10% of the pregnancies were associated with a permanent deterioration in the patient's renal status. Fortunately, the resulting degree of renal impairment was moderate in most cases. Three of the 131 women with LN included in **Table 3** died of complications related to SLE occurring during a pregnancy or in the postpartum period.

Three studies describe the patients' status during pregnancy in terms of whether the SLE was active or in remission prior to conception.[20,22,24] In all three, the rate of SLE exacerbation was lower among pregnancies in which the patient was in remission prior to conception. Hayslett and Lynn[20] and Bobrie et al.[24] also found that the rate of renal deterioration was somewhat lower among pregnancies in which the patient was in remission prior to conception. Firm conclusions cannot be reached, since the total number of pregnancies studied was small and the results were not amenable to statistical analysis. However, these data are often used to counsel SLE patients that their disease should be in remission prior to their conception.

Table 3
Deterioration of renal disease during pregnancy in patients with SLE nephropathy[a]

Author	Patients	Pregnancies	No exacerbation	Exacerbation	No deterioration	Deterioration	Permanent deterioration
Hayslett remission PTC[a]							
active PTC	23	31	21/31 (68%)	10/31 (32%)	24/31 (77%)	7/31 (23%)	2/31 (6%)
Fine	24	25	13/25 (52%)	12/25 (48%)	16/25 (64%)	9/25 (36%)	5/25 (20%)
Jungers	13	14	NA	NA	10/14 (71%)	4/14 (29%)	2/14 (14%)
remission PTC	8	11	9/11 (82%)	2/11 (18%)	9/11 (82%)	2/11 (18%)	1/11 (9%)
active PTC	8	15	4/15 (27%)	11/15 (73%)	13/15 (87%)	2/15 (13%)	1/15 (7%)
Imbasciati	6	18	18/18 (44%)	10/18 (56%)	14/18 (78%)	4/18 (22%)	2/18 (11%)
Devoe	14	17	13/17 (76%)	4/17 (24%)	12/17 (71%)	5/17 (29%)	2/17 (12%)
Bobrie	35	53	35/53 (66%)	18/53 (34%)	NA	NA	4/53 (8%)
Total			68/117 (61%)	67/170 (39%)	98/131 (75%)	33/131 (25%)	19/184 (10%)
Median	131	184	66%	34%	77%	23%	10%

[a] PTC, prior to conception.

Pregnancy-induced hypertension and pre-eclampsia

Interpretation of the literature in terms of pregnancy-induced hypertension (PIH) during SLE pregnancies is difficult due to the varying definitions of the disease, the mix of patients with nephropathy in the various studies, and the method of ascertainment. Overall, 20–30% of SLE pregnancies are complicated by PIH.[25] A history of renal disease appears to be particularly ominous. In the prospective study of Lockshin et al., 8 of 11 (72%) pregnancies in women with LN had PIH, compared with 12 of 53 (22%) in SLE patients without LN.[25]

The reason for the increased frequency of PIH among SLE patients is unknown, but may relate to underlying renal disease, a factor recognized to be associated with PIH.[26] Authorities believe that virtually all SLE patients demonstrate some degree of renal abnormality if biopsies are studied by immunofluorescence or electron microscopic methods. The use of high doses (> 30 mg of prednisone daily) of steroids during pregnancy may predispose to PIH.

Fetal Risks

Pregnancy loss

It is generally agreed that pregnancy loss is more common among women with SLE than among normal women. **Table 4** summarizes the pregnancy losses in the more recent series,[4,7,14,27–32] including the only three prospective series. Overall, the median rate of pregnancy loss is 31%, a figure considerably higher than typically found in the normal population. The three best studies indicate an overall pregnancy loss of 22, 31 and 10.5%, respectively.[7,14,27] Unfortunately, none of the studies included appropriately matched, prospectively acquired controls. However, Mintz et al.[7] found a statistically higher rate of pregnancy loss among the SLE patients than among over 100 women followed in a high-risk clinic during the study period. A few retrospective studies did not find a higher than expected rate of pregnancy loss among women with SLE,[22,27,29] and one small retrospective study found no difference in the proportion of pregnancy losses between SLE patients and controls.[33]

It appears that a disproportionate number of pregnancy losses in women with SLE occur as fetal deaths in the second or third trimester, with a median rate of 8% in the nine studies listed in **Table 4**. The well-detailed, prospective study of Lockshin et al. found that over 20% of the pregnancy losses were second or third trimester fetal deaths.[27] In contrast, the study of Wong et al. found no fetal deaths in 19 continuing pregnancies.[14] Unfortunately, the large prospective study of Mintz et al. did not distinguish fetal death from miscarriage in pregnancies lost before 21 weeks gestation.[7]

Among SLE patients, fetal deaths are associated with the presence of antiphospholipid antibodies (see section on Antiphospholipid Syndrome). In one study of 21 women with SLE, antiphospholipid antibodies were found to be the most sensitive indicator of fetal distress or fetal death.[34] In a second study by the same authors, antiphospholipid antibodies were present in 10 or 11 patients with fetal death, and the positive predic-

Table 4
Pregnancy loss in patients with SLE[4,5,7,14,26–30]

Author	Patients (n)	Pregnancies (n)	Miscarriages[a]	Fetal death[b]	Total losses
Fraga	20	42	NA	NA	17 (40%)
Zurier	13	25	7 (28%)	2 (8%)	9 (36%)
Zulman	23	24	0	3 (12%)	3 (12%)
Varner	31	34	3 (9%)	2 (6%)	5 (15%)
Gimovsky	39	65	23 (35%)	7 (11%)	30 (46%)
Lockshin	28	32	3 (9%)	7 (22%)	10 (31%)
McHugh	NA	47	NA	NA	16 (34%)
Mintz	75	92	16 (17%)[c]	4 (4%)[d]	20 (22%)
Wong	17	19	2 (10%)	0	2 (10%)
Median			10%	8%	31%

Only pregnancies occurring after the diagnosis of SLE are included.
[a] Losses before 13 completed weeks gestation are considered miscarriages.
[b] Losses ≥ 14 weeks gestation are considered fetal deaths.
[c] Included all losses < 21 weeks gestation.
[d] Included all stillbirths ≤ 21 weeks gestation.

tive value of antiphospholipid antibodies for fetal death was over 50%.[25] Another recent study indicates that the presence of antiphospholipid antibodies *and* a history of fetal loss predicts over 85% of pregnancy loss in women with SLE.[35] Thus, it appears that antiphospholipid antibodies (perhaps coupled with a history of fetal loss) is an important predictor of fetal loss in SLE patients.

Three other factors may be associated with pregnancy loss in women with SLE. In a retrospective study of women with SLE and LN, Hayslett and Lynn suggested that pregnancy loss might be related to the activity of SLE during the several months prior to conception.[20] They found that live births occurred in only 64% of patients with clinically active SLE in the 6 months prior to conception, whereas 88% of pregnancies were successful if the disease had been quiescent before conception. Other evidence suggests that the onset of SLE during pregnancy may pose a serious threat to the conceptus. Three studies provide enough detail to analyze pregnancy outcome in patients with the onset of SLE during pregnancy.[22,23,30] Of the 21 pregnancies described, five ended in fetal death and one ended in miscarriage, for an overall loss rate of 29%.

Finally, some authors believe that underlying renal disease may have an adverse effect on pregnancy survival in patients with SLE. **Table 5** summarizes the pregnancy outcomes in 199 pregnancies in 123 women with a diagnosis of LN prior to conception.[10,20,22–24] Excluding therapeutic abortions, a median of 13% of

the pregnancies ended in miscarriage and a median of 7.5% ended in fetal death, figures not remarkably different from those for all patients with SLE shown in **Table 4**. However, in one study, the rate of fetal death was higher after the diagnosis of SLE and LN than before the diagnosis in the same patients.[31] Also, the degree of renal impairment is important. Hayslett and Lynn found that a serum creatinine ≥ 1.5 mg/dl, indicating moderate to severe renal insufficiency, was associated with fetal losses in 50% of 10 cases.[20] Fine *et al.* found fetal loss in 38 and 46% of pregnancies complicated by proteinuria (< 300 mg/24 h) or a creatinine clearance < 100 ml/min respectively.[21] Even without SLE, moderate to severe renal insufficiency may be associated with an increased rate of pregnancy loss, especially in patients with chronic hypertension. Only one small study addresses the important issue of how the renal biopsy findings might influence the pregnancy outcome.[36] Seventeen pregnancies in 14 women with biopsy proven LN were described. There were seven pregnancies among women with mesangial or membranous GN; six ended in viable live births and one ended as a first trimester miscarriage. There were five pregnancies among women with diffuse or focal proliferative lesions; three of these ended in success and two were lost as first trimester miscarriages. Although the number of patients with more benign *vs* more severe lesions is quite small, the authors concluded that there was no consistent correlation between renal biopsy findings and pregnancy outcome.

Table 5
Pregnancy outcomes among women with SLE nephropathy [10,20–24]

Author	Patients	Pregnancies	Therapeutic abortions	Miscarriages	Fetal deaths[a]	Preterm live-borns[a]	Term live-borns[a]	All live-borns[a]
Hayslett								
remission PTC[b]					2			
active PTC	23	31	7	1 (4%)	(8%)[c]	1 (4%)	20 (84%)	21/24 (88%)
Jungers	24	25	3	3 (14%)	5 (23%)	0	14 (64%)	14/22 (64%)
remission PTC	8	11	0	0	0	1 (9%)	10 (91%)	11/11 (100%)
active PTC	8	15	3	3 (25%)	0[d]	2 (17%)	7 (58%)	9/12 (75%)
Imbasciati	6	18	2	0	4 (25%)	10 (62%)	2 (12%)	12/16 (75%)
Gimovsky	19	46	6	16 (40%)[d]	5 (12%)	9 (22%)	10 (25%)	19/40 (48%)[e]
Devoe	14	17	2	2 (13%)	1 (7%)	3 (20%)	9 (60%)	12/15 (80%)
Bobrie	35	53	15	5 (13%)	0	5 (13%)	28 (74%)	33/38 (87%)
Total				28 (17%)	16 (10%)	28 (17%)	91 (56%)	119/163 (73%)
Median	123	199	36	13%	7.5%	15%	62%	77.5%

[a] Percentages calculated excluding therapeutic abortions.
[b] PTC, prior to conception.
[c] Only fetal deaths ≤ 20 weeks are described.
[d] No losses listed as ≤ 13 weeks.
[e] Includes one infant that died of prematurity.

Preterm delivery

Preterm delivery is more likely in SLE pregnancies than in normal pregnancies. In series where the gestational age at delivery is described,[7,14,20–23,27,30,31,35,37] a median of 30% of births are before 37 weeks gestation (range 3–73%). Certainly there are many confounding variables to consider, not the least of which is the tendency for obstetricians to move to delivery as soon as the fetus is considered mature or the potential for neonatal morbidity is thought to be minimal. In the three studies in which indications for preterm delivery are discussed,[30,31,35] 28–66% were for pre-eclampsia and 12–33% were for fetal distress. Thus, about 30–50% of the preterm deliveries in SLE pregnancies are due to maternal or fetal indications for delivery. Preterm labor is probably not more common among SLE patients than in the general population, but preterm delivery is probably more likely if the pregnancy is complicated by SLE flare. The best data indicate that 59% of women whose SLE flared during pregnancy delivered prematurely, compared with a 39% preterm birth rate among those without exacerbations.[7]

Fetal growth impairment

Given the fact that pregnant SLE patients may have pregnancy-induced hypertension, antiphospholipid syndrome or both, it is not surprising that fetal growth impairment may occur. However, few studies document the occurrence of fetal growth impairment. The best data come from the study of Mintz et al.[7] These investigators found that 20 of 86 (23%) pregnancies progressing beyond 20 weeks gestation were delivered of growth-impaired fetuses, including four stillbirths. Only 4% of controls were delivered of growth-impaired fetuses. Other series indicate that 12–32% of neonates are growth-impaired.[14,21,30,35,38]

Neonatal lupus erythematosus

Neonatal lupus erythematosus (NLE) is a rare (approximately 1 : 20000 live births) condition of the fetus and neonate that is characterized by dermatological, cardiac or hematological abnormalities. Probably NLE is due to maternal autoantibodies, particularly anti-Ro/SSA, that cross the placenta and cause the lesions typical of the condition. About half of the mothers who deliver an infant with NLE have SLE or another autoimmune disease, but about half have no autoimmune diagnosis. The most common presentation is probably dermatological. Cardiac disease is less common, but is disproportionately represented in case reports. Hematological abnormalities are the least frequently recognized or reported.

The typical skin lesions are erythematous, scaling annular or elliptical plaques occurring on the face or scalp. They are analogous to the subacute cutaneous lesions in adults, and are probably induced by exposure of the skin to ultraviolet light. The lesions first appear within the first several weeks after delivery and last for up to 6 months. Hypopigmentation may persist for up to 2 years. Skin biopsy shows histopathology and immunofluorescence typical of that of cutaneous lupus.

The cardiac lesions associated with NLE are congenital complete heart block (CCHB) and endocardial fibroelastosis, with the latter being less frequently reported and perhaps uncommon. CCHB associated with NLE is not associated with anatomic malformations of the heart. The usual presentation is a fixed fetal bradycardia in the range 60–80 beats/min detected between 16 and 25 weeks gestation. Ultrasonographic examination of the fetal hearts shows a structurally normal heart with atrio-ventricular dissociation. Hydrops fetalis may develop in utero, and is perhaps dependent upon the degree of endomyocardial fibrosis and myocardial dysfunction. The histological lesion is one of fibrosis and interruption of the conduction system, especially in the area of the atrio-ventricular node. Because the lesion is permanent, a pacemaker may be necessary for neonatal survival. The hematological abnormalities of NLE are less well-established as part of the condition. They include autoimmune hemolytic anemia, leukopenia, thrombocytopenia and hepatosplenomegaly.

The diagnosis of NLE is confirmed by testing for autoantibodies associated with the condition. In total, 75–95% of cases are associated with maternal anti-Ro/SSA, an autoantibody directed against ribonucleoprotein found in about 30% of patients with SLE.[39] A smaller percentage have anti-La/SSB, and some have both. Cutaneous NLE has also been associated with anti-U$_1$RNP without anti-Ro/SSA or anti-La/SSB.[40] Substantial indirect evidence suggests that these maternal autoantibodies are transported across the placenta where they bind to fetal tissue antigens and cause immunological damage resulting in NLE. Immunoglobulin has been demonstrated in the heart and skin of affected infants,[41] and sera from the majority of mothers who deliver an infant with CCHB contain IgG that binds to fetal cardiac tissue.[42] Furthermore, intravenously injected affinity-purified anti-Ro/SSA binds in human skin transplanted onto immunodeficient mice.[43]

The risk of a mother with anti-Ro/SSA and/or anti-La/SSB having a fetus or neonate with NLE remains the subject of investigation. Most mothers with anti-Ro/SSA or anti-La/SSB have normal fetuses and neonates. Among all mothers with SLE, the risk of NLE is low, probably less than 5%.[44] Among mothers with SLE and anti-Ro/SSA, the risk of skin lesions indicative of definite NLE is about 15%.[44] Fortunately, the risk of CCHB, the only seriously morbid or mortal aspect of NLE, is quite low among women with SLE, even if they have anti-SSA. The risk may be higher in women who have previously delivered an infant with CCHB, with some investigators estimating that 25–60% of these mothers will have another fetus with CCHB.[45] In these cases, some authors suggest prophylactic treatment using glucocorticoids and plasmapheresis[45,46] or glucocorticoids and intravenous immune globulin,[47] but such treatments carry risks and are controversial.

There are three reports wherein fetuses with established CCHB and evidence of cardiac failure or serositis appear to have improved after maternally administered prednisone and betamethasone[48,49] or maternally administered dexamethasone and plasmapheresis.[50] In all cases, the CCHB persisted (as one would expect), but serous effusions regressed. This suggests that the treatments either improved fetal cardiac function or effectively treated fetal serositis.

Management Options

Prepregnancy

Ideally, a woman with SLE who is contemplating pregnancy will seek preconceptional counsel. At that time, she should be informed of the potential obstetrical problems, including the risk of pregnancy loss, preterm delivery, pregnancy-induced hypertension and fetal growth impairment. Special concerns related to antiphospholipid syndrome and neonatal lupus should also be discussed. Ideally, the patient should be in remission and discontinue cytotoxic drugs and non-steroidal anti-inflammatory drugs prior to conception. She should also be assessed for evidence of anemia or thrombocytopenia, underlying renal disease (urinanalysis, serum creatinine and 24-h urine for creatinine clearance and total protein), and antiphospholipid antibodies (lupus anticoagulant and anticardiolipin). It is also common to obtain anti-Ro/SSA and anti-La/SSB antibodies on all patients with SLE, but the cost-effectiveness of these tests is not proven.

Prenatal

Once pregnant, the patient with SLE should be seen by a physician at least every 2 weeks in the first and second trimesters and every week thereafter. At each visit, the patient should be questioned about signs or symptoms of SLE activity and her urine should be examined for evidence of blood or protein. Of course, the patient should be urged to notify the physician immediately if she develops evidence of an SLE flare. Optimal management does not require serological evaluation for hypocomplementemia, circulating immune complexes or autoantibody levels, as long as the patient remains asymptomatic. Some obstetricians obtain urine and hematological studies once each trimester in pregnant SLE patients.

Antirheumatic drugs and pregnancy

Glucocorticoids are the mainstay of treatment for SLE during pregnancy. In general, the doses of glucocorticoids used in pregnancy are similar to those used in non-pregnant patients. While an increased frequency of cleft palate has been found in the offspring of glucocorticoid-treated laboratory animals,[51] a wealth of human experience and several studies indicate that the risk for human teratogenesis is very low.[52] The risk of neonatal adrenal suppression following maternal treatment with hydrocortisone or prednisolone is very low, having been only rarely reported. One reason for the relative safety of these glucocorticoids in the human may be the abundance of 11-β-ol dehydrogenase in the human placenta. This enzyme converts these drugs to the relatively inactive 11-keto forms, leaving no more than 10% of the active drug to reach the fetus. Glucocorticoids with fluorine at the 9α position are considerably less well metabolized by the placenta and should not be administered chronically during pregnancy. The possible adverse maternal risks of glucocorticoids are numerous, including weight gain, striae, acne, hirsutism, immunosuppression, osteonecrosis and gastrointestinal ulceration. Also, the combination of pregnancy and glucocorticoids doubtlessly increases the likelihood of glucose intolerance. Patients on moderate or high doses of glucocorticoids should be screened for gestational diabetes at 22–24, 28–30 and 32–34 weeks gestation. Glucocorticoids also cause sodium and water retention, and moderate to high doses are associated with hypertension. In turn, this may predispose to pregnancy-induced hypertension,[25] and might be responsible indirectly for the increased frequency of fetal growth impairment in pregnancies treated with glucocorticoids.[53]

Some physicians place all pregnant SLE patients on prophylactic doses of prednisone.[7,14] No controlled studies have shown this practice to be prudent or necessary, and good maternal and fetal outcomes are reported without prophylactic steroids.[8] Current recommendations are to use glucocorticoids only as necessary to treat the symptoms of SLE. Although pregnancy *per se* is by no means an indication to reduce the dose of glucocorticoids, carefully monitored reduction of the dose of medication during pregnancy is reasonable and safe when the patient's disease appears in remission.

Several other immunosuppressive drugs may be encountered in the pregnant woman with SLE. Three of these agents – azathioprine, methotrexate and cyclophosphamide – are cytotoxic drugs. Limited data suggest that azathioprine, a derivative of 6-mercaptopurine, is not a teratogen in humans. However, it is associated with fetal growth impairment[54] and evidence of impaired neonatal immunity.[55] Ideally, patients should not be treated with azathioprine during pregnancy unless the benefits clearly outweigh the risks. Limited data suggest that methotrexate and cyclophosphamide are teratogenic in the human. They should be avoided during the first trimester and used only in unusual circumstances thereafter. One such circumstance in which cyclophosphamide might be indicated is severe, progressive proliferative glomerulonephritis.

Antimalarial drugs used in the treatment of SLE, such as chloroquine and hydroxychloroquine, cross the placenta and have been associated with several fetal abnormalities. These drugs have an affinity for melanin-containing tissues such as those in the eye, and case reports suggest that these drugs can cause dose-related eye damage in the human.[56] Chloroquine has also been associated with ototoxicity in one case report.[57] However, most infants born to women taking antimalarials during pregnancy are apparently normal, suggesting that the risks of ocular or ototoxicity are small.[58]

The most common types of analgesics used in SLE are non-steroidal anti-inflammatory drugs (NSAIDs). Unfortunately, there are serious fetal and neonatal concerns related to the use of these medications in pregnancy; NSAIDs cross the placenta readily and can block prostaglandin synthesis in a wide variety of fetal tissues. They may affect feto-neonatal clotting through the inhibition of platelet aggregation. In the case of aspirin, the inhibition of platelet function lasts the lifespan of the platelet, since aspirin irreversibly binds to the pertinent platelet enzymes. Maternal ingestion of typical adult doses of aspirin in the week prior to delivery has been associated with increased frequency of intracranial hemorrhage in premature infants.[59] Indomethacin, a NSAID, has been associated with constriction of the fetal ductus arteriosus,[60] which might result in pulmonary artery thrombosis, hypertrophy of the pulmonary vasculature, impaired oxygenation, and congestive heart failure. In a recent trial of indomethacin for the treatment of preterm labor, three neonates had pulmonary hypertension diagnosed soon after birth.[61] Also, NSAIDs have been associated with a decrease in fetal urinary output, and oligohydramnios[62] and neonatal renal insufficiency[63] have been described in association with indomethacin. Given the risks, full-dose aspirin and NSAIDs should be avoided if at all possible during pregnancy. Acetaminophen and codeine are acceptable alternatives for analgesia in the pregnant woman with SLE.

Obstetric management

The obstetrical management of the patient with SLE is guided by the potential risks to the mother and fetus. As mentioned, the pregnant SLE patient should be seen by a physician at least every 2 weeks in the first and second trimesters and every week thereafter. A primary goal of the antenatal visits after 20 weeks gestation is the detection of hypertension and/or proteinuria. Because of the risk of uteroplacental insufficiency, fetal ultrasonography should be performed every 4–6 weeks starting at 18–20 weeks gestation. In the usual case, fetal surveillance (daily fetal movement counts and once weekly non-stress tests and amniotic fluid volume measurements) should be instituted at 30–32 weeks gestation. More frequent ultrasonography and fetal testing is indicated in patients with SLE flare, hypertension, proteinuria, clinical evidence of fetal growth impairment, or antiphospholipid syndrome. In the patients with antiphospholipid syndrome, fetal surveillance as early as 24–25 weeks may be justified.[64]

Because pregnancy-induced hypertension occurs in a substantial proportion of pregnant women with SLE, it may be prudent and reasonable to treat SLE patients with low-dose aspirin (LDA) during pregnancy. There are now five prospective, controlled studies indicating the efficacy of LDA in the prevention or amelioration of PIH in patients at risk to develop the disease.[65] Although none of these studies specifically focused on patients with SLE, some authorities feel that patients with SLE, especially those with pre-existing renal disease, should be considered for treatment with LDA to prevent pre-eclampsia.

Some authors have advocated the prophylactic treatment of mothers who have previously delivered infants with NLE and CCHB, using glucocorticoids and/or plasmapheresis.[45–47] The efficacy and safety of this treatment remain unproven. However, more frequent assessment of the fetal heart rate and serial ultrasound examinations to exclude the development of fetal hydrops would appear reasonable in such cases. In newly discovered cases of CCHB *in utero*, evaluation should include sonographic assessment of the fetal heart and determination of maternal anti-SSA and anti-SSB status.

Labor/delivery

The management of the SLE gravida during labor and delivery represents a continuation of her antenatal care. Exacerbations of SLE can occur during labor, and may require the acute administration of steroids. Regardless, 'stress doses' of glucocorticoids should be given during labor or at the time of cesarean delivery to all patients who have been treated with chronic steroids within the year. This compensates for the anticipated relative endogenous adrenal insufficiency in these patients. Intravenous hydrocortisone, given in doses of 100 mg every 8 h for three doses is an acceptable regimen. Complications such as pregnancy-induced hypertension or fetal growth restriction should be dealt with based on obstetric concerns, and not specifically altered because of the SLE. Neonatology support may be needed at delivery for problems associated with neonatal heart block or other neonatal lupus manifestations.

Postnatal

The data are unclear as to the patient's true predisposition for SLE exacerbation following delivery. Regardless, care should be taken to examine for these 'flares' in the symptomatic parturient. If pregnancy-induced hypertension complicates the intrapartum process, the patient should be anticipated to clear these acute effects in a similar manner as others with this condition. Maintenance medications should be

---

SYSTEMIC LUPUS ERYTHEMATOSUS
Summary of Management Options

Prepregnancy

- Establish good control of SLE; adjust maintenance medications

- If possible, discontinue azathioprine, methotrexate and cyclophosphamide therapy before conception. This should be done only under careful supervision

- Do laboratory assessment for anemia, thrombocytopenia, underlying renal disease and antiphospholipid antibodies

- Counsel patient regarding potential for SLE exacerbations, pregnancy-induced hypertension risks, and fetal/neonatal risks

Prenatal

- Encourage early prenatal care

- Get accurate dating criteria

- Close follow-up every 2 weeks in first and second trimesters; every week in third trimester

- Watch for signs or symptoms of SLE flare, superimposed pregnancy-induced hypertension, fetal growth restriction

- For SLE patients with renal involvement, perform monthly 24-h urine collections for creatinine clearance and total protein

- Serial ultrasonography examinations for fetal growth

- Begin prenatal testing at 30–32 weeks gestation (earlier in patients with worsening disease, evidence of fetal compromise, or with a history of poor pregnancy outcome)

- Consider low-dose aspirin therapy

Labor/delivery

- Deliver at term; avoid postdates

- Continuous electronic fetal monitoring

- Steroid boluses at delivery for patients on chronic steroid therapy

- Pediatric and anesthesiology notification

Postnatal

- Watch for SLE exacerbation

- Restart maintenance therapy

- Evaluate neonate for SLE-associated manifestations

restarted immediately following delivery, at similar doses as during the pregnancy. Further dose adjustments can be handled in the out-patient setting.

ANTIPHOSPHOLIPID SYNDROME

Antiphospholipid syndrome (APS) is a recently described autoimmune condition characterized by the production of moderate to high levels of antiphospholipid antibodies (aPL) and certain clinical features. Most authorities now agree that the most specific clinical features are thrombotic phenomena (venous or arterial, including stroke), autoimmune thrombocytopenia, and pregnancy loss.[66] More debatable clinical features include livedo reticularis, Coombs' positive hemolytic anemia, cardiac valvular lesions, and others. Probably APS occurs most commonly in patients with other underlying autoimmune diseases such as SLE. In this setting, the syndrome is known as *secondary* APS. However, the condition is also diagnosed in women with no other recognizable autoimmune disease. This expression of the syndrome is known as *primary* APS and appears to be what obstetrician-gynecologists encounter most frequently. To be classified as having APS, the patient must have at least one clinical feature of the syndrome along with moderate to high levels of aPL (**Table 6**).

Diagnosis

Unfortunately, laboratory testing for aPL remains somewhat difficult and confusing. The primary problem at present is the limited number of laboratories that perform high-quality testing. Underlying this problem is the fact that reliable testing for aPL is modestly difficult even in the hands of interested investigators. Although many of the problems related to aPL testing will be resolved over time, the best advice for the clinician is that he or she identify and use a reliable laboratory with a special interest in aPL testing.

There are three aPL for which well-established assays are available:

- the biological false-positive test for syphilis (BF-STS)

- lupus anticoagulant (LA)

- anticardiolipin antibody (aCL)

All three aPL bind moieties on negatively charged phospholipids or the moieties formed by the interaction of negatively charged phospholipids with other lipids and phospholipids. Both BF-STS and aCL are detected by conventional immunoassay methods. The assay for aCL is standardized using sera obtainable from the Antiphospholipid Standardization Laboratory in Louisville, Kentucky, USA. Results calibrated against these standards are measured as 'GPL' (IgG aCL) or 'MPL' (IgM aCL) units. However, results should be reported and interpreted in semi-quantitative terms as either negative, low-positive, medium-positive or high-positive.[67] Low-positive results and isolated IgM aCL results (i.e. IgM positive, but LA negative and IgG aCL negative) are of questionable clinical significance and should be interpreted carefully in the light of the clinical situation.

Lupus anticoagulant is detected in plasma using phospholipid-dependent clotting assays such as the activated partial thromboplastin time (APTT), dilute Russell viper venom time or kaolin clotting time. Because LA binds to the phospholipid portion of the clotting tests, the clotting time is prolonged, even though the patients have a thrombotic, not a bleeding tendency. More than one clotting assay is required to determine that the prolonged clotting time is due to LA, but the clinician need only know whether the laboratory detected LA or not. Because the sensitivity of the various clotting assays for LA varies considerably, the clinician should use a laboratory known to perform reliable and sensitive LA testing.

At least two groups of investigators find that LA and aCL may be separated in the laboratory, suggesting that they are different immunoglobulins.[68,69] Others believe that LA and aCL are the same immunoglobulin being detected by different methods. This controversy notwithstanding, LA and aCL are associated with the same set of clinical problems and therefore seem likely

Table 6
Suggested clinical and laboratory criteria for the antiphospholipid syndrome (APS)

Clinical features	Laboratory features

Pregnancy loss
  fetal death
  recurrent pregnancy loss
	Lupus anticoagulant (LA)

Thrombosis
  venous
  arterial, including stroke
	Anticardiolipin antibodies
	IgG, medium- or high-positive

Autoimmune thrombocytopenia	

Other
  Coombs' positive hemolytic
  anemia
  Livedo reticularis
	Anticardiolipin antibodies
	IgM, medium- or high-positive and LA

Patients with APS should have at least one clinical and one laboratory feature at some time in the course of their disease. Laboratory tests should be positive on at least two occasions more than 8 weeks apart.

to be members of the same 'family' of autoantibodies. The majority of patients with APS have LA and IgG aCL. However, given the state of the controversy about whether LA and aCL are the same immunoglobulin and the wide variety of assays used in the past to detect LA or aCL, it is not surprising that many studies have found patients with APS to have either aCL or LA, but not both. *Both* tests should be obtained when considering the diagnosis of APS. The relative contribution of the BF-STS to APS is unclear at this time. Tests for other aPL (e.g. antiphosphatidylserine, antiphosphatidylethanolamine) are performed in the research setting, but should not be used for the diagnosis of APS or related clinical decision making.

Maternal Risks

Thrombosis and stroke

Numerous retrospective studies confirm a link between aPL and venous or arterial thrombosis.[70,71] Venous thrombosis accounts for about 65–70% of episodes. The lower extremity is the single most common site of involvement, but no part of the vasculature is spared. Antiphospholipid antibodies are the only identifiable predisposing factor in 4–28% of cases of stroke in otherwise healthy patients under age 50.[72] The prospective risk of thrombosis or stroke in women with aPL is unclear. In the single prospective study,[73] 50% of patients with SLE and LA had a thrombotic episode during the study period. The authors estimated that the annual risk of venous thrombosis and arterial thrombosis was 13.7 and 6.7%, respectively, both figures being significantly greater than among SLE patients without LA.

In summaries of data from the University of Utah, well over half of thrombotic episodes in patients with APS occurred in relation to pregnancy or the use of combination oral contraceptives.[74] This raises the question as to whether the risk of thrombosis in pregnancy in women with APS is substantial enough to warrant prophylactic treatment with heparin. However, the prospective risk of thrombosis in pregnancy is unknown.

Postpartum syndrome

A retrospective review of patients with significant levels of aPL at the University of Utah turned up three cases wherein the patients had suffered similar postpartum complications that may represent an autoimmune exacerbation.[75] None of the women were known to have underlying autoimmune disease, but all developed fever, pulmonary infiltrates and pleural effusions in the postpartum period. Two of the three also had thrombosis in the postpartum period, and one developed a cardiomyopathy. Fortunately, this syndrome is rare.

Pre-eclampsia

An unusually high rate of pre-eclampsia has been noted in series of patients with APS,[74,76,77] and pre-eclampsia contributes to the high rate of preterm delivery in this condition. The rate of pre-eclampsia does not appear to be markedly diminished by treatment with either glucocorticoids and LDA or heparin and LDA. In the largest series of treated APS pregnancies, half of the cases developed pre-eclampsia.[77]

Two studies have attempted to determine the rate of aPL among patients with pregnancy-induced hypertension. In the first, the rate of aPL was not increased among all patients with PIH, including those near term.[78] However, another study found that a small but significant proportion (16%) of patients with severe pre-eclampsia occurring before 34 weeks gestation had LA or medium to strong positive IgG aCL.[79]

Underlying renal disease may play a role in the apparent association between aPL and pre-eclampsia. In one study of patients with SLE and renal disease, the presence of aPL correlated with a glomerular lesion characterized by thrombosis.[80] At the University of Utah, one patient with APS and severe pre-eclampsia at 20 weeks gestation was found to have focal glomerular scarring and interstitial fibrosis on renal biopsy.

Fetal Risks

Pregnancy loss

Early case reports focused attention on a possible relationship between aPL and pregnancy loss. In particular, fetal death (death of the conceptus after 10–12 weeks gestation) appears to be specific for aPL-related pregnancy loss. In a recent summary of data, over 90% of women with APS presenting with pregnancy loss had suffered at least one fetal death.[74] It is uncommon, though not unheard of, for APS to present with recurrent first trimester pregnancy loss.

Most studies linking aPL to pregnancy loss have found aPL in highly selected patients with underlying autoimmune disease, a history of fetal death, or a history of thrombosis. Studies of less highly selected populations have led to the emergence of two important facts. First, significant levels of aPL may be found, albeit infrequently, among otherwise normal women. In the best study, less than 2% of over 1000 unselected obstetric patients were found to have IgG aCL; 4% had IgM aCL.[81] Over 80% of the positive results were in the low-positive range, with only 0.2% of IgG results and 0.7% of IgM results being in the medium- or high-positive range. Only one investigation found unselected patients with positive aPL results to have pregnancy complications.[82] Two of 723 (0.3%) unselected patients were found to have LA, and both suffered a second trimester fetal death. However, taken together, the available data indicate that aPL testing in the general population as a screening test for pregnancy loss or complications is unwarranted.

The second important finding is that APS is not a common 'cause' of recurrent pregnancy loss (RPL). **Table 7** summarizes five studies[83–87] that determined the frequency of aPL in women with RPL. The median frequency of LA or aCL IgG in women with RPL is 11% (vs 2.5% for controls). The studies by Petri et al. and Parke et al. found that women with predominantly recurrent first trimester losses were not statistically more likely than controls to have LA and/or aCL.[83,86] The other three studies in **Table 7** found aPL to be statistically more frequent among women with RPL than among controls. Given that APS is not a common cause of RPL, only larger series, like that of Parrazzini et al.[85] are likely to test statistical significance. The study of Out et al. compared the frequency of positive tests for LA and/or aCL in patients with fetal death (> 12 weeks gestation) to those with only first trimester miscarriages.[87] Although a trend was found, the figures were not statistically different from each other in this small study. Finally, one study found a statistically higher prevalence of aPL in women with ≥ three pregnancy losses compared with those with < three pregnancy losses,[88] again indicating the importance of the selection of the patients tested. At the University of Utah, 4–5% of patients with ≥ three consecutive pregnancy losses and no more than one live birth have APS.[74]

It is also clear that sporadic miscarriage or fetal death is infrequently 'due to' aPL, a finding that is not surprising given the infrequency of APS. Haddow et al. found only one medium to high positive IgG aCL among 309 cases of sporadic second or third trimester fetal death (all after 14 weeks gestation).[89] Tests for LA were not done. Another study of 331 women with their first pregnancy loss found no relationship between aPL and miscarriage when results were compared with 993 controls.[42] These two studies suggest that APS is not the 'cause' of pregnancy loss in a large proportion of unselected cases, much as parental karyotype abnormalities or uterine malformations are not the 'cause' of pregnancy loss in a large proportion of unselected cases. The importance of identifying APS lies not in its prevalence, but in its implications for the patient and the fact that it is a potentially treatable cause of pregnancy loss.

Fetal growth impairment and fetal distress

Several investigators have noted that aPL are associated with fetal growth impairment.[34,74,77,90] Even in treated pregnancies, the rate of fetal growth impairment along live-born infants approaches 30%.[77] In one recent study, 9 of 37 mothers (24%) who delivered growth-impaired infants had medium or high positive

Table 7
Frquency of antiphospholipid antibodies in patients with recurrent pregnancy loss (RPL) and controls[77–81]

Author	Lupus anticoagulant		Anticardiolipin IgG		Total	
	RPL	Controls	RPL	Controls	RPL	Controls
Petri[a]	4/44 (9%)	0/40 (0%)	5/44 (11%)	1/40 (2%)	7/44 (16%)	1/40 (2%)
Barbui[b]	7/49 (14%)	0/141 (0%)	4/49 (8%)	0/141 (0%)	7/49 (14%)	0/141 (0%)
Parazzini[c]	16/220 (7%)	0/193 (0%)	11/99 (11%)	4/157 (3%)	10/99 (10%)	4/157 (3%)
Parke[d]	4/81 (5%)	4/88 (5%)	6/81 (7%)	0/88 (0%)	8/81 (10%)	4/88 (5%)
Out[e]	5/102 (5%)	NA	8/102 (8%)	2/102 (2%)	11/102 (11%)	NA
Median (%)	7%	0%	8%	2%	11%	2.5%
Range (%)	5–14%	0–5%	7–11%	0–3%	10–16%	0–5%

[a] RPL defined as ≤ 3 consecutive pregnancy losses. Other causes of RPL evaluated, but did not exclude patients from the study.
[b] RPL defined as ≤ 2 consecutive pregnancy losses. Other causes of RPL excluded.
[c] RPL defined as ≤ 2 consecutive pregnancy losses. Other causes of RPL excluded.
[d] RPL defined as ≤ 3 consecutive pregnancy losses. Evaluation for other causes of RPL incomplete in some cases.
[e] RPL defined as ≤ 3 consecutive first trimester losses or at least one unexplained fetal death > 12 weeks gestation. Not all patients had other causes of RPL excluded.

tests for aCL antibodies (four IgG and five IgM), significantly more than among controls.[90]

Fetal distress also appears to be relatively common in APS pregnancy.[34,74,77] Here again, treatment does not appear to markedly diminish the rate. Half of all treated, successful pregnancies in 54 women with APS were complicated by fetal distress in one recent series.[77]

Preterm birth

Primarily because of the above-mentioned complications of aPL pregnancies, preterm delivery is very common among patients with APS.[34,74,77] Treatment with either glucocorticoids and LDA or heparin and LDA does not appear to prevent the need for preterm delivery in many cases. In the largest series of treated APS pregnancies, term delivery was uncommon and one-third of patients were delivered at or before 32 weeks gestation.[77]

Management Options

Prepregnancy

Ideally, patients with APS will seek prepregnancy counsel. At that time, the presence of significant levels of aPL should be confirmed, and the patient should be informed of the potential maternal and obstetrical problems, including a possible (but unknown) risk of thrombosis or stroke, the risk of pregnancy loss, preterm delivery, pregnancy-included hypertension and fetal growth impairment. If the patient also has SLE, the issues related to exacerbation of SLE can be discussed. Primary APS patients, like patients with SLE, should be assessed for evidence of anemia, thrombocytopenia and underlying renal disease (urinanalysis, a serum creatinine, 24 h urine for creatinine clearance and total protein).

The two non-obstetrical issues related to APS that require serious consideration are that of thrombosis (including stroke) and thrombocytopenia. As discussed above, the prospective risk of thrombosis or stroke in pregnancy is unknown. Some physicians believe that the risk of thrombosis in pregnancy is increased in patients with APS. Pending further data, the author believes that treatment with heparin or heparin and LDA may be warranted on the basis of the maternal thrombotic risk; however, the reader should note that this is a controversial point. If heparin therapy is used, it seems reasonable and prudent to continue prophylactic treatment with anticoagulants through the first month postpartum to prevent postpartum thrombosis.

Prenatal

The pregnant APS patient should be seen by a physician every 2 weeks in the first half of pregnancy and every week thereafter. Pre-eclampsia may develop as early as 15–17 weeks gestation! Fetal ultrasonography every 3–4 weeks after 15–18 weeks gestation will aid in identifying early evidence of fetal growth impairment or oligohydramnios. In most cases, fetal surveillance (daily fetal movement counts and once-weekly non-stress tests with amniotic fluid volume measurements) are started at 26–28 weeks gestation. More frequent ultrasound examinations and more frequent or earlier fetal testing may be indicated in selected cases. The presence of subtle late decelerations has been noted in the second trimester in some cases.[64]

Since the early 1980s, clinicians have suggested that women with APS and previous pregnancy loss could be treated during pregnancy to improve the chance of delivering a live infant. The initial reports used prednisone and low-dose aspirin (PRED/LDA).[76,91] The larger series of APS pregnancies treated with this regimen are summarized in **Table 8**.[77,92–97] None of the series included untreated, appropriately selected controls, but the majority of authors concluded that PRED/LDA was beneficial. The single exception is the study of Lockshin et al.[95] in which the outcome of PRED/LDA treated pregnancies was very poor. Direct comparison of these studies is impossible due to the nature of the patients (e.g. SLE vs no SLE; numbers of previous fetal deaths), the autoantibody diagnoses included (e.g. LA and aCL vs LA alone or aCL alone) and differences in the treatments used (e.g. dose of glucocorticoids). Treatment with glucocorticoids is potentially complicated by numerous minor adverse effects and several serious adverse effects. In addition, gestational diabetes is rather common among women treated with high doses of glucocorticoids.

The most attractive alternative to PRED/LDA is subcutaneous heparin treatment, with or without low-dose aspirin (**Table 9**). The first published series was that of Rosove et al.[98] Using a mean dose of 24 700 units of heparin daily started in the first trimester, 14 of 15 pregnancies (93%) were successful. Cowchock and colleagues have recently completed a randomized trial comparing treatment with glucocorticoids and heparin.[96] The mean dose of heparin used was 17 000 units daily. Although only 20 patients were randomized, the results suggest that the two treatments are of similar efficacy in achieving a successful pregnancy. Moreover, treatment with glucocorticoids was associated with an increased neonatal morbidity (preterm delivery and low birth weight) and maternal morbidity (gestational diabetes and pregnancy-induced hypertension).

The experience at the University of Utah using heparin and low-dose aspirin includes 19 pregnancies. The

Table 8
Summary of APS pregnancies treated with prednisone and low-dose aspirin[86,92–97]

Author	Patients (n)	Pregnancies (n)	Miscarriages	Fetal deaths[a]	Live births
Lubbe	19	19	NA	NA	15 (78%)
Gatenby	27	27	NA	NA	17 (63%)
Ordi	7	9	0	2 (22%)	7 (78%)
Lockshin	10	11	3 (27%)	6 (55%)	2 (18%)
Cowchock	19	19	NA	NA	13 (68%)
Reece	18	18	3 (17%)	1 (5%)	14 (78%)
Branch	33	23	8 (21%)	8 (21%)	23 (59%)[b]

[a] Fetal deaths defined as intrauterine death of a fetus proven to be alive after 10 weeks gestation.
[b] Includes two neonates that subsequently succumbed to complications of prematurity.

Table 9
Summary of APS pregnancies treated with heparin or heparin and low-dose aspirin[86,96,98]

Author	Patients (n)	Pregnancies (n)	Miscarriages	Fetal deaths[a]	Live births
Rosove	14	15	NA	NA	14 (93%)
Cowchock	8	8	NA	NA	6 (75%)
Branch	17	19	1 (5%)	2 (11%)	16 (84%)[b]

[a] Fetal deaths defined as intrauterine death of a fetus proven to be alive after 10 weeks gestation.
[b] Includes two neonates that subsequently succumbed to complications of prematurity.

median first trimester dose of heparin used was 15 000 units per day and the median second trimester dose of heparin used was 20 000 units per day. Sixteen of 19 pregnancies have been successful, but two infants died of complications of prematurity. Although not proven to be necessary, the author feels that anticoagulation doses of heparin are justified, and possibly more efficacious than prophylactic doses. Patients with LA can be monitored for anticoagulation using the thrombin time, which is not affected by LA. It seems prudent to start the heparin only after the demonstration of a live embryo ultrasound (usually 5–7 weeks gestation). As long as the patient's platelet count is normal, the author continues to use low-dose aspirin in the treatment regimen, since it may prevent or ameliorate pre-eclampsia in patients at risk.[65]

Heparin treatment is by no means benign. The most common significant risk is heparin-induced osteoporosis. In an attempt to avoid severe osteoporosis, patients treated with either glucocorticoids or heparin should take at least 1 g calcium daily (vitamin D is contained in the prenatal vitamins) and walk for 1 h daily. Heparin is also associated with an uncommon idiosyncratic thrombocytopenia. This phenomenon is independent of the route of administration or dose and may have its onset from several days to several weeks after starting heparin. The frequency is difficult to determine, but probably occurs in less than 5% of pati-

ents treated with heparin. In its severest form, heparin-induced thrombocytopenia is associated with antibodies directed against vascular endothelial cells. Occasionally, thromboembolic events or disseminated intravascular coagulation occur with the thrombocytopenia, and either may be fatal. This complication of heparin may be less frequent in pregnant patients, but formal data are not available. The concomitant use of glucocorticoids and heparin should be avoided because the combination of these two medications has not been shown to be better than either alone in achieving a live infant. The author is aware of several cases of severe osteoporosis with fractures occurring in women with APS treated with this latter regimen.

The use of high-dose intravenous immune globulin has generated interest because of anecdotal reports of successful pregnancy outcomes.[99] The experience at the University of Utah includes three women with APS treated with immune globulin and glucocorticoids. Only one had a successful pregnancy; the other two had fetal losses despite the treatment. These preliminary results suggest that immune globulin may not be better than other regimens.

The chance of a successful pregnancy outcome with treatment appears to depend in part upon the number of pregnancy losses or fetal deaths suffered in the past.[74,77] For clinicians experienced in the evaluation and treatment of women with recurrent pregnancy loss, these observations come as no surprise. Regardless of etiology, the more consecutive pregnancy losses a woman has had, the worse her prognosis for future pregnancies. The reason for this is unknown, but the observation may influence a patient's decision as to whether to attempt a treated pregnancy.

Some patients with APS have had successful pregnancy without specific medical therapy, and this has focused attention on the medical necessity of treatment. It is possible that the recognition of the fetal risk in APS pregnancies has improved the fetal outcome by focusing increased attention on the fetus, resulting in timely delivery. Trudinger et al. successfully managed six untreated pregnancies in women with APS using close fetal surveillance with Doppler velocimetry.[100] While there is no doubt that close fetal surveillance is key to successful pregnancy, the relative contribution of fetal surveillance (vs treatment) is yet to be determined. Even careful, frequent fetal surveillance cannot prevent fetal or neonatal death before 22–24 weeks gestation.

Do patients with APS, but no history of fetal loss, need medical therapy during pregnancy? There are too few data from which to draw conclusions. As previously suggested, some women with APS are likely to have a live birth with close obstetrical observation and fetal surveillance. Unfortunately, there is no way to identify these patients prospectively, and instituting treatment after the recognition of fetal compromise would seem unlikely to save the pregnancy in many cases.

RHEUMATOID ARTHRITIS

RA is a debilitating, chronic arthritic disease of the synovial joints that affects about 1 : 10 000 people in the USA. The ratio of females to males suffering with RA is 3 : 1 and the peak prevalence is age 35–45 years. The disease tends to involve primarily the joints of the wrists, knees, shoulders and metacarpal–phalangeal joints in an erosive arthritis that typically follows a slowly progressive course marked by exacerbations and remissions. Eventually, joint deformities may occur; these are especially obvious at the metacarpal–phalangeal joint and proximal and distal interphalangeal joints of the hands. Fatigue is a prominent symptom. Other extra-articular manifestations include pleurisy, pericarditis, subcutaneous nodules (rheumatoid nodules) and pulmonary fibrosis.

Diagnosis

The etiology of the disease is unknown. Histologically, the synovium is infiltrated with inflammatory cells, particularly lymphocytes. The characteristic autoantibody is rheumatoid factor (RA), which reacts with antigens on the Fc portion of immunoglobulin. In part, this specificity contributes to the extravascular immune complexes found in the synovial and pleural fluids of patients with RA. Inflammatory damage at the synovium eventually leads to typical erosive joint changes, which help to establish the diagnosis of RA on a clinical basis. There is an increased incidence of HLA-DR4 among patients with RA and the disease appears to be polygenic in inheritance.

Juvenile rheumatoid arthritis (JRA) is a somewhat different, but related arthritis. It is probably a heterogeneous group of diseases. By definition, JRA has its onset in individuals less than 16 years of age. Males and females are equally represented. One prominent subgroup is comprised of individuals with Still's disease. This condition is initially systemic in nature and includes fever, skin rash, serositis and lymphadenopathy. Arthritis occurs late in the course of disease and tends not to be as destructive or chronic as classic RA. Nearly three-quarters of patients have a spontaneous and permanent remission by the time they reach adulthood.

ANTIPHOSPHOLIPID SYNDROME
Summary of Management Options

Prepregnancy

- Counseling regarding risks

- Check for:
  - anemia
  - thrombocytopenia
  - renal compromise

Prenatal

- Low-dose aspirin AND EITHER:
  - subcutaneous heparin OR
  - steroids (NOT BOTH)
- Increased frequency of attendance

- Surveillance of fetal growth and health

- Screen for pre-eclampsia

Maternal Risks

The relationship between RA and pregnancy is fascinating even if the basic scientific understanding of the relationship remains elusive. The observation that RA dramatically improves during pregnancy[101] in many patients eventually led Philip Hench to discover cortisone. Numerous studies show that at least 50% of patients with RA demonstrate improvement in their disease in at least 50% of their pregnancies.[101–106] Several of these studies are summarized in **Table 10**. For a majority of patients, the improvement in RA starts in the first trimester heralded by a reduction in joint stiffness and pain.[105] The peak improvement in symptoms generally occurs in the second or third trimester. Other aspects of the disease may also improve during pregnancy, with studies indicating that the subcutaneous nodules associated with RA may disappear during pregnancy.[106] Even with the overall improvement in symptoms, the clinical course of RA during pregnancy is characterized by short-term fluctuations in symptoms as in the non-pregnant state. Most patients who experience an improvement in RA during pregnancy will have a similar improvement in subsequent pregnancies. However, this is not a given, and some patients will have relatively less improvement in a second or third pregnancy. There are no laboratory or clinical features that predict improvement of RA in pregnancy.

A quarter of RA patients have no improvement in their disease during pregnancy, and in a small number of cases the disease may actually worsen. Unfortunately, nearly three-quarters of patients whose disease has improved during pregnancy will suffer a relapse in the first several postnatal months.[105,106] The level of disease during the first postnatal year generally returns to that of a year before conception, but may be worse.[104] In contrast to SLE, there are no data to suggest that RA in remission is likely to have a better course during pregnancy than active RA. The long-term prognosis for RA patients undertaking pregnancy appears to be similar to those that avoid pregnancy. Oka and Vainio compared 100 consecutive pregnant RA patients with age- and disease-matched controls and found no significant differences between the groups in terms of the severity of their disease.[104] There are few studies of juvenile RA, but one study found that only 1 case in 20 had a worsening or reactivation of their disease associated with pregnancy.[107]

The mechanism(s) by which pregnancy favorably affects RA is unknown. Plasma cortisol, which rises during pregnancy to peak at term, was initially thought to be important to the amelioration of RA.[101] However, there is no correlation between cortisol concentrations and disease state.[108] Some studies suggest that estrogens or estrogens and progestagens favorably affect arthritis,[109] but there are conflicting studies[110] and a double-blind crossover trial found that estrogen did not benefit RA.[111] More promising data suggest that certain proteins circulating in higher concentrations during pregnancy or unique to pregnancy are associated with improvement of RA. These include pregnancy-associated alpha$_2$-glycoprotein[112] and gamma-globulins eluted from placenta.[113] Other investigators feel that the placenta may modify RA by clearing immune complexes[114] or that modification of immune globulins during pregnancy alters their inflammatory activity.[115]

Fetal Risks

Rheumatoid arthritis probably does not affect fertility.[116] About 15–25% of pregnancies in women with RA end in miscarriage,[33,116–118] a figure that may or may not be slightly higher than in normal women. The only controlled study found that women with RA have a significantly higher frequency of miscarriage than normal women, even before the onset of their disease (25 vs 17% before disease, 27 vs 17% after disease).[116] However, another controlled study did not find that women with RA have a higher proportion of miscarriage prior to the onset of disease.[119] Interestingly, the same study found that the frequency of fetal death was higher in patients who later develop RA than in nonaffected relatives. There are scant data available, but women with RA do not appear to be at significant risk for preterm birth, pre-eclampsia or fetal growth impairment.

Table 10
Improvement of rheumatoid arthritis in pregnancy[101–103,106,107]

Author	Patients (n)	Patients with improvement	Pregnancies (n)	Pregnancies with improvement
Hench	22	20 (91%)	37	33 (89%)
Oka	93	73 (78%)	114	88 (77%)
Betson	21	13 (62%)	21	13 (62%)
Ostensen	10	8 (90%)	10	9 (90%)
Ostensen[a]	51	NA	76	35 (46%)

[a]Study of patients with juvenile rheumatoid arthritis.

Management Options

Prepregnancy

The prepregnancy management of rheumatoid arthritis is similar to that of any of the other autoimmune disorders. This includes stabilization of the underlying disease process, reducing maintenance medications to minimize early fetal risks, and avoidance of known teratogenic agents.

Prenatal

As with SLE, each patient should be seen by a physician every 2–4 weeks throughout the pregnancy, especially if she is having trouble with her disease. Rest is an important part of the management of RA, and the patient should be counseled to plan adequately for this. Physical therapy can be helpful in patients whose disease does not improve with pregnancy.

Antirheumatic drugs and pregnancy

It is best to use acetaminophen for simple analgesia. If possible, the patient should avoid NSAIDs and aspirin (see discussion in SLE section). If this is not possible, the minimum dose necessary to control inflammation should be used. To avoid the use of large doses of salicylates or other NSAIDs, glucocorticoids should be considered for patients whose RA does not improve during pregnancy. Relatively low doses of prednisone are quite effective in RA, even though glucocorticoids are not often used in long-term management. Intra-articular steroids can also be used if necessary in pregnancy.

RA patients with progressive disease are eventually treated with medications that are aimed at modifying the disease. These include hydroxychloroquine, sulfasalazine, gold salts, D-penicillamine and methotrexate. The antimalarial hydroxychloroquine, discussed above under SLE, may have fetal toxicity, but the risks are apparently small. Sulfasalazine is also used to treat inflammatory bowel disease, and data from this literature suggest no recognizable adverse fetal effects when the drug is used in pregnancy.[120] Gold salts may be very beneficial in controlling RA, but have the potential for serious adverse effects. These compounds cross the placenta to a modest degree,[121] and thus may have adverse effects or immunosuppressant effects on the fetus or newborn. The small number of fetal exposures reported suggest that gold salts may be safe in pregnancy,[122] but definite conclusions cannot be formulated at this time. D-Penicillamine is contraindicated in pregnancy because it has been reported to impair fetal connective tissue formation.[123] Methotrexate is absolutely contraindicated during the first trimester and relatively contraindicated thereafter.

Labor/delivery

Since RA has little, if any, adverse effect on pregnancy outcome, there are no special prenatal obstetrical concerns. In a rare case, severe deforming RA can pose a problem to the mechanics of vaginal delivery; such cases are obvious and require individualized care.

RHEUMATOID ARTHRITIS
Summary of Management Options

Prepregnancy

- Counseling regarding risks

- Review of therapy to improve disease control

- Reduce dosages to lowest levels achieving therapeutic effect

- Avoid known teratogens

Prenatal

- Regular review (joint obstetric and rheumatology surveillance)

- Rest (general and local)

- Physiotherapy
  - try and avoid full-dose aspirin and NSAIDs if possible (or use minimum doses to control inflammation)
  - steroids for worsening disease
  - avoid methotrexate in first trimester
  - d-penicillamine contraindicated

Labor/delivery

- Individualize care according to physical abilities

Postnatal

Postpartum management of the RA parturient is similar to that of patients with other autoimmune disorders (see Lupus erythematosus).

SYSTEMIC SCLEROSIS

Systemic sclerosis (SSc), also known as scleroderma, is characterized by fibrosis of connective tissues and a progressive obliterative vasculopathy. The disease is uncommon, occurring in no more than 10–15 individuals per million per year. The ratio of females to males is 10 : 1 in the 15–44 year age group. The etiology of SSc is unknown, but a major target of the disease appears to be the endothelial cell. A serum factor toxic for endothelial cells has been described in some patients with the disease.[124] Although the exact mechanism of endothelial injury is unknown, disruption of the endothelium seems a primary, early factor in the pathogenesis of SSc.

Diagnosis

Clinically, the expression of SSc varies considerably and the morbidity depends upon the extent of skin or internal organ involvement. Raynaud's phenomenon is common, especially so in patients with CREST syndrome (calcinosis of involved skin, Raynaud's phenomenon, esophageal dysmotility, sclerodactyly and telangiectasias), a more limited form of scleroderma. Patients who eventually develop diffuse disease involving the internal organs are more likely to present with arthritis, finger and hand swelling, and skin thickening. The skin thickening, which usually starts on the fingers and hands, eventually involves the neck and face. In severe, progressive disease, much of the skin may be involved and marked deformities of the hands and fingers may occur. Raynaud's phenomenon and internal organ damage are attributed to fibrosis of arterioles and small arteries. In these circumstances, the normal vasoconstrictor response to various stimuli, including cold, causes near complete obliteration of the vessel. As a result, digital ischemia may occur. A similar vasculopathy is probably responsible for internal organ involvement. Lower esophageal dysfunction is most common. Other portions of the gastrointestinal tract may be involved, producing malabsorption, diarrhea and/or constipation. A variety of pulmonary lesions may occur, with the most common being progression interstitial fibrosis. Pulmonary hypertension, a problem of special interest to the obstetrician, may also occur in longstanding disease. Nearly half of the patients with well-established SSc have evidence of myocardial involvement. Dysrhythmias are probably

the most common sign encountered. Renal disease occurs to some extent in many patients, and is a major cause of mortality among patients with SSc. Severely involved cases may present with proteinuria and renal insufficiency, hypertension, or both. Sudden onset of severe hypertension and progressive renal insufficiency with microangiopathic hemolysis is known as 'scleroderma renal crisis'. These crises usually occur in cold weather, suggesting that the pathophysiology is similar to that of Raynaud's phenomenon.

ANA are present in most patients with SSc, but anti-DNA antibodies are not. About half of patients have serum cryoglobulins. Antibodies to centromere detected by indirect immunofluorescence are common among patients with limited scleroderma (CREST syndrome), but not among those with diffuse disease. Up to 40% of patients have antibody to an extractable nuclear antigen designated ScI. The biological significance of these autoantibodies is unclear.

Maternal Risks

The incidence of SSc in pregnancy is unknown, but it is uncommon, with no more than 150 involved pregnancies in the literature. In an excellent recent review, Black identified 23 case reports, four small series and four case-controlled studies of patients with SSc and pregnancy.[125] Of the case reports, 19 patients with diffuse SSc and four patients with limited SSc had a total of 29 pregnancies. The status of SSc was not recorded in one study, and in one case the SSc had its onset during pregnancy. Of the remaining 27 pregnancies, the SSc appears to have been unchanged during pregnancy in 10 pregnancies (37%), worse in 14 (52%) and better in three (11%). In these highly selected cases, nine of the patients died; eight of the deaths were related or probably related to SSc. Five of the deaths were attributable to renal disease.

Black points out that the reported series differ from the case reports in that most of the patients in the series had limited, rather than diffuse, SSc. These series included 103 pregnancies.[125–128] In nine pregnancies, the onset of SSc occurred during pregnancy and information is lacking in 17 pregnancies. Of the remaining 77 pregnancies, the SSc was unchanged in 35 (45%), worsened in 32 (41%) and improved in 11 (14%). There were two maternal deaths in the 103 pregnancies. These figures are only slightly more encouraging than those from the single case reports.

There are three case-controlled series of scleroderma and pregnancy in the literature.[129–131] The British study[130] is not very helpful in determining how pregnancy influences the course of SSc because it included many pregnancies occurring before the onset of SSc. The case-controlled study of Steen et al.[131] provides the best data and included 69 women with SSc, 48 of

whom were available to be matched with two control groups (patients with RA and neighborhood controls). Only 7% of the patients with SSc reported worsening of their disease during pregnancy, a figure similar to that among patients with RA. Of the patients having at least one pregnancy after the onset of their disease, two (3%) had a serious complication during a pregnancy. In both instances, the complication was renal crisis; one patient suffered renal failure with malignant hypertension and the other died of malignant hypertension with seizures. No patients suffered cardiac or pulmonary complications in pregnancy. There was no difference between SSc patients who had been pregnant or who had never been pregnant in regard to disease-related morbidity or mortality.

Because of the biases inherent in the case reports and small series, one must be cautious in drawing conclusions about the course of SSc in pregnancy from these data. The all-important question of the risk of serious maternal morbidity or mortality cannot be answered with certainty. Data from case reports and small series without controls suggest that SSc worsens in nearly half of the cases and the maternal mortality rate may be as high as 2%. But the case-controlled study of Steen et al.[131] suggests that, overall, maternal outcomes are more salubrious. Pregnancy is probably safest in SSc patients without obvious renal, cardiac or pulmonary disease, and such patients can be counseled using the data of Steen et al. There may be an increased risk of renal crisis in patients with early diffuse SSc;[132] therefore, some authorities suggest that such patients delay pregnancy.[131] Patients with cardiac or pulmonary disease doubtlessly face a substantial risk for serious morbidity or mortality and should not undertake pregnancy. SSc patients with moderate to severe renal disease and hypertension probably face a substantial risk for pre-eclampsia, and perhaps for mortality due to renal crisis. The author feels that pregnancy should be discouraged in such patients, even if good data are lacking.

Two of three case-controlled studies that addressed the issue of fertility suggested an increased rate of infertility among women destined to develop SSc.[129,130] However, in one of these studies, 'fertility problems' occurred in a statistically similar number of cases and controls.[130] It is clear that reproductive aged women with SSc can and do become pregnant and that the rate of infertility, if increased, appears to be only slightly higher than that in normal women.

Fetal Risks

Among the 29 pregnancies accumulated in case reports,[125] there were two miscarriages (7%), two fetal deaths (7%) and one neonatal death attributable to prematurity. Two other infants died because of mul-

tiple anomalies. Among the 103 pregnancies in the small series,[125-128] there were 24 miscarriages (23%), three fetal deaths (3%) and two neonatal deaths due to prematurity. Thus, non-controlled reports suggest that 72–83% of pregnancies among women with SSc are successful (excluding perinatal deaths due to anomalies). In the case-controlled study by Giordano et al.[129] 80 SSc patients had 299 pregnancies. Of these, 50 ended in miscarriage (17%), significantly higher than the rate of miscarriage in the matched controls (10%). There was no difference in the miscarriage rate between patients with diffuse vs limited SSc. The study of Steen et al. included 86 pregnancies after the onset of SSc.[131] Of these, 15% ended in miscarriage and 2% ended in mid-trimester fetal deaths. These percentages were not significantly different from those in RA controls or neighborhood controls. Taken together, the available data suggest that the rate of miscarriages and fetal deaths in patients with SSc might be slightly increased compared with controls.

Recent data suggest that an increased rate of pregnancy loss predates the onset of SSc. Silman et al. analyzed the reproductive histories of 154 patients who eventually developed SSc and 115 matched controls (39 cases did not have controls).[130] A significantly greater number of cases had a history of at least one miscarriage (29 vs 17%). However, only three of the cases had a history of recurrent miscarriage. Similarly, Black reports that Englert and colleagues have analyzed the pregnancy outcome in 204 women destined to develop SSc, 189 normal controls and 233 women who developed Raynaud's phenomenon.[125] Those destined to develop SSc had a higher rate of fetal death and neonatal death. One implication of these findings is that pregnancy may play a role in the development of SSc in patients predisposed to the disease.[125] However, the large case-controlled study by Steen et al. did not find an increased rate of miscarriage or fetal death in patients destined to develop SSc.[131]

Given the microvascular nature of the condition and the relative frequency of renal involvement in SSc, one might speculate that pre-eclampsia and fetal growth impairment would occur significantly more often in SSc pregnancies. In the case reports, 11 of the 23 cases (48%) had pre-eclampsia; the rate of fetal growth impairment and preterm birth cannot be ascertained with certainty.[125] In the small series, only 6% of the pregnancies were reported to involve pre-eclampsia.[125-128] Again, the rate of fetal growth impairment cannot be ascertained with certainty. Only one case-controlled series analyzed obstetrical complications.[131] Patients with SSc delivered growth-deficient infants in 10% of pregnancies, a rate statistically higher than in normal patients or patients with RA.

Neonatal involvement with skin sclerosis possibly attributable to SSc has been described in three case reports.[125] The risks of this condition, as well as its relationship to SSc itself, remain unclear.

Management Options

Prepregnancy

Prior to pregnancy, management of SSc follows the basic guidelines set out for the other autoimmune disorders. Patients with diffuse scleroderma, and with significant cardiopulmonary involvement or severe renal disease, should be counseled against getting pregnant.

Prenatal

SSc patients considering pregnancy, and any patient with SSc who presents for medical care already pregnant, should have her clinical situation thoroughly investigated. Special attention should be given to the evaluation of possible renal or cardiopulmonary involvement. It is prudent to recommend pregnancy termination in patients with diffuse SSc and cardiopulmonary involvement or moderate to severe renal involvement.

Even in the non-pregnant state, there is no satisfactory therapy for SSc. Patients with limited disease are usually managed with vasodilators and anti-inflammatory agents. As discussed above, NSAIDs should be avoided if at all possible during pregnancy. Oral vasodilators for the prevention and treatment of Raynaud's phenomenon may be continued, although substantial data to prove fetal safety are not available. Patients with diffuse SSc may be taking glucocorticoids; these are discussed under SLE in this chapter. Other immunosuppressive or cytotoxic agents should be avoided.

Angiotensin-converting enzyme inhibitors appear to be particularly efficacious in treating SSc-related hypertension. These drugs have been associated with feto-neonatal renal insufficiency in a small number of cases. However, in SSc-related hypertension, the benefits of these medications probably outweigh the risks of discontinuing them.[133]

Patients with continuing pregnancies should be seen by a physician every 1–2 weeks in the first half of pregnancy and once weekly thereafter. Although serial laboratory testing is not necessary, laboratory assessment of unusual or suspicious symptoms or signs may be helpful. The possible risk of fetal growth impairment and fetal death require serial examination of the fetus by sonography. Fetal surveillance should be instituted by 30–32 weeks gestation, or sooner if the clinical situation demands.

SYSTEMIC SCLEROSIS
Summary of Management Options

Prepregnancy

- Counseling regarding risks

- Review of therapy to improve disease control

- Assess cardiopulmonary and renal function (? if significance compromise identified advise against conception)

Prenatal

- Frequent visits

- Monitor cardiopulomonary and renal function (consider termination of pregnancy if severe compromise)

- Drugs for moderate disease:
  - anti-inflammatory for joint problems
  - vasodilators for pulmonary problems
  - steroids for worsening disease

- Vigilance for pre-eclampsia

- Use of ACE inhibitors is a dilemma if hypertension present

- Check fetal growth and health

Labor/delivery

- Intensive/high dependency care may be necessary

- Special precautions to ensure wound healing if cesarean section needed

Postnatal

- Review dosage of drugs

Labor/delivery

In patients with mild to moderate disease, few additional precautions are needed during the labor and delivery process. Again, signs of pre-eclampsia should be sought, since this complication is more likely with scleroderma. Wound healing may be a problem in patients with advanced disease, or on steroids. Therefore, operative interventions require meticulous attention to this issue. In patients with significant pulmonary, cardiac or renal impairment, intensive care management may be needed.

Postnatal

This represents a continuation of the intrapartum management plan. Most often, reinstitution of maintenance medication is all that is required. Complications of scleroderma, as previously outlined, require individualization of care.

MYASTHENIA GRAVIS (see also Chapter 26)

Myasthenia gravis (MG) is an autoimmune disorder characterized by variable weakness and fatiguability of skeletal muscle. Increasing weakness with repetitive use of the muscle(s) is an outstanding feature. Myasthenia gravis is uncommon, occurring in 2–10 individuals per 100 000. It is probably seen in about twice as many women as men, and usually has its onset in the second or third decade in women. The immediate cause of the disease is probably an autoimmune attack of the acetylcholine receptor complex of the neuromuscular junction. Ocular muscle weakness resulting in diplopia or eyelid ptosis is the usual presenting problem. Some patients present with difficulty with chewing or talking. In a large majority of patients, MG progresses from ocular to generalized skeletal muscle involvement over a 1–2 year period. Any trunk or limb muscle may be involved, but the neck flexors, deltoids and wrist extensors are notable. Death results from severe respiratory muscle fatigue. Muscle weakness varies throughout the day, but is usually worse toward the end of the day. The long-term course of disease is likewise variable and is characterized by periodic fluctuations in severity. For unclear reasons, MG tends to be worsened by emotional distress, systemic illness and increased temperature (fever, hot weather).

Diagnosis

Autoantibodies to the human acetylcholine receptor or receptor-decamethonium complex (anti-AChR) are found in the serum of over three-quarters of patients with MG.[134,135] The disease can be transferred passively to laboratory animals by the injection of IgG from affected individuals.[134] It is apparent that the pathophysiology of disease is not simply the 'blockade' of AChRs by antibody. The muscle endplate, wherein the AChRs reside, is misshapen and bears a reduced number of AChRs.[136] This is presumed to be due to autoimmune damage, perhaps mediated through complement destruction. The net result is a diminished depolarization response to acetylcholine at the postsynaptic membrane.

Abnormalities of the thymus are found in most patients with MG. In total, 75% have lymph follicle hyperplasia and 10–15% have lymphoblastic or epithelial thymic tumors. Thymectomy results in improvement in most patients. These observations suggest that MG may be due to (1) an autoimmune attack on the antigens common to the thymus and motor endplate, or (2) abnormal clone(s) of immune cells in the thymus.

The diagnosis of MG rests on the clinical presentation, physical examination, and confirmatory diagnostic procedures. Repetitive use of the muscle under study results in apparent exhaustion. The muscle vigor can be dramatically restored with short-acting anticholinesterase drugs, such as edrophonium in doses of 2–10 mg given by intravenous injection. More sophisticated tests are now available, including single fiber electromyography and repetitive nerve stimulation studies.

Maternal Risks

Several pregnancy-related factors can influence the course of MG. Nausea, vomiting, altered gastrointestinal absorption, expanded plasma volume and increased renal clearance may require that anticholinesterase medication be adjusted during pregnancy. For some mothers, the emotional stress of pregnancy might adversely affect MG. For all mothers, there is increased exertion required to carry the second or third trimester gestation. Finally, the enlarging uterus elevates the maternal diaphragm, resulting in relative hypoventilation of the lower portions of the lungs. This can pose an added problem to patients with respiratory compromise. The stress imposed by serious infections, such as pyelonephritis, can precipitate an exacerbation of MG. Weakness due to MG may be increased by the exertion required in the course of labor and delivery, especially the second stage of labor. In turn, exertion leading to exhaustion may lead to respiratory embarrassment.

It appears that the course of MG during pregnancy is not predictable. In an extensive review, Plauché found that about 40% of women with MG had exacerbation of their disease during pregnancy and about 30% had no change.[137] Also, 30% had an exacerbation postpartum, and these were frequently sudden and serious in nature. Moreover, of the approximately 30% of MG patients whose disease remained unchanged during the pregnancy, several had significant postpartum exacerbations. Plauché found an overall maternal mortality of 4% (9 of 225 reported cases). The majority of these (7 of 9) were due to refractory MG. One author found that the risk of maternal death was greatest in the first year after diagnosis,[138] but others disagree.[137]

Fetal Risks

Plauché's literature review indicates that the miscarriage rate (4.7%) and fetal death rate (2.7%) among women with MG is probably no different from that of the normal population.[137] However, the rate of preterm birth may be high. His own series of 10 patients is the largest; 6 of these delivered prematurely.[139] In three other series of 5–6 patients each, 60–66% of pregnancies delivered prematurely.[140–142] However, in one series of five patients, there were no preterm births.[143] One theoretical reason for an increased rate of preterm labor is that anticholinesterase drugs have an oxytocic action.[144]

The transplacental passage of anti-AChR antibodies can lead to fetal or neonatal MG. Arthrogryposis, presumably resulting from poor fetal movement, has been reported in three infants delivered of two mothers with MG.[145,146] But arthrogryposis is uncommon, unusual, and most mothers with MG report normal fetal movement.[143] Hydramnios, presumably resulting from altered fetal swallowing, is described in a few cases.[146,147] Donaldson et al. suggested that the relative infrequency "of fetal involvement was due to alpha-fetoprotein,[143] which has been shown to inhibit the binding of anti-AChR to AChR.[148]

In contrast, neonatal MG is rather common. Plauché found that 52 of 276 (19%) newborns had symptoms of neonatal MG.[137] Most infants with neonatal MG have high concentrations of anti-AChR in their circulation. The symptoms usually develop within the first several days of life, but are often absent initially, perhaps because of the presence of alpha-fetoprotein.[143] The diagnosis of neonatal MG is made by observation of poor sucking, feeble cry and respiratory difficulties that respond to edrophonium (1 mg i.m.). Neonatal MG is transient, usually abating over a period of 1–4 weeks. When properly recognized, the disease is easily managed with supportive care and anti-acetylcholinesterase drugs.

Management Options

Prepregnancy

Adjustment of medication to establish quiescence/control of the disease process is vital prior to pregnancy.

Patients should be appropriately consulted regarding the need for close supervision, the expected increase in fatigue and the potential for respiratory compromise (especially late in pregnancy); the fetal risks of preterm delivery, the potential for associated anomalies, and the transient nature of neonatal MG should be discussed.

Prenatal

The treatment of MG during pregnancy does not differ remarkably from that used in the non-pregnant state, except that alterations in drug absorption, increased renal clearance and expanded plasma volume may require that the treatment regimen be altered to maintain adequate drug levels. The first line of therapy is quaternary ammonium compounds with anti-acetylcholinesterase activity. Although neostigmine (Prostigmine®) was the first such drug to be used, its short half-life was a major drawback. Pyridostigmine (Mestinon®), which has a longer half-life, is the most popular long-acting medication currently used for maintenance therapy of MG. There is now a sustained-release form of the drug (Mestinon Timespan®, 180 mg), but its popularity is limited by concerns about irregular absorption and drug preparation. Oral pyridostigmine is typically given in doses of 240–1500 mg/day in divided doses at 3–8 h intervals. When used, the sustained-release preparation is typically given as a single bedtime dose of 180–540 mg. If the patient requires more drug, as is often the case with advancing pregnancy, it is best to first shorten the interval between doses. If this fails to control symptoms, the dose of pyridostigmine should be increased by increments of 15–30 mg. Such maneuvers usually lead to adequate control of MG during pregnancy. The most common side-effects of these medications are due to the accumulation of acetylcholine (muscarinic effects). These include gastrointestinal symptoms (nausea, vomiting, cramping, diarrhea) and increased oral and bronchial secretions. Overdose of anti-acetylcholinesterase drugs results in the rare so-called 'cholinergic crisis', including paradoxical muscle weakness and respiratory failure.

Glucocorticoids are effective in most patients with MG. Most authorities prefer high doses (prednisone 60–80 mg/day) to start; the dose is tapered over many months after improvement is noted. The disease may transiently worsen soon after the steroids are started and, for this reason, patients should be hospitalized for steroid therapy. Unfortunately, remission appears to be maintained only if the patient continues on steroids, and withdrawal of steroids may cause myasthenic exacerbations. For these reasons, pregnant MG patients on glucocorticoids should be maintained on them through pregnancy and the postpartum period. Some authors believe that glucocorticoid-induced remission is a particularly good time for pregnancy in patients with MG.[137]

Plasmapheresis has been used with success in severe MG. Most patients were also taking glucocorticoids. There is one case report of using plasmapheresis to successfully treat MG in pregnancy.[149] It may be that maternal plasmapheresis might be the treatment of choice in MG pregnancies in which the fetus had markedly reduced or absent fetal movement that predisposed it to arthrogryposis.

Thymectomy may result in improvement in more than half of the patients with MG by mechanisms that are unknown. However, resorting to thymectomy during pregnancy would seem imprudent because of frequent long delays before improvement and perioperative maternal and fetal concerns.

Patients with MG should be seen relatively frequently throughout pregnancy, every 2 weeks in the first and second trimester, and every week in the third trimester. Undue emotional and physical stress are to be avoided, since they may result in exacerbation of MG. The patient and physician should be alert to the possibility of preterm labor, and appropriate preventative steps instituted. Although care must be individualized, limiting exercise and work is probably in order for many patients. Infections may also result in exacerbation of MG. Respiratory and urinary tract infections must be identified and treated promptly.

Fetal involvement with MG is suspected by poor fetal movement and hydramnios. This is not treatable *in utero*. Differentiating poor fetal movement due to MG from that due to fetal hypoxemia may be difficult, but normal fetal heart rate tests, especially a negative contraction stress test, and a normal biophysical profile score (BPS), are reassuring.

Labor/delivery

The course of the first stage of labor in patients with MG is not altered since MG does not affect smooth muscle.[150] The second stage of labor could be affected by the weakened material expulsive efforts, although the average duration of labor in MG patients is normal.[150]

The management of labor and delivery in patients with MG requires limitation of emotional and physical stress and the appropriate use of parenteral anticholinesterase drugs. Neostigmine (Prostigmine®) can be given subcutaneously, intramuscularly or intravenously. As a rough guide, 60 mg oral pyridostigmine is equivalent to 0.5 mg i.v. neostigmine and 1.5 mg s.c. neostigmine. The usual dose of parenteral neostigmine is 0.5–2.5 mg. Maximal effects on skeletal muscle may occur 20–30 min after i.m. injection; the effects last for about 2.5–4 h. Pyridostigmine (Mestinon®) can be given intramuscularly or very slowly intravenously. The usual dose is 2 mg (approximately 1/30 of the usual oral dose) every 2–3 h.

It is very important to recognize that certain medications that may be used in the management of obstetrical concerns are contraindicated in patients with MG. These are listed in **Table 11**. Magnesium sulfate is absolutely contraindicated because it further interferes with the neuromuscular blockade of MG. Preterm labor can probably be treated weith beta-sympathomimetics,[145] but the associated hypokalemia should be carefully avoided. A small number of patients with MG have an associated cardiomyopathy which could increase the risks of beta-sympathomimetics.

Since the patient with MG is particularly sensitive to neuromuscular drugs, analgesic and anesthetic considerations are important prior to the onset of labor. All patients with MG should be seen in consultation by an anesthesiologist early in the course of pregnancy. Epidural anesthesia is probably best because it limits the need for analgesia, may help prevent anxiety and fatigue, and is excellent for forceps procedures.[53] Some authors recommend general endotracheal anesthesia for cesarean section in patients with respiratory involvement.[53] Myasthenic crises requiring ventilatory support may be precipitated by the stress of labor and delivery, an inadvertent change in medication, or surgery. Rarely, cholinergic crises may result from overdosage with anticholinesterase drugs. These patients have prominent muscarinic symptoms in addition to respiratory weakness. In all patients with MG, labor and delivery management should include the immediate availability of personnel and equipment for ventilatory support and airway maintenance. Postoperative care may be best accomplished in an intensive care setting.

Postnatal

It would be difficult to find a patient, following delivery, who is not fatigued and weakened. Differentiating this normal state of affairs from exacerbation of MG may be difficult, without objective testing. Drug dos-

Table 11
Medications that may exacerbate or cause muscle weakness in patients with MG

Magnesium salts	Cholistin
Aminoglycosides	Polymyxin B
Halothane	Quinine
Propranolol	Lincomycin
Tetracycline	Procainamide
Barbiturates	Ether
Procainamide	Lithium salts
Penicillamine	Trichloroethylene

MYASTHENIA GRAVIS
Summary of Management Options (see also Chapter 26)

Prepregnancy

- Counseling regarding risks

- Review of therapy to improve disease control

- Consider thymectomy

Prenatal

- Continue pre-existing drugs:
  - anticholinesterases
  - steroids
  - azathiaprine

- Plasmapheresis for drug-resistant cases

- Fetal surveillance, especially activity (? boiphysical profile score)

Labor/delivery

- Minimize stress

- Continue anticholinesterase drugs (parenteral)

- Steroid cover if on steroids

- Regional analgesia preferable to narcotics for pain relief and general anesthesia

- Experienced anesthetists if general anesthesia (advisable to consult in prenatal period)

- Assisted second stage more likely

- Avoid magnesium sulfate in patients with pre-eclampsia

Postnatal

- Review dosage of drugs

- Special care and surveillance of newborn; may need short-term anticholinesterases

ages may need to be rapidly adjusted, in particular downward, as the effects of the volume expansion of pregnancy clears. Neonatal management, as previously outlined, should be carried out to minimize the transient effects of the maternal disease on the infant.

REFERENCES

1 Tan EM, Cohen AS, Fries JF *et al.* (1982) The 1982 revised criteria for the classification of systemic lupus erythematosus. *Arthritis and Rheumatism* **25**: 1271–1277.

2 Garenstein M, Pollach VE, Kark RM (1962) Systemic lupus erythematosus and pregnancy. *New England Journal of Medicine* **267**:165–169

3 Estes D, Larson DL (1965) Systemic lupus erythematosus and pregnancy. *Clinics in Obstetrics and Gynecology* **8**:307–321.

4 Zurier RB, Argyros TG, Urman JD, Warren J, Rothfield NF (1978) System lupus erythematosus. *Obstetrics and Gynecology* **51**:178–180.

5 Lockshin MD, Reinits E, Druzin ML, Murrman M, Estes D (1984) Case-control prospective study demonstrating absence of lupus exacerbation during or after pregnancy. *American Journal of Medicine* **77**:893–898.

6 Meehan RT, Dorsey JK (1987) Pregnancy among patients with systemic lupus erythematosus receiving immunosuppressive therapy. *Journal of Rheumatology* **14**:252–258.

7 Mintz R, Niz J, Gutierrez G, Garcia-Alonso A, Karchmer S (1986) Prospective study of pregnancy in systemic lupus erythematosus: Results of a multidisciplinary approach. *Journal of Rheumatology* **13**:732–739.

8 Lockshin MD (1989) Pregnancy does not cause systemic lupus erythematosus to worsen. *Arthritis and Rheumatism* **32**:665–670.

9 Petri M, Howard D, Repke J (1991) Frequency of lupus flare in pregnancy. The Hopkins lupus pregnancy center experience. *Arthritis and Rheumatism* **34**:1538–1545.

10 Devoe LD, Taylor RL (1979) Systemic lupus erythematosus in pregnancy. *American Journal of Obstetrics and Gynecology* **135**:473–479.

11 Devoe LD, Loy GL (1984) Serum complement levels and perinatal outcome in pregnancies complicated by systemic lupus erythematosus. *Obstetrics and Gynecology* **63**:796–800.

12 Buyon JP, Cronstein BN, Morris M, Tanner M, Weissman G (1986) Serum complement values (C3 and C4) to differentiate between systemic lupus activity and preeclampsia. *American Journal of Medicine* **81**:194–200.

13 Lockshin MD, Qamar T, Redecha P *et al.* (1986) Hypocomplementemia with low C1s–C1 inhibitor complex in systemic lupus erythematosus. *Arthritis and Rheumatism* **29**:1467–1472.

14 Wong KL, Chan FY, Lee CP (1991) Outcome of pregnancy in patients with systemic lupus erythematosus. *Archives of Internal Medicine* **151**:269–273.

15 Adelsberg BR (1983) The complement system in pregnancy. *American Journal of Reproductive Immunology* **4**:38–44.

16 Haeger M, Unander M, Bengtsson A (1990) Enhanced anaphylatoxin and terminal C5b-9 complement complex formation in patients with the syndrome of hemolysis, elevated liver enzymes, and low platelet count. *Obstetrics and Gynecology* **76**:698–702.

17 Buyon JP, Tamerius J, Ordorica S *et al.* (1989) Activation of the alternative complement pathway accompanies disease flares in systemic lupus erythematosus during pregnancy. *Arthritis and Rheumatism* **35**:55–61.

18 Lockwood CJ, Peters JH (1990) Increased plasma levels of ED1$^+$ cellular fibronectin precede the clinical signs of preeclampsia. *American Journal of Obstetrics and Gynecology* **162**:358–362.

19 Bear R (1976) Pregnancy and lupus nephritis: A detailed report of six cases with a review of the literature. *Obstetrics and Gynecology* **47**:715–718.

20 Hayslett JP, Lynn RI (1980) Effect of pregnancy in patients with lupus nephropathy. *Kidney International* **18**:207–220.

21 Fine LG, Barnett EV, Danovitch GM *et al.* (1981) Systemic lupus erythematosus in pregnancy. *Archives of Internal Medicine* **94**:667–677.

22 Jungers P, Dougados M, Pelissier C *et al.* (1982) Lupus nephropathy and pregnancy. *Archives of Internal Medicine* **142**:771–776.

23 Imbasciati E, Surian M, Bottino W *et al.* (1984) Lupus nephropathy and pregnancy. *Nephron* **36**:46–51.

24 Bobrie G, Liote F, Houillier P, Grunfeld JP, Jungers P (1987) Pregnancy in lupus nephritis and related disorders. *American Journal of Kidney Disease* **9**:339–343.

25 Lockshin MD, Qamar T, Druzin ML (1987) Hazards of lupus pregnancy. *Journal of Rheumatology* (Suppl. 13) **14**:214–217.

26 Fisher KA, Luger A, Spargo BH *et al.* (1981) Hypertension in pregnancy: Clinical-pathologic correlations and remote prognosis; *Medicine* **60**:267–276.

27 Lockshin MC, Harpel PC, Druzin ML *et al.* (1985) Lupus pregnancy II. Unusual pattern of hypocomplementemia and thrombocytopenia in the pregnant patient. *Arthritis and Rheumatism* **28**:58–66.

28 Fraga A, Mintz G, Orozco J, Orozco JH (1974) Sterility and fertility rates, fetal wastage and maternal morbidity in systemic lupus erythematosus. *Journal of Rheumatology* **1**:293–298.

29 Zulman JI, Talal N, Hoffman GS, Epstein WV (1979) Problems associated with the management of pregnancies in patients with systemic lupus erythematosus. *Journal of Rheumatology* **7**:37–49.

30 Varner MW, Meehan RT, Syrop CH, Strottman MP, Goplerud CP (1983) Pregnancy in patients with systemic lupus erythematosus. *American Journal of Obstetrics and Gynecology* **145**:1025–1040.

31 Gimovsky ML, Montoro M, Paul RH (1984) Pregnancy outcome in women with systemic lupus erythematosus. *Obstetrics and Gynecology* **63**:686–692.

32 McHugh NJ, Reilly PA, McHugh LA (1989) Pregnancy outcome and autoantibodies in connective tissue disease. *Journal of Rheumatology* **16**:42–46.

33 Siamopoulou-Mavridou A, Manoussakis MN, Mavridis AK, Moutsopoulos HM (1988) Outcome of pregnancy in patients with autoimmune rheumatic disease before the disease onset. *Annals of Rheumatic Diseases* **47**:982–987.

34 Lockshin MD, Druzin ML, Goei S *et al.* (1985) Antibody to cardiolipin as a predictor of fetal distress or death in pregnant patients with systemic lupus erythematosus. *New England Journal of Medicine* **313**:152–156.

35 Englert HJ, Derue GM, Loizou S *et al.* (1988) Pregnancy and lupus: Prognostic indicators and response to treatment. *Quarterly Journal of Medicine* **66**(250):125–136.

36 Devoe LD, Loy GL, Spargo BH (1983) Renal histology and pregnancy performance in systemic lupus erythematosus. *Clinical and Experimental Hypertension* **B2**:325–340.

37 Houser MT, Fish AJ, Tagatz GE, Williams PP, Michael AF (1980) Pregnancy and systemic lupus erythematosus. *American Journal of Obstetrics and Gynecology* **138**:409–413.

38 Nossent HC, Swaak TJG (1990) Systemic lupus erythematosus. VI. Analysis of the interrelationship with pregnancy. *Journal of Rheumatology* **177**:771–776.

39 Scott JS, Maddison PJ, Taylor MV *et al.* (1983) Connective tissue disease, antibodies to ribonucleoprotein and congenital heart disease. *New England Journal of Medicine* **309**:209–212.

40 Provost TT, Watson R, Ganmmon WR *et al.* (1987) Neonatal lupus syndrome associated with U$_1$RNP (nRNP) antibodies. *New England Journal of Medicine* **316**:1135–1138.

41 Taylor PV, Scott JS, Gerlis LM, Path FRC, Esscher E, Scott O (1986) Maternal antibodies against fetal cardiac antigens in congenital complete heart block. *New England Journal of Medicine* **315**:667–672.

42 Infante-Rivard C, David M, Gauthier R, Rivard G-E (1991) Lupus anticoagulants, anticardiolipin antibodies, and fetal loss: A case-controlled study. *New England Journal of Medicine* **325**:1063.

43 Lee LA, Gaither KK, Coulter SN *et al.* (1989) Pattern of cutaneous immunoglobulin G deposition in subacute cutaneous lupus erythematosus is reproduced by infus-

ing purified anti-Ro (SSA) autoantibodies into human skin-grafted mice. *Journal of Clinical Investigation* **83**:1556–1562.

44 Lockshin MD, Bonfa E, Elkon D, Druzin ML (1988) Neonatal lupus risk to newborns of mothers with systemic lupus erythematosus. *Arthritis and Rheumatism* **31**:697–701.

45 Buyon J, Roubey R, Swersky S *et al.* (1988) Complete congenital heart block: Risk of occurrence and therapeutic approach to prevention. *Journal of Rheumatology* **15**:1104–1108.

46 Barclay CS, French MAH, Ross LD, Sokol RJ (1987) Successful pregnancy following steroid therapy and plasma exchange in a women with anti-Ro (SS-A) antibodies: Case report. *British Journal of Obstetrics and Gynaecology* **94**:369–371.

47 Kaaja R, Julkunen H, Ammala P *et al.* (1991) Congenital heart block: Successful prophylactic treatment with intravenous gamma globulin and corticosteroid therapy. *American Journal of Obstetrics and Gynecology* **165**:1333–1334.

48 Richards DS, Wagman AJ, Cabaniss ML (1990) Ascites not due to congestive heart failure in a fetus with lupus-induced heart block. *Obstetrics and Gynecology* **76**:957–959.

49 Bierman FZ, Baxi L, Jaffe I, Driscoll J (1988) Fetal hydrops and congenital complete heart block: Response to maternal steroid therapy. *Journal of Pediatrics* **112**:646–648.

50 Buyon JP, Swersky SH, Fox HE *et al.* (1987) Intrauterine therapy for presumptive fetal myocarditis with acquired heart block due to systemic lupus erythematosus. *Arthritis and Rheumatism* **30**:44–49.

51 Melnick M, Jaskoll T, Slavkin HC (1981) Corticosteroid-induced cleft palate in mice and H-2 haplotype: maternal and embryonic effects. *Immunogenetics* **13**:443–450.

52 Bongiovanni AM, McPadden AJ (1960) Steroids during pregnancy and possible fetal consequences. *Fertility and Sterility* **11**:181–186.

53 Rolbin SH, Levinson G, Shnider SM *et al.* (1978) Anesthetic considerations for myasthenia gravis and pregnancy. *Anesthesia and Analgesia* **57**:441–447.

54 Scott JR (1977) Fetal growth retardation associated with maternal administration of immuno-suppressive drugs. *American Journal of Obstetrics and Gynecology* **128**:668–676.

55 Cote CJ, Meuwissen HJ, Pickering RJ (1974) Effects on the neonatare of prednisone and azathioprine administered to the mother during pregnancy. *Journal of Pediatrics* **85**:324–328.

56 Nylander U (1967) Ocular damage in chloroquine therapy. *Acta Ophthalmologica (Copenhagen)* **45**:5 (suppl. 92), 1–71.

57 Hart C, Naughton RF (1964) The ototoxicity of chloroquine phosphate. *Archives of Otolaryngology* **80**:407–412.

58 Parke A (1988) Antimalarial drugs and pregnancy. *American Journal of Medicine* **85**:30–33.

59 Rumack CM, Guggenheim MA, Rumack BH (1981) Neonatal intracranial haemorrhage and maternal use of aspirin. *Obstetrics and Gynecology* **52**:52S–56S.

60 Moise KJ, Huhta JC, Sharif DS *et al.* (1988) Indomethacin in the treatment of premature labor: Effects of the fetal ductus arteriosus. *New England Journal of Medicine* **319**:327–331.

61 Besinger RE, Niebyl JR, Keyes WG, Johnson TRB (1991) Randomized comparative trial of indomethacin and ritodrine for the long-term treatment of preterm labor. *American Journal of Obstetrics and Gynecology* **164**:981–998.

62 Hickok DE, Hollenbach KA, Reilley SF *et al.* (1989) The association between decreased amniotic fluid volume and treatment with non-steroidal anti-inflammatory agents for preterm labor. *American Journal of Obstetrics and Gynecology* **160**:1525–1531.

63 Vanhaesebrouck P, Thiery M, Leroy JG *et al.* (1988) Oligohydramnios, renal insufficiency, and ileal perforation in preterm infants after intrauterine exposure to indomethacin. *Journal of Pediatrics* **113**:738–743.

64 Druzin ML, Lockshin M, Edersheim TG *et al.* (1987) Second trimester fetal monitoring and preterm delivery in pregnancies with systemic lupus erythematosus and/or circulating anticoagulant. *American Journal of Obstetrics and Gynecology* **157**:1503–1510.

65 Imperiale TF, Petrulis AS (1991) A meta-analysis of low-dose aspirin for the prevention of pregnancy-induced hypertensive disease. *Journal of the American Medical Association* **266**:260–264.

66 Harris EN (1986) Syndrome of the black swan. *British Journal of Rheumatology* **26**:324–326.

67 Harris EN (1990) The second international anti-cardiolipin standardization workshop/The Kingston anti-phospholipid antibody study (KAPS) group. *American Journal of Clinical Pathology* **94**:476–484.

68 Exner T, Sahan N, Trudinger B (1988) Separation of anticardiolipin antibodies from lupus anticoagulant on a phospholipid-coated polystyrene column. *Biochemical and Biophysical Research Communications* **155**:1001–1007.

69 Chamley LW, Pattison NS, McKay EJ (1991) Separation of lupus anticoagulant from anticardiolipin antibodies by ion-exchange and gel filtration chromatography. *Haemostasis* **21**:25–29.

70 Lechner K, Pabinger-Fasching I (1985) Lupus anticoagulants and thrombosis: A study of 25 cases and review of the literature. *Haemostasis* **15**:254–262.

71 Gastineau DA, Kazmier FJ, Nichols WL *et al.* (1985) Lupus anticoagulant: An analysis of the clinical and laboratory features of 219 cases. *American Journal of Hematology* **19**:265–275.

72 Hart RG, Miller VT, Coull BM *et al.* (1987) Cerebral infarctions associated with lupus anticoagulant. *Stroke* **18**:257–263.

73 Glueck HI, Kant KS, Weiss MA *et al.* (1985) Thrombosis in systemic lupus erythematosus: Relation to the presence of circulating anticoagulant. *Archives of Internal Medicine* **145**:1389–1395.

74 Branch DW, Scott JR (1990) Clinical implication of anti-phospholipid antibodies: The Utah experience. In Harris EN, Exner T, Hughes GRV, Asherson RA (eds) *Phospholipid-binding Antibodies*, pp. 335–346. Boca Raton, FL: CRC Press.

75 Kochenour NK, Branch DW, Rote NS, Scott JR (1987)

A new postpartum syndrome associated with antiphospholipid antibodies. *Obstetrics and Gynecology* **69**:460–468.

76 Branch DW, Scott JR, Kochenour NK, Hershgold E (1985) Obstetric complications associated with lupus anticoagulant. *New England Journal of Medicine* **313**:1322–1326.

77 Branch DW, Silver RM, Blackwell JL, Reading JC, Scott JR (1992) Outcome of treated pregnancies in women with antiphospholipid syndrome: An update of the Utah experience. *Obstetrics and Gynecology* **80**(4):614–620.

78 Scott RAH (1987) Anti-cardiolipin antibodies and pre-eclampsia. *British Journal of Obstetrics and Gynaecology* **94**:604–605.

79 Branch DW, Andres R, Digre KB *et al.* (1990) The association of antiphospholipid antibodies with severe pre-eclampsia. *Obstetrics and Gynecology* **73**:541–545.

80 Kant KS, Pollack VE, Weiss MA *et al.* (1981) Glomerular thrombosis in systemic lupus erythematosus: Prevalence and significance. *Medicine* **60**:71–86.

81 Harris EN, Spinnato JA (1991) Should anticardiolipin tests be performed in otherwise healthy pregnant women? *American Journal of Obstetrics and Gynecology* **165**:1272–1277.

82 Lockwood CJ, Romero R, Feinburg RF *et al.* (1989) The prevalence and biologic significance of lupus anticoagulant and anticardiolipin antibodies in a general obstetric population. *American Journal of Obstetrics and Gynecology* **161**:369–373.

83 Petri M, Golbus M, Anderson R *et al.* (1987) Antinuclear antibody, lupus anticoagulant, and anticardiolipin antibody in women with idiopathic habitual abortion: A controlled prospective study of 44 women. *Arthritis and Rheumatism* **30**:601–606.

84 Barbui T, Cortelazzo S, Galli M *et al.* (1988) Antiphospholipid antibodies in early repeated abortions: A case-controlled study. *Fertility and Sterility* **50**:589–592.

85 Parrazzini F, Acaia B, Faden D *et al.* (1991) Antiphospholipid antibodies and recurrent abortion. *Obstetrics and Gynecology* **77**:854–858.

86 Parke AL, Wilson D, Maier D (1991) The prevalence of antiphospholipid antibodies in women with recurrent spontaneous abortion, women with successful pregnancies, and women who have never been pregnant. *Arthritis and Rheumatism* **34**:1231–1235.

87 Out HJ, Bruinse HW, Christiaens GCML *et al.* (1991) Prevalence of antiphospholipid antibodies in patients with fetal loss. *Annals of Rheumatic Diseases* **50**:553–557.

88 Creagh MD, Malia RG, Cooper SM *et al.* (1991) Screening for lupus anticoagulant and anticardiolipin antibodies in women with fetal loss. *Journal of Clinical Pathology* **44**:45–47.

89 Haddow JE, Rote NS, Dostal-Johnson D *et al.* (1991) Lack of an association between late fetal death and antiphospholipid antibody measurements in the second trimester. *American Journal of Obstetrics and Gynecology* **165**:1308–1312.

90 Polzin WJ, Kopelman JN, Robinson RD *et al.* (1991) The association of antiphospholipid antibodies with pregnancy complicated by fetal growth restriction. *Obstetrics and Gynecology* **78**:1108–1111.

91 Lubbe WF, Palmer SJ, Butler WS *et al.* (1983) Fetal survival after prednisone suppression of maternal lupus anticoagulant. *Lancet* **1**:1361–1363.

92 Lubbe WF, Liggins GC (1988) Role of lupus anticoagulant and autoimmunity in recurrent pregnancy loss. *Seminars in Reproductive Endocrinology* **6**:181–190.

93 Gatenby PA, Cameron K, Shearman RP (1989) Pregnancy loss with phospholipid antibodies: Improved outcome with aspirin containing treatment. *Australia and New Zealand Journal of Obstetrics and Gynaecology* **29**:294–298.

94 Ordi J, Barquinero J, Vilardelli *et al.* (1989) Fetal loss treatment in patients with antiphospholipid antibodies. *Annals of Rheumatic Diseases* **48**:798–802.

95 Lockshin MD, Druzin ML, Qamar T (1989) Prednisone does not prevent recurrent pregnancy fetal death in women with antiphospholipid antibody. *American Journal of Obstetrics and Gynecology* **160**:439–443.

96 Cowchock FS, Reece EA, Balaban D, Branch DW, Plouffe L (1992) Repeated fetal losses associated with antiphospholipid antibodies: A collaborative randomized trial comparing prednisone with low-dose heparin treatment. *American Journal of Obstetrics and Gynecology* **166**(5):1318–1323.

97 Reece EA, Gabrielli S, Cullen MT *et al.* (1990) Recurrent adverse pregnancy outcome and antiphospholipid antibodies. *American Journal of Obstetrics and Gynecology* **163**:162–169.

98 Rosove MH, Tabsh K, Wasserstrum N *et al.* (1990) Heparin therapy for pregnant women with lupus anticoagulant or anticardiolipin antibodies. *Obstetrics and Gynecology* **75**:630–634.

99 Scott JR, Branch DW, Kochenour NK *et al.* (1988) Intravenous globulin treatment of pregnant patients with recurrent pregnancy loss due to antiphospholipid antibodies and Rh disease. *American Journal of Obstetrics and Gynecology* **159**:1055–1056.

100 Trudinger BH, Stewart GJ, Cook CM *et al.* (1988) Monitoring lupus anticoagulant-positive pregnancies with umbilical artery flow velocity waveforms. *Obstetrics and Gynecology* **72**:215–218.

101 Hench PS (1938) The ameliorating effect of pregnancy on chronic atrophic (infectious) rheumatoid arthritis, fibrositis, and intermittent hydrarthritis. *Proceedings of the Mayo Clinic* **13**:161–167.

102 Oka M (1953) Effect of pregnancy on onset and course of rheumatoid arthritis. *Annals of Rheumatic Diseases* **12**:227–229.

103 Betson JR, Dorn RV (1964) Forty cases of arthritis and pregnancy. *Journal of the International College of Surgeons* **42**:521–526.

104 Oka M, Vainio V (1966) Effect of pregnancy on the prognosis and serology of rheumatoid arthritis. *Acta Rheumatologica Scandinavica* **12**:47–52.

105 Persellin RH (1977) The effect of pregnancy on rheumatoid arthritis. *Bulletin of Rheumatic Diseases* **27**:922–927.

106 Ostensen M, Husby G (1983) A prospective clinical study of the effect of pregnancy on rheumatoid arthritis

and ankylosing spondylitis. *Arthritis and Rheumatism* **26**:1155–1159.

107   Ostensen M (1991) Pregnancy in patients with a history of juvenile rheumatoid arthritis. *Arthritis and Rheumatism* **34**:881–887.

108   Oka M (1958) Activity of rheumatoid arthritis and plasma 17-hydroxycorticosteroids during pregnancy and following parturition. *Acta Rheumatologica Scandinavica* **4**:243–248.

109   Royal College of General Practitioners (1974) *Oral Contraceptives and Health: Interim Report*. London: Pitman.

110   Gilbert M, Rotstein J, Cunningham C (1964) Norethynodrel with mestranol in the treatment of rheumatoid arthritis. *Journal of the American Medical Association* **190**:235.

111   Bijlsma WJ, Huger-Bruning O, Thijssen JHH (1987) Effect of estrogen treatment on clinical and laboratory manifestations of rheumatoid arthritis. *Annals of Rheumatic Diseases* **46**:777–779.

112   Kasukawa R, Ohara M, Yoshida H, Yoshida T (1979) Pregnancy-associated α_2-glycoprotein in rheumatoid arthritis. *International Archives of Allergy and Applied Immunology* **58**:67–74.

113   Sany J, Clot J, Borneau M, Ardary M (1982) Immunomodulating effect of human placenta-eluted gamma globulins in rheumatoid arthritis. *Arthritis and Rheumatism* **25**:17–24.

114   Klippel GL, Cerere FA (1989) Rheumatoid arthritis and pregnancy. *Rheumatic Diseases Clinics of North America* **15**:213–329.

115   Mannik M, Nardella FA (1985) IgG rheumatoid factor and self-association of these antibodies. *Clinics in Rheumatic Diseases* **11**:551–572.

116   Kaplan D (1986) Fetal wastage in patients with rheumatoid arthritis. *Journal of Rheumatology* **13**:875–877.

117   Morris WIC (1969) Pregnancy in rheumatoid arthritis and systemic lupus erythematosus. *Australia and New Zealand Journal of Obstetrics and Gynaecology* **9**:136–144.

118   Ostensen M, Aune B, Husby G (1983) Effect of pregnancy and hormonal changes on the activity of rheumatoid arthritis. *Scandinavian Journal of Rheumatology* **12**:69–72.

119   Silman AJ, Roman E, Beral V, Brown A (1988) Adverse reproductive outcomes in women who subsequently develop rheumatoid arthritis. *Annals of Rheumatic Diseases* **47**:979–981.

120   Newman NM, Correy JF (1983) Possible teratogenicity of sulphasalazine. *Medical Journal of Australia* **1**:528–529.

121   Rocker I, Henderson MJH (1976) Transfer of gold from mother to foetus. *Lancet* **2**:1246.

122   Cohen DL, Orzel J, Taylor A (1981) Infants of mothers receiving gold therapy. *Arthritis and Rheumatism* **24**:104–105.

123   Solomon L, Abrams G, Dinner M, Berman L (1977) Neonatal abnormalities associated with D-penicillamine treatment during pregnancy. *New England Journal of Medicine* **296**:54–55.

124   Cohen S, Johnson AR, Hurd E (1983) Cytotoxicity of sera from patients with scleroderma: Effects on human endothelial cells and fibroblasts in culture. *Arthritis and Rheumatism* **26**:170–178.

125   Black CM (1990) Systemic sclerosis and pregnancy. *Baillière's Clinics in Rheumatology* **4**:105–124.

126   Johnson TR, Banner EA, Winkelmann RK (1964) Scleroderma and pregnancy. *Obstetrics and Gynecology* **23**:467–469.

127   Slate WG, Graham AR (1968) Scleroderma and pregnancy. *American Journal of Obstetrics and Gynecology* **101**:335–341.

128   Weiner RS, Brinkman CR, Paulus HE (1986) Scleroderma, CREST syndrome and pregnancy. *Arthritis and Rheumatism* **29**:51 (suppl.).

129   Giordano M, Valentini G, Lupoli S (1985) Pregnancy and systemic sclerosis. *Arthritis and Rheumatism* **28**:237–238.

130   Silman AJ, Black C (1988) Increased incidence of spontaneous abortion and infertility in women with scleroderma before disease onset: A controlled study. *Annals of Rhenmatic Diseases* **47**:441–444.

131   Steen VD, Conte C, Day N *et al.* (1989) Pregnancy in women with systemic sclerosis. *Arthritis and Rheumatism* **32**:151–157.

132   Steen VD, Medsger TA, Osial TA *et al.* (1984) Factors predicting the development of renal involvement in progressive systemic scleroderma. *American Journal of Medicine* **76**:779–786.

133   Baethge BA, Wolf RE (1989) Successful pregnancy with scleroderma renal disease and pulmonary hypertension in a patient using angiotensin converting enzyme inhibitors. *Annals of Rheumatic Diseases* **48**:776–778.

134   Lindstrom J (1977) An assay for antibodies to human AChR in serum from patients with myasthenia gravis. *Clinics in Immunology and Immunopathology* **7**:36–43.

135   Vernet-der Garbedian B, Eymard B, Bach JF *et al.* (1989) Alpha-bungarotoxin blocking antibodies in neonatal myasthenia gravis: Frequency and selectivity. *Journal of Neuroimmunology* **21**:41–47.

136   Engle AG, Santa T (1971) Histometric analysis of ultrastructure of the neuromuscular junction in myasthenia gravis and in the myasthenic syndrome. *Annals of the New York Academy of Sciences* **183**:46–63.

137   Plauché WC (1991) Myasthenia gravis in mothers and their newborns. *Clinics in Obstetrics and Gynecology* **34**:82–99.

138   Scott JF (1977) Immunologic disease in pregnancy. *Progress in Allergy* **23**:321–366.

139   Plauché WC (1979) Myasthenia gravis in pregnancy: An update. *American Journal of Obstetrics and Gynecology* **135**:691–697.

140   McNall PG, Jafarnia MR (1965) Management of myasthenia gravis in the obstetrical patient. *American Journal of Obstetrics and Gynecology* **92**:518–525.

141   Chambers DC, Hall JE, Boyce J (1967) Myasthenia gravis and pregnancy. *Obstetrics and Gynecology* **29**:597–603.

142   Hay DM (1967) Myasthenia gravis in pregnancy. *British Journal of Obstetrics and Gynaecology* **76**:323–324.

143   Donaldson JO, Penn AS, Lisak RP *et al.* (1981) Anti-acetylcholine receptor antibody in neonatal myasthenia

gravis. *American Journal of Diseases of Children* **135**:222–226.

144 Catanzarite VA, McHargue AM, Sandberg EC *et al.* (1984) Respiratory arrest during therapy for premature labor in a patient with myasthenia gravis. *Obstetrics and Gynecology* **64**:819–822.

145 Shepard MK (1971) Arthrogryposis multiplex congenita in sibs. *Birth Defects* **7**:127.

146 Holmes LB, Driscoll SG, Bradley WG (1979) Multiple contractures in newborn of mother with myasthenia gravis. *Pediatrics Research* **13**:486.

147 Morel E, Erymard B, Vernet-der Garabedian B *et al.* (1988) Neonatal myasthenia gravis: A new clinical and immunological appraisal on 30 cases. *Neurology* **38**:138–142.

148 Brenner T, Beyth Y, Abramsky O (1980) Inhibitory effect of α-fetoprotein on the binding of myasthenia gravis antibody to acetycholine receptor. *Proceedings of the National Academy of Sciences, USA* **77**:3635–3639.

149 Levine, SE, Keesey JC (1986) Successful plasmapheresis for fulminant myasthenia gravis during pregnancy. *Archives of Neurology* **42**:197–198.

150 Plauché WC (1983) Myasthenia gravis. *Clinics in Obstetrics and Gynecology* **26**:592.

28

Renal Disease

TAMEROU ASRAT, MICHAEL P. NAGEOTTE

INTRODUCTION

The renal system undergoes striking alterations during pregnancy. An understanding of these changes is essential if kidney problems occurring in pregnancy are to be detected and managed correctly. This chapter will review

- normal functional alterations of the renal system in pregnancy

- chronic renal disease

- pregnancy with need for dialysis

- renal allograft patients

- acute renal failure during pregnancy.

A discussion of anatomic alterations associated with pregnancy, along with a review of infection-associated diseases of the renal system, can be found in Chapter 30.

CHANGES IN RENAL SYSTEM DURING NORMAL PREGNANCY

Because of methodological difficulties involved in establishing accurate clearance data and a lack of serial studies, the magnitude, timing and duration of the increases in renal plasa flow (RPF) and glomerular filtration rate (GFR) during pregnancy remain controversial. A review of the available data would suggest that GRF and RPF increase by at least 50% during pregnancy, starting soon after conception and lasting until term (as long as measurements are made with the gravida in the lateral recumbent position).[1,2] The increase in GFR lowers serum creatinine and blood urea nitrogen (BUN) levels and is at least partially responsible for the increased excretion of amnio acids, proteins, and several water-soluble vitamins during normal pregnancies. Glucosuria is frequently a normal finding in pregnancy, although it should precipitate diabetic screening. This is thought to result from a marked increase in filtered load with overriding of the renal tubular reabsorption capacity for glucose.[10–12] Selective aminoaciduria develops during pregnancy with losses of certain amnio acids (glycine, histidine, threonine, serine and alanine). This has been suggested to be substantial enough to cause severe maternal malnutrition in less developed countries.[3]

Control of volume homeostasis in pregnancy is also controversial. The best estimates suggest an increase in body water of 7.5 – 9.0l by term. The bulk of this is concentrated in the extracellular compartment distributed between the plasma and interstitium. Plasma volume starts increasing early in the first trimester, accelerates in the second trimester, peaks at around 32 weeks, and stays elevated until term, with an average gain of 1100–1300 ml in singleton gestations. The increase in interstitial fluid makes up the balance of the change in total body water, with most of this increase normally occurring in the third trimester.[4,5]

Management of total body sodium by the renal system is the critical determinant in normal pregnancy volume homeostasis. Pregnancy results in a net sodium gain of 950 mEq, the majority of which is stored in the maternal compartment.[6,7] As GFR increases, the filtered load of sodium increases by 5000–10 000 mmol/day. However, this is accompanied by a parallel increase in tubular reabsorption, sufficient not only to handle the increased filtered load but also to allow an additional 3–5 mmol/day in fetal and maternal stores.[6,7] Plasma sodium concentration is modulated by a poorly understood interplay of factors tending to promote excretion with those favoring reabsorption. The increased GFR and filtered load, the high concentrations of natriuretic hormones (e.g. progesterone, arginine vasopressin and 'natriuretic hormone'), and the increased levels of the vasodilatory prostaglandin, PGE, and PGI_2, augment sodium excretion. However, several antinatriuretic hormones are found in considerably higher concentrations in pregnancy and may serve to blunt the effects of the natriuretic factors. Primarily, they are aldosterone and deoxycorticosterone.[8,9] Others, such as estrogens, prolactin, placental lactogen and growth hormone (ACTH) still have an undefined role.[2,5,10–12] It is unclear if the renin–angiotensin system plays as major a role in volume regulation in gravid women as it does in non-gravid women. There is normally a marked increase in the circulating level of renin and angiotensin II during pregnancy, although most of the renin is in inactive form.[13,14] The trigger mechanism for the increased renin–angiotensin system activity is unknown. Despite these changes, renal handling of acute salt water loads in pregnancy is normal. Most pregnant women respond to salt restriction by increasing renin and aldosterone secretion. However, severe sodium restriction may result in marked natriuresis and weight loss, despite the elevated renin and aldosterone levels.[13]

Pregnancy is associated with a net gain of approximately 350 mEq of potassium, which is primarily incorporated in the growing fetus. Kaliuresis does not occur despite marked increases in the concentration of potent mineralocorticoids in pregnancy.[15] This is attributed to progesterone blocking the mineralocorticoid activity at the level of the renal tubules. Consequently, certain potassium-wasting states, such as Bartter's syndrome and primary hyperaldosteronism, may improve during pregnancy.

During pregnancy, there is a true decrease in plasma osmolality by an average of 8–10 mOsm/kg. This results largely from the relative decrease in plasma concentration of sodium and associated anions. Unlike in non-pregnant subjects, this decreased body fluid tonicity does not cause a vasopressin-mediated water

diuresis, thus suggesting a resetting of the osmotic threshold for both vasopressin secretion and thirst.[7]

CHRONIC RENAL INSUFFICIENCY

Maternal/Fetal Risks (General)

Chronic renal disease is often clinically 'silent' until in advanced stage. The diagnosis is based on decreased creatinine clearance, increased 24-h urine protein excretions, and abnormal microscopic examinations of the urine sediment with red blood cells (RBCs) and RBC casts. One should not rely upon the serum creatinine or BUN, since little change in the serum creatinine or BUN is seen until the creatinine clearance falls below 50 ml/min. There are numerous causes for chronic renal insufficiency, including systemic lupus erythromatosus, diabetic nephropathy, polycystic renal disease, periarteritis nodosa, scleroderma, reflux nephropathy, and acute and chronic glomerulonephritis.

The majority view holds that, with the exception of certain specific disease entities such as systemic lupus erythromatosus (SLE), renal polyarteritis nodosa and scleroderma, obstetric outcome is usually successful provided renal function is at most moderately compromised and hypertension is minimal or absent. Furthermore, pregnancy does not appear to affect adversely the natural history of the renal disease.[16] There are three entities about which controversy exists. Some investigators believe that pregnancy affects adversely the course of IgA nephropathy, membranoproliferative glomerulonephritis and reflux nephropathy.

Maternal risks associated with renal insufficiency are invariably linked to the degree of renal compromise. Fertility is diminished as renal function deteriorates. When preconception serum creatinine and BUN levels are over 3 mg/dl and 30 mg/dl, respectively, pregnancy is rare. Pre-existing hypertension may worsen, particularly in patients with moderate (serum creatinine 1.4–2.5 mg/dl) and severe (serum creatinine > 2.5 mg/dl) disease.[16] Overall, renal function deterioration may also accelerate in those with moderate to severe renal insufficiency.[17,18]

Proteinuria may increase in as many as 50% of pregnancies complicated by renal insufficiency, sometimes reaching amounts exceeding 3 g in 24 h. Nephrotic edema may be a result of this excessive oncotic loss.[16,29] A significantly higher incidence of superimposed pre-eclampsia has also been reported, occurring in 25–30% of these patients.[16] Differentiating this latter condition from an isolated increase in baseline proteinuria can at times be difficult.

Preterm delivery has been associated with 25–50% of pregnancies in renal insufficiency patients.[16,18–20] Most of these early deliveries are due to worsening maternal or fetal complications necessiatating intervention, and not spontaneous preterm labor. The incidence of pyelonephritis is increased in some series. Anemia of chronic disease is usually aggravated by pregnancy; therefore, blood transfusion may be needed.

Fetal risks are less well defined, and are usually a reflection of maternal compromise. Prematurity is increased, as suggested above. Perinatal mortality and intrauterine growth deficiency rates are higher, as is the fetal loss rate.

Maternal/Fetal Risks (Specific)

Lupus nephritis

Primarily SLE occurs in women of child-bearing age.[21] The early literature on lupus during pregnancy variably suggested that there was a tendency to improvement, deterioration, or no change in the clinical status of these patients. In addition, early authors observed a higher incidence of relapse in the postpartum period. However, recent reports challenge these concepts.[22,23] The majority of pregnancies of women with SLE succeed, particularly when the patient has been in complete clinical remission for at least 6 months prior to conception. Prognosis is enhanced if renal function is normal and hypertension is absent.[22,24] Patients with evidence of disease activity before pregnancy have a higher pregnancy loss rate and experience more exacerbations or progression of disease.[21] Overall, two-thirds of patients with SLE have no change in their clinical status during pregnancy. Since suppression of disease activity improves the obstetrical outcome, appropriate therapy with steroids or cytotoxic drugs should not be withheld for the pregnant SLE patient.

Other connective tissue diseases

In contrast to SLE, in patients with periarteritis nodosa and systemic scleroderma, both of which have a high degree of renal involvement, the outcome of pregnancy is very poor, resulting in a high perinatal and maternal mortality. These appear to be caused by hypertensive complications.

Diabetic nephropathy

The majority of long-standing insulin-dependent diabetics who become pregnant most likely have microvascular and subclinical renal disease.[25] The patients do not appear to have deterioration of renal function during pregnancy and most show the normal adjustments in renal function. They do have an increased incidence of urinary tract infections during pregnancy. Further, superimposed pre-eclampsia often occurs, frequently resulting in a need to effect delivery prematurely.[26]

Polycystic kidney disease

Most women with this disease are in their fourth decade and have completed their child-bearing. Pregnant patients with polycystic kidney disease usually have an uneventful course, except for a slightly higher incidence of pre-eclampsia and severe pyelonephritis. Genetic counseling of the patient and her family is critical, since this disease is an autosomal dominant syndrome that often progresses to end-stage renal disease, requiring dialysis or transplantation. DNA probe techniques are now being developed so that early prenatal diagnosis will become available, allowing selective pregnancy termination of the affected fetus.[26]

Management Options

Prepregnancy

Ideally, pregnancy is probably best restricted to women whose preconception serum creatinine levels are less than 2 mg/dl and diastolic blood pressure is 90 mmHg or less. Some extend this arbitary limit of serum creatinine to 2.5 mg/dl, whereas others believe it should be no higher than 1.5 mg/dl.[16,20,27] Risks as outlined above should be discussed with the prospective parents.

Prenatal

Patients should be seen at 2–4 week intervals until 32 weeks gestation. After this, antepartum assessments should most likely be weekly, although these decisions can be individualized to the patient's condition. Careful monitoring of blood pressure for early detection of hypertension is critical. Uncontrolled hypertension is an extremely important factor in the assessment of overall maternal deterioration.[20,28,29] Similarly, early screening for superimposed pre-eclampsia should be instituted. Some have suggested the prophylactic use of low-dose aspirin, beginning at the end of the first trimester, to decrease the incidence of superimposed pre-eclampisa.[30] Routine serial prenatal assessments of renal function, with 24 h creatinine clearance and protein excretion assays, should be done on a monthly basis. Early screening for asymptomatic bacteriuria should also be part of the antepartum evaluation.

Frequent fetal assessments should be included in the monitoring of the gravida with renal insufficiency. Early on, this would be accomplished with the ultrasonographic evaluation of the fetus for structural abnormalities and growth deficiency. Later, starting at around 26–28 weeks gestation, antepartum fetal heart rate monitoring should be incorporated into the management scheme.

If renal function deteriorates, one should look for reversible causes, such as urinary tract infection, dehydration or electrolyte imbalances. Near term, a 15–20% decrement in renal function (which may be reflected in a small rise in serum creatinine) is permissible. Failure to detect a reversible cause for a significant decrease in renal function is reason for hospitalization, and probably delivery. However, increasing proteinuria, in the face of preserved renal function and absent hypertension, is not necessarily an indication to end the pregnancy.

Control of hypertension is important in these patients. Methyldopa, clonidine, beta-blockers and calcium channel blockers can be used with careful monitoring of these agents. Angiotensin-converting enzymes are contraindicated in pregnancy, since they have been associated with fetal deformity syndrome, neonatal renal failure, intrauterine growth restriction and a significant reduction in placental blood flow.[31] Salt restriction and diuretic therapy do not appear to be beneficial. For massive debilitating edema, some investigators have advocated the concomitant use of colloids and diuretics, with careful and frequent monitoring of electrolytes. Delivery is indicated when there is uncontrollable hypertension, superimposed pre-eclampsia, decreased renal function or abnormal antepartum fetal testing.[32]

Renal biopsy is rarely indicated, particularly after 34 weeks gestation. The most likely clinical dilemma necessitating renal biopsy in a pregnant woman would be the development of unexplained severe nephrotic syndrome and severe hypertension between 22 and 32 weeks.[33] Recent reports indicate that in the absence of a coagulopathy, the morbidity from a renal biopsy

---

CHRONIC RENAL INSUFFICIENCY
Summary of Management Options

Prepregnancy

- Careful advice about undertaking pregnancy when serious compromise of renal function (? serum creatinine >2 mg/dl and diastolic BP >90 mmHg)

Prenatal

- Frequent monitoring of:
  - blood pressure
  - renal function
  - bacteriuria
  - fetal growth and health

- Strict control of hypertension

- Consider low-dose aspirin

- Consider hospital admission if renal function deteriorates

- Renal biopsy only very rarely indicated (? unexplained nephrotic syndrome and hypertension between viability and 32 weeks)

Labor/delivery

- Indications for delivery (similar to pre-eclampsia):
  - uncontrollable hypertension
  - deteriorating renal function
  - superimposed pre-eclampsia with either:
    — mature gestation
    — imminent eclampsia
    — liver involvement
    — DIC
    — acute fetal compromise

- Control blood pressure perinatally

Postnatal

- Control blood pressure

- Re-establish maintenance therapy

should be no greater than that observed in non-pregnant patients.[34]

Labor/delivery and postnatal

Labor and delivery issues are routine for the gravida with renal insufficiency, provided that pre-eclampsia or hypertension have not complicated the picture. There are no contradictions to epidural anesthesia, although care should be taken to avoid rapid shifts in blood pressure or blood volume. Obstetrical decisions should dictate the route of delivery. Postpartum care centers on blood pressure control, avoiding hypotension via excessive blood loss, and re-establishing maintenance drug therapy.

CHRONIC DIALYSIS PATIENTS AND PREGNANCY

Maternal/Fetal Risks

Patients on chronic hemodialysis can have successful pregnancies.[35–41] Recently, isolated reports have appeared of women on chronic ambulatory peritoneal dialysis becoming pregnant.[40] It is difficult to establish the true incidence of unsuccessful pregnancies in women on dialysis, since it is unlikely that most clinicians will publish pregnancy failures or disasters. There is a high surgical abortion rate in these patients, indicating that those who become pregnant do so accidentally, probably because they are unaware that pregnancy is a possibility. For this reason, women on dialysis should use appropriate contraception if they wish to avoid pregnancy.

The previously outlined maternal and fetal risks for chronic renal insufficiency patients also apply to these patients. Specific risks to the mother include anemia, fluid imbalances, electrolyte difficulties, dietary restrictions and hydramnios. These patients are usually severely anemic. This is aggravated further by pregnancy. They may therefore require blood transfusions, especially before delivery.

Risks to the fetus include a high incidence of pregnancy wastage, preterm labor and delivery, intrauterine growth deficiency and sudden intrauterine death.

Management Options

Prepregnancy

There are substantial arguments against pregnancy in the patient undergoing dialysis and these should be pointed out and discussed prior to conception. There is,

at best, only a 20% likelihood of successful outcome. It may be advisable for the patient to attempt pregnancy after transplantation.[36,40,42]

Prenatal

As is the case for chronic renal insufficiency patients, a successful outcome of pregnancy depends on scrupulous control of blood pressure. In addition, meticulous attention should be paid to fluid balance, increased frequency of dialysis and provision of good nutrition.[38,42]

The aim of dialysis in these patients should be to maintain the BUN < 80 mg/dl, though some would argue < 60 mg/dl. Intrauterine fetal death is more common if the BUN is > 80 mg/dl. The following technical issues should be stressed:

- Hypotension should be avoided during dialysis.[41]

- The dialysis should be performed in the lateral recumbent position and in the late third trimester continuous fetal monitoring should be employed.[41]

- Rigid control of blood pressure is mandatory. Avoid sudden fluid shifts and limit volume changes, since these can result in hypotension and consequent fetal distress.[43]

Preterm births occur more frequently in dialysis patients. Progesterone is removed during dialysis, increasing the likelihood of preterm contractions and one group of investigators has advocated parenteral progesterone during dialysis.[41,44] Special attention must be paid to electrolyte balance, particularly hypercalcemia and hyperkalemia. Pregnant patients are in a state of chronic compensated respiratory alkalosis and large drops in serum bicarbonate should be prevented. Dialysates containing glucose and bicarbonate are preferred, and those containing citrates should be avoided. Interdialysis weight gain should be limited to about 0.5–1.0 kg until late pregnancy. This means a 50% increase in hours and frequency of dialysis.[36,41] Hydramnios appears to be a frequent complication of women undergoing hemodialysis, although the pathophysiologic mechanisms have yet to be clearly elucidated.[32,45]

A continuous ambulatory peritoneal dialysis (CAPD) has been successfully used in pregnancies.[40,46] The advantages of CAPD over hemodialysis include a more constant chemical and extracelluar environment for the fetus, higher hematocrit levels, infrequent episodes of hemodialysis and no heparin requirements. For diabetic patients, intraperitoneal insulin may facilitate the management of their blood glucose. Magnesium sulfate given intraperitoneally may reduce the

CHRONIC HEMODIALYSIS
Summary of Management Options

Prepregnancy

- Careful counseling about risks
  (? advise against conception until
  successfully transplanted)

Prenatal

- Careful attention to fluid balance

- Increased frequency of dialysis

- Ensure good nutrition

- Offer screening for hepatitis and HIV

- Frequent monitoring of:
  - blood pressure
  - renal function
  - electrolyte balance
  - bacteriuria
  - hemoglobin
  - fetal growth and health

- Strict control of hypertension

- Repeated blood transfusions may
  be necessary

- Consider low-dose aspirin

- During dialysis:
  - avoid hypotension
  - fetal monitoring after 26–28 weeks
  - control blood pressure
  - avoid sudden fluid shifts

Labor/delivery

- Indications for delivery are similar to
  those for chronic renal failure

- Control blood pressure

Postnatal

- Review frequency of dialysis

---

likelihood of preterm labor.[39] These patients, however, are at risk of developing peritonitis, which accounts for the majority of therapy failures.

Chronic anemia is often a difficult problem in dialysis patients. Transfusions with packed RBCs are often needed. These patients should be screened for hepatitis B and C as well as human immunodeficiency virus (HIV). The goal is to keep the hematocrit above 25%. In non-pregnant chronic renal failure patients, synthetic erythropoietin (EPO) has been used successfully, thus reducing the need for transfusions. The safety and efficacy of EPO use in pregnancy, however, has not been established.

Free dietary intake should be discouraged despite more frequent dialysis. A daily oral intake of 70 g protein, 1500 mg of calcium, 50 mmol potassium and 80 mmol sodium is advised with supplements of dialyzable vitamins.[36,41]

Blood pressure tends to be labile and hypertension is a common problem. Hypertension can be controlled to some extent by dialysis. If not satisfactory, antihypertensive treatment should be instituted rapidly. There

is a significant risk of developing superimposed pre-eclampsia and recently low-dose aspirin therapy has been advised in such patients to decrease the risk of developing superimposed pre-eclampsia.

Labor/delivery and postnatal

Fetal surveillance is similar to the scheme outlined for chronic renal failure patients. Cesarean delivery should be done only for obstetrical indications. Dialysis should be continued as needed during the postpartum period.

RENAL TRANSPLANT PATIENTS AND PREGNANCY

Maternal/Fetal Risks

Pregnancy following renal transplantation has become increasingly common. About 1:50 women of child-bearing age with a functioning renal transplant becomes pregnant. Of the conceptions, 40% do not go beyond the initial trimester because of spontaneous or therapeutic abortions. Of the remaining 60% that continue beyond the first trimester, 90% will end successfully.[47,48]

Patients should be aware of the higher risk for ectopic pregnancy because of pelvic adhesions from previous urologic surgery, peritoneal dialysis or pelvic inflammatory disease. The incidence is reported at 0.5% of all conceptions. Significant renal function impairment occurs in about 15% of patients, and this may persist after delivery.[47,49] Serious rejection episodes occur in 9% of pregnant women. This incidence of rejection is no greater than that expected for non-pregnant patients.[47]

Pre-eclampsia is diagnosed clinically in approximately 30% of pregnancies. There is a higher incidence of cesarean delivery, due to the occurrence of pelvic osteodystrophy secondary to previous renal failure and dialysis or prolonged steroid therapy.[50] Premature labor and delivery complicate 40–50% of pregnancies.

Fetal risks include a high incidence of first trimester fetal wastage,[47] prematurity,[47,49] intrauterine growth retardation,[51] and rarely adrenocortical insufficiency in the newborn.[52] Chromosomal aberrations in lymphocytes, due to azathioprine therapy, usually clears within 20–32 months after birth. There is some animal data to suggest that *in utero* exposure to azathioprine may affect the fertility of female offsprings. However, the long-term effects of immunosuppressive therapy remain largely uninvestigated.[53]

Management Options

Prepregnancy

Extensive counseling regarding the risks of pregnancy should be undertaken in all patients with renal transplants contemplating pregnancy. Many previously anovulatory patients begin ovulating postoperatively and regain fertility as renal function normalizes.[54] Consequently, as in the case of women on dialysis, many transplant recipients fail to realize they are pregnant until well into the second trimester. This finding underscores the need for effective contraception counseling and implementation in these patients.

Individual centers have their own specific guidelines that must be met prior to proceeding with pregnancy. In general, the following guidelines are advised.[47,49]

- Whenever possible, patients with allografts should wait at least 2 years after transplantation before becoming pregnant. This time period allows the

patient to recover from surgery, graft rejection will have stabilized and immunosuppression will be at maintenance levels. Usually, if function is well maintained at 24 months, there is a high probability of allograft survival at 5 years.[47]

- Good general health for about 2 years since transplantation.

- No or minimal proteinuria.

- Absence of hypertension.

- No graft rejection.

- Absence of pelvicalyceal dilatation on a recent IVP.

- Stable renal function with plasma cretinine of 2 mg/dl or less.

- Drug therapy reduced to maintenance levels: prednisone 15 mg/day or less, azathioprine 2 mg/kg body weight or less, cyclosporin A 10 mg/kg body weight or less.[54]

Prenatal

Patients should be monitored as high-risk pregnancies. Prenatal visits should be every 2 weeks until 32 weeks, and weekly thereafter. Serial ultrasound measurements are needed to assess fetal growth. Antepartum fetal surveillance should begin at 26–28 weeks gestation. Monthly, the following laboratory studies should be performed: full blood count, BUN, creatinine, electrolytes, 24 h creatinine clearance and protein excretion, midstream urine culture and sensitivity, liver function tests, plasma protein, calcium and phosphates.

Immunosuppressive therapy is usually maintained at prepregnancy levels but adjustments may be needed if maternal leucocyte or platelet counts decrease. The most sensitive method of monitoring azathioprine dosage and bioavailability is by measuring red blood cell 6-thioguanine nucleotides (6-TGN). Azathioprine liver toxicity has been noted occasionally during pregnancy and responds to dose reduction.

Renal allograft rejection may be difficult to diagnose since pregnant patients do not always exhibit the clinical hallmarks of rejection – fever, oliguria, tenderness, decreasing renal function. Occasionally, rejection may mimic pyelonephritis, pre-eclampsia or cyclosporin nephrotoxicity. Renal biopsy may be indicated before aggressive antirejection therapy is begun.

Labor/delivery

During labor, aseptic techniques, fluid balance monitoring, cardiovascular status assessment and temperature evaluations are mandatory. Augmentation of steroids is necessary to cover delivery and the postpartum period. Vaginal delivery should be the aim in these patients. However, allograft recipients have an increased incidence of cephalopelvic disproportion from pelvic osteodystrophy. The transplanted kidney,

---

RENAL TRANSPLANT
Summary of Management Options

Prepregnancy

- Ensure adequate contraception until evidence of successful transplant (? 2 years)

- Avoid combined oral contraceptives and possibly IUD

- Guidelines for suitability for pregnancy are given in text

Prenatal

- Increased frequency of hospital attendance

- Frequent monitoring of:
  - blood pressure
  - renal function
  - bacteriuria
  - liver function
  - hemoglobin, white cell and platelet counts
  - fetal growth and health

- Maintain immunosuppressive therapy at prepregnancy levels; consider reduction if signs of marrow suppression

- Consider renal biopsy if rejection suspected and before aggressive antirejection therapy commenced

Labor/delivery

- Steroid augmentation

- Cesarean section more likely (pelvic osteodystrophy) though transplanted kidney rarely obstructs vaginal delivery

Postnatal

- Avoid combined oral contraceptives and possibly IUD

- Data concerning breast-feeding and immunosuppressive drugs is lacking

however, rarely obstructs vaginal delivery despite its pelvic location.

Postnatal

Rejection has been known to occur during the puerperium when maternal immune competence returns to its prepregnancy level. There are very few data available about azathioprine and cyclosporine A and their metabolites in breast milk. Until the many uncertainties are resolved, breast-feeding is not recommended.

Even though the present consensus is that pregnancy has no effect on graft rejection or survival, parents need to be informed that 10% of mothers with renal allografts die within 1–7 years following the birth of one or more children.[55] More studies are needed to answer the long-term prognosis of these patients, particularly in light of the newer immunosuppressive drugs that are currently available.

Oral contraceptives may cause or aggravate hypertension or thromboembolism and can produce subtle changes in the immune system. The intrauterine device (IUD) is associated with an increased incidence of pelvic infections, which makes its use problematic in immunosuppressed patients. The efficacy of the IUD may be reduced by immunosuppressive and anti-inflammatory agents, possibly because of modification of the leucocyte response.[56]

ACUTE RENAL FAILURE IN PREGNANCY

Maternal/Fetal Risks (General)

Acute renal failure is an unusual complication of pregnancy, occurring in about 1:10000 pregnancies in Western societies.[57,58] In contrast to this situation, in developing nations, the incidence of acute renal failure in pregnancy remains high, with excessively high mortality rates surpassing 50%.[59] In the 1950s and 1960s, as many as 22% of all cases of acute renal failure were obstetric in origin, with mortality rates up to 48%.[57] Since that time, there has been a dramatic decrease in the incidence as well as the mortality of acute renal failure in pregnancy. This marked improvement in incidence and survival appears to be due both to the significant decrease in septic abortions and more successful early intervention in the management of complicated pregnancies.

Acute renal failure is characterized by a sudden decrease in renal function accompanied by rapidly worsening azotemia and often, but not always, oliguria. There is no uniform definition of what constitutes a rapid rise in creatinine and urea nitrogen, or the definition of oliguria. Generally speaking, increments in serum creatinine of at least 0.5 mg/dl, in urea nitrogen of 10 mg/dl or a reduction in urine output below 400 ml/24 h, are considered diagnostic of acute renal failure. Several subsets of acute renal failure in pregnancy exist (**Table 1**). First, there are the many causes of acute renal failure that occur without a relation to pregnancy but are simultaneous occurrences. A second group of patients are those with underlying chronic renal disease that worsens during pregnancy, suggesting the development of acute renal failure superimposed on their chronic diseases, such as chronic glomerular diseases, lupus nephritis, diabetic nephropathy and the chronic interstitial nephritides. Finally, there are those causes of acute renal failure unique to pregnancy which include pre-eclampsia/eclampsia, the HELLP syndrome, acute fatty liver of pregnancy and also postpartum renal failure. Traditionally, acute renal failure has been subcategorized into 'prerenal' (hypoperfusion, volume depletion states), intraparenchymal or intrinsic renal disorders, and 'post-renal' (obstructive).

When renal failure occurs during the first two trimesters, the urinalysis plays a central role in helping the clinician initiate his evaluation. During the third trim-

Table 1
Causes of acute obstetric renal failure

1. Volume contraction, hypoperfusion ('prerenal')
    Antepartum hemorrhage due to placenta previa
    Postpartum hemorrhage
    Miscarriage
    Hyperemesis gravidarum
    Adrecortical failure; usually due to inadequate steroid coverage for delivery in patients on long-term therapy

2. Volume contraction, hypotension and coagulopathy
    Abruptio placenta
    Pre-eclampsia/eclampsia
    Amniotic fluid embolism
    Incompatible blood transfusion
    Drug reaction
    Acute fatty liver of pregnancy
    Hemolytic uremic syndrome

3. Volume contraction, hypotension and coagulopathy
    Septic abortion
    Chorioamnionitis
    Pyelonephritis
    Puerperal sepsis

4. Urinary tract obstruction
    Hydramnios
    Damage to ureters
    Pelvic hematoma
    Broad ligament hematoma
    Calculus or clot in ureters

ester and postpartum period, the clinical presentation along with evaluation of liver functions, peripheral smear and coagulation factors are important in the initial evaluation (see Management section).

The maternal risks are dependent on, and specific to, the underlying disorder causing the acute renal failure. In general, sudden renal failure predisposes the mother to acid/base and electrolyte disturbances; volume overload problems, dehydration; a propensity to develop infection; premature labor and delivery; and coagulopathies. Fetal risks include prematurity, and rapid dehydration in the neonate due to increased levels of urea and other solutes within the fetal circulation that precipitate an osmotic diuresis shortly after birth.

Maternal/Fetal Risks (Specific)

Renal failure in septic abortion (see also Chapter 7)

Where liberalized abortion laws exist, the incidence of septic abortions and acute renal failure (ARF) have decreased dramatically. Septic abortions, especially those infected with *Escherichia coli* and *Clostridia*, present with a striking clinical syndrome. The onset may be sudden, from several hours to 2 days after attempted abortions. There is an abrupt rise in temperature (40°C or above) and the presence of myalgia, vomiting and diarrhea is common.

Once signs and symptoms develop, the patients usually progress to hypotension, dyspnea and frank shock rapidly. The patient is usually jaundiced and has a peculiar bronze color ascribed to the association of jaundice with cutaneous vasodilatation, cyanosis and pallor. Despite fever, the extremities are often cold and purplish areas, the precursors of small patches of necrosis on the toes, fingers or nose, may be present. Characteristic laboratory findings include severe anemia as a result of hemolysis, elevated direct bilirubin levels, striking leucocytosis (25 000/mm^3), thrombocytopenia and other evidence of disseminated intravascular coagulation. Severe oliguria is usually present and the urinalysis demonstrates proteinuria, hemoglobin and red blood cells casts in the sediment. Death occurs only hours after the attempted abortion in about 7% of patients, but in most fever and symptoms usually respond to aggressive antibiotic treatment and volume replacement, leaving a patient who requires management of her renal failure.

The etiology of ARF with septic abortion may have multiple causes, including volume depletion from vomiting and diarrhea, hemoglobinuria which is nephrotoxic, or the agents used to provoke the abortion which may also be nephrotoxic. The organism responsible for the septic shock, *Clostridia*, may produce a specific nephrotoxin which leads to renal failure.

The clinical course of the renal failure is usually that of acute tubular necrosis, although bilateral or patchy cortical necrosis may occur, which may result in permanent, irreversible renal failure. Although the vast majority of these patients respond readily to high-dose antibiotic treatment and evacuation of the contents of the uterus, some advocate rapid removal of the uterus, believing the uterus to be a huge culture medium for bacterial growth and continued toxin production.[60,61]

Renal failure in pre-eclampsia/eclampsia (see also Chapters 18 and 73)

Pre-eclampsia is accompanied by a number of renal changes. 'Glomerular endotheliosis' is the histologic description of the most characteristic renal lesion associated with pre-eclampsia. The glomerulus in these patients appears swollen and distorted. In addition, there is generalized vasoconstriction leading to renal ischemia, proteinuria and a reduction in glomerular filtration. In view of the aforementioned changes, it is not surprising that on occasion pre-eclampsia will lead to frank acute renal failure. This acute renal failure accompanying pre-eclampsia is usually caused by tubular necrosis; however, pre-eclampsia/eclampsia has been known to progress to cortical necrosis.[59,62]

In pre-eclamptic patients, the intravascular volume is severely decreased due to marked vasoconstriction and hemoconcentration. These patients are very susceptible to fluid shifts and to the adverse renal effects of diuretic therapy, salt restriction, antepartum and or intrapartum blood loss than are normal gravidas. However, recent studies have shown that oliguria in pre-eclamptic patients does not necessarily reflect hypovolemia. Additionally, urinary diagnostic incidences do not appear to reliably reflect the intravascular volume status. In oliguric pre-eclamptic patients, an important pathophysiological mechanism appears to be selective vasoconstriction of the renal vascular bed, and aggressive fluid challenges may lead to volume overload and pulmonary edema. Invasive hemodynamic monitoring will provide valuable information regarding the volume status and allow the clinician to tailor the management individually.[63] In general, expectant conservative management, while keeping the patient 'fluid restricted', is all that is needed for resolution of the oliguria. In the presence of prolonged oliguria, and in the face of normal pulmonary capillary wedge pressure, the clinician may consider treating the patient with agents known selectively to improve renal perfusion.[64,65]

Renal failure and acute fatty liver of pregnancy (see also Chapter 25)

Acute renal failure is associated with almost all cases of acute fatty liver of pregnancy.[66–69] Typically, these patients present with persistent nausea and vomiting in late pregnancy associated with varying degrees of liver failure. Jaundice, encephalopathy, disseminated intravascular coagulopathy, renal failure and death may all be seen in this condition. The incidence is believed to be less than 1:13 000 deliveries. The cause for renal failure is unknown and is often of the acute tubular necrosis type.

Acute fatty liver of pregnancy is believed to be one of the microangiopathic hemolytic diseases of pregnancy, which include severe pre-eclampsia, the HELLP (hemolysis, elevated liver enzymes, low platelets) syndrome, and idiopathic postpartum renal failure. An abnormal ratio of prostacyclin to thromboxan A_2 has been postulated as one of the pathophysiologic mechanisms of this disease.

Idiopathic postpartum renal failure

Idiopathic postpartum renal failure, first described in 1968, is characterized by the onset of renal failure, usually in the puerperium after an uneventful pregnancy. It may occur as early as the first trimester and up to 2 months postpartum.[62,70,71] It has even been reported following an ectopic pregnancy.[72] Typically, the patients present with oliguria, or at times, anuria, rapidly progressive azotemia and frequently microangiopathic hemolytic anemia and consumption coagulopathy. Blood pressure may be normal or elevated, although severe accelerated hypertension has been reported.[73,74]

The etiology for this disease is obscure and suggestions include a viral illness, retained placental fragments or drugs such as ergotamine compounds, oxytocic agents or oral contraceptives. Several patients have demonstrated hypocomplementemia, suggesting an immunologic cause. Deficiencies in prostacyclins have also been implicated as an etiology of this disease.[62,70–75] The renal lesions seen in this entity resemble those seen in hemolytic uremic syndrome and arteriolar lesions reminiscent of malignant nephrosclerosis or scleroderma.[70,75]

The prognosis for this disease is guarded with a mortality rate of 60–70%.[73] Most women have either succumbed, required chronic dialysis or have survived with severely reduced renal functions with only a few having recovered completely. Treatment consists of a reduction of high blood pressure if present and general supportive measures as for all patients with acute renal failure. Some investigators have used anticoagulant therapy with heparin, antiplatelet therapy, infusion of blood products, or exchange transfusions and plasmapheresis with no proof of efficacy in general.[76–79] Several patients have received kidney allografts and most have done well after transplantation.

Renal cortical necrosis (see also Chapter 9)

Renal cortical necrosis is a morphologic diagnosis characterized by tissue death throughout the cortex with sparing of the medullary portions of the kidney.[59,80] This is quite an uncommon finding, but when it occurs it is more likely to be associated with pregnant patients. Cortical necrosis is seen more commonly in older multigravidas (over 30 years of age) and tends to be associated most frequently with placental abruption and occurs in the third trimester or the puerperium. It is also less commonly associated with prolonged intrauterine death. When cortical necrosis occurs in association with pre-eclampsia/eclampsia, it is secondary to placental abruption and hemorrhage leading to sustained severe renal ischemia.[81] Although cortical necrosis may involve the entire renal cortex, resulting in irreversible renal failure, it is the incomplete or 'patchy' variety that occurs more often in pregnancy.

The diagnosis of renal cortical necrosis should be suspected when the oliguria or even anuria lasts considerably longer than that of uncomplicated acute tubular necrosis. The definitive diagnosis is based on renal biopsy and/or selective angiography. Arteriography reveals the absence of a cortical nephrogram in complete necrosis and a heterogeneous appearance in the 'patchy' variety. Cortical calcification is a late sign appearing 6 weeks or later after the onset of the disease.[80] It is not known why pregnant women are more susceptible to cortical necrosis than their non-gravid counterparts. Some investigators attribute the pathogenesis to severe and prolonged 'selective' renal vasospasm, which may be followed by local activation of coagulation, while others attribute a primary role to the coagulopathies.

Management Options

In the first two trimesters of pregnancy, the management greatly depends on the urinalysis. If the urinalysis shows proteinuria, hematuria, RBC casts and the patient is hypertensive, the diagnosis is that of underlying renal disease or acute glomerulonephritis. The patient's hypertension should be treated and consideration given to renal biopsy. If the urinalysis is normal, however, the urinary sodium level is low, the patient has prerenal azotemia due to volume loss, commonly through vomiting and diarrhea. The treatment consists of aggressive parenteral fluid replacement and management of the underlying cause. Granular casts seen in the urine sediment, along with hypotension, fever, chills and vaginal bleeding, signify septic abortion. This usually results in acute tubular necrosis and rarely in cortical necrosis. The patient needs hemodynamic support, antibiotics and possibly dialysis. Pyuria, fever, and positive urine culture indicate acute pyelonephritis. The patient should be hospitalized for parenteral antibiotics and fluid replacement. Pyuria and hematuria, along with a skin rash, fever and recent change in medication, may indicate acute interstitial nephritis which is frequently caused by administration of any of a number of medications, particularly non-steroidal anti-inflammatory drugs and a variety of antibiotics. The treatment consists of cessation of drug therapy and consideration of steroid therapy.

When the urinalysis is normal, or shows hematuria, an obstructive process should be suspected. Uterine incarceration, hydramnios or nephrolithiasis may all lead to obstruction. It is distinctly unusual for uterine compression of the ureters to result in renal failure, although this has been reported. The patient should be evaluated for the underlying cause and treated appropriately.

When acute renal failure occurs in the third trimester and in the puerperium, the clinician should look for disease states specific to pregnancy as outlined previously: pre-eclampsia/eclampsia, the HELLP syndrome, acute fatty liver of pregnancy, and postpartum renal failure. Obstetric catastrophe, such as abruptio placenta, intrauterine fetal demise and amniotic fluid embolism, will also lead to acute tubular necrosis and cortical necrosis.

Clinically, patients with reversible acute renal failure first experience a period of oliguria of variable duration. Polyuria then occurs. In this polyuric phase, serum creatinine and BUN may continue to rise and during the recovery phase urine output returns to normal. In the polyuric phase, patients are prone to electrolyte imbalances and electrolytes should be checked frequently and any abnormalities treated.

The main goal of treatment is the elimination of the underlying cause. Invasive hemodynamic monitoring is useful and lessens the need for clinical guesswork, especially in the polyuric phase. Early in the course of the disease, the urine to plasma osmolality ratio and the fractional excretion of sodium should be determined to distinguish between prerenal azotemia and acute tubular necrosis. Central hyperalimentation may also be required if renal failure is prolonged. Acidosis occurs

---

ACUTE RENAL FAILURE
Summary of Management Options

Determine cause (See Table 1)

- Clinical features

- Urinalysis

- Blood pressure

- Temperature

- Urine culture

- Renal function

- Liver function

- Coagulation status

- ? Renal biopsy

Treat/eliminate cause

- Fluid/blood replacement for hypovolemia

- Control hypertension

- 'Empty uterus' with septic abortion and many late pregnancy causes

- Antibiotics for infective causes

- Surgery for obstructive causes

Supportive therapy

- Antibiotics

- Attention to fluid and electrolyte balance

- Consider hyperalimentation if prolonged disease

- Dialysis in severe cases

- Monitor fetal growth and health

- Delivery when reasonable chances of survival

frequently in cases of acute renal failure; therefore, arterial blood gases should be monitored frequently and acidosis treated promptly to prevent hyperkalemia, which develops rapidly and may be fatal. Absolute restriction of potassium intake should be instituted immediately. Since urea, creatinine and probably other metabolites that accumulate in uremia cross the placenta, dialysis should be undertaken early and 'prophylactically' in pregnant women. The aim of treatment is to keep the urea nitrogen levels at or below 30 mg/dl. Peritoneal dialysis and hemodialysis have both been used in patients with obstetric renal failure with equal success.

Fetal surveillance should be instituted immediately and delivery effected as soon as the mother's condition has stabilized and the fetus is near maturity or at a weight that carries a high probability of survival.

Prognosis for survival is significantly better in obstetric ARF patients than in patients with surgical or medical causes of ARF. Maternal mortality has declined markedly over the last two decades. The remote prognosis for these patients also seems to suggest a normal renal as well as reproductive function.[82,83]

REFERENCES

1 Davison JM, Dunlop W (1980) Renal hemodynamics and tubular function in normal human pregnancy. *Kidney International* **13**:152.

2 Lindheimer MD, Katz AL (1981) The renal response to pregnancy. In Brenner BM, Rector FC (eds) *The Kidney*, 2nd edn, p. 1762. Philadelphia, PA: W.B. Saunders.

3 Dure-Smith P (1970) Pregnancy dilatation of the urinary tract: The iliac sign and its significance. *Radiology* **96**:545.

4 Barron WM, Lindheimer MD (1985) Renal function and volume homeostasis during pregnancy. In Gleicher N (ed.) *Principles of Medical Therapy in Pregnancy*, pp. 779–790. New York: Plenum Press.

5 Hytten FE (1981) Weight gain in pregnancy. In Hytten F, Chamberlain G (eds) *Clinical Physiology in Obstetrics*, pp. 193–233. New York: Blackwell.

6 Chesley LC (1972) Plasma and red cell volumes during pregnancy. *American Journal of Obstetrics and Gynecology* **112**:440.

7 Lindheimer MD, Barron WM, Durr J *et al.* (1987) Water homeostasis and vasopressin release during rodent and human gestation. *American Journal of Kidney Disease* **9**:270.

8 Kass E (1956) Asymptomatic infections of the urinary tract. *Transactions of the Association of American Physicians* **60**:56.

9 Savage W, Hajj S, Kass E (167) Demographic and prognostic characteristics and bacteriuria in pregnancy. *Medicine (Baltimore)* **46**:385.

10 Hytten FE (1973) The renal excretion of nutrients in pregnancy. *Postgraduate Medical Journal* **49**:625.

11 Dunlop W, Davison JM (1977) The effect of pregnancy on the renal handling of uric acid. *British Journal of Obstetrics and Gynaecology* **83**:13.

12 Davison JM, Hytten FE (1975) The effect of pregnancy on the renal handling of glucose. *British Journal of Obstetrics and Gynaecology* **82**:374.

13 Kunin C (1970) The natural history of recurrent bacteriuria in schoolgirls. *New England Journal of Medicine* **282**:1443.

14 Whalley P (1967) Bacteriuria of pregnancy. *American Journal of Obstetrics and Gynecology* **97**:723.

15 Campbell-Brown M, McFadyen IR, Seal DV *et al.* (1987) Is screening for bacteriuria in pregnancy worthwhile? *British Medical Journal* **294**:1579.

16 Katz AI, Davison JM, Hayslett JP *et al.* (1980) Pregnancy in women with kidney disease. *Kidney International* **28**:192.

17 Bear R (1976) Pregnancy in patients with renal disease: A study of 44 cases. *Obstetrics and Gynecology* **48**:13.

18 Hou S, Grossman S, Madias N (1985) Pregnancy in women with renal disease and moderate renal insufficiency. *American Journal of Medicine* **78**:185.

19 Packham DK, North RA, Fairley KF *et al.* (1989) Primary glomerulonephritis and pregnancy. *Quarterly Journal of Medicine* **71**:537.

20 Surian M, Imbasciati E, Banfi G *et al.* (1984) Glomerular disease and pregnancy. *Nephron* **36**:101.

21 Mor-Yosef S, Navot D, Rabinowitz R *et al.* (1982) Collagen disease in pregnancy. *Obstetrical and Gynecological Survey* **39**:67.

22 Hayslett JP, Lynn RI (1980) Effect of pregnancy in patients with lupus nephropathy. *Kidney International* **18**:207.

23 Lockshin MD, Reintiz E, Durzin NL *et al.* (1984) Lupus pregnancy: Case control prospective study demonstrating absence of lupus exacerbations during or after pregnancy. *American Journal of Medicine* **77**:893.

24 Jungers P, Dougados M, Pelissies C *et al.* (1982) Lupus nephropathy and pregnancy. *Archives of Internal Medicine* **142**:771.

25 Hayslett JP, Reece EA (1987) Managing diabetic patients with nephropathy and other vascular complications. *Clinics in Obstetrics and Gynecology* **1**:939.

26 Kitzmiller JL, Brown ER, Phillippe M *et al.* (1981) Diabetic nephropathy and perinatal outcome. *American Journal of Obstetrics and Gynecology* **141**:741.

27 Kincaid-Smith P, Whitworth JA, Fairley KF (1980) Mesangial IgA nephropathy in pregnancy. *Clinics of Experimental Hypertension* **2**:821.

28 Hou SH, Grossman SD, Madias NE (1985) Pregnancy in women with renal disease and moderate renal insufficiency. *American Journal of Medicine* **78**:185.

29 Jungers P, Forget D, Henry-Amar M *et al.* (1986) Chronic kidney disease and pregnancy. *Advances in Nephrology* **15**:103.

30 Benigni A, Gregorini G, Frusca T *et al.* (1989) Effect of low dose aspirin or fetal and maternal generation of thromboxane by platelets in women at risk for pregnancy induced hypertension. *New England Journal of Medicine* **321**:357.

31 Broughton-Pipkin F, Turber SR, Symonds EM (1980) Possible risk with catopril in pregnancy. *Lancet* **1**:1256.

32 Thacker SB, Berkelman RL (1986) Assessing the diag-

nostic accuracy and efficacy of selected antepartum fetal surveillance techniques. *Obstetrical and Gynecological Survey* **41**:121.

33 Lindheimer MD, Davison JM (1987) Renal biopsy during pregnancy: 'To b--- or not to b---?' *British Journal of Obstetrics and Gynaecology* **94**:932.

34 Lindheimer M, Fisher K, Spargo B, Katz A (1988) Hypertension in pregnancy: A biopsy study with long term follow-up. *Contributions to Nephrology* **25**:71.

35 Ackrill P, Goodwin F, Marsh F *et al.* (1975) Successful pregnancy in patients on regular dialysis. *British Medical Journal* **2**:172.

36 Kobayashi H, Matsumoto Y, Otsubo O *et al.* (1981) Successful pregnancy in a patient undergoing chronic hemodialysis. *Obstetrics and Gynecology* **57**:382.

37 Savdie E, Caterson R, Mahony J, Clifton-Bligh P (1983) Successful pregnancies in women treated by haemodialysis. *Medical Journal of Australia* **2**:9.

38 Cohen D, Frenkel Y, Maschiach S, Eliahou HE (1988) Dialysis during pregnancy in advanced chronic renal failure patients: Outcome and progression. *Clinics in Nephrology* **29**:144.

39 Redrow M, Cherem L, Elliott J *et al.* (1988) Dialysis in the management of pregnancy patients with renal insufficiency. *Medicine* **67**:199.

40 Hou S (1987) Pregnancy in women requiring dialysis for renal failure. *American Journal of Kidney Disease* **9**:368.

41 Yasin SY, Doun SWB (1988) Hemodialysis in pregnancy. *Obstetrical and Gynecological Survey* **43**:655.

42 Challah S, Wing AW, Broyer M *et al.* (1986) Successful pregnancy in women on regular dialysis treatment and women with a functioning transplant. In Andreucci VF (ed.) *The Kidney in Pregnancy.* Boston, MA: Martinus Nijhoff.

43 Rodriguez S, Leikin S, Hiller M (1964) Neonatal thrombocytopenia associated with ante-partum administration of thiazide drugs. *New England Journal of Medicine* **270**:881.

44 Johnson TR, Korenz RP, Merron KMJ *et al.* (1979) Successful outcome of a pregnancy requiring dialysis. *Journal of Reproductive Medicine* **22**:217.

45 Nageotte MP, Grundy HO (1988) Pregnancy outcome in women requiring chronic hemodialysis. *Obstetrics and Gynecology* **72**:456.

46 Kioko M, Shaw KM, Clarke AD *et al.* (1983) Successful pregnancy in a diabetic patient treated with chronic ambulatory peritoneal dialysis. *Diabetes Care* **6**:298.

47 Davison JM (1987) Renal transplantation in pregnancy. *American Journal of Kidney Disease* **9**:374.

48 Davison J, Lind T, Uldall P (1976) Planned pregnancy in a renal transplant recipient. *British Journal of Obstetrics and Gynaecology* **83**:518.

49 Davison JM, Lindheimer MD (1984) Pregnancy in women with renal allografts. *Seminars in Nephrology* **4**:240.

50 Huffer W, Kuzela D, Popovtzer M (1975) Metabolic bone disease in chronic renal failure. II. Renal transplant patients. *American Journal of Pathology* **78**:385.

51 Scott J (1977) Fetal growth retardation associated with maternal administration of immunosuppressive drugs.

American Journal of Obstetrics and Gynecology* **128**:668.

52 Penn I, Makowski E, Harris P (1980) Parenthood following renal transplantation. *Kidney International* **18**:221.

53 Price H, Salaman J, Laurence K, Langmaid H (1976) Immunosuppressive drugs and the fetus. *Transplantation* **21**:294.

54 Merkatz I, Schwartz G, David D *et al.* (1971) Resumption of female reproductive function following renal transplantation. *Journal of the American Medical Association* **216**:1749.

55 Whetam JCG, Cardelle C, Harding M (1983) Effect of pregnancy on graft function and graft survival in renal cadaver transplant recipients. *American Journal of Obstetrics and Gynecology* **145**:193.

56 Murray S, Hickey J, Houang E (1987) Significant bacteremia associated with replacement of intrauterine contraceptive device. *American Journal of Obstetrics and Gynecology* **156**:698.

57 Beaman M, Turney JH, Rodger RSC *et al.* (1987) Changing pattern of acute renal failure. *Quarterly Journal of Medicine* **231**:15.

58 Lindheimer MD, Katz AI, Ganeval D *et al.* (1983) Acute renal failure in pregnancy. In Brenner BM, Lazarus JM (eds) *Acute Renal Failure*, pp. 510–526. Philadelphia, PA: W.B. Saunders.

59 Chugh KS, Singhal PC, Sharma BK *et al.* (1976) Acute renal failure of obstetric origin. *Obstetrics and Gynecology* **48**:642.

60 Bartlett RH, Yahia C (1969) Management of septic abortion with renal failure: Report of five consecutive cases with five survivors. *New England Journal of Medicine* **281**:747.

61 Hawkins OF, Sevitt LH, Fairbrother DF *et al.* (1975) Management of chemical septic abortion with renal failure: Use of a conservative regimen. *New England Journal of Medicine* **292**:722.

62 Grunfeld JP, Ganeval D, Vournerias F (1980) Acute renal failure in pregnancy. *Kidney International* **18**:179.

63 Lee W, Gonik B, Cotton DB (1987) Urinary diagnostic indices in preeclampsia associated oliguria: Correlation with invasive hemodynamic monitoring. *American Journal of Obstetrics and Gynecology* **156**:100.

64 Gerstner G, Grunberger W (1980) Dopamine treatment for prevention of renal failure in patients with severe preeclampsia. *Clinical and Experimental Obstetrics and Gynecology* **7**:217.

65 Huss R, Hancock KW, Cope GF, Lee MR (1983) Urine dopamine during normotensive and hypertensive pregnancies and the puerperium. *Clinical and Experimental Hypertensive* **2**:317.

66 Burroughs AK, Seong NGH, Dojunov DA *et al.* (1982) Idiopathic acute fatty liver of pregnancy in 12 patients. *Quarterly Journal of Medicine* **204**:481.

67 Davies MH, Wilkinson SP, Hanid MA *et al.* (1980) Acute liver disease with encephalopathy and renal failure in late pregnancy and the early puerperium: A study of 14 patients. *British Journal of Obstetrics and Gynaecology* **87**:1005.

68 Riely CA, Latham PS, Romero R *et al.* (1987) Acute fatty liver of pregnancy: A reassessment based on obser-

vations in nine patients. *Annals of Internal Medicine* **106**:703.

69 Pockros PH, Peters RL, Reynolds TB (1984) Idiopathic fatty liver of pregnancy: Findings in ten cases. *Medicine* **63**:1.

70 Hayslett JP (1985) Postpartum renal failure. *New England Journal of Medicine* **312**:1556.

71 Lazebnik N, Jaffa AJ, Peyeser MR (1985) Hemolytic-uremic syndrome in pregnancy: Review of the literature and report of cases. *Obstetrical and Gynecological Survey* **40**:618.

72 Creasey GW, Morgan J (1987) Hemolytic uremic syndrome after ectopic pregnancy: postectopic nephrosclerosis. *Obstetrics and Gynecology* **69**:448.

73 Segonds A, Louradour N, Suc J, Orfila C (1979) Postpartum hemolytic uremic syndrome: As study of three cases with a review of the literature. *Clinics in Nephrology* **12**:229.

74 Wagoner R, Holley K, Johnson W (1968) Accelerated nephrosclerosis and postpartum acute renal failure in normotensive patients. *Annals of Internal Medicine* **69**:237.

75 Webster J, Rees A, Lewis P, Hensby C (1980) Prostacyclin deficiency in haemolytic uraemic syndrome. *British Medical Journal* **281**:271.

76 Conte F, Mewroni M, Battini G *et al.* (1988) Plasma exchange in acute renal failure due to postpartum hemolytic-uremic syndrome: Report of a case. *Nephron* **50**:167.

77 Remuzzi G, Misiani R, Marchesi D *et al.* (1979) Treatment of hemolytic uremic syndrome with plasma. *Clinics in Nephrology* **12**:279.

78 Poesmans, W, Eeckels R (1974) Has heparin changed the prognosis of the hemolytic-uremic syndrome? *Clinics in Nephrology* **2**:169.

79 Vitacco N, Avalos JS, Gianantonio CA (1973) Heparin therapy in the hemolytic-uremic syndrome. *Journal of Pediatrics* **83**:271.

80 Kleinknecht D, Grunfeld J-P, Gorney PC *et al.* (1973) Diagnostic procedures and long-term prognosis in bilateral renal cortical necrosis. *Kidney International* **4**:390.

81 Stratt P, Canavese C, Colla L *et al.* (1987) Acute renal failure in preeclampsia-eclampsia. *Gynecological and Obstetrical Investigations* **24**:225.

82 Turney JH, Ellis CM, Parsons FM (1989) Obstetric acute renal failure 1956–1987. *British Journal of Obstetrics and Gynaecology* **96**:679.

83 Sibai BM, Villar MA, Mabie BC (1990) Acute renal failure in hypertensive disorders of pregnancy: Pregnancy outcome and remote prognosis in thirty-one consecutive cases. *American Journal of Obstetrics and Gynecology* **162**:777.

29

Viral Diseases

JOSEPH G. PASTOREK II

INTRODUCTION

The reader is advised to consult Chapter 49 for additional fetal considerations of viral diseases in pregnancy.

RUBEOLA (MEASLES)

Maternal/Fetal Risks

Rubeola, also called red measles or first disease, is a highly infectious, acute febrile illness caused by a paramyxovirus that commonly attacks children. The viral syndrome, arising after an incubation period of 10–14 days after respiratory droplet inoculation, includes high fever, rash, cough and rhinorrhea, conjunctivitis, and pathognomonic Koplik's spots on the oral buccal epithelium. In a child, the infection is usually self-limiting, resolving over several days.[1] Immunity to natural infection is lifelong; therefore, the high infectivity of the virus during the childhood years leaves few adults susceptible to the disease. It is the adult, however, who suffers more severe illness when affected. In particular, pneumonia and encephalitis are uncommon but severe complications of measles infection. Pneumonia, especially secondary bacterial infection after a primary measles bronchitis/pneumonitis, is the primary cause of death. Also, the older patient often exhibits hepatitis due to measles infection, sometimes with clinical jaundice.[2] Besides acute measles encephalomyelitis, a chronic disease entity, subacute sclerosing panence-

phalitis, is also associated with measles viral antigen and particles in brain tissue.

Since effective vaccine was introduced in 1963, cases of measles in the USA have decreased markedly. However, due primarily to laxity in the vaccination of children, a sudden recent increase in the annual rate of infection has occurred in the USA (**Figure 1**). In 1990, there were nearly 28 000 cases, over a 50% increase over the previous year. Almost half of these cases occurred in children under 5 years of age, and over 80% of patients had not been vaccinated. The deaths of 89 patients were reported, 81 of whom were unvaccinated. Overall, 21.1% of patients required hospitalization, and the 22.7% complication rate included

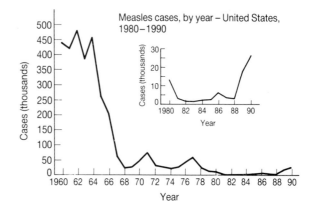

Figure 1. Rubeola (measles) cases: USA, 1960–1990 (from Centers for Disease Control[3]).

diarrhea in 9.4%, otitis media in 6.6%, pneumonia in 6.5% and encephalitis in 0.1%.[3]

Analysis of the distribution of rubeola cases, at least in the USA, indicates that outbreaks of measles are focal in nature. That is, the majority of counties reported no cases of the disease in the most recent decade. Those areas reporting measles outbreaks had higher populations, higher population densities and higher percentages of minority citizens. Also, the higher rates occurred in areas with larger numbers of unvaccinated preschool children in the population.[4]

Measles during pregnancy is not generally associated with increased maternal or fetal death rates,[5] although placental damage from the infection has been implicated in stillbirths,[6] and infection of mothers in developing countries has been associated with an increase in perinatal mortality.[7] As with any febrile illness, though, measles infection in the mother may incite premature uterine activity, leading to premature delivery and its effect upon the neonate. Also, there is no specific syndrome described with intrauterine rubeola infection, as there is with rubella. However, the neonate delivered of a gravida with active disease may develop severe neonatal measles, with pneumonia being the primary cause of mortality. (The outcome is more severe in the case of the premature infant, compared with the term baby.)

Diagnosis

The clinical diagnosis of rubeola is not difficult. Although the rash is not unlike that of other childhood exanthematous diseases, the photophobia and upper respiratory symptomatology are fairly characteristic as a syndrome. However, there are serologic tests which will identify the viral etiology of a measles infection. In particular, hemagglutination inhibition antibody may be measured at the onset of the rash and is positive practically for life; compliment fixation antibody rises somewhat later but becomes undetectable after a decade or so (**Figure 2**).[8]

Management Options

Prepregnancy

Measles, like most viral illnesses, is best treated by prevention. One dose of live measles virus vaccine should be given to all children after 15 months of age on a routine basis; this should result in long-lasting immunity in over 95% of recipients. If a patient anticipating pregnancy has a negative (or questionable) history of measles or proper vaccination, or if she has laboratory evidence of susceptibility, she should receive a dose of live, attenuated virus vaccine if there

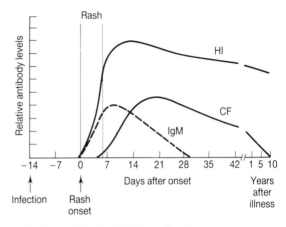

HI – Hemagglutination inhibition antibody
CG – Complement fixation antibody

Figure 2. Immune response to an acute rubeola infection (from Centers for Disease Control[8]). HI, Hemagglutination inhibition antibody; CF, complement fixation antibody.

are no contraindications, followed by a booster dose not less than 1 month later. Patients who received killed virus vaccine prior to 1967, or who were vaccinated earlier than 1 year of age, should also receive two doses of vaccine. In cases of an acute local epidemic of measles, vaccine should be effective even if given within 72 h *after* exposure to the disease.[9]

Prenatal

Acute measles infection is treated symptomatically. The upper respiratory discomfort may be ameliorated somewhat with cough suppressants and other such remedies. Fever, especially if high, is treated aggressively with acetominophen in the gravida. Measles pneumonia when it occurs is addressed as well with respiratory support. Superimposed bacterial pneumonia, which accounts for the major portion of mortality, is treated with antibiotics selected for the appropriate antimicrobial spectrum, depending upon available cultures and local bacterial sensitivity patterns. Even when there is no life-threatening disease in the pregnant patient, however, she should be closely monitored in the acute phases of the illness for signs of uterine contractions. These can be handled in the usual fashion (e.g. magnesium sulfate, beta-adrenergic agents) until systemic illness has subsided.

Pregnant women are not candidates for vaccination with any live virus vaccine, although accidental vaccination of a gravida with rubeola vaccine is not a cause for alarm, certainly not for pregnancy termination. However, immune serum globulin (ISG) may be given to a susceptible pregnant woman exposed to rubeola in an attempt to prevent or modify the clinical expression of the disease (theoretically preventing the severe complications and any resultant premature uterine activity).[10] The intramuscular preparation is given at a dose of 0.25 ml/kg (maximum dose of 15 ml) within 6 days after exposure.[11]

Labor/delivery and postnatal

There are no specific management recommendations for these intervals, since acute disease is unlikely to occur. Clinicians, however, should be aware of appropriate isolation precautions instituted for rubeola in hospital.

MEASLES (RUBEOLA)
Summary of Management Options

Prepregnancy

- Prevention by childhood vaccination

- Serological evaluation and, if negative, vaccination of woman enquiring about status prepregnancy

Prenatal

- Treat acute infection symptomatically

- Antibiotics if secondary bacterial infection suspected

- Vigilance for uterine activity

- Immunoglobulin should be considered for the susceptible woman exposed to the infection

Labor/delivery and postnatal

- Appropriate isolation precautions when in hospital

RUBELLA

Maternal/Fetal Risks

Rubella, also called German measles, three-day measles and third disease, is an exanthematous disease caused by a single-stranded RNA virus of the togavirus family. Like rubeola, rubella is acquired via respiratory droplet exposure and manifest after a 2–3 week incubation period. Unlike red measles, however, German measles is only modestly contagious, leaving many children uninfected after epidemic outbreaks.

Patients becoming ill develop a rash which spreads from the face to the trunk and extremities, lasting about 3 days. Fever, arthralgias, and postauricular and suboccipital lymphadenopathy are characteristic. Rubella infection, both in adults and children, is usually a mild illness; rare but severe complications include encephalitis, bleeding diathesis, and arthritis. Besides the fact that the maculopapular rash resembles that caused by other viruses, overt clinical symptoms occur in only 50–75% of rubella-infected patients, thus invalidating clinical history as a useful method of documenting prior illness.[12]

If rubella produces only mild or subclinical illness in the (pregnant) woman, infection in the fetus is a different story. Congenital rubella syndrome, first described by an Australian ophthalmologist in 1941,[13] is the prototypical embryopathic infection. For over 50 years now, rubella infection *in utero* has been known to produce transient abnormalities, including purpura, splenomegaly, jaundice, meningoencephalitis and thrombocytopenia; structural and permanent anomalies, including congenital cataracts, glaucoma, heart disease, deafness, microcephaly and mental retardation; and late findings, such as diabetes, thyroid abnormalities, precocious puberty and progressive rubella panencephalitis.[14,15]

Rubella vaccine became available in the USA in 1969. Since vaccination produces long-term immunity in 95% of vaccinees, the rates of rubella dropped precipitously after the introduction of the vaccine. By the 1980s, annual counts of rubella infections, including congenital rubella syndrome, had decreased to a mere fraction of prevaccine numbers. However, much the same as with rubeola, rates started rising again in the late 1980s, though not to the high levels reported in the 1960s (**Figure 3**). The largest increases occurred in persons over 15 years or under 1 year of age. Outbreaks were primarily associated with settings where unvaccinated adults were allowed to congregate, e.g. colleges, prisons and in isolated religious communities with poor vaccine coverage (e.g. the Amish communities in three northeastern states). During 1990, ten infants with confirmed congenital rubella syndrome were reported (with six other US cases pending investigation and verification, along with three imported

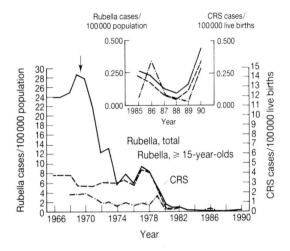

Figure 3. Rubella cases: USA, 1966–1990 (from Centers for Disease Control[16]).

cases), compared with only three confirmed cases during the two previous years combined.[16]

Diagnosis

Clinical diagnosis of rubella infection is extremely difficult, since a large portion of the infection is subclinical, and the rash is not particularly specific (if present at all). Therefore, serologic testing is the primary mode of diagnosis. In a patient with exposure or a suspect illness, seroconversion demonstrated with paired acute and convalescent specimens is indicative of acute infection. Serologic testing for immunity, as is performed routinely in pregnant women, is based upon the assumption that rubella-specific antibodies of the IgG class are present for life after natural infection or vaccination. The hemagglutination inhibition test has traditionally been used to demonstrate immunity, though latex agglutination, fluorescent immunoassay and enzyme immunoassay techniques have been developed in recent years to supplant the older method. In any case, all pregnant women should be surveyed to document seropositivity, whatever the test employed by the local laboratory.

Management Options

Prepregnancy

Widespread vaccination of children and susceptible adults will prevent outbreaks of rubella, thus reducing the possibility of congenital rubella infection. It is recommended that all children receive a single dose of live, attenuated rubella vaccine, usually given at age 15 months, in a trivalent preparation of measles, mumps and rubella strains. Vaccination is recommended for adults who are found to be susceptible by serologic testing, or who do not have documentation of vaccination after their first birthday. In particular, susceptible women receiving health care, including family planning, postpartal care, premarital screening, or hospitalization for any reason, should be vaccinated as long as they are not pregnant and refrain from becoming pregnant for 3 months. Evidence of immunity should be required of applicants for work in places where women of child-bearing age are gathered (including health care facilities) or students seeking admission to colleges/universities.[17] After vaccination, antibody to rubella virus should be detectable for up to 16 years, according to ongoing studies.[18] It should be noted, however, that individuals with low levels of antibody after vaccination may be susceptible to viremia and clinical infection.[19] Indeed, there has been a report of congenital rubella syndrome after previous maternal rubella vaccination.[20]

Prenatal

Documentation of rubella infection in the pregnant woman prompts little concern for her welfare, since infection is usually mild. The fetus, however, is at risk for congenital damage from intrauterine infection. Various methods of *in utero* diagnosis have been attempted, including chorion villus sampling and fetal blood sampling for measurement of fetal levels of rubella-specific IgM.[21] However, documentation of fetal serologic status gives no specific indication of fetal damage, nor does it allow any fetal treatment (other than abortion). Clearly, prevention of maternal infection is the best therapy.

Rubella vaccine is a live virus preparation and should not be administered to pregnant women for theoretical reasons. The Centers for Disease Control monitored inadvertent rubella vaccination during pregnancy, collecting over 500 cases between 1971 and 1989. No case of congenital rubella syndrome was documented due to vaccine virus, even though virus was isolated from the conceptus in several cases. For this reason, patients accidentally vaccinated during pregnancy, or those becoming pregnant shortly after vaccine administration, should be reassured and counseled that the risk of fetal effects is negligible.[22]

PARVOVIRUS B19

Maternal/Fetal Risks

Human parvovirus B19 (HPV B19) is a DNA virus of the family Parvoviridae and the etiologic agent of a

RUBELLA
Summary of Management Options

Prepregnancy

- Prevention by childhood vaccination

- Vaccination programs for girls in their early teens contribute to prevention

- Assess serologic status and offer vaccination in susceptible women:
  - who enquire prepregnancy
  - who are receiving infertility treatment

Prenatal

- Routine check of rubella immunity status at first visit for all women is standard practice in many centers

- Accidental vaccination in early pregnancy is not an indication for termination

- If suspected exposure in woman with 'immunity':
  - confirm presence of rubella specific IgG (if immediately after exposure)
  - confirm failure of appearance of IgM (acute phase) antibodies with two serum samples 2–3 weeks apart
  - reassure

- If suspected exposure in susceptible woman:
  - establish validity of diagnosis serologically in index case if possible
  - check for appearance of IgM (acute phase) antibodies
  - if no serologic evidence of infection, reassure patient
  - if maternal infection confirmed serologically, options will depend on gestation at time of infection:
    - in early pregnancy, termination should be discussed; either immediately or only after confirmation by invasive procedure (see Chapter 49)
    - in late pregnancy, confirmation of fetal infection by invasive procedure can be considered; fetal growth and health should be monitored if infection suspected or confirmed

Labor/delivery and postnatal

- If fetal infection suspected, cord blood should be sent for serologic confirmation

- If fetal infection confirmed, careful pediatric assessment and follow-up

number of human illnesses. The virus was only serendipitously isolated in the mid-1970s during hepatitis B testing of patient sera.[23] However, information relevant to clinical disease caused by HPV B19 has only been seriously accumulated within the past decade or so. Since 1981, the virus has been found to be causative of aplastic crisis in patients with sickle cell disease[24] and other hemolytic states,[25] chronic bone marrow fail-ure in patients with immunodeficiency,[26] a form of chronic arthropathy[27] and the childhood illness erythema infectiosum.[28]

Fifth disease, or erythema infectiosum, a febrile, exanthematous illness of childhood which is characterized by high fever and a peculiar rash which leaves a 'slapped cheek' appearance, is moderately infectious, with an incubation period of 4–14 days. Transmitted by respiratory droplets, the virus causes mild illness in children, who may not even manifest the rash. The rash, when present, is not always clinically distinguishable from rashes of the other childhood exanthems. Infection in adults is often somewhat more serious, with adenopathy and mild arthritis as common complications. Adults may also suffer fatigue and depression for several weeks after the acute infection. Generally, the illness may be confused with various types of measles, scarlet fever and enterovirus infections.[25]

Fifth disease is of special import to the obstetrician, since transplacental infection of the fetus is associated in some cases with non-immune hydrops fetalis.[29,30] It is felt that the parvovirus, having a particular affinity for rapidly dividing erythrocytes in the host,[31] causes a sudden hemolytic anemia in the infected fetus, resulting in cardiac failure, edema and possibly death (conceptually similar to the effect of Rhesus isoimmunization). This influence is apparently limited to the bone marrow, as there have not been any specific teratogenic changes attributed to fetal infection with HPV B19, and 1 year follow-up of children documented to have been infected *in utero* has been normal.[32]

Erythema infectiosum is distributed worldwide and most commonly encountered in children younger than 14 years. The illness is less infectious than measles or chickenpox, though surveys indicate that 60% of adults have serologic evidence prior infection.[33] Transmission of virus to the fetus during maternal infection occurs in approximately one-third of cases.[32] However, HPV B19 related pregnancy losses occur very rarely when gravidas are infected, especially if appropriate care is given to the infant before and after delivery.[32,34]

Diagnosis

The clinical syndrome of fever and characteristic rash makes recognition of the classic case of fifth disease fairly direct. However, the variability of the symptomatology, especially in adults, confounds the clinical diagnosis. Laboratory demonstration of seroconversion using paired acute and convalescent sera, or the demonstration of IgM antibodies specific for HPV B19, are indicative of acute infection. IgM antibodies develop in 90% or more of infected patients within 1 week after the onset of symptoms, lasting up to 4 months. IgG antibodies are detectable within 7–10 days and last for years, probably indicating lifelong immunity.[35]

Management Options

Prepregnancy

There is no specific treatment for acute HPV B19 infection, and therefore supportive and symptomatic care are in order. In the immunocompetent host with a normal hematopoietic system, clinical illness is of minor consequence. The patient at risk for sudden hemolysis must be appropriately monitored and transfused as necessary. Immunoincompetent patients may need prolonged support, due to protracted illness. There are no absolute recommendations when a person can safely become pregnant after acute infection, although empirically one should wait until the clinical symptoms have resolved and an appropriate antibody response is demonstrable.

Prenatal

The pregnant patient with acute HPV B19 infection is supported and treated symptomatically. However, in view of the possibility of non-immune hydrops fetalis in infected fetuses, serial ultrasonographic examinations are indicated to detect evidence of fetal decompensation, e.g. ascites, pericardial effusion.[30,32,34] If fetal jeopardy is detected, the fetus may be delivered, if gestational age permits, for appropriate extrauterine therapy. Otherwise, fetal anemia may be corrected by intrauterine transfusion with fair confidence of success.[36,37] It must be noted, however, that fetal hydrops has recently been shown to resolve spontaneously in some cases.[38,39] Thus, the obstetrician must carefully

---

PARVOVIRUS B19
Summary of Management Options

Prepregnancy

- If diagnosis confirmed before pregnancy, pregnancy should be avoided until clinical cure and antibody response

Prenatal

- If infection is diagnosed:
  - symptomatic treatment of patient
  - screen serially for fetal hydrops

- If hydrops develops, consider fetal blood transfusion (see Chapter 45)

weigh the risks of the available forms of intervention against the condition and prognosis of the fetus.

Labor/delivery and postnatal

There are no specific management recommendations for these intervals.

VARICELLA

Maternal/Fetal Risks

Varicella-zoster virus (VZV) is a DNA virus of the herpes family which produces two distinct clinical syndromes. In temperate climates, VZV is responsible for the childhood exanthematous disease commonly known as chickenpox. Clinical chickenpox develops 10–20 days after respiratory exposure and consists of fever, malaise, and a pruritic rash which develops initially as crops of maculopapules which rapidly vesiculate and finally crust over. Lesion usually begin on the face and scalp, spreading to the trunk as the disease progresses; patients are contagious from 48 h before the onset of the rash until all of the ruptured vesicles have crusted over. Chickenpox in children is a highly infectious but mild infection which causes few sequelae other than occasional skin scars, or pock marks. Primary VZV infection in adults, however, is occasionally more severe, leading to such complications as pneumonia, encephalitis, myocarditis, pericarditis, bacterial superinfection of skin lesions, and adrenal insufficiency.[40]

Like many DNA viruses, VZV has the ability to remain dormant in the host for an indefinite time, surfacing in times of physiologic, hormonal or immunologic stress or insufficiency. It peculiarly recurs as a patch of painful and pruritic vesicles, on a erythematous base, characteristically distributed along the course of a cutaneous nerve in a dermatomal pattern. This manifestation of VZV infection is known as zoster,[41] or shingles in common parlance. There are usually no remarkable systemic symptoms from an outbreak of shingles, although serious disability may occur if the particular nerve affected happens to correspond to a delicate or vulnerable tissue, e.g. the cornea of the eye. Rarely, however, visceral involvement, including hepatitis, pneumonitis, myocarditis, pericarditis and colonic lesions, is reported; these complications are far and away more highly associated with patients who are suffering significant immunosuppression.[42]

The pregnant woman represents at least a mildly immunocompromised patient and, as such, is more susceptible to severe illness from primary VZV infection. Pulmonary complications occur in roughly 10% of gravidas during a bout of chickenpox and represent a major cause of mortality in these circumstances. Respiratory symptoms occur within 1 week of the skin lesions, accompanied by cough, tachypnea, dyspnea and chest pain. In such disseminated cases, oral lesions are more common, fever may be higher than usual, and auscultatory and radiographic findings referable to the lungs are often present. These symptoms may gradually abate over 7 days, while respiratory insufficiency, pneumothorax, bacterial superinfection (as with rubeola) and pulmonary parenchymal fibrosis are the most probable causes of death.[42,43]

In the pregnant woman VZV infection has a number of possible ramifications for the fetus. Zoster, being a localized outbreak in the face of humoral immunity, has no effect on the intrauterine patient. Generally, acute chickenpox in the gravida, if systemic symptoms are significant, may incite premature uterine activity and possible subsequent premature delivery, as may any such febrile illness.[44] More specifically, however, a syndrome of intrauterine VZV infection has been described which includes a number of structural abnormalities which conceptually correspond to effects of cutaneous vesicles occurring in a small fetus (**Table 1**).[44–48] This constellation of effects is thought to occur in as many as 10% of fetuses of women who are infected in the first trimester, with more severe damage found in babies infected at earlier gestational age, and more subtle findings in those infected later. In addition, babies who have been infected with VZV *in utero* may develop zoster within the first 2 years of life.

Finally, significant morbidity may be suffered by babies born to mothers with active chickenpox developing within 4 days – before or after – delivery. Up to 30% of such infants may develop disseminated varicella, due to acquisition of maternal virus near delivery in the absence of passively (transplacentally)

Table 1
Fetal abnormalities associated with congenital (intrauterine) varicella infection

Cutaneous scarring
Limb hypoplasia
Missing/hypoplastic digits
Limb paralysis/muscle atrophy
Psychomotor retardation
Convulsions
Microcephaly
Cerebral cortical atrophy
Chorioretinitis
Cataracts
Chorioretinal scarring
Optic disc hypoplasia
Horner's syndrome
Early childhood zoster

acquired maternal antibody, which would otherwise modify the course of the disease.[49]

Chickenpox is a highly contagious disease which, like rubeola, infects primarily infants and children in high percentages, leaving few patients to reach adulthood without protective antibodies. Over 90% of members of the adult population in temperate areas are seropositive and therefore immune to active systemic disease (although zoster may occur in later years, especially if significant immunosuppression arises). Among children primarily, yearly outbreaks of chickenpox occur, thus immunizing significant segments of society on a regular basis. In the USA, these mini-epidemics arise in the spring, peaking in the early summer (**Figure 4**).[50] In the gravida VZV infection occurs at a rate of approximately five cases per 10 000 pregnancies.

Diagnosis

The clinical presentations of chickenpox acutely, and zoster in the recurrent case, are very characteristic and pose little diagnostic dilemma. In most cases, simple observation of the patient for several days will allow the development of the easily recognizable rash. Occasionally, laboratory methods may be necessary, including viral culture, for more obscure presentations. Most troublesome has been the case of intrauterine varicella, which has been documented indirectly by the ultrasonographic detection of associated fetal anomalies in the appropriate clinical circumstance,[51] direct detection of specific anti-VZV IgM antibodies in fetal blood collected by funipuncture,[52] and by polymerase chain reaction methods applied to chorionic villus specimens.[53]

Due to the fetal implications of acute VZV infection during pregnancy, the obstetrician is often called upon to investigate the serologic status of a pregnant

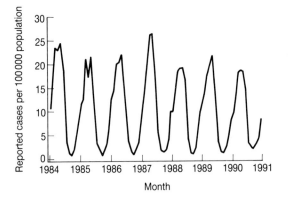

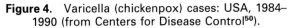

Figure 4. Varicella (chickenpox) cases: USA, 1984–1990 (from Centers for Disease Control[50]).

patient exposed to varicella during a local outbreak. Because the clinical disease is so characteristic, including a few minor but memorable pock marks, a positive history of chickenpox practically insures the presence of immunity. However, the disease is so widespread that even patients with no history of childhood chickenpox may be serologically demonstrated to have been previously infected over 80% of the time.[54] If definitive serologic status needs be determined, the use of the fluorescent antibody test for VZV membrane antigen (FAMA) is appropriate, as well as enzyme-linked immunosorbent assay (ELISA) for anti-VZV IgG antibody. As mentioned, these antibodies are protective of future infection, and therein lies their significance. Of course, artificial induction of protective anti-VZV with effective vaccine is desirable. However, although work with such a vaccine is in progress,[55] no preparation has yet been released for general use.

Management Options

Prepregnancy

Under most circumstances, patients desiring pregnancy do not need to undergo routine antibody screen for VZV to confirm immunity. However, if a family member or close contact has recently been diagnosed to have acute infection, or if the patient anticipates such contact during the pregnancy, testing should then be offered.

Prenatal

Acute chickenpox in the younger patient is generally benign, requiring merely symptomatic relief of the itching and other minor discomforts and attention to the possibility of bacterial superinfection of the raw skin lesions. The adult, including the pregnant woman, with acute VZV infection, should be monitored more carefully for evidence of severe illness and dissemination. In particular, the immunosuppressed patient or the patient otherwise at higher risk for severe illness may be given VZV immune globulin (VZIG) to prevent or lessen the clinical manifestations of the disease. VZIG is given as an intramuscular dose of 125 U/10 kg body weight, with a maximum dose of 625 U (higher doses may be needed in severely immunocompromised patients).[56] The use of VZIG in the pregnant patient to prevent severe maternal disease or congenital infection is problematic. Since supplies of VZIG are limited and expensive, indiscriminant use of the preparation is discouraged. It is suggested that pregnant women be evaluated and treated in the same manner as other adults.[56]

Any evidence of visceral or pulmonic involvement in the patient with acute VZV infection should prompt the appropriate evaluation and supportive care. Also, antiviral chemotherapy with acyclovir is to be recommended for patients with life-threatening VZV infection, including neonates with evidence of disseminated disease acquired near the time of birth. Multiple reports dealing with the use of acyclovir in cases of severe maternal chickenpox, primarily pneumonia, attest to the utility of the drug in this situation.[43,57,58] Doses of 5–10 mg/kg i.v. every 8 hours have been used successfully without untoward maternal or fetal effects. The medication is discontinued when the patient is clinically improved, usually after 7 days of therapy. Of course, during such a severe and life-threatening illness, it should be expected that the gravida will experience premature contractions; the physician should be alert for premature labor and treat it appropriately,

---

VARICELLA-ZOSTER VIRUS
Summary of Management Options

Prenatal

- If mother exposed to VSV, check immunity status (serially if susceptible)

- If patient develops chickenpox:
  - counsel about risks
  - only give VZIG to immunosuppressed patient
  - monitor for dissemination to severe systemic form of illness
  - consider acyclovir with severe illness
  - vigilance for uterine activity

Labor/delivery and postnatal

- Appropriate infection control measures

- Evaluate newborn clinically and serologically

- Prophylactic measures if not infected (e.g. passive or active immunization, acyclovir)

- Acyclovir and supportive therapy if infected

---

predicated on the gestational age and other usual parameters.

Labor/delivery

In the event the parturient has recently demonstrated evidence of acute VZV infection, plans must be made immediately to evaluate and treat the infant after delivery. These efforts should be coordinated with the appropriate pediatric consultant services. Under most circumstances, some combination of passive immunization, acyclovir therapy and vaccination (when available) should be offered to the infant at risk (see Risk section above).

Postnatal

Acute VZV infection is highly contagious and therefore appropriate infection control measures should be instituted during the remainder of the hospitalization.

CYTOMEGALOVIRUS

Maternal/Fetal Risks

Cytomegalovirus (CMV) is a DNA virus, a member of the herpes family of viruses, which causes a number of infectious syndromes in man. However, since CMV is apparently highly efficient, as a virus, in remaining dormant or silent in the host, the most common manifestation of CMV infection in the human is a lack of any demonstrable disease at all. There are three important disease syndromes, though, that are clinically important: heterophile-negative mononucleosis, intrauterine and neonatal infection, and infection in the immunocompromised patient.

The normal adult infected with CMV for the first time (i.e. the initially seronegative patient) may develop a syndrome of fever, atypical lymphocytosis, some malaise, mild lymphadenopathy, but generally a benign course. This illness is clinically indistinguishable from Epstein-Barr mononucleosis, save that the heterophile-agglutinin test is negative in patients with CMV infection; CMV may be cultured from the urine, and patients with CMV mononucleosis tend to be slightly older than patients with Epstein-Barr infection. This manifestation of CMV infection is generally self-limiting, although the fever may last for over a month in a few cases. Rarely, serious complications of the acute infection may occur, including interstitial pneumonitis, hepatitis, the Guillain-Barré syndrome, meningoencephalitis, myocarditis, thrombocytopenia and hemolytic anemia.[59]

In the immunosuppressed patient, CMV infections may be more serious, depending upon the type and degree of immunosuppression. Patients taking immunosuppressive drugs because of such conditions as renal transplantation, or those patients with AIDS, most commonly exhibit the mononucleosis syndrome. The next most frequent manifestation is interstitial pneumonia, which may be relatively asymptomatic to rapidly fatal and often associated with *Pneumocystis* infection in AIDS patients. A large percentage of persons suffering primary CMV infection exhibit chemical hepatitis; severely immunosuppressed patients may develop clinical symptoms, including malaise, nausea and vomiting. Gastrointestinal disease, including ulceration leading to hemorrhage and perforation, is another effect of CMV on the immunocompromised. The AIDS patient may again suffer co-existent CMV infection with the usual cryptosporidiosis and *Mycobacterium avium-intracellulare* infestations. In fact, endoscopic examination of the AIDS patient with colitis and the like due to CMV may demonstrate lesions which resemble Kaposi's sarcoma. Finally, in the AIDS patient specifically, CMV infection of the eye may produce the retinitis typically noted in neonates with the disease, and miscellaneous effects on endocrine organs, including adrenals, pancreas, parathyroids, pituitary and ovaries.[60]

By far the most notable disease complex attributable to CMV is the spectrum of *in utero*/congenital infection. CMV is the most frequent such infection in humans, found in roughly 1% of all newborn infants. In the USA, this results in an estimated 33 000 infected newborns annually;[59] in the UK, CMV is acknowledged to cause much more neonatal disease than rubella.[61] Of the 1:100 infants born infected, only 5–10% will demonstrate clinical illness at birth. This, the most severe manifestation of congenital CMV infection, is one of the classic TORCH syndromes, consisting of hepatosplenomegaly, microcephaly, hyperbilirubinemia, petechiae, thrombocytopenia and often intrauterine growth deficiency. Mortality in these neonates may be as high as 20–30%, with 90% of survivors suffering late complications (**Table 2**). Of the infected neonates delivered without demonstrable disease, 5–15% are at risk of developing some abnormality attributable to CMV before their second birthday, primarily sensorineural hearing loss.[62]

Although CMV may be transmitted by such routes as transfused blood[63] and marrow,[64] the usual routes of acquisition of the virus are perinatal transmission and sexual transmission. Early in life, the infant may be infected transplacentally, by exposure to virus from the cervix and birth, and from virus excreted in breast milk.[65] Another source of childhood infection is exposure to other babies in nurseries and day care centers,[66,67] since infected children tend to shed virus for a prolonged period of time from the urine and respiratory tract (unlike infected but otherwise healthy adults). Rates of infection increase steadily after the first year

Table 2
Early and late neonatal abnormalities associated with symptomatic congenital cytomegalovirus infection

Hepatomegaly
Splenomegaly
Jaundice
Thrombocytopenia
Petechiae
Hemolytic anemia
Intrauterine growth deficiency
Microcephaly
Ventriculomegaly
Cerebral atrophy
Mental retardation
Psychomotor delay
Seizures
Expressive language delays
Learning disabilities
Chorioretinitis
Optic atrophy
Intracranial calcifications
Long bone radiolucencies
Dental abnormalities
Pneumonitis

or two of life. The prevalence is higher in underdeveloped countries[68] and in lower socioeconomic patient populations,[69] though this higher infection rate in the young adults (hence mothers) does not necessarily lead to higher congenital infection rates.[70]

Venereal spread of CMV is conceptually attributed to cervical shedding and the presence of virus in the semen. Aside from the fact that differences in rates of cervical shedding are noted among different patient groups throught the world, it is fairly clear that sexual activity, in particular higher numbers of sexual partners and earlier age at onset of sexual activity, is positively correlated with CMV isolation from the cervix.[71] Heterosexual transmission has been clinically demonstrated by outbreaks of CMV mononucleosis among populations of sexual partners.[72] With respect to carriage and infection in males, CMV may be isolated from semen in both heterosexual and homosexual men,[73] and sexually active homosexual males who are seronegative become infected in a short period of time when prospectively followed.

Unlike other viral infections discussed above, CMV, on the basis of its latency and intermittent shedding from the female genital tract, may infect a fetus or neonate even in the face of maternal antibody. In fact, it would appear that the virus is specially designed to be transmitted during pregnancy, since the infected gravida sheds virus more readily as gestation progresses. Viral shedding from the cervix occurs in about 1–2% of women in the first trimester, 6–10% in the second trimester and 11–28% in the third trimester.[60] The infection rates at birth are higher in babies whose mothers excrete virus. The most severe neonatal disease, however, usually occurs in children born to women who experience primary infection (i.e. who were initially seronegative) during pregnancy. These women transmit the virus to their babies *in utero* approximately a third of the time.

The rate of this primary infection during pregnancy is about 1–2%, with approximately 40–50% of women of child-bearing age being serologically determined to be susceptible to such primary infection.[74] Although severe transplacental infection (i.e. the TORCH syndrome) is not usually seen in children of women with pre-existing antibody,[75] subsequent pregnancies in women with one affected infant have resulted in mildly infected neonates.[76]

Diagnosis

Human CMV is readily grown in cell cultures specifically in cell lines of human fibroblasts. In patients with symptoms suggestive of acute CMV infection, viral culture from urine, nasopharynx or blood may document the presence of the organism. Pathologic specimens (biopsy, necropsy) may also be evaluated for isolation of virus or detection of characteristic histologic changes due to CMV infection. However, since many patients excrete the virus intermittently throughout their lives depending upon certain circumstances (e.g. pregnancy, AIDS), the mere presence of CMV in a specimen does not guarantee that the illness in question was caused by this particular virus. The physician must be extremely careful with the interpretation of such findings.

Serologic testing by older compliment fixation (CF) methods or more current indirect fluorescent antibody (IFA) and anti-compliment immunofluorescent (ACIF) tests are possible. In a primary infection, the IFA and ACIF tests become positive sooner in the disease (because of higher sensitivity) than the CF test.[60] More recently, ELISA methods and radioimmunoassay have been used to detect CMV-specific IgM antibodies,[77] which are important in that reactivation of latent CMV in pregnancy is usually not accompanied by development of IgM antibodies, thus partially helping to differentiate patients with new infection.[78]

Diagnosis of *in utero* CMV infection may be accomplished in a number of ways. Pathologic examination of the products of conception after miscarriage may give hisologic evidence of CMV-associated viral changes.[79] Ultrasonographic demonstration of significant fetal abnormalities (e.g. intracranial calcifications, growth deficiency) in the appropriate clinical circumstance; isolation of the virus from fluid collected by amniocentesis; and demonstration of hematologic, viral or serologic information in fetal blood are all methods of elucidation of CMV and its effects on the unborn.[79–81]

Management Options

Prepregnancy

There are no absolute answers when dealing with CMV counseling during the pre-pregnancy period. Few authorities advocate routine CMV antibody screening prior to pregnancy. However, under some circumstances, baseline studies may be of benefit, such as when a woman anticipating pregnancy enters a work environment placing her at increased risk for CMV exposure. Presence of a positive antibody screen should not be alarming, since a high background positivity rate can be anticipated in many communities. Perhaps more troublesome are issues surrounding the timing of pregnancy after a known subclinical or overt CMV infection. Viral shedding can continue for extended periods of time, and no data are available to extrapolate a 'safe' waiting interval. Again, empiric reasoning suggests that risks for fetal infection should diminish when clinical signs and symptoms have cleared (if present), and the patient has initiated an appropriate immune response to the infection.

Prenatal

Treatment of acute CMV infection in the immunocompetent, normal individual is symptomatic at most, especially since the vast majority of infections are asymptomatic and the rest mild. In so far as CMV is a DNA virus which remains dormant within the host, eradication of the virus is beyond the capacity of modern medicine. In the patient with compromised immunity, (e.g. the transplant patient or the patient with AIDS), the antiviral drug ganciclovir gives at least temporary relief from such severe effects as retinitis.[60] There is no accepted therapy for acute maternal or neonatal infection,[82] although future avenues of research include prenatal use of antiviral drugs to prevent or modify intrauterine infection.

Prevention of infection in the mother is an attractive strategy to avert prenatal or intgrauterine infection. Although work is in progress on a specific CMV vaccine to effect active immunization against the virus,[83,84] there are a number of real and theoretic obstacles to its fruition. Passive immunization with specific anti-CMV immunoglobulin only appears to be useful as prophylaxis in cases of renal and marrow transplantation.[85] The obstetrician is left with the maneuver of avoidance of infection in the seronegative mother during pregnancy. This may take the form of counseling pregnant

CYTOMEGALOVIRUS
Summary of Management Options

Prepregnancy

- Advice about risks for women working in high-risk environment (e.g. child care)

- Counseling about planning pregnancy in women with history of proven CMV infection is difficult; establishing their 'shedding status' may help

Prenatal

- Advice about risks for women working in high-risk environment (e.g. child care)

- If patient is diagnosed to have CMV infection in pregnancy
  - careful counseling about fetal risks
  - consider invasive procedure to establish fetal risk
  - check fetal growth and health
  - consider pregnancy termination (if early gestational age)

Labor/delivery and postnatal

- If patient is diagnosed to have CMV infection in pregnancy
  - infection control measures
  - clinical and serological evaluation of the newborn with pediatric follow-up if infection confirmed

---

women working in high-risk situations (e.g. the day-care center housing young children[86]) or avoiding transfusion-related CMV infection by the use of CMV-negative blood in the gravida.[87] It is not appropriate, however, to screen all pregnant women either for anti-CMV IgG or viral excretion with the aim of isolating them for the duration of the pregnancy. The most reasonable course is to screen women in high-risk areas (e.g. day-care workers) and recommend to susceptible individuals that they pay attention to hygienic measures when coming in contact with possibly infectious clients, fomites and body secretions.

Labor/delivery and postnatal

The only issues surrounding these periods of time relate to infection control measures for the known viral shedder. Universal precautions in place at many health care facilities reduce these risks.

HERPES SIMPLEX VIRUS
Maternal/Fetal Risks

The herpes simplex virus (HSV) is a DNA virus of the herpes family, several types of which cause significant disease in man. HSV-1 has classically been considered the cause of orolabial herpes, referred to commonly as 'fever blisters'; HSV-2 has been considered the cause of genital herpes infection, a well-known STD. Although these two types of HSV are generally thought to be segregated in this way, there is a great deal of overlap, i.e. HSV-2 causing oral disease and HSV-1 causing genital infection. In fact, up to a third of genital infections may be due to HSV-1 in some populations. However, HSV-1 tends to be somewhat less prone to produce recurrent infection than HSV-2. Generally, though, the two viruses may be considered identical in the clinical circumstance of a patient with characteristic ulcerative lesions.[88]

Primary orolabial herpes is mainly a disease of childhood, children acquiring the infection from family members through close contact. While 90–95% of primary oral infections are asymptomatic, a few may consist of a rather florid vesiculoulcerative outbreak in the oropharynx and lips about 1 week after exposure. Adenopathy and viremia, along with fever and malaise, may persist for 1–2 weeks, with viral shedding for up to 6 weeks. Thereafter, antibody production limits the virus such that it remains dormant, occasionally flaring up as localized blisters on the lips in times of stress, sunburn or febrile systemic illness (hence the term 'fever blisters'). During recurrent disease, viral shedding lasts up to 1 week.[89] It should be noted that adults with recurrent oral herpes may transmit the illness through orogenital contact, causing such infections as generally thought to arise from sexual contact.

Genital herpes may occur after sexual contact with an infectious person, or after orogenital contact as mentioned above. The incubation period is less than 1 week, and persons transmitting the virus may actually be asymptomatic themselves,[90] thus confusing the issue as to the origin of the infection. If the patient possesses pre-existing anti-HSV antibody, perhaps from HSV-1 infection in early life, the infection may be all but asymptomatic. Certainly, there will be fewer constitutional symptoms, fewer lesions, shorter duration of lesions, shorter time of viral shedding and fewer complications.[88] In the absence of circulating antibody, primary HSV genital infection may be quite severe, with systemic symptoms of fever, malaise, myalgias and aseptic meningitis. Cases of encephalitis[91] and hepatitis[92] have proven fatal. Lower motor neuron and autonomic dysfunction may contribute to bladder atony and urinary retention. Lesions in extragenital sites may be present in a quarter of women with primary disease, perhaps by auto-inoculation rather than viremia. Viral shedding is present for nearly 3 weeks in the most severe cases. Finally, local recurrent disease may occur weeks or months later, especially if the offending virus is HSV-2, which recurs much more frequently than does HSV-1, especially in the genital area.[93]

HSV infection in the pregnant woman has two important components: primary infection in the mother, and transmission of infection (either primary or recurrent) to the neonate and subsequent disseminated infection. Primary HSV infection in the gravida severe enough to cause systemic illness and fever may stimulate premature uterine contractions. Thus, premature labor and delivery may be serious complications of HSV infection in pregnancy, depending upon the stage of gestation. Also, because of the relative immunosuppression of pregnancy,[94] dissemination of HSV during pregnancy may lead to death from hepatitis, encephalitis and general viral dissemination.[95] The fetus acquiring HSV in the perinatal period, especially likely if the mother suffers an acute, primary infec-

tion,[96] may suffer severe neonatal morbidity, including dissemination leading to chorioretinitis, meningitis, encephalitis, mental retardation, seizures and death. Primary infection early in pregnancy, perhaps due to a viral endometritis ascending from cervical infection, may end in miscarriage. However, there are no consistent reports of a congenital syndrome due to intrauterine infection with HSV, as there is with CMV. Therefore, the spectrum of fetal/neonatal infection includes miscarriage, prematurity and intrapartum infection with resultant disseminated HSV infection.[97]

As mentioned, HSV-1 infection is common in children, whereas HSV-2 is more common in teenagers and older patients who are sexually active. Epidemiologic studies have been hampered by the fact that the two viruses cross-react in a number of serologic tests used for this purpose. Confounding this technical difficulty is the latency of the virus, such that patients who have been infected and who may even be infectious are for the most part asymptomatic.

In the past, non-specific tests for HSV (i.e. not differentiating betwwen HSV-1 and HSV-2) have demonstrated a 90% seropositivity rate by the fourth decade of life.[98] Over the most recent decade or two, however, industrialized countries have reported a decrease in seropositivity rates of HSV-1, due perhaps to increasing sanitation measures, and increasing rates of HSV-2, due to increasingly permissive sexual behaviour.[99] At any rate, since the 1960s, rates of clinical genital HSV infection have been rising dramatically in the USA,[100] in the UK and other parts of Europe.[99]

The rate of HSV carriage in pregnant women is of interest, since transmission to the neonate is of primary concern. Studies of gravidas in labor have demonstrated culture positive rates of 0.35%[101] in a general population, with rates of 0.96%[102] to 2.4%[103] in asymptomatic women with known positive histories of genital HSV infection. The rate of neonatal disease is much lower, from 0.01 to 0.04%, due to variability in maternal antibody (and thus passively acquired fetal antibody) levels and viral inoculum (i.e. primary, severe infection *vs* mild, recurrent infection in the mother). Roughly 75% of neonatal infections are due to HSV-2 and 25% due to HSV-1.[104] Of extreme interest is the finding that the majority of infants developing neonatal HSV infection are born to mothers without sympoms or even a history of genital herpes infection.[102,105]

Diagnosis

It is relatively easy to culture HSV, and tissue culture techniques are the gold standard for diagnosis. Since rapid diagnosis is desirable, fluorescent antibody (FA) staining performed on short incubation tissue culture slides has allowed identification within 48 h, especially in cases of large viral numbers in the original specimen. Also, in high inocula situations, direct FA staining of the original specimen may give the appropriate diagnosis, though it is not as sensitive or specific as tissue culture.[106,107] More recently, ELISA tests have been developed which aid in the rapid diagnosis of viral shedding, including asymptomatic shedding from the cervix with reasonable sensitivity.[108,109]

Although serologic methodology is extensively utilized in epidemiologic studies, serologic identification of HSV in pregnancy is minimally useful. Since a large proportion of the pregnant population is positive for HSV-1, HSV-2 or both, a positive test is basically worthless. If the husband is known to have a history of HSV infection on the one hand and the wife is known to be seronegative on the other, the risk of primary transmission during pregnancy may be addressed.[110] Also, in the case that a patient has what may be a primary HSV infection, seroconversion may be documented, as well as the presence of HSV-specific IgM, to insure the diagnosis. In most cases, though, the patient will be at risk for recurrent disease and merely have static levels of IgG, which will not be particularly helpful clinically.

Management Options

Prepregnancy

Avoidance of pregnancy during primary infections seems intuitively obvious; this is less practical during recurrences, since they tend to be unpredictable. Baseline screening for antibody status appears to be of little value given the high background rate.

Prenatal

Recurrent HSV infection in the pregnant woman is handled symptomatically. Most recurrent infections are mild and short-lived, and therefore little therapeutic intervention is necessary for the mother herself. Although the non-pregnant patient may use oral acyclovir to modify recurrent outbreaks of the disease, as well as for 'prophylaxis' against frequent recurrences,[111–113] the drug is probably not indicated for (oral) use during pregnancy, on the theoretic basis that it does have some small affinity for human thymidine kinase and may have some effect on the fetus *in utero*. Many practitioners, however, recommend topical acyclovir ointment for their pregnant patients on the grounds that it is not significantly absorbed, although the benefits of this approach are unclear.

The gravida with a severe case of primary HSV infection is at risk for premature uterine activity, based on the systemic manifestations of the disease, and dissemination of the infection, based upon her relative immunosuppression. Accordingly, women with significant primary HSV infection during pregnancy should be monitored for signs of premature labor and appropriately treated if this should arise. Also, she should be observed for evidence of visceral involvement indicative of dissemination, including hepatic transaminase levels to detect liver involvement and neurologic status to warn of encephalitis. If there is any doubt as to her well-being, oral or even intravenous acyclovir should be initiated to prevent serious morbidity. (It also goes without saying that she should be hospitalized during the most harrowing part of her illness.) Acyclovir is given orally at a dose of 200 mg five times a day for 7–10 days, or until clinical resolution, and intravenous acyclovir is given at 5 mg/kg every 8 h for the same time period.[114]

Labor/delivery

Conduct of pregnancy in the woman with active or historic herpes is governed by the desire to prevent neonatal infection and subsequent dissemination. Heretofore, it was recommended that such women have weekly genital cultures for HSV in the latter weeks of pregnancy and be delivered abdominally if the most recent cultures were positive.[115] However, with the realization that there was little correlation between prenatal HSV shedding and shedding at delivery,[102] that most women whose infants develop HSV infection have no lesions or history,[106] and that women with recurrent HSV infection (as opposed to primary) pose little risk to their neonates,[116] the recommendations for weekly cultures were abandoned.[117] It is currently the practice in the USA[104] to culture only for HSV to document a new case (i.e. not to search for viral shedding during pregnancy), to allow vaginal delivery in the absence of visible lesions in the genital area at the onset of labor, and to proceed with cesarean delivery if lesions are present at the time of labor. Cases of preterm premature rupture of the membranes in the face of active lesions are to be considered individually, depending upon gestational age and other factors, with input being sought from the patient after appropriate dialog. Finally, fetal scalp electrodes are used in labor if necessary for obstetric indications, even though fetal infection has been attributed to their use.[118]

Postnatal

Management recommendations are similar to those pertaining to CMV infection.

HERPES SIMPLEX VIRUS (GENITAL)
Summary of Management Options

Prepregnancy

- Avoidance of pregnancy during primary infection

Prenatal

- Symptomatic treatment of infections

- Vigilance for dissemination

- Vigilance for uterine activity

- Acyclovir (oral and topical) has been used in pregnancy without adverse outcome, though not generally advocated unless disseminated disease

- Serial viral cultures in the last trimester for patients who are asymptomatic are *no longer recommended*

Labor/delivery

- Allow vaginal delivery if no active lesions and no prodromal symptoms at time of labor

- Active lesions at time of labor is considered to be an indication for cesarean section by most obstetricians, though the risk of fetal infection is less with recurrent disease

- Counseling about the benefits of cesarean section in preventing fetal infection with membrane rupture is difficult

Postnatal

- Infection control measures with active lesions

- Clinical, microbiological and serologic evaluation of the newborn with active maternal lesions

---

HEPATITIS B

Maternal/Fetal Risks

Hepatitis B, or serum hepatitis, is a viral liver disease caused by hepatitis B virus (HBV), a member of the Hepadnaviridae family of DNA viruses. Hepatitis B was only virologically distinguished in the 1960s, although clinical differentiation between HBV and hepatitis A infection was made earlier. HBV is primarily tropic for human hepatocytes, thus the major clini-

cal disease caused by the virus is hepatitis. Clinical illness is generally manifest after a 2–6 month incubation period (thus, the synonym 'long incubation hepatitis'), though virus may be detected in the blood within the first month of infection.

It is estimated that 60–68% of acute HBV infections are either subclinical and asymptomatic, or associated with a mild influenza-like illness which goes unrecognized. Symptoms, if present, include nausea, vomiting, anorexia and perhaps right upper quadrant pain. Commonly, fever is low or absent, and mild diarrhea may occur. Roughly half of HBV cases are anicteric, with only mild bilirubin elevations noted if appropriate laboratory testing is performed. If present, jaundice peaks during the first 10 days of the syndrome and lasts for several weeks, while malaise and anorexia may go on for weeks.[119]

In the normal adult, 90% of acute HBV infections resolve completely within 6 months. In the other 10% of individuals, hepatitis B surface antigen (HBsAg) remains in the serum, the patient being considered a chronic carrier. While a few of these patients will clear the antigen after another 6 months, most will develop chronic active hepatitis (characterized by ongoing symptoms of the disease), chronic persistent hepatitis (characterized by mild or absent symptoms in the face of abnormal liver enzyme levels) or, rarely, fulminant HBV infection which prgresses rapidly to hepatic failure and death. Of significance is the fact that infection in the neonate, as a result of vertical transmission from the mother, gives exactly the reverse in terms of percentages; if immunization does not prevent infection in the baby, nearly 90% will go on to develop chronic HBV carriage and one form or other of the chronic HBV syndromes.[120] The importance of this phenomenon is that infants infected at brith form a large population which suffers the late sequelae of chronic HBV infection, namely post-infectious hepatic cirrhosis and primary hepatocellular carcinoma, which occurs frequently in chronically HBV-infected patients.[121,122]

In developed countries acute HBV infection in pregnancy is roughly of the same severity as in the non-pregnant state, with the exception that the symptoms may be exaggerated due to the gastrointestinal discomfort common to pregnancy in the first instance. In the third world, nutritional deprivation and the co-existence of other diseases and parasites tend to worsen outcome. By the same token, miscarriage, stillbirth and other adverse pregnancy outcomes are not attributable to acute and chronic hepatitis in pregnancy *per se*.[123] Recent studies have found no adverse pregnancy events in HBsAg carriers,[124] nor abnormalities in babies resulting from HBV-contaminated *in vitro* fertilizations.[125]

HBV infection, both acute and chronic, is more prevalent in tropical climes and in developing countries. In such environments, vertical transmission to the neonate is the major mode of spread, and chronic disability due to cirrhosis and hepatocellular carcinoma is common. In industrialized countries, however, HBV is classically transmitted by blood and blood products ('serum hepatitis') and by sexual activity. It has long been recognized that parenteral drug abusers and male homosexuals were at increased risk of HBV exposure, and recent investigations have indicated that heterosexual activity may be involved in the dissemination of the virus.[126–128] In the USA, HBV infection has steadily risen since it was first identified a quarter of a century

ago (**Figure 5**).[129] More recently, the rate of rise in prevalence has leveled out somewhat, due to some extent to changing sexual practices among male homosexuals fearing AIDS; however, rates continue to rise among heterosexuals, particularly among drug users.[128]

Acute HBV infection complicates pregnancy at a rate of roughly 0.1%. However, the major health care problem in industrialized countries is HBsAg carriage during pregnancy. HBV carriage has been reported as occurring in 0.09–1.5% of gravidas in the USA,[130–133] 0.34% in Canada,[134] 1.81% in France[135] and 2.2% in Australia.[136] The risk of HBsAg carriage is to the fetus, rather than the mother. Roughly 5% of fetuses are infected *in utero* due to transplacental hemorrhage near the end of gestation.[137] The remaining infants may be infected at birth from maternal blood and body fluids. Therefore, roughly 1% of pregnant women, depending upon the population in question, are potential risks to their newborns.

Diagnosis

If it is symptomatic and recognized at all, acute HBV infection is difficult to distinguish from any of the other hepatic illnesses (e.g. hepatitis A). Especially elusive is the chronic HBsAg carrier, who cannot be identified by serologic testing. The standard for HBV testing is detection of the various antibodies and antigens specific to the virus, including: (1) HBsAg, antigen from the surface capsule of the virus indicating infectivity; (2) hepatitis Be antigen (HBeAg), antigen from the core of the virus indicating high infectivity; (3) antibody to HBsAg (anti-HBs), indicating immunologic response to infection and cure; (4) anti-HBe, which may be present before anti-HBs and indicates partial immune response and lessens infectivity; and (5) antibody to hepatitis B core antigen (anti-HBc), which rises early in the course of the immune response

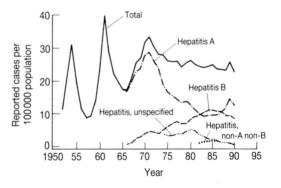

Figure 5. Hepititis cases: USA, 1952–1990 (from Centers for Disease Control[129]).

(HBcAg is not measured in serum). The time-course of these serologic markers is depicted in **Figure 6**.[120]

The patient presenting with signs and symptoms of acute hepatitis should be screened with the so-called 'hepatitis panel', which usually consists of HBsAg, anti-HBs, anti-HBc, HBeAg, anti-HBe, hepatitis A specific IgM and IgG, and perhaps serologic studies for hepatitis C. Of course, the physician should keep in mind that other causes of hepatic disease occur during pregnancy, including viral illnesses such as infectious mononucleosis due to Epstein-Barr virus, and also pregnancy-specific illnesses such as pre-eclampsia/ HELLP syndrome/gestosis. In any event, if the appropriate markers for HBV are found, the diagnosis is achieved. It should be underscored that patients with HBsAg in their serum are infectious, patients with HBeAg are *highly* infectious, and patients with anti-HBs are immunologically cured. Also, chronic HBV infection is defined as HBsAg carriage for greater than 6 months (though, as mentioned above, some patients ultimately take up to 1 year to clear the antigen).

Management Options

Prepregnancy

Patients known to be HBsAg carriers should be counseled regarding the neonatal risks for vertical transmission of HBV, and the need for immediate neonatal intervention to reduce these risks.

Prenatal

The gravida presenting with acute HBV infection should be assessed in the usual fashion, with attention to hydration, control of nausea and vomiting, and concern for degree of liver involvement. As mentioned above, pregnancy-specific maladies such as pre-eclampsia must not be mistaken for hepatitis, as therapy is obviously much different and delay in diagnosis possibly deadly.[138] It is not unreasonable to hospitalize the patient who is experiencing moderate to severe symptoms to insure hydration and monitor for signs of uterine activity. As such time, evaluation of liver status and education as to diet and sanitation may be accomplished. Also, the family and close (especially sexual) contacts may be counseled, tested and, perhaps, vaccinated as appropriate. The patient may also be reassured that, should the fetus survive the acute maternal illness (i.e. without delivering prematurely), there will be no teratogenic effects or congenital anomalies. The patient is then followed for evidence of resolution of her HBsAg and development of anti-HBs. As noted above, 6 months is the arbitrary boundary which determines chronic carriage.

Since roughly half of HBsAg carriers during pregnancy are not identifiable with risk assessment,[130–136] it is recommended that all pregnant women be screened for HBsAg as part of their routine laboratory evaluation during pregnancy.[139] Recommendations from the USA are listed in **Table 3**; these are basically in agreement with the thoughts of experts in Europe and Canada,[140,141] as well as a committee of the American College of Obstetricians and Gynecologists.[142] It is felt that such a strategy, though adding an extra laboratory

Table 3
Recommendations for hepatitis B screening during pregnancy

All pregnant women should be screened for HBsAg at the same time that other routine prenatal screening is accomplished, and health care personnel be informed if a HBsAg-positive mother presents for delivery so as to insure prompt treatment of the infant

In special circumstances (e.g. exposure to HBV, acute hepatitis, or high-risk behavior), additional testing may be warranted later in pregnancy

Unscreened women presenting for delivery should be screened at that time, and the hospital should make arrangements for 24 h turn-around of the results

Infants born to HBsAg-positive mothers should receive HBIG (0.5 ml i.m.) within 12 h of birth and an initial dose of HBV vaccine (5 μg recombinant vaccine i.m.) within 7 days

Infants receive their second and third doses of vaccine at 1 and 6 months, and are tested for HBsAg at 12–15 months of age

Family members of HBsAg-positive women (and infants) are counseled appropriately

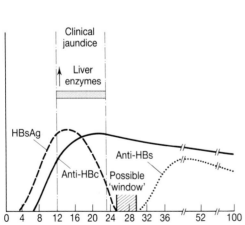

Figure 6. Serologic markers in acute hepatitis B infection (from Pastorek[120]).

HEPATITIS B
Summary of Management Options

Prepregnancy

- In known HBV positive patients, risks for fetus and preventative measures after birth should be discussed

Prenatal

Acute disease

- Supportive care

- Dietary advice

- Monitor liver function

- Assess fetal growth and health

- Vigilance for uterine activity

- Infection control measures

- Contact tracing, testing and vaccination where appropriate

Chronic carriers

- Assessment of carrier status varies (some perform screening on all women, others only on those 'at risk'; see **Table 3** for US recommendations)

- Infection control measures with body products

Labor/delivery and postnatal

- Infection control measures

- Advice about breast-feeding is controversial

- Newborn should receive passive (HBIG) and active (three-dose vaccine) immunization

test to the prenatal patient's battery, ultimately proves cost-effective, as well as prevents the ravages of chronic liver disease in a majority of neonates of HBsAg-positive mothers.[143]

Labor/delivery and postnatal

Because of the implications of neonatal HBV infections, as well as the fact that only a small percentage of neonates have been infected *in utero*, the newborn of a mother carrying HBsAg has been the target of preventive measures involving active and passive immunoprophylaxis. It has been demonstrated that the adminstration of hepatitis B immunoglobulin (HBIG) at birth, followed by the initiation of the three-dose hepatitis B vaccine, is protective in over 90% of such cases.[144–147]

HUMAN IMMUNODEFICIENCY VIRUS

Maternal/Fetal Risks

The human immunodeficiency virus (HIV) is a small RNA retrovirus which causes the clinical disease termed the acquired immunodeficiency syndrome (AIDS), which has only been described since 1981.[148,149] (More specifically, AIDS in the USA and Europe is primarily caused by HIV-1; a similar virus, HIV-2, is responsible for a proportion of the disease in Africa, but has yet to significantly reach the industrialized nations.) However, of all viral agents – indeed, among medical diseases generally – HIV almost single-handedly has radically changed the way the world thinks about medicine, and STDs in general. Some have even bandied about the idea that HIV and the resultant AIDS are somehow a manifestation of 'divine justice' for certain activities and deficiencies of modern humanity.[150] Whatever the case, it is clear that the syndrome of immunosuppression leading inexorably to death has caused massive shifts in health care allocation, psychosocial activities and research endeavors in the industrialized world of the 1980s and 1990s.

Human infection with HIV results after percutaneous inoculation with infected material, usually blood or bodily fluids. Infection at the time of sexual activity is generally thought of as occurring through minute cracks and fissures in the skin exposed to the infectious materials. Use of contaminated drug paraphernalia (e.g. needles) involves rather straightforward injection of virus into the recipient's bloodstream. Upon gaining access to the circulation, HIV preferentially infects cells with CD4+ receptors on the cell's surface, including helper T-lymphocytes, macrophages, some central nervous system cells, and apparently the placenta. The decimation of the population of helper T-lymphocytes, along with some derangement of humoral immunity and macrophage function, ultimately leads to severe immune deficiency and susceptibility to a variety of opportunistic infections, including *Pneumocystis carinii* and atypical *Mycobacterium* spp. (especially *M. avium-intracellulare* and *M. kansasii*), unusually invasive or indolent HSV and *Candida* infections, and rare malignancies, such as Kaposi's sarcoma and primary lymphoma of the brain.[151]

The initial HIV infection may be asymptomatic, or a flu-like or mononucleosis-like syndrome may ensue. Within 3 months or so, occasionally longer, the patient will develop antibodies to the virus and remain asymptomatic for years, though infectious. After a variable time period, immunological disturbance is manifest by generalized lymphadenopathy, fever, cachexia, malaise and neurologic dysfunction. Such common and generally localized infections as HSV and *Candida* become chronic, spread to uncharacteristic areas, and are resistant to the usual remedies. The patient's downhill course prgresses to more severe infections, such as *Pneumocystis carinii* pneumonia (PCP), other disseminated bacterial or fungal infections, and ultimately death from one of the infections or aforementioned malignancies. Roughly one-third of infected patients will develop clinical AIDS within the first 5 years after inoculation.[152]

HIV infection in the pregnant patient is a topic still undergoing much scrutiny. Since the initial populations of HIV/AIDS patients in the early to mid-1980s were primarily male homosexuals and hemophiliacs, few pregnancies occurred in patients with advanced disease. Even now, most pregnant HIV patients formally reported in the literature are asymptomatic carriers, and it is difficult to make definitive statements about the course of HIV and co-existing gestation. Some studies hint that the progression of the immunosuppression, as measured by decreasing helper T-lymphocyte numbers, is accelerated by pregnancy.[153] Others have shown a rather high rate of progression of maternal disease.[154] In addition, these uncontrolled studies demonstrated a high rate of pregnancy complications (e.g. premature rupture of the membranes, preterm labor, low birthweight, sexually transmitted diseases) in the HIV-infected women. However, properly controlled study of HIV-infected gravidas indicates that low birthweight and other complications are due to such confounding circumstances as drug use, smoking and socioeconomic variables, and not the HIV itself.[155,156] At the present level of medical knowledge, then, it is reasonable to say that asymptomatic HIV carriers (living in developed countries) have pregnancies as normal as the population they represent; any effect HIV has on the

pregnancy is predicated upon actual symptomatic AIDS (e.g. PCP) and not the virus *per se*.

Although conceptually similar to HBV due to its blood-borne character, HIV is transmitted from the gravida to her fetus nearly four times as often, perhaps due to the virus' tropism for the placenta. Transplacental passage of HIV occurs in about 30% of affected pregnancies, enhanced by low helper T-lymphocyte numbers (less than 400/mm^3) or advanced maternal illness. Currently, research is underway to identify reasons some infants are protected; perhaps some types of maternal antibody are protective of the baby.[151]

HIV (or more properly, clinical AIDS) was originally discovered in among male homosexuals in 1981. It was soon recognized in hemophiliacs and immigrants from Haiti. In the ensuing decade, cases of clinical AIDS have increased exponentially in number, topping 200 000 in the USA by 1992.[157] Because the disease is sexually transmitted and also associated with contaminated drug materials, however, it did not remain confined to those original populations. Currently, in the USA at least, male homosexuals make up roughly half of the AIDS population; drug addicts and others, including those whose only known risk for infection was heterosexual activity, constitute the rest.[158] It is clear now, in the 1990s, that HIV/AIDS is an infection of the popoulation in general.

As young women of child-bearing age become infected with HIV, either by association with infected partners or through illicit drug use, it is logical to expect that HIV infection rates among children will rise through vertical transmission. This is precisely the case. The exponential rise in AIDS cases in the USA since 1981 is parallelled (though at a much lower level) by a rise in pediatric cases (**Figure 7**).[159] Whereas in the early years of the diseases's history, children with hemophilia and others with a history of blood product transfusion represented the HIV-infected pediatric cohort, today it is the neonate whose mother is a car-

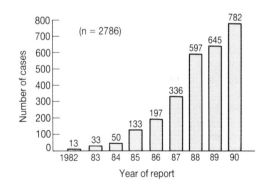

Figure 7. Acquired immunodeficiency syndrome (AIDS), pediatric cases: USA, 1982–1990 (*n* = 2786) (from Centers for Disease Control[159]).

rier. These days, it is not unusual for an asymptomatic gravida to give birth to the unfortunate baby who develops symptomatic disease and dies before his or her second birthday.

Diagnosis

HIV may be cultured from patients with infection. However, methods are predictably labor-intensive, exposure to live virus is hazardous to laboratory personel, and ease of viral recovery is proportional to the severity of the illness (i.e. severely ill patients with low helper T-lymphocyte counts have a higher viral load and are easier to detect, while asymptomatic carriers may be culture negative). Polymerase chain reaction (PCR) methodology has also been utilized to detect minute amounts of HIV nucleic acid in the serum (or tissue), thus documenting the presence of virus. This is highly accurate and sensitive, so much so that contamination from previous specimens is problematic. Hence, this technology is usually reserved for research and reference laboratories, useful in problem cases when screening tests are equivocal or otherwise bear verification. Thus, screening for antibody produced by the patient against the virus has been the mainstay of diagnostic methodology.[160]

Since 1985, ELISA screening tests have been available in the USA for detection of specific viral core and envelope antigens (technically, antigens p24, gp120 and gp4), which are produced by the patient within a few months after infection. Standard practice includes a repeated ELISA test to confirm an initial positive, followed by a confirmatory electrophoresis test for a multitude of specific viral proteins, usually the Western blot.[161] This protocol has been found to have a specificity of 99.4% and a false-positive rate of less than 0.001%, when used with the modern ELISA and Western blot methods.[162]

Problems encountered with standard ELISA screening for HIV include neonates who are positive by virtue of passively acquired maternal IgG antibody which may persist for up to 15 months, and patients with HIV-2 which does not entirely cross-react with antibody tests for HIV-1. The latter is not a serious problem in the industrialized West, though specific HIV-2 ELISA tests are now available and being put in place in blood banks and other laboratories, either as separate HIV-2 tests or as combination HIV-1/HIV-2 tests.[160] Neonates, on the other hand, have traditionally been serially tested for the first year or two of life to document the waning of maternal antibody or the persistence of the child's own antibody due to HIV infection. Of course, earlier diagnosis is desirable, by IgA and IgM testing, direct viral culture of neonatal blood, and PCR detection of antigen in the infant.[163] This remains an important and actively evolving field.

Management Options

Prepregnancy

Female patients recognizably at risk for HIV carriage are generally thought of as intravenous drug users; prostitutes or otherwise sexually promiscuous persons; blood product recipients before 1986 (when screening of blood products for HIV was initiated); bisexuals; persons indigenous to countries with high endemic HIV prevalence; patients with disease symptoms suggestive of HIV infection; or patients with a history of, or current, STDs.[151] This prejudice is well-founded, since patients within high-risk populations have decidedly higher rates of infection than those without known risks, sometimes in the range of 50%.[164,165] Such risk assessment is often misleading, however. In particular, in pregnant populations screened for HIV seropositivity with background HIV rates of less than 2%, 50–70% of HIV-positive individuals give no self-identified risk factors which would single them out for testing.[166,167] This has led to recommendations for routine HIV screening of all women seeking prenatal care (or when possible preconceptually), at least with patient consent, appropriate counseling confidentiality, and availability of expert care and consultation.[168–170] Even inner-city, lower socioeconomic status patients have been fairly amenable to this strategy.[171]

Prenatal

The pregnant woman with HIV infection should be provided appropriate counseling about the disease, its implications for herself and her baby, and the importance of medical care. Of course, HIV is an STD, and persons found to be positive at screening should be treated in a fashion similar to other STDs with regards their sexual activity and testing for other STDs (e.g. syphilis). Additionally, baseline serology for CMV and *Toxoplasma gondii* are recommended, as these organisms are commonly associated with HIV infection and are possible fetal pathogens. Helper T-lymphocyte (CD4+) counts should be serially monitored, perhaps in each trimester. Counts below 500/mm^3 suggest that the patient be seen in consultation by an HIV expert. CD4+ counts below 200/mm^3 require antimicrobial prophylaxis against PCP, either with trimethoprim/ sulfamethoxazole or aerosolized pentamidine, and antiviral therapy with zidovudine, to slow the rate of progression of clinical AIDS. The effects of the above medications on the fetus are theoretic only and do not justify withholding maternal therapy until after delivery. And, finally, treatment of any other overt opportunistic infection in the HIV-infected gravida should be undertaken just as in the non-pregnant woman by the most expedient means.[151,172,173]

Labor/delivery

Questions which still remain include the use of antiviral therapy to interrrupt fetal transmission of HIV and influence of mode of delivery on neonatal disease. There are currently a number of centers actively studying HIV infection in the pregnant woman, with trials of zidovudine underway to prevent fetal infection.[174] What the results of these studies will be is uncertain at present. And although reports suggest that cesarean delivery is somewhat protective against neonatal infection,[175] comparative studies must be formally undertaken before operative delivery, with its hazards to the mother, is advocated on a routine basis.

HUMAN IMMUNODEFICIENCY VIRUS
Summary of Management Options

Prepregnancy

- Careful counseling and offer of screening for at-risk women

- In HIV positive women, careful counseling of risks and prognosis for the patient and fetus/baby, and consideration of whether pregnancy should be avoided

Prenatal

- Counseling and offer of screening for at-risk women; most centers require informed consent before testing can occur

- All at-risk women should be managed as if they were HIV positive in terms of infection control measures with blood and other body products (preventative measures should be employed when handling blood from *all* women in pregnancy, e.g. wearing gloves, spectacles for delivery, etc.)

- For HIV positive women:
  - counseling and support
  - consideration of termination of pregnancy
  - screen for other STDs (see Chapter 30)
  - monitor CD4+ counts serially
    - if $< 500/mm^3$, liaise with HIV specialist
    - if $< 200/mm^3$, commence antibiotic prophylaxis and antiviral therapy
  - treat opportunistic infection
  - role of zidovudine in reducing fetal risk is not yet clear

Labor/delivery and postnatal

- Role of cesarean section in reducing fetal risk is not yet clear

- Dosage of antibiotic, antiviral and immunosupportive therapy may need review after delivery

- Contraceptive advice

- Advise against breast-feeding in developed countries

Postnatal

Management goals following delivery should include reinstitution of immunosupportive and prophylactic agents. Because of changes in volumes of distribution, the dosages of some of these drugs may need to be adjusted and patients should be observed for early evidence of toxicity. Adequate contraception should be recommended. In most developed countries, breastfeeding has been discouraged because of concerns of viral transmission.

REFERENCES

1   Modlin JF (1984) Measles virus. In Belshe RB (ed.) *Human Virology*, pp. 333–360. Littleton, MA: PSG Publishing.

2   Gavish D, Kleinman Y, Morag A, Chajek-Shaul T (1983) Hepatitis and jaundice associated with measles in young adults: An analysis of 65 cases. *Archives of Internal Medicine* **143**:674–677.

3   Centers for Disease Control (1991) Measles – United States 1990. *Morbidity and Mortality Weekly Report* **40**(22):369–372.

4   Hersh BS, Markowitz LE, Maes EF, Funkhouser AW, Baughman AL, Sirotkin BI, Hadler SC (1992) The geographic distribution of measles in the United States, 1980 through 1989. *Journal of the American Medical Association* **267**:1936–1941.

5   Young NA, Gershon AA (1983) Chickenpox, measles and mumps. In Remington JS, Kelein JO (eds) *Infectious Diseases of the Fetus and Newborn Infant*, 2nd edn, pp. 375–427. Philadelphia, PA: W.B. Saunders.

6   Moroi K, Saito S, Durata T, Sata T, Yanagida M (1991) Fetal death associated with measles virus infection of the placenta. *American Journal of Obstetrics and Gynecology* **164**:1107–1108.

7   Aaby P, Bukh J, Lisse IM, Seim E, De Silva MC (1988) Increased perinatal mortality among children of mothers exposed to measles during pregnancy. *Lancet* **i**:516–519.

8   Centers for Disease Control (1982) Serologic diagnosis of measles. *Morbidity and Mortality Weekly Report* **31**(29):396–402.

9   Centers for Disease Control (1991) Update on adult immunization: Recommendations of the Immunization Practices Advisory Committee (ACIP). *Morbidity and Mortality Weekly Report* **40** (No.RR–12):19–22.

10 Amstey MS (1992) Measles. In Gleicher N (ed.) *Principles and Practice of Medical Therapy in Pregnancy*, 2nd edn, pp. 659–661. Norwalk, CN: Appleton and Lange.

11 Centers for Disease Control (1991) Update on adult immunization: Recommendations of the Immunization Practices Advisory Committee (ACIP). *Morbidity and Mortality Weekly Report* **40**(No.RR–12):48.

12 Gershon AA (1990) Rubella virus (German measles). In Mandell GL, Douglas RG, Bennett JE (eds) *Principles and Practice of Infectious Diseases*, 3rd edn, pp. 1242–1247. New York: Churchill Livingstone.

13 Gregg NM (1942) Congenital cataract following German measles in the mother. *Transactions of the Ophthalmological Society of Australia* **3**:35.

14 Cochi SL, Edmonds LE, Dyer K, Greaves WL, Marks JS, Rovira EZ, Preblud SR, Orenstein WA (1989) Congenital rubella syndrome in the United States, 1970–1985. *American Journal of Epidemiology* **129**:349–361.

15 Grossman JH (1990) Why congenital rubella continues to occur. *Contemporary OB/GYN* **36**:50–54.

16 Centers for Disease Control (1991) Incease in rubella and congenital rubella syndrome – United States, 1988–1990. *Morbidity and Mortality Weekly Report* **40**:93–99.

17 Centers for Disease Control (1991) Update on adult immunization: Recommendations of the Immunization Practices Advisory Committee (ACIP). *Morbidity and Mortality Weekly Report* **40**(No.RR–12):24–26.

18 Chu Sy, Bernier RH, Stewart JA, Hermann KL, Greenspan JR, Henderson AK, Liang AP (1988) Rubella antibody persistence after immunization: Sixteen-year follow-up in the Hawaiian islands. *Journal of the American Medical Association* **259**:3133–3136.

19 O'Shea S, Best JM, Banatvala JE (1983) Viremia, virus excretion, and antibody responses after challenge in volunteers with low levels of antibody to rubella virus. *Journal of Infectious Diseases* **148**:639–647.

20 Enders G, Calm A, Shaub J (1984) Rubella embryopathy after previous maternal rubella vaccination. *Infection* **12**:96–98.

21 Daffos F, Forestier F, Grangeot-Keros L, Pavlovsky MC, Lebon P, Chartier M, Pillot J (1984) Prenatal diagnosis of congenital rubella. *Lancet* **ii**:1–3.

22 Centers for Disease Control (1989) Rubella vaccination during pregnancy – United States, 1971–1988. *Morbidity and Mortality Weekly Report* **38**:289–291.

23 Cossart YE, Field AM, Cant B, Widdows D (1975) Parvovirus-like particles in human sera. *Lancet* **i**:72–73.

24 Serjeant GR, Topley JM, Mason K, Serjeant BE, Pattison JR, Jones SE, Mohamed R (1981) Outbreak of aplastic crises in sickle cell anaemia associated with parvovirus-like agent. *Lancet* **ii**:595–597.

25 Thurn J (1988) Human parvovirus B19: Historical and clinical review. *Review of Infectious Diseases* **10**:1005–1011.

26 Kurtzman GJ, Ozawa K, Cohen B, Hanson G, Oseas R, Young NS (1987) Chronic bone marrow failure due to persistent B19 parvovirus infection. *New England Journal of Medicine* **317**:287–294.

27 White DG, Woolf AD, Mortimer PP, Cohen BJ, Blake DR, Bacon PA (1985) Human parvovirus arthropathy. *Lancet* **i**:419–421.

28 Anderson MJ, Lewis E, Kidd IM, Hall SM, Cohen BJ (1984) An outbreak of erythema infectiosum associated with human parvovirus infection. *Journal of Hygiene (London)* **93**:85–93.

29 Anand A, Gray ES, Brown T, Clewley JP, Cohen BJ, (1987) Human parvovirus infection in pregnany and hydrops fetalis. *New England Journal of Medicine* **316**:183–186.

30 Rodis JF, Hovick TJ, Quinn DL, Rosengren SS, Tat-

tersall P (1988) Human parvovirus infection in pregnancy. *Obstetrics and Gynecology* **72**:733–738.

31 Anderson MJ, Pattison JR, (1984) The Human parvovirus: Brief review. *Archives of Virology* **82**:137–148.

32 Public Health Laboratory Service Working Party on Fifth Disease (1990) Prospective study of human parvovirus (B19) infection in pregnancy. *British Medical Journal* **300**:1166–1170.

33 Young N (1988) Hematologic and hematopoietic consequences of B19 parvovirus infection. *Seminars in Hematology* **25**:159–172.

34 Rodis JF, Quinn DL, Gary W, Anderson LJ, Rosengren S, Cartter ML, Campbell WA, Vintzileos AM (1990) Management and outcomes of pregnancies complicated by human B19 parvovirus infection: A prospective study. *American Journal of Obstetrics and Gynecology* **163**:1168–1171.

35 Mortimer PP, Luban NLC, Kelleher JF, Cohen BJ (1983) Transmission of serum parvovirus-like virus by clotting-factor concentrates. *Lancet* **ii**:482–484.

36 Peters MT, Nicolaides KH (1990) Cordocentesis for the diagnosis and treatment of human fetal parvovirus infection. *Obstetrics and Gynecology* **75**:501 504.

37 Sahakian V, Weiner CP, Naides SJ, Williamson RA, Scharosch LL (1991) Intrauterine transfusion treatment of nonimmune hydrops fetalis secondary to human parvovirus B19 infection. *American Journal of Obstetrics and Gynecology* **164**:1090–1091.

38 Pryde PG, Nugent CE, Pridjian G, Barr M, Faix RG (1992) Spontaneous resolution of nonimmune hydrops fetalis secondary to human parvovirus B19 infection. *Obstetrics Gynecology* **79**:859–861.

39 Weinbaum PJ, Keenan K, Samelson R, Pinheiro S (1992) Nonimmune hydrops fetalis: Spontaneous resolution after intrauterine infection with parvovirus B19. *Journal of Maternal and Fetal Medicine* **1**:96–99.

40 Whitley RJ (1990) Varicella-zoster virus. In Mandell GL, Douglas RG, Bennett JE (eds) *Principles and Practice of Infectious Diseases*, 3rd edn, pp. 1153–1159. New York: Churchill Livingstone.

41 Reuler JB, Chang MK (1984) Herpes zoster: Epidemiology, clinical features, and management. *Southern Medical Journal* **77**:1149–1156.

42 Harris RE, Rhoades ER (1965) Varicella pneumonia complicating pregnancy: Case report and review of the literature. *Obstetrics and Gynecology* **25**:734–736.

43 Hankins GD, Gilstrap LC, Patterson AR (1987) Acyclovir treatment of varicella pneumonia in pregnancy. *Critical Care Medicine* **15**:336–337.

44 Paryani SG, Arvin AM (1986) Intrauterine infection with varicella-zoster virus after maternal varicella. *New England Journal of Medicine* **314**:1542–1546.

45 Savage MO, Moosa A, Gordon RR (1973) Maternal varicella infection as a cause of fetal malformations. *Lancet* **i**:352–354.

46 Fuccillo DA (1977) Congenital varicella. *Teratology* **15**:329–330.

47 DeNicola LK, Hanshaw JB, (1979) Congenital and neonatal varicella. *Journal of Pediatrics* **94**:175–176.

48 Lambert SR, Taylor D, Kriss A, Holzel H, Heard S (1989) Ocular manifestations of the congenital varicella syndrome. *Archives of Ophthalmology* **107**:52–56.

49 Meyers JD (1974) Congenital varicella in term infants: Risk reconsidered. *Journal of Infectious Diseases* **129**:215–217.

50 Centers for Disease Control (1990) Summary of notifiable diseases – United States, 1990. *Morbidity and Mortality Weekly Report* **39**(53):51.

51 Byrne JLB, Ward K, Kochenour NK, Dolcourt JL (1990) Prenatal sonographic diagnosis of fetal varicella syndrome. *American Journal of Human Genetics* **47**:A270 (abstract no. 1062).

52 Cuthbertson G, Weiner CP, Giller RH, Grose C (1987) Clinical and laboratory observations: Prenatal diagnosis of second-trimester congenital varicella syndrome by virus-specific immunoglobulin M. *Journal of Pediatrics* **111**:592–595.

53 Isada NB, Paar DP, Johnson MP, Evans MI, Holzgreve W, Qureshi F, Straus SE (1991) *In utero* diagnosis of congenital varicella zoster virus infection by chorionic villus sampling and polymerase chain reaction. *American Journal of Obstetrics and Gynecology* **165**:1727–1730.

54 McGregor JA, Mark S, Crawford GP, Levin MJ (1987) Varicella zoster antibody testing in the care of pregnant women exposed to varicella. *American Journal of Obstetrics and Gynecology* **157**:281–284.

55 Weibel RE, Kuter BJ, Neff BJ, Rothenberger CA, Fitzgerald AJ, Connor KA, Morton D, McLean AA, Scolnick EM (1985) Live Oka/Merck varicella vaccine in healthy children: Further clinical and laboratory assessment. *Journal of the American Medical Association* **254**:2435–2439.

56 Centers for Disease Control (1991) Update on adult immunization: Recommendations of the Immunization Practices Advisory Committee (ACIP). *Morbidity and Mortality Weekly Report* **40**(No.RR–12):49–50.

57 Landsberger EJ, Hager WD, Grossman JH (1986) Successful management of varicella pneumonia complicating pregnancy: A report of three cases. *Journal of Reproductive Medicine* **31**:311–314.

58 Eder SE, Apuzzio JJ, Weiss G (1988) Varicella pneumonia during pregnancy: Treatment of two cases with acyclovir. *American Journal of Perinatology* **5**:168.

59 Stagno S, Pass RF, Dworsky ME Alford CA (1983) Congenital and perinatal cytomegalovirus infections. *Seminars in Perinatology* **7**:31–42.

60 Ho M (1990) Cytomegalovirus. In Mandell GL, Douglas RG, Bennett JE (eds) *Principles and Practice of Infectious Diseases*, 3rd edn, pp. 1159–1172. Edinburgh: Churchill Livingstone.

61 Griffiths PD, Campbell-Benzie A, Heath RB (1980) A prospective study of primary cytomegalovirus infection in pregnant women. *British Journal of Obstetrics and Gynaecology* **87**:308–314.

62 Stagno S, Whitely RJ (1985) Herpesvirus infections of pregnancy. Part I: Cytomegalovirus and Epstein-Barr virus infections. *New England Journal of Medicine* **313**:1270–1274.

63 Yeager AS, Grumet FC, Hafleigh EB, Arvin AM, Bradley JS, Prober CG (1981) Prevention of trans-

fusion-acquired cytomegalovirus infections in newborn infants. *Journal of Pediatrics* **98**:281–287.

64   Hersman J, Meyers JD, Thomas ED, Buckner CD, Clift R (1982) The effect of granulocyte transfusions on the incidence of cytomegalovirus infection after allogeneic marrow transplantation. *Annals of Internal Medicine* **96**:149–152.

65   Stagno S, Reynolds DW, Pass RF, Alford CA (1980) Breast milk and the risk of cytomegalovirus infection. *New England Journal of Medicine* **302**:1073–1076.

66   Gurevich I, Cunha BA (1981) Nonparental transmission of cytomegalovirus in a neonatal intensive care unit. *Lancet* **ii**:222–224.

67   Pass RF, Little EA, Stagno S, Britt WJ, Alford CA (1987) Young children as a probable source of maternal and congenital cytomegalovirus infection. *New England Journal of Medicine* **316**:1366–1370.

68   Krech U (1973) Complement-fixing antibodies against cytomegalovirus in different parts of the world. *Bulletin of the World Health Organization* **49**:103–106.

69   Stagno S, Pass RF, Cloud G, Britt WJ, Henderson RE, Walton PD, Veren DA, Page F, Alford CA (1986) Primary cytomegalovirus infection in pregnancy: Incidence transmission to fetus, and clinical outcome. *Journal of the American Medical Association* **256**:1904–1908.

70   Preece PM, Tookey P, Ades A, Peckham CS (1986) Congenital cytomegalovirus infection: Predisposing maternal factors. *Journal of Epidemiology and Community Health* **40**:205–209.

71   Chandler SH, Handsfield HH, McDougall JK (1987) Isolation of multiple strains of cytomegalovirus from women attending a clinic for sexually transmitted diseases. *Journal of Infectious Diseases* **155**:655–660.

72   Chretien JH, McGinnis CG, Muller A (1977) Venereal causes of cytomegalovirus mononucleosis. *Journal of the American Medical Association* **238**:1644–1645.

73   Lang DJ, Kummer JF (1972) Demonstration of cytomegalovirus in semen. *New England Journal of Medicine* **287**:756–758.

74   Yow MD, Williamson DW, Leeds LJ, Thompson P, Woodward RM, Walmus BF, Lester JW, Six HR, Griffiths PD (1988) Epidemiologic characteristics of cytomegalovirus infection in mothers and their infants. *American Journal of Obstetrics and Gynecology* **158**:1189–1195.

75   Fowler KB, Stagno S, Pass RF, Britt WJ, Boll TJ, Alford CA (1992) The outcome of congenital cytomegalovirus infection in relation to maternal antibody status. *New England Journal of Medicine* **326**:663–667.

76   Kumar ML, Nankervis GA (1979) Cytomegalovirus infections. *Southern Medical Journal* **72**:854–861.

77   Demmler G, Six H, Hurst M, Yow M (1986) Enzyme-linked immunosorbent assay for the detection of IgM-class antibodies against cytomegalovirus. *Journal of Infectious Diseases* **153**:1152–1155.

78   Griffiths PD, Stagno S, Pass RF, Smith RJ, Alford CA (1982) Infection with cytomegalovirus during pregnancy: Specific IgM antibodies as a marker of recent primary infection. *Journal of Infectious Diseases* **145**:647–653.

79   Schwartz DA, Walker B, Furlong B, Breding E, Someren A (1990) Cytomegalovirus in a macerated second trimester fetus: Persistent viral inclusions on light and electron microscopy. *Southern Medical Journal* **83**:1357–1358.

80   Grose C, Weiner CP, (1990) Prenatal diagnosis of congenital cytomegalovirus infection. Two decades later. *American Journal of Obstetrics and Gynecology* **163**:447–450.

81   Hohlfeld P, Vial Y, Maillard-Brignon C, Vaudaux B, Fawer C-L (1991) Cytomegalovirus fetal infection: Prenatal diagnosis. *Obstetrics and Gynecology* **78**:615–618.

82   Centers for Disease Control (1989) Sexually transmitted diseases treatment guidelines. *Morbidity and Mortality Weekly Report* **38**(No.S–8):39.

83   Gehrz RC, Christianson WR, Kinner KM, Groth KE, Balfour HH (1980) Cytomegalovirus vaccine: Specific humoral and cellular immune responses in human volunteers. *Archives of Internal Medicine* **140**:936–939.

84   Fleisher GR, Starr SE, Friedman HM, Plotkin SA (1982) Vaccination of pediatric nurses with live attenuated cytomegalovirus. *American Journal of Diseases of Children* **136**:294–296.

85   Centers for Disease Control (1991) Update on adult immunization: Recommendations of the Immunization Practices Advisory Committee (ACIP). *Morbidity and Mortality Weekly Report* **40**(No.RR–12):69.

86   Adler SP (1989) Cytomegalovirus and child day care: Evidence for an increased infection rate among day-care workers. *New England Journal of Medicine* **321**:1290–1296.

87   McGregor JA, Rubright G, Ogle JW (1990) Congenital cytomegalovirus infection as a preventable complication of maternal transfusion: A case report. *Journal of Reproductive Medicine* **35**:61–64.

88   Landy HJ, Grossman JH (1989) Herpes simplex virus. *Obstetric and Gynecologic Clinics of North America* **16**(3):495–515.

89   Baker DA, Amstey MS (1983) Herpes simplex virus: Biology, epidemiology, and clinical infection. *Seminars in Perinatology* **7**(1):1–8.

90   Rooney JF, Felser JM, Ostrove JM, Straus SE (1986) Acquisition of genital herpes from an asymptomatic sexual partner. *New England Journal of Medicine* **314**:1561–1564.

91   Whitley RJ, Soong S-J, Linneman C, Liu C, Pazin G, Alford CA (1982) Herpes simplex encephalitis: Clinical assessment. *Journal of the American Medical Association* **247**:317–320.

92   Rubin MH, Ward DM, Painter CJ (1985) Fulminant hepatic failure caused by genital herpes in a healthy person. *Journal of the American Medical Association* **253**:1299–1301.

93   Lafferty WE, Coombs RW, Benedetti J, Critchlow C, Corey L (1987) Recurrences after oral and genital herpes simplex virus infection: Influence of site of infection and viral type. *New England Journal of Medicine* **316**:1444–1449.

94   Gonik B, Loo LS, West S, Kohl S (1987) Natural killer cell cytotoxicity and antibody-dependent cellular cytotoxicity to herpes simplex virus-infected cells in

human pregnancy. *American Journal of Reproduction, Immunology and Microbiology* **13**:23–26.

95 Lagrew DC, Furlow TG, Hager WD, Yarrish RL (1984) Disseminated herpes simplex virus infection in pregnancy: Successful treatment with acyclovir. *Journal of the American Medical Association* **252**:2058–2059.

96 Brown ZA, Vontver LA, Benedetti J, Critchlow CW, Sells CJ, Berry S, Corey L (1987) Effects on infants of a first episode of genital herpes during pregnancy. *New England Journal of Medicine* **317**:1246–1251.

97 Whitley RJ, Corey L, Arvin A, Lakeman FD, Sumaya CV, Wright PF, Dunkle LM, Steele R, Soong S-J, Nahmias AJ, Alford CA, Powell DA, Joaquin VS (1988) Changing presentation of herpes simplex virus infection in neonates. *Journal of Infectious Diseases* **158**:109–116.

98 Nahmias AJ, Roizman B (1973) Infection with herpes-simplex virus 1 and 2. *New England Journal of Medicine* **289**:667–674, 719–725, 781–789.

99 Corey L, Spear PG (1986) Infections with herpes simplex virus. *New England Journal of Medicine* **314**:686–691, 749–757.

100 Becker TM, Blount JH, Guinan ME (1985) Genital herpes infections in private practice in the United States, 1966 to 1981. *Journal of the American Medical Association* **253**:1601–1603.

101 Brown ZA, Benedetti J, Ashley R, Burchett S, Selke S, Berry S, Vontver LA, Corey L (1991) Neonatal herpes simplex virus infection in relation to asymptomatic maternal infection at the time of labor. *New England Journal of Medicine* **324**:1247–1252.

102 Arvin AM, Hensleigh PA, Prober CG, Au DS, Yasukawa LL, Wittek AE, Palumbo PE, Paryani SG, Yeager AS (1986) Failure of antepartum maternal cultures to predict the infant's risk of exposure to herpes simplex virus at delivery. *New England Journal of Medicine* **315**:796–800.

103 Catalano PM, Merritt AO, Mead PB (1991) Incidence of genital herpes simplex virus at the time of delivery in women with known risk factors. *American Journal of Obstetrics and Gynecology* **164**:1303–1306.

104 American College of Obstetricians and Gynecologists (1988) Perinatal herpes simplex virus infections. *ACOG Technical Bulletin* No. 122, November.

105 Stone KM, Brooks CA, Guinan ME, Alexander ER (1989) National surveillance for neonatal herpes simplex virus infections. *Sexually Transmitted Diseases* **16**:152–156.

106 Volpi A, Lakeman AD, Pereira L, Stagno S (1983) Monoclonal antibodies for rapid diagnosis and typing of genital herpes infections during pregnancy. *American Journal of Obstetrics and Gynecology* **146**:813–815.

107 Nerurkar LS, Namba M, Sever JL (1984) Comparison of standard tissue culture, tissue culture plus staining, and direct staining for detection of genital herpes simplex virus infection. *Journal of Clinical Microbiology* **19**:631–633.

108 Warford AL, Levy RA, Rekrut KA, Steinberg E (1986) Herpes simplex virus testing of an obstetric population with an antigen enzyme-linked immunosorbent assay. *American Journal of Obstetrics and Gynecology* **154**:21–28.

109 Baker DA, Gonik B, Milch PO, Berkowitz A, Lipson S, Verma U (1989) Clinical evaluation of a new herpes simplex virus ELISA: A rapid diagnostic test for herpes simplex virus. *Obstetrics and Gynecology* **73**:322–325.

110 Kulhanjian JA, Soroush V, Au DS, Bronzan RN, Yasukawa LL, Weylman LE, Arvin AM, Prober CG (1992) Identification of women at unsuspected risk of primary infection with herpes simplex virus type 2 during pregnancy. *New England Journal of Medicine* **326**:916–920.

111 Straus SE, Takiff HE, Seidlin M, Bachrach S, Lininger L, DiGiovanna JJ, Western KA, Smith HA, Lehrman SN, Creagh-Kirk T, Alling DW (1984) Suppression of frequently recurring genital herpes: A placebo-controlled double-blind trial of oral acyclovir. *New England Journal of Medicine* **310**:1545–1550.

112 Reichman RC, Badger GJ, Mertz GJ, Corey L, Dichman DD, Connor JD, Redfield D, Savoia MC, Oxman MN, Bryson Y, Tyrrell DL, Portnoy J, Creigh-Kirk T, Keeney RE, Ashikaga T, Dolin R (1984) Treatment of recurrent genital herpes simplex infections with oral acyclovir: A controlled trial. *Journal of the American Medical Association* **251**:2103–2107.

113 Baker DA, Blythe JG, Kaufman R, Hale R, Portnoy J (1989) One-year suppression of frequent recurrences of genital herpes with oral acyclovir. *Obstetrics and Gynecology* **73**:84–87.

114 Centers for Disease Control (1989) Sexually transmitted diseases treatment guidelines. *Morbidity and Mortality Weekly Report* **38**(No.S–8):16.

115 Boehm FH, Estes W, Wright PF, Growdon JF (1981) Management of genital herpes simplex virus infection occurring during pregnancy. *American Journal of Obstetrics and Gynecology* **141**:735–740.

116 Prober CG, Sullender WM, Yasukawa LL, Au DS, Yeager AS, Arvin AM (1987) Low risk of herpes simplex virus infections in neonates exposed to the virus at the time of vaginal delivery to mothers with recurrent genital herpes simplex virus infections. *New England Journal of Medicine* **316**:240–244.

117 Gibbs RS, Amstey MS, Sweet RL, Mead PB, Sever JL (1988) Management of genital herpes infection in pregnancy (Editorial). *Obstetrics and Gynecology* **71**:779–780.

118 Goldkrand JW (1982) Intrapartum inoculation of herpes simplex virus by fetal scalp electrode. *Obstetrics and Gynecology* **59**:263–265.

119 Robinson WS (1990) Hepatitis B virus and hepatitis delta virus. In Mandell GL, Douglas RG, Bennett JE (eds) *Principles and Practice of Infectious Diseases*, 3rd edn, pp. 1204–1231. New York: Churchill Livinstone.

120 Pastorek JG, (1989) Hepatitis B. *Obstetric and Gynecologic Clinics of North America* **16**(3):645–657.

121 Chen DS, Sung JL (1978) Hepatitus B virus infection and chronic liver diseases in Taiwan. *Acta Hepatogastroenterologica* **25**:423–430.

122 Popper H, Gerber MA, Thung SN (1982) The relation of hepatocellular carcinoma to infection with hepatitis

B and related viruses in man and animals. *Hepatology* **1**:1s–9s.

123 Hieber JP, Dalton D, Shorey J, Combes B (1977) Hepatitis and pregnancy. *Journal of Pediatrics* **91**:545–549.

124 Pastorek JG, Miller JM, Summers PR (1988) The effect of hepatitis B antigenemia on pregnancy outcome. *American Journal of Obstetrics and Gynecology* **158**:486–489.

125 van Os HC, Drogendijk AC, Fetter WPF, Heijtink RA, Zeilmaker GH (1991) The influence of contamination of culture medium with hepatitis B virus on the outcome of *in vitro* fertilization pregnancies. *American Journal of Obstetrics and Gynecology* **165**:152–159.

126 Baddour LM, Bucak VA, Somes G, Hudson R (1988) Risk factors for hepatitis B virus infection in black female attendees of a sexually transmitted disease clinic. *Sexually Transmitted Diseases* **15**:174–176.

127 Alter MJ, Coleman PJ, Alexander WJ, Kramer E, Miller JK, Mandel E, Hadler SC, Margolis HS (1989) Importance of heterosexual activity in the transmission of hepatitis B and non-A, non-B hepatitis. *Journal of the American Medical Association* **262**:1201–1205.

128 Alter MJ, Hadler SC, Margolis HS, Alexander WJ, Hu PY, Judson FN, Mares A, Miller JK, Moyer LA (1990) The changing epidemiology of hepatitis B in the United States. *Journal of the American Medical Association* **263**:1218–1222.

129 Centers for Disease Control (1990) Summary of notifiable diseases – United States, 1990. *Morbidity and Mortality Weekly Report* **39** (53):25.

130 Malecki JM, Guarian O, Hulbert A, Brumback CL (1986) Prevalence of hepatitis B surface antigen among women receiving prenatal care at the Palm Beach County Health Department. *American Journal of Obstetrics and Gynecology* **154**:625–626.

131 Summers PR, Biswas MK, Pastorek JG, Pernoll ML, Smith LG, Bean BE (1987) The pregnant hepatitis B carrier: Evidence favoring comprehensive antepartum screening. *Obstetrics and Gynecology* **69**:701–704.

132 Cruz AC, Frentzen BH, Behnke M (1987) Hepatitis B: A case for prenatal screening of all patients. *American Journal of Obstetrics and Gynecology* **156**:1180–1183.

133 Kuller JA, Meyer MP, Leonhard KR, Harger JH (1991) Efficacy of hepatitis B screening in a private obstetrical population. *Journal of Perinatology* **9**: 164–168.

134 Delage G, Montplaisir S, Rémy-Prince S, Pierri E (1986) Prevalence of hepatitis B virus infection in pregnant women in the Montreal area. *Canadian Medical Association Journal* **134**:897–901.

135 Descos B, Scotto J, Fayol V, Huet J-Y, Pichoud C, Hermier M, Ville G, Charvet F, Dargent D, Thoulon J-M, Trepo C (1987) Anit-HBc screening for the prevention of perinatal transmission of hepatitis B virus in France. *Infection* **15**:434–439.

136 Pesce AF, Crewe EB, Cunningham AL (1989) Should all pregnant women be screened for hepatitis B surface antigen? *Medical Journal of Australia* **150**:19–21.

137 Ohto H, Lin H-H, Kawana T, Etoh T, Tohyama H (1987) Intrauterine transmission of hepatitis B virus is closely related to placental leakage. *Journal of Medical Virology* **21**:1–6.

138 Goodlin RC (1976) Severe pre-eclampsia: Another great imitator. *American Journal of Obstetrics and Gynecology* **125**:747–753.

139 Immunization Practices Advisory Committee (1988) Prevention of perinatal transmission of hepatitis B virus: Prenatal screening of all pregnant women for hepatitis B surface antigen. *Morbidity and Mortality Weekly Report* **37**:341–353.

140 González L, Roses A, Alomar P, Del Valle JM, Garau A, Ferrer P, Maimó M, Llinares R, Blanco I, Lardinois R (1988) The maternal–infant center in the control of hepatitis B. *Acta Obstetrica et Gynecologica Scandinavica* **67**:421–427.

141 Infectious Diseases and Immunization Committee (1986) Hepatitis B: Update on perinatal management. *Canadian Medical Association Journal* **134**:883–886.

142 American College of Obstetricians and Gynecologists (1992) Guidelines for hepatitis B virus screening and vaccination during pregnancy. *ACOG Committee Opinion*, Washington, DC. American College of Obstetricians and Gynecologists, May, No. 111.

143 Arevalo JA, Washington AE (1988) Cost-effectiveness of prenatal screening and immunization for hepatitis B virus. *Journal of the American Medical Association* **259**:365–369.

144 Tada H, Yanagida M, Mishina J, Fujii T, Baba K, Ishikawa S, Aihara S, Tsuda F, Miyakawa Y, Mayumi M (1982) Combined passive and active immunization for preventing perinatal transmission of hepatitis B virus carrier state. *Pediatrics* **70**:613–619.

145 Kanai K, Takehir A, Noto H, Nishida M, Takahashi K, Kawashima Y, Igarashi Y, Matsushita K, Shimizu M (1985) Prevention of perinatal transmission of hepatitis B virus (HBV) to children of antigen-positive HBV carrier mothers by hepatitis B immunoglobulin and HBV vaccine. *Journal of Infectious Diseases* **151**:287–290.

146 Chen D-S, Hsu NH, Sung J-L, Hsu T-C, Hsu S-T, Kuo Y-T, Lo K-J, Shih Y-T (1987) A mass vaccination program in Taiwan against hepatitis B virus infection in infants of hepatitis B surface antigen-carrier mothers. *Journal of the American Medical Association* **257**:2597–2603.

147 Hsu H-M, Chen D-S, Chuang C-H, Lu JC, Jwo D-M, Lee C-C, Lu H-C, Cheng S-H, Wang Y-F, Wang CC, Lo K-J, Shih C-J, Sung J-L (1988) Efficacy of a mass hepatitis B vaccination program in Taiwan: Studies on 3464 infants of hepatitis B surface antigen-carrier mothers. *Journal of the American Medical Association* **260**:2231–2235.

148 Gottlieb MS, Schroff R, Schanker HM *et al.* (1981) *Pneumocystis carinii* pneumonia and mucosal candidiasis in previously healthy homosexual men. *New England Journal of Medicine* **305**:1425–1431.

149 Masur H, Michelis MA, Greene JB *et al* (1981) Outbreak of community-acquired *Pneumocystis carinii* pneumonia. *New England Journal of Medicine* **305**:1431–1438.

150 Bryan CS (1990) Is there divine justice in AIDS? Why

now, and not before? *Southern Medical Journal* **83**:199–202.

151 American College of Obstetricians and Gynecologists (1992) Human immunodeficiency virus infections. *ACOG Technical Bulletin*, Washington DC. American College of Obstetricians and Gynecologists, March, No. 165.

152 Lifson AR, Rutherford GW, Jaffe HW (1988) The natural history of human immunodeficiency virus infection. *Journal of Infectious Diseases* **158**:1360–1367.

153 Biggar RJ, Pahwa S, Minkoff H, Mendes H, Willoughby A, Landesman S, Goedert JJ (1989) Immunosuppression in pregnant women infected with human immunodeficiency virus. *American Journal of Obstetrics and Gynecology* **161**:1239–1244.

154 Minkoff H, Nanda D, Menez R, Fikrig S (1987) Pregnancies resulting in infants with acquired immunodeficiency syndrome or AIDS-related complex: Follow-up of mothers, children, and subsequently born siblings. *Obstetrics and Gynecology* **69**:288–291.

155 Selwyn PA, Schoenbaum EE, Davenny K, Robertson VJ, Feingold AR, Shulman JF, Mayers MM, Klein RS, Friedland GH, Rogers MF (1989) Prospective study of human immunodeficiency virus infection and pregnancy outcomes in intravenous drug users. *Journal of the American Medical Association* **261**:1289–1294.

156 Minkoff HL, Henderson C, Mendez H, Gail MH, Holman S, Willoughby A, Goedett JJ, Rubinstein A, Stratton P, Walsh JH, Landesman SH (1990) Pregnancy outcomes among mothers infected with human immunodeficiency virus and uninfected control subjects. *American Journal of Obstetrics and Gynecology* **163**:1598–1604.

157 Centers for Disease Control (1992) The second 100,000 cases of acquired immunodeficiency syndrome – United States, June 1981–December 1991. *Morbidity and Mortality Weekly Report* **41**:28–29.

158 Centers for Disease Control (1990) Summary of notifiable diseases – United States, 1990. *Morbidity and Mortality Weekly Report* **39**(53):16.

159 Centers for Disease Control (1990) Summary of notifiable diseases – United States, 1990. *Morbidity and Mortality Weekly Report* **39**(53):15.

160 Sloand EM, Pitt E, Chiarello RJ, Nemo GJ (1991) HIV testing: State of the art. *Journal of the American Medical Assocation* **266**:2861–2866.

161 Food and Drug Administration (1989) *Guidelines for the Prevention of Human Immunodeficiency Virus (HIV) Transmission by Blood Products*. Rockville, MD: Food and Drug Administration.

162 Centers for Disease Control (1988) Update: Serologic testing for antibody to human immunodeficiency virus. *Morbidity and Mortality Weekly Report* **36**:833–845.

163 Conner E (1991) Advances in early diagnosis of perinatal HIV infection. *Journal of the American Medical Association* **266**:3474–3475.

164 Ciraru-Vigneron N, Lung RNT, Brunner C, Barrier J, Wautier J-L, Boizard B (1987) HIV infection among high-risk pregnant women. *Lancet* **i**:630.

165 Shapiro CN, Schulz SL, Lee NC, Dondero TJ (1989) Review of human immunodeficiency virus infection in women in the United States. *Obstetrics and Gynecology* **74**:800–808.

166 Lindsay MK, Peterson HB, Feng TI, Slade BA, Tillis S, Klein L (1989) Routine antepartum human immunodeficiency virus infection screening in an inner-city population. *Obstetrics and Gynecology* **74**:289–294.

167 Wenstrom KD, Zuidema LJ, (1989) Determination of the seroprevalence of human immunodeficiency virus infection in gravidas by non-anonymous versus anonymous testing. *Obstetrics and Gynecology* **74**:558–561.

168 Minkoff HL, Landesman SH (1988) The case for routinely offering prenatal testing for human immunodeficiency virus. *American Journal of Obstetrics and Gynecology* **159**:793–796.

169 Duff P (1989) Prenatal screening for human immunodeficiency virus infection: Purpose, priorities, protocol, and pitfalls. *Obstetrics and Gynecology* **74**:403–404.

170 Working Group on HIV Testing of Pregnant Women and Newborns (1990) HIV infection, pregnant women, and newborns: A policy proposal for information and testing. *Journal of the American Medical Association* **264**:2416–2420.

171 Lindsay MK, Adefris W, Peterson HB, Williams H, Johnson J, Klein L (1991) Determinants of acceptance of routine voluntary human immunodeficiency virus testing in an inner-city prenatal population. *Obstetrics and Gynecology* **78**:678–680.

172 Sperling RS, Stratton P (1992) Treatment options for human immunodeficiency virus-infected pregnant women. *Obstetrics and Gynecology* **79**:443–448.

173 Sperling RS, Stratton P, O'Sullivan MJ, Boyer P, Watts DH, Lambert JS, Hammill H, Livingston EG, Gloeb DJ, Minkoff H, Fox HE (1992) A survey of zidovudine use in pregnant women with human immunodeficiency virus infection. *New England Journal of Medicine* **326**:857–861.

174 Stratton P, Mofenson LM, Willoughby AD (1992) Human immunodeficiency virus infection in pregnant women under care at AIDS clinical trials centers in the United States. *Obstetrics and Gynecology* **79**:364–368.

175 Goedert JJ, Duliége A-M, Amos CI, Felton S, Biggar RJ (1991) High risk of HIV-2 infection for first-born twins. *Lancet* **338**:1471–1475.

30

Other Infectious Conditions

MICHAEL G. GRAVETT, JONE E. SAMPSON

INTRODUCTION

Infections are an important contributor to maternal and perinatal morbidity and mortality. Maternal immunosuppression that occurs during pregnancy may alter the natural course of many infectious diseases. Higher attack rates are seen in pregnancy for a variety of bacterial and viral infections. Some microorganisms indigenous to the female genital tract, i.e. Group B streptococci, are seldom associated with infection in the non-pregnant patient but are an important cause of infectious morbidity during pregnancy. Other infections, such as toxoplasmosis, are largely asymptomatic in the non-pregnant or pregnant patient, but may have a devastating effect upon the fetus. Thus, an understanding of infectious processes during pregnancy is important for those providing health care to pregnant patients.

Included in this chapter are a large group of infectious diseases not discussed in other chapters. These include common clinical infectious syndromes (urinary tract infection, intra-amniotic infection, sexually transmitted infections and vaginitis) which may be caused by a wide variety of microorganisms, and specific infections with variable clinical manifestations but which are caused by specific microorganisms (including Group B streptococcal infections, toxoplasmosis, tuberculosis and malaria).

Some aspects of fetal risk are covered in Chapter 49.

URINARY TRACT INFECTION

Urinary tract infection (UTI) is the most common bacterial infection in women of developed countries.[1–4] Furthermore, UTI is the second most common medical complication of pregnancy, second only to anemia, and without proper management may have a significant effect on the outcome of pregnancy. Urinary tract infection is 14 times more common in females than in males.[2] Non-gender related factors associated with bacteriuria in women include sickle cell trait/disease, and diabetes mellitus, as well as specific pathogenic factors of the infecting bacteria. Physiologic and anatomic changes occur in pregnancy which contribute to an even greater risk of UTI in pregnancy.[3]

The most noteworthy change in the urinary tract during pregnancy is pyelo-calyceal dilation. A combination of mechanical and hormonal factors contributes to this physiologic hydronephrosis/hydroureter. Compression of the ureters on the pelvic brim by the enlarging uterus and ovarian vein result in progressive dilation of the calyces, renal pelves and ureters. This condition begins at the end of the first trimester and can persist as late as 12 weeks postpartum.

Hormonal influences may play a role in decreased ureteral muscle tone and peristalsis, but cannot explain why hydronephrosis is more marked on the right side, nor why it does not occur below the pelvic brim. Bladder capacity increases during pregnancy, probably as a result of progesterone effect on the smooth muscle. Upward displacement of the bladder into the abdomen results in the elongation of the urethra. Finally, incomplete emptying of the bladder predisposes the pregnant female to vesicoureteral reflux and contributes to urinary stasis, facilitating ascending bacterial migration.

Physiologic alterations of the urinary tract in pregnancy include changes in renal hemodynamics and fluid and electrolyte regulation. The 50% increase in blood volume and concurrent increase in cardiac output during pregnancy significantly increase the demands placed on the kidney. Increasing renal blood flow and glomerular filtration rate compensate for the volume expansion. The urine becomes more alkaline during pregnancy due to increased excretion of bicarbonate. There is increased glycosuria and proteinuria as well as increased levels of estrogen excretion, all of which have been shown to enhance the growth of bacteria, especially *Escherichia coli*.

Maternal/Fetal Risks

Four major forms of UTI are recognized: asymptomatic bacteriuria, cystitis, pyelonephritis and acute urethral syndrome. Regardless of the terminology, the basic disease process, causative organisms and therapeutic goals remain the same.

Asymptomatic bacteriuria is among the most common of the clinical entities seen in pregnancy. The prevalence of asymptomatic bacteriuria in pregnant women is approximately 6%, with a range of 2–11%.[2,5–8] If untreated, 30–50% of pregnant women with asymptomatic bacteriuria will develop pyelonephritis.[5,6,8] The relationship between asymptomatic bacteriuria and preterm and low-birthweight infants remains controversial. There exist numerous studies to support the role of asymptomatic bacteriuria in the development of preterm labor and the delivery of small-for-gestation age infants.[5,8,9] Conversely, many workers have failed to confirm an association between asymptomatic bacteriuria and preterm delivery or low-birthweight infants.[6,7] An association between bacteriuria and congenital anomalies has been suggested but the establishment of a causal relationship awaits further investigation.[5]

Acute cystitis complicates less than 2% of all pregnancies and presents most often in the second trimester, usually in patients with a negative initial screen for bacteriuria. The diagnosis of acute cystitis is based on urinary urgency and frequency, dysuria and suprapubic discomfort in the absence of systemic symptoms such as fever, and costovertebral-angle tenderness. Hematuria may be present. Cases with symptoms of UTI but without evidence of bacteriologic infection may be called the acute urethral syndrome, which is usually associated with chlamydia infection. There does not appear to be a correlation between cystitis in pregnancy and pyelonephritis.

Acute pyelonephritis has a reported incidence of 1–3% of all obstetric patients and is heralded by fever,

chills, nausea, vomiting and flank pain. The estimated recurrence rate of pyelonephritis during the same pregnancy is between 10 and 18%.[2,10] Pregnant women with acute pyelonephritis are at increased risk for preterm labor and delivery and associated intrauterine growth deficiency and perinatal mortality.[2,5,11,12]

The microorganisms generally responsible for UTI are representative of the normal fecal flora. *Escherichia coli* accounts for approximately 80–90% of all acute UTIs. Additional Gram-negative organisms responsible for UTIs include *Klebsiella* sp., *Proteus* sp. (especially in diabetics), *Enterobacter* sp. and *Pseudomonas* sp. The remainder of UTIs are caused by Group B streptococci, *Enterococcus* sp. and *Staphylococcus saprophyticus*. The latter is felt to be the second most common cause of UTI in young sexually active women. Additionally, *Chlamydia trachomatis* has been implicated as the major cause of acute urethral syndrome among patients with dysuria and pyuria but with negative urine cultures. *Gardnerella vaginalis* is also increasingly documented as a pathogen in UTI in women.

Access to the urinary tract may be gained in separate ways by pathogenic microorganisms. Bacteria from the intestinal mucosa or other septic focus may be transmitted hematologically, or from lymphatic communication between the bowel and urinary tract. However, the most likely source appears to be ascending infection from microorganisms inhabiting the perineum, vaginal vestibule, periurethral and terminal urethral areas. Post-coital voiding has been recommended as a method of decreasing the likelihood of UTI.

Diagnosis

The concepts of etiology, pathogenesis and treatment of UTIs were revolutionized by the introduction of quantitative cultures into clinical practice.[13] It is now recognized that a colony count of greater than 100 000 colony forming units (CFU) per milliliter in midstream voided urine specimen represents a true infection as opposed to sample contamination. Controversy exists with regard to intermediate numbers of aerobic Gram-negative bacilli.[14,15] This criterion for diagnosing infection remains the same during pregnancy.

Microbiologic confirmation of the pathogenic bacteria in the urinary tract should be accomplished. The presence of pyuria alone suggests infection but is not diagnostic of UTI. The diagnosis of asymptomatic bacteriuria is defined as the presence of greater than 10^5 colonies of bacteria per milliliter of urine, on two consecutive clean catch midstream voided specimens or one catheterized specimen without signs or symptoms of a urinary tract infection. Rapid alternative screening methods for pyuria and bacteriuria are currently available. The presence of leucocyte esterase is associated with specific byproducts of leucocytes within the urine. Additionally, the presence of bacteria which reduce urinary nitrates to nitrites may be confirmed by the Greiss test. The first morning specimen should be used for this test as bacteria must incubate in the bladder for at least 4 h to cause this reaction to occur. When compared with quantitative cultures, these rapid diagnostic tests show unacceptable specificity and sensitivity and therefore should not be used alone to diagnose UTI.[16]

Management Options

Prepregnancy

In patients with risk factors for UTI, a prepregnancy urinalysis may be helpful in identifying asymptomatic bacteria. Treatment of this condition, and symptomatic cases, prior to pregnancy is warranted.

Prenatal

Urinalysis should be an initial screening test for any new obstetrical patient. A urine culture should be performed only when the presence of pyuria, bacteriuria and nitrites are present. Studies have shown that the presence of pyuria alone has a low predictive value of a positive urine culture, as does the presence of bacteriuria alone. The presence of nitrites alone or in combination with pyuria or bacteriuria has a 75% accuracy in predicting positive cultures.

Prenatal screening programs include the use of urethral catheterization, clean catch midstream sampling, and suprapubic aspiration when evaluating for bacteriuria. The least invasive of these approaches is the clean catch method, which involves cleansing of the introitus and voiding into a sterile container after discarding the first and last few milliliters of urine. The use of catheterization minimizes the risk of contamination by vaginal flora but may introduce infection in 1–2% of out-patient cases and significantly more in hospitalized cases. Suprapubic aspiration is generally reserved for cases in which equivocal results have been obtained or in which it is the only method to obtain an acceptable sample.

In the majority of pregnant women, UTI develops from covert bacteriuria which antedates gestation. If untreated, greater than one-third of these women will go on to develop acute pyelonephritis, the most common reason for prenatal hospitalization in pregnancy. On the other hand, if the silent infections are treated, approximately 80% of upper urinary tract infections can be prevented. A small number of women (perhaps 1%) will acquire bacteriuria during pregnancy, with about one-third developing pyelonephritis. Thus it may

be beneficial to include repeat urinalysis at the beginning of the third trimester.

Treatment

Multiple strategies for the treatment of UTIs have been proposed. Since treatment of asymptomatic bacteriuria reduces the risk of developing acute pyelonephritis from 30 to 3%, the primary goal in the management of asymptomatic bacteriuria is prevention of serious complications. Multiple strategies for treatment of these entities have been proposed. A treatment regimen should be designed to maintain sterile urine throughout pregnancy, and also to minimize toxicity of the therapy to mother and fetus. The shortest possible course of antimicrobial drugs should be administered. Although it is agreed that all pregnant women should be screened and treated for bacteriuria, the treatment of choice and the duration of treament have remained controversial.

In the past, the treatment of asymptomatic bacteriuria was given for periods ranging from 10 days to 6 weeks. However, recent data indicate that single dose therapy utilizing any one of a number of antimicrobials will cure a large majority of the cases in pregnancy.[8,9,17] The most commonly recommended agents include nitrofurantoin, ampicillin and sulfonamides (except in the third trimester) and all seem to have equal efficacy (**Table 1**). Additionally, beta-lactam antibiotics have no known fetal risks and thus can be used safely at any time during pregnancy. Due to an increasing resistance rate to oral penicillins, oral cephalosporins are utilized in UTI and asymptomatic bacteriuria in obstetric patients, particularly those with penicillin allergies. The newly introduced quinolones, although effective, are not approved for use in pregnancy.

Single dose therapy for the treatment of symptomatic cystitis has not been studied in pregnancy. Pregnant patients with acute cystitis should be treated with a 7–14 day course of therapy with the same agents

Table 1
Treatment of UTI in pregnant women

Agent	Therapeutic regimen	
	7–10 days	Single-dose therapy[a]
Nitrofurantoin	100 mg nightly or 2 times daily	200 mg
Ampicillin	500 mg 4 times daily	2 g with 1 g probenecid
Sulfisoxazole	1 g 4 times daily	2 g

[a] Studied in asymptomatic bacteriuria only.

used in asymptomatic bacteriuria. All patients should receive a test-of-cure culture following therapy. Sensitivity testing should also be routinely used, since in some series, common uropathogens such as *E. coli* demonstrate a greater than 50% resistance to ampicillin. Recurrent infections are common and cultures should be repeated throughout the course of pregnancy.

Urinary tract prophylaxis should be considered in all pregnancies with urologic complications (i.e. ileal conduits, ureteral re-implantations and renal transplants). These patients are more prone to develop upper urinary tract and chronic infections. Antiseptic, antimicrobial agents such as nitrofurantoin may be used under these circumstances, although one should be aware of the potential for the development of hemolytic anemia in patients with G6PD deficiency. Urinary tract infection suppression should also be considered in cases of recurrent asymptomatic bacteriuria, cystitis or bacteriuria following treatment for cystitis and in cases of upper tract infection. A significant reduction in the recurrence of upper urinary tract infections can occur with suppression; nitrofurantoin is recommended for suppressive therapy. In the event that recurrent bacteriuria is frequent or if there is difficulty in eradicating an infection of the urinary tract, an intravenous pyelogram may be indicated to look for signs of obstructive uropathy.[1]

The initial choice of antimicrobial agents for the treatment of pyelonephritis is empiric. The most common pathogens recovered from pregnant women with pyelonephritis are *E. coli*, *Klebsiella*, *Enterobacter* and *Proteus* species. Management should include hospitalization and the administration of intravenous antibiotics as well as intravenous hydration and careful monitoring. Serious maternal complications can include septic shock, respiratory insufficiency (ARDS) and transient renal dysfunction. Contracted blood volume should be corrected with aggressive intravenous hydration and laboratory monitoring should be performed including a complete blood cell count, serum electrolytes, creatinine levels, as well as urine and blood culture levels.

Because of the high prevalence of ampicillin-resistant uropathogens, intravenous therapy with second- and third-generation cephalosporins is now frequently utilized for initial therapy of acute pyelonephritis. Regimens include 2 g cefotetan i.v. every 12 h and 2 g cefoxitin i.v. every 6 h. If ampicillin is utilized, it is frequently given in combination with an aminoglycoside. The recommended dose for aminoglycosides is 3–5 mg/kg/day in three divided doses for gentamicin or tobramycin, and 15 mg/kg/day in three divided doses for amikacin. Anyone receiving an aminoglycoside should have serum levels monitored to ensure adequate dosage. Additionally, renal function should be followed by measurement of creatinine. Alternatively, aztreonam, given as a 1 g dose i.v. every 8 h,

may be substituted for an aminoglycoside. Aztreonam, a monobactam antibiotic, avoids the potential toxicity seen with the aminoglycosides and provides excellent coverage for Gram-negative facultative bacteria. Empiric therapy with ampicillin is 1–2 g intravenously every 6 h; total daily dosage may be increased to 12 g if necessary.

Obstetrical patients with pyelonephritis who fail to show rapid improvement after therapy should be evaluated for urinary tract obstruction. Failure to improve clinically after 72 h of therapy is felt by some authors to be an indication for adding an aminoglycoside to the intravenous antibiotic regimen. Urinary tract obstruction is evaluated with ultrasonography or with plain abdominal radiography as the majority of obstructions will be caused by urolithiasis and these simple tests will confirm 90% of these cases. If these tests are negative, then a 'one shot' intravenous pyelogram after contrast injection will usually permit detection of urolithiasis or structural abnormalities.

Current management of pyelonephritis in pregnancy mandates hospitalization with intravenous antibiotic therapy continued until the patient is afebrile with clinical improvement. This is followed by oral antibiotic therapy to complete a full 10–14 day course. The cost of this therapy is considerable and it has been suggested that oral therapy alone may be effective in patients who are not bacteremic, and who can tolerate oral medication.[18] Because of the potentially serious consequences of pyelonephritis in pregnancy, this regimen cannot be recommended until large studies demonstrate safety and efficacy.

Labor/delivery

Rarely does a clinician have to deal with UTI during the intrapartum period, unless preterm labor has been precipitated by this infectious process. Aggressive parenteral therapy is probably indicated, although oral antibiotics may be continued postpartum (or when labor is arrested) with lower tract infections. Of late, there has been a suggested association between infection, treatment of preterm labor, and the subsequent development of pulmonary edema. Caution should therefore be exercised in the management of these various confounding factors.

Postnatal

Repeated catheterizations, or an indwelling urethral catheter, during the labor and delivery process has been recognized to increase the risk of subsequent UTI. Although the routine use of a 'terminal urinalysis' with discontinuation of a catheter is not particularly useful, patients should be carefully questioned regarding urinary symptoms during the postpartum period.

URINARY TRACT INFECTION
Summary of Management Options

Prepregnancy

- Investigate renal function before pregnancy if recurrent infection (see Chapter 28)

- In such patients, treat and eliminate asymptomatic bacteriuria

Prenatal

Screening

- Regular surveillance for asymptomatic bacteriuria for all women in pregnancy

Treatment

- Asymptomatic bacteriuria (see **Table 1**)

- Acute cystitis
  - 7–14 day course of same antibiotics as in **Table 1**

- Acute pyelonephritis
  - hospitalization
  - i.v. hydration
  - i.v. antibiotics (change to oral when infection controlled)
    Options are ampicillin, a cephalosporin, an aminoglycoside, a monobactam
  - monitor clinical condition, CBC, urea, creatinine, electrolytes, urine and blood culture

- Frequent testing for recurrence of bacteriuria after treatment of any form of infection

- Investigate renal function, renal ultrasound and even i.v. urogram if recurrent or resistant infections

Prophylaxis

- Consider in all pregnancies with urological complications

Postnatal

- Investigate women with recurrent infection or pyelonephritis
  (? ideally after 12 weeks)

INTRA-AMNIOTIC INFECTION/CHORIOAMNIONITIS

Intra-amniotic infection (IAI) is an acute clinical infection of the amniotic fluid and intrauterine contents during pregnancy which occurs in 1–2% of all deliveries.[19,20] Other terms used to describe IAI include amniotic fluid infection, amnionitis and clinical chorioamnionitis. Intra-amniotic infection is a clinical diagnosis characterized by maternal fever, leucocytosis, uterine tenderness or other signs and must be distinguished from histologic chorioamnionitis. Histologic chorioamnionitis is a histopathologic diagnosis characterized by inflammatory cell infiltration of the membranes. Histologic chorioamnionitis occurs much more frequently than IAI, with an incidence of approximately 5% with term deliveries and greater than 50% in preterm deliveries and is usually not accompanied by signs of clinical infection. Unfortunately, many studies have not distinguished between these two distinct entities. The subject is also discussed in Chapter 12.

Maternal/Fetal Risks

Intra-amniotic infection usually results from the ascending spread following rupture of membranes and labor of microorganisms indigenous to the cervix and vagina. Recognized risk factors for the development of IAI include increasing duration of rupture of membranes and labor, use of internal fetal monitoring, number of vaginal exams in labor, nulliparity and the coexistence of bacterial vaginosis.[21,22] Intra-amniotic infection may also rarely result either from the transplacental hematogenous spread secondary to maternal bacteremia, especially for infections attributed to *Listeria monocytogenes*, or from the iatrogenic introduction of bacteria into the amniotic fluid following amniocentesis or cordocentesis. Additionally, subclinical IAI has recently been described in approximately 10% of women in preterm labor with intact fetal membranes.[23]

Since most cases of IAI represent ascending infections following rupture of the membranes, the bacteria recovered are representative of the flora of the lower genital tract (**Table 2**). The majority of these infections are polymicrobial in nature and usually involve both facultative and anaerobic microorganisms.[24] In one case control study, a mean of 2.2 microorganisms was recovered from the amniotic fluid of patients, with IAI.[24] Microorganisms associated with bacterial vaginosis, including *Bacteroides* sp., *Fusobacterium* sp., *Gardnerella vaginalis* and *M. hominis*, are frequently recovered from the amniotic fluid of infected patients in association with one another.[22] Among the facultative bacteria, Group B streptococci and *E. coli* are two of the most common isolates, and also account for over 60% of maternal or neonatal bacteremia.[20]

Intra-amniotic infection may result in significant perinatal mortality, particularly among low-birthweight neonates. In general, there is a three- to four-fold increase in perinatal mortality among low-birthweight neonates born to women with IAI.[19,25,26] There are also increases in the rate of respiratory distress syndrome, intraventricular hemorrhage and clinical neonatal sepsis.[27] In contrast to low-birthweight neonates, term neonates do surprisingly well in developed countries. There is little or no increase in perinatal mortality and the risk of sepsis or pneumonitis is also small among term neonates born to women with IAI. In some developing countries, however, intra-amniotic infection leading to congenital pneumonia is reported to be one of the most common causes of death among term neonates.[28]

Although IAI rarely results in maternal mortality, it may lead to significant maternal morbidity. Maternal bacteremia occurs in 2–6% of patients with IAI and postpartum infectious morbidity is increased. In addition, there is an increased risk of cesarian delivery among patients with intra-amniotic infection. Duff and associates reported a 75% incidence of dysfunctional labor and a 34% incidence of cesarian delivery because of failure to progress among patients with spontaneous labor who developed intra-amniotic infection.[29] The mechanisms by which infection leads to dysfunctional labor remain speculative.

Diagnosis

The diagnosis of intra-amniotic infection is primarily based upon clinical criteria. The most important feature is maternal fever that cannot be attributed to other recognized causes. Maternal fever is almost always present. Other clinical features include maternal peripheral leucocytosis, maternal or fetal tachycardia, uterine tenderness, or foul odor of the amniotic fluid.[19,30,31] However, these other clinical features occur inconsistently when compared with maternal fever and their absence does not necessarily exclude the diagnosis of intra-amniotic infection.

Because of the inconsistency of clinical features or maternal leucocytosis, various other adjunctive laboratory tests have been used to aid in the diagnosis of intra-amniotic infection. These have included measurements of maternal serum C-reactive protein, direct examination of amniotic fluid for leucocytes or bacteria on Gram stain, amniotic fluid culture, measurement of amniotic fluid glucose concentration, detection of amniotic fluid leucocyte esterase, detection of bacterial organic acids by gas-liquid chromatography, and assessment of fetal activity (biophysical profile) by ultrasonography. The efficiency of all these tests in the diagnosis of intra-amniotic infection has been extensively reviewed.[32] While all have reasonable sensitivity, specificity and predictive value, none are sufficiently sensitive or specific to be utilized independently of clinical signs and symptoms in the diagnosis of intra-amniotic infection. With the exceptions of C-reactive protein measurements and ultrasonography, these tests require amniotic fluid for analysis. Amniotic fluid may be obtained by aspiration through a transcervical intrauterine catheter in laboring women. However, for women with premature rupture of membranes not in labor, an amniocentesis is required to obtain amniotic fluid and is successful in only 50% of

Table 2
Microorganisms most frequently associated with intra-amniotic infection

---

Facultative
  Gardnerella vaginalis
  Group B streptococcus
  Escherichia coli
  Enterococcus

Anaerobic
  Prevotella bivia
  Bacteroides fragilis sp. or group
  Peptostreptococcus sp.
  Peptococcus sp.
  Fusobacterium sp.

Mycoplasma
  Mycoplasma hominis
  Ureaplasma urealyticum

Adapted from references 22, 24, 31.

these patients. Thus, amniotic fluid analysis may not be feasible or necessary for many patients with clinically apparent intra-amniotic infection. Amniocentesis and amniotic fluid analysis may be clinically more useful in those patients in preterm labor with intact fetal membranes and suspected infection.

Management Options

Prepregnancy

Not applicable.

Prenatal, labor/delivery

Women with intra-amniotic infection should receive antimicrobial therapy and be delivered. Since intra-amniotic infection is frequently a polymicrobial infection involving both facultative and anaerobic microorganisms, broad-spectrum parenteral antibiotics should be used. For most infections, single agent therapy is usually effective. Recommended intravenous regimens include cefoxitin (2 g every 6 h), cefotetan (2 g every 12 h), piperacillin or mezlocillin (3–4 g every 6 h), ampicillin/sulbactam (2 g/1 g every 6 h) or ticarcillan/clavulanate (3 g/0.1 g every 6 h). For more serious cases when maternal sepsis or severe anaerobic infections with foul amniotic fluid exist, combination antimicrobial therapy with a penicillin or ampicillin, an aminoglycoside, and a specific anaerobic agent such as clindamycin should be utilized. Under such circum-stances, many authors advocate initial therapy with a penicillin and an aminoglycoside, with the addition of clindamycin following delivery of the neonate. A reasonable alternative to this triple therapy may be sin-gle agent therapy with imipenam/cilastatin, a new car-bapenam antibiotic, given as 500 mg intravenously every 6 h, although its use in pregnancy has not been well studied.

Antibiotic therapy should begin in the intrapartum period, as soon as the diagnosis of intra-amniotic infec-tion is confirmed. Therapy should not be deferred until after delivery, unless delivery is imminent. Recent studies comparing intrapartum with postpartum treat-ment for intra-amniotic infection have consistently reported a lower incidence of neonatal sepsis with intrapartum therapy.[25,33,34] In the only randomized, pro-spective trial of intrapartum vs postpartum treatment, Gibbs et al. found significant reductions in neonatal sepsis or pneumonia in those receiving intrapartum treatment (0% vs 32% among those with postpartum treatment) and also found a 2-day reduction in the average neonatal hospital length of stay.[34] Maternal postpartum febrile morbidity was also reduced by intrapartum treatment. It is clear that the benefits of intrapartum therapy outweigh the potential disadvan-tage to the pediatrician in ability to culture the neonate without the presence of antibiotics.

Delivery should be accomplished vaginally when-ever possible in accordance with standard obstetrical practices. There is no advantage to cesarian delivery per se, and cesarian delivery increases maternal risk of postpartum febrile morbidity. When cesarian delivery

---

INTRA-AMNIOTIC INFECTION (CHORIOAMNIONITIS)
Summary of Management Options

Prenatal, labor/delivery

- Once intra-amniotic infection (chorioamnionitis) is diagnosed, management is:
  - give parenteral antibiotics (broad-spectrum or combination if severe sepsis)
    and
  - deliver (cesarean only for normal obstetric indications)
  - no clear evidence whether a time limit for delivery is advisable

Postnatal

- Continue antibiotic therapy (duration determined by clinical course and severity)

is necessary, there is no benefit to an extraperitoneal cesarian. There are few data regarding the effect of the duration of the time interval from the diagnosis of infection until delivery upon neonatal infectious morbidity. Several studies have found no increase in neonatal infections for an interval of at least 12 h from diagnosis to delivery in patients receiving intrapartum therapy.[19,26,30] Whether intervals longer than 12 h increase the risk of neonatal infection has not been determined. Until the safety of longer intervals has been determined, it may be prudent to consider cesarian delivery if vaginal delivery is not imminent after a 12 h interval from diagnosis of intra-amniotic infection.

Postnatal

The ideal duration of antibiotic therapy following delivery has yet to be defined. Recent observations have suggested that shortening the total duration of parenteral therapy to 1–2 days postpartum, without the addition of subsequent oral therapy, is efficacious. This presumes, of course, that a rapid defervescence has occurred, the patient is clinically well and that adequate out-patient follow-up care is available.

SEXUALLY TRANSMITTED DISEASES

Sexually transmitted infections are ubiquitous to all societies and countries. They are caused by a wide variety of bacteria, viruses and protozoa. In pregnancy, sexually transmitted infections may be associated with maternal infectious morbidity, fetal infections or stillbirth, and neonatal infections. A large body of evidence suggests that sexually transmitted infections may also be an important potentially preventable cause of prematurity. The importance of these infections in prematurity is supported by the correlation between chorioamnionitis and prematurity and by a large number of studies linking specific infections with chorioamnionitis or prematurity or both. The maternal demographic characteristics most strongly associated with high prematurity rates are young age, low socioeconomic status, non-White race, and primigravidity, all of which are also associated with increased risk of sexually transmitted infections.

Viral sexually transmitted infections, with the exception of human papilloma virus, are discussed in Chapter 29. This section will focus upon the commonly occurring bacterial sexually transmitted infections and also upon human papilloma virus.

SYPHILIS

Syphilis is a chronic infectious disease caused by the spirochete *Treponema pallidum*. In contrast to many other sexually transmitted diseases, syphilis is a systemic infection. *T. pallidum* can cross the placenta to infect the fetus at any stage of the infection, resulting in congenital disease or stillbirth. Thus, recognition and treatment of syphilis in pregnancy is extremely important.

The incidence of syphilis in the USA has steadily increased since the mid-1980s and was reported as 14.6 cases per 100 000 population by 1987.[35] There has been a concurrent increase in the cases of congenital syphilis as well. From 1978 to 1987, the USA reported a four-fold increase in the number of cases of congenital syphilis.[35] The greatest increase in the incidence of syphilis has been among urban minorities who, unfortunately, may not receive prenatal care.

Maternal/Fetal Risks

Syphilis is divided into three stages: primary, secondary and tertiary. After an average incubation period of 3 weeks (10–90 days), the primary lesion appears as a painless, ulcerated chancre. In women, this may appear on the cervix and therefore may not be detected. The primary chancre spontaneously represses after 2–6 weeks. Following this, there is a secondary stage during which widespread systemic dissemination of the spirochetes occurs. During this stage, the patient may have a generalized maculopapular rash involving the palms and soles, generalized lymphadenopathy and genital condyloma lata. These findings resolve spontaneously in 2–6 weeks and the patient enters a latent period in which clinical manifestations of the disease are absent. The latent period is divided into early latent (duration of disease less than 1 year) and late latent (duration greater than 1 year). Although latent syphilis is generally not sexually transmissible, transplacental transmission of *T. pallidum* may occur even during the latent period. If untreated, approximately one-third of patients ultimately develop tertiary syphilis characterized by involvement of the cardiovascular, central nervous and musculoskeletal systems. Manifestations include aortic aneurysm, tabes dorsalis, paresis, optic atrophy and gummas.

Transplacental transmission of *T. pallidum* leading to congenital syphilis may occur at any stage of the disease, although it is less common with late syphilis. Untreated maternal primary and secondary syphilis lead to symptomatic congenital syphilis in 50% of the neonates and also leads to a striking increase in premature births and stillbirths.[36] In untreated early latent syphilis, approximately 40% of the offspring have congenital syphilis and in late latent syphilis only 10%

have congenital syphilis, but the perinatal mortality rate is still increased tenfold.[36] Although it was previously thought that congenital infection does not occur until after 18 weeks gestation, *T. pallidum* has been identified in fetal tissue as early as 8 weeks gestation.[37] The clinical spectrum of congenital infection includes stillbirth, intrauterine non-immune hydrops, early congenital syphilis and late congenital syphilis. Most infants with early congenital syphilis are asymptomatic at birth and develop incidence of disease at 10–14 days of life. Characteristic findings include a maculopapular rash or petechiae, rhinitis or 'snuffles', hepatosplenomegaly, jaundice, lymphadenopathy, chorioretinitis and osteochondritis, which may lead to pseudoparalysis. Chancres do not occur. If untreated, late congenital syphilis will develop. The characteristics of late congenital syphilis include Hutchinson's teeth, mulberry molars, interstitial keratitis, eighth nerve deafness, saddle nose, saber shins and cardiovascular lesions.

Diagnosis

The diagnosis of syphilis is based upon the observation of *T. pallidum* spirochetes in infected lesions or upon serologic tests. Cultures for *T. pallidum* are not available. Direct examination of a smear taken from a lesion with darkfield microscopy with observation of the typical spirochetes is diagnostic for syphilis. Unfortunately, most pregnant women do not have lesions at the time of prenatal care, or may have an undetected chancre on the cervix. The diagnosis of syphilis in pregnancy usually depends upon serologic screening. All pregnant patients should be screened as early in pregnancy as possible, and in patients at high risk to contract syphilis screening should be repeated in the third trimester and again at delivery.[38] The two most commonly utilized serologic screening tests are the RPR (rapid plasma reagin) test and the VDRL (venereal disease research laboratory) test and detect non-treponemal antibodies.[39] These tests are positive in virtually all patients with secondary or latent syphilis and in most patients with primary syphilis. However, these tests may be non-reactive when the primary syphilitic chancre first appears and should be repeated 2–4 weeks later for patients with suspicious lesions. Specific antitreponemal antibody tests are used to confirm all positive screening tests. These specific tests include the fluorescent treponemal antibody-absorption (FTA-ABS) test, the microhemagglutination assay (MHA) and the *T. pallidum* immobilization (TPI) test. Most commonly used is the FTA-ABS test, which is positive earlier in the course of the infection than the RPR or VDRL and remains positive for the patient's lifetime even with adequate treatment.

Management Options

Prepregnancy

It is important to identify and treat patients with proven syphilis prior to pregnancy. Firm data are not available on the time period needed from initiation of therapy until conception can be safely undertaken. Empirically, the fetus should be adequately protected soon after the first injection. Serial RPR or VDRL measurements (monthly) should give an indication as to the successful eradication of this organism (see below).

Prenatal

The treatment of syphilis in pregnancy is directed toward both cure of the infection in the mother and

Table 3
Guidelines for treatment of syphilis

Early syphilis (pregnancy, secondary or latent syphilis of less than 1 year duration)

Recommended:
  Benzathine penicillin G, 2.4 million units i.m. in one dose

Alternatives (*not* recommended in pregnancy):
  Tetracycline HCL 500 mg orally 4 times daily for 2 weeks
  Erythromycin 500 mg orally 4 times daily for 2 weeks
  Ceftriaxone 250 mg i.m. daily for 10 days

Late latent syphilis (more than 1 year duration and cardiovascular syphilis)

Recommended:
  Benzathine penicillin G, 2.4 million units i.m. weekly for 3 consecutive weeks

Alternative (*not* recommended in pregnancy):
  Tetracycline HCL 500 mg orally 4 times daily for 4 weeks

Neurosyphilis

Recommended:
  Aqueous crystalline penicillin G, 2–4 million units i.v. every 4 h for 10–14 days, followed by benzathine penicillin G, 2.4 million units i.m. weekly for 3 consecutive weeks

Alternative:
  Aqueous procaine penicillin G, 2.4 million units i.m. daily and probenecid 500 mg orally 4 times daily, both for 10–14 days, followed by benzathine penicillin G, 2.4 million units i.m. weekly for 3 consecutive weeks

---

Adapted from reference 38.

prevention of congenital syphilis in the fetus or neonate. The mainstay of therapy is benzathine penicillin G, in accordance with CDC guidelines (**Table 3**).[38] Retrospective data suggest that benzathine penicillin G cures maternal infection and prevents congenital infection in 98% of cases.[40] Alternative therapy with other non-penicillin regimens is not recommended for pregnant patients because of treatment failures in preventing congenital infection, especially with erythromycin.[38] Tetracycline (500 mg orally 4 times daily for 15 days) is not recommended because of discoloration of fetal teeth and bones, but may represent a reasonable choice if no other alternatives are available. Ceftriaxone 250 mg intramuscularly for 10 days is also effective in adults for the treatment of early syphilis, but there is no information about its efficacy in preventing congenital syphilis. If non-penicillin alternative regimens are used during the pregnancy, the neonate should be very carefully evaluated for active disease and treated with benzathine penicillin G 50 000 units/kg intramuscularly as a one time dose.[38]

Patients with a history of penicillin allergy should receive skin testing for the presence of anaphylactic antibodies to both the major determinant antigen, penicilloyl polylysine, and to the minor determinant antigens, benzylpenicillin G and benzylpenicilloric acid.[41] Ninety percent of patients giving a history of 'penicillin allergy' do not, in fact, have a true Ig-E mediated anaphylactic reaction and can be treated with penicillin. Patients who do have an Ig-E mediated allergic reaction should be offered penicillin desensitization, as proposed by Wendel *et al.*[42] Their regimen is based upon increasing doses of oral phenoxymethyl penicillin to the endpoint of developing a temporary tolerance to penicillin (**Table 4**). Penicillin desensitization requires hospitalization and the availability of resuscitative equipment and results in only temporary tolerance to penicillin, but is, nevertheless, still preferable to treatment with alternative non-penicillin regimens. Occasionally, pregnant patients with early syphilis may experience a Jarisch-Herxheimer reaction after therapy which may initiate premature labor. Hospitalization is recommended for women beyond 20 weeks gestation when initiating therapy to permit early recognition and treatment of premature labor.

The role of lumbar puncture for examination of cerebrospinal fluid is controversial. Lumbar puncture is required for any patient with clinical evidence of neurologic involvement and strongly encouraged for patients with co-existent HIV infection or with latent syphilis of greater than 1 year's duration.

Following treatment, quantitative RPR or VDRL titers should be followed monthly until negative (or stable at a low titer of generally less than 1 : 4 for late latent syphilis). In general, the quantitative titer should decline four-fold by the third or fourth month after therapy for primary and secondary syphilis. Patients should be evaluated for neurosyphilis and re-treated for persistently high titers after 3 months, or for a fourfold increase in titer. Sexual contacts should be treated. In addition, because of the frequency of HIV infection among patients with syphilis, HIV counseling and screening should be offered for infected patients and their sexual contact.

Table 4

Oral-desensitization protocol in patients with allergies to penicillin

Dose[a]	Penicillin-V elixir (units/ml)	Amount[b] (ml)	Amount[b] (units)	Cumulative dose (units)
1	1000	0.1	100	100
2	1000	0.2	200	300
3	1000	0.4	400	700
4	1000	0.8	800	1500
5	1000	1.6	1600	3100
6	1000	3.2	3200	6300
7	1000	6.4	6400	12700
8	10000	1.2	12000	24700
9	10000	2.4	24000	48700
10	10000	4.8	48000	96700
11	80000	1.0	80000	176700
12	80000	2.0	160000	336700
13	80000	4.0	320000	656700
14	80000	8.0	640000	1296700

Adapted with permission from reference 42.

[a] Interval between doses, 15 min; elapsed total time, 3 h 45 min.

[b] The specific amount of drug is diluted in 30 ml water and then given orally.

Labor/delivery

Unfortunately, many pregnant women with syphilis still present for the first time to the hospital in labor. Direct examination of suspicious lesions with darkfield microscopy should be undertaken. Serologic screening should be done, but is not helpful acutely. Emergent treatment of the mother if delivery is imminent will be of no major benefit to the neonate. Therefore, a careful work-up of the infant after delivery, with direct therapy, is recommended. Maternal therapy, either intrapartum or following delivery, is of course needed.

Postnatal

The most critical feature of the management of the patient with syphilis is follow-up care. Serial serologic titer determinations are needed to confirm eradication of this disease. There is no contradiction to breast-feeding in the treated patient.

GONORRHEA

Gonorrhea is a common sexually transmitted disease caused by *Neisseria gonorrhoeae*, a Gram-negative diplococci. The prevalence of gonococcal infection in pregnancy varies, depending upon the population studied, from 0.5 to 7.4% in the USA.[43,44] Risk factors for gonococcal infection include multiple sexual partners, young age, non-White race, low socioeconomic status and being unmarried.

Maternal/Fetal Risks

The most prevalent type of gonococcal infection in pregnancy is asymptomatic infection of the cervix. *N. gonorrhoeae* may also cause acute cervicitis, proctitis, pharyngitis and disseminated systemic infection. The rate of pharyngeal gonococcal infection increases during pregnancy, possibly as a result of altered sexual practices.[45] Disseminated gonococcal infection (DGI) also occurs more frequently in pregnant than non-pregnant women.[46] DGI is characterized by a bacteremic phase associated with malaise, fever and a pustular hemorrhagic rash, and a secondary septic arthritis stage usually with asymmetric involvement of the knees, wrists or ankles. Acute salpingitis secondary to gonococcal infection may rarely occur during the first trimester but is rare after 12 weeks gestation because obliteration of the endometrial cavity by the pregnancy prevents ascending infection. In pregnancy, gonococcal cervicitis has been associated with premature rupture of the membranes, premature delivery, chorioamnionitis, and both post-abortion and postpartum endometritis.[47,48] In addition, gonococcal ophthalmia neonatorum may develop in up to 40% of newborns exposed to maternal infection and who did not receive ocular prophylaxis.

Diagnosis

Since it is estimated that up to 80% of women with gonococcal infection of the cervix are asymptomatic, prevention of sequelae of gonorrhea depends upon prenatal screening to detect infected parturient. Diagnosis depends upon the demonstration of Gram-negative intracellular diplococci within leucocytes of a smear obtained from an exudate, if present, or upon culture. Cultures should be inoculated immediately after collection onto a selective medium such as Thayer-Martin.

Management Options

Prepregnancy

Guidelines are similar for most STDs with regard to the identification and treatment of these diseases prior to pregnancy. Test of cure cultures should be done, as well as partner notification and treatment.

Prenatal

Uncomplicated gonorrhea in pregnancy should be treated with ceftriaxone 250 mg intramuscularly in a single dose or spectinomycin 2 g intramuscularly in a single dose (**Table 5**). In areas where penicillin-resistant strains represent less than 1% of the total isolates, therapy with aqueous procaine penicillin G 4.8 million units intramuscularly, or amoxicillin 3 g orally (both with 1 g probenecid orally) is an acceptable alternative. Because concurrent cervical infection with *Chlamydia trachomatis* is frequent,[49] erythromycin base 500 mg orally four times daily for 7 days should also be added, unless specific testing for *C. trachomatis* has been done. For disseminated gonococcal infection, hospitalization and parenteral therapy is recommended for initial therapy.[38] Recommended regimens include 1 g ceftriaxone i.m. or i.v. once daily, 1 g ceftizoxime i.v. every 8 h or 1 g cefotaxime i.v. every 8 h. Parenteral therapy should be continued until 24–48 h after symptoms resolve, and then converted to oral therapy for a total of 1 week of antibiotics. In areas where penicillin-resistant strains are uncommon, 1 g parenteral ampicillin i.v. every 6 h may be used. Identification, screening and treatment of sexual contacts of patients with gonococcal infection is recommended.

Tetracyclines and the quinolone antibiotics are also highly effective in gonococcal infections, but are

Table 5
Treatment of uncomplicated gonococcal or
chlamydial infections in pregnancy

Gonococcal infections
Recommended:
  Ceftriaxone 250 mg i.m.

Alternative:
  Spectinomycin 2 g i.m.
  Aqueous procaine penicillin G, 4.8 million units i.m., or
  amoxicillin 3 g orally, both with probenecid 1 g orally[a]

All regimens followed by erythromycin base 500 mg
  orally 4 times daily for 7 days

Chlamydial infections
Recommended:
  Erythromycin base 500 mg orally 4 times daily for
    14 days

Alternative:
  Erythromycin base 250 mg orally 4 times daily for
    7 days
  Erythromycin ethylsuccinate 800 mg orally 4 times
    daily for 14 days
  Amoxicillin 500 mg orally 3 times daily for 7 days
  Clindamycin 450 mg orally 4 times daily
  Azithromycin 1 g orally once

[a] Recommended only if infection source known not to have
penicillin-resistant gonorrhea.

contraindicated in pregnancy because of possible
adverse fetal effects.

Labor/delivery

Rapid diagnostic screening tools such as Gram-stain
and immune-based assays are available in most larger
institutions. These can be useful in evaluating the laboring patient with a suspicious history or lesion. Intrapartum treatment of the mother may reduce the neonate's risk for infection, although specific treatment of
the infant after delivery is usually done.

Postnatal

See the section on syphilis. Test of cure cultures should
be done. Careful counseling is needed regarding contraception and avoidance of this and other STDs.

CHLAMYDIA TRACHOMATIS

Chlamydia trachomatis is one of the most prevalent
sexually transmitted bacterial infections in the world,
and may be the most prevalent sexually transmitted

bacteria in the USA.[50] Chlamydia are obligate intracellular organisms. *Chlamydia trachomatis* may be differentiated into 15 serotypes. Serotypes A, B and C
cause endemic trachoma, a chronic ocular infection
considered to be the leading cause of blindness in the
world. Serotypes L1, L2 and L3 cause lymphogranuloma venereum (discussed below). Serotypes D through
K cause genital and ocular infections, discussed in this
section. The prevalence of genital infection in pregnant
women in the USA has been reported as between 2
and 37%, with an average estimate of 5–7%.[51–53] Risk
factors for cervical infection include young age, non-
marital status, multiple sexual partners and previous
history of sexually transmitted disease.[50]

Maternal/Fetal Risks

The majority of infected patients have asymptomatic
cervical infection. In the non-pregnant female, chlamydial infections may cause mucopurulent cervicitis,
endometritis, acute salpingitis, infertility and ectopic
pregnancy, or acute urethral syndrome. The role of
maternal chlamydial infection in pregnancy is more
controversial. Several studies have found an association between maternal cervical infection and preterm
delivery, premature rupture of the membranes, low
birthweight, perinatal death and late onset postpartum
endometritis.[54–57] Two prospective studies have found
that only those women with recently acquired infection, as detected by the presence of IgM serum antibody to *C. trachomatis*, are at increased risk for premature rupture of membranes, preterm delivery and low
birthweight.[53,58] Treatment and eradication of maternal
cervical chlamydial infection reduced the risk of
premature rupture of the membranes and premature
delivery in one study.[59] Thus, the available data suggest an association between maternal chlamydial infection and adverse pregnancy outcome. The magnitude
of this association is probably modest and may depend
upon maternal immune status.

Maternal chlamydial infection also poses significant
risk to the neonate. Approximately 50–60% of the neonates delivered vaginally to women with chlamydial
cervicitis will be colonized with *C. trachomatis*.[52] The
most common manifestations of neonatal infection are
inclusion conjunctivitis and pneumonia. Altogether,
18–50% of exposed infants develop conjunctivitis
within the first 2 weeks of life, and 11–18% will
develop pneumonia in the first 4 months of life.

Diagnosis

The diagnosis of chlamydial infections is based upon
isolation of the organism, detection by monoclonal
antibody tests, and serology. Because chlamydia are

obligatory intracellular bacteria, isolation by culture requires inoculation onto a susceptible tissue culture cell line. Cell cultures are both labor-intensive and expensive and are not readily available to most clinicians. Antigen detection kits are widely available to detect chlamydia and represent a less costly alternative to culture. Two types of antigen detection tests are currently available. One utilizes direct fluorescent-labeled monoclonal antibody staining of smears prepared from clinical samples for microscopic examination. The other uses an enzyme-linked immunoassay to detect chlamydia antigen. Both tests are sufficiently sensitive and specific, when compared with cell culture, to be utilized as a substitute for cell culture. A microimmunofluorescent antibody test of sera is also available to detect recent or past infection, but is more useful as a research tool than for the clinical diagnosis of chlamydial infection.

Management Options

Prepregnancy

Chlamydia trachomatis is susceptible to a wide range of antibiotics. For the non-pregnant patient, doxycycline 100 mg orally twice a day for 7 days, or tetracycline 500 mg orally four times a day for 7 days is recommended. Ofloxacin, a quinoline antibiotic, given as 300 mg orally twice a day is also highly effective in the non-pregnant patient.

Prenatal

In pregnancy, erythromycin base 500 mg orally four times a day for 7 days, or erythromycin ethylsuccinate 800 mg orally four times a day for 7 days is recommended (**Table 5**). If gastrointestinal intolerance occurs, these doses may be reduced by half, and therapy given for 14 days. Erythromycin estolate should probably not be used, since it may be associated with hepatotoxicity when given during pregnancy. Because erythromycin therapy is frequently associated with gastrointestinal intolerance in pregnancy, alternative regimens have been proposed. Therapy with either amoxicillin 500 mg orally three times a day for 7 days, or clindamycin 450 mg orally four times a day for 14 days, results in cure rates (98 and 93%, respectively) comparable to cure rates with erythromycin base therapy, and are better tolerated by the patient.[60,61] A single 1 g oral dose of azithromycin, a new macrolide antibiotic, is also very effective in the eradication of *C. tractromatis*, but experience with this drug during pregnancy is limited. Sexual contacts within the previous 30 days should be examined and treated.

Labor/delivery

See sections on gonorrhea and syphilis.

Postnatal

The incidence of neonatal inclusion conjunctivitis can be reduced by ocular prophylaxis at birth with 0.5% erythromycin ocular ointment or 1% tetracycline ointment, but not as well by 1% silver nitrate drops. Conjunctivitis that does occur, or pneumonia, should be treated with oral erythromycin for 2 weeks.

HUMAN PAPILLOMAVIRUS

Human papillomavirus (HPV) is the causative agent of condylomata acuminata (genital warts), juvenile laryngeal papillomatosis, and many cases of cervical intra-epithelial neoplasia (CIN) or cervical cancer. HPV contains a double-stranded DNA genome which persists as a latent provirus in epithelial cells after infection. Nucleotide sequencing of the DNA has identified over 60 types of HPV. Types 6 and 11 are found in greater than 90% of condylomata acuminata and also in laryngeal papillomatosis. Types 16, 18, 31, 33 and 35 are found in CIN and invasive cervical cancer.

Maternal/Fetal Risks

Epidemiologic data suggest that HPV infection is the most prevalent sexually transmitted disease. Although the occurrence of grossly visible genital warts is infrequent, sensitive detection tests utilizing dot blot DNA analysis or the polymerase chain reaction for detection of HPV DNA indicate that as many as 30% of sexually active women in the USA may be infected.[62] The prevalence of HPV infection in pregnancy is similar.[63] HPV infection in pregnancy is important for three reasons:

- genital warts may enlarge rapidly in pregnancy and mechanically obstruct labor;

- the association with cervical intra-epithelial neoplasia;

- perinatal exposure may result in the development of juvenile laryngeal papillomatosis.

Juvenile laryngeal papillomatosis represents the most common neoplasm of the larynx in infants and young children and usually occurs by age 5.[64] The symptoms range from hoarseness to complete upper airway obstruction. Laryngeal papillomatosis is thought to be acquired by perinatal transmission from an infected mother. A history of genital warts can be obtained from over 50% of women whose infants subsequently develop laryngeal papillomatosis.[65] However, the absolute risk of laryngeal papillomatosis following exposure to maternal infection is extremely low. Conservative estimates suggest the risk of papillomatosis developing in an offspring of a mother with HPV genital infection is approximately 1:400.[64] Thus, cesarean delivery to prevent infection cannot be advocated at this time, unless genital warts which obstruct the birth canal are present.

Diagnosis

The diagnosis of condylomata acuminata can be made visually by the appearance of white or pink verrucous friable growths. However, most cases of HPV infection are subclinical. Cytologic evaluation of the Pananicolaou smear may reveal evidence of infection in 10–30% of cases. If koilocytosis is noted on the Pap smear, liberal use of colposcopy and directed biopsies is warranted, given the association of HPV infection and intra-epithelial neoplasia. Colposcopy may identify up to 70% of infected cases.[62] Newer methods of detection utilizing DNA technology are very sensitive and specific, but are used primarily in research.

Management Options

Prepregnancy

Identification and treatment of these lesions in the female genital tract may be of some benefit, although recurrences are common. Patient counseling as to the potential risks as indicated above is recommended.

Prenatal

There is no single definitive treatment for HPV infection in pregnancy. Treatment is dependent on the size, location and number of identified lesions and entails the removal or ablation of all visible lesions. Due to the subclinical and multifocal nature of HPV infection, recurrences are common. Certain treatment modalities effective in the non-pregnant patient are contraindicated during pregnancy. Podophyllum resin, 5-fluorouracil, and intradermal injection of interferon should not be used in pregnancy because of concerns of fetal toxicity.

Topical application of 80% trichloroacetic acid (TCA) can be used for small lesions and is the least expensive treatment. It is not absorbed systemically and can be used in pregnancy. However, it has a cure rate of only 20–30% after a single application and, therefore, weekly applications may be required until the lesions are resolved. Cryotherapy with liquid nitrogen has also been successfully utilized in pregnancy and is a reasonable first-line treatment modality. Laser vaporization has been used successfully in pregnancy, although recurrence rates of 10–14% have been reported.[66] Since laser therapy usually requires regional or general anesthesia, it should be reserved for those patients with large or multiple lesions or with lesions refractory to TCA application or cryotherapy.

Labor/delivery

If patients present to labor and delivery with large, obstructive lesions, cesarean delivery may be necessary. There is no place for the elective debulking of these lesions at the time of delivery for two reasons: first, most lesions will regress to some degree after pregnancy; second, these lesions may be very vascular and obstetric hemorrhage may ensue.

Postnatal

Large lesions should be observed for secondary infection if they involve the episiotomy site. Sitz baths may be particularly useful in comforting and cleansing the perineal area with multiple HPV lesions.

GENITAL MYCOPLASMAS

Maternal/Fetal Risks

Mycoplasmas are a ubiquitous group of microorganisms that inhabit the mucosa of the genital and respiratory tracts. They differ from bacteria in that they lack a cell wall, but they are susceptible to antibiotics that inhibit protein synthesis. The two most common genital mycoplasmas are *Mycoplasma hominis* and *Ureaplasma urealyticum*. The prevalence of these two microorganisms in the lower genital tract in sexually active women has been reported as 40–95% for *U. urealyticum* and 15–70% for *M. hominis*. Their high prevalence rates among otherwise healthy women make it difficult to determine their role in adverse pregnancy outcomes. In general, *M. hominis* has been associated in some, but not all, studies with septic abortion, postpartum endometritis and postpartum fever.[58,67,68] *Ureaplasma urealyticum* has been associated with histologic chorioamnionitis, low birthweight and perinatal death.[69–72]

Serologic evidence of infection with *M. hominis* has been found in 50% of febrile abortions (*vs* 17% of afebrile abortions).[67] In a recent study of early postpartum endometritis among women, genital mycoplasmas, including *M. hominis*, accounted for 30% of the total endometrial isolates and 19% of the total blood isolates, but were usually recovered in association with other pathogenic bacteria, suggesting a mixed infection.[68] Also *M. hominis* has been isolated from the amniotic fluid of patients with amniotic fluid infection, but almost always in association with other bacteria, again implying a mixed infection.[73] Significantly, infected patients from whom *M. hominis* is recovered almost always respond to therapy with beta-lactam antibiotics which have no activity against genital mycoplasmas.

A number of studies have found an association between *U. urealyticum* and chorioamnionitis[70,72] and with perinatal death.[71,74] In one study, *U. urealyticum* was isolated as the sole isolate from fetal lungs in 24 of 290 (8%) perinatal deaths.[74] Twenty-two of these deaths occurred *in utero* and all but one were associated with pneumonia and chorioamnionitis, implying an ascending intrauterine infection. Some studies have also found decreased birthweight among offspring of women colonized with *U. urealyticum*,[69] but this association has not been confirmed by others.[58] Intervention treatment trials have also been inconclusive. McCormack *et al*. demonstrated an increase in birthweight among the offspring of women colonized with *U. urealyticum* treated with erythromycin in the third trimester when compared with colonized women treated with placebo.[75] Since the presence of other potential genital pathogens was not ascertained, their potentially confounding influence upon birthweight cannot be excluded. In contrast, Eschenbach *et al*. found no beneficial effect of erythromycin taken for up to 14 weeks by a large cohort of women colonized for *U. ureaplasma* upon birthweight, gestational age at delivery, frequency of premature rupture of membranes, or neonatal outcome.[76] In this study, women also colonized with either *Chlamydia trachomatis* or Group B streptococci were excluded from analysis, eliminating any potential confounding bias from co-infection.

Management Options

Taken collectively, the data linking either *M. hominis* or *U. urealyticum* to adverse pregnancy outcome are inconclusive. At present, prenatal vaginal cultures for either of these mycoplasmas cannot be recommended. Current evidence does not support the treatment of colonized patients for the prevention of adverse pregnancy outcomes. If treatment is deemed necessary,

tetracycline is effective against both *M. hominis* and *U. urealyticum* but should not be used in pregnancy. *U. urealyticum* is also sensitive to erythromycin but is resistant to clindamycin; *M. hominis* is resistant to erythromycin but sensitive to clindamycin. Since the mycoplasmas lack a cell wall, they are resistant to beta-lactam antibiotics.

CHANCROID

Maternal/Fetal Risks

Chancroid is an acute ulcerative disease, usually of the genitals, caused by infection with *Haemophilus ducreyi*, a facultative Gram-negative bacillus. Although rare in North America and Europe, it remains an important public health concern in developing countries. Chancroid is spread only through sexual contact, and is much more prevalent in men than in women. The incubation period after transmission is usually between 4 and 7 days. A chancre then develops at the site of entry, beginning as a small papule which over the course of 1–2 days becomes eroded and ulcerated. Although the ulcer is usually quite painful in men, it is frequently not painful in women. In women, the majority of ulcers are on the fourchette, vestibule or labia minora. The classic ulcer of chancroid is shallow with an irregular border surrounded by erythema. The base of the ulcer is frequently covered with a necrotic exudate. Painful inguinal adenopathy develops in about 50% of cases and may lead to suppuration and spontaneous rupture if untreated. These buboes appear 7–10 days after the initial ulcer and are unilateral in two-thirds of cases.

Haemophilus ducreyi has not been shown to cause systemic infection or spread to distant sites and poses no special risk to pregnancy.

Management Options

The diagnosis of chancroid is based upon clinical characteristics and Gram-stain and culture of the ulcer or aspirated bubo. The Gram-stain may reveal Gram-negative rods which form chains but has a sensitivity of only 50%.[77] Cultures should be taken from the base of the ulcer and placed on selective media. Cultures are both sensitive and specific in the diagnosis of *H. ducreyi* infection, but may not be readily available. An enzyme-linked immunosorbent assay (ELISA) has been developed that is both sensitive and specific and may represent a good alternative when culture is not available.

Haemophilus ducreyi is susceptible to a variety of antibiotics, although resistance to sulfonamides and tetracycline has emerged which precludes their use.

Quinolones, which are very active against *H. ducreyi*, are contraindicated during pregnancy. Current recommended regimens which may be given in pregnancy include: (1) erythromycin base 500 mg four times daily for 7 days; (2) ceftriaxone 250 mg intramuscularly as a single dose; (3) trimethoprim/sulfamethoxazole 160/800 mg orally two times daily for 7 days; and (4) amoxicillin/clavulonic acid 500/125 mg orally three times a day for 7 days. Although evidence of fetal toxicity is lacking, trimethoprim/sulfamethoxazole is generally not recommended for use in pregnancy if other alternatives are available because it is a folic acid antagonist. Treatment of sexual partners is recommended.

LYMPHOGRANULOMA VENEREUM

Maternal/Fetal Risks

Lymphogranuloma venereum (LGV) is a sexually transmitted disease caused by *Chlamydia trachomatis* serovars L1, L2 and L3. It is characterized by inguinal lymphangitis, anogenital lesions and fibrosis with gross distortion of the perineal tissues. Although LGV occurs sporadically in North America, Europe and Australia, it is endemic in Africa, India, South-East Asia and parts of South America.[78] LGV is predominantly a disease of lymphatic tissue characterized by thrombolymphangitis and spread of the inflammatory process into the adjacent tissues. Three stages of infection are recognized: primary, secondary and tertiary. The primary lesion is characterized by a small shallow genital ulcer which appears at the site of infection after an incubation period of 3–12 days and heals rapidly and is associated with few symptoms. The secondary stage occurs 10–30 days later and is characterized by inguinal lymphadenitis, buboes, inflammatory mats of contiguous lymph nodes and loculated abscesses. The tertiary stage is characterized by a chronic inflammatory response with progressive tissue destruction, ulceration, fistula formation and lymphatic obstruction. Antibiotic treatment during the secondary stage will prevent these tertiary complications.

The course of the disease is not dramatically altered by pregnancy, and transmission to the fetus does not occur. However, infection may be acquired during birth and passage through the infected birth canal.

Management Options

The diagnosis of LGV is based upon clinical appearance, serology and recovery of *C. trachomatis* from infected tissue or its identification by the direct immun-

ofluorescent antibody test. The Frei intradermal antigen test, formerly used in the diagnosis of LGV, has now largely been replaced by the compliment-fixation test for *Chlamydia* group antibodies. This test is very sensitive and titers greater than 1:64 are diagnostic of infection.

A variety of antibiotics have been used to treat LGV. Non-pregnant patients and sexual partners of pregnant patients should be treated with tetracycline 500 mg orally four times a day or doxycycline 100 mg orally two times a day for 21 days. Alternative regimens which may be used in pregnancy include erythromycin base 500 mg orally four times a day for 21 days or sulfisoxazole 500 mg orally four times a day for 21 days. Late sequelae such as fistulae or strictures may require subsequent surgical repair.

GRANULOMA INGUINALE (DONOVANOSIS)

Maternal/Fetal Risks

Granuloma inguinale (GI) is a rare, chronic genital infection characterized by granulomatous ulcers. It is common in tropical climates and developing countries, but extremely rare in temperate climates.[79] Granuloma inguinale is caused by infection with *Calymmatobacterium granulomatis*, a facultative, Gram-negative bacillus. Although most infections probably result from sexual transmission, auto-inoculation and non-sexual transmission also occur. The infection is only mildly contagious and repeated close physical contact is necessary for transmission.[80] Following infection, the incubation period varies from 8 to 80 days. The disease begins as a subcutaneous nodule which erodes through the skin and slowly enlarges to form an exuberant, granulomatous heaped ulcer which is usually painless. Redundant, beefy-red granulation tissue may be present, giving an exophytic appearance to the lesion. In the female, these lesions are most commonly on the labia.

Pregnancy may accelerate the growth of these lesions. The effects of GI upon the fetus are not completely understood, but perinatal transmission at the time of birth through an infected birth canal has been reported.[81]

Management Options

The diagnosis of GI is based upon the clinical appearance of the disease. The diagnosis is readily confirmed by examination of a smear of a crushed tissue preparation of the lesion. The smear is stained with Wright or Giemsa stain and examined for Donovan bodies.

SEXUALLY TRANSMITTED DISEASES
Summary of Management Options

SYPHILIS

Prepregnancy

- Identify and treat prior to pregnancy
- Contact tracing and treatment
- Confirm response with serial serology

Prenatal

- Routine serological screening of all pregnancies
- Treat all with *T. pallidum* positive lesions (rare)
- Probably safer to treat all women with positive serology even if history suggests they have been treated in past
- Treatment guidelines in **Table 3**
- Consider desensitization for penicillin allergy (**Table 4**)
- Contact tracing and treatment
- Confirm response with serial serology

Postnatal

- Baby requires pediatric evaluation for evidence of infection
- Continued surveillance for maternal response to therapy

GONORRHEA

Prepregnancy

- Identify and treat prior to pregnancy
- Contact tracing and treatment
- Confirm response with follow-up cultures

Prenatal

- Give antibiotics (see **Table 5**)
- Contact tracing and treatment
- Confirm response with follow-up cultures
- Exclude chlamydial infection

Postnatal

- Screening of newborn for infection, though most units treat anyway

CHLAMYDIA

Prepregnancy

- Identify and treat with doxycycline or ofloxacin
- Contact tracing and treatment

Prenatal

- If diagnosed give antibiotics (see **Table 5**)
- Contact tracing and treatment

Postnatal

- Prophylactic antibiotic eye ointment to newborn (erythromycin or tetracycline)

HUMAN PAPILLOMA VIRUS

Prepregnancy

- Identify and treat lesions
- Counseling about risks

Prenatal

- Treatment options (depending on size, site and number):
  - topical 80% TCA
  - cryotherapy
  - electrodiathermy
  - laser vaporization
  - excision
- Contraindicated preparations:
  - podophyllum
  - 5-fluorouracil
  - interferon

Labor/delivery

- Avoid treatment at delivery
- Cesarean section may be necessary

Postnatal

- Vigilance for secondary infection

MYCOPLASMA

- If treatment necessary, use erythromycin

CHANCROID

- Treatment of patient and partner with either
  - erythromycin
  - a cephalosporin
  - ampicillin/clavulonate

LYMPHOGRANULOMA VENEREUM

- Erythromycin if diagnosed in pregnancy
- Fistulae/strictures may need repair after pregnancy

GRANULOMA INGUINALE

- Erythromycin or co-trimoxazole for a minimum of 3 weeks

Donovan bodies are the darkly stained organisms within cytoplasmic inclusions contained in infected mononuclear cells. Their presence is diagnostic for GI. Neither cultures nor serologic tests are available.

The treatment of GI for non-pregnant patients is tetracycline 500 mg orally four times a day for a minimum of 3 weeks. Chloramphenicol or gentamicin have been used successfully for resistant cases. In pregnancy, erythromycin base 500 mg orally four times a day or co-trimoxazole two tablets orally twice a day are effective. Treatment should be for a minimum of 3 weeks and until lesions are completely healed to prevent recurrence. Treatment of asymptomatic sexual partners is generally not recommended.

VAGINITIS

Vaginal discharge is one of the most common complaints of pregnant patients. The discharge may be the result of normal physiologic adaptations of pregnancy, or may result from infectious vaginitis, with a possible increased risk for pregnancy complications. The vagina has both a nutrient-rich biochemical mileau and a complex microbial flora. A normal vaginal discharge consists of water (primarily as a serum transudate), desquamated epithelial cells, microorganisms, electrolytes and organic compounds including organic acids, fatty acids, proteins and carbohydrates (primarily glycogen).[82] Normal vaginal fluid contains 2–9 species of facultative and anaerobic bacteria in concentrations of 10^9 CFU/ml.[83] Normally, facultative lactobacillus species account for the majority of the total organisms present. These microorganisms utilize the available glycogen, producing lactic acid which serves to acidify the vaginal pH to less than 4.5, inhibiting the growth of non-acid tolerant potentially pathogenic microorganisms and also producing hydrogen peroxide, a potent antimicrobial toxin to other microorganisms including Candida albicans, Gardnerella vaginalis and anaerobic bacteria.[83,84] When this complex relationship is changed, potentially pathogenic microorganisms indigenous to the vagina such as C. albicans or G. vaginalis and the anaerobes, may proliferate and cause vaginal discharge. Alternatively, sexually transmitted exogenous microorganisms, such as Trichomonas vaginalis, may disrupt the normal vaginal ecosystem and lead to vaginitis.

Pregnancy may also lead to physiologic changes of the lower genital tract which may predispose to vaginitis. During pregnancy, the vaginal walls become engorged with blood, lead to increased transudation, and the glycogen content of the vagina increases.[83] Elevated levels of progesterone seen during pregnancy enhance the adherence of C. albicans to vaginal epithelial cells. Finally, cell-mediated immunity is impaired during pregnancy, predisposing to candidal infections.

The three most commonly occurring causes of infectious vaginitis in pregnancy are bacterial vaginosis, candidiasis and trichomoniasis. Although frequently asymptomatic, these infections have recently been implicated in a variety of adverse pregnancy outcomes. Bacterial vaginosis has been associated with premature rupture of the membranes, preterm labor and delivery, amniotic fluid infection, chorioamnionitis and postpartum endometritis.[22,55,68,72,85,86] Trichomonas vaginalis has been associated with premature rupture of the membranes and a reduction in gestational age at delivery,[51,87] and Candida albicans has been associated with intra-amniotic infection.[86]

The diagnosis of vaginitis is based in large part upon the appearance of the discharge and microscopic examination of the discharge. However, microscopic examination is somewhat insensitive and accurately identifies only 60–70% of women with symptomatic infection. Cultures for Candida sp. and T. vaginalis are both highly sensitive and specific but are not widely available, and vaginal cultures for anaerobes or G. vaginalis are not useful in the identification of bacterial vaginosis. Other adjunctive diagnostic tests, as described below, are therefore frequently utilized in confirming the diagnosis of vaginitis.

CANDIDA VAGINITIS

Maternal/Fetal Risks

Candida vaginitis may be caused by many species of Candida, but the predominant species is Candida albicans, which is responsible for 80–90% of infections. The remainder are caused by Candida (Torulopsis) glabrata and other Candida species. These are saprophytic fungi which may be recovered from the vagina in 25–40% of asymptomatic women. Candida also accounts for approximately 25% of all symptomatic vaginitis among non-pregnant patients and up to 45% of vaginitis in pregnancy. In pregnancy, alterations in the vaginal microflora, glycogen availability and a depression in material cellular immunity may all contribute to an increased risk of Candida overgrowth leading to vaginitis. While infrequent, C. albicans has been reported as a cause of amniotic fluid infection.[86]

Diagnosis

Women with vaginal candidiasis experience vulvar and vaginal pruritis, external dysuria, and a non-malodorous flocculent discharge. Examination usually reveals an erythematous vulvar rash and a characteristic white 'cottage cheese' discharge that adheres to the vaginal walls. The vaginal pH is usually < 4.5 and no odor is present. Microscopic examination of material suspended in 10% potassium hydroxide reveals typical mycelial forms and pseudohyphae in 80% of patients with symptomatic infection. Because *Candida* species may exist in the vagina in low concentrations among normal asymptomatic patients, cultures are usually not indicated. Cultures should be limited to women in whom candidiasis is suspected, but cannot be confirmed by microscopic examination.

Management Options

Treatment by local application of antifungals results in relief of symptoms and eradication of the yeasts in 70–90% of patients. The mainstay of treatment has been with imidazoles. These are broad-spectrum antifungals which include miconazole, clotrimazole, teraconazole and butaconazole. These agents inhibit fungal ergosterol synthesis, resulting in disruption of the cell membrane. These may be given as a one-time intravaginal suppository or as either 3 day or 7 day courses of intravaginal suppositories or creams given once daily at bedtime. In recognition of the immunosuppression of pregnancy, most clinicians prefer a 7 day course of either suppositories or cream. These imidazoles are not absorbed systemically and are safe to use in pregnancy. Boric acid powder, in 600 mg capsules, placed intravaginally daily for 14 days are also 90% effective in eradicating symptomatic vaginal candidiasis and have the advantage of being very inexpensive.[88] While borate is poorly absorbed systemically in non-pregnant women, its absorption during pregnancy is uncertain. Thus boric acid should probably not be used during pregnancy if alternative therapies with topical imidazoles are available. Other antifungal agents which are systemically absorbed after oral or intravenous administration are also available and include ketoconazole, an imidazole, and fluconazole, a triazole. Both have superb activity against *Candida* species and are useful in treating systemic fungal infections or chronic, recurrent vaginal candidiasis in non-pregnant women. However, because of their systemic absorption and unknown fetal effects, these agents should generally not be used in pregnancy in the absence of systemic infection. Similarly, amphotericin B should only be used for serious systemic infection during pregnancy.

TRICHOMONIASIS

Maternal/Fetal Risks

Trichomoniasis is caused by *Trichomonas vaginalis*, a sexually transmitted anaerobic protozoa which may be recovered from 40% of women screened in sexually transmitted disease clinics, and from the prostatic fluid of 70% of the male contacts of the women with symptomatic trichomoniasis.[89,90] The prevalence of trichomoniasis in pregnancy has been reported as ranging from 12 to 27%.[91] Risk factors associated with *T. vaginalis* colonization include Black race, cigarette smoking, greater number of sexual partners and a history of gonorrhea.[91] It is estimated that approximately 50% of women harboring *T. vaginalis* are asymptomatic.[89]

In addition to vaginitis, *T. vaginalis* may also cause other infections of the lower genito-urinary tract including Bartholinitis, urethritis, periurethral gland infection and cystitis. While risk of infection to the neonate is low (less than 1%), vaginitis and cystitis may occur as manifestations of neonatal disease. *Trichomonas vaginalis* has also been rarely suspected as a cause of neonatal pneumonitis. Although the relationship between vaginal trichomoniasis and adverse pregnancy outcome has not been well studied, two prospective studies have found a decrease in mean gestational age at delivery and an increase in premature rupture of membranes among women infected with *T. vaginalis*.[51,87] Further studies are necessary to confirm these relationships.

Diagnosis

Women with trichomoniasis characteristically complain of a profuse and sometimes frothy malodorous, pruritic vaginal discharge. Dysuria and lower abdominal tenderness may also be present. On examination, a gray or yellow-green purulent discharge is frequently present. The pH of the discharge is usually > 4.5 and may have an amine odor after addition of 10% potassium hydroxide. Small submucosal punctate hemorrhages of the cervix, the so-called 'strawberry cervix', are present inconsistently. Microscopically, motile trichomonads may easily be identified on a saline wet mount by their characteristic pear shape, flagella, and rapid, jerking motility. Polymorphonuclear leucocytes are also present on saline wet mount microscopy and may be so abundant that they obscure the trichomonads. The sensitivity of the saline wet mount when compared with culture is 60%, but its specificity is near 100%.[92] *Trichomonas* cultures are easily performed utilizing Diamond's media and are highly sensitive (92–95%) and specific. However, cultures have limited practicality in the clinical setting, since 3–7 days are needed for growth before the diagnosis can be confirmed. Trichomonads can also be seen on a Papanicolaou smear with a similar sensitivity to the wet mount, but with a higher rate of false-positives. Other sensitive and specific rapidly performed diagnostic tests have recently been developed, including direct immunofluorescence assay, enzyme-linked immunoassay and latex-particle agglutination. These are not, however, in widespread use currently. All women with trichomoniasis, whether symptomatic or not, should have a culture taken for *Neisseria gonorrhoeae* because of the frequency of co-infection which exists.

Management Options

Because *T. vaginalis* resides not only in the vagina but in the urethra and bladder, systemic therapy is necessary for treatment. The only effective therapy for trichomoniasis is the nitroimidazole antibiotics, including metronidazole, ornidazole and tinidazole. Metronidazole is the only nitroimidazole available in the USA. Standard treatment with metronidazole consists of either 250 mg orally three times daily for 7 days or, alternatively, a single 2 g oral dose. Both result in a 90% cure rate and which regimen is followed depends upon the physician and patient. With tinidazole, a single 1.5 g oral dose is usually adequate to eradicate *T. vaginalis*. Patients should be advised not to drink ethanol for 24 h after the last dose because of a disulfiram-like effect of the medication. Simultaneous treatment of the male consort is required to prevent recurrent trichomoniasis in the female.

The treatment for patients who do not respond to the initial therapy is controversial. Metronidazole-tolerant and metronidazole-resistant strains of *T. vaginalis* do occur, but infrequently. Low to moderate levels of resistance (metronidazole-tolerant strains) occur in one of every 200–400 cases of trichomoniasis and highly metronidazole-resistant strains occur in one in every 2000–3000 cases.[92] Most cases associated with low to moderate resistant strains can be cured by oral administration of 2.0–2.5 g metronidazole per day, in divided doses, for 7 days. Most cases caused by highly resistant strains can be cured by increasing the dose of metronidazole to 3 g daily, orally, in divided doses, for 14 days. Alternatively, cures have been reported with the use of intravenous metronidazole, 2 g given every 6–8 h for 3 days.[93] Metronidazole-associated neurotoxicity may occur with longer courses of therapy.

Although cross-resistance to other nitroimidazoles among metronidazole-resistant strains occurs, it is usually incomplete. Altogether, 65–70% of metronidazole highly resistant strains are susceptible to tinidazole (not available in the USA). For those cases, treatment with oral tinidazole 2 g daily for 7–14 days has been highly effective in eradicating *T. vaginalis*.[92]

There has been some concern about the use of nitroimidazoles in pregnancy. Nitroimidazoles cross the placenta, and are mutagenic in bacteria and carcinogenic in some animals. However, human studies have not revealed any increase in the expected frequency of congenital anomalies among the offspring of mothers treated with metronidazole during the pregnancy.[94] Further, long-term surveillance studies of women treated for trichomoniasis have not found any increase in

the occurrence of cancer attributable to metronidazole.[95] Although evidence of fetal or maternal harm is lacking, the nitromidazoles should probably be avoided during the first trimester. As an alternative treatment in the first trimester, treatment with intravaginal 100 mg clotrimazole suppositories (a chemically related non-absorbed imidazole antifungal) daily for 14 days provides symptomatic relief in approximately 50% of patients with trichomoniasis. Beyond the first trimester, treatment of trichomoniasis with a single 2 g oral dose of metronidazole is probably warranted, given the possible association between *T. vaginalis* and adverse pregnancy outcome.

BACTERIAL VAGINOSIS

Maternal/Fetal Risks

Bacterial vaginosis is the most frequent vaginal infection of sexually active women; it occurs in approximately 20% of pregnant women.[55,86,96] In contrast to other vaginal infections, bacterial vaginosis cannot be attributed to a single pathogenic microorganism. Rather, the symptoms associated with bacterial vaginosis result from an increase in the prevalence and concentration of certain facultative and anaerobic bacteria normally found as part of the vaginal microflora. Specifically, there is an increased prevalence of *Gardnerella vaginalis*, selected anaerobes (*Bacteroides* sp., *Peptostreptococcus* sp. and *Mobiluncus* sp.) and *Mycoplasma hominis*, and a decreased prevalence of hydrogen-peroxidase producing *Lactobacillus* sp.[84,97] Additionally, there is a 100-fold increase in the intravaginal concentration of *G. vaginalis* and a 1000-fold increase in the concentration of the anaerobes.[97] Thus, the diagnosis of bacterial vaginosis does not depend upon the recovery or identification of any single microorganism from the vagina, but rather requires the recognition of the altered vaginal microbial mileau.

A relationship between bacterial vaginosis and adverse pregnancy outcome has been reported in several studies. Bacterial vaginosis has been associated with preterm labor or delivery, amniotic fluid infection, chorioamnionitis and postpartum endometritis. This assocation is based upon:

- case-control and cohort studies demonstrating an approximate two-fold increase in preterm labor or delivery among women with bacterial vaginosis;[55,86,96]

- the recovery of bacterial vaginosis-associated microorganisms from the amniotic fluid of 30% of women with intact fetal membranes in preterm labor and subclinical amniotic fluid infection (see reference 85 for a review);

- the frequent recovery of BV-associated microorganisms from amniotic fluid of women with overt clinical amniotic fluid infection[22] or from the chorioamnion of women with histologic chorioamnionitis or preterm delivery;[72]

- the recovery of *Gardnerella vaginalis* or anaerobes associated with bacterial vaginosis from the endometrium in over 60% of women with early postpartum endometritis.[68]

Little is known about the mechanisms by which bacterial vaginosis may cause prematurity. The increased intravaginal concentrations of bacteria may simply overwhelm the local host defenses, allowing for ascending infection. Alternatively, these bacteria could also produce protease or phospholipases which weaken the membranes or stimulate prostaglandin production.[99] Although the magnitude of the increased risk for prematurity noted in these studies is modest (approximately a two-fold increased risk compared with patients without bacterial vaginosis), the total impact upon prematurity may be much greater given the high prevalence (20%) for bacterial vaginosis in pregnancy. However, routine prenatal screening for bacterial vaginosis and treatment of asymptomatic cases cannot be recommended until adequate randomized prospective treatment trials have been performed to ascertain whether treatment reduces the risk of adverse pregnancy outcome. Until such studies have been performed, treatment during pregnancy should be reserved for symptomatic cases.

Diagnosis

The most common symptom among women with vaginosis is thin, watery non-pruritic discharge with a fishy odor. However, 50% of women with bacterial vaginosis are asymptomatic.

The criteria for the clinical diagnosis of bacterial vaginosis are well established.[98] These criteria include: (1) the presence of a thin, homogeneous discharge which adheres to the vaginal walls; (2) a vaginal pH of > 4.5; (3) the release of a fishy odor upon alkalinization with 10% potassium hydroxide; and (4) clue cells on a saline wet mount. The diagnosis of bacterial vaginosis requires the presence of three of these four criteria. The diagnosis of bacterial vaginosis can also be made by direct Gram-stain of the vaginal discharge. The Gram-stain is both highly sensitive (97%) and specific (79%) when compared with the clinical diagnosis, and offers the advantages of being easily per-formed, readily available and inexpensive with high inter-observer reproducibility.[98] Other diagnostic methods include gas-liquid chromatography and the proline aminopeptidase assay, but these are not routinely available.

Management Options

The treatment of choice for symptomatic bacterial vaginosis is metronidazole given orally in a dose of 500 mg twice daily for 7 days. This results in cure rates of 90%. A single 2 g oral dose of metronidazole is also effective.[100] However, as discussed in the previous section, there is concern and reluctance to use the nitroimidazoles during pregnancy, particularly in the first trimester. Treatment with other antimicrobial agents, including sulfa cream, amoxicillin or ampicillin, and erythromycin have resulted in very disappointing cure rates of 14–56% and cannot be recommended.

VAGINITIS
Summary of Management Options

CANDIDA

- Treat topically with an imidazole (miconazole, clotrimazole, teraconazole, butaconazole)

- Ketoconazole and fluconazole are best avoided in pregnancy except for severe systemic infection

TRICHOMONAS

- Treat patient and partner systemically with a nitroimidasole antibiotic (metronidazole, ornidazole, tinidazole)

BACTERIAL VAGINOSIS

- Intravaginal 2% clindamycin cream

- Intravaginal 0.75% metronidazole gel

Of late, clindamycin, an antibiotic with excellent activity against anaerobic bacteria, has been found to be highly effective in the treatment of bacterial vaginosis. Clindamycin given orally as a dose of 300 mg twice daily for 7 days has been reported to result in a 94% cure rate.[101] Two topical intravaginal preparations are also now available for the treatment of bacterial vaginosis. These include 0.75% metronidazole intravaginal gel, used twice daily for 5 days, and 2% clindamycin cream, used once daily for 7 days. Both preparations result in cure rates comparable with either oral metronidazole or clindamycin.[102,103] Since significant systemic absorption does not occur with either, it is likely that they will become the treatment of choice for bacterial vaginosis during pregnancy. Other agents such as acid lactate gel have been used in a limited fashion to help restore a more acidic environment to the vagina and may be useful when used prophylactically among patients with recurrent bacterial vaginosis.

GROUP B STREPTOCOCCUS

Maternal/Fetal Risks

The Group B streptococcus (*Streptococcus agalactiae*) has become recognized over the past two decades as one of the most important causes of neonatal infection. Although early reports in the 1930s and 1940s linked Group B streptococcus (GBS) with postpartum infections and neonatal meningitis, it was not until the early 1960s that the scope of perinatal and neonatal GBS infections became evident.[104] Currently, in the USA 11 000 neonates annually have invasive Group B streptococcal infections, with an estimated mortality rate of 20%. Additionally, maternal genital tract colonization with GBS leads to maternal infectious morbidity in approximately 50 000 women in the USA annually.

Group B streptococci are one of many serologically distinct species within the genus *Streptococcus*. Streptococci are facultatively anaerobic Gram-positive cocci, usually arranged in chains on Gram stain. The most important pathogenic streptococcal species for man include Group A (*Streptococcus pyogenes*), Group B (*Streptococcus agalactiae*), Group D (*enterococci*), *Streptococcus pneumoniae*, and *Streptococcus viridans*. Definitive identification is based on the presence of a polysaccharide group-specific antigen common to all Group B streptococcal strains as determined by serologic testing. Group B streptococci can be further subdivided into types Ia, Ib, Ic, II, and III on the basis of distinctive type-specific polysaccharide antigens. About 99% of strains can be typed into one of these five antigen types. Group B streptococci can be recovered from the vagina or cervix in 6 to 30% of pregnant women at some point during gestation. The rate of colonization does not vary with gestational age. There is evidence that the gastrointestinal tract is the major primary reservoir and that vaginal or cervical contamination and colonization occurs form a gastrointestinal source. The frequency of GBS isolation increases as one proceeds from the cervix to the introitus, and GBS can be recovered twice as frequently from rectal cultures as from vaginal cultures. Group B streptococci can also be recovered from the urethra of 45–63% of the male consorts of female carriers, implying that sexual transmission may also occur (see reference 105 for a review).

Neonatal GBS colonization may occur either by vertical transmission from a colonized mother as the neonate passes through the birth canal or by horizontal transmission, including both nosocomial spread in the nursery from colonized nursery personnel or other colonized neonates and acquisition from community sources. Overall, 3–12% of all neonates are colonized with GBS in the first week of life. Also, 40–70% of neonates born to colonized mothers become colonized, usually with the same serotype that is present in the mother.[105] In contrast, only 1–12% of neonates born to non-colonized mothers will become culture-positive. Several additional factors may modify or enhance the risk of GBS vertical transmission. Higher neonatal transmission rates occur when women are persistently culture-positive carriers or when women are heavily colonized with GBS as demonstrated by semi-quantitative vaginal cultures.[106] The site of maternal carriage is also important; vertical transmission is more likely to occur with cervical GBS carriage than with rectal carriage.[106]

The most important determinant of susceptibility to invasive infection after colonization may be maternal antibodies directed against the capsular polysaccharide antigens of GBS. Immunity to GBS is medicated by antibody-dependent phagocytosis. Mothers of infants with type III GBS invasive disease have lower serum levels of type-specific antibodies than women giving birth to asymptomatically colonized infants. This antibody, which has some broad reactivity to all Group B streptococcal types, is an IgG immunoglobin that readily crosses the placenta. When measured in mother–infant pairs, an excellent correlation exists between maternal and cord antibody levels. Baker *et al.* showed that 73% of 45 GBS-colonized mothers with healthy neonates had high serum levels of type III antibody in contrast to only 19% of 32 GBS-colonized mothers whose neonates developed early-onset septicemia or meningitis ($P < 0.001$).[107] Strain virulence is also an important determinant of disease. Although type III strains of GBS represent approximately one-third of isolates from symptomatically colonized infants, they account for over 85% of the isolates from early-onset meningitis or late-onset disease. Overall, type III strains account for more than 60% of isolates from infants with all varieties of invasive GBS infections.

Although most research has focused on GBS neonatal infection, GBS is also an important pathogen for maternal intrapartum and postpartum infections. Puerperal septicemia due to GBS occurs with an incidence of approximately 1–2 per 1000 deliveries, and accounts for up to 15% of positive blood cultures from postpartum patients.[108] Postpartum endometritis is reported to be more frequently observed among GBS-colonized parturients than among non-colonized parturients. GBS is also associated with clinical intra-amniotic infection, and is one of the most frequent isolates from amniotic fluid of patients with intra-amniotic infection.[25]

GBS has also been associated with premature rupture of the membranes and with preterm delivery prior to 32 weeks gestation in some, but not all, studies.[109] Recent studies have indicated that this association may be strongest for patients with GBS bacteriuria.[110] Thomsen et al. have demonstrated significant reductions in premature rupture of the membranes and preterm labor among patients with asymptomatic GBS bacteriuria who were treated with penicillin.[111] However, antepartum antibiotic treatment to eradicate GBS from patients with asymptomatic vaginal colonization without bacteriuria has not been demonstrated to alter pregnancy outcome. Thus, a causal relationship between GBS colonization and prematurity still remains to be established.

In the past decades, GBS has become a leading cause of septicemia and meningitis during the first 2 months of life in neonates. From reported current GBS neonatal attack rates, it has been estimated that 11 000 neonates develop invasive disease in the USA annually; 20% of infected infants will die, and many of the survivors with meningitis will develop neurologic sequelae. Two distinct clinical syndromes occur among neonates with GBS infections. These differ in the age at onset, pathogenesis and outcome. The first clinical syndrome, early-onset infection, occurs within the first 5 days of life. The mean age at onset is 20 h of life. A significant portion of these infections are apparent at birth or become symptomatic within the first 90 min of life, indicating that in-utero GBS exposure and infection often occur. Early infection attack rates range from 1 to 4 per 1000 for all live births. Among offspring of maternal GBS carriers, however, the attack rate is much higher, ranging from 10 to 60 per 1000. In total, 70–80% of these early-onset neonatal infections occur among low-birthweight neonates (less than 2500 g) and among women with obstetric complications such as preterm labor, prolonged rupture of membranes, intrapartum fever and multiple gestations.

Early neonatal infection results from vertical transmission of GBS from a colonized mother. There is a direct relationship between neonatal attack rates and the size of the inoculum and number of colonized neonatal sites. Early-onset infection usually manifests as septicemia or pneumonia with a rapidly progressive course. In addition, approximately 30% of infected neonates have concomitant meningitis.

The second type of infection, a late-onset infection, occurs in infants after the first week of life. The overall attack rate is estimated to be 1.3–1.6 per 1000 live births. In contrast to early-onset infection, nosocomial transmission may be as important as vertical transmission. The serotype distribution of strains recovered from late-onset infection does not reflect the serotypes present in the maternal genital tract; over 90% of late-onset infection is caused by type III GBS. Over 80% of late-onset infection manifests as meningitis, and it has an overall mortality rate of about 20%. Approximately 50% of survivors will have neurologic sequelae, including cortical blindness, diabetes insipidus, deafness or other cranial nerve deficits, and spasticity. Although the majority of late-onset infection occurs as meningitis, other manifestations of late-onset infection may also occur. These manifestations include septic arthritis, osteomyelitis, empyema, endocarditis, cellulitis and otitis media.

Diagnosis

Group B streptococci can be easily grown on selective or non-selective media. Most Group B streptococcal colonies appear on blood plates as small (1–2 mm), gray-white colonies surrounded by a zone of beta-hemolysis, although 2% of strains are non-hemolytic. Preliminary identification and distinction of GBS from other streptococci is based on biochemical reactions including resistance to bacitracin, hydrolysis of sodium hippurate, and production of a soluble hemolysin that acts synergistically with beta-lysin of Staphylococcus aureus to produce beta-hemolysis (CAMP test). Although GBS can be recovered after overnight growth on non-selective media such as blood agar, use of a selective broth medium such as Todd-Hewitt broth with nalidixic acid and colistin or gentamicin greatly enhances the isolation rate of GBS from any culture site.

A major limitation of cultures is the length of time necessary for growth and identification. A number of more rapid screening tests have been developed to detect GBS directly in either body fluids or in cervical–vaginal secretions. These culture-independent tests include Gram-stain,[112–116] latex particle agglutination (LPA)[117–123] and enzyme immunoassay.[115,122–124] The latter two tests are commercially available kits to detect group-specific antigen in body fluids. A large number of studies have evaluated the ability of these indirect tests to rapidly detect GBS colonization of the maternal lower genital tract (Table 6). Such identification is important to interrupt maternal-to-neonatal vertical transmission that leads to early-onset neonatal disease.

Table 6
Rapid, culture-independent tests for the detection of genital tract colonization by Group B streptococci

Test	Prevalence of GBS colonization (%)	Sensitivity (%)	Specificity (%)	Positive predictive value (%)	Negative predictive value (%)
Gram-stain					
Feld and Harrigan[112]	13	100	67	30	100
Holls et al.[113]	14	93	69	33	98
Sandy et al.[114]	14	38	61	13	86
Towers et al.[115]	15	45	63	18	86
Carey et al.[116]	18	28	69	17	81
Latex particle agglutination					
Isada and Grossman[117]	4	58	93	28	98
Wald et al.[118]	11	40	99	87	93
Lotz-Nolan et al.[119]	11	62	99	92	95
Brady et al.[120]	5	88	100	92	99
Kontnick and Edberg[121]	15	19	99	92	88
Skoll et al.[122]	10	15	99	67	92
Greenspoon et al.[123]	2	33	95	15	98
Enzyme immunoassay					
Towers et al.[115]	15	60	92	57	93
Skoll et al.[122]	10	21	99	62	93
Greenspoon et al.[123]	2	33	99	40	98
Gentry et al.[124]	10	33	95	43	93

Most recent studies have not confirmed the initially encouraging results. On balance, none of these rapid tests is sufficiently sensitive or predictive to replace cultures in the identification of GBS colonization of the genital tract. This is particularly true for vaginal Gram-stain to detect Gram-positive cocci. Because of the very low predictive value and lack of sensitivity of vaginal Gram-stain for GBS, this test cannot be recommended.[116]

Management Options

Prepregnancy

There is no current evidence to suggest that the identification of a GBS carrier prior to pregnancy is predictive of the eventual outcome. Similarly, treatment of asymptomatic women found to be GBS-positive prior to pregnancy does not impart any recognized benefit. Positive results may be of some limited value in patient counseling, but the cost-effectiveness of this approach is questionable.

Prenatal, labor/delivery

Although, in general, the attack rate for neonatal GBS infection is low, a variety of prevention strategies have been advocated because of the high mortality and morbidity seen in neonatal GBS disease. These strategies have involved chemoprophylaxis, aimed at eradicating the organism from the mother or the neonate, or immunoprophylaxis, aimed at inducing humoral immunity.

Antibiotic chemoprophylaxis has been advocated for the pregnant patient in either the antepartum or intrapartum period, or for the neonate in the immediate neonatal period. Attempts to eradicate GBS colonization with antepartum treatment have been unsuccessful, and early neonatal prophylaxis is also frequently unsuccessful because many neonates are already septic at birth as a result of in-utero infection.[125] Most chemoprophylactic prevention strategies have therefore focused upon selective intrapartum treatment.[126,127] Boyer et al. have demonstrated that 74% of neonates with early-onset disease and 94% of those infections with a fatal outcome occur among neonates with one or more of the perinatal risk factors of birthweight $\geq$ 2500 g, rupture of membranes of greater than 18 h or intrapartum fever.[125] These investigators performed vaginal–rectal cultures on 13 381 women at 26–28 weeks gestation and found a prevalence of GBS colonization of 23%.[126] Those GBS-colonized patients who experienced premature labor or prolonged rupture of membranes of greater than 12 h at the time of enrolment were randomized to receive either 2 g ampicillin i.v., followed by 1 g ampicillin every 4 h until delivery, or placebo. No neonate born to 85 women receiving ampicillin developed bacteremia. In contrast, 5 neonates born to 79 women receiving placebo developed bacteremia ($P = 0.04$). By selective prophylaxis of only those patients with both GBS colonization and a risk factor for infection, this reduction in neonatal infection was achieved by intrapartum prophylaxis of only 3% of the total study population. Despite these impressive results, this approach has not been widely adopted because of the need for universal GBS screening at 26–28 weeks, as recommended by the authors. In addition to the expense of such a program, the overall predictive value of a positive prenatal culture is only 67%. Further, 8% of patients initially culture-negative acquire GBS by term.[128]

An alternative approach has been suggested by Minkoff and Mead which focuses only upon patients at risk for preterm delivery and does not require universal prenatal screening.[129] In this approach, all women with premature rupture of the fetal membranes of preterm labor are cultured for GBS upon admission to the hospital and empirically treated with intravenous ampicillin (2 g every 6 h) if delivery is anticipated before culture results are available. If the culture results become available and the patient has not delivered, then antibiotics are discontinued in those patients with negative cultures. Culture-positive patients are treated for 24 h with intravenous ampicillin and then switched to oral ampicillin (500 mg every 6 h) for 2 weeks, and then recultured. Erythromycin 500 mg orally every 6 h may be used in pencillin-allergic patients.

While this protocol would not identify or offer prophylaxis to colonized patients at term who are also at some risk for neonatal infection, it would identify, culture and treat the 7–10% of pregnant patients who deliver prematurely and who account for over 90% of all fatal neonatal early-onset infections. In addition, many authors recommend intrapartum ampicillin for those patients who have had a previous child with early-onset GBS disease. Given the severity of these infections and the patient's fear that surrounds them, this seems a reasonable approach.

Culture-independent rapid screening tests, described previously, may be helpful in identifying patients with heavy vaginal colonization.[121,124] With the exception of vaginal Gram-stain, these tests are sufficiently specific (few false-positives) to permit timely prophylaxis when positive. However, in the absence of heavy vaginal colonization, none of these rapid tests currently available is sufficiently sensitive or predictive to be used as a substitute for culture at the present time.

An alternative approach to intrapartum chemoprophylaxis is to immunize pregnant women. As noted previously, women delivering neonates with invasive early-onset disease usually have very low (less than 2 μg/ml) serum concentrations of type III GBS antibody.[107] A type III GBS capsular polysaccharide vaccine has recently been developed, and initial immunization trials of non-immune pregnant patients utilizing this vaccine has led to the development of protective levels of antibody in 20 of 35 (57%) patients.[130] Further, 62% of the vaccine-induced immunoglobulin was IgG, which readily crossed the placenta and provided protective levels of antibody to the neonate. Larger trials are necessary to evaluate the efficacy and safety of vaccination in the prevention of neonatal disease. Ultimately, the development of effective immun-

---

GROUP B STREPTOCOCCAL INFECTION
Summary of Management Options

Prepregnancy

- No evidence that identification or treatment of GBS carrier before pregnancy has any benefit

Prenatal, labor/delivery

- No evidence that generalized chemoprophylaxis for mother or newborn is of benefit

- Some evidence that *selective* intrapartum chemoprophylaxis may help GBS-positive women with an additional risk factor for low birthweight or preterm delivery

- Many routinely offer intrapartum chemophrophylaxis to women with previous severe GBS infection

- Immunization against GBS needs to be further evaluated

Postnatal

- Chemoprophylaxis need not be continued after delivery

- Diagnosis of postpartum endometritis in a GBS-positive woman should be treated with broad-spectrum antibiotics

oprophylaxis may obviate the need for prenatal screening cultures or intrapartum chemoprophylaxis.

Postnatal

In the asymptomatic parturient receiving antimicrobial prophylaxis for GBS intrapartum, there is no need to continue this therapy following delivery. Conversely, in the symptomatic GBS patient, intra-amniotic therapy should be continued as prescribed in earlier sections of this chapter. Since GBS can be a causative pathogen in postpartum endometritis, known carriers should be observed for this condition, and treated accordingly. It should be recognized, however, that postpartum endometritis is frequently a polymicrobial infection and therefore broad-spectrum agents should be used in these GBS-positive subjects as well.

TOXOPLASMOSIS

Toxoplasma gondii, the causative agent of toxoplasmosis, is one of the most common protozoan parasites of man, found worldwide. *T. gondii* infection is usually acquired by ingestion of oocysts in the feces of infected cats, or tissue cysts in undercooked or raw meats. Epidemiologic evidence suggests that 25–50% of the world's population has been infected, with serologic evidence of infection ranging from 15 to 90% of certain selected populations.[131] Most toxoplasmosis infections in humans are inapparent, resulting in failure to clinically diagnose primary infection. The high prevalence coupled with minimal symptoms making clinical diagnoses difficult, and the implications of primary infection in pregnancy which may lead to severe infectious sequelae in the fetus, make it necessary for the practicing obstetrician to be aware of preventive measures and screening programs available to pregnant patients.

T. gondii is an obligate intercellular protozoan parasite for which the definitive host is the domestic or wild cat. The organism exists in three forms – the trophozoite or tachyzoite, the tissue cyst and the oocyst. *T. gondii* undergoes a sexual cycle in the cat leading to the production of oocysts which are shed in the feces. These oocysts become infectious after incubation for 2–4 days, and remain infective for as long as 13–18 months depending upon the climate. Ingested cystozoites or oocysts invade the host's intestinal epithelium, where trophozoites, the invasive form of the organism, develop. These trophozoites spread to the regional lymph nodes, gaining access to the circulation via the thoracic duct. They are then capable of infecting, replicating and forming cysts in mammalian tissue, particularly tissues of the central nervous system, and striated and skeletal muscle.

Exposure to cat feces containing oocysts, and eating uncooked meats with toxoplasmosis cyst, are the main sources for infection. Such cysts can be found in as much as 10% of lamb, 25% of pork and 10% of beef samples. Other modes of transmission in humans include transplacental passage, blood or leucocyte transfusions, organ transplantations, lab accidents and ingestion of raw eggs or milk.[131]

Maternal/Fetal Risks

The majority of persons infected with *T. gondii* remain asymptomatic. However, five clinical syndromes have been described:[132]

- acute febrile toxoplasmosis

- lymphadenopathy

- encephalitis, especially in the immunocompromised patient

- neonatal jaundice and encephalitis and

- chorioretinitis.

The most common clinically apparent manifestation of adult toxoplasmosis is asymptomatic lymphadenopathy, usually involving the posterior cervical nodes. This may be accompanied by a mild mononucleosis-like syndrome with malaise, fever and sore throat. Spontaneous resolution occurs in several months in the vast majority of patients. Acute toxoplasmosis in the immunologically compromised host may be fatal. The infection may be primary or recrudescence of a chronic infection. A fulminant clinical course characterized by central nervous system involvement with necrotizing encephalitis leads to a mortality rate of about 50%.[133] Such patients do not have normal immunologic responses and therefore serologic testing may not reveal IgM or IgG. Clinical suspicion may necessitate a biopsy for definitive diagnosis.

When a primary infection with *T. gondii* occurs during pregnancy, the parasite may infect the placenta and fetus. Maternal parasitemia leads to a congenital infection in 40–50% of fetuses ranging from a transmission rate of 17% in the first trimester to 63% in the third trimester. Of the infected children, approximately 15% will have severe clinical damage, 19% will have mild disease and the remainder will be asymptomatic.[134]

The classical tetrad of congenitally acquired toxoplasmosis consists of chorioretinitis, microcephaly or hydrocephaly, cerebral calcifications, and clinically evident cerebral damage. Spontaneous abortion and stillbirth are more common with first trimester infection as are serious sequelae including fever, seizures, spinal fluid abnormalities, hepatosplenomegaly, jaundice and mental retardation. Overall, 75% of infected infants are asymptomatic at birth, but 40% of these experience low intelligence quotients, developmental delay and/or eye findings consistent with congenital infection.

Currently, there is no reliable way to predict the outcome in neonates with asymptomatic infection at birth, although a correlation may exist between high maternal antibody and pediatric findings of bilateral deafness, microcephaly and low IQ (a score less than 70).[135]

Diagnosis

The diagnosis of toxoplasmosis can be confirmed by culture of the organism in inoculated mice, by histologic examination of a lymph node, or by serologic test. A positive antibody titer against toxoplasmosis is indicative of previous infection, but pinpointing the time of infection can be difficult, particularly if the patient has been asymptomatic.

There are two groups of serologic tests in use. Group 1 includes the Sabin–Feldman dye test, the direct agglutination test and the indirect fluorescent antibody test. These tests employ whole cellular antigens to detect antibody against cell membrane antigens. Group 2 tests include the indirect hemagglutination test, the compliment fixation test and the enzyme-linked immunoabsorbent assay (ELISA), which use antigen extracts and test for antibodies directed against endocystoplasmic antigens.

Group 1 tests closely parallel one another and probably measure the same antibody. There is a rapid rise in titer after a primary infection, peaking about 2–3 months after infection. The level of antibody may plateau for 6 months and then titers slowly decrease; however, some patients will have persistently high titers. The dye test is the most specific, sensitive and most reproducible test. This test is based on the absence of staining of living parasites exposed to the combined action of anti-toxoplasma antibodies and a complement-like factor and does not distinguish between IgG and IgM. Therefore, confirmation of infection depends on paired and convalescent samples. The indirect fluorescent antibody test can be modified to demonstrate IgM antibodies, which begin to increase within the first week of infection.

The agglutination test is widely used to screen women for toxoplasmosis antibody during pregnancy because it is easy to perform, inexpensive and accurate. The test employs formalin-preserved whole parasites and detects IgG antibody.

The indirect hemagglutination test is not useful for screening pregnant women. It has been negative in documented cases of congenital toxoplasmosis, and can be negative for a long period after infection. It is more useful for diagnosis of chronic or recurrent infections.

The new ELISA technology provides an alternative method for toxoplasmosis sero-diagnosis. Both IgG ELISA and IgM ELISA tests are available. Demonstration of the antibodies of the IgM class not only confirms early infection in most cases, but also isolates those antibodies to the fetus if obtained by fetal blood sampling without contamination.

The double sandwich IgM ELISA is more sensitive and specific than the IgM-specific indirect fluorescent antibody test because it avoids false-positive results due to the presence of rheumatoid factor, or antinuclear antibody and false-negative results from high levels of IgG antibody. A second IgM titer should be performed in 3 weeks in any patient with suspicious symptomatology whose initial titer is negative. Likewise, initial high titers should be repeated; some people have persistent high titers and if there is no rise it may not be indicative of an acute infection.

Diagnosis of acute infection by serology is complicated by the high prevalence of antibody in the normal population, sometimes at significantly elevated levels. Confirmation of an acute infection requires demonstration of sero-conversion, a four-fold increase in the IgG titer in samples drawn 3 weeks apart, or the presence of high titers of IgG and IgM concurrently. Specifically, this means an IgG titer on the dye test or the indirect fluorescent test or greater than 1:1000, an IgM titer as measured by the indirect fluorescent test of greater than or equal to 1:64, or an ELISA assay for IgM at greater than or equal to 1:256. Negative dye test or indirect fluorescent antibody tests exclude the diagnosis of acute toxoplasmosis. A negative IgM ELISA also excludes the possibility of acute toxoplasmosis; however, the IgM indirect fluorescent antibody test may be falsely negative if the IgG level is very high.[136]

Familiarity with these various tests, their limitations and their accuracy in local laboratories is essential for the proper diagnosis of toxoplasmosis.

Management Options

Prepregnancy

Ideally, the public should be educated about toxoplasmosis and pregnancy and preventative measures for patients at risk prior to conception. Women anticipating pregnancy should be counseled to avoid ingestion of raw meat, to heat meat to at least 66°C, freeze it to minus 20°C, smoke it, or cure it. If the patient has a cat, the litter should be changed daily (if possible by someone else), and the litter box should be routinely washed with household bleach diluted with 10 parts of water. Women should wear gloves while gardening and should wash their hands thoroughly after handling raw meat, gardening, or changing the cat litter. All vegetables should be washed prior to consumption. Patients considered at high risk should be screened. This would include women with cats, women who work outdoors, such as on farms or in zoos, and women who eat raw or undercooked meats. Dining out frequently has also been considered to be a risk factor.[137] If a patient demonstrates a positive IgG titer prior to pregnancy, it can be assumed that she has been infected in the past and no further action is required.

Prenatal

Most patients do not obtain a titer prior to conception, and are first offered screening during pregnancy. If the patient has a low positive IgG titer, an IgM titer is done and a repeat IgG titer is done in 3 weeks. If the IgM is negative, the patient is asymptomatic, and if the repeated IgG titer is unchanged, it can be assumed that the patient was previously infected. If there is any clinical evidence of active infection, an IgM titer should be repeated as well.

As previously stated, an initially high IgG or IgM may indicate active infection and repeat studies are indicated. There have been cases of persistent levels of IgM at high titers for years. If the patient's initial test for IgG is negative, the patient should be reassured and counseled regarding preventative measures. Titers should then be repeated. Some recommend repeat titers every 1–2 months for patients at risk,[136] whereas others recommend a repeat titer just prior to 20 weeks and then in the third trimester.[138]

Since therapeutic pregnancy termination may be considered in patients with documented maternal infection, retesting prior to 20 weeks allows evaluation of the possibility of fetal infection. Maternal infection in the first and second trimester, with early infection of the fetus, is more frequently associated with severe manifestations of congenital toxoplasmosis than infection in the third trimester. Therefore, if direct studies can be done on the fetus to document infection, the parents can be more accurately counseled regarding outcome. Desmonts *et al.* recommend the following protocol once there is serologic evidence of primary maternal infection in early pregnancy:[139]

- Prenatal ultrasound to look for non-specific findings such as intracranial calcifications, microcephaly, hydrocephaly and hepatosplenomegaly.

- Fetal blood sampling for the detection of fetal toxoplasma-specific IgM at approximately 20 weeks of gestation. This test has a sensitivity of 52% and a specificity of 97%. This low sensitivity results from the inability of the fetus to mount an antibody response to infection until 18–20 weeks gestation. Infection with toxoplasmosis may also interfere with the immune response. Fetal blood

can also be obtained for LDH, eosinophil count, white blood count, platelet count and gammaglutamyl transferase. Abnormalities in these chemical markers are non-specific but cumulatively can raise the positive predictive value of a test.

- Amniotic fluid and blood should be inoculated into tissue culture or mice for definitive diagnosis.

Other methods allowing prenatal detection of congenital toxoplasmosis at an earlier stage are currently under investigation.[140]

Treatment

If the fetal IgM is negative, the other blood chemistries are normal, and there are no abnormalities noted on ultrasound, the patient may be counseled that there is no evidence of current fetal infection, although the risk of having an affected fetus cannot be totally excluded. Empiric treatment of the mother with a primary infection in pregnancy may theoretically prevent infection of the fetus, and is recommended.

If the fetal IgM is positive and/or other lab work is abnormal, or if there are abnormal ultrasound findings consistent with congenital infection, termination of the pregnancy may be offered. In cases where termination is not a legal or moral option, the mother is offered treatment. However, knowledge of the efficacy of treatment of congenital toxoplasmosis is meager. It is believed that anti-parasitic therapy of acute toxoplasmosis begun immediately after confirmation of maternal infection can reduce but not eliminate the risk of congenital infection.[141]

Treatment of toxoplasmosis includes the use of a sulfonamide such as sulfadiazine, sulfamerazine, sulfamethazine or sulfapyrazine, administered orally in combination with pyrimethamine. However, the use of these antibiotics in pregnancy is not without risk. They inhibit DNA synthesis and should be given with folic acid supplementation. Pyrimethamine has been associated with Stevens-Johnson syndrome or erythema multiforme, with an incidence of severe reactions estimated at 1:5000 to 1:8000. Pyrimethamine is purported to be teratogenic when used in the first trimester by some authors, but most studies have found it to be safe during pregnancy.

Severe jaundice in the newborn has been related to maternal sulfonamide ingestion at term and may theoretically lead to kernicterus. However, this is rarely, if ever, seen clinically. Administration of sulfonamides to a fetus with G6PD deficiency can also cause hemolytic anemia.

The macrolide antibiotic spiramycin has also been utilized in the treatment of toxoplasmosis, but may be less active than the combination of pyrimethamine/sulfadiazine. Spiramycin has less toxicity than pyrimethamine/sulfadiazine and has been widely used in Europe. Spiramycin therapy is reported to reduce the risk of fetal infection by as much as 50%.[142] Spiramycin reaches high concentrations in the placenta and therefore has been used when maternal infection is proved to reduce transmission to the uninfected fetus as determined by fetal blood sampling and culture.[138] It does not appear to have any teratogenic effects and side-effects are minimal, although they include drug rash, gastrointestinal upset and elevated liver enzymes (see **Table 7** for dosages of these drugs).

In summary, it seems appropriate that any woman with serologic evidence of acute toxoplasmosis infection during pregnancy should be counseled regarding the risk to her fetus. If she chooses, the fetus may be evaluated by the methods outlined. Termination can be offered, or treatment *in utero* with pyrimethamine and sulfadiazine, or spiramycin, available in the USA only through the CDC. The debate concerning universal routine prenatal screening continues. A more important focus may be implementation of preventive measures through patient education about the disease, the risk to the fetus, and simple precautionary measures.

Labor/delivery

In the patient with known toxoplasmosis infection during pregnancy, preparations should be made at delivery for pediatric consultation, and acute management of the neonate. Prenatal ultrasonography may be useful in anticipating specific neonatal complications associated with this transplacental infection.

Postnatal

There are no specific management requirements related to the postpartum period.

TOXOPLASMOSIS
Summary of Management Options (see also Chapter 49)

Prepregnancy

- General education of the public and specific counseling of individuals about risks, preventative measures
- Women expressing great concern can be reassured if IgG titer is positive

Prenatal

Screening

- Decisions about routine serological screen will depend on prevalence (most countries do not offer screening)
- Serological screening for those at risk; opinions as to optimum frequency vary

Documented maternal infection

- Assess fetal risk
  - ultrasound for stigmata
    intracranial calcification
    microcephaly
    hydrocephaly
    hepatosplenomegaly
  - fetal blood sampling
    specific IgM
    LDH
    white cell count
    platelet count
    gamma-GT
  - amniotic fluid culture

Maternal infection but no fetal infection

- Counseling of mother and offer prophylactic treatment with a sulfonamide or spiramycin (see **Table 7**)

Documented fetal infection

- Termination of pregnancy is one option to discuss if before viability
- If termination not an option, offer antibiotic treatment with careful counseling about benefits and risks

Table 7
Oral drug regimens for *T. gondii*

Pyrimethamine[a]	Loading dose of 75–200 mg in 2 equal doses, then 25 mg four times a day
and	
Sulfadiazine	75–100 mg/kg/day in 4 divided doses for 28 days
or	
Spiramycin	3 mg/day continuously throughout pregnancy or alternating 3 weeks of therapy with 2 weeks off, until delivery

[a] Given with folic acid supplementation.

TUBERCULOSIS

With the advent of effective anti-tuberculosis antibiotic regimens and screening programs, the number of reported tuberculosis (TB) cases in the USA decreased by greater than 70% in the years 1953–1984. However, beginning in 1985, this decline halted, and since 1986 there has been a steady increase in the annual incidence of TB, especially among hispanics and Blacks aged 22–44 years. A portion of this increase is attributable to the current spread of the human immunodeficiency virus (HIV).[143] Approximately 10 million infectious cases of TB occur each year in developing countries with at least 3 million dying from the disease.[144] In light of this, it is important that the clinician be more aware of the clinical signs and symptoms of active disease, risk factors for screening purposes and current recommended regimens for treatment and prophylaxis.

Maternal/Fetal Risks

Human tuberculosis is a bacterial infection caused by *Mycobacterium tuberculosis* and rarely *Mycobacterium bovis* (transmitted to humans from cows through ingestion of contaminated milk products). The bacillus is carried on droplet nuclei expelled when people with pulmonary tuberculosis sneeze, spit or cough. The small size of the droplet nuclei enables circumvention of normal mucociliary clearance. Thus, the organisms penetrate to distal airways where they multiply locally.

The development of tuberculosis from its onset is an interplay between multiplication of the bacilli and host response. Only about 5% of all newly infected people develop a clinically active disease. The risk for development of active disease is greatest in the first 1–2 years following primary infection and then it varies with age, being more prevalent in the very young and the very old. Immunosuppression also exacerbates infectivity.

The mid- or lower-lung fields are the initial foci of infection, with subsequent hematogenous spread to the apical and posterior regions where the bacilli grow best. Within 6–8 weeks after initial infection, a delayed cutaneous reaction develops, coincident with the development of a cell-mediated immune response to the tuberculosis antigen. This forms the basis for the tuberculin skin test. At this point, host responses can halt the disease process or the disease can progress to its active state.[145]

Active tuberculosis most often presents as pulmonary disease, with fewer than 15% of patients presenting with extra pulmonary disease. When the tubercle bacilli settle in the lung, the cell-mediated host response causes localized tissue inflammation (the primary or Ghon complex) and necrosis producing the characteristic lesion with a caseous center and surrounding granulation tissue. Airborne dissemination occurs if this complex accesses the alveolar/bronchoalveolar tree forming a cavity.

Miliary TB results from the erosion of a blood vessel by a necrotic focus, releasing a massive dose of bacilli into the blood stream to seed multiple organs simultaneously. Fortunately, this is uncommon unless the host is severely immunocompromised. Foci elsewhere in the body can be sites of progression even if the pulmonary site is not clinically evident. Asymptomatic renal, genital tract, bone and joint involvement are most common. Pericardial and peritoneal TB are uncommon, as are TB meningitis or mastitis.[146,147]

Progression of the primary or Ghon complex to caseation necrosis of lung tissue is usually accompanied by the development of the characteristic signs and symptoms of pulmonary tuberculosis. These include generalized weakness, malaise, night sweats, anorexia, hemoptosis, cough and sputum production, although up to 20% will have minimal symptoms at the time of diagnosis.[148] If the primary complex heals, viable bacilli can remain dormant for long periods of time in the untreated host and can reactivate. The predominance of minimal disease in active tuberculosis, as well as the prevalence of the carrier dormant state, make it essential that the clinician ask a detailed history and consider epidemiologic risk factors in evaluation of patients at risk.

Disease due to atypical mycobacterium is relatively uncommon in otherwise healthy adolescents and adults, but may occur in HIV-infected patients. Clinical manifestations and specific treatment regimens depend on the bacteria isolated and drug susceptibility and will not be considered in this discussion.

The incidence of tuberculosis in pregnancy as well as the incidence of neonatal or congenital tuberculosis is low. A higher birth rate among women of lower socioeconomic groups, coupled with the AIDS epidemic, may lead to an increased rate of infection in these pregnant populations. Other risk factors for infection in pregnancy are poor living conditions, crowded housing, poor nutrition and lack of adequate prenatal care. While it is controversial whether or not pregnancy alters the course of tuberculosis, it is clear that effective anti-tuberculosis treatment leads to the same excellent prognosis for recovery as in non-pregnant patients.

Congenital tuberculosis is rare; fewer than 300 cases have been reported in the literature. However, congenital and neonatally acquired tuberculosis are frequently under-diagnosed, and may result in delayed treatment and a mortality rate approaching 50%.[149] The criteria for making the diagnosis of congenital TB were defined in 1935 by Beitzki and include:[150]

- a proven bacteriologic diagnosis

- a primary complex in the infant or fetal liver

- manifestation of disease during the first few days of life

- exclusion of the possibility of extrauterine infection.

Fetal ingestion of infected amniotic fluid, aspiration of infected amniotic fluid, and hematogenous infection via the umbilical vein are proposed mechanisms of infection. Congenital infection is more common in offspring of women with miliary TB, particularly with involvement of the endometrium.[151] Although rare, the devastating consequences of missing the diagnosis emphasize the great importance of screening for TB in pregnancy.

Diagnosis

Tuberculin skin testing is the cheapest, safest and most productive means for detecting tuberculosis. There are two types of tuberculin in existence: old tuberculin (OT) and purified protein derivative (PPD). The intracutaneous administration of 5 units of PPD (the Mantoux test) is the best means for detecting infection, and this is the standard for reading the tuberculin skin test referred to in this text. The antigen is injected intracutaneously as a single dose of 0.1 ml (5 units) of PPD on the volar aspect of the forearm, producing a wheal 6–10 mm in diameter. The material is Tween stabilized, but should not remain in the syringe for longer than 1 h prior to use. An interpretive reading should be done in 48–72 h after infection, although positive readings beyond 96 h are significant. The margins of induration should be measured by touch and not sight and erythema should be ignored. A reaction of equal to or greater than 10 mm is usually considered positive.

However, there are some clinical situations where this is altered, which will be discussed subsequently. The test is safe and reliable in pregnant women and should be used as the primary screening tool.[152]

Management Options

Prepregnancy

On the basis of recent medical literature on epidemiologic surveillance data, the advisory committee for the elimination of tuberculosis recommend that the following groups be screened for tuberculosis and tuberculin infection:[153]

- persons infected with the HIV virus

- close contacts of persons known or suspected to have tuberculosis, sharing the same household or enclosed environment.

- persons with medical risk factors known to increase risk of disease or infection (**Table 8**)

- foreign born persons with high TB prevalence which include most countries in Africa, Asia and Latin America

- medically under-served low-income populations, including high-risk racial or ethnic minority populations

- alcoholics and i.v. drug abusers

- residents of long-term and residential care facilities.

Although some clinicians routinely screen all pregnant women, screening should be targeted to popu-

Table 8
Medical risk factors for tuberculosis

Silicosis
Gastrectomy
Jejunoileal bypass
Weight of 10% or more less than ideal body weight
Chronic renal failure
Diabetes mellitus
Chronic high-dose corticosteroid therapy
Immunosuppressive therapy
Leukemia or lymphoma
Other malignancies

lations with risk factors in order to maximize detection of disease in a cost-effective manner. The most problematic aspects of screening involve access to care and compliance. Some of the most indigent patients do not receive adequate prenatal care and when they do receive the skin test, 20–50% do not return to have it read at the appropriate time.

Factors which modify the standard reading of the Mantoux test include:

- persons with HIV infection

- close contacts of persons with newly diagnosed infectious tuberculosis

- persons with abnormal chest x-rays that show a fibrous lesion likely to represent old healed TB.

These people should be considered candidates for preventive therapy if they have a tuberculin test greater than or equal to 5 mm at 48–72 h, unless they have a history of prior therapy.[153]

False-negative tests do occur, most commonly in patients with concurrent acute viral illness or in anergic individuals. If this is suspected, another common antigen such as mumps or candida may be placed at the same time. Some patients have previously been given BCG, the bacillus of Calmette and Guerin derived from a strain of *Mycobacterium bovis* and used as a TB vaccine in many parts of the world. In general, it is usually prudent to administer the test regardless of previous BCG exposure, and to consider significant reactions in BCG-vaccinated persons as indicative of infection.

Prenatal

PPD-positive pregnant women with a prior negative reaction, time of conversion unknown, or with a suspicious history (regardless of PPD status), should be evaluated with a chest radiograph and three sputum samples sent for a stain for acid fast bacilli and for culture and sensitivity. If the PPD test is positive, the patient is asymptomatic and the chest x-ray is normal, chemotherapeutic prophylaxis, consisting of isoniazid 300 mg orally once a day for 6 months, should be postponed until after delivery. However, if the PPD conversion occurred within the previous 1–2 years, prophylaxis with isoniazid should be started after the first trimester.[149,154,155] All patients less than 35 years of age should be treated. However, there is an increased incidence of hepatotoxicity with isoniazid after the age of 35. Beyond age 35, prophylactic treatment is given only to patients with risk factors including HIV infection, recent skin test conversion, a history of i.v. drug

use, and medical risk factors listed previously.[153] Baseline liver function studies and monthly monitoring for symptoms of hepatotoxicity should be followed for patients receiving isoniazid prophylaxis.

Because of the slow growth rate of mycobacteria, regimens for treatment of active disease must contain multiple drugs to which the organism is susceptible, and drug ingestion must be continued for a sufficient period of time. Promoting and monitoring compliance are essential for successful treatment. First-line antituberculous drugs are used for initial therapy. These include isoniazid, rifampin, pyrazinamide, streptomycin and ethambutol. Second-line drugs are usually reserved for cases of treatment failure and/or drug resistance and include aminosalicylate sodium (sodium PAS), ethionamide, cycloserine, kanamycin and capreomycin. These drugs are not recommended for use during pregnancy.

Retrospective studies suggest that isoniazid (INH), rifampin and ethambutol can safely be utilized during pregnancy. Isoniazid has many therapeutic advantages and appears to be the safest agent to use during pregnancy. Since isoniazid is known to produce central nervous system toxicity, pyridoxine (vitamin B_6) should be given concurrently. Both ethambutol and rifampin have been used during pregnancy without evidence of teratogenicity. Rifampin may be associated with diminished limb size, but the number of case reports is too small to draw conclusions.[156] Therapy should be continued for a minimum of 9 months with the two agents (see **Table 9** for dosages).[152,155]

Izoniazid resistance is prevalent in several areas of the world including Taiwan, Indochina and Haiti. Immigrants from these areas with active tuberculosis should have susceptibility studies done and should empirically be treated with isoniazid, rifampin and ethambutol for the 9 months course.[155]

Routine follow-up of tuberculosis includes smears and cultures until they become negative, as well as clinical monitoring for adverse hepatotoxic effects due

Table 9
Tuberculosis treatment in pregnant women

1. Two-drug regimens	
Isoniazid[a] and rifampin	300 mg orally once daily 600 mg orally once daily
or	
Isoniazid[a] and ethambutol	2.5 g orally once daily 15–25 mg/kg/day up to 2.5 g maximum dose
2. Three-drug regimen	
Isoniazid,[a] rifampin and ethambutol	

[a] Must be taken with pyridoxine 50 mg orally once daily.

TUBERCULOSIS
Summary of Management Options

Prepregnancy

- Screen those at increased risk (see text for list)

- Treat those who are positive

Prenatal

- Confirm diagnosis with:
  - PPD
  - chest x-ray
  - three sputum samples

- If positive PPD, and clinically and radiologically positive, commence treatment (see **Table 9**)

- Follow-up cultures and clinical monitoring for response to therapy

- If PPD positive but negative clinically and radiologically, consider INH prophylaxis (risk factors, age, liver function and medical history will influence decision)

- Monitor liver function in patients taking INH

Labor/delivery

- Special anesthetic precautions if general anesthesia

Postnatal

- Continue treatment until course completed

- Breast-feeding not contraindicated

- If mother has been treated, baby receives INH-resistant BCG and a course of prophylactic INH

- Some antituberculosis agents may reduce efficacy of oral contraceptives

---

to INH therapy. Within 2 weeks of initiating therapy, patients are considered non-infectious.

Labor/delivery

There are no special management recommendations for the intrapartum care of the TB patient unless significant pulmonary compromise is a part of the clinical presentation. Here, consultation with the anesthesiology and pulmonary services will be important if the need for general anesthesia arises.

Postnatal

Patients should be continued on their prepregnancy (or antepartum) medications as recommended by the primary care physician. Breast-feeding is not specifically contraindicated once the patient has been determined to be non-infectious. Adequate contraception should be recommended, with awareness of the literature that suggests oral contraceptives may be less reliable when taken with some anti-tuberculosis agents.

MALARIA

Malaria remains a challenging parasitic disease, both in terms of prevalence with greater than 200 million cases per year, and in morbidity and mortality, resulting in greater than 1 million deaths per year.[157] Malaria is caused by four species of the protozoan genus *Plasmodium*: *P. vivax*, *P. falciparum*, *P. malariae* and *P. ovale*. The infection is maintained in nature by female mosquitoes of the genus *Anopheles*, in which sporogony occurs. Malaria is an endemic disease in parts of Asia, Africa, Oceania, and Central and South America. The mosquito feeds on human blood, in which the *Plasmodium* life-cycle is completed.

When a female anopheles mosquito bites an infected human, male and female gametocytes are ingested into the mosquito stomach. The sexual reproductive cycle produces sporozoites in about 2 weeks, which accumulate in the mosquito salivary glands and are infectious for humans. When the mosquito bites again, the sporozoites are injected into the blood stream and gametocytes may again be ingested by the mosquito if the person has been infected previously. The sporozoites infect liver parenchymal cells during this clinically inapparent pre-erythrocytic or exoerythrocytic phase. After several days, merozoites are released into the blood stream. This form of the parasite is capable of red blood cell invasion and multiplication, a process called schizogony, which leads to red blood cell lysis. When enough parasites are in synchrony, periodic fevers manifest themselves coincident with rupture of red blood cells and release of merozoites. This cycle takes 36–48 h for *P. falciparum*, 48 h for *P. vivax* and *P. ovale*, and 72 h for *P. malariae*.[158]

The severity of disease is related to the species of plasmodium, the level of parasitemia, and the immune status of the individual specifically to malaria. *Plasmodium falciparum* is the most virulent species, invading erythrocytes of any age, whereas *P. vivax* infects younger red blood cells (reticulocytes) and *P. malariae* infects older red blood cells. Therefore, *P. falciparum* multiply faster and generally produce a more dense parasitemia.

Certain hemoglobinopathies and erythrocyte enzyme defects render patients less susceptible to severe complications of malaria. Patients with sickle hemoglobin acquire falciparum malaria as frequently, but the clinical disease is attenuated, possibly because the parasite is less able to divide in the abnormal erythrocyte. Certain Black populations are less susceptible to *P. vivax* infections because of the absence of Duffy blood group antigen, which acts as an erythrocyte receptor for *P. vivax* merozoites.[159]

Immunity to clinical malaria is acquired gradually as a result of repeated exposure to the infection. In endemic areas, this process takes 5–10 years to develop and immunity is partial, meaning that the parasites are present intermittently in the blood of semi-immune subjects. Both cellular and humoral factors are involved in the development and maintenance of this condition, known as premunition.[160] Intra- and inter-species antigenic variation, stage-specific immunity and different host responses all complicate the picture, particularly as they relate to clinical manifestations of the disease, and research and development of potential vaccines for malaria.[161]

Diagnosis

Clinical manifestations of malaria vary from acute attacks to development of a chronic form. Acute malaria occurs in non-immune subjects, who are usually either visitors to endemic areas, or non-immune children living in those same areas. These attacks are particularly virulent and account for the major morbidity and mortality.

Patients with acute malaria usually present with chills and fever, often associated with headache and myalgia. Early on, these fevers may be erratic before developing a synchronous periodicity related to timing of schizogony. Between the paroxysms of chills and fever, the patient often feels well. Other presenting non-specific symptoms include malaise, dry cough, abdominal pain, nausea, anorexia or vomiting. Physical exam reveals a tachycardia, hepatomegaly, splenomegaly (more common in *P. vivax* and *P. ovale* infections), and sometimes jaundice. Identification of plasmodia in fixed, stained blood thick or thin smears is diagnostic, and may be identified by an alert technician during an examination of the differential white blood cell count. A thin smear fixed in methanol and stained with Giemsa, or fixed and stained with Wright stain, is preferred for the identification of the species. The highest level of parasitemia will be demonstrable several hours after a chill and serial thick and thin slides may be needed to demonstrate parasitemia.

Fever and related symptoms gradually subside over several weeks in untreated *P. vivax*, *P. ovale* and *P. malariae* malaria. Months or years after initial exposure, dormant forms of the parasite (hypnozoites) may emerge from the liver and cause relapses. With *P. falciparum*, serious complications such as coma, severe hemolytic anemia, disseminated intravascular coagulation, acute renal failure and acute pulmonary edema may develop rapidly in the non-immune host; however, once eradicated from the blood, *P. falciparum* does not relapse.

The development of antibodies and cell-mediated immunity contribute to the pathogenesis of some of the clinical features of chronic malaria like nephrotic syndrome and tropical splenomegaly. Disruption of the host–parasite balance by malnutrition, pregnancy, or introduction of new strains of parasite, may precipitate recrudence and clinical manifestations in the semi-immune host.

Maternal/Fetal Risks

Parturient malaria in tropical Africa was described as early as 1925 by Blacklock and Gordon.[162] Women living in endemic areas demonstrate an increased prevalence in the severity of malarial infection during pregnancy, particularly in the second trimester. Recrudescence of infection is a major cause of anemia, preterm labor and low-birthweight infants, particularly among primigravidae. These effects are related to the degree of pre-existing immunity and therefore differ in hyperendemic, mesoendemic and hypoendemic areas.[163-165]

In areas of unstable endemicity, mesoendemic areas, a state of premunition is not attained by adulthood and symptomatic malaria can be seen at all ages, as well as during pregnancy. Effective anti-malarial prophylaxis, or avoidance of exposure, are the only measures likely to protect pregnant women and their offspring.

In areas where malaria is hyperendemic and where substantial protective immunity has been developed by the inhabitants, the effect on pregnancy is less dramatic and may be confined to transient asymptomatic parasitemia and/or placental infection. Incidences of placental malaria have been estimated to range from 15 to 60%.[166] Congenital malaria is rare in the immune individual because there is passive transfer of protective immunoglobulin G across the placenta to the fetus. Primiparous women in endemic areas seem to be more susceptible to recrudescent infections than multiparous women.

Acute malaria in the unexposed, pregnant host is a medical emergency requiring immediate treatment to prevent maternal sequelae, as well as miscarriage, fetal death and premature labor. Congenital malaria has been documented in non-immune infected mothers. Women travelling to malarious areas should therefore be counseled to take prophylaxis.

Management Options

Prepregnancy

Travel to areas with endemic malaria should be discouraged in patients attempting to get pregnant. This relates to the potential acuteness of the disease process and to the prophylactic agents needed to prevent infection. If travel cannot be avoided, prophylactic agents should not be withheld.

Prenatal

Both quinine and chloroquine have been used during pregnancy. Quinine is ototoxic, mildly oxytocic and can cause profound hypoglycemia. Its use in pregnancy has been limited to acute severe attacks. Chloroquine can cause retinal and cochlea-vestibular damage to both mother and fetus in very high doses. However, its use in prophylaxis during pregnancy has not been associated with any increased incidence of birth defects.[167]

The combination of a diaminopyrimidine and a long-acting sulfonamide was developed because the mechanism of action of the individual components proved to be complementary against malaria, and there was a theoretical advantage against development of resistance. Pyrimethamine, a dihydrofolate reductase inhibitor, is a slow-acting blood schizonticide for all plasmodia species with some exoerythrocytic stage activity. Sulfadoxine is also a slow-acting blood schizonticide against *P. falciparum* with weaker activity against the erythrocytic stages of the other species. Multiple-dose regimens of pyrimethamine/sulfadiazine have been associated with severe adverse cutaneous reactions. As with all sulfonamides, the drug should be avoided in the last month of pregnancy because of the possibility of kernicterus in the infant. When given during pregnancy, folic acid supplementation should be provided.

Mefloquine is a 4-quinolinemethanol compound for which there is effective oral absorption in acute malaria. It is an effective blood schizonticide against *P. falciparum*, *P. vivax* and *P. malariae*, and may be used in the areas of chloroquine-resistant *P. falciparum* both for treatment and prophylaxis. It has been used to treat pregnant women, but its use in pregnancy has not been adequately evaluated and it is not currently recommended by the CDC.[168]

A new anti-malarial agent, artemisinine, is a derivative of the plant *Artesmisia annua* from traditional Chinese medicine pharmacopeia. This drug is not commercially available, although it has been well tolerated in clinical trials in China. Limited use during human pregnancy has not shown any toxicity, but this class of drugs has caused embryotoxicity in rats and mice.

The tetracycline group of antibiotics and clindamycin have a place treating of multiple drug-resistant *P. falciparum* infections. The tetracyclines are slow-acting, blood schizonticides, also effective against the exoerythrocytic stage of *P. falciparum*. In acute infections, they must be combined with a more rapid-acting agent such as quinine, and their use is contraindicated in pregnancy. Clindamycin is a slow-acting blood schizonticide of *P. falciparum* which may be used in children and pregnant women with quinine for the treatment of multiple drug-resistant *P. falciparum*.

Primaquine, an 8-amino quinoline, is effective in eradicating hypnozoites in the liver, thus preventing relapses of *P. vivax* and *P. ovale*. The drugs are contraindicated in patients with G6PD deficiency and in persons with hereditary NAD methemoglobin-reductase deficiency. Treatment is generally withheld until after pregnancy as its effects on the fetus are unknown.

Drug resistance has become a major epidemiologic concern in malaria treatment and prophylaxis. Chloroquine resistance has not been reported in infections with *P. vivax*, *P. ovale* or *P. malaria*. However, *P. falciparum* resistance to chloroquine is widespread. Although quinine-resistant *P. falciparum* has been reported, significant resistance to this drug is limited mainly to South-East Asia, and may necessitate larger dosing or the addition of a second agent. Pyrimethamine/sulfadoxine (Fansidar®) resistance is common among *P. falciparum* as well as *P. vivax* and this regimen is never recommended as monotherapy. Mefloquine, the newest anti-malarial in the armamentarium, has limited resistance, mostly confined to South-East Asia.

Severe malaria is almost always caused by *P. falciparum*. However, *P. vivax* may be complicated by splenic rupture, thrombocytopenia, anemia and hepatic dysfunction with jaundice. The diagnosis of malaria must be considered in any febrile patient who has visited an endemic area, or immigrants, and returning long-term residents from those areas. Early diagnosis is important in treatment and a strong clinical suspicion should prompt a therapeutic trial of anti-malarial drugs. Parental therapy must be started quickly using a rapidly acting schizonticidal drug effective against the suspected strain (**Tables 10** and **11**).

Before initiating treatment, it is important to con-

Table 10
Treatment of acute chloroquine-sensitive malaria in pregnancy[a]

Oral	
Chloroquine phosphate	1 g, then 500 mg in 5 h, then 500 mg each day for 2 days
Quinine sulfate	600 mg every 8 h for 5–7 days
Intravenous	
Chloroquine phosphate	8.3 mg/kg loading dose over 4 h repeated every 12 h until a total dose of 41.7 mg/kg
Quinine dihydrochloride[b]	20 mg/kg loading dose over 4 h, then 10 mg/kg infused over 2–4 h repeated every 8 h until the patient can tolerate oral therapy
Quinine gluconate[b]	15 mg/kg loading dose over 4 h, then 5–7 mg/kg infused over 4 h repeated every 8 h until the patient can tolerate oral therapy
Intramuscular	
Quinine dihydrochloride[b]	20 mg/kg load, then 10 mg/kg every 8 h until the patient can tolerate oral therapy

[a] For hepatic stages of *P. vivax* and *P. ovale*, primaquine phosphate 15 mg 4 times a day must be given postpartum for 14 days.

[b] If therapy is necessary for greater than 72 h, maintenance dose should be decreased by 50% and total therapy should be given for 7 days.

Table 11
Treatment of acute chloroquine-resistant malaria in pregnancy

Oral	
Quinine sulfate[a] and pyrimethamine/sulfadoxine	3 tablets on day 3
Quinine sulfate[a] *and* clindamycin	10 mg/kg every 8 h for 5 days
or	
mefloquine	15 mg/kg single dose
Intravenous	
Quinine dihydrochloride[a]	
or	
Quinidine gluconate[a] and clindamycin	10 mg/kg every 8 h for 5 days

[a] Dosages previously recommended in **Table 1**.
[b] Administration may be delayed until oral intake is possible.

sider the possibility of chloroquine-resistant strains, to find out if the patient has been taking any anti-malarial agents, and if there is any past history of heart disease, arrhythmias or hypersensitivity to anti-malarial drugs. A stable patient with *P. vivax*, *P. ovale* or *P. malariae* may be treated with oral agents. Severe acute malarial attacks should be managed in an intensive care unit. Close monitoring of temperature, blood pressure, pulse, urine output and weight are necessary in order to calculate drug dosages and follow hydration status. Antipyretics are useful for hyperpyrexia, which may cause confusion, delirium, convulsion or fetal distress. Some clinicians recommend prophylactic low-dose phenobarbital (3.5 mg/kg) to reduce the incidence of convulsions.[169]

Anemia may be acute and severe, necessitating transfusion or exchange transfusion in patients who are fluid overloaded or have pulmonary edema. Fresh whole blood or concentrates of clotting factors and platelets may be used in patients with coagulopathy. Hypoglycemia is common in patients receiving quinine or quinidine and in pregnant patients with malaria. Careful monitoring of glucose levels and glucose replacement by 50% dextrose bolus or 10% dextrose solution may be used. Glucagon and somatostatin analog (SMS) have been used in limited settings with some success.

Cerebral malaria is best managed as above. There are no data supporting the use of osmotic or diuretic agents or dexamethasone. Hyperkalemia, fluid overload, metabolic acidosis and uremia may necessitate hemodialysis in the patient with black water fever

MALARIA
Summary of Management Options

Prepregnancy

- If possible, women trying to conceive should avoid travel to endemic areas

- If such travel is unavoidable, prophylaxis should be taken

Prenatal

- If possible, pregnant women should avoid travel to endemic areas, especially those with drug-resistant strains

- If such travel is unavoidable, prophylaxis should be taken

- Prophylaxis (see **Table 12**)

- Treatment
  - anti-malarial agents (see **Tables 10** and **11**)
  - supportive therapy (fluids, blood, glucose, anticonvulsants)
  - monitor electrolytes, renal and liver function, hematology
  - monitor fetal growth and health

Table 12
Prophylactic agents

Chloroquine-sensitive malaria	
Chloroquine phosphate	300 mg each week taken 1 week prior to travel, during visit, and for 4 weeks after leaving
Chloroquine-resistant malaria	
Chloroquine phosphate	(same as above)
and	
pyrimethamine/sulfadoxine[a]	3 tablets if malarial symptoms occur and seek doctor immediately
or	
proguanil[a,b]	200 mg per day
Mefloquine	250 mg each week for 4 weeks, then every 2 weeks, to continue for 4 weeks after leaving

[a] Need to take supplemental folic acid 1 mg/day.
[b] Currently not available in the USA.

(renal failure). Patients with acute malaria are more prone to Gram-negative septicemia and should be placed on appropriate empiric antibiotic therapy.

Acute malaria in early mid-trimester pregnancy may result in fetal death and a miscarriage. In the third trim-ester, monitoring may reveal uterine contractions, a fetal tachycardia and late decelerations. Correction of fever and hypoglycemia may correct the transient fetal hypoxia; however, persistent deceleration may reflect impairment of the intensely parasitized placenta and necessitate delivery.

With regard to prophylaxis against malaria, travel to areas with endemic malaria should of course be discouraged during pregnancy. Pregnancy is a contraindication to travel in areas known to have drug-resistant *P. falciparum*. However, if life-events dictate travel to these areas, the risk of chemoprophylaxis must be weighed against the risk of complications of severe malaria, as well as intrauterine growth deficiency, spontaneous abortion and intrauterine fetal death, secondary to malarial infection. Mechanical means of protection must not be discounted. Long sleeve clothing and mosquito repellant are important and effective measures. Chloroquine prophylaxis is safe during pregnancy.

In areas where there is chloroquine-resistant *P. falciparum*, pregnant women may take proguanil hydrochloride (not available in the USA). There do not seem to be any adverse effects during pregnancy, though conclusive studies are limited. Likewise, pyrimethamine sulfadiazine (Fansidar®) or mefloquine have been used during pregnancy, but as before, Fansidar® should be avoided in the third trimester and there are no studies proving safety for use of these drugs during pregnancy (see **Table 12** for prophylactic dosage).

Labor/delivery and postnatal

No specific recommendations apply to the intrapartum and postpartum periods.

REFERENCES

1 Sanford JP (1976) Urinary tract symptoms and infections. *Annual Review of Medicine* **26**:485–498.

2 Sweet RL (1977) Bacteriuria and pyelonephritis during pregnancy. *Seminars in Perinatology* **1**:25–40.

3 Sabath LD, Charles D (1980) Urinary tract infections in the female. *Obstetrics and Gynecology* **55**:162–169.

4 Nicolle LE, Harding GKM, Preiksaitis J, Ronald A (1982) The association of urinary tract infection and sexual intercourse. *Journal of Infectious Diseases* **146**:579–583.

5 Whalley PJ, Martin FG, Peters PC (1965) Significance of asymptomatic bacteriuria detected during pregnancy. *American Journal of Obstetrics and Gynecology* **193**:879–883.

6 Kass EH (1962) Pyelonephritis and bacteriuria: a major problem in preventive medicine. *Annals of Internal Medicine* **56**:46–53.

7 Low J, Johnston E, McBride R, Tuffnell P (1964) The significance of asymptomatic bacteriuria in the normal obstetric patient. *American Journal of Obstetrics and Gynecology* **90**:897–906.

8 Romero R, Oyarzun E, Mazor M *et al.* (1989) Meta-analysis of the relationship between asymptomatic bacteriuria and preterm delivery/low birth weight. *Obstetrics and Gynecology* **73**:576–582.

9 Bryant RE, Windom RE, Vineyard JP Jr *et al.* (1964) Asymptomatic bacteriuria in pregnancy and its association with prematurity. *Clinical Medicine* **63**:224–231.

10 Gilstrap LC III, Cunningham FC, Walley PF (1981) Acute pyelonephritis in pregnancy: Retrospective study. *Obstetrics and Gynecology* **57**:409–413.

11 Harris RE, Thomas VI, Shelekov A (1976) Asymptomatic bacteriuria of pregnancy: Antibiotic-coated bacteria, renal function, and intrauterine growth retardation. *American Journal of Obstetrics and Gynecology* **126**:20–26.

12 Kass EH (1973) The role of unsuspected infection in the etiology of prematurity. *Clinics in Obstetrics and Gynecology* **16**:134–152.

13 Kass EH, Finland M (1956) Asymptomatic infections of the urinary tract. *Transactions of the Association of American Physicians* **60**:56–65.

14 Stamm WE, Counts GW, Latham RH *et al.* (1982) Diagnosis of coliform infection in acute dysuric women. *New England Journal of Medicine* **307**:463–468.

15 Latham RH, Wong ES, Larson A *et al.* (1985) Laboratory diagnosis of urinary tract infection in ambulatory women. *Journal of the American Medical Association* **254**:3333–3336.

16 Plauche WS, Janney FA, Curole DN (1981) Screening for asymptomatic bacteriuria in pregnant patients: 3 of 5 screening systems versus quantitative culture. *Southern Medical Journal* **74**:1227–1233.

17 Harris RE, Gilstrap LC, Pretty A (1981) Single dose antimicrobial therapy for asymptomatic bacteriuria during pregnancy. *Obstetrics and Gynecology* **59**:546–549.

18 Angel JL, O'Brien WF, Finan MA *et al.* (1990) Acute pyelonephritis in pregnancy: A prospectus study of oral versus intravenous antibiotic therapy. *Obstetrics and Gynecology* **76**:28–32.

19 Gibbs RS, Castillo MS, Rogers PJ (1980) Management of acute chorioamnionitis. *American Journal of Obstetrics and Gynecology* **136**:709–713.

20 Gibbs RS, Duff P (1991) Progress in pathogenesis and management of clinical intraamniotic infection. *American Journal of Obstetrics and Gynecology* **164**:1317–1326.

21 Soper DE, Mayhall CG, Dalton HP (1989) Risk factors for intraamniotic infection: A prospective epidemicologic study. *American Journal of Obstetrics and Gynecology* **161**:562–568.

22 Silver HM, Sperling RS, St Clair PJ (1989) Evidence relating bacterial vaginosis to intraamniotic infection. *American Journal of Obstetrics and Gynecology* **161**:808–812.

23 Romero R, Avila C, Brekus CA, Morotti R (1991) The role of systemic and intrauterine infection in preterm parturition. *Annals of the New York Academy of Science* **622**:355–375.

24 Gibbs RS, Blanco JD, St Clair PJ, Castaneda YS (1982) Quantitative bacteriology of amniotic fluid from women with clinical intraamniotic infection at term. *Journal of Infectious Diseases* **145**:1–8.

25 Gilstrap LC, Leveno KJ, Cox SM *et al.* (1988) Intrapartum treatment of acute chorioamnionitis: Impact on neonatal sepsis. *American Journal of Obstetrics and Gynecology* **159**:579–583.

26 Garite TJ, Freeman RK (1982) Chorioamnionitis in the preterm gestation. *Obstetrics and Gynecology* **59**:539–545.

27 Morales WJ (1987) The effect of chorioamnionitis on the developmental outcome of preterm infants at one year. *Obstetrics and Gynecology* **70**:183–186.

28 Naeye RL, Tafari N, Judge D *et al.* (1977) Amniotic fluid infections in an African city. *Journal of Pediatrics* **90**:965–970.

29 Duff P, Sanders R, Gibbs RS (1983) The course of labor in term pregnancies with chorioamnionitis. *American Journal of Obstetrics and Gynecology* **147**:391–395.

30 Hauth JC, Gilstrap LC, Hankins, GDV, Connor KD (1985) Term maternal and neonatal complications of acute chorioamnionitis. *Obstetrics and Gynecology* **66**:59–62.

31 Yoder PR, Gibbs RS, Blanco JD *et al.* (1983) A prospective, controlled study of maternal and perinatal outcome after intra-amniotic infection at term. *American Journal of Obstetrics and Gynecology* **145**:695–701.

32 Ohlsson A, Wang E (1990) An analysis of antenatal tests to detect infection in preterm rupture of the membranes. *American Journal of Obstetrics and Gynecology* **162**:809–818.

33 Sperling RS, Ramamurthy RS, Gibbs RS (1987) A comparison of intrapartum versus immediate postpartum treatment of intraamniotic infection. *Obstetrics and Gynecology* **70**:861–865.

34 Gibbs RS, Dinsmoor MJ, Newton ER, Ramamurthy RS

(1988) A randomized trial of intrapartum versus immediate postpartum treatment of women with intra-amniotic infection. *Obstetrics and Gynecology* **72**:823–828.

35 Centers for Disease Control (1988) Syphilis and congenital syphilis – United States, 1985–1988. *Morbidity and Mortality Weekly Report* **37**:486–489.

36 Fiumara NJ, Fleming WL, Downing JG *et al.* (1952) The incidence of prenatal syphilis at the Boston City Hospital. *New England Journal of Medicine* **247**:48–52.

37 Harter CA, Benirschke K (1976) Fetal syphilis in the first trimester. *American Journal of Obstetrics and Gynecology* **124**:705–711.

38 Centers for Disease Control (1989) 1989 Sexually transmitted diseases treatment guidelines. *Morbidity and Mortality Weekly Report* **38**:1–43 (suppl. 8).

39 Larsen SA, Hunter EF, McGrew BE (1984) Syphilis. In Wentworth BB, Judson FN (eds) *Laboratory Methods for the Diagnosis of Sexually Transmitted Diseases*, pp. 1–42. Washington, DC: American Public Health Association.

40 Thompson SE (1976) Treatment of syphilis in pregnancy. *Journal of the American Venereal Diseases Association* **3**:159–166.

41 Beall GN (1987) Penicillins. In Saxon A (ed.) Immediate hypertensitivity reactions to beta lactam antibiotics. *Annals of Internal Medicine* **107**:204–215.

42 Wendel GD, Stark BJ, Jamison RB *et al.* (1985) Penicillin allergy and densensitization in serious maternal/fetal infections. *New England Journal of Medicine* **312**:1229–1232.

43 Charles AG, Cohens S, Kass MB *et al.* (1970) Asymptomatic gonorrhea in prenatal patients. *American Journal of Obstetrics and Gynecology* **108**:595–599.

44 Spence MR (1973) Gonorrhea in a military prenatal population. *Obstetrics and Gynecology* **42**:223–226.

45 Corman LC, Levison ME, Knight R *et al.* (1974) The high frequency of pharyngeal gonococcal infection in a prenatal clinic population. *Journal of the American Medical Association* **230**:568–570.

46 Holmes KK, Counts GW, Beaty HN (1971) Disseminated gonococcal infection. *Annals of Internal Medicine* **74**:979–993.

47 Edwards L, Barrada MI, Hamann AA *et al.* (1978) Gonorrhea in pregnancy. *American Journal of Obstetrics and Gynecology* **132**:637–641.

48 Burkman RT, Tonascia JA, Atienza MF *et al.* (1976) Untreated endocervical gonorrhea and endometritis following elective abortion. *American Journal of Obstetrics and Gynecology* **126**:648–651.

49 Christmas JT, Wendel GD, Bawdon RE *et al.* (1989) Concomitant infection with *Neisseria gonorrhoeae* and *Chlamydia trachomatis* in pregnancy. *Obstetrics and Gynecology* **74**:295–298.

50 Centers for Disease Control (1985) *Chlamydia trachomatis* infection: Policy guidelines for prevention and control. *Morbidity and Mortality Weekly Report* **34**:53S–74S (suppl. 3).

51 Hardy PH, Hardy JB, Nell EE *et al.* (1984) Prevalence of six sexually transmitted disease agents among pregnant inner-city adolescents and pregnancy outcome. *Lancet* **2**:333–337.

52 Schachter J, Grossman M, Sweet RL *et al.* (1986) Prospective study of perinatal transmission of *Chlamydia trachomatis*. *Journal of the American Medical Association* **255**:3374–3377.

53 Sweet RL, Landers DV, Walker C, Schachter J (1987) *Chlamydia trachomatis* infection and pregnancy outcome. *American Journal of Obstetrics and Gynecology* **156**:824–833.

54 Martin DH, Koutsky L, Eschenbach DA *et al.* (1982) Prematurity and perinatal mortality in pregnancies complicated by maternal *Chlamydia trachomatis* infection. *Journal of the American Medical Association* **247**:1585–1588.

55 Gravett MG, Nelson HP, DeRowen T *et al.* (1986) Independent associations of bacterial vaginosis and *Chlamydia trachomatis* infection with adverse pregnancy outcome. *Journal of the American Medical Association* **256**:1899–1903.

56 Alger LS, Lovchik JC, Hebel JR *et al.* (1988) The association of *Chlamydia trachomatis*, *Neisseria gonorrhoeae*, and Group B streptococci with preterm rupture of the membranes and pregnancy outcome. *American Journal of Obstetrics and Gynecology* **159**:397–404.

57 Wager GP, Martin DH, Koutsky L *et al.* (1980) Puerperal infectious morbidity: Relationship to route of delivery and to antepartum *Chlamydia trachomatis* infection. *American Journal of Obstetrics and Gynecology* **138**:1028–1033.

58 Harrison HR, Alexander ER, Weinstein L *et al.* (1983) Cervical *Chlamydia trachomatis* and mycoplasmal infections in pregnancy: Epidemiology and outcomes. *Journal of the American Medical Association* **250**:1721–1727.

59 Cohen I, Veille J, Calkins BM (1990) Improved pregnancy outcome following successful treatment of chlamydia infection. *Journal of the American Medical Association* **263**:3160–3163.

60 Crombleholme WR, Schachter J, Grossman M *et al.* (1990) Amoxicillin therapy for *Chlamydia trachomatis* in pregnancy. *Obstetrics and Gynecology* **75**:752–756.

61 Alger LS, Lovchik JC (1991) Comparative efficacy of clindamycin versus erythromycin in eradication of antenatal *Chalmydia trachomatis*. *American Journal of Obstetrics and Gynecology* **165**:375–381.

62 Osborne NG, Adelson MD (1990) Herpes simplex and human papillomavirus genital infections: Controversy over obstetric management. *Clinics in Obstetrics and Gynecology* **33**:801–811.

63 Kemp EA, Hakenewerth AM, Laurent SL *et al.* (1992) Human papillomavirus prevalence in pregnancy. *Obstetrics and Gynecology* **79**:649–656.

64 Kashima HK, Shah K (1987) Recurrent respiratory papillomatosis: Clinical overview and management principles. *Obstetrical and Gynecological Clinics of North America* **14**:581–588.

65 Hallden C, Majmudar B (1986) The relationship between juvenile laryngeal papillomatosis and maternal condylomata acuminata. *Journal of Reproductive Medicine* **31**:804–807.

66 Schwartz DB, Greenberg MD, Daoud Y, Reid R (1988) Genital condylomas in pregnancy: Use of trichloroacetic

acid and laser therapy. *American Journal of Obstetrics and Gynecology* **158**:1407–1416.

67 Harwick HJ, Purcell RH, Iuppa J *et al.* (1970) *Mycoplasma hominis* and abortion. *Journal of Infectious Diseases* **121**:260–268.

68 Watts DH, Eschenbach DA, Kenny GE (1989) Early postpartum endometritis: The role of bacteria, genital mycoplasmas, and *Chlamydia trachomatis*. *Obstetrics and Gynecology* **73**:52–60.

69 Braun P, Lee YH, Klein JO *et al.* (1971) Birth weight and genital mycoplasmas in pregnancy. *New England Journal of Medicine* **284**:167–171.

70 Shurin PA, Alpert S, Rosner B *et al.* (1975) Chorioamnionitis and colonization of the newborn infant with genital mycoplasmas. *New England Journal of Medicine* **293**:5–8.

71 Kundsin RB, Iriscoll SG, Monson RR *et al.* (1984) Association of *Ureoplasma urealyticum* in the placenta with perinatal morbidity and mortality. *New England Journal of Medicine* **310**:941–945.

72 Hillier SL, Martius J, Krohn M *et al.* (1988) Case-control study of chorioamnionitis infection and chorioamnionitis in prematurity. *New England Journal of Medicine* **319**:972–978.

73 Blanco JD, Gibbs RS, Malherbe H *et al.* (1983) A controlled study of genital mycoplasmas in amniotic fluid from patients with intra-amniotic infection. *Journal of Infectious Diseases* **147**:650–653.

74 Tafari N, Ross S, Naeye RL *et al.* (1976) Mycoplasma T strains and perinatal death. *Lancet* **1**:108–109.

75 McCormack WM, Rosner B, Lee YH *et al.* (1987) Effect on birth weight of erythromycin treatment of pregnant women. *Obstetrics and Gynecology* **69**:202–207.

76 Eschenbach DA, Nugent RP, Rao V *et al.* (1991) A randomized placebo-controlled trial of erythromycin for the treatment of *Ureaplasma urealyticum* to prevent premature delivery. *American Journal of Obstetrics and Gynecology* **164**:734–742.

77 Hammond GW, Chang JL, Walt JC, Ronald AR (1978) Comparison of specimen collection and laboratory techniques for isolation of *Haemophilus ducreyi*. *Journal of Clinical Microbiology* **7**:39–43.

78 Willcox RR (1975) International aspects of the venereal diseases and nonvenereal treponematosis. *Clinics in Obstetrics and Gynecology* **18**:207–222.

79 Kuberski T (1980) Granuloma inguinale (donovanosis). *Sexually Transmitted Diseases* **7**:29–36.

80 Sowmini CN (1983) Donovanosis. In Holmes KK, Mardh PA (eds) *International Perspectives on Neglected Sexually Transmitted Diseases*, pp. 205–217. Washington, DC: Hemisphere.

81 Scott CW, Harper G, Jason R *et al.* (1953) Neonatal granuloma inguinale. *American Journal of Diseases of Children* **85**:308–315.

82 Huggins GR, Preti G (1981) Vaginal odors and secretions. *Clinics in Obstetrics and Gynecology* **24**:355–377.

83 Redondo-Lopez V, Cook RL, Sobel JD (1990) Emerging role of lactobacillus in the control and maintenance of the vaginal bacterial microflora. *Reviews of Infectious Diseases* **12**:856–872.

84 Eschenbach DA, Davick PR, Williams BL *et al.* (1989) Prevalence of hydrogen peroxide producing *Lactobacillus* species in normal women and women with bacterial vaginosis. *Journal of Clinical Microbiology* **27**:251–256.

85 Martius J, Eschenbach DA (1990) The role of bacterial vaginosis as a cause of amniotic fluid infection, chorioamnionitis and prematurity – a review. *Archives of Gynecology and Obstetrics* **247**:1–13.

86 Gravett MG, Hummel D, Eschenbach DA, Holmes KK (1986) Preterm labor associated with subclinical amniotic fluid infection and with bacterial vaginosis. *Obstetrics and Gynecology* **67**:229–237.

87 Minkoff H, Grunebaum AN, Schwarz RH *et al.* (1984) Risk factors for prematurity and premature rupture of membranes: A prospective study of the vaginal flora in pregnancy. *American Journal of Obstetrics and Gynecology* **150**:965–972.

88 Van Slyke KK, Michel VP, Rein MF (1981) Treatment of vulvovaginal candidiasis with boric acid powder. *American Journal of Obstetrics and Gynecology* **141**:145–148.

89 McLellan R, Spence MR, Brockman M *et al.* (1982) The clinical diagnosis of trichomoniasis. *Obstetrics and Gynecology* **60**:30–34.

90 Block E (1959) Occurrence of trichomonas in sexual partners of women with trichomoniasis. *Acta Obstetrica et Gynecologica Scandinavica* **38**:398–401.

91 Cotch MF, Pastorek JG II, Nugent RP *et al.* (1991) Demographic and behavioral predictors of *Trichomonas vaginalis* infection among pregnant women. *Obstetrics and Gynecology* **78**:1087–1092.

92 Lossick JG, Kent HL (1991) Trichomoniasis: Trends in diagnosis and management. *American Journal of Obstetrics and Gynecology* **165**:1217–1222.

93 Dombrowski MP, Sokol RJ, Brown WJ *et al.* (1987) Intravenous therapy of metronidazole-resistant *Trichomonas*. *Obstetrics and Gynecology* **69**:524–525.

94 Rosa FW, Baum C, Shaw M (1987) Pregnancy outcomes after first-trimester vaginitis drug therapy. *Obstetrics and Gynecology* **69**:751–755.

95 Beard CM, Noller KL, O'Fallon WM *et al.* (1979) Lack of evidence for cancer due to use of metronidazole. *New England Journal of Medicine* **301**:519–522.

96 Martius J, Krohn MJ, Hillier SL *et al.* (1988) Relationships of vaginal *Lactobacillus* species, cervical *Chlamydia trachomatis* and bacterial vaginosis to preterm birth. *Obstetrics and Gynecology* **71**:89–95.

97 Spiegel CA, Amsel R, Eschenbach DA *et al.* (1980) Anaerobic bacteria in nonspecific vaginitis. *New England Journal of Medicine* **303**:601–607.

98 Eschenbach DA, Hillier S, Critchlow C *et al.* (1988) Diagnostic and clinical manifestations of bacterial vaginosis. *American Journal of Obstetrics and Gynecology* **158**:819–828.

99 Bejar R, Curbelo V, Davis C, Gluck L (1981) Premature labor. II. Bacterial sources of phospholipase. *Obstetrics and Gynecology* **57**:479–482.

100 Lugo-Miro VI, Green M, Mazur L (1992) Comparison of different metronidazole therapeutic regimens for bacterial vaginosis: A meta-analysis. *Journal of the American Medical Association* **268**:92–95.

101 Greaves WL, Chungafung J, Morris B *et al.* (1988) Clindamycin versus metronidazole in the treatment of bacterial vaginosis. *Obstetrics and Gynecology* **72**:799–802.

102 Hillier S, Krohn MA, Watts DH *et al.* (1990) Microbiologic efficacy of intravaginal clindamycin cream for the treatment of bacterial vaginosis. *Obstetrics and Gynecology* **76**:407–413.

103 Hillier SL, Lipinski C, Briselden AM, Eschenbach DA (1993) Efficacy of intravaginal 0.75% metronidazole gel for the treatment of bacterial vaginosis. *Obstetrics and Gynecology* **81**:963–967.

104 Eickhoff TC, Klein JO, Daly AK *et al.* (1964) Neonatal sepsis and other infections due to Group B beta-hemolytic streptococci. *New England Journal of Medicine* **271**:1221–1228.

105 Gravett MG (1985) Specific bacterial infections: Group B streptococcus. In Sciarra JW (ed.) *Gynecology and Obstetrics, Vol. III: Maternal and Fetal Medicine*, pp. 1–10. Philadelphia, PA: Harper and Row.

106 Hoogkamp-Korstanje JAA, Gerards LJ, Cats BP (1982) Maternal carriage and neonatal acquisition of Group B streptococci. *Journal of Infectious Diseases* **145**:800–805.

107 Baker CJ, Edwards MS, Kasper DL (1981) Role of antibody to native type III polysaccharide of Group B *streptococcus* in infant infection. *Pediatrics* **68**:544–549.

108 Blanco JD, Gibbs RS, Costaneda YS (1981) Bacteremia in obstetrics: Clinical course. *Obstetrics and Gynecology* **58**:621–626.

109 Romero R, Mazor M, Oyarzun E *et al.* (1989) Is there an association between colonization with Group B *streptococcus* and prematurity? *Journal of Reproductive Medicine* **34**:797–801.

110 Moller M, Thomsen AC, Borch K *et al.* (1984) Rupture of fetal membranes and premature delivery associated with Group B streptococci in urine of pregnant women. *Lancet* **2**:69–70.

111 Thomsen AC, Morup L, Brogaard-Hansen K (1987) Antibiotic elimination of Group B streptococci in urine in prevention of preterm labour. *Lancet* **1**:591–593.

112 Feld SM, Harrigan JT (1987) Vaginal Gram stain as an immediate detector of Group B streptococci in selected obstetric patients. *American Journal of Obstetrics and Gynecology* **156**:446–448.

113 Holls WM, Thomas J, Troyer V (1987) Cervical Gram stain for rapid detection of colonization with beta-streptococcus. *Obstetrics and Gynecology* **69**:354–357.

114 Sandy EA, Blumenfeld ML, Ianis JD (1988) Gram stain in the rapid determination of maternal colonization with Group B beta-streptococcus. *Obstetrics and Gynecology* **71**:796–798.

115 Towers CV, Garite TJ, Friedman WW *et al.* (1990) Comparison of a rapid enzyme-linked immunosorbent assay test and the Gram stain for detection of Group B streptococcus in high risk antepartum patients. *American Journal of Obstetrics and Gynecology* **163**:965–967.

116 Carey JC, Klebanoff MA, Regan JA (1990) Evaluation of the Gram stain as a screening tool for maternal carriage of Group B beta-hemolytic streptococci. *Obstetrics and Gynecology* **76**:693–697.

117 Isada NB, Grossman JH III (1987) A rapid screening test for the diagnosis of endocervical Group B streptococci in pregnancy: Microbiologic results and clinical outcome. *Obstetrics and Gynecology* **70**:139–141.

118 Wald ER, Dashefsky B, Green M *et al.* (1987) Rapid detection of Group B streptococci directly from vaginal swabs. *Clinics in Microbiology* **25**:573–574.

119 Lotz-Nolan L, Amato R, Iltis J *et al.* (1989) Evaluation of a rapid latex agglutination test for detection of Group B streptococci in vaginal specimens. *European Journal of Clinical Microbiology and Infectious Diseases* **8**:289–293.

120 Brady K, Duff P, Schilhab JC, Herd M (1989) Reliability of a rapid latex fixation test for detecting Group B streptococci in the genital tract of parturients at term. *Obstetrics and Gynecology* **73**:678–681.

121 Kontnick CM, Edberg SC (1990) Direct detection of Group B streptococci from vaginal specimens compared with quantitative culture. *Journal of Clinical Microbiology* **28**:336–339.

122 Skoll MA, Mercer BM, Baselski V *et al.* (1991) Evaluation of two rapid Group B streptococcal antigen tests in labor and delivery patients. *Obstetrics and Gynecology* **77**:322–326.

123 Greenspoon JS, Fishman A, Wilcox JG *et al.* (1991) Comparison of culture for Group B streptococcus versus enzyme immunoassay and latex agglutination rapid tests: Results in 250 patients during labor. *Obstetrics and Gynecology* **77**:97–100.

124 Gentry YM, Hillier SL, Eschenbach DA (1991) Evaluation of a rapid enzyme immunoassay test for detection of Group B *streptococcus*. *Obstetrics and Gynecology* **78**:397–401.

125 Boyer KM, Gadzala CA, Burd LI *et al.* (1983) Selective intrapartum chemoprophylaxis of neonatal Group B streptococcal early-onset disease. I. Epidemiologic rationale. *Journal of Infectious Diseases* **148**:795–801.

126 Boyer KM, Gotoff SP (1986) Prevention of early-onset neonatal Group B streptococcal disease with selective intrapartum chemoprophylaxis. *New England Journal of Medicine* **314**:1665–1669.

127 Tuppurainen N, Hallman M (1989) Prevention of neonatal Group B streptococcal disease: Intrapartum detection and chemoprophylaxis of heavily colonized parturients. *Obstetrics and Gynecology* **73**:583–587.

128 Boyer KM, Gadzala CA, Kelly PD *et al.* (1983) Selective intrapartum chemoprophylaxis of neonatal Group B streptococcal early-onset disease. II. Predictive value of prenatal cultures. *Journal of Infectious Diseases* **148**:802–809.

129 Minkoff H, Mead P (1986) An obstetric approach to the prevention of early-onset Group B beta-hemolytic streptococcal sepsis. *American Journal of Obstetrics and Gynecology* **154**:973–977.

130 Baker CJ, Rench MA, Edwards MS *et al.* (1988) Immunization of pregnant women with a polysaccharide vaccine of Group B streptococcus. *New England Journal of Medicine* **319**:1180–1185.

131 Chowdhury MN (1986) Toxoplasmosis: A review. *Journal of Medicine* **17**:373–395.

132 Frenkel JK (1971) Toxoplasmosis: Mechanisms of infection, laboratory diagnosis and management. *Current Topics in Pathology* **54**:28–35.

133 Ruskin J, Remington JS (1976) Toxoplasmosis in the compromised host. *Annals of Internal Medicine* **84**:193–199.

134 Joss AW, Chatterton JM, Ho-Yen DO (1990) Congenital toxoplasmosis: To screen or not to screen? *Public Health* **104**:9–20.

135 Sever JL, Ellenberg JH, Ley AC et al. (1988) Toxoplasmosis: Maternal and pediatric findings in 23,000 pregnancies. *Pediatrics* **82**:181–192.

136 Remington JS, Desmonts G (1990) Toxoplasmosis. In Remington JS, Klein JO (eds) *Infectious Diseases of the Fetus and Newborn Infant*, pp. 89–195. Philadelphia, PA: W.B. Saunders.

137 Jeannel D (1989) The risk of contamination by toxoplasma during pregnancy in the Parisian area. *Tenth International Meeting of Clinical Biostatistics*, Maastricht, Netherlands.

138 Ghidini A, Sirtori M, Spelta A, Jergani P (1991) Results of a preventative program for congenital toxoplasmosis. *Journal of Reproductive Medicine* **36**:270–273.

139 Desmonts G, Daffos F, Forestier R et al. (1985) Prenatal diagnosis of congenital toxoplasmosis. *Lancet* **1**:500–504.

140 Foulon W, Naessens A, Mahler T et al. (1990) Prenatal diagnosis of congenital toxoplasmosis. *Obstetrics and Gynecology* **76**:769–772.

141 Daffos F, Forestier F, Capella-Pavlovsky M et al. (1988) Prenatal management of 746 pregnancies at risk for congenital toxoplasmosis. *New England Journal of Medicine* **318**:271–275.

142 Couvreur J, Desmonts G, Thulliez P (1988) Prophylaxis of congenital toxoplasmosis: Effects of spiramycin on placental infection. *Journal of Antimicrobial Chemotherapy* **22**:193–200 (suppl. B).

143 Reider HL, Cauthen GM, Kelly GD et al. (1989) Tuberculosis in the United States. *Journal of the American Medical Association* **262**:385–389.

144 Joint IUAT/WHO Study Group (1982) Tuberculosis control. *Tubercle* **63**:157–159.

145 Benson CA (1992) Mycobacterial infections. In Gleicher N (ed.) *Principles and Practice of Medical Therapy in Pregnancy*, pp. 575–82. East Norwalk, CT: Appleton and Lange.

146 Schaefer G et al. (1954) Extrapulmonary tuberculosis and pregnancy. *American Journal of Obstetrics and Gynecology* **67**:605–615.

147 Golditch IM (1971) Tuberculous meningitis and pregnancy. *American Journal of Obstetrics and Gynecology* **110**:1144–1146.

148 Good JT Jr, Iseman MD, Davison PT et al. (1981) Tuberculosis in association with pregnancy. *American Journal of Obstetrics and Gynecology* **140**:492–498.

149 Jacobs RF, Abernathy RS (1988) Management of tuberculosis in pregnancy and the newborn. *Clinics in Perinatology* **15**:305–319.

150 Beitzki H (1935) Über die angioborne tuberkulose Infektion. *Ergebnisse der Gesamten Tuberkulose Forschung* **7**:1–30.

151 Ramos AD, Hibbard LT, Graig JR (1974) Congenital tuberculosis. *Obstetrics and Gynecology* **43**:61–64.

152 Snider D (1984) Pregnancy and tuberculosis. *Chest* **86**:105–135.

153 Centers for Disease Control (1990) The use of preventive therapy for tuberculosis infection in the United States. *Morbidity and Mortality Weekly Report* **39** (RR8):9–12.

154 Schaefer G, Zercondakis IA, Fuchs FF et al. (1975) Pregnancy and pulmonary tuberculosis. *Obstetrics and Gynecology* **46**:706–715.

155 Weinstein L, Murphy T (1974) The management of tuberculosis during pregnancy. *Clinics in Perinatology* **1**:395–405.

156 Holdiness MR (1987) Teratology of the antituberculous drugs. *Early Human Development* **15**:61–74.

157 Marshall E (1991) Malaria parasite gaining ground against science. *Science* **254**:190.

158 Spencer HC, Strickland GT (1984) Malaria. In Strickland GT (ed.) *Hunter's Tropical Medicine*, pp. 516–527. Philadelphia, PA: W.B. Saunders.

159 Lee RV (1992) Protozoan and helminthic infections. In Gleicher N (ed.) *Principles and Practice of Medical Therapy in Pregnancy*, pp. 702–704. East Norwalk, CT: Appleton and Lange.

160 Playfair JHL (1982) Immunity to malaria. *British Medical Bulletin* **38**:153–159.

161 Mitchell GH (1989) An update on candidate malaria vaccines. *Parasitology* **98**:529–547.

162 Blacklock B, Gordon RM (1925) Malaria parasites in the placental blood. *Annals of Tropical Medicine and Parasitology* **19**:37–45.

163 Bruce-Chwatt LJ (1983) Malaria and pregnancy. *British Medical Journal* **286**:1457–1458.

164 McGregor IA (1984) Epidemiology, malaria and pregnancy. *American Journal of Tropical Medicine and Hygiene* **33**:517–525.

165 Brabin BJ (1983) An analysis of malaria in pregnancy in Africa. *Bulletin of the World Health Organization* **61**:1005–1016.

166 McGregor IA (1983) Malaria infection of the placenta in the Gambia, West Africa. *Transactions of the Royal Society of Tropical Medicine and Hygiene* **77**:232–244.

167 Wolfe MS, Cordero JF (1985) Safety of chloroquine in chemosuppression of malaria during pregnancy. *British Medical Journal* **290**:1466–1467.

168 Centers for Disease Control (1990) Recommendations for the prevention of malaria among travelers. *Morbidity and Mortality Weekly Report* **39** (RR3):1–10.

169 Warrell DA (1989) Treatment of severe malaria. *Journal of the Royal Society of Medicine* **82**:44–59 (suppl. 17).

31

Dermatological Problems

CAMERON THOMAS CAMPBELL KENNEDY

INTRODUCTION

The pregnant woman is likely to notice many changes in the skin as a result of pregnancy. Many of these conditions will provoke concern and a request for therapy. Others will be noted by the women and/or her physician and accepted without intervention. The dermatologist or attending physician caring for a woman with skin disease will need to be aware of changes in the natural history of that disease due to pregnancy and possible consequences of drug therapy on the pregnancy. Dermatologic problems in pregnancy can present in the following ways:

- pre-existing skin disorder

- pruritus and/or rash

- miscellaneous skin complaints which are either pathological or non-pathological and are secondary to changes associated with pregnancy.

PRE-EXISTING SKIN DISORDERS

Many pre-existing dermatoses may be altered during pregnancy; in most cases, very probably either because of the profound immunological or endocrine changes that prevail. This section focuses on dermatologic concerns associated with these pre-existing disorders.

INFECTIONS

Risks and Management Options

A detailed consideration of the effects of pregnancy on certain infections and consequences for the mother and fetus is given in Chapters 29, 30 and 49. The dermatologist may be involved when there are exacerbations of the following:

- genital human papilloma virus infection

- candidiasis

- herpes simplex

- trichomoniasis

- leprosy[1]

- pityrosporum follicullitis

Certain disseminated infections are more likely in pregnancy, may present with generalized eruptions, and result in death of the fetus or confer serious complications.[2] Some of these are summarized in **Table 1**.

Table 1
Pregnancy and infection-related dermatoses: high risk for transfer to the fetus

Disease (causative agent)	Maternal skin lesions	Distribution	Other features (maternal)	Diagnostic tests
Syphilis (*Treponema pallidum*)	*Primary*: chancre – a painless ulcer with induration	Genital, oral		Dark ground microscopy
	Secondary: coppery-red maculopapular slightly scaly lesions; eroded plaques on the genitals and ulcers in the mouth; patchy hair loss may occur	Widespread, including palms and soles	Malaise, fever lymphadenopathy, hepatitis; occasional lymphocytic meningitis, iritis	FTA-ABS, VDRL, TPHA
Lyme disease (*Borrelia burgdorferi*)	Centrifugally expanding erythematous ring (*Erythema chronicum migrans*)	At site of tick bite	History of tick bite	ELISA, then specific immunoblotting
	Secondary annual lesions (mostly North America)	Widespread	*Early*: low-grade fever, regional lymphadenopathy, meningitis *Late*: Neurological rheumatic and cardiac complications	PCR (where available)
Gonococcal septicemia (*Neisseria gonorrhoea*)	Inflammatory vesico-pustules may have purpuric base	Extremities	Fever, arthritis, cardiac complications, meningitis occasionally	Culture (specialized medium) blood and pustule
Erythema infectiosum (human parvovirus B19)	Macnular erythema (slapped cheeks)	Face (early)	Fever, malaise before rash; arthritis, especially hands, wrists and knees	Serial IgG titers and specific IgM
	Reticulate or morbilliform	Trunk and limbs	Anemia, especially in immunocompromised and hemolytic anemia patients	
Chicken pox (varicella zoster)	Crops of papules evolving to vesicles, pustules, crusts then scars	Centripetal (trunk and face, proximal more than distal limbs)	Occasional encephalitis, hepatitis, pneumonia	EM for virus; culture; CF antibody
Measles (rubeola)	*Mouth*: Koplik spots *Skin*: pink macules become confluent and papular	Rash spreads from forehead and behind ears to face then trunk and limbs	Prodrome; malaise, fever, conjunctivitis, coryza, cough; occasional pneumonia, encephalitis	Specific Ag by IF; CF antibody
German measles (rubella)	Pink macules become confluent	Face to trunk and limbs	Prodrome; lymphadenopathy, especially suboccipital; arthritis of large joints	Serial IgG titers and specific IgM
Enterovirus (echo, coxsackie B)	Erythematous and papular eruption	Face to trunk	Stomatitis common; occasional meningitis myocarditis, hepatitis, pneumonia	Culture (throat, stool); CF antibody
Infectious mononucleosis (Epstein–Barr)	Erythematous, occasionally purpuric maculopapular eruption; rash aggravated by some antibiotics, especially ampicillin	Trunk and limbs	Prodrome; fever, often prolonged; sore throat, posterior cervical lymphadenopathy ± hepatosplenomegaly; occasional neurological, cardiac, hematological complications	Atypical mononuclear cells on blood smear; heterophile antibody; EBV Ab. (capsid)
AIDS (human immuno-deficiency virus)	Seborrheoic dermatitis Folliculitis Orogenital candidosis Herpes simplex Molluscum contagiosum Kaposi sarcoma: purplish macules and plaques (uncommon in women)	Face, ears, trunk Trunk Vaginal and oral mucosa Mouth and/or genitalia Widespread Widespread, can be generalized, often aligned along skin creases	Lymphadenopathy, weight loss, hairy leucoplakia of tongue, pneumocystis, pneumonia, atypical mycobacterial infections, neurological disease, lymphomas	HIV Ab

COLLAGEN VASCULAR DISEASE: LUPUS ERYTHEMATOSUS

Risks and Management Options

In the absence of active multi system disease, pregnancy does not, in general, adversely affect systemic lupus erythematosus (SLE).[3] When exacerbations do occur, they mainly involve the skin and joints (**Figure 1**) and respond to an increased dose of prednisolone.[4]

The general consequences for the fetus are described in Chapter 27. The major cutaneous complication is neonatal lupus erythematosus. This is an auto-immune disease due to transplacental passage of antibody, usually anti-Ro. The incidence is about 1:20 000 live births, 1:20 in women with the Ro (SS-A) antibody and perhaps 1:60 for all SLE pregnancies.[5] In total, 75% of reported infants are female.[6] There is an association with HLA DR2 and DR3 in the mothers.

The skin lesions of neonatal lupus erythematosus are apparent within the first 2 months of life and predominate on the face, scalp and other exposed sites.[7] Sometimes it is evident that they have been triggered by UV exposure, a common feature in Ro-positive adults with cutaneous lupus erythematosus. Occasionally, phototherapy for neonatal jaundice may play a role. Erythematous macules, papules and plaques, often with slight scaling and central hypopigmentation giving an annular appearance, are characteristic. Unlike discoid lupus erythematosus, there is no follicular plugging,

atrophy or scarring. The inflammatory lesions have generally cleared by 6 months, although the hypopigmentation may last 1–2 years. About 10% of cases with skin lesions also have congenital heart block, about 50% of which need a pacemaker, and occasionally hepatitis and/or thrombocytopenia will be present.

The mothers of these neonates may have a history of rash with photosensitivity, rheumatic symptoms, dry mouth and eyes, i.e. mild lupus erythematosus and/or Sjogrens syndrome. At the outset, about 50% of mothers have no symptoms of connective tissue disease but with follow-up many do become symptomatic. The risk for the mother, who has had a baby with neonatal lupus, of further affected children is about 25%.[8]

Diagnosis is often made by clinical evaluation. The skin biopsy shows basal cell damage and a superficial perivascular mononuclear cell infiltrate. Direct immunofluorescence is usually positive in the epidermis. Nearly all infants with neonatal lupus and their mothers have anti-Ro (SSA) antibodies;[9] some have anti-La (SS-B) and this may be of such a high titer as to mask anti-Ro. A few have anti-U-1 RNP. Antinuclear antibodies may in addition be present. Thus, anti-Ro, anti-La and anti-RNP status should be documented in mother and infant. The baby should be screened for heart block including an electrocardiogram (ECG), and also have liver function tests and a platelet count.

Attempts have been made to prevent damage *in utero* using plasmapheresis and high-dose corticosteroids, but this cannot yet be recommended as a routine. The rash is self-limiting. Topical steroids may have a role. Protection from UV light during the first year of life is important, with appropriate use of clothing, avoidance of unnecessary sun exposure and high SPF sun screens. Long-term survivors of neonatal lupus are at risk of developing connective tissue disease in adulthood but there are insufficient data at present to quantify this risk.

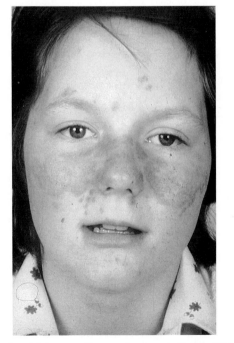

Figure 1. Malar erythema in a pregnant woman with SLE.

COLLAGEN VASCULAR DISEASE DERMATOMYOSITIS/ POLYMYOSITIS (DM/PM)

Risks and Management Options

This connective tissue disease (**Figure 2**) is much less common than lupus erythematosus, with an incidence of 5 cases per million. Although it can occur at any age, it is rare in the reproductive years. Nevertheless, there are serious risks for mother and child if it does occur.[9] If the disease is in remission at the outset of pregnancy, there is much less likelihood of an adverse outcome than when the outset is during pregnancy. Any exacerbation can usually be controlled by increas-

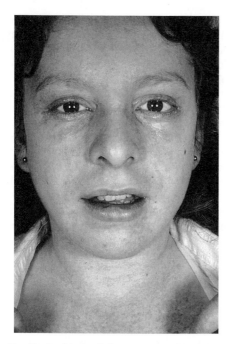

Figure 2. Periorbital violaceous erythema characteristic of dermatomyositis in a teenager.

ing the dose of prednisolone. A reduction of the steroid dose should be done cautiously, particularly in the postpartum period, when recurrences are especially likely. When DM/PM begins in pregnancy, there is a perinatal mortality of 57% and an increased risk of death for the mother.[9] Immunosuppressants such as methotrexate may be required if steroids alone do not control the disease with an attendant high incidence of fetal malformations if given early in pregnancy. If DM/PM is diagnosed in the first trimester, the possibility of therapeutic abortion can be discussed in the light of the poor prognosis.

There is a high incidence of high intrauterine growth deficiency and premature labor, so intensive prenatal care is essential. If the myositis is still active at the time of labor, an assisted vaginal delivery may be required.

COLLAGEN VASCULAR DISEASE: SYSTEMIC SCLEROSIS

Risks and Management Options

Although there is a marked female preponderance in this condition, the concurrence of systemic sclerosis[10,11] and pregnancy is uncommon (**Figure 3**) and there is very limited information from controlled case studies. Furthermore, systemic sclerosis is a heterogeneous disorder ranging from mildly affected cases with Raynaud's phenomenon, dysphagia and sclerodactyly to the diffuse type with widespread skin sclerosis and life-threatening multisystem involvement. Management of the pregnancy in a patient with systemic sclerosis is discussed in detail in Chapter 27.

There is a risk of increased small-for-dates babies and neonatal deaths, even in those with Raynaud's phenomenon alone at the time of pregnancy.[6] Those with diffuse disease fare badly, with the likelihood of deterioration in renal, cardiac and lung function. The

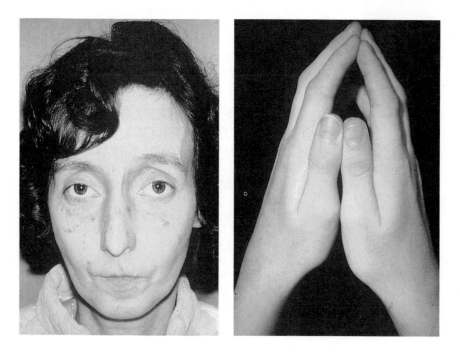

Figure 3. (a, left) Systemic sclerosis: a 35-year-old woman showing tight facies and small mouth. (b, right) Systemic sclerosis: the prayer sign – stiffening of the skin preventing complete apposition of the hands.

greatest danger is during the third trimester and post-partum period, when hypertension and renal failure can develop suddenly, sometimes with fatal consequences for the mother. There is no evidence of transmission of the disease to the fetus.

COLLAGEN VASCULAR DISEASE: PEMPHIGUS

Risks and Management Options

Pregnancy can aggravate pemphigus.[12] There is an increased fetal death rate[13] and the newborn can have skin lesions because of transplacental transfer of antibody. Thus, fetal growth and well-being should be monitored. The neonate should be examined carefully for lesions. If at all possible, pemphigus should be controlled with steroids alone during pregnancy.

DISORDERS OF CONNECTIVE TISSUE: EHLERS DANLOS SYNDROME

Risks and Management Options

Women with types I or IV Ehlers Danlos syndrome are very susceptible to postpartum bleeding, poor wound healing, wound dehiscence, uterine lacerations and abdominal hernias.[9,14,15] Rupture of the major arteries, the bowel or uterus can also occur mainly with type IV,[16] and in this gropup maternal mortality may be as high as 25%. The risks are such that women with Ehlers Danlos syndrome type I or IV should be counseled against pregnancy. However, if they are pregnant, vigilance for the above problems should be maintained. Intravenous access and crossmatch of blood is advisable in advance of vaginal delivery. Operative delivery should be undertaken with as little tissue trauma as possible. Non-absorbable sutures are advisable for cesarean section.

DISORDERS OF CONNECTIVE TISSUE: PSEUDOXANTHOMA ELASTICUM

Risks and Management Options

The main complication of this condition is massive hematemesis necessitating blood transfusion. Careful monitoring of blood pressure during pregnancy and prompt treatment if elevated are essential.[17]

TUMORS: MALIGNANT MELANOMA

Risks and Management Options

Much controversy has surrounded the relationship between pregnancy and melanoma. A World Health Organization prospective study has shown a reduced 5 year survival (66%) for women who develop stage 1 disease during pregnancy, compared with those in whom the melanoma begins before (80%) or between (78%) pregnancies.[18] Transplacental transmission of malignant melanoma is extraordinarily rare. The treatment of choice is prompt excision of the tumor. For a more detailed discussion, see Chapter 32.

OTHER TUMORS

Risks and Management Options

Mycosis fungoides can worsen in pregnancy,[19] as can Langerhans' cell histiocytosis.[20] There are several potential hazards for patients with neurofibromatosis including hypertension, renal artery rupture, eruption of new skin lesions and enlargement of existing ones, particularly plexiform neuromas.

METABOLIC DISEASES: PORHYRIA

Risks and Management Options

The prophyrias can present problems in pregnancy both with acute attacks (acute intermittent porphyria)[21] and an exacerbation of skin fragility (porphyria cutanea tarda and porphyria variegata). These problems usually occur in the first trimester. In treating patients, venesection is acceptable but it is important that chloroquine is avoided.

METABOLIC DISEASES: ACRODERMATITIS ENTEROPATHICA

Risks and Management Options

This disorder of zinc metabolism typically worsens during pregnancy.[22] It may even make its initial presentation in pregnancy with a widespread pustular and erosive eruption. Serum zinc levels are low and the condition responds to supplementation. Occasional

PRE-EXISTING SKIN DISORDERS
Summary of Management Options

INFECTIONS
(see Chapters 29, 30 and 49)
COLLAGEN VASCULAR DISEASE
(see also Chapter 27)

Systemic lupus erythematosus

- Maternal skin and joint exacerbations respond to prednisolone

Neonatal lupus erythematosus

- Skin biopsy if diagnosis uncertain

- Document maternal and neonatal anti-Ro, anti-La and anti-RNP status

- EKG, liver function, platelets in newborn

- Topical steroids, protect from UV

- Congenital heart block (see Chapter 47)

Dermatomyositis/polymyositis

- First attack in pregnancy
  - poor prognosis
  - prednisolone (metrotrexate as second line)
  - vigilance for IUGR and preterm labor
  - consider assisted vaginal delivery

- Pre-existing disease
  - prednisone for exacerbation

Systemic sclerosis

- See also Chapter 27

- Vigilance for IUGR

- Monitor maternal BP, renal, cardiac and pulmonary function

Pemphigus

- Control maternal lesions with steroids

- Monitor fetal growth and well-being

- Examine newborn for lesions

CONNECTIVE TISSUE DISORDERS

Ehlers Danlos syndrome

- Prepregnancy counsel against conception

- Vigilance for PPH, wound dehiscence, rupture of viscera

- I.V. access and crossmatch blood for delivery

- Avoid excessive trauma at operative delivery

- Non-absorbable sutures for cesarean section

Pseudoxanthoma elasticum

- Monitor BP and prompt treatment for hypertension

TUMORS
Malignant melanoma

- Prompt excision

Others

- Monitor BP in patients with neurofibromatosis

METABOLIC DISEASES

Porphyria

- Vigilance for recurrence/exacerbation

- Consider venesection

- Avoid chloroquine in first trimester

Acrodermatitis enteropathica

- Zinc supplementation

- Careful screening for fetal normality

Psoriasis

Generalized pustular psoriasis

- Monitor maternal cardiac and renal function

- Monitor fetal well-being

- High-dose corticosteroids

- Metrotrexate and cyclosporin A are second line drugs

- Consider termination of pregnancy

OTHER SKIN DISEASES
Eczema

- Emollients, soap substitutes, 1% hydrocortisone cream

Epidermolysis bullosa

- Offer fetal skin biopsy for severe heredity forms

- Avoid skin trauma/irritation

cases of fetal abnormalities have been reported; thus careful screening for fetal normality is important.

METABOLIC DISEASES: PSORIASIS

Risks and Management Options

Pregnancy may improve, worsen, or have no effect on the natural history of psoriasis. If there is an effect, it is often repeated with successive pregnancies. Generalized pustular psoriasis can occur in pregnancy, and there is controversy as to whether impetigo herpetiformis is a variant or a distinct disease (see below). The diagnosis of generalized pustular psoriasis is suggested by an antecedent and/or family history of psoriasis; a generalized inflammatory dermatosis with myriads of sterile, often coalescing pustules (**Figure 4**), associated with high fever and toxicity. Untreated, death can occur from cardiac or renal failure and fetal prognosis is very poor. There is usually a prompt response to high-dose corticosteroid therapy, although termination of pregnancy is usually required. If this also fails to control the disease, systemic methotrexate or cyclosporin A may prove successful. A mestranol/ethynodiol combination has been used.[23]

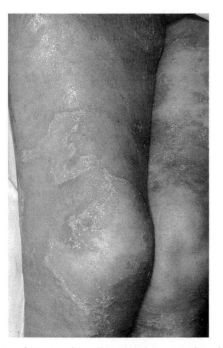

Figure 4. Sheets of sterile pustules associated with widespread erythema: generalized pustular psoriasis or impetigo herpetiformis.

OTHER SKIN DISEASES: ECZEMA

Risks and Management Options

Atopic dermatitis often improves in pregnancy but in some it worsens. The breast-feeding mother often has problems after delivery with cracked, itchy, sore and ezematous nipples. Emollients, use of soap substitutes such as aqueous cream BP (British Pharmacopoeia) and a mild topical steroid such as 1% hydrocortisone ointment is usually helpful.

OTHER SKIN DISEASES: EPIDERMOLYSIS BULLOSA

Risks and Management Options

This is a heterogeneous group of disorders in which blistering occurs after minor trauma. For epidermolysis bullosa letalis, and the severely scarring hereditary forms, prenatal diagnosis by fetal skin biopsy analysis has been successful (see Chapter 56). For the mother with a severe form of epidermolysis, there are special concerns for the anesthetist, e.g. avoidance of adhesive tape, care to avoid pressure and friction from the mask and with intubation. Padding of the face mask and well-lubricated, smaller than usual endotracheal tubes are recommended, as is regional anesthesia when this is feasible.[24]

PRURITUS IN PREGNANCY

Since about 15% of pregnant women complain of pruritus,[25] the following are some general guidelines for evaluating the patient:

- Careful clinical evaluation, supported, if necessary, by appropriate laboratory investigations, will identify specific skin conditions such as scabies and systemic disorders with associated dermatological manifestations. Some of these diseases have already been discussed.

- In the patient with itching and no rash (or solely excoriations), one should consider other systemic disorders such as lymphoma, liver and thyroid disease.[26]

- In the remaining women, when a rash is present, a pregnancy-specific dermatosis should be considered (see below).

- Goodlin and colleagues have developed the concept that an overactive placenta, as measured by elevated hCG, can be associated with pruritus,[27] provided other causes have been excluded. Confirmation from other centers is needed to establish the identity of this condition.

- The women who has no rash, no systemic disorder and no specific non-pregnancy skin disorder should be considered to have pruritus gravidarum (see below).

PRURITUS GRAVIDARUM

Risks and Management Options

The term 'pruritus gravidarum' (obstetric cholestasis)[28] is best applied to itching secondary to pregnancy-related intrahepatic cholestasis. It occurs in about 0.2% of pregnancies,[29] with a higher incidence in Swedes and Chilean Indians. It is recurrent in about 40% of affected women, and some data suggest an autosomal dominantly inherited genetic trait.[30] Although the mother remains well, there are risks for the fetus. These include an increased incidence of prematurity and stillbirth,[31] and intrapartum fetal distress.[32,33]

The biliary obstruction is probably related to changes in the canaliculi induced by altered estrogen metabolism,[34] and this produces an elevation in circulating bile salts. Itching begins in the second half of pregnancy, often over the abdomen, but may become widespread, and can be severe in intensity. The woman remains well, in contrast to cases of pruritus secondary to other types of liver disease.[29] If jaundice occurs, it is slight and develops late. The symptoms resolve rapidly after delivery.

To make the diagnosis of pruritus gravidarum, the best laboratory correlation is elevation of serum bile acids, especially cholic acid, which may well rise 10–100 times normal. This may precede any symptoms. Bilirubin may be raised, as may alkaline phosphatase; but the latter is typically elevated anyway in pregnancy. Standard liver function tests are normal in about 25% of cases.[29] The transaminases may be slightly elevated; much higher levels suggest other hepatic pathology. An ultrasound of the gallbladder will help to exclude gallstones. Fetal growth and well-being should be carefully monitored during pregnancy.

The definitive treatment is parturition. The timing of this will be determined by factors such as gestational age, progressive deterioration of liver function, fetal conditions and perhaps fetal pulmonary maturity.[29] During labor, careful monitoring of the fetal condition is advised.

Symptomatic control of the pruritus has been

PRURITUS IN PREGNANCY
Summary of Management Options

Establish the diagnosis

- Specific disorders and systemic diseases with skin involvement (see previous sections)

- Other systemic diseases with pruritus (lymphoma, liver, thyroid)

- If rash present, consider pregnancy-specific dermatoses (see following section)

- Pruritus gravidarum

- ?Hyperplacentosis

Management (depends on the cause)

For pruritus gravidarum

- Monitor fetal growth and well-being

- Delivery is the definitive treatment

- Monitor fetal well-being in labor

- Maternal treatment

  - phenobarbitone

  - cholestyramine (+ vitamin K)

  - hydroxyethylrutosides

- UV-B radiation

---

attempted by a variety of means. Antihistamines and topical therapies are of little value. Phenobarbitone, to induce hepatic secretion of bile salts, has been shown to be unsuccessful in controlled trials.[35,36] Cholestyramine 12 g daily helps, but only those with moderately elevated bile acids.[36] If it is used, vitamin K supplements should be given to the mother. Hydroxyethylrutosides, which have been used in primary biliary cirrhosis to reduce bile leakage from dermal capillaries,[37] may also be of some value in pruritis gravidarum,[29] but further studies are needed. Finally, suberythema doses of ultraviolet B radiation three times weekly can be effective and safe.[38]

RASHES IN PREGNANCY

A woman who develops a rash in pregnancy will have either:

- a pre-existing skin condition which has the rash as a recognized feature (see original section of this chapter)

- a specific dermatosis of pregnancy (see below).

THE SPECIFIC DERMATOSES OF PREGNANCY

It is clear that there are inflammatory dermatoses found exclusively in pregnancy, but there remains some confusion about their terminology. The system adopted by Holmes and Black.[39] is used here with some of the many alternatives listed for individual diseases. With the exception of pemphigoid gestationis, for which there are confirmatory immunopathological findings, diagnosis is based on clinical observation.

SPECIFIC DERMATOSES: POLYMORPHIC ERUPTION OF PREGNANCY

Risks and Management Options

This condition has many alternative names, including pruritic and urticarial papules and plaques of pregnancy, toxemic rash of pregnancy, toxemic erythema of pregnancy, late onset prurigo of pregnancy, prurigo gestationis and erythema multiforme of pregnancy. It is a common problem, affecting 1:160 pregnancies,[40] mainly primigravida. There are no associations with auto-immune or other disease, no known inherited tendency, geographical variation, or relationship to hormonal balance.

The rash (**Figures 5, 6**) may begin between 17 weeks gestation and up to 1 week postpartum, with a mean of 36 weeks. It is usually itchy, sometimes severely so, and typically begins in the abdominal striae as erythematous edematous papules. Other sites often affected are the thighs and extensor surfaces of the

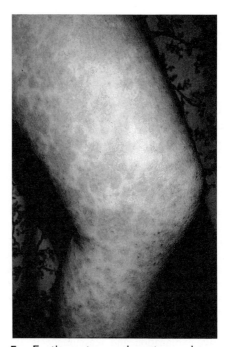

Figure 5. Erythematous edematous plaques and papules on the thighs.

arms. The eruption may become widespread, but usually spares the scalp, face, palms and soles. It does not involve mucous membranes. Plaques, polycyclic lesions, small vesicles, and some degree of scaling often occur and in some cases there are target lesions. It may be more common in twin pregnancies[41] and manifestations more severe.[42] The pathogenesis is uncertain.[40,43] There are no serious risks for the mother or fetus.[40] If it does recur in a subsequent pregnancy, it is usually with reduced severity.

Because there can be overlap in clinical appearances with pemphigoid gestationis, a skin biopsy for direct immunofluorescence should be considered,[44] particularly if there are atypical features such as presentation before the third trimester or if the condition is severe. Occasionally, drug eruption, scabies and eczema will need to be excluded as differential diagnoses. On biopsy there is a lympho-histiocytic infiltrate in the upper – and sometimes lower – dermis, with variable numbers of eosinophils, dermal edema and sometimes spongiosis of the epidermis.[45,46] Direct immunofluorescence is usually negative, in contrast to pemphigoid (herpes) gestationis. One case has been reported of a pemphigus-like pattern of epidermal intercellular IgG[47] and occasional cases of weak positivity with C3 but no IgG have been recorded.[41,48] There are no consistent serological or hematological abnormalities.

Reassurance should be given as to the expectation of resolution after parturition and the lack of any harmful effect on the fetus. If treatment is needed, moderate potency topical corticosteroids and sedative antihistamines are often sufficient to control pruritus. In severe cases, oral prednisolone (e.g. 30 mg daily) can be rapidly effective.[49]

SPECIFIC DERMATOSES: PRURITIC FOLLICULITIS OF PREGNANCY

Risks and Management Options

The frequency of this disorder is unknown, but it is probably not uncommon.[50] The condition begins in the second or third trimester. The lesions (**Figure 6**) are pruritic and erythematous follicular papules which may involve trunk and limbs, and become excoriated. They resemble steroid acne. Resolution occurs after delivery. In two of the original six cases, the condition had occurred with previous pregnancies.[51] There are no risks for the mother and baby.

Usually, explanation and reassurance is all that is required. If the diagnosis is uncertain or the symptoms are severe, skin biopsies may be considered and will show intrafollicular pustules with variable numbers of eosinophils and that direct immunofluorescence is negative.[51] If treatment is necessary, topical 10% benzoyl peroxide together with 1% hydrocortisone cream is said to be helpful.[28]

SPECIFIC DERMATOSES: PRURIGO OF PREGNANCY

Risks and Management Options

This itchy papular eruption occurs in about 1:300 pregnancies.[52] It has been suggested that prurigo of pregnancy is the result of pruritus gravidarum occuring in women with an atopic diathesis, but as yet this is unproven. A condition termed 'papular dermatitis of pregnancy' was first described in 1962 by Spangler[53] as occurring in 1:2400 pregnancies; the current status of this entity is now uncertain and it is probably best regarded on review as a variant of prurigo of pregnancy.[45,50] There are no risks for the mother or baby.

Eruption (**Figure 7**) usually begins at 25–30 weeks gestation. There are discrete itchy papules, most numerous over the extensor aspect of the upper arms and thighs, on the abdomen and sometimes elsewhere. There are no urticaria-like lesions or vesicles. The lesions become excoriated and usually persist for several weeks postpartum. Recurrence with subsequent pregnancies in unusual. Skin biopsy may be considered in severe cases and should reveal non-specific epidermal thickening, parakeratosis and a predominantly lymphocytic upper dermal infiltration. Immunofluorescence is negative. Moderately potent topical steroids and oral sedative antihistamines are effective treatment.

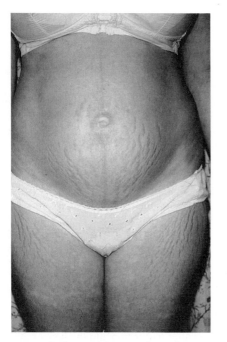

Figure 6. Polymophic eruption of pregnancy.

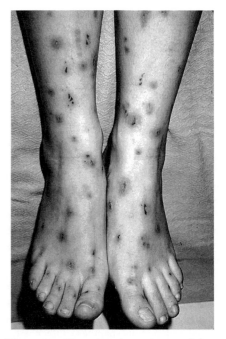

Figure 7. Excoriated prurigo nodules.

SPECIFIC DERMATOSES: PEMPHIGOID (HERPES) GESTATIONIS

Risks and Management Options

The best characterized of the specific inflammatory dermatoses of pregnancy was initially named herpes gestationis by Milton in 1872.[54] The term herpes, which comes from the Greek 'to creep', dates back to Galen, and has been used for skin conditions in which there are clusters of vesicles which tend to extend at the periphery. On the grounds that this pregnancy-associated bullous dermatosis has much in common with the immunologically mediated disorder bullous pemphigoid and is not caused by any herpes virus, Holmes and Black have championed the term 'pemphigoid gestationis'.[39,45] It is a rare condition, occurring in about 1:50 000 pregnancies.[55] and probably rarer still among non-white patients.[56] It is significantly associated with other auto-immune diseases such as Grave's disease, alopecia areata and vitiligo,[57,58] and there is an increased incidence of HLA-B8, HLA-DR3 and in particular the paired haplotype HLA-DR3, DR4.[54] As well as being associated with normal pregnancy, pemphigoid gestationis has been described with hydatidiform mole[59] and choriocarcinoma.[60]

Provided there is the same consort, recurrences in further pregnancies are usual, with further episodes beginning earlier in pregnancy and being more severe, suggesting that paternal antigenicity is critical.[61,62] As well as the immunological and genetic background, the hormonal milieu is important, recurrences sometimes being seen well after parturition in association with oral contraceptives and the menstrual cycle.[61] The evidence points strongly towards pemphigoid gestationis being an auto-immune disease. The antigenic trigger is likely to be of paternal origin, expressed on placental cells and cross-reactive with a maternal skin basement membrane site.[63]

The condition usually begins in the second or third trimester with an average onset at 21 weeks, although about 20% of patients first manifest the disease in the postpartum period.[58] When recurrent, the onset is usually earlier. Itching may occur before any rash. Lesions often develop initially within or around the umbilicus and then become widespread on the trunk, buttocks and extremities (**Figure 8**), involvement of the palms and soles being quite common. Oral lesions occur occasionally. Pemphigoid gestationis is a polymorphic disorder, with urticaria-like papules and plaques, annular and polycyclic lesions, vesicles and bullae. The latter arise both on inflamed and clinically normal skin. The most distinctive lesion is the urticated plaque with tense vesicles and bullae arising peripherally and then crusting. Pruritus is the main symptom, liable to disturb

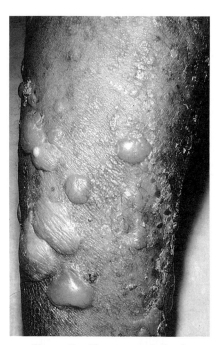

Figure 8.   Herpes gestationis.

sleep. Without secondary infection, healing occurs without scarring.

The clinical course may improve spontaneously towards the end of the third trimester but in 50–75% of cases there are exacerbations within 24–48 h of delivery which may persist for weeks to several months. The bullae settle before the inflammatory plaques. A case has been reported with the disease still active 12 years postpartum.[64] Breast-feeding may contribute to shortening the course of the disease after delivery.[58] As stated above, minor flares may be associated with oral contraception,[54] menstruation and less commonly ovulation.[61,65] For the mother, the main hazard is the high likelihood of recurrence with greater severity and a more protracted course in subsequent pregnancies. A few infants, probably less than 5%, develop transient vesicular-bullous lesions after birth and the condition is clinically mild.

There is controversy about overall fetal outcome in the literature. Holmes and Black[66] reported an increased incidence of small-for-dates babies and infant mortality suggesting placental insufficiency in pemphigoid gestationis, although Shornick reported no increase in fetal complications.[55] It would seem prudent that babies of affected mothers should be delivered in centers with full neonatal facilities. If there is any doubt about the diagnosis, skin biopsy is advisable. The histology shows upper dermal edema with perivascular inflammation showing variable proportions of lymphocytes, histiocytes and eosinophils. In the epidermis, there may be spongiosis, sometimes with eosino-

Table 2
Comparison of pemphigoid gestationis and
polymorphic eruption of pregnancy

	Pemphigoid gestationis	Polymorphic eruption of pregnancy
Incidences per 100 000	2	625
Morphology		
urticarial lesions	+	+
vesicles	++	+
bullae	++	−
Prominently in striae	3%	81%
Umbilical lesions	87%	12%
Postpartum exacerbations	75%	15%
C3 at basement membrane zone by direct immunofluorescence	100%	0%

Modified from Holmes et al.[68]

phils, and the bullae are subepidermal. Electron microscopy reveals a lamina lucida split.[67]

Direct immunofluorescence shows C3 in a linear distribution at the basement membrane zone in all patients. A circulating basement membrane-specific complement binding IgG can be found in 25% of cases by indirect immunofluorescence,[68] and perhaps all cases with more sensitive immuno-electron microscopic techniques.[69] Using immunoblotting techniques, it has been shown that the major antigen recognized by the basement membrane zone-specific IgG is a 180 kD protein, with some sera also detecting a 240 kD protein characteristic of bullous pemphigoid.[70]

Examination of cryostat sections of perilesional skin for the distinctive linear pattern of C3 immunofluorescence is diagnostic. The major differential diagnosis is polymorphic eruption of pregnancy (see **Table 2**). Other diseases such as urticaria, erythema multiforme, contact dermatitis and non-pregnancy related bullous dermatoses can usually be easily distinguished.

With early mild cases, it is reasonable to initiate therapy with moderately potent topical corticosteroids and a sedative antihistamine. If this fails, and with more severe disease, prednisolone 40 mg daily should be instituted, reducing 7–10 days after control is achieved to the minimal effective dose. Most cases can be maintained on 10 mg prednisolone daily or less. The dose should be increased around the time of delivery to cover for the frequent postpartum flare.[58] Occasionally, patients do not respond to 40 mg prednisolone daily. Initially, a higher dose (e.g. 80 mg) should then be tried, but if this is unsuccessful after a few days, plasmapheresis is an alternative that can be considered and may also be appropriate for the patient in whom corticosteroids are contraindicated.[71]

Despite the controversy over fetal risk, it is prudent to screen for placental dysfunction by monitoring fetal growth and well-being. The baby should be examined for the transient vesicular-bullous lesions after birth (see above).

SPECIFIC DERMATOSES: IMPETIGO HERPETIFORMIS

Risks and Management Options

Until recently,[72] this rare condition had been assumed to be generalized pustular psoriasis modified by pregnancy and many authorities do not recognize it as a distinct entity.[39,73,74] Some of the differences are shown in **Table 3**. Onset is usually in the third trimester. With subsequent pregnancies it is recurrent, often with an earlier onset and with greater severity. The eruption begins in the major flexures and may spread to the trunk and extremities (**Figure 4**). It consists of rounded or arcuate erythematous patches studded with minute pustules which remain discrete and may be concentric in arrangement. Patients are often toxic, febrile and hypocalcemic, as are those with generalized pustular psoriasis. There are serious risks for mother and fetus. Maternal death can occur from cardiac or renal failure. There is a high risk of intrauterine or early postnatal death.

If there is any doubt about whether the eruption is generalized pustular psoriasis or impetigo herpetiformis a short course of high-dose prednisolone can be tried, since generalized pustular psoriasis usually responds in a few days. The maternal condition needs to be monitored carefully with special attention to cardiac and renal function. The fetal condition should also be monitored. Termination of the pregnancy is usually required, and in most cases promptly cures the disorder. The timing will be determined by the maternal and fetal conditions.

MISCELLANEOUS SKIN COMPLAINTS ASSOCIATED WITH PHYSIOLOGICAL CHANGES IN PREGNANCY

Risks and Management Options

These are generally assumed to be due to the endocrine milieu of pregnancy but precise evidence for a mechanism is usually lacking.[75,76] None of these changes have any harmful effect on the health of the mother or the fetus. The management options are summarized in **Table 4**.

Table 3
Comparison of generalized pustular psoriasis with impetigo herpetiformis

	Generalized pustular psoriasis	Impetigo herpetiformis
Antecedent psoriasis	+	−
Family history of psoriasis	+	−
Strictly limited to pregnancy	±	++
Flexures only	±	++
Fever, malaise	+	+
Pustules remain discrete	±	++
Atypical mononuclear cells in infiltrate[60]	−	+
Responsive to high-dose steroid therapy	+	±
Improvement after delivery	+	++

Table 4
Management of miscellaneous skin complaints associated with physiological changes in pregnancy

Complaint	Comment	Management
Spider naevi	Five-fold increase in pregnancy, appear in first half and fade after pregnancy	No treatment (electrodesiccation) unless present 3 months postpartum
Palmar erythema	In two-thirds of Caucasian, and one-third of Afro-Caribbean women	Explanation/reassurance
Varicosities	50% of women have these in various sites	(a) *Legs*: elevation when resting, elastic support stockings (b) *Hemorrhoids*: stool softeners, anesthetic creams and suppositories
Non-pitting edema	Present in ankles of 70% and face of 50%	Exclude hypertensive disease; leg elevation, stockings; diuretics only if severe
Striae gravidarum	Present in 90% of Caucasian women (less in Asian and Afro-Caribbean)	Explanation/reassurance; topical 1% hydrocortisone if symptoms severe
Gum hypertrophy and gingivitis	Present in most pregnancies	Explanation/reassurance
Eruptive oral hemangioma	Present in 27% of women; smooth red nodule arising in mouth in early pregnancy	Explanation/reassurance; good dental hygiene; excision of excess bleed
Skin tags	Occur on upper body in late pregnancy; mostly resolve spontaneously	Explanation/reassurance; physical treatments if persist postnatally
Pigmentation	Noted in 90% (especially dark skinned)	Explanation/reassurance; avoid excess sun exposure
Hair growth	Increase in pregnancy is common	Exclude pathological androgen production if excessive
	Alopecia can occur, but usually recovers postnatally	
Sweat and sebaceous glands	Eocrine sweating increases; apocrine sweating is reduced; sebum secretion increases to worsen acne in some	Severe axillary sweating controlled by 20% solution of aluminum hydrochloride at night

---

RASHES IN PREGNANCY
Summary of Management Options

Establish the cause

- Specific skin disorders and systemic diseases with skin involvement (see first section)

- Dermatoses of pregnancy

FOR DERMATOSES OF PREGNANCY

Polymorphic eruption of pregnancy

- Consider skin biopsy (if atypical or severe)

- Explanation and reassurance

- If treatment is required
  - oral antihistamine (e.g. chlorpheniramine)
  - topical corticosteroids (moderate potency)
  - oral prednisolone

Pruritic folliculitis of pregnancy

- Consider skin biopsy (if severe)

- Explanation and reassurance

- If treatment is required, topical 10% benzoyl peroxide or 1% hydrocortisone

Prurigo of pregnancy

- Explanation and reassurance

- If treatment is required:

  - topical corticosteroids (moderate potency)

  - oral antihistamine

Pemphigoid gestationis

- Skin biopsy if doubt about diagnosis

- Oral antihistamines

- Topical corticosteroids (moderate potency)

- If severe/resistant form, oral prednisolone

- Plasmapheresis if prednisolone fails

Impetigo herpetiformis

- Try high-dose oral prednisolone

- Monitor maternal cardiac and renal function

- Delivery is usually curative

REFERENCES

1 Duncan ME, Pearson JMH, Ridley DS *et al.* (1982) Pregnancy and leprosy: The consequences of alteration of cell-mediated and humoral immunity during pregnancy and lactation. *Leprosy Review* **55**:129–142.
2 Smith LG, and Faro S (1990) Cutaneous manifestations of bacterial and viral disorders in pregnancy. *Clinics in Obstetrics and Gynecology* **33**:792–800.
3 Out HJ, Derksen RHWM, Christiaens GCML (1989) Systemic lupus erythematosus and pregnancy. *Obstetrical and Gynecological Survey* **44**:585–591.
4 Anonymous (1991) Systemic lupus erythematosus in pregnancy. *Lancet* **338**:87–88.
5 Ramsay-Goldman R, Horn D, Deng J *et al.* (1986) Anti-SS-A antibodies and fetal outcome in maternal systemic lupus erythematosus. *Arthritis and Rheumatism* **29**:1269–1273.
6 Lee LA, Weston WL (1986) Lupus erythematosus in childhood. *Dermatologic Clinics* **4**:151–160.
7 Provost TT, Watson R, Gaither KK, Harley JB (1987) The neonatal lupus syndrome. *Journal of Rheumatology* **14**:199–205.
8 Lee LA (1990) Maternal autoantibodies and pregnancy.

II: The neonatal lupus syndrome. *Ballière's Clinics in Rheumatology* **4**:69–84.

9　Rosenzweig BA, Rotmensch S, Binelte SD, Philippe M. (1989) Primary idiopathic polymyositis and dermatomyositosis complicating pregnancy: Diagnosis and management. *Obstetrical and Gynecological Survey* **44**:162–170.

10　Black CM (1990) Systemic sclerois and pregnancy. *Ballière's Clinics in Rheumatology* **4**:105–120.

11　Maymon R, Fejgin M (1989) Scleroderma in pregnancy. *Obstetrical and Gynecological Survey* **44**:530–533.

12　Honeyman JF, Equiguren G, Pinto A *et al.* (1981) Bullous dermatoses of pregnancy. *Archives of Dermatology* **117**:264–267.

13　Ross MG, Kaut B, Frieder R *et al.* (1986) Pemphigus in pregnancy: A re-evaluation of fetal risk. *American Journal of Obstetrics and Gynecology* **155**:30–33.

14　Rivera-Alsina ME, Kwan P, Zavisca FG *et al.* (1984) Complications of the Ehlers Danlos Syndrome in pregnancy: A case report. *Journal of Reproductive Medicine* **29**:757–759.

15　Snyder RR, Gilstrop LC, Hauth JC (1983) Ehlers Danlos syndrome and pregnancy: *Obstetrics and Gynecology* **61**:649–651.

16　Rudd NL, Nimrod C, Holbrook KA *et al.* (1983) Pregnancy complications in type IV Ehlers Danlos syndrome. *Lancet* **1**:50–53.

17　Berde C, Willis DC, Sandberg EC (1983) Pregnancy in women with pseudoxanthoma elasticum. *Obstetrical and Gynecological Survey* **38**:339–344.

18　Mackie RM, Bufalino R, Sutherland C (1990) The effect of pregnancy on melanoma prognosis. *British Journal of Dermatology* **123**:40 (suppl. 37).

19　Vonderheid EC, Dellatorre DL, Van Scott EJ (1981) Prolonged remission of tumour-stage mycosis fungoides by topical immunotherapy. *Archives of Dermatology* **117**:586–589.

20　Growden WA, Cline, Tesler A *et al.* (1986) Adverse effects of pregnancy on multifocal eosinophilic granuloam. *Obstetrics and Gynecology* **67**:2–6s.

21　Kanaan C, Veille JC, Larkin M (1989) Pregnancy and acute intermittent porphyria. *Obstetrical and Gynecological Survey* **44**:244–249.

22　Bronson DM, Barsky R, Barsky S (1983) Acrodermatitis enteropattica: Recognition at long last during a recurrence in pregnancy. *Journal of the American Academy of Dermatologists* **9**:140–144.

23　Gligora M, Kolacio Z (1982) Hormonal treatment of impetigo herpetiformis. *British Journal of Dermatology* **107**:253.

24　Price T, Katz VL (1988) Obstetrical concerns of epidermolysis bullosa. *Obstetrical and Gynecological Survey* **43**:445–449.

25　Furhoff WR Itching in pregnancy: A 15 year follow up study. *Acta Medica Scandinvavica* **196**:403–410.

26　Dacus JV (1990) Pruritis in pregnancy. *Clinics in Obstetrics and Gynecology* **33**:738–745.

27　Goodlin RC, Anderson JC, Skiles TL (1985) Pruritis and hyperplacentosis. *Obstetrics and Gynecology* **66**:36–38s.

28　Kater RMH, Mistilis SP (1967) Obstetric cholestasis and pruritis of pregnancy: *Medical Journal of Australia* **1**:638–640.

29　Fisk NM, Bye WB, Storey GNB (1988) Maternal features of obstetric cholestasis: 20 years experience at King George V Hospital. *Australia and New Zealand Journal of Obstetrics and Gynaecology* **28**:172–176.

30　Holzbach RT (1982) Familial recurrent intrahepatic cholestasis of pregnancy: Evidence for a dominant, possible autosomal trait. *Hepatology* **2**:149.

31　Reid R, Ivey KJ, Rencoret RH, Storey B (1976) Fetal complications of obstetric cholestasis. *British Medical Journal* **1**:870–872.

32　Laatkainen T, Ikonen E (1977) Serum bile acids in cholestasis of pregnancy. *Obstetrics and Gynecology* **50**:313–318.

33　Shaw D, Frohlick J, Wittman BAK, Wilms M (1982) A prospective study of 18 patients with cholestasis of pregnancy. *American Journal of Obstetrics and Gynecology* **142**:621–625.

34　Reyes H, Ribalta J, Gonzalez MC *et al.* (1981) Sulfobromophthalein clearance tests before and after ethinyl oestradiol administration in women and men with family history of intrahepatic cholestasis of pregnancy. *Gastroenterology* **81**:226–231.

35　Heikkinen J, Meintausta O, Ylostalo P, Janne O (1982) Serum bile acid levels in intrahepatic cholestasis of pregnancy during treatment with phenobarbitone or cholestyramine. *European Journal of Obstetrics, Gynaecology and Reproductive Biology* **14**:153–162.

36　Laatkainen T (1978) Effect of cholestyramine and phenobarbital on pruritus and serum bile acid levels in cholestasis of pregnancy. *American Journal of Obstetrics and Gynecology* **132**:501–506.

37　Hishun S, Rose JD, Hunter JO (1981) The relief of pruritis in primary biliary cirrhosis by hydroxyethylrutosides. *British Journal of Dermatology* **105**:457–460.

38　Greenberger P, Patterson R. (1978) Safety of therapy for allergic symptoms during pregnancy. *Annals of Internal Medicine* **89**:234–237.

39　Holmes RC, Black MM (1982) The specific dermatoses of pregnancy: A reappraisal with special emphasis on a proposed simplified clinical classification. *Clinical and Experimental Dermatology* **7**:65–73.

40　Charles-Holmes R (1988) Polymorphic eruption of pregnancy. *Seminars in Dermatology* **8**:18–22.

41　Yancey KB, Hall RP, Lawley TJ (1984) Pruritic urticarial papules and plaques of pregnancy: Clinical experience in 25 patients. *Journal of the American Academy of Dermatologists* **10**:473–480.

42　Bunker CB, Erskine K, Rustin MHA, Gilkes JJH (1990) Severe polymorphic eruption of pregnancy occurring in twin pregnancies. *Clinical and Experimental Dermatology* **15**:228–231.

43　Ingber A, Alcalay J, Sandbank M (1988) Multiple dermal fibroblasts in patients with pruritic urticarial papules and plaques of pregnancy: A clue to the etiology? *Medical Hypotheses* **26**:11–12.

44　Saurat J-H (1989) Immunofluorescence biopsy for pruritic urticarial papules and plaques of pregnancy. *Journal of the American Academy of Dermatologists* **20**:711.

45　Holmes RC, Black MM (1983) The specific dermatoses

of pregnancy. *Journal of the American Academy of Dermatologists* **8**:405–412.

46 Moreno A, Noguera J, de Moragas JM (1985) Polymorphic eruption of pregnancy: Histopathologic study. *Acta Dermato Venereologica* **65**:313–318.

47 Trattner A, Ingber A, Sandbank M (1991) Antiepidermal cell surface antibodies in a patient with pruritic urticarial papules and plaques of pregnancy. *Journal of the American Academy of Dermatologists* **24**:306–308.

48 Alcalay J, Ingber A, David M *et al.* (1987) Pruritic urticarial papules and plaques of pregnancy: Clinical experience in 24 patients. *Journal of Reproductive Medicine* **32**:315–316.

49 Lawley TJ, Hertz KC, Wade TR *et al.* (1979) Pruritic urticarial papules and plaques of pregnancy. *Journal of the American Medical Association* **241**:1696–1699:

50 Black MM (1989) Prurigo of pregnancy, papular dermatitis and pruritic folliculitis of pregnancy. *Seminars in Dermatology* **8**:23–25.

51 Zoberman E, Farmer ER (1981) Pruritic folliculitis of pregnancy. *Archives of Dermatology* **117**:20–22.

52 Nurse DS (1968) Prurigo of pregnancy. *Australian Journal of Dermatology* **9**:258–267.

53 Spangler AS, Reddy W, Bardawill WA *et al.* (1962) Papular dermatitis of pregnancy. *Journal of the American Medical Association* **181**:577–581.

54 Shornick JK (1987) Herpes gestationis. *Journal of the American Academy of Dermatologists* **17**:539–556.

55 Shornick JK, Bangert JL, Freeman RG, Gilliam JN (1983) Herpes gestationis: Clinical and histologic features of 28 cases. *Journal of the American Academy of Dermatologists* **8**:214–224.

56 Shornick JK, Meek TJ, Nesbitt LT, Gilliam JN (1984) herpes gestationis in blacks. *Archives of Dermatology* **120**:511–513.

57 Holmes RC, Black MM (1980) Herpes gestationis. *Journal of the American Academy of Dermatologists* **3**:474–477.

58 Holmes RC, Black MM (1983) Herpes gestationis. *Dermatologic Clinics* **1**:195–203.

59 Tindall JG, Rea TH, Shulman I *et al.* (1981) Herpes gestationis in association with hydatidiform mole. *Archives of Dermatology* **117**:510–512.

60 Slazinski L, Degefu S (1981) Herpes gestationis associated with choriocarcinoma. *Archives of Dermatology* **118**:425–428.

61 Holmes RC, Black MM, Jurecka W *et al.* (1983) Clues to the aetiology and pathogenesis of herpes gestationis. *British Journal of Dermatology* **109**:131–139.

62 Kajii T, Ohama K (1977) Androgenetic origin of hydatidiform mole. *Nature* **268**:633–634.

63 Kelly SE, Black MM (1989) Pemphigoid gestationis: Placental interactions. *Seminars in Dermatology* **8**:12–17.

64 Holmes RC, Williamson DM, Black MM (1986) Herpes gestationis persisting for 12 years post-partum. *Archives in Dermatology* **122**:375–376.

65 Lawley TJ, Stingl G, Katz SI (1978) Fetal and maternal risk factors in herpes gestationis. *Archives in Dermatology* **114**:552–555.

66 Holmes RC, Black MM (1984) The fetal prognosis in pemphigoid gestationis (herpes gestationis). *British Journal of Dermatology* **10**:67–72.

67 Schaumberg-Lever G, Safford OE, Orfanos CE *et al.* (1973) Herpes gestationis: Histology and ultrastructure. *Archives of Dermatology* **107**:888–892.

68 Holmes RC, Black MM, Dann J *et al.* (1982) A comparative study of toxic erythema of pregnancy and herpes gestationis. *British Journal of Dermatology* **106**:499–510.

69 Jurecka W, Holmes RC, Black MM *et al.* (1983) An immuno-electron microscopy study of the relationship between herpes gestationis and polymorphic eruption of pregnancy. *British Journal of Dermatology* **108**:147–151.

70 Morrison LH, Labib RS, Zone, JJ *et al.* (1988) Herpes gestationis autoantibodies recognise a 180 kD human epidermal antigen. *Journal of Clinical Investigation* **81**:2023–2026.

71 Van de Wiel A, Hart H, Flinterman J *et al.* (1980) Plasma exchange in herpes gestationis. *British Medical Journal* **281**:1041–1041.

72 Lotem M, Katzenelson V, Rotem A *et al.* (1989) Impetigo herpetiformis: A variant of pustular psoriasis or a separate entity? *Journal of the American Academy of Dermatologists* **20**:338–341.

73 Baker H, Ryan TJ (1968) Generalised pustular psoriasis – a clinical and epidemiological study of 104 cases. *British Journal of Dermatology* **80**:771–793.

74 Camp RDR (1991) Psoriasis. In Champion RH, Burton JL, Ebling FJG (eds) *Textbook of Dermatology*, 5th edn, pp. 1391–1457. Oxford: Blackwell.

75 Wong RC, Ellis CN (1984) Physiological skin changes in pregnancy. *Journal of the American Academy of Dermatologists* **10**:929–940.

76 Wong RC, Ellis CN (1989) Physiological skin changes in pregnancy. *Seminars in Dermatology* **8**:7–11.

32

Malignant Disease

CHARLES O. SLOCUMB, JOSEPH G. PASTOREK, II

INTRODUCTION

Cancer occurs in approximately 1:1000 pregnancies and has been reported to account for one-third of maternal deaths. Cancer of the cervix, breast cancer, melanoma, ovarian cancer, colorectal cancer, leukemia and lymphoma, in decreasing frequency, are the most common malignancies found in pregnancy (**Table 1**).

This chapter primarily deals with malignancies which occur during pregnancy. As a general rule, cancers identified prior to conception should be adequately treated, with appropriate follow-up, before attempting pregnancy. Once successfully treated, few if any malignant diseases (other than those which require

Table 1
Incidence of cancer in pregnancy

Site/type	Estimated incidence per 1000 pregnancies
Cervix uteri	
non-invasive	1.3
invasive	1.0
Breast	0.33
Melanoma	0.14
Ovary	0.10
Thyroid	unknown
Leukemia	0.01
Lymphoma	0.01
Colorectal	0.02

Taken from Allen and Nisker.[1]

extirpation of the reproductive organs) absolutely mandate against future pregnancies.

GENERAL CONSIDERATIONS PERTAINING TO MATERNAL AND FETAL RISKS
(see also Chapter 23)

CHEMOTHERAPY

All antineoplastic drugs are theoretically teratogenic and mutagenic; their use can result in miscarriage, fetal death, malformations and growth deficiency. The long-term effects on the fetus are unknown, and the need for long-term observation has been emphasized dramatically with the recognition of diethyl stilboestrol (DES) related adenocarcinomas of the vagina and cervix in young women exposed *in utero* to this drug during the first trimester of pregnancy.

In the first 2 weeks of life, the blastocyst is resistant to teratogens; if it is not killed, a surviving blastocyst will not manifest any organ-specific abnormalities as a result of that teratogen. From the third to the eight week of development (5–10 weeks gestation age), susceptibility to teratogenic agents is maximum. In the human fetus, the period of organogenesis usually ends by 13 weeks gestation. However, brain and gonadal tissue are exceptions, since they continue to differentiate beyond week 13.

Most available data suggesting teratogenicity and mutagenicity of chemotherapeutic agents have been derived from experiments in laboratory animals. The first trimester is that time at which the fetus is most vulnerable to cancer chemotherapeutic agents.[2,3,4,5,6] The risk of alkylating agents given during pregnancy would appear to be small, with no increased risk of congenital anomalies if given after the first trimester.[2,3,5,6]

The antifolics aminopterin and methotrexate, when given in the first trimester of pregnancy, almost invariably result in spontaneous miscarriage or an abnormal fetus. A small amount of data indicate that aminopterin and methotrexate do not cause harm when given after the first trimester of pregnancy.

Although most of the other cancer chemotherapeutic agents, including 6-mercaptopurine, azathioprine, 5-fluorouracil, alkylating agents, vinca alkaloids and procarbazine, are known to be teratogenic in animal experiments, there have been surprisingly few case reports of human fetal abnormalities resulting from the use of these drugs in the first trimester of pregnancy. The same is true for doxorubicin and cisplatin.[7,8] Many reports of the use of combination chemotherapy for acute leukemia during pregnancy have noted no fetal congenital anomalies, and the fetuses have survived.

Because ovarian and testicular functions are characterized by rapid turnover of cells, these cells are similar to tumor cells in that both are prime targets for anticancer agents. Direct evidence of the possible gonadal effects of these drugs can be sought in mothers who become pregnant while receiving immunosuppressive therapy after renal transplantation. These gravidas appear to deliver healthy babies, barring prematurity and other obstetric problems. In addition, men father normal children when receiving immunosuppressive therapy.

Most comparable data for patients on cytotoxic drug therapy concern those with gestational trophoblastic disease (GTN) treated with methotrexate or actinomycin and those receiving alkylating agents. Drugs used to treat GTN do not appear to damage human oocytes in the doses and time periods used.[9] However, the possibility that recessive mutations are induced but undetected still exists. The effect of alkylating agents, such as chlorambucil, melphalan, busulfan, nitrogen mustard and especially cyclophosphamide, on the ovary is similar to that of radiotherapy. These drugs cause amenorrhea through direct ovarian depression; the severity of follicular depletion seems to be a function of the number and the activity of follicles present at the initiation of chemotherapy. Quiescent prepubertal ovaries not yet under cyclic hormonal control seem protected against destruction from chemotherapy. The younger the patient, the larger the reserve of oocytes that can be recruited after chemotherapy, making the return of menses and ovulation a function of age.

Alkylating agents, especially procarbazine, are also the most implicated drugs in testicular failure. The loss of testicular function is related to total drug dose and the length of time of administration. It is interesting that spermatogenesis may be abnormal before chemotherapy, so the usefulness of sperm cryopreservation has therefore been questioned. The exact cause of depressed semen count in males with malignancy is unknown, but it would appear the chance of future fertility using semen cryopreservation is not as simple as it first appeared.[8]

In additon to teratogenesis, effects on fertility and long-term effects including carcinogenesis and recessive mutations, chemotherapeutic administration can be associated with an increased risk of miscarriage, fetal growth deficiency, impaired mental and physical development, and transmission of maternal toxicity to the fetus (hematopoietic depression, infection, hemorrhagic phenomena, myocardial toxicity, etc.). However, when cure is a reasonable goal, therapy should be instituted as soon as possible and, with the exception of antifolate therapy in the first trimester, the incidence of fetal abnormalities is low. Alkylating agents should not be used in the first trimester unless the patient's life is threatened and therapeutic abortion may be considered if antifolate therapy is used in the first trimester.

RADIATION

The embryo undoubtedly represents the most radiosensitive stage of human life, and there are varying sensitivities within the tissues in the human embryo. Any irradiation of gonadal tissue involves genetic damage with no threshold below which mutations do not occur. It is estimated that 1 rad produces 5 mutations in every 1 million genes exposed. Most mutants are recessive and not expressed for many generations, until two people with the same mutation mate. The maximum permissible fetal dose of radiation is considered to be 5 rad.[10,11,12,13]

For the fetus, the most sensitive period is days 18–38 In the pre-implantation period, radiation produces an all-or-none effect in that it either destroys the fertilized egg or does not affect it significantly.[14] During days 18–38, doses of 10–40 rad may cause visceral organ or somatic damage.[15] Microcephaly, anencephaly, eye damage, growth deficiency, spina bifida and foot damage are reported with doses of 4 rad or less, but cause and effect has not been proven with these lower doses. After day 40, larger doses are prone to produce external malformations, but organ systems, especially the nervous system, may still be damaged. Doses more than 50 rad may produce significant mental retardation and microcephaly even in the second trimester.

A chest x-ray film only delivers 0.08 rad to the fetus, whereas a barium enema will result in a total dose to the gonads and pelvis of 6 rad. Evidence suggests that even an exposure of 3–5 rad can result in an increase in benign and malignant tumors in the child after birth. In addition, possible detrimental genetic consequences remain a matter of concern. Also of importance for patients planning child-bearing after significant exposure of gonadal tissue to irradiation is that the genetic effect of radiation on the gonad may be minimized by delaying conception after exposure. In humans, pregnancy should be delayed 12–14 months after significant exposure.

The ovary is sensitive to radiation at higher doses than the testis and younger women at higher doses than older women. Oophoropexy can be performed to displace the ovaries laterally out of the radiation field or medially behind the uterus where they are shielded during treatment.

SURGERY

Cancers of the breast, ovary, bowel and thyroid, and malignant melanoma are potentially curable with operative intervention. Of the available therapeutic options, surgery is least likely to affect pregnancy, as opposed to chemotherapy and radiotherapy. Teratogenicity of anesthesia is minimal, and minor procedures using local anesthesia are essentially without risk to the fetus.[11,16]

The pregnant state requires several special considerations. Supine positioning is to be avoided during surgery.[17,18] Due to a decrease in plasma fibrinolytic activity, an increase in all coagulation factors except XI and XIII and a pregnancy-associated decrease in lower extremity venous flow, the risk of thromboembolism is 5–6 times that of a non-pregnant patient.[18,19,20,21] The perioperative use of minidose heparin and/or sequential compression stockings is advocated. Perioperative infection and extensive surgery potentiates preterm labor.[16,22] The prophylactic use of tocolytics remains controversial, as beta-mimetics may cause tachycardia and pulmonary edema. However, close observation for increased uterine activity is always appropriate in such cases.

Overall, surgery can usually be safely performed during pregnancy with minimal risk to the mother and fetus, especially in the second and third trimesters. Fetal heart rate and tocodynamietric monitoring are easily employed and may provide an early warning of impending complications.

FETAL AND PLACENTAL METASTASES

Fetal Risks

Fortunately, metastases of maternal malignancies to the fetus or placenta are extremely rare. Melanoma is by far the most likely to do so, accounting for 50% of all tumors metastasizing to the placenta and nearly 90% of those to the fetus. It is rare for the fetus to be involved if there is invasion only of the maternal side of the placenta, which is true in 90% of cases.[23,24,25] The reported low incidence of tumor metastases to products of conception probably is due to a number of factors, including the unexplained resistance of the placenta to invasion of maternal cancer that has been demonstrated in many animal studies.

Leukemia may develop postnatally in the child of a mother with acute leukemia,[26] but it is extremely unlikely. Some infants with metastatic melanoma have demonstrated complete tumor regression and have survived. Breast cancer has also metastasized to the placenta.[24]

MALIGNANCIES

CERVICAL CANCER

Maternal Risks

Carcinoma of the uterine cervix is the most frequently diagnosed invasive neoplasm in pregnancy, reported in 1:1240 pregnancies.[27] Stage for stage, frankly invasive carcinoma discovered during pregnancy is associated with survival rates that are similar to those found in the non-pregnant population.[27] In general, cancer patients under the age of 35 tend to have a poorer prognosis than those in whom disease is diagnosed later, and cervical cancer in pregnancy usually occurs in the younger group of patients. This has led to incorrect suggestions that pregnancy might accelerate the growth of carcinoma of the cervix.[13,27,28] The age range of pregnant cervical cancer patients was 19–46 years, with a mean of 33 years, in one series.[28] Age at diagnosis had no influence on the prognosis of the lesion within a given stage. Prognosis is not related to parity either, as long as the patients are compared within a given stage. In 30% of patients there were no symptoms when the diagnosis of cervical cancer was established, but vaginal bleeding was the most common symptom whether or not the patient was pregnant.

Management Options

The methods of diagnosis and treatment of this lesion in the pregnant or postpartum woman are the same as in the non-pregnant patient. As part of every first prenatal visit, the physician should obtain a Papanicolaou smear from both the cervix and endocervical canal. Biopsy of suspicious lesions should be done even in the presence of a normal Papanicolaou smear. The incidence of abnormal Papanicolaou smears in one large study of pregnant patients was 1.2%.[29]

Most cervical cancers detected during gestation are at an early stage and have a relatively good prognosis. Over 40% are stage I lesions.[30] There should be no hesitancy to do colposcopically directed cervical biopsy during gestation. A diagnosis of microinvasion made by colposcopically directed biopsy must be followed as soon as possible by a cone biopsy to rule out frankly invasive disease. This is the only absolute indication for conization during pregnancy, as the risk of miscarriage may be as high as 30% during the first trimester. Hemostatic sutures should be utilized (**Figure 1**). Endocervical curettage is not performed during pregnancy because of the risk of bleeding and ruptured membranes. A conization during pregnancy should be envisioned as excising a 'coin' of tissue rather than a 'cone' of tissue (**Figure 2**). This is due to eversion of the squamocolumnar junction which occurs during gestation, thereby limiting the need for sampling tissue high in the endocervix.

Patients with intra-epithelial neoplasia of the cervix may deliver vaginally with subsequent reassessment performed postpartum. Microinvasive lesions, or those not penetrating the stroma more than 3 mm below the basement membrane, not manifesting vascular or lymphatic invasion, free of confluent tongues of tumor and not extending to the margins of the surgical specimen, do not prevent the patient from continuing her pregnancy safely to term. The route of delivery should be determined by obstetric indications. Postpartum hysterectomy is not essential in those women who desire to bear more children.

Treatment of invasive cervical cancer requires consideration of both the stage of disease and duration of

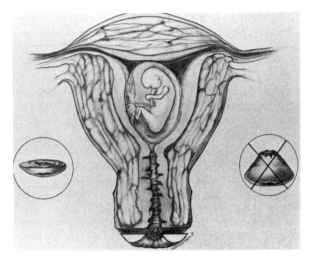

Figure 2. Excision of a coin of tissue rather than a cone of tissue.

pregnancy. Short delays of several weeks in definitive therapy, until the fetus has reached viability, are appropriate. However, patients in the first and second trimesters are often advised to undergo definitive therapy immediately. For stage I and IIa lesions, radical hysterectomy with bilateral lymphadenectomy is technically acceptable during any trimester. Radiation therapy is equally efficacious in stage I and IIa lesions and is the treatment of choice in more advanced stages. In the first and second trimesters, if the fetus is to be disregarded, treatment should begin with whole pelvic radiation. Up to 16 weeks gestation, spontaneous miscarriage will usually occur during therapy.[31] If spontaneous miscarriage does not occur by completion of the external beam therapy, a modified radical or extended extrafacial hysterectomy without pelvic lymphadenectomy should be done to excise the remaining central neoplasm. An alternative approach to the patient who has not miscarried is to evacuate the uterus by means of hysterotomy, followed by conventional intracavitary irradiation delivered within 1–2 weeks. Conventional intracavitary irradiation is also used after whole pelvic irradiation in those patients who miscarry.

Patients who have therapy delayed until fetal viability undergo cesarean section when tests of lung maturity indicate viability, usually at 34 weeks gestation. Stages Ib and IIa can be treated with either surgery or radiation. There is a lack of conclusive evidence that either approach offers increased survival over the other. Wertheim-type radical hysterectomy with pelvic lymphadenectomy at the time of cesarean section can be performed safely, allowing the patient to return home with her infant without needing further therapy; this also preserves ovarian function. If radiation is preferred or the stage is greater than IIa, whole pelvic irradiation is begun 10–14 days following cesarean section; intracavitary radiation is then adminis-

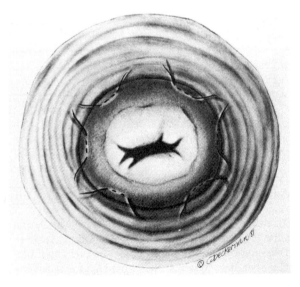

Figure 1. Hemostatic sutures.

tered at the completion of whole pelvic irradiation.

In a report of 96 cases of cervical cancer occurring in pregnancy of which 87 patients were available for disease-free survival rate analysis, 92.3% of stage Ia, 68.2% of stage Ib, 54.5% of stage II and 37.5% of stage III survived.[32] Although controversial, cesarean delivery does not seem to confer any survival benefit

as opposed to vaginal delivery.[1,28] As mentioned earlier, pregnancy does not affect the prognosis of cervical cancer and, stage for stage, the 5-year survival rate is the same for pregnant and non-pregnant patients.[13,27,28] The overall 5-year survival rate for those patients with invasive carcinoma of the cervix associated with pregnancy was reported to be 49.2% which compares favorably with the 51% rate quoted for non-pregnant patients (**Table 2**).[27] The later in pregnancy that carcinoma of the cervix is diagnosed, the worse the prognosis (**Table 3**). This is because cases discovered later in gestation are of more advanced stage.

CARCINOMA OF THE CERVIX
Summary of Management Options

Prenatal

Diagnosis

- Take cervical smear at first visit if
  - at-risk group
  - no smear for 3 years

- Colposcopic directed biopsy of suspicious lesions

- Cone biopsy if microinvasion diagnosed on directed biopsy; avoid endocervical curettage

Treatment

- Intra-epithelial neoplasia: colposcopic review through pregnancy and definitive management after pregnancy

- Microinvasive: careful counseling; options are:
  - as for intra-epithelial neoplasia
  - as for invasive

- Invasive: careful counseling with options depending on stage of disease and duration of pregnancy (see **Tables 2** and **3**):
  - in late pregnancy: wait until fetus viable with use of steroids if necessary, then deliver and implement definitive therapy
  - in early pregnancy: implement definitive treatment immediately with termination of the pregnancy

---

Table 2
Cervical cancer: 5-year survival by clinical stage[a]

Stage	Treated	Survival	%	Annual report 1954–1963 (%)
Ib	474	348	74.5	76.5
II	449	214	47.8	55.0
III/IV	326	53	16.2	27.9
Total	1249	615	49.2	51.0

Taken from Hacker et al.[27]
[a] Survival for all cases of cervical cancer.

Table 3
Cervical cancer: 5-year survival by stage of gestation

Trimester	Treated	Survival	%
First	137	94	68.6
Second	51	32	62.7
Third	87	45	51.7
Postpartum	621	289	46.3
Total	896	460	51.3

Taken from Hacker et al.[27]

BREAST

Maternal Risks

Breast cancer is the most common cancer in women, with 1:11 women developing the disease. Breast cancer is first detected in approximately 1:2000 pregnancies,[34,35] accounting for 2–3% of all cases. Multiparous women, particularly those who breast-feed, have a lower incidence. Late menarche and early menopause, absence of benign breast disease, and an initial pregnancy before the age of 34 also lower the incidence. Daughters of women who developed bilateral cancer premenopausally have a nine-fold increase in risk.

Although the overall survival rate for breast cancer is about 50%, in pregnancy the overall rate is reported by some to be only 15%–20%. Pregnant patients tend to have a higher incidence of positive nodes.[33,34,35] This more advanced stage of disease is sometimes attributed to delayed diagnosis secondary to the changes in breast density which occur during pregnancy. However, the low incidence of stage I lesions in pregnancy strongly suggests an acceleration of the disease process in the preclinical period. Cell kinetic studies of breast cancer suggest that lesions are harbored within the breast for 2–5 years before becoming clinically detected. Since the period of gestation is no longer than 9 months, it is difficult to believe that the sole explanation for the high incidence of advanced disease in pregnancy is related to late diagnosis caused by the engorged breast. There may be increased vascularity and lymphatic drainage from the pregnant breast, assisting the metastatic process to regional lymph nodes. Increased secretion of hormonal substances in pregnancy might influence neoplasms in the breast. The increased production of glucocorticoids may reduce cellular immunity and perhaps promote the implantation and growth of malignancies. Similarly, elevated quantities of prolactin produced by the hypophysis and human placental lactogen by the placenta late in pregnancy and during milk production might affect breast cancer adversely.

Prolactin promotes the growth of diethylene anthracin-induced mammary tumors in mice. The observation that women with bone pain from metastatic breast cancer sometimes obtain relief from prolactin suppression implicates prolactin as a possible promoter of breast cancer in humans. Pure concentrations of all three major estrogen fractions (estrone, estradiol and estriol) rise from 4 µg/100 ml early in pregnancy to means of 8–22 mg/100 ml at term, at least a 2000-fold increase. The ability of estrogens to promote growth of breast cancer in animals and humans has been amply illustrated. Whether the disproportionate rise of estriol, a relatively weak estrogen and a possible antagonist of estrone and estradiol, confers some measure of protection is unknown.

Whether the advanced stage of the disease at the time of discovery in pregnancy reflects an increase in the rate of growth and spread of subclinical lesions is a crucial question. In a small study of 28 patients diagnosed in the first trimester, interruption of pregnancy did not seem to affect the survival rate.[36] Some investigators have suggested that patients treated during the second half of pregnancy seem to have a poorer prognosis when compared with those treated early in gestation or during the puerperium.[35,37] These reports, however, may be flawed by bias in the selection of patients for treatment. It has been pointed out that treatment of small and slowly growing tumors may have been postponed until after delivery, while aggressive tumors were more promptly treated.[34,38] This suggests prompt treatment during the second half of pregnancy to prevent even small lesions from growing and reaching an inoperable stage. Stage for stage, survival rates for pregnant women and non-pregnant, premenopausal women are equal; but if pregnancy affects the stage at which the disease is discovered, pregnancy has a significant effect on prognosis.[37]

Management Options

The hyperplastic breast of pregnancy is characterized by an increase in radiographic density, limiting the value of mammography. However, mammography should not be avoided, since radiation exposure to the fetus is negligible.[39] Fine-needle aspiration of a mass for cytologic study is recommended during pregnancy. Equivocal cytologic diagnoses require excision of the tumor under local anesthesia. The majority of breast carcinomas are infiltrating ductal carcinomas, and the variety is the same as in non-pregnant women. Because inflammatory carcinoma can be mistaken for mastitis, a biopsy should be taken when incision and drainage are performed.

Staging of breast cancer currently employs a complicated system jointly recommended by the International Union Against Cancer and the American Joint Committee. The Haagensen clinical staging for breast cancer is more useful in pointing out the unfavorable prognostic indicators in this disease process (**Table 4**).

The extent and timing of surgery for breast cancer is controversial. Most authorities recommend a radical or modified radical mastectomy for patients with stage I or stage II disease. Although many clinicians feel that localized breast cancer in the first trimester of pregnancy is a valid reason to recommend termination, therapeutic abortion has not been found to increase survival, and the presence of a fetus does not compromise proper therapy in early stages. Similarly, therapy of localized disease in later pregnancy can be carried out without pregnancy termination when the diagnosis is made. Therapeutic abortion is no longer believed to be an essential component of effective treatment of early disease.[37,40]

In cases of advanced breast cancer, therapeutic abortion is usually felt to be a necessity to achieve effective palliation. Surgical castration is generally acknowledged as the appropriate first step in managing premenopausal women with disseminated mammary cancer and castration would be useless unless accompanied by therapeutic abortion to remove the placental source of hormones. When pregnancy enters the third trimester, the decision for preterm delivery depends heavily on the patient's wishes and the urgency for palliation.

In rare instances, tumors lack estrogen receptors and

Table 4
Breast cancer staging

Stage A

No skin edema, ulceration, or solid fixation to chest wall; axillary nodes clinically negative

Stage B

As in stage A, clinically involved nodes not more than 2.5 cm in transverse diameter and not fixed to skin or deeper structures; are palpable

Stage C

Any one of five grave signs present:
1. Edema of skin of limited extent (involves less than one-third of breast surface)
2. Skin ulceration
3. Solid fixation to chest wall
4. Massive axillary nodes (more than 2.5 cm transverse diameter)
5. Fixation of axillary nodes to skin or deep structures

Stage D

All more advanced carcinomas including:
1. Any combination of two or more grave signs
2. Extensive edema (more than one-third breast surface)
3. Satellite skin nodules
4. Inflammatory carcinoma
5. Clinically involved supraclavicular nodes
6. Parasternal tumor of internal mammary nodes
7. Edema of the arm
8. Distant metastases

From Haagensenm.[41]

tion of selection, because most women will wait at least 2 years following treatment, during which time many tumors destined to recur will do so. In addition, only women with a good prognosis are likely to achieve counsel recommending subsequent pregnancies. There appears to be no justification for recommending pregnancy termination in a patient without recurrence, the pregnant patient with advanced disease might elect to undergo cytotoxic chemotherapy without therapeutic abortion or castration. When this occurs after the first trimester, risk to the fetus is small, and pregnancy can be allowed to proceed.

If distant metastases occur after pregnancy, oophorectomy will produce a remission in 50% of patients with previous advanced disease positive for estrogen receptors. If a patient fails to respond to oophorectomy, she will not respond to androgen or other hormonal manipulations either, but if there is a response and relapse later, androgen or other hormonal manipulations will result in remission in about 25% of patients.

Subsequent pregnancies after mastectomy have no influence on the disease, and a few reports have even suggested that future pregnancies might be protective. Such patients should wait at least 3 years after their mastectomy and undergo bone and liver scans, chest-x-rays and mammography of the remaining breast prior to becoming pregnant. Breast-feeding is discouraged to avoid vascular enrichment in the opposite breast, which may also contain a neoplasm. This phenomenon of a favorable outcome for patients who become pregnant following treatment for a breast cancer may be a func-

---

CARCINOMA OF THE BREAST
Summary of Management Options

Prenatal

Diagnosis

- Can be difficult and delayed

- Mammography is not contraindicated

- Fine-needle aspiration if carcinoma suspected

- Equivocal results require open biopsy

- Staging (see **Table 4**)

Treatment

- Termination is controversial if diagnosis is in early pregnancy

- Definitive treatment as for non-pregnant patient should be offerred with the main difficulties in management options being where oophorectomy or chemotherapy are indicated

Postnatal

- Advise against breast-feeding in index or subsequent pregnancy

- Avoid pregnancy for at least 3 years and confirmation of disease-free status

but termination may be considered when a recurrence exists. Prophylactic castration does not reduce the incidence of recurrence.[42]

Patients who are candidates for wide local excision and axillary node sampling followed by radiation are most often advised to terminate the pregnancy. In such cases, the amount of radiation delivered to the fetus must be calculated and is usually about 30 rad. This dose presents an unacceptable risk to the fetus.

For very advanced disease, chemotherapy has been used after the first trimester. Alkylating agents, 5-fluorouracil and vincristine are relatively safe, but methotrexate should be avoided if possible. It appears that the premenopausal patient is the best candidate for aggressive adjuvant chemotherapy and that this approach might result in improved survival when used at the time of the initial procedure.

MELANOMA

Maternal Risks

Many case reports have indicated that pregnancy adversely affects the course of melanoma. Partial or complete regressions of melanoma after delivery have been reported. Many observations have given support to this assumption. Melanocyte-stimulating hormone (MSH) of the pituitary has been measured and noted to increase after the second month of pregnancy. Pregnancy is also associated with increased ACTH production, which results in heightened intrinsic MSH activity. All melanomas masquerade as nevi before diagnosis, and potentially dangerous nevi, such as those on the feet, palms, genitals and areas of persistent irritation, should be removed during childhood. Studies of the effect of pregnancy on the course of melanoma have produced conflicting data.[43,44,45] Despite this, most authorities recommend that patients who have histories of malignant melanomas are best advised to avoid pregnancy for about 3 years after complete surgical excision.

Management Options

The standard criteria for staging melanoma are given in **Table 5**. The Clark microstaging classification (**Table 6**) is based on the level of penetration of the melanoma under the epidermis and dermis. Data indicate that Clark level 1, which refers to the rare lesion located entirely above the basement membrane of the epidermis, should be viewed as an *in situ* lesion requiring no lymph node dissection. Clark level II involves penetration down to the papillary dermis with lymph node metastases seen in 1–5% of patients, not justifying an elective lymph node dissection. Clark level III involves no invasion of the reticular layer, but filling

Table 5
Criteria for staging melanoma

Stage 0	Superficial melanoma

Stage 1	No metastases: primary melanoma only
A.	Intact primary melanoma
B.	Primary melanoma locally excised
C.	Multiple primary melanomas

Stage II	Local recurrence or metastasis

All melanotic lesions within 3 cm of primary site (satellitosis)

Stage III	Regional metastases (3 cm from primary site)
A.	Intradermal (in transit metastasis)
B.	Regional lymph nodes
A–B.	Intradermal and regional nodes

Stage IV	Distant hematogenous metastases
A.	Cutaneous
B.	Visceral
C.	Lymph nodes
A–C.	Combination of the above

and widening of melanoma cells of the papillary dermis at its interface with the reticular dermis. Clark level IV extends into the reticular dermis and involves regional lymph node metastasis in 40% of patients. Clark level V extends into the subcutaneous tissue and involves regional lymph nodes in 70% of patients. Clark levels IV and V require lymphadenectomy as part of critical therapy (**Table 6**).

Table 6
Clark's five levels of cutaneous invasion

Level 1
Melanoma located above the basement membrane (basal lamina) of the epidermis. These lesions essentially present no danger

Level II
Melanoma invades through the basement membrane down to the papillary dermis

Level III
Melanoma at this level is characterized by filling and widening by melanoma cells of the papillary dermis at its interface with the reticular dermis
Characteristically, there is no invasion of the underlying reticular layer

Level IV
These lesions show melanoma penetration into reticular dermis

Level V
Melanoma at this level is evident by its presence in the subcutaneous tissue

Modified from Goldsmith.[46]

MALIGNANT MELANOMA
Summary of Management Options

Prenatal

Diagnosis

- By biopsy or excision

- Staging (see **Tables 5** and **6**)

Treatment

- As for non-pregnant patient

Stage 0 refers to melanomas with invasion of the dermis confined to the adjacent subepidermal zone. Stage 1 refers to invasion into the papillary dermis (level II) to a maximum depth or into the papillary–reticular interface (level III) but not to the reticular dermis and/or a maximum thickness measurement of 1.5 mm. Stage II refers to invasion to a maximum depth of the reticular dermis or subcutaneous tissue (levels IV and V) and/or thickness measurement of more than 1.5 mm. This includes all local recurrences or metastases and all melanotic lesions within 3 cm of a primary site. Stage III refers to regional metastases (more than 3 cm from primary site). Stage IV refers to distant, hematogenous metastases (**Table 5**).

Breslow's classification is a simple micrometer measurement of lesion thickness. Lesions 1.5–4.0 mm in size have a 57% incidence of regional node involvement and a 15% incidence of distant metastases. Lesions between 0.76 and 1.5 mm have a 25% incidence of regional node involvement and an 8% incidence of distant metastasis. Lesions less than 0.76 mm are usually not associated with any spread. Almost half of all tumors metastasizing to the placenta and nearly 90% metastasizing to the fetus are melanomas, but this situation is rare.

OVARY

Maternal Risks

Most ovarian cysts in pregnant patients are follicular or corpus luteum cysts and usually not more than 5 cm in diameter; some rarely are as large as 11 cm in diameter. More than 99% of these functional cysts are undetectable by 14 weeks gestation. If the cyst remains unchanged or increases in size, the patient should be explored at 16 weeks gestation, when the exploration is associated with negligible fetal wastage. If the patient is symptomatic or the ovarian mass is solid or cystic and larger than 8 cm in diameter, an observation period is not required.[47] In non-pregnant patients, about 20% of ovarian tumors are malignant; in pregnancy, this percentage is 5%.

The differential diagnosis of adnexal masses in pregnancy includes retroverted pregnant uterus, pedunculated uterine fibroid, carcinoma of the rectosigmoid, pelvic kidney and a uterine congenital anomaly such as an accessory uterine horn. Complications include pelvic impaction, obstructed labor, torsion, hemorrhage into the cyst, rupture of the cyst and infection. Diagnostic studies can include ultrasonography, intravenous pyelogram and a limited barium enema. Radiologic studies should be avoided during the first trimester, whenever possible.

Torsion occurs in 10–15% of ovarian tumors in pregnancy. Most torsions occur when the uterus is enlarging at a rapid rate (8–16 weeks) or when the uterus is involuting (in the puerperium). About 60% of cases occur at or before 20 weeks and 40% in the puerperium. The usual sequence of events is sudden lower abdominal pain, nausea, vomiting and, in some cases, shock-like symptoms. The abdomen is tense and tender, and there is rebound tenderness with guarding.

Cancer of the ovary occurs in 1:18 000 to 1:25 000 pregnancies.[48,49] Approximately 60% of malignant ovarian tumors diagnosed during pregnancy are epithelial, the remainder being germ cell and gonadal stromal tumors. The majority of these epithelial lesions are of low malignant potential or are stage I, as commonly found in non-pregnant patients in the reproductive age group.

Management Options

If an ovarian malignancy is found at the time of abdominal exploration, the surgeon's first obligation is to stage the patient properly. Stage Ia lesions may be treated with unilateral salpingo-oophorectomy, provided a thorough exploration of the abdominal cavity has been carried out. More advanced lesions should not be treated this conservatively unless the tumor is of the borderline variety, in which case definitive surgical therapy can sometimes be deferred until fetal viability is achieved. The decision regarding the degree of surgical intervention, which might include hysterectomy while the fetus is still immature, ultimately rests with the patient. However, pregnancy does not appear to adversely affect the prognosis for the patient who has an ovarian malignancy.

Fortunately, ovarian germ cell neoplasms are usually benign. Dermoid cysts are by far the most common neoplastic cysts found in pregnancy. They should be removed at 16 weeks gestation to avoid torsion, rupture or obstruction of the birth canal during parturition. The uninvolved ovarian tissue usually can be preserved, because mature teratomas are well encapsulated and can be easily dissected off the remainder of the ovary.

Malignant germ cell neoplasms usually can be managed with a unilateral salpingo-oophorectomy because they are usually stage Ia; the prognosis for this stage is not improved with more extensive surgery. Adjuvant chemotherapy in this group of highly malignant tumors plays an important role in treating all except the dysgerminoma. The high success rate obtained with adjuvant chemotherapy has been recorded using this modality in the immediate postoperative period. The effect of postponing adjuvant chemotherapy until the fetus has reached viability has not been tested adequately and incomplete data are available, but these tumors grow rapidly and recur within months when therapy is withheld.

Initiation of adjuvant chemotherapy during pregnancy is a subject that is controversial and for which little experience exists. Although retrospective studies have not shown frequent congenital abnormalities in patients treated in the second and third trimesters, many newer agents have not been used frequently in pregnancy, and all chemotherapeutic agents are theoretically teratogenic. Delay in, or withholding of, chemotherapy for patients with more advanced stages of these tumors is definitely not warranted. As in earlier stages, the uterus and opposite ovary can be preserved if metastatic tumor is not found in these locations.

Ovarian dysgerminomas are unique among the malignant germ cell tumors because of their overall good prognosis in stage I treated by surgery alone, their apparent lack of responsiveness to chemotherapy, and their exquisite sensitivity to radiation therapy. Dysgerminomas account for 30% of ovarian malignancies in pregnancy. Dysgerminomas metastasize primarily via the lymphatic system to the ipsilateral pelvic and periaortic lymph nodes; therefore, staging should include a pelvic and periaortic lymphadenectomy on the side of the tumor mass. Stage Ia dysgerminomas can be managed with a unilateral adnexectomy and continuation of pregnancy without additional therapy. Torsion and incarceration are common, and contralateral ovarian biopsy is necessary because dysgerminomas are often bilateral. A 30% recurrence rate in 23 stage Ia dysgerminomas has been reported, but the extent of exploration was not known in most cases.[50] Most authors quote a recurrence rate of 10% for stage Ia dysgerminomas. Because radiation therapy is successful in curing more than 75% of patients even with metastatic and/or recurrent dysgerminoma, most

authors recommend patients continue their pregnancies with completion of their proper evaluation in the puerperium. Recent data suggest that multiagent chemotherapy can be curative and is an important new therapeutic tool in the management of this disease.

Rarely, ovarian tumors of stromal origin, such as granulosa-theca cell tumors and Sertoli Leydig cell tumors, are found in pregnancy. It is recommended that these be managed conservatively as in the young non-

---

CARCINOMA OF THE OVARY
Summary of Management Options

Prenatal

Diagnosis

- Most likely by identification of ovarian tumor on ultrasound which is biopsied or removed at subsequent laparotomy; decision to perform laparotomy is dependent on clinical and ultrasound features

- At laparotomy for unexplained severe abdominal pain (see Chapter 34)

Treatment

- Most cases will have the diagnosis made after the laparotomy when histological results are available; diagnosis will only be made or strongly suspected without laparotomy in a few cases

- Thus definitive treatment and risks have to be discussed carefully with patient

- Factors that will influence the management include:
  - gestation
  - histological type
  - stage of disease
  - need for adjuvant chemotherapy
  - patient's wishes

pregnant patient, because these are neoplasms of low malignant potential.

The possibility of an ovarian cancer must be kept foremost in the mind of the physician caring for pregnant patients and abdominal exploration should not be resisted because of the fear of precipitating fetal loss. Most dangers seem those created by acts of omission rather than commission.

THYROID

Maternal Risks

Thyroid cancer associated with pregnancy is rare, but the peak incidence of most epithelial carcinomas of the thyroid is between ages 30 and 34, so it may occur. Most frequently observed, in descending order of appearance, are papillary, follicular and anaplastic histologic types. Medullary carcinoma, arising from the parafollicular C cells, comprise approximately 5% of thyroid carcinomas and may be associated with the syndrome of multiple endocrine neoplasias. In this patient population, papillary and follicular carcinomas of the thyroid tend to be well localized, well differentiated and indolent, in contrast to anaplastic and medullary carcinomas, which are very aggressive. Anaplastic carcinoma of the thyroid is a uniformly lethal disease.

During pregnancy, there is clinical enlargement of the thyroid gland secondary to follicular cell hyperplasia and abundant colloid formation. Serum thyroxin and total triiodothyronine are elevated in normal pregnancy, while TSH levels remain normal.[51] The T_3 uptake test is usually decreased in pregnancy due to increased thryoid finding globulin.[51]

Carcinoma of the thyroid gland usually manifests as a relatively asymptomatic solitary nodule in the thyroid gland, but is multifocal as seen on careful sectioning in approximately 30–40% of patients. Fortunately, only 5% of these become clinically evident if thyroid tissue remains after surgery. Regional lymphatics are involved microscopically in 50–70% of patients, but this subclinical involvement does not affect the prognosis. Clinical evidence of recent enlargement of an anterior neck nodule, cervical lymphadenopathy and fixation to local tissues are features suggestive of malignancy. Laboratory indices of thyroid function are contributory only if they indicate a hyperthyroid state, thus supporting the diagnosis of a toxic adenoma. Radioisotope scanning using any radionuclide is contraindicated, although ultrasound is permissible, and fine-needle aspiration of a solitary module is 90% reliable. If the results of cytologic examination are benign, a course of thyroid suppression using 0.2 mg L-thyroxine daily is indicated for the duration of the pregnancy. As in the non-pregnant population, 40% of aspirated nodules will be malignant.[52,53]

Management Options

Papillary and follicular carcinomas of the thyroid are best treated surgically by subtotal thyroidectomy, but in the late second and third trimesters, suppression with exogenous thyroxine and delay of surgery until after delivery may be safely accomplished. Preservation of the parathyroid glands is essential, as hypoparathyroidism during pregnancy is a dangerous situation. When a medullary carcinoma is suspected either by history, needle cytology or elevated thyrocalcitonin levels, thyroidectomy with neck dissection is the only known effective therapy and results in a 50% survival at 5 years. This extensive surgery is associated with a high incidence of fetal wastage and a delay of a few weeks to allow the fetus to mature should be considered. The

---

CARCINOMA OF THE THYROID
Summary of Management Options

Prenatal

Diagnosis

- By needle or open biopsy

Treatment

- Depends on gestation, histological type and patient's wishes

- Options
  - allow the pregnancy to continue until fetal viability achieved before definitive treatment
  - terminate the pregnancy immediately and commence definitive therapy

- Extensive neck surgery during pregnancy is associated with high fetal loss

- Airway obstruction is the only indication for commencing radiotherapy during pregnancy

standard treatment for patients with anaplastic carcinoma of the thyroid gland is radical total thyroidectomy followed by radiation therapy. Frequently, the main concern is merely to keep the mother alive until the pregnancy has come to term. Chemotherapy may be used when the pace of metastatic disease progression threatens the likelihood of the mother delivering a healthy child.[52] Lesions compromising the upper airway are the only indication for radiotherapy during pregnancy.

Younger patients have a better prognosis than older ones. The effect of pregnancy on the growth and spread of these lesions is negligible, and it is not necessary to avoid or abort subsequent pregnancies.[54,55] Fortunately, cancer of the thyroid in pregnancy tends to be of low grade and very slowly progressive with 95% survival even when cytologic examination is inconclusive and subclinical nodal metastasis is present.

HODGKIN'S DISEASE (see also Chapter 23)

Maternal Risks

The incidence of Hodgkin's disease complicating pregnancy is about 1:6000.[56] It commonly affects young people, but is now cured or controlled for long periods with irradiation and chemotherapy. Non-Hodgkin lymphomas are uncommon in younger women and have rarely been reported in pregnancy. In one report, placental involvement led to disseminated disease in the newborn, who died at 5 months of age.[25] Pregnancy does not appear to adversely affect the course of the maternal disease.

In up to 90% of cases, Hodgkin's disease presents as an enlarged cervical or axillary lymph node. Systemic symptoms consist of fever, night sweats and weight loss. The diagnosis is established by biopsy and histologic examination of suspected nodes. Two histologic variants, nodular sclerosis and lymphocyte predominant, have a better prognosis than mixed cellularity and lymphocyte-depleted specimens. Women have a better prognosis than men, and patients over age 40 have a poorer prognosis than younger patients.

Management Options

The importance of staging in Hodgkin's disease was recognized by Peters as early as 1950, when she devised the first clinical staging classification. Then, lymphangiography made possible the earlier detection of retroperitoneal lymph node involvement, and it became important to distinguish two subgroups: those with widespread disease confined to lymphatic organs

and those with spread of disease beyond the lymph nodes, thymus, spleen and Waldeyer ring to one or more extralymphatic organs or tissues. The latter is now recognized as stage IV disease (**Table 7**). The major difference in the staging workup of the pregnant patient lies with the last three diagnostic procedures in **Table 8**. Surgical staging after the week 14 of pregnancy avoids some of the diagnostic tecnniques that might be harmful to the fetus, such as lower extremity lymphangiography, intravenous pyelography, and bone and liver scans. Splenectomy is not contraindicated and is frequently performed at these staging procedures.

The stage of disease is the most important factor in planning therapy and estimating prognosis. Magnetic resonance imaging has proved to be helpful in demonstrating intra-abdominal adenopathy. Thomas and Beckham have described the use of a modified lymphangiographic technique in which a single film is obtained 24 h after the injection of contrast. This probably results in an exposure of less than 1 rad to the

Table 7
Clinical staging of Hodgkin's disease

Stage I
Disease localized to a single lymph node, or a single lymph node-bearing area, either above or below the diaphragm

Stage IE
Disease confined to a single focus in an extralymphatic organ other than liver or bone marrow

Stage II
Disease confined to two or more lymph node-bearing areas on the same side of diaphragm

Stage IIE
Involvement of one or more lymph node regions on either side of the diaphragm, plus a localized solitary area of contiguous spread to an extralymphatic organ other than liver or bone marrow

Stage III
Disease confined to lymph nodes but involving both sides of the diaphragm

Stage IIIS
Stage III involvement of the spleen

Stage IIIE
Stage III with solitary area of contiguous spread to an extralymphatic organ other than liver or bone marrow

Stage IIISE
Stage IIIS plus IIIE

Stage IV
Disease with disseminated extranodal involvement (e.g. to liver, lung, bone, marrow, skin)

Table 8
Staging workup for Hodgkin's disease

1. Careful clinical history
2. Thorough physical examination with careful description of all superficial lymph node areas
3. Roentgenographic examination of chest, including tomograms; CT scan if necessary
4. Liver function tests, particularly alkaline phosphatase
5. Biopsy of bone marrow, needle or open
6. Complete blood counts and urinalysis
7. Serum electrophoresis
8. Lower extremity lymphangiograms
9. Abdominal CT scan with intravenous contrast
10. Bone and liver scans in symptomatic patients

HODGKIN'S DISEASE
Summary of Management Options
(see also Chapter 23)

Prenatal

Diagnosis, staging and assessment

• See **Table 8**
Treatment

• See **Table 9**

---

fetus, which is well below the acceptable doses reported in the literature.[52]

The mainstay of treatment for early-stage Hodgkin's disease is radiation therapy. Multiple-agent chemotherapy is employed for the treatment of advanced stage disease with organ involvement (**Table 9**). The most widely used combination of drugs is the MOPP regimen (nitrogen mustard, vincristine, procarbazine and prednisone). Most investigators agree that treatment should not be withheld during pregnancy except in early-stage disease, particularly if it is discovered

Table 9
Hodgkin's disease: Treatment

Treatment group	Patient included	Procedure
1	Ia IIa, IIIa (spleen and/or upper abdominal nodes are the only intra-abdominal involvement); patients must have no mediastinal mass or one that is less than one-third of chest diameter; no E stage of lung (may be E stage elsewhere, such as thyroid or bone)	Extended field radiotherapy alone; nodes need not be treated
2	Any I, II or IIIa patient with E stage of lung or a mediastinal mass greater than one-third of chest diameter; all IB and IIb patients; all III2a patients (lower abdominal nodal involvement)	Extended field radiotherapy followed by six courses of MOPP with a month between modalities; pelvic nodes irradiated only for stage III2a
3	IIIb, IVa, IVb	MOPP alone

late in pregnancy. However, if the patient and her family absolutely refuse any intervention or treatment until the natural termination of the pregnancy, one has no choice but to wait. In patients with stage I or II disease with or without symptoms and irrespective of the length of gestation, vigorous therapy is strongly indicated. Delay should be minimal, and termination of pregnancy appears prudent unless the patient is well into her third trimester.[57,58] Patients in the third trimester can begin the upper portion of the mantle technique of radiotherapy with proper shielding of the uterus. Combination chemotherapy including the MOPP regimen is definitely contraindicated in the second and third trimesters. Termination of pregnancy may be necessary, as delaying therapy has been associated with progression of this disease in pregnant patients.[59]

Therapeutic irradiation alone does not appear to jeopardize post-treatment reproduction in fertile Hodgkin's disease patients, but in patients who receive both irradiation and chemotherapy, spontaneous miscarriages and abnormal offspring are increased compared with controls.[59,60,61,62] Oophoropexy at the time of surgical staging and shielding the ovaries during radiation has resulted in two-thirds of the patients retaining ovarian function with many pregnancies in which no abnormalities were observed.[63] Combination oral contraceptives have also been employed to preserve ovarian function in patients receiving cytotoxic therapy.[64] Because recurrent disease within the first 2 years of treatment carries with it poor prognosis, patients should not plan pregnancy during this time period.

LEUKEMIA (see also Chapter 23)

Maternal/Fetal Risks

Acute leukemia accounts for one-half of all leukemia cases during pregnancy occuring in less than 1:75 000 pregnancies. Despite many cures in children with acute lymphocytic leukemia (ALL), acute leukemia in adults has a 5-year survival rate of only about 25–30%.[65] Acute non-lymphocytic leukemia (ANLL) is slightly more common than acute lymphocytic leukemia (ALL).[66] Newer techniques, including bone marrow transplantation, show some promise for improving the survival in these cases, but these therapeutic modalities continue to have many biologic and practical limitations.

The diagnosis of acute leukemia is rarely difficult; pallor, fatigue, fever, infection, and easy bleeding with petechiae usually prompt evaluation with a complete blood and platelet count which reveals anemia, granulocytopenia and thrombocytopenia. Patients with ALL have a normal or elevated white blood cell count, but only 25% exceed 50 000/mm³. In contrast, patients with ANLL usually have a white blood cell count in excess of 50 000/mm³, although one-third will initially be leukopenic.[65] The diagnosis of leukemia should always be confirmed by bone marrow biopsy and aspirate.

The frequent need for immediate institution of chemotherapy raises the question of the potential effects of such therapy on the developing fetus, but exposure to single drugs or combination therapy during the second and third trimesters has generally not been associated with gross fetal abnormalities.[2,3] Never-

---

LEUKEMIA
Summary of Management Options (see also Chapter 23)

Acute leukemias

Prepregnancy

- Counsel about prognosis

- Advise against conception until in remission and on no chemotherapy

Prenatal

- Start chemotherapy as for non-pregnant

- Supportive therapy (blood, platelets, antibiotics, etc.)

- Careful counseling, especially if treatment commenced in first trimester

- Monitor fetal growth and health

Labor/delivery

- Expedite if normal obstetric indications

- Ideally when mother in remission and fetus mature

- Steroids if preterm delivery contemplated

Postnatal

- Contraceptive advice

- Counseling about long-term prognosis

Chronic leukemias

Prepregnancy

- Counsel about prognosis both for pregnancy and in long-term

- Give contraceptive advice

Prenatal

- Hematologic screening for blast phase

- Manage blast phase as for AML

- Avoid busulfan in first trimester

- Monitor fetal growth and health

theless, there are several reports of neonatal bone marrow depression resulting from agents commonly employed to treat leukemia during pregnancy, and there are few reports of long-term follow-up in offspring of treated women.[67] The incidence of healthy live births in pregnancies treated with chemotherapy for acute leukemia varies widely, from 40 to 90%[68,69,111] Remission of the disease is achieved in at least 75% of cases.[69] Catanzarite collected 14 pregnancies reported in patients cured of acute lymphocytic leukemia, of which there was one early spontaneous miscarriage and there were 13 term infants. All the mothers survived.[68]

Management Options

Pregnancy exerts no specific effect on the course of acute leukemia, except that early gestation poses an obstacle to vigorous treatment of leukemia.[70] Prophylactic intrathecal chemotherapy and whole-brain radiation may be safely performed in pregnancy; however, craniospinal radiation should be avoided.[71] Treatment of acute leukemia should be initiated quickly, as delay may compromise any chance of cure and may prove to be rapidly fatal. Measures to avoid conception are strongly advocated for young women with acute leukemia requiring chemotherapy, and a solid case for interruption of pregnancy in this same group of patients can be made. However, this advice is not acceptable to all patients.

Chronic leukemia accounts for approximately 50% of the cases of leukemia during pregnancy, with the overwhelming majority of these being patients with chronic myelocytic leukemia.[66] Chronic lymphocytic leukemia (CLL) is generally an indolent disease, and treatment should be withheld until after delivery unless complications such as severe systemic symptoms, autoimmune hemolytic anemia, recurrent infection or symptomatic lymphatic enlargement occur. The usual therapy includes prednisone and an alkylating agent such as chlorambucil. Chlorambucil is teratogenic in laboratory animals and humans, although its use has been associated with normal outcomes if administered during the second and third trimesters.[72] Steroids in high doses may be used as the sole therapy for autoimmune hemolytic anemia.

Chronic myelogenous leukemia (CML) accounts for approximately 90% of the chronic leukemias complicating pregnancy.[73] The disease is marked by excessive production of mature myeloid cell elements, with granulocyte counts averaging 200 000/dl. Most patients have a thrombocytosis and a mild normochromic, normocytic anemia. Platelet function is often abnormal, although hemorrhage is usually limited to patients with marked thrombocytosis.[73] About 75% of these patients have splenomegaly. Localized radiation therapy can be utilized to reduce the spleen size if discomfort, recurrent infarction or perisplenitis occur. Many patients are treated with busulfan, an agent often responsible for amenorrhea and ovarian failure; on this account pregnancy in a patient with established and treated CML is very rare. Cures are virtually non-existent unless marrow transplantation is performed. Even then, the good outcomes have usually been limited to young patients whose donors were HLA-identical siblings.[74]

Several reports have shown that pregnant patients with chronic granulocytic leukemia treated during the first trimester with chemotherapy and radiation therapy to the spleen will usually delivery apparently healthy, viable babies if the uterus is protected with lead shields.[75] However, because the life-threatening complications so common in acute leukemia (hemorrhage secondary to thrombocytopenia and infection) are rarely encountered in the early months in patients with CML, the pregnancy can usually be carried to term without the use of chemotherapy or other modalities. In this way, the risks to the fetus of potentially mutagenic or teratogenic interventions can be avoided.

COLORECTAL CANCER

Maternal Risks

Cancer of the colon or rectum occurs in 1:50 000 to 100 000 pregnancies and has been reported in pregnant women age 19–48, with a mean of 32 years.[76,77,78] The distribution is felt to be the same as in the non-pregnant population, with 57% arising in the rectum, and 20% scattered throughout the remaining colon.[32,79] There has been speculation that increasing parity and early childbirth may exert a protective influence.[80]

Early colorectal cancer may be asymptomatic. Delay in diagnosis is common and symptoms, when present, are often attributed to normal bowel changes in pregnancy.[78] Severe constipation, weight loss, anorexia, abdominal pain, distention, rectal bleeding and bloody diarrhea may be presenting symptoms and always require investigation. Althogether, 75% of colorectal cancers are detected at the time of rectal examination during pregnancy or early labor.[32] Carcinoembryonic antigen (CEA) is of dubious value as a tumor marker in pregnancy. Patients with unexplained hypochromic microcytic anemia should be evaluated with stool guaiac testing.

Management Options

Management of these tumors in pregnancy is the same as in the non-pregnant state. Radical surgery, during the first trimester, is frequently followed by abortion, but resectable lesions should be operated expeditiously unless fetal pulmonary maturity is shortly forthcoming. If the patient is at 12–20 weeks gestation, Barber and Brunschwig advocated routine hysterectomy to provide better exposure for an adequate margin of resection around the rectosigmoid tumors.[81] However, multiple successful pregnancies have been reported by O'Leary after definitive surgery for colorectal carcinoma.[82] Oophorectomy is recommended for all low-lying colonic tumors because of the high incidence of metastasis to the ovaries. According to Graffner 3–8% of women operated for colorectal carcinoma have macroscopic evidence of metastasis in their ovaries.[83] Autopsy studies using microscopic review of the ovarian tissue reveal an incidence of about 14%. With advanced or metastatic disease, surgical intervention should be delayed until delivery, unless a palliative procedure (e.g. colostomy in the presence of obstructive symptoms) is necessary.

The treatment of colorectal cancer during the third trimester is controversial. Some surgeons believe that with adequate exposure, the neoplasm can be removed without disturbing the uterus and its contents. Others believe that the resection should be done 2 weeks after cesarean section, when the patient has regained strength and when the uterus and the vasculature of the pelvis are less troublesome to the surgeon. Cesarean delivery may be indicated if the lesion is still present at the time of delivery and it arises below the pelvic brim; otherwise, the route of delivery is determined by the usual obstetric indications. Definitive surgery can then be done a few days postpartum because the vaginal vault will not likely be opened by the removal of this lesion, and the increased morbidity from changes in vaginal flora will not be a factor.

There is no apparent role for radiotherapy in the treatment of pregnancy associated colorectal cancer. Chemotherapy does not appear to offer sufficient benefit to warrant the risk to the fetus.[11] As in cancer of the cervix, ovary and bladder, colon cancer appears to have equivalent prognoses, stage for stage, in pregnant and non-pregnant patients.

COLORECTAL CARCINOMA
Summary of Management Options

Prenatal

Surgery is the mainstay of treatment. Management options include:

- In early pregnancy:
  - consideration of termination before surgery
  - surgery without termination has high miscarriage risk
  - hysterectomy is considered for rectosigmoid tumors

- In late pregnancy:
  - elective delivery when fetus viable followed by definitive surgery; hysterectomy is determined by surgical access
  - definitive surgery without disturbing uterus and contents

- Oophorectomy for all low-lying tumors because of high metastasis rate

---

GESTATIONAL THROPHOBLASTIC NEOPLASIA
(see also Chapter 7)

Maternal Risks

Gestational trophoblastic neoplasia (GTN) represents a spectrum of pregnancy-related trophoblastic proliferative disorders which are classified principally by clinical findings and serial determinations of chorionic gonadotropin. For many years, these abnormalities were classified histologically as hydatidiform mole, chorioadenoma destruens and choriocarcinoma, but what they constitute are a spectrum rather than separate and distinct entities.

Hydatidiform mole occurs in 1:1200 pregnancies in the USA, but in 1:120 pregnancies in the Far East. Molar pregnancies occur more frequently in the early teens and perimenopausally. Parity does not influence the incidence and neither age nor parity affects the clinical outcome. Spontaneous remission is common in 80–85% of all patients with hydatidiform mole. A deficiency of animal fat and the fat-soluble vitamin carotene may contribute to the disease.[84] Goldstein et al. reported that 9 of 1339 patients (1:150) had at least two consecutive molar pregnancies.[85] Other centers have reported incidences as high as 1:50 women. With recurrent molar pregnancies, there is an increased risk of malignant sequelae.

Essentially, all patients with hydatidiform mole have delayed menses, and most patients are considered to be pregnant. Vaginal bleeding occurs usually during the first trimester, ranging from a brown discharge to brisk hemorrhage. Hyperemesis is present in one-third of patients. Pre-eclampsia in the first trimester of pregnancy has been said to be almost pathognomonic of a hydatidiform mole, although this occurs in only 12% of cases.[86] Hyperthyroidism occurs rarely but can precipitate a medical emergency. Blood values are affected in 10% of patients, but clinical manifestations occur in only 1%.[86] Hyperthyroidism results from the production of thyrotropin by molar tissue and disappears once the molar pregnancy is evacuated, but antithyroid therapy may be indicated for a short period. Classically, uterine size is excessive for gestational age, and this is found in 50% of patients with moles, but one-third of patients will have uteri that are smaller than expected for gestational age. About 5% of patients have enlarged theca lutea cysts which are associated with a higher incidence of malignant sequelae. The combination of enlarged ovaries and an enlarged for gestational age uterus results in a 57% risk of malignant sequelae.

The first evidence to suggest the presence of hydatidiform mole is usually passage of vesicles per vagina. A urinary quantitative hCG determination greater than 1 million IU/l is suggestive, but a single determination is not diagnostic. Occasionally, a single determination will be high in a normal single or erythroblastic pregnancy and, conversely, a normal hCG titer will be seen in a molar pregnancy. Ultrasonography can be used to make a definitive diagnosis in almost all cases. This has almost eliminated amniography. Rarely, a fetus coexists with a mole, thereby confusing the ultrasonographic findings.

The classic (complete) mole is well recognized histologically by the presence of trophoblastic proliferation and hydropic degeneration, and the absence of vasculature. The embryo dies before the stage of organogenesis and no fetus, cord or amniotic fluid is identified. A normal karyotype (usually $46X^PX^P$ but rarely 46XY) is present. This results from fertilization of an 'empty egg' by a single sperm which duplicates itself, or an 'empty egg' may be fertilized by two sperm. In contrast, the partial mole consists of both placenta and fetus and usually has a triploid karyotype. This is due to a normal egg being fertilized by two sperm. Patients with partial moles tend to be older with longer gestational age and uteri which are not enlarged for gestational age. Pre-eclampsia occurs less frequently and not until well into the second trimester. HCG titers are lower in patients with partial moles, luteal cysts are less common, and malignant sequelae are less frequent.

Patients with a complete mole and a normal size or larger uterus have a 25% chance of developing malignancy compared with only 11% in patients with small for date uterus.[86] Patients with enlarged ovaries, irrespective of uterine size, have a 49% chance of developing malignancy in the future.[86] With both enlarged ovaries and a large for date uterus, 57% develop malignancy.[86] If time of evacuation was less than 10 weeks, only 4% developed malignancy. But between 11 and 15 weeks, the incidence increased to 29%, than fell to 19% if more than 16 weeks. The method of evacuation has limited, if any, influence on the incidence of malignant sequelae.[87,88]

Management Options

Before the use of suction curettage for the evacuation of molar pregnancy, hysterotomy was frequently used on those uteri that were greater than 14 weeks in size. Suction curettage is now the method of choice on all sizes unless major hemorrhage is present, although a laparotomy set-up must be available for all patients with large uteri. Pitocin is begun after a moderate amount of tissue has been removed and uterine contractions can no longer cause trophoblastic tissue to be engulfed by the large venous sinusoids in the uterus and embolize to the lungs. When the suction curettage has been completed and involution has begun, a sharp curettement is done and this tissue is submitted separately for pathologic evaulation. A primary hysterectomy may be selected as the method of evacuation if the patient is not desirous of future pregnancies, but the patient must be followed in the same manner as when other evacuation techniques are used. The ovaries can be left undisturbed even when theca-luteum cysts are encountered, as they will regress when hCG is no longer present in the serum.

Since hCG is produced by viable trophoblastic cells in the body, the clinical course of the disease and the response to therapy can be followed accurately by this marker. Radioimmunoassay for beta-hCG must be used rather than less sensitive biologic or immunologic assays. After evacuation, the patient should have serial radioimmune beta-hCG determinations at 1–2 week intervals until there are two normal determinations, then bimonthly for at least 1 year. Contraception is essential during this year, as subsequent normal pregnancy would make it impossible to follow up a molar pregnancy with beta-hCG determination. Oral contraceptives are the preferred method of contraception after evacuation of a hydatidiform mole.[89] Regular pelvic examinations should be done at 2 week intervals until the hCG titers return to normal levels, then at 3 month intervals for 1 year. When titers, examinations and chest films are negative for 1 year, contraception may be stopped. The risk of recurrence in subsequent pregnancies is about 1%. In total, 65% of patients will develop normal titers within 60 days and another 16% by 110 days.[90] Nineteen percent will require chemotherapy, but only 3% will have disease outside of the uterus.[90] If the hCG plateaus for 3 consecutive weeks, or rises, or metastases are seen on a chest film, or examination reveals enlargement, chemotherapy must be started promptly. Prophylactic chemotherapy reduces the incidence of persistent trophoblastic disease in patients at high risk, but it also increases tumor resistance and morbidity.[91] Therefore, it is not indicated.[91]

Malignant choriocarcinoma is preceded by hydatidiform mole in 50% of cases, normal pregnancy in 25% of cases, and miscarriage or ectopic pregnancy in 25% of cases. Invasive mole is always preceded by a hydatidiform mole. If choriocarcinoma occurs many years after a pregnancy, a biopsy may be read as anaplastic malignant disease and diagnostic hCG determinations may not be obtained, resulting in unnecessary thoracotomy, craniotomy, or worse.

It has been common practice to perform a diagnostic uterine curettage when beta-hCG plateaus or rises but this procedure is unnecessary, rarely helpful and occasionally results in uterine perforation, massive hemorrhage and the need for a hysterectomy. Malignant tissue is often deep in the myometrium and unobtainable by curettage. Thus the need for chemotherapy is not altered either by the presence or absence of molar tissue or choriocarcinoma on repeat uterine curettage. In many cases, patients have metastases in the absence of disease within the uterus.

The workup for a diagnosis of persistent gestational trophoblastic neoplasia should consist of a history and physical exam, chest x-ray and CT scan of the lungs, liver and brain scans or CT scans, serum chemistries, hematologic survey, pretreatment hCG titer, and ultrasound of the pelvis if indicated (**Table 10**). Once these tests have been obtained, categorization of disease can be performed and specific therapy begun. Several authors have suggested that the use of HCG has made the histologic diagnosis unnecessary. The categories are non-metastatic and metastatic with the latter divided between good prognosis disease and poor prognosis disease (**Table 11**). Staging and scoring systems also exist (**Tables 12** and **13**).

Non-metastatic trophoblastic disease is usually a diagnosis of exclusion, since metastasis cannot be identified. Particularly if subsequent fertility is desired, a pelvic arteriogram can be performed and disease

Table 10
Workup of gestational trophoblastic neoplasia

History and physical examination
Chest film
Liver scan
Hematologic survey
Serum chemistries of renal and liver function
Pretreatment hCG titer
CT of brain
Ultrasound of pelvis if indicated

Table 11
Classification of gestational trophoblastic neoplasia

Non-metastatic disease: no evidence of disease outside uterus
Metastatic disease: any disease outside uterus

1. Good prognosis metastatic disease

   short duration (last pregnancy <4 months)
   low pretreatment hCG titer (<100 000 IU/24 h or <40 000 mIU/ml)
   no metastasis to brain or liver
   no significant prior chemotherapy

2. Poor prognosis metastatic disease

   long duration (last pregnancy >4 months)
   high pretreatment hCG titer (>100 000 IU/24 h or >40 000 mIU/ml)
   brain or liver metastasis
   significant prior chemotherapy
   term pregnancy

Table 12
International Federation of Gynecologists and Obstetricians (FIGO) clinical stages in gestational trophoblastic neoplasia

Stage I
GTN strictly contained to the uterine corpus

Stage II
GTN extends to the adnexa outside the uterus but is limited to the genital structures

Stage III
GTN extends to the lungs with or without genital tract involvement

Stage IV
All other metastatic sites

identified within the uterus. This may be a guide, especially if chemotherapy is unsuccessful. Patients with non-metastatic trophoblastic disease are treated with single-agent chemotherapy. Recently, the use of high-dose methotrexate with folinic acid rescue has been tested with excellent results (**Table 14**).[92] If patients have abnormal liver function, dactinomycin should be used rather than methotrexate. In the Far East, 5-fluorouracil has been used successfully as a single agent.[93] Actinomycin-D has the advantages of ease of administration, greater patient convenience and improved cost-effectiveness.

Therapy should be repeated at 7 day intervals if at all possible, but the WBC must be greater than 3000/mm³, polymorphonuclear count must be greater than 1500/mm³, platelets must be greater than 100 000/mm³ and BUN, SGOT and SGPT must be essentially normal (**Table 15**). Severe oral or gastrointestinal ulceration

Table 13
World Health Organization (WHO) scoring system for gestational trophoblastic neoplasia

Prognostic factor	Score			
	0	1	2	4
Age	≤39	>39		
Antecedent pregnancy		Abortion	Term	
Months from last pregnancy	4	4–6	7–12	12
hCG (IU/l)	10^3	10^3–10^4	10^4–10^5	10^5
ABO (female × male)	0 × A A × 0	B AB		
Largest tumor (cm)	3–5	5		
Site metastases	Spleen Kidney	GI Liver	Brain	
No. of metastases	1–4	4–8	8	
Prior chemotherapy	None	Single drugs	2 or more drugs	

Note: ≤4: low risk; 5–7: middle risk; ≥8: high risk.

Table 14
Single agent chemotherapy for gestational trophoblastic neoplasia

1. Methotrexate 20–25 mg i.m. every day for 5 days (repeat every 7 days if possible)
2. Dactinomycin 10–12 mg/kg i.v. every day for 5 days (repeat every 7 days if possible)
3. Methotrexate 1 mg/kg i.m. on days 1, 3, 5 and 7; folinic acid 0.1 mg/kg i.m. on days 2, 4, 6 and 8 (repeat every 7 days if possible)

Table 15
Management of single-agent chemotherapy in gestational trophoblastic neoplasia

1. Chemotherapy as noted in **Table 14** repeated at 7–10 day intervals depending on toxicity contraception begun (oral if not contraindicated)
2. Drug continued as above until hCG titer is normal
3. Chemotherapy changed if:
   titer rises (10-fold or more)
   titer plateaus
   evidence of new metastasis
4. Laboratory values – chemotherapy not repeated unless:
   WBC >3000/mm³
   polys >1500/mm³
   platelets > 100 000/mm³
   BUN, SGOT, SGPT essentially normal
5. Other toxicity mandating postponement of chemotherapy
   severe oral or gastrointestinal ulceration
   febrile course (usually present only when leukopenia)
6. Remission defined as three consecutive normal weekly hCG titers

Table 16
Remission and follow-up in gestational trophoblastic neoplasia

1. Three consecutive normal weekly hCG assays (1–3 courses after normal)
2. hCG titers every 2 weeks for 3 months
   then monthly for 3 months
   then every 2 months for 6 months
3. Frequent pelvic examination
4. Contraception for 1 year

Table 17
Role of therapy in non-metastatic gestational trophoblastic neoplasia

	Patients	Days hospitalized	No. of courses of chemotherapy
Chemotherapy + 1⁰ hysterectomy	17	32.8	2.2
Chemotherapy only (cure)	106	50.8	4.0
Chemotherapy + 2⁰ surgery	16	121.2	8.3

1⁰: primary, 2⁰: secondary.
Based on data from Hammond et al.[94]

and fever are also reasons to postpone chemotherapy. The therapy should be continued until three consecutive normal weekly hCG titers are obtained. However, if a patient's hCG titer rises or if there is a titer plateau after two courses of chemotherapy, an alternate drug should be tried. Evidence of new metastasis while the patient is being treated is also an indication for changing the chemotherapy. Once the hCG titers have returned to normal levels, appropriate follow-up is mandatory (**Table 16**). This entails hCG titers every 2 weeks for 3 months, then monthly for 3 months, then ever 2 months for 6 months. Frequent pelvic exams are also required. Contraception is essential for 1 year and oral contraceptives, unless otherwise contraindicated, may be used.

Treatment of non-metastatic GTN has been 100% successful (**Tables 17** and **18**). Failure of either methotrexate or actinomycin-D warrants switching to the other of these two drugs. Subsequent failure of the

Table 18
Role of therapy in non-metastatic gestational
trophoblastic neoplasia

Therapy	Remission
Chemotherapy only	106/122
Chemotherapy + hysterectomy (2^0)	9/9　122/122
Chemotherapy + pelvic infusion	3/7
Chemotherapy + pelvic infusion + hysterectomy 3^0	4/7
Chemotherapy + 1^0 hysterectomy	17/17
Total	139/139 (100%)

1^0: primary, 2^0: secondary, 3^0: tertiary.
Based on data from Hammond *et al.*[94]

second drug can still be treated successfully either with intra-arterial infusion of the drug into the uterus, multiple agent chemotherapy as described later for metastatic disease with poor prognosis, or hysterectomy. When either hysterectomy or intra-arterial chemotherapy is contemplated, a pelvic arteriogram should be done to verify a resistant focus of tumor within the uterus. Fertility after treatment is reported in **Table 19**.

Patients with GTN who hae metastases are categorized as having a good prognosis when none of the following is present:

- brain or liver metastasis

- urinary hCG titer greater than 100 000 IU/24 h or serum beta-hCG titer greater than 40 000 mIU/ml;

- previous chemotherapy;

- interval since last pregnancy greater than 4 months

There is no general agreement in the literature whether patients who had an antecedent term pregnancy and developed GTN should be placed on the poor prognosis category. Therapy for good prognosis metastatic

Table 19
Fertility after metastatic gestational trophoblastic
neoplasia

Desired fertility	109/122 (89%)
Subsequent pregnancies (47 patients)	57
Normal infants	45 (2 sets of twins)
Spontaneous abortion	7
Therapeutic abortion	3
Mole	2

Based on data from Hammond *et al.*[94]

GTN can be the same as described for non-metastatic disease. When negative titers have been achieved, one additional course is routinely given. Complete, sustained remission can be achieved in 100% of this category, but more courses of chemotherapy are required.[95]

Multiple-agent chemotherapy is recommended in this disease if at least one of the above 'poor' prognostic features are present. These patients should be treated in centers that have special interests and expertise in this disease. Most patients require months of hospitalization with life-threatening toxicity from therapy. Remission rates are described in **Tables 20** and **21**.

Beginning in 1969, a combination of methotrexate, actinomycin-D and cyclophosphamide (MAC) was utilized every 12–14 days as permitted by bone marrow toxicity. Cerebral or hepatic metastases were treated concurrently with 2000–3000 rad in 10–15 days to the whole brain or liver. Concurrently, Bagshawe developed a complex seven-drug regimen believed to be less toxic but it proved to be more toxic. Since 1979, Bagshawe's group has employed a five-drug regimen of etoposide, methotrexate and actinomycin-D (EM-A), plus vincristine and cyclophosphamide (CO) alternating the two- and three-drug regimens weekly (**Table 22**).

Bagshawe's group has reported an 84% overall survival rate, including patients in whom prior chemotherapy had failed and a 94% survival rate in those who had not received prior chemotherapy. At least four

Table 20
Role of therapy in poor prognosis metastatic
gestational trophoblastic neoplasia

Therapy	Remission
Chemotherapy + radiation therapy	20/23 (87%)
Chemotherapy + 1^0 surgery	17/29 (57%)
Chemotherapy + 2^0 surgery	5/11 (45%)
Total	42/63 (66%)

1^0: primary, 2^0: secondary.
Based on data from Hammond *et al.*[94]
Note: 16 patients died of disease; 5 patients died of toxicity.

Table 21
Results of treatment of GTN

Disease	Remission
Non-metastatic	139/139 (100%)
Good prognosis metastatic	55/55 (100%)
Poor prognosis metastatic	42/63 (66%)
Total	236/257 (92%)

Modified from Hammond *et al.*[94]

<table>
<tr><td>

GESTATIONAL TROPHOBLASTIC NEOPLASIA
Summary of Management Options
(see also Chapter 7)

Prenatal and postnatal

Diagnosis, assessment and staging

- See **Tables 10**, **11**, **12** and **13**

Treatment

- Suction curettage for primary disease (laparotomy and hysterectomy only for severe uncontrollable hemorrhage)

- Tissue should be sent for
  - histology
  - karyotype

- Monitor response by hCG assay

- If titers fail to fall or rise secondarily, commence single-agent chemotherapy (see **Table 14**) and monitor response, toxicity and hematological, renal and liver function (see **Table 15**)

- Once titers have returned to normal values, the follow-up is as in **Table 16**

</td></tr>
</table>

Table 22
EMA-CO chemotherapy[a]

Course 1 (EMA)

Day 1
Etoposidem 100 mg/m^2, i.v. infusion in 200 ml saline
Dactinomycin 0.5 mg, i.v. stat
Methotrexate 100 mg/m^2, i.v. stat 200 mg/m^2, i.v. infusion over 12 h

Day 2
Etoposide 100 mg/m^2, i.v. infusion in 200 ml saline over 30 min
Dactinomycin 0.5 mg, i.v. stat
Folinic acid 15 mg, i.m. or orally every 12 h for 4 doses beginning 24 h after start of methotrexate

---

Course 2 (CVO)

Day 8
Vincristine 1.0 mg/m^2, i.v. stat
Cyclophosphamide 600 mg/m^2, i.v. infusion

---

[a] This regimen consists of two courses. Course 1 is given on days 1 and 2. Course 2 is given on day 8. These courses can usually be given on days 1 and 2, 8, 15 and 16, 22, etc., and the intervals should not be extended without cause.

metastatic, 5.4% of good prognosis metastatic and 21% of poor prognosis metastatic GTN, but GTN remains the most curable of all gynecologic malignancies.

BONE

Maternal Risks

Benign bone tumors rarely cause a problem during pregnancy, but enchondromas and benign exostoses can obstruct labor when they occur at the pelvic brim. The most frequently encountered malignant bone tumors are Ewing's sarcoma, osteogenic sarcoma and osteocystoma. The most frequent locations are the spine, rib cage and long bones. Myelitis can be produced by primary sarcoma of the spine and this causes severe pain when the nerve roots are involved. Metastases are usually from the breast, uterus, thyroid or adrenals and are usually found in the lower thoracic and lumbar regions.

Management Options

Primary bone cancer is aggressive, frequently metastasizing by the hematogenous route at the time of diagnosis. Treatment of oesteogenic sarcoma has been more successful since utilizing adjuvant chemotherapy with prompt but more limited surgery than advocated previously. Because the risk of fetal malformations

courses of chemotherapy are administered after the first negative hCG titer. Follow-up evaluation after complete remission is the same as described earlier for mole and non-metastatic GTN. Either brain or liver metastases are associated with less than 50% overall survival and lower yet if both are involved. Altogether, 97% of women treated with chemotherapy were able to conceive, and 80% achieved at least one live birth.[96] Women who had received combination chemotherapy were found to be less likely to have a live birth than those treated with methotrexate alone. There was no excess of congenital malformations in the offspring of these women as compared with that expected for women of comparable age who had never received chemotherapy. Recurrences occur in 2.1% of non-induced by chemotherapy during the second half of pregnancy is low, continuation of pregnancy despite administration of a methotrexate-containing multiple-drug regimen can be considered. However, termination of pregnancy may be recommended for patients whose cancer is discovered in the first or early second trimesters. Further pregnancy should not be anticipated until 3 years after initial therapy, at which time most recurrences will have occurred. Pregnancy has no effect on the clinical behavior of bone sarcomas.[97]

PITUITARY

Maternal Risks

An increasing number of prolactin-secreting pituitary adenomas are now being detected in women. With the use of ovulation induction and suppression of prolactin synthesis by dopaminergic agents such as bromocriptine, pregnancy has become increasingly common in patients with prolactinomas. Much of the pituitary enlargement found during pregnancy is thought to be secondary to hyperplasia of the lactotropin cells of the anterior pituitary that are stimulated by estrogen.[98] However, most patients with a microadenoma have an uneventful pregnancy and in those who do become symptomatic, regression usually follows delivery.[99,100,101]

Evaluation for possible prolactin-secretary tumors is made difficult during pregnancy by the physiologic rise in serum prolactin that accompanies normal gestation. Furthermore, prolactin levels do not always rise during pregnancy in women with prolactinomas, and they do not always rise with pregnancy-induced tumor enlargement.[102] Therefore, radiologic diagnosis is necessary for the pregnant patient who develops severe headaches or a visual field defect.[101] Symptoms requiring therapy occur in 20% of patients who have untreated tumors, but in only 1% of women with previously treated adenomas.[100] In all, 15:5% of patients with macroadenomas experience symptomatic tumor enlargement.[101]

Management Options

When complications arise during pregnancy and fetal maturity is present, induction of labor or cesarean section for obstetric indications should be performed. Earlier in gestation, if radiologic evidence suggests tumor enlargement, therapy should not be delayed. Bromocriptine appears to be safe in early pregnancy, as evidenced by its use for induction of ovulation without an increased incidence of congenital malformations.[103,104] Other treatment modalities employed during pregnancy include trans-sphenoidal surgery and, in one case, hydrocortiscone therapy.[99,100,101]

Following delivery, radiologic assessment of tumor size and a serum prolactin assay should be performed at the first postpartum visit. Breast-feeding is not contraindicated in the presence of a prolactin-secreting microadenoma.[99] Patients should not attempt further pregnancies unless progression of tumor growth has not occurred. Subsequent pregnancies are not associated with an increased frequency of symptoms.[98]

SARCOMA

Maternal Risks and Management Options

Most sarcomas discovered during pregnancy are neurofibrosarcomas or similar lesions and their course depends greatly on the grade of the neoplasm. Therapy for low-grade sarcomas can be deferred to the postpartum period, when resection should technically be much easier. Cesarean delivery is often required due to obstruction. High-grade lesions have a poor prognosis, and therapy must be individualized acording to the length of gestation and preference of the patient.

VAGINA

Maternal Risks

Cancer of the vagina is extremely uncommon, although clear cell adenocarcinoma of the vagina or cervix has been described in pregnant women who were, themselves, exposed *in utero* to diethylstilbestrol. Among patients with stage I and stage II tumors (73% vaginal and 27% cervical), the overall 5- and 10-year age-adjusted survival rates did not differ significantly between pregnant and non-pregnant individuals.[105] Primary squamous cell carcinoma of the vagina is especially rare with a poor prognosis.[106] Even more rare is the occurrence of sarcoma botryoides of the vagina and cervix in pregnancy.

Management Options

When these latter sarcomatous lesions occur in the upper half of the vagina with or without cervical involvement, the most appropriate therapy has been a radical hysterectomy, upper vaginectomy and bilateral pelvic lymphadenectomy followed by postoperative adjuvant chemotherapy. A similar procedure is indicated for clear cell adenocarcinoma of the upper vagina and cervix. The pregnancy is disregarded in the first and second trimesters. In the third trimester, surgery can be delayed until the fetus is mature if the patient insists, but the patient must be aware of the risk she is assuming. With extensive involvement of the vagina by any lesion, including squamous cell carcinoma, one should seriously consider evacuation of the uterus by hysterotomy or cesarean section and beginning appropriate radiation therapy. Radical surgery appears to be appropriate only for early lesions involving the upper vagina and/or cervix. The prognosis appears to be unaffected by the pregnancy.

VULVA

Maternal Risks

Cancer of the vulva occurring during pregnancy is extremely rare, but invasive epidermoid carcinomas, melanomas, sarcomas and adenoid cystic adenocarcinomas have been described. Vulvar intraepithelial neoplasia is common and, as with cervical intraepithelial neoplasia, therapy can be delayed until the postpartum period. Vaginal delivery is appropriate.

Management Options

Vulvar malignancy diagnosed during the first and second trimesters is usually treated by radical vulvectomy with bilateral groin dissection after the 14 weeks gestation.[102,108] When diagnosed in the third trimester, wide local excision can be performed followed by definitive surgery within 1 week post-delivery.[102] Survival of these patients, stage for stage, is similar to that of non-pregnant patients. Several patients have become pregnant and delivered normally after radical vulvectomy and bilateral inguinal lymphadenectomy. Usually, delivery can be performed vaginally, but a high degree of stenosis or other fibrosis demands a cesarean delivery.

BLADDER

Maternal Risks

Carcinoma of the bladder is rarely seen during pregnancy. About 95% of cases are transitional cell carcinomas originating in the trigone area and spreading by direct extension, by lymphatics and, less commonly, by the hematogenous route to regional and distant sites. Metastasis to bone, especially the pelvis and lumbar spine, is common and may be the source of intractable pain. The prognosis is directly related to the extent of disease and grade of tumor.

Management Options

Well-differentiated lesions that are superficial can be managed by local fulguration laser therapy, or intravesical chemotherapy, whereas others require partial or total urinary bladder removal with lymphadenectomy for cure. Radiation therapy can be curative, but the fetus complicates the situation. The mode of delivery of the fetus depends on the length of gestation as well as patient and physician preference. Both cystectomy and pelvic irradiation have resulted in high rates of fetal wastage.

FALLOPIAN TUBE

Maternal Risks and Management Options

Cancer of the fallopian tube associated with pregnancy is extremely rare, but has been reported. The usual, sometimes profuse, serosonguinous vaginal discharge seen with carcinoma of the fallopian tube in non-pregnant patients is not seen after 12 weeks gestation in the pregnant patient. This makes diagnosis even more difficult than in the non-pregnant patient. Usually, it is discovered at laparotomy, at which time appropriate treatment is total abdominal hysterectomy with bilateral salpingo-oophorectomy and postoperative radiation therapy or chemotherapy as indicated. When the carcinoma is discovered incidentally in specimens from tubal ligation, total abdominal hysterectomy with bilateral salpingo-oophorectomy is appropriate.

UTERUS

Maternal Risks and Management Options

Authorities disagree whether adenocarcinoma of the endometrium occurs during pregnancy. Some feel the reported cases represent misdiagnosed Arias-Stella phenomena. However, a well-documented case with deep myometrial invasion had been described, which lends credence to the previous reports.[109,111] Those described in the literature have usually been local, well-differentiated and non-invasive or minimally invasive. Appropriate therapy is total hysterectomy with bilateral salpingo-oophorectomy and adjuvant radiotherapy where indicated.

Leiomyosarcoma and carcinosarcoma of the uterus have also been reported as incidental findings noted in surgical specimens.

OTHER MALIGNANT CONDITIONS
Summary of Management Options

Bone sarcoma

- In early pregnancy, consider termination followed by surgery and adjuvant chemotherapy

- In late pregnancy, chemotherapy can be commenced and definitive surgery deferred until fetal viability and delivery is achieved

- Further pregnancy should be avoided for 3 years to reduce likelihood of relapses/recurrences

Prolactinoma (see also Chapter 22)

- If there is enlargement during pregnancy, bromocriptine should be given; other treatment (surgery/radiotherapy) will depend on tumor size and response

- Delivery is an option if fetal viability has been reached

Sarcoma

- Treatment should be individualized according to grade and site

Vagina

- Termination of the pregnancy before implementing definitive therapy will depend on patient's wishes and gestation

- Radical surgery, radiotherapy and chemotherapy all have a place in definitive treatment depending on tumor type and location

Vulva

- In early pregnancy, consider termination followed by radical vulvectomy and bilateral groin dissection

- In late pregnancy, definitive surgery can be deferred until fetal viability and delivery is achieved

Bladder

- Treatment (laser ablation, radical surgery with or without adjuvant chemotherapy or radiotherapy will depend on size and degree of differentiation of tumor)

- Termination of the pregnancy (abortion or elective delivery) will depend on gestation and patient preference

Fallopian tube

- Rare; often chance finding at laparotomy

- Total abdominal hysterectomy and bilateral salpingo-oophorectomy is the definitive operation followed by adjuvant radiotherapy or chemotherapy

- Termination of the pregnancy (abortion or elective delivery) will depend on gestation and patient preference

REFERENCES

1 Allen H, Nisker J (eds) (1986) *Cancer in Pregnancy: Therapeutic Guidelines.* New York: Futura.

2 Doll DC, Ringenberg QS, Yarbro JW (1989) Antineoplastic agents and pregnancy. *Seminars in Oncology* **16**:337–346.

3 Nicholson HO (1968) Cytotoxic drugs in pregnancy. *Journal of Obstetrics and Gynaecology of the British Commonwealth* **75**:307.

4 Schapira DV, Chudley AE (1984) Successful pregnancy following continuous treatment with combination chemotherapy before conception and throughout pregnancy. *Cancer* **54**:800.

5 Sokal JE, Lessman EM (1960) The effects of cancer chemotherapeutic agents on the human fetus. *Journal of the American Medical Association* **172**:1765.

6 Sweet DL, Kinzie J (1976) Consequence of radiotherapy and antineoplastic therapy for the fetus. *Journal of Reproductive Medicine* **17**:241.

7 Roboz J *et al.* (1979) Does doxorubison cross the placenta? *Lancet* **2**:1382.

8 Sanger WG, Armitage JO, Schmidt MA (1980) Feasibility of semen cryopreservation in patients with malignant disease. *Journal of the American Medical Association* **244**:789.

9 Van Theil DH, Ross GT, Lipsett MB (1970) Pregnancies after chemotherapy of trophoblastic neoplasms. *Science* **169**:1326.

10 Brent RL (1986) The effects of embryonic and fetal exposure to x-ray, microwaves, and ultrasound. *Clinical Perinatology* **13**:615.

11 Doll D, Ringenberg Q, Yarbro J (1988) Management of cancer in pregnancy. *Archives of Internal Medicine* **148**:2058–2064.

12 Hammer-Jacobson E (1959) Therapeutic abortion on account of x-ray examination during pregnancy. *Danish Medical Bulletin* **6**:113–122.

13 Sall S, Rini S, Pineda A (1974) Surgical management of invasive carcinoma in pregnancy. *American Journal of Obstetrics and Gynecology* **118**:1–5.

14 Timothy A (1986) Radiation and pregnancy. In Allen H, Nisker J (eds) *Cancer in Pregnancy: Therapeutic Guidelines*, pp. 9–34. New York: Futura.

15 Sutcliffe S (1985) Treatment of neoplastic disease during pregnancy: Maternal and fetal effects. *Clinical Investigation and Medicine* **8**:333–338.

16 Barron W (1984) The pregnant surgical patient: Medical evaluation and management. *Annals of Internal Medicine* **101**:683–691.

17 Awe R, Nicotra M, Newsom T *et al.* (1979) Arterial oxygenation and alveolar–arterial gradients in term pregnancy. *Obstetrics and Gynecology* **53**:182–186.

18 Pritchard J, MacDonald P, Gant N (1985) Maternal adaption to pregnancy. In Pritchard J, MacDonald P, Gant N (eds) *Williams' Obstetrics*, pp. 181–210. Norwalk: Appleton-Century-Crofts.

19 Hathaway W, Bonnar J (1978) *Perinatal Coagulation.* Philadelphia, PA: Grune and Stratton.

20 Laros R, Alger L (1984) Thromboembolism in pregnancy. In Depp R, Eschenbach D, Sciarra J (eds) *Gynecology and Obstetrics*, pp. 1–12. New York: Harper and Row.

21 Ueland K (1984) Cardiorespiratory physiology of pregnancy. In Depp R, Eschenbach D, Sciarra J (eds) *Gynecology and Obstetrics*, pp. 1–12. New York: Harper and Row.

22 Schnider S, Webster G (1965) Maternal and fetal hazards of surgery during pregnancy. *American Journal of Obstetrics and Gynecology* **92**:891–900.

23 Holland E (1949) A case of transplacental metastasis of malignant melanoma from mother to fetus. *J. Obstet Gynec Br Eurp* **56**:529.

24 Potter JF, Schoeneman M (1970) Metastasis of maternal cancer to the placenta and fetus. *Cancer* **25**:380–388.

25 Rothmore LA, Cohen CJ, Astarloa J (1973) Placenta and fetal involvement by maternal malignancy: A report of rectal carcinoma and review of the literature. *American Journal of Obstetrics and Gynecology* **116**:1023–1034.

26 Cramblett HG, Friedman JL, Najjao S (1958) Leukemia in an infant born to a mother with leukemia. *New England Journal of Medicine* **259**:727.

27 Hacker NF, Berek JS, Lagasse LD *et al.* (1982) Carcinoma of the cervix associated with pregnancy. *Obstetrics and Gynecology* **59**:735.

28 Creasman W, Rutledge F, Fletcher G (1970) Carcinoma of the cervix associated with pregnancy. *Obstetrics and Gynecology* **36**:495–501.

29 Lurain JR, Gallop DG (1979) Management of abnormal Papanicolaou smears in pregnancy. *Obstetrics and Gynecology* **53**:184.

30 Lee RB, Neglia W, Park RC (1981) Cervical carcinoma in pregnancy. *Obstetrics and Gynecology* **58**:584.

31 Prem K, Makowski E, McKelvey J (1966) Carcinoma of the cervix associated with pregnancy. *American Journal of Obstetrics and Gynecology* **95**:99–108.

32 Allen H, Nisker J (1986) Colorectal cancer in pregnancy. In Allen H, Nisker J (eds) *Cancer in Pregnancy: Therapeutic Guidelines*, pp. 281–285. New York: Futura.

33 King RM, Welch JS, Martin JK Jr, Coulaun CB (1985) Carcinoma of the breast associated with pregnancy. *Surgery Gynecology Obstetrics* **160**:228.

34 Donegan WL (1977) Breast cancer and pregnancy. *Obstetrics and Gynecology* **50**:244.

35 White TT, White WC (1956) Breast cancer and pregnancy: Report of 49 cases followed five years. *Annals of Surgery* **144**:384.

36 Holleb AI, Farrow JH (1962) The relation of carcinoma of the breast and pregnancy in 283 patients. *Surgery Gynecology Obstetrics* **115**:65.

37 Peters MV (1968) The effect of pregnancy in breast cancer. In Forrest APM, Kunkler PB (eds) *Prognostic Factors in Breast Cancer*, p. 120. Baltimore, MD: Williams and Wilkins.

38 Sommer RG, Young GP, Kaplan NJ *et al.* (1985) Fine needle aspiration biopsy in the management of solid breast tumors. *Archives of Surgery* **120**:673.

39 Parente JT, Amsel M, Lerner R, Chivea F (1988) Breast cancer associated with pregnancy. *Obstetrics and Gynecology* **71**:861.

40 Rosemond GP, Maier WP (1970) *In Breast Cancer: Early and Late.* Chicago, IL: Year Book Medical Publishers.

41 Haagensenm CD (1971) *Diseases of the Breast.* Philadelphia, PA: W.B. Saunders.

42 Radvin RG, Lewison EF, Slock NH *et al.* (1970) The results of a clinical trait concerning the worth of prophylactic oophorectomy for breast cancer. *Surgery Gynecology Obstetrics* **131**:1055.

43 Pack GT, Scharnazel LM (1951) The prognosis for malignant melanoma in the pregnant woman. *Cancer* **4**:324.

44 Reintgen DS *et al.* (1985) Malignant melanoma and pregnancy. *Cancer* **55**:1340.

45 White LP *et al.* (1961) Studies on melanoma: The effect of pregnancy on survival in human melanoma. *Journal of the American Medical Association* **117**:235.

46 Goldsmith HS (1979) Melanoma: An overview. *CA-A Cancer Journal for Clinicians* **29**.

47 Hogstan P, Lilford RJ (1986) Ultrasound study of ovarian cysts in pregnancy: Prevalence and significance. *British Journal of Obstetrics and Gynaecology* **93**:625.

48 Ghung A, Birnbaum S (1973) Ovarian cancer associated with pregnancy. *Obstetrics and Gynecology* **41**:211–214.

49 Munnell E (1963) Primary ovarian cancer associated with pregnancy. *Clinics in Obstetrics and Gynecology* **6**:983–993.

50 Karlen JR, Akfari A, Cook WA (1979) Dysgerminoma associated with pregnancy. *Obstetrics and Gynecology* **53**:330.

51 Burrow G (1975) The thyroid in pregnancy. *Medical Clinics of North America* **59**:1089–1098.

52 Kavanagh J (1988) Thyroid cancer in pregnancy. In *Proceedings of the Second International Conference on Cancer in Pregnancy*, Clearwater, FL, February.

53 Rosen I (1986) Pregnancy as a predisposing factor in thyroid neoplasin. *Archives of Surgery* **121**:1287–1290.

54 Hill CS, Clark RL, Wolf M (1966) The effect of subsequent pregnancy in patients with thyroid carcinoma. *Surg Gynecol Obstet* **122**:1219.

55 Rosvoll RV, Winship J (1965) Thyroid carcinoma and pregnancy. *Surgery Gynecology Obstetrics* **121**:1039.

56 Stewart HL, Monto RM (1952) Hodgkin's disease and pregnancy. *American Journal of Obstetrics and Gynecology* **63**:570.

57 Thomas PRM, Peckham MJ (1976) The investigation and management of Hodgkin's disease in the pregnant patient. *Cancer* **38**:1443.

58 Jacobs C, Donaldson SS, Rosenberg SA, Kaplan HS (1981) Management of the pregnant patient with Hodgkin's disease. *Annals of Internal Medicine* **95**:649.

59 Barry RM, Diamond HD, Craver LF (1962) Influence of pregnancy on the course of Hodgkin's disease. *American Journal of Obstetrics and Gynecology* **84**:445.

60 Holmes GE, Holmes FF (1978) Pregnancy outcome of patients treated for Hodgkin's disease: A controlled study. *Cancer* **41**:1317.

61 McKeen EA, Mulvill JJ, Rosiver F, Zarrari MH (1979) Pregnancy outcome in Hodgkin's disease. *Lancet* **2**:590.

62 Sweet DL Jr (1976) Malignant lymphoma: Implications during the reproductive years and pregnancy. *Journal of Reproductive Medicine* **17**:198.

63 LeFloch O, Donaldson SS, Kaplan HS (1976) Pregnancy following oophoropexy and total modal

irradiation in women with Hodgkin's disease. *Cancer* **38**:2263.

64 Chapman RM, Sutcliffe SB, Leeg LH (1979) Cyclical combination chemotherapy and gonadal function. *Lancet* **1**:285.

65 Wiernik PH (1982) Acute leukemias of adults. In DeVita VJR, Hellman S, Rosenberg SA (eds) *Cancer: Principles and Practice of Oncology*, p. 302. Philadelphia, PA: J.B. Lippincott.

66 O'Dell R (1979) Leukemia and lymphoma complicating pregnancy. *Clinics in Obstetrics and Gynecology* **22**:859–870.

67 Okum DB, Grancy RK, Sieger L (1979) Acute leukemia in pregnancy: Transient neonatal myelosuppression after combination chemotherapy in the mother. *Med Pediatr Oncol* **7**:315.

68 Catanzarite VA, Ferguson JE (1984) Acute leukemia and pregnancy: A review of management and outcome, 1972–1982. *Obstetrical and Gynecological Survey* **39**:663.

69 Reynoso EE, Shepherd FA, Messner HA *et al.* (1987) Acute leukemia during pregnancy: The Toronto leukemia study group experience with long-term follow-up in children exposed *in utero* to chemotherapeutic agents. *Journal of Clinical Oncology* **5**:1098.

70 Frenkel EB, Meyers MC (1960) Acute leukemia and pregnancy. *Annals of Internal Medicine* **53**:656.

71 Sutcliffe S, Chapman R (1986) Lymphomas and leukemias. In Allen H, Nisker J (eds) *Cancer in Pregnancy: Therapeutic Guidelines*, pp. 135–190. New York: Futura.

72 Barber HRK (1981) Fetal and neonatal effects of cytotoxic agents. *Obstetrics and Gynecology* **58**:41.

73 McClain CR (1974) Leukemia in pregnancy. *Clinics in Obstetrics and Gynecology* **17**:185.

74 Champlin RE, Goldman JM, Gale RB (1988) Bone marrow transplantation in chronic myelogenous leukemia. *Semin Hernatal* **25**:74.

75 Levine AM, Collea JV (1979) When pregnancy complicates chronic granulocytic leukemia. *Contemporary Obstetrics and Gynecology* **13**:47.

76 Byers T, Graham S, Swanson M (1982) Parity and colorectal cancer risk in women. *Journal of the National Cancer Institute* **69**:1059–1062.

77 Levin B (1976) Aspects of gastrointestinal tumors during the reproductive years. *Journal of Reproductive Medicine* **17**:233–240.

78 Nesbit JC, Moise KJ, Sawyers JL (1985) Colorectal carcinoma in pregnancy. *Archives of Surgery* **120**:636.

79 Hill J, Kassam S, Talledo O (1984) Colonic cancer in pregnancy. *Southern Medical Journal* **77**:375–378.

80 Armentano G (1988) Colorectal carcinoma in pregnancy. *European Journal of Gynecology and Oncology* **9**:178–181.

81 Barber HRK, Brunschwig A (1963) Gynecologic cancer complicating pregnancy. *American Journal of Obstetrics and Gynecology* **85**:156.

82 O'Leary JA, Pratt JH, Symmonds RE (1967) Rectal carcinoma in pregnancy. *Obstetrics and Gynecology* **30**:862.

83 Graffner HOL, Alm POA, Oscarson JEA (1983)

Prophylactic oophorectomy in colorectal cancer. *American Journal of Surgery* **146**:233.

84 Berkowitz RS, Cramer DW, Bernstein NR (1985) Risk factors for complete molar pregnancy from a case control study. *American Journal of Obstetrics and Gynecology* **152**:1016.

85 Goldstein DP, Berkowitz RS, Bernstein NR (1984) Reproduction performance after molar pregnancy in gestational trophoblastic tumors. *Clinics in Obstetrics and Gynecology* **27**:221.

86 Curry SL *et al.* (1975) Hydatidiform mole: Diagnosis, management, and long-term follow-up of 347 patients. *Obstetrics and Gynecology* **45**:1.

87 Ho Yuen B, Burch P (1983) Relationship of oral contraceptives and the intrauterine contraceptive devices to the regression of concentrations of the beta-subunit of human chorionic gonadotropins and invasive complications after molar pregnancy. *American Journal of Obstetrics and Gynecology* **145**:214.

88 Stone N *et al.* (1976) Relationship of oral contraception to development of trophoblastic tumor after evacuation of a hydatidiform mole. *British Journal of Obstetrics and Gynaecology* **83**:913.

89 Curry SL, Schlaerth JB, Kohorn EI, Boyce JB, Gore H, Twiggs LB, Blessing JA (1989) Hormonal contraception and trophoblastic sequelae after hydatidiform mole (Gynecologic Oncology Group study). *American Journal of Obstetrics and Gynecology* **60**:805–809; discussion 809–811.

90 Lurain JR *et al.* (1982) Gestational trophoblastic disease: Treatment results at the Brewer Trophoblastic Disease Center. *Obstetrics and Gynecology* **60**:354.

91 Kim DS *et al.* (1986) Effects of prophylactic chemotherapy for persistent trophoblastic disease in patients with complete hydatidiform mole. *Obstetrics and Gynecology* **67**:690.

92 Berkowitz RS, Goldstein DP, Bernstein NR (1986) Ten-year experience with methotrexate and folinic acid as primary treatment for gestational trophoblastic disease. *Gynecologic Oncology* **23**:111.

93 Sung AC, Wu FC, Wang YB (1984) Reevaluation of 5 FU as a single agent for gestational malignant trophoblastic disease. *Adv Exp Med Biol* **176**:355.

94 Hammond CB, Weed JC, Currie JL (1980) *American Journal of Obstetrics and Gynecology* **136**:844.

95 Hammond CB, Borchert LG, Tyrey L *et al.* (1973) Treatment of metastatic trophoblastic disease: Good and poor prognosis. *American Journal of Obstetrics and Gynecology* **115**:4.

96 Rustin GJ, Booth M, Dent J *et al.* (1984) Pregnancy after cytotoxic chemotherapy for gestational trophoblastic tumors. *British Medical Journal (Clinical Research)* **14**:288.

97 Simon MA, Phillips WA, Bonfiglio M (1984) Pregnancy and aggressive or malignant primary bone tumors. *Cancer* **53**:2564.

98 Gemzell O, Wang CF (1979) Outcome of pregnancy in women with pituitary adenoma. *Fertility and Sterility* **31**:363.

99 Jewelewicz R, Van De Wiele RL (1980) Clinical course and outcome of pregnancy in twenty-five patients with pituitary microadenomas. *American Journal of Obstetrics and Gynecology* **136**:339.

100 Maygar DM, Marshall JR (1978) Pituitary tumors and pregnancy. *American Journal of Obstetrics and Gynecology* **132**:739.

101 Molitch ME (1984) Pregnancy and the hyperprolactinemic woman. *New England Journal of Medicine* **312**:21.

102 Divers W, Yen SSC (1983) Prolactin producing microadenomas in pregnancy. *Obstetrics and Gynecology* **62**:425.

103 Jewelewicz R, Zimmerman EA, Carmel PW (1977) Conservative management of a pituitary tumor during pregnancy following induction of ovulation with gonadotropins. *Fertility and Sterility* **28**:35.

104 Turkalj I, Braun P, Krup P (1982) Surveillance of bromocriptine in pregnancy. *Journal of the American Medical Association* **247**:1589.

105 Senekjian EK *et al.* (1986) Clear cell adenocarcinoma (CCA) of the vagina and cervix in association with pregnancy. *Gynecology and Oncology* **24**:207.

106 Collins CG, Barclay DL (1972) Cancer of the vulva and cancer of the vagina in pregnancy. *Clinics in Obstetrics and Gynecology* **6**:927.

107 Barclay DL (1974) Surgery of the vulva, perineum, and vagina in pregnancy. In Barber HRK, Graber EA (eds) *Surgical Disease in Pregnancy*. Philadelphia, PA: W.B. Saunders.

108 Lutz MH *et al.* (1977) Genital malignancy in pregnancy. *American Journal of Obstetrics and Gynecology* **129**:536.

109 Karlen JR, Sternberg LB, Abbott JN (1972) Carcinoma of the endometrium coexisting with pregnancy. *Obstetrics and Gynecology* **40**:334.

110 Sandstrom RE, Welch WR, Green JH (1979) Adenocarcinoma of the endometrium in pregnancy. *Obstetrics and Gynecology* **53**:73.

111 Lilleyman JS, Hill AS, Anderton KJ (1977) Consequences of acute myelogenous leukemia in early pregnancy. *Cancer* **40**:1300.

FURTHER READING

1 Antunez de Mayolo J, Ahn YS, Temple JD, Harrington WJ (1989) Spontaneous remission of acute leukemia after the termination of pregnancy. *Cancer* **63**:1621–1623.

2 Aviles A, Diaz-Maqueo JC, Talovera A, Guyman R, Garcia EL (1991) Growth and development of children of mother treated with chemotherapy during pregnancy. *American Journal of Perinatology* **36**:243.

3 Aviles A, Niz J (1988) Long-term follow-up of children born to mothers with acute leukemia during pregnancy. *Med Pediatr Oncol* **16**:3.

4 Bagshawe KD (1976) Risk and prognostic factors in trophoblastic neoplasia. *Cancer* **38**:1373.

5 Barnavon Y, Wallack MK (1990) Management of the pregnant patient with carcinoma of the breast. *Surgery Gynecology, Obstetrics* **171**:347–352.

6 Berkowitz RS, Goldstein DP, Bernstein NR (1991) Evolving concepts of molar pregnancy. *Journal of Reproductive Medicine* **36**:40–44.

7 Bokhman JV, Urmancheyeva AF (1989) Cervix uteri cancer and pregnancy. *European Journal of Gynecology and Oncology* **10**:406–411.

8 Byrne J (1990) Fertility and pregnancy after malignancy. *Seminars in Perinatalogy* **14**:423–429.

9 Caligiuri MA, Mayer RJ (1989) Pregnancy and leukemia. *Seminars in Oncology* **16**:388–396.

10 Clement PB, Young RH, Scully RE (1989) Nontrophoblastic pathology of the female genital tract and peritoneum associated with pregnancy. *Seminars in Diagnostic Pathology* **6**:372–406.

11 Cunnah D, Besser M (1991) Management of prolactinomas. *Clinical Endocrinology (Oxford)* **34**:231–235.

12 Currie TH (1990) Gestational trophoblastic neoplasia. *Semin Oncol Nurs* **6**:228–236.

13 Dildy GA, Moise KJ Jr, Carpenter RJ Jr *et al.* (1989) Maternal malignancy metastatic to the products of conception: A review. *Obstetrical and Gynecological Survey* **44**:535–540.

14 Dow KH (1990) Breast cancer and fertility. NAACOGS Clin Issu Perinat Womens *Health Nurs* **1**:444–452.

15 Egan PC *et al.* (1985) Doxorubicin and cisplatin excretion into human milk. *Cancer Treat Rep* **69**:1387.

16 Escrich E (1990) Hormone-dependence of experimental mammary tumors. *Rev Esp Fisiol* **46**:89–94.

17 Farahmand SM, Marchetti DL, Asirwatham JE, Dewey MR (1991) Ovarian endodermal sinus tumor associated with pregnancy: Review of the literature. *Gynecology and Oncology* **41**:156–160.

18 Finkler NJ (1991) Placental site trophoblastic tumor: Diagnosis, clinical behavior and treatment. *Journal of Reproductive Medicine* **36**:27–30.

19 Franceschi S (1989) Reproductive factors and cancers of the breast, ovary and endometrium. *Eur J Cancer Clin Oncol* **25**:1933–1943.

20 Franceschi S, Barion AE, LaVecchia C (1990) The influence of female hormones on malignant melanoma. *Tumori* **76**:439–449.

21 Gallenberg MM, Loprinzi CL (1989) Breast cancer and pregnancy. *Seminars in Oncology* **16**:369–376.

22 Garner PR, Tsang R (1989) Insulinoma complicating pregnancy resenting with hypoglycemic coma after delivery: A case report and review of the literature. *Obstetrics and Gynecology* **73**:847–849.

23 Gilman EA, Wilson LM, Kneale GW, Waterhouse JA (1989) Childhood cancers and their association with pregnancy drugs and illnesses. *Pediatric and Perinatal Epidemiology* **3**:66–94.

24 Gormley DE (1990) Cutaneous surgery and the pregnant patient. *Journal of the American Academy of Dermatologists* **23**:269–279.

25 Greene JP, Guay AT (1989) New perspectives in pheochromocytoma. *Urologic Clinics of North America* **16**:487–503.

26 Hannigan EV (1990) Cervical cancer in pregnancy. *Clinics in Obstetrics and Gynecology* **33**:837–845.

27 Harper MA, Murnaghan GA, Kennedy L, Hadden DR, Atkinson AB (1989) Pheochromocytoma in pregnancy.

Five cases and a review of the literature. *British Journal of Obstetrics and Gynaecology* **96**:594–606.

28 Hod M, Sharony R, Friedman S, Ovadia J (1989) Pregnancy and thyroid carcinoma: A review of incidence, course, and prognosis. *Obstetrical and Gynecological Survey* **44**:774–779.

29 Hoover HC Jr (1990) Breast cancer during pregnancy and lactation. *Surgical Clinics of North America* **70**:1151–1163.

30 Huang CC, Lee CC (1991) Thymoma and myasthenia gravis in pregnancy: Report of a case. *Taiwan I Hsueh Hui Tsa Chih* **90**:206–208.

31 Huff BC (1990) Gestational trophoblastic disease. *NAACOGS Clin Issu Perinat Womens Health Nurs* **1**:453–458.

32 Jacob JH, Stringer CA (1990) Diagnosis and management of cancer during pregnancy. *Seminars in Perinatology* **14**:79–87.

33 Jolles CJ (1989) Gynecologic cancer associated with pregnancy. *Seminars in Oncology* **16**:417–424.

34 King LA, Nevin PC, Williams PP, Carson LF (1991) Treatment of advanced epithelial ovarian carcinoma in pregnancy with cisplatin-based chemotherapy. *Gynecology and Oncology* **41**:78–80.

35 Klimek R (1990) Nuclear magnetic resonance in obstetrics and gynecology. *International Journal of Gynecology and Obstetrics* **32**:199–205.

36 Kohorn EI (1991) Single-agent chemotherapy for nonmetastatic gestational trophoblastic neoplasia: Perspectives for the 21st century after three decades of use. *Journal of Reproductive Medicine* **36**:49–55.

37 Kommoss JF, Mercer L, Schmidt RA, Talerman A (1989) Granular cell tumor of the breast mimicking carcinoma in pregnancy. *Obstetrics and Gynecology* **73**:898–900.

38 Koren G, Weiner L, Lishner M, Zemelickes D, Finegen J (1990) Cancer in pregnancy: Identification of unanswered questions on maternal and fetal risks. *Obstetrical and Gynecological Survey* **45**:509–514.

39 Kozlowski RD, Steinbrunner JV, Mackenzie AH, Clough JD, Wilke WS, Segal AM (1990) Outcome of first-trimester exposure to low-dose methotrexate in eight patients with rheumatic disease. *American Journal of Medicine* **88**:589–592.

40 Kutteh WH, Albert T (1991) Mature cystic teratoma of the fallopian tube associated with an ectopic pregnancy. *Obstetrics and Gynecology* **78**:984–986.

41 Lala PK (1989) Similarities between immunoregulation in pregnancy and in malignancy: The role of prostaglandin E2. *American Journal of Reproductive and Immunology* **20**:147–152.

42 Larkin KR (1990) Cancer and pregnancy. *NAACOGS Clin Issu Perinat Womens Health Nurs* **1**:255–261.

43 MacKie RM, Bufalino R, Morabito A, Sutherland C, Cascinelli N (1991) Lack of effect of pregnancy on outcome of melanoma. *Lancet* **337**:653–655.

44 Maged DA, Keating HJ (1990) Noncystic liver mass in the pregnant patient. *Southern Medical Journal* **83**:51–53.

45 Mills G (1986) Immunology of cancer in pregnancy. In Allen N, Nisker J (eds) *Cancer in Pregnancy: Therapeutic Guidelines*, pp. 9–34. New York: Futura.

46 Molitch ME (1989) Management of prolactinomas. *Annual Review of Medicine* **40**:225–232.

47 Nader S (1990) Pituitary disorders and pregnancy. *Seminars in Perinatalogy* **14**:24–33.

48 Ory SJ (1991) Chemotherapy for ectopic pregnancy. *Obstetrics and Gynecology Clinics of North America* **18**:123–134.

49 Pajor A, Zimonyi I, Koos R, Leghocky D, Ambrus C (1991) Pregnancies and offspring in survivors of acute lymphoidleukemia and lymphoma. *European Journal of Obstetrics and Gynecology and Reproductive Biology* **40**:1–5.

50 Pricolo VE, Monchik JM, Prinz RA, DeJong S, Chadwick DA, Lamberton RP (1990) Management of Cushing's syndrome secondary to adrenal adenoma during pregnancy. *Surgery* **108**:1072–1077; discussion 1077–1078.

51 Raney DJ (1991) Malignant spinal cord tumors: A review and case presentation. *J Neurosci Nurs* **23**:44–49.

52 Ringenberg QS, Doll DC (1989) Endocrine tumors and miscellaneous cancers in pregnancy. *Seminars in Oncology* **16**:445–455.

53 Sadat-Ali M, Ibrahim EM (1989) Malignant bone tumors in pregnancy: A report of two cases and review of literature. *Indian Journal of Cancer* **26**:151–155.

54 Sawada M, Yamasaki M, Urabe T, Katayama S, Yamane T (1990) A case of ovarian cystadenocarcinoma associated with pregnancy. *Japanese Journal of Clinical Oncology* **20**:199–203.

55 Singhal S, Sharma S, De S, Kumar L, Chander S, Rath GK, Gupta SD (1990) Adult embryonal rhabdomyosarcoma of the vagina complicating pregnancy: A case report and review of the literature. *Asia and Oceanic Journal of Obstetrics and Gynecology* **16**:301–306.

56 Smith RA, Hawkins MM (1989) Pregnancies after childhood cancer. *British Journal of Obstetrics and Gynaecology* **96**:378–380.

57 Suzuki A *et al.* (1984) A case of grade II adenocarcinoma of the endometrium in pregnancy. *Gynecology and Oncology* **18**:261.

58 Sweet DL, Kinzie J (1989) Consequences of radiotherapy and antineoplastic agents and pregnancy. *Seminars in Oncology* **16**:337.

59 Titcomb CL (1990) Breast cancer and pregnancy. *Hawaii Medical Journal* **49**:18, 20–22, 24.

60 Tokunaga T, Miyazaki K, Okamura H (1991) Pathology of the fallopian tube. *Current Opinions in Obstetrics and Gynecology* **3**:574–579.

61 Van Voorhis B, Cruikshank DP (1989) Colon carcinoma complicating pregnancy: A report of two cases. *Journal of Reproductive Medicine* **34**:923.

62 Vander Vange N, Van Dongen JA (1991) Breast cancer and pregnancy. *Eur J Surg Oncol* **17**:1–8.

63 Vejerslev LO, Larsen G, Jackobsen M (1991) Partial hydatidiform mole with subsequent trophoblastic tumor: A case report. *European Journal of Obstetrics and Gynecology and Reproductive Biology* **40**:73–77.

64 Ward FT, Weiss RB (1989) Lymphoma and pregnancy. *Seminars in Oncology* **16**:397–409.

65 Weed JC Jr, Hunter VJ (1991) Diagnosis and management of brain metastasis from gestational trophoblastic disease. *Oncology (Williston Park)* **5**:48–50; discussion 50, 53–54.

66 Weeks DD (1990) Acute leukemia and pregnancy. *NAACOGS Clin Issu Perinat Womens Health Nurs* **1**:437–443.

67 Wile AG, DiSaia PJ (1989) Hormones and breast cancer. *American Journal of Surgery* **157**:438–442.

68 Wong DJ, Strassner HT (1990) Melanoma in pregnancy. *Clinics in Obstetrics and Gynecology* **33**:782–791.

33

Thromboembolism

MICHAEL DE SWIET

INTRODUCTION

This chapter will consider venous thromboembolism (i.e. deep vein thrombosis (DVT) and pulmonary embolism (PE)), management of the acute event if it occurs in pregnancy and prophylaxis for those who have had venous thromboembolism in the past. For a general review, see Reference 2.

Arterial thromboembolism, which usually occurs in relation to heart disease and in particular to artificial heart valves, is considered in Chapter 20.

The maternal mortality from pulmonary embolus is about 1 : 100 000 pregnancies in the developed world, making pulmonary embolism and hypertension the leading causes of maternal mortality in the UK.[1] The data concerning maternal mortality are precise because they almost invariably relate to autopsy evidence. The data concerning incidence of DVT and PE are much less satisfactory because of imprecision in diagnosis (see below) and because patients may have no symptoms. However, quoted figures for the incidence of PE range between 0.3 and 1.2% and for DVT range between 0.5 and 0.7%, increasing to 1.4% if superficial thrombophlebitis is included.[2] In general, these data relate to patients presenting clinically rather than to screening tests applied to all patients and the diagnosis may not have been established objectively.

The factors associated with an increased risk of venous thromboembolism in pregnancy include:

- increasing maternal age
- increasing parity
- operative delivery
- bedrest or other immobolization (e.g. air travel)
- obesity
- congestive cardiac failure
- malignant disease
- estrogen therapy
- dehydration
- previous thromboembolism
- blood group other than O
- Caucasian race
- sickle cell disease
- thrombophilia syndrome (see **Table 1**).

Maternal Risks

The risk to the mother from pulmonary embolus is death. It has been estimated that untreated pulmonary

Table 1
Factors to be considered in a thrombophilia screen

Antithrombin III deficiency
Protein S deficiency
Protein C deficiency
Abnormal fibrinogen
Homocystinuria
Paroxysmal nocturnal hemoglobinuria
Cardiolipin/lupus anticoagulant syndrome

embolus has a maternal mortality of 13%.[3] As indicated above, pulmonary embolism is a leading cause of maternal mortality. Studies in the non-pregnant state indicate that recovery from pulmonary embolism if it does occur is usually complete, though there may be subtle residual effects only detectable by lung function testing.[4]

The risks from deep vein thrombosis are the risks of pulmonary embolus and the post-phlebitic syndrome. It is difficult to assess the true risk of pulmonary embolus, since once detected, deep vein thromboses are treated. However, in the original placebo-controlled trial of anticoagulants for the treatment of pulmonary embolism (not in pregnancy), the incidence of recurrent pulmonary embolus in the placebo treated group was 26% (5/19) and a further 26% died.[5]

Deep vein thrombosis destroys the valves in the deep veins as they recanalize. The valves are responsible for maintaining venous flow toward the heart. As a result of their destruction, patients may suffer from symptoms varying from simple swelling to skin ulceration. At follow-up of 104 patients 11 years after deep vein thrombosis in pregnancy, only 22% of women were symptom-free and 4% had frank skin ulceration.[6]

The risk of thromboembolism in pregnancy in patients who have had thromboembolism in the past must also be considered, especially related to prophylaxis. Badarraco and Vessey's follow-up studies suggested that this risk is about 13% in patients who have had a single episode of deep vein thrombosis in the past, whether the original episode was in patients taking the oral contraceptive or not.[7] However, this was a postal survey and was not based on objective tests regarding the diagnosis of the second thromboembolism in pregnancy. Our own data relating to the use of prophylaxis (see below) would suggest the risk of *prenatal* thromboembolism in otherwise low-risk patients is far lower (0 in 70 patients; de Swiet and Letsky, unpublished).

There are also the risks to the mother relating to the treatment of thromboembolism. Because of the fetal risks of oral anticoagulants (see below), heparin is used throughout pregnancy in patients who present with thromboembolism in pregnancy. In the short term, the major risk is of hemorrhage from overdosing. With proper control of heparin, the risk of this is small.

Also, long-term heparin therapy (at least 10 000 units per day for at least 3 months) can cause a form of osteoporosis.[8,9] It presents clinically with fractured vertebrae and ribs. Fortunately, such patients are rare, less than 1 : 100 patients treated as above. But radiological studies of bone density suggest that many patients treated as above may have subclinical bone demineralization;[10] the significance of this is uncertain, since the bone demineralization may improve spontaneously on stopping heparin. The mechanism of bone demineralization is also unknown, as is the effect of possible prophylactic measures such as supplemental vitamin D and dietary calcium.

Heparin may also cause thrombocytopenia by two mechanisms, either platelet aggregation in the first few days of treatment or interaction between platelets, heparin and a specific IgG antibody[11,12] after the first week. Thrombocytopenia and alopecia are very rare.

Oral anticoagulants may also cause maternal hemorrhage, but as indicated they are not used in pregnancy for venous thromboembolism because of the fetal risks.

Fetal Risks

The fetal risks of maternal thromboembolism almost entirely relate to maternal therapy, though if the mother does not survive, the fetus is clearly at risk. There are a variety of teratogenic risks associated with maternal warfarin therapy, the best known of which is chondrodysplasia punctata, where the cartilage of the face in particular is misshapen and abnormally calcified.[13]

In addition, the asplenia syndrome[14] and diaphragmatic herniae[15] have also been reported. Warfarin crosses the placenta; the fetus has an immature clotting system, so full maternal anticoagulation is likely to cause a bleeding problem in the fetus. This was certainly the case in those women who delivered when fully warfarinized. There was a high risk of fetal intracerebral and retroplacental hemorrhage.[16] At one time it was thought that this risk was confined to the late third trimester and that there might be a 'window' of safety for the fetus after 12 weeks when there was no longer a perceived teratogenic risk, until 36 weeks when the fetus was at risk from hemorrhage at delivery. Unfortunately, this does not seem to be true, since even the fetus exposed to warfarin only after 12 weeks is at risk of abnormality, typically optic atrophy, microcephaly and other central nervous system defects.[17] These are thought to be due to repeated intracerebral hemorrhage in the fetus. It is not known how the risk of these problems relates to the intensity of warfarin treatment. In general, they have only been seen in patients who have been maintained with aggressive anticoagulation using warfarin to give levels equivalent to an International Normalized Ratio for prothrombin (INR) of 4. But because of the adverse fetal effects of warfarin, the drug is not usually used for the treatment or prophylaxis of venous thromboembolism in pregnancy.

There are no known fetal risks from heparin, since heparin does not cross the placenta.

Management Options

Prepregnancy

Prepregnancy counseling is necessary for the patient who has had thromboembolism in the past. Such counseling will involve discussion of the risks to mother and fetus from thromboembolism and its treatment as described above plus discussion of management options. In addition, it can be very helpful to assess bone density by scanning or radiologically, since longterm heparin treatment may well be one of the management options and since such investigations are contraindicated in pregnancy.

It is now clear that some inherited and acquired conditions increase the risk of thromboembolism. The increased risk has been named 'thrombophilia', in contrast to the bleeding risk of hemophilia.[18,19] At prepregnancy counseling, a thrombophilia screen should also be performed for those conditions indicated in **Table 1**: partly to counsel the patient about any additional risks of thromboembolism due to thrombophilia; partly because the cardiolipin syndrome has implications for pregnancy independent of the risk of thromboembolism (see Chapter 27); and partly because it is easier to diagnose conditions in the non-pregnant state – for example, protein S deficiency is a recognized cause of thrombophilia and the level of free Protein S decreases in rather variable ways during pregnancy. The management of patients with thrombophilia is highly specialized. For example, patients may require antithrombin III or Protein C concentrate and the induction of oral anticoagulation with Protein C or S deficiencies is dangerous because of the risk of purpura fulminans. These patients should be managed in cooperation with hematologists with a special interest in thrombosis.[19]

Prenatal

Diagnosis

● *Deep vein thrombosis*

Deep vein thrombosis (DVT) is traditionally diagnosed on the basis of an acutely painful swollen leg in the absence of trauma. The calf, and thigh if affected, are turgid and tender. Dorsiflexion of the calf causes pain in the calf (Homan's sign). Tender hard veins may be palpable in the deep tissues. Altogether, 30% of such patients do not have DVT when assessed objectively using venography.[20] Therefore, it is essential to have an objective form of diagnosis that is more accurate than subjective clinical impression.

Ultrasonography has now replaced venography for the diagnosis of DVT in many centers. Ultrasonography has been compared with venography in the non-pregnant state and found to be accurate using the criteria of imaging the clot, lack of compressibility of the vein in the presence of clot and lack of dilatation of the vein during a Valsalva maneuver.[21] In pregnancy, the first two features are more helpful together with relatively small veins distal to the clot on the affected side. Doppler and particularly color Doppler assessment of blood flow may also be very helpful.

Ultrasonography cannot be used to diagnose DVT with accuracy much above the inguinal ligament or in the calf. But calf vein thromboses rarely embolize and the procedure can be repeated as frequently as necessary if there is clinical concern that a calf vein thrombosis may be extending to the thigh.

An alternative to ultrasonography that is also non-invasive is venous occlusion plethysmography; but this also has not been compared with venography in pregnancy. Venous flow is particularly likely to be affected by pregnancy and this latter technique requires specialized equipment.

● *Pulmonary embolism*

The clinical features of pulmonary embolus are well known. However, patients with minor pulmonary embolus may present with less specific features such as fever, syncope, cough or pleuritic pain. The latter should not be diagnosed as pleurisy (a rare condition in pregnancy) without exclusion of pulmonary embolism. For investigation, chest X-ray, ECG and blood gas analysis all have a place, but none can be relied upon for exclusion or confirmation of diagnosis if the clinical presentation is anything but obvious. It is in these circumstances that a perfusion and if necessary ventilation lung scan should be performed. The radiation dose, about 50 mrem, is about one-tenth of the maximum recommended in the USA for pregnancy and false-negatives are unlikely to be clinically significant. For example, in a non-pregnant series of 515 patients clinically suspected of pulmonary embolus but with a negative lung scan, anticoagulant therapy was withdrawn from all except those who have objective evidence of DVT. There was only one subsequent asymptomatic pulmonary embolism.[22]

Treatment

• Acute phase

The aim of therapy in the acute phase is to produce as high an anticoagulant level as possible without putting the patient at risk of spontaneous bleeding. Conventional monitoring is by the partial thromboplastin time; the target is to double the control level. This is usually achieved by an initial dose of about 40 000 units heparin/24 h given by continuous intravenous infusion. The partial thromboplastin time is difficult and unpredictable to use in pregnancy. An alternative is to monitor the heparin level in the blood by the protamine sulfate neutralization test, aiming for a target of 0.8–1.0 unit ml.

The few patients who remain hypotensive and oliguric 1 h after the acute event have a high risk of dying. Their management is controversial even in the nonpregnant state. Possibilities are pulmonary embolectomy with either circulatory standstill or cardiopulmonary bypass if the facilities are available on site.[23,24] If they are not, thrombolytic therapy with streptokinase or tissue plasminogen activator (TPA) should be used in this life-threatening situation, despite its potential for causing bleeding in the pregnant patient. TPA has also been successfully used in a patient with massive pulmonary embolus who was subsequently found to be AT-III deficient.[25]

However, Brady et al.[26] have recently redescribed the use of catheter fragmentation and distal dispersion of proximal pulmonary embolus in three patients with severe pulmonary embolus. The technique involves fragmentation of the clot using a standard cardiac catheter following its identification by pulmonary angiography. Formal angiography is not necessary. Hand injection of non-ionic contrast medium and simple radiographic screening as used for placing temporary pacing wires is adequate. This seems a good procedure to try before thrombolysis or more aggressive surgical therapy. It could certainly be used in pregnant patients.

Even though there is significant long-term morbidity following DVT (see above), there is no evidence at present that this is reduced by surgical intervention or thrombolysis. Because of the additional risks of these procedures in pregnancy, they are not advised except possibly for recurrent events (see below).

• Chronic phase

After about 1 week, the risks of further thromboembolism are less and it is reasonable to aim for a lower level of anticoagulation. For the reasons given above and because heparin does not cross the placenta, heparin is preferred to warfarin for chronic phase treatment in pregnancy. The standard prophylactic dose of heparin in pregnancy is 10 000 units given subcutaneously twice daily. This should be started after 1 week of intravenous therapy. The simplest way to monitor this form of heparin therapy is by the thrombin time. If the thrombin time is not prolonged more than a few seconds beyond the control (usually 12–14 s), the patient is not excessively anticoagulated and will not bleed spontaneously or because of heparin in labor, at cesarean section or with epidural anesthesia. If the thrombin time is prolonged in chronic phase treatment, the heparin dose should be reduced. It is not necessary to increase the heparin dose to more than 10 000 units twice daily to achieve a given level of anticoagulation. A more precise test of low-dose heparin activity is the heparin assay, which is based on heparin's anti-Xa activity. The recommended upper limit of the heparin assay is 0.2 units/ml; but the heparin assay is much more expensive and time-consuming than the thrombin time. One of these tests, together with a platelet count (because of the risk of thrombocytopenia; see above), should be performed whenever the patient attends the prenatal clinic in the standard pattern of prenatal care, and also at least once after delivery.

Treatment failure

• Deep vein thrombosis

Patients sometimes develop worse symptoms (pain and swelling of the leg) despite anticoagulation. If anticoagulation is adequate, delivery should be considered because the symptoms are likely to be caused by obstruction to venous flow from the pregnant uterus.

• Pulmonary embolus

Patients may develop recurrent pulmonary embolus despite anticoagulation in the presence of DVT. If anticoagulation was again judged to be adequate at the time that the pulmonary embolus reoccurred, placing a filter or obstruction in the inferior vena cava should be considered.[27] This is usually done under local anesthesia by percutaneous puncture of the unaffected femoral vein, lodging the obstruction above the bifurcation of the inferior vena cava but below the renal veins.

• Septic thrombophlebitis

This is a rare association with pulmonary embolus. The patient presents with pulmonary embolus which is recurrent despite adequate anticoagulant therapy. The source is usually considered to be the pelvic veins, since the patient does not have DVT in the legs. There may be signs to suggest sepsis, such as high fever and secondary bronchopneumonia. The patient responds to antibiotics in addition to anticoagulant therapy.

Prophylaxis

Prophylaxis of thromboembolism is usually considered in relation to patients who are pregnant and have a history of thromboembolism in the past. It could be considered for those at particular risk without a past history (e.g. the elderly multigravida having an emergency cesarean section), but there has been little formal evaluation in this or similar situations.

Because of the concern about bone demineralization and other maternal side-effects of heparin (see above), patients with a past history of thromboembolism may be divided into a low-risk group who have only had a single episode of thromboembolism and who do not have any additional risk factors and a high-risk group.[28] Patients in the high-risk group have either had multiple thromboembolic episodes or have an additional risk factor such as the lupus/cardiolipin syndrome, other causes of thrombophilia (see **Table 1**) or a strong family history of thromboembolism, suggesting that they may have a yet undiscovered cause of thrombophilia. There is no evidence that venography, whether performed before pregnancy or prenatally, predicts patients at risk of a recurrent DVT.

Because of the maternal risks of heparin therapy, low-risk patients start heparin at the onset of labor or delivery and continue prophylactic treatment until 6 weeks post-delivery (**Table 2**). However, in high-risk patients, the risk of recurrence prenatally seems too great and they should start heparin as soon as practicable in early pregnancy (**Table 2**) after they have been counseled about the risks of bone demineralization. Of course, the policy cannot be rigidly enforced and informed patients may opt to choose either prophylactic strategy.

The policy of withholding anticoagulant prophylaxis from patients with a single episode of thromboembolism and no other risk factors was originally reported in 1985.[28] There were 30 patients in the study and none had a recurrence prenatally. Since then, more than 70 patients have been managed in this way without any problem (de Swiet and Letsky, unpublished observations). Nevertheless, this form of prophylaxis does remain a compromise and patients who are presumed to be at some risk – albeit a small risk – are being left unprotected for the majority of their pregnancies. In the future, low-dose aspirin may be used to decrease the risk still further once its safety has been assessed by current clinical trials for the prevention of pre-eclampsia.[29] Alternatively, it may be possible to use the new low molecular weight heparins, which are said not to affect the bones so much, and which may have the additional patient advantage of daily rather than twice daily injection.[30] However, the efficacy of single daily injections of low molecular weight heparins has not been proven in pregnancy.

Labor/delivery

Patients who develop thromboembolism prenatally should continue subcutaneous heparin throughout labor and for at least 1 week after delivery. Because of the reduction in circulating blood volume at the time of delivery, the dose is reduced to 7500 units every 12 h at the onset of labor or at elective delivery. In the unlikely event that the patient bleeds and this is due to or associated with heparin treatment (i.e. the thrombin time is prolonged), heparin can be reversed by giving a dose of protamine calculated from the protamine sulfate neutralization test.[31]

Postnatal

It is difficult to know for how long patients remain at excess risk for thromboembolism following delivery. The usual advice is to continue treatment for 6 weeks after delivery, but this is an arbitrary recommendation. One week after delivery, it is reasonable to change to warfarin if the patient so wishes; she needs to decide which is the less inconvenient form of therapy – twice daily heparin injections (usually self-administered) but without the need for hematological monitoring, or warfarin tablets that need frequent hospital visits to establish the correct dose. It is unwise to switch to heparin before 1 week after delivery because of the risks of secondary postpartum hemorrhage and wound hematoma. Only minute quantities of warfarin are excreted in milk (in contrast to Dindevan®) and breast-feeding should be encouraged in patients taking warfarin.[32]

Table 2
Treatment and prophylaxis of thromboembolism in pregnancy

1. Confirm diagnosis objectively
2. Start heparin 40 000 units/day by i.v. infusion. Adjust dose to achieve a heparin level of 0.8–1.0 unit/ml (protamine sulfate neutralization test) or to double partial thromboplastin time
3. After 5–7 days, change to 10 000 units heparin s.c. twice daily. Decrease dose if thrombin time prolonged or heparin assay > 0.2 units/ml. *High-risk prophylaxis starts here*
4. In labor, decrease dose to 7500 units heparin s.c. twice daily. Epidural anesthesia, surgery OK if thrombin time not prolonged. *Low-risk prophylaxis starts here*
5. Continue heparin for at least 1 week after delivery
6. Switch to warfarin or continue heparin for a further 5 weeks depending on patient choice. Breast-feeding OK on warfarin and heparin

THROMBOEMBOLISM
Summary of Management Options

Prepregnancy

- Counsel regarding risks in those with history of thromboembolism in past or at greater risk (**Table 1**)

- Consider bone density assessment if long-term heparin therapy planned

Prenatal

Diagnosis

- Maintain high index of clinical suspicion

- Venogram or ultrasonography (DVT) and ventilation/perfusion scan or angiography (PE) are the definitive investigations to confirm diagnosis

Treatment

- Acute phase
  - i.v. heparin therapy (see **Table 2**)
  - Severe, life-threatening PE may require further measures to be considered:
    - thrombolytic therapy (streptokinase or TPA)
    - pulmonary embolectomy
    - cardiopulmonary bypass

- Failure of improvement after acute treatment may require:
  - delivery if DVT
  - inferior vena cava plication or filter if PE

- Chronic phase
  - Commence s.c. heparin 1 week after starting i.v. therapy (see **Table 2**)

Prophylaxis (depends on risk)

- High risk (multiple emboli or condition in **Table 1**):
  - Start s.c. heparin early in pregnancy (see **Table 2**) and continue until 6 weeks after delivery

- Low risk (single embolic event):
  - start s.c. at labor/delivery (see **Table 2**) and continue for 6 weeks after delivery

Labor/delivery

- Continue prophylaxis (see above and **Table 2**)

Postnatal

- Continue prophylaxis until 6 weeks after delivery, changing to warfarin if patient wishes after 1 week

- Breast-feeding *not* contraindicated with heparin or warfarin

REFERENCES

1 (1991) *Report on Confidential Enquiries into Maternal Deaths in the United Kingdom* 1985–1987, pp. 37–45. London: HMSO.
2 de Swiet M (1989) Thromboembolism. In de Swiet M (ed.) *Medical Disorders in Obstetric Practice*. 2nd edn, pp. 166–197. Oxford: Blackwell Scientific Publications.
3 Quilligan EJ, Zuspan FP (1990) *Current Therapy in Obstetrics and Gynaecology*, 3rd edn. Philadelphia, PA: W.B. Saunders.
4 Sharma GVRK, Burlesco VA, Sasahara AA (1980) Effect of thrombolytic therapy on pulmonary-capillary blood volume in patients with pulmonary embolism. *New England Journal of Medicine* **303**:842–845.
5 Barrit DW, Jordan SC (1960) Anticoagulant drugs in the treatment of pulmonary embolism: A controlled trial. *Lancet* **i**:1309–1312.

6 Bergqvist A, Bergqvist D, Lindhagen A, Matzsch T (1990) Late symptoms after pregnancy-related deep vein thrombosis. *British Journal of Obstetrics and Gynaecology* **97**:338–341.

7 Badaracco MA, Vessey M (1974) Recurrence of venous thromboembolism disease and use of oral contraceptives. *British Medical Journal* **1**:215–217.

8 Griffiths HT, Liu DTY (1984) Severe heparin osteoporosis in pregnancy. *Postgraduate Medical Journal* **60**:424–425.

9 Griffith GC, Nichols G, Asher JD, Hanagan B (1965) Heparin osteoporosis. *Journal of the American Medical Association* **193**:91–94.

10 de Swiet M, Dorrington Ward P, Fidler J, Horsman A, Katz D, Letsky E, Peacock M, Wise PH (1983) Prolonged heparin therapy in pregnancy causes bone demineralisation (heparin induced-osteopenia). *British Journal of Obstetrics and Gynaecology* **90**:1129–1134.

11 Bergqvist D, Hedner U (1983) Pregnancy and venous thromboembolism. *Acta Obstetrica et Gynecologica Scandinavica* **62**:449–453.

12 Wolf H, Wick G (1986) Antibodies interacting with, and corresponding binding site for, heparin in human thrombocytes. *Lancet* **ii**:222–223.

13 Shaul WL, Emery H, Hall JG (1975) Chondrodysplasia punctata and maternal warfarin use during pregnancy. *American Journal of Diseases of Children* **89**:916–923.

14 Cox DR, Martin L, Hall BD (1977) Asplenia syndrome after fetal exposure to warfarin. *Lancet* **2**:1134.

15 O'Donnel D, Sevitz H, Seggie JL, Meyers AM, Botha JR, Myburgh JA (1985) Pregnancy after renal transplantation. *Australia and New Zealand Journal of Medicine* **15**:320–325.

16 Villasanta U (1965) Thromboembolic disease in pregnancy. *American Journal of Obstetrics and Gynecology* **93**:142–160.

17 Holzgreve W, Carey JC, Hall BD (1976) Warfarin-induced fetal abnormalities. *Lancet* **2**:914–915.

18 The British Committee for Standards of Haematology (1990) Guidelines on the investigation and management of thrombophilia. *Journal of Clinical Pathology* **43**:703–709.

19 Walker ID (1991) Management of thromboembolism in pregnancy. *Blood Reviews* 1–6.

20 Sandler DA, Martin JF, Duncan JS, Blake GM, Ward P, Ramsay LE, Lamont AC, Ross B, Sherriff S, Walton L (1984) Diagnosis of deep-vein thrombosis: Comparison of clinical evaluation, ultrasound, plethysmograph and venoscan with X-ray venogram. *Lancet* **ii**:716–719.

21 Lensing AWA, Prandoni P, Bueller HR *et al.* (1990) Lower extremity venography with iohexol: Results and complications. *Radiology* **1771**:503–505.

22 Hull RD, Raskob GE, Coates G, Panju AA (1990) Clinical validity of a normal perfusion lung scan in patients with suspected pulmonary embolism. *Chest* **97**:23–26.

23 Clarke DB, Abrams LD (1986) Pulmonary embolectomy: A 25 year experience. *Journal of Thoracic and Cardiovascular Surgery* **92**:442–445.

24 Gray HH, Miller GAH (1989) Pulmonary embolectomy is still appropriate for a minority of patients with acute massive pulmonary embolism. *British Journal of Hospital Medicine* **41**:467–468.

25 Baudo F, Caimi TM, Redaelli R, Nosari AM, Mauri M, Leonardi G, de Cataldo F (1990) Emergency treatment with recombinant tissue plasminogen activator of pulmonary embolism in a pregnant woman with antithrombin III deficiency. *American Journal of Obstetrics and Gynecology* **163**:1274–1275.

26 Brady AJB, Crake T, Oakley CM (1991) Percutaneous catheter fragmentation and distal dispersion of proximal pulmonary embolus. *Lancet* **338**:1186–1189.

27 McCollum C (1987) Vena cava filter: Keeping big clots down. *British Medical Journal* **294**:1566.

28 Lao TT, de Swiet M, Letsky E, Walters BNJ (1985) Prophylaxis of thromboembolism in pregnancy: An alternative. *British Journal of Obstetrics and Gynaecology* **92**:202–206.

29 de Swiet M, Fryers G (1990) The use of aspirin in pregnancy: Possible adverse effects during pregnancy parturition and the puerperium? *Journal of Obstetrics and Gynaecology* **10**:467–482.

30 Levin MN, Planes A, Hirsh J, Goodyear M, Vochelle N, Gent M (1989) The relationship between anti-factor Xa level and clinical outcome in patients receiving enoxaparine low molecular weight heparin to prevent deep vein thrombosis after hip replacement. *Thrombo-Haemost* **62**:940–944.

31 Letsky EA (1985) *Coagulation Problems During Pregnancy.* Edinburgh: Churchill Livingstone.

32 Orme ML-E, Lewis PJ, de Swiet M, Serlin MJ, Sibeon R, Baty JD, Breckenbridge AM (1977) May mothers given warfarin breast-feed their infants? *British Medical Journal* **1**:1564–1565.

34

Abdominal Pain

WILLIAM H. CLEWELL

INTRODUCTION

Abdominal pain is a common complaint in pregnancy. If mild symptoms are included, then nearly all women experience some pain at some time during pregnancy prior to the onset of labor. The problem for the clinician is to distinguish physiological pain or discomfort from pathological pain. One must also distinguish pain due to problems intrinsic to the pregnancy from pain due to processes incidental to the pregnancy. These later processes may be influenced and modified by the anatomic and physiological changes of pregnancy. The general approach to abdominal pain in pregnancy is the same as that in the non-pregnant patient, except that the pregnancy-specific conditions must be included in the differential diagnosis and the influence of the pregnancy on extrinsic disease processes must be considered. The risk to the mother and the fetus depends on the diagnosis. Because of increased difficulty of diagnosis and reluctance to carry out some diagnostic procedures and laparotomy during pregnancy, there may be delay in diagnosis and treatment of the pregnant woman. This may lead to more morbidity associated with many conditions in pregnancy than in non-pregnant women.

The initial step in evaluation of abdominal pain is a detailed history and physical examination, including the pregnancy history and, unless contraindicated, a pelvic examination. Additional investigations such as ultrasonography, x-rays and laboratory studies are used to confirm, exclude or refine diagnoses as indicated by the initial history and physical examination (**Tables 1–**

5). Details of this process will be covered in sections devoted to specific causes.

PREGNANCY-SPECIFIC CAUSES: PHYSIOLOGICAL

ROUND LIGAMENT PAIN

Women frequently complain of lower quadrant abdominal pain, which is variably described as cramp-like or stabbing and influenced by movement. This most commonly occurs in the middle of the second trimester. It is often ascribed to 'round ligament stretching'. There is little objective evidence to prove that this is the source of the pain, but patients with the complaint often report tenderness over the area of the round ligaments. When the pain is on the right side, it must be distinguished from appendicitis. The complaint of mild-to-moderate pain, which is ultimately attributed to the round ligament, occurs in 10–30% of pregnancies.

Risks

The principal risk in this condition is to erroneously attribute the pain of appendicitis, urinary tract infection or stone, preterm labor or abruptio to round ligament stretching.

Table 1
Pregnancy-specific causes: physiological

History				
Pain	Cramp-like; posture-dependent	Mild/irregular	Mild/varied	Recurrent attacks, increasing severity
Urinary				Retention ±
Trimester	2nd	3rd > 2nd	3rd	3rd
Previous disease			Fibroids	Uterine anomaly, surgery
Examination				
Shock				+
Uterus		Irregular contractions		Tender + +, tender adnexa anterior
Extrauterine tenderness	Round ligament insertion			
Others		No cervical change		Vagina distorted/ changed
Investigations				
All	Negative or normal	Negative or normal	Negative or normal	Negative or normal
Diagnosis	Round ligament pain	Braxton–Hicks contractions	Mild discomfort	Uterine torsion

Management Options

Prenatal

Since there is no specific diagnostic test for this condition, diagnosis depends on history and physical examination. Occasionally, it may be necessary to perform additional tests to rule out more serious conditions. Measures like local heat, decreased physical activity and reassurance are usually sufficient. Failure of the pain to respond to these approaches – or worsening of the symptoms – are grounds for further investigation.

ROUND LIGAMENT PAIN
Summary of Management Options

- Exclude pathological causes of pain

- Reassure

- Reduce physical activity

- Local heat

BRAXTON–HICKS CONTRACTIONS

Many women experience Braxton–Hicks contractions[1] in the latter half of pregnancy, especially during the third trimester. While in the majority of women these are painless, some women find them painful. They are, however, irregular in frequency and inconsistent in intensity.

Risks

The main danger is to mistake the uterine activity of true preterm labor for Braxton–Hicks contractions.

BRAXTON–HICKS CONTRACTIONS
Summary of Management Options

- Confirm no evidence of labor with vaginal examination if necessary

- Reassure

Table 2
Pregnancy-specific causes: pathological

	Ectopic pregnancy	Abortion/miscarriage	Uterine fibroids	Placental abruption	Preterm labor	Severe pre-eclampsia	Uterine rupture
History							
Pain	++ Shoulder tip	±	++	±	+	Epigastric	±
Vaginal bleeding	±	++	±	±	'Show'		±
Alimentary			Vomiting			Vomiting	
Urinary							Hematuria ±
Trimester	1st > 2nd	1st > 2nd	3rd > 2nd	3rd > 2nd	3rd > 2nd	3rd > 2nd	3rd
Previous disease	±		+	Previous bleed BP +			Uterine scar
Others					Membrane rupture	Headache	
Examination							
Shock	±	±		±			±
Pyrexia			Low-grade				
Hypertension				±		++	
Uterus		Tender	Tender fibroid	Tender ±; contractions ±	Contractions		Tender ++
Extrauterine	Tender mass ±					Liver tender	Fetus extrauterine
Fetal heart		±		±		±	±
Proteinuria				±		++	
Others						Clonus	
Investigations							
Full blood count	Low Hb ±		Raised white cells ±	Low platelets ±; low Hb ±		Low platelets ±	
Ultrasound abnormality	+ (vaginal)	+	+	Retroplacental; chorionic bleed ±		Growth-deficient ±	±
Others	+ ve beta-HCG			Positive Kleihauer ±; abnormal clotting ±		Abnormal renal and liver function	
Diagnosis	Ectopic pregnancy	Abortion/miscarriage	Uterine fibroids	Placental abruption	Preterm labor	Severe pre-eclampsia	Uterine rupture

Management Options

A careful history and examination should be undertaken to exclude genuine labor. The absence of a 'show' and/or membrane rupture together with an unengaged fetal head would be reassuring. Vaginal examination, perhaps repeated after 3–4 h, may be the only satisfactory way to assess the significance of uterine contractions. Once the diagnosis is made, reassurance is all that is necessary.

MISCELLANEOUS DISCOMFORT IN LATE PREGNANCY

During the third trimester, most pregnant women will experience varying degrees of symptoms, which some will describe as 'discomfort' and others as 'pain'.[1] Normal events causing such symptoms include vigorous fetal activity, engagement of the fetal head, pressure effects from the fetal head with a breech presentation, abdominal wall distension and Braxton–Hicks contractions (see p. 606).

Table 3
Incidental causes: physiological

History			
Pain	Retrosternal	Epigastric ±	Colicky
Alimentary	Vomiting ±	Vomiting + +; hematemesis ±	Constipation + +
Trimester	2nd/3rd > 1st	1st > 2nd/3rd	All
Previous disorder			Iron therapy
Examination			
Extrauterine tenderness		Epigastric	Left flank, iliac fossa
Others	Negative or normal	Negative or normal	Negative or normal
Investigations			
All	Negative or normal	Negative or normal	Negative or normal
Diagnosis	Heartburn	Excess vomiting	Constipation

MISCELLANEOUS DISCOMFORT LATE IN PREGNANCY
Summary of Management Options

- Exclude pathological cause

- Reassure

Risks

The main risk is to miss a pathological cause for the pain, erroneously ascribing a woman's symptoms to these events.

Management Options

Once pathological causes for the pain have been excluded, reassurance is all that is necessary.

SEVERE UTERINE TORSION

Mild asymptomatic axial rotation of the uterus, usually to the right, is observed in the majority of pregnancies.[2]

This normally is by no more than 40°.[3,4] However, very rarely this natural rotation progresses beyond 90° to produce subacute or acute torsion of the uterus – an uncommon but serious cause of abdominal pain in the latter half of pregnancy. In 80–90% of cases, there is a predisposing factor such as a fibroid, congenital anomaly, adnexal mass or a history of pelvic surgery.[5]

SEVERE UTERINE TORSION
Summary of Management Options

Conservative

- Bed rest

- Analgesia

- Altering maternal position

- Monitor fetal well-being

Surgical (diagnosed at laparotomy)

- Correct the torsion

- Delivery by cesarean section

Table 4
Incidental causes: common pathological

History								
Pain	+	+	+	+	+	+	+	+
Alimentary	±	+	+		+	+	+	
Urinary				+				
Trimester		3rd/postnatal						
Previous disease		±		±	+	Alcohol, gall-stones	+	+
Others			Jaundice	±				
Examination								
Shock							+ if perforation	
Pyrexia	±	±	±	±				
Extrauterine	Tender	Tender, distended	Tender	Tender	Tender ±, distended ±	Tender	Tender	Tender mass
Preteinuria				±				
Others				Rigors				
Investigations								
Full blood count	Raised white cells ±			Raised white cells if sepsis				
Midstream urine	Pyuria ±			+ if sepsis				
Ultrasound abnormality			+	±				±
x-Ray abnormality		+		±			+ if perforation	
Others					Endoscopy, biopsy	Amylase +	Endoscopy	
Diagnosis	Appendicitis	Bowel obstruction	Cholecystitis	Renal disease	Inflammatory bowel disease	Pancreatitis	Peptic ulcer	Torsion of adnexa

Risks

Maternal shock and possible fetal asphyxia are the main risks of severe uterine torsion.

Management Options

If the diagnosis is made before laparotomy, conservative measures such as bed rest, analgesia and altering the position of the mother can be used to try and produce a spontaneous correction of the torsion. The well-being of the fetus should be assessed and monitored.

However, the true diagnosis is rarely made before laparotomy. At operation, the torsion often of 180°, will be discovered with the posterior surface of the uterus presenting in the wound.[5] In such circumstances, delivery of the fetus by cesarean section is probably advisable, especially if the risks of preterm delivery are not considered to be great. Technically, most would probably untwist the uterus first and then perform a conventional lower segment procedure. However, some have advocated delivery of the baby through the posterior wall first and then correcting the torsion.[5] Because the condition is very uncommon and generally occurs late in pregnancy, there is no evidence to suggest that it is reasonable to only untwist the uterus and close the abdominal incision. If the diagnosis is made at laparotomy and if the fetus is extremely preterm (such as less than 28 weeks) and otherwise well, untwisting might be considered.

Table 5
Incidental cases: rare pathological

History					
Pain	+	+	±	+	+
Vaginal bleeding			±		
Alimentary			±		±
Urinary			±	±	
Previous disease		+	±	Precipitating factors	±
Others	Trauma/cough	Precipitating factor		Psychological, autonomic	
Examination					
Shock					++
Pyrexia			±		
Uterine					Tender if uterine vein rupture
Extrauterine	Tender		± Mass/tender ±		
Others			Ascites, cachexia, etc.		
Investigations					
Full blood count		Low Hb	±		
Midstream urine			±		
Ultrasound abnormal			+		±
x-Ray abnormal	±				
Others		Hb S, sickling	Specific	Urinary porphyrins	
Diagnosis	Rectus hematoma	Sickle crisis	Malignant disease	Porphyria	Arterial hemorrhage

PREGNANCY-SPECIFIC CAUSES: PATHOLOGICAL

ECTOPIC PREGNANCY (see Chapter 7)

Incidence and Risks

The reported frequency varies from 1:80 to 1:230 pregnancies. Different patient populations appear to have different rates and this may be due to both the rate of reproductive tract disease in these populations and contraceptive practices. The maternal death rate from ectopic pregnancy is reported at between 1:500 and 1:1000. It may be declining with improved diagnostic techniques such as transvaginal sonography, laparoscopy and better appreciation of the role of serial beta-HCG assays in the diagnosis of the condition. It remains a significant cause of maternal morbidity.[6]

Management Options

The risks and management of ectopic pregnancy are discussed in detail in Chapter 7.

MISCARRIAGE AND ITS VARIANTS (see Chapter 7)

Incidence and Risks

The most common pathological cause of pain in the first trimester is miscarriage, especially when this is the inevitable type. If the miscarriage is complete, the pain can subside, but may persist if it is incomplete or septic.

Management Options

The risks and management of these conditions are discussed in detail in Chapter 7.

UTERINE FIBROIDS

Incidence

Leiomyomas are relatively common (0.5–5.0% incidence, which varies with the population studied) and increase in prevalence with advancing maternal age. While their presence may interfere with conception and maintenance of pregnancy, usually their presence is incidental. Approximately 10% of women with uterine myomas will experience acute abdominal pain associated with 'red' or 'carneous degeneration' of a fibroid.[7,8] Histologically, this is hemorrhagic infarction of the tumor. Occasionally, the pain may be due to torsion of a pedunculated fibroid.

Risks

Maternal and fetal risks are related to incorrect diagnosis. Since the signs and symptoms can be almost identical to those of acute appendicitis, pyelonephritis and placental abruption, the greatest hazard to both the mother and fetus is incorrect diagnosis and either unnecessary operation or delay of correct diagnosis and treatment.

Management Options

Prepregnancy

Asymptomatic uterine fibroids rarely require treatment. With large tumors, patients may show symptoms of pelvic pressure, and urinary or bowel symptoms due to the enlarged uterus. They may also experience irregular or heavy uterine bleeding. If such symptoms are severe, then myomectomy with preservation of the uterus can be performed. The removal of multiple fibroids can distort the uterine cavity and increase the risk of infertility. Extensive surgical disruption of the uterine wall may weaken it and predispose to uterine rupture during pregnancy. These risks must be considered when deciding whether to perform a myomectomy prior to pregnancy. In some infertile women, the presence of fibroids is thought to be a contributing factor. In others, the presence of large or multiple fibroids may distort the uterine cavity and impinge on the endometrium, increasing the risk of preterm labor, abruptio placenta or fetal deformation. The balancing of these various risks is difficult and counseling and management of the prepregnant patient must be individualized (see also Chapter 8).

Prenatal

The presenting complaint in red degeneration is the sudden onset of severe pain with local tenderness over the tumor. There may be slight temperature elevation and signs of local peritoneal irritation. There are usually minimal or no gastrointestinal symptoms. Differentiating this condition from acute appendicitis, placental abruption, ureteral stone and pyelonephritis can be very difficult. Ultrasonography examination which demonstrates a fibroid, especially if it is located in the area of maximal tenderness, is very helpful. If that sonogram can be compared with a previous study and demonstrates a change in sonolucency of the tumor, it is even more supportive of the diagnosis.

Management is conservative with the use of narcotic analgesics recommended as needed until the pain resolves. Local ice packs may produce symptomatic improvement. The most important aspect of care is to differentiate it from other conditions such as appendicitis, pyelonephritis and abruptio placenta, which require immediate and specific treatment. Spontaneous resolution of the symptoms generally occurs within 4–7 days. If more myomas are present, they too may undergo degeneration and the patient may have a recurrence of symptoms.

Labor/delivery

Leiomyomata may be obstructive to normal labor and delivery, in which case cesarean delivery is needed. One should delay making the decision for cesarean delivery until term. With the normal development of the lower uterine segment in the third trimester, myomas which initially appear to be obstructive often move out of the true pelvis and at the time of labor are no longer a problem for vaginal delivery. Vaginal examination and ultrasonography may be necessary to determine the mode of delivery. Degeneration occurring at the time of labor can be very confusing and may mimic placental abruption or uterine rupture.

Postnatal

Leiomyomata generally undergo some regression in size following delivery. Degeneration can occur for the first time in the puerperium. Fibroids which have undergone degeneration during pregnancy may dramatically shrink following delivery and often calcify. This involution can be painful and analgesia may be necessary.

UTERINE FIBROIDS
Summary of Management Options

Prepregnancy

- The majority of women with fibroids will have no problem either in conceiving or during pregnancy

- Myomectomy should only be cautiously considered in cases with uterine cavity distortion and problems such as menorrhagia, recurrent miscarriage and/or infertility. Even then it should be undertaken only after careful counseling

Prenatal

- If asymptomatic, reassure

- If associated with pain, exclude other diagnoses first

- Red degeneration:
  - bed rest
  - analgesia
  - ? local ice packs

- Review mode of delivery at 36–38 weeks
  (? malpresentation, possible dystocia)

Postnatal

- Vigilance for red degeneration

- Analgesia if excessive pain with involution

PLACENTAL ABRUPTION

Placental abruption occurs in between 0.5 and 1.0% of all pregnancies. Since characteristically it is accompanied by vaginal bleeding, it is discussed in detail in Chapter 9. The risks are also described in detail in Chapter 9. However, when abruptio placenta presents without external bleeding, there is the additional risk of missed or delayed diagnosis.

PRETERM LABOR

Since abdominal pain is often the first symptom of preterm labor, it must be included in the differential diagnosis of abdominal pain in pregnancy. The risks and management are discussed in Chapter 11.

SEVERE PRE-ECLAMPSIA

Fulminating pre-eclampsia may be associated with upper abdominal pain and liver tenderness. It is thought to be due to liver edema and subsequent stretching of its capsule.

Management Options

The risks and management of this condition are discussed in detail in Chapters 18 and 73.

UTERINE RUPTURE

Incidence

Rupture of the unscarred uterus prior to labor is extremely uncommon. It occurs in cases of pregnancy developing in a malformed uterus such as a rudimentary horn, in obstructed labor, with excessive oxytocin dosage and in patients with very high parity. Rupture of the scarred uterus may occur either before or during labor. In an era when the cesarean section rate in some centers is approaching 25%, the risk of uterine rupture is bound to increase. While the low transverse cesarean section scar is relatively strong and not prone to failure even under the stress of labor, a significant minority of cesearian incisions are of the classical or vertical type. These do have a low but significant risk of rupture both before and during labor. With prior classical uterine incision, the risk of rupture is approximately 2%. While the lower segment incision is less likely to rupture, the true risk is difficult to determine. It has been estimated that approximately half of these will rupture prior to labor and even prior to the time that cesarean section would normally be done.[9]

Risks

Maternal risks from uterine rupture are hypovolemic shock and its consequences, including death. It is reported as the ninth most common cause of maternal death in England and Wales. In third world countries, it may be an even more common cause of death due to the lack of prenatal and intrapartum care. The fetal risks are shock, anemia, hypoxia and death. It is clear that in the rare case of rupture of the unscarred uterus, the risk to both the mother and fetus is much higher than with rupture of the previously scarred uterus. Once a patient has suffered a uterine rupture, she appears to be at very high risk of having it occur again in subsequent pregnancies.

Management Options

Prepregnancy

The woman with a history of uterine rupture in a previous pregnancy should be carefully counseled about the risks of proceeding with another. Sterilization may be considered.

Prenatal

Patients at high risk for prenatal uterine rupture must be informed of this risk and the symptoms. This should include patients with a history of rupture, prior vertical incision cesarean sections or any other extensive uterine scarring. These patients should be evaluated immediately for any symptoms suggestive of rupture or impending rupture. In many cases, uterine rupture is an acute event accompanied by severe abdominal pain and the rapid onset of shock. The only other condition which could be confused with it is placental abruption and the only management is laparotomy, delivery, and control of hemorrhage as soon as possible. In other cases, complete rupture is preceded by lower abdominal pain, which is less severe and not accompanied by shock or fetal distress. In these cases, meticulous evaluation with fetal well-being testing and serial examinations may provide the only chance to intervene before catastrophic rupture occurs. Management decision making is complicated by the fact that these symptoms may occur at an immature gestational age, when delivery is not an attractive option. In suspicious cases, near term consideration must be given to amniocentesis for fetal maturity testing and delivery.

Labor/delivery

During labor, the patient with a uterine scar is at risk of rupture as is the grand multiparous woman, the patient with an over-distended uterus, the patient with prolonged or obstructed labor, and the patient receiving excessive oxytocin dosage. Risk of rupture of the low transverse cesarean section scar seems quite low and when it does occur it is generally a relatively benign event. Rarely is there extensive hemorrhage or shock. It is often an incidental finding at cesarean section for failure to progress or other reason. Occasionally, scar dehiscence is completely asymptomatic and is found in manual uterine exploration of the uterus following a vaginal delivery.

Catastrophic rupture in labor can present as a sudden increase in abdominal pain with shock and fetal distress. Hematuria may appear and suprapubic tenderness

---

UTERINE RUPTURE
Summary of Management Options

Prepregnancy

- Discuss sterilization in the patient with a history of uterine rupture.

Prenatal

- Careful counseling and vigilance in those with risk factors

- Consider delivery by cesarean section if diagnosis is suspected

Labor/delivery

- In women at 'high risk' (uterine scar, high parity, prolonged oxytocic stimulation), vigilance for uterine rupture with:
  - continuous fetal heart rate monitoring
  - regular vaginal examinations to ensure normal progress

- If the diagnosis is suspected, proceed to laparotomy, delivery by cesarean section and uterine repair (hysterectomy may occasionally be necessary)

- Correct blood loss (see Chapter 73)

may be noted. On other occasions it may present as a cessation of labor and the fetus may be noted to move up from a previously observed pelvic station. If rupture is diagnosed, immediate laparotomy for delivery and control of bleeding is needed.[9] In the majority of cases, the uterine dehiscence can be repaired. However, in a few cases, a hysterectomy may be necessary.

INCIDENTAL CAUSES: PHYSIOLOGICAL

HEARTBURN, EXCESS VOMITING, CONSTIPATION

These are common causes of mild abdominal discomfort or pain during pregnancy. The management options are summarized below.

INCIDENTAL CAUSES: COMMON PATHOLOGICAL

APPENDICITIS

Incidence

Acute appendicitis is the most common surgical condition to accompany pregnancy. It complicates approximately 1:2000 pregnancies. Its frequency in pregnant women is the same as in non-pregnant women.[10,11]

Risks

When acute appendicitis complicates pregnancy, in addition to the risks of perforation with peritonitis and sepsis, there is substantial risk of miscarriage, fetal demise and preterm labor. This risk is greatest in cases with perforation and peritonitis. For example, when perforation has occurred, maternal and fetal mortality

---

HEARTBURN, EXCESS VOMITING, CONSTIPATION
Summary of Management Options

Heartburn

- Reassure

- Avoid bending

- Avoid lying flat in bed (more pillows/raise head of bed)

- Antacids

- H-2 antagonists if severe

Excess vomiting

- Exclude pathological cause

- Reassure

- Dietary adjustment

- Rectal antiemetics (? avoid first trimester)

- Consider hospital admission (especially if dehydration/ketosis):
  - nil, else as first measure
  - consider i.v. fluids and i.v. antiemetics if continued problem

Constipation

- Dietary adjustment, increase fiber

- Stop iron therapy unless absolutely indicated

- Consider laxatives

- Consider suppositories/enema only if severe

rates as high as 17 and 43%, respectively, have been reported, whereas when no perforation has occurred the rates are virtually zero.[12]

The anatomical and physiological changes of pregnancy complicate diagnosis. These, combined with some reluctance to perform a laparotomy on a pregnant woman, make delays in diagnosis and definitive surgical treatment the greatest risk of appendicitis in pregnancy.

Management Options

Prenatal

The distortion of abdominal anatomy by the enlarged pregnant uterus complicates the diagnosis of appendicitis. The cecum and appendix are displaced upward and to the right with advancing gestation. By term, the appendix is generally in the right flank and well above the iliac crest. With peri-appendiceal or pelvic adhesions, however, it may remain in the right lower quadrant or it may be found in the vicinity of the kidney or ureter. Since the pain of appendicitis is largely due to the irritation of the surrounding parietal peritoneum and organs, it is not surprising that the pain in appendicitis in pregnancy would be atypical. It can occur in the right lower quadrant as in non-pregnant women or the right flank or even mimic right pyelonephritis. If the appendix is in proximity to the ureter, it may cause pyuria which can further complicate the diagnosis. If it remains in the pelvis, it may be so isolated from the anterior peritoneum by the pregnant uterus as to make the pain difficult to locate and the diagnosis very confusing.

The other symptoms of appendicitis such as anorexia, nausea, vomiting, fever and chills may be less evident in pregnancy or even attributed to normal symptoms of pregnancy or urinary tract infection. Normal pregnant women may have a mild leukocytosis. For these reasons, it is often necessary to observe the patient over a period of hours and obtain serial white blood cell counts, temperatures and repeat examinations. Ultrasonography contributes little to the diagnosis other than to help rule out such things as a degenerating fibroid, ruptured adnexal cyst, ureteric obstruction and abruptio placenta.

Laparotomy can be performed in pregnancy with little risk to mother and fetus. Care must be taken to avoid maternal hypotension and hypoxia. Since the location of the appendix is variable in pregnancy, the incision used must be individualized. In the first trimester, since the appendix remains in its usual location and the uterus does not obstruct access to it, a low transverse or McBurney incision can be used. In the second and third trimesters, a right paramedian incision over the area of maximal pain allows better access to the appendix and the option of easily extending the incision if needed. It is preferable to extend the incision to gain adequate exposure than to extensively compress or manipulate the pregnant uterus.

During the postoperative period, one must be alert for the signs of developing preterm labor. Since the patient is receiving analgesics for postoperative pain, one cannot rely on her to report uterine contractions. Continuous or intermittent monitoring for contractions is needed in this period. It is also essential that the patient has had a cervical examination prior to surgery so that progressive cervical effacement and dilatation can be detected if it should occur in the postoperative period. Some advocate the use of an intravenous tocolytic during the first few days following surgery when the risk time for preterm labor is greatest. Once this period is passed, further tocolysis is rarely needed.[10]

Postnatal

Appendicitis occurring in the postpartum or post-cesarean patient can be particularly difficult to diagnose. It is essential to distinguish the pain, nausea, fever and leucocytosis of appendicitis from normal post-cesarean recovery or recovery complicated by endometritis. This diagnostic difficulty often results in delay of surgery and excessive morbidity in the postpartum patient.

APPENDICITIS
Summary of Management Options

Prenatal or postnatal

- Diagnosis is not easy; however, risk to mother and fetus greatly increased with perforation

- Laparotomy with right paramedian incision at site of maximal tenderness

- ? Use of prophylactic tocolysis postoperatively for 2–3 days

---

BOWEL OBSTRUCTION

Intestinal obstruction complicates approximately 1:3000 pregnancies.[13] The underlying causes include adhesions (from preceding appendicectomy, ovarian cyctecomy, tubal surgery, classical cesarean section, bowel surgery or pelvic inflammatory disease), volvulus, intussusception, internal and external hernias and neoplasms.

The presentation is usually in the second or third trimester with colicky abdominal pain, nausea, vomiting, constipation and abdominal distension being the most common features. As with appendicitis, diagnosis is not easy. Diffuse extrauterine abdominal tenderness may be a useful additional sign as would an increase (characteristic of obstruction) or absence (characteristic of secondary paralytic ileus) of bowel sounds. If the diagnosis is suspected, an erect abdominal x-ray will reveal the characteristic distended loops of bowel with fluid levels.

Risks

The maternal mortality from intestinal obstruction in pregnancy has been quoted as varying between 10 and 20% and the fetal loss rate between 30 and 50%.[8] Such high figures are especially likely if strangulation and/or perforation occur or the mother's condition is complicated by fluid and electrolyte disturbance.

Management Options

Prenatal or postnatal

When the diagnosis is made, the management options are either conservative or surgical. Some advocate that, provided there are no signs of strangulation, conservative management of nasogastric aspiration and intravenous fluids may be tried for a few hours, followed by a surgical approach if there is no improvement.[1] Others maintain that because the risks of strangulation/perforation are so great for mother and fetus (see above), then early recourse to laparotomy is the safest course for mother and child.[8] In either case, close attention should be paid to fluid and electrolyte balance. If or when a laparotomy is undertaken, it is probably advisable for the operation to be performed by an obstetrician and a general surgeon. A vertical midline incision is usually necessary and should be of adequate size. Occasionally, a cesarean section is required if the pregnancy is sufficiently far advanced in order to gain adequate access to the surgical field. However, if division of adhesions, correction and stabilization of a volvulus or bowel resection can be carried out without disturbing the pregnancy, this is preferable.[8] As with appendicectomy in pregnancy, if delivery has not occurred as part of the laparotomy, some would advocate the use of tocolysis for 2–3 days after surgery.

BOWEL OBSTRUCTION
Summary of Management Options

Prenatal or postnatal

- Once diagnosis is made, conservative *vs* surgical approach is cause for debate:
  - conservative (nasogastric suction and i.v. fluids) may be considered for a few hours if no strangulation/perforation
  - surgical approach (laparotomy and surgical correction of obstruction) always if strangulation/perforation, though some would advocate early surgery for all cases

- If surgical option chosen:
  - obstetrician and surgeon operating is advisable
  - have adequate vertical incision
  - cesarean section may be necessary for adequate surgical field in late pregnancy

- Careful attention to fluid and electrolyte balance

- ? Tocolysis for 2–3 days after surgery

CHOLECYSTITIS

Incidence

Gall-stones grow more rapidly during pregnancy than in non-pregnant patients.[8] Acute cholecystitis complicates about 1:1000 pregnancies. Many women will have their first gall-bladder attack during pregnancy. Also women with a history of gall-bladder disease before pregnancy have a high risk of worsening disease during pregnancy and many need surgery before delivery.[14]

Risks

Pregnancy poses a risk of worsening pre-existent gall-bladder disease. If the problem cannot be managed conservatively, surgery may be needed during pregnancy. The risk of such surgery to the fetus is very small. If possible, the surgery should be performed in the second trimester. This avoids exposure of the developing embryo to anesthetic agents and may reduce the risk of miscarriage following surgery. The enlarged uterus in the third trimester and its increased irritability makes surgery late in pregnancy technically more difficult and thus carries a higher risk of preterm delivery.

Management Options

Prepregnancy

The patient with symptomatic gall-stones should be counseled to consider surgery prior to conception. As noted above, pregnancy appears to exacerbate the problem and there is approximately a 50% risk of her needing surgery prior to delivery. Laparoscopic cholecystectomy has significantly reduced the morbidity and discomfort associated with uncomplicated gall-bladder surgery, so it should be an attractive option to many patients.

Prenatal

The management of cholecystitis during pregnancy is similar to that in non-pregnant women. Ultrasound examination of the gall-bladder and common duct reliably demonstrates gall-stones and can detect common duct dilation. Once the diagnosis is made, conservative treatment with analgesics, intravenous fluids and nasogastric suction is initiated. Antibiotics are sometimes required, but chenodeoxycholic acid is contraindicated because of possible teratogenicity. Often the attack rapidly subsides and with proper dietary management may not recur. Recurrent attacks, jaundice, liver function abnormalities, empyema of gall-bladder or common duct dilation indicative of obstruction are indications for surgery. If pancreatitis occurs, then surgery is indicated.[15] As noted above, it is preferable to perform surgery in the second trimester or postpartum. In the first trimester, laparoscopic surgery is relatively simple. In later pregnancy, open cholecystectomy is generally performed but laparoscopic removal of the gall-bladder has been described in the third trimester.[16] Laparotomy is also mandatory if there is doubt about the diagnosis and appendicitis cannot be ruled out.

It is important to distinguish cholecystitis from HELLP syndrome and severe pre-eclampsia. Both can present with right upper quadrant pain, nausea, vomiting, liver function abnormalities and jaundice. Both may initially appear to respond to conservative ther-apy. Severe pre-eclampsia inevitably gets worse and only resolves following delivery. Erroneously diagnosing it as cholecystitis could critically delay appropriate treatment and delivery at great risk to both the mother and baby. In addition to liver function abnormalities, HELLP syndrome is accompanied by renal function abnormalities, especially elevated serum uric acid and hematologic abnormalities, especially decreased platelet counts and hemoconcentration. In evaluating any patient for cholelithiasis, particularly in the second half of pregnancy, one should consider the possibility of

---

CHOLECYSTITIS
Summary of Management Options

Prepregnancy

- Consider cholecystectomy prior to conception with symptomatic gall-stones

Prenatal

- Conservative approach in the first instance:
  - bedrest
  - analgesia/sedation
  - i.v. fluids
  - nasogastric suction
  - antibiotics (such as amoxicillin, cefradine or co-amoxiclav) (chenodeoxycholic acid is contraindicated because of possible teratogenic effects)

- Dietary adjustment after attack has subsided (avoiding fatty foods, etc.)

- Indications for cholecystectomy (preferably in second trimester):
  - recurrent attacks of cholecystitis
  - jaundice
  - abnormal liver function
  - empyema of gall-bladder
  - bile duct dilatation suggestive of obstruction
  - pancreatitis
  - laparotomy is also indicated if appendicitis cannot be excluded

severe pre-eclampsia and perform appropriate tests to rule it out.

Labor/delivery

Recent cholecystectomy does not complicate normal labor and delivery. A cesarean delivery should only be performed for usual obstetric indications.

Postnatal

No different from the care of the non-pregnant woman.

RENAL DISEASE

Incidence

Infection is the most common and arguably the most important renal cause of abdominal pain in pregnancy. In total, 5% of pregnant women will have bacteriuria at their first visit; 25% of these will develop symptomatic urinary tract infection subsequently in the pregnancy if not treated.[1,8] Other renal causes of abdominal pain in pregnancy include calculi (approximate incidence 1:1500 pregnancies), pelviureteric obstruction (e.g. due to calculi, fibrosis or congenital obstruction) and hydronephrosis.

Management Options

The risks and management of these conditions are discussed in detail in Chapter 28.

INFLAMMATORY BOWEL DISEASE

Both ulcerative colitis and Crohn's disease may cause abdominal pain and diarrhea during pregnancy. Pain is characteristically a more marked feature of Crohn's disease except in the uncommon acute toxic dilatation of ulcerative colitis.[1]

Management Options

The risks and management of these conditions are discussed in detail in Chapter 28.

ACUTE PANCREATITIS

Incidence

Although pancreatitis is rare in pregnancy (1:4000), some have suggested that it is more common in preg-

nancy because of the higher incidence of gall-stones. Certainly if acute pancreatitis occurs in pregnancy, gall-stones are more likely to be the cause than alcohol or thiazide diuretics.[1,8] Acute pancreatitis tends to occur in late pregnancy or soon after delivery with central or upper abdominal pain often radiating to the back and epigastric tenderness. Recurrent vomiting is often found, often so severe as to produce dehydration and even shock. Confusion with hyperemesis gravidarum is a common error. Ultrasonography will reveal gall-stones in over 50% of cases. The pathognomonic investigation is a raised serum amylase concentration. However, some maintain that occasionally false-negative results can be obtained if the blood is taken 24–72 h after the attack or in acute hemorrhagic pancreatitis with massive necrosis.[8]

Risks

The main risks are, first, of delay in diagnosis assuming that the patient merely has hyperemesis gravidarum. Secondly, the mother may become grossly dehydrated and even shocked. The reported maternal mortality in the third trimester is 37%;[1] however, this may be overly pessimistic with modern intravenous therapy (see below).

Management Options

Treatment is as in the non-pregnant patient with the underlying principles being prevention and treatment of shock, suppression of pancreatic activity, relief of pain, prevention and treatment of infection, and prompt recognition and treatment of surgical complications.[8] Careful attention must be paid to intravenous fluid replacement with close monitoring of electrolyte, calcium and glucose concentrations being especially important.

Some authors argue against the traditional use of nasogastric suction in such patients, claiming that is of no proven benefit and indeed may produce a further increase in serum amylase levels. The same workers also itemize the various therapeutic agents used to inhibit pancreatic secretion, including anticholinergic drugs, steroids, prostaglandins, glucagon, cimetidine and trypsin inhibitors.[17] None of these are of proven benefit in randomized clinical trials; however, all have been associated with clinical improvement when used uncontrolled in individual cases.[8]

Laparotomy should only be considered if conservative measures fail. Cholecystectomy can be considered as an early option when acute pancreatitis occurs in association with gall-stones unusually in the first or second trimesters. The decision to perform the operation when the disease occurs in the third trimester is

---

ACUTE PANCREATITIS
Summary of Management Options

Prepregnancy

- Discuss specific measures in women with risk factors:
  - cholecystectomy in women with known gall-stones and previous attacks of cholecystitis or pancreatitis
  - various strategies in women with alcohol abuse (see Chapter 5)
  - change treatment in women taking thiazide diuretics

Prenatal

- Prevention and treatment of shock with i.v. fluids and monitoring electrolyte, calcium and glucose concentrations

- Analgesia

- Prophylactic antibiotics (such as amoxicillin, cefradine or co-amoxiclav)

- Suppression of pancreatic activity;
  - use of nasogastric suction is questioned
  - the following, though advocated, have not been subjected to controlled study:
    —anticholinergic drugs
    —steroids
    —prostaglandins
    —glucagon
    —cimetidine
    —trypsin inhibitors

- Prompt recognition and treatment of surgical complications:
  - laparotomy usually with cholecystectomy if conservative measures fail
  - cholecystectomy as an early option when pancreatitis occurs with gall-stones in first or second trimesters

Postnatal

- Cholecystectomy if pancreatitis with gall-stones successfully treated conservatively in pregnancy

---

more difficult, but generally it would seem reasonable only to consider the operation at that time if conservative treatment fails. Certainly it can be performed as a planned procedure soon after delivery if the pancreatitis settles with conservative measures. There is no evidence that ending the pregnancy will influence the course of the disease.[8]

PEPTIC ULCER

Gastric and duodenal ulcer rarely occur for the first time in pregnancy. Patients with known pre-existing ulcers tend to improve during their pregnancy.[1] There is a tendency for relapse after delivery. Abdominal pain can be associated with the conditions either as a chronic feature or as an acute event following perforation.

Management Options

The risks and management of these conditions are discussed in detail in Chapter 28.

TORSION OF ADNEXA

Torsion of the ovary can occur in pregnancy and is almost always associated with an ovarian cyst or tumor. Torsion presents as severe, perhaps intermittent, lower quadrant abdominal pain with nausea and vomiting. Due to enlargement of the uterus, adnexal torsion is rare in the third trimester of pregnancy. If the process involves the right adnexa, it must be distinguished from acute appendicitis. In the first trimester, ectopic pregnancy must be considered in the differential diagnosis.

Incidence

While ovarian cysts are relatively common, torsion of the adnexa is rare. Most ovarian cysts in pregnancy are presumed to be corpus luteum cysts. Since they are generally asymptomatic and resolve spontaneously in most cases, the diagnosis is rarely confirmed. Cysts which are large and persist or are complex with solid and cystic areas need to be further evaluated. In addition to the risk for torsion or rupture, a small but significant number are ovarian neoplasms and some of these will be malignant.

Risks

Torsion of the adnexa is an acute surgical problem. It can lead to miscarriage or, in later pregnancy, premature labor. It is often included in the differential diagnosis of lower abdominal pain in pregnancy.

Management Options

Prenatal

Torsion presents with the acute onset of lower quadrant abdominal pain, often accompanied by nausea and vomiting. The pain may be constant or intermittent but generally increases in intensity with time. There may be tachycardia, slight temperature elevation and leucocytosis. It may be difficult to differentiate torsion from appendicitis, ruptured adnexal cyst or ectopic pregnancy. Sonographic demonstration of an ovarian cyst is helpful in this situation.

Once the condition is strongly suspected, laparotomy is the only effective treatment. In removing the twisted adnexa, care should be taken to avoid untwisting the pedicle if the adnexa appears to be either necrotic or the vessels appear thrombosed. In this case, the pedicle should be clamped and the entire adnexa removed. If the adnexa appears to be viable and is not twisted at the time of surgery, the cystectomy can be performed with preservation of the tube and ovary.

Following surgery, the patient should be watched for signs of miscarriage or preterm labor. Some would advocate the use of intravenous tocolytic therapy. If the removed ovary contained the corpus luteum of pregnancy, and the surgery was performed in the first 8 weeks, the patient will need progesterone support for the pregnancy until after 8–10 weeks of amenorrhea. This can be provided in the form of sublingual lozenges, suppositories/pessaries or intramuscular injections.

> **TORSION OF ADNEXA**
> **Summary of Management Options**
>
> **Prenatal**
>
> - Laparotomy: untwisting and then deciding on ovarian cystectomy *vs* oophorectomy depending on viability
>
> - ? i.v. tocolysis
>
> - If corpus luteum removed before 8 weeks for progesterone support until 8–10 weeks

INCIDENTAL CAUSES: RARE PATHOLOGICAL

RECTUS HEMATOMA

Bleeding into the rectus muscle and hematoma formation from rupture of a branch of the inferior epigastric artery may occur following a bout of coughing or direct trauma in late pregnancy. A large unilateral painful swelling may be confused with an ovarian cyst, a degenerating fibroid, uterine rupture or abruption.

Management Options

Diagnosis may only be made at laparotomy when surgical treatment comprising evacuation of the hematoma and ligation of the bleeding artery should be performed. However, if the diagnosis is made before surgery, conservative management of bed rest and analgesia should be tried first. In the majority of cases, the problem should improve with this approach. In a few cases, surgery will be necessary.

SICKLE CRISIS

Women who have homozygous SS or SC disease can present in pregnancy with abdominal pain due to a crisis.

Management Options

The risks and management of this condition are discussed in detail in Chapter 23.

MALIGNANT DISEASE

Rarely, malignancy can cause abdominal pain in pregnancy. In many such cases, the diagnosis and subsequent management is often delayed because of the pregnancy.

Management Options

The risks and management of this disease are discussed in detail in Chapter 32.

PORPHYRIA

Acute porphyria presents with abdominal pain, psychiatric disturbance and autonomic effects. Pregnancy itself can precipitate an attack and so porphyria may present for the first time in pregnancy.

Management Options

Any drug which precipitated the attack should be stopped. Analgesics and antiemetics should be prescribed.

ARTERIAL HEMORRHAGE

Miscellaneous, very rare conditions resulting in intraabdominal hemorrhage can cause abdominal pain in pregnancy. These include rupture of the liver in preeclampsia, rupture of the utero-ovarian veins and rupture of aneurysms (splenic, hepatic, renal, aortic). In addition to the abdominal pain, rapidly progressing shock is a feature.

Risks

The main risks of these conditions are maternal and fetal demise.

Management Options

Speed of action is imperative in these cases and even then death may not be avoided. In all conditions, the principles of management are the same; namely, surgical control of the hemorrhage, correction of shock and specific measures for specific problems (such as splenectomy with splenic rupture or insertion of a graft with aortic rupture). Obviously, if the patient survives long enough for such definitive measures to be considered, practical assistance from a general or vascular surgeon is mandatory.

Procedure: Laparotomy in Pregnancy

Indications

Indications for laparotomy are discussed above. In general, they are the same as in the non-pregnant patient. Obstetricians often find that they are more comfortable with the idea of operating on the pregnant woman than are general surgeons. They are also often more familiar with the alterations in disease presentation and differential diagnosis in pregnancy than general surgeons. For these reasons, it is essential that obstetricians do not simply turn the care of their patients over to surgical specialists for diagnosis and treatment, but rather remain actively involved in their patients' management throughout the period of evaluation, treatment and postoperative care.

Procedure description

Anesthetic considerations

The choice of anesthetic for surgery during pregnancy depends on the operation proposed, the skill of the anesthesiologist, the preference of the surgeon and the patient. While it has been suggested that chronic exposure of operating room personnel to anesthetic agents leads to an increased rate of miscarriage, the hazard associated with acute general anesthetic administration is not well characterized. It seems likely that the risk is very small. It is probably more important that meticulous attention is paid to maintenance of maternal homeostasis. The fetus is totally dependent on maternal oxygenation and uterine perfusion for respiration. Any compromise of maternal oxygenation will be reflected in the fetus. Both conduction or regional anesthesia and general anesthesia can be used in pregnancy with safety for both the mother and fetus.

Operation

Abdominal incisions in pregnancy are the same as those used in non-pregnant patients. McBurney and low transverse incisions are best used in the first trimester. Later in pregnancy, the enlarged uterus so completely fills the lower abdomen that access to organs other than the anterior, lower uterine segment (as for cesarean section) is extremely difficult. It is generally advisable to make a generous incision which can be extended if necessary, rather than attempting to use a small and poorly placed incision and being forced to manipulate the uterus in an attempt to accomplish the operation. Midline or paramedian incisions work well. Healing in pregnancy is generally without complications, though there may be some skin scar spreading as the pregnancy progresses due to the rapidly enlarging uterus. If labor occurs shortly after surgery, the fresh incision may inhibit maternal expulsive efforts during the second stage. It would probably be advisable to assist delivery in these circumstances with either vacuum extractor or forceps.

Complications

There is an increased risk of miscarriage in association with laparotomy performed during early pregnancy. This risk exists especially in the first trimester and is considerably reduced on planned procedures carried out in the second trimester.[18,19] Preterm delivery and technical difficulty are problems encountered when laparotomy is carried out during the third trimester.[19] However, while the risks of laparotomy carried out during pregnancy should not be minimized, as a generalization the risks of the condition for which the surgery is required are greater than the risks of the operation itself to mother and baby.[12,19]

REFERENCES

1   Setchell M (1987) Abdominal pain in pregnancy. In Studd J (ed.) *Progress in Obstetrics and Gynaecology*, Vol. 6, pp. 87–99. London: Churchill Livingstone.

2   Smith CA (1975) Pathological uterine torsion: A catastrophic event in late pregnancy. *American Journal of Obstetrics and Gynecology* **123**:32–33.

3   Nowoelski PF, Henderson H (1960) Axial torsion of the pregnant uterus. *American Journal of Obstetrics and Gynecology* **80**:272–273.

4   Graber EA (1974) Surgery of the uterus in pregnancy. In Barber HRK, Graber EA (eds) *Surgical Diseases in Pregnancy*, pp. 428–439. Philadelphia, PA: W.B. Saunders.

5   Taylor ES (1985) Editorial comment. *Obstetrical and Gynecological Survey* **40**:81.

6   Pisani BJ (1982) Ectopic pregnancy. *The Female Patient* **71**:1.

7   Hasan F, Arugugam K, Sivanesaratnam V (1990) Uterine leiomyomata in pregnancy. *International Journal of Gynaecology and Obstetrics* **34**:45.

8   Amias AG (1989) Abdominal pain in pregnancy. In Turnbull A, Chamberlain G (eds) *Obstetrics*, pp. 605–621. Edinburgh: Churchill Livingstone.

9   Phelan JP (1990) Uterine rupture. *Clinics in Obstetrics and Gynecology* **33**:432.

10 Tamir IL, Bongard FS, Klein SR (1990) Acute appendicitis in the pregnant patient. *American Journal of Surgery* **160**:571.

11 McGee TM (1989) Acute appendicitis in pregnancy. *Australia and New Zealand Journal of Obstetrics and Gynaecology* **29**:378.

12 Horowitz MD, Gomez GA, Santiesbastian R, Burkitt G (1985) Acute appendicitis during pregnancy. *Archives of Surgery* **120**:1362–1367.

13 Welch JP (1990) Miscellaneous causes of small bowel obstruction. In Welch JP (ed.) *Bowel Obstruction: Differential Diagnosis and Clinical Management*, pp. 454–456. London: W.B. Saunders.

14 van Beek EJR, Farmer KCR, Millar DM, Brummelkamp WH (1991) Gallstone disease in women younger than 30 years. *Netherlands Journal of Surgery* **43**:60.

15 Block P, Kelly TR (1989) Management of gallstone pancreatitis during pregnancy and the postpartum period. *Surgery Gynecology and Obstetrics* **168**:426.

16 Pucci RO, Seed RW (1991) Case report of laparoscopic cholecystectomy in the third trimester of pregnancy. *American Journal of Obstetrics and Gynecology* **165**:401.

17 Fagan EA, Chadwick VS (1984) Disorders of gastrointestinal tract, pancreas and hepato-biliary system. In de Swiet M (ed.) *Medical Disorders in Obstetric Practice*, pp. 322–325. Oxford: Blackwell Scientific.

18 Kammerer WS (1979) Non-obstetric surgery during pregnancy. *Medical Clinics of North America* **6**:1157–1163.

19 Dixon NP, Green J, Rogers A, Rubin L (1983) Fetal loss after cholecystectomy during pregnancy. *Canadian Medical Association Journal* **88**:576–577.

35

Gynecological Disease (Non-Malignant)

JOHN HUTTON

SUBFERTILITY

Although 1:6 couples of fertile age present to the medical practitioner with difficulty in conceiving, about half of these will ultimately conceive with or without medical help. The medical treatments available for couples who are found to have a male factor contributing to their infertility are donor insemination and intrauterine insemination. With regard to female factors contributing to infertility, anovulation is the most common and is usually due to hypothalamic dysfunction, hyperprolactinemia, polycystic ovarian disease syndrome or some degree of primary ovarian failure. The medical treatments of anovulation include clomiphene, Pergonal® or pure FSH with or without a GnRh analog. Bromocriptine is the usual treatment for hyperprolactinemia due to a pituitary microadenoma. Severe tubal dysfunction is now only usually treated by some form of *in vitro* fertilization (IVF). Rarely, cervical factors may be a cause of infertility, and probably the best treatment then is intrauterine insemination.

Risks Associated with Pregnancy after Subfertility

The pregnancy outcome depends mostly on the age of the woman, presumably because older women are more likely to have chromosomal and endocrine problems that lead to miscarriage or defective ovulation. Specific risks to the mother and the fetus associated with subfertility are better related to the cause of the infertility and/or the treatment, as follows.

Donor insemination

The pregnancy risk of donor insemination is a slightly increased rate of spontaneous miscarriage in the first trimester. The procedure seems to be associated with more ovulatory dysfunction, possibly because of the stress. There is no proven risk from the use of frozen semen. The use of fresh semen is not now possible because of the need to quarantine semen for at least 3 months because of the HIV risk. There are no other risks to the mother or the fetus during the pregnancy provided Rh negative donors are used in Rh negative mothers.

Intrauterine insemination

This is carried out using only a small volume of about 0.4 ml so that there is no risk from the procedure. Intrauterine insemination, like donor insemination, may be associated with an increased risk of spontaneous miscarriage in the first trimester.

Polycystic ovarian syndrome (PCO)

This syndrome is arguably characterized by a blood LH:FSH ration >2.5:1 and/or >8 microcysts of 2–8 mm size visualized ultrasonically and arranged peripherally just beneath the capsule in each ovary. Up to 10% of the population may have this disorder, though many of these women have no difficulty in conceiving. The risks of pregnancy in women with PCO relate to the association of PCO with disordered carbohydrate metabolism due to insulin resistance, pre-existing hypertension or the need for drugs to stimulate ovulation.

Hypothalamic anovulation

Pregnancy induced by drugs in women with anovulation due to a weight-related disorder is complicated by premature labor, growth deficiency and a poor infant outcome. Maternal hypoalbuminemia and edema can also occur. Consequently, the use of drugs is now contraindicated in women with a ponderal (body mass) index <19. Should such women conceive spontaneously, they must continue to eat normally and put on weight to ensure there is a good outcome to the pregnancy.

Treatment of women with other causes of hypogonadotrophic hypogonadism by either clomiphene or Pergonal® can be associated with hyperstimulation, multiple pregnancy, or an increased fetal abnormality rate – this latter risk occurs particularly with multiple pregnancy.

In vitro fertilization (IVF)

The major pregnancy risk from IVF or gamete intrafallopian transfer (GIFT) is multiple pregnancy associated with the hyperstimulation and the transfer of more than one embryo or ovum. However, even singleton pregnancies appear to be complicated by an increased risk of premature labor, growth deficiency or problems in labor requiring cesarean section. Some studies have also suggested an increased rate of congenital heart defect.

Tubal disease

Women with previous tubal infection or tubal surgery are at increased risk of ectopic pregnancy. The chance of an intrauterine pregnancy after conservative surgery for a previous ectopic pregnancy is at least twice the chance of a recurrence of the ectopic. Women with tubal disease associated with a ureaplasma or Chlamydia infection appear to have an increased chance of premature labor – the urea plasma organism can be cultured in about 10% of women with premature rupture of the membranes.

Management Options

Prepregnancy

The physician is bound to ensure that all women presenting with infertility are safe to sustain a pregnancy.

Thus all women with infertility should be tested for rubella and, if not immune, given vaccination and advised to take contraceptive precautions, probably for 3 months. Similarly, the diagnosis of medical disorders, such as hypertension, renal disease or Chlamydia, at the onset of a pregnancy rather than at the time of presentation with infertility is suboptimal care.

Prenatal

The first and probably most important management step is to confirm that the missed period is associated with at least one viable intrauterine pregnancy. The pregnancy is usually best diagnosed by quantitative serum beta-HCG assay, although quantitative assays may improve the prognostic value. Determining viability in the uterus depends on ultrasound – a visible yolk sac at 6 weeks is optimistic with the viability being confirmed by a fetal heart, usually at the end of the sixth week of pregnancy.

Once viability is proven, the risk of miscarriage is less than 5%. If the pregnancy is associated with hyperstimulatory drugs, corpora luteal cysts are commonly seen until 12 weeks – under no circumstances should surgical therapy or aspiration be considered. Sometimes the need for ovulation stimulation is associated with an endocrine dysfunction in early pregnancy such as a progesterone defect; high-dose progestagen therapy has been advocated, but should only be initiated in women whose progesterone levels are less than the fifth percentile for their gestation. Interestingly, only half the women with low serum progesterones actually miscarry, suggesting that the endometrial or myometrial roles of progesterone are still uncertain.

Women with polycystic ovarian disease should be screened for gestational diabetes during the pregnancy or earlier if there is glycosuria.

In these more 'precious' pregnancies in women with a previous history of infertility, it is difficult to resist the use of ultrasound to check fetal growth and welfare. Such testing helps allay (couple and doctor) anxiety, especially as many of these women are also older and therefore have little chance or time to rectify a mistake or misadventure.

The prenatal management of the woman with twins is that of multiple pregnancy (see Chapter 10). However, should there be more than two fetuses, and certainly if there are more than three fetuses, the risk of prematurity is so high that selective reduction needs to be considered (see Chapter 57).

Ideally, the number of people caring for such women in pregnancy should be restricted, especially so that consistent information and advice is given to the anxious couple. Some specialist checking in early pregnancy and again at 32 weeks, when adequate growth should be checked, is probably advisable. Occasion-

SUBFERTILITY
Summary of Management Options

Prepregnancy

- Check for underlying medical disease (e.g. hypertension or diabetes)

- Ensure rubella immune

- Try and avoid hyperstimulation and multiple pregnancy

Prenatal

- Check viability and number of intrauterine pregnancies

- Diagnose ectopic pregnancy early

- Check progesterone levels until at least 12 weeks in those requiring clomid or Pergonal®

- Screen for gestational diabetes in patients with PCO

- Check fetal normality and growth in IVF pregnancies

- Multiple pregnancy (see Chapters 10 and 55)

- Reassure

Labor/delivery

- Continuous fetal heart rate monitoring

- Increased risk of operative delivery because of failure to progress or fetal heart irregularity

Postnatal

- Contraception not usually an issue

- Length of subsequent birth interval probably not important

ally, the couple believe that their only difficulty was conception and, once assisted in achieving this, that no extra surveillance or intervention is necessary. The author does not support this choice for the care of such 'precious' pregnancies.

Labor/delivery

The 'preciousness' of these pregnancies with the associated anxiety and stress, results in more operative deliveries. In addition, catecholamines released with the anxiety may inhibit the labor or affect the fetus leading to increased numbers of cesarean sections for failure to progress or fetal distress. Continuous fetal heart monitoring is, nevertheless, advisable or, if not undertaken, is usually demanded by the women. Immediate use of fetal scalp pH is important when any fetal heart irregularities occur, otherwise doctor or midwife anxiety results in an unnecessary cesarean section.

Postnatal

Contraception is not usually an issue in such couples; requests for sterilization should initially be regarded as 'reactive relief'. The use of IUCDs and depot progestogens should be avoided.

OVARIAN CYSTS
(see also Chapter 34)

The apparent incidence of ovarian cysts in pregnancy has risen with the increased use of ultrasound to determine viability, maturity or normality of the fetus during the first 20 weeks of pregnancy. A sonolucent adnexal mass > 6 cm can be identified in about 1% of pregnancies. Smaller cysts are not significant and require no further observation, as they are usually associated with the corpus luteum.

Risks

The major risk of ovarian cysts in pregnancy is to the mother; the cyst may undergo torsion (and then infarction), rupture with hemorrhage or be malignant. If the cyst is big enough to obstruct labor and is impacted in the pelvis, then the mother is at risk of an abdominal delivery. The important fetal risk is miscarriage or prematurity that is usually induced as a reaction to surgical removal. Thus, it is important first to ascertain the nature of the cyst and avoid undertaking surgery to remove a functional corpus luteum cyst – the cause of 90% of ovarian cysts in pregnancy.

Management Options

Prepregnancy

The management of adnexal masses detected prior to pregnancy is very similar to that in the pregnant state; thus cysts 8 cm or more in size that contain echogenic material and persist for more than 4 weeks, or are symptomatic, must be examined laparoscopically. If they are then noted not to be due to endometriosis or tuberculosis that might be treated medically, then some form of surgical treatment, either cystectomy or oophorectomy, is advisable. Aspiration of cysts, either laparoscopically or ultrasonically, with cytological examination of the fluid, is now no longer favored as cystadenomas or cystadenocarcinomas can be misdiagnosed.

Prenatal

The most common cysts (approximately 90%) in pregnancy are corpus luteum cysts, which invariably begin to regress by 16 weeks. Asymptomatic cysts that persist, and are of a significant size (>6–8 cm), should be removed at about 18–20 weeks. The most usual reason for a persistent sonolucent cyst is an ovarian cystadenoma or a paraovarian cyst. Dermoid cysts usually have echogenic material, as do tubovarian abscesses. Endometriotic cysts mimic the other forms, but if found at laparotomy, surgical removal should not be attempted as premature labor is more likely. Malignant cysts are rare but should be suspected if there is no regression.

If the patient develops symptoms such as torsion from an ovarian cyst, this should be operated on immediately.

Labor/delivery

Occasionally, an ovarian cyst may present as an obstructed labor. Cesarean section is then necessary before undertaking treatment (ovarian cystectomy) of the tumor at the same operation. The cyst is usually impacted in the Pouch of Douglas. Aspiration is probably not advisable because of the small risk of malignancy (probably about 2%). Fortunately, the routine use of ultrasound means that such 'chance' findings are now uncommon.

OVARIAN CYSTS
Summary of Management Options

Prepregnancy

- Treat symptomatic cysts or persistent sonolucent cysts or echogenic cysts measuring 8 cm or more

Prenatal

- Expect most cysts to be functional corpus luteum cysts that regress by 16 weeks

- Remove symptomatic cysts acutely

- Perform laparotomy (not laparoscopy) to examine echogenic cysts 8 cm or more in size. Leave endometriotic cysts, TB, but remove others. Ideal time for operation in asymptomatic women is 18–20 weeks

Labor/delivery

- Perform LSCS and ovarian cystectomy rather than aspirate cysts impacted in Pouch of Douglas

---

Procedure: Ovarian Cystectomy in Pregnancy

Indications

1. Symptomatic cyst, e.g. torsion, hemorrhage, rupture

2. Asymptomatic cyst recognized ultrasonically if:

(i) does not regress by 16 weeks, or

(ii) has echogenic material suggestive of dermoid, or

(iii) is septate or multilocular

Gestation

Best done at 18–20 weeks (earlier gestation could still be corpus luteum

Description

Preoperative preparations: thromboembolic stockings ± heparin 5000 IU subcut

Anesthesia

General anesthetic

Incision

Longitudinal midline from below umbilicus to just above pubic bone (actual size will depend on cyst size)

Method

*Retract uterus gently to one side. The ovary with cyst is usually very mobile unless cyst is associated with infection, endometriosis or malignancy. Gently draw ovary and cyst through incision. Identify mesenteric border. Put two Allis forceps on anti-mesenteric border near each pole of the ovary (**Figure 1a***).*

*Incise ovarian capsule only (not cyst) along anti-mesenteric border between the two forceps (being careful not to puncture cysts). (**Figure 1b***).*

*Use handle of scalpel or closed scissor blades to bluntly dissect capsule away from cyst using tissue forceps on margin of capsule as countertraction (**Figure 1c***). Continue blunt dissection close to cyst including along mesenteric aspect. Cyst can then be removed and sent for histology.*

Hemostasis

Spot diathermy to bleeding points arising from mesenteric aspect of ovarian substance

Repair of ovary

Using atraumatic 2-0 chromic catgut on a

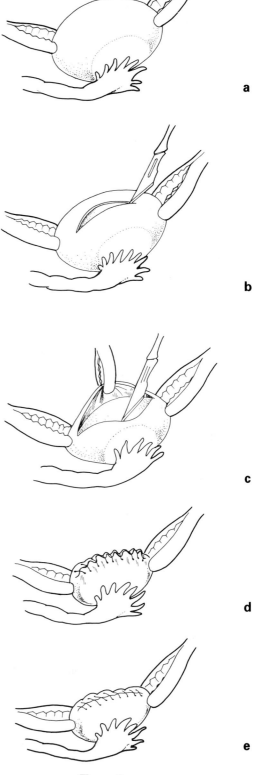

Figure 1.

*trocar needle (T10 or T25), approximate the substance of the ovary, thereby obliterating much dead space (**Figure 1d**).*

Avoid penetrating the capsule.

*The capsule is then repaired using a similar suture but inverting the edges; care with tissue handling of the capsule is required and microsurgical techniques (i.e. forceps) should be preferred to gross handling (**Figure 1e**).*

The abdominal wall is closed in layers, with dexon or vicryl being preferred for the sheath, especially as there will be pressure on this layer in the next few weeks with the expanding pregnancy. It is probably advisable to use three or four interrupted sutures in the sheath as well as the standard continuous suture.

Postop management

Use narcotic analgesia
Check for uterine activity: if excessive, start tocolysis
Check fetal heart
Check histology

Complications

The major complication of ovarian cystectomy in pregnancy is miscarriage or premature labor; this probably depends on the amount of inflammation the operation generates.

If there are adhesions, a representative biopsy should be undertaken rather than attempting a radical operation for what is subsequently proven to be tuberculosis or endometriosis, and possibly therefore better managed medically rather than surgically. Infection and wound dehiscence occur and probably relate to hemostasis and surgical technique.

Tubal adhesions of the fimbria to the incision in the ovarian capsule may theoretically occur and thereby impair future fertility. This is not usually recognized until a subsequent laparoscopic examination.

If the lesion does not appear to be a dermoid, and is possibly a mucinous or serous cystadenoma, oophorectomy is probably not the treatment of choice, as malignancy is rare. In young women, it is probably better to repeat the laparotomy to remove the ovary rather than remove an ovary for what is subsequently shown to be a benign condition.

Rarely, the patient may develop an ileus, but usually there is no need to handle bowel, and hence the risk is low.

FIBROIDS
(see also Chapters 8 and 34)

Fibroids in pregnancy are rare. The major predisposing factors to the development of fibroids are increasing age of the women, relatively unopposed estrogen stimulation previously, and/or increased tissue sensitivity to estrogen such as occurs in Negroid women, at least in comparison with Caucasian women. Thus fibroids are most common in older Negroid women and least common in Caucasian or Asian women.

Risks

The risks of fibroids in pregnancy depend on the size of the fibroid and its position; it is very rare for there to be more than one fibroid in the uterus affecting the pregnancy.

A submucous fibroid polyp, if large, may affect fertility; if it protrudes through the cervix, it may even cause bleeding, including postcoital bleeding. Submucous fibroid polyps have also been implicated in miscarriages in the first and second trimesters of pregnancy.

Fibroids arising in the lower segment of the uterus obstruct labor and/or predispose to an abnormal lie of the fetus. Intramural fibroids in the upper segment of the myometrium may predispose to an abnormal presentation, or affect uterine contractility such that there is failure to progress in labor or a primary postpartum hemorrhage.

Subserous fibroids are usually of no significance in pregnancy unless they become impacted in the Pouch of Douglas. Fibroids may undergo degeneration during pregnancy, causing pain and uterine activity; classically, this occurs about 20–22 weeks gestation.

Management Options

Prepregnancy

All endometrial fibroid polyps should be removed before a pregnancy. Transvaginal ultrasound is excellent at identifying them. Their removal is simply achieved by hysteroscopic evaluation, avulsion and, if necessary, cautery to the base (a CO_2 medium must then not be used). Other fibroids should only be removed if they are symptomatic and even then only after careful counseling of the patient. Myomectomy is now always a simple operation and a hysterectomy may become necessary if there is excessive bleeding. Preoperative GnRH analog therapy may reduce this operative risk of hemorrhage. Furthermore, uterine rupture and delivery by cesarean section are at increased risk in subsequent pregnancies. If performed for infertility or recurrent miscarriage, there is no guarantee of success.

Prenatal

Most fibroids are asymptomatic during pregnancy and only diagnosed at the time of a routine ultrasound examination. If degeneration occurs causing pain, then analgesia is necessary. Local heat or ice packs to the abdomen may produce relief. Prostaglandin inhibitors may also be useful but should be prescribed for only a few days because of their theoretical adverse fetal effects (premature closure of ductus).

If a cervical fibroid polyp is causing symptoms, it may be removed by avulsion; this can be done in the ward by simply grasping the polyp with sponge forceps and twisting until it avulses. If a fibroid (usually a lower segment fibroid) results in an abnormal lie of the fetus after 36 weeks gestation, then elective abdominal delivery at 38–39 weeks gestation is advisable.

Labor/delivery

The management of a woman in labor with a fibroid depends really on whether the fibroid is obstructing delivery. If it is not, then problems with uterine contractility should be anticipated. Postpartum hemorrhage, resulting sometimes from difficulty in effecting complete shearing off of the placenta, should be anticipated. Adequate oxytocic therapy should be prescribed and blood transfusion anticipated by having blood grouped and held on admission in labor in case urgent crossmatch is required. A wide-bore intravenous cannula should be *in situ*.

Should a fibroid, and even a subserous fibroid, be found at a cesarean section, it should be *noted*, but *not* removed, as excessive hemorrhage is almost inevitable.

Procedure: Cesarean Section with a Lower Segment Fibroid

Indication

A lower segment fibroid that:

(i) causes an abnormal lie at 38 weeks or,

(ii) is >6 cm at 38 weeks and palpable below the fetal head, either abdominally or vaginally (smaller fibroids are usually soft and 'drawn' or 'pressed' out of the way during labor).

The ultrasonic dimensions may not accurately reflect the actual dimensions of the fibroid, so clinical evaluation is more important than the ultrasonic assessment.

Description

Preoperative preparation:

(i) blood crossmatched

(ii) antibiotics

(iii) thromboembolic stockings

Anesthetic

General or epidural

Skin incision

Midline suprapubic skin incision is advisable if the fibroid is large or a classical procedure is anticipated. However, if the fibroid is small or is known to be a posteriori, a routine lower segment cesarean section can be performed.

Uterine incision

This depends on the observed site of the fibroid. If the lower segment is well-formed around the fibroid and a transverse lower segment incision can be made, allowing a 2–3 cm margin with the fibroid, then a lower segment approach should be used. If access through the lower segment with a 2–3 cm margin is not possible, then a classical cesarean section should be performed, again ensuring a 2–3 cm safety margin with the fibroid (see Chapter 67). Under no circumstances should any attempt be made to remove a fibroid at the time of cesarean section.

Complications/postnatal care

There are no complications aside from the usual complications of cesarean section. Normally, with the hypoestrogenic state of the puerperium, the fibroid regresses

---

FIBROIDS
Summary of Management Options

Prepregnancy

- Remove endometrial fibroid polyps

- Consider myomectomy for other fibroids if symptomatic, but only after careful counseling

Prenatal

- Bed rest, analgesia, local heat/ice for red degeneration

- Avulse symptomatic cervical fibroid polyps

- Consider elective cesarean section at 38–39 weeks if:
  - lower segment/cervical fibroids causing unstable lie
  - previous myomectomy for intramural fibroids

Labor/delivery

- Cesarean section if fibroid produces obstructed labor

- Vigilance for third-stage complications

- Do not remove fibroids at cesarean section

- If delivery is by cesarean section, only consider classical approach if access through the lower segment with a 2–3 cm margin of normal tissue is not possible

Postnatal

- Analgesia if excessive involutional pain (? GnRH in extreme cases)

---

and degenerates and this may cause some pain. Occasionally, this involution does not occur in the puerperium, in which case medical therapy such as GnRH analogs can be tried in an effort to induce regression. If myomectomy then becomes indicated, there is evidence to suggest that hemorrhage is less likely with the prior use of a GnRH analog.

Previous myomectomy

If women have had a previous myomectomy in which the endometrial cavity has been opened, then the standard advice is to perform elective cesarean section, especially if the implantation site is likely to be over the previous myomectomy incision scar. However, if the myomectomy or myomectomies have been performed for subserous fibroids only, there is less risk of uterine rupture during the labor and so conservative management is usually advised, though the labor should be managed as in a woman who has had a previous cesarean section.

PROLAPSE

During pregnancy, many women will suffer from stress incontinence. A few will develop more troublesome prolapse with herniation of the bladder or the cervix through the introitus. This may improve as pregnancy advances.

Risks

The major problem from a cystocoele in pregnancy is a urinary tract infection resulting from urinary stasis or incomplete emptying. Coitus is also difficult for these women. Ulceration of the prolapsed cervix is very rare, although bleeding may sometimes occur. There appear to be no fetal risks.

Management Options

Prepregnancy

In women planning further children, medical treatment by pelvic floor exercises should be encouraged. This usually requires specific instruction by a physiotherapist. There are also various aids, such as vaginal cones, which may assist in focusing the exercises. Definitive surgery arguably should be deferred until a women considers her family is complete.

Prenatal

Urinary tract infection should be treated when asymptomatic, thus regular bacteriological examination of urine specimens is required. Symptomatic prolapse of the cervix can sometimes be effectively treated with a ring pessary. Usually at least an 80 mm pessary is required and it will only be effective if there is some body to the perineum, otherwise it will drop out. Other pessary types, such as the Hodge pessary, have also been advocated. Whenever a pessary is used, physiotherapy exercises must also be encouraged, as the pelvic floor muscles with their insertion into the perineum are critical in holding the pessary in place.

Surgical treatment of a prolapse is generally not undertaken during pregnancy, because the symptoms often improve after delivery, trauma and blood loss are more likely, and delivery by elective cesarean section becomes necessary.

Labor/delivery

This is rarely a problem. Vaginal delivery is not contraindicated in the absence of previous surgery for prolapse.

Postnatal

Occasionally, a prolapse may be aggravated puerperally; physiotherapy exercises should be encouraged. If symptoms persist several months after delivery, and have not responded to medical treatment, surgical treatment of the prolapse can be considered.

Management of Pregnancy in Women with a Previous Successful Repair Operation

Pregnancy may occasionally cause a relapse of symptoms in women who have otherwise appeared to have had successful surgical treatment. Physiotherapy exercises for the pelvic floor musculature should be encouraged from the outset.

Labor/delivery

There is general consensus that allowing a vaginal delivery of a term baby may jeopardize the success

---

PROLAPSE
Summary of Management Options

Prepregnancy

- Conservative management if possible; definitive surgery arguably best deferred until after family complete

Prenatal

- Screen for urinary infection

- Consider physiotherapy and ring or other pessaries if troublesome

- Avoid surgery to correct prolapse during pregnancy

Labor/delivery

- Elective cesarean section if previous successful surgery for prolapse

Postnatal

- Encourage physiotherapy and exercises

- Review 3–6 months after delivery for a long-term management plan

---

of a repair operation; consequently, most obstetricians advocate elective cesarean section in such women. However, should premature labor occur, vaginal delivery is often allowed, presumably because the premature fetus will not traumatize the lower genital tract and pelvic musculature in the same way as a term fetus.

OTHER GYNECOLOGICAL DISEASES AND PROBLEMS
Congenital Disorders

A few women have congenital abnormalities of their genital tract that affect the pregnancy or labor/delivery.

The most common disorder is the vaginal septum, which is fenestrated superiorly such that labor may be obstructed. This is simply managed acutely by division of the septum in the second stage, usually under epidural or local anesthesia. Hemostatic measures are not usually required.

Cervical Stenosis from Previous Cone Biopsy

Rarely, the fibrosis associated with a cone biopsy may inhibit the progress of labor. Usually, such fibrosis actually inhibits fertility. If pregnancy occurs, the fibrosis then becomes evident during the vaginal examination in labor. Rather than incise the cervix, and risk lateral extension and hemorrhage, a cesarean section is a safer alternative.

Previous Third-degree Tear Repair

If there has been a previous third-degree repair, a generous mediolateral episiotomy to avoid the sphincter and perineum should be undertaken. However, if healing of the previous third-degree repair was complicated, and especially if there was a fistula, elective cesarean section is advisable.

Vaginal Infection

Herpetic infections are a particular risk to the fetus, and can be distressing to the mother. They can cause urinary retention, which is best managed symptomatically or by suprapubic catheterization (the pain causes spasm of the pelvic floor musculature and consequently micturition cannot be initiated).

Recurrent thrush infection in pregnancy suggests some altered immunity or disordered carbohydrate metabolism. Apart from relieving the vaginal irritation, it is important to 'reduce' infection prior to delivery so that the infant does not suffer from oral thrush at a time when feeding should be becoming established.

Diffuse congenital condylomatous lesions can complicate vaginal deliveries, usually by causing bleeding. The fetus may also acquire the disease prenatally or during passage through the birth canal; perineal or laryngeal papilloma in the neonate may be difficult to treat.

Treatment of the condylomata is arguably best done using cryosurgery rather than electro-cautery or CO_2 laser, since bleeding, necrosis and secondary infection are less frequent. Podophyllin is contraindicated during pregnancy.

Vulval Varicosities

Vulval varicosities are unsightly and sometimes uncomfortable. Medical treatment by injections should be avoided during pregnancy. Bed rest and support tights may produce symptomatic improvement. They should be avoided during episiotomies as they can bleed profusely. Occasionally, vaginal varicosities are traumatized during delivery, but primary surgery repair and hemostasis are usually effective.

FURTHER READING

Subfertility

1 Yovich JL, Matson PL (1988) The treatment of infertility by the high intrauterine insemination of husband's washed spermatozoa. *Human Reproduction* **3**:939–943.
2 Tuck SM, Yukin PL, Turnbull AC (1988) Pregnancy outcome in elderly primigravidae with and without a history of infertility. *British Journal of Obstetrics and Gynaecology* **95**:230–237.
3 AIH National Perinatal Statistics Unit (1991) *Assisted Conception Australia and New Zealand 1989*. Sydney: AIH.

Ovarian Cysts

1 Lavery JP, Koontz WL, Layman L, Shaw L, Gumpel U (1986) Sonographic evaluation of the adnexa during pregnancy. *Surg Gynecol Obstet* **163**:319–323.
2 Nelson MJ, Cavalieri R, Graham D, Saunders RC (1986) Cysts in pregnancy discovered by sonography. *Journal of Clinical Urology* **14**:509–512.
3 Thornton JG, Wells M (1987) Ovarian cysts in pregnancy: Does ultrasound make traditional management inappropriate? *Obstetrics and Gynecology* **69**:717–721.
4 Allen JR, Helling TS, Langenfeld M (1989) Intrabdominal surgery during pregnancy. *American Journal of Surgery* **158**:567–569.
5 Granberg S, Norstrom A, Wikland M (1991) *Journal of Ultrasound in Medicine* **10**:9–14.

Fibroids

1 Valle RF (1990) Hysteroscopic removal of submucous leiomyomas. *J Gynecol Surg* **6**:89–96.
2 Lev-Toaff AS, Coleman BG, Arger PH, Mintz MC, Arenson RL, Toaff ME (1987) Leiomyomas in pregnancy: Sonographic study. *Radiology* **164**:375.
3 Marut EL (1989) Etiology and pathophysiology of fibroid tumour disease: Diagnosis and current medical and surgical treatment alternatives. *Obstetrical and Gynecological Survey* **44**:308–310.

Prolapse

1   MacDonald D (1982) Previous obstetrical or gynaeco-
    logical surgery. *Clinics in Obstetrics and Gynaecology*
    9:147–159.
2   Finn WF (1948) The outcome of pregnancy following
    vaginal operations. *American Journal of Obstetrics and
    Gynecology* **56**:291–299.

Other Gynecological Diseases

1   Baker DA (1990) Herpes and pregnancy: New manage-
    ment. *Clinics in Obstetrics and Gynecology* **33**:253–256.
2   Patsner B, Baker DA, Orr JW Jr (1990) Human papil-
    lomavirus genital tract infections during pregnancy. *Clin-
    ics in Obstetrics and Gynecology* **33**:258–267.
3   Vin F (1990) Vulvar varices. *J Mal Vasc* **15**:406–409.

36

Chorionic Villus Sampling and Placental Biopsy

WOLFGANG HOLZGREVE, PETER MINY

INDICATIONS

Chorion frondosum or placental tissue sampled by catheter or needle aspiration or biopsy is an alternative to amniotic fluid and fetal blood sampling for prenatal diagnosis of genetic disorders throughout gestation.[1] It is the method of choice for the second trimester diagnosis of monogenic disorders which require a large amount of DNA or where a rapid karyotype is required.

Chorionic Villus Sampling (CVS) in the First Trimester of Pregnancy

Direct chromosome preparations from the cytotrophoblast and rapid culture techniques using the mesenchymal core of the villi permit early and rapid karyotyping during the first trimester. Exclusion of maternal age-related aneuploidy is by far the most frequent indication for CVS, followed by a history of either a previous aneuploid child or a monogenic disorder. The distribution of indications in **Table 1** summarizes our experience. CVS can be more acceptable than conventional amniocentesis to some women, especially in high-risk situations like a parental balanced structural chromosomal abnormality or when a late termination of pregnancy has already been experienced due to aneuploidy. In addition to classic cytogenetic indications, villi can also be used for the diagnosis of chromosomal breakage syndromes, fragile X, and for rapid sexing in pregnancies at risk for X-linked diseases.

Chorionic villi are an excellent source of DNA, sup-

Table 1
Indications for CVS[a]

	n	%
Maternal age	3678	82.6
Previous child with aneuploidy	273	6.1
Risk for monogenic disorder	270	6.1
Parental chromosome rearrangement	44	1.0
Suspicious ultrasound findings	27	0.6
Others	163	3.7
Total	4455	100.1

[a]As of 31 December 1992.

plying sufficient amounts for most molecular genetic techniques without prior culture. The frequent high recurrence risks (25% with autosomal recessive disease, 50% in male fetuses of carriers for X-linked conditions) also favor an early diagnostic test which allows, if chosen by the parents, a termination of pregnancy prior to 12 weeks. Some conditions which have been diagnosed using CVS samples are listed in **Tables 2** and **3**. Today, biochemical testing of a CVS sample is possible for almost all metabolic diseases that can be diagnosed from amniotic fluid cells. Due to the rapid progress in molecular genetics, the number of diagnosable, monogenic disorders is increasing steadily. However, an increased risk for neural tube defects remains an indication for amniocentesis because alpha-fetoprotein testing cannot be performed on chorionic tissue. In

Table 2
X-linked diseases as indication for CVS
or placental biopsy (CVS program, Münster)

Indication	n	Test
Duchenne muscular dystrophy	59	DNA
Hemophilia A/B	19	DNA
Menke syndrome	6	copper determination
MPS II Hunter	6	enzyme
Chorioideremia	3	DNA
X-linked hydrocephalus	3	ultrasound
Adrenoleukodystrophia	3	long-chained fatty acids
Wiskott-Aldrich syndrome	3	fetal blood sampling
Norrie syndrome	4	DNA
X-linked thrombocytopenia	1	fetal blood sampling
Fragile X	3	DNA, chromosomes
Lowe syndrome	3	DNA
Incontinentia pigmenti	1	fetal skin biopsy
OTC deficiency	3	DNA, fetal liver biopsy
Pelizaeus Merzbacher syndrome	1	DNA
Total	118	

Table 3
Autosomal recessive diseases as indication for
CVS or placental biopsy (CVS program, Münster)

Indication	n	Test
Thalassemia/hemoglobinopathy	55	DNA
Cystic fibrosis	37	DNA
MPS I Pfaundler-Hurler	13	enzyme
MPS III Sanfilippo A-C	8	enzyme
MPS IV Morquio	2	enzyme
AGS	9	HLA, DNA
Krabbe disease	4	enzyme
Cystinosis	3	cystine determination
Gaucher disease	2	enzyme
Niemann-Pick disease	3	enzyme
Zellweger syndrome	5	long-chained fatty acids
Alpha-1-antitrypsine deficiency	3	DNA
Fructose intolerance	1	enzyme
Tay-Sachs disease	5	enzyme
G_{M1}-gangliosidosis	4	enzyme
G_{M2}-gangliosidosis	2	enzyme
Propionic acidemia	1	enzyme
HMG-CoA lyase deficiency	2	enzyme
Hypophosphatasia	2	enzyme
Chondrodysplasia punctata	1	enzyme
Spinal muscular atrophy SMA II	3	DNA
Total	165	

case of doubt, a geneticist should be consulted as early as possible.

Placental Biopsy in the Second and Third Trimesters of Pregnancy

Despite a decreasing mitotic index in the cytotrophoblast of the aging placenta, both rapid karyotyping by direct chromosome preparation and culture are feasible throughout gestation.[2] Frequent indications for third trimester CVS include ultrasound findings suspicious of fetal aneuploidy, followed by women with other indications such as late registration, failed amniotic fluid cell cultures, or late maternal serum screening results (**Table 4**). As compared with lymphocyte cultures after fetal blood sampling, direct chromosome preparation after placental biopsy is, in some laboratories, available on the same day. A placental biopsy may be easier to perform than cordocentesis in women with hydramnios. A representative distribution of the gestational ages at the time of placental biopsy from

Table 4
Indications for placental biopsy[a]

	n	%
Suspected rubella infection, IUD removal	11	1.2
Confirmation	46	5.2
Late booking		
failure to obtain result	29	3.3
maternal serum screening	120	13.5
DNA diagnosis	19	2.1
others (e.g. maternal age)	54	6.1
Suspicious ultrasound findings	609	68.6
Total	888	100

[a]As of 31 December 1992.

Number of procedures

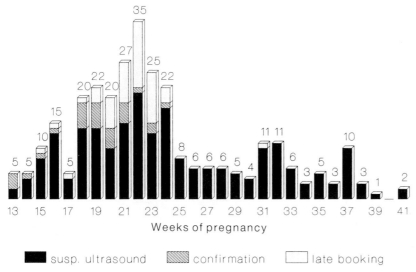

Weeks of pregnancy

■ susp. ultrasound   ▨ confirmation   □ late booking

Figure 1. Distribution of gestational ages at the time of placental biopsies.[3]

Table 5
Results of placental biopsies in 609 women with suspicious ultrasound findings (University of Münster, 31 December 1992)

Result	n	%
46,XY or 46,XX	486	79.8
Chromosomal anomaly (structural or aneuploidy)		
45,X	29	4.8
47,+18	25	4.1
Triploidy	20	3.3
47,+21	20	3.3
47,+13	15	2.5
46,XX/47,XX,+13	1	0.2
47,XX,+9	1	0.2
46,XX/47,XX,+9	1	0.2
47,XX,+21/48,XX,+18,+21	1	0.2
46,XX,13q–	1	0.2
45,X/46,Xr(X)46,XX	1	0.2
46,XY,del(7q)	1	0.2
47,XYY	1	0.2
47,XXY	1	0.2
45,X/46,XY	1	0.2
46,XY/47,XY,+i(12p)	1	0.2
46,XY,t(12;16)(p12;q11)	1	0.2
46,XX/47,XX,+21	1	0.2
46,XX/47,XX,+16 (uniparental mat. disomy 16 in the fetus)	1	0.2
Total	123	100.6

our series[3] is depicted in **Figure 1**. There is a clear peak shortly before the 24th week of gestation, which is the legal limit for termination of pregnancy for genetic indications in Germany. **Table 5** summarizes a recent account of the cytogenetic results after placental biopsies in more than 500 women with suspicious ultrasound findings indicating a 20% risk of aneuploidy in this group.

Procedure: CVS in the First Trimester of Pregnancy

*Of the 10 plus different techniques proposed for CVS in the first trimester, only two are adopted on a large scale.[4,5] Until today, most procedures were performed transcervically.[6] A bendable polyethylene catheter with a metal obturator or angled metal aspirator is introduced through the cervix and guided to the chorion frondosum under continuous simultaneous ultrasound guidance (**Figures 2a** and **b**). With an attached syringe partly filled with medium, a vacuum is applied and approximately 10–50 mg of tissue are aspirated and rinsed into a sterile Petri dish. Some workers use a curved biopsy forceps to obtain the material. The transvaginal approach is not generally used after 13 weeks.*

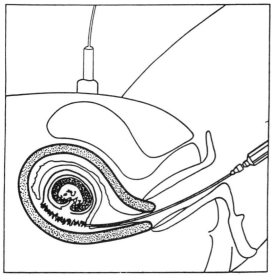

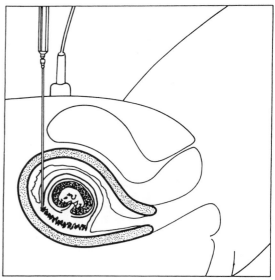

a

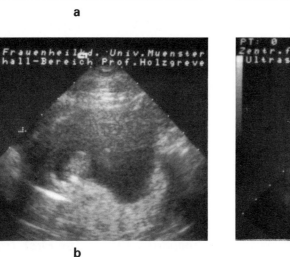

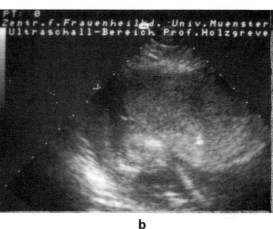

b

Figure 2. Transcervical CVS: (a, upper) schematic depiction; (b, lower) ultrasound picture.

Figure 3. Transabdominal CVS: (a, upper) schematic depiction (b, lower) ultrasound picture.

*The transabdominal technique was first developed in Denmark by Smid-Jensen and Hahnemann.[7] It can be applied either as a free-hand, ultrasound-guided, fine-needle aspiration or with a needle guide ultrasound transducer (**Figures 3a** and **b**). In either case, continuous simultaneous ultrasound is mandatory. By minimizing unintended lateral movement, placental trauma should be reduced. The aspirated tissue needs to be carefully separated under a dissection microscope in order to exclude contamination with maternal cells (decidua, blood).* **Figure 4** *illustrates a Petri dish with clean chorionic villi, a villus and decidua. The main advantage of CVS performed for advanced maternal age is the rapidity of the result. However, not all cytogenetics laboratories have been successful in producing high-quality direct preparations. In those centers where a culture must be awaited before giving a normal result, CVS has little advantage over early amniocentesis (see Chapter 40).*

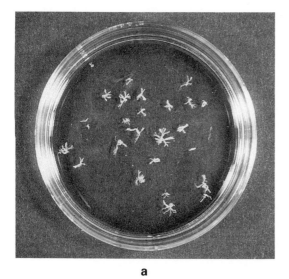

a

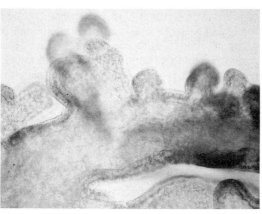

b

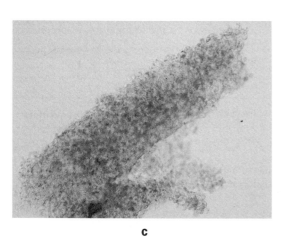

c

Figure 4. (a, upper) Chorionic villi after separation; (b, middle) chorionic villus under dissection microscope; (c, bottom) decidua under dissection microscope.

Procedure: Placental Biopsy in the Second and Third Trimesters of Pregnancy

Placental biopsies in late gestation are only performed transabdominally by applying the same techniques used in the first trimester. **Figure 1** *illustrates that placental biopsies can be performed as late as 41 weeks when immediate perinatal decisions are required in the presence of suspicious ultrasound findings. Some investigators use a 'double needle' technique where a guide needle is advanced through the uterine wall and an inner needle then placed for aspiration of villi. Others apply a 'single needle' approach, usually with a 20-gauge spinal needle.[3] A transabdominal placental biopsy forceps is also used by some workers; this is introduced through an outer guide needle.*

COMPLICATIONS

Procedure-related risks

The medical risks of pregnancy termination are considerably higher as gestational age advances.[8] Various studies[9,10] confirm that women would prefer an early diagnosis compared with a late diagnosis provided the risks of both procedures are equal. In one study, women aged 35 years or more were asked after extensive counseling to choose between no test, amniocentesis or joining a trial. The majority chose to have some test and CVS was a more popular choice than amniocentesis.[11] Similar findings have been reported by others.[12]

Randomized[13,14] and controlled[15] trials have been published that compare first trimester CVS and conventional amniocentesis (i.e. after 15 weeks gestation). Whereas the randomized Canadian and the controlled American trials did not reveal a significant difference in fetal loss rates, the randomized MRC European trial showed a significantly higher rate of live-birth infants who survived in the amniocentesis group. There is no clear explanation for the difference. Altogether, 31 centers participated in the MRC trial, contributing variable numbers of cases. The number of repeat procedures was significantly higher in the CVS group compared with the amniocentesis group. Recently, concern was raised that CVS may cause severe limb deficiencies.[16] However, after reviewing the international literature and taking our own experience of more than 3500 cases into account, we could not confirm the initial report.[17] An informal survey conducted in September 1991 among the members of the so-called 'Fetoscopy Group' indicated that the risk for limb reduction defects after CVS may be higher if the procedure is performed before 9 weeks gestation (**Table 6**).

Table 6
Limb reduction defects after CVS[a]

	< 9 weeks	≥ 9 weeks
Limb reductions	9/2971 (0.302%)[b]	33/49 731 (0.066%)[b]

[a]Fetoscopy Group Meeting, Hong Kong, September 1991.
[b]$P < 0.01$.

One randomized clinical trial, which compared transcervical and transabdominal CVS, did not reveal a significant difference between the techniques regarding safety and efficiency.[18] However, Smid-Jensen and Philip found a higher risk of a loss in their transcervical CVS group compared with their transabdominal CVS and amniocentesis group.[19] Analogous to the relationship between incidence and timing of pregnancy losses and maternal and gestational ages,[20] Jahoda et al.[21] observed that the fetal loss rates of older women after transcervical and transabdominal sampling was between 5.8 and 6.2% but dropped to 2.4% after 12 weeks. Similar losses have been reported by others.[22] The safety and reliability of late placental biopsies have been established in several individual series,[3,23,24] as well as in a large international survey.[25] There is no data to suggest biopsy is more dangerous than aspiration when carried out by the same route.

Diagnosis-related Risks

The contamination of chorionic cell cultures with maternal cells causing a false-negative diagnosis is a possible hazard of CVS or placental biopsies. This issue is especially critical in DNA diagnosis using polymerase chain reaction amplification and in some biochemical examinations. In our experience (**Figure 5**), the risk of maternal cell contamination is clearly related to the experience of the person separating the tissue microscopically.

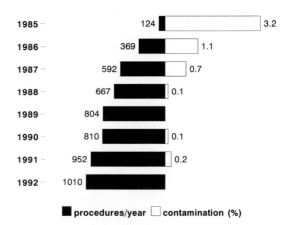

■ procedures/year □ contamination (%)

Figure 5. Maternal cell contamination in the CVS program, Münster.

There have been occasional diagnostic errors due to incorrect interpretations of apparent placental mosaicism. The large-scale use of chorionic and placental cells for diagnostic purposes has greatly increased our understanding of early human development.[26] Today, it is well established that aneuploidy (mosaic and, rarely, non-mosaic) may be confined to extra-embryonic or extrafetal tissues, while the fetus proper has a normal chromosome count. A number of so-called false-positive (aneuploidy not confirmed in the fetus) and a few false-negative results (fetal aneuploidy not detected in chorionic or placenta cells) have been reported after CVS or placental biopsy.[27] In larger series, true mosaicism is found in about 1% of samples (**Table 7**). Most of these instances represent mosaicism which is confined to the chorion or placenta. In these cases, confirmation of aneuploidy by examination of another tissue (either fetal blood or amniotic fluid cells) is mandatory before termination of pregnancy is

Table 7
Mosaicism

	Not confirmed	Confirmed
Low *a priori* risk (n = 4736) (maternal age, screening etc.)	43 (0.9%)	7 (0.1%)
High *a priori* risk (n = 636) (suspicious ultrasound findings)	12 (1.9%)	5 (0.8%)

As of 31 December 1992

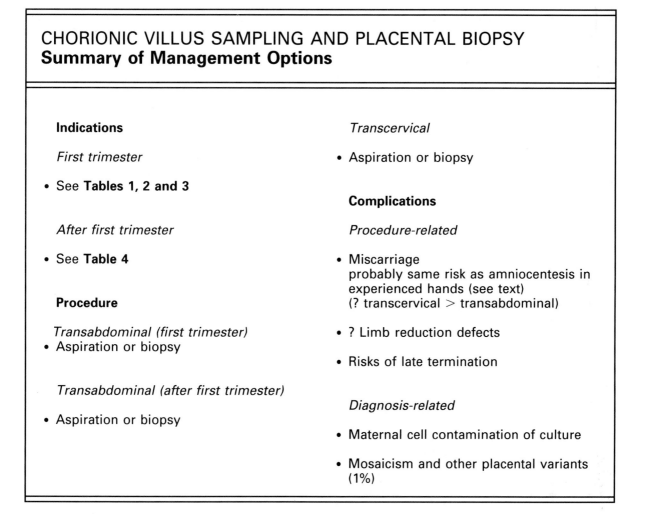

CHORIONIC VILLUS SAMPLING AND PLACENTAL BIOPSY
Summary of Management Options

Indications

First trimester

- See **Tables 1, 2 and 3**

After first trimester

- See **Table 4**

Procedure

Transabdominal (first trimester)
- Aspiration or biopsy

Transabdominal (after first trimester)
- Aspiration or biopsy

Transcervical

- Aspiration or biopsy

Complications

Procedure-related

- Miscarriage
  probably same risk as amniocentesis in experienced hands (see text)
  (? transcervical > transabdominal)

- ? Limb reduction defects

- Risks of late termination

Diagnosis-related

- Maternal cell contamination of culture

- Mosaicism and other placental variants (1%)

---

considered. There is evidence now that confined placental mosaicism may lead to intrauterine growth deficiency and an increased risk for miscarriage. In some cases, uniparental disomy has been demonstrated in newborns after the diagnosis of confined placental mosaicism,[28] presumably originating from mitotic chromosomal loss during the early cleavage of a trisomic zygote.

So-called false-negative results after CVS or placental biopsy originate from mosaicism in the fetus and/or placenta and are – with only a very few exceptions – restricted to cases where direct preparation is performed exclusively. The simultaneous analysis of cultured cells reliably prevents diagnostic errors by raising the likelihood of detecting mosaicism in both the placenta and fetus. Of course, culture also increases the time before an answer is available. As in any other tissue used for prenatal diagnosis of aneuploidy, it has to be kept in mind that any realistic number of cells used for chromosome analysis still represents an extremely narrow sample, and that low-grade mosaicism may remain undiagnosed.

CONCLUSIONS

Placental biopsy is an acceptably safe alternative to either amniocentesis or cordocentesis from the late first trimester onward. Because culture may be avoided, placental biopsy specimen shortens the time necessary for the diagnosis of monogenic disorders which require a sizable amount of DNA. It may be performed either transvaginally up until 13 weeks or transabdominally throughout gestation. The most common indication for placental biopsy is to rule out a karyotypic abnormality in a woman over age 35 years. For this indication, there are alternatives, including traditional and early amniocentesis. The inability of the cytogenetics laboratory to produce high-quality direct preparations counters some of the inferred advantages of placental biopsy, since a culture must be performed. True mosaicism is observed in approximately 1% of samples. Most are confined to the placenta and/or the chorion. Any abnormality observed on the direct preparation should be confirmed by a culture, except in the presence of diagnostic ultrasound findings.

REFERENCES

1   Holzgreve W, Tercanli S, Schneider HPG, Miny P (1992) Prenatal karyotyping: When, whom, and how? *Journal of Ultrasound in Obstetrics and Gynecology* **2**:64–69.

2   Simoni G, Gimelli G, Cuoco C, Romitti L, Terzoli G, Guerneri S, Rossella F *et al.* (1986) First trimester fetal karyotyping: one thousand diagnoses. *Human Genetics* **72**:203–209.

3   Holzgreve W, Miny P, Gerlach B, Westendorp A, Ahlert D, Horst J (1990) Benefits of placental biopsies for rapid karyotyping in the second and third trimesters (late chorionic villus sampling) in high-risk pregnancies. *American Journal of Obstetrics and Gynecology* **162**:1188–1192.

4   Ward RHT, Modell B, Petrou M, Karagözlu F, Douratsos E (1983) Method of sampling chorionic villi in the first trimester of pregnancy under guidance of real time ultrasound. *British Medical Journal* **286**:1542.

5   Holzgreve W, Miny P (1987) Chorionic villi sampling with an echogenic catheter: experiences with the first 500 cases. *Journal of Perinatal Medicine* **15**:244.

6   Jackson L (1991) *CVS Newsletter* 31 (Jan 28th).

7   Smid-Jensen S, Hahnemann N (1984) Transabdominal fine needle biopsy from chorionic villi in the first trimester. *Prenatal Diagnosis* **4**:163.

8   Fletcher JC (1986) Ethical issues in clinical trials of first trimester prenatal diagnosis. In Brambati B, Simoni G and Fabro S (eds) *Chorionic Villus Sampling* pp. 275–301. New York: Dekker.

9   Lippman A, Perry TB, Mandel S, Cartier L (1985) Chorionic villi sampling: women's attitudes. *American Journal of Medical Genetics* **22**:395–401.

10 McGovern MM, Goldberg JD, Desnick RJ (1986) Acceptability of chorionic villi sampling for prenatal diagnosis. *American Journal of Obstetrics and Gynecology* **155**:25–29.

11 Abramsky L, Rodeck CH (1991) Women's choices for fetal chromosome analysis: *Prenatal Diagnosis* **11**:23–28.

12 Brandenburg H, Van der Zwan L, Jahoda MGJ, Stijnen TH, Wladimiroff JW (1991) Prenatal diagnosis in advanced maternal age. Amniocentesis or CVS, a patient's choice or lack of information? *Prenatal Diagnosis* **11**:685–690.

13 Canadian Collaborative CVS-Amniocentesis Clinical Trial Group (1989) Multicentre randomised clinical trial of chorion villus sampling and amniocentesis. *Lancet* **1**:16.

14 MRC Working Party on the Evaluation of Chorion Villus Sampling. (1991) Medical Research Council European Trial of chorion villus sampling. *Lancet* **1**:1491–1499.

15 Rhoads GG, Jackson LG, Schlesselman SI *et al.* (1989) The safety and efficacy of chorionic villus sampling for early prenatal diagnosis of cytogenetic abnormalities. *New England Journal of Medicine* **320**:609.

16 Firth HV, Boyd PA, Chamberlain P, MacKenzie IZ, Lindenbaum RH, Huson SM (1991) Severe limb abnormalities after chorion villus sampling at 56–66 days' gestation. *Lancet* **1**:762–763.

17 Schloo R, Miny P, Holzgreve W, Horst J, Lenz W (1991) Limb reduction defects following chorionic villus sampling. *American Journal of Medical Genetics* **42**:404–413.

18 Brambati B, Terzian E, Tognoni G (1991) Randomized clinical trial of transabdominal versus transcervical chorionic villus sampling methods. *Prenatal Diagnosis* **11**:285–293.

19 Smid-Jensen S, Philip J (1991) Comparison of transabdominal and transcervical CVS and amniocentesis: sampling success and risk. *Prenatal Diagnosis* **11**:529–537.

20 Simpson JL (1990) Incidence and timing of pregnancy losses: Relevance to evaluating safety of early prenatal diagnosis. *American Journal of Medical Genetics* **35**:165–173.

21 Jahoda MGJ, Brandenburg H, Reuss A, Cohen-Overbeek TE, Wladimiroff JW, Los FJ, Sachs ES (1991) Transcervical (TC) and transabdominal (TA) CVS for prenatal diagnosis in Rotterdam: experience with 3611 cases. *Prenatal Diagnosis* **11**:559–561.

22 Young SR, Shipley CF, Wade RV, Edwards JG, Waters MB, Cantu ML, Best RG, Dennis EJ (1991) Single center comparison of results of 1000 prenatal diagnoses with chorionic villus sampling and 1000 diagnoses with amniocentesis. *American Journal of Obstetrics and Gynecology* **165**:255–263.

23 Hogdall CK, Doran TA, Shime J *et al.* (1988) Transabdominal chorionic villus sampling in the second trimester. *American Journal of Obstetrics and Gynecology* **158**:345–349.

24 Chieri PR, Aldini AJR (1989) Feasibility of placental biopsy in the second trimester for fetal diagnosis. *American Journal of Obstetrics and Gynecology* **160**:581.

25 Holzgreve W, Miny P, Schloo R (1990) "Late CVS" International registry compilation of data from 24 centres. *Prenatal Diagnosis* **10**:159–167.

26 Kalousek DK, Barrett IJ, Gärtner AB (1992) Spontaneous abortion and confined chromosomal mosaicism. *Human Genetics* **88**:642–646.

27 Miny P, Hammer P, Gerlach B, Tercanli S, Horst J, Holzgreve W, Eiben B (1991) Mosaicism and accuracy of prenatal cytogenetic diagnoses after chorionic villus sampling and placental biopsies. *Prenatal Diagnosis* **11**:581–589.

28 Purvis-Smith SG, Saville T, Manass S, Yip M-Y, Lam-Po-Tang PRL, Duffy B, Johnston H, Leigh D, McDonald B (1992) Uniparental disomy 15 resulting from "correction" of an Initial trisomy 15. *American Journal of Human Genetics* **50**:1348–1349.

37

Abnormalities of Alpha-fetoprotein and Other Biochemical Tests

ROGER A. WILLIAMSON

INTRODUCTION

Maternal serum screening in pregnancy is a process of identifying patients whose fetuses are at greater risk for disorders amenable to prenatal detection. Screening is the first step leading to one or several more definitive tests and/or procedures. The first test to achieve widespread acceptance and utilization was the maternal serum assay for a fetal-specific protein termed alpha-fetoprotein (AFP). Transudation of AFP across open neural tube defects (NTDs) was first shown in 1972 to elevate the maternal serum (MSAFP) and amniotic fluid (AFAFP) concentrations.[1]

Today, MSAFP screening has become the framework upon which other pregnancy screening tests have been added. Most of these latter protocols have taken advantage of the modestly reduced levels of MSAFP[2] and the marked association of higher levels of human chorionic gonadotropin[3] with Down's syndrome. Unconjugated estriol is also decreased and has been incorporated into some screening protocols.[4] Other serum markers and other screening modalities show promise and could be applied in the future.

The attitude of different countries toward biochemical screening is evolving and reflects their resources and perceived needs. If testing is to be done, it should be within an organized and efficient program with prompt access to follow-up services. The laboratory aspects of these programs are critical: '[a] screening program should be established only when there is linked excellent interdisciplinary support among obstetrician, laboratory, clinical geneticist, ultrasonographer, and an identified program coordinator'.[5]

MATERNAL SERUM ALPHA-FETOPROTEIN SCREENING (MSAFP)

Physiology of AFP

Alpha-fetoprotein, a glycoprotein similar in molecular weight and structure to albumin, is made first in the fetal yolk sac and then primarily in the fetal liver. Its function is unknown. The rare fetus who makes no AFP because of a presumed mutation of the gene on chromosome 4 is otherwise normal.[6]

Fetal serum AFP concentration peaks at about 13 weeks. It enters the amniotic fluid largely via fetal urination after renal filtration. Amniotic fluid AFP rises until approximately 12 weeks and thereafter declines. In contrast, MSAFP continues to rise until 30–32 weeks before declining. The AFP enters the maternal circulation by diffusion across the placenta and amnion. During the period of testing from 15 to 20 weeks, MSAFP rises about 15% per week and the gradient of levels between amniotic fluid and maternal serum is 100:1 to 200:1. A similar gradient exists between fetal serum and amniotic fluid.

Neural Tube Defects

Neural tube defects (NTDs) are common major birth defects, second in frequency only to congenital heart disease (see Chapter 50). The birth prevalence of NTDs varies by geographic locale, race and certain maternal conditions. In the USA, the prevalence in Caucasians is 1–2 per 1000 but varies four-fold from regions of lowest to highest prevalence.[7] In some parts of the UK, the rate is about three times greater than the overall rate in the USA.[8] Blacks have about one-half the incidence of Caucasians.[7] Maternal risk factors are shown in **Table 1**.[9–16]

Most NTDs are isolated and presumed multifactorial in causation. About half are defects in spinal closure and half anencephaly. A recurrent NTD tends to be concordant, i.e. open spina bifida more likely to again be spina bifida and anencephaly to recur as anencephaly.[10] Ten percent of spinal NTDs are skin covered and hence do not leak AFP. Encephaloceles represent 5–7% of NTDs and greater than 50% of these are closed. NTDs can be a component of chromosome abnormalities such as trisomies 13, 18 and triploidy and of a single gene disorder such as Meckel-Gruber syndrome.[9] The heterogeneity of NTDs is illustrated by a study of more than 100 stillborn or live-born infants with an NTD where only 12% had a definable cause.[17]

A positive family history increases the risk. For countries with a birth prevalence of 1–2 per 1000, if a couple has previously had a child with a neural tube defect, or if one or other parent is affected, the risk is 1–3%; for two affected children, the risk rises to approximately 6%.[9–11] Since males are not as frequently affected as females, the recurrence risk after an affected male is somewhat higher. A higher prevalence of the disorder in the population increases the risk.[18] **Table 2** illustrates the risk for recurrence of a neural tube defect in families with a positive history in the USA and the UK. Affected family members more remote than first-degree relatives variably increase a fetus' chance,[19] as do combinations of affected family members.

Why Screen for NTDs?

At least 90% of infants with an NTD are born to couples with a negative family history. Prenatal AFP testing began in the UK in the early 1970s. A large collaborative study demonstrated that screening could

detect the majority of open neural tube defects.[20] Screening was found to be most accurate between 16 and 18 weeks; the accuracy dropped significantly prior to 15 weeks. A further multicenter study in the UK demonstrated that 98% of open neural tube defects had an amniotic fluid AFP (AFAFP) which exceeded their defined cut-offs, increasing from 2.5 times the median at 13–15 weeks gestation to 4.0 times the median at 22–24 weeks.[21]

Subsequent to the studies in the UK, other countries, including the USA and Germany, reported favorable experiences with MSAFP screening in large pilot or regional projects.[5,22–24] A consensus conference was convened in 1983 to consider the important elements of MSAFP program development.[25] The signatories from the USA, UK, Canada, Germany, Switzerland, Sweden, Finland and Denmark concluded that MSAFP screening was cost-effective and that laboratories should perform at least 400 serum AFP tests per month to maintain proficiency.

Acetylcholinesterase (AChE) is a neural tissue specific enzyme which has proven helpful in distinguishing open NTDs from most other causes of elevated AFAFP.[26] Although AChE is present in high concentrations in fetal cerebrospinal fluid and low concentrations in fetal serum, it is not detectable by gel electrophoresis in amniotic fluid of normal gestations. The AChE assay should be performed when the AFAFP level is ≥ 2.0 MoM (multiple of the median).[27]

Usually AFP is expressed as the multiple of the median (MoM). An MoM is obtained by dividing an individual's MSAFP value by the median for the relevant gestational week. Using the MoM to normalize AFP values allows information from different laboratories to be interpreted in a common manner, allows for the rising MSAFP and declining AFAFP during the period of screening, and can be readily adjusted for the variables which affect AFP determinations such as diabetes, weight and race. It also provides a more precise parameter for setting screening cut-offs as opposed to standard deviations and percentile ranks.[28]

When an NTD has been discovered prenatally, counseling and pregnancy management issues arise for which the reader is referred to Chapter 50. Of great significance for couples who have had a fetus/child with an NTD is the protective effect of periconceptional folate in reducing the recurrence risk.[29]

Other Abnormalities Detected by MSAFP Screening

MSAFP is elevated by a number of other fetal and placental abnormalities which require specialized attention (**Table 3**).[30] Other fetal body openings, principally gastroschisis and omphalocele (combined birth

Table 1
Risk factors for neural tube defects

Positive family history: first- to third-degree relation[9–11]
Maternal insulin-dependent diabetes mellitus[12]
Maternal valproic acid therapy[13]
Maternal gastric bypass surgery[14]
Prior birth of a child with hydrocephalus or multiple
   vertebral defects[15,16]

Table 2
Fetal risk for NTD

Relation with NTD	Prevalence per 100 births	
	USA	UK
Parent	1–3	4–5
One sibling	2–3	5
Two siblings	5–6	10–12
Half-sibling	0.8	
Maternal aunt's child	1	
Other first cousins	0.3	

Adapted from Refs 8–11, 18.

Table 3
Conditions associated with elevated MSAFP levels

Neural tube defects
Abdominal wall defects
Fetal growth deficiency and death
Congenital nephrosis
Certain skin disorders
Upper fetal bowel obstruction
Obstructive uropathy and other renal abnormalities
Sacrococcygeal teratoma
Congenital cystic adenomatoid malformation
Amniotic band disruption
Placental and umbilical cord tumors
Other placental abnormalities, including fetomaternal
    hemorrhage and oligohydramnios
Multiple gestation
Gestation more advanced than suspected
Maternal liver disease

prevalence about 1:3000), are associated with elevated MSAFP and AFAFP. Of the two abdominal wall defects (AWDs), the uncovered gastroschisis has the highest MSAFP values. When testing for AChE in the presence of an AWD, there is often a dense pseudo-cholinesterase (PChE) band and a weak AChE band. These findings are more common with gastroschisis than omphalocele. The death of a co-twin can also produce these biochemical findings, but in these circumstances there may also be multiple bands of non-specific cholinesterases from the degrading tissues.

The rare autosomal recessive condition of congenital nephrosis is associated with striking elevations of AFP in maternal serum and amniotic fluid.[31] The cases of which we have personal experience have shown a mean MSAFP of 13 MoM and a mean AFAFP of 38 MoM. The AChE assay is negative and this condition can only be suspected after the exclusion of others. Because fetal swallowing regulates a portion of AFAFP, upper fetal bowel interruptions or obstructions may be associated with elevated AFP levels and can occasionally produce a positive AChE band.[32] The mechanism for this finding is unclear.

Several rare skin disorders mimic findings seen with NTDs, including elevated MSAFP, AFAFP and a strong positive AChE band.[33] These conditions encompass several genetic forms of epidermolysis bullosa and cutis aplasia. MSAFP testing cannot, however, be relied upon as a screen for these disorders. If, for instance, a couple has had a child with the autosomal recessive lethal epidermolysis bullosa, a fetal skin biopsy is required for definitive diagnosis (see Chapter 56).

Other fetal conditions which have shown a relationship, though inconsistent, with an increased MSAFP, include fetal obstructive uropathies and other renal disorders, sacrococcygeal teratoma, congenital cystic adenomatoid malformation, amniotic band disruption, and placental and umbilical cord tumors. Turner's syndrome has been mentioned as one condition which can be associated with an elevated AFAFP. However, more recent experience suggests the reported elevations were probably associated with an inadvertent puncture of large cystic hygroma at amniocentesis.[34] Finally, maternal liver disease can be a rare cause for significant elevations in MSAFP. Maternal liver function tests and occasionally other diagnostic evaluations may be indicated.

In the absence of fetal structural abnormality, the most important risk/consequences of an elevated MSAFP are fetal growth deficiency and death, oligohydramnios, placental abruption and preterm delivery (see below).

Description of an MSAFP Screening Program

The author has been associated with the state of Iowa MSAFP Screening Program since its inception in 1984. MSAFP testing is restricted to the laboratory designated by the Birth Defects Institute of the State Health Department. Test interpretation and follow-up are coordinated by members of the Prenatal Genetics Division of the state's medical school. The laboratory participates in the New England Regional Genetics Group sponsored External Quality Assessment Program for Pregnancy AFP.[35]

Figure 1 illustrates the protocol followed which assumes a prevalence of NTDs of 1:1000.[7] Screening cut-offs are determined to maximize detection while keeping false-positives at an acceptable rate. An initial serum is considered elevated if it is $\geq$ 2.2 MoM. If so, an ultrasound is performed locally for dating and a

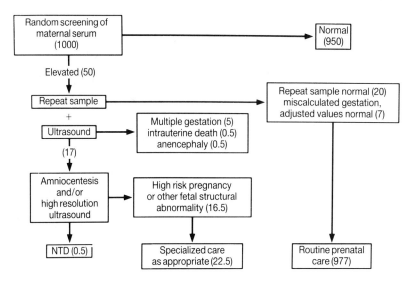

Figure 1. Expected outcomes of 1000 women undergoing MSAFP screening. The accuracy for NTD detection is optimal between 16 and 18 weeks. Modified from American College of Obstetrics and Gynecology Technical Bulletin No. 154, April 1991.

repeat serum sample obtained at least 7 days after the first sample. Combining an ultrasound with the second sample rather than performing this study only if the repeat MSAFP is still elevated, hastens the screening process and hence the resolution of anxiety. If one value is $\geq$ 2.2 MoM and the other $\geq$ 2.5 MoM, the local physican is advised to refer the patient to a tertiary center. It is reasonable to forego a second sample if the first specimen is quite elevated or the gestation is more advanced.

Patients are referred to our Fetal Diagnosis and Treatment Unit because of the availability of higher resolution equipment and the increasing sophistication of sonologists in recognizing spinal and cranial signs of a fetal NTD (see Chapter 50). A normal scan eliminates at least 95% of any MSAFP-associated risk.[36] Amniocentesis may be elected if suboptimal views of the fetus are obtained or for added reassurance despite a normal scan. The use of amniocentesis with an elevated MSAFP varies between centers. Each center has to make policy decisions based on the quality of its ultrasound equipment and skill and experience of its sonographers. Some units rarely resort to amniocentesis, whereas others frequently do so.

A technical consideration of some importance is the performance of the amniocentesis (see Chapter 40). Ultrasound guidance or direction doubtless decreases the fetal loss rate and will substantially reduce the number of specimens contaminated with fetal blood.[37] Fetal blood contamination has been the major cause of

a false-positive AFAFP. If the fluid has greater than 60×10^6 fetal RBCs/ml, the AChE will also be falsely positive.[38]

The performance of a fetal karyotype is another issue when considering an amniocentesis for elevated MSAFP. Accumulated studies suggest that the risk of a chromosome abnormality with elevated MSAFP levels when the scan is normal and the woman less than age 35 is about 0.6%. About one-third of these are sex chromosome aneuploidy.[36] The risk for Down's syndrome is lowered by an elevated MSAFP. If a woman is age 35 or older, the consideration for a karyotype is stronger. All of these factors become a part of counseling a woman contemplating amniocentesis for elevated MSAFP. If the fetus has a structural abnormality, or there are alterations of fluid volume or fetal growth, a karyotype is indicated. In such circumstances, the incidence of a chromosome abnormality is substantial.[39] NTDs are associated with a chromosome abnormality in a small percentage of cases and a karyotype is desirable to provide more definitive counseling.

Applying the protocol illustrated in **Figure 1**, there should be a 5–6% initial positive rate. Ultimately, about 1.5% of the screened population require tertiary level services as described. Within this latter group, one in 30 women have a fetus with an open spina bifida. When a program is in place, periodic monitoring of these variables should be undertaken. If the numbers of false-positives and/or women referred for tertiary level services and/or fetal abnormalities detected show a trend away from the expected yield, efforts should be made to determine the cause. Any physician who is screening gravidas should be able to obtain this information readily. However, it is essential for physicians and their patients to understand that about 15% of open spina bifida will not be detected.

The issue of using cut-offs to trigger a tertiary level referral as opposed to stating a woman's risk for an NTD or AWD based on her level of MSAFP and other relevant factors[40] is largely philosophical. There are proponents of both approaches. Most programs have adopted a binary approach to MSAFP screening, i.e. a woman is or is not at risk based on defined cut-offs without indicating the magnitude of risk. However, stating a patient-specific risk has become common when screening for fetal chromosome abnormalities, though a woman may be called 'positive' or 'negative' based on a cut-off.

Laboratory Aspects

There are a number of kits for MSAFP determination which perform reliably over the range of values important for detecting NTDs (50–100 ng/ml). Some are radioimmunoassays and others enzyme-immunoassays. There are advantages and disadvantages to both, but either can be reliable for screening. The same kits used for MSAFP testing can be used for AFAFP deter-

mination after dilution of the sample. This must be by the diluent provided by or recommended by the kit manufacturer.

Normative data should be established in the population served by a laboratory.[25,41] One hundred samples per gestational week from unaffected pregnancies will suffice to set the medians for screening. *Using inappropriate reference data is a common cause of error in screening recommendations.*[35]

Once stable medians have been established for a laboratory, assay precision and accuracy must be monitored using carefully defined internal and external controls.[42] Precision refers to the coefficient of variation (CV) when performing replicate assays on the same samples. The greater the assay CV, the greater is the overlap of MSAFP distribution curves of affected and unaffected. **Figure 2** shows the expected distribution of these curves. If the CV becomes unacceptably large, the false-positive rate rises commensurately without an appreciable effect on NTD detection. Accuracy refers to the laboratory result compared with a known external standard. Participation in a well-designed external quality control program will help ensure accuracy. Using rigorous internal and external quality control methods will also protect against assay drift, a tendency for there to be a change in medians over time as compared with the original reference data which have been collected.[43,44] Assay drift will produce an effect similar to assay imprecision.

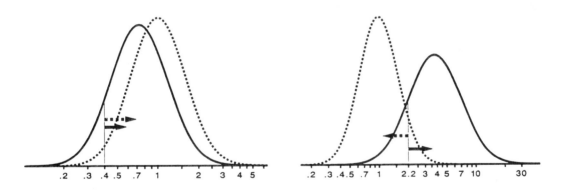

Figure 2. (Left) The distribution of MSAFP in multiples of the median (MoM) in pregnancies associated with Down's syndrome (DS: solid line) and unaffected pregnancies (dotted line). For pregnancies associated with a DS fetus and for normals, a second value will tend to move toward the mean of the population from which that sample was obtained and in the same direction. Thus, a woman who is carrying a DS fetus and is called 'positive' at 0.4 MoM, for example, may be removed from this risk category upon repeat sampling. In contrast, a repeat sample if the MSAFP is initially elevated does help to distinguish those fetuses who do have an NTD from those who do not. (Right) The distribution of MSAFP values in pregnancies associated with an open spina bifida (solid line) and unaffected pregnancies (dotted line). The repeat specimens after an initial elevation of 2.2 MoM, for example, will tend to move in opposite directions and toward the mean of the populations they represent, thus enhancing detection of NTDs. Distribution curves reproduced from Knight *et al.*[80] with permission.

Several variables are known which influence MSAFP values (see **Table 4**). Blacks have about 10% higher levels of MSAFP than do Caucasians, Orientals and Hispanics,[45] and a lower incidence of NTDs. For regions with Black populations, adjustments are appropriate.[46] Insulin-dependent diabetics have lower levels of MSAFP,[47] but they also have an incidence of NTD about four times the background.[12] Appropriate adjustments need to be made for these factors. In the Iowa program, an MSAFP value from a diabetic is called positive if it is $\geq$ 1.5 MoM after dividing her MoM by 0.8. The class of diabetes does not seem to influence MSAFP levels, nor does glucose control as judged by glycosylated hemoglobin values.[48] Weight correction is another important laboratory consideration.[49] For lighter women with relatively greater levels and heavier women with lesser levels, most authorities agree that weight correction is indicated. This will result in a gain in specificity with no sacrifice in sensitivity.[50]

Twins have, on the average, twice the level of MSAFP as singletons. Data exist to estimate NTD risk in twins.[51] A cut-off of $\geq$ 4.0 MoM will detect 58% of NTDs in twins with a false-positive rate of 7.8%. At a cut-off of $\geq$ 5.0 MoM, 39% of NTDs will be detected with a false-positive rate of 3.3%. More recent data from a small study revealed a detection rate of open spina bifida of 85% in twins with a cut-off of 4.5 MoM.[52] In our screening program, referral is initiated for a value $\geq$ 4.5 MoM.

If an amniocentesis is to be performed in a twin gestation, zygosity and resultant placental anatomy can influence amniotic fluid values when one twin is affected and the other is not.[53] Whether monozygous or dizygous, if the placenta is dichorionic, diamnionic the amniotic fluid values are usually reliable. *However, if the placenta is monochorionic, diammionic the fluid from the sac of the unaffected twin can often show a falsely elevated AFP and positive AChE.* This also applies to abdominal wall defects in twin gestation. Again, detailed ultrasound will be of aid in this circumstance. Concordance for NTD in twins is about 7%.[54]

Table 4
Factors which influence MSAFP concentrations

Blacks have 10% higher MSAFP levels than do Caucasians, Orientals or Hispanics and a lower incidence of NTDs

Insulin-dependent diabetic patients have lower MSAFP levels but four times the incidence of NTD than non-diabetic patients

Maternal weight <115 lb (52 kg) or >175 lb (80 kg)

Women with a twin gestation have, on average, twice the level of AFP found in women with singleton pregnancies.

Other Approaches to NTD Detection

Targeted screening

In some countries, organized MSAFP programs targeting the entire pregnant population do not exist. In this circumstance, reasonable attempts can be made to specifically study those pregnancies at highest risk by ultrasound or a combination of ultrasound and MSAFP. For example, a family history of NTD is rather frequent and data are available to estimate the risk if a second- or third-degree relative of a fetus is affected.[19] The highest risk is for a fetus whose maternal aunt has an affected child (about 1%).

Ultrasound

Ultrasound is a particularly important modality for some at-risk pregnancies, such as for insulin-dependent diabetes where the risk is not only for NTDs, but also for heart, renal defects and other central nervous system disorders.[12] The anticonvulsant, valproate, significantly increases the risk for an NTD. *Many of the NTDs caused by valproate are skin-covered and will not be detectable by MSAFP.* MSAFP screening may miss Meckel-Gruber, which is characterized by encephalocele, polydactyly and polycystic kidneys, if the encephalocele is skin-covered. For each, ultrasound is the only other readily available diagnostic tool.

The question is whether NTD detection would be better served by routine ultrasound. The cost of ultrasound in many countries is very high. Further, it is not practical because there are insufficient trained personnel to carry out the task. One potential advantage of MSAFP screening is that an elevated MSAFP distinguishes a group of pregnancies at greater risk for numerous adverse outcomes, including the structural malformations discussed.

Other Adverse Pregnancy Outcomes with Elevated MSAFP Levels

Several investigations have clarified the previously known association between an elevated MSAFP unassociated with a structural malformation and an adverse pregnancy outcome.[55–58] The principal risks are fetal death, intrauterine growth deficiency, first trimester and late pregnancy bleeding, and preterm delivery. One study observed an adverse outcome in 24, 41 and 91% if a woman's second trimester MSAFP was 2.5–2.9 MoM, 3.0–5.0 MoM, or $\geq$ 5.0 MoM, respectively.[56] In a case-control study, women with MSAFP levels $\geq$ 3.0 MoM had a 10.4 odds ratio of fetal death; this ratio was 2.4 if the levels were between 2.0 and 2.9 MoM.[57]

Elevated MSAFP is not a reliable screen for the subsequent development of pre-eclampsia.

A particularly ominous finding is the presence of oligohydramnios and high MSAFP. The initial task is to determine whether the urinary tract is present and normal. In many such cases, the urinary tract is structurally normal. Despite this, the outlook for a successful pregnancy is severely compromised.[59,60] An abdominal pregnancy may also explain these findings.[59]

An elevated MSAFP level also predicts pregnancy complications in twin gestations. In 145 gestations where neither twin had a structural defect, an MSAFP of $\geq$ 4.0 MoM was associated with a mean gestation at delivery of 32.5 weeks, mean birthweights of 1963 and 1523 g, and a perinatal mortality of 400 per 1000. In contrast, if the MSAFP was less than 2.0 MoM, the mean gestation was 37 weeks, the birthweights 2507 and 2443 g, and the perinatal mortality rate 32.6 per 1000.[61] An MSAFP $\geq$ 5.0 MoM was associated with a loss in greater than 50% in another study.[62]

Knowledge of an elevated MSAFP unassociated with a fetal structural malformation should trigger a change in prenatal care. Careful fetal surveillance is indicated. The frequency and intensity of follow-up is dictated by many factors, including the MSAFP levels, amniotic fluid volume, fetal size, length of gestation, placental appearance, and fetal well-being testing. It is presently unknown whether such alterations will improve the perinatal outcome, though they may provide the insights which will allow effective intervention strategies to be developed.

A prominent feature of MSAFP screening is the anxiety generated by an elevated MSAFP level. Anxiety levels do return to baseline when follow-up studies suggest the fetus does not have a structural defect.[63] Yet, as indicated, some of these pregnancies remain at higher risk for complications. One reason to continue to follow at-risk pregnancies in a specialized unit is that an ongoing dialogue can be maintained. In other situations, increased medical contact has appeared to decrease the risk of an adverse outcome.

MSAFP Screening: Conclusion

The measurement of the maternal serum concentration of alpha-fetoprotein has proven a cost-effective screening tool for the detection of open spine defects. Targeted screening based on recognized risk factors will lead to identification of a minority of cases. MSAFP screening also leads to the identification of fetuses with a variety of other malformations including abdominal wall defects and trisomy 21. Pregnancies complicated by an elevated MSAFP unassociated with a fetal malformation are at increased risk for perinatal morbidity and mortality. The greater the increase, the greater the

---

MATERNAL SERUM ALPHA-FETOPROTEIN SCREENING
Summary of Management Options

see Figure 1

The decision to use high-resolution ultrasound rather than amniocentesis to identify fetuses with structural abnormalities will depend on:

- The quality of the ultrasound equipment

- The skill and expertise of the sonographers

- The ease with which the fetal anatomy can be visualized

---

risk of an untoward outcome. For maximal efficiency and to minimize unnecessary parental concern, the screening program requires planning, the hiring of skilled personnel, and strict laboratory quality controls.

MATERNAL SERUM SCREENING FOR FETAL CHROMOSOME ABNORMALITIES

In some countries MSAFP screening has become an integral part of routine obstetric practice. The same status is beginning to be achieved in some locales or countries for one or more of the screening tests which enhance detection of fetal chromosome abnormalities. For the previously established MSAFP program, the addition of other tests can be accomplished without major logistic or laboratory problems. The principal effort is instructional. Continuing education for practitioners and their patients is essential.

For many programs, screening for fetal chromosome abnormalities has progressed in stages. The first test shown to be altered with a chromosome abnormality was MSAFP and its association with Down's syndrome (DS). Thus, many programs began fetal aneuploidy screening with this marker. As other markers have shown an association, one or more have been incorporated. This chapter is written during a period of intense research activity relating to fetal- and placental-specific markers which may allow screening to become more effective.

MSAFP and Down's Syndrome

The overall risk for Down's syndrome (DS) at the time of amniocentesis in women age 35 and older is 1:140. Because age 35 has been the standard time in many countries when amniocentesis is recommended, the detection rate for screening programs has been compared with this group. These programs are usually thought of as DS screening programs because this is the most common chromosomal condition (birth prevalence about 1:700) and because of its clinical significance in terms of severity and compatibility with life. DS is also the condition for which these screening protocols are relatively more effective.

A 1984 retrospective study revealed an association between lower levels of MSAFP and DS.[2] This decrease has been repeatedly confirmed and is, on average, 25% less than the level in women with chromosomally normal fetuses and not maternal age dependent.[64] Prospective trials were begun to validate the use of MSAFP screening in women less than age 35. The first study combining age-related risk with a low level of MSAFP in women less than age 35 revealed a detection rate below that achieved using age 35 and above as the criterion for amniocentesis.[65] In this study, individual risks were assigned based on a weight-corrected MSAFP level, gestation and maternal age, and about 5% of screened women were identified with a risk equal to or greater than that of a 35-year-old woman.

A more recent prospective study of 77 000 women conducted in the New England region of the USA revealed that MSAFP could be made more efficient than using age 35 and older as the criterion for amniocentesis.[66] The study criteria included maternal age less than 35, weight-adjusted MSAFP, individualized risk figure based on age and MSAFP level, analysis of only one serum, ultrasound to confirm or correct dates, and amniocentesis for a DS risk equal to or greater than 1:270 (the midgestational risk for a 35-year-old woman). Ultrasound corrected 40% of initial positives; 2.7% of screened women remained at risk after ultrasound. Down's syndrome was detected in 1:89 at-risk pregnancies. Four trisomy 18 fetuses were also detected, raising the yield to 1:64. Other studies have confirmed that this screening protocol will detect chromosome abnormalities other than DS. These include trisomy 13, trisomy 18, Turner's syndrome, and some chromosomal deletions.[67]

If all women age 35 or older (5% of the pregnant population) underwent amniocentesis, 20% of all fetuses with DS would be detected. If all women less than age 35 were to be screened with MSAFP and amniocentesis performed for a calculated risk equal to or greater than a 35-year-old woman, another 25% of DS cases would be detected. Thus, a maximum of 45% of DS cases could potentially be detected with MSAFP alone.

Other Maternal Serum Markers: Unconjugated Estriol (MSuE₃) and Human Chorionic Gonadotropin (MShCG)

It is not apparent why women carrying Down's syndrome fetuses have a lower concentration of MSAFP. In one small study, fetal serum AFP from normal and Down's syndrome fetuses did not differ.[68] Nonetheless, there was reason to speculate that another product of the feto-placental unit, unconjugated estriol (uE_3), might be similarly decreased because the fetal liver is the source of AFP. Synthesis of uE_3 requires a key fetal precursor from liver, 16-alpha OH-dehydroepian-drosterone. Indeed, $MSuE_3$ levels were found to be about 27% lower for DS pregnancies.[69] An expanded study concluded that screening sensitivity for fetal trisomy 21 could be doubled by adding $MSuE_3$ to the established MSAFP screening protocol and performing an equivalent number of amniocenteses.[70] Though one study did not find an association between lower levels of $MSuE_3$ and DS,[71] all other published studies have revealed this difference.[72] *The principal benefit of incorporating $MSuE_3$ into screening protocols is its effect on lowering the rate of false-positives.*

The most effective marker demonstrated to date has been human chorionic gonadotropin (hCG). This placental-specific product is elevated about twice normal in DS pregnancies[3,4] and several other chromosome abnormalities.[3] The reason for the increase is unknown. Whereas both MSAFP and $MSuE_3$ rise between weeks 14 and 21, the latter increasing 25% per week, MShCG falls. **Figure 3** illustrates the effect of gestation on these three markers. The concentrations of the three markers with DS approximate those of a normal fetus 2–3 weeks earlier in gestation. Thus, some have surmised the levels reflect functional 'immaturity' of DS fetal organs.

Screening for Chromosome Abnormalities Based on Multiple Markers and Maternal Age

A three-center collaborative effort between groups in London, UK and the New England region of the USA has demonstrated that combined maternal age and the measurement of the triple markers improves screening sensitivity for DS compared with previously described

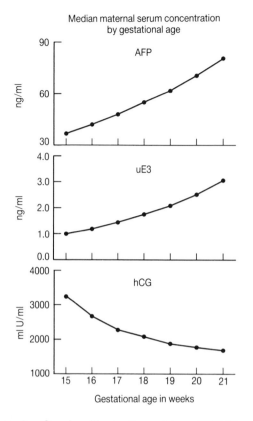

Figure 3. Graphs illustrating rising MSAFP and MSuE$_3$ and falling MShCG levels during the period of testing from 15 to 20 weeks. Provided courtesy of the University Hygienic Laboratory, Oakdale, Iowa.

DS protocols.[4] The London group posesses the world's largest bank of second trimester sera, ($n = 77$) from women across the age spectrum carrying a DS fetus. The above study verified the Down's syndrome–hCG relationship and indicated a method of calculating risk. Maternal age is independent of the three markers and can therefore be used to define a risk *a priori*. Since the three markers are not completely independent of each other, a trivariate Gaussian distribution has been successfully fitted to the data and the necessary parameters to calculate an individual's risk based on age, MSAFP, MSuE$_3$ and MShCG derived. A software package, Alpha Program (Logical Medical Systems, London, UK), is available to assist these calculations.

Table 5 illustrates the increased sensitivity achieved when screening is based on age alone as the criterion for amniocentesis *vs* less than 35 and MSAFP *vs* age-related risk and the multiple markers. Along with the increasing detection efficiency, both the cost–benefit ratio and the number of procedure-related losses of normal fetuses for each DS case detected are reduced. Another feature of Table 5 is the relatively large number of initial elevations secondary to an overestimation

of gestational age. When a gestational dating error has occurred, overestimation is slightly more common than underestimation. *An underestimation of gestational age is a frequent reason for a false-positive MSAFP elevation.*

Table 6 reveals the fact that triple-hormone screening can 'spread out' the calculated risk. This distribution of potential risk figures is much greater than that achievable by using MSAFP and age as the screening variables, or age alone. This ability to expand the numbers may have the greatest relevance for programs choosing to offer the amniocentesis option based not on a screening cut-off, but rather on a woman's perceived risk when comparing her age-related risk before screening with that after screening.

Table 7 shows the effect of choosing two cut-offs currently in use in different centers. If one chooses a risk cut-off of 1:190, about 1:20 women are candidates

Table 5
Clinical sensitivity and specificity of major screening categories

	Maternal age 35 and above	Maternal age <35 and MSAFP[a]	Maternal age MSAFP + MSuE$_3$ + MShCG[b]
Sensitivity (detection rate)	20%	25%	60%
Initial positive rate	5%	4.7%	6%
Amniocentesis recommended after ultrasound	NA	2.7%	4.5%

[a]Assumes 1:270 cut-off. Adapted from Palomaki *et al.*[66]
[b]Assumes 1:190 cut-off. Adapted from Wald *et al.*[4]

Table 6
Risk distribution by various combinations of multiple-marker values for a 35-year-old woman

	MoM	MoM
MSAFP	0.4	2.5
MDSuE$_3$	0.4	1.4
MShCG	2.0	0.5
Combined risk	1:16	1:52 000

The midtrimester risk before screening for a 35 year old woman is 1:270. A woman with the median value, 1.0 MoM, for each marker receives a substantial reduction of risk, 1:1400. Adapted from Wald *et al.*[4]

Table 7
Estimated effects of selecting two commonly used
cut-offs for screening

Risk cut-off	False-positive rate	Detection rate
1:190	4.5%	60%
1:270	8%	68%

Data adapted from Wald *et al.*[4]

for amniocentesis with an estimated 60% detection
rate. In this circumstance, about 1:50 amniocenteses
would show DS. Using a 1:270 cut-off, there is a false-
positive rate of about 8%, with only a modest gain in
detection rate. As data with triple-hormone screening
has accumulated, it is evident that a majority of cases
of DS will be found when the calculated risk is 1:100
or greater.

As stated, the test with the greatest benefit is hCG.
Thus, some programs have utilized two markers,
MSAFP and MShCG. MSAFP is included because of
its ability to detect NTDs. One relatively small retrospective study documented that the use of these two
could yield a DS detection rate and amniocentesis rate
similar to that projected with triple-hormone testing.[73]
Thus, the issue of adding MSuE$_3$ presents itself. The
best available data suggest that the principle benefit of
adding this assay is its effect of reducing the false-
positive rate.[4,74] Improving the detection rate is a more
modest effect of MSuE$_3$. **Tables 8** and **9** illustrate these
points. Studies which claim equivalent or greater benefit from one group of markers (i.e. MSAFP and
MShCG) as opposed to triple-hormone screening, or
claim one hCG assay (i.e. free beta) is more sensitive
than another,[75] must be viewed critically. A proper
study would compare these assays within the same

Table 8
Influence on false-positive rate of adding MSuE$_3$ to
screening protocols

Detection rate	False-positive rate using age, MSAFP and MShCG	False-positive rate using age, MSAFP MShCG and MSuE$_3$	Difference
50%	3.7%	2.5%	−33%
60%	6.7%	4.7%	−30%
70%	12%	8.6%	−28%

Data adapted from Wald *et al.*[4]
A commonly stated endpoint of triple hormone is a 60%
detection rate with a false-positive rate about 5%. For these
screening levels, MSuE$_3$ decreases the false-positive rate by
approximately one-third.

Table 9
Influence on detection rate of adding MSuE$_3$ to
screening protocols

False-positive rate	Detection rate using age, MSAFP and MShCG	Detection rate using age, MSAFP, MShCG and MSuE$_3$	Difference
5%	55%	61%	+11%
6.5%	59%	65%	+10%
8.0%	64%	69%	+8%

Data adapted from Wald *et al.*[4]
MSuE$_3$ has a lesser effect on detection rate than it does on
decreasing the false-positive rate. At a 5% false positive rate,
the increase in detection rate is about 11%, as shown.

population instead of comparing outcomes for different
populations which may differ in maternal age distribution and other relevant factors.

When contemplating multiple-marker screening,
there are a number of approaches. Some program direc-
tors will feel more comfortable allowing time for
analysis of the currently accumulating prospective data
before initiating this form of screening. MSAFP has
been shown to be a valid screen for aneuploidy, and
in areas with established MSAFP programs it may be
elected to begin with this marker.

Prospective data on triple-hormone screening is
accumulating as this chapter is being prepared, and the
data from many centers, including ours, suggest the
benefits projected. A large prospective study in the
New England region of the USA has demonstrated that
triple marker screening performed somewhat better
than predicted,[4] with a lower false-positive rate (4.5%
vs 3.8%) and comparable detection rate.[76]

Risk Assessment Using MSAFP and Other Laboratory Considerations

In the USA, commercially available AFP kits were
approved for NTD screening and were not optimized
for measurements of MSAFP in the range associated
with DS (10–25 ng/ml). Nonetheless, some kits proved
reliable and others were made reliable by modification.
External quality control programs not only aid in
determining kit performance but also in assisting the
correction of a problem when found.[35] Notably, the
measurements obtained using one kit were consistently
lower in the Down's syndrome range, leading to an
excessive number of false-positives until discovered
through quality assurance testing and corrected.[77]
Other data suggest that maternal ingestion of medication such as aspirin may lower MSAFP values. Care-

ful external quality testing has shown that aspirin does not have this property. *There is currently no solid evidence that any drug significantly alters MSAFP levels.*

One laboratory consideration which has caused some confusion is the recommendation that only one specimen (if drawn at the appropriate time) be analyzed to assign a DS risk. The rationale for this practice is illustrated in **Figure 2** and involves the concept of regression to the mean.[78] Repeat specimens enhance screening for NTDs. However, screening efficiency is decreased if a second sample is used to assign a DS risk. Risk calculations could be modified to accommodate a second sample, but no gain would be realized in doing so. Even when using three markers, two of which are lower but one higher than normal with DS, it is valid to test a single sample.

There are a number of ways by which risk may be assigned when screening with MSAFP alone. A set MoM cut-off may be utilized, say less than 0.4 MoM or less than 0.5 MoM, to offer amniocentesis for anyone less than age 35. Others have assigned cumulative risks for groups of women of a certain age range at a specified MSAFP cut-off.[79] Both of these methods may significantly underestimate or overestimate an individual's true risk. Since age and MSAFP level are independent predictors of risk, it is a relatively simple matter to calculate an individual's risk which is specific to her age and her MSAFP MoM. A thorough treatment of these concepts as they involve MSAFP and DS screening has been provided.[80] Some of these same concepts apply when multiple markers are used, though, as mentioned, the mathematical treatment of risk is more sophisticated because the levels of the multiple markers are not completely independent of one another.

Triple-marker screening has been shown to be valid without yet applying the potential effects of race, weight and/or maternal conditions to the interpretatation of $MSuE_3$ and MShCG. These adjustments may not need to be made, but insufficient data are available to make definitive recommendations.

Maternal weight does affect MShCG concentration and some have advised weight correction.[81,82] $MSuE_3$ is less affected by weight, though a correction formula has been derived for this parameter.[82] There are data to suggest that weight-corrected MShCG levels are higher in Orientals and Black women than in Caucasians or Hispanic women.[81] There is no evidence that the incidence of aneuploidy varies by race.

Presently, an aneuploidy risk is not assigned for twins because there is insufficient data from twin pregnancies discordant for DS. Several studies have documented that MShCG, like MSAFP, is about two-fold higher in twin gestations compared to singletons.[83,84] However, $MSuE_3$ levels were significantly less than 2.0 MoM in twins in one study.[83]

Also remaining to be explored in greater depth are adverse pregnancy outcomes which may be predicted by altered levels of MShCG not associated with aneuploidy.[81] One pattern, consisting of a high hCG and undetectable MSAFP and $MSuE_3$, is correlated with hydatidiform mole. Perhaps higher or lower levels of $MSuE_3$ may be found to be associated with certain adverse outcomes. It is known that undetectably low levels of maternal serum estriol can occur with anencephaly or rare conditions such as congenital adrenal hypoplasia or placental steroid sulfatase deficiency.

Down's Syndrome Screening in a Statewide Program

The state of Iowa initiated DS screening based on lower levels of MSAFP in 1987; triple-hormone screening was begun in 1990. **Figure 4** illustrates the protocol followed.[85]

We elected the following parameters for screening: three markers measured in a single sample drawn at an appropriate time, ultrasound to correct or confirm gestational age, a risk cut-off of 1:190, weight correction for the MSAFP value, and use of day-specific medians (risk can be refined by utilizing day-specific rather than week-specific medians). Though these calculations can be done by recording LMP or fetal biparietal diameter (BPD), the BPD is accurate for DS screening[86] and actually enhances NTD detection.[87] The BPD of fetuses with a NTD is generally smaller than normal, causing the MSAFP level to be artificially elevated.

Much debate centers on whether to use a 'screen-positive/screen-negative' approach with an arbitrary cut-off value (e.g. 1:190) as illustrated in **Figure 4** or merely to quote the risk calculated and let the patient decide for herself whether that figure constitutes a 'high' or 'low' risk (perhaps using her age-related risk for comparison).

To tighten the screening process, we have urged that a dating ultrasound accompany the first specimen unless a woman has regular cycles, a reliable LMP, and confirmatory uterine size on physical examination.

Screening protocols such as the one outlined in **Figure 4** substantially increase detection of DS and some other chromosome abnormalities. Because this screening is a second trimester endeavor, abnormalities are inevitably detected at a later stage of pregnancy than would be the case if found by chorionic villus sampling, an early amniocentesis, or even the traditional time for amniocentesis of 16 weeks. Thus, if an abnormality is found, the emotional cost may be greater.[88] It is incumbent upon programs to ensure sensitive and medically competent abortion services which may be required at greater than 20 weeks in some cases. Counseling services which extend beyond the period of ter-

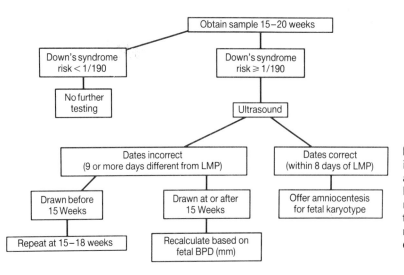

Figure 4. Triple-hormone screening protocol for risk assessment and detection of fetal aneuploidy. Low values are not routinely repeated because of regression to the mean (see **Figure 2**). LMP, last menstrual period; BPD, biparietal diameter. Reproduced from Williamson[85] with permission.

mination, if elected, have become an integral component of our program. It is also important not to neglect a couple who have chosen to continue the pregnancy of an affected fetus, but to provide ongoing support and counseling. The practitioner should select a screening program which readily provides the necessary information (e.g. the percentage of screened women offered amniocentesis and the ratio of abnormalities detected to procedures performed) indicating the screening process is accomplishing the stated goals.

Screening for Trisomy 18

It has become evident that trisomy 18 may present with a unique maternal serum profile which can become the basis of a specific screen for this severe disorder.[89] Trisomy 18 is associated with lower levels of MSAFP and $MSuE_3$, as in DS, but the hCG level is also reduced rather than elevated. We have participated in a study where an amniocentesis was recommended if a woman's serum profile showed $MSAFP \leq 0.75$ MoM, $MSuE_3 \leq 0.60$ MoM, and $MShCG \leq 0.55$ MoM.[90] A specific risk figure is not assigned. Preliminary data indicate that about 50% of trisomy 18 fetuses can be detected with an increase in the amniocentesis rate of only 0.4%. About 1:16 procedures will be associated with trisomy 18, making this a remarkably effective screen.

Trisomy 18 fetuses may be undergrown even at 15–20 weeks, and ultrasound biometry suggesting a younger gestation was one cause of missing such cases when MSAFP alone was used as the screen.[91] With all three markers depressed, the current recommendation is to proceed directly to amniocentesis without obtaining a dating ultrasound at that time.

The hormone profile unique to trisomy 18 can also be applied in selected cases. For instance, the finding

of a choroid plexus cyst in the second trimester is common and it usually represents a benign finding (see Chapter 50). However, it may be associated with

---

MATERNAL SERUM SCREENING FOR FETAL CHROMOSOMAL ABNORMALITY
Summary of Management Options

See Figure 4

It should be noted that different centers have different approaches to reporting the risk for Down's syndrome based on maternal serum screening:

- Some take an arbitrary cut-off point and report all values that fall above that value as 'screen-positive' and those that fall below that value as 'screen-negative'. The actual cut-off point varies, e.g. 1:190; 1:200; 1:250; 1:300;

- Others prefer to report the actual calculated risk (e.g. 1:237) and allow the patient to decide whether that is an acceptable risk, perhaps in comparison with her age-related risk.

trisomy 18 in about 1% of such cases.[92] If the fetal growth by ultrasound is normal and no other anomalies are seen, the triple hormone screen may provide reassurance to forego amniocentesis.

Maternal Serum Screening for Chromosome Abnormalities: Conclusion

Once established, an MSAFP screening program can be expanded with reasonable cost for the detection principally of trisomy 21. Fetuses with trisomy 21 have lower MSAFP and serum unconjugated estriol (uE_3), and higher serum human chorionic gonadotropin (hCG) concentrations. Combined with knowledge of the maternal age and gestational age, these factors may be combined to predict the likelihood of the fetus having trisomy 21. Their accuracy is such that three times the number of fetuses with trisomy 21 will be identified as would be using maternal age alone as an indication for testing. Further, less normal fetuses are subjected to the risks of second trimester amniocentesis.

FUTURE DEVELOPMENTS

Ultrasound

A number of studies, which will not be reviewed in detail, have suggested that ultrasound may be a useful screen for DS because of the findings of a shortened femur, increased nuchal skinfold thickness, and hypoplasia of the middle phalanx of the fifth finger producing an incurving (clinodactyly). While these findings have been replicated, they are rather operator- and equipment-dependent. Even when these factors are optimized, the sensitivity and specificity are not such that these findings could be used as a unique screen.[93] It may be, however, that ultrasound will become one component of a DS screen, perhaps helping to refine a risk assigned from maternal age and triple-hormone screening. Nuchal skinfold thickness may become an important parameter if first trimester screening becomes feasible (see below).

Triple Hormone Screening at Age 35 and Above

Despite cautions voiced from many quarters, it is inevitable that some women age 35 and older will desire to use triple-hormone screening to modify their risk. Some investigators feel the detection rate is not high enough to offset the value of universally offering amniocentesis for this age group and/or that chromosomal

abnormalities other than DS may not be detected as predictably as might be desired.[94]

A prospective trial coordinated by principal investigators from the Foundation for Blood Research and the California MSAFP program is ongoing to answer this important question. Samples are being contributed by multiple centers. It is projected that at a screening cut-off of 1:270, 90% of DS cases will be detected with an amniocentesis rate of 30% of the screened women.

Other Hormone Markers

At present, about 40 pregnancy-specific proteins have been found. The function of most is obscure. Several have been studied for a possible association with fetal aneuploidy. Placental-specific products including progesterone, human placental lactogen, and SP_1 (pregnancy-specific $beta_1$-glycoprotein) are elevated with DS.[95] None is as elevated as hCG, and factoring these assays into a risk calculation does not significantly enhance screening. Other placental products are currently being investigated, such as Pap A or pregnancy-associated plasma protein A. From these studies, markers superior to hCG may be found.

First Trimester Screening

It would be an obvious advantage if screening could be performed as reliably in the first trimester as in the second. From several studies, it appears that MSAFP is lower in the first trimester of DS pregnancies.[96, 97] $MSuE_3$ was also lower in one study.[98] However, hCG does not discriminate DS from normal in the first trimester,[97,98] though trisomies 13 and 18 have lower levels of hCG in the first trimester.[97,99] From the information thus far gathered, it appears that for the foreseeable future fetal aneuploidy screening will remain a second trimester option.

Other combinations of pregnancy markers may prove feasible for first trimester screening. One promising approach is the 'aneuploidy index' obtained by multiplying the ratios of progesterone/hCG and free alpha-hCG/hCG.[99] This calculation may provide a reasonable first trimester screen by taking advantage of trends of these multiple markers. Further study is required.

Another test which has shown the greatest sensitivity yet reported is an activity measurement of urea-resistant neutrophil alkaline phosphatase.[100] For 72 women with DS fetuses, this test detected 79% with a 5% false-positive rate at the cut-off selected. Two of three tests from the first trimester were clearly elevated, with the third close to the cut-off. Whether this test will be clinically useful is unknown as the test will require automation and the interpretation is subjective.

CONCLUSIONS

These screening programs are complex, requiring constant communication between physician offices, program coordinators and laboratory personnel. Abnormal screens must be resolved as rapidly as possible; thus the need for centralized, efficient and comprehensive services. In addition, readily accessible genetic counseling for an individual at any stage of the screening process is critically important.

Because of the deeply felt sensitivities about tests which can lead to the detection of abnormalities for which there is no prenatal treatment, this form of prenatal testing should be voluntary.[25,41] A specimen should be obtained only after fully informed consent. To draw these tests because they are 'standard of care' with the view that one will deal with the abnormals as they arise is to invite trouble.

Finally, there is concern among some that prenatal testing has become a euphemism for modern-day eugenics, an attempt to rid society of 'undesired' members. As long as the decision to have or not to have such testing, or to elect a pregnancy termination or not if an abnormality is found, remains with an informed woman or couple, this concern will largely be obviated. Nonetheless, one must be constantly vigilant against any coercive influences, however subtle and from whatever source.

REFERENCES

1   Brock DJH, Sutcliffe RG (1972) Alpha-fetoprotein in the antenatal diagnosis of anencephaly and spina bifida. *Lancet* **ii**:197–201.
2   Merkatz IR, Nitowsky HM, Macri JN, Johnson WE (1984) An association between low maternal serum alpha-fetoprotein and fetal chromosome abnormalities. *American Journal of Obstetrics and Gynecology* **148**:886–894.
3   Bogart MH, Pandian MR, Jones OW (1987) Abnormal maternal serum chorionic gonadotropin levels in pregnancies with chromosome abnormalities. *Prenatal Diagnosis* **7**:623–630.
4   Wald NJ, Cuckle HS, Densem JW, Nanchahal K, Royston P, Chard T, Haddow JE, Knight GJ, Palomaki GE, Canick JA (1988) Maternal serum screening for Down's syndrome in early pregnancy. *British Medical Journal* **297**:883–887.
5   Milunsky A, Alpert E (1984) Results and benefits of a maternal serum α-fetoprotein screening program. *Journal of the American Medical Association* **252**:1438–1442.
6   Greenberg F, Faucett WA, Rose E, Alpert E, Bancalari L, Kardon NB, Mizjewski G, Knight GJ, Haddow JE (1989) Congenital deficiency of alpha-fetoprotein. *Pediatric Research* **25**:52A.
7   Greenberg F, James LM, Oakely GP Jr (1983) Estimates of birth prevalence rates of spina bifida in the United States from computer generated maps. *American Journal of Obstetrics and Gynecology* **145**:570–573.
8   Kirke PN, Elwood JH (1984) Anencephaly in the United KIngdom and Republic of Ireland. *British Medical Journal* **289**:1621.
9   Main DM, Mennuti MT (1986) Neural tube defects: Issues in prenatal diagnosis and counselling. *Obstetrics and Gynecology* **67**:1–16.
10 Cowchock S, Ainbender E, Prescott G, Crandall B, Lau L, Heller R, Muir WA, Kloza E, Feigelson M, Mennuti M, Cederquist L (1980) The recurrence risk for neural tube defects in the United States: A collaborative study. *American Journal of Medical Genetics* **5**:309–314.
11 Crandall BF, Matsumoto M (1984) Routine amniotic fluid alpha-fetoprotein measurement in 34,000 pregnancies. *American Journal of Obstetrics and Gynecology* **149**:744–747.
12 Kŭcera J (1971) Rate and type of congenital anomalies among offspring of diabetic women. *Journal of Reproductive Medicine* **7**:61–69.
13 Lindhout D, Schmidt D (1986) *In-utero* exposure to valproate and neural tube defects. *Lancet* **i**:1392–1393.
14 Martin L, Chavez GF, Adams MJ Jr, Mason EE, Hanson JW, Haddow JE, Currier RW (1988) Gastric bypass surgery as maternal risk factor for neural tube defect. *Lancet* **i**:640–641.
15 Cohen T, Stern E, Rosenmann, A (1979) Sib risk of neural tube defect: Is prenatal diagnosis indicated in pregnancies following the birth of a hydrocephalic child? *Journal of Medical Genetics* **16**:14–16.
16 Wynne-Davies R (1975) Congential vertebral anomalies: Aetiology and relationship to spina bifida cytica. *Journal of Medical Genetics* **12**:280–288.
17 Holmes LB, Driscoll SG, Atkins L (1976) Etiologic heterogeneity of neural tube defects. *New England Journal of Medicine* **294**:365–369.
18 Carter CO (1974) Recurrence risk of common congential malformations. *Practitioner* **213**:667–674.
19 Lippman-Hand A, Fraser FC, Cushman Biddle CJ (1978) Indications for prenatal diagnosis in relatives of patients with neural tube defects. *Obstetrics and Gynecology* **51**:72–76.
20 Wald NJ, Cuckle H, Brock DJH, Petro R, Polani PE, Woodford FP (1977) Maternal serum alpha-fetoprotein measurement in antenatal screening for anencephaly and spina bifida in early pregnancy: Report of UK Collaborative Study on Alpha-fetoprotein in Relation to Neural Tube Defects. *Lancet* **i**:1323–1332.
21 Second Report of the UK Collaborative Study on Alpha-fetoprotein in Relation to Neural Tube Defects: Amniotic Fluid Alpha-fetoprotein Measurement in Antenatal Diagnosis of Anencephaly and Open Spina Bifida in Early Pregnancy (1979). *Lancet* **ii**:651–661.
22 Macri JN, Weiss RR (1982) Prenatal alpha-fetoprotein screening for neural tube defects. *Obstetrics and Gynecology* **59**:633–639.
23 Burton BK, Sowers SG, Nelson LH (1983) Maternal serum alpha-fetoprotein screening in North Carolina: Experience with more than twelve thousand pregnancies. *American Journal of Obstetrics and Gynecology* **146**:439–444.
24 Fuhrmann W, Weitzel HK (1985) Maternal serum

alpha-fetoprotein screening for neural tube defects: Report of a combined study in Germany and short overview on screening in populations with low birth prevalence of neural tube defects. *Human Genetics* **69**:47–61.

25 Maternal serum alpha-fetoprotein screening for neural tube defects: Results of a consensus meeting (1985). *Prenatal Diagnosis* **5**:77–83.

26 Amniotic fluid acetylcholinesterase as a secondary test in the diagnosis of anencephaly and open spina bifida in early pregnancy: Report of the Collaborative Acetylcholinesterase Study (1981). *Lancet* **ii**:321–324.

27 Wald N, Cuckle H, Nanchahal K (1989) Amniotic fluid acetylcholinesterase measurement in the prenatal diagnosis of open neural tube defects: Second Report of the Collaborative Acetylcholinesterase Study. *Prenatal Diagnosis* **9**:813–829.

28 Wald NJ, Cuckle HS (1980) Cut-off levels in AFP screening. *Lancet* **i**:542.

29 Medical Research Council (1991) Prevention of neural tube defect: Results of the Medical Research Council Vitamin Study. *Lancet* **338**:131–137.

30 Burton BK (1988) Elevated maternal serum alpha-fetoprotein (MSAFP): Interpretation and follow-up. In Pitkin RM, Scott JR (eds) *Clinical Obstetrics and Gynecology*, Vol 31 (2), pp. 293–305. Philadelphia, PA: J. B. Lippincott.

31 Wiggelinkhuizen J, Nelson MM, Berger GMB, Kaschula ROC (1976) Alpha-fetoprotein in the antenatal diagnosis of the congenital nephrotic syndrome. *Journal of Pediatrics* **89**:452–455.

32 Holzgreve W, Golbus MS (1983) Amniotic fluid acetylcholinesterase as a prenatal diagnostic marker for upper gastrointestinal atresias. *American Journal of Obstetrics and Gynecology* **147**:837.

33 Bick DP, Balkite EA, Baumgarten A, Hobbins JC, Mahoney MJ (1987) The association of congenital skin disorders with acetylcholinesterase in amniotic fluid. *Prenatal Diagnosis* **7**:543–549.

34 Brock DJH, Barron L, Bedgood D, Rodeck C (1985) Distinguishing hygroma and amniotic fluid. *Prenatal Diagnosis* **5**:363–366.

35 Knight GJ, Palomaki GE, Haddow JE (1987) Assessing reliability of AFP test kits. *Contemporary Obstetrics and Gynecology* **37** (October): 37–52.

36 Watson WJ, Chescheir NC, Katz VL, Seeds JW (1991) The role of ultrasound in evaluation of patients with elevated maternal serum alpha-fetoprotein: A review. *Obstetrics and Gynecology* **78**:123–128.

37 Williamson RA, Varner MW, Grant SS (1985) Reduction in amniocentesis risks using a real time-needle guide procedure. *Obstetrics and Gynecology* **65**:751–755.

38 Barlow RD, Cuckle HS, Wald NJ (1982) False positive gel-acetylcholinesterase results in blood-stained amniotic fluids. *British Journal of Obstetrics and Gynaecology* **89**:821–826.

39 Williamson RA, Weiner CP, Patil S, Benda J, Varner MW, Abu-Yousef MM (1987) Abnormal pregnancy sonogram: Selective indication for fetal karyotype. *Obstetrics and Gynecology* **69**:15–20.

40 Adams MJ Jr, Windham GC, James LM, Greenberg F, Clayton-Hopkins JA, Reimer CB, Oakley GP Jr (1984) Clinical interpretation of maternal serum α-fetoprotein levels. *American Journal of Obstetrics and Gynecology* **148**:241–254.

41 American Society of Human Genetics (1987) Policy Statement for Maternal Serum Alpha-fetoprotein Screening Programs and Quality Control for Laboratories Performing Maternal Serum and Amniotic Fluid Alpha-Fetoprotein Assays. *American Journal of Human Genetics* **40**:75–82.

42 Wald NJ, Cuckle HS, Catz C, Dayton D, Reimer CB (1981) Alpha-fetoprotein screening and diagnosis of fetal open neural tube defects: The need for quality control. *American Journal of Obstetrics and Gynecology* **141**:1–4.

43 Macri JN, Kasturi RV, Krantz DA, Hu MG (1987) Maternal serum alpha-fetoprotein screening. II. Pitfalls in low volume decentralized laboratory performance. *American Journal of Obstetrics and Gynecology* **156**:533–535.

44 Strickland DM, Butzin CA, Wians FH Jr (1991) Maternal serum α-fetoprotein screening: Further consideration of low volume testing. *American Journal of Obstetrics and Gynecology* **164**:711–714.

45 Crandall BF, Lebherz TB, Schroth PC, Matsumoto M (1983) Alpha-fetoprotein concentrations in maternal serum: Relation to race and body weight. *Clinical Chemistry* **29**:531–533.

46 Johnson AM, Palomaki GE, Haddow JE (1990) Maternal serum α-fetoprotein levels in pregnancies among black and white women with fetal open spina bifida: A United States collaborative study. *American Journal of Obstetrics and Gynecology* **162**:328–331.

47 Wald NJ, Cuckle H, Boreham J, Stirrat GM, Turnbull AC (1979) Maternal serum alpha-fetoprotein and diabetes mellitus. *British Journal of Obstetrics and Gynaecology* **86**:101–105.

48 Greene MF, Haddow JE, Palomaki GE, Knight GJ (1988) Maternal serum alpha-fetoprotein levels in diabetic pregnancies. *Lancet* **ii**:345–346.

49 Johnson AM, Lingley L (1984) Correction formula for maternal serum alpha-fetoprotein. *Lancet* **ii**:812.

50 Haddow JE, Kloza EM, Knight GJ, Smith DE (1981) Relationship between maternal weight and serum alpha-fetoprotein concentration during the second trimester. *Clinical Chemistry* **27**:133–134.

51 Cuckle H, Wald N, Stevenson JD, May HM, Ferguson-Smith MA, Ward AH, Barbour HM, Laurence KM, Norgaard-Pedersen B (1990) Maternal serum alpha-fetoprotein screening for open neural tube defects in twin pregnancies. *Prenatal Diagnosis* **10**:71–77.

52 Lustig L, Feuchtbaum L, Cunningham G (1991) MSAFP screening for open neural tube defects in twin pregnancies. *American Journal of Human Genetics* **49**:A1214 (suppl.).

53 Stiller RJ, Lockwood CJ, Belanger K, Baumgarten A, Hobbins JC, Mahoney MJ (1988) Amniotic fluid α-fetoprotein in twin gestations: Dependence on placental membrane anatomy. *American Journal of Obstetrics and Gynecology* **158**:1088–1092.

54 Janerich DT, Piper J (1978) Shifting patterns in anencephaly and spina bifida. *Journal of Medical Genetics* **15**:101–105.

55 Killam WP, Miller RC, Seeds JW (1991) Extremely high maternal serum alpha-fetoprotein levels at second trimester screening. *Obstetrics and Gynecology* **78**:257–261.

56 Crandall BF, Robinson L, Grau P (1991) Risks associated with an elevated maternal serum α-fetoprotein level. *American Journal of Obstetrics and Gynecology* **165**:581–586.

57 Waller DK, Lustig LS, Cunningham GC, Golbus MS, Hook EB (1991) Second-trimester maternal serum alpha-fetoprotein levels and the risk of subsequent fetal death. *New England Journal of Medicine* **325**:6–10.

58 Bernstein IM, Barth RA, Miller R, Capeless EL (1992) Elevated maternal serum alpha-fetoprotein: Association with placental sonolucencies, fetomaternal hemorrhage, vaginal bleeding and pregnancy outcome in the absence of fetal anomalies. *Obstetrics and Gynecology* **79**:71–74.

59 Stirrat GM, Gough JD, Bullock S, Wald NJ, Cuckle HS (1981) Raised maternal serum AFP, oligohydramnios and poor fetal outcome. *British Journal of Obstetrics and Gynaecology* **88**:231–235.

60 Richards DS, Seeds JW, Katz VL, Lingley LH, Albright SG, Cefalo RC (1988) Elevated maternal serum alpha-fetoprotein with oligohydramnios: Ultrasound evaluation and outcome: *Obstetrics and Gynecology* **72**:337–341.

61 Redford DHA, Whitfield CR (1985) Maternal serum α-fetoprotein in twin pregnancies uncomplicated by neural tube defect. *American Journal of Obstetrics and Gynecology* **152**:550–553.

62 Ghosh A, Woo JSK, Rawlinson HA, Ferguson-Smith MA (1982) Prognostic significance of raised serum α-fetoprotein levels in twin pregnancies. *British Journal of Obstetrics and Gynaecology* **89**:817–820.

63 Burton BK, Dillard RG, Clark EN (1985) The psychological impact of a false positive elevation of maternal serum α-fetoprotein. *American Journal of Obstetrics and Gynecology* **151**:77–82.

64 Cuckle HS, Wald NJ, Lindenbaum RH (1984) Maternal serum alpha-fetoprotein measurement: A screening test for Down syndrome. *Lancet* **i**:926–929.

65 DiMaio MS, Baumgarten A, Greenstein RM, Saal HM, Mahoney MJ (1987) Screening for fetal Down's syndrome in pregnancy by measuring maternal serum alpha-fetoprotein. *New England Journal of Medicine* **317**:342–346.

66 Palomaki GE, Williams J, Haddow JE (1989) The New England Regional Genetics Group Collaborative Study of Down Syndrome Screening: Combining maternal serum alpha-fetoprotein measurements and age to screen for Down syndrome in pregnant women under age 35. *American Journal of Obstetrics and Gynecology* **160**:575–581.

67 Drugan A, Dvorin E, Koppitch FC, Greb A, Krivchenia EL, Evans MI (1989) Counseling for low maternal serum alpha-fetoprotein should emphasize all chromosome anomalies, not just Down syndrome! *Obstetrics and Gynceology* **73**:271–274.

68 Nicolini U, Hubinont C, Santoyala J, Fisk NM, Rodeck CH, Johnson RD (1988) Fetal serum alpha-fetoprotein in fetuses with chromosomal abnormalities. *Lancet* **ii**:1316–1317.

69 Canick JA, Knight GJ, Palomaki GE, Haddow JE, Cuckle HS, Wald NJ (1988) Low second trimester maternal serum unconjugated oestriol in pregnancies with Down syndrome. *British Journal of Obstetrics and Gynaecology* **95**:330–333.

70 Wald NJ, Cuckle HS, Densen JW, Nanchahal K, Canick JA, Haddow JE, Knight GE, Palomaki GE (1988) Maternal serum unconjugated oestriol as an antenatal screening test for Down's syndrome. *British Journal of Obstetrics and Gynaecology* **95**:334–341.

71 Macri JN, Kasturi RV, Krantz DA, Cook EJ, Sunderji SG, Larson JW (1990) Maternal serum Down syndrome screening: Unconjugated estriol is not useful. *American Journal of Obstetrics and Gynecology* **162**:672–673.

72 Haddow JE, Palomaki GE, Knight GJ, Canick JA (1990) Maternal serum unconjugated estriol levels are lower in the presence of fetal Down syndrome. *American Journal of Obstetrics and Gynecology* **163**:1372–1373.

73 Suchy SF, Yeager MT (1990) Down syndrome screening in women under age 35 with maternal serum hCG. *Obstetrics and Gynecology* **76**:20–24.

74 MacDonald ML, Wagner RM, Slotnick RN (1991) Sensitivity and specificity of screening for Down syndrome with alpha-fetoprotein, hCG, unconjugated estriol and maternal age. *Obstetrics and Gynecology* **77**:63–68.

75 Macri JN, Kasturi RV, Krantz DA, Cook EJ, Moore ND, Young JA, Romero K, Larsen JW Jr (1990) Maternal serum Down syndrome screening: Free β-protein is a more effective marker than human chorionic gonadotropin. *American Journal of Obstetrics and Gynecology* **163**:1248–1253.

76 Haddow JE, Palomaki GE, Knight GJ, Williams J, Pulkkinen A, Canick JA, Saller DN, Bowers GB (1992) Prenatal screening for Down's syndrome with use of maternal serum markers. *New England Journal of Medicine* **327**:588–593.

77 Knight GJ, Palomaki GE, Haddow JE (1986) Maternal serum alpha-fetoprotein: A problem with a test kit. *New England Journal of Medicine* **314**:516.

78 Haddow JE, Palomaki GE, Wald NJ, Cuckle HS (1986) Maternal serum alpha-fetoprotein screening for Down syndrome and repeat testing. *Lancet* **ii**:1460.

79 Hershey DW, Randall BF, Perdue S (1986) Combining maternal age and serum alpha-fetoprotein to predict risk of Down's syndrome. *Obstetrics and Gynecology* **68**:177–180.

80 Knight GJ, Palomaki GE, Haddow JE (1988) Use of maternal serum alpha-fetoprotein measurements to screen for Down's syndrome. In Pitkin RM, Scott JR (eds) *Clinical Obstetrics and Gynecology*, Vol. 31(2), pp. 306–344. Philadelphia, PA: JB Lippincott.

81 Bogart MH, Jones OW, Felder RA, Best RG, Bradley L, Butts W, Crandall B, MacMahon W, Wians FH Jr, Loeh PV (1991) Prospective evaluation of maternal serum human chorionic gonadotropin levels in 3428 pregnancies. *American Journal of Obstetrics and Gynecology* **165**:663–667.

82 Schmidt D, Weyland B, Rose E, Greenberg F (1991) Maternal weight and levels of β-hCG and unconjugated

estriol in mid-pregnancy. *American Journal of Human Genetics* **49**:A1255 (suppl.).

83 Nieb B, Joyce A, Burton BK (1991) Mid-trimester hCG and uE₃ levels in twin gestations. *American Journal of Human Genetics* **49**:A1197 (suppl.).

84 Nebiolo LM, Adams WB, Miller SL, Milunsky A (1991) Maternal serum human chorionic gonadotropin levels in twin pregnancies. *Prenatal Diagnosis* **11**:463–466.

85 Williamson RA (1991) Enhanced screening for fetal chromosome abnormalities. *Postgraduate Obstetrics and Gynecology* **11**:1–5.

86 Perry TB, Benzie RJ, Cassar N, Hamilton EF, Stocker J, Toftager-Larsen K, Lippman A (1984) Fetal cephalometry by ultrasound as a screening procedure for the prenatal detection of Down syndrome. *British Journal of Obstetrics and Gynaecology* **91**:138–143.

87 Wald NJ, Cuckle HS, Boreham J (1980) Small biparietal diameter of fetuses with spina bifida: Implications for antenatal screening. *British Journal of Obstetrics and Gynaecology* **87**:219–221.

88 Brown J (1989) The choice. *Journal of the American Medical Association* **262**:2735.

89 Staples AJ, Robertson EF, Ranieri E, Ryall RG, Haan EA (1991) A maternal serum screen for trisomy 18: An extension of maternal serum screening for Down syndrome. *American Journal of Human Genetics* **49**: 1025–1033.

90 Palomaki GE, Knight GJ, Haddow JE, Canick JA, Saller DN, Panizza DS, Grant SS, Wenstrom KD, Hudson JD (1991) Prospective trial of a screening protocol to identify trisomy 18 using maternal serum alpha-fetoprotein, unconjugated estriol and human chorionic gonadotropin. *American Journal of Human Genetics* **49**:A1238 (suppl.).

91 Albright SG, Lingley LH, Seeds JW, Lincoln-Boyea B (1988) Pitfalls of gestational age reassignment in evaluation of low maternal serum α-fetoprotein levels. *American Journal of Obstetrics and Gynecology* **159**:369–370.

92 Achiron R, Barkai G, Katznelson MB, Mashiach S (1991) Fetal lateral ventricle choroid plexus cysts: The dilemma of amniocentesis. *Obstetrics and Gynecology* **78**:815–818.

93 Lockwood CJ, Lynch L, Berkowitz RL (1991) Ultrasonographic screening for the Down syndrome fetus. *American Journal of Obstetrics and Gynecology* **165**:349–352.

94 Heyl PS, Miller W, Canick JA (1990) Maternal serum screening for aneuploid pregnancy by alpha-fetoprotein, hCG and unconjugated estriol. *Obstetrics and Gynecology* **76**:1025–1031.

95 Knight GJ, Palomaki GE, Haddow JE, Johnson AM, Osathanondh R, Canick JA (1989) Maternal serum levels of the placental products hCG, hPL, SP₁, and progesterone are all elevated in cases of fetal Down syndrome. *American Journal of Human Genetics* **45**:A263.

96 Milunsky A, Wands, J, Brambati B, Bonacchi I, Currie K (1988) First-trimester maternal serum α-fetoprotein screening for chromosome defects. *American Journal of Obstetrics and Gynecology* **159**:1209–1213.

97 Johnson A, Cowchock FS, Darby M, Wagner R, Jackson LG (1991) First-trimester maternal serum alpha-fetoprotein and chorionic gonadotropin in aneuploid pregnancies. *Prenatal Diagnosis* **11**:443–450.

98 Cuckle HS, Wald NJ, Barkai G, Fuhrmann W, Altland K, Brambati B, Knight G, Palomaki G, Haddow JE, Canick J (1988) First-trimester biochemical screening for Down syndrome. *Lancet* **ii**:851–852.

99 Kratzer PG, Golbus MS, Monroe SE, Finkelstein DE, Taylor RN (1991) First trimester aneuploidy screening using serum human chorionic gonadotropin (hCG); free α-hCG, and progesterone. *Prenatal Diagnosis* **11**:751–765.

100 Cuckle HS, Wald NJ, Goodburn SF, Sneddon J, Amess JAL, Dunn SC (1990) Measurement of activity of urea resistant neutrophil alkaline phosphatase as an antenatal screening test for Down's syndrome. *British Medical Journal* **301**:1024–1026.

38

The Routine 18–20 Week Ultrasound Scan

CHRIS HARMAN

INTRODUCTION

Growing evidence suggests midtrimester ultrasound provides enough benefit to justify routine use. The economics of such application, and non-obstetric factors which must influence such allocations, are public problems of broad range. From the perspective of fetal medicine, the theory, principles and ideal practise are clear and well-established. Measuring the benefits of practical application of routine midtrimester ultrasound, however, is more problematic.

A precise role of 'routine' obstetric ultrasound remains in debate. This is easy to appreciate, considering the ways fetal examination may impact on the fetus, the pregnancy, the mother, her family, her health care-givers, and the community in general (**Table 1**). Public awareness and a growing need to establish unique fetal ethics and fetal law, are logical results of detailed fetal visualization.

WHO SHOULD BE SCANNED IN MIDTRIMESTER? SELECTING SUBJECTS

There are enough potential advantages to midtrimester ultrasound examination (**Table 2**), that most pregnancies will have direct, obvious benefits. Within the context of a wanted pregnancy, psychological benefits may expand this list to virtually *all* pregnancies. The principal benefit may be seen in one of three general areas:

- obstetrics/fetal
- maternal/family
- prospective aspects.

Table 1
Impact of obstetric ultrasound

General
    timing pregnancy events

Fetal
    diagnosis
    prognosis
    monitoring
    therapy

Obstetric
    planning

Maternal/family
    bonding
    prenatal education
    participation

Societal
    education
    fetal ethics

Several series have detailed the positive effects of obstetric ultrasound on pregnancy management in large populations.[1–3] Examples in the discussion which follows include:

- opportunities to adjust plans for timed events

- initiation of fetal investigation or treatment

- intervention for non-viable pregnancy

- planning of preventive monitoring or therapy within the context of risk prediction.

Most pregnancies are normal, needing neither investigation nor intervention in a medical sense. The benefits in this population may be of less intensity in the individual case, but ultimately of significant impact. The normal pregnancy scan demystifies fetal life.[4,5] Bonding is facilitated, the family is involved, and a rightful atmosphere of acquisition to information about 'the baby' is established. In single teenage mothers, notorious for non-compliance, the routine midtrimester scan can be a powerful motive for adherence to prenatal care.[6]

Decisions later in pregnancy are emphatically enhanced when, for example, detailed baseline measurements, anatomic review, proof of normal renal function/amniotic fluid volume are available. This planning benefit is significant to the family, too, as many uncertainties about third trimester management – that is, factors which can confuse informed choices in

Table 2
Potential advantages of midtrimester obstetric ultrasound exam

---

Confirm potentially viable intrauterine pregnancy
   (exclude hydatidiform mole, ectopic pregnancy, etc.)

Certify pregnancy dating

Identify multiple gestation

Identify major congenital anomalies (general)

Exclude specific malformation (risk-based)

Assign baseline morphometric values

Review fetal function/behavior

Document placental location

Review uterine and adnexal structures

Initiate maternal–fetal bonding

Initiate/reinforce routine prenatal care and education

Initiate fetal investigation/treatment

High- or low-risk discrimination

Planning value

Adjunctive (genetic amnio, cervical cerclage)

Specific problems (e.g. absent fetal heart tones, APH)

---

treatment – are eliminated by the detailed knowledge of the pregnancy obtained at 20 weeks.

The 18–20 week scan may occur in the context of a pregnancy 'event' such as genetic testing, elevated maternal serum alpha-fetoprotein or a specific problem such as antepartum bleeding, delayed quickening or absent fetal heart tones. While maternal anxiety mandates increased sensitivity here, the scan, the scanners and the scannee (the fetus) are usually the same as in the 'routine' situation. The author agrees with recent opinions that an incomplete or 'partial' scan is inappropriate for any of these situations.[7]

Integration of obstetric ultrasound in prenatal care is complicated, as one would expect from a detailed physical examination of any individual in any health care setting. The information produces a ripple effect of answers and opportunities for recognition, understanding, learning and correction, concerning virtually all aspects of fetal life. Why this depth of appreciation should be confined to high-risk/complicated cases is hard to argue. As confidence increases in results and safety, official statements have shifted from 'non-mandatory, indication-based' applications (NIH consensus, 1984)[8] to a 'scan if mother wants it' approach (American Medical Association, 1992).[7]

Since this liberalized approach places pressure on resources, one response has been to advocate 'selected' scans. Routine (i.e. universal) midtrimester obstetric ultrasound vs selected (i.e. specifically indicated) examination has been evaluated in two large non-randomized studies.[9,10] In summary, diagnosis-based, 'selected' scanning is better than no ultrasound, but it misses substantial opportunities compared with systematic, universal application. Accurate pregnancy dating provides much of this benefit, but incidental observation of the many variants of pregnancy provides benefit in another large group. Obviously, if a major function of the 18–20 week scan is screening for adverse possibilities, 'selecting' subjects is inappropriate: 'selective screening' is an absolute oxymoron in this context.

Pressure to adopt universal scanning comes from obstetricians (who want/need the data to 'manage' pregnancy appropriately), perinatologists (whose dilemmas spring just as often from absent information as from present complications), families (who want to see the baby), the medicolegal climate ('Exactly why did you deny the patient a routine ultrasound, doctor?'), and the mothers. In some jurisdictions, women consider obstetric ultrasound an essential, desirable component of high-grade care. Their attitudes to this highly informative study mean that the days of the mute technician and the hidden screen are long past. Despite the serious work of trialists[11] and the hesitation of some reviewers,[12] the trend is to use ultrasound in 'almost all' pregnancies. It might well be that the expense is least when a single scan is done at 18–20 weeks.

WHY IS MIDTRIMESTER ULTRASOUND DONE? A STATEMENT OF GOALS

Many priorities are population-dependent. If prenatal care is poorly attended, pregnancy dating is critical. With a high rate of teratogen exposure, high-risk ethnicity, or in many situations where risk factors are 'concentrated' by referral patterns, specific anatomic concerns may be more important. In general, however, the positive goals of this systematic program are:

- Maximize the advantages of midtrimester ultrasound (**Table 2**).

- Obtain as much information as possible in a single examination.

- Benefit mother and family as much as possible during the process.

- Limit health care costs while improving health care results.

These goals are addressed as follows:

- A full, detailed, systematic, routine approach, according to the description below ('Content') is carried out for *all* scans.

- With prerequisite information and consultative orientation, highly trained obstetrically oriented personnel do the examination.

- The examination is interactive with mother, coordinated with referring agent, flexible to family concerns, with appropriate ancillary contact.

- Mandatory repeat visits and elaborate modalities are not required. Continued updating, remote outreach, streamline the program. Nurse ultrasonographers can be the primary scanners.

The first three points are addressed in detail in this chapter. The fourth varies so much from one area to another, it is not possible to address it comprehensively. The ability of any health care system to bear the cost of universal deployment of sophisticated technology is limited, and economies are necessary. *Reductions in unnecessary, less informative scans, both too early and too late (i.e. first and third trimester), will result from the systematic application of midtrimester scans and lead to the argument that the program will pay for itself.*

WHEN SHOULD THE MIDTRIMESTER SCAN BE DONE? THE CASE FOR AN 18–20 WEEK EXAMINATION

This is not a question of the failures of earlier (or later) scans to detect twins, assign dates and so on, but a question of common sense and efficiency. If routine obstetric ultrasound is accepted, one important economy will be to maximize the information available at each visit. The larger, more developed fetus compared with 12 weeks, for example, affords views of anatomic detail from which detailed diagnosis is possible.

The margin of error in assignment of dates at 10 weeks is ±2–4 days. At 18 weeks, it is three or four times that variance, but this difference is not clinically important. In fact, being able to visualize the subject precisely at 18 weeks provides numerous opportunities to correct errors made when a curved embryo was measured in an incomplete straight line at a very early stage.[13] Twins are rarely missed on ultrasound at 18 weeks, but more commonly so either much earlier or much later. Though endovaginal ultrasound can reveal surprising detail at 8–10 weeks when the transducer is brought within 1–2 cm of the embryo, the utility of routine early endovaginal scanning (as opposed to the novelty of it) has not been asserted, let alone proven. The advantages of early *abdominal* ultrasound, also capable of high resolution at early gestation, are debatable.[14] Though there are specific advantages in pregnancy complicated by abnormal bleeding when endovaginal ultrasound can lead to earlier and safer intervention for molar or ectopic pregnancy, 18–20 weeks is optimal diagnostically in the apparently normal, asymptomatic woman.

Integration of the scan in overall obstetric care also suggests 18–20 weeks. Maternal serum alpha-fetoprotein (MS-AFP) results are known, early pregnancy failure has been revealed, the critical 'second wave' of placentation has taken place, the fetus controls amniotic fluid volume, organogenesis is complete, and teratogenicity is a fading concern. Maternal medical complications are often quiescent (or at least quite well defined), intrauterine growth deficiency has not yet complicated assessment of size and age, fetal movements are beginning to be felt, and most of the fetus still fits on the screen. Thus, for all areas of interest, 18–20 weeks seems most satisfactory.

Limitations to the 18–20 weeks scan are highlighted in **Table 3**. These are examples only; there are times when significant problems are found only after serial observation. Documentation of normal anatomy in those at risk for an anomaly is often done in two stages (18 and 24 weeks) to allow 'second-looks' at face and heart. Unusual findings, such as absent umbilical artery end-diastolic velocities (AEDV), might be highly significant later in pregnancy but are mainly a source of anxiety if over-interpreted at 18–20 weeks. Follow-up at 24 and 28 weeks will sort these fetuses. Another example is the moving placenta, which often seems obviously placenta previa at 18 weeks and almost fundal at 36 weeks. This should be noted, but is not a reason for re-scanning an asymptomatic woman without other risk factors (previous placenta previa, uterine anomaly, malpresentation or previous uterine infection).

Most fetal anomalies evolve graphically during prenatal life. For example, diaphragmatic hernias and gastroschisis may slide, arrhythmias may be intermittent, aortic valve obstruction may not be manifest, and hydrocephalus may be gradually progressive. Thus, while ultrasound is highly successful (>90%) at major anomaly detection over the course of pregnancy, a single exam at 18–20 weeks has much lower sensitivity. And while this exam provides a baseline for fetal growth evaluation, late growth disturbances such as macrosomia or severe growth deficiency cannot necessarily be anticipated. On the other hand, for the 18–20 week fetus with absent end diastolic velocities, marginal amniotic fluid, and elevated MS-AFP, severe early onset growth deficiency requiring intervention as early as 27–28 weeks is fairly common and early evaluation may be life-saving.

Finally, the impacts of findings at this gestation must be a reasonable compromise. The discovery of a lethal anomaly might be 'best' if fetal movements have not yet been felt, but in many instances (especially cardiac anomalies) our diagnostic abilities are stretched to the maximum to be sure of anomaly this early. Clearly, the basis for irrevocable action must be unequivocal visualization. The 18–20 week time-frame allows for this degree of certainty, as well as a short interval for considering options, second opinions and consultation.

HOW IS THE 20–WEEK SCAN DONE? METHODS

Prerequisites

These include:

- maternal serum alpha-fetoprotein (MS-AFP) result
- prenatal database and routine testing completed
- prepregnancy/periconceptual risk factors identified
- relevant serology, genetic concerns, etc., specified
- pre-scan interview.

Maternal Preparation

Bladder-filling hurts and is usually unnecessary. For a detailed examination of the lower uterine segment, or to dislodge a low-lying back-down fetus, several glasses of water will usually suffice. Later in pregnancy, time interval since a meal, cigarette smoking and inherent periodicity all influence fetal behavior and thus performance of biophysical profile scoring (see Chapter 39). At 18–20 weeks, however, fetal activity is less discreet in cyclicity, and less influenced by short-term maternal behaviors.

Pre-scan counseling for those with specific risk factors necessitates close coordination with prenatal programs (**Table 4**). Even for the unscheduled patient, such resources can be readily available in university-based, tertiary-level centers (or collaborating secondary-level centres). For most routine scans, preparation is begun by the referring agent (obstetrician, family doctor, midwife, remote nursing station, etc.) and is completed with the intake interview at the Fetal Assessment Unit.

Table 3
Some limitations of the 18–20 week scan

Structural review may be incomplete
  face (lips)
  heart (ventricular development, leaflets)
  genitalia (some fetuses)
  peripheral vessels (too small)

Uncertain significance
  umbilical artery flow velocity waveforms
  subjectively reduced amniotic fluid volume
  'low-lying' placenta
  unusual placental anatomy

Deficit not yet manifest
  late obstructive defects (hydrocephalus, hydronephrosis,
    some posterior urethral valves, duodenal atresia, etc.)
  intermittent/incomplete abnormality
  fetal growth disturbances
  fetal behavior disorders

Evolution of maternal status

Therapy limited to extrauterine regimes

Table 4
Pre-scan counseling at 18–20 weeks

Factor	Content	Personnel[a]
Elevated MS-AFP	Specific patient literature, detailed AFP counseling, scan explained, intra-scan counseling, postscan counseling	AFP program, FAU perinatologist
Advanced maternal age (Down syndrome risk)	Risk assessment, testing options, re-evaluation of risk (intra-scan, preprocedure)	Prenatal geneticist, FAU perinatologist
Anomaly recurrence risk	Detailed explanation of goals and limitations (immediately prescan)	Prenatal geneticist, FAU perinatologist
Maternity anxiety	Explanation of scan procedure, establishment of rapport	FAU personnel, primary health care provider
'Routine' scan	Receptive attitude during prescan database acquisition may detect underlying/unrevealed anxieties, risk factors, or symptoms	Primary health care; FAU personnel, family
Alloimmunization	Pathophysiology, risk evaluation, management options	Rh program, FAU personnel
Cultural/physical barriers	Detailed prescan explanation	Interpreter, family, social worker and FAU personnel

[a]Team approach emphasized. FAU, Fetal Assessment Unit.

Equipment

The basic tool for the examination is a high-resolution, real-time gray scale ultrasound unit. Continued advances in ultrasound technology have made most of the choices between various instruments of economic and cosmetic concern. Within the framework of standardized energy output, service costs and requirements, portability, ease of operation and operator preference, a wide range of instruments is available to the potential purchaser. Most of the maneuvers required can be accomplished using a single transducer. In our laboratory, a 13 cm linear phased array, 3.5 mHz transducer suffices. Useful adjuncts include a small-footprint transducer (e.g. annular array, sector scan head), endovaginal ultrasound probe, and pulsed Doppler/duplex. Equipment occasionally used this early in gestation includes a fetal heart rate monitor with autocorrelation and computerized numerical analysis,[15] and ready access to equipment necessary for invasive fetal monitoring, including installation of artificial amniotic fluid.[16] Image-recording requirements are discussed below. While this is an evolving issue, we do not invite videotaping, still photography or copying of images by parents/family. Finally, a number of components may appear trivial, but produce an aura of security, comfort and cooperation which greatly facilitate a complete examination: variable-intensity lighting, variable-position bed, individual linen, privacy screens, lockable doors (for vaginal scanning, specific procedures), large auxiliary video screen visible by mother and family members and, last but not least, body-temperature ultrasound gel warmers at the bedside.

Readiness

This heading emphasizes the 18–20 week scan should not be done in a peripheral unit without backup. Close collaboration, and hopefully close geographic proximity, is necessary with those agencies detailed in **Table 4**, as well as the individuals identified as part of the Fetal Assessment Unit team in **Table 8**, (see below). Such backup facilities, which include being able to embark virtually immediately on invasive fetal testing and treatment (for example, if an unexpected hydropic fetus is found in an alloimmunized mother) would most likely be on site at tertiary-level centers. Close collaboration with such a center also provides ample benefit in the areas of continuing education and standards maintenance.

Documentation

Radiologists who have progressed toward obstetric ultrasound may find this topic self-evident. Obstetricians who have become 'sono-literate' may be unclear on how much documentation is required. Requirements vary from one geographic region to another, one medicolegal climate to another, and may be limited by economics. Much of the exam is based on real-time observation: hard copy of still images may not prove a detailed examination was done. An emphasis on potential medicolegal consequences might suggest a full videotape record of every examination – clearly beyond the scope of most units. A reasonable compromise might be a formatted series, detailing measurements, amniotic fluid volume, and Doppler/M-mode evidence of fetal heart rate. This information can fit on six full-field images, stored in digitized format. Whereas many units developed previously were connected directly to x-ray film-based multiformat cameras, that system is clearly not cost-effective today.

Performance of the Scan

Mother is semi-recumbent. The video monitor is placed so the image is not hidden from the mother's view by the examiner. Family members are able to see the screen from the side of the mother's bed. Mother's clothing is protected with reusable towels (laundry expense is generally less than that of single-use replacements), and she is not required to disrobe before the exam. With an average opening interview of 5–8 min, the examination detailed below (including measurements, detailed anatomic and functional review, and a short segment for questions and answers) can be concluded and the report generated within the allotted 30 min schedule.

WHAT IS DONE IN THE 18–20 WEEK SCAN?[17]

That this is not a checklist emphasizes the importance of integrating the scan within the health care context of the woman concerned, *and* within the family context of what is most likely (85–90%) to be a series of normal events with a normal result. Keeping this in mind reduces the pomposity of predictive accuracy and the secrecy of special techniques. This section addresses the advantages in **Table 2**. This is representative only; for more detailed descriptions, a variety of texts are available.[18–20] Measurement principles (see also Chapter 42) and congenital anomalites (see also Chapters 50–54) are discussed below.

Confirm Potentially Viable Intrauterine Pregnancy

If the pregnancy is of 20 weeks duration, this is straightforward. When they are together in the same pregnancy at 20 weeks, normal anatomy, good activity, normal amniotic fluid volume, significant diastolic

velocities in umbilical arterial flow, normal AFP, normal fetal size, and a normally situated placenta confer a chance of intact survival of >95% in our population. The order of these factors is not accidental: they are arranged in descending order of their importance, when absent, in predicting poor outcome. Among structurally normal fetuses, amniotic fluid volume and skeletal size are the most powerful predictors of viability.[21] Conversely, the highest mortality (95% or more) is seen in the group with absent amniotic fluid and elevated AFP: almost all either have, or soon develop, inadequate growth. Among maternal findings, continued antepartum hemorrhage (APH) (**Figure 1**) confers increased risk of loss. In most pregnancies at 20 weeks, however, loss related to APH is associated with other intrauterine factors. Knowing what to expect may determine the relative wisdom of maternal interventions, offer opportunities for detailed obstetric and non-obstetric planning, and may allow precise application of experimental therapies such as maternal hyperoxygenation, low-dose aspirin and amniotic fluid instillation.

Certify Pregnancy Dating

Combining the fetal head measurements biparietal diameter (BDP) occipitofrontal diameter (OFD) and computed head circumference (HC) (**Figure 2**) with femur length (FL) measurement is often enough to confirm reliably reported menstrual history.[22,23] Measurement of the abdominal circumference (AC) establishes a nutritional baseline, noting that most fetuses (even those destined to lie below the 5th percentile at 32–34 weeks) fall in a narrow range. If there is a discrepancy

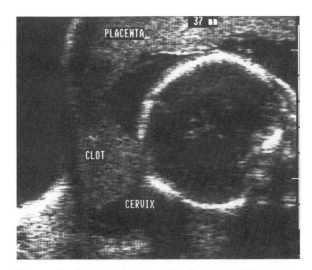

Figure 1. Marginal abruptio placentae 20+ weeks gestation, mild cramps, bright red bleeding. Maternal bladder (L), fetal head (R).

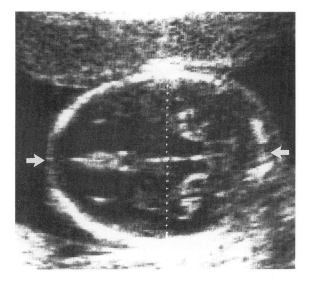

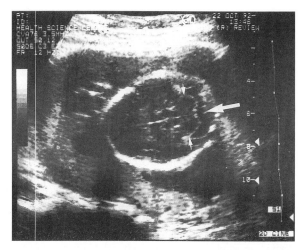

Figure 4. The transcerebellar diameter (between small arrows) measuring 21.1 mm at 20 weeks 6 days gestation. Posterior fossa (large arrow) is also normal, 4 mm in this plane.

Figure 2. Standard measurements at the level of the biparietal diameter. BPD 40 mm compatible with sure gestation by LMP, 18 weeks. Normal skull symmetry with OFD (between arrows) = 50 mm. The cephalic index' (BPD/OFD) is 0.80 (normal = 0.73 – 0.85).

between the BPD and OFD (caphalic index), e.g. dolicocephaly with breech presentation, HC is usually still reliable (**Figure 3**). An alternative to skull measurements is the transverse cerebellar diameter, TCbD (**Figure 4**),[24] although it requires some experience and caution in obtaining the correct plane. The TCbD in millimeters approximates the weeks of gestation, from 14 to 24 weeks.

Despite the enormous effort put into measurements

of various bones in the human fetus and several non-bony structures (e.g. kidney, ear, colon), these are only novelties in a routine ultrasound exam. With a significant HC:FL discrepancy, fetal foot length may provide an additional reference of skeletal size (**Figure 5**).[25] Dates are adjusted appropriately if the consensus of measurements is equal to or greater than 10–11 days at variance with mother's dates and if there is the clinical possibility of the dates being less than certain. When the fetus is >11 days smaller than allowed by history,

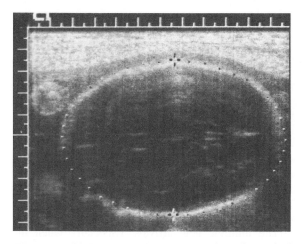

Figure 3. Dolichocephaly due to reduced amniotic fluid volume, breech. BPD is less than expected, but head circumference is within normal limits.

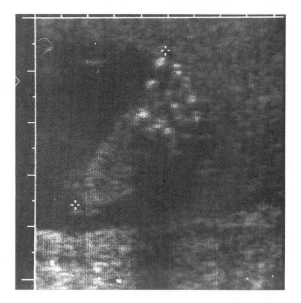

Figure 5. Right foot, size 34, compatible with stated gestation of 20 weeks.

and the mother (in solitary confidence) refutes alternative conception dates, investigation and monitoring for early, severe fetal growth deficiency is initiated. If the dates are not reassigned, the smaller-than-average 20 week fetus might be expected to go beyond '42 weeks' with increased frequency. In the context of advanced maternal age and low MS–AFP, finding a generally small fetus would *not* suggest reassigning the expected date of delivery – it may well fulfil an increased risk of Down syndrome (see Chapter 37).[26–28] Before using the automatic EDC calculation in your scanner's software package, be sure it does not simply average out values (such as FL appropriate for 18 weeks with a BPD suggesting 24 weeks computes as an average gestational age of 21 weeks) without narrow tolerance for variance. A useful discussion of the derivation (and dangers) of such calculations may be found in Jeanty.[29]

In summary, it is advisable to measure multiple parameters at multiple sites until a clear *consensus* is established. If none of the measurements makes sense, trust the TCbD, the femur length and foot length and follow the others serially.

Identify Multiple Gestation

The 20 week scan should be nearly flawless in correct assignment of number of fetuses likely to reach a viable gestational age. The 'vanishing twin' (which in most cases was probably *not* another gestational sac but a cystic space of other origin) has vanished in most cases.[30,31] There is space for both to show up effectively, and the uterus is usually completely erect.[32] We have seen one example of a missed twin due to a folded uterus, the fundus (containing one fetus) remaining in the cul-de-sac while the lower half of the uterus grew anteriorly, showing an apparently normal singleton on abdominal ultrasound as late as 18 weeks. A clue to this possibility is an abrupt superior disappearance of the uterus without the usual myometrical rim. The best time to scan triplets and higher numbers of fetuses is at 20 weeks before all the body parts are difficult to determine. Often, the positions seen clearly at 20 weeks are more or less maintained throughout the course of subsequent monitoring (**Figure 6**).

A separate empty sac or the skeletal remains of a dead co-twin is not an uncommon finding at this gestation, especially with elevated MS-AFP.[33] Intact survival of the other fetus to 20 weeks confers a near-normal prospect.[34] The other extreme, severe discordance – the 'stuck twin' complex – this early, suggests a very poor prognosis and justifies radical intervention.[35–37] Other discordance, especially size, cardiac anatomy and non-immune hydrops, found on the 18–20 week scan, may benefit from prompt diagnostic steps to explain the discordance (infection, aneuploidy,

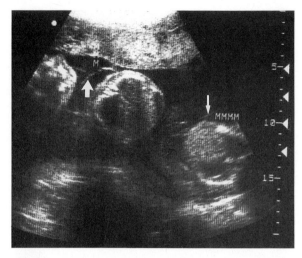

Figure 6. Triplets. Thick membrane (large arrow) separates girl from her two indentical brothers (thin membrane, small arrow).

lethal anomaly, non-communicating hemodynamic disorders), leading to therapy to salvage the normal twin.

It remains unclear what the best prenatal management for triplets constitutes,[38,39] but the nihilist-trialists certainly cast doubt on the benefits of the early diagnosis of twins.[40] Bed rest, frequent pelvic exams, cerclage, progesterone injections, and tocolytics probably do not improve outcome in twins. However, a broader variety of interventions is now available for which early detection may be key. Repeated reduction amniocenteses,[36] indomethacin therapy (for amniotic fluid reduction and/or reversal of effacement)[37] or short-term tocolysis to allow maternal steroid administration, all are greatly facilitated by early diagnosis and monitoring. Division of the *in-situ* placenta with intrauterine laser, selective feticide, transfusion of the donor twin in twin-to-twin transfusion and many other examples, are innovative therapies which merit investigation. All are more likely to succeed if diagnosis is early. Even the randomized disproval of bed rest as an intervention capable of altering outcome in twins may have produced different results if the 20 week scan had been used; these trials did not put mothers of twins to bed until well into the third trimester.[41–43] Remembering twin gestations most often result in delivery of two normal survivors, the benefits of early diagnosis would include initiating third trimester monitoring, planning the site of delivery and, perhaps most important, planning home and family renovations required to accommodate multiple new arrivals. Especially when the mother is first seen to resolve elevated MS-AFP, the high anxiety level may not be dispelled by the information that two babies are expected.

Fetal Anatomy Review

Incidental detection of a major congenital anomaly at 20 weeks averages 1–2% depending on the population scanned.[44] Serendipitous detection does not constitute proof of benefit, of course; **Table 5** shows the majority are either (a) lethal or (b) non-progressive, not life-threatening and require no intervention, except organizing delivery at an appropriate tertiary center (though this in itself may be lifesaving).

Our prenatal system has routine MS-AFP screening, genetic testing ≤ age 35, and a high compliance with universal Rh program. Since defects or abnormalities in this group are detected at 18–20 weeks as the result of *directed* scans done in the same units by the same personnel, the benefit of incidental detection is reduced. Second, with prior anomalous fetuses, the rate of detection of recurrence for referred families approaches 100%. Again, such scans are 'directed' and not included in incidental detection. Third, some anomalies are obvious later but not detectable at 18–20 weeks (see those items labelled *b* in **Table 5**, and others remain undetectable until after birth. Overall detection of major anomalies in our population is 80–85% at 20 weeks, >90% by 28 weeks. Finally, there *are* several fetuses whose detection in the random sample shown in **Table 5** was instrumental in effecting definitive therapy with measurable benefit.

Detection and management of anomalies or abnormalities of fetal condition are described in detail elsewhere.[20,45–50] What follows is a sketch of the anatomic survey needed to exclude major anomalies, including the first examination of women referred for elevated MS-AFP, risk of recurrent anomaly, alloimmunization, and so on.[17]

Head and neck

Orientation is established by identifying the midline, an exact horizontal axial plane is determined by identifying the orbits, and the standard measurements made. Rotating the transducer occipitally, without altering the plane, brings the transverse cerebellar diameter into view. *This structure is important: the normal views shown in Figure 7a effectively exclude an open neural tube defect.* Cerebellar abnormalities are associated with a large variety of fetal structural problems, and should suggest karyotype determination, detailed review of fetal anatomy, and a follow-up examination.[24,47–49] Absolute adherence to measurement criteria, frequent referencing to the midline and true horizontal/transverse orientation achieve reliable views.

The head *shape* may account for many differences between expected and measured values and provides

Table 5
100 Consecutive fetal anomalies discovered at routine midtrimester scan (normal MS-AFP)[a]

Primary anomaly		Frequency
Central nervous system		13
isolated hydrocephalus	4	
holoprosencephaly	4	
neural tube defect	2	
hydranencephaly	1	
other non-lethal brain defect	2	
Cardiovascular system		16
hypoplastic ventricle	6	
critical aortic stenosis	3	
other lethal malformation (cardiac hydrops)	3	
fetal arrhythmia requiring treatment	3	
fetal pericarditis	1	
Pulmonary-thoracic		5
diaphragmatic hernia[b]	3	
pleural effusion[b]	2	
Gastrointestinal		7
GI obstruction	2	
ascites NYD (cystic fibrosis)	1	
hepatic tumor	1	
other GI non-lethal	3	
Genitourinary tract		20
non-progressive UPJ/renal cyst	7	
unilateral multicystic dysplastic	6	
bilateral dysplasia – lethal	2	
fetal polycystic kidneys – lethal	2	
posterior urethral valves	2	
ovarian cyst[b]	1	
Musculoskeletal system		6
Lethal short limb dystrophy[b]	3	
arthrogryposus multiplex congenita	2	
non-lethal skeletal dysplasia	1	
Lymphatic obstruction		8
cystic hygroma, trisomy	4	
cystic hygroma, normal karyotype	2	
other lethal lymphatic	2	
Multiple congenital anomaly (MCA) complexes		16
MCA, trisomy proven	7	
MCA, normal chromosomes	2	
cloacal exstrophy	1	
hydrops fetalis – infectious	3	
hydrops fetalis – idiopathic	3	
Unanticipated fetal demise		1
Twin discordance		4
twin-to-twin transfusion	2	
anomaly discordance	2	
Oligohydramnios/absent renal function		4

MS-AFP, Maternal serum alpha-fetoprotein; UPJ, ureteropyeloric junction obstruction.
[a]During a randomly chosen period in 1990.
[b]At least one additional case had no apparent anomaly at 18–20 weeks, anomaly seen/apparent at 24–26 weeks.

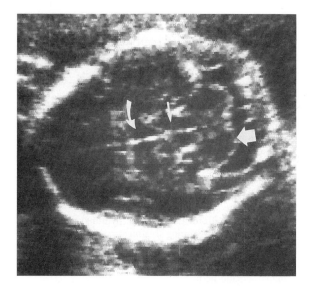

Figure 7a. Axial plane, level of the cerebellar hemispheres (large arrow). This plane is 5–7° down/occipitally from BPD, illustrates thalami (curved arrow) and cerebral peduncles (small arrow). This image puts an end to fears of spina bifida.

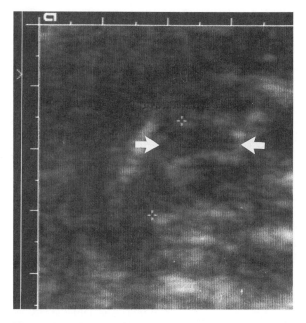

Figure 7c. 20+ weeks. 'Banana sign' posterior herniation of the cerebellum with large spina bifida, results in marked elongation of cerebellum (arrows); abnormally small TCbD = 15.8 mm.

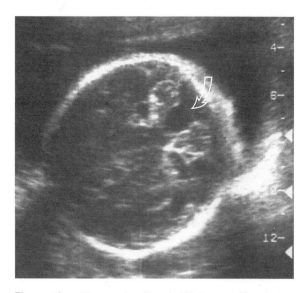

Figure 7b. 20+ weeks. Dandy-Walker malformation with absent cerebellar vermis, typical defect. Note round head, cephalic index = 0.90.

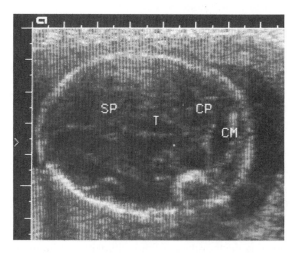

Figure 8a. Normal head shape, 19+ weeks. SP, Septum cavum pellucidum; CM, cisterna magna; T, thalami. CP, cerebellum.

clues to underlying malformation (**Figure 8**). Detailed study of the fetal brain at 18–20 weeks is not only possible, but also mandatory. In families at risk for a facial or intracranial anomaly recurrence, specific measurements such as orbital diameter (**Figure 9**) are helpful in determining facial proportions. Ventricu-

lar:hemisphere ratio, cephalic index, axial diameter of the insula and transverse occipital horn diameter also have use in particular situations. But in general, if overall measurements and symmetry are within normal ranges, and bone density is normal (anterior skull table more reflective than the falx), minute quantification is not necessary in the routine examination.

Imaging of the fetal face is particularly rewarding

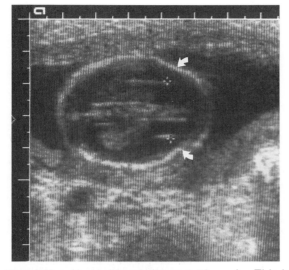

Figure 8b. Normal head shape at 18 weeks. This is *not* the 'lemon sign' – the slight depression of the frontal bones (curved arrows) is normal when the axial plane is *above* the thalami. The calipers are positioned on the lateral walls of the bodies of the lateral ventricles (normal width).

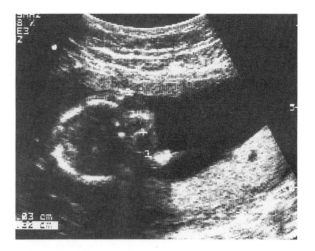

Figure 9. Normal facial proportions at 20 weeks gestation exclude recurrence of cryptophthalmos in a family with Fraser's syndrome. Interocular distance of one-third of binocular distance excludes hypertelorism.

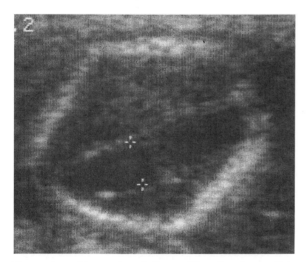

Figure 8c. Bizarre head shape ('Reverse lemon') in microcephalic fetus with trisomy 18. Occiput is on the *left*. Ventriculomegally is apparent.

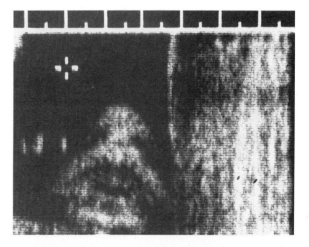

Figure 10. This facial view rules out cleft lip; better than average detail for 20 weeks.

in identifying the human character of the images on the screen (**Figure 10**). Reasonably detailed views can be seen at this age, allowing the examiner to exclude gross malformations. By 24 weeks, however, proportional enlargement of facial bones permits a repeat examination which will exclude cleft lip or other less obvious facial problems. Seeing the face is often not that critical to the examiner but when the fetus moves to where the face is plainly visible, the operator should

pause for the less formal aspects of the scan because one cannot rely on the fetus to be in the right position at the end of the appointment, so mother can 'see the baby'.

The head gives many helpful hints, directing detailed study of other regions for a corresponding anomaly (**Figure 11**). Functional assessment may also be useful. Thumb-sucking, mouthing movements, swallowing, wide 'yawning' and eye movements are all illustrated by the active 20 week fetus. There is interest in fine movements such as grimaces, grins and gentle sucking, in the novel field of fetal neurology. Carotid and/or intracranial arterial velocimetry is of uncertain signifi-

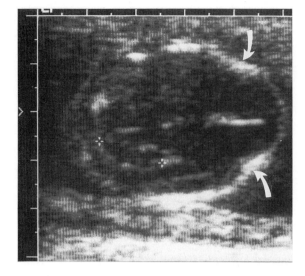

Figure 11a. Lemon sign' collapse of frontal bones (curved arrows) due to posterior herniation in spina bifida. Calipers = banana sign.

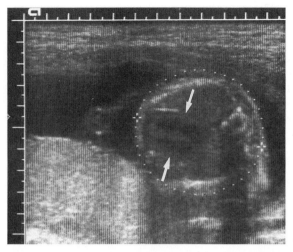

Figure 12a. Normal chest proportions at 20 weeks. The heart is oriented to the left of the chest, and occupies approximately one-third of the internal area of the thorax. Four-chamber view with A-V septum running in the 10 o'clock direction, parallel to a line between the caliper marks. The BVOD (between arrows) is 21 mm (normal, see text).

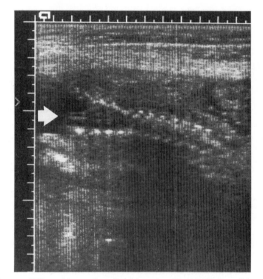

Figure 11b. Huge lumbosacral spina bifida of fetus in Figure 11a. MS-AFP = 6.6 MOM.

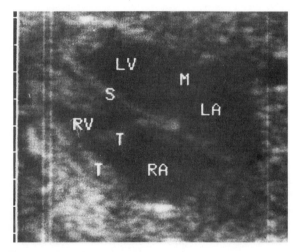

Figure 12b. Same fetus 4 weeks later, repeat visit to complete cardiac assessment – previous sibling with lethal congenital heart disease. V, Ventricles; A = atria; S, intraventricular septum; T, tricuspid valve; M, mitral valve.

cance at this gestation. The unknown potential of high-energy insonation of the early fetal brain may mean Doppler interrogation in this area is considered experimental.

Thorax

At 18–20 weeks, the four-chamber heart view is usually clear, the primary ultrasound landmark in the chest

(**Figure 12**). While this view is seen as early as 16 weeks gestation on most fetuses, detailed study of fetal cardiac anatomy is a two-stage process.[51] Examination at 18 and 24 weeks excludes lethal malformations on the first visit, and lethal or morbid connections and function at the second (**Figure 12**). Interim examinations are done if initial cardiac anatomy is unsatisfac-

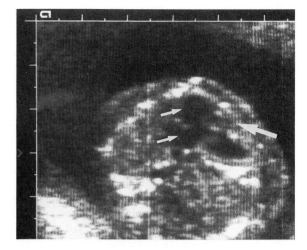

Figure 12c. Previous affected sibling, 19+ weeks gestation with right ventricular hypoplasia. Fetal spine at 7 o'clock position. Atria (small arrows) have normal proportions, normal orientation. Right ventricle (closest to chest wall, large arrow) had no measurable cavity at autopsy.

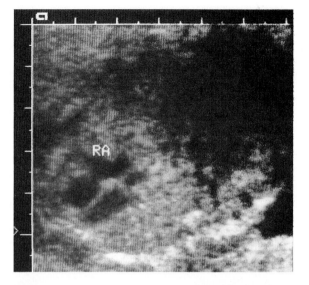

Figure 13. Lethal pulmonary hamartoma replaces normal lungs, distorts chest. Fetal chest is pointing to 11 o'clock position; cardiac axis to 7 o'clock = gross levorotation. RA, Right atrium (small for 18 weeks).

tory, or the family history is significant (**Figure 12c**). Fetal heart rate (FHR) and rhythm are usually within a narrow range.[52] Note that the normal 20 week fetus may be asystolic for up to 5 s, and that transducer pressure on the uterus, especially in a multigravid woman, easily produces significant FHR deceleration. Both occurrences are quite normal, but are readily seen by the parents watching the screen, so one must be ready to explain, and repeat the monitoring later in the examination.[53,54]

Normal lung anatomy is difficult to quantify at 18–20 weeks, except to note the relative proportions of heart and lungs ($\frac{1}{3} : \frac{2}{3}$). Gross lung abnormality can be obvious at this gestation (**Figure 13**); an association with fetal hydrops would be an indication to consider pregnancy termination.[55,56] Formal thoracic measurements are unrewarding at this gestation. These include chest:abdomen ratio, relation of clavicles to rib circumference and internal lung diameter, and they are not useful in predicting pulmonary status 3 or 4 months hence. Serial values such as in oligohydramnios may be predictive.[57,58] Marked asymmetry and flattening of the fetal chest in various skeletal dysplasias, leaving a chest with only the cardiac silhouette, would be highly predictive of lethal disease.

Fetal echocardiography is limited by the size of the heart, but it is possible to perform detailed fetal heart examination even at 20 weeks.[51,59–61] Rhythm is easily assessed in real time. Atrial-ventricular association, relative chamber size and a subjective appreciation of ventricular wall motion can all be established. A rule of thumb for heart size is that the biventricular outer diameter (BVOD; **Figure 12a**) is normally within 110% of the number of weeks gestation (e.g. ≤22 mm at 20 weeks). Quantification of valvular integrity, ejection fractions, virtual cardiac output, and so on, are beyond the scope of the routine examination, but can in fact be done this early by experienced fetal cardiologists. Referral would be based on any abnormality of the above general assessment, or as directed by specific risk factors. Cardiac malformation or malfunction indicate detailed anatomic review, reappraisal of family and environmental risks, and invasive testing for fetal karyotype, evidence of infection, and so on.[47,53,54]

Fetal breathing movements (FBM) are intermittent but not episodic[62] so that evaluation of diaphragmatic movement, effectively eliminating all but a very small diaphragmatic hernia, is readily done. On the other hand, diaphragmatic hernias (and other hernias) can slide – it may be absolutely not visible at 20 weeks, but obvious at 24 weeks; follow-up visits may be necessary in specific risk groups. FBM themselves are similar in character and mechanism throughout gestation. Fluid flux down the trachea in 'inspiration' is limited by closure of the glottis, but new techniques using color Doppler have illustrated that the glottis is not held completely closed; fluid may move in and out to some degree.[62] During vigorous FBM, when much fluid is moving through the respiratory tract, the larynx and trachea may be outlined (**Figure 14**). FBM is associated with the so-called respiratory arrhythmia, even at gestations as early as 20 weeks (**Figure 15**), and may also affect umbilical artery velocimetry.

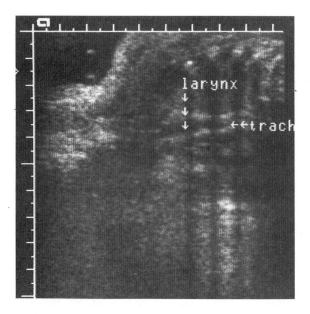

Figure 14. Longitudinal view of thoracic inlet shows larynx and upper third of trachea.

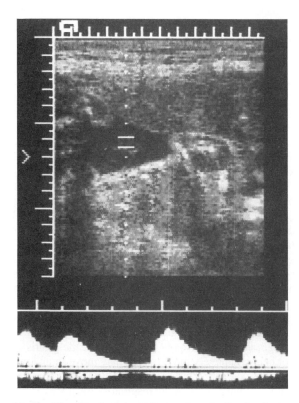

Figure 15. Marked 'respiratory' arrhythmia during vigorous fetal breathing movements. Arterial waveforms (above line) are irregularly irregular; waves below line reflect changes in venous flow.

Abdomen

At 20 weeks, the relative density of abdominal structures is similar. The fetal liver is different from the intestines, for example, but one often has to rely on one's imagination to differentiate the liver from the spleen, or the small from the large bowel.[63,64] Visualization of the fetal pancreas is not possible at 18 weeks. Demonstrating the undistended fetal stomach completely within the abdominal cavity[65] is a reasonable goal (**Figure 16**), but even this is open to overinterpretation – if the stomach appears unusually large, it is advisable to keep watching and normal motility will usually empty it in a few minutes. Similarly, finding the kidneys may be relatively straightforward, but unequivocal measurement at this gestation may be difficult.[66,67] During FBM, paraspinal longitudinal visualization will illustrate the kidneys by their up and down movement. The fetal bladder (**Figure 17**) is usualy obvious, but its presence does not mean that the fetal kidneys will continue to work. The maintenance of normal amniotic fluid volume to this gestation, likewise, does not mean that the renal function will be sustained until birth; in those at risk for recurrent renal disease, serial follow-up examinations are thus recommended.

Even in the 20 week fetus, the abdomen is much more pliable than the chest, so that restricted amniotic fluid volumes may preclude examination of the ventral abdominal wall. More than once, the presence of oligohydramnios has prevented detection of an overt defect made visible by transcutaneous ultrasound-guided instillation of normal saline.[16]

The external genitalia may be examined during this

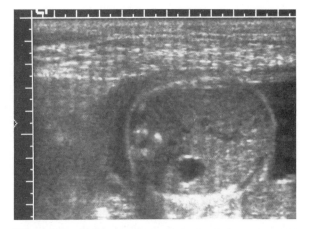

Figure 16. Cross-section of fetal abdomen at 20 weeks, showing single stomach bubble, bifurcation of umbilical vein. The landmarks for the measurement of abdominal circumference, shown here, are the same as those used at later gestation. This AC was on the 50th percentile, a level maintained throughout gestation.

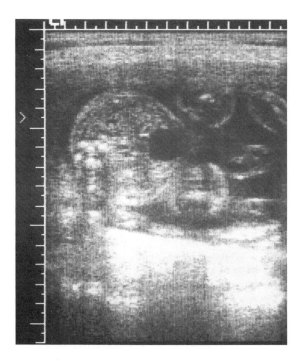

Figure 17. Transverse section, lower fetal abdomen, at 20 weeks. Note full fetal bladder, 3 o'clock position, normal amniotic fluid volume.

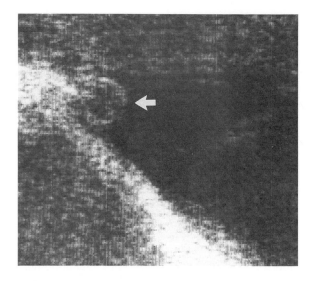

Figure 18b. Round structure on perineum (arrow) at 20+ weeks, ultimately shown to be due to severe clitoromegaly with atretic labia, Fraser's syndrome.

gestational age interval, but one must be cautious about interpretation.[68] Unless the male genitalia are unequivocally demonstrated (**Figure 18a**), one should be quite reserved about announcing fetal sex before 18–20 weeks. When one is attempting to exclude a recurrent disorder featuring ambiguous genitalia, it is best not to offer any comments unless there is absolute certainty

(**Figure 18b**); the same would apply to x-linked disorders.

Functional assessment of gastrointestinal motility may be helpful when the stomach is distended, but frequently is normal even in cases subsequently shown to be small bowel atresias of varying location. Unusual intra-abdominal echoes are not uncommon at this gestation (**Figure 19a**), often being associated with a history of flu-like illness, or defined viral exposure. Overt calcification of intra-abdominal structures may also be

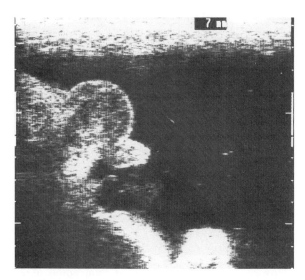

Figure 18a. Unambiguous male genitalia.

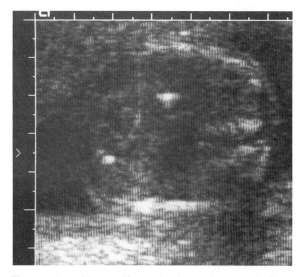

Figure 19a. Non-artifactual echogenic areas in fetal liver at 19 weeks. Term delivery, normal infant. Normal at 2 years.

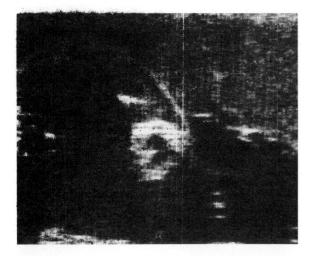

Figure 19b. Bright mass in RUQ of fetal abdomen, 20+ weeks. Spine at 9 o'clock, ? mass at 3 o'clock. At delivery, asymptomatic infant had 'calcified' colonic serosa at hepatic flexure. All cystic fibrosis markers negative on DNA hybridization; no functional deficit in gastrointestinal tract.

detected at this gestation (**Figure 19b**). It may sometimes be the result of fetal infection. While these cases should be followed serially, progressive resolution is often demonstrated, and a normal fetus/newborn results. Dire predictions about cystic fibrosis, short-gut syndrome or lethal digestive abnormalities, or the need for invasive 'testing' in the face of such non-specific findings, are clearly unwarranted. On the other hand, finding a ventral wall defect at this gestation, considering the neonatal consequences of gastroschisis/oomphalocoele, offers an ideal opportunity for appropriate fetal testing (i.e. karyotype by amniocentesis), and initiating steps leading to near-term vaginal delivery in a tertiary center, with mother and family thoroughly introduced and educated in neonatal/surgical management (see Chapter 52).[69]

A final point about fetal abdominal examination deserves emphasis. When absolute oligohydramnios presents at premature gestation, a decision must be made as to whether urgent delivery will result in a small, but potentially viable, infant, or whether the fetus has a lethal malformation justifying no invasive maneuvers. At the 20 week scan, then, one must be absolutely certain of an intact, functioning urinary tract and normal amniotic fluid volume, as can be seen in **Figure 17**.

Axial skeleton

The 18–20 week scan is *the* pivotal event in a pregnancy complicated by an elevated maternal serum AFP

(see Chapter 37). Our MS-AFP screening program has functioned since 1987 without reliance on amniocentesis, based on the high-resolution ultrasonic demonstration of normal intracranial and spinal anatomy at 18–20 weeks.[19,24] Over 2000 single, live fetuses of appropriate gestational age with elevated levels have been scanned in detail at 18 weeks to exclude neural tube defects without false-negative or false-positive scan. Obtaining proper fetal views (**Figures 7, 11, 20**) is absolutely mandatory before invasive testing can be excluded.[70] Application of this principle may account for the differences in success of an 'ultrasound only' approach.[71,72]

Well-defined landmarks are established for the study of all long bones (**Figure 21**), and many other aspects of the fetal skeleton.[73] It is worth noting that many fetuses ultimately shown to have severe skeletal dysplasia, have apparently normal bone length, ossification, density, and anatomic landmarks, when viewed at 20 weeks. Obvious bony malformation, or marked asymmetry between groups of long bones and the rest of the skeleton at this stage in gestation would be predictive of *severe* skeletal dysplasias.[74]

Integument

Fetal epidermalization nears completion at 18–20 weeks, resulting in enhanced visualization of superficial fetal structures. The hair, nails and adipose tissue are not yet visible. The fetal breast may go through a

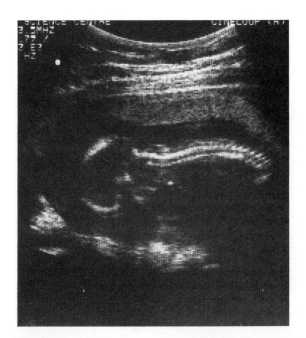

Figure 20. Longitudinal view of fetal spine at 20 weeks.

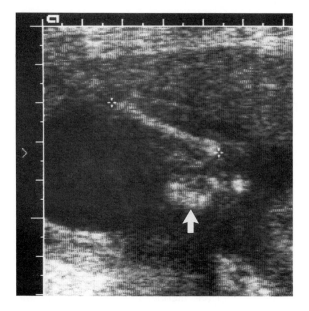

Figure 21. Femur length measured at 19+ weeks. Note iliac wing (arrow).

temporary period of growth at this time, with regression a few weeks later (**Figure 22**).[17]

Amniotic Fluid

Quantitative assessment of amniotic fluid volume in midtrimester has not been well correlated with ultimate outcome.[75] The significance of normal amniotic fluid

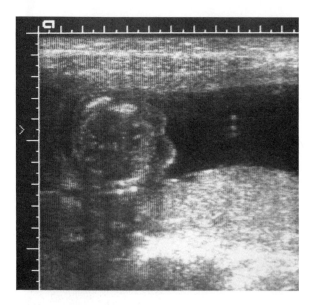

Figure 22. Routine scan at 20 weeks showed bilateral masses on the anterior chest. The ?breast enlargement resolved over the next 2 weeks. A normal girl delivered 18 weeks later.

volumes at this gestation has been emphasized, and the distinction between 'subjectively reduced', absolute oligohydramnios, marginal fluid volume, and so on, is not important here. The fetus ordinarily occupies about one-third of the intrauterine volume, the flanks of the uterus are compressible, the contour of the uterus is oval rather than tense and round, and the maximum depth from anterior to posterior is not more than 8 cm and usually less than 6 cm.

Reduced amniotic fluid volume (a maximum pocket depth <3 cm) is alarming, and should invoke a specific review of fetal status, urine production, relevant maternal history, and so on. *This finding, if conclusive, should not be deferred until a later gestation.* Presuming fetal kidney function can be proven, early therapy may have a defined role. Overtly increased amniotic fluid volume should be the cause of a number of immediate steps, further detailed in Chapter 48. In general, hydramnios suggests the possibility of fetal anomalies, or serious derangement of fetal–placental perfusion and fluid regulation.

Copious particulate matter may be seen at this gestation. The mother should be advised that this may indicate a *previous* intra-amniotic bleed, but obviously the fetus has survived that 'event'. Such advice is tempered by clinical data, and/or documentation of definite intra-amniotic clot or placental abnormality. Surveillance of amniotic fluid pocket contours at this gestation may reveal the presence of amniotic bands, and irregularities in the uterine wall (**Figure 23**).

Fetal Behavior

By 20 weeks, fetal movements are well-established, and are not strikingly different in character from the term fetus. There are many differences in the frequency, velocity, cyclicity and distribution of individual types of movements, but if you are patient, you will see virtually all the repertoire of the fully mature infant at this early stage. The 20 week fetus, unlike the mature baby, should not have discreet periods of quiescence of any length – longest 'rest cycle' <5 min.[76] Similarly, a clustering of activities analagous to behavioral states, is not seen until much later. Circadian rhythms, however, with fetal activity intensifying late in the evening, are normally present, often as early as 16 weeks.

In practical terms, one expects the fetus to be active through most of the scan. Biophysical profile scoring *per se*, has not been studied at 18–20 weeks, but all normal fetuses will easily satisfy those criteria, noting that FBM are less common, and hiccups more common, at this stage. Fetal posture will be relaxed, but not flaccid, with limbs in a position of moderate flexion, depending on the position in the uterus. Even at this stage, fixed postures and rigid or rachitic movements may signify underlying neurologic deficit.

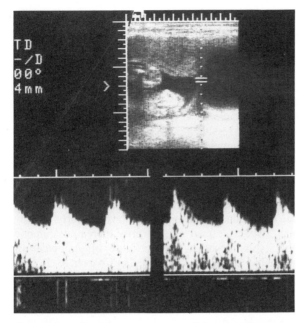

Figure 23. Duplex sonogram of intrauterine septum. In upper frame, two-dimensional image shows placenta and fetus on left, vacant amniotic fluid on right, Doppler gate (double white dashes) on septum in between. Doppler velocimetry (bottom image) of uterine artery.

Maternal and Fetal Doppler Studies

Umbilical artery velocimetry is easy to do at 20 weeks, but its significance has not yet been determined in large longitudinal studies.[77–79] A systolic:diastolic ratio within normal limits (<4 at 20 weeks) likely places the fetus in the normal group, prognostically, but this is not sufficient to disregard prenatal care.[80,81] Within the context of the routine examination, complete Doppler interrogation of all available fetal vessels at this gestation is a waste of time. On the other hand, severe growth deficiency may already be manifest at 20 weeks in the fetus showing oligohydramnios and is associated with a mortalty of up to 95%. In these fetuses, the absence of end-diastolic velocities may be helpful in excluding spontaneous premature rupture of membranes and absent renal function in anomalous fetuses even at this early stage.[82] True prospective studies are pending. In the face of a completely normal examination, any elevated *S:D* ratio, or even absent end-diastolic velocities, at this gestation, should not be used for prognosis, but would indicate continued follow-up. Color Doppler flow mapping is a visually exciting, entertaining modality. It delights parents and visitors as a novel way of showing heart activity and umbilical flow. It has marginal utility in identifying the cord insertion (to avoid it) during genetic amniocentesis and at cordocentesis (to hit it), but no other value

at the routine 18–20 week scan. Similarly, the value of documenting Doppler blood flow within the uterine circulation is not yet established. These issues are discussed further in Chapter 43.

The Placenta

Placental localization at 20 weeks has pitfalls. Since most uterine development from 20 to 40 weeks is in the lower segment, early prediction of placenta previa is full of false-positives.[83] Vaginal ultrasound may prove a reliable means of differentiation of the extent of placenta previa. This is undoubtedly true at term, but there are many errors in extrapolating from early vaginal ultrasound just as there are with abdominal examination.[84,85]

In an asymptomatic woman not at high risk (previous placenta previa, uterine anomaly, malpresentation or previous uterine infection), repeating the scan is not necessary. When the cervix is clearly identified on a suspicious ultrasound exam, or when the patient is at risk, more precise localization suggesting placenta previa may be possible this early; a repeat scan at 26–28 weeks will be more definitive.

On the other hand, documentation of abnormal placental structure (**Figure 24**), aberrant vessels within the

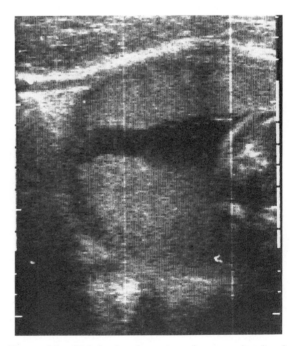

Figure 24. Bi-lobed placenta shown clearly in longitudinal view at 18 weeks. Required manual removal of placenta after spontaneous delivery of healthy infant at term.

membranes (**Figure 25**), and correlation of abnormal placental anatomy with elevated MS-AFP[86] is quite possible, and may have real impact. This simply emphasizes a principle of ultrasound examination at 20 weeks: *it never hurts to look, it only hurts to make an absolute prediction.*

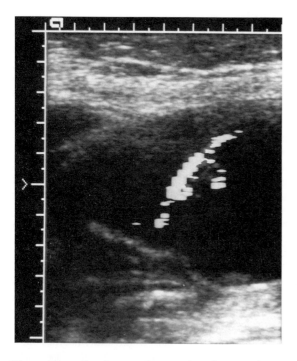

Figure 25a. Fetal vessels running in membranes identified at 20 weeks during detailed fetal/placental examination regarding elevated MS-AFP.

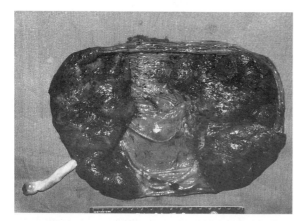

Figure 25b. Continued follow-up showed persistent, unequivocal vasa previa. Photograph of placenta after elective cesarean section, which confirmed ultrasound diagnosis. Note major umbilical vessels running through bare membranes, positioned directly over internal cervical os.

Uterine and Adnexal Structures

Normal uterine position and orientation are documented. Uterine septa may be visible, receding as pregnancy progresses (**see Figure 23**). Functional ovarian cysts have usually regressed by this gestation; if a cystic structure is visible, its appearance should arouse clinical suspicion (**Figure 26**). Customary parameters apply for invasive *vs* observational responses. As discussed above, uterine arterial Doppler interrogation may have significance in specific situations, but is currently not a component of 20 week examinations in most units. The potential advantages of these techniques are reviewed in Chapter 43.

WHOSE SCAN IS IT ANYWAY? ATTITUDES

Among the advantages attributed to the midtrimester scan detailed in **Table 2**, were references to the initiation or reinforcement of prenatal care and maternal–fetal bonding. This is not reserved for a specific parcel of time during the routine of the scan. It is, rather, a question of attitude *throughout* the examination, emphasizing that this fetus belongs to the *mother* who is the 'target' the transducer rests on. While the ultrasonographer is inputting data, information is also being acquired by the mother, who is watching the screen with a completely different eye. The *experience* of the examination is far more important to mother, her baby-to-be, her family and society in general, than it is to the caregivers *per se*. The data, the decimal

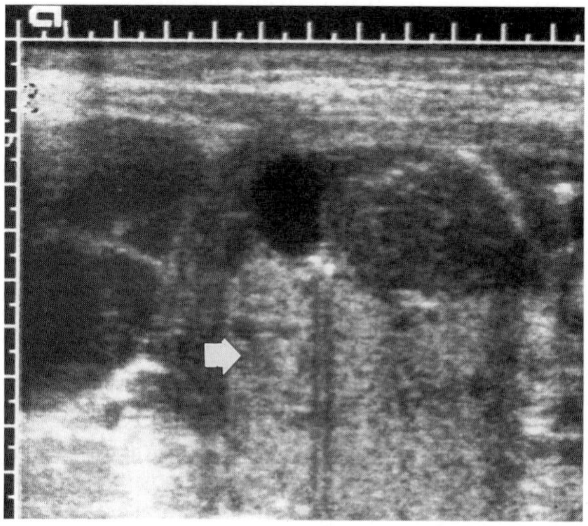

Figure 26. Transverse sonogram, 20+ weeks, shows very large corpus luteum cyst on left, abnormally large, partially hydropic placenta (arrow) and abnormally small fetus (above placenta). Triploidy.

points, the frozen planar images, the predictive accuracy, the physics of ultrasound, all belong to the clinician. The images, the swallowing, the thumb-sucking, the strength of the kicks, *the baby* belong to the family. The dividing line between data and information is impossible to discern: no aspect of the scan is private/exclusive to the ultrasonographer.

An interactive process requires the ultrasonographer to be both knowledgeable and open about fetal physiology and developmental processes, applying these with common sense. This may be highly beneficial in ongoing prenatal care. In general, women are coming to expect routine ultrasound, and believe the information provided in the scan will be reassuring for the remainder of their pregnancy.[4,5,87] Maternal response to 'open' ultrasound examinations is emphatic, demonstrable in randomized trials. These trials, done in the early and mid 1980s, found that women responded much more positively when the scan procedure included being able to see the screen throughout the examination, and a receptive attitude existed between the individual performing the scan and the mother.[88–91]

On receipt of the introduction, explanation and information detailed above, a high degree of parental interest in the scan, and satisfaction with the service provided, go hand in hand. Systematic measurement of the *impact* of such involvement is ongoing. In situations such as with elevated MS-AFP, anxiety reaches a peak at the start of the scan and declines successively from that point. It is not completely alleviated, however, until delivery.[92–94] It is interesting that these randomized trials have demonstrated maternal psychological benefit to the satisfaction of the National Perinatal Epidemiology Unit in Oxford.[11] Yet the same text suggests that the benefits currently documented do not 'provide a basis for recommending routine use of ultrasound for screening in either early or late pregnancy'. One wonders how demonstration of these maternal psychological benefits can be separated from routine application of midtrimester ultrasound.

Not only is the examination and associated interchange valued by the mother and family, it also determines ongoing planning by all levels of care givers. Though discrimination of high from low risk never ends, the process logically begins with the 18–20 week scan. Successful trials of early detection of fetal growth deficiency have utilized the midtrimester scan as baseline.[95–99] As one might expect from observational data, diagnosis of growth deficiency was greatly enhanced, while modalities of therapy in practice at the time did not result in any benefit from the diagnosis. These trials convincingly demonstrated, in randomized fashion, that if there was a successful treatment, early ultrasound would be key to its initiation. Since those trials were performed, the worldwide effort has been to study the benefits of low-dose ASA in pregnancy in pre-

venting, or in some cases actually treating, proteinuric pre-eclampsia and/or growth deficiency. Data from these trials is beginning to show a reduction in the incidence of growth deficiency, even among moderate-risk, and certainly among high-risk, pregnancies. Combining these data with the increasing support of the use of Doppler velocimetry to predict growth deficiency,[100–103] creates a logical connection between establishment of risk and successful early intervention.

Planning regarding site of delivery, necessary consultation, even arrangements as mundane as when grandparents should come, begin at this point as well. The interplay of procedures such as genetic amniocentesis, cordocentesis, and even fetal therapy also happens at this time: the examiner should take the opportunity to complete this comprehensive examination. For example, when a woman presents for her first Rh-amniocentesis at 19–20 weeks, the full examination is completed. Ideally, this routine would also be completed on referral for specific problems such as absent fetal heart tones, antepartum hemorrhage, persistent hyperemesis, and so on.

FOLLOW-UP ULTRASOUND EXAMINATIONS

This is a matter of common sense, and many examples have already been given. Follow-up visits are determined by a combination of factors, including previous and current obstetric risks, fetal and maternal indications, developments as pregnancy progresses, and the availability of successful interventions to address documented problems or risk factors.

A few aspects deserve specific comment. Follow-up examinations are not mandatory. Further ultrasound examination is not necessary if all aspects of the 18–20 week scan are normal, and clinical performance is satisfactory, judged by the primary caregivers. Routine third trimester ultrasound for detection of growth deficiency, for example, has not been validated in women with no risk factors, no associated maternal conditions and normal prenatal physical examinations. On the other hand, there are many instances when follow-up is necessary and the need well known at the 18–20 week scan.

The Fetal Assessment Unit (FAU) where the 18–20 week scan is delivered is ideally situated to coordinate follow-up with other agencies. The network of collaborating ultrasound/perinatal units will vary from place to place, but in Manitoba includes secondary-level ultrasound/obstetric units in urban areas, radiology-based ultrasound units in smaller centers, and the Obstetric Ultrasound Outreach program. The latter provides regular visits to local centers as distant as 600 km, by a team of two nurse-ultrasonographers with a portable ultrasound unit. At regular intervals, an FAU perinatologist will also travel, providing on-site continuing education, consultation services and program updates. This program is highly cost-effective in reducing the costs regarding remote patients, complicated pregnancy in rural women and duplication of services. Adequate documentation is essential, and information must be transmitted in detail, if secondary referral centers are used. Indications for follow-up, the potential outcomes, and reassurance as to ongoing communication with the primary caregiver are emphasized to the mother.

CONSEQUENCES OF THE ABNORMAL 18–20 WEEK SCAN

The discovery of an abnormality is full of obligation, virtually all of it belonging to the team doing the 18–20 week 'routine' scan. The ultrasound 'team' includes a wide variety of resources (**Table 6**). If an abnormality is discovered, intensive counseling and ongoing support are essential regardless of whether the abnormality is lethal, repairable, non-progressive or of no material consequence. The perinatologist on site in the unit throughout the working day, is available for immediate consultation. In the scanning room, the pathophysiology of the anomaly, including real-time demonstration of its ultrasound features to the parents, is explained. Then the parents (with a pause for the

Table 6
The Fetal Assessment Unit team

Group 1	Mother and fetus Patient-specific nurse ultrasonographers Perinatologist in the unit
Group 2	Prenatal counselor (AFP, Genetics, etc.) Fetal testing lab (on call to unit) Social worker (anomaly/grieving specialist)

Group 3	Fetal/neonatal consultants
	   fetal hematology (Rh laboratory)
	   infectious diseases
	   ethics consultation team
	   genetics/dysmorphology
	   neonatology
	   pediatric subspecialties:
	     surgery, cardiology, urology, nephrology,
	     dermatology, etc.
	   infectious diseases

Group 4	Family Interpreters Culture-based support Diagnosis-related support groups Attending physicians Community resources (including other ultrasound units) Labor and delivery unit

spouse to come to the unit after making arrangements for babysitting, attendance of other significant family members, etc.) move to a 'counseling' room. Ideally, such a room is private, with access to outside telephone facilities, has a comfortable non-institutional atmosphere, but includes facilities for diagrams and clear, defined explanations.

In cases of unequivocal lethal anomalies where management might include pregnancy termination, second opinion is always obtained from a consultant perinatologist, ideally at the same visit. Second opinions may not be considered mandatory in other situations, but are freely offered. A factual explanation, using illustrations as appropriate in plain language is imperative. Experience suggests that euphemisms frequently result in absolute misunderstanding: 'your baby will die' is blunt but not subject to misinterpretation. 'You will lose your baby', 'the baby won't have a heart beat', 'the baby will not survive outside the uterus', all have been misinterpreted by parents faced with absolutely certain lethal fetal anomaly.

The mother is not simply left at the exit with knowing she caries a baby with a lethal anomaly. Referral mechanisms must be in place for discussion of pregnancy termination, as appropriate to the situation.[104] The consultant concerned would ideally be highly skilled in the dilatation and evacuation (D&E) procedure, and in midtrimester termination using a combination of laminaria and local or systemic prostaglandins. In most cases, D&E techniques are less desirable in cases of lethal malformation, from the point of view of the pathologist, the geneticist, the perinatologist who will do the counseling in the next pregnancy, and not least, the parents. Just as with photographs of stillborn infants, giving the parents pictures of the ultrasound of their fetus may be an extremely valuable tool in the ongoing counseling and support of families grieving after the loss of a wanted child.

The same team is available to these parents as would be available to the parents experiencing a term stillbirth of a normal baby. This requires the availability at short notice, and the ongoing participation in all Fetal Assessment Unit programs, of a highly skilled anomaly/grieving counselor, in our case a dedicated, specifically trained social worker.

The process is even more complicated when the lethality of the anomaly is less certain, or when the anomaly is severe but not lethal. In such cases, consultation with other appropriate medical resources may prove of great value. Consultation does not end there, however. Valuable resources may be discovered within the institution in other departments, from Social Work to Nutrition. Community resources should not be overlooked, and may include the relevant specific parent/family support groups, or specific individuals within such groups. For example, many parents in the Spina Bifida Association have technical knowledge of factors such as urinary tract problems, feeding, postural problems and skin care, which is very valuable to other parents.

Counseling about anomalies deserves long and complicated explanation, beyond the function of this chapter. The fundamentals include a multidisciplinary team; a human, plain-language approach which does not seek protection in medical jargon; the appropriate invasive or other ongoing testing to clarify recurrence risk, typically including early mention that this was not the fault of the parents and, if appropriate, that future pregnancies are not doomed; a clear assignment of roles of those involved in this resolution, including the parents; and exact definition of an ongoing plan for support, contact and follow-up. Do not underestimate the importance of this process.

WHO SHOULD DO THE SCAN? PERSONNEL AND TRAINING

A number of ideals are apparent in statements issued by any of the principal ultrasound and/or radiologic societies. Examples are shown in **Table 7**, but in the expanding field of comprehensive fetal assessment, it is artificial to adhere rigidly to standards such as those set by a national association in the mid-1980s, established for contact scanners in a non-real-time context with interpretation at the end of the day at a viewing box. Often, common sense and an obstetric orientation are more useful than any number of didactic courses.

Course lengths may vary, but it takes at least a year of 'hands-on' scanning of referral patients to gain independent competence in practice. Following strict measurement criteria is important; patience and high standards for 'normal' combine to make anatomic review a meticulous process; manual dexterity and a

light but firm touch on the transducer are valued skills. Sensitivity to the patient extends beyond showing the parents the scan; it includes being receptive to new medical/fetal information which may be critical in ongoing management. As these qualities mature with experience, a curious 'three-dimensional' facility evolves. This learned skill includes visualizing the three-dimensional fetus as comprised of the two-dimensional planes on the screen, assembling them in logical sequence. *The continuous referencing supplied by subtle angulations in transducer attitude, means that this three-dimensional 'assembly' can only be done in real time and not at the end of the day by the review of static pictures.*

Randomized comparisons of ultrasonographers of different background have not appeared in the literature. Previous divisions of scan content (Level 1,2,3) are really no longer relevant – all patients should have at least one *complete* scan.[7] Our nurse-ultrasonographers function competently at this level, detecting >80% of major fetal anomalies present at the 18–20 week scan and >90% on follow-up at 22–24 weeks, while carrying out the complete survey in an average 20-min scan.[105] Certain scans are carried out electively by the perinatologist (**Table 8**) The nurse-ultrasonographers are also primary educators – nutritional counseling, lifestyle advice and basic perinatal/maternal physiology are favourite topics. Many changes – ligament laxity, postural shifts, abdominal stretching, fatigue, cardiovascular demands – are impacting at the time of the 18–20 week scan. Many complications – invasive monitoring, even intrauterine fetal transfusions for serious alloimmunization, for example – will be initiated at this time, and the basic educational components of these processes are critical. So, while the 'scan' may seem like a simple test, it offers a unique opportunity to consolidate a comprehensive, holistic approach to pregnancy. Who does the scan, and who is immediately available to collaborate, may well determine the success of that approach.

Table 7
The ideal 'fetal assessor': Aptitudes

Perinatal orientation

Common sense

Three-dimensional real-time ultrasonographer[a]

Technical skills/attitudes
    methodical approach
    adherence to measurement criteria
    detailed observational skills
    manual dexterity
    awareness of mother
    receptive to patient information

Knowledge base
    didactic training – ultrasound
    didactic training – perinatal/obstetric

[a]See text.

Table 8
Scan review in real-time by perinatologist

Elevated MS-AFP (all)
Size–dates discrepancy > 10 days
Referred by genetics (previous abnormality)
Multiple gestation
All invasive fetal testing (↑ Down risk,
    alloimmunized, etc.)
Anomaly suspected
Abnormal amniotic fluid, abnormal fetal behavior
Abnormal placenta, membranes, uterus
Maternal medical disorders (e.g. LAC[+] with losses)

MS-AFP, Maternal serum alpha-fetoprotein; LAC[+], lupus anticoagulant positive.

WHY NOT SCAN AT 18–20 WEEKS?

One should always weigh the advantages of scanning against individual relative contraindications as listed in **Table 9**. The law of diminishing returns suggests very limited benefit to women with exemplary obstetric history, dating, performance so far, prohibitions against any action in case of abnormal findings and 'faith' in the goodness of this baby (so there would be no additional positive psychological benefit). If there was an element of hardship involved in achieving the scan (long distance, financial inability, severe anxiety, etc.) an equilibrium *against* scanning might be achieved.

These are relative issues and are usually sorted out by the primary caregiver. They may be revisited, however, when there is further inconvenience (waiting a long time, bladder-filling required, vaginal ultrasound indicated), when follow-up examinations or tests are indicated, when there is an adverse outcome despite a satisfactory examination, or when hidden agendas (most often identification of fetal sex) cannot be satisfied for technical reasons. Carefully considered responses, based on local factors, should be available to all personnel performing ultrasound examinations. *'Discuss it with your doctor when he gets the report' is no longer a sufficient response.*

This point deserves emphasis. Increasingly, popular exposure to the abilities and expectations of ultrasound means that patients/mothers are often unimpressed with the technological 'wonder' of seeing their half-grown baby on the screen. As attitudes evolve, blanket acceptance previously 'enjoyed' by ultrasonographers is giving way to a high level of technical expectation, and lower tolerance to the negative aspects of ultrasound examination. For, not only are there relative reasons not to have a scan, there are several areas where the scan may produce a perceived 'harm' (**Table 10**).

Safety of Midtrimester Ultrasound

Historically, safety concerns were based on the physical properties of sound, animal experimentation, individual case reports, or uncontrolled, selected groups with independent association of ultrasound exposure and adverse outcomes (e.g. children scanned for clini-

Table 10
Potential negative impacts of ultrasound

Fetal effects
  safety
  behavioral (immediate)

Maternal effects
  Ultrasound exam
  anxiety
  secondary morbidity

Family

Physician

Perinatal team

Health care system

Table 9
Reduced benefits of routine 18–20 week ultrasound exam

Limited value	Increased 'cost'

Asymptomatic mother with all of:
    certain pregnancy dating (IVF, ovulation, induction,
    artificial insemination, etc.)
Normal MS-AFP
Normal obstetric risk factors
No relevant positive history
No interest in fetal normality
Normal 12–14 week scan
Maximally bonded
	Self-paying patient with limited resources
	Long-distance travel required
	Scarce ultrasound resources
	Test-based or location-based maternal anxiety

Predetermined nihilism	Inappropriate expectations

No tests, no treatment, no action allowed by parents'
    decision
	'Rule out' growth deficiency, placenta previa, determine
	    mode of delivery, etc.
	Absolutely determine risk category assignment

cal growth deficiency are smaller at age 2 than their unscanned, normally grown peers). There is no evidence in the ongoing follow-up of large non-randomized populations or smaller randomized trials, of cavitation, sister chromatid exchanges, free radical generation, membrane interface motion, intrauterine heating or cell death, from intrauterine ultrasound exposure, producing detectable neonatal or pediatric injury.[106–111] Considering the *millions* of people who have been scanned, the absence of injury is reassuring.

This 'safety' is not surprising. Total sound exposure is low, considering the time the scanner is on, the tiny fraction of time sound is actually being *sent* ('duty cycle') during a total transducer cycle, distance of the fetus from the energy source, low energy emission in the first place, reduced susceptibility (organogenesis long since complete), fetal movement in and out of the scan, and insonation of individual structures for short periods of time.[112] Laboratory experiments showing cell or organ injury are not in general applicable to human experience. Reviews demonstrating the absence of adverse effects are numerous and deal with concerns about hearing, neurologic function, malignancy, birthweight and growth, and many other factors, in large populations.[113] Further, 4-year follow-up of children exposed to much higher energy sounds of much less-refined quality (i.e. a blast of 99–129 dB, across 30–10 000 Hz, peak 500 Hz, for 3 s up to 27 times in a pregnancy!) during acoustic stimulation, showed no hearing or neurologic deficit.[114]

Several factors have changed over time which justify confidence about safety: positive cases would likely have been reported by now, energy outputs have fallen progressively with each generation of ultrasound instruments, quality control has improved, and initial worrisome experimental data have failed reproducibility. This 'safety' may be overstated, however, due to: low frequency of effects, long exposure–effect interval (e.g. at reproductive ages, 20–40 years later), absence of appropriate controls, unexpected (and therefore unmeasured) effects, and other theoretical concerns. Finally, the current technology (Doppler ultrasound, vaginal ultrasound) and practice (very early pregnancy scans, multiple repeat scans, prolonged periods of observation/insonation) are different from that upon which 'safety' predictions have been based. There may be concern, for example, that detailed study of embryonic (i.e. susceptible to organ injury) cerebral circulation (i.e. subject to unique vascular effects) with vaginal (i.e. very close) Doppler (i.e. higher energy) might well deliver ultrasound with characteristics not experienced by any of the subjects currently being reported in follow-up studies.

A final statement on safety cannot be issued. At present, there is no evidence of any injury of any kind due to midtrimester obstetric ultrasound.

Maternal and 'Other' Negative Effects

Bladder-filling is a painful and unnecessary experience for the 18–20 week scan. Other physical unpleasantness, however, includes transducer pressure on the lower abdomen, ultrasonographer's arm resting on the woman's chest or abdomen, vaginal ultrasound, manual vaginal manipulation to displace a low-lying fetus, and many other technical side-effects. These side-effects are much more likely when extreme detail is required (e.g. elevated MS-AFP), when mother is very obese, or when other factors interfere with imaging.

Obstetrical orientation and training is emphasized in dealing with the anxious mother/parents. In some situations, it would be anticipated (previous lethal malformation), but many 'routine' examinations can be sources of ongoing anxiety and conflict if the examiner is inflexible. In addition to this 'psychological morbidity', finding a problem in the routine setting inevitably leads to further, 'secondary' morbidity – repeat examinations, invasive testing, or even pregnancy termination. Another risk for negative impact on family and attending physician alike may be *isolation*. Being secretive about ultrasound and the data derived from it is counterproductive. Even in the case of grievous malformation, ultrasound terminology (like medical jargon everywhere) ought to give way to clear language.

This comprehensive, humane approach to the midtrimester exam makes significant new demands on the perinatal team: one skilled fetal medicine specialist-ultrasonographer must be immediately available for invasive testing, parent counseling and consultation as described above. As well as these constraints, the scan/equipment/personnel have to be paid for. It is in this context that the benefits of midtrimester ultrasound need to be measured.

Measuring the Benefits

The 20 week scan provides detailed visualization of the potential intrauterine patient. Identification of a treatable problem, or a hopeless anomaly, would be both significant and timely. In the large majority, however, outcome was destined to be normal – 'proving' that normal outcome by midtrimester ultrasound, produces no objective obstetric benefit, but has a significant cost. The evolution of obstetric ultrasound has not been preceded by the kind of research and supervised trials demanded of the pharmaceutical industry. Broadly based acceptance/application, fortified with confidence in safety, is no proof of efficacy, of course. Obstetric ultrasound has become entrenched *despite* many difficulties in identifying and evaluating the 'benefits'.

Detailed analysis possible through the Oxford Database of Perinatal Trials, for example, suggested that the only benefits were those ascribable to accurate pregnancy dating.[11] These included a reduced incidence of intervention for postdatism (most women with corrected dates managed to labor spontaneously before intervention was scheduled) in the routinely scanned group, and the presence of morbidity from inappropriate intervention (for mistaken postdatism) in the non-scanned group. Obviously, if postdatism was 'managed' with observation alone, and/or induction was a straightforward process with little liability, the 'benefits' of scanning would be faint. In fact, both of these conditions have been shown in a recent trial of postdates management.[115]

Many factors in the cost–benefit equations for ultrasound are changing. Longer, improved follow-up has validated safety. Better resolution, improved training and higher standards have all reduced errors and omissions, while magnifying the obvious benefits. Public acceptance of the application of technology, and the popular 'entertainment' value of ultrasound images of the baby, mean there is little resistance to universal application. These factors support propagation of routine obstetric ultrasound.

Obstetric practices have changed. Many centers have no problem deciding what to do about postdatism, and little morbidity arises. Waiting for spontaneous labor and allowing a trial of vaginal birth after previous cesarean section means 'precise' dating is of little benefit if the newer approach (i.e. doing nothing) is in place. A better understanding of fetal conditions may suggest early diagnosis is of no advantage: there is no effective treatment (renal agenesis); new intrauterine therapies have been replaced by even newer, more effective neonatal treatment (congenital diaphragmatic hernia); or even that the prenatal treatment produced worse results than waiting for newborn therapy (most hydrocephalus). In some cases, early ultrasound produces impressions which cause anxiety, expense and intervention erroneously: placental site and fetal presentation can be pitfalls here. These changes continue to complicate the measurement of the benefits of ultrasound in pregnancy.

Psychological impacts are receiving increasing attention, and they are not unipolar either. While information and preparation (including prenatal family bonding) are admirable goals, delivery of the necessary data often adds large components of anxiety and uncertainty. Hope, love, expectation, responsibility, remorse, grief are increasingly nurtured and magnified in the direction of the fetal image on the video screen.

The demand that an intervention should produce altered (i.e. improved) outcome is a primary justification of perinatal trialists: this approach has produced several critical reviews of routine ultrasound in pregnancy.[12,96,97,116,117] Additional trials have since been published, with some clarification of the issue (summarized in **Table 11**).[95,118,119] Not all trials are

constructed equally; there are different schemes of application and different definitions of outcome. 'Trialists' regard success differently. For example, earlier detection of placenta previa was defined by the authors of the Helsinki Trial[119] as an attribute; the numbers were too few to compare with the four unscreened patients (all of whom hemorrhaged). Knowing placenta previa was present did not alter the outcome of cesarean section, and so on: meta-analysis might judge that there is 'no benefit' in this regard.

Comparing routine, systematized ultrasound to 'selected', demand-based ultrasound makes this discussion even more problematic. In the trials noted, 60–80% of the 'controls' had obstetric ultrasound, many before or at the same time as the experimental group.[9,10] Many of the benefits of ultrasound are inherent in having one detailed examination, not in that examination being on a specific day in the pregnancy – randomization obscures such benefits. Further, negative findings are often overlooked.[120] For example, ultrasound in obstetrics has eliminated placental angiography and radionucleotide placental scans, almost eliminated placental hormone testing (conjugated estriols, HPL, etc.) and dramatically reduced prenatal radiography. These benefits are so obvious that they may be overlooked because a proper 'control' population, which receives *no* prenatal ultrasound but does experience *all* of the other aspects of optimal prenatal care, is (a) not available historically and (b) not ethically possible prospectively.

Cost savings from such a program may also be hard to measure. Several trials have shown decreased use of third trimester scans when answers were sought in advance at 20 weeks. The number of general prenatal visits may be fewer under some circumstances, but may rise when admission is required to deal with specific complications found by the 18–20 week scan: the net result may be 'no change', even though quality of care rises substantially. Direct cost-benefit analyses are limited and inexact. One trial claimed the 18–20 week program could be paid for by the unnecessary third trimester scans it precluded. Others suggested reduced cesarean section rate, reduced hospital admissions, reduced amount of expensive neonatal care, etc., as ways of effectively financing routine midtrimester obstetric ultrasound programs. Overall, the impact of Fetal Assessment Units is measurable and very cost-effective;[121] the exact proportion of that saving which is derived primarily from keeping high-risk care on an out-patient basis due to routine 18–20 week ultrasound is hard to quantify.

This discussion cannot be considered complete without mention of the reverse argument, i.e. what are the costs of not doing routine ultrasound? Initially, there are a host of omissions – all the advantages of **Table 2** disappear. More than that, however, is the abrogation of women's rights, and perhaps fetal 'rights' as well.[122]

Table 11
Benefits demonstrated in randomized trials

Benefit	Ref. 118 (1986–1988)	Ref. 119 (1986–1987)	Ref. 95 (1985–1987)	Ref. 96 (1979–1981)	Ref. 97 (1979–1980)	Ref. 116 (1979–1980)	Ref. 117 (1977–1987)
			Trials				
Reduced prenatal visits	NT	+	+[b]	NT	—	NT	NT
Improved twin management	—	+	—	NT	+	+	NT
Improved management of placenta previa	NT	+	NT	NT	NT	NT	NT
Reduced third trimester scans[a]	NT	+	+	NT	+	NT	NT
Reduced hospital admission	+	—	—	—	+	+	NT
Fewer interventions: postdatism	—	—	+	NT	—	+	NT
Fewer interventions: overall	+	—	+	—	—	NT	—
Birthweight <2500 g	+	—	+	—	+	NT	—
Fewer NICU admissions	—	—	—	NT	—	+	NT
Perinatal mortality	+	+	—	—	—	—	—

+, Benefit demonstrated with routine ultrasound; —, no benefit proven; NT, not tested; NICU, neonatal intensive care unit.
[a]Required by attending physician, i.e. excluding screening scan(s); [b]in specific circumstances only.

Without an opportunity to consider the information available, the family of a grievously handicapped newborn may suffer beyond the range of any randomized trial's ability to detect.[123] It may be considered that a woman's right to pregnancy termination, fetal therapy, safer site of delivery, even the right to begin 'knowing' her baby is curtailed by withholding this scan; so much so, it might be expected that a woman who understood the potential of this exam, would (by that understanding alone) be deemed to have an indication for it.[124] The same authors have not yet made a case for the fetus in this regard, perhaps a less secure area of perinatal ethics.[125] It seems likely, however, that the progress of fetal ethics, advocacy and, ultimately, fetal law, will soon lead to the suggestion that proper physical examination, a component of any basic medical care, is a fetal right as well.[126]

CONCLUSIONS

An overwhelming trend (perhaps most dominant in affluent/medicolegally sensitive health care jurisdictions, but prevalent in almost all medical cultures) is the broad application of ultrasound in obstetrics. The number of scans per pregnancy varies with reports, but averages more than two per delivery in many areas. It would seem sensible, in health care budget terms, to ensure that at least one examination be allocated routinely to each fetus on a routine basis, with the remainder to be applied on a risk-related, 'indicated' basis. The decision to do this is influenced by many factors, but the most important must be that there is significant benefit to routine obstetric ultrasound.

Proving the benefit of routine obstetric ultrasound may be difficult. This may be because there is little or no advantage, i.e. no benefit exists. There are enough illustrations in individual cases, specific risk groups, specific fetal disorders, and in the randomized trials, to show that routine ultrasound is not without benefit. The second, more likely explanation is that the benefits are multiple: some achieve statistical significance based on obstetric practice at the moment, others require much larger population bases, and some are so obvious as not to be counted by statisticians.

This chaper has illustrated one pragmatic approach to the routine application of a thorough but efficient ultrasound examination at 18–20 weeks gestation. This examination addresses a broad range of objectives and is effective only when applied in the context of effective care of both mother and fetus in a fully comprehensive fashion. Ultrasound imparts very little energy – it does not, therefore, have any direct therapeutic effect of its own; its only benefit must derive from a detailed

THE ROUTINE 18–20 WEEK ULTRASOUND SCAN
Summary of Management Options

Prerequisites

- Maternal serum AFP result

- Basic details of history and examination for pregnancy and routine investigations completed

- Relevant risk factors identified

- Relevant serology and genetic concerns specified

- Pre-scan interview and counseling

Contraindications (relative)

- See **Table 9**

Preparation

- High-resolution real-time gray scale US machine

- Experienced ultrasonographer

- Semi-recumbent with screen visible to mother and ultrasonographer

Content

- Viability

- Gestational age

- Fetal number

- Anatomy
  - head and neck
  - thorax
  - abdomen
  - axial skeleton
  - integument

- Amniotic fluid

- Fetal activity/behavior

- ? Doppler studies

- Placenta

- Uterus and adnexal structures

Documentation (varies with centers)

- Written

- Hard copy

- Video

Appropriate follow-up of problems

background of awareness of fetal medicine and developmental obstetrics. In plain language, ordering an 18–20 week scan cannot substitute for sensitive, interactive prenatal care.

The midtrimester scan presents an ideal opportunity to document milestones, to detect significant variance, to alleviate anxiety or to initiate specific care. The care which may be initiated varies from fetal, to fetal/maternal, to maternal only, and beyond, to the family in general. The importance of the care given may not be in its medical significance but in the ownership of information about the pregnancy being given to the mother and her family, a private intelligence which is bound to effect responsible decision-making before and after birth. In fact, the greatest benefits derived from our ongoing, improving awareness of the fetus as a patient (an awareness which can be started effectively and efficiently at the 18–20 week scan), may lie in enhanced social attitudes (a public intelligence) about the *life* of the human fetus.

REFERENCES

1   Grennert L, Persson PH, Gennser G (1978) Benefits of ultrasonic screening of a pregnant population. *Acta Obstetrica et Gynecologica Scandinavica* **78**:5–14 (suppl).

2   Persson PH, Kullander S (1983) Long-term experience of general ultrasound screening in pregnancy. *American Journal of Obstetrics and Gynecology* **146**:942–947.

3   Manning FA, Morrison I, Harman CR *et al.* (1987) Fetal assessment based on biophysical profile scoring: Experience in 19,221 referred high-risk pregnancies. II. An analysis of false-negative fetal deaths. *American Journal of Obstetrics and Gynecology* **157**:880–884.

4   Milne LS, Rich OJ (1981) Cognitive and affective aspects of the responses of pregnant women to sonography. *Maternal and Child Nursing Journal* **10**:15–39.

5   Hyde B (1986) An interview study of pregnant women's attitudes to ultrasound scanning. *Social Science in Medicine* **22**:587–592.

6   Morris M, Arnett J, Harman CR (1994) Ultrasound fetal assessment in the adolescent pregnancy clinic. *American Journal of Obstetrics and Gynecology* (in press).

7   Evans MI, Chervenak FA, Eden RD (1991) Report of the Council on Scientific Affairs of the American Medical Association: Ultrasound evaluation of the fetus. *Fetal Diagnosis and Therapy* **6**:132–147.

8   Consensus Report (1984) The Use of Diagnostic Ultrasound Imaging During Pregnancy (Committee: F Frigoletto, R. Auerbach, A Brickler *et al.*). *Journal of the American Medical Association* **252**:669–672.

9   Cochlin DL (1984) Effects of two ultrasound scanning regimens on the management of pregnancy. *British Journal of Obstetrics and Gynaecology* (1987) **91**:885–890.

10 Belfrage P, Fernstrom I, Hallenberg G (1987) Routine or selective ultrasound examinations in early pregnancy. *Obstetrics and Gynecology* **69**:747–750.

11 Neilson J, Grant A (1991) Ultrasound in pregnancy. In Chalmers I, Enkin M, Keirse MJNC (eds), *Effective Care in Pregnancy and Childbirth*, Vol. 1, pp. 419–439. Oxford: Oxford University Press.

12 Thacker SB (1985) Quality of controlled clinical trials: The case of imaging ultrasound in obstetrics: A review. *British Journal of Obstetrics and Gynaecology* **92**:437–444.

13 Goldstein SR (1991) Embryonic ultrasonographic measurements: Crown-rump length revisited. *American Journal of Obstetrics and Gynecology* **165**:497–501.

14 Kossoff G, Griffiths KA, Dixon CE (1991) Is the quality of transvaginal images superior to transabdominal ones under matched conditions? *Ultrasound in Obstetrics and Gynecology* **1**:29–35.

15 Dawes GS, Moulden M, Redman CWG (1991) System 8000: Computerized antenatal FHR analysis. *Journal of Perinatal Medicine* **19**:47–51.

16 Gembruch U, Hansmann M (1988) Artificial instillation of amniotic fluid as a new technique for the diagnostic evaluation of cases of oligohydramnios. *Prenatal Diagnosis* **8**:33–45.

17 Harman CR (1989) Comprehensive examination of the human fetus. *Fetal Medicine* **1**:125–176.

18 Romero R, Pilu G, Jeanty P, Ghidini A, Hobbins JC (eds) (1988) Normal sonographic anatomy of the fetal central nervous system: The central nervous system. In *Prenatal Diagnosis of Congenital Anomalies*, pp. 1–21. Norwalk, CT: Appleton and Lange.

19 Chervenak FA, Isaacson G, Lorber J (eds) (1988) Normal anatomy. In *Anomalies of the Fetal Head, Neck and Spine: Ultrasound Diagnosis and Management*, pp. 1–37. Philadelphia, PA: W.B. Saunders.

20 Manning F (1994) *Fetal Medicine*. Norwalk, CT: Appleton and Lange. (in press).

21 Dombrowski MP, Bottoms SF, Zador I *et al.* (1991) Ultrasound findings in gestations destined for unanticipated fetal demise. *Ultrasound in Obstetrics and Gynecology* **1**:269–271.

22 Reece EA, Gabrielli S, Degennaro N, Hobbins JC (1989) Dating through pregnancy: A measure of growing up. *Obstetrical and Gynecological Survey* **44**:544–555.

23 Campbell S, Warsof SL, Little D, Cooper DJ (1985) Routine ultrasound screening for the prediction of gestational age. *Obstetrics and Gynecology* **65**:613–620.

24 Nicolaides KH, Campbell S, Gabbe SG, Guidetti R (1986) Ultrasound screening for spina bifida: Cranial and cerebellar signs. *Lancet* **ii**:72–74.

25 Mercer BM, Sklar S, Shariatmadar A *et al.* (1987) Fetal foot length as a predictor of gestational age. *American Journal of Obstetrics and Gynecology* **156**:350–355.

26 Lockwood CJ, Lynch L, Berkowitz RL (1991) Ultrasonographic screening for the Down syndrome fetus. *American Journal of Obstetrics and Gynecology* **165**:349–352.

27 Reynolds TM, Penney MD, Hughes H (1992) Ultrasonographic dating of pregnancy causes significant errors in Down syndrome risk assessment that may be minimized by use of biparietal diameter-based means. *American Journal of Obstetrics and Gynecology* **166**:872–877.

28 Winston YE, Horger EO (1988) Down syndrome and femur length. *American Journal of Obstetrics and Gynecology* **159**:1018.

29 Jeanty P (1990) Fetal biometry. In Fleischer AC, Romero R, Manning FA, Jeanty P, James AE Jr (eds), *The Principles and Practice of Ultrasonography in Obstetrics and Gynecology*, 4th edn, pp. 93–108. Norwalk, CT: Appleton and Lange.

30 Sulak LE, Dodson MG (1986) The vanishing twin: Pathologic confirmation of an ultrasonographic phenomenon. *Obstetrics and Gynecology* **68**:811–815.

31 Chitkara U, Berkowitz RL (1991) Multiple gestations. In Gabbe SG, Niebyl JR, Simpson JL (eds), *Obstetrics: Normal and Problem Pregnancies*, 2nd edn, pp. 881–921. New York: Churchill Livingstone.

32 Levi CS, Lyons EA, Lindsay DJ, Gratton D (1990) The sonographic evaluation of multiple gestation pregnancy. In Fleischer AC, Romero R, Manning FA, Jeanty P, James AE Jr (eds), *The Principles and Prac-*

tice of Ultrasonography in Obstetrics and Gynecology, 4th edn, pp. 359–379. Norwalk, CT: Appleton and Lange.

33 Winsor EJT, St John Brown B, Luther ER, Heifetz SA, Welch JP (1987) Decreased co-twin as a cause of false positive amniotic fluid AFP and AchE. *Prenatal Diagnosis* **7**:485–489.

34 Hanna JH, Hill JM (1984) Single intrauterine fetal demise in multiple gestation. *Obstetrics and Gynecology* **63**:126–130.

35 Mahony BS, Petty CN, Nyberg DA *et al.* (1990) The 'stuck twin' phenomenon: Ultrasonographic findings, pregnancy outcome, and management with serial amniocenteses. *American Journal of Obstetrics and Gynecology* **163**:1513–1522.

36 Urig MA, Clewell WH, Elliott JP (1990) Twin–twin transfusion syndrome. *American Journal of Obstetrics and Gynecology* **163**:1522–1526.

37 Lange IR, Harman CR, Ash KM *et al.* (1989) Twins with hydramnios: Treating premature labor at source. *American Journal of Obstetrics and Gynecology* **160**:552–557.

38 Crowther CA (1982) Hospitalisation for bed rest in triplet pregnancy. In Chalmers I (ed.), *Oxford Database of Perinatal Trials*. Version 1.3, Disk Issue 8, Autumn 1982, Record 3377.

39 Alvarez M, Berkowitz R (1990) Multifetal gestation. *Clinics in Obstetrics and Gynecology* **33**:79–87.

40 Crowther C, Chalmers I (1991) Bed rest and hospitalization during pregnancy. In Chalmers I, Enkin M, Keirse MJNC (eds), *Effective Care in Pregnancy and Childbirth*, Vol. 1, pp. 624–632. Oxford: Oxford University Press.

41 Saunders MC, Dick JS, Brown IMcL (1985) The effects of hospital admission for bed rest on the duration of twin pregnancy: A randomised trial. *Lancet* **ii**:793–795.

42 Hartikainen-Sorri AL (1986) Is routine hospitalisation of twin pregnancy necessary? *Acta Geneticae Medicae Gemellologicae* **34**:189–192.

43 Crowther CA, Verkuyl DAA, Neilson JP, Bannerman C, Ashurst HM (1990) The effects of hospitalization for rest on fetal growth, neonatal morbidity, and length of gestation in twin pregnancy. *British Journal of Obstetrics and Gynaecology* **97**:872–877.

44 Chitty LS, Hunt GH, Moore J, Lobb MO (1991) Effectiveness of routine ultrasonography in detecting fetal structural abnormalities in low risk population. *British Medical Journal* **303**:1165–1169.

45 Fleischer AC, Romero R, Manning FA, Jeanty P, Kames AEJr (eds) (1990) *The Principles and Practice of Ultrasonography in Obstetrics and Gynecology*, 4th edn. Norwalk, CT: Appleton and Lange.

46 Graham JM Jr, Otto C (1990) Clinical approach to prenatal detection of human structural defects. *Clinics in Perinatology* **17**:513–547.

47 Chueh J, Golbus MS (1989) Diagnosis and management of the abnormal fetus. *Fetal Medical Review* **1**:61–78.

48 Holzgreve W (1990) Sonographic screening for anatomic defects. *Seminars in Perinatology* **14**:504–513.

49 Nicolaides KH, Snijders RJM, Gosden CM *et al.*

(1992) Ultrasonographically detectable markers of fetal chromosome abnormalities. *Lancet* **340**:704–707.

50 Benacerraf BR (1991) Prenatal sonography of autosomal trisomies. *Ultrasound in Obstetrics and Gynecology* **1**:66–75.

51 Allan LD (1986) *Manual of Fetal Echocardiography*. Lancaster: MTP Press.

52 Pillai M, James D (1990) The development of fetal heart rate patterns during normal pregnancy. *Obstetrics and Gynecology* **76**:812–816.

53 Berg KA, Clark EB, Astemborski JA, Boughman JA (1988) Prenatal detection of cardiovascular malformations by echocardiography: an indication for cytogenetic evaluation. *American Journal of Obstetrics and Gynecology* **159**:477–481.

54 Crawford DC, Chita SK, Allan LD (1988) Prenatal detection of congenital heart disease: Factors affecting obstetric management and survival. *American Journal of Obstetrics and Gynecology* **159**:352–356.

55 Dolkart L, Reimers FT, Helmuth WV *et al.* (1992) Antenatal diagnosis of pulmonary sequestration: A review. *Obstetrical and Gynecological Survey* **47**:515–520.

56 Mayden KL, Tortora M, Chervenak FA *et al.* (1984) The antenatal sonographic detection of lung masses. *American Journal of Obstetrics and Gynecology* **148**:349–351.

57 D'Alton M, Mercer B, Riddick E, Dudley D (1992) Serial thoracic versus abdominal circumference ratios for the prediction of pulmonary hypoplasia in premature rupture of the membranes remote from term. *American Journal of Obstetrics and Gynecology* **166**:658–663.

58 Nimrod C, Nicholson S, Davies D, Harder J, Dodd G, Sauve R (1988) Pulmonary hypoplasia testing in clinical obstetrics. *American Journal of Obstetrics and Gynecology* **158**:277–280.

59 Copel JA, Hobbins JC, Kleinman CS (1991) Doppler echocardiography and color flow mapping. In Platt LD (ed.), *Obstetrics and Gynecology Clinics of North America* **18**:845–851.

60 Carpenter RJ, Edmondson S, Ayres N (1993) Management of fetal cardiac dysrhythmias. In Harman CR (ed.), *Invasive Fetal Testing and Treatment*. Oxford: Blackwell Scientific Publications (in press).

61 Allan LD, Chita SK, Al-Ghazali W, Crawford DC, Tynan M (1987) Doppler echocardiographic evaluation of the normal human fetal heart. *British Heart Journal* **57**:528–533.

62 Pillai M, James D (1990) Hiccups and breathing in human fetuses. *Archives of Diseases of Children* **65**:1072–1075.

63 Zilianti M, Fernandez S (1983) Correlation of ultrasonic images of fetal intestine with gestational age and fetal maturity. *Obstetrics and Gynecology* **62**:569–573.

64 Schmidt W, Yarkoni S, Jeanty P *et al.* (1985) Sonographic measurements of the fetal spleen: Clinical implications. *Journal of Ultrasound in Medicine* **4**:667.

65 Goldstein I, Reece EA, Yarkoni S *et al.* (1988) Growth of the fetal stomach in normal pregnancies. *Obstetrics and Gynecology* **70**:256–260.

66 Arger PH, Coleman BG, Mintz MC *et al.* (1985) Rou-

tine fetal genitourinary tract screening. *Radiology* **156**:485–489.

67 Jeanty P, Dramaix-Wilmet M, Elkhazen N *et al.* (1982) Measurement of fetal kidney growth on ultrasound. *Radiology* **144**:159.

68 Elejalde BR, de Elejalde MM, Heitman T (1985) Visualization of the fetal genitalia by ultrasonography: A review of the literature and analysis of its accuracy and ethical implications. *Journal of Ultrasound in Medicine* **4**:633.

69 Nakayama DK, Harrison MR, Gross BH *et al.* (1984) Management of the fetus with an abdominal wall defect. *Journal of Pediatric Surgery* **19**:408–413.

70 de Elejalde MM, Elejalde BR (1985) Visualization of the fetal spine: A proposal of a standard system to increase reliability. *American Journal of Medical Genetics* **32**:445–456.

71 Neven P, Ricketts NEM, Geirsson RT, Smith R, Crawford JW (1991) Screening for neural tube defect with maternal serum alpha-fetoprotein and ultrasound without the use of amniocentesis. *Journal of Obstetrics and Gynaecology* **11**:5–8.

72 Nadel AS, Green JK, Holmes LB, Frigoletto FD, Benacerraf BR (1990) Absence of need for amniocentesis in patients with elevated levels of maternal serum alpha-fetoprotein and normal ultrasonographic examinations. *New England Journal of Medicine* **323**:557–561.

73 Mahony BS, Filly RA (1984) High-resolution sonographic assessment of the fetal extremities. *Journal of Ultrasound in Medicine* **3**:489–498.

74 Romero R, Pilu G, Jeanty P, Ghidini A, Hobbins JC (eds) (1988) Normal anatomy of the fetal skeleton: Skeletal dysplasia. In *Prenatal Diagnosis of Congenital Anomalies*, pp. 311–332. Norwalk, CT: Appleton and Lange.

75 Manning FA (1990) Dynamic ultrasound-based fetal assessment: The fetal biophysical profile score. In Fleischer AC, Romero R, Manning FA, Jeanty P, James AE Jr (eds), *The Principles and Practice of Ultrasonography in Obstetrics and Gynecology*, 4th edn, pp. 417–428. Norwalk, CT: Appleton and Lange.

76 Pillai M, James D (1990) Development of human fetal behaviour: A review. *Fetal Diagnosis and Therapy* **5**:15–32.

77 Low JA (1991) The current status of maternal and fetal blood flow velocimetry. *American Journal of Obstetrics and Gynecology* **164**:1049–1063.

78 Thompson RS, Trudinger BJ, Cook CM, Giles WB (1988) Umbilical artery velocity waveforms: Normal reference values for *A/B* ratio and Pourcelot ratio. *British Journal of Obstetrics and Gynaecology* **95**:589–591.

79 Arduini D, Rizzo G, Mancuso S, Romanini C (1987) Longitudinal assessment of blood flow velocity waveforms in the healthy human fetus. *Prenatal Diagnosis* **7**:613–617.

80 Arduini D, Rizzo G, Romanini C (1991) Doppler ultrasonography in early pregnancy does not predict adverse pregnancy outcome. *Ultrasound in Obstetrics and Gynecology* **3**:180–185.

81 Jauniaux E, Jurkovic D, Campbell S, Hustin J (1992) Doppler ultrasonographic features of the developing placental circulation: Correlation with anatomic findings. *American Journal of Obstetrics and Gynecology* **166**:585–587.

82 Hackett GA, Nicolaides KH, Campbell S (1987) Doppler ultrasound assessment of fetal and uteroplacental circulations in severe second trimester oligohydramnios. *British Journal of Obstetrics and Gynaecology* **94**:1074–1077.

83 Oppenheimer LW (1992) The classification of placenta praevia – time for a change? *Fetal and Maternal Medical Review* **4**:73–78.

84 Lim BH, Tan CE, Smith APM, Smith NC (1989) Transvaginal ultrasonography for diagnosis of placenta praevia. *Lancet* **i**:44.

85 Leerentveld RA, Gilberts ECAM, Arnold MCWJ, Wladimiroff JW (1990) Accuracy and safety of transvaginal sonographic placental localization. *Obstetrics and Gynecology* **76**:759–762.

86 Bernstein IM, Barth RA, Miller R, Capeless EL (1992) Elevated maternal serum alpha-fetoprotein: Association with placental sonolucencies, fetomaternal hemorrhage, vaginal bleeding, and pregnancy outcome in the absence of fetal anomalies. *Obstetrics and Gynecology* **79**:71–74.

87 Berwick DM, Weinstein MC (1985) What do patients value? Willingness to pay for ultrasound in normal pregnancy. *Medical Care* **23**:881–893.

88 Reading AE, Platt LD (1985) Impact of fetal testing on maternal anxiety. *Journal of Reproductive Medicine* **30**:907–910.

89 Field T, Sandberg D, Quetel TA, Garcia R, Rosario M (1985) Effects of ultrasound feedback on pregnancy anxiety, fetal activity, and neonatal outcome. *Obstetrics and Gynecology* **66**:525–528.

90 Campbell S, Reading AE, Cox DNA, Sledmere CM, Mooney R, Chudleigh P, Beedle J, Ruddick H (1982) Ultrasound scanning in pregnancy: The short-term psychological effects of real-time scans. *Journal of Psychosomatic Obstetrics and Gynaecology* **1**:5761.

91 Cox DN, Wittman BK, Hess M, Ross AG, Lind J, Lindahl S (1987) The psychological impact of diagnostic ultrasound. *Obstetrics and Gynecology* **70**:673–676.

92 Chodirker BN, Evans JA (1992) MS-AFP Screening Programmes: The Manitoba Experience. A Report prepared for the Royal Commission on New Reproductive Technologies, April.

93 Evans MI, Bottoms SF, Carlucci T, Grant J, Belsky RL, Solyom AE, Quigg MH, LaFerla JJ (1988) Determinants of altered anxiety after abnormal maternal serum alpha-fetoprotein screening. *American Journal of Obstetrics and Gynecology* **159**:1501–1504.

94 Keenan KL, Basso D, Goldkrand J, Butler WJ (1991) Low level of maternal serum alpha-fetoprotein: Its associated anxiety and the effects of genetic counseling. *American Journal of Obstetrics and Gynecology* **164**:54–56.

95 Waldenstrom U, Axelsson O, Nilsson S, Eklund G, Fall O, Lindeberg S, Sjodin Y (1988) Effects of routine one-stage ultrasound screening in pregnancy: A randomized controlled trial. *Lancet* **ii**:585–588.

96 Neilson JP, Munjanja SP, Whitfield CR (1984) Screen-

ing for small for dates fetuses: A controlled trial. *British Medical Journal* **289**:1179–1182.

97   Bakketeig LS, Eik-Nes SH, Jacobsen G, Ulstein MK, Brodtkorb CJ, Balstad P, Eriksen BC, Jorgensen NP (1984) Randomised controlled trial of ultrasonographic screening in pregnancy. *Lancet* **i**:207–210.

98   Rosendahl H, Kivinen S (1988) Routine ultrasound screening for early detection of small for gestational age fetuses. *Obstetrics and Gynecology* **71**:518–521.

99   Larsen T, Larsen JF, Petersen S, Greisen G (1992) Detection of small-for-gestational age fetuses by ultrasound screening in a high risk population: A randomized controlled study. *British Journal of Obstetrics and Gynaecology* **99**:469–474.

100 Hendricks SK, Sorensen TK, Wang KY, Bushnell JM, Seguin EM, Zingheim RW (1989) Doppler umbilical artery waveform indices: Normal values from fourteen to forty-two weeks. *American Journal of Obstetrics and Gynecology* **161**:761–765.

101 Steel SA, Pearce JM, McParland P, Chamberlain GVP (1990) Early doppler ultrasound screening in prediction of hypertensive disorders of pregnancy. *Lancet* **i**:1548–1551.

102 Steel SA, Pearce JMF, Chamberlain GVP (1988) Doppler ultrasound of the uteroplacental circulation as a screening test for severe pre-eclampsia with intra-uterine growth retardation. *European Journal of Obstetrics and Gynecology and Reproductive Biology* **28**:279–287.

103 McParland P, Pearce JM, Chamberlain GVP (1990) Doppler ultrasound and aspirin in recognition and prevention of pregnancy-induced hypertension. *Lancet* **i**:1552–1555.

104 Pryde PG, Isada NB, Hallak M, Johnson MP, Odgers AE, Evans MI (1992) Determinants of parental decision to abort or continue after non-aneuploid ultrasound-detected fetal abnormalities. *Obstetrics and Gynecology* **80**:52–56.

105 Manning FA, Harman CR, Menticoglou S, Morrison I (1991) Assessment of fetal well-being with ultrasound. In Platt LD (ed.), *Obstetrics and Gynecology Clinics of North America* **18**:891–905.

106 British Institute of Radiology Working Group (1987) The safety of diagnostic ultrasound. *British Journal of Radiology* **20** (suppl.).

107 Mole R (1986) Possible hazards of imaging and doppler ultrasound in obstetrics. *Birth* **13**:29–37.

108 Royal College of Obstetricians and Gynaecologists (1984) *Report of the Working Party on Routine Ultrasound Examinations in Pregnancy*. London: Royal College of Obstetricians and Gynaecologists.

109 Goss SA (1984) Sister chromatid exchange and ultrasound. *Journal of Ultrasound in Medicine* **3**:463–470.

110 Cartwright RA, McKinney PA, Birch JM, Hartley AL, Mann JR, Waterhouse JAH, Johnston HE, Draper GJ, Stiller C (1984) Ultrasound exposure in pregnancy and childhood cancer. *Lancet* **ii**:999–1000.

111 Stark CR, Orleans M, Haverkamp AD, Murphy J (1984) Short and long-term risks after exposure to

diagnostic ultrasound *in utero*. *Obstetrics and Gynecology* **63**:194–200.

112 Andrews M, Webster M, Fleming JEE, McNay MB (1987) Ultrasound exposure time in routine obstetric scanning. *British Journal of Obstetrics and Gynaecology* **94**:843–846.

113 Salvesen KA, Bakketeig LS, Eik-Nes SH, Undheim JO, Okland O (1992) Routine ultrasonography *in utero* and school performance at age 8–9 years. *Lancet* **339**:85–89.

114 Nyman M, Barr M, Westgren M (1992) A four-year follow-up of hearing and development in children exposed *in utero* to vibro-acoustic stimulation. *British Journal of Obstetrics and Gynaecology* **99**:685–688.

115 Hannah ME, Hannah WJ, Hellmann J, Hewson S, Milner R, Willan A (1992) Canadian Multicenter Post-term Pregnancy Trial Group: Induction of labor as compared with serial antenatal monitoring in post-term pregnancy. A randomized controlled trial. *New England Journal of Medicine* **326**:1587–1592.

116 Eik-Nes SH, Okland O, Aure JO, Ulstein M (1984) Ultrasound screening in pregnancy: A randomised controlled trial. *Lancet* **i**:1347.

117 Bennett MJ, Little G, Dewhurst J, Chamberlain G (1982) Predictive value of ultrasound measurement in early pregnancy. A randomized controlled trial. *British Journal of Obstetrics and Gynaecology* **89**:338–341.

118 Ewigman B, LeFevre M, Hesser J (1990) A randomized trial of routine prenatal ultrasound. *Obstetrics and Gynecology* **76**:189–194.

119 Saari-Kemppainen A, Karjalainen O, Ylostalo P, Heinonen OP (1990) Ultrasound screening and perinatal mortality: Controlled trial of systematic one-stage screening in pregnancy. The Helsinki Trial. *Lancet* **336**:387–391.

120 Neilson JP (1992) Routine ultrasonography in early pregnancy. In Chalmers I (ed.), *Oxford Database of Perinatal Trials*, Version 1.3, Issue 8, Autumn 1992, Record 3872.

121 Soothill PW, Ajayi R, Campbell S, Gibbs J, Chandran R, Gibb D, Nicolaides KH (1991) Effect of a fetal surveillance unit on admission of antenatal patients to hospital. *British Medical Journal* **303**:269.

122 Foster DC, Guzick DS, Pulliam RP (1992) The impact of prenatal care on fetal and neonatal death rates for uninsured patients: A 'natural experiment' in West Virginia. *Obstetrics and Gynecology* **79**:40–45.

123 Chervenak FA, McCullough LB (1991) Ethics, an emerging subdiscipline of obstetric ultrasound, and its relevance to the routine obstetric scan. *Ultrasound in Obstetrics and Gynecology* **1**:18–20.

124 Chervenak FA, McCullough LB, Chervenak JL (1989) Prenatal informed consent for sonogram: An indication for obstetric ultrasonography. *American Journal of Obstetrics and Gynecology* **161**:857–860.

125 Jennings JC (1989) Ethics in obstetrics and gynecology: A practitioner's review and opinion. *Obstetrical and Gynecological Survey* **44**:656–661.

126 Harman CR (1987) Bioethical issues in perinatology – is the future now? *Fetal Therapy* **1**:217–222.

39

Prenatal Fetal Monitoring: Abnormalities of Fetal Behavior

CHRIS HARMAN, SAVAS MENTICOGLOU, FRANK MANNING, HASSAN ALBAR, IAN MORRISON

INTRODUCTION

The loss of a wanted baby, especially term stillbirth of a structurally normal infant of good size, is shattering. This is an experience all of us – parents and caregivers alike – strive to avoid. That loss may be superseded (in some eyes) only by the survival of a horribly damaged baby, and the years of family grief which follow. These are melancholy thoughts, but they form at least part of the rationale for prenatal monitoring.

A second cluster of motivating influences is similar, although even more highly focused: prevention of *recurrent* stillbirth. The anxiety which attends the entire pregnancy is dispelled (perhaps not entirely) only after the neonatal period has passed. When offered prenatal monitoring, women with previous stillbirth in uncomplicated pregnancy usually select it. The most common frequency chosen is biweekly, with weekly monitoring next in preference, regardless of cause of the previous loss. Women with previous stillbirth comply with complicated regimes, and are unlikely to accept reassurance based on epidemiology alone, or statements on fetal well-being which exclude detailed ultrasound monitoring.

A third group of emotions prompting monitoring is responsibility/guilt/blame, founded on the principle that such deaths are 'ideally preventable' and that 'someone' – mother/midwife/attending physician/public educator – might have been able to prevent it.[1] Obstetrics disciplines accept this principle in focusing on maternal 'risks' (such as diabetes or hypertension) and fetal risks (intrauterine growth deficiency or twins) as designating higher likelihood and therefore responsibility to attempt prevention of these adverse events. At least part of the motivation for monitoring, then, is to demonstrate a response to apparent perils.

A fourth, although uncommonly promoted motive, may be more positive – the aspect of caring. Significant maternal–fetal bonding may be initiated by routine mid-trimester ultrasound; this may also be true of other facets of paying attention to the fetus. The participation of the father and family in 'feeling the baby', hearing the heart beat on office Doppler, and so on, is likely to make the impending family addition more concrete. Further, a defined role of mother in *caring* for her baby is likely to enhance participation in all aspects of pregnancy care. Anecdotal evidence, for instance, suggests that women conducting formal movement counting and seeing their fetus on ultrasound examination in an interactive format, have more success in smoking cessation. Fetal monitoring, then, addresses motives of caring, parenting and teamwork, while reinforcing maternal autonomy.

From an obstetric perspective, fetal monitoring addresses a fifth concern – the need to understand. To date, no consistent data have arisen from literally years of fetal monitoring to demonstrate *precursors* to injury, factors which predict cerebral palsy in structurally normal fetuses, or preconditions to sudden intrauterine death in uncomplicated pregnancy. There are strata of fetal risk – severe growth deficiency, abruptio placentae, maternal disorders such as eclampsia or ketoacidosis, environmental issues such as drugs or infection – but in a large proportion of pregnancies, recognition of signs of impending disaster have not been clearly quantified. Only through continued observation and meticulous data acquisition are we 'scientists' likely to satisfy that motive.

There are many motives, therefore, underlying the enormous effort generated toward fetal monitoring. We believe that there are reasons to monitor, both *against* bad events and *for* good things, but what exactly are we looking for? Detailed inquiry into the nature of pregnancy loss may help.

THE NATURE OF STILLBIRTH

There may be a subtle differentiation by parents between miscarriage (<20 weeks) and stillbirth (>20 weeks) in terms of the degree of grieving/loss, but in many instances the distinction is odd to their point of view. The continuum in causes of 'late miscarriage' (i.e. 16–19 weeks) and mid-trimester stillbirth (20–26+ weeks) means the traditional boundary of 20 weeks is also artificial from an obstetric viewpoint[2] **Table 1** shows data on intrauterine deaths in the second half of pregnancy[2] but less artificial demarcations might be 18 weeks (quickening) or 24 weeks (first viability).

Such surveys are invariably retrospective – factors are 'isolated' by multivariate analysis – and are not very helpful in themselves in choosing among women (few of whom will have had a previous loss) for prospective monitoring. **Table 2**, for example, identifies

ways in which care might have been applied to alter outcome. Despite disclaimers, many of these surveys which appear in the literature, do appear to be catalogs of blame-assignment, as though 'ideally preventable' stillbirths are necessarily more clearly understood than 'unexplained' ones.[3–7] In fact, among women with 'preventable' disorders, factors which single out some for prenatal fetal death are not well defined. Selecting women with any of these factors generates a very large population for monitoring! On the other hand, even for women with more than one (e.g. essential hypertension with a history of eclampsia), the likelihood (60–70% in the example) is that there will be a satisfactory outcome. Thus even for identified, high-risk situations, fetal monitoring of a multitude of normal pregnancies is necessary to ensure monitoring of the few ultimately 'abnormal' ones.

Table 2
'Preventable' elements in stillbirth (for stillbirths >1000 g, no anomaly)

Inadequate prenatal care	8%
Mother/family at fault	10%
Physician error in judgment	24%
Physician error in technique	7%
Intercurrent disease	8%
Unavoidable	44%

Table 1
Stillbirth characteristics 1980–90

Stillbirth proportion of total PNM	55%
proportion of PNM 500–1000 g	68%
proportion of PNM >1000 g	50%
Stillbirth weight (% of total stillbirths)	
500–1000 g	36%
1000–1500 g	15%
1500–2000 g	11%
2000–2500 g	10%
>2500 g	28%
Time of death	
before admission	75%
on hospital[a]	13%
on labor[a]	12%
Ideally preventable (% of all stillbirths)	33%
Unavoidable	62%
Unclassifiable	5%
Avoidable (% of stillbirths > 1000 g, no anomaly)	56%

[a]90% <26 weeks gestation.

Table 3
Emerging risk factors for stillbirth[a]

Fetal anomalies
    Chromosomal (e.g. non-lethal translocations)
    Structural (e.g. pleural effusions)
    Functional (e.g. neurologic deficits)

Severe maternal disorders
    autoimmune (e.g. lupus anticoagulant)
    chronic disease (e.g. renal failure on dialysis)
    coagulation abnormality (e.g. AT-III deficiency)

Bleeding: fetus to mother, fetus to fetus

Infections, e.g. syphilis, parvovirus, *Listeria*

Platelet, atypical red cell alloiummunization

Maternal (? and paternal) cigarette smoking

Inadequate nutrition

Maternal drug (cocaine) ingestion

Toxic exposure, environmental stress

Inadequate parental participation in pregnancy care

[a]As overall rates fall (e.g. for growth deficiency, diabetes, etc.), these factors become relatively more important and influence the type of monitoring.

Many factors associated with an exaggerated frequency of stillbirth have newly been identified and are more clearly defined on an ongoing basis. Some of these (**Table 3**) reflect advances in understanding, or in diagnostic techniques, while some reflect changes in the pregnant population. Application of a detailed 'stillbirth protocol' may disclose causes for as many as 70% of all losses. Nevertheless, this still limits *prospective* identification of pregnancies at risk to 40–60% when 'medical' factors alone are utilized.

Some of the 'non-medical' factors which identify increased risk of stillbirth are included in **Table 3**. While all deserve detailed attention, a focused discussion on cigarette smoking in pregnancy will illustrate why risk assessment and monitoring may not achieve optimal results.

SMOKING IN PREGNANCY: RISK MULTIPLICATION

The pervasive effects of cigarette smoking on reproduction are the subject of a major portion of Chapter 5. The statistical arguments relating cigarette smoking to the adverse outcomes in **Table 4** number in the hundreds.[8–14] The acceptance of cigarette smoking as a risk factor contributing to multiple adverse outcomes is recognized in a multitude of scoring systems with different end-points.[15] By virtue of the length of this list, cigarette smoking may be *the* most important prenatal factor influencing the prenatal antecedents for perinatal loss or injury. Data are emerging suggestive of deleterious effects of second-hand or 'passive' cigarette smoking as well.[16–18]

There are many examples of cigarette smoking as a *mediator* of adverse effects; for example, both stress[19] and alcohol consumption[20] may exert their detrimental effects via increased tobacco consumption. In short, cigarette smoking would appear to have all the characteristics of a Category X substance as defined by the US Food and Drug Administration: 'studies in animals or human beings have demonstrated fetal abnormalities or there is evidence of fetal risk based on human experience or both, and the risk of the use of the (substance) in pregnant women, clearly outweighs any possible benefit.' Impacts of cigarette smoking may not be apparent when the *primary* antecedents of pregnancy loss (e.g. abruption, prematurity, preterm premature rupture of the membranes, etc.) are data *endpoints*. Further, the effects of cigarette smoking may be so broad that individual associations seem vague or minor: a small increase in stillbirth rate, added by cigarette smoking to each of the factors in **Table 4**, would achieve statistical significance in *none*, while contributing in overwhelming fashion to *all*!

Many studies upon which dogmatic statements about monitoring are based did not stratify cigarette

Table 4
Documented adverse outcomes associated with cigarette smoking in pregnancy

Maternal
Periodic hypertension
Respiratory complications[a]
Stroke[a]
Myocardial infarction[a]
Hemorrhage[a] (hysterectomy, transfusions)
Chronic inflammatory bowel disease
Ectopic pregnancy
Failed tubal ligation
Anorexia and altered bone metabolism
Mediator of stress
Failure to decrease ethanol intake

Fetal–neonatal
Spontaneous abortion
Intrauterine death
Prematurity[b]
Premature rupture of membranes[b]
Abnormal adrenal function
Reduced brain size
Intrauterine growth deficiency[b]
Reduced intellectual function[b]
Impaired newborn lung function
Reduced childhood stature[b]
Sudden infant death syndrome

Placental
Abruptio placentae
Abnormal vascular resistance
Placenta previa
Infarction

[a]Some lethal; [b]in combination *and* individually.

intake/exposure. There is some evidence (although much is contradictory) that acute cigarette smoking can influence the biophysical parameters commonly used in fetal monitoring.[21–24]

Direct maternal vascular effects are not debatable, but the exact mechanism of cigarette action in contributing to its adverse associations is not known. Perhaps the combination of tar, nicotine and metabolites, smoke and pulmonary responses, carbon monoxide, chromium, etc., produces such a variety of effects that no single pathway will show them clearly. For example, we have documented five unusual cases in which oligohydramnios (maximum pocket depth <2 cm throughout the uterus) resolved (minimum pocket depth >4 cm in all four quadrants) after the cessation of smoking.

The thread of multiplying risk factors can also be seen in poor nutrition, absent prenatal care, first pregnancy, socioeconomic deprivation, and so on. Such non-obstetric factors obviously make risk assignment, and correct selection of monitoring candidates, very difficult. *Such factors illustrate the complexity of risk assignment: simply picking out 'previous stilbirths' or 'renal disease' for monitoring is no help in knowing what to look for.*

EVALUATING IMPACTS OF FETAL MONITORING ON PERINATAL LOSS

There are *many* considerations which are likely to interfere with monitoring the fetus to prevent intrauterine death/damage.

No Monitoring Produces Good Results

Since pregnancy is by odds a normal, uncomplicated and positive event, *any* monitoring system is likely to have excellent results. In fact, a monitoring system consisting only of pregnancy termination for lethal abnormality at 18–20 weeks would likely achieve healthy babies going home with mother in >90% of cases. The argument has been made thoroughly elsewhere,[25] that the pertinent statistics for the evaluation of apparent benefits of monitoring lie within the positive and negative predictive values of the system, rather than the specificity and sensitivity. Further, this means that any comparison of systems – especially in low-risk populations with a low incidence of fetal death/damage – must study *enormous* numbers of pregnancies if the intervention is to be measured at all.

Time Passing Produces Good Results

As displayed in **Figure 1**, the stillbirth rate has shown a gradual decline over the past two decades. This has not been at the cost of death/damage in the residual neonatal population. In fact, the decline in stillbirth may be due to enhanced neonatal performance; previously unacceptable nursery candidates who were simply allowed to die *in utero* may now be intact survivors with delivery. Virtually all the studies of prenatal monitoring discussed later took place over several years and therefore have this bias.

Changes in Obstetric Practice

Iatrogenic perinatal deaths have been eliminated in several areas. These include ultrasound for all amniocentesis procedures, pregnancy dating and/or waiting longer in pregnancy for scheduled events (such as elective delivery in insulin-dependent diabetics), and 'allowing' spontaneous onset of labor and vaginal

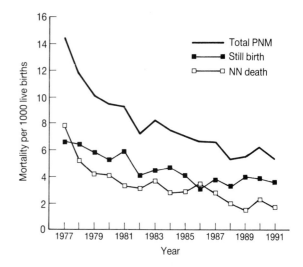

Figure 1. The declining rate of perinatal loss, Manitoba, 1977–91.

delivery in patients with previous cesarean section. *Not* included in positive effects on stillbirths have been programs such as symphysis–fundal height measurement[26] and routine screening for Group B beta-hemolytic streptococcus.[27] These and many other programs have failed to impact upon prenatal fetal loss.

Changes in Screening/Prophylaxis Programs

Rh-disease accounted for approximately 10% of stillbirths prior to 1945, i.e. a perinatal mortality rate of 4:1000 from alloimmunization alone.[28] Today, it is less than 1% of total stillbirths, due to a combination of effective prophylaxis and successful intrauterine treatment. Such programs, especially the prenatal (28 weeks) component of anti-D immune globulin administration, have been widespread only in the past 7–10 years. Rh-disease is the most striking example of such prophylaxis; other examples include Rubella and other immunization programs, atypical antibody screening and toxoplasmosis in high-risk populations.

Improved Risk Assessment

Early ultrasound (see Chapter 38), preventative programs in women at risk for prematurity, nutritional and smoking-cessation interventions, and many other examples, are developing. While the impact of individual components of improved prenatal care may be substatistical, it is possible that successful interventions will prevent compromise, removing fetal candidates from prenatal detection, making it even harder to know if prenatal monitoring works.

Fetal Cyclicity

Enhanced knowledge of the behavior patterns of the human fetus explains why single variable-testing is not uniformly successful. Any given behavioral pattern is present only part of the time, varying from one gestation to another. This is perhaps the most important factor in considering the ideal testing scheme from the aspect of reducing unwarranted interventions, and is discussed in detail later (see the section: Patterns of Fetal Behaviour).

Changes in Public Awareness

The impact of the presence of a trial on the behavior of the control population is well-documented.[29] Public education may alter substantially the frequency of fetal compromise available for detection, if advertising programs against drinking alcohol, smoking cigarettes and drug ingestion, or for fetal movement counting in pregnancy, are successful. Mothers demanding Rh-antibody screening, or ultrasound for decreased movement with normal fetal heart tones, or second opinions regarding antepartum bleeding at term, are examples.

Fetal Monitoring

The benefits of fetal monitoring in segments of the population may obscure or trivialize the benefits in the overall population. In particular, if the combination of risk evaluation and accurate intervention are properly applied, fetal monitoring may work so well as to appear of little benefit in the majority of pregnancies. Further, it may be that those who apply the methods, rather than the methods themselves, are critical factors. This undoubtedly accounts in part for the wide range of opinions about the 'best' approach to use.

Many distracters, then, interfere with the intention to monitor at-risk fetuses, recognize the pattern of fetal compromise and intervene in time. Before proceeding further on the trail of compromise, one must appreciate the patterns of normality.

NORMAL FETAL BEHAVIOR

Evolution of the Study of Fetal Behavior

Many maternally perceived movements are now understood to be indicative of discrete types of behavior

(**Table 5**). These observations stem from the application of animal research, carried out by Dawes and associates in the early 1970s at Oxford, which demonstrated that breathing movements were present in normal fetal sheep.[30] This acute fetal biophysical activity was suppressed or abolished in the presence of experimental fetal hypoxemia.[31] Boddy and Dawes extended these observations to the human fetus using gated single line A-scan methodology, undoubtedly extremely crude, and prone to artifact and observer bias. Despite these limitations, this breakthrough in conceptualizing the human fetus was the first to record cyclic behavior, and demonstrated that in some complicated pregnancies there was an alteration in the frequency and pattern of this normal behavior.[32] This may seem quite logical in retrospect and, in fact, quantifies what mothers were certainly capable of observing. From a scientific point of view, however, this represented the first recognition that there might be means other than the fetal heart rate for the systematic monitoring of

Table 5
The range of human fetal behavior

Basal functions
    precise homeostatic balance
    maternal manipulations
    adaptive changes
    growth and maturation

'Non-essential' functions
    urine production
    digestion
    fetal breathing, hiccups

General movement
    gross trunk/limb
    fine motor control
    stretching, rolling, jiggling

State-related activity
    mouthing
    rapid eye movements
    heart rate – CNS linkage

Cyclic behavior
    circadian
    rest/activity
    behavioral states

Responsive behavior
    acoustic startle
    glucose breathing
    adjusting to maternal position

'Purposeful' behavior
    sucking, spitting, yawning, swallowing, sighing,
      grimacing, ? crying, hand-play, tongue-play
    learning/adaptive mentation

fetal health, and that there might be methods for grading fetal condition, based on the incidence and character of fetal behaviors. Throughout that decade, experiments in chronic fetal sheep preparations showed a wide range of physiological activities, under normal circumstances, including the normal organization of such behaviors into discrete patterns which mirrored a sleep/wake cycle.[33,34]

In the mid-1970s, real time ultrasound technology progressed to the point of routine human application. The initial work on fetal breathing was not in direct line with clinical decision-making which was based completely upon fetal heart rate monitoring. This situation allowed the observation in both health and disease of the distribution and nature of many fetal behaviors. While preliminary work was directed toward the characterization of human fetal breathing movements, and the alteration of normal patterns with regard to the performance of the non-stress test and oxytocin stimulation test, it soon evolved into a much broader study of many aspects of fetal behavior.[35–37] The branch of fetal observation which developed from that group has concerned itself primarily with the application of these principles to fetal testing (Biophysical Profile Scoring, see below).[38]

Observations which now include assessment of all patterns of fetal behavior, depended in part on the evolution of more sophisticated ultrasound technology. While the association of amniotic fluid volume with fetal condition was a chance observation among compromised fetuses,[39] this was substantially affected by the poor resolution of the equipment available. The detailed longitudinal studies of fetal behavior, maturational patterns, and the demonstration of fetal behavioral states, followed a decade later as a result of detailed work with further generations of ultrasound instruments.[40,41] While this evolution may not be complete, it has reached a decidedly mature stage, where several interacting factors may now be interpreted in order to achieve an accurate assessment of fetal condition.[42]

Patterns of Fetal Behavior

As the fetus progresses from whole-body twitches to the discrete and varied, fine motor movements of the term fetus, a series of stages may be apparent at which the organization of acute biophysical activities becomes obvious. The concept of fetal neurologic milestones[43] reached fulfilment with the advent of the perinatal science of fetal neurology.

Acute periodicity of fetal activity

Different fetal behaviors apparently arise at different stages. By 10–12 weeks gestation, these may be compartmentalized into periods of quiet (seldom lasting more than 5 min) and periods in which some movements seem to be repeated, with the exclusion of others. For example, total body movement vs isolated limb movements vs periodic spasmodic movements similar to hiccups.[44] While the wiggling movements apparent at 8–10 weeks become less frequent, the 'star jumps' continue to 18 weeks or so.[45] The repertoire of the 18–20 week fetus includes virtually all the activities which his or her term counterpart displays, although these are grouped in very different concentrations. Nevertheless, there is already discernible alteration between one kind of activity and another toward the end of the first trimester.

Diurnal patterns[46]

By 18–20 weeks, there are periods of high and low activity, which are discernible from one another. In most fetuses, the periods of higher activity are in late evening, in accord with concepts of circadian fetal rhythms, in opposition to maternal rhythms. This represents the initial organization of acute activities in discrete episodes of rest and activity of significant duration.

Behavioral states

Even later in pregnancy, at approximately 30 weeks gestation, the longest intervals of complete quiescence begin to increase from the mean of 220 s or so which is maintained throughout the mid-trimester.[44] This is reflected by the clear establishment in most (80%) fetuses of defined behavioral states by 33–34 weeks. These behavioral states are constellations of fetal biophysical activities, which are stable over some significant period of time, and recur in recognizable patterns, not only in individual fetuses, but also reproducibly in all normal fetuses.[47] The behavioral states in the fetus defined by Nijhuis et al.[40] are similar to the neonatal states described by Prechtl,[48] designated with the F to indicate fetal state. An excellent and detailed review of this subject is found in Pillai and James.[44] The influence of such diurnal, rest/activity and behavioral state variations upon the chance observation of any number of fetal behaviors, in the context of fetal monitoring, is obvious.

Specific Coupling of Behaviors

The first clinical observation of coupled behavior was that of fetal heart rate acceleration coupled to fetal movement, the primary basis of the non-stress test (NST) and the principal factor in the development of the cardiotocogram.[49] This is not universally apparent until 24–26 weeks gestation, although more sophisticated use of numerical analysis of fetal heart rate suggests the onset of significant variability prior to this.[50–52] Fetal breathing movements and glucose administration, cyclic variation in both heart rate variability and vascular Doppler analysis due to episodes of fetal breathing, and the ability to provoke state changes by vibroacoustic stimulation, all mature at varying gestations. This has obvious implication in any system designed to detect impending fetal trouble: absence of a given coupling prior to its routine observation in the normal fetus would render it an inappropriate association for monitoring.

Absence of Normal Behavior: Distribution

As the third trimester progresses, the paucity of behaviors during quiet 'sleep' (fetal behavioral State IF) becomes profound. This quiescent state is characterized by : a low-frequency, high-voltage brain electrical pattern; infrequent gross body movements, consisting mainly of startle-type, sporadic (if any) fetal breathing movements; a stable, almost flat fetal heart rate pattern; uncoupling of gross body movements from fetal heart rate accelerations; and absent fetal eye movements. Rhythmic mouthing movements, on the other hand, occur in bursts more common during State IF.[53]

In the early days of fetal heart rate monitoring,[53] this profound change in fetal heart rate variation, and the uncoupling of movement and acceleration, resulted in many errors of commission. The 'non-reactive NST' (**Figure 2**) was one impetus for the development of the formal fetal biophysical profile score (BPS).[36] The large number of term fetuses who may be incorrectly described as being compromised on the basis of extreme inactivity associated with a flat heart rate tracing, was effectively dealt with in a diagnostic sense by

the observation of multiple fetal variables which usually show transition into other fetal states, not necessarily determined by changes in fetal heart rate recording. Thus, although State IF usually lasts less than 45 min,[40] occasionally up to 75 min,[57] the non-reactive NST may last up to 100 min.[54] Further, although the major proportion of fetal activity occurs in Stage 2F (active sleep), lasting for about 50% of fetal time near term, there is a significant overlap during the state changes, so that periods of *total* inactivity still only average 15–20 min at the longest in the term fetus.

Taken in concert, the varying schedules of development and persistence of different behaviors mean that any individual single behavior may give a false impression of fetal condition (i.e. absence indicating fetal compromise), but the likelihood of all indicators of fetal normality being absent on a sustained basis in a normal fetus is extremely small.

FETAL ADAPTATION TO HYPOXEMIA

First, the sequential development of fetal behavior means that hypoxemia has the potential for modifying fetal behavior in different ways at different gestations. Second, the physiology of oxygen and blood flow distribution evolve throughout pregnancy. Third, since early animal models are very difficult to manipulate without causing pregnancy wastage, there is a dearth of experimental data. Further, since the clinical ability to do anything about it is limited, observations of asphyxiated human fetuses at early gestations are not very detailed. In addition, even though observations in animals and humans correspond, their mechanisms and amplitudes are usually profoundly different (for example, the baboon aborts, the rhesus monkey develops IUGR, the ewe dies, and the pregnant woman takes little notice of sustained severe environmental acoustic

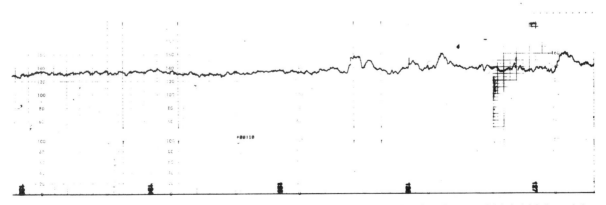

Figure 2. Normal cycling between (left) low activity, low variability and quiet sleep and (right) high activity, high variability and active sleep.

stress). Many of the landmark observations of cerebral hypoxemia in the primate model now seem of limited application in mechanisms of hypoxemia in humans.[55–57] In other words, what follows is substantially hypothetical, theoretical and the result of significant extrapolation. It may well be that continued observations utilizing invasive fetal testing such as cordocentesis, oxygen administration to the mother, and even direct fetal nutritive supplements, will further elucidate these mechanisms.

The Compromised Fetus

We believe that the fetus makes a series of compromises in order to remain alive in a hostile intrauterine environment. These compromises are in the opposite direction from those made by the newborn, pediatric or adult patient. Because the fetus can do *nothing* to impact the blood flow and oxygen delivery to the placental bed, which is clearly established by 16–18 weeks, fetal responses to compromise are always *conservative*. A cascade of reflexes (probably very well organized) as early as 18–20 weeks, reduces energy expenditure, diverts blood flow and oxygenation to vital, central organs, and may even subvert much in the way of normal development in order to preserve life.[58,59] Little is known about these mechanisms. As a result of these compromises, the fetus may appear relatively 'normal' (i.e. well-compensated), especially in terms of acute behaviors, until the final abrupt decline to acidosis and death. Several characteristics of this adaptive cascade influence fetal monitoring and are discussed here.

Onset

If compromise is early, the fetus will use total-body economies to allow a relatively normal course in pregnancy, resulting in a healthy, but symmetrically small, fetus with low normal values for virtually all behaviors. Whether there is a specific limit beyond which such fetuses show a marked increase in risk of acute deterioration, has not been demonstrated. Conversely, later insults may be serious enough to cause asymmetric growth deficiency, or an even less obvious shortfall in reaching fetal growth potential, but more obvious compromise in terms of shorter-term behaviors.

Duration

Acute insult is unlikely to affect growth, especially if it is severe enough, whereas a chronic, slowly progresive insult may allow substantial time for accommodation.

A sudden drop in oxygen supply may result in severe damage, such as hydranencephaly. The same drop, when extended over a number of weeks, may be reflected only as growth restriction.

Periodicity

The intermittent compromise, perhaps such as that seen with cigarette smoking, may produce very subtle changes, whereas a continuous deficit (e.g. following non-lethal abruption) produces an abrupt stoppage of some behaviors.

Extent

Obviously, a moderate degree of compromise is tolerated by every fetus who delivers vaginally. The severity of the compromise multiplied by the above factors will determine the ability of the fetus to withstand, and then adapt to, hypoxemia.

Origin

Maternal: If hypoxemia has its origin in the *mother*, as in maternal cyanotic heart disease, no amount of adaptive response by the fetus can achieve improvement. If supplemental oxygen is not available, the natural history is fetal death.

Placental origins of hypoxemia, the most common pathway for maternal disorders to affect the fetus, feature a high frequency of fetal growth deficiency with or without obvious placental indicators. Chronic, repeated abruptions may show stepwise compromise, but in general, placental bed/placental hypoxemia results in a gradual series of adaptations which have become the standard model for intrauterine compromise. This does not mean, however, that they are the most common series of events.

Acquired forms of hypoxemia include fetal infection, hydrops fetalis (both alloimmune and non-immune), metabolic (e.g. the macrosomia–hyperinsulinemia–hypoxemia triad in unregulated diabetes), chronic fetal anemias of many causes, and so on.

Intrinsic disorders (multiple congenital anomalies), specific anomalies involving vital vascular structures (e.g. omphalocoele), or chromosome abnormalities with an intrinsic inability to respond appropriately/sufficiently to even ordinary degrees of challenge, all contribute.

Serendipitous: This miscellaneous collection of factors which may cause severe, even lethal, acute hypoxemia without allowing any time for adaptation, includes: massive acute fetal–maternal hemorrhage, acute feto-fetal hemorrhage, cord accidents, acute intrauterine pneumonia and fetal abruption.

All of these factors are further conditioned by the gradual development of cardiovascular control by the fetus. These systems mature gradually, such that regulation of blood flow distribution is first evident by 14–16 weeks, and is clearly established by the end of the second trimester. As the autonomic nervous system becomes more sophisticated, the potential for selective perfusion of essential organ systems improves, and the ability to withstand greater stresses follows. An example of this maturational effect may be seen in oligohydramnios with serious hypoxemia. Prior to 20 weeks gestation, fetal hypoxemia of severity sufficient to kill the fetus is rarely associated with reduced amniotic fluid, even though fetal urine production is a major contributor to amniotic fluid volume from at least 16 weeks gestation on. Only by 20–22 weeks does decreased amniotic fluid volume become an accurate marker of compromise. To further complicate matters, there is evidence that in the growth-deficient fetus, maturational patterns are also delayed.[60]

We have not reviewed the delicate work with carefully controlled hypoxemia under many clinically applicable situations in fetal sheep.[58,61-63] First, that work is of exquisite detail and beyond the scope of this *clinical* chapter. Second, however, is a growing conviction that human fetuses are significantly more adaptive than sheep, and early *warning* of *impending* compromise may be perceived in humans enabling conservatism *before* any impairment takes place. The first of several detailed case studies will highlight this aspect.

Case Study 1

A 22-year-old primigravida had accurate menstrual dates with ultrasound confirmation at 12 weeks gestation. She attended prenatal care regularly and had no abnormal events whatsoever. Clinical growth was adequate, the fetus was vigorous, with movements readily felt by mother, father and attending physician. It was part of that physician's routine to use movement counting for fetal monitoring in his general population. Beginning at 34 weeks, mother noted that movements were less strong and less frequent, as well as being grouped in definite activity cycles. By 36 weeks gestation, she frequently took longer than 90 min to obtain 10 fetal movements, but always managed to achieve 10 movements within 2 h. At 36 weeks 6 days, she counted fetal movements for 3 h, but there were only 6 movements. The following day, at 37 weeks exactly, mother felt only one movement during her morning counting interval, and was referred to our tertiary-level center for investigation. A fetal heart rate monitor was applied immediately, which disclosed the pattern shown in **Figure 3**. When this persisted for more than 90 min, consultation was obtained with the perinatologist on call. Forty-min ultrasound examination showed: the fetus was

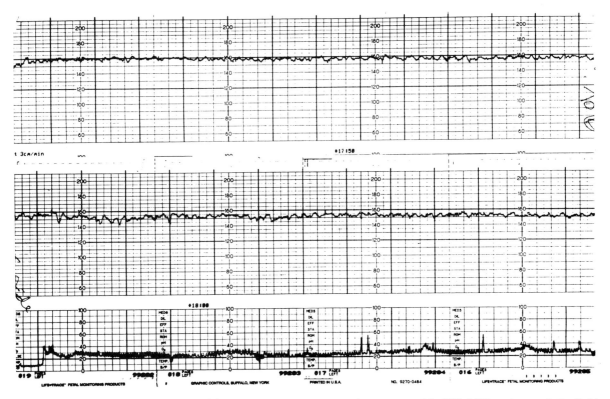

Figure 3. Reduced variability, repetitive, monotonous sawtooth pattern, with BPS 2/10; only amniotic fluid was normal.

vertex, in a very relaxed posture, with the neck in a partly deflexed position, hands and feet open. There was no discernible fetal movement, other than one facial grimace. Breathing movements were absent, and the fetal heart rate was high for this gestation at 155–165. Cardiac contractility was subjectively reduced, and although the cardiac diameter measurement fell within normal limits, the heart appeared distended. The umbilical cord was visibly pulsatile (excursions of >4 mm) in the generous amniotic fluid.

There was no evidence of abruption or external bleeding, the mother was absolutely stable and had a normal hemoglobin. The biophysical profile score was 2/10, only amniotic fluid volume being normal. As per protocol, induction of labor was commenced by ARM, disclosing clear liquor. The externally recorded fetal heart rate pattern was duplicated on study with a scalp clip. Despite supplementary oxygen, continuation of adequate maternal hydration and the presence of very mild contractions, there was further evidence of fetal compromise with reduction in variability, and a single mixed late variable-type bradycardia (**Figure 4**). The decision to proceed with cesarean section was based on probable fetal asphyxia (cause undefined), cervical dilatation of only 2 cm in a primigravida, with fetal intolerance of uterine activity at an early stage. A normal-weight female infant at the birthweight centiles predicted by the ultrasound measurements was delivered. The baby cried vigorously within 2 min of delivery, and had Apgar scores of 5 and 9. She was extremely pale, with a central hemoglobin concentration of 53 g/l. There was evidence of low-grade fetal–maternal hemorrhage, with approximately 3 ml of fetal blood present in the weight-adjusted calculated maternal circulating volume, on Kleihauer testing. Fetal–maternal, A/O incompatibility suggested that the Kleihauer would be a significant underestimation of the volume of fetal cells, but based on serial testing following delivery, this degree of underestimation was not more than 100% (i.e. the fetus did *not* have a sudden massive hemorrhage causing exsanguination). After two simple transfusions, the baby was well, and was discharged home in care of the mother.

Comment

This case illustrates two factors. First, that fetal–maternal hemorrhage can be severe enough to cause profound fetal anemia, but over a long enough duration allowing time for successful fetal adaptation. Second and more importantly, this case illustrates a finding which is not at all uncommon among infants with an abnormal set of biophysical variables. Because birth in this case resulted in a baby who functioned normally, vigorously and apparently without compromise, it points to the 'voluntary' nature of fetal adaptive quiescence. This fetus did not become immobile because she was hypoxemic (UVpO$_2$ 32) or acidotic (UVpH 7.40). She undoutedly was able to 'perceive', either centrally or via cardiac receptors, increasing anemia, and responded by reducing oxygen utilization. This is not a unique situation. In summary, the serious and recognizable stress produced complete fetal shutdown, not on the basis of the stress *per se*, but on the basis of protective responses well in advance of metabolic compromise.

It is clear, therefore, that well-researched animal models of asphyxia may not explain findings in human fetuses. It may very well be that relatively subtle changes, readily reversible at the time of delivery (or following the extremely noxious vibroacoustic stimulation of the nearly asphyxiated fetus), are markers of impending compromise in the non-growth deficient near-term human fetus.

An ideal monitoring system must take into account *all* of these potential variables, and one can only do this if a wide range of information is available. Such information is highly observational, and may indeed be highly individual, and is not based on a detailed understanding of the mechanisms of hypoxemia/

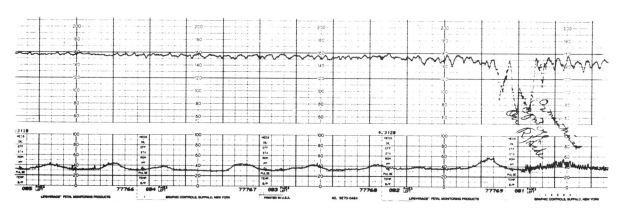

Figure 4. Induction of labor was commenced, but when this single deceleration occurred, the continued complete absence of complete fetal movement justified cesarean section.

compromise. We simply do not yet have the data to know why such challenges initiate central adaptive responses. Several things should be clear: fetal monitoring is desirable from a number of points of view; the multiplicity of fetal behavior suggests a group of parameters which could be assessed regarding response to compromise; compromise may come from a variety of directions, with a variety of characteristics, and with varying ease of prospective identification. We can therefore define the ideal requirements of a system which could address these concerns.

PRINCIPLES OF FETAL MONITORING

The ideal prenatal monitoring system should:

- detect impending intrauterine damage with: (a) specificity, (b) sensitivity, (c) utility, (d) timeliness;

- exclude the possibility of stillbirth or injury with high assurance over a reasonable length of time;

- exclude lethal malformation as the cause of testing abnormalities;

- exclude normal cyclicity of fetal behavior as the cause of deficits in testing;

- detect specific causes of fetal compromise;

- be practicable in large numbers while consuming limited resources;

- produce *measureable benefits* in reduction of perinatal death and injury.

Following the previous discussion, *implications* for such a monitoring system are respectively:

- Correlation with 'gold standards' of fetal compromise must exist. Such gold standards *might* include pH (pre-labor), Apgar scores, intensive neonatal care requirements, and so on. Extreme abnormalities would likely show an increase in permanent injury or death. Detection of this 'condition' of compromise would have to be highly unlikely in the normal fetus, very common in the compromised fetus, soon enough to allow prompt reversal on delivery of the baby, yet late enough

in pregnancy to allow successful care of the newborn.

- A normal, reassuring test, must be reliable for more than the instant, in most clinical applications. Seven days is a convenient interval for several reasons.

- Only a system with at least one detailed real-time ultrasound examination (see Chapter 38) can address this point.

- Only a system with multiple parameters can avoid a time-consuming wait for fetal behavior cycles.

- Only a system which includes observations of multiple systems (e.g. CNS, cardiovascular, fluid regulation, spinal innervation) within the context of real-time ultrasound can hope to recognize non-uteroplacental causes of fetal compromise dysfunction. This includes several of the causes of stillbirth often included among 'unavoidable, not preventable', discussed below ('serendipity').

- Non-physician-based, rapid, easily taught, sequential testing, stratified according to risk factor and actual disorder appraisal, is the goal here.

- The *measurement* of benefits as discussed previously will be difficult.

ONE SYSTEM FOR DETAILED FETAL MONITORING: THE BIOPHYSICAL PROFILE SCORE

Apology

This text has the mandate to present representative views and options for the practitioner. In this regard, some systems are more or less equivalent to biophysical profile scoring. These include any system using real-time ultrasound on a regular basis to study fetal behavior and amniotic fluid, while relying on instantaneous confirmation of fetal well-being through the detailed and computer-assisted assessment of a minimum 20-min cardiotocogram (CTG). In women who require definitive fetal monitoring, we do not feel an acceptable option can restrict information to a single modality. We advocate the comprehensive approach. We do not, therefore, endorse the use of non-stress testing or the CTG *alone*, contraction stress testing alone, or Doppler umbilical vessel velocimetry alone, as viable options to this program of fetal monitoring. Second, whereas the argument was acceptable 10 years ago that real-time ultrasound was a limited resource unavailable for widespread application, this is no longer the case. Where secondary or tertiary level fetal–maternal units exist, real-time ultrasound *must* be an integral, available and practical resource. On the other hand, it is clear that such monitoring is not necessary for a large proportion of the population. The means by which pregnancies may be assigned relatively low risk, and monitored with a less intensive regime, are discussed in a later section (Monitoring the Normal Pregnancy).

Methodology

The origins of the biophysical profile score (BPS), and the serendipitous nature of the parameters which were welded together, has been well reviewed.[64–66] The basic parameters of the BPS are shown in **Table 6**. Vibroacoustic stimulation has been added to biophysical profile scoring in some scenarios. We are reluctant to endorse this particular modification, because it may be may be unreliable prior to 32 weeks[67] and, second, it clearly causes marked disruption of CNS behavioral states, even if it is not dangerous.[68,69] It may be possible to get a response out of the almost-asphyxiated

fetus by use of this noxious stimulation, resulting in false reassurance.[70] Vintzelios has added placental grading to this system to give a maximum of 12 points.[71] Others have replaced single-pocket depth with the amniotic fluid index, which simply measures the maximum pocket available in four quadrants.[72] While as yet there are limited published reports, it is common practice in many units to supplement the information available by biophysical profile scoring with umbilical artery Doppler velocimetry.[73] It is notable that none of these systems *ignores* information. All use the basic criteria of the BPS, and strive to further enhance predictive accuracy by *adding* information.

Biophysical profile scoring appears, based on our experience with over 70 000 referred high-risk cases, to satisfy the criteria set forth above.

Detection of Fetal Compromise

Biophysical profile scoring detects impending intra-uterine injury with precision. The statistical performance parameters of the biophysical profile scoring system, which has been applied to high-risk pregnancies over more than a decade in our institution, are shown

Table 6
Parameters of biophysical profile scoring

Fetal variable	Normal behavior (score = 2)	Abnormal behavior (score = 0)
Fetal breathing movements	More than 1 episode of 30 s duration, intermittent within a 30 min overall period. Hiccups count. (Not continuous throughout the observation time)	Repetitive or continuous breathing without cessation. Completely absent breathing or no sustained episodes
Gross body/limb movements	Four or more discrete body/movements in a 30 min period. Continuous active movement episodes are considered as a single movement. Also included are fine motor movements, positional adjustments, and so on	Three or fewer body/limb movements in a 30 min observation period
Fetal tone and posture	Demonstration of active extension with rapid return to flexion of fetal limbs, brisk repositioning/trunk rotation. Opening and closing of hand, mouth, kicking, etc.	Only low-velocity movements, incomplete return to flexion, flaccid extremity positions; abnormal fetal posture. Includes score = 0 when FM absent
Fetal heart rate reactivity	Greater than 2 significant accelerations associated with maternally palpated fetal movement during a 20 min cardiotocogram. (Accelerations graded for gestation: 10 beats/min for 10 s before 26 weeks; 15 beats/min for 15 s >26 weeks; 20 beats/min for 20 s at term)	Fetal movement and accelerations not coupled. Insufficient accelerations, absent accelerations, or decelerative trace. Mean variation <20 on numerical analysis of CTG
Amniotic fluid volume evaluation	One pocket of >3 cm without umbilical cord loops. More than 1 pocket of >2 cm without cord loops. No elements of subjectively reduced amniotic fluid volume	No cord-free pocket >2 cm, or elements of subjectively reduced amniotic fluid volume definite

in **Table 7**. Detailed studies both in our population and in several other centers, indicate several beneficial aspects of BPS performance.[74-78]

Corrected stillbirth rates (*in utero* death of fetuses >1000 g without anomalies) are shown in **Table 8**. There are now three studies in which the total population studied exceeds 1500 fetuses (1845–55 661 fetuses).[66,74,75] These studies demonstrate similar results. Perinatal mortality ranges from 1.86:1000 to 3.1:1000 in populations managed completely by biophysical profile scoring. Even in populations where biophysical profile scoring was applied on a 'selected basis', the perinatal mortality fell drastically within 2 years, to an average rate of 3.6:1000. It must be emphasized, that although these results are highly statistically signficant, this does not represent a randomized trial.

Table 7
BPS performance statistics

Normal score 8/8	Completion mean 11 min
Current population	>60 000 high-risk pregnancies >130 000 BPS tests

Negative predictive value
(normal score, still healthy at
7 days)   99.935%

Positive predictive values
(vary with test score, intervention, outcome measure)

For example:

BPS	Outcome measure	PPV
0/10	Perinatal mortality	100% without intervention
0/10	Neonatal mortality	43% despite intervention
0/10	Perinatal mortality[a]	100%
4/10	Perinatal mortality	12.5%
6/10	Perinatal morbidity[a]	35%

[a]Perinatal morbidity is defined as any occurrence of: 5-min Apgar score <7, umbilical venous pH <7.20, intrapartum fetal distress, or fetal growth deficiency.

Table 8
Corrected stillbirth rates in large BPS studies

Author(s)	No. of fetuses	Corrected perinatal mortality (per 1000)[a]
Manning *et al.*[66]	55 661	1.86
Basket *et al.*[75]	5 034	3.1
Chamberlain[74]	1 845	3.0

[a]Lethal anomalies excluded.

Correlation with 'Gold Standards'

The relationship of biophysical profile scoring to outcome has been documented in numerous reports, from several centers. **Figure 5** demonstrates the relationship of overall score and various fetal morbidities.[42] The fact that this is curvilinear is reassuring in a biological sense; undoubtedly, fetuses move up and down between various scores as they cycle between different activities during the day. Thus, a normal fetus may have a score of 10 on one occasion, 8/10 on another occasion, and perhaps as low as 6/10 based on coincidence of different factors. As long as normal amniotic fluid is present, it is possible (although increasingly unlikely as observation time is extended) that a normal fetus may have a score of 2 or 4. At the same time, the compromised fetus may well illustrate variations in behavioral patterns, such that a score of 2/10, 4/10 or even 6/10 during coincidence of excellent activity is possible in the fetus with reduced amniotic fluid volume and an unsatisfactory CTG. These observations of cyclic behavior, even in the face of some compromise, disappear in the obviously asphyxiated fetus with scores of 0/10 and 2/10, and in most fetuses with a score of 4/10.[79]

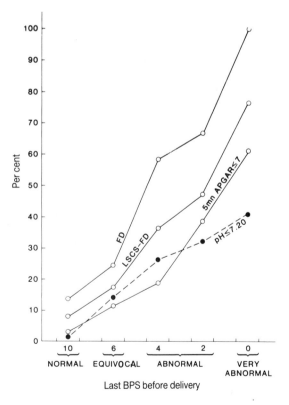

Figure 5. Last BPS *vs* perinatal morbidity. %, percent of fetuses with respective morbidity; FD, fetal distress.

Recently, we have been able to review a large number of fetuses where cordocentesis was necessary, either in the investigation of alloimmune disease, or in the investigation of intrauterine growth deficiency.[80] **Figure 6** shows the correlation between pH and BPS as an example.

The issue of the actual gold standard is important. Various scores of well-being (e.g. Apgar score in infants delivered by cesarean section prior to labor) correlate well with outcome, but do not necessarily fit the pH and blood gases observed in the cord blood.[81] Which of these elements, fetal behavior and ultimate outcome, or pH as plotted against a normative distribution, should be taken as a gold standard? Similarly, with biophysical profile scoring, it might be that the true gold standard of fetal status is in fact the normality of fetal behaviors, and not the biochemical representation of status. This question deserves significant attention in the future.

In the studies currently in the literature correlating fetal blood gases and pH with biophysical profile scoring, several consistencies are apparent.[82–87] A more detailed review of these studies is available,[66] but the collected information suggests the following generalizations:

- Among structurally normal fetuses, there is a direct relationship between prenatal fetal pH and base deficit, and the BPS.[81–84]

- The relationship between biophysical profile scoring and fetal PO_2 and pCO_2 is more variable.

- In the structurally abnormal fetus, behavior may also be significantly abnormal, despite normal fetal blood gas and pH parameters.

- While a direct relationship between fetal blood gas and/or pH values and the individual components of the BPS is suggested, results are variable.

More subjective, but commented upon by various authors, is a reduction in the overall frequency and amplitude of behaviors of all descriptions, while remaining above the threshold. In other words, there may well be a progressive reduction on a more or less continuous scale in total fetal activity. Because of the binary nature of the BPS, these gradual declines are not measured until the threshold is crossed. These observations are consistent with the model of fetal adaptation to hypoxemia. In the face of hypoxemia, or the progression of the underlying placental abnormality, the conservative fetal response would be a loss of the acute biophysical variables, and if the disease process were sustained long enough, a resulting decrease in amniotic fluid volume. Further compensation by the fetus may well allow return of more or less normal activity despite an overall reduction in oxygen supply, as redistribution of cardiac output enables resumption of some of the suppressed behaviors. Thus, one would expect the correlation between BPS and fetal blood gases to have substantial variation between individuals.

Finally, the conclusion inevitable from a review of these studies and our own data is that the 'weighting' of an individual variable is not appropriate.[80,88] The BPS is truly composite (see also Case Study 7). The composition of equivocal or overtly abnormal BPS is not restricted to one or two of the possible combinations.[80,89] While one might predict a series of orderly steps (e.g. first the loss of fetal breathing, then reduction in tone, then abolition of the CTG variables, then loss of fluid and, finally, loss of movement), there is in fact no exclusive path for the loss of fetal biophysical variables in the course of deterioration.[90,91] For example, with a score of 6/10 there are 10 possible combinations of variables being present and absent. First, nine out of the ten possible combinations were observed. Second, each individual combination had a similar predictive accuracy relative to the whole. It would appear in this group of fetuses, that there is *not* a single pathway to the demonstration of a fetal compromise. This is disappointing to the purists who wish to define a single mechanism by which the fetus compensates. It is likely, however, to be closer to what happens in the real fetus, namely a diversity of fetal responses to disease in general and to hypoxemia in particular. Predicting the full range of possible adverse perinatal outcomes is only achieved by considering all variables and all combinations.

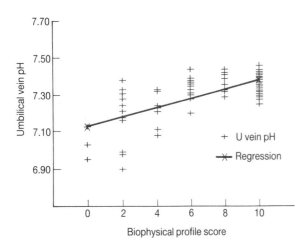

Figure 6. Biophysical profile score measured at the time of obtaining umbilical venous pH in alloimmunized and growth-deficient groups.

Utility

Utility of the system is evident by the fact that virtually all prenatal monitoring of high-risk pregnancy in our health care jurisdiction is done by biophysical profile scoring; the large number of fetuses supervised with BPS has continued to grow despite no significant increase in physical resources; the program is largely administered by nurse ultrasonographers, and the quality of results has not changed with the increasing demands on the system (**Figure 7**).[92]

Timeliness of Interventions

Timeliness of interventions described by biophysical profile scoring is difficult to prove to the sceptical observer. The absence of a preponderance of neonatal and early pediatric sequelae, combined with the encouraging mortality results, suggest that in general interventions are not at the 'last minute'.[92] This point deserves further clarification, as numerous commentaries (none of which were substantiated by data in the literature) have been offered that the acute biophysical variables (tone, movement and fetal breathing) are only truly absent in the almost-dead fetus. As illustrated in Case Study 1, this is clearly not so. Because many interventions are based on oligohydramnios (especially post-term), and in other instances of fetal compromise with normal fetal size at term, the fetus is not given time to decompensate, these interventions are also timely. As with any successful intervention, the result is absent morbidity, and therefore it is impossible to prove that the intervention was necessary in the given individual.

Stillbirth or severe fetal compromise are extremely unlikely within 7 days of a normal score. Biophysical profile scoring has the lowest false-negative rate of any contemporary antepartum testing scheme. The false-negative fetal death rate (fetal death within a week of a final normal biophysical score) is 0.6:1000, i.e. one in greater than 1500 pregnancies.[92–93] False-negative results are diverse, including clinical accidents such as acute abruption, true knots in the cord, intrapartum deaths (almost always preventable), and fetal infection. In some situations, however, it is true that the methodology employed failed to detect apparent fetal hypoxemia. The decrease in corrected stillbirth rate suggests that additional modalities such as Doppler and retesting frequently in specific disorders prone to accelerated change (e.g. proteinuric pre-eclampsia), important in selected individuals, may also influence the overall results.

As observed, only real-time ultrasound examination in a highly detailed and formatted way can exclude lethal malformation. This is a very significant beneficial benefit of biophysical scoring. In all series reporting biophysical profile scoring, a substantial contributor to residual mortality is lethal anomaly: more than 90% are diagnosed by the nurse ultrasonographers performing the BPS.[94]

Being fooled by the normal fetus is most common when the score is equivocal (6/10) compared with an overtly abnormal score. As indicated by the test score distribution (**Table 9**), the concept of multiple parameter testing is highly effective in excluding the lazy baby from the population of truly abnormal fetuses. All large studies of this methodology report distributions similar to those shown in **Table 9**. These are strikingly different than those reported for non-stress testing, in which 5–20% are reported as non-reactive, the vast majority of these on the basis of cyclic fetal behavior.[77]

In the area of detecting individual cases of compromise from non-chronic and/or non-asphyxial causes,

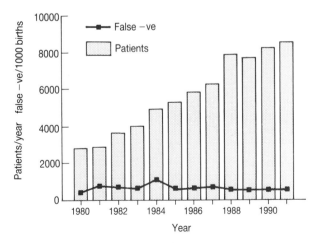

Figure 7. False-negative deaths (structurally normal fetuses who died within 7 days of last normal score) have not changed significantly despite a progressive increase in demands on resources.

Table 9
BPS test score distribution (*n* = 110 000)

Normal score		
10/10	All parameters normal	
8/10	All ultrasound parameters normal	
8/10	Not oligohydramnios[a]	97.52%
Equivocal score		
6/10	Multiple combinations	1.72%
Abnormal scores		
4/10	Only 2 parameters normal	0.52%
2/10	Only 1 parameter normal	0.18%
0/10	No parameters normal	0.06%

[a]In selected populations, 8/10–oligohydramnios has a significant distribution (e.g. post-dates pregnancy 6.8%).

real-time ultrasound observation by experienced observers achieves extraordinary success. In the literature, this is largely discounted as a collection of individual cases, and not indicative of the benefits of monitoring for asphyxia. There is no argument about this. However, a cause of death does not have to be asphyxia to be important to fetus and family. Thus prenatal detection of imminent cord prolapse,[95] a true knot in the cord, asymptomatic abruptio placenta, vasa previa, multiple nuchal loops of cord, undiagnosed alloimmunization, asymptomatic complete placenta previa, and many more examples, undoubtedly contribute to the enhanced statistics when real-time ultrasound is employed effectively.[96]

To summarize, biophysical profile scoring fulfils the demands of the optimal fetal evaluation process. That process includes multiple steps; in specific instances, simply detecting abnormalities of fetal behavior is only the initial step. Resources must be available for urgent delivery, or urgent fetal investigation and therapy. There is an obvious need for detailed collaborative arrangements with a high-risk obstetric center. On the other hand, given modern transportation methodology, the location of the BPS does not have to be within the same building.

INDIVIDUAL COMPONENTS OF THE BIOPHYSICAL PROFILE SCORE

While score variables appear in different combinations with different overall scores and are somewhat limited in terms of logical constraints (for example, fetal tone cannot be the only variable present when the BPS is 2/10), it is the overall score which correlates best with ultimate outcome (**Figure 8**).[97,98] Specific comments may be helpful as to the interpretation, interrelationship and, occasionally, relative weighting of different factors.

Amniotic Fluid Volume[99–102]

The score has not been modified to reflect the altered impact of gross hydramnios (**Figure 9**). This in part reflects the diverse nature of hydramnios, relative to twin pregnancy and other normal fetal anatomic combinations, versus structural abnormalities, versus acquired disease, versus a poorly understood group of miscellaneous central nervous system disorders. Cases of overt hydramnios (largest pocket depth >8 cm, fetus free-floating from three sides of the uterus, free range of movement of extended limbs), also shows a graded difference relative to the fetus with gross hydramnios (fetus free-floating from all four walls of the uterus,

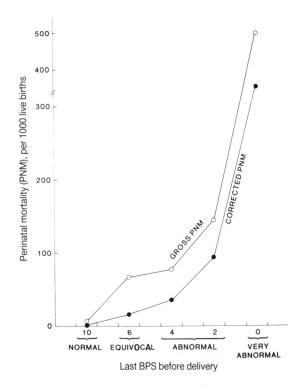

Figure 8. The curvilinear relationship between final BPS and perinatal mortality (gross or uncorrected, and corrected for lethal anomalies).

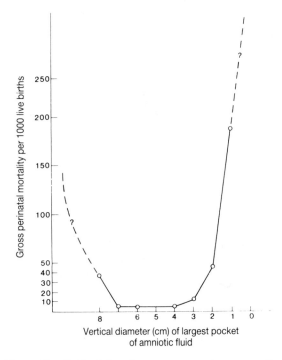

Figure 9. Perinatal outcome *vs* maximum vertical amniotic fluid pocket depth.

pocket depth >12 cm, clinically distended maternal abdomen). While oligohydramnios may also have a similar list of associated anomalies or serious conditions (including previously undiagnosed spontaneous rupture of membranes, this entity may also have several measurement variations. One must be absolutely certain that there is no vertical column of umbilical cord present in the supposed amniotic fluid pocket (**Figure 10**). Second, a group of subjective criteria may be useful, even when a pocket can be found which measures >2 cm in maximum depth. The subjective characteristics of reduced amniotic fluid include:

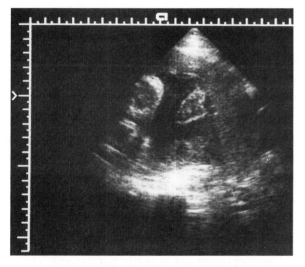

Figure 10a. Identification of an apparently satisfactory amniotic fluid pocket on linear ultrasound.

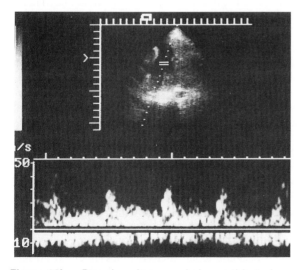

Figure 10b. Doppler ultrasound shows this to be a vertical loop of umbilical cord, rather than amniotic fluid.

uterus molded to the fetus, including molding of the uterus at the nape of the neck, around an elbow, and so on; no amniotic fluid pocket >3 cm in depth; need to measure between loops of cord in order to reach the normal criteria for amniotic fluid pocket depth; presence of small decelerations when the fetus moves indicating minor cord compression; restricted range of movement despite normal tone and frequency; uterine contour round and firm as opposed to the usual oval and flexible (often including uterine contractions stimulated by the transducer 'massaging' the abdomen during the exam). It is our policy to increase the frequency of surveillance (twice per week, up to daily if the clinical situation warrants) when amniotic fluid is in the subjectively reduced category. Absolute oligohydramnios at any viable gestation is an indication for intervention.

Cardiotocogram[103,104]

The reader will be familiar with the major impact of fetal heart rate tracing throughout monitoring, both antepartum and intrapartum. During the intrapartum period, lengthy tracings, with the additional information available from repetitive contractions, mean that over time a picture of fetal well-being can be assembled. The same may be true of CTG, with recording over a long period of time, but in general an hour or more to demonstrate state changes, or document a period of relatively high fetal activity in the less mature individual, places undue strain on resources intended to monitor large numbers of pregnancies at risk. Numerical analysis utilizing systems such as the System 8000[105] may be of value, when traditional criteria of accelerations are complemented by more confidence in baseline variability.

Perhaps more than any other of the parameters of biophysical profile scoring, the data available from cardiotocography must be interpreted with strict guidelines relative to gestational age. *At gestational ages <28 weeks, the traditional criteria for accelerations need to be scaled down from 15 beats/min × 15 s to a more realistic goal of 10 beats/min × 10 s.*[106] The tracing in **Figure 11**, for instance, might be acceptable if the fetus was only 20 weeks, but for the gestational age of 29 weeks, this was a markedly flat tracing, noting as well the presence of a shallow late deceleration with the contraction. This fetus had a BPS of 2/10, with normal (although subjectively reduced) amniotic fluid volume (AFV), and was delivered within an hour of this tracing, with umbilical vein pH of 7.01.

A wealth of information is available from cardiotocography. One emphasizes this by referring to the prenatal heart rate record as a CTG, as opposed to a 'nonstress test',[107] which because of its narrow parameters, and the purposeful neglect in analyzing variability,

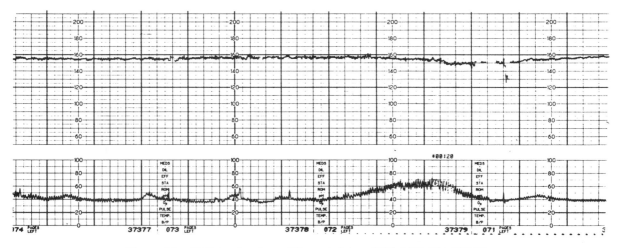

Figure 11. FHR tracing from 29 week fetus: BPS 4/10; UVpH 7.01.

contractile pattern, and so on, has traditionally excluded much of this information. Fetal movements and fetal breathing movements will often show up on the tocodynameter, as well as the classic irregularity of fetal heart rate associated with fetal breathing movements (**Figure 12**).[108] Further, even in the presence of extremely mild contractions, decelerative patterns can be highly suggestive (**Figure 13**). When contractions are present, the contraction stress test may be interpreted according to the standardized criteria.[109]

Our current rate of oxytocin challenge tests (OCT) is 1:8000 biophysical profile scores. The 10% or so of false-alarm non-reactive NST notwithstanding, the

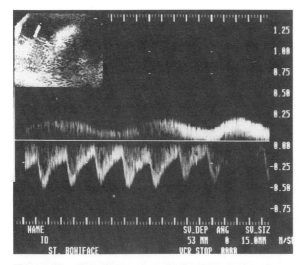

Figure 12. Respiratory arrhythmia depicted on Doppler ultrasound. Large excursions in venous wave (top) reflect pressure changes in fetal chest. Careful comparison of R-R interval shows significant irregularity on arterial side.

CTG has significant drawbacks. On occasion, oligohydramnios is suggested by the presence of overt variable decelerations, or more often, the 'minimal variable' (**Figure 14**), but the majority of CTGs in the face of overt oligohydramnios fail to make the diagnosis. Second, even when fetal impairment is obvious, illustrated by severe growth deficiency, overt oligohydramnios, few fetal movements and no fetal breathing movements, correlated with an umbilical venous pH by cordocentesis of 7.20, the tracing shown in **Figure 15** is not uncommon. This is reassuring from the point of view of indicating continued linkage between the central nervous system and heart rate, but obviously would be erroneous in terms of planning management. Also, it is our opinion that monitoring of twin gestations, especially when there is evidence of discordance, maternal complication, and at any gestation beyond 28 weeks, cannot be done with the CTG alone (see Case Studies 3 and 4). The fetal behavior during decelerative traces can be fascinating when followed on real-time ultrasound. The fetus with the enormous deceleration shown in **Figure 16** had complete cessation of movement during and for the 5 min following the deceleration, although normal variability and vigorous fetal activity were associated prior to the deceleration. The incongruities clearly make this an abnormal tracing: the 18–20 week fetus may have such a deceleration from time to time and be completely normal, but would not have the variability illustrated on the left-hand portion of the tracing. In fact, this was a 30-week fetus without growth deficiency but with a BPS of only 4/10 (normal movement and tone, but no fluid and no FBMs with this equivocal tracing).

Our response to any abnormalities in fetal heart rate in non-laboring women where monitoring is by external Doppler fetal heart rate (FHR) monitor, is to perform a BPS which we consider to be the definitive

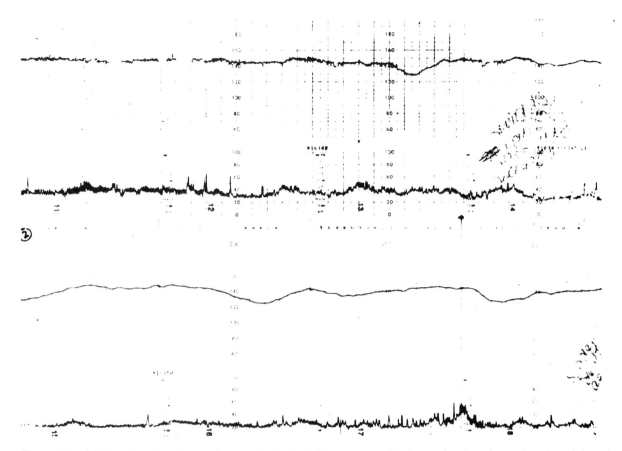

Figure 13. Minimal contractions of a modestly irritable uterus with large decelerations showing delayed recovery.

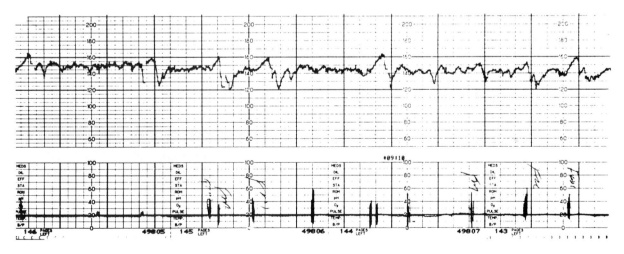

Figure 14. The 'minimal variable' pattern. Biophysical profile score 6/10 with no amniotic fluid pocket measurable and these small decelerations associated with each fetal movement. Induction of labor was unsuccessful due to repetitive decelerations associated with the oligohydramnios, ultimately progressing to reduction of variability.

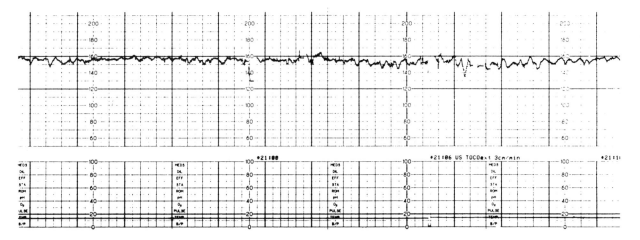

Figure 15. Reasonable variability in a 34 week fetus, but without accelerations. No decelerative pattern apparent on prolonged monitoring. Biophysical profile score, however, 0/10, with no movement of any kind, no measurable amniotic fluid. Baby delivered by cesarean section was flat with Apgars of 2, 5 and 7 at 1, 5 and 10 min, respectively. Umbilical venous pH 7.20 markedly low for an unlabored fetus at this gestation.

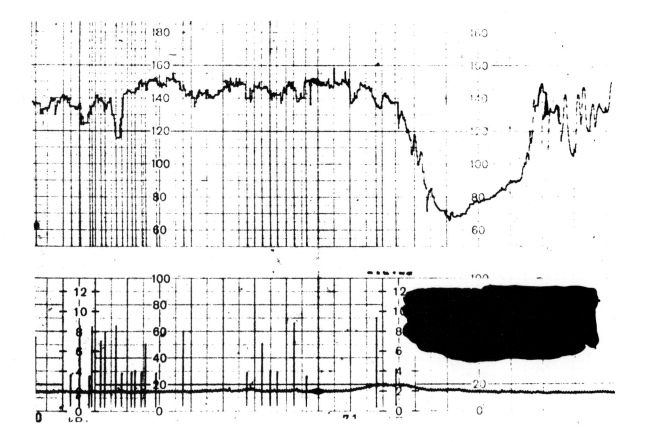

Figure 16. Spontaneous large deceleration in small fetus with maternal proteinuric pre-eclampsia. Not related to uterine activity, repeated approximately once per hour.

examination for fetal well-being. Finding a bizarre pattern such as in **Figure 17** may be associated with a moribund hydropic fetus from unsuspected severe anemia or other non-immune causes. Similarly, a fetus with an aberrant heart rate on routine office monitoring should be assessed with ultrasound, including a detailed cardiac scan. The fetus illustrated in **Figure 18** was in fact having decelerations with almost every small movement, owing to absolute oligohydramnios. The diagnosis of lethal renal agenesis with pulmonary hypoplasia averted emergency delivery on the basis of this tracing. Fetal cardiac abnormalities are reviewed in detail elsewhere, but the CTG often offers significant insight as to the frequency and regulatory context in which an arrhythmia takes place. In **Figure 19**, the monitor is trying to reconcile wildly discrepant intervals between excursions of the interventricular septum with its electronic parameters. The result is a 'searching pattern', which rejects the observed data and either multiplies or divides the frequency, depending on the exact direction of the impulse. This fetus has trigeminy, associated with transplacental passage of anticardiolipin antibodies. Although biophysical profile scoring both prenatally and while in labor formed the basis for reassurance of normal respiratory status of this fetus, a CTG was helpful in indicating the relative frequency of these bursts of arrhythmia.

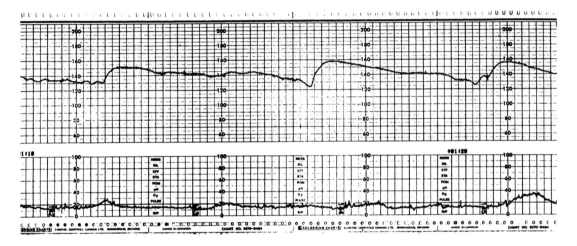

Figure 17. Reverse late decelerations or overshoots. Bizarre decelerative pattern associated with hydropic fetus, failing heart. Intrauterine death was confirmed approximately 6 h later. The parents had refused intrauterine investigation/treatment.

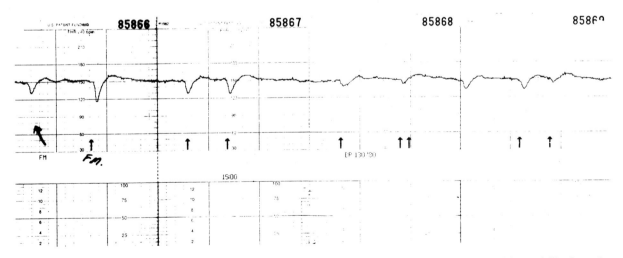

Figure 18. Active fetus with no amniotic fluid; BPS 6/10. This tracing indicates a vulnerable umbilical cord.

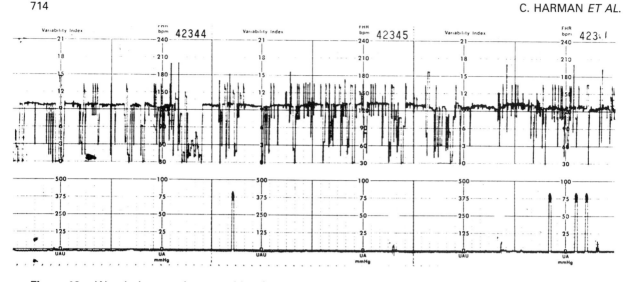

Figure 19. Wandering monitor searching for consistent heart rate in a fetus with persistent arrhythmia (see text).

Fetal Breathing Movements

Fetal breathing movements (FBMs) and hiccups are interchangeable in terms of their use in the BPS. While it is clear that hiccups are more prominent at earlier gestations, comprising at least 50% of diaphragmatic movements at 16–18 weeks, their frequency gradually declines and periods of fetal breathing become more dominant by 28 weeks or so. This has been used by some to argue against the value of biophysical profile scoring at earlier gestations, and it has been argued by others that a sliding scale needs to be imposed on BPS which recognizes different likelihoods of breathing.[110] In fact, the mean performance of normal behaviors in normal fetuses is no longer in the 28 week fetus (mean time 10.1 min *vs* 9.6 min in the 36 week fetus). Similarly, the frequency of absent FBM in scores of 8/10 is no more common at earlier gestations than at later gestations. It is notable, however, that these data include very few fetuses in the 20–24 week range, when such limitations in amount of FBM may be observed. A further qualifier here must be that the criteria for the BPS (sustained breathing for 30 s or more) are relatively generous, in that most fetuses will have some periods of breathing lasting this long, even if they are very premature. Since fetal breathing is more common after 26–28 weeks, this relative deficit in the early normal fetus has a reduced impact on the population most commonly targeted for prenatal monitoring.

Under specific circumstances, FBM may be helpful in indicating other problems (e.g. see Case Study 7 which shows continuous FBM with acidosis). On other occasions, however, statistical associations have been exaggerated with regard to fetal behavior. Since FBM is episodic, the likelihood of it overlapping with observation time is significantly less than unity (as opposed to fetal movements during a 30 min scan, which in the normal fetus are 'guaranteed' to be present). Thus, various trials of small numbers of patients in preterm premature rupture of membranes,[111,112] preterm labor,[113,114] suspected intrauterine infection, [115,116] pulmonary hypoplasia, and so on, have found associations with either present or absent FBMs. As the group which has the consistently largest population studied in various conditions with fetal breathing observations, we remain firm in our conviction that fetuses can breathe when in labor, that they breathe when infected, and often do not when not infected, and that fetal breathing movements are not only not deficient, they are frequently exaggerated, in cases of pulmonary hypoplasia.[117,118] Because of intrinsic cyclicity, FBM are the factor most likely to be absent in a normal or equivocal core ultimately associated with normal outcome. It is possible to 'correct' this by maternal glucose infusion,[119] but this seems unnecessary interference.

Fetal Movement and Tone

There has always been theoretical objection to giving 4 points for movement, which is essentially one way of looking at these two variables. For, if fetal movement (FM) is completely absent, points cannot be given for fetal tone (FT) in the standard BPS. Thus the current statements about biophysical profile scoring which have used a modification whereby position is judged to be normal (and therefore FT is scored as normal), *despite the fact the fetus is totally immobile.* We do not agree with this modification. This modification has led to the mistaken assignment of a score of 4/10 in a moribund fetus with no movement of any kind, normal fluid, a flat trace and pH 7.00. In the study cited,[85] four such examples (FM 0 but FT 2) were 'incorrectly' assigned. Correction of such technical misunderstandings would markedly alter the correlations, receiver–operator curves, and sweeping conclusions of such small studies.[120] Fetal movements include virtually any movement the fetus can make, with the possible exception of staccato mouthing movements, or rhythmic contractions of paraspinous muscles (intrauterine seizures). We include all ranges of fine motor movement, rapid eye movement, swallowing, grimacing, sucking, yawning, opening and closing of the hand, all the way to thumping kicks with the classic rapid extension and a quick return to the flexed position. *Fetal tone is judged on a combination of the velocity of movement, the return to the flexed position, and the resting position of the fetus.* The open hand shown in **Figure 20** is an extreme example of absent tone in an asphyxiated baby. Most often, however, the compromised fetus will be in a curled position, with partial flexion and a relatively normal fetal position. Putting together a mental image of the three-dimensional position, attitude and orientation of the fetus, is essential to establishing whether or not the fetal lie is appropriate. For example, we have seen several instances where 'standard' measurements and observations were obtained despite the fact that the fetus was in a completely hyperextended face presentation, basically with the heels on either side of the head, the back being virtually a complete circle!

PRACTICAL APPLICATION OF BIOPHYSICAL PROFILE SCORING

Many factors influence successful application of BPS (**Table 10**). Integration, collaboration, obstetric orien-

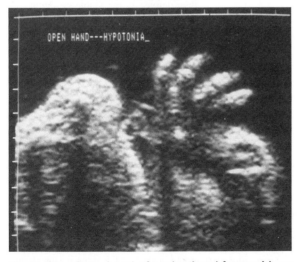

Figure 20. Open hand of asphyxiated fetus with no tone, normal amniotic fluid.

Table 10
Factors altering BPS application

Agent	Fetal effect
Drugs	
Sedatives/sedative side-effects (e.g. Aldomet®)	Diminished activity of all varieties; abolition of none
Excitatory (e.g. theophylline)	Continuous, 'picket fence' FBM
Street drugs (e.g. crack cocaine)	Rachitic, rigid, furious, bizarre FM
Indomethacin	Oligohydramnios
Maternal cigarette smoking	Various observations: diminished fetal breathing, diminished but not abolished gross body movement, abolished FBM, no effect
Maternal hyperglycemia (iatrogenic or unregulated)	Sustained FBM/acidosis, diminution or abolition of FM/FT/CTG-R
Maternal hyperglycemia (e.g. poor nutrition, insulin excess)	Abnormal paucity of all behaviors, normal AFV
Single parameter removed by perinatal condition	
Persistent fetal arrhythmia	Uninterpretable CTG
Spontaneous premature rupture of membranes	Obligatory oligohydramnios
Periodic decelerations (e.g. in preeclampsia PET)	CTG defined as non-reactive
Acute disasters (eclampsia, abruptio placentae, ketoacidosis)	Invalidates BPS predictive accuracy

tation, holistic family-centered care, all describe the effective fetal monitoring program. Receptivity to mother's questions, complaints or observations is a frequent source of course-altering information. A consultative role, similarly, maintains continuous communication between all providers of health care: we do not 'take over' management of mothers and fetuses referred for assessment. Management decisions (except for matters of life-threatening urgency) are always the purview of the referring consultant. In practical terms, a complementary division of roles has evolved based on trust and absence of professional possessiveness.

The Fetal Assessment Unit at a women's hospital is often the site of restrained chaos – family members, women on beds in street clothing with their boots on, attending physicians coming to see individual fetal exams, or to share the facilities in examining the mother, women having blood drawn, blood pressure checked and so on – not the calm, clean atmosphere of the 'ultrasound department'. Fetal examinations are scheduled in 08:00–11:30 and 13:00–16:00 blocks, which is not as arbitrary as it may seem; these are the times when maternal blood sugars are unlikely to be particularly low regarding FBMs. The mother-friendly physical and philosophical approach has been explored in Chapter 38. Smokers are encouraged to abstain for at least 1 h prior to BPS; the data suggesting decreased FBM is arguable.

The philosophy of accepting as much information as the fetus offers, means we make liberal use of endovaginal, Doppler, fetal heart rate monitor and invasive fetal testing modalities, but the core of this information is the orthodox application of biophysical profile scoring (**Table 11**). We accept that some aspects of success may be experience-related and, further, that the application may have as much to do with it as the actual method. Thus, the following series of 'helpful hints' will illustrate that BPS is not applied in a rigid format. These are principles of biophysical profile scoring, which condition the application of the generalized responses in **Table 11** and preclude dogmatic imposition.

A Score of '6/8' Does Not Exist

The CTG *is* used selectively.[121,122] If all four ultrasound variables are present within 30 min, the score is 8/8, and the CTG is not done (*exceptions*: fetal arrhythmia, macrosomia in uncontrolled diabetes, proteinuric pre-eclampsia at premature gestation, and other unstable situations where 'score out of 10' is a standing order). If one of the dynamic variables is absent, however, the score is completed by performance of a formatted CTG, including, in our unit, a numerical analysis using the System 8000.

Table 11
Clinical action in response to biophysical profile scoring

Test score	Significance	Predicted perinatal mortality[a]	Recommended management
10/10 8/8 8/10 (AFV-normal)	No evidence of fetal asphyxia present	Less than 1:1000	No active intervention on a fetal basis. Serial testing as per disorder-specific protocol
8/10-OLIGO	Chronic fetal compromise likely	89:1000	For absolute oligohydramnios, prove normal urinary tract, disprove asymptomatic rupture of membranes, then deliver at any viable gestation
6/10 (AFV-normal)	Equivocal test, fetal asphyxia is not excluded	Depends on progression	Repeat testing immediately, before assigning final value. If score is 6/10 and 10/10 in two adjacent 30 min periods, manage as 10/10. If score continues 6/10, deliver the mature fetus. In the immature fetus, repeat test within 24 h, deliver if less than 6/10
4/10	Acute fetal asphyxia likely. If AFV-OLIGO, acute or chronic asphyxia very likely	91:1000	Deliver by obstetrically appropriate method, with continuous monitoring
2/10	Acute fetal asphyxia, most likely with chronic decompensation	125:1000	Deliver for fetal indications (cesarean section)
0/10	Severe, acute asphyxia virtually certain	600:1000	Deliver *immediately* by cesarean section

[a]Per 1000 live births, within 1 week of the test result shown, if no intervention. For scores of 0, 2 and 4, intervention should commence virtually immediately.

8/10–OLIGO is an Indication for Intervention

Regardless of the presence of the other variables in normal character, oligohydramnios (maximum fluid pocket depth <2.0 cm, amniotic fluid index[72] <8) should lead to a consideration of delivery at any gestation >26 weeks. This case illustrates the clinical significance of oligohydramnios.

Case Study 2

An 18-year old nullipara, at 28 weeks gestation by reliable dates confirmed by a 12 week ultrasound scan, presented to the labor floor because of an episode of postcoital bleeding. The uterus was non-tender and non-contracting. The symphyseal fundal height was only 23 cm. The cardiotocogram showed a reactive pattern but there were some variable decelerations to 80 beats/min. Ultrasound examination revealed nothing to suggest previa or abruption. The abdominal circumference was on the 20th percentile. The fetus was making breathing movements and vigorous trunk and limb movements. The striking finding was the absence of any visible pockets of amniotic fluid; furthermore, three different observers over the course of the next several hours were unable to visualize the fetal bladder or kidneys. An amnioinfusion was not carried out. The conclusion was that the fetus had renal agenesis, and the mother was sent home. Three days later, the mother reported that the fetus had stopped moving and fetal death was established. Delivery of an 850 g fetus occurred 1 week later. Autopsy revealed no evidence of chromosomal abnormality or structural defect; specifically, the kidneys were of normal shape and size.

Comment

Oligohydramnios that cannot be ascribed to ruptured membranes or structural defect indicates the fetus is producing less urine and less lung fluid, presumably due to the redistribution of cardiac output away from the kidneys and lungs consequent to chronic hypoxemia.[123,124] Persistent non-visualization of the fetal bladder and kidneys, in the presence of normal FBM, FM and FT, suggested this was not hypoxemic in cause, but due to renal agenesis, so delivery was not recommended. In retrospect, the fetus was seen at a time when it had so severely restricted renal perfusion as to produce no urine at all,[125] but at a time when there was still enough cerebral oxygen delivery to maintain normal activity. Such an error could have been avoided in one of several ways. First, normal routine ultrasound examination at 18–20 weeks would eliminate renal agenesis as the cause, if oligohydramnios and non-visualized bladder/kidneys present later in pregnancy (see Chapter 38). Doppler waveforms from the fetal descending aorta have been reported to be reliable in distinguishing between severe oligohydramnios due to

renal agenesis/dysplasia and that due to hypoxemia.[126] Transabdominal amnioinfusion can also be used to minimize the chances of a false-positive diagnosis of renal agenesis.[127] Finally, a fetal blood sample showing no evidence of hypoxemia or acidosis would tip the diagnosis toward renal agenesis. In any event, all necessary steps should be taken to disprove the diagnosis of renal agenesis, lest a salvageable fetus be 'written off'.

When the fetus is structurally normal at a viable gestation, but there is oligohydramnios and no bladder filling is seen (exceptions would be iatrogenic oligohydramnios-indomethacin, ACE inhibitors), the situation has reached a perilous state and delivery should be effected, even if fetal behavior is normal.[128] The situation is more problematic if there is oligohydramnios, the fetus is behaving appropriately, and bladder filling and emptying is seen. We believe that in these cases, delivery is still the best choice, but concede that this management is not universally accepted, especially at very early gestations (say, 26–30 weeks); it is also possible that maternal oxygen therapy may be a reasonable alternative in some instances.[129,130] If the decision is made not to deliver in these cases of severe oligohydramnios, then one is compelled to watch the fetus carefully once or several times a day.

Twins and BPS

While the normal population includes twins or other multiple gestations in only 1.5%, the referred population usually includes *all* multiple pregnancies in the referral area, based on risk. Twin gestation, especially where discordance is suspected, *cannot* be monitored without serial multiple-parameter ultrasound surveillance (whether one calls this 'BPS' or not, is immaterial).[131,132]

Case Study 3

This 28-year-old primigravida had twin gestation known from her early scan following elevated MS-AFP on screening. At 28 weeks, she noted increased swelling – the diagnosis of proteinuric pre-eclampsia was soon complete. She was admitted to hospital, and had detailed maternal monitoring and biochemical surveillance. Despite antihypertensive therapy, her pre-elampsia gradually worsened. Fetal monitoring was by thrice-daily movement counting and daily CTG of both fetuses. After 20 days in hospital, mother's blood pressure settled, proteinuria fell from 2.5 g/day maximum, to 400 mg/day and the antihypertensives were withdrawn. On day 21 of admission, the CTG in **Figure 21** was obtained by an experienced midwife, with the transducers placed (a) in the lower left pole of the uterus, pointing right/posteriorly and (b) at the fundus, held pointing cephalad, midline (transverse lie). As part of a study of introduction of ultrasound monitoring, BPS was done prior to discharge, her pre-

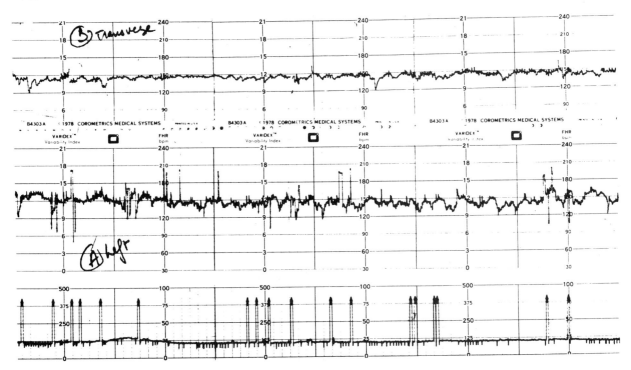

Figure 21. CTGs obtained from the twins in the case study, immediately prior to ultrasound examination which demonstrated the smaller twin (upper trace) had died.

eclampsia having subsided. The clinical presentation vertex/transverse was confirmed. The transverse twin was dead without evidence of maceration, with oligohydramnios, 40 percentile points lower (5th *vs* 45th) than his apparently healthy sibling, who had BPS 10/10 weekly until spontaneous onset of labor and normal vaginal delivery at 38 weeks. There was no recurrence whatsoever of the pre-eclampsia.

Case Study 4

A 22-year-old woman, G3P1SA1, had twins diagnosed on referral for size >dates discrepancy at 26 weeks. Initial ultrasound assessment showed a very thin membrane separating same-sex twins with size discordance (right:left 40th *vs* 15th percentiles), who were otherwise normal, active, with BPS 10/10, and UA Doppler indices normal for gestation. On weekly visits, there was modest broadening of the size difference, with BPS 8/8 for both, and maintenance of normal amniotic fluid pockets (5.0 cm both sides of the membrane at 31 weeks). At the routine 32 week visit, Twin Right had BPS 4/10 with *continuous* FBM, AFV 8.4 cm, no FM or FT, a distended bladder, a distended heart (Biventricular outer diameter 43.8 mm!, appropriate for a 40 week singleton), tricuspid regurgitation and umbilical artery Doppler indices suggestive of hypervolemia. Twin Left had BPS 6/10 (good activity, cyclic FBM, no accelerations on CTG, *absolute oligohydramnios*), no visible bladder, no visible stomach, very small heart, a bounding cord, umbilical artery velocities of severe downstream resistance (*new* absent end-diastolic

velocities). Thus, within 1 week of normal examination, the apparent cardiovascular/volume changes were so dramatic that *acute* twin–twin transfusion was the diagnosis. At emergency cesarean section, the following results were obtained:

Twin	Right	Left
Weight (g)	2345	1385
Apgar 5	9	8
UA pH	7.30	7.28
UA pO$_2$	26	24
Cord Hb (g/l)	188	109
Mean BP (mm)	30	48

Twin Right was plethoric and needed 2 days of phototherapy for moderate hyperbilirubinemia. Twin Left was pale, required two simple transfusions, glucose supplement, transient nasal C-PAP, and stayed an extra 3 weeks in the intermediate nursery for feeding. Both were structurally normal, with the same blood type, and were neurologically intact.

Comment

In these two very similar situations, two very different outcomes are apparent. There are details of interest: the resolution of pre-eclampsia after demise of the compromised twin in the first case; the documentation of an *abrupt* change in a previously balanced situation in the second. While many twin pregnancies are not this complicated, assigning relative risk among multi-fetal pregnancies is not rewarding. The mandate of BPS in such cases seems obvious.

Decreased Fetal Movement is an Indication for Prompt BPS

This case illustrates that acidemia need not be accompanied by oligohydramnios, while suggesting the potential importance of maternal fetal movement monitoring.

Case Study 5

The mother was 22 years old, G3P2. Her first pregnancy ended with antepartum asphyxial fetal death at 28 weeks gestation (Case Study 2). The second pregnancy resulted in a vaginal delivery of a healthy 3300 g baby at 40 weeks. During the third pregnancy, she was seen fortnightly in the Fetal Assessment Unit starting at 24 weeks. At the 30 week visit, abdominal circumference was on the 10th percentile. Amniotic fluid volume was normal, the NST was reactive, and fetal tone, breathing and trunk movements were all appropriate: BPS 10/10. History and small fetal size called for weekly assessments at that point, and the mother was reminded to report promptly should she notice a change in fetal movement. Five days later, the mother reported that the fetus was moving much less. Ultrasound examination over a 50 min period showed a normal volume of amniotic fluid, no fetal breathing movements, normal tone, but only eight short-lived trunk and lower-limb movements. A non-stress test was non-reactive. Two hours later, the fetus was re-examined. Over a 1 h observation, the fetus made only one trunk movement and no fetal breathing movements. A cesarean section was performed 90 min later. The baby weighed 970 g. The Apgars were 4 and 8. The umbilical vein pH was 7.22 and artery pH was 7.18. The baby did well.

Comment

The important lesson here is that in some cases an extended margin of safety cannot be guaranteed with any test, be it contraction stress test, non-stress test, BPS, or even fetal blood gas analysis. It is vital that the mother be instructed about monitoring fetal movements, not in a pro-forma way, but with emphasis that this is an important responsibility on her part.

Also of interest is that amniotic fluid volume did not warn of the asphyxia. The amniotic fluid volume represents several days of urine output: an acute onset of hypoxemia, even if it results in no perfusion of the kidneys, may not be reflected for some time in an obvious diminution of the AFV. It is possible that, in selected cases, a more accurate reflection of the current state of fetal oxygenation is to estimate actual urine output per hour by ultrasound observation by changing bladder volumes.[133] All biophysical variables should be taken together in assessing fetal health.

The Complete Clinical Picture

The following case study illustrates that the complete clinical picture has to be considered when evaluating fetal condition.

Case Study 6

A 22-year old-woman, G5P1A3, 29 weeks gestation, was brought to the labor floor by ambulance. She had 'sniffed' paint thinner for about 60 min, 5 h earlier. She complained of nausea, vomiting, abdominal pain, headache and double vision. She was very lethargic, could be roused to answer questions but was somnolent when undisturbed. Although the maternal pulse was 120–130, she was well perfused, and all other vital signs were normal. There was no vaginal bleeding and the uterus was relaxed. Fetal tachycardia, 175–195 beats/min, persisted with minimal variability, and no accelerations, over more than 12 h.

Ultrasound exam showed a fetus of appropriate size without evident anomalies. The placenta showed no abruption. The amniotic fluid volume was normal. During a 60-min observation, there were no FBM and no trunk or limb movements. There were some hiccups, some small hand and face movements. Bladder filling was seen.

Ten hours later, the cardiotocogram was still non-reactive with minimal variability, but it was not terminal or decelerative.[134] There were now a few trunk movements evident. Twenty-four hours after the initial scan, the fetus was moving vigorously with about 20 trunk movements in a 30-min period. At 36 h after the first scan (48 h after the solvent inhalation), the fetal behavior was entirely normal and the CTG was reactive.

Comment

At the first ultrasound examination of the fetus, 12 h after the solvent inhalation, there was a difficult diagnostic dilemma. A fetus at 29 weeks does not go 60 min without making either breathing or trunk movements unless there is something wrong. The three possibilities considered were: (1) a hypoxemic fetus, in which case prompt delivery would be required; (2) a non-hypoxemic fetus, intoxicated with solvent, in which case delivery at 29 weeks would be bad; and (3) a fetus that was not hypoxemic now, but may have suffered severe brain damage beforehand. Cordocentesis to evaluate fetal oxygenation and acid-base status may have distinguished between the first two, but the mother's lack of cooperation made one reluctant to put a needle in the vicinity of the umbilical cord! Ultimately we reasoned that since the solvent intoxication had clearly depressed the maternal central nervous system, and since volatile organic substances easily cross the placenta, it was likely that the fetal brain was similarly affected.

Hypoxemia causing acidemia is the most common cause of prolonged ($\geq$ 60 min) fetal inactivity. Another cause is fetal intoxication as above. A more common situation is the initation of maternal medication (notably alpha-methyldopa) where maternal 'sedation' is mirrored by a quiet, but not immobile, fetus. Fetal anemia, either from a large transplacental hemorrhage or from alloimmune hemolysis, can also present as fetal inactivity, and not necessarily with hydrops if the anemia is of sudden or late onset (see Case Study 1). Fetal bacterial infection, fetal head injury or fetal brain death[135,136] are also possible explanations. Maternal disorders such as myotonic dystrophy or myasthenia gravis can markedly reduce fetal activity. Fetal neurologic disease (e.g. Vertnig-Hoffman disease) is a rare cause.

Antepartum testing must be interpreted in the context of the entire clinical situation.

Biophysical Profile Scoring is Truly Composite

A low score is a low score, and a powerful indicator of real compromise, no matter which variables are individually present/absent (perhaps with the exclusion of a reactive heart rate tracing).

Case Study 7

The mother was a 32-year-old with two previous vaginal deliveries of healthy babies at term. The current pregnancy was entirely unremarkable except there was less movement than usual for 2 days previous, and no movement at all for 8 h on the day of evaluation. She felt well and denied abdominal pain, vaginal bleeding, ruptured membranes or fever. The vital signs and physical examination were normal. Ultrasound showed no fetal anomaly, a normal placenta and normal AFV. Most striking was the behavior of the fetus. During one full hour of observation, not a single trunk or limb movement was seen. However, during that same time, there were continuous, unremitting, monotonous breathing movements of about 40 per min. A CTG showed no accelerations during a 40 min observation and spontaneous decelerations were noted: BPS 4/10.

Membranes were ruptured artificially revealing thick meconium and a scalp clip was applied. The fetal heart rate was 140 but the baseline was flat and decelerations occurred after spontaneous contractions. Cesarean section was performed 80 min after the scan. The baby weighed 2540 g, large amounts of thick meconium were suctioned from below the vocal cords. The Apgar scores were 3 and 7. The baby was extubated at 20 min, but by 30 min of age, indrawing and

nasal flaring were noted and clinical and chest x-ray findings were consistent with meconium aspiration. On 65% FiO_2, an arterial blood gas at 50 min of life showed a pH of 7.07, pCO_2 23 mmHg, pO_2 95 mmHg, HCO_3 meq/l, and a base deficit of -22. The hemoglobin was 194 g/l, the WBC 24 000, and the platelet count 70 000. It was at this point that the pediatric team became aware of the results from the cord umbilical vein: pH 6.93, pCO_2 46 mmHg, pO_2 26 mmHg, HCO_3 10 meq/l and base deficit -24.

Appropriate cultures were obtained, antibiotics begun, bicarbonate given and supplemental O_2 continued. Increasing respiratory fatigue necessitated ventilator assistance at 10 h of age. From then on, there was steady improvement in condition. The baby was discharged in good health at 1 week of age without ever displaying cardiovascular instability or neurologic disturbance. All cultures were negative. The discharge diagnosis was severe intrauterine asphyxia of unknown cause with meconium aspiration.

Comment

The total absence of any trunk or limb movements during a full hour of observation, the terminal fetal heart rate pattern, and the severe metabolic acidosis at delivery all indicated that the fetus was very sick, if not dying, at the time of the scan. Nevertheless, this fetus breathed continuously for an hour, 80 min before delivery by cesarean section, without preceding labor. In this case, the simple combination of normal AFV and FBM did *not* indicate fetal well-being, in contrast to the claims of other writers.[137]

Laboratory observations in sheep and monkeys and clinical observations in humans show that most fetuses are 'apneic' for many hours before death. However, in some animal fetuses, the apneic period is followed by continuous breathing movements that can last hours and continue until a few minutes before death; these fetuses are hypoxemic and acidemic.[138,139] In animal fetuses, infusions of HC1 or NH_4C1 that lower pH levels to 6.80 result in continuous fetal breathing for as long as 8 h.[140,141] The most likely explanation for the continuous breathing activity in this fetus was the marked metabolic acidosis, which overcame the inhibitory effects of hypoxemia, and may also have contributed to *in-utero* aspiration of meconium, a phenomenon observed in baboons and humans.[142–144] It is notable that in the experimental animal, and in the woman,[145] monotonous FBM provoked by acidosis *does* feature absent FM, abnormal FT and a non-reactive trace. Although this combination (leading to an *abnormal* score of 4/10) has been known for several years,[146] interpretive errors still occur.[147]

Finally, there was nothing in this mother's history or pregnancy course to make her 'high risk'. In our population, the paradoxical situation has occurred where there is now a higher stillbirth rate in the untested 'low-risk' population than in the tested 'high-risk' group. For this 'low-risk' population, the greatest benefit would likely come from instituting a program of maternal recording of fetal movements, with BPS as the gold standard for non-movers.

Unstable Fetal or Maternal Situations Demand Frequent Testing

Case Study 8

The mother was a 32-year-old nullipara, with rheumatic mitral stenosis and mitral regurgitation. She was on heparin because of previous cerebral emboli, and quinidine for ventricular ectopy. She had no congestive heart failure. At 20 weeks gestation, the fetus was examined for elevated maternal serum AFP; anatomy was normal and size was consistent with dates. However, by 24 weeks there was poor interval growth, with both abdominal and head circumference below the 10th percentile. Umbilical artery end-diastolic flow was absent. The fetus was appropriately active and AFV was normal. At 26 weeks, no interval fetal growth was evident, but fetal activity and fluid volume were still appropriate. Again, no umbilical artery end-diastolic flow was seen.

Since a gestational age had now been reached (26:2 weeks) at which intervention on fetal behalf would be considered, mother was admitted to hospital to allow more intense fetal monitoring (as well as to permit complete evaluation of the mother's health by the appropriate consultants). The fetus was examined with biophysical profile scoring twice a day. At 28 weeks, BPS was 10/10 at 09:00 h. At 17:00 h, FM were fewer than at any time the examiner had ever seen, although it still made six trunk movements in 30 min. The mother herself reported a marked decrease in fetal movement. Between 22:20 and 22:55 h, the fetus was examined again and this time only moved *once* during the entire observation. After the mother was prepared, a classical cesarean section was performed 4 h later. The baby weighed 570 g, had Apgars of 5 and 9. (Unfortunately, no blood could be obtained from the umbilical cord for evaluation of gases and acid base.) The baby had an uncomplicated course of considerable length due to the severe growth deficiency.

Comment

Antepartum testing is made appropriate to the individual fetus, not done by a predetermined schedule appropriate to the population as a whole. In this case, absent umbilical artery end-diastolic flow and lack of fetal growth over a period of several weeks, convinced us this fetus had no oxygen reserve and could deteriorate very quickly. The sicker the fetus, the more intensive is the observation.

The easiest way to monitor the very premature fetus is with ultrasound observations using the BPS.[148] However, allowances have to be made for the early gestational age. Interpretation of the early NST can be problematic.[149-151] Furthermore, whereas it may be normal for the fetus beyond 30 weeks to make only four or five trunk movements in a 30-min period, or even go up to 60 min without a trunk movement,[152] the situation is different before 30 weeks. The healthy premature fetus makes an average of about one trunk movement a minute. *Indeed, absence of body movements for more than 15 min is extremely rare before 30 weeks.*[153,154]

Biophysical Profile Scoring is Flexible and Interpretive

Case Study 9

A 31-year-old woman had one previous pregnancy, delivered by induction of labor at 39 weeks gestation for a clinical diagnosis of growth deficiency. That child showed substantial 'catch-up' growth as a baby, rising from the 9th percentile to the 60th by 12 months, with normal developmental milestones. In this pregnancy, clinical growth deficiency was obvious much earlier: ultrasound showed a fetus <10th percentile for all standard measurements. She was referred to our team for fetal blood sampling to exclude aneuploidy at 32 weeks.

The BPS was 8/10: there were good-quality FM of broad variety; cyclic FBM were present. The CTG was non-reactive, but not decelerative and had acceptable variability. The fetus was much below the 3rd percentile for all measurements. Estimated fetal weight by multiple parameters was <750 g. Although normal, AFV was subjectively reduced (uterus hugging the fetal back, small decelerations with fetal movement, maximum cord-free pocket <3 cm). Umbilical artery Doppler velocimetry showed an elevated *S:D* ratio, but maintained diastolic velocities, 'suggestive' of increased downstream resistance. The placenta was bizarre in appearance (**Figure 22**). There were no apparent structural anomalies on detailed review, but the fetal bowel was modestly distended and peristalsis was absent (a very unusual finding at 32 weeks). Umbilical venous blood sampling showed a pO_2 of 18 (very low for an unlabored fetus at this gestation) and a pH 7.27 with a pCO_2 of 36 suggesting the base deficit of 9.0 was at least partly metabolic in nature. The needle was maintained in place while oxygen was administered by 10 liter rebreathe mask, tightly sealed to the mother's face. At 10 min, the pO_2 had risen to 26, while an associated uterine contraction resulted in a pCO_2 rise to 54 mmHg. Sequential contractions following needle removal constituted a positive contraction stress test, with the decelerations resolving once the contractions abated. The circulating hemoglobin level of 133 was modestly elevated for this gestation, but the red cell smear showed a dramatic surge of erythropoiesis – nucleated red cell count >1900 per 100 WBC (normal 8–10). The MCV was normal. The diagnosis was compensated uteroplacental dysfunction.

Maternal oxygenation was continued a further 4 h. Prelabor cesarean section produced a 710 g female, structurally intact, with Apgars of 4 and 8. A cord vein pO_2 of 30 and pH of 7.30 suggested further (modest) improvement by maternal

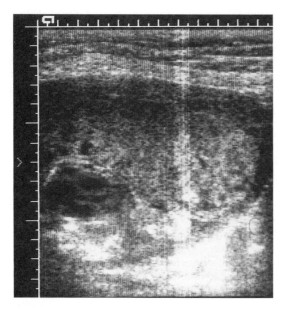

Figure 22. Unusual placental appearance, associated with severe growth deficiency and acidosis/hypoxemia as described in the text; 95% of functioning villi were replaced by dense fibrinization.

hyperoxygenation. The neonate required short-term, non-ventilator supplemental oxygen. *Consequent to the fetal abdominal findings, she was not fed for 7 days, during which moderate abdominal distension arose and resolved.*

Comment

The BPS is there to be flexible. If the data are equivocal or contradictory, repeat the testing, add modalities, consider invasive confirmation in order to achieve maximum precision. These principles are applied more frequently in the growth deficient fetus than the appropriately grown fetus. The 'oxygen uptake test' illustrated here is in the process of development, but in addition to the initial data confirming hypoxemia and acidosis, may help differentiate intrinsic (e.g. infectious, chromosomal) fetal problems from true uteroplacental dysfunction. Note that the *normal* fetus (at 32 weeks, for example) will show a rise from 40 to 80 torr in as little as 3 min, under the same circumstances. Finally, the elements of BPS may also be useful reflections of the *range* of impairment even in the clearly compromised individual. **Figure 23** shows the results of the BPS among a highly selected group of fetuses whose mothers had pre-eclampsia prior to 36 weeks and who themselves had repetitive decelerations without labor on daily CTG. Even in these unstable

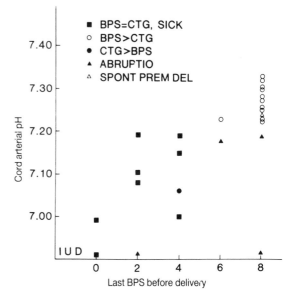

Figure 23. Biophysical profile score in fetuses with repetitive decelerations, not in labor. All mothers had proteinuric pre-eclampsia. All CTGs were decelerative, therefore maximum BPS was 8/10. Even among these severely compromised fetuses, there was good correlation between limits of activity and outcome. The individual cases are characterized as showing agreement between BPS and CTG, the two systems differing in their appraisal with BPS giving a more reliable estimate of fetal well-being, the CTG being more reliable than BPS, acute abruptio placenta intervening, and spontaneous premature delivery ensuing, respectively. In this population of compromised fetuses, there were three intrauterine deaths shown at the bottom of the ordinate scale: BPS 0, 2, 8, respectively. No scoring system should expect to be perfect, especially when acute events intervene. As in all similar studies, the *combination of BPS and CTG information coupled with ultrasound observations and careful clinical appraisal, give the most accurate impression.*

situations, the overall impression derived from ultrasound variables was a good reflection of fetal 'respiratory' status.[155] The generation of such data is essential if our understanding of the progression of asphyxia in human fetuses is to grow.

BPS is not a Panacea

Case Study 10

In her first pregnancy, this 19-year-old obese woman underwent cesarean section for fetal distress in labor, for a

4700 g baby. Glucose tolerance testing done because of this history of macrosomia showed: fasting blood sugar 6.7; 1 h 7.0; 2 h 6.5; 3 h 3.6 mmol/l. Because only one result of four was abnormal, this was recorded as normal on the prenatal sheet. However, the high fasting sugar indicated there was a problem with glucose tolerance. At 38 weeks, the fetus was clinically and sonographically large. A repeat 1 h postprandial glucose was normal (6.5). At 40 weeks, ultrasound estimate of fetal weight was >5000 g. BPS was 10/10 with hydramnios and marked anatomic evidence of fetal macrosomia. The 1 h postprandial glucose was high (8.8). A repeat elective cesarean section was booked for 3 days later. The fetal heart rate was unobtainable 30 min before scheduled cesarean section. A 6100 g stillborn baby was delivered. At autopsy, the striking findings were organomegaly and marked pancreatic islet-cell hypertrophy.

Comment

A macrosomic fetus in a mother with impaired glucose tolerance is an unstable clinical combination. Delivery *was* indicated but taking long-term reassurance from the BPS is *not* appropriate in such a situation. Antepartum tests, which are ideally suited to detect chronic hypoxia, are less reliable in predicting outcome in such instances. Because of constant glucose oversupply to the fetus, there is pancreatic islet-cell hypertrophy and hyperplasia, and in some instances fetal insulin production may far exceed maternal production. In the last weeks of pregnancy, exaggerated glucose siphoning by the fetus due to fetal hyperinsulinemia may make the mother's metabolic situation, as reflected by her blood glucose levels, appear quite good, when in fact the fetal metabolic situation is worsening.[156] In our view, when a macrosomic fetus is identified in a woman with diabetes, delivery should be effected at 37 or 38 weeks with *stable* peripartum maternal glucose levels, regardless of the antepartum test result.

Disease-Specific Testing

Several examples have already been given in the case studies. The broad variety of conditions which can lead to fetal compromise suggest that: (a) multivariable testing will give the most accurate description of fetal status and that (b) different variables, and different testing intervals, will have an enhanced effect in certain conditions. For example, in chronic placental dysfunction leading to asymmetrical growth deficiency, the 'disease' progression may be gradual, with maintenance of normal behaviors over a long period of time, and additional information supplied by considering fetal size, fetal growth parameters, Doppler umbilical artery velocimetry, and so on. On the other hand, is the fetus who has passed an optimal functional state, such as seen in the post-mature fetus, and who may

show compromise over a few days, manifest first by oligohydramnios.

Because BPS is based on an assessment of both acute behavioral indices and more chronic variables such as fluid volume, and includes the ability to follow growth parameters on a regular basis, the potential exists for detection of compromise on many timescales. Other ultrasound-based observations, which correlate with fetal outcome, can be observed during the process of biophysical profile scoring and continue to 'set the mood' upon which variable testing is performed. For example, if end-diastolic velocities are zero or the systolic and diastolic components of flow are out of proportion, scoring can be done more often, *although the BPS is the only tool we use to decide management.*

While the mechanism of fetal compromise in the infant of a diabetic mother remains incompletely clear, there is no doubt that biophysical profile scoring enhances the overall outcome in such populations.[157] Modification of the protocol is based not only on disease, but tailored to severity of disease, with scoring done as frequently as is necessary to minimize any chance of a sudden change in fetal status between tests (even as often as three times daily). It is essential that each group evaluates and develops protocols individual to the post-term pregnancy, the uncontrolled diabetic pregnancy, the growth-deficient fetus and others, based on its population of referred patients. Details of such reviews are beyond the scope of this chapter, but include the overall observation that biophysical profile scoring can be adapted while allowing progression of pregnancy and reduction of maternal morbidity from unnecessary interference.[158–161]

An example is the standard management of the post-term pregnancy, according to biophysical profile scoring, and the sensible application of obstetric principles.[162] The general scheme for this approach is outlined in **Figure 24**; and this management plan has been applied to more than 5000 women referred with reliable pregnancy dating beyond 42 weeks 0 days. In this situation, BPS twice weekly allows observation of the dynamic variables, as well as monitoring of amniotic fluid volumes, cervical assessment, reviewing fetal movement counting with mother, and documenting significant changes in maternal status. The use of prostaglandin gel to ripen the cervix, and moving ahead with induction as soon as ARM is favorable according to cervical condition, are also vital components of this scheme. In other words, the system does not advocate passive watching in every woman, only in those women whose cervix suggests a high likelihood of failed induction and cesarean section.

A recent randomized trial of induction *vs* observation[163] has satisfied many reviewers that the policy of interference according to the clock (induction of labor for all patients once 41+ weeks has been reached)

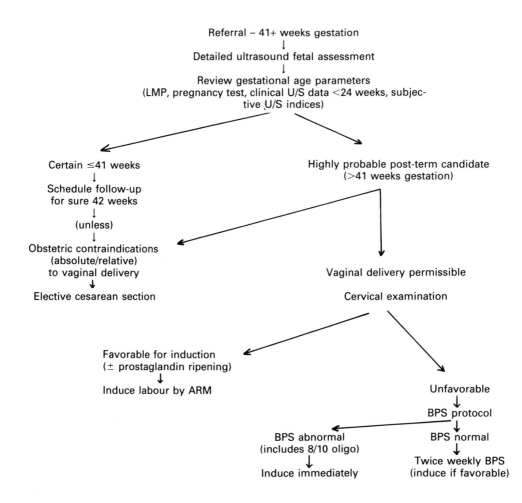

Referral – 41+ weeks gestation
↓
Detailed ultrasound fetal assessment
↓
Review gestational age parameters
(LMP, pregnancy test, clinical U/S data <24 weeks, subjec-
tive U/S indices)

Certain ≤41 weeks
↓
Schedule follow-up
for sure 42 weeks
↓
(unless)
↓
Obstetric contraindications
(absolute/relative)
to vaginal delivery
↓
Elective cesarean section

Highly probable post-term candidate
(>41 weeks gestation)

Vaginal delivery permissible

Cervical examination

Favorable for induction
(± prostaglandin ripening)
↓
Induce labour by ARM

Unfavorable
↓
BPS protocol
↓
BPS normal
↓
Twice weekly BPS
(induce if favorable)

BPS abnormal
(includes 8/10 oligo)
↓
Induce immediately

Figure 24.   Schematic diagram of management of the post-term pregnancy, using biophysical profile scoring
and induction of labor when the cervix is favorable.

is justified. This study has several failings when viewed in the light of biophysical profile scoring. First, patients were monitored in that trial with NST (an ineffective tool in post-term pregnancy), as opposed to biophysical profile scoring.[162] Second, the major discriminant between the two groups was the incidence of cesarean section. The group in whom mandatory induction of labor took place at 41 weeks were part of a second trial reviewing the benefits of prostaglandin gel. They therefore received, as part of their induction protocol, prostaglandin gel ripening of the cervix prior to induction of labor. In the group being induced for fetal reasons, or because the cervix was judged to be favorable at 42+ weeks (i.e. the conservative management group), prostaglandin gel was not allowed under the conditions of the trial. One might judge that the rate of cesarean section was bound to be higher in the group refused access to prostaglandins, therefore determining the outcome of the trial. The cesarean sec-

tion rate observed in that randomized controlled trial, for patients induced at 41 weeks, is much higher than that observed in women whose fetuses behave normally, and are allowed to progress beyond 42 weeks.

The BPS must remain flexible and is not to be rigidly applied without recognition of other clinical input. As such, the BPS is the obtaining of a number of vital signs from the fetus. As with the extrauterine patient, simply obtaining the vital signs at a moment in time is not sufficient for comprehensive total care. The BPS is meant to function within the framework of a comprehensive and integrated approach to maternal and fetal health.

Summary of Clinical Application of BPS

We believe that biophysical profile scoring addresses the theoretical objectives of monitoring of high-risk women and high-risk fetuses. The overall score is a reliable indicator of health when normal, of compromise when overtly abnormal, and shows a graded relationship to metabolic standards and outcome.

Once BPS was established as the primary means of evaluating fetuses in high-risk pregnancy, perinatal mortality in the tested population fell, and has remained constant, at a gross rate of 6.7:1000 and a corrected total perinatal mortality of 1.9:1000. The gross stillbirth rate has remained relatively unchanged over several years due to an increase in the absolute frequency of lethal anomalies in our monitored population. The corrected stillbirth rate has fallen marginally, possibly due to continued improvements in biophysical profile scoring, the addition of other technologies, and recognition of fetal problems related to ultrasound data, not based on biophysical variables. The corrected neonatal death rate has fallen dramatically during this decade.[164]

Table 12 shows the contrasting statistics in the untested population within our health care jurisdiction. Although showing the decrease in overall perinatal mortalities common in most health care jurisdictions, these values have remained consistently higher in the untested portion of our population than in our study groups. The difference in performance during the 1980s illustrates the magnitude of efficacy of biophysical profile scoring. During that 10-year period, 55 661 pregnancies were monitored with antepartum fetal assessment by biophysical profile scoring (including single and serial observations), while another 104 337 were not. Corrected perinatal mortality showed a significant difference between the two groups, being 1.9:1000 in the monitored group and 7.7:1000 in the unmonitored group. This comparison may be misleading in that many patients in the untested group were not monitored because of their presentation in premature labor, which of course contributes heavily to their mortality. *The stillbirth rate, however, is not so subject to prematurity, and also supports the benefits of monitoring. The corrected stillbirth rate for the tested group (1.23:1000) is highly significantly lower than that for the untested group (4.57:1000).*

This is *not* a randomized controlled trial. It is, however, a worthwile experimental situation. Women were diverted to biophysical profile scoring on the basis of observable risk (they cannot therefore be classified as being at *lower* risk for fetal problems, i.e. the difference in mortality is not based on inherent qualities of the subjects). The consistent results over the long term of *clinical application* demonstrate that this is a practicable system, too.

At the same time, even in this environment, when a proven system is fully integrated into the high-risk scene, resources are not available to monitor *everyone* this way. What of the women and fetus with no apparent risk; what about the 'normal' pregnancy?

MONITORING THE NORMAL FETUS IN A NORMAL PREGNANCY

The formatted ultrasound exam for 18–20 weeks is detailed in Chapter 38: when 'everything' is normal at that point (normal MS-AFP, size = dates, normal fluid, normal anatomy, normal placental location, well-developed diastolic velocities), and standard prenatal monitoring proceeds without major disruption in maternal status, any unsatisfactory outcome is *extremely* unlikely (<5%). Addressing that extreme, in which a remote fraction results in unexplained stillbirth, is frustrating. It would not be a cost-effective venture to monitor thousands of carefully screened normal women. A proposal for surveillance of pregnancies at no apparent risk is shown in **Figure 25**. The central intervention in this scheme is fetal movement counting.

Fetal Movement Counting (FMC)[7,165–169]

That this is efficacious in the individual case is clear from previous application examples. That fetal movement counting is a tool which requires reasonable precision in application is highlighted by the following case:

Case Study 11

A 32-year-old woman had ultrasound-verified pregnancy dating and meticulous prenatal care, including instructions from her family physician on twice-daily FMC routine. The previous pregnancy resulted in normal term vaginal delivery after spontaneous onset of labor. There was no intercurrent illness, and the current planned, welcome, cigarette-free, alcohol-free pregnancy progressed well until 37+ weeks gestation. Before retiring, the mother realized she had not felt many movements during the day, although the morning FMC had been her normal (eight kicks in <20 min). As was her

Table 12
BPS effects on Manitoba obstetric population

	Unmonitored population	Monitored with BPS
Number of pregnancies	104 337	55 661
Gross perinatal mortality/1000	9.79	6.71
Corrected perinatal mortality/1000	7.69	1.86
Gross stillbirth/1000	5.2	3.21
Corrected stillbirth/1000	4.57	1.23

First visit: 'No apparent risk' classification – subject to regular review

Maternal serum alpha-fetoprotein 15–16 weeks = normal
Detailed 20 week ultrasound (see Chapter 38) = normal
Includes introduction to fetal activity, smoking-cessation etc.

24–26 weeks: Fetal movement (FM) surveillance

Routine, protocol enquiry re: FM, at each office visit.
Trial of 'count to 10' method: Count *all* palpable FMs
                                Count twice daily – early and late
                                Tally average time to 10 for 1 week
                                Review results by phone after 7 days

EVALUATE METHOD IN FAMILY CONTEXT

Method satisfactory	**Method unsatisfactory**
1. Reinforce at A/N visits	**1. No/FEW FM:** Try semi-prone, 'comfort' or semi-recumbent positions, with firm hand on abdomen. Repeat scan if required, to educate mother.
2. Written directions	
3. Alarm **A. No FM for 60 min** (vs established pattern) Attend hospital/clinic for immediate biophysical profile	**2. Too long to 10: count *all* FM.** Exclude distractions. Change position, time, intake. Reduce to 8 FM threshold, scan to exclude anomalies if low activity persists.
B. >50% increase time to 10 Review by phone: 1–4 FM/h = **Biophysical profile** 4–8/h = review daily >8 FM/h = reassure	**3. Poor compliance:** Patient, family education, family FM counting. R/O social or other problems. Ultimately, reduce demands.

Full biophysical profile score is the gold standard for all sudden declines in fetal movement. Management is determined by the actual score. At full term, bona fide significant decrease in total fetal activity suggests cervical assessment and consideration of elective induction of labor.

Back-up, cooperation by staff is ensured by in-service education. As term approaches, mother is reminded that while FM may become more clustered, more sophisticated, gentler, the time to 10 is unlikely to change drastically, even if labor is close.

Figure 25. A monitoring scheme for low-risk pregnancy, concentrating on fetal movement counting, with biophysical profile scoring as the gold standard.

routine, she timed the interval required for eight kicks that evening. This took more than 90 min, but was achieved. In the morning, she had only one movement in the first hour, so reported immediately to the Fetal Assessment Unit. The tracing shown in **Figure 26** was associated with a BPS of 2/10 – only amniotic fluid was within normal limits. Acute feto-maternal hemorrhage was suspected on the basis of the small, hyperdynamic fetal heart, pyknotic umbilical cord, and movement history.

The fetus was judged unsuitable for induction of labor. Immediate cesarean section produced a pale, shocky, moribund boy weighing 3100 g. Apgar scores assessed by a neutral observer at 1, 5, 10 and 15 min were: 1, 5, 7 and 8. Cord gases, umbilical vein: pO_2 45, pCO_2 77, pH 7.15, base excess -2. Hemoglobin measurement was not possible because there was only 0.4 ml blood in the entire cord, and there was no neonatal blood pressure. *After* rapid transfusion of 75 ml packed red cells, the baby's hemoglobin concentration measured just 53 g/l; calculations using a standard blood volume predicted a *rise* of 60 g/l should result from the transfusion, i.e. the pretransfusion hemoglobin concentration was negli-

gible. The maternal Kleihauer test commenced during preanesthesia oxygenation was reported during the resuscitation as indicating transplacental hemorrhage of approximately 400 ml.

Although the resuscitation appeared successful, optimism was premature: after 24 h, the baby began uninterrupted seizures, was anuric, hypotensive and died at the end of the third day.

Comment

The case recognizes several weaknesses of fetal movement counting:

- Complete cessation of maternal perception of fetal movement may be a pre-mortem event, rather than a warning of danger on the horizon.

- The actual warning may be a sharp *change* in rou-

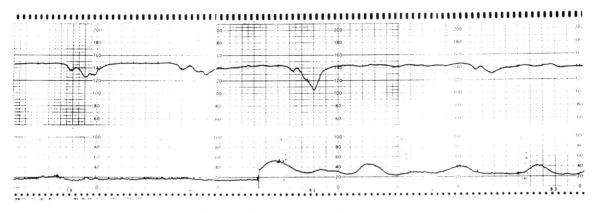

Figure 26. CTG of fetus described in case study.

tine, or even the subconscious maternal message 'things are pretty quiet here', as opposed to the numerical limits suggested by the attending physician.

- Such events are critically rare, but when they occur, unreasonable responsibility may be left with the mother – 'victim blaming' at its worst.

- What might be considered normal for one woman/pregnancy/fetus/gestational age combination would be unattainable by many women; the average kicks per hour in many studies is 4–6, not the 20 or more this mother was accustomed to!

The definitive study of FMC took place in a multicenter trial, which studied the 'count to 10' method[169] in 68 654 women, in the late 1980s.[29] The study, and the parallel commentary by the trial coordinators,[7] are mandatory reading for the student of fetal monitoring, and of 'RCT' (randomized controlled trial) methodology. A summary of the problems with FMC is displayed in **Table 13**.[170–173] The penultimate statement in the RCT report is not particularly encouraging: 'Routine daily counting by women, followed by appropriate action when movements are reduced, seems to offer no advantage over informal inquiry about movements during standard antenatal care, and selective use of formal counting in high-risk cases.'

Table 13
Factors impairing fetal surveillance by movement counting

Factors	Effect
Highly variable methodology	Confusion and inconsistent instructions
? Efficacy	Physician non-compliance

Fetal/maternal variation:
  Different activity between fetuses
  Changing activity in the same fetus
  Different perceptions between mothers
  Different perceptions by same mother
	These factors require flexible, individualized FMC methodology

Public misinformation (e.g. the baby stops moving before labor, it's OK)	Failure to follow protocol directions, in given unusual circumstances
Poor maternal compliance	Up to 20% of women do not count, but may falsify records
Faulty clinical response	Despite proper maternal performance, no definitive testing/intervention is undertaken. Biophysical profile scoring is the only acceptable response to bona fide decreased fetal movement

PRENATAL FETAL MONITORING
Summary of Management Options

Indications

General

- Pregnancies where 'high risk' rather than 'low risk' of fetal compromise

- Where there is a risk of chronic hypolemia

- ? Fetal movement counting for 'low risk'

Maternal

- Cyanotic heart disease

- ? Diabetes

Placental

- 'Idiopathic' growth deficiency

- Recurrent abruption

- Pre-eclampsia

Fetal

- Acquired
  - infection
  - hydrops
  - metabolic
  - anemia

- Congenital (*Note*: fetal monitoring is unlikely to be implemented for these)
  - syndromes
  - structural anomalies
  - chromosomal

Principles

Integrated comprehensive fetal evaluation with monitoring and

Maternal factors

- Clinical, e.g. hypertension, diabetes

- Laboratory, e.g. Kleihauer, renal function

Fetal factors

- Normality

- Growth/size

- Doppler velocimetry

- Invasive procedures, e.g. karyotype

Select test appropriate for pathology (if possible)

Overall, BPS gives best prediction of acute or chronic fetal compromise

---

Success, it seems, is in the eye of the beholder. The results achieved in experimental and study groups were nearly identical, indicating *either* (as the authors concluded) that formal FMC probably did not alter outcome, *or* that the monitoring routinely performed by the control group (who all attended prenatal care, who were allowed to do formal FMC when the physician requested it – only 8.9% did, however – who could be asked about fetal movements as part of routine prenatal

visits, who had free access to the high rate of obstetric ultrasound utilized in the centers concerned, whose physicians were participating in the trial, and who knew themselves of the intense interest in fetal movement!) actually constituted a detailed and helpful form of fetal surveillance.

In strong support of the *second* alternative is the low stillbirth rate among 'controls' (2.9:1000 normally formed singleton births), which was much lower than the trial supervisors had predicted. Second, compliance among the experimental group was lower than in previous trials. Third, 11 women in the counting group reported decreased FMC, had a living fetus at that point, but ultimately experienced stillbirth – none of these had delivery prescribed, reflecting 'false reassurance, from diagnostic testing, especially cardiotocography' – allowing improvement if BPS were utilized.

The change in stillbirth rate achieved by formal FMC was judged ineffective within the context of the trial; it appears to be proof of superior prenatal monitoring when compared with our unmonitored population in Manitoba. We recommend further study, with the model shown in **Figure 25**. This emphasizes several critical points. Biophysical profile scoring is the gold standard for assessment of fetal activity – the resources must be available to respond virtually immediately to documented significant decline (50% fewer movements than normal for the individual). 'Compliance' must be reinforced on regular prenatal vists, supplemented by public education to eliminate myths such as the idea that movements dropping to zero is a good sign for impending labor and, consequently, nothing to worry about. Compliance includes early, prompt and meticulous reporting when the 'alarm' threshold is reached – that day/night, not next morning. This scheme calls for a high level of fetal activity in a short period of time, emphasizing its application to *low-risk* fetuses who are expected to be quite active. Various thresholds have been tried by various groups, though none have been systematically tested against one another (nor are they likely to be, considering the numbers of subjects required). In fact, one really has no idea what 'normal' will be for a given patient, thus the emphasis on defining normal for that individual at a time when activity is typical for that fetus and applying time (no more than 50% longer to reach average counts) or number (no fewer than one-third the number in the given time) constraints.

CONCLUSION

The integrated application of the principles illustrated here has produced clear, definite, reproducible and clinically meaningful reductions in stillbirth in the Manitoba population in which it has been used for over 13 years. Risk assignment, and re-evaluation on a regular basis throughout the pregnancy, remain the cornerstones of initiating the highly specific, highy sensitive, flexible system of fetal assessment by real-time ultrasound described here. These modalities may not yet be perfect, but the principle of multiple-variable testing is beyond challenge, in our view. The need to focus on the *majority* of normal women without apparent risk, with a practicable, sensitive system for averting intrauterine injury or death, will be the task of the 1990s.

REFERENCES

1   Vincent CA, Martin T, Ennis M (1991) Obstetric accidents: The patient's perspective. *British Journal of Obstetrics and Gynaecology* **98**:390–395.

2   Hogston P, James DK (1990) Total perinatal wastage: A clarification of priorities. *British Journal of Obstetrics and Gynaecology* **97**:999–1002.

3   Magani IM, Rafla NM, Mortimer G, Meehan FP (1990) Stillbirths: A clinicopathological survey (1972–1982). *Pediatric Pathology* **10**:363–374.

4   Pitkin RM (1987) Fetal death: Diagnosis and management. *American Journal of Obstetrics and Gynecology* **157**:583–589.

5   Kirkup B, Welch G (1990) Normal but dead: Perinatal mortality in non-malformed babies of birthweight 2.5 kg and over in the Northern Region in 1983. *British Journal of Obstetrics and Gynaecology* **97**:381–392.

6   McIlwaine GM, Dunn FH, Howat RCL, Smalls M, Wyllie MM, Macnaughton MC (1984) *The Scottish Perinatal Mortality Survey 1977–81.* Glasgow: University of Glasgow.

7   Grant A, Elbourne D (1991) Fetal movement counting to assess fetal well-being. In Chalmers I, Enkin M, Keierse MJNC (eds), *Effective Care in Pregnancy and Childbirth*, Vol. 1, 28, pp. 440–454 Oxford: Oxford University Press.

8   Special Report: Mothers who smoke and their children (Committee: Ball KP, Andrews J, Hytten FE, Kelnar CJH, Ross EM) (1980) Report of the Committee appointed by Action on Smoking and Health. *The Practitioner* **224**:735–740.

9   Ferraz EM, Gray RH (1991) A case-control study of stillbirths in Northeast Brazil. *International Journal of Gynecology and Obstetrics* **34**:13–19.

10 Rush D, Andrews J, Kristal A (1990) Maternal cigarette smoking during pregnancy: Adiposity, social class, and perinatal outcome in Cardiff, Wales, 1965–1977. *American Journal of Perinatology* **7**:319–326.

11 Benowitz NL (1991) Nicotine replacement therapy during pregnancy. *Journal of the American Medical Association* **266**:3174–3177.

12 Williams MA, Lieberman E, Mittendorf R, Monson RR, Schoenbaum SC (1991) Risk factors for abruptio placentae. *American Journal of Epidemiology* **134**:965–972.

13 Procianoy RS, Giacomini CB (1991) The influence of maternal cigarette smoking on fetal adrenal function. *International Pediatrics* **6**:331–334.

14 Lagerstrom M, Bremme K, Eneroth P, Faxelius G, Magnusson D, Smedler AC (1991) WISC-test scores at the age of 10 for children born to women with risk pregnancies. *Journal of Perinatal Medicine* **19**:269–283.

15 Alexander S, Keirse MJNC (1991) Formal risk scoring during pregnancy. In Chalmers I, Enkin M, Keierse MJNC (eds), *Effective Care in Pregnancy and Childbirth*, Vol.1, 22, pp. 345–365. Oxford: Oxford University Press.

16 Ahlborg G, Bodin L (1991) Tobacco smoke exposure and pregnancy outcome among working women. *American Journal of Epidemiology* **133**:338–347.

17 Sarnet JM (1991) Editorial commentary: New effects of active and passive smoking on reproduction? *American Journal of Epidemiology* **133**:348–350.

18 Mantel N (1992) Re: 'Tobacco smoke exposure and pregnancy outcome among working women: A prospective study at prenatal care centers in Orebro County, Sweden'. *American Journal of Epidemiology* **135**:837–838.

19 Newton RW, Hunt LP (1984) Psychosocial stress in pregnancy and its relation to low birth weight. *British Medical Journal* **288**:1191–1194.

20 Walpole I, Zubrick S, Pontre J (1989) Confounding variables in studying the effects of maternal alcohol consumption before and during pregnancy. *Journal of Epidemiology and Community Health* **43**:153–161.

21 Socol ML, Manning FA, Murata Y, Druzin ML (1982) Maternal smoking causes fetal hypoxia: Experimental evidence. *American Journal of Obstetrics and Gynecology* **142**:214–218.

22 Thaler I, Goodman JD, Dawes GS (1980) Effects of cigarette smoking on fetal breathing and fetal movements. *American Journal of Obstetrics and Gynecology* **138**:282–287.

23 Goodman JDS, Visser FGA, Dawes GS (1984) Effects of maternal cigarette smoking on fetal trunk movements, fetal breathing movements and the fetal heart rate. *British Journal of Obstetrics and Gynaecology* **91**:657–661.

24 Bocking AD (1989) Observations of biophysical activities in the normal fetus. *Clinics in Perinatology* **16**:583–594.

25 Mohide P, Grant A (1991) Evaluating diagnosis and screening during pregnancy and childbirth. In Chalmers I, Enkin M, Keierse MJNC (eds), *Effective Care in Pregnancy and Childbirth*, Vol.1, 3, pp. 66–80. Oxford: Oxford University Press.

26 Lindhard A, Nielsen PV, Mouritsen LA, Zachariassen A, Sorensen HU, Roseno H (1990) The implications of introducing the symphyseal–fundal height-measurement: A prospective randomized controlled trial. *British Journal of Obstetrics and Gynaecology* **97**:675–680.

27 Gardner SE, Yow MD, Leeds LJ, Thompson PK, Mason EO, Clark DJ (1979) Failure of penicillin to eradicate Group B streptococcal colonization in the pregnant woman. *American Journal of Obstetrics and Gynecology* **135**:1062–1065.

28 Harman CR (1987) Alloimmune disease. In *Clinical Obstetrics*, Vol.21, pp. 441–469. New York: John Wiley.

29 Grant A, Elbourne D, Valentin L, Alexander S (1989) Routine formal fetal movement counting and risk of antepartum late death in normally formed singletons. *Lancet* **ii**:345–349.

30 Dawes GS, Fox HE, Leduc BM *et al.* (1972) Respiratory movements and rapid eye movement sleep in the foetal lamb. *Journal of Physiology (London)* **220**:119.

31 Boddy K, Dawes GS, Fisher R, Pinter S, Robinson JS (1974) Foetal respiratory movements, electrocortical and cardiovascular responses to hypoxemia and ypercapnia in sheep. *Journal of Physiology (London)* **243**:599–618.

32 Boddy K, Dawes GS (1975) Fetal breathing. *British Medical Bulletin* **31**:1.

33 Dalton KJ, Dawes GS, Patrick JE (1977) Diurnal, respiratory and other rhythms of fetal heart rate in lambs. *American Journal of Obstetrics and Gynecology* **127**:414.

34 Ruckebusch Y, Gaujoux M, Eghbali B (1977) Sleep cycles and kinesis in the fetal lamb. *Electroencephalography and Clinical Neurophysiology* **42**:226.

35 Platt LD, Manning FA, LeMay M, Sipos L (1978) Human fetal breathing: Relationships to fetal condition. *American Journal of Obstetrics and Gynecology* **132**:514.

36 Manning FA, Platt LD, Sipos L, Keegan KA Jr (1979) Fetal breathing movements and the nonstress test in high-risk pregnancies. *American Journal of Obstetrics and Gynecology* **135**:511–515.

37 Manning FA, Platt LD, Sipos L (1980) Antepartum fetal evaluation: Development of a fetal biophysical profile score. *American Journal of Obstetrics and Gynecology* **136**:787.

38 Manning FA, Baskett TF, Morrison I *et al.* (1981) Fetal biophysical profile scoring: A prospective study in 1184 high-risk patients. *American Journal of Obstetrics and Gynecology* **140**:289.

39 Manning FA, Hill LM, Platt LD (1981) Qualitative amniotic fluid volume determination by ultrasound: Antepartum detection of intrauterine growth retardation. *American Journal of Obstetrics and Gynecology* **139**:254–258.

40 Nijhuis JG, Prechtl HFR, Martin CB Jr *et al.* (1982) Are there behavioural states in the human fetus? *Early Human Development* **6**:177–195.

41 Nijhuis JG (1992) Fetal behavioural states. In Chervenak FA, Isaacson GC, Campbell S (eds), *Ultrasound in Obstetrics and Gynecology*, Vol.1, 42, pp. 447–455. Boston, MA: Little, Brown.

42 Manning FA (1990) Dynamic ultrasound-based fetal assessment: The fetal biophysical profile score. In Fleischer AC, Romero R, Manning FA, Jeanty P, James AE Jr (eds), *The Principles and Practice of Ultrasonography in Obstetrics and Gynecology*, 4th edn, Vol.7, pp. 93–108. Norwalk CT: Appleton & Lange.

43 Birnholz JC, Stephens JC, Faria M (1978) Fetal movement patterns: A possible means of defining neurologic developmental milestones *in utero. American Journal of Roentgenology* **130**:537–540.

44 Pillai M, James D (1990) Development of human fetal behaviour: A review. *Fetal Diagnosis and Therapy* **5**:15–32.

45 de Vries JIP, Visser GHA, Prechtl HFR (1988) The emergence of fetal behaviour. III. Individual differences and consistencies. *Early Human Development* **16**:85–104.

46 de Vries JIP, Visser GHA, Mulder EJH *et al.* (1975) Diurnal and other variations in fetal movement and heart rate patterns at 20 to 22 weeks. *Early Human Development* **15**:333–348.

47 Martin CB Jr (1981) Behavioral states in the human fetus. *Journal of Reproductive Medicine* **26**:425–432.

48 Prechtl HFR (1974) The behavioural states of the newborn infant (A review). Brain Research **76**:185–212.

49 Lee CY, DiLoreto PC, O'Lane JM (1975) A study of fetal heart rate acceleration patterns. *Obstetrics and Gynecology* **45**:142.

50 Dawes GS, Moulden M, Redman CWG (1991) The advantages of computerized fetal heart rate analysis. *Journal of Perinatal Medicine* **19**:39–45.

51 Pillai M, James D (1990) The development of fetal heart rate patterns during normal pregnancy. *Obstetrics and Gynecology* **76**:812–816.

52 Snijders RJM, McLaren R, Nicolaides KH (1990) Computer-assisted analysis of fetal heart rate patterns at 20–41 weeks' gestation. *Fetal Diagnosis and Therapy* **5**:79–83.

53 Pillai M, James D (1991) Human fetal mouthing movements: A potential biophysical variable for distinguishing state IF from abnormal fetal behaviour: Report of 4 cases. *European Journal of Obstetrics and Gynecology and Reproductive Biology* **38**:151–156.

54 Brown R, Patrick J (1981) The nonstress test: How long is enough. *American Journal of Obstetrics and Gynecology* **151**:646–651.

55 Myers RE (1977) Experimental models of perinatal brain damage: Relevance to human pathology. In Gluck L (ed.), *Intrauterine Asphyxia and the Developing Brain*, p. 378. Chicago: Yearbook Medical Publishers. 37–97.

56 Myers RE, de Courten-Myers GM, Wagner KR (1984) Effect of hypoxia on fetal brain. In Beard RW, Nathanielsz PW (eds), *Fetal Physiology and Medicine: The Basis of Perinatology*, pp. 419–458. New York: Marcel Dekker.

57 Rurak DW, Selke P, Fisher M *et al.* (1987) Fetal oxygen extraction: Comparison of the human and sheep. *American Journal of Obstetrics and Gynecology* **156**:360–366.

58 Richardson BS (1989) Fetal adaptive responses to asphyxia. *Clinics in Perinatology* **16**:595–611.

59 Natale R, Clewlow F, Dawes GS (1981) Measurement of fetal forelimb movements in the lamb *in utero*. *American Journal of Obstetrics and Gynecology* **140**:545–551.

60 an Vliet MAT, Martin CB Jr, Nijhuis JG *et al.* (1985) Behavioural states in growth retarded human fetuses. *Early Human Development* **12**:183–197.

61 Sheldon RE, Peeters LLH, Jones MD *et al.* (1979) Redistribution of cardiac output and oxygen delivery in the hypoxemic fetal lamb. *American Journal of Obstetrics and Gynecology* **135**:1071–1078.

62 Anderson DF, Parks CM, Faber JJ (1986) Fetal O_2 consumption in sheep during controlled long-term reductions in umbilical blood flow. *American Journal of Physiology* **250**:H1037–H1042.

63 Milley JR (1987) Protein synthesis during hypoxia in fetal lambs. *American Journal of Physiology* **252**:E519–E524.

64 Manning FA (1990) The fetal biophysical profile score: Current status. *Obstetrics and Gynecology Clinics of North America* **17**:147–162.

65 Patrick J (1989) The physiological basis for fetal assessment. *Seminars in Perinatology* **13**:403–408.

66 Manning FA (1993) *Fetal Medicine* (Fetal biophysical profile scoring: Theoretical considerations and clinical application.) Norwalk, NJ: Appleton and Lange.

67 Gagnon R (1989) Acoustic stimulation: Effect on heart rate and other biophysical variables. *Clinics in Perinatology* **16**:643–660.

68 Gagnon R, Hunse C, Carmichael L *et al.* (1986) Effects of vibratory acoustic stimulation on human fetal breathing and gross body movements near term. *American Journal of Obstetrics and Gynecology* **155**:1227.

69 Nyman M, Barr M, Westgren M (1992) A four-year follow-up of hearing and development in children exposed *in utero* to vibro-acoustic stimulation. *British Journal of Obstetrics and Gynaecology* **99**:685–688.

70 Schwartz DB, Sherman SJ, Goyert GL, Fields P, Simkins S, Daoud Y (1991) An evaluation of antenatal fetal acoustic stimulation. *European Journal of Obstetrics and Gynecology and Reproductive Biology* **40**:97–103.

71 Vintzileos AM, Campbell WA, Ingardia CJ, Nochimson DJ (1983) The fetal biophysical profile and its predictive value. *Obstetrics and Gynecology* **62**:271–278.

72 Moore TR (1990) Superiority of the four-quadrant sum over the single-deepest-pocket technique in ultrasonographic identification of abnormal amniotic fluid volumes. *American Journal of Obstetrics and Gynecology* **163**:762–767.

73 James DK, Parker MJ, Smoleniec JS (1992) Comprehensive fetal assessment with three ultrasonographic characteristics. *American Journal of Obstetrics and Gynecology* **166**:1486–1495.

74 Chamberlain PF (1991) Later fetal death – Has ultrasound a role to play in its prevention? *Irish Journal of Medical Science* **160**:251–254.

75 Baskett TG, Allen AC, Gray JH *et al.* (1987) Fetal biophysical profile and perinatal death. *Obstetrics and Gynecology* **70**:357–360.

76 Vintzileos AM, Campbell WA, Rodis JF (1989) Fetal biophysical profile scoring: Current status. *Clinics in Perinatology* **16**:661–689.

77 Jackson GM, Forouzan I, Cohen AW (1991) Fetal well-being: Nonimaging assessment and the biophysical profile. *Seminars in Roentgenology* **26**:21–31.

78 Manning FA, Harman CR, Menticoglou S, Morrison I (1991) Assessment of fetal well-being with ultrasound. *Obstetrics and Gynecology Clinics in North America* **18**:891–905.

79 Manning FA, Morrison I, Harman CR, Menticoglou SM (1990) The abnormal fetal biophysical profile score. V. Predictive accuracy according to score composition. *American Journal of Obstetrics and Gynecology* **162**:918–927.

80 Manning FA, Snijders R, Harman CR, Nicolaides K (1993) The relationship between fetal biophysical profile score and fetal pH. In *Proceedings of the Society of Perinatal Obstetricians' Annual Meeting*, February (abstract).

81 Ruth VJ, Raivio KO (1988) Perinatal brain damage: Predictive value of metabolic acidosis and the Apgar score. *British Medical Journal* **297**:24–27.

82 Ribbert LSM, Snijders RJM, Nicolaides KH, Visser GHA (1990) Relationship of fetal biophysical profile

and blood gas values at cordocentesis in severely growth-retarded fetuses. *American Journal of Obstetrics and Gynecology* **163**:569–571.

83 Arabin B, Nicolaides KH (1993) The relationship between fetal blood gases obtained by cordocentesis and the fetal biophysical profile score. *American Journal of Obstetrics and Gynecology* (in press).

84 Okamura K, Watanabe T, Endo H, Tanigawara S, Iwamoto M, Murotsuki J, Uehara S, Yajima A (1991) Biophysical profile and its relation to fetal blood gas level obtained by cordocentesis. *Acta Obstetrica et Gynaecologia Japonica* **43**:1573–1577.

85 Bo-Hyun-Yoon, Hee-Chul-Syn, Sying-Wook-Kim (1992) The efficacy of Doppler umbilical artery velocimetry in identifying the fetal acidosis: A comparison with fetal biophysical profile. *Journal of Ultrasound in Medicine* **11**:1–6.

86 Walkinshaw S, Cameron H, MacPhail S, Robson S (1992) The prediction of fetal compromise and acidosis by biophysical profile scoring in the small for gestational age fetus. *Journal of Perinatal Medicine* **20**:227–232.

87 Vintzileos AM, Flemming AD, Scorza WE, Wolf EJ, Balducci J, Campbell WA, Rodis JF (1991) Relationship between fetal biophysical activities and umbilical cord blood gas values. *American Journal of Obstetrics and Gynecology* **165**:707–713.

88 Devoe LD, Youssef AA, Gardner P, Dear C, Murray C (1992) Refining the biophysical profile with a risk-related evaluation of test performance. *American Journal of Obstetrics and Gynecology* **167**:346–352.

89 Platt LD, Manning FA (1980) Fetal breathing movements: An update. *Clinics in Perinatology* **7**:423–433.

90 Manning FA, Harman CR, Morrison I, Menticoglou SM, Lange IR, Johnson JM (1990) Fetal assessment based on fetal biophysical profile scoring. IV. An analysis of perinatal morbidity and mortality. *American Journal of Obstetrics and Gynecology* **162**:703–709.

91 Manning FA, Harman CR, Morrison I, Menticoglou S (1990) Fetal assessment based on fetal biophysical profile scoring. III. Positive predictive accuracy of the very abnormal test (biophysical profile score = 0). *American Journal of Obstetrics and Gynecology* **162**:398–402.

92 Manning FA, Morrison I, Harman CR, Lange IR, Menticoglou S (1987) Fetal assessment based on fetal biophysical profile scoring: Experience in 19,221 referred high-risk pregnancies. II. An analysis of false-negative fetal deaths. *American Journal of Obstetrics and Gynecology* **157**:880–884.

93 Manning FA, Morrison I, Lange IR *et al.* (1985) Fetal assessment based on fetal biophysical profile scoring: Experience in 12,620 referred high-risk pregnancies. I. Perinatal mortality by frequency and etiology. *American Journal of Obstetrics and Gynecology* **151**:343–350.

94 Manning FA, Baskett TF, Morrison I, Lange I (1981) Fetal biophysical profile scoring: A prospective study in 1,184 high-risk patients. *American Journal of Obstetrics and Gynecology* **140**:289–294.

95 Lange IR, Manning FA, Morrison I *et al.* (1985) Cord

prolapse: Is antenatal diagnosis possible? *American Journal of Obstetrics and Gynecology* **151**:1083–1085.

96 Harman CR (1989) Comprehensive examination of the human fetus. In Dunlop W (ed.), *Fetal Medicine* **1**:125–176.

97 Manning FA, Morrison I, Lange IR, Harman C (1982) Antepartum determination of fetal health: Composite biophysical profile scoring. *Clinics in Perinatology* **9**:285–296.

98 Baskett TF, Gray JH, Prewett SJ *et al.* (1984) Antepartum fetal assessment using a fetal biophysical profile score. *American Journal of Obstetrics and Gynecology* **148**:630–633.

99 Chamberlain PF, Manning FA, Morrison I *et al.* (1984) Ultrasound evaluation of amniotic fluid volume. I. The relationship of marginal and decreased amniotic fluid volumes to perinatal outcome. *American Journal of Obstetrics and Gynecology* **150**:245–249.

100 Chamberlain PF, Manning FA, Morrison I *et al.* (1984) Ultrasound evaluation of amniotic fluid volume. II. The relationship of increased amniotic fluid volume to perinatal outcome. *American Journal of Obstetrics and Gynecology* **150**:250–254.

101 Whittle MJ (1991) Amniotic fluid volume – does it really help us? *Ultrasound in Obstetrics and Gynecology* **1**:383.

102 Bastide A, Manning F, Harman CR *et al.* (1986) Ultrasound evaluation of amniotic fluid: Outcome of pregnancies with severe oligohydramnios. *American Journal of Obstetrics and Gynecology* **154**:895–900.

103 Druzin ML (1989) Antepartum fetal heart rate monitoring – state of the art. *Clinics in Perinatology* **16**:627–642.

104 Martin CB Jr (1978) Regulation of the fetal heart rate and genesis of FHR patterns. *Seminars in Perinatology* **2**:131–145.

105 Dawes GS, Moulden M, Redman CWG (1991) System 8000: Computerized antenatal FHR analysis. *Journal of Perinatal Medicine* **19**:47–51.

106 Baser I, Johnson TRB, Paine LL (1992) Coupling of fetal movement and fetal heart rate accelerations as an indicator of fetal health. *Obstetrics and Gynecology* **80**:62–66.

107 Lavery JP. Nonstress fetal heart rate testing. *Clinics in Obstetrics and Gynecology* **25**:689–705.

108 Fouron J-C, Korcaz, Y, Leduc B (1975) Cardiovascular changes associated with fetal breathing. *American Journal of Obstetrics and Gynecology* **123**: 868–876.

109 Pircon RA, Freeman RK (1990) The contraction stress test. *Obstetrics and Gynecology Clinics of North America* **17**:129–146.

110 Pillai M, James D (1990) The importance of the behavioural state in biophysical assessment of the term human fetus. *British Journal of Obstetrics and Gynaecology* **97**:1130–1134.

111 Vintzileos AM, Feinstein SJ, Lodeiro JG *et al.* (1986) Fetal biophysical profile and the effect of premature rupture of the membranes. *Obstetrics and Gynecology* **67**(6):818–823.

112 Fleming AD, Salafia CM, Vintzileos AM, Rodis JF, Campbell WA, Bantham KF (1991) The relationships among umbilical artery velocimetry, fetal biophysical

profile, and placental inflammation in preterm premature rupture of the membranes. *American Journal of Obstetrics and Gynecology* **164**:38–41.

113 Castle BM, Turnbull AC (1983) The presence or absence of fetal breathing movements predicts the outcome of preterm labour. *Lancet* **2**:471–473.

114 Boylan P, O'Donovan P, Owens OJ (1985) Fetal breathing movements and the diagnosis of labor: A prospective analysis of 100 cases. *Obstetrics and Gynecology* **66**:517–520.

115 Roussis P, Rosemond RL, Glass C, Boehm FH (1991) Preterm premature rupture of membranes: Detection of infection. *American Journal of Obstetrics and Gynecology* **165**:1099–1104.

116 Vintzileos AM, Campbell WA, Nochimson DJ *et al.* (1986) Fetal biophysical profile versus amniocentesis in predicting infection in premature preterm rupture of the membranes. *Obstetrics and Gynecology* **68**:488–494.

117 Manning FA, Platt LD (1980) Human fetal breathing monitoring – clinical considerations. *Seminars in Perinatology* **4**:311–318.

118 Menticoglou SM, Morrison I, Harman CR, Manning FA, Lange IR (1992) Maximum possible impact of tocolytics in preventing preterm birth: A retrospective assessment. *American Journal of Perinatology* **9**:394–397.

119 Natale R, Richardson B, Patrick J (1981) Effect of intravenous glucose infusion on human fetal breathing activity. *Obstetrics and Gynecology* **59**:320–324.

120 Vintzileos AM, Campbell WA, Nochimson DJ, Weinbaum PJ (1987) The use and misuse of the fetal biophysical profile. *American Journal of Obstetrics and Gynecology* **156**:527–533.

121 Manning FA, Lange IR, Morrison I, Harman CR (1984) Fetal biophysical profile score and the nonstress test: A comparative trial. *Obstetrics and Gynecology* **64**:326–331.

122 Manning FA, Morrison I, Lange IR *et al.* (1987) Fetal biophysical profile scoring: Selective use of the nonstress test. *American Journal of Obstetrics and Gynecology* **156**:709–712.

123 Peeters LLH, Sheldon RE, Jones MD, Makowski EL, Meschia G (1979) Blood flow to fetal organs as a function of arterial oxygen content. *American Journal of Obstetrics and Gynecology* **135**:637–646.

124 Sheldon RE, Peeters LLH, Jones MD, Makowski EL, Meschia G (1979) Redistribution of cardiac output and oxygen delivery in the hypoxemic fetal lamb. *American Journal of Obstetrics and Gynecology* **135**:1071–1078.

125 Steele BT, Paes B, Towell ME, Hunter DJS (1988) Fetal renal failure associated with intrauterine growth retardation. *American Journal of Obstetrics and Gynecology* **159**:1200–1202.

126 Hackett GA, Nicolaides KH, Campbell S (1987) Doppler assessment of fetal and uteroplacental circulations in severe second trimester oligohydramnios. *Brish Journal of Obstetrics and Gynaecology* **94**:1074–1077.

127 Fisk NM, Ronderos-Dumit D, Soliani A, Nicolini U, Vaughan J, Rodeck CH (1991) Diagnostic and therapeutic transabdominal amnioinfusion in oligohydramnios. *Obstetrics and Gynecology* **78**:270–278.

128 Groome LJ, Owen J, Neely CL (1991) Oligohydramnios: Antepartum fetal urine production and intrapartum fetal distress. *American Journal of Obstetrics and Gynecology* **165**:1077–1080.

129 Battaglia C, Artini PG, D'Ambrogio G, Galli PA, Segre A, Genazzani AR (1992) Maternal hyperoxygenation in the treatment of intrauterine growth retardation. *American Journal of Obstetrics and Gynecology* **167**:430–435.

130 Bekedam DJ, Mulder EJH, Snijders RJM, Visser GHA (1991) The effects of maternal hyperoxia on fetal breathing movements, body movements and heart rate variation in growth retarded fetuses. *Early Human Development* **27**:223–232.

131 Lodeiro JG, Vintzileos AM, Feinstein SJ *et al.* (1986) Fetal biophysical profile in twin gestations. *Obstetrics and Gynecology* **67**:824–827.

132 Jones JM, Sbarra AJ, Cetrulo CL (1990) Antepartum management of twin gestation. *Clinics in Obstetrics and Gynecology* **33**(1):32–41.

133 Nicolaides KH, Peters MT, Vyas S, Rabinowitz R, Rosen DJD, Campbell S (1990) Relation of rate of urine production to oxygen tensions in small-for-gestational-age fetuses. *American Journal of Obstetrics and Gynecology* **162**:387–391.

134 Visser GHA, Redman CWG, Huisjer HJ, Turnbull AC (1980) Nonstressed antepartum heart rate monitoring: Implications of decelerations after spontaneous contractions. *American Journal of Obstetrics and Gynecology* **138**:429–435.

135 Nijhuis JG, Crevels AJ, van Dongen PWJ (1990) Fetal brain death: The definition of a fetal heart rate pattern and its clinical consequences. *Obstetrical and Gynecological Survey* **45**:229–232.

136 Awoust J, Levi S (1984) New aspects of fetal dynamics with a special emphasis on eye movements. *Ultrasound in Medicine and Biology* **10**:107–116.

137 Vintzileos AM, Goffrey SE, Salinger LM, Kontopoulos VG, Campbell WA, Nochimson OJ (1987) The relationship among the fetal biophysical profile, umbilical cord pH, and Apgar scores. *American Journal of Obstetrics aqnd Gynecology* **157**:627–631.

138 Patrick JE, Dalton KJ, Dawes GS (1976) Breathing patterns before death in fetal lambs. *American Journal of Obstetrics and Gynecology* **125**:73–78.

139 Chapman RLK, Dawes GS, Rurak DW, Wilds PL (1978) Intermittent breathing before death in fetal lambs. *American Journal of Obstetrics and Gynecology* **131**:894–898.

140 Hohimer AR, Bissonnette JM (1981) Effect of metabolic acidosis on fetal breathing movements *in utero*. *Respiration Physiology* **43**:99–106.

141 Molteni RA, Melmed MH, Sheldon RE, Jones MD, Meschia G (1980) Induction of fetal breathing by metabolic acidemia and its effect on blood flow to the respiratory muscles. *American Journal of Obstetrics and Gynecology* **136**:609–620.

142 Manning FA, Schreiber J, Turkel SB (1978) Fatal meconium aspiration '*in utero*': A case report. *American Journal of Obstetrics and Gynecology* **132**:111–113.

143 Block MF, Kallenberger DA, Kern JD, Nepveux RD (1981) *In utero* meconium aspiration by the baboon fetus. *Obstetrics and Gynecology* **57**:37–40.

144 Brown BL, Gleicher N (1981) Intrauterine meconium aspiration. *Obstetrics and Gynecology* **57**:26–29.

145 Benacerraf BR, Frigoletto FD Jr (1986) Fetal respiratory movements: Only part of the biophysical profile. *Obstetrics and Gynecology* **67**:556–557.

146 Manning FA, Heaman M, Boyce D, Carter LJ (1991) Intrauterine fetal tachypnea. *Obstetrics and Gynecology* **58**:398–400.

147 Yaffe H, Kreisberg GA, Gale R (1989) Sinusoidal heart rate pattern and normal biophysical profile in a severely compromised fetus. *Acta Obstetrica et Gynecologica Scandinavica* **68**:561–563.

148 Smith CV (1992) Antepartum fetal surveillance in the preterm fetus. *Clinics in Perinatology* **19**:437–448.

149 Baskett TF (1988) Gestational age and fetal biophysical assessment. *American Journal of Obstetrics and Gynecology* **158**:332–334.

150 Castillo RA, Devoe LD, Arthur M, Searle N, Metheny WP, Rendwick DA (1989) The preterm nonstress test: Effects of gestational age and length of study. *American Journal of Obstetrics and Gynecology* **160**:172–175.

151 Ribbert LSM, Fidler V, Visser GHA (1991) Computer-assisted analysis of normal second trimester fetal heart rate patterns. *Journal of Perinatal Medicine* **19**:53–59.

152 Patrick J, Campbell K, Carmichael L, Natale R, Richardson B (1982) Patterns of gross fetal body movements over 24-hour observation intervals during the last 10 weeks of pregnancy. *American Journal of Obstetrics and Gynecology* **142**:363–371.

153 Nasello-Peterson C, Natale R, Connors G (1988) Ultrasonic evaluation of fetal body movements over twenty-four hours in the human fetus at twenty-four to twenty-eight weeks gestation. *American Journal of Obstetrics and Gynecology* **158**:312–316.

154 Drogtrop AP, Ubels R, Nijhuis JG (1990) The association between fetal body movements, eye movements and heart rate patterns in pregnancies between 25 and 30 weeks of gestation. *Early Human Development* **23**:67–73.

155 Harman CR (1984) Antepartum decelerative fetal heart rate patterns: The role of biophysical profile scoring. Presented at the *Annual Meeting of the Society of Obstetricians and Gynecologists of Canada*, Montreal, June (abstract).

156 Weiss PAM (1988) Gestational diabetes: A survey and the Gray approach to diagnosis and therapy. In Weiss PAM, Coustan DR (eds), *Gestational Diabetes*, pp. 1–55. New York: Springer-Verlag.

157 Johnson JM, Lange IR, Harman CR, Torchia MG, Manning FA (1988) Biophysical profile scoring in the management of the diabetic pregnancy. *Obstetrics and Gynecology* **72**:841–846.

158 Phelan JP (1988) Antepartum fetal assessment: Newer techniques. *Seminars in Perinatology* **12**:57–65.

159 Devoe LD, Ramos-Santos E (1991) Antepartum fetal assessment in hypertensive pregnancies. *Clinics in Perinatology* **18**:809–832.

160 Ajayio RA, Soothill PW, Campbell S, Nicolaides KH (1992) Antenatal testing to predict outcome in pregnancies with unexplained antepartum haemorrhage. *British Journal of Obstetrics and Gynaecology* **99**:122–125.

161 Ambrose SE, Petrie RH (1989) Antenatal detection of fetal compromise. *Fetal Medicine Review* **1**:27–41.

162 Johnson JM, Harman CR, Lange IR, Manning FA (1986) Biophysical profile scoring in the management of the postterm pregnancy: An analysis of 307 patients. *American Journal of Obstetrics and Gynecology* **154**:269–273.

163 Hannah ME, Hannah WJ, Hellman J, Hewson S, Milner R, Willan A (1992) Canadian Multicenter Postterm Pregnancy Trial Group: Induction of labor as compared with serial antenatal monitoring in post-term pregnancy. A randomized controlled trial. *New England Journal of Medicine* **326**:1587–1592.

164 Wiens HA (1991) *Perinatal and Maternal Welfare Committee 1990 Report*. College of Physicians and Surgeons of Manitoba.

165 Sadovsky E, Yaffe H (1973) Daily fetal movement recording and fetal prognosis. *Obstetrics and Gynecology* **41**:845–850.

166 Valentin L, Lofgren O, Marsal K, Gullberg B (1984) Subjective recording of fetal movements. I. Limits and acceptability in normal pregnancies. *Acta Obstetrica et Gynecologica Scandinavica* **63**:223–228.

167 Valentin L, Marsal K (1987) Pregnancy outcome in women perceiving decreased fetal movements. *European Journal of Obstetrics and Gynecology and Reproductive Biology* **24**:23–32.

168 Moore TR, Piacquadio K (1989) A prospective evaluation of fetal movement screening to reduce the incidence of antepartum fetal death. *American Journal of Obstetrics and Gynecology* **160**:1075–1080.

169 Pearson JF (1979) Fetal movement recording: A guide to fetal well-being. *Nursing Times* **75**:1639–1641.

170 Ahn MO, Phelan JP, Smith CV, Jacobs N, Rutherford SE (1987) Antepartum fetal surveillance in the patient with decreased fetal movement. *American Journal of Obstetrics and Gynecology* **157**:860–864.

171 Baskett TF, Liston RM (1989) Fetal monitoring. *Clinics in Perinatology* **16**:613–625.

172 Draper J, Field S, Thomas H (1986) Women's views on keeping fetal movement charts. *British Journal of Obstetrics and Gynaecology* **93**:334.

173 Neldam S (1983) Fetal movements as an indicator of fetal well-being. *Danish Medical Bulletin* **30**:274–278.

40

Amniocentesis

PHILIPPA A. RAMSAY, NICHOLAS M. FISK

INTRODUCTION

Amniocentesis is the removal of fluid which contains cells and biochemical products of fetal origin from the amniotic cavity. Amniocentesis was the first technique for access to the intrauterine environment and remains the most commonly performed invasive procedure for prenatal diagnosis. Amniocentesis should be performed only under ultrasound guidance (**Figure 1**).

INDICATIONS

Prenatal Diagnosis

Chromosome analysis

The performance of a fetal karyotype is the most common reason for amniocentesis, and is offered in the same circumstances as chronic villus sampling (CVS): advanced maternal age (≤35 years old), previous fetal aneuploidy and parenteral balanced translocation. Additional indications include ultrasonic features suggestive of aneuploidy (See Chapter 38), a positive biochemical screen for Down's syndrome (See Chapter 37) and mosaicism on CVS (See Chapter 36).

Metaphase analysis until recently required 2–3 weeks culture of amniotic fluid cells desquamated from fetal skin, the gastrointestinal, urogenital and respiratory tracts, and the amnion. Approximately 0.5% of cultures fail, while maternal contamination muddles the diagnosis in <0.2%.[1] Though level 2 mosaicism (multiple cells with the same abnormality in the single flask) occurs in 0.7% of amniocentesis and level 3 (multiple cells with the same abnormality in the multiple flasks) in 0.2%,[2–4] they are confirmed in the fetus in only 20 and 60% of cases, respectively. Thus culture of a second tissue may occasionally be necessary to confirm a karyotype from the amniocytes.

New culture techniques permit faster results (**Figures 2, 3**). When grown in an enriched media such as Chang[5] culture, duration is reduced to an average of 9.5 days,[6] and by growing the amniocytes on a cover slip, an adequate number of colonies can be available in 6–7 days (**Figures 1** and **2**). The recent development of fluorescein-labeled *in situ* hybridization techniques for direct DNA probing of interphase chromosomes (i.e. 21, 18, 13, X and Y) without preliminary culture may further expedite results in the future, although culture confirmation will probably still be required.

DNA diagnosis

DNA analysis can be performed on nuclear material from amniotic fluid cells, although the time taken to grow a sufficient mass of cells means that either the chorion or fetal blood are usually preferred.

Biochemistry

Enzyme assay

Prenatal diagnosis is now possible for over half the 200 or so inborn errors of metabolism in which the enzymatic defect is known. The enzyme in question can often be measured in amniotic fluid cells after 3–4 weeks culture and that level compared to known normal and homozygous-deficient amniotic fluid cells and with fibroblasts from the proband and parents. Maternal contamination, which could result in spuriously high activity levels in an affected fetus, must be avoided (See Chapter 56) for related information).

Metabolite analysis

Cell-free amniotic fluid can also be used for the biochemical diagnosis of certain diseases. Fetal gut microvillar enzymes (chiefly alkaline phosphatase and beta-glutamyl transpeptidase) have low acitivity in fetuses homozygous for cystic fibrosis (CF). However, substantial false-positive (2.5%) and false-negative (5%) rates, coupled with the availability of more accurate DNA-based techniques applicable to 80%, have led to a decline in their usage.[7] Low levels of 17 alpha-hydroxyprogesterone may indicate a fetus homozygous for 21-hydroxylase-deficient congenital adrenal hyperplasia as early as 11 weeks gestation.[8]

Some inborn errors such as the urea cycle disorders cannot be diagnosed by amniocentesis because the affected protein is not expressed in cultured fibroblasts and excess metabolite accumulation is prevented by transplacental passage into the mother. Prenatal diagnosis for these disorders requires fetal liver biopsy (see Chapter 56).

Alpha-fetoprotein

Amniocentesis at 16–20 weeks has been widely performed for the measurement of alpha-fetoprotein (AFP) and acetyl cholinesterase (ACh) to diagnose neural tube defects (NTD) following an elevated maternal serum AFP, a previous fetus with an NTD or an abnormal ultrasound (see Chapter 37). However, amniocentesis is now less often performed for this indication because of the high degree of accuracy that is possible with high-resolution ultrasound[9,10] and because false-positive AFP and ACh results could lead to unwarranted terminations of unaffected pregnancies.[11] Nevertheless, some centers still advocate amniocentesis for raised maternal serum AFP to avoid a misdiagnosis in the presence of a small defect and suboptimal visualization.[12,13]

Fetal infection

Amniotic fluid can be inoculated into mice, for the diagnosis of congenital toxoplasmosis, but this is done only in combination with other tests on fetal blood and an ultrasound of the fetal brain.[14] More recently, polymerase chain reaction amplification of toxoplasmosis

gene sequences in amniotic fluid cells has yielded higher sensitivities than any of the above tests alone.[15]

Fetal cytomegalovirus (CMV) infection can be reliably diagnosed by culturing the virus in amniotic fluid as the virus is excreted in the fetal urine.[16] Detection of CMV antigen in the amniotic fluid with the sheel vial assay will yield a result in 24 h, but should be confirmed by culture (for related information, see Chapter 49).[17]

Fetal Welfare

Maternal RBC alloimmunization

The spectrophotometry of amniotic fluid for the $\Delta OD450$ gives an indirect measurement of the level of bilirubin present in pregnancies complicated by maternal RBC alloimmunization reflecting the degree of fetal hemolysis in the third trimester.[18] This is reviewed extensively in Chapter 44.

Lung maturity

Fetal pulmonary maturity can be assessed by a variety of amniotic fluid tests, including the A650 and the measurement of the lecithin/sphingomyelin ratio or phosphatidyl glycerol (see Chapter 11). However, there are considerable regional differences in the use of these tests and improvements in neonatal care and the use of early unltrasound to confirm gestational age has led to a reduction in the need for confirmation of fetal lung maturity before delivery.[19]

Chorioamnionitis

After the recognition of an association between amniotic fluid colonization, premature rupture of the membranes and preterm labor (see Chapter 12),[20] amniocentesis was advocated by some for Gram-stain, microscopy, culture and assessment of pulmonary maturity in women with ruptured membrane prior to labor. Amniocentesis is successful in up to 97% of cases of premature rupture of the membranes when performed with ultrasound guidance.[21] In large series, amniotic fluid cultures are positive in 17–34% of asymptomatic women with premature rupture of the membranes[21] and 9–11% of women in premature labor with intact membranes.[22,23] Though advocates of amniocentesis in these settings argue that it allows earlier diagnosis of intra-amniotic infection than clinical signs and identification of the responsible organism and its sensitivities,[24] there are no large randomized controlled trials to support this practice. In fact, spontaneous labor

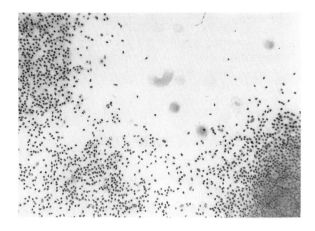

Figure 1. Low power (×2.5) of three adjacent amniocyte clones growing on the floor of a petrie dish. Each clone is derived from a single cell or a closely apposed group of cells from the fetus.

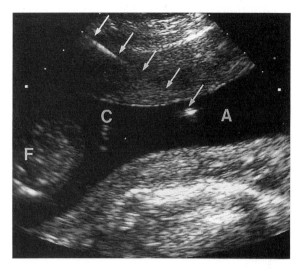

Figure 3. Insertion of needle (arrows) into amniotic cavity (A) under continuous ultrasound guidance, avoiding fetus (F) and cord (C).

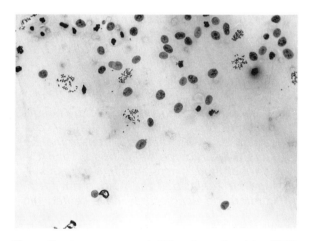

Figure 2. Low power (×10) of analysable GTG banded metaphase spreads in a single amniocyte clone. Metaphases at the edge of the clone are chosen for harvesting as those deep within the clones are often underspread.

within 24 h of rupture in the face of amniotic fluid colonization is the rule rather than the exception.

Obstetric cholestasis

Intrahepatic cholestasis of pregnancy is associated with risks of meconium-stained fluid and fetal death *in utero* not predicted by conventional fetal welfare monitoring techniques.[25] Accordingly, intensive fetal surveillance including weekly amniocentesis to check for meconium discoloration and fetal lung maturity has been recommended to facilitate timing of delivery and reduce the stillbirth rate.[26] The utility remains to be confirmed.

Fetal Therapy

Amniocentesis has also been used therapeutically for uterine decompression in hydramnios (see Chapter 48), amnioinfusion in oligohydramnios (see Chapter 48), multifetal pregnancy reduction (see Chapter 57) and intra-amniotic thyroxine treatment of fetal goitrus hypothyroidism (see Chapter 55).

Procedure: Amniocentesis

Role of ultrasound

Before the development and wide availability of real-time ultrasound amniocentesis was performed blindly. Ultrasound enables placement of the needle with greater precision and is now considered the standard. First, a sonographic examination is performed to confirm fetal viability and gestational age, to detect fetal anomalies and multiple gestation, and to assess amniotic fluid volume and placental position.

Approach

The transabdominal approach is used almost universally. Transvaginal amniocentesis is associated with infection and miscarriage,[27] yet it and transcervical amniocentesis continue to have their advocates.[28,29]

Asepsis

Aseptic techniques are used with sterile gloves, povidone iodine to prepare the skin, and a 'no-touch technique'. Breaches of technique may result in chorioamnionitis and/or contamination of the sample with subsequent culture failure.

Needle

A 22-gauge, 7–10 cm sterile disposable spinal needle is used. The stilette reduces the chance of maternal tissue contamination.

Needle insertion *(Figure 3)*

After locating a suitable pocket of fluid, the approach is chosen to avoid the fetus, placenta and cord. Even with an extensive anterior placenta, a small window can usually be found. We favor the fundus whenever possible. The needle is inserted dexterously to minimize maternal discomfort. Local anesthetic is usually not necessary.

Preliminary scan technique

An accessible pool of amniotic fluid is identified with ultrasound, the site for needle insertion selected, and marked on the maternal abdomen. The needle is then inserted semi-blind.

Ultrasound guided technique

This is performed in one of two ways. In the first, a sterile needle guide attached to the transducer allows the needle to be introduced along a fixed, predetermined path and visualized as it enters the amniotic cavity. Alternatively, in the freehand technique, the operator holds the ultrasound transducer in one hand and the needle in the other with the ultrasound beam directed across the planned needle path allowing visualization of the needle. Compared with the semi-blind approach, continuous ultrasound monitoring reduces the number of dry and bloody taps.[30,31]

Aspiration of fluid

After connecting the syringe to the needle hub, the first 1–2 ml of aspirate is discarded to avoid maternal contamination should a karyotype be planned. Then 15–20 ml of fluid is aspirated into a fresh syringe for analysis. If the fluid is not forthcoming the needle may have tented the

Table 1
Summary of collaborative studies

	US study[37]		Canadian study[38]	UK study[39]			
	Cases	Controls	Cases	Cases	Controls	Supplementary cases	Supplementary controls
Patients	1040	992	1020	1402	1402	1026	1026
Fetal losses	36(3.5%)	32(3.2%)	33(3.2%)	38(2.7%)	20(1.4%)	27(2.6%)	11(1.1%)
Needle injuries	1(0.1%)	—	—	4(0.3%)	3(0.2%)	—	—
Infants with respiratory distress syndrome	30(3.1%)	20(2.1%)	–	17(1.2%)	6(0.4%)	13(1.3%)	3(0.3%)
Infants with severe orthopedic postural abnormalities	—	—	—	20(1.4%)	0(0.0%)	4(0.4%)	4(0.4%)

After Elias and Simpson.[48]

membranes and not perforated the amniotic cavity or be up against the fetus. In such cases, the needle is rotated to redirect the bevel, or reoriented under ultrasound guidance until amniotic fluid flows freely. Twisting or advancing the needle will usually pierce membranes which have tented away from the anterior uterine wall. Alternatively, advancing the needle into the posterior myometrium to transfix obstructing membranes has also been suggested.[32] This is not usually necessary.

Multiple pregnancy

Amniocentesis is performed for the same indications in multiple gestation as singletons except for amniotic fluid AFP and ACh estimation in monochorionic twins, as these equilibrate across the membranes.[33] Many regard amniocentesis as the procedure of choice for fetal karyotyping in multiple pregnancies, since chorion cannot always be sampled reliably from each placental site. Difficulties include ensuring that separate samples are obtained in dizygotic pregnancies and identifying which specimen represents which fetus in case the results prove discordant (see Chapter 57). Separate puncture sites are usually needed. In the past, dyes such as indigo carmine were instilled into the first sac so that the absence of dye-stained fluid from the second indicates successful sampling of the second sac. Indigo carmine (1.5ml) is preferred to methylene blue which has been associated with congenital small bowel atresias and methhemoglobinemia.[34] Methylene blue is also an inhibitor of guanylate cyclase, which plays a crucial role in the regulation of fetal blood flow. Ultrasonic guidance now renders dye-labeling unnecessary for most patients in experienced hands.

Jeanty and co-workers suggested a single needle insertion technique. Following aspiration of fluid from the first sac, the dividing membrane is punctured to allow sampling of the second sac.[35] Theoretical risks include amnion rupture resulting in pseudo-monoamniotic twins and the amniotic band syndrome.[36]

Table 2
Complications of ultrasound-guided mid-trimester genetic amniocentesis in a randomized controlled trial of 4606 low-risk women

	Study group	Control group	Odds ratio (95% CI)
Early pregnancy complications (within 6 weeks)			
Abdominal pain	184(8.1%)	67(3.0%)	2.72(2.11–3.51)
Amniotic fluid leakage	39(1.7%)	10(0.4%)	3.35(1.91–5.89)
Vaginal bleeding	55(2.4%)	58(2.6%)	0.96(0.66–1.39)
Pregnancy outcome			
Miscarriage (after 16 weeks)	34(1.5%)	9(0.4%)	3.24(1.78–5.91)
Stillbirth	10(0.4%)	12(0.5%)	0.83(0.36–1.93)
Preterm delivery	85(3.7%)	72(3.1%)	1.19(0.86–1.63)
Neonatal outcome			
Very low birthweight	21(0.9%)	9(0.4%)	2.27(1.11–4.65)
Postural deformities of lower limbs	39(1.7%)	46(2.0%)	0.86(0.56–1.32)
Respiratory distress syndrome	25(1.1%)	12(0.5%)	2.06(1.08–3.93)
Pneumonia	15(0.7%)	6(0.3%)	2.40(1.02–5.65)

After Tabor et al.[40] and Grant et al.[63].

HAZARDS (Tables 1 and 2)

Fetal Loss

Older studies are flawed by lack of data on the background miscarriage rate, by their failure to confirm fetal viability before amniocentesis and by the absence of ultrasound guidance. There are no large studies which have defined the risks of amniocentesis after 20 weeks gestation. Regarding amniocentesis performed prior to 20 weeks, there are three large collaborative studies. It is assumed that amniocentesis after 20 weeks is subject to the same types of complications.

One of the three major collaborative case-control/cohort studies, the US NICHD, reported a 3.5% fetal loss rate compared with 3.2% for controls,[37] which was unrelated to previous miscarriage, volume of fluid removed, or number of attempts. The Canadian Collaborative Study[38] found a loss rate of 3.2%. Factors which increased the risk of a loss were a needle gauge larger than 19 and failed attempts. However, there was no control group. The British Working Party on Amniocentesis[39] reported a 2.4% fetal loss rate <28 weeks (1.2% in controls), a 1.2% stillbirth rate (0.8% in controls) and a 1.1% neonatal death rate (0.5% in controls). They attributed the fetal wastage rate of 1.5% directly to amniocentesis. However, some of the matched controls who miscarried were replaced with fresh controls and many controls were recruited into the study at a later gestation than their counterparts, thus reducing the likelihood of miscarriage. Furthermore, the indication for amniocentesis in 110 cases was an elevated AFP, which is associated with an increased risk of miscarriage (see Chapter 37).

Our patients are quoted a risk of miscarriage attributable to amniocentesis of 1%, based on the results of the only randomized controlled trial.[40] Some have attributed this high rate to the use of large gauge needles, although based on subsequent correspondence from the authors it appears that 20-gauge needles were used in the majority of patients.[41] Transplacental insertions have been linked with an increased miscarriage rate, though all were done free-handed and many without ultrasound guidance.[40,42]

The risks of amniocentesis in multiple pregnancies are greater than in singletons,[37,38] with a loss rate <28 weeks in one study of 3.6% compared with 0.6% in singletons.[43] This result compares favorably with the natural loss rate in multiple gestation.[44]

Respiratory Distress

A small but significant increase in neonatal respiratory morbidity has been reported in some [39,40] but not all studies[37,45] after second trimester amniocentesis, consistent with a study in monkeys showing decreased alveolar number after a single amniocentesis.[46] However, the fact that these changes were also seen when the membranes were punctured but no fluid removed, that single needle puncture in rats causes chronic leakage and oligohydramnios,[47] and that up to 2% of amniocentesis in humans are complicated by chronic leakage of fluid[40] raises the possibility that any respiratory sequelae which follows a single amniocentesis may be due to chronic oligohydramnios.

Orthopedic Postural Abnormalities

The British collaborative study also implicated amniocentesis in the etiology of postural deformities of the newborn. Specifically, talipes equinovarus, congenital dislocation and subluxation of the hip were observed in 24/2389 (1%) subjects compared with 4/2413 (0.2%) controls.[39] This observation was not supported by the findings of the other two trials.

Needle Injuries

Neonatal lesions such as ileocutaneous fistula, ileal atresia, corneal perforation and umbilical cord hematoma have been attributed to amniocentesis needle injury.[48] Such injuries are rare and are related to the 'blind' technique. However, so-called needle injuries have also been reported in controls with similar frequency.[39]

Alloimmunization

Sensitization of Rh-negative women has been documented after amniocentesis,[39] the attributable risk being approximately 1% greater than the background risk of 1.5%.[49] This is minimized by avoiding transplacental approaches and using small-gauge needles.[50] Unsensitized Rh-negative patients should be given anti-D immunoglobulin intramuscularly after the procedure (see Chapter 44).

EARLY AMNIOCENTESIS

Traditionally, genetic amniocentesis has been done between 15 and 17 weeks when the fundus is readily accessible transabdominally, the volume of amniotic fluid (150–200 ml) permits removal of 20 ml with relative impunity, and abormal results may be known in time to allow termination of pregnancy before 20 weeks. Recognition of the disadvantages of CVS[51] has focused interest on alternatives, such as early amniocentesis, which would still have the advantages of first trimester diagnosis.

Using ultrasound guidance, early amniocentesis is technically easy with a failure rate of only 2% in a review of 2200 procedures at 11–14 weeks.[52] Some operators use 22-gauge needles to avoid stripping the membrane from the uterine wall,[53] aspirate slowly to prevent the amniotic sac from collapsing[54] and remove only 10–12 ml of fluid in view of the smaller volume present at earlier gestations.

Using standard cytogenetic techniques, culture success rates at 12–14 weeks gestation are usually well above 95%,[52,55–60] with mean times to cell harvest (12 days) only 1–2 days longer than in those performed at 16 weeks.[56,57] However, between 9 and 11 weeks, only 68–70% of samples yield a karyotype,[56,60] suggesting that culture of amniotic fluid <12 weeks is not yet practical. Early amniocentesis is associated with lower rates of maternal contamination and pseudomosaicism than CVS.[61]

The safety of early amniocentesis has not yet been established. Penso and co-workers, in a study of 407 amniocenteses at 11–14 weeks, found no obvious increase in fetal loss rates (3.9%), prematurity (6.6%) or low-birthweight rates (6.1%) when compared with those in the literature for procedures at 16–20 weeks. The frequency of neonatal pulmonary complications (6.1%) and orthopedic deformities (2.2%),[58] however, were high. Smaller studies report lower loss rates and no increase in respiratory or orthopedic complications.[59,60] As the theoretical risks of oligohydramnios and neonatal respiratory distress are greater after early amniocentesis, some authors advocate sampling a smaller volume of amniotic fluid: 1 ml/week until 14 weeks.[54,61] Amniofiltration has also been suggested as a way of increasing the number of cells without significantly depleting amniotic fluid volume. Approximately 40 ml of amniotic fluid is removed and then returned to the amniotic cavity without its component cells. Early work has shown that filtering a greater volume produces a larger number of cell clones but a similar time to harvest.[62] Details on the failure rates and loss rates are as yet unknown.

CONCLUSIONS

Amniocentesis, when performed with a narrow-gauge needle and ultrasound guidance, is a safe, simple,

---

AMNIOCENTESIS
Summary of Management Options

Indications

Prenatal diagnosis

- Chromosome analysis

- DNA analysis

- Biochemistry

- Fetal infection

Fetal welfare

- Maternal red cell alloimmunization

- Lung maturity

- Chorioamnionitis

- Maternal obstetric cholestasis

Fetal therapy

- Hydramnios and oligohydramnios (see Chapter 48)

- Fetal reduction (see Chapter 57)

- Hypothyroidism (see Chapter 55)

Complications

- Fetal loss

- Preterm labor and delivery

- Respiratory distress

- Postural deformities

- Trauma

- Alloimmunization

reliable and well-tolerated procedure for prenatal diagnosis. Its applications are diverse and will likely continue with the application of molecular techniques to prenatal diagnosis. Despite its simplicity, complications inherent to all percutaneous, intrauterine procedures occur. These include rupture of the amniotic membranes, chorioamnionitis, fetal trauma and maternal red blood cell alloimmunization. Rh-women should receive anti-D immunglobulin after each procedure.

Acknowledgement

We thank Dr A. Daniel of the Cytogenetics Unit, Westmead Hospital for assistance with Figs 1 and 2.

REFERENCES

1 Thirkelsen AJ (1979) Cell culture and cytogenetic technique. In Murken JD, Stengel-Rutkowski S, Schwinger EN (eds) *Prenatal Diagnosis: Proceedings of the 3rd European Conference on Prenatal Diagnosis of Genetic Disorders*, pp. 258–270. Stuttgart: Ferdinand Enke.

2 Bui TH, Iselius L, Lindsten J (1984) European collaborative study on prenatal diagnosis: Mosaicism, pseudomosaicism and single abnormal cells in amniotic fluid cell cultures. *Prenatal Diagnosis* 4:145–162.

3 Hus LYF, Perlis TE (1984) The United States survey on chromosome mosaicism and pseudomosaicism in prenatal diagnosis. *Prenatal Diagnosis* 4:97–130.

4 Worton RG, Stern R (1987) A Canadian collaborative study of mosaicism in amniotic fluid cell cultures. *Prenatal Diagnosis* 4:131–144.

5 Chang HC, Jones W (1981) A new growth medium for human amniotic fluid cells. *Karyogram* 7:4.

6 Evans MI, Bhatia RK, Bottoms SF, Koppitch FC (1988) Effects of karyotype, gestational age and medium on the duration of amniotic fluid cell culturing. *Journal of Reproductive Medicine* 33:765–767.

7 Brock DJH (1986) DNA probes or microvillar enzymes or both for prenatal diagnosis of cystic fibrosis. *Med Genet* 23:376–377.

8 Raux-Demay M, Mornet E, Boue J, Couillin P, Oury JF, Ravise N, Deluchat C, Boue A (1989) 17-Hydroxyprogesterone determination and probes. *Prenatal Diagnosis* 9:457–466.

9 Richards DS, Seeds JW, Katz VL, Lingley LH, Albright SG, Cefalo RC (1988) Elevated maternal serum alphafetoprotein with normal ultrasound: Is amniocentesis always appropriate? A review of 26069 screened patients. *Obstetrics and Gynecology* 71:203–207.

10 Nadel AS, Green JK, Holmes LB, Frigoletto FD, Benacerraf BR (1990) Absence of need for amniocentesis in patients with elevated levels of maternal serum alphafetoprotein and normal ultrasonographic examinations. *New England Journal of Medicine* 323:557–561.

11 Chitayat D, Kalousek DK, McGillivary BC, Applegarth DA (1991) A co-twin fetus papyraceus as a cause of elevated AFP and acetyl-cholinesterase in the amniotic fluid of the normal co-twin. *Pediatric Pathology* 11:487–491.

12 Drugan A, Zador IE, Syner FN, Sokol RJ, Sacks AJ, Evans MI (1988) A normal ultrasound does not obviate the need for amniocentesis in patients with elevated serum alpha-fetoprotein. *Obstetrics and Gynecology* 72:627–630.

13 Thornton JG, Lilford RJ, Newcombe RG (1991) Tables for estimation of individual risks of fetal neural tube and ventral wall defects, incorporating prior probability, maternal serum alpha-fetoprotein levels and unltrasonographic examination results. *American Journal of Obstetrics and Gynecology* 164:154–160.

14 Daffos F, Forestier F, Capella-Pavlovsky M, Thullilez P, Aufrent C, Valenti D, Cox W (1988) Prenatal management of 746 pregnancies at risk for congenital toxoplasmosis. *New England Journal of Medicine* 381:271–275.

15 Grover CM, Tyhulliez P, Remington JS, Boothroyd JC (1990) Rapid prenatal diagnosis of congenital toxoplasma infection by using polymerase chain reaction and amniotic fluid. *Journal of Clinical Microbiology* 28:2297–2301.

16 Weiner CP, Grose C (1990) Prenatal diagnosis of congenital cytomegalovirus infection by virus isolation from amniotic fluid. *American Journal of Obstetrics and Gynecology* 163:1253–1255.

17 Hohlfeld P, Maillard-Brighton C, Fawer CL (1991) Cytomegalovirus fetal infection: Prenatal diagnosis. *Obstetrics and Gynecology* 78:615–618.

18 Liley AW (1961) Liquor amnii analysis in the management of pregnancy complicated by rhesus sensitisation. *American Journal of Obstetrics and Gynecology* 82:1359–1370.

19 James DK, Tindall VR, Richardson T (1983) Is the lecithin/sphingomyelin ratio outdated? *British Journal of Obstetrics and Gynaecology* 90:995–1000.

20 Dodson MG, Fortunato SJ (1988) Microorganisms and premature labour. *Journal of Reproductive Medicine* 33:87–95.

21 Dudley J, Malcolm G, Ellwood D (1991) Amniocentesis in the management of preterm premature rupture of the membranes. *Australia and New Zealand Journal of Obstetrics and Gynaecology* 31:331–336.

22 Romero R, Sitori M, Oyarzun E *et al.* (1988) Infection and labor: V. Prevalence, microbiology and clinical significance of intra-amniotic infection in women with preterm labor and intact membranes. *American Journal of Obstetrics and Gynecology* 161:817.

23 Morales WJ, Angel JL, O'Brien WF *et al.* (1988) A randomized study of antibiotic therapy in idiopathic preterm labour. *Obstetrics and Gynecology* 72:829.

24 Fisk NM (1988) Modifications to selective conservative management in preterm premature rupture of the membranes. *Obstetrical and Gynecological Survey.* 43:328–334.

25 Reid R, Ivey KJ, Rencoret RH, Storey B (1976) Fetal complications of obstetric cholestasis. *British Medical Journal* i:870–872.

26 Fisk NM, Storey GNB (1988) Fetal outcome in obstetric cholestasis. *British Journal of Obstetrics and Gynaecology* 95:1137–1143.

27 Scrimgeour JB (1973) Amniocentesis: Technique and complications. In Emery AEH (ed.) *Antenatal Diagnosis of Genetic Disease*. Baltimore, MD: Williams and Wilkins.

28 Shalev E, Dan U, Machiach S, Chaki R, Shalev J, Barkai G, Goldman B (1990) First trimester transvaginal amniocentesis for genetic evaluation of multiple gestation [Letter]. *Prenatal Diagnosis* 10:344–345.

29 Evans E, Drugan A, Koppitch FC et al. (1989) Genetic diagnosis in the first trimester: The norm for the 1990s. *American Journal of Obstetrics and Gynecology* 160:1332–1339.

30 de Crespigny L, Robinson HP (1986) Amniocentesis: A comparison of 'monitored' versus 'blind' needle insertion technique. *Australia and New Zealand Journal of Obstetrics and Gynaecology* 26:124–128.

31 Romero R, Jeanty P, Reece EA, Grannum P, Bracken M, Berkowitz R, Hobbins JC (1985) Sonographically monitored amniocentesis to decrease intraoperative complications. *Obstetrics and Gynecology* 65:426–430.

32 Bowerman RA, Barclay ML (1987) A new technique to overcome failed second trimester amniocentesis due to membrane tenting. *Obstetrics and Gynecology* 70:806–808.

33 Stiller RJ, Lockwood CJ, Belanger K, Baumgarten A, Hobbins JC, Mahoney MJ (1988) Amniotic fluid alpha-fetoprotein concentrations in twin gestations: Dependence on placental membrane anatomy. *Prenatal Diagnosis* 158:1809–1092.

34 Nicolini U, Monni G (1990) Intestinal obstruction in babies exposed *in utero* to methylene blue [Letter]. *Lancet* 336:1258–1259.

35 Jeanty P, Shash D, Roussis P (1990) Single-needle insertion in twin amniocentesis. *Journal of Ultrasound Medicine* 9:503–510.

36 Gilbert WM, Davis SE, Kaplan C, Pretorius D, Merritt TA, Benirschke K (1991) Morbidity associated with prenatal disruption of the dividing membrane in twin gestations. *Obstetrics and Gynecology* 78:623–630.

37 National Institutes of Child Health and Human Development National Registry for Amniocentesis Study Group (1976) Amniocentesis for prenatal diagnosis: Safety and accuracy. *Journal of the American Medical Association* 236:1471–1476.

38 Simpson NE, Dallaire L, Miller JR, Siminovich L, Hamerton JL, Miller J, McKeen C (1976) Prenatal diagnosis of genetic disease in Canada: Report of a collaborative study. *Canadian Medical Association Journal* 115:739–746.

39 Medical Research Council (1978) An assessment of the hazards of amniocentesis. *British Journal of Obstetrics and Gynecology* 85:1–41. (suppl.2).

40 Tabor A, Philip J, Madsen M, Bang J, Obel EB, Norgaard-Pederson B (1986) Randomised controlled trial of genetic amniocentesis in 4606 low risk women. *Lancet* i:1287–1293.

41 Tabor A, Philip J, Madsen M, Obel EB, Norgaard-Pedersen B (1988) Needle size and risk of miscarriage after amniocentesis (Letter). *Lancet* i:183–184.

42 Kappel B, Nielsen J, Hansen KB, Mikklesen M, Therkelsen AAJ (1987) Spontaneous abortion following mid-trimester amniocentesis: Clinical significance of placental perforation and blood stained amniotic fluid. *British Journal of Obstetrics and Gynecology* 94:50–54.

43 Anderson RL, Goldberg JD, Golbus MS (1991) Prenatal diagnosis in multiple gestation: 20 years' experience with amniocentesis: *Prenatal Diagnosis* 11(4):263–270.

44 Naeye RL, Tafari N, Judge D, Marboe CC (1978) Twins: Causes of perinatal death in 12 United States cities and one African city. *American Journal of Obstetrics and Gynecology* 31:267.

45 Hunter AGW (1987) Neonatal lung function following mid-trimester amniocentesis. *Prenatal Diagnosis* 7:431–441.

46 Hislop A, Fairweather DVI, Blackwell RJ, Howard S (1984) The effect of amniocentesis and drainage of amniotic fluid on lung development in Macaca Fascicularis. *American Journal of Obstetrics and Gynecology* 91:835–842.

47 Moessinger AC, Bassi GA, Ballantyne G, Collins MH, James S, Blane WA (1983) Experimental production of pulmonary hypoplasia following amniocentesis and oligohydramnios. *Early Human Development* 8:343–350.

48 Elias S, Simpson JL (1986) Amniocentesis. In Milunsky A (ed.) *Genetic Disorders and the Fetus: Diagnosis, Prevention and Treatment*, 2nd edn. New York: Plenum Press.

49 Murray JC, Karp LE, Williamson RA et al. (1983) Rh isoimmunization related to amniocentesis. *American Journal of Medical Genetics* 16:527.

50 Tabor A, Bang J, Norgaard-Pederson B (1987) Feto-maternal haemorrhage associated with genetic amniocentesis: Results of randomized trial. *British Journal of Gynaecology* 194:528–534.

51 Canadian Collaborative CVS–Amniocentesis Clinical Trial Group (1989) Multicentre randomized clinical trial of chorionic villus sampling and amniocentesis. *Lancet* i:1–6.

52 Johnson A, Godmilow L (1988) Genetic amniocentesis at 14 weeks or less. *Clinics in Obstetrics and Gynecology* 31:345–352.

53 Stripparo L, Buscaglia M, Longatti L, Ghisoni L, Dambrosio F, Guerneri S, Rosella F, Cordones M, De Biasio P, Passamonti U, Gimelli G, Cuoco C (1990) Genetic amniocentesis: 505 cases performed before the sixteenth week of gestation. *Prenatal Diagnosis* 10:359–364.

54 Hanson FW, Zorn EM, Tennant FR, Marianos S, Samuels S (1987) Amniocentesis before 15 weeks gestation: Outcome, risks and technical problems. *American Journal of Obstetrics and Gynecology* 156:1524–1531.

55 Benacerraf BR, Greene MF, Saltzman DH, Barss VA, Penso CA, Nadel AS, Heffner LJ, Stryker JM, Sandstrom MM, Frigoletto FD (1988) Early amniocentesis for prenatal cytogenetic evaluation. *Radiology* 169:709–710.

56 Rooney DE, MacLachlan N, Smith J, Rebello MT, Loeffler FE, Beard RW, Rodeck C, Coleman DV (1989) Early amniocentesis: A cytogenetic evaluation. *British Medical Journal* 299:25.

57 Rebello MT, Gray CTH, Rooney DE, Smith JH, Hackett GA, Loeffler FE, Horwell DH, Beard RW, Coleman DV (1991) Cytogenetic studies of amniotic fluid taken before the 15th week of pregnancy for earlier prenatal

diagnosis: A report of 114 consecutive cases. *Prenatal Diagnosis* **11**:35–40.

58 Penso CA, Sandstrom MM, Garber MF, Ladoulis M, Stryker JM, Benacerraf BB (1990) Early amniocentesis: Report of 407 cases with neonatal follow-up. *Obstetrics and Gynecology* **76**:1032–1036.

59 Nevin J, Nevin NC, Dornan JC, Sim D, Armstrong MJ (1990) Early amniocentesis: Experience of 222 consecutive patients, 1987–1988. *Prenatal Diagnosis* **10**:79–83.

60 Hackett GA, Smith JH, Rebello MT, Gray CTH, Rooney DE, Beard RW, Loeffler FE, Coleman DV (1991) Early amniocentesis at 11–14 weeks' gestation for the diagnosis of fetal chromosome amnormality: A clinical evaluation. *Prenatal Diagnosis* **11**:311–315.

61 Godmilow L, Weiner S, Dunn LK (1987) Genetic amniocentesis performed between 12 and 14 weeks (Abstract). *American Journal of Human Genetics* **41**:A275 (suppl.).

62 Choo V (1991) Conference: Early amniocentesis. *Lancet* **ii**:750–751.

63 Grant AM (1991) Genetic amniocentesis at 16 weeks gestation. In Chalmers I (ed.) *Oxford Database of Perinatal Trials*, Version 1.2, Disc Issue 6, Autumn 1991.

41

Fetal Blood Sampling Before Labor

PETER W. SOOTHILL

INTRODUCTION

Fetal blood was first obtained from the capillary circulation of the presenting part after cervical dilation and rupture of the membranes.[1] This transcervical approach is only possible after a commitment to delivery has been made. Fetal blood sampling before labor requires a transabdominal approach and was initially undertaken for the prenatal diagnosis of severe inherited disease with a view to pregnancy termination if the fetus was affected. More recently, a medical approach to diseases of the unborn has developed, and the role of phlebotomy in fetal medicine is now comparable to its place in postnatal medicine.

INDICATIONS

It is increasingly difficult to list discrete indications for fetal blood sampling since it has become part of the process of diagnosis, treatment and, in several instances, monitoring of fetal disease. However, the indications for accessing the fetal circulation can be grouped into diagnostic and therapeutic areas. In general, a fetal blood sample is indicated when a judgment of the potential benefits of changes in management outweigh the procedure-related risks.

Diagnostic

Chromosome abnormalities

The rapid division rate of white blood cells allows the preparation of a karyotype with good-quality chromo-

some banding within 48–72 h in most centers. The most common indication for a rapid karyotype by fetal blood sampling is further investigation of malformation or early-onset fetal growth deficiency as detected by ultrasound scanning (see Chapters 38 and 42). Other problems which can be resolved by fetal blood cytogenetic analysis include a mosaic result or culture failure after either amniocentesis or placental biopsy, late registration for prenatal care of women requesting fetal karyotyping, and the prenatal diagnosis of fragile X mental retardation.

Single gene defects

Fetal blood sampling is now performed less often for prenatal diagnosis of these disorders, since many can be diagnosed earlier in pregnancy using DNA techniques (see Chapter 36). The diseases that can be diagnosed using a fetal blood sample include hemoglobinopathies, coagulopathies, severe combined immunodeficiency, chronic granulomatous disease and some metabolic disorders.[2] Fetal blood sampling remains important for patients at risk and who register late, and in families in which DNA analysis is not possible.

Anemia

Although there are various indirect methods of assessing fetal anemia (see Chapters 43 and 44), the definitive investigation in medicine before and after birth is measurement of the hemoglobin concentration.

This may be required in maternal red cell alloimmuniz-ation[3] or some cases of non-immune hydrops.[4]

Thrombocytopenia

Severe fetal thrombocytopenia may lead to cerebral hemorrhage before, during or after birth, leading to death or mental handicap. The fetal platelet count can be measured to guide diagnosis and treatment (see Chapter 46).

Hypoxia/acidosis

Suspected fetal hypoxemia or acidemia can be con-firmed or refuted by fetal blood gas analysis.[5,6] This may become increasingly important with emerging evi-dence that chronic fetal acidemia is associated with poor long-term neuro-development.[7] However, evi-dence that interventions (such as preterm delivery) based on this assessment of fetal blood acid/base status improves the outcome is awaited.

Fetal infection

Whether maternal infection has led to fetal infection can be assessed by appropriate fetal blood investi-gations (e.g. infection-specific fetal IgM at 22 weeks gestation). However, the difference between being infected and affected (i.e. damaged) must not be for-gotten (see Chapter 49). Fetal blood tests are increas-ingly being used in conjunction with ultrasound scan-ning signs.[8]

Monitoring of transplacental therapy

Some fetal diseases can be treated by therapeutic agents given to the mother so that they cross the pla-centa. Examples include anti-arrythmic agents to cor-rect fetal tachyarrhythmias, gamma-globulin and ster-oids to improve low fetal platelet counts, antithyroid agents for women with thyroid-stimulating immune globulin (TSIG) and maternal hyper-oxygenation to increase fetal pO_2 levels. In many instances, assess-ment of placental transfer and monitoring the success of therapy may require repeat fetal blood sampling.[9–11]

Therapeutic

Injection into the fetal circulation has proved dramati-cally effective therapy for some conditions and shows promise in others.

Anemia

Fetal anemia of any cause can be treated by intravascu-lar blood transfusion (see Chapter 44).

Thrombocytopenia

Platelet transfusion is more controversial than blood transfusion because platelets have a short half-life and repeated transfusions at frequent intervals are required to maintain the fetal platelet count[12,13] (see Chapter 46). Thrombocytopenic fetuses may have a greater chance of hemorrhage at the time of a blood sam-pling procedure.

Drug adminstration

Fetal arrhythmias leading to hydrops fetalis and not responding to transplacental treatment can be corrected by injection of anti-arrhythmic drugs into the fetal cir-culation (see Chapter 47).[11,14]

Fetocide

Intravascular injection of strong potassium solutions can be used when a handicapping abnormality is found in a fetus of multiple pregnancy or when the number of fetuses is so great that the survival of any is unlikely (see Chapter 57). It can also be used during late abor-tion of singleton pregnancies and especially for termin-ation of viable fetuses with handicapping conditions in countries in which this is legal.[15]

PROCEDURAL OPTIONS

When considering a fetal blood sample, the operator must first choose the intended sampling site and tech-nique. There are several possible options.

Sampling Site

Umbilical cord vessels (cordocentesis)

A variety of terms with alternative meanings have been used to describe this technique (e.g. 'funi-centesis' or 'PUBS'), but they have added confusion to the litera-ture and made computer searches more difficult. The consensus view is in favor of the word 'cordocentesis' for aspiration of blood from the umbilical cord, and the author recommends this word for future publications.

Cordocentesis was first performed under fetoscopic guidance,[16] but fetoscopy carried a 2–5% risk of serious complications[17] and the maternal sedation used changed fetal blood gas measurements[18]. There is agreement that ultrasound-guided needling is safer and is the preferred technique.[19–21]

The placental umbilical cord insertion is usually the easiest site to puncture. Puncture of a free loop, though useful for placental avoidance, requires pinning the cord and fetal paralysis and is more likely to result in hemorrhage. The author strongly discourages transfusion into the cord at any site other than the placental insertion. Although cordocentesis is usually done after 18 weeks gestation, some groups have reported successful cordocentesis as early as 12 weeks, but with a marked increase in fetal risk.[22,23]

Fetal heart

The heart is larger than the umbilical cord vessels, making ultrasound-guided needling relatively easy. Despite fears of damaging this organ, it appears that it can be needled relatively safely.[24,25] Since the fetal heart contains blood of different origins, it is not suitable for blood gas assessment.[26] However, the heart is an alternative sampling site in the unusual event that either the placental cord insertion cannot be used safely or when fetal blood must be obtained at a gestational age less than 17–18 weeks. It can also be useful if an emergency blood transfusion is required (e.g. to treat procedure-related bleeding) or for fetocide (see **Figure 1**).

Fetal intrahepatic vessels

Blood can be obtained from vessels within the substance of the liver.[27–29] It is now usually done with fetal paralysis (intramuscular injection of pancuronium[30]) and good results have been reported. However, most suggest its use when cordocentesis is difficult and some practitioners prefer to sample the heart in this event (see **Figure 2**).

Needling Technique

Needle guide

A needle guide technique uses a sector ultrasound transducer with a guide attached containing a needle channel. Lines on the ultrasound screen indicate the path the needle will follow when inserted down the guide. The transducer is moved until these lines cross the intended target. This approach has several advantages. First, it allows needles which are thinner (i.e. 22–26 gauge) than those needed for a free-hand technique. Second, it prevents lateral movement of the needle, thus minimizing trauma to the uterus, placenta or cord. However, it limits the operator's ability to

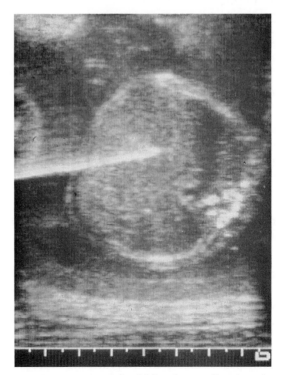

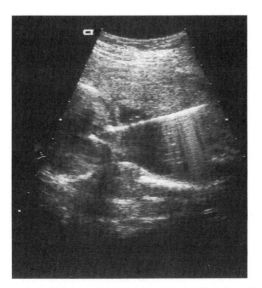

Figure 1. Picture of fetal blood sampling by ultrasound-guided needling of the heart.

Figure 2. Picture of fetal blood sampling by ultrasound-guided needling of the intrahepatic vein.

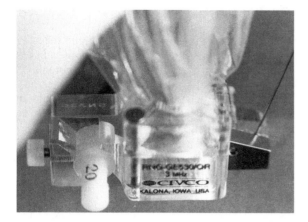

Figure 3a. A typical needle guide used for the performance of cordocentesis. Note that the small footprint allows the needle to enter the sonographic plane shortly after it penetrates the skin.

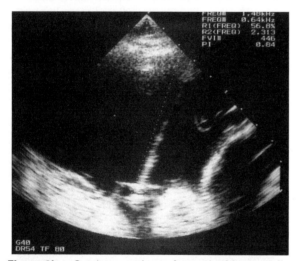

Figure 3b. Cordocentesis performed with a needle guide on a free loop of umbilical cord. The needle is the bright white echoes crossing the amniotic fluid diagonally. The predicted track of the needle can be seen as a dotted line immediately adjacent to the needle.

adjust to difficulties or changes that may occur during the procedure (see **Figure 3**).

Free-hand

A free-hand technique uses a curvilinear or linear ultrasound transducer. The ultrasound transducer is moved until the intended sampling site is identified and appears on one side of the ultrasound screen. This needle path is then nearly perpendicular to the ultrasound beam and so good imaging of the whole needle length will be achieved (see **Figure 4**). The advantage of the free-hand technique is that it allows the operator to compensate for contractions or fetal movement. Controversy continues whether one technique is safer than the other but the author prefers the flexibility of the free hand technique.

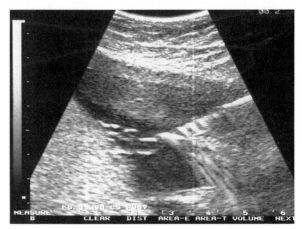

Figure 4. Picture of cordocentesis using the free-hand technique.

One or two operators?

Some prefer to have a different person controlling the scanning transducer, but this loses the operator's control over the intended needle path (which is fixed by the transducer as described above). However, since a 'single operator' means one hand holding the needle and the other the ultrasound transducer, an assistant is inevitably required to withdraw the needle stilette, fix a syringe, aspirate at the right time and place the blood into containers, with the correct anticoagulant quickly without spillage, contamination or mislabelling.

Procedure: Fetal Blood Sampling

Fetal blood sampling should only be undertaken by operators with considerable experience in other obstetric ultrasound-guided needling procedures (e.g. amniocentesis and transabdominal (CVS). Units offering this service should have a sufficient throughput of appropriate cases to maintain expertise, which would usually be a center with a considerable number of referrals from other hospitals for anomaly scanning and fetal medicine opinions.[31] Twelve procedures per year would seem to be a reasonable absolute minimum.

Step 1: Preparation

Maternal supine hypotension, hyperventilation and sedation must be avoided (especially for studies of fetal oxygenation). Therefore, the approach should be relaxed and informal. Anything that gives the patient an image of an 'operation' (surgical masks, hats, gloves, drapes, etc.) can be replaced by a scrupulous 'no-touch' technique. The length of needle required depends on obesity, amniotic fluid volume and fetal and placental positions, but the distance can be measured on the ultrasound screen before starting and a 12 cm needle is usually sufficient.

Step 2: Needle path selection

After identifying the chosen target and keeping it visualized on the screen, the transducer is rotated through 180° until a path which avoids fetal parts and maternal vessels is identified. With the free-hand technique the best skin insertion point is identified by observing sonographically the effect of digital pressure on the maternal abdomen and the transducer is adjusted until the sampling site and the skin inserting point are on opposite sides of the screen. The transplacental approach is usually the easiest route to the placental cord insertion unless the placenta is entirely posterior. However, in red cell alloimmunized pregnancies, placental puncture, as with amniocentesis, can boost the maternal antibody titer as a result of feto-maternal hemorrhage.[32] In the instance of modest alloimmunization it is best to avoid the placenta when possible (see **Figure 5**)

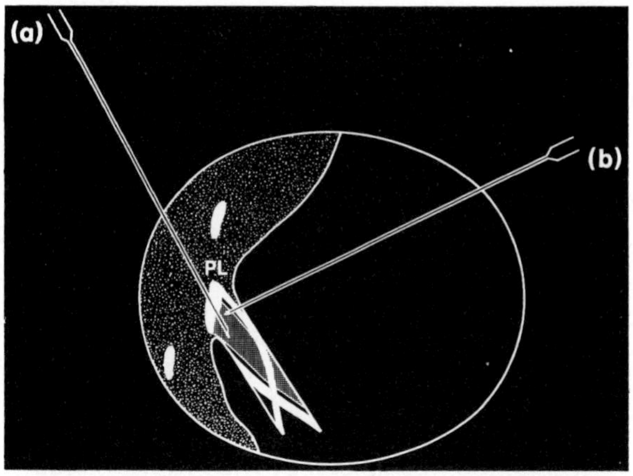

Step 3: Antiseptic and anesthetic

The skin insertion site is scrupulously cleaned with an antiseptic solution, such as chlorhexidine or popovidene. If a local anesthetic agent is to be used, it should be injected into the skin and the abdominal and uterine peritoneum. When using the free-hand technique, the anesthetic injection can help to confirm the needle angle required to follow the intended path and so can reduce the need to change the sampling needle direction during the procedure. However, patients who have had cordocentesis repeatedly (e.g. for rhesus

Figure 5. Schematic diagram of (a) transplacental and (b) transamniotic fetal blood sampling from the placental insertion of the umbilical cord (cordocentesis).

disease) say the local anesthetic may be more painful than the procedure if done quickly without anesthetic. Furthermore, by the time the anesthetic has been given time to work, it can produce a contraction in the needle path and move the position of the cord insertion.

Step 4: Needle insertion

With the needle guide technique, the needle path is fixed approximately 30° off from the ultrasound beam. Though the length of the needle is not always seen, the needle tip appears as a bright dot. The needle is advanced the correct distance while observing the tip. With the freehand technique the length of the needle can be seen clearly (**Figure 4**).

Step 5: Target puncture

Cordocentesis The best sampling site is usually about 1 cm from the placental insertion where blood obtained must be fetal. To enter the umbilical cord, the needle is brought close to the cord in line with the umbilical vein, and then advanced sharply the remaining distance. A slow advance can push the tissues away even at this relatively fixed sampling site. After confirming that the needle tip is in the umbilical cord, the stilette is withdrawn and, if the needle is ideally sited, blood will be seen filling the needle hub. A syringe is applied tightly to the hub and the desired volume of blood withdrawn. At 18 weeks, 2 ml can be taken safely and larger volumes at later gestations. Often no blood is obtained initially and the operator must assess whether the needle tip is through the vessel or not far enough into the cord. The needle is sharply advanced or gently withdrawn and rotated through 180° between the operator's finger and thumb while suction is maintained with the syringe.

Sometimes amniotic fluid is obtained when the needle appears on the screen to be in the cord. With the free-hand technique, the needle can be moved from side to side, looking for resulting movements of the cord. Should the needle be through the cord, it can be withdrawn until no more amniotic fluid is aspirated, the syringe is changed (even a small amount of amniotic fluid is a very powerful coagulant) and the procedure described above continued. If the needle has passed through or to the side of the cord, the needle is withdrawn a little and the needle path adjusted. A slow careful advance can be used to touch the cord with the needle before the sharp movement to puncture the vessels is repeated.

After aspiration of the required volume of blood, the punctured umbilical vessel should be confirmed as an artery or vein with the flush technique a small volume of fluid (e.g. up to 1 ml normal saline) is rapidly injected and the resulting turbulence allows identification of the vessel ultrasonically.[21] It is essential to identify the vessel if the blood gas results are to be interpretable.

Fetal vessel puncture

If the intrahepatic vein or heart is the intended sampling site, fetal paralysis by intramuscular pancuronium (0.3 mg/kg estimated fetal weight) injection should be considered. The fetus is paralysed rapidly (within minutes) and the effect lasts for 90–120 min. The techniques for needle path selection and guidance are the same as those described for the umbilical cord, only the fetal chest or abdomen is entered first, the direction checked and then the needle advanced into the sampling site as a separate movement.

Some have used a double needle technique, the first to enter the fetal body cavity and a second finer needle passed within the first to puncture the target, but this is not necessary. The fetus appears to feel such needling since, without paralysis, movements can be expected unless the fetus is acutely unwell. The heart should be entered through the anterior chest and through the thick muscle of the ventricles (**Figure 1**) to avoid damage to either the valves or electrical conducting system.

Step 6: Fetal monitoring

After removal of the needle, the puncture site should be observed ultrasonically for bleeding. This is often seen after transamniotic cordocentesis, but is almost always short-lived and apparently without significance. When any bleeding observed has stopped, the fetal heart rate is examined. If the fetus is pre-viable, the patient should wait in the hospital until she feels well and can then return home with no special precautions or restrictions in her activity. If local anesthetic has been used, she is warned to expect a bruised sensation in a few hours and that a simple analgesic may be used safely. If the fetus is viable, heart rate monitoring for about 30 min by cardiotocography may be used before leaving hospital. If pancuronium has been given, the mother should be warned that movements may not return for some hours.

In the rare event that fetal bleeding is prolonged and heavy, maternal blood should be collected into heparinized syringes and emergency fetal transfusion considered. This is probably more likely when sampling thrombocytopenic fetuses as in allo-immune thrombocytopenia.

Step 7: Rhesus prophylaxis

Anti-D in adequate doses (usually 500 IU) is given to D-negative women unless they are already alloimmunized or the fetus in known to be D-negative.

Step 8: Laboratory testing

Various laboratory techniques for rapidly confirming that the blood obtained is fetal and pure have been reported. They are largely unnecessary if the technique described above is used, especially if a 'flush' is seen. Further, they may be impossible if the fetal blood has already been replaced with adult blood by transfusion. However, it is prudent after the procedure to send a small sample of blood for a hematology profile and check that the mean cell volume, hemoglobin concentration, and white cell and platelet counts are normal. Careful arrangements for sample transport and communication of results to both the fetal medicine unit and the patient without delay are an important part of the procedure.

COMPLICATIONS AND RISKS

Fetal

Complications

Complications of fetal blood sampling which threaten the fetus are bleeding or hematoma (and obstruction to flow) at the site of needling,[33] fetal bradycardia[34] (probably secondary to vasospasm after trauma to the umbilical artery[35]) or intrauterine infection. Chorioamnionitis is usually secondary to *Staphylococcus epidermiditis* and may present as myalgia, arthralgia and a low fever 4–10 days after the procedure. A case report of an abruption shortly after cordocentesis has been published.[36] Amniotic fluid leakage or premature membrane rupture seems to be rare but should be expected, with a similar frequency to that after amniocentesis. There is also a theoretical risk of carrying an infection from the mother's blood (e.g. hepatitis or human immunodeficiency virus) to the fetus. Although this has not apparently been documented, it is perhaps prudent to avoid invasive procedures when a mother is known to be infected unless there are more important indications.

Post-procedure loss rates

Several groups using different techniques and of varying experience have reported a post-procedure pregnancy loss rate (excluding elective termination of pregnancy) of about 1% (range 0–2.5%) (**Table 1**). Transfusion carries a considerably higher procedure-related risk than blood sampling.

The use of the term 'procedure-related loss' to mean a fetal death within 2 weeks should be discouraged

Table 1
The number of fetal deaths and serious complications in pregnancies sampled for low risk indications

Authors	Complications/ total	%
Nicolaides* et al.[37]	20/928	2.2
Daffos et al.[38]	4/606	1
Donner et al.[39]	4/391	1
Weiner et al.[48]	1/333	0.3
Boulot et al.[40]	4/322	1
Nicolini et al.[29]	2/214	1
Shalev et al.[41]	2/198	1
Radunovic et al.[42]	0/154	0
Bovicelli et al.[43]	3/123	2.4
Perry et al.[44]	2/100	2
Maxwell et al.[47]	1/76	1.5
Maeda et al.[46]	1/45	2
Pielet et al.[45]	0/27	0
Orlandi et al.[22]	? Number 18 weeks	2.5
Levi et al.[23]	? Number 18 weeks	0.7

*10 within 2 weeks of the procedure, another 10 at 4–20 weeks including intrapartum stillbirths.

since some of these deaths will be the result of the indication for sampling (e.g. non-immune hydrops or hypoxic growth deficiency) rather than the procedure. It is also possible, although less likely, that some complications due to the procedure might first be detected after 14 days. Observed post-procedure loss rates are determined by the procedure risk (intrinsic and operator-skill dependent) added to the pre-procedure risk. This total is then reduced by emergency delivery of viable fetuses. The loss and complication rates are clearly related to the indication.[35,47,48]

In one study of 202 pregnancies which were not electively terminated, the loss rate was 1:76 (1.5%) of fetuses sampled for perinatal diagnosis, 5:76 (7%) sampled for an anomaly, 4:29 (14%) for fetal assessment and 9:35 (25%) for non-immune hydrops. This report is consistent with data from Weiner et al.[35] (**Table 2**).[48]

The gestational age at the time of sampling is an important determinant of observed fetal loss rate because:

- the earlier the pregnancy, the greater the pre-procedure risk of miscarriage

- viable fetuses can be delivered if a complication arises.

Table 2
Major complications of diagnostic cordocentesis
(University of Iowa, March 1992)

Final diagnosis	GA (SD)	Emergency delivery	Perinatal death
RBC allo-immunization	28 (4)	1/296 (0.3%)	1/296 (0.3%)[a]
UP dysfunction	31 (4)	3/59 (5.0%)	1/59 (1.7%)
Chromosome abnormality	28 (6)	3/36 (8.3%)	6/36 (16.7%)
All others	28 (5)	0/333 (0.0%)	1/333 (0.3%)
Total	28 (5)	7/724 (1.0%)	9/724 (1.2%)

[a]Amnionitis; all others associated with bradycardia. UP, uteroplacental; RBC, red blood cell.
From C. Weiner, personal communication.

If a problem occurs, emergency cesarean section may prevent fetal death, but by the time the complication has failed to resolve spontaneously and delivery has been organized, the fetus may survive permanently damaged or die in the neonatal rather than fetal period. Furthermore, a very premature delivery or problems associated with the indication for sampling may also result in neonatal death or permanent handicap. It is possible that units with very low fetal mortality rates may be sampling more mature pregnancies and, as a result of urgent cesarean section, could have a higher incidence of surviving individuals with long-term morbidity. All of these risks, however, may be minimized by performing the procedure adjacent to the surgical suite so that delivery may be accomplished within 15 min if necessary.

Maternal

The main risk to the mother directly from fetal blood sampling is red cell alloimmunization. Therefore, anti-D should be given to D-negative women. However, chorioamnionitis or emergency cesarean section in the interest of the fetus can result in secondary maternal problems. When a fetal blood sample or transfusion is undertaken and the fetus is considered viable, the maternal aspects of emergency delivery should be considered.

Needle injury to maternal intra-abdominal organs such as intestines or vessels may be quite common, but significant morbidity as a result has not been reported after cordocentesis. Maternal intra-abdominal infection and bleeding would be expected to occur at the same rate as after expertly performed amniocentesis (see Chapter 40).

CONCLUSIONS

- Fetal blood sampling is indicated when a judgment of the potential benefits of a change in the clinical management based on the result outweighs the procedure-related risks. As with all obstetric procedures, this includes a balance between the risks and benefits to both fetus and mother.

- Most groups sample fetal blood by ultrasound-guided needling of the umbilical cord (cordocentesis), but the fetal heart and intrahepatic vein are alternative sampling sites.

- The possible techniques are briefly described but these procedures should not be attempted unless the operator has considerable experience of other obstetric needling procedures.

- The best estimate of the overall procedure-related 'serious complication rate' (i.e. leading to fetal death or emergency delivery) is about 1%, but pre-procedure risk must be considered. Indeed, the most important determinant of observed fetal loss rates is the indication for sampling. Insufficient data are currently available to compare the relative risks of the different techniques described.

FETAL BLOOD SAMPLING BEFORE LABOR
Summary of Management Options

Indications

Diagnostic

- Chromosome abnormalities
- DNA abnormalities
- Fetal anemia
- Fetal thrombocytopenia
- Fetal hypoxia/acidosis
- Fetal infection
- Monitoring the effects of fetal therapy

Therapeutic

- Fetal anemia
- Fetal thrombocytopenia
- Fetal drug therapy
- Fetocide

Procedure options

Sampling site

- Umbilical cord vessels ('cordocentesis')
- Fetal heart
- Intrahepatic vessels

Needling

- Needle guide
- Free-hand

Complications

Fetal

- Bleeding/hematoma
- Bradycardia
- Chorioamnionitis
- Amniotic fluid leak or membrane rupture
- Placental abruption
- Delivery/miscarriage
- Death

Maternal

- Alloimmunization
- Chorioamnionitis
- Emergency cesarean
- Maternal trauma
- Effects of fetal loss

REFERENCES

1   Saling E (1963) *Foetal and neonatal Hypoxia* (trans. Loeffler FE). London: Arnold.
2   Nicolaides KH (1988) Cordocentesis. *Clinics in Obstetrics and Gynecology* **31**:123–135.
3   Nicolaides KH, Soothill PW, Clewell CH, Rodeck CH, Mibasham R (1988) Fetal haemoglobin concentration to assess the severity of red cell iso-immunisation. *Lancet* **i**:1073–1075.
4   Soothill PW, (1990) Successful treatment of non-immune hydrops caused by parvo-virus B19. *Lancet* **336**:121–122.
5   Soothill PW (1989) Cordocentesis: Role in assessment

of fetal condition. In Manning F (ed.) *Clinics in Perinatology*, pp. 755–769. Philadelphia, PA: W.B. Saunders.

6   Ajayi RA, Soothill PW (1992) Assessment of fetal oxygenation. In Ludomirski A, Nicolini U, Bhutani VK (eds) *Therapeutic and Diagnostic Interventions in Early Life*. New York: Futura.

7   Soothill PW, Ajayi RA, Campbell S, Ross EM, Candy DCA, Snijders RM, Nicolaides KH (1992) Relationship between fetal acidemia at cordocentesis and subsequent neuro-development. *Ultrasound in Obstetrics and Gynecology* 2:80–83.

8   Hohlfeld P, MacAleese J, Capella-Pavlovski M, Giovangrandi Y, Thulliez P, Forestier F, Daffos F (1991) Fetal toxoplasmosis: Ultrasonographic signs. *Ultrasound in Obstetrics and Gynecology* 1:241–244.

9   Nicolini U, Tannirandorn Y, Gonzalez P, Fisk NM, Beacham J, Letsky EA, Rodeck CH (1990) Continuing controversy in alloimmune thrombocytopenia: Fetal hyper-immunoglobulinemia fails to prevent thrombocytopenia. *American Journal of Obstetrics and Gynecology* 163:1144–1146.

10 Rayburn WF (1991) Fetal drug therapy: An overview of selected conditions. *Obstetrical and Gynecological Survey* 47: 1–9.

11 Hansmann M, Gembruch U, Bald R, Manz M, Redel A (1991) Fetal tachyarrhythmias: Transplacental and direct treatment of the fetus – a report of 60 cases. *Ultrasound in Obstetrics and Gynecology* 1:162–170.

12 Nicolini U, Rodeck CH, Kochenour NK *et al.* (1988) *In utero* platelet transfusion for alloimune thrombocytopenia. *Lancet* ii:506.

13 Murphy MF, Pullen HW, Metcalfe P, Chapman JF, Jenkins E, Waters DH, Nicolaides KH, Mibashan RS (1990) Management of fetal allo-immune thrombocytopenia by weekly *in utero* platelet transfusions. *Vox Sang* 58:45–49.

14 Weiner CP, Thompson MI (1988) Direct treatment of supraventricular tachycardia after failed transplacental therapy. *American Journal of Obstetrics and Gynecology* 158:570–573.

15 Morgan D, Lee RG (1991) *Human Reproduction and Embryology Act 1990: Abortion and Embryo Research – The New Law*. London: Blackstone Press.

16 Rodeck CH, Campbell S (1979) Umbilical cord insertion as a source of pure fetal blood for prenatal diagnosis. *Lancet* i:1244–1245.

17 Soothill PW, Nicolaides KH, Rodeck CH (1987) Invasive techniques for prenatal diagnosis and therapy. *Journal of Perinatal Medicine* 15:117–127.

18 Soothill PW, Nicolaides KH, Rodeck CH, Campbell S (1986) Effect of gestational age on fetal and intervillous blood gas and acid base values in human pregnancy. *Fetal Therapy* 1:168–175.

19 Bang J (1983) Ultrasound guided fetal blood sampling. In Albertini A Crosnani PG (eds) *Progress in Perinatal Medicine*. Amsterdam: Excerpta Medica.

20 Daffos F, Forrestier F, Capella-Pavlovsky M (1983) Fetal blood sampling via the umbilical cord using a needle guided by ultrasound. *Prenatal Diagnosis* 3:271–274.

21 Nicolaides KH, Soothill PW, Rodeck CH, Campbell S (1986) Ultrasound-guided sampling of umbilical cord and placental blood to assess fetal wellbeing. *Lancet* i:1065–1067.

22 Orlandi F, Damiani G, Jahil C, Lairicella S, Bertolini O, Maggie A (1990) The risks of early cordocentesis (12–21 weeks): Analysis of 500 cases. *Prenatal Diagnosis* 10:425–428.

23 Levi-Setti PE, Buscaglia M, Ferrazi E, Zuliani G, Ghisoni L, Pardi G (1989) Evaluation of the fetal risk after each o-guided blood sampling from the umbilical cord in the 2nd trimester of pregnancy. *Ann-Obstet-Ginecol-Med-Perinat* 110:98–104.

24 Bang J (1983) Intrauterine needle diagnosis. In Bang J (ed.) *Interventional Ultrasound*, pp. 122–128. Copenhagen: Munksgaard.

25 Westgren M, Selbing A, Stangenberg M (1988) Fetal intracardiac transfusions in patients with severe rhesus isoimmunisation. *British Medical Journal* 296:885–886.

26 Soothill PW (1990) Cardiac blood sampling for fetal wellbeing. *American Journal of Obstetrics and Gynecology* 162:1636–1637.

27 Bang J, Bock JE, Trolle D (1982) Ultrasound-guided fetal intravascular transfusion for severe rhesus haemolytic disease. *British Medical Journal* 284:373–374.

28 DeCrespigny LCh, Robinson HP, Quinn M, Doyle L, Ross A, Cauchi M (1985) Ultrasound guided fetal blood transfusions for severe red cell isoimmunisation. *Obstetrics and Gynecology* 66:529–532.

29 Nicolini U, Nicolaides P, Fisk N, Tannirandorn Y, Rodeck CH (1990) Fetal blood sampling from the intrahepatic vein: Analysis of safety and clinical experience with 214 procedures. *Obstetrics and Gynecology* 76:47–53.

30 DeCrespigny LCh, Robinson HP, Ross AW, Quinn M (1985) Curarisation of fetus for intrauterine procedures. *Lancet* i:1164.

31 Whittle M (1989) Safety of cordocentesis. *British Journal of Hospital Medicine* 41:511.

32 Weiner CP, Grant S (1989) Effect of diagnostic and therapeutic cordocentesis on maternal serum alpha-fetoprotein concentration. *American Journal of Obstetrics and Gynecology* 161:706–708.

33 Jaineaux E, Douner C, Simon P, Vanesse M, Hustin J, Rodesch F (1989) Pathological aspects of the umbilical cord after percutaneous umbilical blood sampling. *Obstetrics and Gynecology* 73:215–218.

34 Benacerraf B, Baras VA *et al.* (1987) Acute fetal distress associated with percutaneous umbilical blood sampling. *American Journal of Obstetrics and Gynecology* 156:1218–1220.

35 Weiner CP (1987) Cordocentesis for diagnostic indications: Two years experience. *Obstetrics and Gynecology* 70:664–668.

36 Feinkind L, Nanda D, Delke I, Minkoff H (1990) Abruptio placentae after percutaneous umbilical cord sampling: A case report. *American Journal of Obstetrics and Gynecology* 162:1203–1204.

37 Nicolaides KH, Snijder RJM, Abbas A (1992) Cordocentesis. In Iffy L, Apuzzio JJ, Vintzileos AM (eds) *Operative Obstetrics* pp. 82–90. New York: McGraw-Hill.

38 Daffos F, Capella-Pavlovsky M, Forrestier F (1985) Fetal blood sampling during pregnancy with a needle

guided by ultrasound: A study of 606 consecutive cases. *American Journal of Obstetrics and Gynecology* **153**:655–659.

39 Donner C, Simon P, Gosselin F, Verneylen D, Arni F, Liesnard C, Vamos E, Cochaux P, Vassart G, Rodesch F (1990) Cordocentesis: Experience on 391 initial samples. *Rev Med Brux* **11**:211–215.

40 Boulot P, Deschapms F, Lefort G, Sarda P, Mares P, Hedon B, Laffargne F, Viala JL (1990) Pure fetal blood samples obtained by cordocentesis: Technical aspects of 322 cases. *Prenatal Diagnosis* **10**:93–100.

41 Shalev E, Dan U, Weiner E, Romano S, Giselevitz J, Mashiach S (1989) Prenatal diagnosis using sonographic guided cordocentesis. *Journal of Perinatal Medicine* **17**:393–398.

42 Radunovich N, Lazarevic B (1989) Cordocentesis – a new diagnostic approach in modern perinatology. *Jugosl-Ginekol-Perinatol* **29**:161–164.

43 Bovicelli L, Orsimi LF, Grannum PAT, Pittalis MC, Tolfoli C, Dolcini B (1989) A new funi-puncture technique. Two-needle ultrasound and needle biopsy-guided procedure. *Obstetrics and Gynecology* **73**:215–218.

44 Perry KG, Hess LW, Roberts WE, Albert JR, Floyd RC, McCaul JF, Martin RW, Martin JN, Morrison JC (1991) Cordocentesis (Funipuncture) by materno-fetal fellows: The learning curve. *Fetal Diagnosis and Therapy* **6**:87–92.

45 Pielet BW, Socol ML, MacGreggor SV, Ney J, Rooderg L (1988) Cordocentesis: An appraisal of risks. *American Journal of Obstetrics and Gynecology* **159**:1497–1500.

46 Maeda H, Shimokawa H, Satoh S, Yanagudi Y, Hisanaga S, Koyanagi T, Nakano H (1990) Safety of cordocentesis under ultrasound guidance for fetal blood sampling. *Nippon-Sanka-Fujunka-Gakkai-Zasshi* **42**:199–202.

47 Maxwell D, Johnson P, Hurley P, Neales K, Allan L, Knott P (1991) Fetal blood sampling and pregnancy loss in relation to indication. *British Journal of Obstetrics and Gynecology* **98**:892–897.

48 Weiner CP, Wenston KD, Siper SL, Williamson RA (1991) Risk factors for cordocentesis and fetal intravascular transfusion. *American Journal of Obstetrics and Gynecology* **165**:1020–1025.

42

Fetal Growth Deficiency and its Evaluation

CARL P. WEINER

DEFINITION

Body Weight vs Mass

Growth deficiency may be defined either by body weight or mass. Birthweight, by virtue of its ease and availability, is most popular worldwide. Neonates below the third or tenth percentile for gestation are generally considered growth-deficient. The phrase 'growth deficiency' is preferred to 'growth retardation', which has undesirable connotations to the lay public. The assignment of a birthweight percentile requires an accurate assessment of gestational age and the availability of tables appropriate for the population with adjustments for gender, race and birth order.[1] Neonates classified as growth-deficient by birthweight percentile may indeed be malnourished, but they may also be misdated or well-nourished and short. The thin but tall neonate may have a birthweight percentile above that used to define growth deficiency, yet still be malnourished and at risk for perinatal morbidity and mortality.

The diagnosis of growth deficiency is best made by an index of body mass like the Ponderal Index [Birthweight (g)/crown heel length^3) × 100].[2] The Ponderal Index is independent of gender, race, birth order and, to a certain extent, gestational age. And while a fetus who is proportionally thin and short may have a normal Ponderal Index, it can usually be identified by a small head circumference.

These two definitions of growth deficiency identify different groups of neonates. In one study, 40% of the infants with a birthweight percentile less than the tenth were not growth-deficient by their Ponderal Index;[3] 50% of infants identified as growth-deficient by the Ponderal Index had average birthweight percentiles. From a clinical perspective, the Ponderal Index is more closely correlated with perinatal morbidity and mortality than is the birthweight percentile.[4] Appropriate categorization of growth deficiency is essential if accurate postnatal follow-up studies are to be completed.

ETIOLOGY AND RISK FACTORS

Normal fetal growth occurs by a sequential process of cellular hyperplasia, hyperplasia plus hypertrophy and, lastly, by hypertrophy alone.[5] Growth deficiency is the end result of numerous pathologies which reduce fetal cell size and, when early and severe enough, cell number. The loss of cell number is not generally corrected after delivery and these children remain small. Broadly categorized, causes of growth dediciency include fetal, maternal, uterine and placental disorders (**Figure 1**). Risk factors for growth deficiency common to any obstetric practice include smoking and maternal vascular disease.

PATHOPHYSIOLOGY OF FETAL GROWTH DEFICIENCY

While a large number of animal studies over the past two decades have provided important background

757

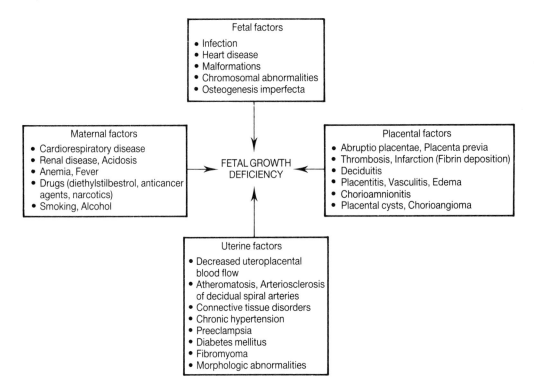

Figure 1. Causes of growth deficiency.

information on fetal growth deficiency, they were conducted upon intrinsically normal fetuses growing within an intrinisically normal uterus. Growth deficiency was produced variously by uterine artery banding, microsphere embolization of the placenta via either the fetal or maternal circulation, surgical reduction of the number of ovine placentomes or chronic maternal hypoxia (reviewed in reference **6**). The degree of hypoxemia which developed was small and not generally accompanied by hypercapnia. Fetal hypoglycemia occurred, but the lactate concentration was low or normal.[7,8]

Recently, it has become possible to study the moderate to severely growth-deficient human fetus at steady-state using both non-invasive and invasive techniques. Non-cardiac and cardiac Doppler studies demonstrate an initial increase in cardiac output coupled with a redistribution of blood to organs essential for fetal survival.[9–13] When oxygen transport is also hindered, the fetal cerebral vasculature dilates and blood flow increases. These protective responses fail with time and cardiac output falls.[14] Head growth, which had been relatively spared, slows. The decreasing resistance to cerebral blood flow ultimately causes shunting of desaturated blood away from the trunk (and therefore placenta) to the brain. *There is no animal model for growth deficiency which parallels the spontaneous human event.* As a rule, the earlier the onset of the

disease process, the more likely the fetus will be symmetrically small (decreased cell number) and the more likely the etiology is either a severe maternal vascular disorder, a fetal infection or chromosome disorder.[15]

Blood specimens obtained by cordocentesis reveal that 40–60% of fetuses with detectable growth deficiency prior to 34 weeks have hypoxemia.[16–18] There is a strong correlation between fetal hypoxemia and the Doppler measured flow resistances of the uterine arcuate artery, umbilical artery, internal carotid artery, and descending fetal aorta (see Management Options).[9–13] There are also significant correlations between fetal hypoxemia and hypercapnia, hypoaminoacidemia, hypoglycemia and hyperlactic acidemia.[19,20] This suggests that placental dysfunction which results in early-onset growth deficiency alters both substrate and gas transport. The observation that intravenous glucose adminstration *in utero* causes a significant decline in blood pH of growth-deficient but not appropriately grown fetuses, indicates that placental oxygen transport is fixed and cannot be increased acutely in response to a sudden increase in substrate availability.[21] There are other abnormalities which accompany human fetal growth deficiency which may affect the distribution and resistance to blood flow. These include significant increases in the circulating concentrations of arginine, vasopressin, norepinephrine, epinephrine and PGF_{2a} (reference **22** and unpublished observations). Many are directly related to the severity of acid-base disturbance. These studies of growth-deficient human fetuses confirm that the animal models currently available are not necessarily reflective of the naturally occurring human disorder and demonstrate that birth asphyxia is not always due to parturition, but frequently precedes labor by many weeks.

Once hypoxemia develops, it is progressive in the absence of an intervention which alters the intrauterine milieu. Fetal heart rate abnormalities are the norm when the umbilical venous pH declines much below 7.33, an extremely abnormal pH for the fetus at steady state (**Figure 2**). Further, recent studies suggest that the chronically hypoxemic fetus suffers childhood deficits in intellectual development proportional to the severity of the prenatal acidemia.[23]

The cause of the increased resistance to placental blood flow in many fetuses with growth deficiency is unknown. Elevated resistance may be secondary to ultrastructural damage (e.g. fibrosis, placentitis), loss of adaptive mechanisms secondary to chronic hypox-

emia, the presence of elevated concentrations of circulating substances like AVP or PGF_{2a} which increase placental and fetal resistance and speed decompensation, or a combination of the three. The observation that low-dose aspirin slows the rate of 'placental deterioration' in fetuses with modestly but not severely elevated Doppler resistances is potentially consistent with any of the possibilities.[24]

SCREENING OPTIONS FOR GROWTH DEFICIENCY

Biochemical

At least three hormone/protein markers measured in the maternal sera have been suggested as markers of growth deficiency: estriol, human placental lactogen and alpha-fetoprotein (AFP). Each of these is reviewed in Chapter 37. In summary, the maternal serum AFP

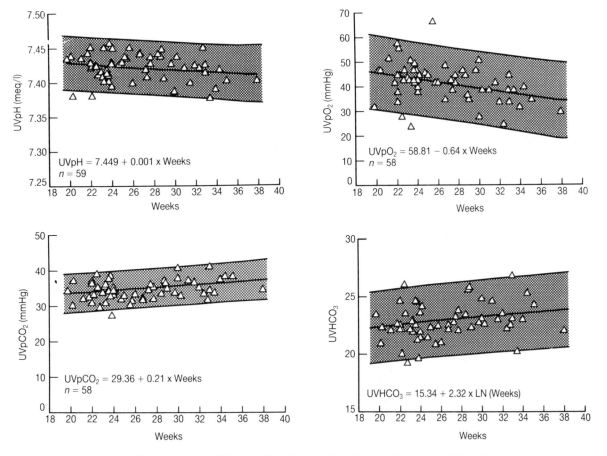

Figure 2. Normal umbilical venous pH (top left), pO_2 (top right), pCO_2 (bottom left) and base excess (bottom right), illustrated as the 95% prediction interval across gestation. Reproduced with permission from Weiner *et al.*[55]

is most useful clinically. In most studies, a single unexplained elevated value raises the risk of growth deficiency five- to ten-fold.

Clinical

As detailed in Chapter 3, the maternal uterine fundus should be objectively measured and charted during each prenatal visit. After 20 weeks gestation, the normal fundal height in centimeters approximates the number of weeks gestation after appropriate allowances for maternal height and the fetal station are made. However, the measurement of fundal height is only a low-cost screening tool. Its accuracy for the overall prediction of growth deficiency is not good; for example, the reported figures for fundal-symphysial height measurements vary between 60–85% for sensitivity, 80–90% for specificity and 20–80% for positive predictive value. Though a small fundus does not necessarily mean a small fetus, a significant size less than dates discrepancy is associated with growth deficiency. Further, the accuracy of a sonographic prediction is enhanced if there is a clinical suspicion of growth deficiency.

Ultrasound

The interpretation of a growth study is based upon the absolute measurement, the percentile rank for the assigned gestational age, and the interval growth since the last study. Each is important. For example, uteroplacental dysfunction is an unlikely explanation for the fetus whose measurements are in a low percentile but whose interval growth over time remains appropriate. This pattern is more consistent with a genetically small but appropriately nourished fetus. The use of percentiles in the evaluation of fetal growth renders table selection critical. Since the goal is to identify the malnourished or poorly growing fetus, the table selected should be based on uncomplicated pregnancies delivered at term.

The adequacy of fetal growth cannot be determined by a single sonographic examination without a preexisting estimate of gestational age. Even after several examinations, the assessment of fetal growth is facilitated by knowledge of the likely gestational age, since the rate of growth for several parameters varies with age. Because fetal morphology varies with both the timing of onset and etiology of the growth deficiency, no single sonographic method can possibly suffice for diagnosis. Likewise, knowledge of the fetal morphology can provide clues as to how the diagnostic workup should proceed.

All commonly used sonographic tables are based on women with a known last menstrual period rather than the date of ovulation or conception. It is essential to remember that the accuracy of menstrual dates is ±3 weeks, and that the last menstrual period is uncertain in 20–40% of gravidas who state recall of the day.[25,26] This reflects both the normal physiologic variation in the ovulatory cycle and misinterpretation of implantation bleeding as menses by either patient or caregiver. The sonographic estimate of fetal age in a patient with regular menses (and thus the diagnosis of growth deficiency) cannot be more accurate than the data from which the ultrasound tables were derived. Other potential and common variables such as oral contraception, breast-feeding or a limited number of coital exposures should be promptly sought when differences arise between the menstrual and sonographic estimates. Since the normal variation among fetuses increases as gestation advances, the accuracy of the sonographic age estimate must diminish. *If the sonographic estimate of age is within the predictive error of the ultrasound measurement for that gestational age, the assigned age is the menstrual age.* Once the estimated date of confinement (EDC) is set by an adequate early ultrasound examination (whether or not it agrees with the stated menses), it does not change even if subsequent measurements deviate from those expected. There is no reason to confuse either the physician, the patient or the growth study by altering the assigned EDC after each examination or by listing several different EDCs in the data column of the report.

It has been suggested that the performance of ultrasound routinely twice during pregnancy will greatly enhance the identification of growth-deficient fetuses and thus improve outcome.[27] In many parts of the world, this is already standard practice. Though it is argued that the number of growth-deficient fetuses identified is increased, the costs and benefits of the practice are less clear.[28,29]

Measurements

Biparietal diameter

Though popular and easy to measure, the biparietal diameter (BPD) is far from ideal. The physiologic variation with advancing gestation is high, the fall off in cranial growth with nutritional deficiency late, and the shape of the cranium readily altered by external forces (oligohydramnios, breech presentation, etc.).[30] Further, a technically adequate BPD cannot be had if the fetal head is oriented in a direct anterior/posterior position.

Head circumference (**Table 1**)

The head circumference is not subject to the extrinsic variability of the BPD. Most of the current generation of ultrasound equipment permits either the calculation

Table 1
Normal head circumference measurements across gestation

	Percentile ranks of head circumference (cm)[a]				
Week[b]	10	25	50	75	90
18	14.0	16.5	16.0	17.0	17.5
19	15.0	16.0	17.0	17.5	18.0
20	16.0	17.0	18.0	18.5	19.0
21	17.0	18.0	19.0	19.5	20.0
22	18.0	19.0	20.0	20.5	21.0
23	19.5	20.0	21.0	21.5	22.0
24	21.0	21.5	22.0	22.5	23.0
25	22.0	22.5	23.0	23.5	24.0
26	23.0	23.5	24.0	24.5	25.0
27	24.0	26.0	26.0	26.5	27.0
28	25.5	26.0	27.0	27.5	28.0
29	26.5	27.0	28.0	29.0	29.5
30	27.0	27.5	28.5	29.0	30.5
31	27.0	28.0	29.0	30.0	31.0
32	27.5	28.0	29.0	30.0	31.5
33	28.0	28.5	29.5	30.5	32.0
34	28.5	29.0	30.5	31.5	32.5
35	29.5	30.0	31.5	32.0	33.0
36	30.0	31.0	32.0	33.0	34.0
37	30.5	31.5	32.5	33.5	35.0
38	30.5	31.5	32.5	34.0	35.0
39	31.0	32.0	33.0	34.5	35.0
40	31.5	32.5	33.5	34.5	35.5
41	32.0	33.0	34.0	34.5	36.0

Reproduced with permission from Sabbagha.[31]
[a]Measured directly from tracings in the screen of ultrasound machines or, alternatively, by digitizer from photographs.
[b]Menstrual weeks of pregnancy (adapted from Tamura et al.[56]).

of, or on-screen measurement of, the circumference. The method by which the HC is determined is important, since calculated HCs are systematically smaller than those measured directly.[31]

Abdominal circumference (**Table 2**)

Encompassing the liver, the abdominal circumference (AC) is the single best and clinically most useful reflection of fetal nourishment.[32] Of any growth parameter, the abdominal circumference percentile has both the highest sensitivity and greatest negative predictive value for the prenatal diagnosis of growth deficiency, whether defined by the birthweight percentile or the Ponderal Index.[3] Because of its high sensitivity, some type of abdominal measurement should be part of each sonographic examination. *But since the abdominal circumference reflects the fetal nutrition, it should be excluded as a parameter in the gestational age estimate after the early second trimester.*

The most accurate AC is the smallest one obtained between fetal respirations at the level of the hepatic vein, since the smallest perimeter will be that closest to the plane perpendicular to the spine. A measured circumference is preferable to either a calculated circumference or the sum of several diameters, since the shape of the fetal abdomen is often irregular.[33] Like bony measurements, the circumference of the healthy fetus usually grows within a fixed percentile range. Any abrupt change in the percentile, especially an increase, should be viewed with suspicion, and the possibility of an oblique cut through the abdomen considered.

If a table based exclusively on healthy women delivering appropriately nourished neonates at term is used (**Table 2**), an AC > 2.5 percentile for gestational age is inconsistent with growth deficiency no matter how defined postnatally.[3] Unfortunately, the positive predictive value of an AC percentile 52.5 for growth deficiency is about 50% in any given population. Thus, we are loath to label these fetuses 'growth-deficient' unless the circumference is *considerably* below the 2.5 percentile or another parameter such as the sonographic estimate of weight is also abnormal. The managing physician is informed that the biometric parameters are consistent with, but not necessarily diagnostic of, intrauterine growth deficiency. If less than 36 weeks gestation, an additional growth study is obtained in 2–3 weeks. A closer interval will not yield additional information on growth. If there has been continued growth but the AC is still below the 2.5 percentile, the study is repeated 2–3 weeks later.

Transverse cerebellar diameter

The transverse cerebellar diameter is one of the few soft tissue measurements which correlates well with gestational age,[34] being relatively spared from the effects of mild to moderate malnourishment. Whether its measurement offers any advantage over bone measurements in the assessment of compromised fetal growth remains controversial.[35,36]

Ratios

In 1977, Campbell and Thomas reported that some 70% of neonates with asymmetric growth deficiency had an HC/AC ration 2 SDs above the norm.[37] However, subsequent study revealed that both the sensitivity and the positive predictive value of this parameter for growth deficiency is worse than either the AC percentile or the sonographic estimated fetal weight (SEFW).[3,27,38] In light of the superiority of the AC percentile and SEFW, it is difficult to justify reliance on this ratio as either a screen for, or the diagnosis of, growth deficiency.

Table 2
Normal abdominal circumference measurements across gestation

Weeks of gestation	Percentile								
	2.5	5	10	25	50	75	90	95	97.5
18	9.8	10.3	10.6	11.8	13.1	14.2	14.5	15.9	16.4
19	11.1	11.6	12.3	13.3	14.4	15.6	15.9	17.2	17.8
20	12.1	12.6	13.3	14.3	15.4	16.6	16.9	18.2	18.8
21	13.7	14.2	14.8	15.9	17.0	18.1	18.4	19.8	20.3
22	14.7	15.2	15.8	16.9	18.0	19.1	19.4	20.8	21.3
23	16.0	16.5	17.1	18.2	19.3	20.4	20.7	22.1	22.6
24	17.2	17.7	18.3	19.4	20.5	21.6	21.9	23.3	23.8
25	18.0	18.5	19.1	20.2	21.3	22.4	22.7	24.1	24.6
26	18.8	19.3	19.9	21.0	22.1	23.2	23.5	24.9	25.4
27	25.4	20.9	21.5	22.6	23.7	24.8	25.1	26.5	27.0
28	22.0	22.5	23.1	24.2	25.3	26.4	26.7	28.1	28.6
29	23.6	24.1	24.7	25.8	26.9	28.0	28.3	29.7	30.2
30	24.1	24.6	25.2	26.3	27.4	28.5	28.8	30.2	30.7
31	24.7	26.2	25.8	26.8	28.0	28.1	29.4	30.0	31.3
32	25.4	25.9	20.0	27.0	28.7	30.8	30.1	31.5	32.0
33	25.7	20.2	20.0	27.0	20.0	30.1	30.4	31.8	32.3
34	26.8	27.3	27.9	29.0	30.1	31.2	31.5	32.0	33.1
35	28.9	29.4	30.0	31.1	32.2	33.3	33.3	35.0	36.5
36	30.0	30.5	31.1	32.2	33.3	34.4	34.7	36.1	36.6
37	31.1	31.6	32.2	33.3	34.4	35.5	35.8	37.2	37.7
38	32.4	32.9	33.5	34.6	35.7	36.8	37.1	38.5	39.0
39	32.6	33.1	33.7	34.8	35.9	37.0	37.3	38.7	39.2
40	32.8	33.3	33.9	35.0	36.1	37.2	37.5	38.9	39.4

Reproduced with permission from Tamura and Sabbagha.[32]

The cephalic index is the ratio of the BPD/occipito-frontal diameters. Proposed as an age-independent aid for the identification of dolichocephaly and brachiocephaly,[32] its current practical value is limited. Dolichocephaly is rare prior to the third trimester, and the ability to measure the head circumference easily has eliminated the need to recognize mild degrees of either dolichocephaly or brachiocephaly as it relates to the prediction of gestational age. It has also been proposed as an aid for the diagnosis of trisomy 21. The sonographic signs of aneuploidy will not be reviewed here.

The ratio of femur length to head circumference (FL/HC) was originally proposed as a tool to identify either short-limbed dwarfism, hydrocephaly or microcephaly.[39] However, enhanced sonographic capabilities have rendered it unnecessary for the diagnosis of hydrocephaly, unnecessary for the diagnosis of dwarfism since the fetal limbs are well below the tenth centile for gestation, and unnecessary for the diagnosis of microcephaly which is most accurately made when the HC is 3 SDs or more below the mean. Because the sonographic FL correlates with the neonatal crown heel length (CHL), it would be attractive if the FL could be used to generate an index of fetal mass. Unfortu-

nately, all attempts to date have failed to yield clinically useful results.

The FL/AC ratio was suggested as a poor man's *in utero* Ponderal Index,[40,41] but in prospective trials has had lower sensitivity, specificity, positive and negative predictive values for the diagnosis of a malnourished fetus than either the AC percentile or the sonographic estimate of fetal weight.[3]

Sonographic estimated fetal weight

A large number of general-purpose and special application formulas have been devised. Several of the more reliable ones are listed in **Table 3**. The accuracy of most (±2 SDs) is 10%. An estimation of the fetal weight does not routinely add to the abdominal circumference percentile for the diagnosis of growth deficiency. It does, however, add a graphic image easy for both patient and referring physician to conceptualize. And while its sensitivity for the identification of the malnourished fetus is considerably lower than the AC percentile, the positive predictive value of a fetal weight estimate below the tenth percentile is gre-

Table 3
Example formulas validated prospectively for the sonographic estimate of fetal weight

Parameters		Formula	Reference
General			
BPD, AC	$\log_{10}$ BW =	$-1.7492 + (0.166/(BPD) + 0.46(AC) - 2.646(AC \times BPD)/1000$	**52**
AC, FL	$\log_{10}$ BW =	$1.3598 + 0.051(AC) + 0.1844(FL) - 0.0037(AC \times FL)$	**53**
HC, AC, FL	$\log_{10}$ BW =	$1.5662 - 0.0108(HC) + 0.0468(AC) + 0.171(FL) + 0.00034(HC)^2$	
		$- 0.003685(AC \times FL)$	**53**
<2200 g			
HC, AC, FL	$\log_{10}$ BW =	$1.6961 + 0.02253(HC) + 0.01645(AC) + 0.06439(FL)$	**54**

BPD, biparietal dimaeter; HC, head circumference; AC, abdominal circumference; FL, femur length.

ater. As a rule, the fetus should not be labeled growth-deficient unless both the AC and SEFW percentiles are below their respective norms. Though management will be altered in either instance (see below), it is better not to worry the patient unnecessarily with a label that has a 50% chance of being wrong if only the AC is small.

DIAGNOSIS AND EVALUATION OF FETAL GROWTH DEFICIENCY

The diagnosis of fetal growth deficiency requires three elements. First, the clinician needs an impression of gestational age that whenever possible is not based solely on a sonographic estimate. Second, the clinician needs to understand what constitutes normal and abnormal growth and the *basis* for those standards. The final requirement for the diagnosis of growth deficiency is the measurement of objective fetal parameters.

The postnatal definition of growth deficiency is of pragmatic concern as it impacts upon the accuracy of prenatal diagnosis. For example, the thin fetus whose estimated fetal weight is normal, might still be classified as growth-deficient by the Ponderal Index. Each practitioner must be aware of the diagnostic criteria used in their hospital and encourage their colleagues not to rely exclusively on the birthweight percentiles.

'Asymmetric' or 'symmetric' growth deficiency are descriptive terms and not a diagnosis. More relevant than symmetry is the timing of onset. Late-onset growth deficiency, i.e. that which is detected after 32 weeks gestation unassociated with a fetal structural malformation, is usually the result of uteroplacental dysfunction. These fetuses are slender with a normal head circumference and body length. Dysfunction is chosen over the more frequently used term 'insufficiency', since the later connotes inadequate blood flow which is frequently not the case. It is defined as nutrient and oxygen exchange at the maternal–fetal interface that is inadequate to support normal growth and aerobic metabolism. In contrast to late-onset growth deficiency, early-onset growth deficiency is frequently associated with aneuploidy, congenital infection or severe uteroplacental dysfunction such as that accompanying maternal disease or abnormal placentation (**Table 4**). Though these fetuses may be symmetrically small when delivered weeks or months later, they often are not when first identified. Based on that understanding, it may be assumed that the symmetrically small fetus identified at 34 weeks is likely to have early-onset growth deficiency and should be evaluated as such.

Two-dimensional Ultrasound

A fetus is considered at risk for growth deficiency when its AC percentile is less than 2.5, but its estimated weight is still above the tenth percentile. The diagnosis is made when both the AC percentile and the estimated weight are both abnormally low. Since fetuses with suspected growth deficiency and those with the diagnosis are followed similarly, and the accuracy of the diagnosis based on the AC or estimated

Table 4
Etiology of severe intrauterine growth deficiency, University of Iowa, 1984–1992

Diagnosis	n	%
1. Severe uteroplacental dysfunction (diagnosis by exclusion)	62	54.9
2. Chromosome abnormality	22	19.5
3. Associated structural malformations	13	11.5
4. Congenital infection	9	
proven	7	6.2
likely	2	1.8
5. Miscellaneous	7	6.2
Total	113	

weight alone is only about 50%, there is no need to worry the parents unnecessarily by basing the diagnosis on a single parameter.

Fetal Echocardiography

Fetal echocardiography may ultimately serve several roles in the assessment of abnormal fetal growth. The *first* is in the evaluation of severe, early-onset growth deficiency. In approximately 20%, the etiology is a chromosome abnormality. Though half are lethal, the fetus with trisomy 21 may pose philosophic problems for physician and patient. In this instance, knowledge that the fetus has a major atrioventricular canal defect might lead the parents in one direction or another concerning either pregnancy termination or cesarean section for fetal distress.

Second, fetal echocardiography may aid the timing of delivery. A recent cross-sectional and longitudinal study of fetuses with uteroplacental dysfunction has permitted characterization of the fetal cardiac adaptation to hypoxemia.[14] Left cardiac output rises to a point and then begins to decline. Shortly thereafter, the fetal blood gases deteriorate and heart rate patterns usually suggest the need for immediate delivery. Should these pathophysiologic studies be confirmed, the logical time for delivery would be when decompensation is detected.

Doppler Velocimetry

Over the last decade, most uterine and fetal vascular beds of healthy and growth-deficient fetuses have been examined with non-cardiac Doppler ultrasound. There is now abundant evidence that the fetus responds to a variety of pathologic stresses by altering blood flow.[9–14] Though the contribution of these human studies to our understanding of fetal pathophysiology is significant, the clinical role of non-cardiac Doppler ultrasound in the overall evaluation of fetal growth disturbances remains unclear. Part of the clinical problem has been the diffuse nature of the published investigations. Investigators have sought to predict a variety of neonatal outcomes with disparate etiologies using a single parameter such as an umbilical artery resistance index. Not surprisingly, the positive and negative predictive values have been unsatisfactory.

There is an inverse relationship between the fetal pO_2 and the Doppler-measured resistance to flow in the uterine arcuate and umbilical arteries, and a direct relationship in the carotid artery.[9–14] Unfortunately, there is a great deal of overlap between the measurements obtained from normal and growth-deficient fetuses. Because of that overlap, Doppler studies should only be used (with one exception described below) as adjuncts to the growth examination. Thus, the presence of a normal umbilical artery Doppler resistance index is a very reassuring sign from the standpoint of acid–base balance. Further, a normal umbilical artery resistance index associated with severe or early-onset growth deficiency renders aneuploidy or severe uteroplacental insufficiency less likely explanations. Unfortunately, the same cannot be said for an elevated index. The one exception where a Doppler measurement is important for clinical management is the fetus with *persistently* absent or reversed umbilical artery diastolic flow. In the setting of severe fetal growth deficiency, normal anatomy and a heart rate above 100 beats/min, it is predictably associated with hypoxemia. In the absence of intervention, these fetuses usually die within 7 days of the observation.

Management Options

Prenatal

Patients at risk for growth deficiency

A number of women may be identified at increased risk of fetal growth deficiency in early pregnancy (**Figure 1**). Fetuses with a normal sonographic estimated weight but a small AC percentile may be at risk for growth deficiency. It is recommended that these pregnancies be followed in the same way as those complicated by late-onset growth deficiency (see below). Identification of the growth-deficient fetus is the beginning of the task, not the end.

Late-onset growth deficiency

The most frequent etiology of growth deficiency first identified after 32 weeks is mild to moderate uteroplacental dysfunction secondary to a variety of causes. Uteroplacental dysfunction is defined as inadequate nutrient and oxygen supply to support normal growth and aerobic metabolism. The prenatal management of these pregnancies can be summarized as close supervision with delivery for evidence of either acute or chronic fetal compromise, or elective delivery after 36 completed weeks. In the interim, prenatal fetal surveillance of the type locally preferred is initiated. If the membranes are intact, it is usually not necessary to assess the amniotic fluid volume more than once a week, since it is a reflection of chronicity. Oligohydramnios after 34 weeks is an indication for delivery even if the fetal heart rate tracing is appropriate and the cervix not ideal for the induction of labor. The sonographic growth study is repeated at 2-week intervals if discovered prior to 36 weeks.

Therapy: The first step in the treatment of growth deficiency is to reduce or eliminate any potential external contributors such as stress, smoking, etc., and to encourage maternal rest in a lateral position. Though not of proven efficacy, these should maximize uterine blood flow. Low-dose aspirin significantly improves the outcome of fetuses with growth deficiency secondary to uteroplacental dysfunction characterized by an umbilical artery Doppler index greater than 2 but less than 5 SDs above the gestational age norm.[24] Its value in the woman at risk will become clearer after the completion of randomized trials currently taking place.

Early-onset growth deficiency

Early-onset growth deficiency is that identifiable prior to 32 weeks, or symmetric growth deficiency identified at any gestational age. In the absence of maternal systemic or cardiovascular disease, the principle differential diagnoses are:

- congenital infection

- chromosome or other abnormality

- uteroplacental dysfunction (by exclusion).

Determination of the specific etiology prior to delivery is important to both patient and physician. **Figure 3** illustrates a diagnostic and management scheme which

seeks both a definitive diagnosis and delivery under the most optimal circumstances. The decision to perform a cordocentesis and its timing are controversial. Only a fetal blood sample can provide in any tertiary hospital a karyotype within 48 hours, a comprehensive search for fetal infection, and an evaluation of the fetal acid–base staus. Unfortunately, the presence of early-onset growth deficiency also increases the risk of cordocentesis in proportion to the severity of the hypoxemia.[42] There is a 1:5 chance that a severely growth-deficient fetus will experience a bradycardiac episode during cordocentesis. The patient and physician should decide in advance whether an emergency cesarean section is to be performed in the event of a sustained bradycardia. Furthermore, a proportion of these fetuses will be thrombocytopenic. Cordocentesis should be performed in close proximity to a delivery suite and only by individuals trained in surgical delivery. As a rule, fetal heart rate testing is not performed in our unit until karyotype has returned, even if a modest metabolic acidemia is documented. Maternal hyperoxygenation may be used until the karyotype returns (see below). The decision not to monitor and risk an intrauterine demise during the 48–72 hour interval necessary for the karyotype to be completed must ultimately be made by the parents. *Because of its risks in the setting of severe growth deficiency, repetitive cordocenteses are not recommended to monitor acid–base status.*

In our experience, almost 20% of fetuses with early-onset growth deficiency have a chromosome abnor-

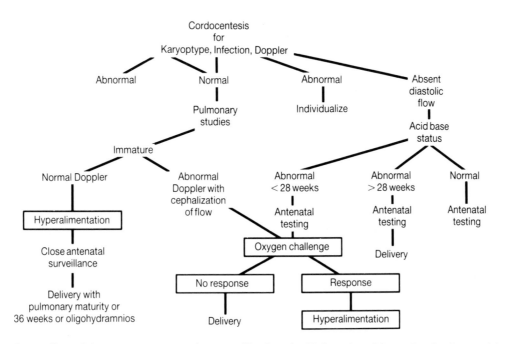

Figure 3. An outline of the management scheme utilized at the University of Iowa for the fetus with severe, early-onset growth deficiency. Those items enclosed in boxes are either of theoretic interest or are presently under investigation and should not be considered mainstream obstetric care.

mality (**Table 4**). The presence of a co-existent structural malformation raises the risk of a chromosome abnormality. Should aneuploidy be the explanation, the cause and risk of recurrence are known, helping to reduce the inevitable parental soul-searching and guilt feelings which accompany a perinatal loss and certainly influence management. *At the very minimum, a karyotype should be obtained on almost every fetus with severe, early-onset growth deficiency.* Some authors have suggested that a placental biopsy is the best way of obtaining this for reasons of speed and safety. Unfortunately, most laboratories still take 5–7 days to obtain a karyotype from a placental biopsy. The diagnosis of a structural anomaly incompatible with survival eliminates the need for extensive prenatal monitoring and the high chance of cesarean section for fetal indications.

In our experience, a viral agent can be identified, in about 5% of fetuses with early-onset growth deficiency. In another 2% of fetuses, congenital infection is suspected, but a specific agent cannot be identified. Considering the population from which the University of Iowa draws its patients, this incidence will likely be higher in urban centers. Congenital viral infection is detailed in Chapter 49. The actual diagnosis of fetal infection remains problematic. The diagnosis of congenital infection is considered a strong possibility when a severely growth-deficient fetus has a normal blood gas in association with either a high or low white blood cell or platelet count. The fetal lactic dehydrogenase (LDH), gamma-glutamyl transpeptidase (GGT) and asparatate transaminase (AST) are often elevated. it is important for the clinician to bear in mind that transaminases are also elevated in hypoxemic, severely growth-deficient fetuses associated with either aneuploidy or uteroplacental dysfunction. While IgM is routinely quantitated when infection is part of the differential diagnosis, the yield is low. IgM may be normal or only transiently elevated in the infected fetus.[43] A low IgM concentration can even be masked by maternal IgG and not revealed until the IgG is separated. The diagnosis of fetal infection may also be made by identifying viral particles by electron microscopy in fetal ascites and serum. If the viral morphology is known, a more selective serologic analysis can be performed. The optimum management if the diagnosis is viral infection is controversial.

Fetuses whose growth deficiency is secondary to either aneuploidy or uteroplacental dysfunction are indistinguishable by their blood gas measurements. Since normally grown aneuploid fetuses do not display the same abnormalities, aneuploidy is not itself the sole cause of the hypoxemia. However, the appropriately grown aneuploid group are less likely to have a trisomy, suggesting that the early-onset growth deficiency associated with aneuploidy reflects an intrinsic abnormality of placental function secondary

to placental trisomy. Fetuses whose growth deficiency is secondary to congenital infection have normal umbilical venous blood gas measurements in the absence of placentitis. Regardless of etiology, growth deficiency is associated with polycythemia. In the absence of an acute viral infection, the reticulocyte counts are low to normal, suggesting a chronic process likely to be stimulated by tissue hypoxia with the release of erythropoietin. Macrocytoses is typical of the trisomic and triploid fetus and a normal mean corpuscular volume renders the diagnosis of trisomy or triploidy extremely unlikely (**Figure 4**).[44,45]

Though specific treatments for fetal infection have yet to be evaluated, prenatal diagnosis is still valuable. Since the fetal response to infection is often transient, the opportunity to identify the etiology may be lost and the neonate inappropriately excluded from specific follow-up if the diagnostic efforts are delayed several weeks until delivery. Further, these neonates are usually actively shedding virus. For the protection of susceptible nursing mothers and staff, they should be isolated. Finally, congenitally infected, growth-deficient fetuses are usually well-oxygenated, thus extensive prenatal testing is usually unnecessary and the need for early intervention in the absence of oligohydramnios less likely.

Treatment: In addition to those measures listed under late-onset growth deficiency, consideration should be given to hospitalized bedrest which has several advantages over bedrest at home. *First*, even the most motivated patient will, after the passage of time, rest less and less. Family support may be so poor that the patient has little chance to rest. In the hospital, there is no such problem. *Second*, hospitalization facilitates daily fetal testing.

Growth deficiency secondary to uteroplacental dysfunction is the most common fetal disorder potentially

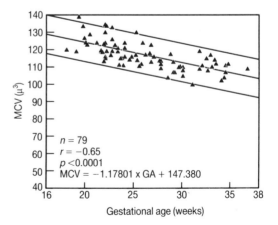

Figure 4. Normal fetal mean corpuscular volume measurements illustrated as the 95% prediction interval across gestation. Reproduced with permission from Sipes *et al.*[45]

amenable to direct fetal therapy. Though a fetus with mild to moderate growth deficiency will not be considered a candidate for the next few decades, the techniques to increase both nutrient and oxygen delivery to the fetus exist now. Whether such activities will be successful in instances of severe growth deficiency are unknown. It is clear that the hypoxemic fetus will not be a candidate unless the supply of oxygen can be increased.

Attempts have been made to prolong the gestation of very premature, acidemic, growth-deficient fetuses by administering oxygen by mask to the women.[46] In several reports, this approach has been associated with a short-term correction of the acidemia but without a clear improvement in outcome.[47–50] Many fundamental issues remain unclear, such as patient selection, efficacy and the requisite testing needed to monitor the fetus during therapy. Until these are resolved maternal oxygen supplementation should be viewed as experimental therapy.

Treatment of the congenitally infected, growth-deficient fetus remains in the distant future. It requires the development of sophisticated diagnostic techniques, the completion of long-term follow-up studies of congenitally infected infants diagnosed prenatally so that the prognosis is clear, and an ability to treat the viral infection itself. Palliative therapy has been tried.[51] One fetus determined prenatally to have non-immune hydrops secondary to viral myocarditis died despite responding initially to treatment with an ionotropic agent. Though the hydrops rapidly resolved, the fetus succumbed from progressive cardiac destruction. Another fetus with cytomegalic virus infection was treated directly with an infusion of gancyclovir. Though the viremia cleared, the fetus died prior to the onset of labor (U. Nicolini, personal communication).

Labor/delivery

Timing

The obstetric management of the patient with either presumed or demonstrated growth deficiency is controversial. Part of the controversy no doubt stems from incomplete categorization by etiology of the growth deficiency. The obstetric management will vary with etiology, the severity, and stage of gestation.

The following discussion pertains to chromosomally normal fetuses presumed to be malnourished. When the diagnosis of growth deficiency is firm, the amniotic fluid volume is within the normal range and the gestational age is 36 completed weeks or more, the patient should probably be delivered electively. The need for prior documentation of fetal pulmonary maturity and an adequate Bishop's score of the cervix is controversial. Because of the risk of an umbilical cord acci-

dent, oligohydramnios at 36 weeks or greater represents a strong indication for delivery. In most instances, delivery should be effected when repetitive late decelerations are demonstrated at any stage in gestation, or after 36 weeks with the appearance of a tracing suggestive of a vulnerable cord. If there has been no growth of a fetus with presumed growth deficiency when the sonogram is repeated in 2–3 weeks, or the estimated fetal weight is now below the tenth percentile for gestation, delivery is a consideration.

Prior to 36 weeks, delivery should be considered under the following sets of circumstances: lack of growth over 3 weeks and mature amniotic lung studies, anhydramnios at 30 weeks gestation or beyond, a persistently abnormal fetal heart rate pattern (see Chapters 39 and 62), or a BPS <6. The observation of compromised intellectual development proportional to the chronic antepartum hypoxemia/acidemia underscores the need for delivery when medically feasible. The efficacy of corticosteroids to ameliorate neonatal respiratory disease in the setting of severe growth deficiency is uncertain. However, if it appears delivery will be necessary prior to 32 weeks gestation, they should be considered. Typically, these very premature fetuses with early-onset growth deficiency are cared for on a day-to-day basis and the decision for delivery made at the last possible moment. Certainly, as the gestation advances, delivery in the absence of frank fetal distress becomes a more desirable option.

Method

Cesarean delivery without a trial of labor is indicated whenever there is evidence of acidemia prior to delivery. Evidence of presumed acidemia includes repetitive late decelerations, absent or reversed umbilical artery diastolic blood flow, or blood gas values obtained at the time of cordocentesis. Otherwise, a trial of labor should be considered first. The likelihood of success may be increased by laboring the woman in a left lateral decubitus position with supplemental oxygen

CONCLUSIONS

Uteroplacental dysfunction is the most common cause of late-onset growth deficiency. These patients are followed with weekly surveillance tests and delivered after 36 weeks unless intervention is indicated earlier. Therapy is limited to bedrest, elimination of extrinsic contributing factors, and low-dose aspirin if the umbilical artery *S/D* ratio is >2 SD but <5 SD below the mean for gestation. Whenever possible, an etiology should be sought for early-onset growth deficiency. Additional treament options are limited and delivery is considered when the risk of severe neonatal surfactant deficiency is low.

FETAL GROWTH DEFICIENCY
Summary of Management Options

Screening

Biochemical

- Most useful clinically is AFP (if raised value with no abnormality, then risk of growth deficiency is increased five- to ten-fold)

Clinical

- Fundal-symphysial height measurement reported accuracy:
     sensitivity = 60–85%
     specificity = 80–90%
     positive predicitive value = 20–80%

Ultrasound

- Controversy whether two ultrasound measurements in late pregnancy will improve detection and outcome

Diagnosis and evaluation

- Diagnosis is by ultrasound

- Exclude abnormality by:
     ultrasound
     karyotype

- Doppler velocimetry may help differentiate causes and assign fetal risk

Management

In those at risk

- Serial ultrasound scans for growth (especially head and abdomen)

Late-onset

- Serial ultrasound growth scans

- Serial biophysical assessment non-stress tests, amniotic fluid volume, biophysical profile score

Early-onset

- Detailed scan to exclude fetal anomaly

- Fetal karyotyping

- Consider fetal blood sampling for blood gases and viral infection

- Serial biophysical assessment (NST, AFV, BPS) if normal fetus

- Steroids to aid pulmonary maturation if needed

- Hospitalization, bedrest, stop smoking, etc.

- Maternal oxygenation and hyperalimentation are experimental

Labor/delivery

- When risks from prematurity are low or when fetal distress is present

- Method will be determined by gestation, fetal well-being and severity of pathology

It is important to differentiate between early- and late-onset growth deficiency. The former has a strong association with either aneuploidy, fetal infection or severe uteroplacental dysfunction. Ultrasound is the key to the diagnosis of growth deficiency, but is greatly aided by an independent assessment of gestational age. The single most sensitive parameter for the detection of fetal growth deficiency is the AC percentile, though its positive predictive value is only 50%. Fetuses with a small AC are considered to be possibly growth-deficient. Doppler ultrasound is an adjunct, of limited value, and not a guide for either diagnosis or management, with one exception: the fetus with absent or reversed diastolic flow in the umbilical artery is hypoxemic and strong consideration for delivery should be given. Many fetuses with growth deficiency are hypoxemic before the onset of labor. Chronic *in utero* hypoxemia acidemia appears to be associated with intellectual impairment postnatally.

REFERENCES

1 Hoffman HJ, Stark CR, Lundin FE, Ashbrook JD (1974) Analysis of birth weight, gestational age, and fetal viability, US births, 1968. *Obstetrical and Gynecological Survey* **29**:651.

2 Miller HC (1972) Fetal growth and neonatal mortality. *Pediatrics* **49**:392–399.

3 Weiner CP, Robinson D (1989) The sonographic diagnosis of intrauterine growth retardation using the postnatal ponderal index and the crown heel length as standards of diagnosis. *American Journal of Perinatology* **6**:380–383.

4 Walther FJ, Ramaekers LHJ (1982) The Ponderal Index as a measure of the nutritional status at birth and its relation to some aspects of neonatal morbidity. *Journal of Perinatal Medicine* **10**:42–47.

5 Winick M, Noble A (1965) Quantitative changes in DNA, RNA, and protein during prenatal and postnatal growth in the rat. *Developmental Biology* **12**:451–466.

6 Monographs in Fetal Physiology 5. *Animal Models in Fetal Medicine*. In Nathanielsz PW (Ed.): Perinatology Press, Ithaca, New York, 1984.

7 Robinson JS, Kingston EJ, Jones CT, Thorburn GD (1979) Studies on experimental growth retardation in sheep: The effect of removal of endometrial caruncles on fetal size and metabolism. *Journal of Developmental Physiology* **1**:379–398.

8 Lafeber HN (1981) Experimental intrauterine growth retardation in the guinea pig. MD thesis, University of Rotterdam.

9 Weiner CP (1990) The relationship between the umbilical artery systolic:diastolic ratio and umbilical blood gas measurements in specimens obtained by cordocentesis. *American Journal of Obstetrics and Gynecology* **162**:1198–1202.

10 Arduini D, Rizzo G, Romanini C, Mancuso S (1989) Are blood flow velocity waveforms related to umbilical cord acid-base status in the human fetus? *Gynecological and Obstetrical Investigations* **27**: 183–187.

11 Jouppila P, Kirkinen P (1984) Increased vascular resistance in the descending aorta of the human fetus in hypoxia. *British Journal of Obstetrics and Gynecology* **91**:853–856.

12 Tonge HM, Wladimiroff JW, Noordam MJ, Van Kooten C (1986) Blood flow velocity waveforms in the descending aorta: Comparison between normal and growth-retarded pregnancies. *Obstetrics and Gynecology* **67**:851.

13 Favre R, Schonenberger R, Nisand I, Lorenz U (1991) Standard curves of cerebral Doppler flow velocity waveforms and predictive values for intrauterine growth retardation and fetal acidosis. *Fetal Diagnosis and Therapy* **6**:113–119.

14 Rizzo G, Arduini D (1991) Fetal cardiac function in intrauterine growth retardation. *American Journal of Obstetrics and Gynecology* **165**:876–882.

15 Weiner CP (1989) Pathogenesis, evaluation, and potential treatments for severe, early onset growth retardation. *Seminars in Perinatology* **13**:320–327.

16 Soothill PW, Nicolaides KH, Bilardo K, Hackett GA, Campbell S (1986) Uteroplacental blood velocity resistance index and umbilical venous pO_2, pCO_2, pH, lactate and erythroblast count in growth retarded fetuses. *Fetal Therapy* **1**:176–179.

17 Pearce JM, Chamberlain GVP (1987) Ultrasonically guided percutaneous umbilical blood sampling in the management of intrauterine growth retardation. *British Journal of Obstetrics and Gynecology* **94**:318–321.

18 Weiner CP, Williamson RA (1989) Evaluation of severe growth retardation employing cordocentesis – hematologic and metabolic alterations by etiology. *Obstetrics and Gynecology* **73**:225–229.

19 Soothill PW, Nicolaides KH, Campbell S (1987) Prenatal asphyxia, hyperlactincaemia, hypoglycaemia, and erythroblastosis in growth retarded fetuses. *British Journal of Medicine* **294**:1051–1053.

20 Economides DL, Nicolaides KH, Gahl WA, Bernardini I, Evans M (1989) Plasma amino acids in appropriate and small-for-gestational-age fetuses. *American Journal of Obstetrics and Gynecology* **161**:1219–1227.

21 Nicolini U, Hubinont C, Santolaya J, Fisk NM, Rodeck CH (1990) Effects of fetal intravenous glucose challenge in normal and growth retarded fetuses. *Hormonal and Metabolic Research* **22**:426–430.

22 Weiner CP, Robillard JE (1988) Atrial natriuretic factor, digoxin-like immunoreactive substance, norepinephrine, epinephrine, and plasma renin activity in human fetuses and their alteration by fetal disease. *American Journal of Obstetrics and Gynecology* **159**:1353–1360.

23 Soothill PW, Ajuyi RA, Campbell S, Ross EM, Candy DCA, Snijders RM, Nicolaides KH (1992) Relationship between fetal acidemia at cordocentesis and subsequent neurodevelopment. *Ultrasound in Obstetrics and Gynecology* **2**:80–83.

24 Trudinger BJ, Cook CM, Thompson RS *et al.* (1988) Low-dose aspirin therapy improves fetal weight in umbilical placental insufficiency. *American Journal of Obstetrics and Gynecology* **159**:681–685.

25 Drumm JE (1977) The prediction of delivery date by

ultrasonic measurement of fetal crown-rump length. *British Journal of Obstetrics and Gynaecology* **84**:1–5.

26 Selbing A, Fjällbrant B (1984) Accuracy of conceptual age estimation from fetal crown-rump length. *Journal of Clinical Ultrasound* **12**:343–346.

27 Warsof SL, Cooper DJ, Little D, Campbell S (1986) Routine ultrasound screening for antenatal detection of intrauterine growth retardation. *Obstetrics and Gynecology* **67**:33–39.

28 Bakketeig LS, Jacobsen G, Brodtkorb CJ, Eriksen BC, Eik-Nes S, Ulstein MK, Balstad P, Jörgensen NP (1984) Randomized controlled trial of ultrasonographic screening in pregnancy. *Lancet* **i**:207–210.

29 Saari-Kemppainen A, Karjalainen O, Ylöstalo P, Heinonen OP (1990) Ultrasound screening and perinatal mortality: Controlled trial of systematic one-stage screening in pregnancy. *Lancet* **336**:387–391.

30 Hadlock FP, Deter RL et al. (1981) Estimating fetal age: Effect of head shape on BPD. *American Journal of Roentgenology* **137**:83–85.

31 Sabbagha RE (1987) Intrauterine growth retardation. In Sabbagha RE (ed.) *Diagnostic Ultrasound applied to Obstetrics and Gynecology*, 2nd edn, pp. 112–131. Philadelphia, PA: J.B. Lippincott.

32 Tamura RK, Sabbagha RE ('1980) Percentile ranks of sonar fetal abdominal circumference measurements. *American Journal of Obstetrics and Gynecology* **138**:475–479.

33 Tamura RK, Sabbagha RE, Pan WH, Vaisrub N (1986) Ultrasonic fetal abdominal circumference: Comparison of direct versus calculated measurement. *Obstetrics and Gynecology* **67**:833–835.

34 Smith PA, Johansson D, Tzannatos C, Campbell S (1986) Prenatal measurement of the fetal cerebellum and cisterna cerebellomedullaris by ultrasound. *Prenatal Diagnosis* **6**:133–141.

35 Reece EA, Goldstein I, Pilu G, Hobbins JC (1987) Fetal cerebellar growth unaffected by intrauterine growth retardation: A new parameter for prenatal diagnosis. *American Journal of Obstetrics and Gynecology* **157**:632–638.

36 Hill LM, Guzick D, Rivello D, Hixson J, Peterson C (1990) The transverse cerebellar diameter cannot be used to assess gestational age in the small for gestational age fetus. *Obstetrics and Gynecology* **75**:329–333.

37 Campbell S, Thomas A (1977) Ultrasound measurement of the fetal head to abdomen circumference ratio in the assessment of growth retardation. *British Journal of Obstetrics and Gynaecology* **84**:165–174.

38 Gray DL, Songster JGS, Parvin CA, Crane JP (1989) Cephalic index: A gestational aged dependent biometric parameter. *Obstetrics and Gynecology* **74**:600–603.

39 Hadlock FP, Harrist RB, Shah Y, Park SK (1984) The femur length/head/circumference relation in obstetric sonography. *Journal of Ultrasound Medicine* **3**:439–442.

40 Hadlock FP, Deter RL, Harrist RB, Roecker E, Park SK (1983) A data-independent predictor of intrauterine growth retardation: Femur length/abdominal circumference ratio. *American Journal of Roentgenology* **141**:979–984.

41 Sarmandal P, Grant JM (1990) Effectiveness of ultra-sound determination of fetal abdominal circumference and fetal ponderal index in the diagnosis of asymmetrical growth reatrdation. *British Journal of Obstetrics and Gynaecology* **97**:118.

42 Weiner CP, Wenstrom KD, Sipes SL, Williamson RA (1991) Risk factors for cordocentesis and intravascular transfusion. *American Journal of Obstetrics and Gynecology* **165**:1020–1023.

43 Weiner CP, Grose CF, Naides SJ (1993) Diagnosis of fetal infection in a patient with an abnormal ultrasound examination and without a positive clinical history. *American Journal of Obstetrics and Gynecology* **168**:6–11.

44 Nicolaides KH, Snijders RJ, Thorpe-Beeston JG, Vanden Hof MC, Gosden CM, Bellingham AJ (1990) Mean red cell volume in normal, anemic, small, trisomic and triploid fetuses. *Fetal Therapy* **4**:1–13.

45 Sipes SL, Weiner CP, Wenstrom KD, Williamson RA, Grant SS (1991) The association between fetal karyotype and mean corpuscular volume. *Obstetrics and Gynecology* **165**:1371–1376.

46 Nicolaides KH, Campbell S, Bradley RJ, Bilardo CM, Soothill PW, Gibb D (1987) Maternal oxygen therapy for intra-uterine growth retardation. *Lancet* **i**:942–945.

47 Rizzo G, Arduini D, Romanini C, Mancuso S (1990) Effects of maternal hyperoxygenation on atrioventricular velocity waveforms in healthy and growth-retarded fetuses. *Biology of the Neonate* **58**:127–132.

48 Arduini D, Rizzo G, Mancuso S, Romanini C (1988) Short-term effects of maternal oxygen administration on blood flow velocity waveforms in healthy and growth-retarded fetuses. *American Journal of Obstetrics and Gynecology* **159**:1077–1080.

49 Rajhvajn B, Dukic V, Zmijanac J (1991) Waveform analysis before and after oxygen therapy in severely growth retarded fetuses. *Ultrasound in Obstetrics and Gynecology* **1**:88 (suppl. 1).

50 Ribbert LSM, van Lingen, Visser GHA (1991) Continuous maternal hyperoxygenation in the treatment of early fetal growth retardation. *Ultrasound in Obstetrics and Gynecology* **1**:331–335.

51 Naides SJ, Weiner CP (1989) Antenatal diagnosis and palliative treatment of non-immune hydrops fetalis secondary to fetal parvovirus B19 infection. *Prenatal Diagnosis* **9**:1–10.

52 Shepard MJ, Richards VA, Berkowitz RL, Warsof SL, Hobbins JC (1982) An evaluation of two equations predicting fetal weight by ultrasound. *American Journal of Obstetrics and Gynecology* **142**:47–54.

53 Hadlock P, Harrist RB, Carpenter RJ, Deter RL, Park SK (1984) Sonographic estimation of fetal weight. *Radiology* **150**:535–540.

54 Weiner CP, Sabbagha RE, Vaisrub N, Socol ML (1985) Ultrasonic fetal weight prediction: Role of head circumference and femur length. *Obstetrics and Gynecology* **65**:812.

55 Weiner CP, Sipes SL, Wenstrom K (1992) The effect of fetal age upon normal fetal laboratory values and venous pressure. *Obstetrics and Gynecology* **79**:713–718.

56 Tamura RK, Sabbagha RE, Pan WH, Hampton D (1993) Ultrasonic fetal head circumference: Comparison of direct versus calculated measurement (in press).

43

Abnormalities of Utero-Placental and Fetal Doppler Studies

PETER W. SOOTHILL

HISTORY AND INTRODUCTION

The non-invasive study of the movement of blood *in vivo* based on the change in frequency of reflected sound (Doppler shift) has been used in medicine for many years.[1] In 1977, the technique was applied to umbilical vessels[2] and over the next few years it was confirmed that abnormalities in umbilical arterial blood velocity were associated with fetal growth deficiency. In 1983, Doppler techniques were applied to the utero-placental circulation,[3] allowing study of both sides of the placenta. Study of vessels within the fetus, such as the aorta[4] and those supplying the brain,[5] permitted investigation of fetal hemodynamic responses to physiologic[6] and pathologic events.[7,8] Despite these important developments, the place of Doppler studies in obstetric management has been difficult to define and remains controversial.

DOPPLER TECHNIQUES

Equipment

Continuous-wave (see **Figure 1**)

These are the simplest (and most economic) systems, but have the disadvantage that movement anywhere along the path of the sound will be detected. Thus, it is impossible to tell how far away a signal is coming from or to determine the angle of insonation. As a result, continuous-wave Doppler can only be used for waveform studies of vessels that are reliably identified by their blood velocity waveform so continuous-wave Doppler equipment cannot be used to study blood vessels within the fetus. It is possible with the umbilical cord vessels. However, where the combination of fetal

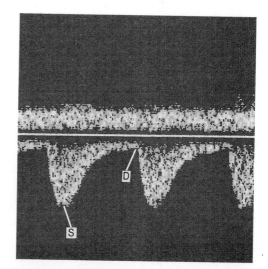

Figure 1. Continuous-wave Doppler ultrasound picture of the umbilical cord. The pulsatile flow in the bottom half is from the umbilical artery and the continuous flow in the upper screen is from the umbilical vein. The peak systolic and trough diastolic points are indicated (S and D, respectively) and these are used to assess the waveform as described in the text.

pulsatile flow in one direction with continuous flow in the opposite direction is sufficiently characteristic. These systems have also been used to study the utero-placental circulation but an abnormal pattern may be confused with another vessel.

Pulsed-wave systems (see **Figure 2**)

These machines emit sound intermittently. By studying only reflections that have taken a known time to return to the receiving transducer, it is possible to study vessels at a known distance. Combining this equipment with an imaging ultrasound transducer ('duplex' systems) allows visual identification of the vessel being studied and makes study of utero-placental and fetal vessels more reliable. Since the angle of insonation can be measured, blood velocity and blood flow estimates are possible. Values obtained by continuous- and pulse-wave systems have a reasonable correlation, especially when the umbilical artery rather than the uterine artery is studied.[8,9]

Color blood flow mapping (see **Figure 3**)

The principle of these machines is similar to the pulsed systems, but the location of any Doppler shift is imaged as either red or blue (depending on whether the direction of flow is toward or away from the transducer). The combination of gray screen imaging with color blood flow mapping makes the identification of vessels much easier. It also allows more accurate assessment of the angle of insonation, especially for small vessels such as those in the fetal cerebral circulation.

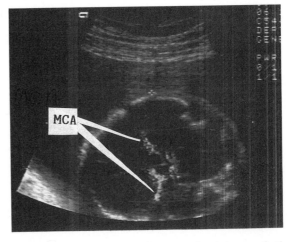

Figure 3. A Doppler ultrasound picture of the fetal cerebral circulation. The circle of Willis can be clearly seen and the middle cerebral artery (MCA) identified.

Assessment of Blood Flow

Blood flow measurement

Blood flow can be measured using Doppler, but it requires knowledge of both the mean blood velocity and the vessel diameter. The latter must be recorded very accurately because even small errors are compounded by a cubic function in the equation. Since current ultrasound imaging equipment cannot measure below 1 mm accurately, determination of blood flow in the small vessels of the fetus is rarely possible and is almost never used in clinical practice. The term 'blood flow' should only be used to describe measurements of the amount of blood traveling down the vessel per unit time (e.g. ml/min) and not the related Doppler assessments such as velocity or waveform patterns.

Blood velocity

Knowledge of both the Doppler shift and the angle between the ultrasound beam and the vessel (angle of insonation) allows for the calculation of blood velocity. It does not require measurement of the vessel diameter and can be averaged over the cardiac cycle to give the mean blood velocity in cm/s. The angle of insonation (which should be <55°) can be determined accurately for long straight vessels such as the fetal aorta (**Figure 2**), but not for curved vessels such as the umbilical artery.

Factors which alter fetal blood velocity include the fetal heart rate,[10,11] behaviour state[12] and maternal smoking,[13] but not maternal exercise.[14] Low blood

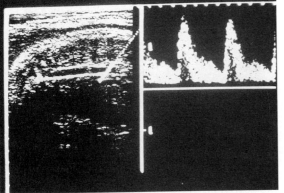

Figure 2. A duplex Doppler and imaging ultrasound picture allowing the Doppler gate to be placed over the fetal aorta.

velocity in fetal vessels is usually associated with high-resistance waveform indices.

Waveform indices

The use of velocity waveform indices has the advantage of near independence of the angle of insonation and therefore can be used with continuous-wave equipment. The peak systolic Doppler shift is either called S or A and the trough diastolic shift D or B (see **Figure 1**). There are three commonly used indices:

$$S/D \text{ ratio} = \frac{S}{D}$$

$$\text{resistance index} = \frac{(S-D)}{S}$$

$$\text{pulsatility index} = \frac{(S-D)}{\text{mean}}$$

where 'mean' represents the average Doppler shift over 1 waveform. The first two have the disadvantage of being unable to quantify waveforms with absent end diastolic flow (D = 0) when they become infinity or 1, respectively. The pulsatility index requires equipment which can digitize the waveform to calculate the mean Doppler shift. American and Australian authors have tended to report the S/D ratio, whereas in the UK the resistance index or pulsatility index are most often quoted. The inter- and intra-observer variation are both <15%. [15–18]

A high value for any of these indices is usually associated with a low blood velocity, and there is strong evidence that this indicates a high resistance to flow in the distal vascular bed. In animal studies, embolization of the feto-placental circulation or constriction of the umbilical vein increases the umbilical artery S/D ratio. [19–21] Analysis of a computerized simulation of the utero-placental circulation suggests that by increasing the resistance to blood flow, both the S/D ratio and the pulsatility index would increase and a dicrotic notch appear. [22] Furthermore, high-resistance indices in the umbilical artery of human pregnancies are associated with a decrease in the number of arteries in the tertiary villi[23–25] compared to pregnancies with normal resistances. All of these measurements change with gestational age in normal pregnancies and so results must be compared with the appropriate normal ranges (**Figures 4** and **5**).

Waveform imaging

It is possible to gain very useful information by simply 'eye-balling' the waveform from the uterine or umbilical arteries. Absent (D = 0 in **Figure 1**) or even reversed flow at the end of diastole makes fetal hypoxia or acidosis extremely likely[26] (for a related discussion, See Chapter 42). In the uterine artery waveform, a dicrotic notch is a sign of high resistance thought to result from the failure of trophoblastic invasion. [3]

DOPPLER TESTS

Utero-placental Vessels

The rapid development of ultrasound equipment has allowed the study of different vessels within the utero-placental circulation. [27] Transvaginal Doppler ultrasonography, especially with color flow mapping, permits the ascending uterine artery near the cervix to be visualized on each side. [28] Uterine artery blood flow estimates suggest a four-fold increase from prepregnancy levels to term. [29] Most investigators have scanned transabdominally using either continuous-wave or pulsed Doppler techniques. The vessels studied include the uterine artery (**Figure 4**),[30] the arcuate artery on both sides of the placental implantation site[3] and the subplacental vessels. [31] However, without color flow mapping, visual identification of a vessel in the lateral wall of the uterus can be difficult or impossible. Furthermore, very different results are obtained from different parts of the uterus[27] if the test is repeated in the same patient. The difference between the highest and lowest

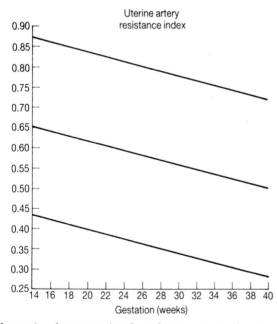

Figure 4. An example of a reference range for uterine artery resistance index. Since this changes with gestational age, results must be assessed using such a chart. Reproduced with permission from Pearce et al.[85.]

waveform index from one pregnancy can be 50% of the measurement.[32] Investigators have reported their results in terms of the highest resistance signal (which usually comes from the non-placental site),[33] from the placental site (usually the lowest) or as an average of several locations.[30]

Despite these major technical problems, there is a consensus about physiological findings and significant correlations with pathology. There is a marked fall in uterine resistance from prepregnancy to 24 weeks gestation, followed by a more gradual fall to term.[29] This decline is thought to reflect trophoblastic invasion changing high-resistance, muscular spiral arteries to low-resistance vessels. High waveform resistance indices or the presence of a dicrotic notch are associated with both growth deficiency and pre-eclampsia.[34] This suggests that, as in animal studies,[35] very large changes in the utero-placental circulation are required before there is any detectable fetal consequence, and that such problems do occur in pathological human pregnancy.

Feto-placental Vessels

Umbilical vein

The flow of blood through the umbilical vein has been calculated to range between 105 and 130 ml/kg/min (reviewed in reference 36). Umbilical blood flow is approximately 50–64% of aortic flow and this proportion seems to remain constant after 24 weeks with advancing gestation.[37] The technical limitations of Doppler blood flow measurement as described previously have resulted in wide reference ranges and restricted the clinical use of this technique. Since blood flow in the umbilical vein is not normally pulsatile, waveform indices cannot be applied.

Umbilical artery

Because the umbilical artery can be studied reliably with continuous-wave equipment, it is the most commonly tested vessel. However, its tortuous path makes blood flow or velocity studies impractical. Umbilical artery blood velocity waveform indices fall with advancing gestation and high resistance patterns are normal before 20 weeks. The pulsatility index (see **Figure 5**) is probably the most versatile of the waveform indices for study of this vessel because absent or reversed end-diastolic blood flow ($D = 0$) is a common pathological finding in this circulation.

Fetal Vessels

Descending thoracic aorta

Since the descending thoracic aorta is a straight vessel,

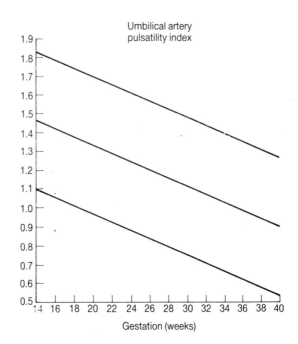

Figure 5. An example of a reference range for the umbilical artery pulsatility index. Since this changes with gestational age, results must be assessed using such a chart. Reproduced with permission from Pearce et al.[85].

estimates of blood flow in the aorta have been made and average 220 ml/kg/min.[36] The mean blood velocity can also be determined reliably. It increases with gestational age, even though the pulsatility index remains constant (**Figure 6**).[6]

Cerebral vessels

Several vessels supplying the fetal brain have been studied. Though the common carotid artery supplies the external tissues of the head through the external carotid artery, it is straight enough to determine the angle of insonation. The mean velocity of blood in the carotid artery rises linearly and the waveform indices fall with advancing gestational age.[6]

Similar results have been obtained from the internal carotid and middle cerebral arteries, but the latter is closer to the fetal brain and is becoming the most commonly used test to assess the cerebral circulation. In these vessels, high-resistance waveforms are found until about 30 weeks gestation, followed by a significant fall in resistance during the rest of pregnancy. It has been suggested that the normal change from high to low resistance in the vessels of the cerebral circulation may indicate a vasodilation response to the normal fall in pO_2 which occurs with advancing gestational age (see Chapter 42).[6]

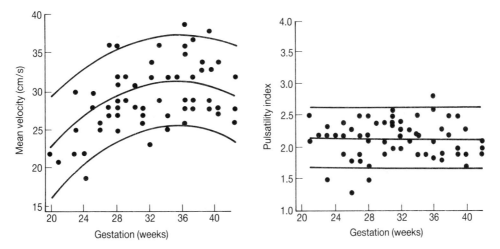

Figure 6. Reference ranges for mean velocity (mean intensity-weighted) and pulsatility index in the fetal descending thoracic aorta. From Bilardo *et al.*[6] Reproduced with permission.

In the sheep fetus, hypoxia causes a redistribution of blood to the most acutely vital organs (such as the brain) and away from the body (such as gut and lower limbs).[38] Hypoxemic human fetuses have a low middle cerebral artery resistance index and high blood velocity, while the resistance index in the aorta is high and the blood velocity low (see **Table 1**). This is though to be indicative of a similar 'brain sparing' redistribution as noted in the animals. Cerebral artery/aorta ratio appears to be the most sensitive predictor of fetal hypoxemia at cordocentesis.[39]

Renal arteries

Renal artery resistance normally falls with advancing gestation.[40] The renal artery pulsatility index is increased in growth-deficient fetuses with hypoxemia. This is probably part of the 'brain sparing' redistribution described above.

Adjusting for Changes with Gestational Age

Since almost all of the Doppler tests change with advancing gestation in normal pregnancies, any result must be interpreted by comparison with a normal range. When results are being compared or correlations with other factors are considered, this effect must be removed. One way to express the results in a clinically useful manner is in multiples of standard deviation from the normal mean (a z score).

CLINICAL INDICATIONS: SPECIFIC

Fetal Growth Deficiency

Utero-placental Doppler studies may become abnormal weeks before the fetal growth rate falls. There is a negative correlation between the utero-placental resistance indices and fetal pH and pO_2 in growth-deficient fetuses (see Chapter 42). However, the waveform can be abnormal up to 18 weeks before any fetal problem is observed. While the sensitivity and specificity are low, there is adequate information to conclude that if utero-placental Doppler studies are abnormal in a pregnancy with a growth-deficient fetus, utero-placental insufficiency is more likely to be the cause of the small size than if these tests are normal.

Abnormal Doppler indices are found in the umbilical artery[41–46] and fetal aorta[47,48] in some growth-deficient fetuses. Initially, birthweight was used as the end-point to measure the success of the tests and reported sensitivities ranged from 17 to 100% (reviewed in reference

Table 1
Abnormalities in Doppler blood velocity studies found in hypoxemic growth deficient and anemic fetuses

	Hypoxia		Anemia	
	PI	Mean velocity	PI	Mean velocity
Uterine	↑		↔	
Umbilical	↑		↔	
Aorta	↑	↓	↓	↑
Cerebral	↓	↑	↓	↑

36). This large range probably relates to differences in the populations studied because normal, healthy, small fetuses have normal Doppler tests. Indeed, it has become clear that abnormal Doppler findings identify only a subgroup of growth-deficient fetuses – those that are hypoxemic and small as a result of inadequate placental function.[7,8] There is strong evidence of an association between abnormal blood velocity waveforms in the aorta[49,50] or umbilical artery [50–59] and subsequent fetal decelerations and operative delivery for fetal distress in labor.

There is controversy as to the order in which feto-placental and fetal Doppler tests become abnormal. The umbilical artery has been used by many groups as the primary Doppler test to detect fetal hypoxemia and other fetal vessels are studied only if this test is abnormal. There is increasing interest in the possibility that a redistribution pattern within the fetus may be the first sign of fetal hypoxemia, even when the umbilical artery studies remain normal.

Management Options

Being small for gestational age is a physical sign of disease not a diagnosis. Distinguishing between

- a normal but small fetus

- a chromosomally abnormal fetus

- a structurally abnormal but euploid fetus

- a starved-hypoxemic small fetus

is an important differential diagnosis. There is a consensus that Doppler studies have an important clinical role in this process. Should utero-placental, feto-placental and fetal Dopplers all be normal, the first or third groups are much more likely to be the cause of the small size than placental failure. Alternatively, if the Dopplers show placental perfusion abnormalities and a hypoxemic-like redistribution of blood flow in the fetus, the fourth cause is likely to be the explanation.[60]

The role of Doppler studies in the subsequent management of a compromised pregnancy remains to be established. Delivery decisions should balance the risks of delivery against those of continuing the pregnancy. Although the growth-deficient fetus with abnormal Dopplers is probably small as a result of placental dys-

function, this does not mean that the fetus is at immediate risk of dying. Instances of fetuses surviving with absent end-diastolic flow for 60 days have been reported.[61] Further, there have been no randomized trials to compare early intervention vs waiting for overt signs of distress. Therefore, if the aim of monitoring is to prevent fetal death, other tests (such as cardiotocography and/or biophysical profile score assessment) almost always give adequate warning. On the other hand, growth-deficient fetuses with abnormal feto-placental Dopplers are likely to be chronically hypoxemic and/or acidemic. Although these fetuses may survive for many weeks, there is now evidence that acidemia is associated with diminished neurodevelopment.[62] Thus, one can make a fairly strong case for delivering mature fetuses with significantly abnormal fetal Doppler studies without waiting for other tests to deteriorate. Indeed, even an equivocal biophysical profile is associated with a ten-fold increase in perinatal mortality rate[63] and so may be too late to prevent some morbidity (see Chapter 39). Only randomized intervention studies with neurodevelopment as an end-point will indicate which is ultimately the better management.

If a small for gestational age fetus is thought to be otherwise normal, intervention should be avoided. Since Doppler tests provide early evidence of fetal hypoxia, monitoring by serial (say weekly) Doppler measurements may be considered if the initial results are normal.

Assessment of Anemia and Other Conditions

In fetal, as in postnatal life, severe anemia is associated with a hyperdynamic circulation. An increase in blood velocity and low resistance patterns are found throughout the fetus and do not show the redistribution pattern typical of growth deficiency (see **Table 1**). These tests have been used to monitor fetuses known to be at risk of anemia as a result of red cell alloimmunization. However, the effects of anemia on the Doppler studies are variable and seem to be most useful when trends are considered. It may ultimately be helpful to 'calibrate' an individual pregnancy by knowing the Doppler results found with a particular hemoglobin concentration.

Reduced amniotic fluid volume is associated with many pathologies and Doppler studies can be useful to detect those associated with placental dysfunction. Continuous-wave Doppler has not been useful when monitoring pregnancies complicated by unexplained antepartum hemorrhage,[64] post-maturity,[65–68] maternal diabetes[69] and hypertension in the absence of proteinuria.[70]

ROUTINE (SCREENING)

There are two completely different approaches to the routine use of Doppler scanning. One attempts to detect pregnancies which have failed to establish a low-resistance utero-placental circulation before it has had any clinical or fetal consequences. It is hoped that by defining a group of patients at high risk for subsequent problems, appropriate monitoring and interventions will improve outcome. The second approach results from the observation that feto-placental Doppler tests can indicate non-invasively which small for gestional age fetuses are associated with placental dysfunction and thus at risk for hypoxemic morbidity. With this approach, it is hoped that problems leading to hypoxemia in appropriately grown fetuses may be detected or mothers with healthy pregnancies will be reassured more effectively than can be done at present. The two concepts will be considered in turn.

Screening for Failed Trophoblastic Invasion

Histopathologic studies have shown that in placental bed biopsies from pregnancies with either fetal growth deficiency or pre-eclampsia, the arteries are often more muscular than the normal, low-resistance vessels.[71] The change from high- to low-resistance vessels normally occurs gradually during the first 24 weeks of pregnancy but at a variable rate. It is suggested that this decline is the result of trophoblastic invasion of the arcuate arteries leading to increased utero-placental blood flow. Doppler studies of utero-placental vessels support this histological hypothesis, since they suggest a drop in blood flow resistance during this stage of pregnancy (**Figure 4**).[29] More important is the observation that pregnancies with several complications have higher utero-placental resistance patterns than normal.

Studies have now confirmed that pregnancies which do not develop a low-resistance utero-placental circulation by 24 weeks are at higher risk of growth deficiency, pre-eclampsia and abruption.[31,33,72–74] However, very different sensitivity and specificity results have been obtained by different groups. In fact, one group could find no significant discriminate ability at all.[75]

Screening for Fetal Hypoxia

Most hypoxic morbidity at birth is found in neonates who weigh within the normal range. If hypoxic morbidity associated with fetal distress in labor and unexplained fetal intrauterine death of well-grown fetuses are caused by placental dysfunction, detecting and preventing its consequences would be important. Since Doppler studies detect hypoxemic growth-deficient fetuses, this approach has been tried, but unfortunately, these studies are hampered by the lack of easily measured, meaningful end-points.

Two studies using Doppler tests in pregnancies during the late second and third trimesters showed poor prediction of growth deficiency as defined by low birthweight.[76,77] This may be partly because a large proportion of fetuses with a birthweight below the tenth centile in an unselected population are small but normal fetuses. Two other population studies revealed an association between umbilical artery blood velocity and fetal distress in labor, but the sensitivity and predictive values were poor.[78–80] Recent work suggests that umbilical artery Doppler tests predict hypoxic morbidity only in growth-deficient but not in appropriately grown fetuses.[81] An explanation for this finding could be that impaired placental function sufficient to produce clinically significant fetal hypoxemia has usually caused the fetus to be small first. If this hypothesis is correct, hypoxic morbidity at birth in well-grown fetuses is usually due to acute changes in labor and will thus be undetectable in advance.

Management Options

Uterine artery screening

Although this is a very promising test, its use for screening all pregnancies is not yet justified. There are two questions which must first be answered:

- Does the test define a group at high enough risk to justify intervention?

- Is there an intervention that can be made before a complication occurs that would be detected clinically which would have a significant benefit?

The most obvious potential therapy that might fulfil the latter criteria is low-dose aspirin and already several trials have suggested this could be effective.[82–84] If these encouraging results are confirmed, utero-placental Doppler screening may be useful.

Fetal Doppler screening

There is no evidence that fetal Doppler tests should be introduced routinely for all pregnancies. Apart from its clear role in the investigation and management of small for gestational age fetuses, these tests have not been shown to be successful in detecting hypoxemia in well-grown fetuses with or without other indications for testing.

CONCLUSIONS

Doppler studies of pregnancy are an important advance in fetal medicine and should be available in every major obstetric unit. They provide information about function rather than structure and enhance our understanding of the pathophysiology of abnormal pregnancy.

There is a consensus that Doppler studies have an important role in helping to identify the cause of a fetus being small for gestational age. There is also a role for fetal Doppler studies in monitoring the well-being of growth-deficient fetuses and for timing delivery.

The role of utero-placental Doppler studies as a routine screening test in pregnancy is promising but not justified by currently available data. Although it can identify a group at increased risk, the sensitivity and predictive values are low and the value of early therapeutic intervention or changed management based on the results remains to be established.

There does not appear to be a role for screening whole populations with feto-placental or fetal Doppler tests. Indeed, their value in pregnancies with indications other than small for gestational age is not yet established.

REFERENCES

1 Satomura S (1959) Study of flow pattern in peripheral arteries by ultrasonics. *Journal of the Acoustical Society of Japan* **15**:151–154.

2 FitzGerald DE, Drumm JE (1977) Non-invasive

DOPPLER STUDIES IN UTERO-PLACENTAL AND FETAL CIRCULATIONS
Summary of Management Options

Utero-placental

- Can predict increased risk of pre-eclampsia and/or growth deficiency.

- Further studies using color flow mapping and intervention trials are needed before recommendations for clinical practice can be made

Feto-placental

Umbilical artery

- Is of value in ascertaining the cause and risk in small for gestational age fetuses; Is helpful in timing delivery of mature growth deficient fetuses

- Not of value for screening in a normal population

Fetal vesels

- May give earlier prediction of fetal risk than umbilical artery recordings

- Clinical value is as for feto-placental studies but more research is needed

measurement of human fetal circulation using ultrasound: A new method. *British Medical Journal* **2**:1450–1451.

3 Campbell S, Diaz-Recasens J, Griffin DR, Cohen-Overbeek TE, Pearce JM, Wilson K, Teague MJ (1983) New Doppler technique for assessing utero-placental blood-flow. *Lancet* **i**:675–677.

4 Eik-Nes SH, Brubaak AO, Ulstein MK (1980) Measurement of human fetal blood flow. *British Medical Journal* **280**:283–284.

5 Wladimiroff JW, Tonge HM, Stewart PA (1986) Doppler ultrasound assessment of cerebral blood flow in the human fetus. *British Journal of Obstetrics and Gynaecology* **93**:471–475.

6 Bilardo CM, Campbell S, Nicolaides KH (1988) Mean blood velocities and flow impedance in the fetal descending thoracic aorta and common carotid arteries in normal pregnancies. *Early Human Development* **18**:213–221.

7 Soothill PW, Nicolaides KH, Bilardo CM, Campbell S (1986) Relation of fetal hypoxia in growth retardation to mean blood velocity in the fetal aorta. *Lancet* **ii**:1118–1120.

8 Weiner CP (1990) The relationship between the umbilical artery systole/diastole ratio and umbilical blood gas measurements obtained by cordocentesis. *American Journal of Obstetrics and Gynecology* **162**:1198–1202.

9 Mahalek KE, Berkowitz GS, Chitkara U, Rosenberg J, Berkowitz RL (1988) Comparison of continuous-wave and pulsed Doppler *S/D* ratios of umbilical and uterine arteries. *Obstetrics and Gynecology* **72**:603–606.

10 Mires G, Gempster J, Patel NB, Crawford JW (1987) The effect of fetal heart rate on umbilical artery flow velocity waveforms. *British Journal of Obstetrics and Gynaecology* **97**:665–669.

11 van den Wijngaard JA, van Eych J, Wadimiroff JW (1988) The relationship between fetal heart rate and Doppler blood flow velocity waveforms. *Ultrasound in Medicine and Biology* **14**:593–597.

12 Marsal K, Lindblad A, Lingman G (1984) Blood flow in the fetal descending aorta: Intrinisic factors affecting fetal blood flow, ie fetal breathing, movements and cardiac arrythmia. *Ultrasound in Medicine and Biology* **10**:339–348.

13 Sindberg Eriksen P, Marsal K (1987) Circulatory changes in the fetal aorta after maternal smoking. *British Journal of Obstetrics and Gynaecology* **94**:301–305.

14 Morrow RJ, Ritchie JW, Bull SB (1989) Fetal and maternal hemodynamic responses to exercise in pregnancy assessed by Doppler ultrasonography. *American Journal of Obstetrics and Gynecology* **160**:138–140.

15 Rasmussen K (1987) Precision and accuracy of Doppler flow measurements: *In vitro* and *in vivo* study of applicability of the method in human fetuses. *Scandinavian Journal of Clinical and Laboratory Investigation* **47**:311–318.

16 Nienhuis SJ, van Vinght JM, Hoogland HJ, Ruissen CJ, de Haan J (1988) Interexaminer variability of fetal Doppler velocity waveforms. *Gynecological and Obstetrical Investigations* **25**:152–157.

17 Spencer JA, Price J (1989) Intraobserver variation in Doppler ultrasound indices of placental perfusion

derived from different numbers of waveforms. *Journal of Ultrasound in Medicine* **8**:197–199.

18 Maulik D, Yarlagadda AP, Youngblood JP, Willoughby L (1989) Components of viability of umbilical arterial Doppler velocimetry: A prospective analysis. *American Journal of Obstetrics and Gynecology* **160**:1406–1409.

19 Trudginger BJ, Stevens D, Connelly AN *et al.* (1987) Umbilical artery flow velocity waveforms and placental resistance: The effect of embolization on the umbilical circulation. *American Journal of Obstetrics and Gynecology* **157**:1443–1448.

20 Morrow RL, Adamson SL, Bull SB, Ritchie JWK (1989) Effect of placental embolization on the umbilical arterial velocity waveform in fetal sheep. *American Journal of Obstetrics and Gynecology* **161**:1055–1060.

21 Fouron JC, Teyssier G, Maroto E, Lessaerd M, Marquette G (1991) Diastolic circulatory dynamics in the presence of elevated placental resistance and retrograde diastolic flow in the umbilical artery: A Doppler echographic study in lambs. *American Journal of Obstetrics and Gynecology* **164**:195–203.

22 Adamson SL, Morrow RL, Bascom PA, Mo LY, Ritchie JW (1989) Effect of placental resistance, arterial diameter, and blood pressure on the uterine arterial velocity waveform: A computer modelling approach. *Ultrasound in Medicine and Biology* **15**:437–442.

23 Giles WB, Trudinger BJ, Baird PJ (1985) Fetal umbilical artery flow velocity waveforms and placental resistance: Pathological correlation. *British Journal of Obstetrics and Gynaecology* **92**:31–38.

24 McCowan LM, Mullen BM, Ritchie K (1987) Umbilical artery flow velocity waveforms and the placental vascular bed. *American Journal of Obstetrics and Gynecology* **157**:900–902.

25 Bracero LA, Beneck D, Kirshenbaum N, Peiffer M, Stalter P, Schulman H (1989) Doppler velocimetry and placental disease. *American Journal of Obstetrics and Gynecology* **161**:388–393.

26 Nicolaides KH, Bilardo CM, Soothill PW, Campbell S (1988) Absence of end diastolic frequencies in umbilical artery: A sign of fetal hypoxia and acidosis. *British Medical Journal* **297**:1026–1027.

27 Bewley S, Campbell S, Cooper D (1989) Utero-placental Doppler flow velocity waveforms in the second trimester: A complex circulation. *British Journal of Obstetrics and Gynaecology* **96**:1040–1046.

28 Deutinger J, Rudelstorfer R, Bernaschek G (1988) Vagino-sonographic velocimetry of both main uterine arteries by visual vessel recognition and pulsed Doppler method during pregnancy. *American Journal of Obstetrics and Gynecology* **159**:1072–1076.

29 Thaler I, Manor D, Itskovitz J *et al.* (1990) Changes in uterine blood flow during pregnancy. *American Journal of Obstetrics and Gynecology* **162**:121–125.

30 Schulman H, Fleischer A, Farmakides G, Bracero L, Rochelson B, Grunfeld L (1986) Development of uterine artery compliance in pregnancy as detected by Doppler ultrasound. *American Journal of Obstetrics and Gynecology* **155**:1031–1036.

31 Trudinger BJ, Giles WB, Cook CM (1985) Utero-placental blood flow velocity–time waveforms in normal

and complicated pregnancy. *British Journal of Obstetrics and Gynaecology* **92**:39–45.

32 Chambers SE, Johnstone FD, Muir BB, Hoskins P, Haddad NG, McDicken WN (1988) The effects of placental site on the arcuate artery flow velocity waveform. *Journal of Ultrasound in Medicine* **7**:671–673.

33 Soothill PW, Nicolaides KH, Bilardo CM, Hackett S, Campbell S (1986) Utero-placental blood velocity resistance index and umbilical venous pO_2, and pCO_2, pH, lactate and erythroblast count in growth retarded fetuses. Fetal *Therapy and Diagnosis* **1**:176–179.

34 Campbell S, Pearce JMF, Hackett G, Cohen-Overbeek T, Hernandez C (1986) Qualitative assessment of utero-placental blood flow: Early pregnancy screening test for high-risk pregnancies. *Obstetrics and Gynecology* **68**:649–653.

35 Wilkening RB, Meschia G (1983) Fetal oxygen uptake, oxygenation, and acid–base balance as a function of uterine blood flow. *American Journal of Physiology* **244**:H749–755.

36 Low JA (1991) The current status of maternal and fetal blood flow velocity. *American Journal of Obstetrics and Gynecology* **164**:1049–1063.

37 Chen HY, Chang FM, Huang HC, Hsieh FJ, Lu CC (1988) Antenatal fetal blood flow in the descending fetal aorta and in the umbilical vein and their ratio in normal pregnancy. *Ultrasound in Medicine and Biology* **14**:263–268.

38 Peeters LLH, Sheldon RF, Jones MD, Makowski EL, Meschia G (1979) Blood flow to fetal organs as a function of arterial oxygen content. *American Journal of Obstetrics and Gynecology* **135**:639–646.

39 Bilardo CM, Nicolaides KH, Campbell S (1990) Doppler measurements of fetal and utero-placental circulations: Relationship with umbilical venous blood gases measured at cordocentesis. *American Journal of Obstetrics and Gynecology* **162**:115–120.

40 Vyas S, Nicolaides KH, Campbell S (1989) Renal artery flow–velocity waveform in normal and hypoxemic fetuses. *American Journal of Obstetrics and Gynecology* **161**:168–172.

41 Erskine RLA, Ritchies JWK (1985) Umbilical artery blood flow characteristics in normal and growth retarded fetuses. *British Journal of Obstetrics and Gynaecology* **92**:605–610.

42 Chambers SE, Hoskins PR, Haddad NG, Johnstone FD, McDicken WN, Muir BB (1989) A comparison of fetal abdominal circumference measurements and Doppler ultrasound in the prediction of small-for-dates babies and fetal compromise. *British Journal of Obstetrics and Gynaecology* **96**:803–808.

43 Trudinger BJ, Giles WB, Cook CM, Bonebardirri J, Collins L (1985) Fetal umbilical artery velocity waveforms and placental resistance: Clinical significance. *British Journal of Obstetrics and Gynaecology* **92**:23–30.

44 Wladimiroff JW, Noordam MJ, van den Wijngaard JA, Hop WC (1989) Fetal internal carotid and umbilical artery blood velocity waveforms as a measure of fetal well-being in intrauterine growth retardation. *Pediatric Research* **24**:609–612.

45 Gaziano E, Knox GE, Wager GP, Bendel RP, Boyce DJ, Olson J (1988) The predictability of the small-for-gestational-age infant by real-time ultrasound-derived measurements combined with pulsed Doppler umbilical artery velocimetry. *American Journal of Obstetrics and Gynecology* **158**:1431–1439.

46 Satoh S, Koyanagi T, Fukuhara M, Hara K, Nakano H (1989) Changes in vascular resistance in the umbilical and middle cerebral arteries in the human intrauterine growth-retarded fetus measured with pulsed Doppler ultrasound. *Early Human Development* **20**:213–220.

47 Griffin D, Bilardo K, Mansini L *et al.* (1984) Doppler blood flow waveforms in the descending thoracic aorta of the human fetus. *British Journal of Obstetrics and Gynecology* **91**:997–1006.

48 Tonge HM, Wladimiroff JW, Noordam MJ, van Kooten C (1986) Blood flow velocity waveforms in the descending fetal aorta: Comparison between normal and growth-retarded pregnancies. *Obstetrics and Gynecology* **67**:851–855.

49 Laurin J, Lingman G, Marsal K, Persson PH (1987) Fetal blood flow in pregnancies complicated by intrauterine growth retardation. *Obstetrics and Gynecology* **156**:655–659.

50 Lingman G, Laurin J, Marsal K (1986) Circulatory changes in fetuses with imminent asphyxia. *Biology of the Neonate* **49**:66–73.

51 Reuwer PJ, Sijmons EA, Rietman GW, van Tiel MW, Bruinse HW (1987) Intrauterine growth retardation: Prediction of perinatal distress by Doppler ultrasound. *Lancet* **2**:415–418.

52 Brar HS, Platt LD, Paul RH (1989) Fetal umbilical blood flow velocity waveforms using Doppler ultrasonography in patients with late decelerations. *Obstetrics and Gynecology* **73**:363–366.

53 Laurin J, Marsal K, Persson PH, Lingman G (1987) Ultrasound measurement of fetal blood flow in predicting fetal outcome. *British Journal of Obstetrics and Gynaecology* **94**:940–948.

54 Rochelson B, Schulman H, Farmakides G *et al.* (1987) The significance of absent end-diastolic velocity in umbilical artery waveforms. *American Journal of Obstetrics and Gynecology* **156**:1213–1218.

55 Berkowitz GS, Mehalek KE, Chitkara U, Rosenberg J, Cogswell C, Berkowitz RL (1988) Doppler umbilical velocimetry in the prediction of adverse outcome in pregnancies at risk for intrauterine growth retardation. *Obstetrics and Gynecology* **71**:742–746.

56 Farmakides G, Schulman H, Winter D, Ducey J, Guzman E, Penny B (1988) Prenatal surveillance using non-stress testing and Doppler velocimetry. *Obstetrics and Gynecology* **71**:184–187.

57 Lowery CL, Henson BV, Wan J, Brumfield CG (1990) A comparison between umbilical artery velocimetry and standard antepartum surveillance in hospitalized high-risk patients. *American Journal of Obstetrics and Gynecology* **162**:710–714.

58 Newnham JP, Patterson LL, James IR, Diepeveen DA, Reid SE (1990) An evaluation of the efficacy of Doppler flow velocity waveform analysis as a screening test in pregnancy. *American Journal of Obstetrics and Gynecology* **162**:403–410.

59 Feinkind L, Abulafia O, Delke I, Feldman J, Minkoff

H (1989) Screening with Doppler velocimetry in labor. *American Journal of Obstetrics and Gynecology* **161**:765–770.

60 Soothill PW, Ajayi RA, Nicolaides KH (1992) Fetal biochemistry of growth retardation. *Early Human Development* **29**: 91–97.

61 Pillai M, James D (1991) Continuation of normal neuro-behavioural development in fetuses with absent umbilical arterial end diastolic velocities. *British Journal of Obstetrics and Gynaecology* **98**:277–281.

62 Soothill PW, Ajayi RA, Campbell S, Ross EM, Candy DCA, Snijders RM, Nicolaides KH (1992) Relationship between fetal acidemia at cordocentesis and subsequent neuro-development. *Ultrasound in Obstetrics and Gynecology* **2**:80–83.

63 Manning FA, Morrison I, Harman CR, Menticoglou SM (1990) The abnormal fetal biophysical profile score. V. Predictive value according to score composition. *American Journal of Obstetrics and Gynecology* **162**:918–927.

64 Ajayi RA, Soothill PW, Campbell S, Nicolaides KH (1992) Antenatal testing to predict outcome in pregnancies with unexplained antepartum haemorrhage. *British Journal of Obstetrics and Gynaecology* **90**: 122–125.

65 Rightmire DA, Campbell S (1987) Fetal and maternal Doppler blood flow parameters in post-term pregnancies. *Obstetrics and Gynecology* **69**:891–894.

66 Brar HS, Horenstein J, Medearis AL, Platt LD, Phelan JP, Paul RH (1989) Cerebral, umbilical, and uterine resistance using Doppler velocimetry in post-term pregnancy. *Journal of Ultrasound in Medicine* **8**:187–191.

67 Guidetti DA, Divon MY, Cavalieri RL, Langer O, Merkatz IR (1987) Fetal umbilical artery flow velocimetry in post-date pregnancies. *American Journal of Obstetrics and Gynecology* **157**:1521–1523.

68 Farmakides G, Schulman H, Ducey J *et al.* (1988) Uterine and umbilical artery Doppler velocimetry in post-term pregnancy. *Journal of Reproductive Medicine* **33**:259–261.

69 Bracero LA, Schulman H (1991) Doppler studies of the utero-placental circulation in pregnancies complicated by diabetes. *Ultrasound in Obstetrics and Gynecology* **1**:391–394.

70 Soothill PW, Khullar V, Campbell S, Nicolaides KH (1993) Prediction of the severity of pre-eclampsia by utero-placental Doppler studies. *Journal of Obstetrics and Gynaecology* **13**: 523–528.

71 Khong TY (1991) The Robertson-Brosens-Dixon hypothesis: Evidence for the role of haemochorial placentation in pregnancy success. *British Journal of Obstetrics and Gynaecology* **98**:1195–1199.

72 Ducey J, Schulman H, Farmakides G, Rochelson B, Bracero L (1987) A classification of hypertension in pregnancy based on Doppler velocimetry. *American Journal of Obstetrics and Gynecology* **157**:680–685.

73 Arduini D, Rizzo G, Romanini C, Mancuso S (1987) Utero-placental blood flow velocity waveforms as predictors of pregnancy of pregnancy-induced hypertension. *European Journal of Obstetrics and Gynaecology and Reproductive Biology* **26**:335–341.

74 Bewley S, Cooper D, Campbell S (1991) Doppler investigation of uteroplacental blood flow resistance in the second trimester: A screening study for pre-eclampsia and intrauterine growth retardation. *British Journal of Obstetrics and Gynaecology* **98**:871–879.

75 Hanretty KP, Whittle MJ, Rubin PC (1988) Doppler utero-placental waveforms in pregnancy-induced hypertension: A reappraisal. *Lancet* **1**:850–852.

76 Beattie RB, Dornan JC (1989) Antenatal screening for intrauterine growth retardation with umbilical Doppler ultrasonography. *British Medical Journal* **298**:631–635.

77 Sijmons EA, Rewer PJ, van Beek E, Hein PR (1987) The validity of screening for small-for-gestational-age and low-weight-for-length infants by Doppler ultrasound. *British Journal of Gynaecology* **96**:557–561.

78 Hanretty KP, Primrose MH, Neilson JP, Whittle MJ (1989) Pregnancy screening by Doppler utero-placental and umbilical artery waveforms. *British Journal of Obstetrics and Gynaecology* **96**:1163–1167.

79 Newnham JP, Patterson LL, James IR, Diepeveen DA, Reid SE (1990) An evaluation of the efficacy of Doppler flow velocity waveform analysis as a screening test in pregnancy. *American Journal of Obstetrics and Gynecology* **162**:403–410.

80 Newnham JP, O'Dea MR, Reid KP, Diepeveen DA (1991) Doppler flow velocity waveform analysis in high risk pregnancies: A randomised controlled trial. *British Journal of Obstetrics and Gynaecology* **98**: 956–963.

81 Soothill PW, Ajayi RA, Campbell S, Nicolaides KH (1993) Prediction of morbidity in small and normally grown fetuses by fetal heart rate variability, biophysical profile and umbilical artery Doppler testing. *British Journal of Obstetrics and Gynaecology* **100**: 742–745.

82 Bower S, Campbell S (1991) Abstract. In *First Meeting of the International Society of Ultrasound in Obstetrics and Gynecology*, Lancs, UK: Parthenon Publishing.

83 McParland P, Pearce JM, Chamberlain GVP (1990) Doppler ultrasound and aspirin in recognition and prevention of pregnancy-induced hypertension. *Lancet* **1**:1552–1555.

84 Uzan S, Beaufils M, Breart G, Bazin B, Capitant C, Paris J (1991) Prevention of fetal growth retardation with low-dose aspirin: Findings of the EPREDA trial. *Lancet* **337**:1427–1431.

85 Pearce JM, Campbell S, Cohen-Overbeek T, Hackett G, Hernandez J, Royston JP (1988) Reference ranges and sources of variation for indices of pulsed Doppler flow velocity waveforms from the utero-placental and fetal circulation. *British Journal of Obstetrics and Gynecology* **95**:248–256.

44

Fetal Hemolytic Disease

CARL P. WEINER

INTRODUCTION

Though manifestations of fetal hemolytic disease have been recognized for hundreds of years, it was not until 1932 that hydrops fetalis, jaundice and anemia of the neonate were recognized to result from a single disease characterized by perinatal hepatosplenomegaly, extramedullary hematopoiesis and the presence of nucleated red blood cells on peripheral smear.[1] Nine years later, Levine and coworkers identified the mechanism for the anemia when they demonstrated Rhesus (Rh) antibodies on the red blood cells of affected neonates and their absence from the red blood cells of unaffected neonates.[2] In 1954, Chown proved transplacental fetal to maternal hemorrhage was a cause of maternal isoimmunization.[3] In 1961, hemolytic anemia became the first treatable fetal disease after Liley first characterized the natural history of the disease and then successfully transfused intraperitoneally a number of ill fetuses with adult red blood cells.[4,5] In 1964, Freda and colleagues demonstrated that passive immunization of Rh negative individuals with Rh positive antibodies prior to purposeful exposure prevented immunization to Rh negative red blood cells.[6] And in 1981, Rodeck et al. achieved a high survival rate using intravascular transfusion to treat hydropic fetuses.[7] Despite these notable advances in understanding, treatment and prevention, fetal hemolytic disease remains a serious and common cause of perinatal morbidity and in some countries perinatal mortality.

INCIDENCE

Though antibodies to the D antigen site remain most common, the development of immunoprophylaxis has diminished its relative importance while enhancing that of the other antigen groups (**Table 1**). Yet, anti-D remains the prototype for maternal red cell alloimmunization and will be used throughout this chapter for illustration.

The incidence of Rh negative individuals varies by race with a low ≤1% in Chinese and Japanese to a high of 30% in the Basques where the mutation probably occurred. In North American Caucasians, the incidence of Rh negative genotype is 15% and in Blacks 7–8%.

Table 1
Antigens causing fetal hemolytic disease requiring treatment

Common
Rhesus family: D, C, E, c, e
Kell
Less common
JK^a (Kidd)
Fy^a (Duffy)
Kp$^{a\ or\ b}$
k
S
Rare
Do^a, Di$^{a\ or\ b}$, Fy^b, Hutch, Jk^b, Lu^a, M, N, s, U, Yt^a
Never
Le$^{a\ or\ b}$, P

PATHOPHYSIOLOGY

Maternal red blood cell alloimmunization results from the exposure and response to a foreign red blood cell antigen. Fetal to maternal transplacental hemorrhage is the most common cause of alloimmunization. Heterologous blood transfusion is second overall, but the most common cause of sensitization to the less common antigens (**Table 1**). It has been estimated that fetal red blood cells can be identified on a Kleihauer-stained peripheral smear in 75% of women at some time either during pregnancy or at delivery.[8] Both the frequency and magnitude of the bleed increase as pregnancy advances from 3% and 0.03 ml respectively in the first trimester, to 45% and up to 25 ml in the third trimester. Miscarriage, too, is associated with fetal to maternal hemorrhage but the incidence is <1% and the volume usually <0.1 ml. In contrast, surgically induced abortion has a 20–25% risk of transplacental hemorrhage of significantly greater volume.

There are three major nomenclatures for the rhesus blood group. Each has its strengths, but that of Fisher and Race works best in clinical practice.[9] They hypothesized three pairs of closely linked Rh antigens, Cc, Dd and Ee, which are inherited one from each parent as two sets of three alleles. An individual may be homozygous or heterozygous for each of the three alleles. The presence or absence of the D antigen site, respectively, determines whether an individual is Rh positive or Rh negative. Because certain combinations are more common than others, the D genotype may be predicted from the phenotype determined using antibody-specific sera for D, C, c, E and e (**Table 2**). The 'd' antigen has never been detected and its existence is questionable.

The Rh blood group includes some 40 other antigens in addition to cCDeE. The most common is the D^u variant of which there appear to be two types. The first (and most common) group of women are actually Rh positive, but their D expression has been weakened by the presence of a C allele on the complementary chromosome (e.g. Cde/cDe). These women are not at risk for D isoimmunization. In the second group of women termed D^u-positive, part of the D antigen is actually missing. These women are at risk for D isoimmunization.[11]

The primary immune response to the D antigen manifests over 6 weeks to 12 months. It is usually weak, consisting predominantly of IgM that is too large to cross the placenta. Thus, the first pregnancy is not usually at great risk. A second antigen challenge generates an amnestic response which is both rapid and almost exclusively IgG. Bowman observed that the longer the duration between challenges, the greater the increase in both the quantity of antibody and the avidity with which it binds to the red blood cell.[12] The presence of both these features increases the chances for more severe fetal disease.

Table 2

Prediction of Rh (D) zygosity based on phenotype

Phenotype CDE	Genotype CDE	Frequency (%)		Likelihood of zygosity for D % Whites		Blacks	
		Whites	Blacks	Homo-	Hetero-	Homo-	Hetero-
CcDe	CDe/cde	31.1	8.8				
	CDe/cDe	3.4	15.0	10	90	50	41
	Cde/cDe	0.2	1.8				
CDe	CDe/CDe	17.6	2.9	91	9	81	19
	CDe/Cde	1.7	0.7				
cDEe	cDE/cde	10.4	5.7	10	90	63	37
	cDE/cDe	1.1	9.7				
cDe	cDE/cDE	2.0	1.2	87	13	99	1
	cDE/cdE	0.3	<0.1				
CcDEe	CDe/cDE	11.8	3.7				
	CDe/cdE	0.8	<0.1	89	11	90	10
	Cde/cDE	0.6	0.4				
cDe	cDe/cde	3.0	22.9	6	94	46	54
	cDe/cDe	0.2	19.4				

Modified from Mourant et al.[10]

Fetal hematopoiesis can be divided into three overlapping phases corresponding to the major hematopoietic organ: mesoblastic, hepatic and myeloid. Erythropoiesis begins in the fetal yolk sac by day 21 of gestation, moves to the liver and ultimately the bone marrow beginning by 16 weeks gestation.[13] The decreasing contribution of the liver is characterized by an exponential decrease in the number of circulating erythroblasts. Contrary to ABO antigens, which are only weakly expressed on fetal red blood cells, the Rh antigens are well developed by day 30 of gestation. Any IgG crossing the placenta may then bind to the fetal red blood cell. The anti-D antibody triggered hemolysis is not complement-mediated. Rather, the anti-D coated fetal red blood cells are destroyed extravascularly by the reticulo-endothelial system at a faster than normal rate. The response of the affected fetus is quite variable and likely reflects the quantity and subclass of IgG antibody, the efficiency of placental passage, the avidity with which the antibody binds the antigen site, and the maturity and efficiency of the reticulo-endothelial system.

The recent application of fetal blood sampling to the evaluation of hemolytic disease has revealed much regarding the natural history. Anemia may develop slowly over several months in association with a gestationally low reticulocyte count and a gestationally normal bilirubin, or within a week in association with a reticulocytosis and hyperbilirubinemia.[14,15] The normal fetal reticulocyte and hematocrit are shown in **Figures 1a** and **b**. Significant fetal anemia is associated with increased erythropoietin, but in the absence of labor, the concentrations are generally orders of magnitude less than those observed in adults with the same hemoglobin deficit.[16] Erythropoiesis may occur anywhere in the fetal–placental unit. Both the fetal liver and spleen are enlarged secondary to extramedullary hematopo-

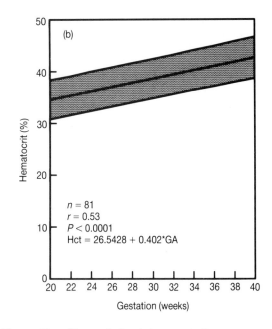

Figure 1b. Normal fetal hematocrit across gestation illustrated as the 95% prediction interval. Reproduced with permission from Weiner *et al.*[14]

iesis and congestion. Nucleated red blood cell precursors, 'erythroblasts' are released into the peripheral circulation, hence the term erythroblastosis fetalis. The greater the number of erythroblasts for gestation, the greater the likelihood prenatal transfusion therapy will be necessary.

All fetal sequelae of hemolytic disease stem from the development of anemia. In general, the fetus tolerates mild to moderate anemia well. However, as the anemia worsens, other metabolic alterations develop. Since the red blood cell is the principle fetal buffer, a metabolic acidemia with hyperlactatemia may be seen with extreme anemia.[18] The precise mechanism underlying the development of hydrops is uncertain, but it probably requires a combination of hematologic and cardiac events. *First*, the hemoglobin deficit must be extreme for the gestational age.[19] Since hemoglobin concentration rises with advancing gestation, hydrops may occur at a higher hemoglobin concentration in late compared with early gestation and is rare prior to 20 weeks gestation. *Second*, hepatomegaly could either hinder blood flow or produce portal hypertension, but this cannot be the sole cause of hydrops in light of the elements which are listed subsequently. Nor is hypoalbuminemia secondary to liver failure a contributing factor as once thought based on postnatal studies,[20] since the albumen concentration is *normal* for gestation in all but premordibund, hydropic fetuses.[16] *Third*, it is now clear that cardiac dysfunction, probably mediated by hypoxemia, occurs in approximately two-thirds of hydropic fetuses. This dysfunction is detect-

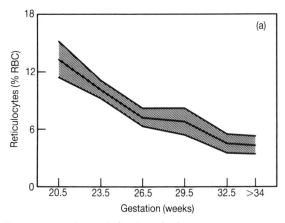

Figure 1a. Normal fetal reticulocyte count across gestation illustrated as the 95% prediction interval. Reproduced with permission from Weiner *et al.*[14]

able immediately prior to the development of hydrops. It is characterized by an increase in the cardiac biventricular diameter, the development of systolic atrioventricular valve regurgitation, and a gestationally elevated umbilical venous pressure (**Figure 1c**).[21] Consistent with ventricular dysfunction, we have found that the umbilical venous pressure rises in the hydropic fetus to a greater extent following the infusion of an intravascular volume compared to a non-hydropic fetus.[22] Within days following the first RBC transfusion and before the hydrops resolves, the umbilical venous pressure declines into the normal range. This reversal is *too* rapid for the occurrence of hydrops to be explained solely by hepatosplenomegaly.

Hyperbilirubinemia is an important part of alloimmune disease and is another element which has its origin in erythrocyte hemolysis. Heme pigment from the hemolyzed red blood cell is converted to biliverdin by heme oxygenase and then to a water-insoluble, lipid-soluble bilirubin (the indirect fraction) by biliverdin reductase. Both the fetus and neonate have reduced levels of glucuronyl transferase, the enzyme necessary for the production of the water-soluble diglucuronide. Indirect bilirubin not bound to albumen can penetrate the lipid neuronal membrane causing cell death. During normal pregnancy, both the fetal serum albumen and bilirubin concentrations rise linearly with advancing gestation (**Figures 1d, e**).[15,23] Virtually all the fetal bilirubin in normal and hemolytic conditions is indirect bilirubin; there is no need to fractionate it routinely. Since placental bilirubin transport is limited, the *normal* fetal total bilirubin is 5–10 times above normal adult levels. The levels rise progressively as the severity of the hemolysis increases. Total bilirubin concentration in fetuses with hemolytic disease often exceeds 3 mg/dl before actual development of the anemia.[15]

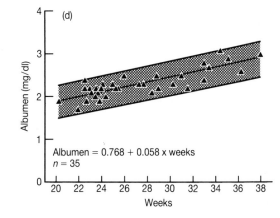

Figure 1d. Normal fetal serum albumen concentration across gestation illustrated as the 95% prediction interval. Reproduced with permission from Weiner *et al.*[17]

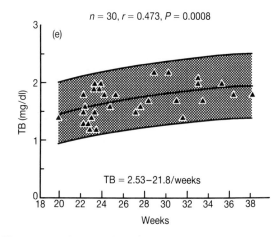

Figure 1e. Normal fetal serum total bilirubin across gestation illustrated as the 95% prediction interval. Reproduced with permission from Weiner.[15]

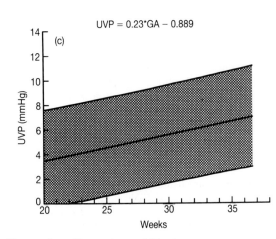

Figure 1c. Normal umbilical venous pressure (corrected for amniotic fluid pressure) across gestation illustrated as the 95% prediction interval. Reproduced with permission from Weiner *et al.*[17]

The neonate with severe hyperbilirubinemia is at risk for an encephalopathy (kernicterus). The concentration of bilirubin necessary for kernicterus rises with advancing gestational age. While a term neonate can tolerate well a total bilirubin of 25 mg/dl, the extremely preterm neonate is at risk when the total bilirubin exceeds levels as low as 12 mg/dl. Affected neonates are initially lethargic and then become hypertonic, lying with their neck hyperextended, their back arched, and their knees, wrists and elbows flexed. They suck poorly and ultimately develop apneic episodes. Fortunately, with modern-day monitoring of bilirubin levels and treatment, these signs of bilirubin toxicity are rarely observed. When severe signs of toxicity are present, the mortality rate approximates 90%. Neural tissue in the auditory center seems particularly sensitive to indirect bilirubin. Survivors usually have profound neurosensory deafness and choreoathetoid spastic cerebral palsy.

Severe anemia leads to hydrops fetalis. The precise mechanism is unclear, but probably combines cardiac and hematologic events. There is clear evidence of cardiac dysfunction in most hydropic fetuses, which precedes the development of hydrops and resolves promptly after fetal transfusion. Postnatally, the affected neonate is at risk for complications of hyperbilirubinemia, which include neural deafness and encephalopathy. All complications of fetal hemolytic anemia are potentially preventable.

DETECTION OF ALLOIMMUNIZATION

Management Options

Antibody detection

The identification and management of potential fetal hemolytic disease employs several methods for the detection of antibodies either in the maternal sera or bound to the fetal red blood cell.

Agglutination test

- *Saline*

Rh positive red blood cells suspended in saline will agglutinate if serum added to the slide contains IgM but not IgG. IgM is too large a molecule to cross the placenta.

- *Colloid*

Rh positive red blood cells suspended in a colloid media (such as bovine albumen) agglutinate if serum containing either IgM or IgG is added to the slide. Thus, if both saline and colloid tests are positive, the antibody may be *either* an IgM or a IgG. IgM can be eliminated by pretreating the serum with dithiothreitol, which disrupts the sulfydryl bonds of IgM preventing binding to the red blood cell. The IgG is unaffected.

Antiglobulin or Coombs' test

- *Indirect*

Red blood cells of specific or mixed antigen type are first incubated with the serum in question. The addition of antihuman antiglobulin causes agglutination if the red cells have adsorbed antibody from the patient's serum. The reciprocal of the highest dilution of serum which causes agglutination is the titer. Indirect antiglobulin titers are 1–3 times more sensitive than colloid agglutination for the detection of alloimmunization.

- *Direct*

Antihuman antiglobulin is added directly to the red blood cells under study. Agglutination indicates the presence of antibody bound to the red blood cell. The antibody may be eluted off the cell and identified by performing an indirect test using type-specific antigen type cells.

- *Enzyme pretreatment*

The red blood cells are incubated with either a proteinase like trypsin or with bromelin to reduce the negative electric potential that normally exists between the cells. When resuspended in saline, the treated cells lie closer together and are more readily agglutinated by the IgG bound to them. These are the most sensitive manual methods for the detection of red blood cell alloimmunization. Variations of the technique have been automated permitting the detection of microgram quantities of antibody.[24] Unfortunately, the automated techniques generate false-positives and are thus not widely used.

Rh NEGATIVE WOMEN DURING PREGNANCY

Management Options

All women, regardless of their past medical and obstetric history, should have blood drawn at their first prenatal visit and after delivery for the determination of ABO and Rh blood type, and for a red blood cell antibody screen (both indirect and direct Coombs' tests). This includes women who have either been previously typed as Rh negative or had a negative antibody screen. Laboratory errors remain a significant contributing cause of anti-D prophylaxis failure and almost 50% of patients managed in our unit since 1983 have an RBC antibody directed against an antigen other than D.[14] Although there is controversy as to how women who are Rh-positive should be managed after the initial screen, the most complete approach would be to repeat the antibody screen at 32 weeks in search of newly developed non-anti-D antibodies. The cost efficacy of this approach is unclear, since the first immunized pregnancy is unlikely to be associated with profound anemia and neonates with significant jaundice will be given a Coombs' test for a blood group incompatibility at birth.

Non-sensitized Rh negative women

The indirect Coombs' test should be repeated at monthly intervals beginning at 18–20 weeks gestation in Rh negative women without evidence of sensitization. In some societies, it may be reasonable to test the father and, if Rh negative, repeat the screen only once between 32 and 34 weeks gestation. Unfortunately, paternity is often only claimed or simply unknown. If the father is tested, the patient should be informed in a non-threatening manner in the privacy of the exam room of the potential risk for a management error. The decision whether to consider paternity in management is best left to the physician's discretion. Even in the socially conservative geographic location of the author, several instances of impossible paternity appear in our Fetal Diagnosis and Treatment unit each year.

Maternal fetal ABO incompatibility has a protective effect on the risk of alloimmunization to D.[12] If the father is heterozygous Rh positive, there is a 50% chance the fetus will be Rh positive. If the father is also ABO incompatible with the mother, there is a 60% chance that the fetus will be ABO incompatible. If the fetus is both Rh positive and ABO incompatible with the mother ($0.5 \times 0.6 = 0.3$ probability), then the risk of maternal Rh alloimmunization is reduced from approximately 16% to 2%.

Women with vaginal bleeding of unknown origin should receive anti-D immunglobulin for prophylaxis. Routine antenatal anti-D immunglobulin therapy is of proven cost benefit and should be administered to all non-sensitized Rh negative women at 28 weeks gestation.[25] Amniocentesis carries a 2% risk of maternal sensitization even when performed under ultrasound guidance and anti-D immunglobulin should be administered if an amniocentesis is performed.[26] At delivery, cord blood is obtained to determine the neonatal ABO and Rh blood type and for the detection of red blood cell bound antibodies. After delivery, the maternal blood should be screened for the occurrence of a fetal to maternal hemorrhage greater than 30 ml. Anti-D immunoglobulin 300 μg (1500 IU) administered to the mother will prevent maternal sensitization secondary to fetal to maternal hemorrhage if the volume has been less than 30 ml of fetal Rh positive blood.[27,28] About 1:400 women experience a bleed of at least this magnitude and will not be protected by the normal dose of anti-D immunglobulin.[28] Both cesarean section and manual removal of the placenta increase fetal to maternal hemorrhage, increasing the risk of Rh sensitization. In such situations, 150–200% of the estimated anti-D immunglobulin requirement is given.

The use of the Kleihauer test at potential sensitization events will indicate whether additional doses of anti-D over and above the 'standard' doses are required. In the UK, the 'standard' or recommended doses of anti-D for potential sensitization events and in the presence of a negative Kleihauser test are 50 μg (250 IU) in the first half of pregnancy and 100 μg (500 IU) in the second half.

Sensitized Rh negative women

Non-invasive evaluation

- *History*

Once an alloimmunized woman is identified, the physician or midwife caring for the mother must make some estimate of the risk of fetal disease. The prediction of fetal risk by a combination of the maternal obstetric history and serologic examination remains at best an imprecise art. While the magnitude of fetal and neonatal disease may remain unchanged from one pregnancy to another, it more commonly progresses in severity. The risk of hydrops in the undiagnosed and untested situation approximates 10% in the first sensitized pregnancy.[12]

- *Antibody titer*

If maternal indirect Coombs' antibody titers are performed in the same hospital using constant techniques, the results are both reproducible and of some value in predicting the risk of severe fetal disease, *especially during the first sensitized pregnancy*. In every laboratory, there will be a critical titer below which severe fetal hemolytic disease does not occur. At the University of Iowa Hospital Blood Bank, this titer over the past 30 years has been 1:8 (~1–2 IU/ml). In other laboratories, it is 1:16 (~2–5 IU/ml). The practitioner must be familiar with his or her laboratory's threshold to avoid clinical error. When the maternal titer is below the critical threshold, it should be repeated at monthly intervals. Any invasive fetal evaluation is deferred until the critical titer is exceeded. The utility of antibody titers above the critical threshold is best during the first sensitized pregnancy. Once the critical threshold is crossed, titer and history are inadequate measures upon which to base management. In 1965, Bowman reported that in a third of severely sensitized fetuses, a potentially lethal management error would have occurred if only the maternal obstetrical history and antibody titer had been relied on.[29]

- *Ultrasound*

The development of high-resolution ultrasound has aided our ability to monitor the fetus at risk for hemolytic anemia. Sonographic findings which may precede the development of hydrops and may be predictive of fetal anemia include amniotic fluid volume, liver length or thickness, placental thickness, increased bowel echogenicity and the cardiac biventricular diameter.[18,30,31] Unfortunately, either the utility or the reproducibility of these findings outside of the initial reporting center has been low.[31] Further, the fetal hematocrit may change rapidly. We have observed on several occasions fetuses with a normal hematocrit who became hydropic over a 7 day period unassociated with a change in the maternal antibody titer. Each had a completely normal ultrasound examination 7 days prior to the detection of hydrops. There is a pragmatic limit upon how often these examinations may be done. Clearly, ultrasound at this time is an adjunct, not a replacement for invasive fetal studies.

Invasive evaluation

The invasive evaluation of fetal hemolytic disease is currently in a state of transition. Two methods, one indirect and the other direct, are available: spectrophotometry ($\Delta OD450$) using a specimen of amniotic fluid obtained by ultrasound-guided amniocentesis, and fetal studies using a blood sample obtained by cordocentesis. Each has potential advantages and disadvantages. Ultimately, the method selected should reflect the facilities available and the physician's experience. As the incidence of maternal alloimmunization is declining, any individual physician's experience with the management will be less than in the past. This makes consultation or referral to a more experienced individual an increasingly important consideration. Once maternal alloimmunization has been confirmed, the patient should be referred to either a Fetal Diagnosis and Treatment Unit or to the individual in the geographic locale with the greatest experience managing fetal hemolytic disease.

• Amniotic fluid spectrophotometry

Frequently, the fetus affected with hemolytic anemia will have an elevated serum bilirubin (**Figure 2**).[15] Since amniotic fluid consists of fetal urine and tracheal/pulmonary effluent by the mid-second trimester, the amniotic fluid bilirubin is also elevated. While William Liley was not the first to employ amniotic fluid spectrophotometry for the management of rhesus disease, he standardized an approach which has remained essentially unchanged since its initial report in 1961.[4] While the $\Delta OD450$ can, when used appropriately, predict the relative fetal hematocrit, it is best at predicting the development of hydrops.

The principal advantage of amniocentesis in the 1990s is that most obstetricians are familiar with the technique and find it simple. The amniotic fluid is obtained by ultrasound-guided amniocentesis (see Chapter 40), transported to the laboratory in a light resistant container to prevent degradation of bilirubin, centrifuged and filtered. The optical density is meas-

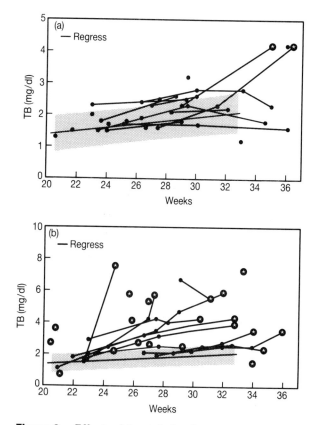

Figure 2. Effect of hemolytic disease on the fetal total bilirubin concentration comparing fetuses who do not (a) to those who do develop anemia (b). *Indicates at which point a hematocrit <30% was first discovered. Reproduced with permission from Weiner.[15]

ured between 700 and 350 nm and plotted on semi-logarithmic graph paper with the wavelength on the x-axis. A line parallel to the y-axis is drawn through 450 nm and the deviation from linearity of the absorption trace measured at that point (**Figure 3**). The result is plotted on semi-logarithmic paper with gestational age on the x-axis and the $\Delta OD450$ on the y-axis (**Figure 4**). Based on the study of 101 single amniotic fluid specimens obtained between 28 and 35 weeks gestation, Liley observed that the $\Delta OD450$ normally declines with advancing gestation (the opposite to fetal serum bilirubin concentration.[4] He divided the graph into three ascending zones.

- zone one represents mild or no fetal disease;

- zone 3 indicates severe disease with the possibility of hydrops developing within 7 days;

- zone 2 is intermediate with the disease severity increasing as zone 3 is approached

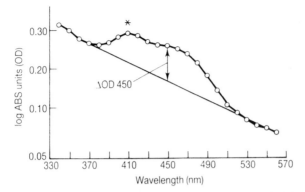

Figure 3. Semi-logarithmic plot of an amniotic fluid ΔOD450. * Illustrates a spike in the absorption of light produced by blood (courtesy of G. Snyder, University of Iowa).

specimens reveal a progressive and rapid rise of the ΔOD450 into the upper 80% of zone 2.

The determination of the severity of fetal alloimmune hemolytic disease by amniotic fluid spectrophotometry has several major disadvantages. First, its application requires the performance of serial invasive procedures over the space of several weeks. In a 20 year experience which included 1027 women, Bowman *et al.* performed a mean of 3.1 procedures per patient.[12] Recall that each procedure is associated with a risk of enhanced maternal sensitization, as well as a loss from either amnionitis or premature rupture of the membranes. Though there are no reports of large numbers of women undergoing amniocentesis after 22 weeks gestation which document the incidence of these complications, series of genetic amniocenteses between 16 and 20 weeks performed under ultrasound guidance demonstrate that amnionitis and rupture of the membranes, both of which are complications of any percutaneous procedure, do occur (in our experience, around 1:400 for second trimester amniocentesis).

Second, amniotic fluid spectrophotometry is an indirect test for fetal anemia. The natural history studies by Liley demonstrate a wide range in disease severity for a single ΔOD450 at any gestational age between 28 and 34 weeks (**Figure 4**). We and others have con-

Amniocentesis is repeated at 1–2 week intervals depending upon the gestation, the zone of the ΔOD450 and the change from the preceding sample. Management is dictated by the trend revealed by serial values. Fetal transfusion (or delivery) is considered when either the ΔOD450 is in zone 3 or serial amniotic fluid

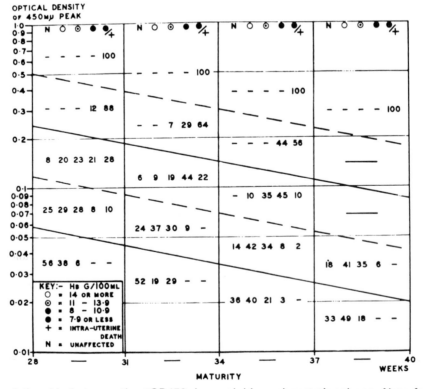

Figure 4. The relationship between the ΔOD450, hemoglobin and gestational age. Note for example, that of fetuses between 28 and 31 weeks and a ΔOD450 in low zone II, 25% are unaffected while 18% are either profoundly anemic or dead. Reproduced from Liley.[5]

firmed that observation using cordocentesis to obtain a fetal blood sample. Though most obvious for zone 2, it is also true for zone 3 measurements. In a series of 11 fetuses with a ΔOD450 in zone 3 followed for several weeks, 30% had a clinically acceptable hematocrit at birth.[32] Bowman *et al.* have opinioned that the 'experience and judgment of the individual assessing the amniotic fluid findings are more important than the method used'.[12] Yet, in their almost unparalleled experience, 9% of the predictions made based on a zone 2 ΔOD450 (which comprised almost 50% of their measurements) were erroneous. Few clinicians in this era of anti-D immunglobulin prophylaxis have their breadth of experience with amniotic fluid spectrophotometry and none are likely to do so in the future.

The third disadvantage of amniocentesis is that there is no clinically useful correlation between ΔOD450 reading and the fetal hemoglobin prior to 28 weeks.[33,34] The normal ΔOD450 in the second trimester is midzone 2 of the Liley curve. Yet, with the advent of high-resolution ultrasound, amniocentesis is often initiated weeks before. Practitioners in this situation rely on the trend of several amniocenteses or the finding of an extraordinarily high ΔOD450 value (e.g. >0.400). However, the published experience is small.

The fourth disadvantage of the ΔOD450 measurement is that it is subject to a variety of extrinsic errors which can interfere with its laboratory measurement, e.g. maternal hyperbilirubinemia and specimen contamination with blood or meconium. The fifth and final disadvantage of amniocentesis is that there is no way of telling whether the fetus is Rh negative when the father is heterozygous. Unnecessary repeat amniocenteses may be performed.

• *Fetal blood sampling*

The accuracy of cordocentesis for the evaluation of fetal anemia has never been an issue. The concerns have been safety (immediate vascular accidents and the longer term risk of worsening sensitization) and how to decide if and when to repeat the cordocentesis. The safety of cordocentesis is detailed in Chapter 41. The pregnancy loss rate reflects the indication for the procedure, the presence of hypoxemia, the vessel actually punctured, and the technique used (needle guide *vs* free hand).[35] If a needle guide is used to eliminate any risk of lateral movement of the needle, the placenta avoided in instances of mild to moderate sensitization (as would be the practice for amniocentesis) by targeting a free loop of cord, and the umbilical vein punctured, the risk of losing an otherwise healthy fetus is <0.3%. This is virtually identical to our experience with second trimester genetic amniocentesis. We have also demonstrated that when a placental puncture is avoided, the magnitude of the fetal–maternal bleed as reflected by the percent increase in the maternal serum alpha-fetop-

rotein concentration after cordocentesis is similar to that found after amniocentesis.[36] Though we continue to measure serial indirect Coombs' titers in patients who begin testing with a titer $\leq$1:128, only two women have shown a 'two-tube' increase in titer and the hematologic status of their fetuses remained stable.

The first cordocentesis is performed when the maternal indirect Coombs' titer has exceeded the critical threshold at the same gestation an amniocentesis would normally be done. In our unit, this is between 24 and 25 weeks unless there is a history of a severely affected fetus earlier in gestation or the initial indirect Coombs titer of a first affected pregnancy is very high or increasing rapidly. The laboratory tests performed on the first and on any subsequent fetal blood sample are listed in **Table 3**. Either a strongly positive direct Coombs test or a manual reticulocyte count outside the 95% confidence interval (**Figure 1a**) are high risk factors for the development of prenatal anemia.

Table 3
Fetal hematologic and serologic
testing for the prediction of anemia

First specimen
ABO and Rh type
Direct Coombs test
Complete blood count (CBC)
Manual reticulocyte count (%RBCs)
Total bilirubin

Subsequent specimens
Complete blood count (CBC)
Manual reticulocyte count
Total bilirubin

The protocol for risk assessment and the timing of any repeat cordocenteses is shown in **Table 4**. There is a significant direct correlation between the reticulocyte count, the strength of the direct Coombs test, the risk of fetal anemia and the trimester during which it will occur.[14] Using direct fetal hematologic and serologic tests, a sensitive and specific assessment of the risk for developing pathologic levels of fetal anemia can be made. Approximately 50% of alloimmunized women require only one cordocentesis (**Figure 5**).

By employing ultrasound as a backup, delivery may be safely deferred until 37–38 weeks with only a 2% risk of unexpected anemia.[37] Eighty percent of pregnancies requiring more than one cordocentesis will ultimately require a fetal transfusion for a hematocrit less than 30%. However, this protocol for assessment is predictive of prenatal anemia only, not postnatal

Table 4
Criteria for repeat cordocentesis if affected fetus

Pattern	Hematocrit	Reticulocytes	&/or Direct Coombs'	Interval for cordocentesis	Scan	Comments
1	Normal	Normal	−/tr	—	4 week interval	Repeat if initial maternal indirect Coombs <1:128 and two-fold increase documented
2	Normal	Normal or <2.5 centile	1+/2+	5–6 weeks	2 week interval	Do not repeat after 32 weeks if studies unchanged; delivery at term
3	Normal	>97.5 centile	3+/4+	2 weeks	1 week interval	Continue through 34 weeks if hematocrit stable; delivery at 37–38 weeks if not transfused
4	<2.5 centile but >30%	Any	Any	1–2 weeks	1 week interval	Repeat as long as hematocrit criteria fulfilled; deliver with pulmonary maturity if not tranfused

Modified from Weiner et al.[38]

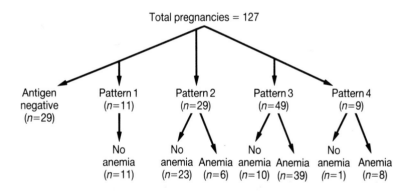

Figure 5. Likelihood of a fetus requiring transfusion based on its hematologic pattern. See **Table 4** for description of pattern type. Reproduced with permission from Weiner et al.[14]

hyperbilirubinemia. Untreated neonates remain at significant risk for postnatal complications (**Table 5**).[37]

Delivery of the non-transfused fetus should occur between 37 and 38 weeks gestation in a center capable of dealing with a potentially ill neonate.

The direct testing of the fetus at risk for hemolytic anemia offers several advantages over amniotic fluid testing. Both sensitivity and specificity for the diagnosis and the prediction of fetal anemia are much greater than the ΔOD450. Direct testing of the fetus for anemia has a zero false-positive rate and a 2% false-negative rate. Fewer invasive procedures are necessary, reducing the overall risk of premature rupture of the membranes, amnionitis and worsening of sensitization.

Treatment by suppression of maternal anti-erythrocyte antibodies

Several methods have been used to suppress or ameliorate either the maternal antibody concentration or its effect on the fetus. None are of documented efficacy and only two appear to have limited potential.

- *Plasmapheresis*

Although plasmapheresis can reduce the antibody concentration by as much as 80%,[39] the decline is transient. At best, plasmapheresis may delay the need for fetal transfusion by a few weeks. Based on the avail-

Table 5
Affected, untreated pregnancies: neonatal complications

	n	(%)	$\bar{x} \pm SD$	Range
			Neonatal outcome	
Gestation weeks	48	(100)	38±2	34–41
Body weight (g)	48	(100)	3176±552	2010–4171
Hematocrit (%)	23	(47)	47±9	24–59
Reticulocytes	10	(21)	9.2±7	2.8–28
Maximum total				
bilirubin (mg/dl)	28	(58)	14.9±5	5–23
Phototherapy (h)				
no	17	(36)	—	
yes	31	(64)	110±60	23–240
DVET	8	(17)	—	
Late transfusion	6	(13)	—	

Modified from Weiner.[37]
DVET, double volume exchange transfusion; late transfusion, performed in the first
3 weeks of life for anemia not present at birth.

able information, this costly procedure is indicated only when there is a history of hydrops prior to 20–22 weeks and the father is homozygous for the offending antigen. In these circumstances, plasmapheresis should be begun at 12 weeks, removing 15–20 l per week. Because of the risk of hepatitis, it should not be undertaken lightly.

- *Immune globulin*

The intravenous infusion of immune globulin (400–500 mg/kg maternal weight × 5 days q 4 weeks) has been reported to reduce the severity of fetal hemolytic disease.[40] Rarely indicated alone in light of the currently available therapies, intravenous immune globulin may be effective as an adjunct to plasmapheresis.

Treatment by fetal transfusion

In the absence of hydrops, fetal transfusion therapy of any kind should not be undertaken without first confirming the fetus does indeed have a significant anemia. We define this as a hematocrit less than 30%, since it is below the 2.5 centile for all gestational ages greater than 20 weeks (see discussion under Intravascular Transfusion). These procedures should be performed only by individuals in units with considerable and regular experience, 8–10 transfusions per year as a minimum, whenever possible.

- *Intraperitoneal*

The original method for fetal transfusion is the intraperitoneal injection of packed red blood cells. The blood is absorbed via the lymphatic vessels and requires fetal respiration. A mean of 10% of the transfused cells are absorbed by the non-hydropic fetus each day. In the presence of hydrops, absorption is poor. The volume infused is a compromise between the estimated hemoglobin deficit and the amount of packed cells that will safely fit into the intra-abdominal cavity. The formula of Bowman is quite practical:

Volume = (weeks gestation −20) × 10 ml

Once absorption is complete, the residual hemoglobin concentration may be estimated by:

Residual = $((0.8 \times x)/(125 \times y)) \times ((120 - z)/120)$

where x is the amount of donor blood in grams transfused, y the estimated fetal weight, z the interval in days since the last transfusion and 120 the estimated life of the transfused blood. The second transfusion is performed when the first has been completely absorbed and thereafter at 3–4 week intervals. If the fetus is both hydropic and survives the first intraperitoneal transfusion, the fetal abdomen is drained as completely as possible at the time of the second transfusion to minimize pressure and maximize the amount of fresh packed cells that may be infused. The last transfusion is performed no later than 32 weeks gestation.

Intraperitoneal transfusion has several drawbacks. In addition to a slow correction of the hemoglobin deficit, it carries a higher risk of trauma and the unique risk of obstructing cardiac return should the intra-abdominal pressure rise too high. Intraperitoneal transfusion has no advantage over intravenous transfusion except when percutaneous access to the fetal vasculature is extremely difficult, such as prior to 18 weeks gestation.

It has been suggested that a combined intravascular and intraperitoneal transfusion will allow a wider interval between procedures. Further study of this approach is needed, since the intravascular route permits routine spacing of 3–5 weeks (see below) and combined transfusion rarely reduces the actual number of required needle punctures. And while there has not been a randomized trial comparing the intraperitoneal and intravascular routes, it is clear that the intravascular approach entails a lower risk of trauma and death for both hydropic and non-hydropic fetuses. The highest reported survival rates with intraperitoneal transfusion are well below those for intravascular transfusion,[41–43] and in a historical comparison from an experienced team in Winnipeg, Canada, the risk of death per transfusion was six times that of intravascular transfusion.[43] Though the method is summarized in **Table 6**, intraperitoneal transfusion is likely soon to become more of historical interest.

- *Intravascular*

In contrast to intraperitoneal transfusion, the goal of intravascular transfusion therapy is the *term* delivery of a healthy, non-anemic neonate. Tranfusions are begun when the fetal hematocrit declines below 30%.[38] This is a pragmatic selection, since the fetus can tolerate a hematocrit 25% or lower without clinically significant sequelae. However, it is reasonable, since:

- 30% is less than the 2.5 centile after 20 weeks gestation (**Figure 1b**);

- many patients referred to a Fetal Diagnosis and Treatment Unit come from a great distance away and cannot be seen on either a twice-weekly or even weekly basis without great hardship;

- it is difficult to predict how fast the fetal hematocrit will decline with great certainty;

- treatment of significant anemia will prevent the development of hydrops which greatly increases the likelihood of an adverse outcome.

Table 6
Protocol for fetal intraperitoneal transfusion

Preparation

Confirm fetal hematocrit <30%
Preparation of donor blood as fresh as possible
   compatible with both mother and fetus
   buffy coat poor
   washed in saline × 3
   irradiated
   final hematocrit 90%
Preparation of two sets of tubing with three-way valves for
   transfusion; filters are mandatory
Diazepam 5–10 mg slow i.v. for maternal comfort
Lateral displacement of the uterus, support lower back
Acetone wipe to remove ultrasound contact gel from the
   skin
Popovidine or alcohol surgical preparation of the skin
Drape as desired and prepare surgical tray
   20 gauge Tuohy needle 25 cm long
   20 ml syringe
   5 ml normal saline
   22 gauge spinal needle
   pancuronium 0.3 mg/kg EFW
Prepare ultrasound transducer

Transfusion

Target fetal abdomen between umbilicus and bladder,
   avoid liver
Administer pancuronium intramuscularly targeting the fetal
   buttock
Insert Tuohy needle into selected site
Confirm intra-abdominal, extravisceral location by
   injecting saline
Infuse donor blood in 10 ml aliquots over 10 min,
   checking the fetal heart rate after each aliquot
Continue transfusion until planned volume infused
   calculated by:
      volume = (weeks gestation −20) × 10 ml

Follow-up

Continuous heart rate monitoring until fetal movement
   resumes
Document complete absorption of donor blood by serial
   ultrasound examinations at 2–3 day intervals
Second transfusion after complete absorption; thereafter,
   repeat at 4 week intervals

Procedure: Intravascular Transfusion

The protocol used for intravascular transfusion is shown in **Table 7**. *Blood for the transfusion should be fresh if available, and compatible with both mother and fetus. Infectious agents routinely tested for include cytomegalovirus, hepatitis A, hepatitis B, hepatitis C and human immune deficiency virus. The blood, prepared the day of transfusion, is rendered leukocyte poor, washed several times in saline to remove particles associated with transmission of viral infection, resuspended in saline to a hematocrit between 70–80%, and irradiated to eliminate the small risk of fetal graft versus host disease.*

The patient is made comfortable with pillows under her knees to take pressure

Table 7
Protocol for fetal intravascular transfusion

Preparation

Confirm fetal hematocrit <30%
Preparation of donor blood as fresh as possible
  compatible with both mother and fetus
  buffy coat poor
  washed in saline × 3
  irradiated
  final hematocrit 70–80%
Preparation of two sets of tubing for transfusion and
  measurement of umbilical venous pressure (UVP); filters
  are mandatory
Diazepam 5–10 mg slow i.v. for maternal comfort
Lateral displacement of the uterus, support lower back
Acetone wipe to remove ultrasound contact gel from the
  skin
Popovidine or alcohol surgical preparation of the skin
Drape as desired and prepare surgical tray
  eight 1 ml tuberculin syringes:
    flush three with heparin (100 U/ml)
    fill one with lidocaine (1%)
    fill one with desired dose of pancuronium
      (0.3 mg/kg SEFW)
    three 3-way valves
    one 5″ 22 gauge needle
    three 4″ × 4″ gauze sponges
Prepare transducer

Transfusion

Puncture vein at most accessible site
Immediately administer pancuronium – paralysis will be
  rapid
Aspirate 1 ml for CBC, Kleihauer stain and reticulocyte
  count; check hematocrit immediately
Aspirate 1 ml for venous blood gases
Measure pressure and confirm puncture is of umbilical
  vein
Begin infusion of packed RBCs after double checking that
  there is no air in the system
Infuse half the estimated requirement (see **Table 8**)
Repeat blood sampling and pressure measurement
Halt transfusion if the rise in the UVP has exceeded
  10 mmHg; check heart rate to rule out bradycardia as an
  explanation
If UVP acceptable, calculate remaining volume necessary
  to achieve a hematocrit of 50%; infuse that volume
Repeat blood sampling and pressure measurement; remove
  needle if UVP at acceptable level
Monitor fetus until spontaneous movement resumes

off her lower back and the uterus laterally displaced to avoid supine hypotension during the transfusion. Because the transfusion takes on average 25–30 min, diazepam 5–10 mg i.v. is given to enhance maternal comfort and cooperation. The abdomen is surgically prepared, draped

and the operator's hands gloved. Neither a surgical mask nor cap are necessary. Nor is their evidence that prophylactic parenteral antibiotic administration is either effective or cost-efficient. The skin is the main source of bacterial contamination. The operator should never touch the shaft of the needle. A new needle is used if one must be removed after insertion into the skin. With this protocol, the incidence of amnionitis at the University of Iowa is <0.5%. The skin is filtrated with 1% lidocaine in deference to the duration of time the needle will be in situ.

The easiest approach to the umbilical vein is selected. In total, 35% of transfusions at Iowa are performed in a free loop of cord. The vein is punctured with a 22-gauge needle as it is adequate for the infusion of 80% hematocrit packed red blood cells. A larger gauge needle unnecessarily increases the risk of premature rupture of the membranes. Immediately following the free return of blood, the fetus is paralyzed with pancuronium (approx 0.3 mg/kg of the estimated fetal weight, EFW, range 0.2–0.6 mg/kg) regardless of the puncture location, since any fetal movement may lacerate the vessel or dislodge the needle. Should the latter occur during transfusion, a catastrophic Whartons jelly hematoma with concomitant decrease in umbilical blood flow could result. Pancuronium, as opposed to other agents for neuromuscular blockade, has the theoretic advantage of causing an increase in heart rate secondary to catecholamine release. Without pancuronium, transfusion decreases the fetal heart rate and cardiac output prolonging the time required to clear the acid contained in the preserved banked donor blood. With pancuronium, the fetal heart rate remains at or above the pre-transfusion rate. The injection of the pancuronium, followed by the measurement of the umbilical venous pressure, allows the definitive identification of the vessel punctured. If the artery is inadvertently entered, the needle is removed, since the risk of a fetal bradycardia is increased five-fold. Though furosemide has been used in the past (3 mg/kg EFW), clinical and laboratory investigations have failed to show a benefit.[44]

*The equipment needed for an intravascular transfusion is illustrated in **Figure 6**.*

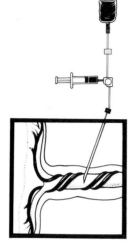

Figure 6. Set-up for an intravascular transfusion.

The blood must be filtered immediately prior to transfusion to remove aggregates which could obstruct the microvasculature. Careful attention is paid to purge the system of air. With a series of three-way valves, an assistant can inject the donor blood while the operator is free to concentrate on the fetus and needle placement which may shift with uterine activity. Prostaglandin synthetase inhibitors are contraindicated, since an increase in the fetal prostacyclin and PGE₂ levels are part of the normal adaptive responses to the abrupt increase in intravascular volume.[45] The assistant must remain poised to halt the infusion if there is any abrupt change in the resistance to flow. To minimize the time the needle is in place, the blood is infused with haste up to 5 ml/min.

Except for the first transfusion of a hydropic fetus, the target for the post-transfusion hematocrit is 48–55%. The volume required will depend upon gestational age, the initial hematocrit and the presence of hydrops. Assuming similar opening and closing hematocrit measurements, the volume infused is strongly dependent on gestational age (see **Table 8**).

• *Fetal hydrops*

Not infrequently, the volume infused equals or exceeds that of the calculated total fetal–placental intravascular volume. Because most hydropic fetuses have evidence

Table 8
Intravascular fetal blood transfusion

Approximate volumes of donor blood (Hct = 72%) required for intravascular transfusion after the first transfusion to raise the Hct to 45–55% from 25%

Gestation	Volume (ml)
≤22.5	25–40
22.5–27.49	45–65
27.5–32.49	75–90
≥32.5	100–120

of myocardial dysfunction which both prevents them from tolerating a significant infusion volume[22] and corrects rapidly with an increase in the oxygen carrying capacity, the target hematocrit after their first transfusion is only 25% (see Pathophysiology). Twenty-four hours later, the hematocrit can (in most instances) be safely brought to 50% by the second transfusion. The decline in UV pH, which normally occurs during transfusion, appears to be especially important in severely anemic fetuses. The red blood cell is the principal fetal buffer and the pH of the banked blood preserved in citrate is approximately 6.98–7.01. We found that our losses of hydropic fetuses from transfusion were associated with a profound acidemia even when the increase in the umbilical venous pressure had been acceptable and there was no acute bradycardia. We speculated that the acidemia aggravated the pre-existing pump failure and began to infuse bicarbonate in 1 meq increments to maintain the UV pH above 7.30. Since that practice was initiated, there have been no further losses and it is now our standard practice for the severely anemic fetus.

Numerous formulas have been proposed for the calculation of the volume of transfused blood necessary (see examples given in Table 8). Though reasonably accurate, none are good enough to remove the needle without first checking the hematocrit. Further, there is a possibility of overtransfusion when any formula is relied upon blindly. We prefer to transfuse half the estimated total and then check the incremental increase. Based on the increase in hematocrit achieved with the first aliquot, the remaining volume necessary can be accurately and rapidly calculated. Contrary to the adult or child, donor blood with a hematocrit below 80% equilibrates rapidly perhaps because of the rapid fluid exchange across the placenta. On many occasions, we have found the hematocrit 24 h after transfusion to be within a few percentage points of the close. Transfused blood with a hematocrit higher than 80% is more viscous and does not equilibrate as rapidly. Volume guidelines across gestation are offered in **Table 8**.

The decline in the hematocrit after transfusion will

be more rapid and variable between the first and second transfusions compared with subsequent procedures. This variability results from the differing rates of destruction of disparate amounts of fetal antigen-positive and banked antigen-negative red blood cells. Except as noted above for the hydropic fetus, the second transfusion is performed 2 weeks after the first. Subsequently, the decline in hematocrit per week, defined as (closing hematocrit transfusion x − opening hematocrit transfusion $x + 1$)/week interval, is quite predictable for any given fetus (**Figure 7**). The rate at which the hematocrit drops declines with advancing gestation, such that by 34–35 weeks, delivery may be safely delayed 4–5 weeks without another transfusion.

The fetus can be monitored during the transfusion by a variety of methods. Many prefer to visualize the fetal heart at periodic intervals to rule out bradycardia. While important, it is of limited value. Umbilical venous pressure measurement is a superior monitoring method for several reasons. First, an occasional non-hydropic fetus (about 6.5% in our experience) with a low hematocrit will not tolerate the transfusion volume necessary. Under such circumstances, an increase in the umbilical venous pressure of more than 10 mmHg may occur and is associated with increased perinatal mortality. If the pressure rises more than 10 mmHg, the transfusion should either be halted or an appropriate volume of blood removed to reduce the umbilical venous pressure into a safe range. Second, fetal brady-

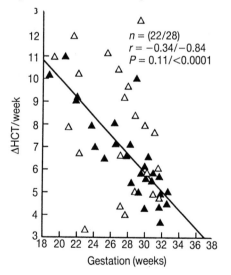

Figure 7. The rate at which the hematocrit declines per week after a transfusion. Open triangles reflect the interval decline between the first and second transfusions. The solid black triangles and the regression line reflect the decline in hematocrit per week between subsequent transfusions. Thus, if the fetus was transfused to 50% hematocrit at 22 weeks, we would expect it to decline approximately 9% per week. Based on this estimate, the transfusion would be repeated in 2.5 weeks.

Table 9

Acute non-hematologic effects of intravascular transfusion

Cardiovascular

Increased intravascular volume
Decreased heart rate (without pancuronium)
Decreased cardiac output (without pancuronium)
Increased umbilical venous pressure
Increased renal blood flow
Decreased placental resistance
Decreased aortic resistance

Biochemical

Acidemia (blood preservative, inadequate fetal buffer capacity)
Increased oxygen carrying capacity
Increased viscosity
Increased atrial naturetic peptide
Increased prostacyclin
Increased prostaglandin E_2
Increased iron stores (chronic)

cardia will increase the umbilical venous pressure. If pulsed Doppler is part of the ultrasound equipment used, the two causes of an elevated umbilical venous pressure can be easily differentiated by dropping a Doppler gate on the umbilical artery. Finally, any resuscitative efforts triggered by a fetal bradycardia will be facilitated with the needle in place.

Intravascular transfusion has many effects on the fetus (**Table 9**) other than raising the hematocrit.[45–47] Many, such as the increase in atrial naturietic factor and prostacyclin, help the fetus to tolerate a volume load that postnatally would be lethal.

It is advantageous to perform at least two transfusions 3 weeks apart prior to delivery, since postnatal complications of hyperbilirubinemia are significantly less likely after two or more prenatal transfusions.[38] In experienced hands, fetal losses are uncommon and confined to the previable fetus. In our view, there is no justification for routine preterm delivery. The last transfusion is performed 34–35 weeks gestation and labor induced at 37–38 weeks.

The obstetric philosophy need not be altered for the non-anemic, transfused fetus. There is no reason to deny either a vaginal birth after cesarean section or the vaginal delivery of the appropriately selected breech just because of a prenatal transfusion. If the final hematocrit at the end of the last transfusion is 50%, it will be in the mid-30s in the umbilical cord at delivery. Typically, the neonatal hematocrit increases 5–15% within 8 h of delivery, reflecting a massive shift of extracellular and intravascular fluid. Over the next few days to weeks, the hematocrit will decline to or below the delivery level.

Postnatally, infants who received *in utero* transfusion therapy do remarkably well with an average hospitalization time of less than 7 days. Their hyperbilirubinemia can usually be managed with phototherapy. Because they are delivered at term, a higher neonatal bilirubin concentration can be tolerated. Double volume exchange transfusion is rarely needed when there have been at least two prenatal transfusions. However, small, simple transfusions are frequently necessary, often beginning at several weeks of age, as the banked blood transfused 5 weeks earlier is at the end of its lifespan and any neonatal blood is hemolyzed by persistent maternal antibody in the neonatal serum and extracellular fluid. This anemia is typified by a low reticulocyte count. The neonatal hematocrit and reticulocyte count should be monitored weekly. If not, severe anemia with resulting high output failure and failure to thrive may occur. The pediatric goal is to keep the neonate asymptomatic but with a modest anemia (>16%) so as to maintain an erythropoietic stimulus. Though the period of neonatal anemia is transient, neonates may go 16 weeks before reticulocytes appear on a peripheral smear. Once a reticulocytosis is noted, further transfusion therapy is generally not needed.

Effect of anemia and treatment on the fetus

It is remarkable how well the fetus tolerates all but the most severe degree of anemia. Fetuses who have a mild, chronic anemia are neither growth-deficient or acidemic. Though mild to moderate anemia is not associated with dramatic prenatal sequelae, severe anemia clearly is so. As dramatic as hydrops fetalis may be, it is for the most part preventable and completely reversible. Hydropic fetuses who are not yet grossly acidemic recover rapidly with appropriate transfusion therapy and on long-term follow-up appear without specific sequelae.[48,49]

Transfusion therapy has a predictable and desirable efefct upon fetal erythropoiesis. With adequate replacement of fetal erythrocytes, the reticulocyte count and percent of circulating red blood cells of fetal origin drops rapidly (**Figure 8**). Part of this decline may be due to consumption of newly formed fetal RBCs as they emerge from the fetal bone marrow and liver, but after two transfusions correcting the hematocrit to 50%, smears of neonatal bone marrow reveal decreased erythrogenic precursors.[50] The greater the number of prenatal transfusions (i.e. the longer the period of fetal erythroid suppression), the less severe the hyperbilirubinemia postnatally and the longer the suppression of erythropoiesis postnatally.[38] These observations, coupled with the decrease in fetal plasma erythropoietin concentrations after several transfusions, are indicative of marrow and liver suppression.[16]

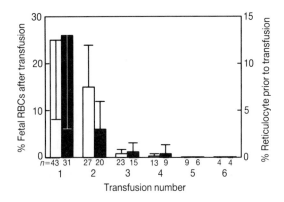

Figure 8. Effect of simple intravascular transfusion on the circulating fetal red blood cell percentage (□) and % RBC which are reticulocytes (□).

Future pregnancies: prepregnancy consultation

Modern approaches to fetal hemolytic disease have drastically reduced the impact of this disease on the family. Though cognisant that it may occur, we do not expect to lose a fetus to hemolytic disease. Several women under our care, after presenting with a hydropic fetus in the first treated pregnancy, have gone on to a second and a third treated pregnancy. Though not unreasonable to suggest in many cases, there is no reason to badger these women toward either an undesired surgical sterilization or a pregnancy by artificial insemination with an Rh negative donor to avoid a recurrence. However, it is essential they understand the time demands that will be placed upon them, the costs and maternal and fetal risks involved. This information is best supplied prior to conception.

CONCLUSIONS

The management of the pregnant alloimmunized woman utilizes both direct and indirect methods of maternal/fetal evaluation. Serial indirect Coombs' tests are performed at monthly intervals after 18 weeks gestation until the critical titer for the laboratory is exceeded. At that time, an invasive evaluation should be initiated by a consultant skilled in the area. During the first sensitized pregnancy, the Coombs' titer correlates with the severity of fetal disease. After the first sensitized pregnancy, they are poorly predictive. Invasive studies may consist of either amniotic fluid spectrophotometry or fetal blood sampling. The method chosen will depend on the facility and consultant, though cordocentesis has many advantages over amniotic fluid studies with a false-negative rate of 2% and a false-positive rate of 0%. No fetal therapy should be

FETAL HEMOLYTIC DISEASE
Summary of Management Options

Routine screening of Rh negative women

- First visit
  - ABO and Rh group and antibody screen (indirect and direct Coombs')

Non-sensitized women

- Recheck antibodies (monthly)

- Most centers would not test paternal genotype

- Cover potential sensitization events with anti-D (50 μg or 250 IU in the first half of pregnancy; 100 μg or 500 IU in the second half of pregnancy); check extra dose not required with Kleihauer test

- Prophylactic anti-D at 28 weeks (? and 34 weeks) reduces the risk of 'spontaneous' sensitization

Sensitized women

Assessment options

- Non-invasive
  - serial antibody titers in first sensitized pregnancy
  - serial ultrasound scans for hydrops

- Invasive options
  - amniocentesis
  - fetal blood sampling
  (variation exists in practice over which method to use and when to perform it)

Treatment options

- Plasmapheresis (? women with history of hydrops before 22 weeks)

- Immune globulin (largely experimental; ? with plasmapheresis)

- Transfusion (intravascular rather than intraperitoneal) – see **Table 4**

Delivery options

- In non-transfused fetus
  - at 37–38 weeks

- In transfused fetus
  - last transfusion at 34 weeks unless dangerous and deliver at 37 weeks

Pediatric surveillance from birth

- Phototherapy

- Exchange transfusions if severe

- Top-up transfusions may be necessary

undertaken without first confirming fetal anemia directly.

The treatment of significant fetal hemolytic anemia prior to 34 weeks gestation is transfusion. Successful transfusion eliminates the prenatal, and to a large extent the postnatal, complications of fetal hemolytic disease. Intravascular transfusion is rapidly becoming the procedure of choice. But whether the transfusion is intravascular or intraperitoneal, it should be performed by the most experienced person or team available. Delivery may be safely delayed until 37 weeks if intravascular transfusion is done. By maintaining the hematocrit at the high end, fetal erythropoiesis is minimized, reducing the risk of postnatal hyperbilirubinemia.

REFERENCES

1 Diamond LK, Blackfan KD, Baty JM (1932) Erythroblastosis fetalis and its association with universal edema of the fetus, icterus gravis neonatorum and anemia of the newborn. *Journal of Pediatrics* **1**:269–274.

2 Levine P, Katrin EM, Burnham L (1941) Isoimmunization in pregnancy: Its posisble bearing on the etiology of erythroblastosis fetalis. *Journal of the American Medical Association* **116**:825–830.

3 Chown B (1954) Anemia from bleeding of the fetus into the mother's circulation. *Lancet* **i**:1213–1215.

4 Liley AW (1961) Liquor amnii analysis and management of pregnancy complicated by rhesus immunization. *American Journal of Obstetrics and Gynecology* **82**:1359–1368.

5 Liley AW (1963) Errors in the assessment of hemolytic disease from amniotic fluid. *American Journal of Obstetrics and Gynecology* **86**:485–494.

6 Freda VJ, Gorman JG, Pollack W (1964) Successful prevention of experimental Rh sensitization in man with an anti-Rh gamma-2-globulin antibody preparation: A preliminary report. *Transfusion* **4**:26–31.

7 Rodeck CH, Holman CA, Karnicki J, Kemp JR, Whitmore DN, Austin MA (1981) Direct intravascular fetal blood transfusion by fetoscopy in severe rhesus isoimmunization. *Lancet* **i**:652–654.

8 Bowman JM, Pollock JM, Penston LE (1986) Fetomaternal transplacental hemorrhage during pregnancy and after delivery. *Vox Sang* **51**:117–125.

9 Race RR (1948) The Rh genotype and Fisher's theory. *Blood* **3**:27.

10 Mourant AE, Kopec AC, Domaniewska-Sobazak K (1976) *The Distribution of Human Blood Groups and Other Polymorphisms*, 2nd edn, pp. 351–505. Oxford: Oxford University Press.

11 Tippett, P, Sanger R (1962) Observations on subdivisions of the Rh antigen D. *Vox Sang* **7**:9–14.

12 Bowman JM (1992) Maternal alloimmunization and fetal hemolytic disease. In Reece EA, Hobbins JC, Mahoney MJ, Petrie RH (eds), *Medicine of the Fetus and Mother*, pp. 1152–1182. Philadelphia, PA: J. B. Lippincott.

13 Knoll W (1949) Der Gang der Erythropoese beim menschlichen Embryo. *Acta Haematologica* **2**:369–377.

14 Weiner CP, Williamson RA, Wenstrom KD, Sipes SL, Grant SS, Widness J (1991) Management of fetal hemolytic disease by cordocentesis: 1. Prediction of fetal anemia. *American Journal of Obstetrics and Gynecology* **165**:546–553.

15 Weiner CP (1992) Human fetal bilirubin and fetal hemolytic disease. *American Journal of Obstetrics and Gynecology* **116**:1449–1454.

16 Widness JA, Harmann CR, Weiner CP *et al.* (in press) Plasma erythropoietin levels and erythropoiesis in anemic fetuses with immune hemolytic anemia.

17 Weiner CP, Sipes SL, Wenstrom K (1992) The effect of fetal age upon normal fetal laboratory values and venous pressure. *Obstetrics and Gynecology* **79**:713–718.

18 Soothill PW, Nicolaides KH, Rodeck CH, Clewell WH, Lindridge J (1987) Relationship of fetal hemoglobin and oxygen content to lactate concentration in Rh sensitized pregnancies. *Obstetrics and Gynecology* **69**:268–271.

19 Nicolaides KH, Warenski JC, Rodeck CH (1985) The relationship of fetal protein concentration and haemoglobin level to the development of hydrops in rhesus isoimmunization. *American Journal of Obstetrics and Gynecology* **152**:341–344.

20 Phibbs RH, Johnson P, Tolley WH (1974) Cardio-respiratory status of erythroblastotic infants. II. Blood volume, hematocrit, and serum albumin concentration in relation to hydrops fetalis. *Pediatrics* **53**:13–26.

21 Weiner CP, Heilskov J, Pelzer G, Grant S, Wenstrom K, Williamson RA (1989) Normal values for human umbilical venous and amniotic fluid pressures and their alteration by fetal disease. *American Journal of Obstetrics and Gynecology* **161**:714–717.

22 Weiner CP, Pelzer GD, Heilskov J, Wenstrom KD, Williamson RA (1989) The effect of intravascular transfusion on umbilical venous pressure in anemic fetuses with and without hydrops. *American Journal of Obstetrics and Gynecology* **161**:1498–1501.

23 Weiner CP, Sipes SL, Wenstrom KD (1992) The effect of gestation upon normal fetal laboratory parameters and venous pressure. *Obstetrics and Gynecology* **79**:713–718.

24 Moore BPL (1969) Automation in the blood transfusion laboratory. I. Antibody detection and quantification in the Technicon AutoAnalyzer. *Canadian Medical Journal* **100**:381–387.

25 Bowman JM, Chown B, Lewis M, Pollack JM (1978) Rh-immunization during pregnancy: Antenatal prevention. *Canadian Medical Journal* **118**:623–629.

26 Bowman JM, Pollack JM (1985) Transplacental fetal hemorrhage after amniocentesis. *Obstetrics and Gynecology* **66**:749–755.

27 Chown B, Duff AM, James J *et al.* (1969) Prevention of primary Rh immunization: First report of the Western Canadian Trial. *Canadian Medical Journal* **100**:1021–1027.

28 Pollack W, Ascari WQ, Kochesky RJ, O'Connor RB, Ho Ty, Tripodi D (1971) Studies on Rh prophylaxis. I. Relationship between doses of anti-Rh and the size of the antigenic stimulus. *Transfusion* **11**:333–339.

29 Bowman JM, Pollack JM (1965) Amniotic fluid spec-

trophotometry and early delivery in the management of erythroblastosis fetalis. *Pediatrics* **35**:815–821.

30 Vintzileos AM, Campbell WA, Storlazzi E *et al.* (1986) Fetal liver ultrasound measurements in isoimmunized pregnancies. *Obstetrics and Gynecology* **68**:162–166.

31 Nicolaides KH, Fontanarosa M, Gabbe SG, Rodeck CH (1988) Failure of six ultrasonographic parameters to predict the severity of fetal anemia in Rhesus isoimmunization. *American Journal of Obstetrics and Gynecology* **158**:920–926.

32 Frigoletto FD, Greene MF, Benecerraf BR, Barss VA, Saltzman DH (1986) Ultrasonographic fetal surveillance in the management of the isoimmunized pregnancy. *New England Journal of Medicine* **315**:430–432.

33 Nicolaides KH, Rodeck CH, Mibashan RS, Kemp JR (1986) Have Liley charts outlived their usefulness? *American Journal of Obstetrics and Gynecology* **155**:90–94.

34 Weiner CP (1987) percutaneous umbilical blood sampling. In Sabbagha RE (ed.), *Diagnostic Ultrasound Applied to Obstetrics and Gynecology*, 2nd edn, p. 419. Philadelphia, PA: J. B. Lippincott.

35 Weiner CP, Wenstrom KD, Sipes SL, Williamson RA (1991) Risk factors for cordocentesis and fetal intravascular transfusions. *American Journal of Obstetrics and Gynecology* **165**:1020–1023.

36 Weiner CP, Grant SS, Hudson J, Williamson RA, Wenstrom KD (1989) Effect of diagnostic and therapeutic cordocentesis upon maternal serum alpha fetoprotein concentration. *American Journal of Obstetrics and Gynecology* **161**:706–708.

37 Weiner CP (in press) Management of fetal hemolytic disease by cordocentesis: Outcome of affected neonates not requiring transfusion. *Fetal Diagnosis and Therapy*.

38 Weiner CP, Williamson RA, Wenstrom KD, Sipes SL, Widness JA, Grant SS, Estle LC (1991) Management of fetal hemolytic disease by cordocentesis: Outcome of treatment. *American Journal of Obstetrics and Gynecology* **165**:1302–1307.

39 Graham-Pole J, Barr W, Willoughby ML (1977) Continuous-flow plasmapheresis in management of severe rhesus disease. *British Medical Journal* **1**:1185–1188.

40 Berlin G, Selbing A, Ryden G (1985) Rhesus haemolytic disease treated with high dose intravenous immunoglobulin. *Lancet* **i**:1153.

41 Watts DH, Luthy DA, Benedetti TJ, Cyr DR, Easterling TR, Hickok D (1988) Intraperitoneal fetal transfusion under direct ultrasound guidance. *Obstetrics and Gynecology* **71**:84–88.

42 Frigoletto FD, Umansky I, Birnholz J *et al.* (1981) Intrauterine fetal transfusion in 365 fetuses during fifteen years. *American Journal of Obstetrics and Gynecology* **139**:781–786.

43 Harman CR, Bowman JM, Manning FA, Menticoglou SM (1990) Intrauterine transfusion: Intraperitoneal versus intravascular approach. A case-control comparison. *American Journal of Obstetrics and Gynecology* **162**:1053–1059.

44 Chestnut DH, Pollack KL, Weiner CP, Robillard JE, Thompson CS (1989) Does furosemide alter the hemodynamic response to rapid intravascular transfusion of the anemic fetal lamb. *American Journal of Obstetrics and Gynecology* **161**:1571–1575.

45 Weiner CP, Robillard JE (1989) Effect of acute intravascular volume expansion upon human fetal prostaglandin concentrations. *American Journal of Obstetrics and Gynecology* **161**:1494–1497.

46 Robillard JE, Weiner CP (1988) Atrial natriuretic factor in the human fetus – effect of volume expansion. *Journal of Pediatrics* **113**:552–555.

47 Weiner CP, Robillard JE (1989) Arginine vasopressin and acute, intravascular volume expansion in the human fetus. *Fetal Therapy* **4**:69–72.

48 Ellis MI (1980) Follow-up study of survivors after intrauterine transfusion. *Developmental Medicine and Child Neurology* **22**:48–54.

49 White CA, Goplerud CP, Kisker CT, Stehbens JA, Kitchell M, Taylor JC (1978) Intrauterine fetal transfusion, 1965–1976, with an assessment of the surviving children. *American Journal of Obstetrics and Gynecology* **130**:933–942.

50 Giller RH, Widness JA, de Alarcon PA, Weiner CP, Johnson KJ (1990) Postnatal anemia following intravascular intrauterine transfusion for isoimmune hemolytic disease: Natural history and possible mechanisms. *Pediatric Research* **27**:265A (abstract 1571).

45

Fetal Hydrops

DAVID JAMES, JOHN SMOLENIEC, CARL P. WEINER

INTRODUCTION

The phrase hydrops fetalis does not refer to a disease; rather, it is a morphologic description which signifies the presence of an underlying problem. Hydrops is defined as edema *plus* a collection of fluid in at least one visceral cavity.

Traditionally, hydrops has been considered under two headings.[1]

- Immune

- Non-immune.

This remains valid today in clinical practice since the evaluation and survival rates for the two differ markedly. The various presumed causes of hydrops are summarized in **Table 1**. It is likely that many of these are associations rather than actual causes of hydrops.

There has been a dramatic reduction in the incidence of immune hydrops secondary to hemolytic disease since the advent of Rhesus Immune Globulin (RhIG) prophylaxis,[1–5] yet 1–2% of susceptible women still become sensitized. In the UK:[3]

- the incidence of new anti-D sensitization approximates 1:1000 births

- the approximate incidence of old cases is 1.5:1000 births

- the approximate incidence of sensitization from other antibodies is 3:1000

- the approximate incidence of fetal hydrops is 2–3% of those women with either anti-D or other antibodies.

The management of red blood cell (RBC) alloimmunization is detailed in Chapter 44.

It has been estimated that the ratio of non-immune to immune hydrops approximates 9:1.[1] While the reported incidence of non-immune hydrops has been as low as 0.3:1000 births, 1:1000 seems a more realistic figure.[6,7]

PRESENTATION

Fetal hydrops may present clinically in one of several ways summarized in **Table 2**.

Fetal Risks

The main risks from fetal hydrops are:

- *Perinatal death*: There is a high perinatal mortality in association with fetal hydrops. Even in immune hydrops where effective treatment by intravascular red blood cell transfusion is available, mortality rates of 25–30% have been reported in the recent past.[1–5] With non-immune hydrops, the reported mortality rates range between 50 and 90%.[8–11]

Table 1
Abnormalities associated with hydrops
(Chapter numbers refer the reader to detailed discussion of management options for specific conditions
within a given group)

Immune (Chapter 44)

Anti-D Rhesus antibodies
Antibodies to K in the Kell system
Antibodies to Fya in the Duffy system
Antibodies to C and E in the Rhesus system

Non-immune

'Idiopathic'/Unknown

Anemia (other than alloimmunization)
  homozygous alpha-thalassemia (Chapter 23)
  chronic fetomaternal transfusion (Chapter 9)
  twin-twin transfusion and variants (Chapters 10, 55)
  erythroleukemia

Cardiovascular (Chapters 47 and 53)
  severe congenital heart disease (ASD, VSD,
    hypoplastic left heart, pulmonary valve insufficiency,
    Ebstein's anomaly, subaortic stenosis, A-V canal
    defect, Tetralogy of Fallot)
  premature closure of foramen ovale
  premature closure of ductus (? indomethacin therapy
    not reported)
  myocarditis (coxsackie, CMV, parvovirus B19)
  large A-V malformation
  tachyarrhythmias (SVT, atrial flutter)
  bradyarrhythmias (heart block)
  Wolff-Parkinson-White
  intracardiac tumors (teratoma, rhabdomyoma)
  cardiomyopathy (e.g. fibroelastosis)
  myocardial infarction
  arterial calcification

Chromosomal (Chapter 2)
  trisomies
  Turner's syndrome (45 XO)
  triploidy

Pulmonary
  cystic adenomatous malformation
  pulmonary lymphangiectasia
  pulmonary hypoplasia
  diaphragmatic hernia (Chapter 52)
  chondrodysplasia
  bronchogenic cyst and other tumors
  pulmonary sequestration
  congenital hydro-/chylo-thorax

Renal (Chapter 51)
  congenital nephrosis (Finnish type)
  renal vein thrombosis
  urethral obstruction (atresia, posterior valves)
  spontaneous bladder perforation
  cloacal malformation
  prune belly

Infection (intrauterine)
  (Chapters 29, 30, and 49)
    parvovirus B19 (either by anemia myocarditis or
      hepatitis)
    syphilis
    cytomegalovirus
    toxoplasmosis
    herpes simplex
    leptospirosis
    Chagas disease

Liver
  hepatic calcifications
  hepatic fibrosis
  congenital hepatitis
  cholestasis
  polycystic disease
  biliary atresia
  familial cirrhosis

Genetic metabolic disease (many have their effect via the
  liver)
  Gaucher disease
  GM1 gangliosidosis
  mucopolysaccharidosis (types IVa and VII)
  iron-storage disease

Anomalies (many associated with fetal immobility)
  achondroplasia (Chapter 54)
  achondrogenesis type 2 (Chapter 54)
  thanatophoric dwarfism (Chapter 54)
  sacrococcygeal teratoma (Chapter 55)
  arthrogryphosis (Chapter 54)
  multiple pterygium syndrome (Chapter 54)
  Neu-Laxova syndrome
  Pena-Shokeir type I syndrome
  Noonan syndrome
  myotonic dystrophy
  neuronal degeneration

Miscellaneous
  cystic hygroma (Chapter 55)
  meconium peritonitis
  fetal neuroblastosis
  tuberous sclerosis
  small bowel volvulus
  amniotic band syndrome
  torsion of ovarian cyst
  polysplenia syndrome

Placental
  umbilical vein thrombosis
  chorangioma
  true cord knots

Maternal
  diabetes mellitus (Chapter 19)
  pre-eclampsia (Chapter 18)
  severe anemia (Chapter 23)
  hypoalbuminemia (Chapter 25)

Data from references **1–16**.

- *Consequences of the underlying cause*: Even if the hydrops is mild or responds to treatment and the child survives the neonatal period, the long-term prognosis will depend on the underlying diagnosis e.g. cardiac anomaly, chromosomal abnormality, or renal disease (see **Table 1**).

- *Complications of the various invasive diagnostic and therapeutic procedures thought indicated*: These include miscarriage, preterm labor, trauma, perinatal death, and maternal red cell alloimmuniz-ation (see Chapters 36, 40, and 41). In general, the likelihood of a serious complication is considered lower than the risk of hydrops (see above). Thus, the application of these diagnostic techniques is justified for both the diagnosis and importantly, the identification of fetuses who may be amenable to prenatal treatment. Nevertheless, careful coun-seling should be undertaken before performing any invasive procedure since the associated mortality rates may be higher than when the procedure is performed for another indication.[12,13]

Table 2
Presentation of fetal hydrops

Routine ultrasonic screening of the patient with Rhesus or other antibodies (see Table 1)

By chance from
   ultrasound examination
   fetal heart rate recording

Hydramnios

'Large-for-dates'

Reduced fetal movements

Placental abruption

Maternal diabetes

Maternal pre-eclampsia

Maternal Risks

These include:

- *Before labor and delivery*: anemia, hydramnios, and placental abruption.[9,14]

- *At labor/delivery*: cesarean delivery, postpartum hemorrhage (primary and secondary) and retained placenta.[9,14]

PATHOPHYSIOLOGIC MECHANISMS OF HYDROPS

There are at least three pathophysiologic mechanisms which may cause hydrops.[15]

- The first is inadequate cardiac output resulting from either obstructed or diverted outflow, inad-equate cardiac return, or inadequate ionotropic force.

- The second possible mechanism for hydrops is a diffuse lymphatic malformation such as that found in association with cystic hygroma, Noonan's syn-drome, pulmonary or peritoneal lymphangiectasia, or a lymphatic-venous anastomosis.[16]

- The third possible mechanism is liver or peritoneal disease causing an exudative ascites and hypoprot-einemia such as that which might result from an overwhelming viral hepatitis or peritonitis.[17]

Identification of the pathophysiologic mechanism both assists the diagnostic evaluation and helps pinpoint those fetuses who might benefit from prenatal therapy.

Management Options

Assessment/Diagnosis

General

Once hydrops is identified, it is reasonable to offer the patient further assessment in order to attempt to make a diagnosis. The reasons for this are:

- to provide an explanation for the condition

- to provide counseling for further management in the current pregnancy

- to provide counseling about the implications for future pregnancies

- to identify those cases where potentially successful treatment may be offered.

At the beginning of the 1980s it was considered possible to make a definitive diagnosis in only 50% of cases.[1] However, more recent reports have shown an improved rate of positive diagnoses.[8,9] Indeed, one recent article reported a series where the 'idiopathic' group was less than 5%.[21]

The range of investigations appropriate for the assessment of mother and fetus when fetal hydrops is diagnosed are given in **Tables 3 and 4**. Arguably the most valuable of these for both diagnosis of the condition and identification of possible cause is real-time ultrasound evaluation. It has been suggested that the underlying pathophysiology may be surmised by the distribution or pattern of fluid accumulation. Unfortunately, the distribution of fluid did not predict the perinatal outcome and the final diagnoses were often based on morphology.

Invasive fetal tests

Unless there is an obvious structural explanation discovered which cannot be secondary to a chromosome abnormality, the next stage of evaluation requires invasive procedures.

If fetal infection is a possibility, amniotic fluid is obtained for the culture of cytomegalovirus (CMV).[18] Next, a cordocentesis is performed, the intravascular pressure (corrected for amniotic fluid pressure) measured, and blood obtained for total IgM, liver enzymes, blood gases, karyotype, and a complete blood profile

Table 3
Maternal investigations for fetal hydrops

Maternal history

Previous fetal hydrops or diagnosis causing hydrops
Previous baby with jaundice
Ethnic origin

Maternal blood

Complete blood count
Blood group and antibody screen (titer if antibodies present)
Electrophoresis (depending upon ethnic background)
G-6-PD and pyruvate kinase carrier status
Alpha-fetoprotein
Serological test for
　syphilis
　parvovirus B19
　toxoplasmosis
　CMV
　herpes simplex
　coxsackie
Urate, urea and electrolytes
Liver function including albumin
Kleihauer (-Betke) test
Test of glucose tolerance
Lupus anticoagulant and anti-Ro if fetal bradycardia

Data from references **1, 6, 7, 10, 11, 15, 21**.

Table 4
Fetal investigations for fetal hydrops

Ultrasound

Detailed real-time ultrasound for congenital abnormality and abnormality of placenta and cord
Fetal echocardiography, color-flow studies and M-mode
Amniotic fluid volume
Fetal activity
Biophysical assessment (non-stress testing or biophysical profile score) will give an indication of the immediate well-being of the fetus

Invasive (mainly fetal blood)

Umbilical venous pressure
Karyotype (blood, placenta, ascitic or pleural fluids are suitable sources)
Complete blood count
Hemoglobin electrophoresis (depending on ethnic background)
Serological tests for acute phase specific IgM antibodies for infection
White cell enzymes (Gaucher's, mucoplysaccharidoses)
Albumin
Blood gas analysis and pH estimation to provide an indication of the immediate well-being of the fetus

Data from References **1, 6, 7, 10, 11, 15, 21**.

(CBC). It is essential that gestationally appropriate laboratory norms be used.[19] An extra 2 ml aliquot should be stored at $-20°C$ in case the need for additional tests becomes apparent after the preliminary laboratory results have been completed.

Though not identical, the umbilical venous pressure (UVP) can be used as a surrogate for the fetal central venous pressure. Its measurement allows for the rapid separation of cardiac and non-cardiac causes of the hydrops. A normal UVP essentially eliminates a cardiac explanation. While an elevated UVP usually indicates that the pathophysiology causing the hydrops has a cardiac etiology, the exact disorder cannot be determined solely by measuring the pressure. The UVP may also be elevated in the absence of hydrops by cardiac malformations such a Tetralogy of Fallot. The pressure of the umbilical artery (UAP) can also be useful if the artery is inadvertently punctured. Like the UVP, the UAP rises with advancing gestation.[20] Case reports indicate that the UAP is reduced by cardiac tamponade from either a pericardial effusion or massive hydrothoraces.[15]

If the heart is displaced from its normal midline position by a unilateral or asymmetrical, bilateral pleural effusion, the fetal chest should be punctured, the intrathoracic pressure measured, the effusion(s) drained, and both the intrathoracic and UV pressure measurements repeated to determine the effect of decompression and restoration of the heart to its normal midline position (**Figure 1**).

Treatment

General

Once the assessment has been completed, careful counseling is required regarding the overall prognosis and whether treatment is possible. The prognosis depends on the following:

- *The diagnosis*: This will reflect both the underlying pathophysiology and the potential for prenatal therapy.

- *The gestation at presentation*: In general, those presenting before 24 weeks have a worse prognosis than those after 24 weeks. Table 5 gives an indication of the prognosis for the main causes of fetal hydrops.[4,14]

The proportion of cases amenable to prenatal treatment varies in each reported series since they are generally small in number and reflect variation in the local referral practices. It is likely that no more than 20–30% are potential therapeutic candidates.[21]

To date, only hydrops associated with inadequate cardiac output (as defined by an elevated UVP) has been amenable to fetal therapy.[15] There are several, relatively common causes of hydrops in this category.

- anemia (hypoxic ventricular dysfunction)

- arrhythmia

- hydrothoraces

- hyperviscosity syndrome (recipient in the twin to twin transfusion syndrome)

Each of these causes of hydrops are associated with an elevated UVP. Fetal therapy that corrects the UVP also reverses the hydrops. Hydrops characterized by an elevated UVP not remedied by either surgical or medical therapy is usually progressive and the fetus either dies *in utero* or requires preterm delivery for postnatal therapy. Infection and arrhythmia are the only causes of spontaneously reversible hydrops clearly documented.

There are presently no therapeutic options available when the hydrops is not cardiac in origin. In the experience of one of the authors, liver disease secondary to viral infection has been the most common cause of non-cardiac hydrops (**Table 6**). Hydrops of non-cardiac origin does not generally progress and preterm delivery is not usually required.

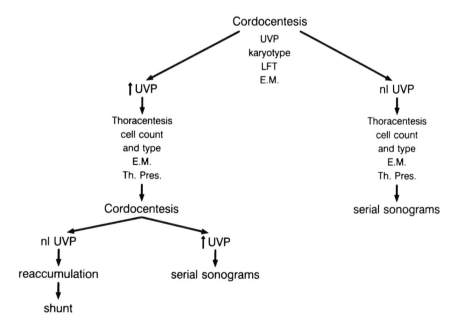

Figure 1. Algorythm for the evaluation of non-immune hydrops associated with hydrothorax. Reproduced from Weiner (1993)[15], with permission.

Table 5
Approximate survival rates (%) for major causes of fetal hydrops

Cause	Gestation at presentation		
	< 24 weeks	>/ = 24 weeks	
Anemia			
alloimmune	24–74	31–92	*a*
non-immune	25	22	*a*
Cardiovascular	7	29	*a*
Chromosomal	0	27	
Pulmonary	0	46	*a*
Renal	0	20	
Infection	50 (2 cases)	11	*a*
Anomalies	0	13	
Miscellaneous	0	25	
'Idiopathic'	0	2	

*a*Potential treatment available.
(Blood transfusion for fetal anemia, correction of fetal cardiac arrhythmia, treatment of twin-twin transfusion syndrome, Shunt insertion for hydro-/chylo-thorax).
Data extracted from references **4, 14**.

Fetal hypoproteinemia/hypoalbuminemia occurs in about a third of non-immune hydrops fetuses, but is distributed with equal frequency in groups with a high and low UVP (the exception being twin-twin transfusion which shall be discussed in Chapters 10, 48 and 55). Clearly, the practice of giving a fetus albumin in the absence of knowing its cardiac status and its albumin level cannot be recommended.[22]

After counseling, the patient may elect to undergo a termination of pregnancy. This decision will no doubt be affected by the gestation at presentation, the prognosis and whether termination is legal. Like much fetal therapy, this is a gray area. A patient may legitimately choose this option even though the condition is potentially amenable to treatment. Termination is more likely to be selected when the diagnosis is made before 24 weeks.

Anemia

Fetal blood transfusion is the only therapeutic option for the treatment of hydrops secondary to anemia. The details of the procedure are provided in Chapter 44. The principles are the same whether the anemia is sec-

Table 6
Causes of non-immune hydrops fetalis by underlying cause

Mechanism	No.	Gestational age (week mean ± 1 SD)	Umbilical venous pressure corrected for amniotic fluid pressure (mmHg)	Comments
Presumed heart failure (elevated UVP)		28 ± 5	13 ± 2	
Cardiac		29 ± 4		
arrhythmia (atrial flutter)	1			UVP 16 mmHg
pericardial effusion (infection)	1			UAP 5 mmHg
Thoracic		31 ± 4	13 ± 1	
chylous thora	4			One UAP 9 mmHg
mediastinal cyst	1			
extralobar sequestration	1			
Polycythemia or anemia		25 ± 5	12 ± 2	
twin-twin transfusion recipient twin	3			
viral infection	1			
fetal-maternal bleeding	1			
No heart failure (normal UVP)		26 ± 6	5 ± 2*a*	
Chylous ascites	2			
Viral infection	3			One UAP 30 mmHg
Cervical teratoma	1			
Unknown	1			Large twin, mild anemia

UVP: Umbilical venous pressure.
UAP: Umbilical arterial pressure.

a$p < 0.05$, compared with value for presumed heart failure.
From reference **15**.

ondary to parvovirus B19 infection or chronic fetomaternal hemorrhage.[23,24] However, the prognosis for both these conditions may be worse than that for hemolytic disease secondary to RBC alloimmunization. This may be because parvovirus B19 can produce, a pancytopenia as well as a myocarditis.[25] Transfusion therapy for parvovirus may not be necessary if the fetus is not acidemic and reticulocytes are present. This suggests spontaneous recovery is underway. In chronic fetomaternal hemorrhage, bleeding tends to continue after transfusion.

The prognosis for homozygous alpha-thalassemia is not nearly as good as for other causes of anemia; the management options are discussed in Chapter 23. There are no effective prenatal treatments for G-6-P-D deficiency and erythroleukemia. Gene therapy may prove possible in the near future and interdisciplinary counseling involving pediatric colleagues and clinical geneticists is advisable.

Cardiovascular

The management options for these conditions are discussed in Chapters 47 and 53. Those hydropic fetuses with an arrhythmia but a structurally normal heart usually respond to either transplacental or direct fetal therapy. The prognosis is good.

Chromosomal

The main therapeutic option is pregnancy termination. Careful counseling of the family is important (see Chapter 2).

Pulmonary

The prognosis for these conditions is generally poor and the therapeutic options limited. Diaphragmatic hernia is discussed in Chapter 52.

The main exception to the above generalization is hydrops associated with hydrothorax causing cardiac displacement. The diagnosis of congenital hydrothorax is a diagnosis of exclusion – excess pleural fluid in the absence of another detectable cause. Hydrothoraces typically present after 24 weeks gestation after human lung development has entered the cannulicular phase. Thus, therapy is aimed at improving cardiac function not pulmonary development. The lymphocyte content of the fluid is not relevant to either the prognosis or the diagnosis.[26] Though it has been known since the early 1980s that the placement of a thoraco-amniotic shunt could reverse hydrops,[27] the rate of success among reported series has been variable.[26] This suggests more than one mechanism may underlie the hydrops. Draining the thorax permits the heart to return to its normal midline position. An initially elevated UVP associated with an elevated intrathoracic pressure which both normalize after the effusion(s) have been drained confirms that the hydrops was secondary to a mechanical impairment of cardiac output.[15] If the effusion recurs, placement of a thoraco-amniotic shunt should be curative. On the otherhand, if the UVP is normal prior to decompression of the chest, or remains elevated after the chest has been drained and the heart has returned to its normal midline position, there is little reason to expect placement of a thoraco-amniotic shunt will be beneficial (**Figure 1**).

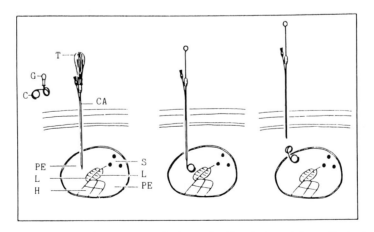

Figure 2. Procedure for insertion of pleuro-amniotic drain. Reproduced from Rodeck *et al.* (1988).[26], with permission. The instruments consist of a double pig-tailed catheter (C) of 6-French nylon tubing with radio-opaque stainless-steel inserts at each end and lateral holes around the coil, a guidewire (G) for straightening, and the trocar (T) and cannula (CA) with two introducers. PE, pleural effusion; H, heart; S, spine; L, lungs.

Procedure: Insertion of Fetal Thoraco-Amniotic Shunt (see **Figure 2**)[26]

Method

The usual preparations for a major invasive procedure (such as fetal blood transfusion) should be followed (see Chapter 44). The practice of using fetal paralysis varies.

In preparation for the procedure, the ultrasound transducer is positioned to give a transverse view of the fetal chest at the level of the maximal fluid collection. The optimal line of approach is chosen to avoid (if possible) crossing the placenta and to enter the anterior-lateral aspect of the fetal chest.

Once the line of approach has been determined, the maternal abdomen is cleaned, draped and a local anesthetic instilled down to the surface of the uterus.

The double pig-tailed catheter with introducing wire is stretched into a more linear shape. A small stab incision is made in the mother's skin and the introducer (trochar and cannula) inserted along the optimal line of approach into the amniotic cavity. The line of entry into the anterior part of the fetal chest is then reviewed and adjusted if necessary. Once this secondary adjustment is made, the introducer is inserted into the pleural cavity with a sharp, stabbing motion.

The trochar is removed and the elongated double pig-tailed catheter with introducing wire carefully inserted down the cannula by an assistant. Pleural fluid will escape through the cannula at this stage.

Once the elongated catheter is completely inside the cannula, the guide wire is removed. After checking that the end of the cannula is still within the fetal chest, the shorter of the two advancing guides is used to advance half the catheter into the fetal chest where it should be seen to adopt its natural shape of a single coil (half of the 'pig-tail').

The introducer cannula is then moved out of the fetal chest into the amniotic cavity. The remainder of the double pig-tailed catheter is extruded from the cannula into the amniotic cavity using the full length guide and the cannula removed from the uterus. If there are bilateral effusions, a second shunt will usually be needed since decompressing only one side can actually worsen cardiac displacement.

A sonographic examination should be performed 8–24 h postoperatively to assess shunt function. Complete resolution of the effusion is to be expected if the shunt is working well. The hydrops itself and the hydramnios may take an additional 10–14 days to resolve. On average, these shunts remain patent for 2–3 weeks. If the pleural fluid reaccumulates, it is either due to blockage or displacement. At this juncture, the decision whether to replace the drain or to deliver will be determined mainly by gestational age.

Complications

Complications of shunt placement include miscarriage, labor and delivery, fetal and maternal trauma, and red blood cell alloimmunization.

Renal

These are discussed in detail in Chapter 51. In general, the absence of amniotic fluid is a poor prognostic sign.

Infection

Apart from parvovirus (see above), very little can currently be done prenatally to treat these conditions once they have produced fetal hydrops. Myocarditis secondary to parvovirus has been treated with fetal digitalization.

Other causes

There are very few therapeutic options available for prenatal treatment of other causes of fetal hydrops. Some workers have used albumin infusions in an attempt to correct the hydrops.[22] These treatments are of gestational scientific value and have thus far proved largely unsuccessful. A more productive approach is to try and discover other causes of fetal hydrops and to reduce this 'idiopathic' group.

<table>
<tr><td>

FETAL HYDROPS
Summary of Management Options

Presentation
See **Table 2**

Management options

Assessment/diagnosis

- Maternal – see **Table 3**

- Fetal – see **Table 4**

Treatment

- Careful counseling about:

  - diagnosis (if known)

  - prognosis

  - possible treatment

- Focus on the identification of potentially treatable causes:

  - blood transfusion for fetal anemia (see Chapters 44, 23, 9, 10, 55)

  - correction of fetal cardiac arrhythmia (see Chapters 47 and 53)

  - treatment of twin-twin transfusion syndrome (see Chapters 10, 48, 55)

  - shunt insertion for hydro-/chylo-thorax

- Termination of pregnancy should be considered in the counseling especially where there is no effective treatment and the gestation is early enough for the procedure to be legal

- Interdisciplinary approach if pregnancy continues

</td></tr>
</table>

CONCLUSIONS

Fetal hydrops is a serious condition which can be caused by a wide range of pathologies carrying, overall, a poor prognosis. The principles of management are:

- Make a diagnosis.

- Offer treatment to those cases where prenatal therapeutic options exist and for whom the prognosis is generally better.

REFERENCES

1 Warsof S, Nicolaides KH, Rodeck C (1986) Immune and non-immune hydrops. *Clinical Obstetrics and Gynecology* **29**: 533–542.

2 Hussey RM, Clarke CA (1991) Death from Rh haemolytic disease in England and Wales in 1988 and 1989. *British Medical Journal* **303**: 445–456.

3 Tovey LAD (1986) Haemolytic disease of the newborn – the changing scene. *British Journal of Obstetrics and Gynaecology* **93**: 960–966.

4 Stangenberg M, Selbing A, Lingman G, Westgren M (1991) Rhesus immunisation: New perspectives in maternal-fetal medicine. *Obstet Gynecol Survey* **46**: 189–195.

5 Rodeck CH, Nicolaides KH, Warsof SL, Fysh WJ, Gamsu HJR, Kemp JR (1984) The management of severe rhesus isoimmunization by fetoscopic intravascular transfusions. *American Journal of Medical Genetics* **150**: 769–774.

6 Holzgreve W, Curry CJR, Golbus MS, Callen PW, Filly RA, Smith JC (1984) Investigation of nonimmune hydrops fetalis. *American Journal of Obstetrics and Gynecology* **150**: 805–812.

7 Machin GA (1989) Hydrops revisited. *American Journal of Medical Genetics* **34**: 366–390.

8 Skoll MA, Sharland GK, Allen LD (1991) Is the ultrasound definition of fluid collections in non-immune hydrops fetalis helpful in defining the underlying cause or predicting outcome? *Ultrasound in Obstetrics and Gynecology* **1**: 309–312.

9 Gough JD, Keeling JW, Castle B, Iliff PJ (1986) The obstetric management of non-immunological hydrops. *British Journal of Obstetrics and Gynaecology* **93**: 226–234.

10 Carlton DP, McGillivray BC, Schreiber MD (1989) Nonimmune hydrops fetalis: A multidisciplinary approach: *Clinics in Perinatology* **16**: 839–851.

11 Holzgreave W, Holzgreave B, Curry CJR (1985) Non-immune hydrops fetalis: diagnosis and management. *Seminars in Perinatology* **9**: 52–67.

12 Maxwell DJ, Johnson P, Hurley P, Neales K, Allan L, Knott P (1991) Fetal blood sampling and pregnancy loss in relation to indication. *British Journal of Obstetrics and Gynaecology* **98**: 892–897.

13 Weiner CP, Wenstrom KD, Sipes SL, Williamson RA (1993) Risk factors for cordocentesis and fetal intravascular transfusion. *American Journal of Obstetrics and Gynecology* **165**: 1020–1025.

14 Hutchinson AA, Drew JH, Yu VYH, Williams ML, Fortune DW, Beischer NA (1982) Nonimmunologic hydrops fetalis: a review of 61 cases. *Obstetrics and Gynecology* **59**: 347–352.

15 Weiner CP (1993) Umbilical pressure measurement in the evaluation of nonimmune hydrops fetalis. *American Journal of Obstetrics and Gynecology* **168**: 817–823.

16 Windebank KP, Bridges NA, Ostman-Smith I, Stevens JE (1987) Hydrops fetalis due to abnormal lymphatics. *Archives of Diseases of Childhood* **62**: 198–200.

17 Bender MD, Ockner RK (1986) Diseases of the peritoneum, mesentery, and diaphragm. In: Sleisenger MH, Fordtran JS (eds), *Gastrointestinal Disease, Pathophysiology, Diagnosis, Management*, Philadelphia: WB Saunders, 1582–1385.

18 Grose C, Itani O, Weiner CP (1989) Prenatal diagnosis of fetal infection: Advances from amniocentesis to cordocentesis. *Pediatric Infectious Diseases Journal* **8**: 459–468.

19 Weiner CP, Heilskov J, Pelzer GD, Grant SS, Wenstrom KD, Williamson RA (1989) Normal values for human umbilical venous and amniotic fluid pressures and their alteration by fetal disease. *American Journal of Obstetrics and Gynecology* **161**: 714–717.

20 Merrill DC, Weiner CP (in press) Intrauterine Pressure: Amniotic and Fetal Circulation: In Ludomirsky A, Nicolini U, Bhutani VK (eds) *Therapeutic and Diagnostic Interventions in Early Life*, Mount Kisco, NY: Futura Publishing Company.

21 Hansmann M, Gembruch U, Bald R (1989) New therapeutic aspects of nonimmune hydrops fetalis based on four hundred and two prenatally diagnosed cases. *Fetal Therapy* **4**: 29–36.

22 Lingman G, Stangenberg M, Legarth J, Rahman F (1989) Albumin transfusion in non-immune fetal hydrops: Doppler ultrasound evaluation of the acute effects on blood circulation in the fetal aorta and umbilical arteries. *Fetal Therapy* **4**: 120–125.

23 Soothill P (1990) Intrauterine blood transfusion for nonimmune hydrops fetalis due to parvovirus B19 infection. *Lancet* **336**: 121–122.

24 Rouse D, Weiner CP (1990) Ongoing fetomaternal hemorrhage treated by serial fetal intravascular transfusions. *American Journal of Obstetrics and Gynecology* **76**: 974–975.

25 PHLS Working Party on Fifth Disease (1990) Prospective study of human parvovirus (B19) infection in pregnancy. *British Medical Journal* **300**: 1166–1170.

26 Rodeck CH, Fisk NM, Fraser DI, Nicolini U (1988) Longterm in utero drainage of fetal hydrothorax. *New England Journal of Medicine* **319**: 1135–1138.

27 Weiner CP, Varner MW, Pringle KC, Hein HA, Williamson RA, Nielsen C (1986) Antenatal diagnosis and treatment of nonimmune hydrops fetalis secondary to pulmonary extralobar sequestration. *Obstetrics and Gynecology* **68**: 275–280.

46

Fetal Thrombocytopenia

MARTIN J. WHITTLE

INTRODUCTION

Fetal thrombocytopenia most often arises secondary to one of two separate disease processes.

- The first results from some form of autoimmune disease in the mother, who may herself have asymptomatic thrombocytopenia or purpura.

- The second results from an alloimmune phenomenon in which the mother produces antiplatelet antibodies which have no effect on her platelet count but cross the placenta and destroy fetal platelets.

In general, hemorrhagic complications are most common in alloimmune, and at the worst, rare with autoimmune disease.

Definitions

Thrombocytopenia is traditionally defined as a platelet count less that $150 \times 10^9/l$ (mild $100–150 \times 10^9/l$, moderate $50–99 \times 10^9/l$ and severe $<50 \times 10^9/l$). However, spontaneous hemorrhage is unlikely as long as the platelet count is greater than $20 \times 10^9/l$.

Incidence

Autoimmune platelet disease, presenting as thrombocytopenia in the mother, occurs with an incidence of 7–8%.[1] The incidence of alloimmune platelet disease is difficult to estimate, but symptomatic newborns result in about 1:5000 pregnancies; it is likely that asymptomatic cases occur more commonly. Unlike red blood cell alloimmunization, about 30% of affected neonates are delivered from nulliparous women.

Risks

Autoimmune disease in the mother

When the mother has asymptomatic thrombocytopenia, the chances that the fetus will develop thrombocytopenia are probably around 4% though the chance of a seriously affected fetus is extremely low ($<0.5\%$).[2] The situation is much less certain when the thrombocytopenia occurs in the presence of purpura, or when it has been necessary for the mother to start corticosteroids or to undergo splenectomy. In these circumstances, the overall risk of fetal/neonatal thrombocytopenia may be as high as 40%,[2] though the risk of serious complications in the fetus may be low. The consequence of thrombocytopenia for the baby when the mother has autoimmune disease is uncertain given the available literature. In one series,[2] the overall risks of bleeding problems was about 12%, although these all occurred postnatally. The most serious risk, because of its immediate and long-term complications, is fetal/neonatal intraventricular hemorrhage (IVH). In this series, IVH occurred in two (2%), one with a platelet count of $7 \times 10^9/l$ and the other $78 \times 10^9/l$ (both delivered by cesarean section). Other, less serious, complications can occur with counts between 100 and $150 \times 10^9/l$. When the count is less than $100 \times 10^9/l$, about 30% of newborns may be expected to have a bleeding problem postnatally.

Alloimmune thrombocytopenia

The chances that subsequent babies will be affected by thrombocytopenia can be estimated from the partner's platelet genotype, but it will lie between 50 and 100%. Alloimmune thrombocytopenia places the fetus at greater risk than that arising from an autoimmune process, possibly because the platelet counts may be lower at an early stage in pregnancy. The risks of a prenatal intracerebral hemorrhage (ICH) in an affected fetus is between 10 and 30%.[3] Intracerebral hemorrhage may occur during delivery but it is the prenatal hemorrhage, a particular feature of alloimmune thrombocytopenia, that is of major concern, since it has the potential to produce mid-brain damage, optic atrophy and secondary hydrocephalus, leaving many survivors with severe mental and physical handicap. Other symptoms that may be distressing but less potentially harmful include bruising, excessive bleeding from puncture sites and rectal bleeding postnatally.

Management Options

Mode of presentation

Autoimmune thrombocytopenia

There are three clues from the mother that the pregnancy may be at risk:

- Asymptomatic thrombocytopenia found on routine testing in pregnancy.

- Present or past idiopathic thrombocytopenic purpura, with or without corticosteroids/ splenectomy.

- Some other disorder associated with thrombocytopenia.

It is likely that the majority of mothers are asymptomatic (65%,[1] 46%[2]). The mothers who are symptomatic

or who have intercurrent disorders are much more likely to have manifestations of their underlying disease, and be on additional therapy such as corticosteroids or to have undergone splenectomy in the past.

Alloimmune disease

Here the method of presentation is entirely different and the history will relate to problems in the fetus or neonate. Some of the neonates with thrombocytopenia will be asymptomatic but identified by a routine blood test taken soon after birth for an unconnected reason. Symptomatic neonates may present either with evidence of damage from a prenatal hemorrhage or with active bleeding. A variation of this presentation would include an unexpected stillbirth.

Laboratory investigations

Autoimmune thrombocytopenia

Maternal platelet counts need to be monitored on a weekly or fortnightly basis depending on the apparent activity of the disease process. The underlying cause of the low platelet count is usually obscure (idiopathic) but conditions like:

- leukemia

- autoimmune disorders, e.g. SLE

- AIDS

- pre-eclampsia

should all be excluded by appropriate testing. A diagnostic bone marrow aspiration is reserved for special circumstances and it is not generally incorporated as a routine test.

The value of testing for platelet-binding or platelet-associated IgG antibody using the indirect antiglobulin test is controversial and highly laboratory-dependent. Overall, it probably has a limited role in the evaluation process (see below).

Alloimmune thrombocytopenia

Once the condition is suspected from the history, the presence of anti-Hpa[1], the most common platelet antibody, or another antiplatelet antibody, should be established in the maternal blood. This is done in a fashion analogous to red blood cell alloimmunization disease, by mixing maternal sera with paternal or donor platelets and observing aggregation. The platelet antigen status of the male partner should be determined to establish zygosity. About 98% of the population are Hpa[1] positive. The absolute level of antibodies in the maternal blood does not correlate well with the severity of disease in the fetus/neonate.

In addition to the immediate parents, other members of the mother's family should be screened, both to establish whether her sisters are at risk and to identify both male or female sibs who may be suitable Hpa[1] negative platelet donors should the need arise for a fetal or neonatal transfusion.

Treatment

Autoimmune thrombocytopenia (**Figure 1**)

In general, corticosteroids should be commenced when the maternal platelet count falls below 50×10^9/l. A falling platelet count as a feature of disease activity (i.e. SLE) may have very serious connotations for the pregnancy and the mother, and is discussed in Chapters 23 and 27. If the platelet count does not increase with steroids, immune globulin may be given at 36 or 37

weeks to obtain a rapid but usually short-lived increase in platelet number prior to delivery.

The management of the delivery of a pregnancy complicated by autoimmune thrombocytopenia remains controversial, with views that range from total non-intervention to cesarean section for all cases. The rationale for non-intervention but avoidance of an operative pelvic delivery is based on the observation that there are few, if any, documented cases of fetal hemorrhage, despite the high incidence of autoimmune thrombocytopenia. The role of fetal blood sampling by either cordocentesis or from the fetal scalp is uncertain.

When maternal thrombocytopenia is an incidental finding, the fetal risk is clearly low. Under these circumstances, and even though the level of the maternal platelet count does not correlate with fetal counts and the presence or absence of platelet-associated antibody do not contribute to the risk calculations, there appears little need to establish the baby's platelet count prior to delivery. However, there are certain factors which may help to identify those babies at particular risk of being severely affected and indicate the need to seek advice from a specialist center. These include:

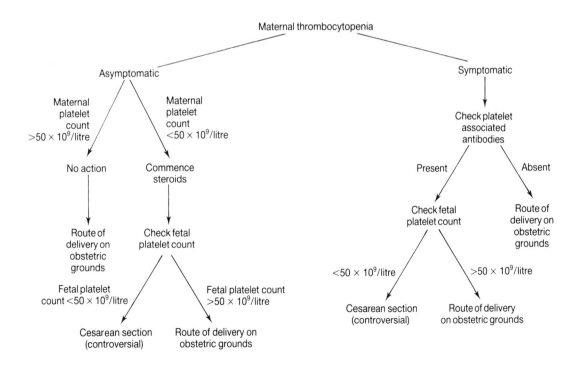

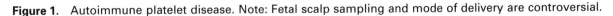

Figure 1. Autoimmune platelet disease. Note: Fetal scalp sampling and mode of delivery are controversial.

- history of ITP

- presence of disease and platelets with a count $<100 \times 10^9/l$, and/or splenectomy, and/or on steroids

- elevated platelet-associated antibodies.

Under these circumstances, the presence of circulating platelet antibodies may help identify a baby at particular risk. In one study,[2] no baby developed thrombocytopenia when circulating antibodies were absent, whereas 50% did so in their presence, with over half of these babies having a platelet count of $50 \times 10^9/l$.

When the risk is substantial, establishing the fetal platelet count prior to delivery seems prudent but is yet unproven. This can be cordocentesis or if the obstetrician prefers, a scalp platelet count can be performed when the cervix has reached about 3 cm dilation. Unfortunately, this tends to give a low result, probably secondary to the sampling method itself. Blood should be collected into EDTA tubes. A level in excess of $50 \times 10^9/l$ is usually recommended if vaginal delivery is contemplated, but the controversies surrounding this issue are discussed above.

If the maternal platelet count is less than $20 \times 10^9/l$ at delivery, platelet transfusion for the mother is advisable.

Alloimmune thrombocytopenia (**Figure 2**)

Management plans are currently undecided and a trial based in the USA is addressing the issue. Cases should be managed in a specialist center. The treatment options include administering dexamethasone and intravenous gammaglobulin to the mother (or, more recently the fetus), backed when necessary by repeated fetal platelet transfusions. Women selected for this type

of treatment usually have had a previous neonate who suffered hemorrhagic complications or has been born with a platelet count below $100 \times 10^9/l$.[3]

The need for treatment depends on the platelet count determined by cordocentesis performed between 20 and 24 weeks. A more aggressive policy might be adopted when a previous baby had suffered an intracerebral hemorrhage than if it had been born with merely reduced platelets.

As well as providing a fetal platelet count, the platelet antigen-type should also be determined. In practice, it may be advisable to commence a platelet transfusion while waiting for the results of the platelet count, since removal of the needle from the cord in the presence of a very low count has been associated with fetal hemorrhage in some centers.

If the fetal platelet count is less than $100 \times 10^9/l$, therapy is indicated. Regimes vary and are currently the subject of randomized trials. One regime includes either intravenous gammaglobulin (IVG) (1 g/kg body weight every week) alone or in combination with 5 mg dexamethasone daily. If either of these regimens fails to produce a rise in the fetal platelet count (checked 2–4 weeks later by cordocentesis), a regimen of either weekly fetal platelet transfusions or direct fetal administration of IVG is commenced. The weekly interval between transfusion of platelets is necessary because of their short life-span. Therapy is a considerable undertaking for the mother and repeated cordocentesis is likely to increase the risk of preterm delivery. However, the prospect of a damaging ICH occurring in fetal life has been claimed to justify the approach, although the risks, costs and inconvenience of the regimens emphasizes the importance of good case selection.

Mode of delivery will depend on the the platelet count at the time of delivery. A trial of labor is reasonable if the platelet count exceeds $50 \times 10^9/l$. If the platelet count is lower than that, labor can be induced after a final platelet transfusion.

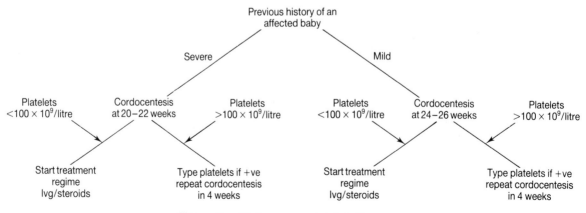

Figure 2. Alloimmune platelet disease.

FETAL THROMBOCYTOPENIA
Summary of Management Options

	AUTOIMMUNE	ALLOIMMUNE
Fetal risk	• Low	• High
Clinically suspected	• Maternal history	• Fetal/neonatal history
Assessment	• Serial maternal platelet counts	• Confirm antiplatelet antibodies in maternal blood (usually anti-Hpa[1])
	• Exclude other causes	• Most centers advocate cordocentesis to assess fetal platelet count before deciding upon therapy (fetal platelet transfusion may be necessary)
	• Value of antibody testing is debated	
	• Fetal blood sampling prior to labor is not indicated	
	• Fetal scalp sampling in labor is controversial	
Treatment	• See **Figure 1**	• See **Figure 2**
	• Options include:	• Manage in specialist center
	• steroids (often if count falls $<50 \times 10^9$/l)	• Ideal management not clear; options include:
	• immunoglobulin (? at 36–37 weeks if steroids fail)	• Maternal therapy:
	• platelet cover for delivery if count ⟨50	• dexamethasone
	• See also Chapters 23 and 27	• i.v. gammaglobulin
	• Pediatric review and surveillance of baby	• Fetal therapy:
		• i.v. gammaglobulin
		• platelet transfusions
		• Cesarean section is likely to be chosen if the fetal platelet count is low

Conclusions

Although the incidence of autoimmune disease is relatively high in women of reproductive age, the chances of the fetus developing significant thrombocytopenia seem fairly low, especially when the condition has been found incidentally in the mother. The situation may be different if the mother suffers from immune thrombocytopenia, particularly if she requires steroids or has had a splenectomy. Even so, the risk of prenatal hemorrhage is remote. Under these circumstances, a fetal scalp platelet count in early labor may provide some reassurance, though this is not a view shared by all.

The situation is different for alloimmune disease. Here, the past history of a child with bleeding problems is important and second trimester investigation of the fetus by cordocentesis should be considered. If affec-ted, the mother can be given either immunoglobulin and/or corticosteroids. Referral to a specialist center is mandatory.

REFERENCES

1 Burrows RF, Kelton JG (1990) Thrombocytopenia at delivery: A prospective survey of 6715 deliveries. *American Journal of Obstetrics and Gynecology* **162**: 731–734.

2 Samuels P, Bussel JB, Braitman LE, Tomaski A, Druzin ML, Mennuti MT, Cines DB (1990) Estimation of thrombocytopenia in the offspring of pregnant women with presumed immune thrombocytopenic purpura. *New England Journal of Medicine* **323**:229–235.

3 Bussel JB, Berkowitz RL, McFarland JG, Lynch L, Chitkara U (1988) Antenatal treatment of neonatal alloimmune thrombocytopenia. *New England Journal of Medicine* **319**:1374–1377.

47

Fetal Arrhythmias

LINDSEY D. ALLAN

INTRODUCTION

The normal baseline fetal heart rate after 24 weeks is approximately 140 beats/min, ranging between 120 and 150 beats/min. The rhythm can be disturbed in one of three ways: tachycardia, bradycardia and irregularity of rhythm. We exclude from this discussion physiological, transient accelerations and decelerations such as those associated with fetal movement, growth deficiency, hypoxia or umbilical cord compression. A tachycardia is defined as a sustained rate over 200 beats/min; a bradycardia is a sustained rate less than 100 beats/min. A rhythm disturbance may be detected during routine ausculation of the fetal heart, ultrasound examination or on cardiotocography. If a fetal heart rate of over 200 or less than 100 beats/min is detected, the pregnancy should be referred to a Fetal Diagnosis and Treatment Unit for further evaluation.

ASSESSMENT

Assessment involves:

- evaluation of the rate and type of rhythm disturbance

- looking for evidence of fetal compromise

- defining any structural cardiac malformations if present.

Evaluation of the Rate and Type of Rhythm Disturbance

In postnatal life, an arrhythmia is assessed by examination of the electrocardiogram to determine the relationship of the P-wave, or atrial contraction, to the QRS complex, which represents ventricular contraction. Before birth, it is not possible to amplify sufficiently the electrical signals from the fetal heart externally in order to distinguish the P-wave clearly, although the QRS complex can be found.[1] However, the mechanical cardiac events can be defined by M-mode or Doppler echocardiography. If the M-mode cursor is positioned through the ventricular and atrial wall, the resulting trace will show the relationship between the atrial and ventricular contractions. Alternatively, the M-mode cursor can be situated through the aortic valve and atrial wall (**Figure 1**). The opening of the aortic valve reflects the timing of systole. An example of M-mode tracing through the aortic valve is shown in **Figure 2**. In the normal fetus, there is a one-to-one relationship between atrial and ventricular contraction, with a fixed time interval of less than 80 ms between the two. Rhythm disturbances can also be evaluated by Doppler echocardiography. Positioning the Doppler sample volume in the left ventricular outflow tract will allow the outflow and inflow velocities to be recorded simultaneously and the relationship between atrial and ventricular contraction can be assessed.[2] We are less experienced with Doppler evaluation of fetal arrhythmias than with M-mode echocardiography.

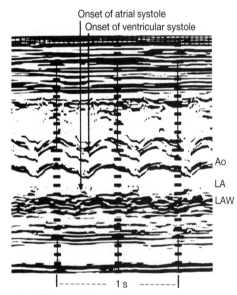

Figure 1. The M-line is positioned through the aorta and the left atrial wall.

Onset of atrial systole
Onset of ventricular systole

Ao
LA
LAW

|--------- 1 s -------|

Figure 2. The aortic valve opening and atrial wall contraction can be seen. The relationship between the two can be determined. This shows a normal tracing.

Tachycardias

Anti-arrhythmic therapy should not be prescribed until the rhythm disturbance has been defined on M-mode echocardiography. These may be either atrial or ventricular in origin. It is important to distinguish them from each other; since the therapy for one would not be appropriate for the other.[3] Atrial tachycardias are much more common than those of ventricular origin.

Examples of a supraventricular tachycardia are seen in **Figures 3** and **4**, on M-mode and on Doppler echocardiography, respectively. There is a rate of 240 beats/min with one-to-one conduction between the atria and ventricles in both examples. In a ventricular tachycardia, the atrial rate is slower than the ventricular rate unless there is retrograde conduction of every ventricular beat, which is unlikely. A supraventricular tachy-

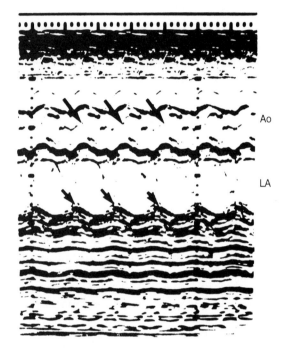

Ao

LA

Figure 3. A supraventricular tachycardia. The distance between the vertical markers represent 1 s and there are four atrial (small arrows) and ventricular (larger arrows) contractions in each second.

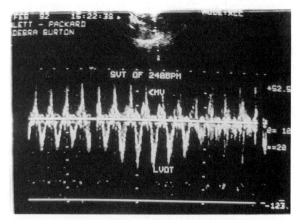

Figure 4. The Doppler sample volume is positioned in the left ventricle to record the inflow and outflow simultaneously. There is a supraventricular tachycardia of 240 beats/min with regular conduction between atria and ventricles.

cardia can also be distinguished from atrial flutter as the M-mode echocardiogram will show an atrial rate, usually of 480 beats/min, with two-to-one block in conduction (**Figure 5**).

Bradycardias

Occasional short episodes of sinus bradycardia are normal in the fetus around 20 weeks gestation but become less frequent as pregnancy advances. A bradycardia is important only if sustained. A sinus bradycardia may indicate the need for urgent obstetric intervention and must be distinguished from complete heart block, which is not usually an indication for emergency delivery. The fetus with complete heart block is usually active and without signs of umbilical cord compression. The M-mode echocardiogram in a sinus bradycardia will show one-to-one atrial to ventricular conduction at a rate of less that 100 beats/min. In complete heart block, the atrial and ventricular contractions are dissociated. The atrial rate is normal, while the ventricular rate is between 45 and 80 beats/min (**Figure 6**). Occasionally, a ventricular bradycardia is due to coupled ectopic beats blocking the sinus beat. In this situation, the atrial ectopic beat will occur close to the sinus beat but not be conducted to the ventricles. There will be a longer interval to the next sinus beat after the ectopic than before it (**Figure 7**). This is referred to as

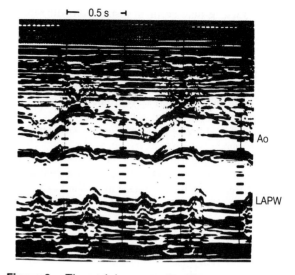

Figure 6. The atrial contractions have no relationship to the aortic valve opening. The atrial rate is 140 beats/min with the ventricles contracting at 60 beats/min. This is complete heart block.

a compensatory pause. It is a self-limiting arrhythmia of no sinister implication. However, it is important to distinguish this arrhythmia from complete heart block.

Complete heart block occurs in two sets of circum-

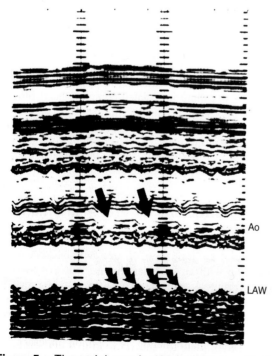

Figure 5. The atrial rate is 480 beats/min with the ventricles responding to every second atrial contraction. The vertical markers represent 0.5 s.

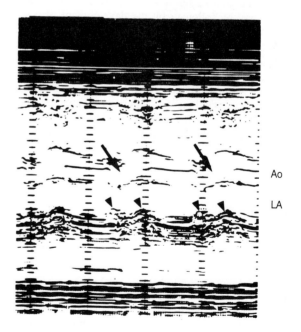

Figure 7. There are coupled atrial ectopics. The ventricle is still refractory when the atrial ectopic occurs such that this beat is blocked. A ventricular bradycardia results.

stances.[4] First, it may occur in association with structural, usually complex, congenital heart disease and second, it may be caused by maternal connective tissue disease with circulating anti-SSA (also known as anti-Ro) antibodies damaging the developing conduction tissue.[5] The underlying maternal disease may be clinically evident (e.g. Sjogren's syndrome or as systemic lupus erythematosis) or the condition may be subclinical. *The appearance of these antibodies may antedate the development of disease by up to 20 years.* It is important to distinguish between the two different etiologies, as the prognosis when there is associated heart disease differs from the prognosis in isolated complete heart block.

Irregular rhythms

These are due to ectopic beats of atrial or ventricular origin. They can be as frequent as every second beat but are usually just occasional. They can be 'regularly irregular' or completely erratic in nature. Some dropped beats are almost invariably found in every fetus between 30 weeks gestation and term. These represent immaturity of the conducting system and can be observed in premature infants. Dropped beats are not associated with morbidity or mortality, and both mother and obstetrician can be reassured once the structure of the fetal heart has been checked.

On occasion (about 1%), frequent premature atrial beats may be followed by the development of a sustained supraventricular tachycardia. Thus, the fetal heart should be auscultated weekly and the mother instructed to telephone if there is an abrupt decrease in fetal activity. Some authors have suggested that there is a causal association between ectopic beats and the presence of an atrial septal aneurysm.[6] However, both ectopic beats and the appearance of a widely bulging atrial septal flap valve are common in late gestation and the association is more likely fortuitous than causative.

Looking for Evidence of Fetal Compromise

When a fetal arrhythmia is found (whether or not there is an associated cardiac malformation), the rest of the fetus should be examined for evidence of cardiac failure. Fetal cardiac failure can be due to complete heart block or a tachycardia, but does not occur as a result of an irregular rhythm. When failure occurs, it worsens the prognosis and alters the management of the pregnancy. One of the earliest signs of failure is the development of cardiomegaly (**Figure 8**), as defined by an increased cardiothoracic ratio compared to normal range.[7] Atrioventricular valve regurgitation may occasionally precede failure and can be documented on

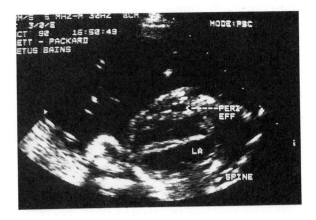

Figure 8. There is cardiomegaly in the context of complete heart block and intrauterine cardiac failure (PERI EFF, pericardial effusion; LA, left atrium).

pulsed Doppler or color flow mapping once cardiac failure has developed. Skin edema, pericardial effusion and abdominal ascites develop later in the course of cardiac failure. Pleural effusions may occur, but are more frequently due to extracardiac causes.[8] The hydramnios associated with failure can precipitate the onset of premature labor. The mechanisms underlying this hydramnios are unknown.

Fetal cardiac failure is more likely to occur in tachycardias with a very fast rate i.e. over 260 beats/min) or in complete heart block when the rate falls below 60 beats/min. It is also likely to occur when the ventricular ionotrophic function is diminished. This can occur in association with both tachycardias and bradycardias. Circulating maternal autoimmune antibodies not only damage the fetal conduction tissues, but also the ventricular myocardium in isolated complete heart block.

The progression of cardiac failure as it develops, or improves during treatment, should be followed by sequential measurement of the cardiothoracic ratio, degree of atrioventricular valve incompetence, the abdominal circumference and skin thickness.

Defining Structural Cardiac Malformation if Present

A structural malformation of any type can occur in association with an irregular rhythm, but this association is fortuitous and occurs with the same frequency as in the general population. Congenital heart disease is uncommon (about 1%) in fetal tachycardias. We have seen one case out of over 80 fetuses with tachycardia. Heart malformation is common in cases of complete heart block, occurring in up to 50% evaluated prenatally. Most typically, the defect includes an atrioventricular septal defect with left atrial isomerism, but other forms can occur. Fetuses with complete heart block and left atrial isomerism commonly present in cardiac failure and frequently die *in utero*.

Management Options

Tachycardias

The treatment of intrauterine tachycardias will depend on:

- whether the fast rate is intermittent or sustained

- the gestational age

- the presence of absence of cardiac failure

- the type of rhythm disturbance.

If a tachycardia occurs late in pregnancy, that is after 37 weeks gestation, it is reasonable to offer no treatment apart from observation on an out-patient basis. However, it is the opinion of the author that all sustained tachycardias prior to 37 weeks should be treated prenatally. I do not advocate delivery prior to 37 weeks gestation. The rationale for treatment is that, if persistent, it may result in intrauterine cardiac failure which will compromise the outlook and potentially the chance of a therapeutic success.[9] The drug of choice will depend on the type of rhythm disturbance and the presence or absence of fetal hydrops. For an atrial tachycardia in the non-hydropic patient, digoxin is a safe drug which can be used while the mother is an out-patient. A dose of 0.75 mg/day is often necessary to maintain the maternal serum digoxin level at 2.0 µg/l. There is controversy over how effective digoxin crosses the placenta. Though it has been reported that the placental transfer of digoxin is between 40 and 60%, much of this is endogenous digoxin-like substance.[10] Further, there are now multiple reports of fetuses with supraventricular tachycardia who failed to respond to adequate maternal digitalization, who did respond to direct administration of digoxin.[11] Weiner observed that the concentration of fetal digoxin as measured with an immunologic assay changed little before, during and after adequate maternal digitalization. If the rhythm fails to convert after 2 weeks of adequate serum levels, or there is evidence of hydrops, verapamil may be added. The starting dose would be 120 mg/day, increasing it weekly until control is achieved. Though there are reports of sudden death from its use in infants, we have had no problems in the fetus, perhaps because placental transfer is as low as 20%. Conversion of the

arrhythmia is usually achieved in those cases of tachycardia without hydrops at presentation. There should be a low morbidity and mortality if these fetuses are carefully managed and delivered at term.

Where a fetus with an atrial tachycardia is in cardiac failure at presentation, the mother should be admitted to the hospital for treatment. A tachycardia with fetal hydrops is more difficult to treat, as digoxin is even less efficiently transferred across the hydropic placenta. Though digoxin or adenosine given directly to the fetus are safe forms of therapy (neither have a negative inotropic effect), we have not been successful maintaining sinus rhythm after conversion with either. Other authors do report success with direct fetal intravenous, intramuscular or intraperitoneal digoxin.[11,12] Weiner *et al.* have measured the elimination half-life of digoxin in several fetuses. It is rapid, being <15 h in all fetuses studied.[19] Flecainide has good placental transfer and can be effective in a maternal oral dose of 300 mg/day.[13] Unfortunately, this drug can be associated with sudden death[14] and preferably *should only be used for the hydropic fetus with an otherwise resistant supraventricular tachycardia*. There is rapid conversion to sinus rhythm in the 70% of fetuses who respond. If conversion has not occurred after 4 days, alternatives should be sought. We have used a combination of digoxin and verapamil with success,[9] and this would be our first line of treatment in atrial flutter.

There have been reports of the successful use of procainamide, quinidine and amiodarone.[11,15–17] If conversion occurs and delivery can be delayed, the hydrops will resolve and the outcome will be good. Resolution of hydrops has been 'encouraged' by draining fluid-filled cavities, such as the abdominal cavity, after the arrhythmia has been controlled, but there is no evidence such an invasive procedure is of value. Symptomatic relief for the mother can be achieved by draining tense hydramnios. Indomethacin has been given to treat the hydramnios, but there is reason for caution. Fetal ductal constriction is a known side-effect of this drug, which could further tax the weakened fetal heart. Although its consequences are as yet unclear, it may be wise to monitor the ductal velocity during the administration of indomethacin.[18] The maximum normal ductal velocity is 1.0–14 m/s. Treatment of the arrhythmias is the best treatment for the hydramnios, which will resolve when the fetus develops a sustained, normal sinus rate. Premature labor, if it starts, often cannot be prevented, particularly if there is hydramnios. A therapeutic amniocentesis would be a consideration here (see Chapter 48). Elective premature delivery should be avoided, as prematurity is the major cause of morbidity and mortality in these babies.

Where the fetus survives a fetal tachycardia, the long-term outlook is good. In the past, we have recommended maintenance of the anti-arrhythmic therapy for 1 year. More recently, we have recommended 3

FETAL ARRHYTHMIAS
Summary of Management Options

Prepregnancy

- Counseling for those mothers of a child with heart disease and complete heart block: the risk of recurrence of left atrium isomerism is slightly higher than is usual in heart disease (about 1:10 to 1:20)

- Counseling for those mothers with known anti-SSA antibodies: if several fetal losses have occurred, preconception steroids may be considered

Prenatal

Complete heart block

- Sequential study of mothers with known anti-SSA antibodies

- Assessment and differentiation of cases of complete heart block into those with and without structural malformation

- Termination of pregnancy in complex heart disease if appropriate

Tachycardias

- Assessment of fetal tachycardias: it is important to identify the arrhythmia

- Controversy remains regarding placental passage of digoxin, but in the absence of hydrops it remains a reasonable first choice (verapamil and flecainide are alternatives in hydropic fetuses)

Irregular rhythms

- Evaluate cardiac structure, and if normal reassure

- Check 2 weeks later to ensure disappearance of arrhythmia and no tachycardia

Labor/delivery

Complete heart block

- Should be delivered in specialist center as close to term as possible

- Early operative delivery may be indicated in the hydropic case not amenable to prenatal therapy

Tacycardia

- Local delivery at term in non-hydropic fetus after arrhythmia control

- Delivery in tertiary center if hydrops is still present or control not established

- Neonatal intensive care if fetus hydropic at delivery

Postnatal

- Assessment of rhythm disturbance on continuous monitoring

- Treat tachycardia if recurrent

- Consider cases of complete heart block for pacing

months. A few children have continuing problems with arrhythmias. Occasionally, an underlying conduction defect such as the Wolff-Parkinson-White syndrome is found.

Bradycardias

In complete heart block, those with structural heart disease must be identified and counseled as to the likely outcome. Because of the complexity of malformation, a poor prognosis should be expected, especially if hydrops is present. Termination of pregnancy offered if the gestational age allows. There is no effective treatment which can be offered during pregnancy and an early or operative delivery is unhelpful. In complete heart block with normal cardiac structure, the outlook depends on whether or not hydrops develops. In the majority of cases, fetal cardiac output is maintained at an adequate level throughout pregnancy and the fetus can be delivered at term. Cesarian section is rarely necessary. Hydrops, if it develops, usually becomes evident between 20 and 30 weeks gestation and presents a difficult management problem. Premature delivery of a hydropic infant before 32–34 weeks is likely to be associated with a very high perinatal morbidity and mortality rate. Direct intrauterine fetal cardiac pacing has been attempted, but has not to date been successful in the long-term.[19] Further, the approach has several theoretical disadvantages. The *first* is that the cardiac failure is probably only partially related to the ventricular rate itself. It is also related to the associated cardiomyopathy which cannot be treated effectively. *Second*, there is an inherent and high risk of infection to the fetus should the pacing be maintained for more than a few days, unless the pacemaker is inserted into the mother. *Third*, the pacing wire needs to pass from the pacing box through the fetal thorax into the fetal heart. The wire stands a high chance of dislodgment during fetal movement. Alternative treatment includes the use of steroids,[20] but we have not been successful with this action. If the fetal condition, despite signs of hydrops, does not deteriorate, early delivery may be appropriate after 30 weeks gestation, especially with the concomitant use of dexamethasone.

Postnatally, the neonate is assessed for cardiac pacing. The need for a pacemaker will depend on the slowest heart rate or the frequency of ventricular ectopics during a 24 h recording. Symptoms in the newborn such as poor feeding and failure to thrive would also be an indication to insert a pacemaker. Pacing has been necessary in about one-third of 30 cases in our series.

Mothers who are known carriers of the anti-SSA antibody are at risk of recurrence of the condition in subsequent pregnancies, though the precise incidence in unknown. However, we have cared for several women where, in their next pregnancy, the fetus was unaffected despite the continuing presence of circulating antibodies. These women may also have an increased rate of early miscarriage. The pregnancy should be monitored throughout gestation, as we have observed complete heart block developing between 18 and 28 weeks gestation.

Irregular rhythms

No treatment or intervention is necessary for ectopic beats, even when they are frequent, since they disappear spontaneously toward term or soon after. Rarely, ectopic beats can trigger the onset of a tachycardia which would require treatment.

REFERENCES

1   Allan LD, Anderson RH, Sullivan ID, Campbell S, Holt DW and Tynan MJ (1983) The evaluation of fetal arrhythmias by echocardiography. *British Heart Journal* **49**:154–156.

2   Strasberger JF, Huhta JC, Carpenter RJ (1986) Doppler echocardiography in the diagnosis and management of persistent fetal arrhythmias. *Journal of the American College of Cardiologists* **7**:1386–1391.

3   Kleinman CS, Copel JA, Weinstein EJ et al. (1985) *In utero* diagnosis and treatment of supraventricular tachycardia. *Seminars in Perinatalogy* **9**:113–129.

4   Machado MVL, Tynan MJ, Curry PVL, Allan LD (1988) Complete heart block in prenatal life. *British Heart Journal* **60**:512–515.

5   McCue CM, Mantakas ME, Tingelstad JB, Ruddy S (1977) Congenital heart block in newborns of mothers with connective tissue disease. *Circulation* **56**:82–89.

6   Rice MJ, McDonald RW, Reller MD (1988) Fetal atrial septal aneaurysm: A cause of fetal atrial arrhythmias. *Journal of the American College of Cardiologists* **12**:1292–1297.

7   Paladini D, Chita SK, Allan LD (1990) Prenatal measurement of cardiothoracic ratio in evaluation of congenital heart disease. *Archives of Diseases of Children* **65**:20–23.

8   Skoll A, Sharland GK, Allan LD (1991) Ultrasound findings in non-immune hydrops. *Ultrasound in Obstetrics and Gynecology* **1**:309–312.

9   Maxwell DJ, Crawford DC, Curry PVM, Tynan MJ, Allan L (1988) Obstetric importance, diagnosis and management of fetal tachycardias. *British Medical Journal* **297**:107–110.

10 Weiner CP, Landas S, Persoon TJ (1987) Digoxin-like immunoreactive substance in fetuses with and without cardiac pathology. *American Journal of Obstetrics and Gynecology* **157**:368–371.

11 Weiner CP, Thompson MIB (1988) Direct treatment of fetal supraventricular tachycardia after failed transplacental therapy. *American Journal of Obstetrics and Gynecology* **158**:570–573.

12 Gembruch U, Hansmann M, Redel DA, Bad R (1988) Intrauterine therapy of fetal tachyarrhythmias: Intraperitoneal administration of anti-arrhythmic drugs to the fetus in fetal tachyarrhythmias with severe hydrops fetalis. *Journal of Perinatal Medicine* **16**:39–44.

13 Allan LD, Chita SK, Sharland G, Maxwell D, Priestley K (1991) Flecainide in the treatment of fetal tachycardias. *British Heart Journal* **65**:46–49.

14 The Cardiac Arrhythmias Suppression Trial Investigators (1989) Preliminary report: effect of encamide and flecamide on mortality in a randomised trial of arrhythmia suppression after myocardial infarction. *New England Journal of Medicine* **321**:406–412.

15 Dumesic DA, Silverman NH, Tobias S *et al.* (1982) Transplacental cardioversion of fetal supraventricular tachycardia with procainamide. *New England Journal of Medicine* **307**:1128.

16 Spinnato JA, Shaver DC, Flinn GS, Sibai BM, Watson DL, Marin-Garcia J (1984) Fetal supraventricular tachycardia: *In utero* therapy with digoxin and quinide. *Obstetrics and Gynecology* **64**:730–735.

17 Arnoux P, Seyral P, Llurens M, Djiane P, Potier A, Unal D, Cano JP, Serradimigni A, Rouault F (1986) Amiodarone and digoxin for refractory fetal tachycardia *American Journal of Cardiology* **59**:166–167.

18 Huhta JC, Moise, KJ, Fisher DJ *et al.* (1987) Detection and quantitation of constriction of the fetal ductus arteriosis by Doppler echocardiography. *Circulation* **75**:406–412.

19 Carpenter RJ, Strasberger JF, Garson A, Smith RT, Deter RL, Engelhardt HT (1986) Fetal ventricular pacing for hydrops secondary to complete atrioventricular block. *Journal of the American College of Cardiologists* **8**:1434–1436.

20 Bierman FZ, Baxi L, Jaffe I, Driscoll J (1988) Fetal hydrops and congenital complete heart block: Response to maternal steroid therapy. *Journal of Pediatrics* **112**:646–648.

48

Hydramnios, Oligohydramnios

SIMON E. MEAGHER, NICHOLAS M. FISK

INTRODUCTION

Clinical assessments of amniotic fluid volume, including bimanual palpation and/or tape measure of the symphysial–fundal height, are unreliable.[1] The excess or depletion of amniotic fluid is usually severe before detection by these methods. Direct quantification of amniotic fluid volume is not performed in clinical practice, since it necessitates two amniocenteses with attendant risks[2] and relies on the questionable supposition that complete mixing of the injected indicator dye occurs within a 15–30 min interval.[2–4] Accordingly, definitions of increased and decreased amniotic fluid volume are based on non-invasive criteria. Semi-quantitative ultrasonic assessment includes the depth of the deepest vertical pool (DP) or the amniotic fluid index (AFI), which is a summation of the deepest vertical pool depth in each of four quadrants and a more reliable estimate of amniotic fluid volume throughout gestation.[5,6] The prevalence of hydramnios and oligohydramnios varies with the diagnostic criteria used. using a DP $\geq$ 8 cm, hydramnios has been reported in 1–3% of pregnancies[7,8] and with a DP $\leq$ 2 cm, oligohydramnios in 4% of pregnancies.[9]

HYDRAMNIOS

Definition

Standard definitions of hydramnios are a deepest vertical pool $\geq$ 8 cm or an AFI above the 95th centile for gestational age (**Figure 1**).[6]

Etiology

The common causes of hydramnios are shown in **Table 1**. Although impairment of fetal swallowing has been implicated in anencephaly,[10] only 65% develop

Table 1
Common causes or associations with hydramnios

Maternal

Diabetes mellitus

Fetal

Obstruction of fluid through the gastrointestinal tract
    intestinal atresias (commonly duodenal)
    esophageal compression secondary to thoracic or
        mediastinal masses (including diaphragmatic hernia)

Neurologic impairment of swallowing
    central nervous system lesions (e.g. anencephaly)
    chromosome abnormalities (e.g. trisomy 21)
    muscular dystrophies

Fetal polyuria
    twin-twin transfusion syndrome
    diabetes insipidus (central or nephrogenic)

High-output cardiac failure
    profound fetal anemia
    sacrococcygeal teratoma
    chorioangioma

Congenital infection (e.g. syphilis, viral heptatitis)

hydramnios. While this may reflect variation in the amount of brain present, alternative mechanisms include fluid transudation across the meninges or vasopressin deficiency resulting in fetal polyuria.[11] Although fetal polyuria secondary to an osmotic diuresis might seem an obvious mechanism in diabetes mellitus, Van Otterlo *et al.*[12] found normal fetal urine production rates in 12 of 13 diabetic pregnancies with mild hydramnios. On the other hand, fetal polyuria has been documented in recipient fetuses in twin-twin transfusion syndrome (TTTS) and is supported by finding enlarged glomeruli and dilated distal convoluted tubules on renal histology.[13–15] Hydramnios in non-hydropic rhesus disease may be explained by the associated hypoxic induced hyperlacticemia;[16] this hypothesis being supported by recent animal data showing the powerful osmotic effects of elevated fetal plasma lactate drawing fluid from the maternal into the fetal compartment.[17] Hyperlacticemia appears to be a late development.

The incidence of idiopathic hydramnios is related to the severity, with a cause being identified in 75–91% with a DP $\geq$ 12 cm *vs* 17–29% with a DP of 8–12 cm.[8,18] The term 'acute hydramnios' refers to a sudden accumulation of amniotic fluid associated with maternal symptoms, which may mimic placental abruption. The fundal height grows in excess of 1 cm a day. This is almost exclusively a manifestation of TTTS with a rapid fluid accumulation in the sac of the recipient twin, usually before 26 weeks gestation.[2,19]

There is argument whether acute hydramnios occurs in singleton pregnancies.[2]

Maternal Risks

Maternal complications reflect uterine distension and include abdominal discomfort, uterine irritability, postpartum hemorrhage and compromised respiratory function secondary to upward diaphragmatic displacement.[20,21] In this regard, intra-amniotic pressure has been shown to be markedly elevated in severe hydramnios (**Figure 2**).[22,23] The incidence of cesarean section is also increased as a result of unstable lie and placental abruption, which may occur with the rapid decrease in intra-uterine volume that accompanies membrane rupture.[24,25] The higher incidence of pre-eclampsia may be a manifestation of the mirror or maternal syndrome in association with fetal hydrops.[26,27] With gross uterine distension, maternal ureteric obstruction may occur.[28,29]

Fetal Risks

The high perinatal mortality rates of 10–30%[10,30] associated with hydramnios are largely due to the presence of congenital malformations, preterm premature rupture of the membranes, or preterm labor and delivery. Asphyxial events secondary to cord prolapse, placental abruption or uteroplacental insufficiency also contribute. In Queenan and Gadow's series,[2] the perinatal morality rate was 87% in anomalous fetuses com-

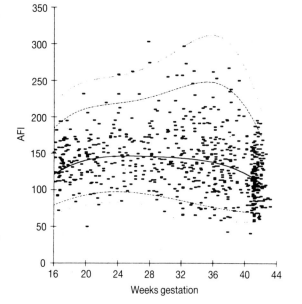

Figure 1. Normal range for AFI from 16 to 44 weeks gestation. Reproduced with permission from Moore and Cayle.[6]

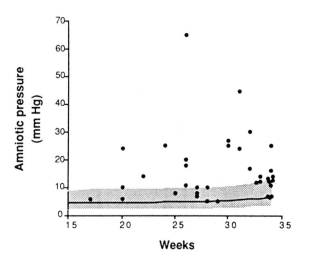

Figure 2. Amniotic fluid pressure in 36 pregnancies complicated by hydramnios shown against the normal pregnancy reference range with the continuous line representing the mean and the upper and lower limits of the shaded area the reference range. From Fisk.[115]

pared with 13% in structurally normal fetuses with idiopathic hydramnios. Similarly, the perinatal mortality rate fell from 13% to 6% in another series[8] when corrected for lethal malformations. These associations, however, do not entirely account for the high perinatal mortality rate, since 6–14% of perinatal deaths occur antepartum in normally formed singletons.[2,18,30] In this regard, hypoxemia and acidemia have been reported *in utero* in fetuses with hydramnios and raised intra-amniotic pressure.[23] As a result, it has been suggested that uteroplacental perfusion is impaired in hydramnios. However, this is refuted by the observation that ovine fetal blood gases do not change when the intra-amniotic pressure is acutely elevated by instillation of a large volume of fluid.[31]

Management Options

Diagnosis

Objectives include assessment of:

- fetal number and chorionicity

- degree of hydramnios

- underlying etiology

- presence of associated anomalies.

The diagnostic approach is outlined in **Table 2**.

Table 2
Diagnostic evaluation of hydramnios

History taking with an emphasis on maternal symptoms, diabetes mellitus, RBC alloimmunization and diabetes insipidus

High-resolution ultrasound to assess the:
degree of hydramnios (AFI, DP)
presence of multiple gestation, growth deficiency or macrosomia
fetal thorax
fetal central nervous system (neural tube, tone)
fetal gastrointestinal system (mouth, stomach, small bowel, abdominal wall)
fetal bladder dynamics
chorionicity in multiple gestation

Fetal karyotype

Maternal serology for syphilis

Kirshon[32] observed that hourly fetal urine production rates (HFUPR) calculated by ultrasonic change in bladder dimensions over 20 min intervals[33] distinguished hydramnios secondary to fetal polyuria from that due to other causes. Recent work suggests that the technique used underestimates fetal urine production by at least 50%.[34] In multiple pregnancy, hydramnios may occur (1) in dichorial pregnancies as a consequence of any of the listed causes for singleton gestation, or (2) in monochorial pregnancies secondary to twin-twin transfusion syndrome or twin reverse arterial perfusion sequence. In the latter, the bladder of recipient fetuses in TTTS remains chronically full, with its size at the upper limit of normal, and therefore there is little benefit in actually calculating HFUPR. The 15–17% of twin gestations with a single placental mass and concordant sexes, the presence of three or four membrane layers or a membrane greater than 2 mm thick have been used to predict dichorial placentation with sensitivities and specificities of up to 90%.[35,36] However, in the presence of severe hydramnios, these parameters are poorly reproducible. In view of the 2–27%[37] association with chromosomal abnormalities, karyotyping is recommended and this may be performed by sampling either fetal blood, chorion or amniotic fluid.

Therapeutic options

General

The therapeutic aims are to relieve maternal symptoms and prolong gestation. Mild asymptomatic hydramnios is managed expectantly. There are no data to support dietary restriction of salts and fluids; similarly, diuretics administered to the mother seem ineffective and may in fact reduce uteroplacental perfusion.[1] They are to be discouraged.

Indomethacin

Indomethacin may be useful in selected cases where fetal polyuria results in hydramnios. Cifuentes *et al.*[38] first noted decreased urinary production rates in neonates receiving indomethacin for closure of the ductus arteriosus. Subsequently, maternally administered indomethacin has been shown not only to reduce fetal urine production,[39] but also to reduce amniotic fluid volume.[40–42] Indomethacin's mechanism of action is unclear, but is believed to reduce fetal urine production either by having a renovascular effect or removing prostaglandin inhibition of antidiuretic hormone on the renal tubule.[43–45]

The dose administered varies widely (50–200 mg/day), depending on the amniotic fluid response assessed ultrasonically. When the patient is symptomatic or there is concern regarding preterm labor, the AFI is recorded and indomethacin 50 mg three times a day commenced. The amniotic fluid volume should be monitored twice weekly. When the AFI falls below the reference range, indomethacin should be either discontinued or tapered. The time interval between commencing treatment and achieving normal amniotic fluid volume ranges from 4 to 20 days.[46,47] The delayed response with indomethacin may be overcome by a therapeutic amniocentesis (amnioreduction) prior to commencing therapy.[48]

Because most reports of neonatal morbidity result from indomethacin prescribed in late gestation, most authors discontinue treatment at 35 weeks.[40,42] While the initial clinical experience with indomethacin is promising, there is growing concern about the risks of:

- premature closure of the ductus[49]

- cerebral vasconstriction in the fetus[50]

- impaired renal function[51]

Ductal constriction occurs in 5–50% depending on gestation. However, proof of a definitive association with neonatal persistent fetal circulation and pulmonary hypertension is lacking. Some authors have recommended that pulsed-wave Doppler of the ductus arteriosis be performed within the first 24 h of starting treatment and once weekly thereafter. When evidence of ductal constriction develops, indomethacin is discontinued.[52] Because complications rarely arise, the value of the practice is currently unclear. Raised serum creatinine has been documented in neonates of mothers who received indomethacin prenatally; while this is of concern, it is usually a transient phenomenon.[53,54] Prior to 30 weeks gestation, these risks are clearly outweighed by the risk of preterm delivery.

Therapeutic amniocentesis (amnioreduction)

Therapeutic amniocentesis (or amnioreduction) describes transabdominal aspiration of amniotic fluid under ultrasound control and was first described by Rivett in 1933[55] for the relief of maternal symptoms. It has been performed occasionally since, but fell into disrepute because of the frequency and rate with which fluid reaccumulated. There has been a recent resurgence of interest in amnioreduction which modern studies suggest prolong gestation in both singleton and multiple pregnancies,[2,56,57,61] and therefore improve perinatal survival rates.[57–61] It may be performed as early as 18 weeks gestation and is generally reserved for those with either:

- severe hydramnios

- symptomatic hydramnios

- In whom indomethacin has failed.

Procedure: Amnioreduction

After local anesthetic (10 ml of 1–2% xylocaine), a 20–22 gauge spinal needle is directed under ultrasound control into the amniotic cavity. The needle is attached to a 50 ml syringe with a three-way tap to facilitate removal of fluid and reduce the procedure duration.[58] Enough fluid is removed to achieve a DP ≤ 8 cm or an AFI within the normal range. The frequency with which the procedure must be repeated will depend upon the rate the fluid accumulates.

Risks of the procedure include:

- premature rupture of the membranes

- chorioamnionitis

- placental abruption

- membranous detachment (**Figure 3**); which follows multiple procedures and which appears to precede membrane rupture by several weeks.

The perinatal mortality rate with untreated mid-trimester TTTS complicated by hydramnios approaches 80–100%. Recent series[57–60] not only report prolongation of pregnancy with a 37–79% perinatal survival rate after serial amnioreduction, but surprisingly note amniotic fluid reaccumulation in the sac of the oligohydramniotic donor. It has been postulated that relief of intra-amniotic pressure in the hydramniotic recipient twin improves the circulation to the 'stuck' donor twin, thus restoring its renal function.[58] There is no direct evidence to support this theory. Tentative explanations include leakage of fluid into the sac of the 'stuck' twin through needle puncture.

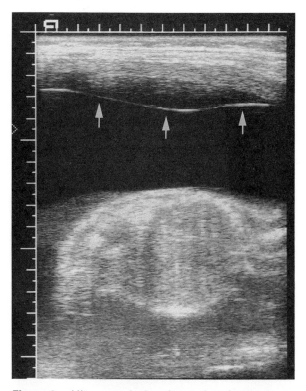

Figure 3. Ultrasound showing a longitudinal section through maternal anterior abdominal wall showing the fetus lying opposed to the posterior uterine surface. The arrows point to membranous detachment from the upper uterine segment.

OLIGOHYDRAMNIOS

Definition

Oligohydramnios has been variously defined as a deepest vertical pool devoid of cord or fetal limbs measuring < 3, 2 or 1 cm,[62,63] the latter of these indicating moderate to severe oligohydramnios. Alternatively, an AFI < 5th centile for gestational age has more recently been used (**Figure 4**).

Etiology

The common causes of oligohydramnios are summarized in **Table 3**. Human data suggest that the oligohydramnios associated with growth deficiency is secondary to fetal oliguria,[64,65] the degree of reduction in the hourly urine rate correlating with the degree of hypoxemia.[66] Recent non-cardiac Doppler studies reveal an increase in downstream resistance in the renal artery.[67, 68] The mechanism is different in postmaturity. Fetal urine production rates decline after 40 weeks.[62,69] In contrast to growth deficiency, Doppler studies do not support a renovascular mechanism with redistribution of blood flow[68] in postmature fetuses.[68]

Premature rupture of the membranes complicates 3–17% of pregnancies[70, 71] and while the clinical diagnosis is obvious in most cases, only 5–44% have ultrasonic evidence of oligohydramnios (see Chapter 12).[72,73] The earlier the gestation, the lower the incidence of PPROM. In one series, PPROM complicated only 0.7% of pregnancies ≤ 25 weeks.[74] Reports of reaccumulation of amniotic fluid volume after occlusion of the cervix with fibrin gel[75] and of fetal urine production being unaltered in the presence of ruptured membranes,[76] support the mechanism of physical leakage through a membranous defect.

Seven percent of pregnancies with oligohydramnios are associated with congenital malformations.[77] The incidence rises to 26–35% if detected in the second trimester.[78,79] Renal anomalies account for 33–57%[80] and include those fetuses with absent renal function such as bilateral renal agenesis or multicystic/ dysplastic kidneys, and those with urinary tract obstruction. Oligohydramnios in these cases is secondary to decreased fetal urination, since normal volume may be restored after vesico-amniotic shunting of an obstructive uropathy (see Chapter 51).[81,82] In fewer than 10% of patients with oligohydramnios, an explanation can not be found. However, the reduction in amniotic fluid volume in these cases is usually mild.

Maternal Risks

Oligohydramnios *per se* does not lead to maternal complications, although its etiological conditions may. Irrespective of etiology, the mother has an increased risk of delivery by cesarean section for fetal distress from growth deficiency, fetal malformation or umbilical cord compression.[63,83,84] Other maternal risks are incurred by the high rates of physician intervention, e.g. induction of labor, termination of pregnancy, and clinical chorioamnionitis in 39–58% of PPROM.[74,85]

Fetal Risks

Perinatal mortality

The increased perinatal mortality associated with oligohydramnios is in part, related to the underlying etiology, such as fetal abnormality or growth deficiency, in part to prematurity, and in part to the sequelae of prolonged oligohydramnios. It is unclear whether the perinatal mortality of pregnancies with mild oligohydramnios at term is increased.[9,85] Poor perinatal outcome in PPROM is principally confined to those with membrane rupture prior to 29 weeks, in whom perinatal

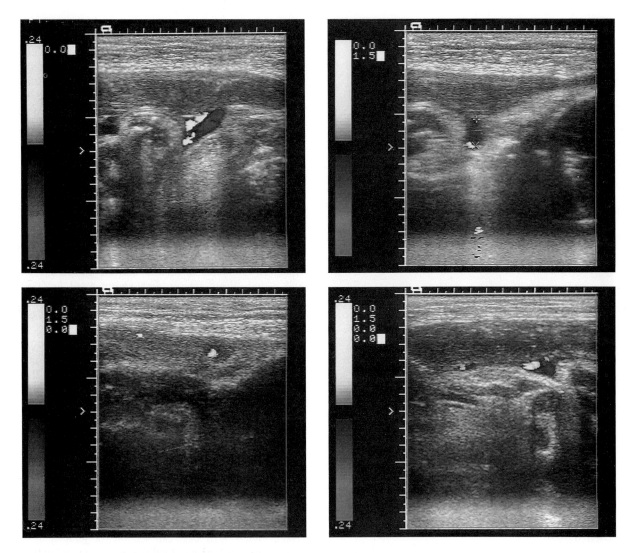

Figure 4. Ultrasound with color Doppler examination showing a four-quadrant amniotic fluid index in a patient with mild to moderate oligohydramnios (AFI 1.5 cm at 30 weeks gestation). Color examination helps to distinguish amniotic fluid from loops of umbilical cord.

Table 3
Common causes or associations with oligohydramnios

Premature rupture of membranes

Intrauterine growth deficiency

Postmaturity

Fetal anomalies
   renal agenesis
   urethral or ureteral obstruction
   renal dysplasia
   polycystic kidneys

---

mortality rates of 37–76% are reported.[87,88] Fetal loss rates of 43–88% have been reported with mid-trimester oligohydramnios.[80,86]

Oligohydramnios sequelae

Pulmonary hypoplasia (PH) is a disorder of impaired lung growth, characterized by diminished size, generational branching and vasculature. It is found in 13–21% of perinatal autopsies,[89–91] with the most common association being oligohydramnios. Pulmonary hypoplasia after oligohydramnios depends on several variables: gestation at onset, severity and duration of oligohydramnios.[92–94] Following multiple regression analysis on 88 mid-trimester cases of prolonged

Table 4
Diagnostic evaluation of oligohydramnios

History taking with an emphasis on maternal symptoms of
hypertension, rupture of membranes and congenital
infection

High-resolution ultrasound to assess the:
degree of oligohydramnios (AFI, DP)
presence of growth deficiency
presence and structure of the kidneys
genitourinary malformations

Fetal intraperitoneal infusion to outline renal beds if
necessary

Amnioinfusion if necessary to improve resolution

Fetal karyotype

Culture of the amniotic fluid for CMV

Maternal serology

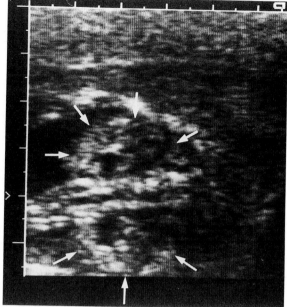

Figure 5. Transabdominal ultrasound showing a coronal section through the lower fetal spine with renal outline (arrowed) highlighted following intra-peritoneal saline infusion.

PPROM, Rotschild *et al.* showed that severity and duration of PPROM were not significantly associated with PH after correction for gestational age.[94] Gestational age at rupture is statistically the most important variable determining pulmonary hypoplasia. In contrast, duration of PPROM was the most significant variable for skeletal deformities.

Management Options

Diagnostic options

The objective is to establish the etiology and determine the presence of associated anomalies (see **Table 4**).

The diagnosis of PPROM is usually obvious from the history and physical examination, with the exception of rupture early in gestation when the small quantities of fluid lost vaginally may go unnoticed.[95] The diagnosis of renal agenesis is especially difficult in view of the associated anhydramnios and lack of an acoustic window. Improved visualization of fetal anatomy with transvaginal ultrasound may reduce errors in diagnosis, and is especially useful when the fetal abdomen overlies the lower uterus.[96,97] Maternal or fetal diuretic administration is no longer used following reports of numerous false-negative diagnoses[96,98] and animal studies indicating that furosemide does not cross the placenta.[99] Fetal intraperitoneal saline infusion is useful to either exclude or outline the renal contours, thus confirming or refuting the diagnosis of renal agenesis (**Figure 5**).[100] Karytotyping is recommended as aneuploidy is found in 5–10% of fetuses, with this number increasing two-fold when the oligohydramnios is detected in the mid-trimester.[101,102]

Diagnostic amnioinfusion

Ultrasonic visualization of fetal anatomy is difficult in instances of severe oligohydramnios/anhydramnios. Resolution is dramatically improved by instillation of fluid into the amniotic cavity.[95,102]

Procedure: Amnioinfusion

Most groups use warmed physiological solutions such as normal saline, Ringers lactate or 5% glucose. The maternal abdomen is prepared aseptically. Broad-spectrum antibiotics are used by some, but are not of demonstrated efficacy. The absence of flow on color Doppler imaging identifies either a pool of amniotic fluid devoid of cord or a potential space. Lidocaine is injected into the tissues overlying the selected site. A 20–22 gauge spinal needle is guided under ultrasound control to the target site and its intra-amniotic position confirmed by either aspiration of fluid or by injecting 1–2 ml of normal saline and visualizing fluid turbulence and dispersal from the needle tip. The needle is attached to tubing, a three-way valve and a 50 ml syringe. Care is taken to avoid the infusion of air.

The volume infused is the minimum volume to improve the ultrasonic view, one group recording a mean DP of 3.2 cm and an AFI of 8.5 cm, using this regime.[95] The fetal heart rate and position of the needle are monitored throughout. Loss of fluid turbulence or a rise in injecting pressure suggest displacement of the needle tip into the neighboring tissues. Fetal tissues for rapid karyotyping can be collected before or after amnioinfusion. Contrary to the suggestion that restoration of amniotic fluid volume facilitiates other invasive procedures,[102] fetal blood sampling is often easier before amnioinfusion if one is willing to sample a free loop of cord. Although in some cases more than one needle insertion is required, amnioinfusion is successfully completed in 95% of cases.[95,102]

This procedure allows confirmation of a suspected diagnosis of fetal malformation and is especially useful in documenting renal agenesis. It also unmasks PPROM in those in whom it has not been previously obvious, by allowing indigocarmine colored normal saline to drain from the vagina and stain a perineal pad. Methyl-ene blue should no longer be used in view of recent reports documenting its association with upper intestinal atresia.[103,104] Membranous detachment can be identified on transvaginal or transabdominal ultrasound and is a useful marker for premature rupture of the membranes (**Figure 6**). Complications, which include infection and failed procedures, occur in less than 5% of cases.[95]

Therapeutic options

Although the mechanism of oligohydramnios-related fetal pulmonary hypoplasia remains unclear, the restoration of amniotic fluid in animal models allows normal lung development.[105,106] Identification of fetuses who are at risk of pulmonary hypoplasia and who theoretically might benefit from amniotic fluid replacement has been based on the ultrasonic measurement of the fetal chest circumference,[107,108] lung length[109] and Doppler studies of the pulmonary vasculature.[110] These parameters, however, are poorly reproducible in the absence of amniotic fluid and are only of predictive value after the end of the canalicular phase of lung development (~25 weeks), indicating established hypoplasia at a time too late for intervention.[107,111,112]

Several treatments have been tried in human midtrimester oligohydramnios to maintain amniotic fluid volume and thus promote lung development throughout gestation. These include:

- vesico-amniotic shunting in obstructive uropathies[81,113]

- infusion of fluid via a transcervical catheter[114]

- cervical canal occlusion with fibrin gel[75]

- serial transabdominal therapeutic amnioinfusions

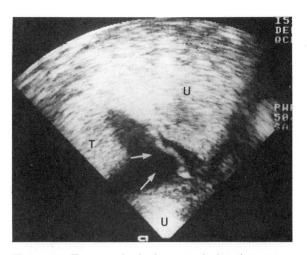

Figure 6. Transvaginal ultrasound showing membranous separation (arrowed) with a wide area of free-floating membrane, in a patient with ruptured membranes. U, Uterine wall; T, fetal trunk.

Despite restoration of amniotic fluid volume after vesico-amniotic shunting, perinatal mortality rates in obstructive uropathies remain high, largely as a result of pulmonary hypoplasia (see Chapter 51).[113] Likewise, cervical occlusion with fibrin gel or a balloon positioned at the internal cervical os has been unsuccessful in preventing continued amniotic fluid leakage. However, restoration of amniotic fluid volume following infusion of normal saline through a balloon catheter has been reported in the third trimester,[114] but awaits evaluation earlier in pregnancy.

In a recent pilot study,[95] where serial amnioinfusion was performed weekly until the end of the canalcular phase of lung development, pulmonary hypoplasia was found in two of nine (22%) pregnancies complicated by severe oligohydramnios diagnosed ≥ 22 weeks, which compared favorably with 60% reported in severe oligohydramnios diagnosed ≥ 28 weeks.[86] If serial amnioinfusion is confirmed by other studies as beneficial, further research is needed to determine:

- optimal gestation at which to commence and cease infusions

- the longevity of infused fluid within the amniotic cavity

- the optimal interval between infusions

- the optimal fluid to maintain amniotic fluid volume

Despite this pilot study and the encouraging animal evidence, there are as yet no controlled data in humans to support the use of serial amnioinfusion, or indeed the other interventions discussed above, to promote lung development.

Until that time, these procedures must be viewed as novel and unproven therapy.

CONCLUSIONS

Aberrant amniotic fluid volume complicates up to 7% of pregnancies, although in many the derangement will be mild, idiopathic, occur in the third trimester and not produce sequelae. In contrast, severe oligohydramnios and hydramnios in the mid-trimester are associated with substantial perinatal morbidity and mortality, reflecting both the underlying etiology and the complications of disordered amniotic volume.

The investigation of hydramnios involves detection of anomalies by ultrasound and karyotyping, and exclusion of carbohydrate intolerance. Transplacental indomethacin reduces fetal urine output and has been used in severe hydramnios to prolong gestation. It is inappropriate in twin–twin transfusion, the most common etiology of acute hydramnios, because it further impairs the donor's renal function. Serial amnioreduction is associated with perinatal survival rates of 37–79% in mid-trimester hydramnios associated with twin pregnancy, representing a considerable improvement on the uniformly poor prognosis associated with conservative management. However, there is no evidence that such therapy reverses the pathological process. Rather, it prolongs gestation.

ABNORMALITIES OF AMNIOTIC FLUID
Summary of Management Options

Hydramnios

- Identity the cause (if possible): see **Table 2**

- Relieve maternal symptoms (if present) and prolong gestation by either

  - indomethacin 25–50 mg t.i.d.

  - therapeutic amniocenteses (aim is to maintain an acceptable/normal amniotic fluid volume)

Oligohydramnios

- Identify the cause (if possible): see **Table 4**

- Management depends on etiology:

  - PROM: see Chapter 12

  - growth deficiency: see Chapter 42

  - prolonged pregnancy: see Chapter 16

  - fetal renal anomalies: see Chapter 51

Severe oligohydramnios, which may be due to ruptured membranes, growth deficiency, absent renal function, or fetal urinary tract obstruction, poses a diagnostic challenge because it impairs ultrasound resolution. Transabdominal amnioinfusion facilitates visualization of fetal anatomy and determines membranous integrity. Karyotyping and transvaginal ultrasound may also be indicated. In order to prevent pulmonary hypoplasia, veslco-amniotic shunting and serial amnioinfusion have been used to maintain amniotic fluid volume in selected euploid fetuses with functioning renal tissue. Despite their valid experimental basis, no controlled data exist to indicate benefit of these procedures in human pregnancies.

REFERENCES

1   Boylan P, Parisi V (1986) An overview of hydramnios. *Seminars in Perinatology* **10**:136–141.

2   Queenan JT, Gadow EC (1970) Polyhydramnios: Chronic versus acute. *Americal Journal of Obstetrics and Gynecology* **108**:349–355.

3   Charles D, Jacoby HE (1966) Preliminary data on the use of sodium aminohippurate to determine amniotic fluid volumes. *American Journal of Obstetrics and Gynecology* **95**:266–269.

4   Brans YW, Andrew DS, Dutton EB, Schwartz CA, Carey KD (1989) Dilution kinetics of chemicals used for estimation of water content of body compartments in perinatal medicine. *Pediatric Research* **25**:377–382.

5   Moore TR (1990) Superiority of the four-quadrant sum over the single-deepest-pocket technique in ultrasonic identification of abnormal amniotic fluid volumes. *American Journal of Gynecology* **163**:762–767.

6   Moore TR, Cayle JE (1990) The amniotic fluid index in normal human pregnancy. *American Journal of Obstetrics and Gynecology* **162**:1168–1173.

7   Chamberlain PF, Manning FA, Morrison I, Harman CR, Lange IR (1984) Ultrasound evaluation of amniotic fluid volume. The relationship of increased amniotic fluid volume to perinatal outcome. *American Journal of Obstetrics and Gynecology* **150**:250–254.

8   Hill L, Breckle R, Thomas ML, Fries JK (1987) Polyhydramnios: Ultrasonically detected prevalence and neonatal outcome. *Obstetrics and Gynecology* **69**:21–25.

9   Philipson EH, Sokol RJ, Williams T (1983) Oligohydramnios: Clinical associations and predictive value for intrauterine growth retardation. *American Journal of Obstetrics and Gynecology* **146**:271–278.

10 Moya F, Apgar V, James LS, Berrien C (1960) Hydramnios and congenital anomalies. *Journal of the American Medical Association* **173**:1552–1556.

11 Naeye RL, Milic AMB, Blane W (1970) Fetal endocrine and renal disorders: clues to the origin of hydramnios. *American Journal of Obstetrics and Gynecology* **108**:1251–1256.

12 Van Otterlo LC, Wladimiroff JW, Wallenburg HCS (1977) Relationship between fetal urine production and amniotic fluid volume in normal pregnancy and pregnancy complicated by diabetes. *British Journal of Obstetrics and Gynaecology* **84**:205–209.

13 Achiron R, Rosen N, Zakut H (1987) Pathophysiologic mechanism of hydramnios development in twin–twin transfusion syndrome. *Journal of Reproductive Medicine* **32**:305–308.

14 Rosen DJ, Rabinowitz R, Beth Y, Fejgin M, Nicolaides K (1990) Fetal urine production in normal and in twins with acute polyhydramnios. *Fetal Diagnosis and Therapy* **5**:57–60.

15 Naeye RL, Milic AM, Blanc W (1970) Fetal endocrine and renal disorders: Clues to the origin of hydramnios. *American Journal of Obstetrics and Gynecology* **108**:1251–1256.

16 Southill PW, Nicolaides KH, Rodeck CH, Clewell WH, Lindridge J (1987) Relationship of fetal hemoglobin and oxygen content to lactate concentration in Rh isoimmunized pregnancies. *Obstetrics and Gynecology* **69**:268–270.

17 Brace RA, Powell TL (1991) Elevated fetal plasma lactate produces polyhydramnios in the sheep. *American Journal of Obstetrics and Gynecology* **165**:1595–1607.

18 Barkin SZ, Pretorius DH, Beckett MK, Manchester DK, Nelson TR, Manco-Johnson ML (1987) Severe polyhdramnios: Incidence of anomalies. *American Journal of Roentgenology* **148**:155–159.

19 Weir PE, Ratten GH, Beischer NA (1979) Acute polyhydramnios: A complication of monozygous twin pregnancy. *British Journal of Obstetrics and Gynaecology* **86**:849–853.

20 Caldreyro-Barcia R, Pose SV, Alvarez H (1957) Uterine contractility in polyhydramnios and the effects of withdrawal of the excess of amniotic fluid. *American Journal of Obstetrics and Gynecology* **73**:1238–1254.

21 Steinberg LH, Hurley VA, Desmedt E, Beischer NA (1990) Acute polyhydramnios in twin pregnancies. *Australia and New Zealand Journal of Obstetrics and Gynaecology* **30**:196–200.

22 Weiner CP, Heilskov J, Pelzer G, Grant S, Wenstrom K, Williamson RA (1989) Normal values for human umbilical venous and amniotic fluid pressures and their alteration by fetal disease. *American Journal of Obstetrics and Gynecology* **161**:714–717.

23 Fisk NM, Tannirandorn Y, Nicolini UM, Talbert DG, Rodeck CH (1990) Amniotic pressure in disorders of amniotic fluid volume. *Obstetric Gynecology* **76**:210–214.

24 Jacoby HE, Charles D (1966) Clinical conditions associated with hydramnios. *American Journal of Obstetrics and Gynecology* **94**:910–919.

25 Pritchard JA, Mason R, Corley M, Pritchard S (1970) Genesis of severe placental abruption. *American Journal of Obstetrics and Gynecology* **108**:22–25.

26 Desmedt EJ, Henry OA, Beischer NA (1990) Polyhydramnios and associated maternal and fetal complications in singleton pregnancies. *British Journal of Obstetrics and Gynaecology* **97**:1115–1122.

27 Kirkinen P, Jouppila P (1978) Polyhydramnios: A clinical study. *Annales Chirugiae et Gynaecologiae* **67**:117–122.

28 Vintzileos AM, Turner GW, Campbell WA, Weinbaum PJ, Ward SM, Nochimson DJ (1985) Polyhydramnios and obstructive renal failure: A case report and review of the literature. *American Journal of Obstetrics and Gynecology* **152**:883–885.

29 Seeds JW, Cefalo RC, Herbert WN, Bowes WA (1984) Hydramnios and maternal renal failure: Relief with fetal therapy. *Obstetrics and Gynecology* **64**:265–295.

30 Carlson DE, Platt LD, Medearis AL, Horenstein J (1990) Quantifiable polyhydramnios: Diagnosis and management. *Obstetrics and Gynecology* **75**:989–993.

31 Fisk NM, Giussani DA, Parkes MJ, Moore PJ, Hanson MA (1991) Amnioinfusion increases amniotic pressure in pregnant sheep but does not alter fetal acid–base status. *American Journal of Obstetrics and Gynecology* **165**:1459–1463.

32 Kirshon B (1989) Fetal urine output in hydramnios. *Obstetrics and Gynecology* **73**:240–242.

33 Campbell S, Wladimiroff JW, Dewhurst CJ (1973) The antenatal measurement of fetal urine production. *British Journal of Obstetrics and Gynaecology* **80**:680–686.

34 Rabinowitz R, Peters MT, Sanjay V *et al.* (1989) Measurement of fetal urine production in normal pregnancy by real-time ultrasonography. *American Journal of Obstetrics and Gynecology* **161**:1264–1266.

35 Hung NW, Gabrielli S, Reece EA, Roberts JA, Salafia C, Hobbins JC (1989) Ultrasonographic criteria for the prenatal diagnosis of placental chorionicity in twin gestations. *American Journal of Obstetrics and Gynecology* **161**:1540–1542.

36 D'Alton ME, Dudley DK (1989) The ultrasonographic prediction of chorionicity in twin gestation. *American Journal of Obstetrics and Gynecology* **160**:557–561.

37 Brady K, Polzin W, Jerime N, Kopelman JN, Read JA (1992) Risk of chromosomal abnormalities in patients with idiopathic polyhydramnios. *Obstetrics and Gynecology* **79**:234–238.

38 Cifuentes RF, Olley PM, Balfe JW, Radde IC, Soldin SJ (1979) Indomethacin and renal function in premature infants with persistent patent ductus arteriosus. *Journal of Pediatrics* **95**:583–587.

39 Kirshon B, Moise KJ, Wasserstrum N, Ou CN, Huhta JC (1988) Influence of short-term indomethacin therapy on fetal urine output. *Obstetrics and Gynecology* **72**:51–53.

40 Mamopoulos M, Assimakopoulos E, Reece EA, Andreou A, Zheng XZ, Manalenakis S (1990) Maternal indomethacin therapy in the treatment of polyhydramnios. *American Journal of Obstetrics and Gynecology* **162**:1225–1229.

41 Lange IR, Harman CR, Ash KM, Manning FA, Menticoglou S (1989) Twins with hydramnios: Treating premature labor at source. *American Journal of Obstetrics and Gynecology* **160**:552–557.

42 Cabrol D, Landesman R, Muller J, Uzan M, Sureau C, Saxena BB (1987) Treatment of polyhydramnios with prostaglandin synthetase inhibitor (indomethacin). *American Journal of Obstetrics and Gynecology* **157**:422–426.

43 Anderson RJ, Berl T, McDonald KM *et al.* (1975) Evidence for an *in vivo* antagonism between vasopressin and prostaglandin in the mammalian kidney. *Journal of Clinical Investigation* **56**:420–426.

44 Seyberth H, Rascher W, Hackenthal R, Wille L (1983) Effect of prolonged indomethacin therapy on renal function and selected vasoactive hormones in very low birth weight infants with symptomatic patent ductus arteriosis. *Journal of Pediatrics* **103**:979–984.

45 Dunn MJ, Zambraski EJ (1984) Renal effects of drugs that inhibit prostaglandin synthesis. *Kidney International* **18**:609–622.

46 Moise KJ, Ou CN, Kirshon B, Cano LE, Rognerud C, Carpenter RJ (1990) Placental transfer of indomethacin in the human pregnancy. *American Journal of Obstetrics and Gynecology* **162**:549–554.

47 Goldenberg RL, Davis RO, Baker RC (1989) Indomethicin induced oligohydramnios. *American Journal of Obstetrics and Gynecology* **190**:1196–1197.

48 Kirshon B, Mari G, Moise KJ (1990) Indomethacin therapy in the treatment of symptomatic polyhydramnios. *Obstetrics and Gynecology* **75**:202–205.

49 Moise KJ, Huhta JC, Sharif DS *et al.* (1988) Indomethacin in the treatment of premature labor: Effects on the fetal ductus arteriosis. *New England Journal of Medicine* **6**:327–330.

50 Cowan F (1989) Indomethacin, patent ductus arteriosus, and cerebral blood flow. *Journal of Pediatrics* **109**:341–344.

51 Hendricks SD, Smith JR, Moore DE, Brown ZA (1990) Oligohydramnios associated with prostaglandin synthetase inhibitors in preterm labour. *British Journal of Obstetrics and Gynecology* **97**:312–316.

52 Huhta JC, Cohen AW, Wood DC (1990) Premature constriction of the ductus arteriosus. *Journal of the American Society of Echocardiography* **3**:30–34.

53 Cantor B, Tyler T, Nelson RM, Stein GH (1980) Oligohydramnios and transient neonatal anuria: A possible association with the maternal use of prostaglandin synthetase inhibitors. *Journal of Reproductive Medicine* **24**:220.

54 Vanhaesebrouck P, Thiery M, Vandewalle J, Defoort P, Van Maele G (1988) Serum creatinine levels in preterm infants after intrauterine exposure to indomethacin. *Medical Science Research* **16**:93.

55 Rivett LC (1933) Hydramnios. *Journal of Obstetrics and Gynaecology of the British Empire* **40**:522–525.

56 Mahoney BS, Petty CN, Nyberg DA, Luthy DA, Hickok DE, Hirsch JH (1990) The 'stuck twin' phenomenon: Ultrasonographic findings, pregnancy outcome, and management with serial amniocenteses. *American Journal of Obstetrics and Gynecology* **163**:1513–1522.

57 Chescher NC, Seeds JW (1988) Polyhydramnios and oligohydramnios in twin gestations. *Obstetrics and Gynecology* **71**:882–884.

58 Elliott JP, Urig MA, Clewell WH (1991) Aggressive therapeutic amniocentesis for treatment of twin–twin transfusion syndrome. *Obstetrics and Gynecology* **77**:537–540.

59 Feingold M, Cetrulo CL, Newton ER, Weiss J, Shakr C, Shmoys S (1986) Serial amniocenteses in the treatment of twin to twin transfusion complicated with acute polyhdramnios. *Acta Geniticae Medicae et Gemellologiae* **35**:107–113.

60 Saunders NJ, Snijders RM, Nicolaides KH (1992) Therapeutic amniocentesis in twin–twin transfusion syndrome appearing in the second trimester of pregnancy. *American Journal of Obstetrics and Gynecology* **166**:820–824.

61 Weiner C, Ludomirsky A (1992) Diagnosis and treatment of twin–twin transfusion syndrome. *American Journal of Obstetrics and Gynecology* **284**: (abstract 23).

62 Crowley P (1980) Non-quantitative measurement of

amniotic fluid volume in prolonged pregnancy. *Journal of Perinatal Medicine* **8**:249–251.

63 Manning FA, Hill LM, Platt LD (1981) Qualitative amniotic fluid volume determination by ultrasound: Antepartum detection of intrauterine growth retardation. *American Journal of Gynecology* **139**:254–258.

64 Wladimiroff JW, Campbell S (1974) Fetal urine production rates in normal and complicated pregnancy. *Lancet* **i**:151–154.

65 Kurjak A, Kirkinen P, Latin V, Ivankovic D (1981) Ultrasonic assessment of fetal kidney function in normal and complicated pregnancies. *American Journal of Obstetrics and Gynecology* **141**:266–270.

66 Nicolaides KH, Peters MT, Vyas S, Rabinowitz R, Rosen DJ, Campbell S (1990) Relation of rate of urine production to oxygen tension in small-for-gestational-age fetuses. *American Journal of Obstetrics and Gynecology* **162**:387–391.

67 Vyas S, Nicolaides KH, Campbell S (1989) Renal flow–velocity waveforms in normal and hypoxemic fetuses. *American Journal of Obstetrics and Gynecology* **161**:168–172.

68 Ardiuni D, Rizzo G (1991) Fetal renal artery velocity waveforms and amniotic fluid volume in growth-retarded and post-term fetuses. *Obstetrics and Gynecology* **77**:370–373.

69 Beischer NA, Brown JB, Townsend L (1969) Studies in prolonged pregnancy: Amniocentesis in prolonged pregnancy. *American Journal of Obstetrics and Gynecology* **103**:496.

70 Gunn GC, Mishell D, Morton DG (1970) Premature rupture of the fetal membranes. *American Journal of Obstetrics and Gynecology* **106**:469–483.

71 Grant J, Keirse MJ (1989) Prelabour rupture of the membranes at term. In Chalmers I, Enkin M, Keirse MJ (eds) *Effective Care in Pregnancy and Childbirth*, Vol. 2. pp. 1112–1117. Oxford: Oxford University Press.

72 Gonik B, Bottoms SF, Cotton DB (1985) Amniotic fluid volume as a risk factor in preterm premature rupture of the membranes. *Obstetrics and Gynecology* **65**:456–459.

73 Robson MS, Turner MJ, Strong JM, O'Herlihy CO (1990) Is amniotic fluid quantitation of value in the diagnosis and conservative management of prelabour membrane rupture at term? *British Journal of Obstetrics and Gynaecology* **97**:324–328.

74 Taylor J, Garite TJ (1984) Premature rupture of membranes before fetal viability *Obstetrics and Gynecology* **64**:615–620.

75 Baumgarten K, Moser S (1986) The technique of fibrin adhesion for premature rupture of the membranes during pregnancy. *Journal of Perinatal Medicine* **14**:43–49.

76 Watson WJ, Latz VL, Seeds JW (1991) Fetal urine output does not influence residual amniotic fluid volume after premature rupture of membranes. *American Journal of Obstetrics and Gynecology* **164**:64–65.

77 Mercer LJ, Brown LG, Petres RE, Messer RH (1984) A survey of pregnancies complicated by decreased amniotic fluid. *American Journal of Obstetrics and Gynecology* **149**:355–361.

78 Mercer LJ, Brown LG (1986) Fetal outcome with oligohydramnios in the second trimester. *Obstetrics and Gynecology* **67**:840–842.

79 Morre TR, Longo J, Leopold GR, Casola G, Gosink BB (1989) The reliability and the predictive value of an amniotic fluid scoring system in severe second trimester oligohydramnios. *Obstetrics and Gynecology* **73**:730–742.

80 Mercer LJ, Brown IG (1986) Fetal outcome with oligohydramnios in the second trimester. *Obstetrics and Gynecology* **67**:840–842.

81 Harrison MR, Golbus M, Filly RA, Nakayama DK, Callen PW, deLorimier AA, Hricak H (1982) Management of the fetus with congenital hydronephrosis. *Journal of Pediatric Surgery* **17**:728–742.

82 Nicolini U, Rodeck CH, Fisk NM (1987) Shunt treatment for fetal obstructive uropathy. *Lancet* **ii**:1338–1339.

83 Crowley P, O'Herlihy C, Boylan P (1984) The value of ultrasound measurement of amniotic fluid volume in the management of prolonged pregnancies. *British Journal of Obstetrics and Gynaecology* **91**:444–448.

84 Moberg LJ, Garite TJ, Freeman RK (1984) Fetal heart rate patterns and fetal distress in patients with preterm premature rupture of membranes. *Obstetrics and Gynecology* **64**:60–64.

85 Lanier LR, Scarbrough RW, Fillingim DW, Baker RE (1965) Incidence of maternal and fetal complications associated with rupture of membranes before onset of labour. *American Journal of Obstetrics and Gynecology* **93**:398–404.

86 Moore TR, Longo J, Leopold GR, Casola G, Gosink BB (1989) The reliability and predictive value of an amniotic fluid scoring system in severe second trimester oligohydramnios. *Obstetrics and Gynecology* **73**:739–742.

87 Moretti M, Sibai BM (1988) Maternal and perinatal outcome of expectant management of premature rupture of membranes in the mid-trimester. *American Journal of Obstetrics and Gynecology* **159**:390–396.

88 Major CA, Kitzmiller JL (1990) Perinatal survival with expectant management of mid-trimester rupture of the membranes *American Journal of Obstetrics and Gynecology* **163**:838–844.

89 Blanc WA (1986) Causes of pulmonary hypoplasia. In *CIBA Foundation Symposium 1986: The Fetus and Independent Life*, p. 332. London: Academic Press.

90 Wigglesworth JS, Desai R (1982) Is fetal respiratory function a major determinant of perinatal survival? *Lancet* **i**:264–267.

91 Knox WF, Barson AJ (1986) *Early Human Development* Pulmonary hypoplasia in a regional perinatal unit. **14**:33–42.

92 Harrison MR, Globus M, Filly RA, Nakayama DK, Callen PW, de Lorimier AA, Hricak H (1982) Management of the fetus with congenital hydronephrosis. *Journal of Pediatric Surgery* **17**:728–742.

93 Nimrod C, Varela-Gittings F, Machin G, Campbell D, Wesenberg R (1984) The effect of very prolonged membrane rupture on fetal development. *American Journal of Obstetrics and Gynecology* **148**:540–543.

94 Rotschild A, Ling EW, Puterman ML, Farquharson D

(1990) Neonatal outcome after prolonged preterm rupture of the membranes. *American Journal of Obstetrics and Gynecology* **162**:46–52.

95 Fisk NM, Ronderos-Dumit D, Soliani A, Nicolini U, Vaughan J, Rodeck CH (1991) Diagnostic and therapeutic transabdominal amnioinfusion in oligohydramnios. *Obstetrics and Gynecology* **78**:270–278.

96 Fisk N, Rodeck C (1990) Detection of congenital abnormalities of the renal and urinary tract by ultrasound. In Chamberlain G (ed.), *Modern Antenatal Care of the Fetus*, pp. 359–387. Oxford: Blackwell Scientific Publications.

97 Benacerraf BR (1990) Examination of the second-trimester fetus with severe oligohydramnios using transvaginal scanning. *Obstetrics and Gynecology* **75**:491–493.

98 Harman CR (1984) Maternal furosemide may not provoke urine production in the compromised fetus. *American Journal of Obstetrics and Gynecology* **150**:322–323.

99 Chamberlain PF, Cumming M, Torchia MG *et al.* (1985) Ovine fetal urine production following maternal intravenous furosemide administration. *American Journal of Obstetrics and Gynecology* **151**:815–819.

100 Nicolini U, Santolaya J, Hubinont C, Fisk NM, Maxwell D, Rodeck CH (1989) Visualisation of fetal intraabdominal organs in second trimester severe oligohydramnios by intraperitoneal infusion. *Prenatal Diagnosis* **9**:191–194.

101 Hackett GA, Nicolaides KH, Campbell S (1987) Doppler ultrasound assessment of fetal and utero-placental circulations in severe second trimester oligohydramnios. *British Journal of Obstetrics and Gynaecology* **94**:1074–1077.

102 Gembruch U, Hansmann M (1988) Artificial instillation of amniotic fluid as a new technique for the diagnostic evaluation of cases of oligohydramnios. *Prenatal Diagnosis* **8**:33–45.

103 Van Der Pol JG, Wolf H, Boer K *et al.* (1992) Jejunal atresia related to the use of methylene blue in genetic amniocentesis in twins. *British Journal of Obstetrics and Gynaecology* **99**:141–143.

104 Nicolini U, Monni G (1990) Intestinal obstruction in babies exposed *in utero* to methylene blue. *Lancet* **336**:1258–1259.

105 Harrison MR, Nakayama DK, Noall R *et al.* (1982) Correction of congenital hydronephrosis *in utero*:

Decompression reverses the effects of obstruction on the fetal lung and urinary tract. *Journal of Pediatric Surgery* **17**:965–974.

106 Nakayama DK, Glick PL, Harrison MR *et al.* (1983) Experimental pulmonary hypoplasia due to oligohydramnios and its reversal by relieving thoracic compression. *Journal of Pediatric Surgery* **18**:347–353.

107 Nimrod C, Davies D, Iwanicki S, Harder J, Persaud D, Nicholson S (1986) Ultrasound prediction of pulmonary hypoplasia. *Obstetrics and Gynecology* **68**:495–497.

108 Chitkara I, Rosenberg J, Chervenak FA *et al.* (1987) Prenatal sonographic assessment of the fetal thorax. *American Journal of Obstetrics and Gynecology* **156**:1069–1074.

109 Roberts AB, Mitchell JM (1990) Direct ultrasonographic measurement of fetal lung length in normal pregnancies and pregnancies complicated by prolonged rupture of the membranes. *American Journal of Obstetrics and Gynecology* **163**:1560–1566.

110 Van Eyck J, Van der Mooren L, Wladimiroff JW (1990) Ductus arteriosus flow velocity modulation by fetal breathing movements as a measure of fetal lung development *American Journal of Obstetrics and Gynecology* **163**:558–566.

111 Songster GS, Gray DL, Crane JP (1989) Prenatal prediction of lethal pulmonary hypoplasia using ultrasonic fetal chest circumference. *Obstetrics and Gynecology* **73**:261–6.

112 D'Alton M, Mercer B, Riddick E, Dudley D (1992) Serial thoracic versus abdominal circumference ratios for the prediction of pulmonary hypoplasia in premature rupture of the membranes remote from term. *American Journal of Obstetrics and Gynecology* **166**:658–663.

113 Manning RA, Harrison MR, Rodeck CH, and members of the International Fetal Medicine and Surgery Society (1986) Catheter shunts for fetal hydronephrosis and hydrocephalus. *New England Journal of Medicine* **315**:336–340.

114 Imanaka M, Ogita S, Sugawa T (1989) Saline solution amnioinfusion for oligohydramnios after premature rupture of the membranes. *American Journal of Obstetrics and Gynecology* **161**:102–106.

115 Fisk NM (1992) *Amniotic pressure in disorders of amniotic fluid volume.* PhD Thesis, University of London.

49

Fetal Infection

Y. GIOVANGRANDI, C.P. WEINER, J. SMOLENIEC, J.P. BRETTES

INTRODUCTION

Fetal infection is a significant cause of perinatal morbidity and mortality. It seems that each year a new organism (parasite or virus) is shown to cause fetal infection. Though some are more virulent than others, only a few have unique effects. In general, the approach to the diagnosis of fetal infection depends upon how the patient presents. In this chapter, we assume that a specific parasite or virus is suspected. However, infection should be part of the differential diagnosis whenever a fetus is found to have:

- hydrops

- an isolated fluid collection

- hydrocephalus

- intracranial calcifications

- early-onset growth deficiency apparently not associated with uteroplacental dysfunction (i.e. normal Doppler velocimetry).

An algorithm is suggested in **Figure 1**.

This chapter should be read in conjunction with Chapters 29 and 30.

TOXOPLASMOSIS

Toxoplasmosis is a worldwide parasitic disease caused by the protozoan parasite, *Toxoplasma gondii*, which infects both animals and humans. The human fetus is at risk for damage when the primary infection occurs during pregnancy. Much work has been done on congenital toxoplasmosis, and its evaluation serves as a template for many congenital infections.

Replication Cycle[1]

The natural host of toxoplasma is a member of the cat family where the sex cycle occurs in the intestine (enteroepithelial cycle) with the formation of gametocytes and excretion of oocysts in feces. Oocysts sporulate and become infectious sporocysts that can remain viable in moist soil for a long time. When ingested by an intermediate host, the asexual phase of the life-cycle occurs with the release of tachyzoites (the proliferative form) into the blood stream and the formation of tissue cysts. These tissue cysts may contain in excess of 1000 bradyzoites (the quiescent form), and can occur in the brain, heart and skeletal muscle. Human infection usually results from the ingestion of sporocysts from a telluric reservoir (e.g. vegetables contaminated by cat's feces) or from bradyzoites contained in raw meat. The life-cycle of the parasite is completed when an infected rodent or bird is eaten by a cat. If the infection occurs during pregnancy, tachyzoites may cross the placenta and infect the fetus.

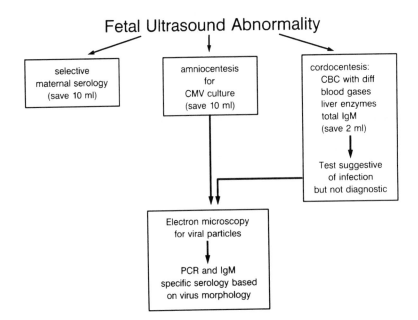

Figure 1. Fetal ultrasound abnormality.

Incidence

The seroprevalence rates increase with age.[1-3] Differences in rates among countries and populations within the same country are explained by variations in exposure to the oocysts and tissue cysts (cat population, the preparation of food, hygienic and eating habits). The overall seropositivity among women of child-bearing age ranges from 20–25% in the UK to 50–60% in Belgium and 70–80% in France. Inner-city rates are usually higher. The incidence of acquired infection during pregnancy is comparable with the incidence of disease among the general population.

The estimated incidence of congenital toxoplasma infection is based like those of most congenital infections on postnatal sero-epidemiological studies. Because a significant percentage of infected fetuses may be IgM-negative, these are likely to be underestimates. The incidence ranges from 0.12 per 1000 births in Birmingham, Alabama, 0.07–0.5 per 1000 births in London, 2.0 per 1000 births in Brussels to 3.22 per 1000 births in Paris.

Clinical Presentation and Risks[4-11]

Adults

In 80–90% of cases, adult toxoplasma infection is either asymptomatic or so mild that most women have forgotten the symptoms. Confirmation of prior exposure requires serologic investigation. In the remaining 10–20%, a mononucleosis-like illness characterized by asthenia, malaise, fever, sore throat, myalgia, headache, localized lymphadenopathy (posterior cervical, supraclavicular, axillary, inguinal areas) occurs which resolves spontaneously.

Fetal

Maternal parasitemia, which occurs during primary infection, is a prerequisite for placentitis and subsequent fetal infection. The rate of transmission to the fetus depends upon the time of pregnancy the maternal infection occurs: the later the maternal infection is acquired, the more frequently the parasite is transmitted to the fetus (**Table 1**). The period of the highest risk for the fetus is 10–24 weeks gestation. When the

Table 1
Timing of maternal toxoplasma, percentage of fetal infection and termination of pregnancy

Maternal infection	*n*	Infected fetuses	Termination of pregnancy
Periconceptional	250	3 (1.2%)	2 (67%)
6–20 weeks	937	62 (6.6%)	32 (52%)
21–35 weeks	83	24 (28.9%)	0 (0%)
Total	1270	89 (7%)	34 (38.2%)

From Daffos *et al.*[9] and Hohlfeld *et al.*[26]

onset of the maternal infection occurs before conception, the risk for fetal infection is extremely low (<1%). Congenital toxoplasmosis secondary to maternal infection preceding pregnancy has also been observed in immunodeficient women.[10] The severity of congenital disease also depends upon the age of the fetus when infected, age of pregnancy at maternal infection plus the delay between maternal infection and transmission to the fetus, i.e. the prenatal incubation period (**Table 2**). The earlier the fetus is infected, the greater the severity of fetal disease.

The clinical spectrum at birth varies from normal in appearance to severe neonatal disease.[8] The clinical findings include generalized acute infection (28%), splenomegaly–hepatomegaly, jaundice, anemia, chorioretinitis, pneumonia, lymphadenopathy, and abnormal cerebrospinal fluid. Neurologic disease is found in 69%. The common neurologic triad consists of hydrocephalus, chorioretinitis and intracranial calcifications. Convulsions commonly result. Classic lesions of the central nervous system and the eye may be delayed and/or progress.[11]

The overall mortality rate of clinically apparent disease is 12%; 85% of the survivors have sequelae (mental retardation, convulsions, spasticity and palsies, deafness) and 50% have severely impaired vision. The asymptomatic group may have lymphocytosis and/or elevated cerebrospinal protein, and persistent serologic test titers. Follow-up of these children may show no sequelae or progressive chorioretinitis with the accompanying risk of visual loss, cerebral calcifications, hydrocephaly or microcephaly, psychomotor and mental retardation, epilepsy, or deafness (whose appearance may be delayed for months or even years).[5] Of 48 children not treated during their first 10 months of life, 18% had chorioretinitis by 4 years of age.[8] Early treatment in the first year of life may limit the sequelae.[7]

Table 2
Pathogenesis of congenital toxoplasmosis

Placenta	Fetus	Infant
Not infected	→ Not infected	→ No congenital infection
Infected (early)	→ Fetal disease	→ Severe congenital toxoplasmosis
Infected (late)	→ Fetal disease	→ Mild or subclinical disease

Diagnosis

Laboratory diagnosis of maternal disease[12]

Serology

The diagnosis of primary toxoplasmosis is based upon the demonstration of rising serologic test titers. The antigenic structure of *Toxoplasma gondii* is complex. Both cytoplasmic antigens, which are liberated when the organism is lysed, and membrane antigens are involved in the immune response. The antibodies formed differ in both their class of immunoglobulin and their specificity. Detection depends on the serologic method used. There is no 'universal' assay applicable to the simultaneous investigation of the pregnant woman, fetus and neonate. We will focus only on those modern tests useful for the diagnosis of primary or congenital infection.

Several methods are based on responses to the whole parasite:

- *The Sabin-Feldman dye test* is based on lysis of living organism when exposed to IgG antibody containing serum in the presence of complement (C'). It can also detect protective antibodies and may reveal IgM if there is excess complement. The performance of this test is generally limited to specialized centers.

- *The agglutination (AG) test* uses the whole parasite preserved in formalin. It is a simple, accurate, inexpensive test. It is also very sensitive to IgM antibodies. A decrease in titer after treatment with 2-mercaptoethanol indicates IgM is present. A variation of this test detects IgG toxoplasma antibodies using acetone-fixed tachyzoites (AG agglutination) and formalin-fixed tachyzoites (HS agglutination). They can be very helpful in differentiating between acute and chronic infection.[13]

- *The indirect fluorescent antibody (IFA) test* uses slide preparations of killed toxoplasma incubated with serial dilutions of the patient's serum. The immune specific reaction is detected under the microscope. To avoid misinterpretation due to naturally occurring IgM antibodies, the fluoresceintagged conjugate should be only anti-IgG and not against total immunoglobulin.

- *The immunosorbent agglutination assay (ISAGA)* uses parasites preserved in formalin. It is both sensitive and specific for the detection of IgM. As simple to perform as the direct agglutination test and read in the same manner, it avoids false-positive results related to the presence of rheumatoid factor and/or antinuclear antibodies in serum samples.

Several methods measure antigen liberated from the lysis of toxoplasma:

- Latex-tagged particles make use of the same principle as the agglutination test and detect IgG and IgM antibodies.

- Enzyme-linked immunosorbent assay (ELISA) tests use enzyme conjugated antibody directed against either human IgG, IgM or total immunoglobulin. The IgG-ELISA correlates fairly well with titers obtained by either the Sabin-Feldman dye or IFA tests. The double sandwich IgM-ELISA is more sensitive and specific than the IgM-ELISA and IgM-IFA, since it is not inhibited by the presence of rheumatoid factor and/or antinuclear antibodies. The Capture ELISA is used for the detection of the IgA antibody anti-P30.[14] Both the double sandwich and the Capture ELISA methods are highly sensitive and specific for the detection of acute, recently acquired, and congenital infections.

- Enzyme-linked immunofiltration assay (ELIFA)[15] allows the simultaneous study of antibody specificity (IgA, IgG, IgE, IgM) by immunoprecipitation and analysis of antibody isotypes with enzyme-labeled antibody. This method is useful for the diagnosis of congenital infection.

Since the symptoms of the toxoplasma infection are not specific and greater than 80% of acquired toxoplasma infections are subclinical, the diagnosis relies on serologic testing. False-positive results (detection of non-specific antibodies) must be avoided. The evolution of the antibody response to acute infection is depicted in **Figure 2**. IgM antibodies are first synthesized at a steep rate after the onset of the disease and peak approximately 2 weeks later. They are usually not detectable after 6 months if the IgM-IFA test is used, but may be high for more than 12 months if either the IgM-ISAGA or the double sandwich IgM-ELISA is employed.

The synthesis and the rise of IgG antibody is initially slow, reaching a peak in 2–3 months when measured by a dye test, and then remain stable or decrease slowly over several years. With whole cell agglutination tests, IgG antibodies reach a steady high titer in 2–6 months. It is important to note that the dye test may be positive, while the agglutination test is still negative. Owing to the greater sensitivity of the agglutination test for detecting low titers of IgG antibodies, it may be positive in chronically infected persons when the dye test is negative.

In France, maternal blood is obtained at the first two prenatal visits. In the absence of immunosuppression,

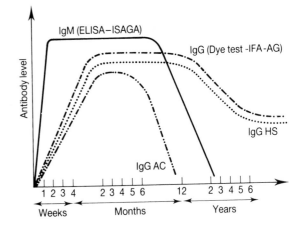

Figure 2. Evolution of antibody response to acute toxoplasma infection.

the risk of the patient giving birth to a congenitally infected infant is very low if the patient is seropositive (defined as a negative IgM and steady IgG titer in two samples obtained 3 weeks apart but tested in parallel). Seronegative women are screened every 5–8 weeks. The diagnosis of acute toxoplasma infection is made if either the patient seroconverts, or there is a significant rise in the IgG titer in association with high and steady titer of IgM in the first two serum samples tested.

Differentiating between acute and chronic infection may be difficult if the antibody titers have peaked by the time the first serum is obtained. Serologically, this is characterized by IgG and IgM-ELISA or an ISAGA as a high and stable titer in the first two serum samples tested. If the first serum was drawn prior to 10 weeks gestation, maternal infection probably occurred before or shortly after conception and the risk to the fetus is quite low. However, if the first serum was obtained later in pregnancy, it is more difficult to exclude seroconversion during pregnancy, particularly if the titer is high (dye test >300 IU/ml or 1:1000). The performance of HS/AC agglutination and/or capture ELISA IgA anti-P30 may be helpful in these circumstances. *Since spiramycin may blunt the rise in IgG antibody if adminstered during the initial antibody response, it should not be prescribed before the second serum sample is drawn 3 weeks later.*

Parasite isolation

Isolation of the parasite provides unequivocal proof of infection.[1] During pregnancy, the parasite can be isolated from amniotic fluid and/or fetal blood, and after birth from non-fixed placenta digested with trypsin, blood and or cerebrospinal fluid from the newborn. Mouse inoculation is very sensitive but takes a long time (40–45 days). Cell culture inoculation is more rapid but less sensitive.[16]

Detection of specific toxoplasma DNA[17,18]

This will overcome the drawbacks of culture in the near future.

Prenatal diagnosis

Prenatal diagnosis of toxoplasmosis requires a multi-faceted approach and is based on ultrasound examination plus tests performed on amniotic fluid and fetal blood obtained no earlier than 20 weeks gestation.[9,29] The tests include:

- Specific IgM in fetal sera tested by ISAGA.

- Parasite isolation from the sediment of fetal blood and amniotic fluid inoculated intraperitoneally into mice, or fibroblast tissue culture (amniotic fluid alone).

- Non-specific laboratory signs of infection: increased total IgM, leucocytosis, eosinophilia, thrombocytopenia, increased gamma-glutamyl-transferase (γGT).

The combination of specific tests allows 96% of infected fetuses to be identified prenatally.[9,19–21] The remaining 4% of infected fetuses are detectable by ultrasound findings[22] and/or non-specific tests and proven by subsequent repeat sampling.

Parasite isolation and specific IgM

Parasite isolation is the single most sensitive and specific test, with tissue culture being less sensitive than mouse inoculation (53 vs 73%). The main drawback to mouse inoculation is the 3–6 weeks required to obtain a result. However, the combination of cell culture and toxoplasma-specific IgM permits a diagnosis within 4 days in 70% of cases. The diagnosis of fetal infection should not be made solely on the presence of specific IgM, since false-positive tests have been reported.[23] Anti-toxoplasma IgM detection is the single least sensitive specific test (29.5%). Specific IgM should be associated with other biological signs (specific or not).

Specific anti-toxoplasma IgM has not in the French experience been detected before 22 weeks gestation. The incidence of a positive specific IgM increases with the gestational age at sampling: 9.5% of infected fetuses sampled between 20 and 24 weeks, 29% sampled between 25 and 29 weeks, and 63% sampled between 30 and 34 weeks.

Certain findings, such as increased total IgM and thrombocytopenia, or leucocytosis associated with increased γGT, have a high value predicting fetal infection.

Specific DNA analysis

In September 1991, Michel Vidaud (Institute of Pueri-culture, Paris) developed a polymerase chain reaction (PCR) based assay for the amplification of B1 and P30 genes of *Toxoplasma gondii* on cells pelleted from amniotic fluid (AF) from 18 weeks gestation onwards. More than 400 specimens have been studied without a false-negative or false-positive result. PCR can be completed within 24 h. It is likely that this test will become the diagnostic method of choice.

Ultrasound examination

In one series of 89 infected fetuses, 33 (37%) showed abnormal morphological signs.[22] The most common finding was symmetrical cerebral ventricular dilation secondary to necrotizing lesions in the region of the Sylvius duct. Other sonographic lesions included intra-cranial densities from focal necrosis, hepatomegaly and intrahepatic densities, ascites, and pleural and pericardial effusions. It should be emphasized that *major cerebral damage (multiple foci of brain necrosis) may exist without ventricular dilation. Simply stated, failure to detect a fetal abnormality does not mean there are none.*

When a maternal infection occurs before 20 weeks gestation with a proven fetal infection, the incidence of brain lesions is high, even when the ultrasound examination is normal. Therefore, it is reasonable to offer termination of pregnancy in such cases (see later). In the future, magnetic resonance imaging (MRI) may prove more sensitive.

Neonatal diagnosis [1]

The diagnosis of congenital toxoplasmosis may be based on either the isolation of the parasite or serology plus other findings.

Isolation of the parasite

Toxoplasma can be isolated from cord or peripheral blood of the neonate if not treated prenatally. A placental tissue culture is positive in >90% of pregnancies yielding infected neonates. It remains positive in 73% of infected children delivered of women treated with spiramycin, but in only 42% of those receiving specific anti-toxoplasma therapy during pregnancy.

Serologic diagnosis

The presence of toxoplasma-specific IgM in cord or peripheral blood of the newborn is diagnostic of congenital infection. It can be demonstrated by the ISAGA method in 70% of congenitally infected children born of a mother treated with spiramycin and in 18% of cases whose mother was administered specific therapy. The diagnosis is far more difficult to confirm in the subclinically infected newborn, with a negative test for IgM antibodies and a negative placental culture. It may be impossible to isolate the parasite from congenitally infected infants when prenatal specific therapy was administered.

Infected newborns can have a negative IgM. High titers of maternal IgG antibody may coat antigenic sites, delaying the fetal synthesis of fetal toxoplasma antibodies. If the fetal antibody level is low, treatment may prevent or reduce antibody formation by the destruction of the tachyzoite. Lastly, it is possible that the fetus fails to maintain IgM antibody production as has been documented in several congenital viral infections. Thus, the IgM might be positive early but not late in the course of the disease.

The half-life of human immunoglobulin-G is approximately 30 days. Thus, the concentration of maternal IgG decreases by one-half per month and should be absent from the infant's circulation by 10 months of age. Therefore, all potentially infected infants (i.e. maternal seroconversion during pregnancy or those suspected to be infected at birth) should be tested at intervals of 2 months until their final status is established.

Other findings

The suspected infected infant must have a long-term follow-up with clinical and ophthalmoscopy examination. At birth, transfontanelle ultrasonography and lumbar puncture must be done to look for pleocytosis, and elevated protein content.

Management Options

Screening and prevention[24,25]

Seronegative and immunodeficient pregnant patients are two populations at risk for *Toxoplasma gondii*. In some countries with a high prevalence of maternal seroconversion (Austria, Belgium, France), women are routinely screened during pregnancy to reduce the inci-

dence of congenital toxoplasma infection. Since 1978, the French government has paid for the serological surveillance of the non-immune pregnant patients. The French national program advises the first screen be performed prior to pregnancy so that the non-immune patient can be appropriately advised. During pregnancy, serum is obtained at first prenatal visit. Seronegative women are told how to avoid toxoplasma (**Table 3**). The serologic tests are then repeated every 4–8 weeks until delivery. Severe cases of congenital toxoplasma are now rare in France, except for the mothers not tested for toxoplasma infection during pregnancy.

Other countries, such as the UK, where the prevalence of toxoplasmosis is low, have chosen a less expensive strategy based on a program of health education. This is a financial decision, since the health information given to at-risk women is only moderately effective in reducing the incidence of infection during pregnancy.

Prenatal (**Figure 3**)

Once a primary maternal infection is identified, spiramycin (3 g/day) is begun to reduce the likelihood of fetal infection.[26] This regimen reduces the risk of transmission by 60%, but does not modify the pattern of infection. At birth, the placental concentration of spiramycin is four times the average maternal blood concentration and six and a half times that of cord blood.[27] The longer the interval between maternal seroconversion and the initiation of spiramycin, the greater the likelihood of fetal damage. Spiramycin therapy carries no significant risk of maternal or fetal toxicity even when administered over a long time.

If an investigation reveals that the fetus is not infected, the spiramycin is continued to prevent late transmission. Monthly ultrasound examinations are performed until delivery.

Table 3
Prevention of toxoplasmosis: advice for non-immune pregnant women

Cook meat to well done (industrial deep-freezing also seems to destroy parasites efficiently)
When handling raw meat, avoid touching mouth and eyes: wash hands thoroughly after handling raw meat, or vegetables soiled by earth
Wash kitchen surfaces that come into contact with raw meat
Wash fruit and vegetables before consumption
Avoid contact with things that are potentially contaminated with cat faeces
Wear gloves when gardening or handling cat litter box
Disinfect cat litter box for 5 minutes with boiling water

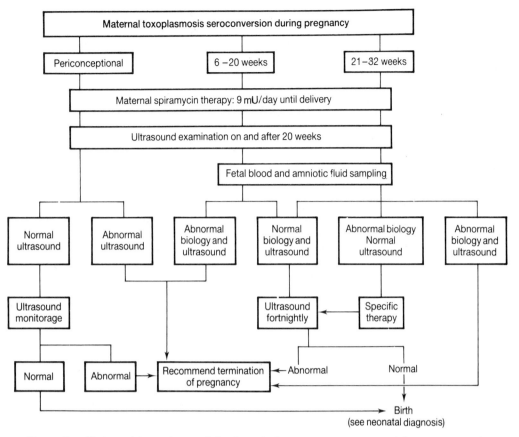

Figure 3. Maternal toxoplasma infection during pregnancy: prenatal management.

If fetal infection is documented prior to 20 weeks, or if the ultrasound examination shows fetal damage, termination of the pregnancy should be considered. However, pregnancy termination was carried out in only 2.7% of 1200 cases of maternal seroconversion.

Specific antiparasitic therapy is indicated when fetal infection is documented and the pregnancy is to continue. Therapy consists of pyrimethamine (50 mg/day) and sulfadiazine (50 mg/kg/day).[28,29] Pyrimethamine is a folic acid antagonist which often causes a reversible bone-marrow toxicity characterized by thrombocytopenia within 7–10 days, anemia and leucopenia. It can be prevented by folinic acid administered as leucovorin calcium 15 mg/day. Leucovorin does not modify treatment efficiency, since the parasite cannot metabolize it. No fetal toxicity secondary to pyrimethamine has been identified. However, high doses of pyrimethamine are teratogenic in several mammalian species. Thus, it is considered ill-advised to initiate pyrimethamine before 16 weeks of pregnancy.

Sulfadiazine is also a folic acid antagonist. The two drugs act synergistically against toxoplasma with a combined activity eight times that which would occur if they were only additive. Sulfadiazine is contraindicated in cases of glucose-6-phosphate dehydrogenase deficiency, sulfonamide allergy or leucopenia.

Typically, the pyrimethamine-sulfadiazine combination is continued for 4 weeks and then alternated with a 2 week course of spiramycin. Fortnightly ultrasound examinations are performed. During a pyrimethamine–sulfadiazine course, folinic acid (50 mg) should be given twice weekly. Maternal bone-marrow function is monitored by a complete blood count obtained at the beginning and the end of each course of pyrimethamine–sulfadiazine therapy. The pyrimethamine-sulfa*doxine* combination (Fansidar®) is effective against toxoplasma, but is not recommended because of its potential toxicity (Lyell syndrome).

The above recommended treatment was employed in 54 cases of proven fetal infection and resulted in 53 healthy children (44 of them had subclinical toxoplasmosis infection and 9 had benign signs). All infants had normal neurological development up to 4 years of age. However, five infants developed peripheral chorioretinitis at 5–17 months of age (without impairment of vision).[26]

In summary, prenatal diagnosis in more than 90% of cases avoids the abortion of an uninfected fetus and fetal treatment limits the sequelae of the disease in pregnancies which continue. Such treatment should not be administered 'blindly', since at birth it will be difficult to differentiate the non-infected from the infected but insufficiently treated neonate. Further, the treatment would have been useless for 90%.

Future Developments

There are two major concerns with the approach outlined in this chapter. The first is the long interval of time between the onset of fetal infection and the beginning of treatment. The earlier treatment is begun after infection, the better the prognosis. The introduction of DNA probes for cells recovered from amniotic fluid should allow earlier accurate diagnosis, leading to earlier treatment of an infected but undamaged fetus, and accurate monitoring of successful fetal treatment by the disappearance of toxoplasma DNA in amniotic fluid after one or two courses of specific therapy. The second is that the long-term prognosis of an infected fetus may be unclear, since lesions may be missed. If magnetic resonance imaging appears to be more reliable than ultrasound for the detection of a fetal brain abnormality, it will be used in the future.

Genomic DNA analysis of *Toxoplasma gondii* may, in the future, identify the loci contributing to virulence of various strains of *Toxoplasma*,[30] which would probably be a factor of prognosis of the fetal disease.

A vaccine for the prevention of *Toxoplasma* infection is under development.[31,32]

CYTOMEGALOVIRUS

Cytomegalovirus (CMV) infects most people at some time during their life. The infection is of little consequence except in the fetus and the immunocompromised subject. After a primary infection, the virus remains latent in the host's body, but can reactivate periodically. Most primary and recurrent infections are subclinical. Regardless of whether or not symtoms are present, the fetus may be infected and damaged.[33]

CMV is a large DNA virus of the Herpesviridae family.[33,34] It replicates in the nucleus of infected cells producing the characteristic nuclear inclusions. Human CMV (HCMV) replicates only in differentiated human cells. Replication stimulates the production of viral proteins on the membrane of the infected cell. These proteins bind IgG to protect the infected cell against humoral and cell-mediated immune lysis. The factors controlling viral reactivation are not well established.

Congenital cytomegalovirus infection has a high incidence compared to other intrauterine viral infections (0.2–2.2% of live births). In total, 10% of congenitally infected neonates will have sequelae; 50% of these are severe (mental retardation, sensorineural hearing loss, cerebral palsy).

Incidence[35–40]

Large sero-epidemiological investigations have been conducted to determine the incidence of congenital CMV infection. However, more recent fetal studies clearly demonstrate that the production of CMV-specific IgM can be transient, ceasing by the time delivery occurs. Thus, these figures are likely to be an underestimate of the true prevalence. CMV seropositivity is age, socioeconomic class and country dependent. In the developing countries, CMV is usually acquired during childhood. In developed countries such as the USA, 40–60% of child-bearing age, middle-class women are seropositive compared with 65–80% of those from lower socioeconomic classes. *Pregnancy does not enhance the risk of seroconversion, which is 2.0–2.5% among susceptible women in the USA.* Seroconversion occurs more frequently in low-income (3.7%) compared with higher-income (1.5%) groups.

The incidence of congenital infection is fairly stable (0.5–2.0% of live births per year in the USA, 0.3% in the UK). During primary maternal infection, the rate of transmission to the fetus is 40% and is not apparently influenced by gestational age. Yet, the severity of congenital infection and its sequelae are higher when the infection occurs during the first half of pregnancy. although pre-existing naturally acquired maternal immunity does not prevent fetal infection,[41] it may protect against overwhelming fetal damage.

Recurrent maternal infection accounts for 20–30% of congenital CMV infections in the UK.[42] Among seropositive pregnant women, CMV reactivation and shedding (in urine, saliva, cervical secretions) are associated with younger age and high parity. The rate of cervical shedding increases from 3% in the first trimester to 8% near term. Shedding can lead to neonatal infection.

Among neonates infected *in utero*, about 10% are symptomatic at birth, of which 15% have classic cytomegalic inclusion disease. Altogether, 15–20% of symptomatic infants die and 90% of the survivors develop sequelae. Among infected but asymptomatic newborns, 5–15% develop sequelae, especially sensorineural hearing loss (**Figure 4**). Thus, among the 4 million live births in the USA each year, 40 000 neonates are congenitally infected and 8000 are damaged. In England and Wales, about 400 neonates will be damaged either at birth or by age 1 year.

Infection is not highly contagious and its transmission requires close and prolonged contact with CMV-infected secretions. Though sexual transmission of CMV is well documented,[43,44] the major source of infection for susceptible reproductive age women is

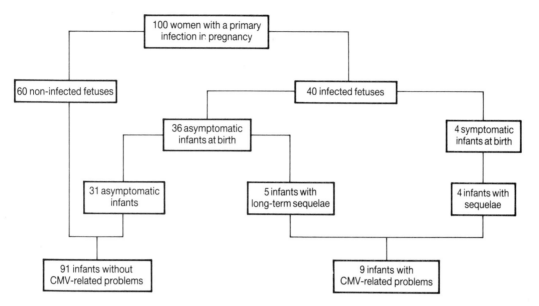

Figure 4. Infant outcome following primary CMV: maternal infection in pregnancy. Adapted from *Congenital, Perinatal and Neonatal Infections.* Greenough A, Osborne J, Sutherland S (eds) (1992). Edinburgh: Churchill Livingstone.

young children.[45–47] The younger the child introducing CMV into the home, the higher the rate of parental infection (45% if the infected child is under 18 months), probably because the exchange of body fluids cannot be avoided.[48] Fifty percent of all susceptible family members will seroconvert within the next 6 months.[49] Restriction endonuclease analyses of viral DNA recovered from mother and offspring confirm transmission of virus from child to mother.[50]

Recent studies warn of high rates of horizontal transmission among daycare providers. The risk of infection parallels the rate of acquisition of infection among children.[51–53] In total, 20–70% of children attending daycare centers acquire CMV infection and shed the virus in their urine and saliva periodically for up to 2 years. Because of the increasing number of women in the workforce and young children in daycare centers, it is likely that the incidence of congenital CMV infection will increase over the next few years. However, *pregnant health care workers are not at increased risk of acquiring CMV infection compared to the general population, even if they work in a pediatric, neonatal intensive care or acute renal unit.*[54,55] This demonstrates the protective efficacy of standard infection control procedures among health care workers.

Clinical Syndromes and Risk

Maternal

Maternal CMV infection is detailed in Chapter 30. In brief, fewer than 10% of primary CMV infections are symptomatic, usually presenting as a mononumcleosis-like illness. The viremia develops simultaneously with clinical symptoms. After a primary infection, CMV shedding from saliva, tears, urine, cervical secretions, etc, may persist for prolonged but intermittent periods. Recurrent infection (viral reactivation) is commonly asymptomatic.

Fetal

Transplacental passage may occur at any time during pregnancy after a primary or recurrent infection causing either symptomatic or asymptomatic fetal infection. Asymptomatic fetal infection carries the risk of chronic postnatal infection and subsequent sequelae. The congenital malformations ascribed to CMV are probably a chance association. The virulence of the CMV infection is not strain-dependent. Rather, the severity of the disease may be due to:

- chronic viral replication in the affected organs

- vasculitis, which may continue after birth leading to disseminated intravascular coagulopathy

- the formation of immune complexes which are deposited in some organs (renal glomeruli)

- abnormalities in cell-mediated immunity.

Table 4
Sequelae in children with congenital CMV infection according to type of maternal infection

	Primary	Recurrent
Symptomatic disease at birth	24/132 (18%)	0/65 (0%)
Any sequela	31/125 (25%)	5/64 (8%)
More than one sequela	7/125 (6%)	0/64 (0%)
Sensorineural hearing loss	18/120 (15%)	3/56 (5%)
Bilateral hearing loss	10/120 (8%)	0/56 (0%)
Microcephaly	6/125 (5%)	1/64 (2%)
Seizures	6/125 (5%)	0/64 (0%)
IQ < 70	9/68 (13%)	0/32 (0%)
Death	3/125 (2%)	0/64 (0%)

From Fowler *et al.*[56]

Most of the classic features of congenital CMV infection postnatally may be detected prenatally. These include growth deficiency, hepatosplenomegaly, microcephaly, intracerebral calcifications, anemia, thrombocytopenia, elevated liver enzymes. Hydrops has a poor prognosis. Other findings may be present at birth: chorioretinitis, central nervous system manifestations, petechiae, hyperbilirubinemia.

A recent study (**Table 4**) indicated that maternal CMV immunity prior to conception may protect an infected fetus from further damage.[57] However, there is no unanimity on this.[42]

Neonatal[56–59]

With the advent of reliable prenatal diagnosis, more information on the long-term effects of fetal CMV infection is needed. In addition to the systemic signs noted under fetal disease, the central nervous system effects now manifest and include microcephaly (about 50% of symptomatic infants), periventricular microcalcifications, vascular hyperechogenicity in the form of a 'branched candlestick', polymicroguria, ocular abnormalities (commonly associated with cerebral calcifications) such as chorioretinitis, optic atrophy, microphthalmia, and cataracts, cerebral palsy, epilepsy (which may appear later) and intellectual impairment. Uni- or bilateral sensorineural hearing loss and chorioretinitis may develop later in childhood after a subclinical infection at birth. Dental defects are common in symptomatic infants. Interstitial pneumonia is less frequent. *The infected newborn is infectious and should be isolated.*

The prognosis for infants with symptomatic congenital CMV infection at birth is not good. A prospective study of 65 symptomatic neonates[57] revealed that whereas 55% were normal or had some minor abnor-

mality, 45% had neurological impairment, of whom 34% had gross motor or psychomotor problems. The remaining 11% had mainly sensorineural deafness. Of the 34% with gross neurological problems, one died at 2 years, and 68% were microcephalic with associated perceptual function impairments. The neonatal clinical factor associated with poor neurological status were abnormal neurological signs (other than microcephaly), hepatomegaly, splenomegaly or purpura.

Term newborns may be infected either from genital tract secretions during birth or while breast- feeding.[60,61] Though usually asymptomatic, they may excrete the virus after 3 weeks of life and for several years. More than 30% of seropositive women intermittently excrete CMV into the breast milk during the first year after delivery. One term breast-fed child in five born to a seropositive woman acquires the infection by 12 months. Preterm infants born to seronegative women may develop severe postnatal CMV infection (usually pneumonia) after blood transfusion.[62] Disease acquired by breast-feeding from a seropositive mother can have the same impact on the preterm infant.

Diagnosis

Laboratory diagnosis of maternal disease[63–68]

Serology

There is wide cross-reactivity of human CMV antibodies to different HCMV strains. Testing should employ a sensitive method – either an enzyme-linked immunosorbent assay (ELISA) or a radioimmunoassay (RIA). The sensitivity of these methods for the detection of anti-CMV IgM is about 70%. IgM antibodies may be detected after a seroconversion (until the 12th week in 25% of cases). The presence of CMV-specific IgM antibodies is a good marker for recent infection, usually primary, but also for reactivation in more than 15% of cases. IgM anti-P60-66 and anti-P100 are potentially good markers of primary infection, but have not as yet been used during pregnancy.

Neither specific IgM nor viremia nor viruria are exclusive features of primary infection. They may develop during reactivation. *The only marker of a primary infection is the confirmed seroconversion after an earlier negative serology.* A significant rise (fourfold or greater) in specific total antibody (IgG and IgM) titer after a 2–3 week interval is an indicator of a recent infection, but it may be either primary or recurrent.

Virus isolation

CMV can be isolated from white blood cells, urine, throat swab, amniotic fluid and placenta. Viral culture in fibroblasts is the traditional method but requires 2–6 weeks for completion. Electron microscopy can be very effective, but requires a critical viral load. There are as yet no well-documented instances of a fetus with congenital CMV infection and a negative amniotic fluid culture. *Thus, amniotic fluid culture is currently the method of choice for the diagnosis of congenital CMV.*

Antigen detection

The development of specific monoclonal antibodies enables the detection of viral antigen in cell cultures performed on flat monolayers. Immediate early protein of CMV may be thus detected within 24–48 h.

DNA hybridization and amplification by polymerase chain reaction

Fetal or neonatal infection may be diagnosed using biotin-labeled probes on cells from amniotic fluid or fetal blood, and postnatally from fetal urine. *In situ* hybridization can detect viral DNA in culture cells or directly in infected tissue.

Prenatal diagnosis [69–81]

Is there a rationale for the prenatal diagnosis of congenital CMV? If one takes the narrow approach that clinical signs of maternal CMV infection are poor, serological screening is not recommended, and there is no safe intrauterine treatment of infected fetuses, it is useless to attempt the diagnosis of fetal infection. This approach cannot be recommended for several reasons. First, fetal production of specific IgM can be transient. To await delivery may be to lose the opportunity to make a definitive diagnosis of a chronic illness whose long-term prognosis is unclear. Second, effective prenatal viral therapy when the fetus is infected but has not any sonographic abnormality in the hope of limiting disease development may be feasible in the near future. Until then, postnatal antiviral therapy for an infected but undamaged infant may help to limit the extent of early CMV-related problems. Treatment is not possible without a diagnosis.

Prenatal diagnosis allows the detection of fetal infection in some circumstances. However, *fetal damage (eye, ear) cannot be ruled out even with normal ultrasonographic examination.* When counseling patients on the risk to their fetus with a normal sonogram, it should be remembered that:

- the risk of a baby having CMV-related damage is 4–9 per 100 after a primary infection (**Table 4**)

- the likelihood of fetal damage is 10–15 per 100 if fetal infection is confirmed, with unilateral or bilateral hearing loss occurring in 50–60% of these cases.

A search for fetal infection should be considered if:

- the mother shows CMV-like clinical signs confirmed by seroconversion

- abnormal fetal ultrasonographic signs consistent with congenital infection are present, e.g. cerebral ventricular dilation or other intracranial abnormalities, parenchymal echodensities, oligohydramnios, echogenic large placenta, ascites, meconium peritonitis.

What fetal samples should be investigated? When the fetus is infected, the virus seems consistently to be found in the amniotic fluid after 21 weeks gestation. Thus amniocentesis alone is a very sensitive diagnostic tool for the diagnosis of fetal CMV. However, fetal blood should also be obtained, not only to measure total and specific IgM (the cause of the sonographic abnormality may be another virus), but also to evaluate the fetal condition. For example, evidence of systemic disease (anemia, thrombocytopenia, elevated liver tests) would worsen the prognosis.

Management Options [47,82–89]

Prepregnancy prevention

Prenatal screening

Routine prenatal screening is not recommended unless the patient expresses a concern, since:

- Everyone is exposed to asymptomatic cytomegalovirus excretors in their professional, family and social life.

- CMV immunity is not completely protective against reactivation or reinfection which can result in fetal damage.

- There is no safe intrauterine treatment at the present time which can be offered to an infected fetus. However, this may change in the future. Ganciclovir is effective treatment for CMV chorioretinitis and prospective studies using ganciclovir for the treatment of congenital CMV disease are under way. There is at least one instance where ganciclovir was adminstered directly to an infected fetus with resolution of the viremia and viruria.

- There are no vaccination programs. An alive, attenuated CMV vaccine (Towne strain) has been developed and tested in renal transplant recipients. Unfortunately, the potential for reactivation or long-term oncogenicity has hampered its use during pregnancy. Moreover, the use of a live vaccine made from a single strain of CMV raises the question of its efficacy against reinfection from another strain. With the successful cloning of the viral genome, a recombinant vaccine which might prove effective for the prevention of congenital disease is possible.

However, if a patient still wishes to be tested, then asymptomatic primary infection is identified by screening at the beginning of the pregnancy and, if negative, again at 28–30 weeks. This assumes the major fetal risk occurs with a first half of pregnancy primary maternal infection. Prenatal diagnosis can then be offered to patients who seroconvert.

Health education policy

Daycare givers, health care workers and especially women of child-bearing age should be warned that a high percentage of young children are excreting CMV. They should be instructed on the modes of transmission and the hygienic procedures available when dealing with young children. Screening children for virus excretion is useless, since virus shedding is intermittent. The following infection control procedures must be applied in daycare centers and pediatric wards:

- handwashing after changing diapers

- proper disposal of used diapers

- preparation of food far from the diaper changing area

- toys which are likely to be contaminated by body secretions should be cleaned

- contacts that might involve the exchange of body fluids should be avoided with any child. Likewise, breast-feeding of a premature infant should not be encouraged if the mother is CMV-positive and, if blood transfusion is required, CMV-negative blood should be given.

Confirmed fetal infection

Termination of pregnancy should be considered, especially if there are abnormalities in either the fetal blood tests or the ultrasound examination. These fetuses are otherwise likely to fall into the 10% with symptomatic disease. Pregnancies which continue are scanned fortnightly. If the ultrasound becomes abnormal, consideration should be given to referral of the patient to a Fetal Diagnosis and Treatment Unit for novel therapy.

No fetal infection

If the woman has evidence of recent infection (either primary or reactivation), but the amniotic fluid culture is negative, the ultrasound examination is repeated fortnightly. If an abnormality develops, the search for fetal infection is repeated, since infection could follow endogenous reactivation after the first set of tests. At birth, a search is made to be sure that fetal infection has not occurred in the interim.

RUBELLA

Rubella is endemic worldwide. In 1941, Gregg described the occurrence of congenital cataracts after maternal rubella.[90] Twenty years later, Weller and Neva[91] and Parkman *et al.*[92] independently isolated the virus from ill patients. Shortly thereafter, live attenuated vaccines were developed.[93] Since Gregg's report, our understanding of rubella's effect on the embryo, fetus and neonate has increased considerably.

Rubella is a small (58 nm) single-stranded RNA togavirus (genus Rubivirus) with hemagglutinin antigens. It infects only humans and is transmitted to seronegative subjects by aerosolized respiratory secretions. The virus replicates in the respiratory system and then enters a viremic phase. The placenta and fetus are infected at that time.

Incidence[94–96]

Rubella seroprevalence is age-related. More than 90% of Caucasian women of child-bearing age have rubella antibodies. *In total, 0.5–2.0% of susceptible pregnant women are infected each year.* Congenital disease occurs in 0.2–0.5 per 1000 births. Localized epidemics occur every 6–9 years, while pandemics take place every 10–30 years. During epidemics, the incidence of congenital disease may reach 4–30% of susceptible pregnancies.

Women whose immunity is vaccine-induced experience reinfection more frequently (50%) than those whose immunity is naturally acquired (5%). Of the 101 confirmed infections during pregnancy reported in England and Wales between July 1988 and June 1989, 35 were probable reinfections.[97]

Clinical syndromes and risks[98–100]

Maternal

Maternal rubella is detailed in Chapter 30. Briefly, rubella is a mild childhood infection of little consequence except when it occurs during pregnancy. One-third of primary infections are subclinical. Prodromal symptons of malaise, headache, low-grade fever, coryza and conjunctivitis may precede the characteristic pinpoint macular rash by 1–5 days. The rash erupts nearly 16 days after exposure to the virus and first appears on the face and behind the ears before spreading down the trunk and the limbs. The contagious period (i.e. viral shedding) extends from 8 days before until 8 days after the onset of the rash. Rubella antibodies are present by the time the rash appears. *The clinical diagnosis of rubella is unreliable because other viral infections (enterovirus, adenovirus, parvovirus B19) can present similarly. Serological confirmation of a clinical diagnosis is essential, especially during pregnancy.*

Fetal[101–107]

Maternal viremia associated with either symptomatic or asymptomatic primary disease is a prerequisite for fetal infection. The likelihood of fetal infection and damage is dependent on the gestation of maternal infection (**Table 5**).[105–107] When maternal infection is acquired during organogenesis (the first 12 weeks), cardiac, eye and ear defects may develop (**Tables 6 and 7**). Hearing defects are common up to 17 weeks gestation. In fact, deafness may be the only anomaly when rubella is acquired after the first trimester. Because the onset can be delayed, progressive and bilateral, children who have no clinical evidence of the disease but persistent rubella antibodies should be carefully evaluated during childhood for hearing loss. The risk of a rubella defect after the 17th week of pregnancy is small but real. At any stage of pregnancy, a multisystem fetal infection with viral persistence and ongoing damage may occur.

The perinatal sequellae of rubella infection are secondary to both vascular damage and decreased mitotic activity of infected cells. Growth deficiency is common and is not corrected by delivery. Viremia is rare during reinfection, though there are several well-documented cases. The risk of fetal infection is probably below 10%, but must be considered, especially in women with vaccine-induced immunity.[97,108,109] It should be stressed that reinfection is asymptomatic. 'rubella-immune' women who report an exposure should probably undergo repeat serological investigation.[110,111]

Diagnosis

Laboratory diagnosis of maternal infection[112,113]

Serology

The hemagglutinin inhibition test (HIA) was the first test used and requires pretreatment of the serum to

Table 5
Consequences of symptomatic maternal rubella during pregnancy

Stage of pregnancy (weeks)	Infection		Defects		Overall risk of defect (rate of infection × rate of defects)
	No. tested	No. positive	No. followed	Rate	
< 11	10	9 (90%)	9	100%	90%
11–12	6	4 (67%)	4	50%	33%
13–14	18	12 (67%)	12	17%	11%
15–16	36	17 (47%)	14	50%	24%
17–18	33	13 (39%)	10		
19–22	59	20 (34%)			
23–26	32	8 (25%)			
27–30	31	11 (35%)			
31–36	25	15 (60%)	53		
> 36	8	8 (100%)			
Total	258	117 (45%)		200%	
			102		

From Miller *et al.*[105]

Table 6
Abnormalities in congenital rubella: Triad of Gregg

Eye

Cataract	Usually bilateral and present at birth
Retinopathy	'Salt and pepper' appearance, may have a delayed onset, frequently bilateral, visual acuity is not affected
Microphthalmia	Often associated with cataract
Glaucoma	Is rare but leads to blindness if not recognized

Heart

Patent ductus arteriosus	Common, often associated with persistence of the foramen ovale
Pulmonary valvular stenosis Pulmonary artery stenosis	Common, due to intimal proliferation and arterial elastic hypertrophy
Coarctation of the aorta	Infrequent
Ventricular septal defects	Rare
Atrial septal defects	Rare

Ear

Commonly damaged	Injury of cells of the middle ear leading to sensorineural deafness may also have a central origin.
Bilateral and progressive	May be present at birth or develop later in childhood. Severe enough for the child to need education at a special school; rare when maternal rubella occurs after the fourth month of pregnancy

Adapted from Freij et al.[99]

Table 7
Other clinical abnormalities encountered in congenitally acquired rubella

IUGR	Associated with other manifestations of congenital rubella syndrome

Central nervous system

Mental retardation	Directly related to postnatal growth deficiency
Meningoencephalitis	Common, transient
Behavioral disorders	Common
Hypotonia	Common
Microcephaly	Uncommon, may be associated with normal intelligence
Chronic panencephalitis	Rare, males affected, late-onset manifestation (second decade of life)

Liver

Hepatosplenomegaly	Common, transient
Hepatitis	Rare, may not be associated with jaundice

Blood

Thrombocytopenic purpura	Common, transient, no response to steroid therapy
Anemia	Infrequent, transient

Immune system

Lymphadenopathy	Uncommon, transient
Hypogammaglobulinemia	Uncommon, transient
Thymic hypoplasia	Uncommon, fatal

Bone

Radiographic lucencies	Common transient

Lung

Interstitial pneumonitis	Infrequent, probably immunologically mediated, may be severe

Endocrine glands

Diabetes mellitus	Common, appears in second decade
Thyroid disease	Infrequent
Growth hormone deficiency	Rare

Skin

'Blueberry muffin' spots	Infrequent, represents dermal erythropoiesis
Chronic rubelliform rash	Usually generalized, appears in infancy, lasts several weeks.

Adapted from Freij et al.[99]

eliminate nonspecific inhibitors of hemagglutination that would yield a false-negative result. The results are expressed as the final dilution of serum which completely inhibits hemagglutination of a viral suspension. A serum titration of 40 is evidence of rubella immunity. Radial hemolysis (RH) is frequently used in the United Kingdom and Northern Europe. This test is an estimate of the lytic effect of serum complement (C') on red blood cells sensitized with rubella virus. Pretreatment of the serum is not necessary. Other tests include the latex agglutination test (LA), which is less reliable than either the HIA or RH.

The detection of rubella-specific IgM antibodies requires a sensitive and reliable test, usually an antibody capture immunoassay (MAC-ELISA: anti-M-IgM capture ELISA). Other viral infections (Ebstein-Barr virus, CMV, parvovirus B19) may produce a false-positive result. The M-antibody capture radioimmunoassay (MAC-RIA) is the most sensitive and reliable IgM assay presently available.[114] Rubella-specific IgM is demonstrable up to 8 weeks after the onset of the rash, when an antibody capture technique is used.

Virus detection

Culture techniques are insensitive, slow and available in only a few laboratories. However, techniques for detecting viral-specific nucleic acid by PCR are both rapid and sensitive and with the proper controls may be used for the diagnosis of fetal rubella infection.[115]

Prenatal diagnosis[116–118]

The diagnosis of fetal infection is made after the detection of specific antirubella IgM (by capture immunoassay) in fetal blood sampled after 22 weeks. Before then, specific IgM may not be detectable, and even after that time false-negative results occur.[119] Further, it is possible that the production of fetal-specific IgM has ceased by the time the sample is obtained. Like many viral infections, a non-specific syndrome including erythroblastemia, mild anemia and thrombocytopenia, increased GGT and acid labile alpha-interferon may be present.[120]

There are three notes of caution:

- Detection of rubella-specific antigen and RNA in a placental biopsy specimen does not prove fetal infection.

- Fetal infection does not always mean fetal damage.

- A negative ultrasound examination does not necessarily mean no damage.

Neonatal diagnosis[121]

Neonates with congenital rubella syndrome excrete virus and are potentially infectious. They should be isolated from other newborns and from non-immune hospital personnel. The diagnosis at birth is made by testing cord blood. Neonatal serum is positive for specific IgM measured by an M-antibody-capture technique in most congenitally infected infants until 3 months of age.

Management Options

Pre- and postpregnancy prevention[121]

Prenatal screening

Rubella serology screening should be offered to all women of child-bearing age. Susceptible subjects (HIA titer < 40) should be encouraged to undergo vaccination before or after pregnancy while using effective contraception. In the USA, the UK and several other countries, all women are tested at the beginning of pregnancy, even if previously seropositive. If such a patient is exposed to rubella in the first trimester of her pregnancy, a search for reinfection should be made. Reinfection is diagnosed on the basis of a significant rise (four-fold) in rubella-specific IgG antibodies with a negative or low-level IgM response.[112,122]

Vaccination[101–122]

The prevention of congenital rubella is based on active immunization. RA 27/3 is the live attenuated rubella vaccine most commonly used. It is administered subcutaneously, either alone or simultaneously with other vaccines. However, if the other vaccine is also a live virus, a different innoculation site should be used. The vaccine is well tolerated, though a transitory rash, arthralgia and lymphadenopathy may occur 15 days after vaccination and the virus is excreted for days or weeks. It is not transmitted to susceptible contacts.

Vaccination is effective. Approximately 95% of vaccines seroconvert and the vaccine-induced antibodies persist at levels above 15 000 IU/l for more than 10 years.[123,124] Rubella vaccine should not be given to immunosuppressed patients or during pregnancy. As a rule, vaccination should be delayed for 3 months after a blood transfusion or a dose of immunoglobulin. Susceptible women given anti-D immunoglobulin, however, may be vaccinated and seroconversion tested up to 8 weeks later.

Two vaccination policies have been applied. The first is to selectively vaccinate women of child-bearing age in order to protect future pregnancies. This strategy limits the use of the vaccine to subjects at risk, and allows the virus to circulate among the population. The second approach is universal childhood vaccination. This strategy rapidly reduces transmission of the virus and thus the risk of an epidemic, and theoretically will lead in the long term to eradication of the wild virus.

Universal childhood vaccination was introduced in the USA in 1969. The RA 27/3 strain vaccine has been used since 1979. The policy appears to have been effective and was susequently introduced in the UK in 1988 by offering measles–mumps–rubella (MMR) vaccination to preschool children of both sexes. Similar

programmes were introduced in Sweden, Finland, and
Norway in the early 1980s. It should be emphasized
that while multiparous women are less likely to be susceptible than primiparas, those who are susceptible are
more likely to be exposed to young children with
rubella. Nearly 60% of infected pregnant women are
multiparous. Vaccination of such seronegative women
in the immediate postpartum period, including those
who breast-feed, would alone reduce by 50% the present number of recorded cases.

Pregnancy is an absolute contraindication for the
administration of rubella (or any other live) vaccine.
Vaccinated women of child-bearing age should be
warned not to become pregnant for 1 month. However,
nearly 500 susceptible women have inadvertently been
vaccinated either within 3 months of conception or during pregnancy and elected to continue the pregnancy.
Of 372 infants tested, 9 (2.4%) had evidence of fetal
infection, but none had abnormalities compatible with
congenital rubella. Although the observed risk of congenital defects was zero, the maximal estimated theoretical risk of rubella-induced major malformation for
women inadvertently vaccinated around conception or
in early pregnancy is 1.2%. Since this figure is lower
than the 2–3% rate of major birth defects in any pregnancy, abortion is not recommended and patients
should be reassured.

Prenatal[105–107,112,116–118]

An evaluation for fetal rubella should be considered
after either exposure to rubella or a rubella-like disease
or the development of a rubella-like rash. Several questions must first be addressed. First, is there serologic
evidence of maternal rubella (either a significant rising
IgG titer or positve IgM)?[125] If yes, what was the precise gestation at exposure? The latter is essential if the
patient is to be counseled accurately (**Table 5**).

The first serum sample should be collected as soon
as possible. After an exposure, the second serum is
collected either 2 weeks later if the first serum HIA
titer was >20, or 4 weeks later if the first titer was
<10. Should a maternal rash trigger the referral, the
second serum sample is collected 2 weeks after the
appearance of the rash. *It is important that both specimens be tested by the same laboratory in parallel.*
When a brief exposure occurs in a child-care setting
for a woman whose immunity is either non-existent or
unknown, it is essential that any repeat exposure be
avoided until the result of the first serology is known.
Seronegative women should be tested 4 weeks after the
last contact.

The administration of normal human immunoglobulin or high-titer rubella immunoglobulin (two doses of
15–30 ml) within 2–3 days of exposure has been suggested by some, but it does not prevent fetal infection.

There are at least three instances where knowledge
of rubella-specific IgM status might prove beneficial.
The first is in the case of a rubella contact where the
first serum (S1) was collected 10–14 days after
exposure and returned positive. If an earlier specimen
is available, it can be tested in parallel with the S1
obtained after the known contact. Otherwise, IgM testing is necessary. The second instance is where a significant rise in rubella antibodies is discovered without
the appearance of the exanthem. The third is in the
case of a rubella-like illness where the patient attends
the clinic 5 or more days after the onset of the rash
and where the HIA rubella antibody titers may have
reached maximum levels. Seropositive (>40 HIA) patients with no rubella specific IgM may be reassured
that they were immune at the time of contact.

Cordocentesis

Considering the fact that reliable prenatal diagnosis
requires relatively late testing, even when maternal
infection occurs early in pregnancy, which patients
should be offered cordocentesis? Daffos[126] tested 119
fetuses after an episode of rubella during the first 18
weeks; 54 seroconverted before 12 weeks. Only 31 of
the 54 fetuses (57%) were serologically positive.
Others have observed a higher percentage of fetal damage.[106] In light of the long wait before fetal blood testing may be accurately accomplished, termination of
pregnancy should be considered without prenatal diagnosis when seroconversion occurs in the first 12 weeks
of gestation.[117] Following this line of reasoning,
cordocentesis would be offered to women who either
decline termination, who seroconvert between 12 and
18 weeks gestation, or who become reinfected during
the first 12 weeks of gestation. If the fetus is infected,
ear and/or eye damage cannot be ruled out with ultrasonography and termination of the pregnancy should
be considered.

PARVOVIRUS B19

Human parvovirus B19 was discovered in 1975 by
Cossart.[127] Since 1980, its pathogenicity and association with many clinical syndromes have been documented.[128–130] Its adverse effect on pregnancy outcome
was first recognized in 1984[131] and the first prenatal
diagnosis was made in 1987 by Naides and Weiner.[132]
Since that time, several reports have confirmed the
pathogenicity of this virus in the human fetus.

B19 belongs to the family Parvoviridae.[129] It is a
small (20–25 nm), non-enveloped, single-stranded
DNA virus. B19 is an autonomous parvovirus (it replicates without 'help' from another virus), infecting only
humans usually via aerosolized droplets. B19 replicates
in the nucleus during the S-phase of active DNA syn-

thesis.[133] Viral replication is restricted to actively dividing cells and the preferential site of replication is erythroid progenitors – either burst-forming unit-erythroid (BFU-E) or colony-forming unit-erythroid (CFU-E).

Incidence

B19 seroprevalence is age-related; about 50% of women of child-bearing age are immune.[134,135] The incidence of a recent infection as determined by the presence of B19 IgM is about 1% of unselected pregnancies in the USA, though there is reason to believe pregnancy may blunt or slow seroconversion. The rate of secondary transmission for school teachers and day-care personnel exposed at work during an epidemic is 20%. The risk of a fetal loss is now estimated to be 1% (estimated risk of susceptibility = 0.5 × rate of secondary transmission = 0.2 × rate of fetal death = 0.1). For the patient exposed in the household to an infected child, the rate of secondary transmission becomes 50% and the calculated risk of fetal death 2.5%. Further studies are needed to determine the true prevalence of this infection in pregnancy.

Clinical Syndromes and Risks[129,130,136,137]

Maternal

Maternal parvovirus infection is detailed in Chapter 30. Briefly, the characteristic B19 infection is *erythema infectiosum* (EI) (fifth disease), which affects children between 4 and 10 years; 25% of adult infections are asymptomatic. Other B19 sydromes include: transient aplastic crisis (TAC), which occurs in patients with either sickle cell disease or chronic hemolytic anemia, thrombocytopenia and severe prolonged anemia due to persistent infection in immunocompromised patients.

The viremia develops 7–8 days postinoculation and has usually ended by the time the rash appears. The contagious period lasts from inoculation to until the rash erupts, and is increased during the 1–4 days of mild fever and myalgias which precede the rash in up to 60% of patients. In adults, and especially women, acute symmetrical peripheral polyarthralgia, which resolves within 2 weeks, may occur in up to 50% of cases. *TAC and chronic B19 infection in immunosuppressed patients are particularly contagious for health care workers.*

Fetal

Fetal infection is explained by the appreciable duration of viremia in the infected pregnant woman. Fetal death may occur in the first, second or third trimester of gestation after symptomatic or asymptomatic parvovirus infection in the mother. A recent prospective study found 30 adverse fetal outcomes in 186 pregnant women with serologically confirmed B19 primary infection.[135] The transplacental transmission rate was estimated to be 33%. Extrapolating from this study, the overall fetal loss due to intrauterine B19 infection is 9–10% with the highest fetal risk probably in the first 18 weeks of pregnancy. The actual transmission rates of the virus to the conceptus and fetal susceptibility with gestational age are unknown.

The effect of B19 infection on the fetus ranges from no effect to growth deficiency to chronic hepatitis with the development of isolated ascites to non-immune hydrops fetalis. Non-immune hydrops can result from either aplastic anemia with high-output cardiac failure or from viral myocarditis.[131,132,138,139] Meconium peritonitis associated with fetal B19 infection has also been reported.[140] *After delivery, these children continue to shed virus for a variably duration.*[141] *It is important that they be isolated from other newborns and health care workers at risk.*

Pathophysiology of fetal infection[133,136]

B19 infects dividing cells. In early pregnancy, most fetal cells are rapidly dividing, which likely accounts for the varied cytopathic effect. It may also account for structural abnormalities. One neonate had a shortened limb and another an ocular abnormality. However, there is inadequate information upon which to conclude that B19 is or is not teratogenic.[142] After the differentiation of most fetal tissues is complete and the development of hepatic hematopoiesis in the second trimester of pregnancy, B19 most commonly infects erythroid cells with a lytic cell cycle in 72 h. The resulting aplastic anemia may lead to hydrops or be self-limited. Transplacental passage of specific maternal IgG and the development of the immune system of the fetus may aid recovery and result in the term delivery of a normal infant, in whom the presence of B19 IgM in cord blood or persistent B19 IgG through the first year of life are the only markers of *in utero* infection. However, the long-term effect of fetal B19 infection is unknown and is likely to be variable.

Diagnosis

The diagnosis of a viral infection is made either by the direct detection of the virus or its protein components, or serologic evidence of infection. The diagnostic tests for B19 infection are not widely available. Difficulty growing the virus *in vitro* has hampered the production of diagnostic reagents. In the near future, recombinant or synthetic B19 antigen should make serological assays more available for routine diagnosis. In each country, diagnostic samples must be tested in a Reference Laboratory.

B19 serology[143,144]

Specific antibodies to B19 virus are detectable using an antibody capture enzyme-linked immunosorbent assay (ELISA) or radioimmune assay (RIA). B19 IgM directed against structural viral protein of the capsid (VP1 and VP2) appears >14 days after inoculation and is present for 3–4 months. The presence of IgM confirms recent primary infection, though its absence in the fetus does not preclude the possibility. B19 IgG directed against VP1 and VP2 appears during the third week and persists life-long, conferring immunity.

Detection of viral particles or its components

Conventional cell culture methods cannot be used for B19 virus. Techniques for identifying B19 virus in clinical samples usually focus on B19 antigen detection and nucleic acid detection by:[145]

- counter-immunoelectrophoresis (CIE) – rapid but insensitive

- RIAs to detect B19 antigens (viral protein VP1 and VP2) with monoclonal antibodies.

The RIAs are far more sensitive than CIE. However. co-existing specific antibodies in serum or tissue samples, or formalin fixation of tissue sampling, may block the reaction and render the antigen undetectable.

B19 nucleic acid can be detected using 'dot blot' or *in situ* hybridization with cloned B19-DNA digoxigenin-labeled probes.[146–151] *In situ* DNA hybridization may also be used on routine paraffin sections. Recently, PCR with specific primers has been used to detect the presence of B19 in samples of amniotic fluid and fetal blood. PCR is rapid, specific and sensitive, capable of detecting as little as 1 fg of viral DNA. Appropriate controls are essential.

Electron microscopy (EM) is a valuable tool for the detection of virus in fetal serum because B19 viremia is intense.[145,152,153] A modification, immune EM, concentrates a great number of viral particles by agglutination with specific serum and improves the detection sensitivity. However, this technique cannot be used on formalin-fixed tissue.

Light microscopic examination of autopsy material reveals diffuse erythroblastosis within vessels of the fetal liver and in the placenta. Many erythroblasts contain the typical central eosinophilic intranuclear inclusion with peripheral chromatin condensation. This sign is a good marker for B19 infection.[152]

Management Options[131,132,138,154–169]

Prenatal

Two circumstances must be considered:

- the pregnant woman who is exposed to B19 infection

- the pregnant woman who develops an illness suggestive of B19 infection.

Such women should be tested for B19 antibodies. Those who are IgG-positive but IgM-negative were infected at least 3 months earlier and are at little risk for fetal B19 infection.

Women with IgM antibodies have recently been infected. The adverse fetal effects may manifest 4–12 weeks after maternal infection. The possibility of fetal infection is monitored by weekly ultrasonography to search for excess amniotic fluid, scalp edema, ascites, pleural effusion, hepatomegaly and echogenic placentomegaly. Maternal serum AFP levels have on occasion been reported to be elevated prior to the onset of hydrops.[131] If abnormal ultrasonographic signs appear, a cordocentesis is indicated to clarify the diagnosis. Since an infected fetus may have negative IgM serology, the diagnosis must be made in fetal blood by B19 antigen or nucleic acid detection and/or B19 virus detection by electron microscopy. A simple test suggestive of infection is the demonstration of eosinophilic inclusions and marginated chromatin in erythroid cells by light microscopy. If the fetus is hydropic with severe aplastic anemia intrauterine blood transfusion is recommended to assist the fetus until the natural recovery begins. Fetuses who show reticulocytes on their peripheral smear have *already begun* to recover and are less likely to benefit from transfusion.

Women susceptible to B19 parvovirus infection (IgG- and IgM-negative) should be advised of routine hygienic practices for control of respiratory secretions (handwashing, disposal of facial tissues containing secretions) which lessen the risk of infection. Intravenous injection of normal immunoglobulin-containing neutralizing antibodies against VP of the B19 capsid is effective in the treatment of persistent B19 infection in immunocompromised patients and may be of value for the prevention of infection after exposure. Fetal ultrasonography is advised. If fetal ascites or hydrops is the sole symptom of the disease and maternal B19 IgM has already disappeared, the etiologic evaluation will be of a non-immune hydrops: chromosomic analysis, virologic assessment for other agents, and analysis for metabolic or hematologic disease (see Chapter 45).

Conclusions[170,171]

Parvovirus B19 infection is not thought to be a significant public health problem and there is no consensus on what constitutes effective management. Prenatal screening is unnecessary except for health care workers who care for patients with hematological and immune disorders.

Pregnant women who are exposed to infected children at work (teachers, daycare workers) or at home are at increased risk of infection with B19. However, a routine policy of exclusion from the workplace when *erythema infectiosum* is present is not recommended because it does not eliminate the risk of infection. Children with EI may attend school or daycare because they are no longer contagious after the rash appears. Patients with TAC are highly infectious and pose a significant risk of transmission to health care workers. It has been recommended that these patients, as well as immunosuppressed patients with chronic red-cell aplasia, should be cared for in contact isolation (including use of gowns and gloves) for the duration of their illness and that pregnant health care workers should not care for them, unless they are immune to B19.

HIV

Human immune deficiency virus is a worldwide problem affecting homosexual, heterosexual, fetus and newborn alike. There are several human immunodeficiency viruses of which type I is the most common. Infection with this DNA retrovirus results in a systemic, degenerative and, ultimately, fatal disease affecting the immune and central nervous systems. The pathognomonic finding is the selective depletion of the $CD4^+$ helper T lymphocytes. The origin of the virus is in dispute. The first cases were recognized in 1976.

Incidence

HIV is a sexually transmitted disease. Women are more likely to contract it than men. The risk factors for HIV are similar to other sexually transmitted diseases – multiple sex partners, sex practices associated with

mucosal tears, poor hygiene (includes parenteral drug abuse), etc. The true incidence is unknown and published statistics are likely to be a gross underestimate.[172] In the inner city, it is on the increase. Approximately 2.5 per 1000 women attending prenatal clinics in Edinburgh and inner London have positive HIV serology (most associated with intravenous drug abuse).[173,174] In neonatal serosurveys conducted in inner London, there has been an increase in the HIV prevalence from 1:2000 in 1988 to 1:500 in 1991. Outside London, the seroprevalence is stable at 1:16 000.[175] In the USA, 1.5 per 1000 women are seropositive at delivery. But, as in most countries, there are marked regional, ethnic and social class differences reflecting sex and drug habits.

Perinatal transmission accounts for over 80% of all cases of AIDS in infants less than 1 year of age. The incidence of intrauterine infection has been reported to range from a low of 13%[176] to a high of 33%.[177] The risk of transmission to the fetus may reflect the stage of maternal disease, since the magnitude of the maternal viremia is greatest during the initial stages and with preterminal disease.

Clinical Presentation and Risks

Maternal

Maternal HIV infection is detailed in Chapter 29. Briefly, the course of HIV infection in the asymptomatic woman appears unaffected by pregnancy. However, women with advanced disease may be at increased risk of severe, opportunistic infections, the most common being *Pneumocystis carinii* pneumonia.[178,179]

Fetal

The mechanisms by which HIV might reach the fetus have recently been reviewed.[180] There is no specific fetal syndrome known to be associated with the HIV virus, but this, too, may be a function of the time during gestation infection occurs. There is no added risk of malformation. Theoretic fetal risks from maternal drug therapy with ziduvodine (AZT) include growth deficiency and anemia.[181] It is unclear whether women taking zidovudine have a lower risk of vertical transmission.[182]

Neonatal

The diagnosis of HIV in the neonate is complicated by the presence of maternal antibodies. However, the application of PCR to amplify viral DNA promises earlier diagnosis.[183] The incidences of prematurity and low birthweight are increased in women who continue to abuse drugs during pregnancy.[184] Whether fetal infection increases this risk is unclear. When there is a safe alternative, breast-feeding should be avoided, since there is a risk of infection.[185] *Cesarean delivery does not reduce the incidence of neonatal disease.* The course of disease in the infected newborn tends to be quite rapid compared with the adult.

Diagnosis

General

The laboratory method of choice in the clinical environment is an ELISA (enzyme-linked immunosorbent assays or antigen-capture sandwich assays). A positive HIV ELISA test must be confirmed with Western blot test. Measurement of p24 antigenemia is available. Unfortunately, the measurement of viral antigen may not correlate well with the state of viral infection, i.e. infected cells may have a low expression of viral antigen. The measurement of viral nucleic acids using PCR may provide a more accurate measure of the extent of infection. An assay for the effect of the retrovirus on an appropriate target cell/animal/virus specific product is available, but it is slow, expensive and relatively insensitive. Laboratory diagnosis in the newborn or infant can present some difficulty, since all children have maternal antibodies which may last up to 15 months after delivery.[186] In the newborn a combination of diagnostic tests is now used: p24 antigen detection, HIV genomic material detection with PCR, which allows the diagnosis to be accurate from birth to 6 months of age.

Prenatal

HIV has been cultured from fetal tissues obtained at the time of therapeutic abortion. HIV genomic sequences as well as viral-specific antigen have also been demonstrated. Though these findings prove that fetal infection may occur early, the frequency of vertical transmission later in pregnancy is unknown though probably more frequent than early transmission. Thus, even if molecular techniques for identification of the virus prove reliable, neonatal disease may not necessarily be excluded by testing early in gestation. *The demonstration of maternal antibody in the fetus by Western blot analysis is of no diagnostic value.*

The prenatal diagnosis of congenital HIV presents technical and ethical problems. First, not all laboratories are equally qualified to perform these tests. They should be done only by laboratories experienced with the range of diagnostic methods to minimize the risk of a false-negative or false-positive result. Controversy exists over the safety and utility of cordocentesis for the diagnosis of HIV. The time of vertical transmission in pregnancy is not known. The major concern is the risk of infecting an uninfected fetus as the needle passes through virus-containing tissue. HIV infection is lethal and some have suggested that cordocentesis be limited to women about to undergo pregnancy termination. Yet, the weight of evidence seems to favor prenatal diagnosis. Cordocentesis entails the same risk of virus transmission for other congenitally acquired active infections, and *there is no evidence it increases the fetal risk of toxoplasmosis and CMV.* Since most neonates of HIV-infected women are themselves not infected, negative prenatal studies might persuade a patient against an undesired pregnancy termination. The opposite would also be true. Finally, the application of future antiviral therapies which either treat or reduce vertical transmission will be best served by prenatal diagnosis.

Management Options

Prenatal

The management of maternal HIV is detailed in Chapter 30. Briefly, numerous studies have demonstrated the futility of relying on patient questionnaires to determine the risk of infection in a high prevalence area.[175] All women attending prenatal clinics in a high-risk area (e.g. the inner city) should be screened for HIV; in low risk areas, only those patients with known or acknowledged risk factors are currently tested and all pregnant women who give consent are tested. Infected women are given the option of pregnancy termination if at a stage in gestation where it is legal in that locale. Other sexually transmitted diseases should be routinely sought. It is important that infected women are monitored closely for evidence of disease progression, such as an opportunistic infection or weight loss. Should the $CD4^+$ count fall below 300 mm^3, the administration of zidovudine (AZT), an inhibitor of the viral reverse transcriptase, is a reasonable option; if it falls below 200 mm^3, prophylaxis against *Pneumocystis carinii* with pentamidine or sulfamethoxazole and trimethaprim is indicated.[187] *Pregnancy is not a contraindication to antiretroviral therapy for those patients with advanced HIV infection.*

Labor/delivery

The fetus is managed as if uninfected. Scalp blood sampling and electrodes are to be avoided. After delivery, the infant's skin should be cleansed of all maternal secretions before being punctured by a needle.

Postnatal

The prevention of the horizontal spread of the disease is primary. Breast-feeding should be avoided in locales where a safe, alternative form of nutrition is available. Mothers must be comprehensively educated on techniques to minimize the risk of transmission, e.g. prevent exposure to maternal secretions. There is no evidence that household contact leads to infection and mother–child interaction is specifically encouraged.

Neonatal

All children have maternal antibodies which may last up to 15 months after delivery. Most infected children develop symptoms within the first 2 years of life. Bacterial infections, chronic parotitis, fevers, lymphadenopathy, hepatosplenomegaly, chronic or recurrent diarrhea, failure to thrive, and recurrent or persistent candidiases are all common clinical events.

LISTERIA MONOCYTOGENES

Listeria monocytogenes is a small, Gram-positive, non-spore-forming bacillus widely distributed in nature.

Incidence

The sources of human infection are poorly understood. Food-borne outbreaks have been traced to dairy products such as soft cheeses and ice cream, raw vegetables and shellfish. Asymptomatic vaginal or fecal carriage may be responsible for sporadic cases. Pregnancy-related cases comprise approximately 25% of the total incidence.[188] In England, Northern Ireland and Wales, the number of reported cases increased dramatically between 1965 and 1988 (50 cases in 1965–77; 291 cases in 1988, 93 of which were perinatal), but then decreased sharply in 1989 after government health warnings. The incidence since then, including the first 6 months of 1992, has been similar to that before the 1987 rise.

Clinical Presentation and Risks

Maternal

In the otherwise healthy adult, *Listeria* infection is either asymptomatic or manifests as a non-specific influenza-like illness. In contrast, most infected pregnant women present with fever, preterm labor and brown-stained amniotic fluid. *Listeria* can cause a fatal septicemia in immunocompromised women.

Fetal

Fetal infection follows hematogenous spread of the bacillus early in pregnancy and may end in miscarriage. Later in pregnancy, septicemia causes multi-organ morbidity, e.g. intraventricular hemorrhage, pneumonia, hepatitis, neurological handicap and death. The fetal mortality may exceed 75%.[189]

Neonatal

Neonatal disease may either manifest early (within 2 days of birth) or late. Early disease results from transplacental spread, whereas late-onset disease is thought to result from infection acquired during delivery. Neonates with early-onset disease are typically premature, appropriately grown, and have evidence of congenital pneumonia. In late-onset disease, meningitis is the prominent feature.

Diagnosis

Prenatal

Maternal listeriosis should be suspected in any pregnant woman with a flu-like illness associated with pyrexia, uterine irritability and bloody vaginal discharge.[190] Blood, vaginal and amniotic fluid cultures are indicated in the evaluation of such a patient. The demonstration of the organism on Gram-stain provides presumptive evidence adequate to initiate therapy. However, the microbiologist should be informed that listeria is part of the differential diagnosis, since the rod can easily be mistaken for diptheroids and ignored.

Labor/delivery

Fetal biophysical abnormalities are common. A non-reactive fetal heart rate pattern, absence of fetal movement, poor tone, and abnormal umbilical Doppler have each been reported in infected fetuses. Serological tests on maternal or umbilical bloods are unhelpful.

Management Options

The prevention of epidemic disease is best accomplished through maternal education: avoid dairy products made from unpasturized milk and uncooked or undercooked meat and poultry; thoroughly recook, precooked meals; avoid raw vegetables which have been stored cool after preparation (e.g. coleslaw) and paté.

There have been no controlled trials of therapy and

all series reported have been small. The current consensus favors a combination of long-term ampicillin and gentamicin or tobramycin.*[191] In the absence of fetal infection, gentamicin should perhaps be avoided initially because of potential fetal ototoxicity. Other reported successful agents are intravenous chloramphenicol** and co-trimoxazole. Treatment failures have occurred when cephalosporins and penicillins were used alone. The drugs are given for 3–6 weeks (especially in neonates), since recurrences have been reported after 2 week courses.

SYPHILIS

Syphilis is a chronic, debilitating infectious disorder characterized by infrequent but severe exacerbations caused by the spirochete *Treponema pallidum*. *Treponema pallidum* is morphologically indistinguishable from the other treponemes that cause non-venereal human diseases such as pinta, yaws and bejel (endemic syphilis).

Incidence

Syphilis has been on the increase worldwide in areas with large numbers of HIV infected women. In the USA, the urban Hispanic and Black heterosexual populations have also experienced an acute increase. The result of this re-emergence has been an increase in congenital syphilis typically in young, non-White, poor, single, inner-city dwellers with inadequate prenatal care. Of 437 infants with congenital syphilis born in the USA between 1983 and 1985, only 48% had any prenatal care. For those who did receive prenatal care, it began on average at 22 weeks gestation.[192]

Clinical Presentation and Risks

Maternal

Maternal syphilis is detailed in Chapter 30. Briefly, syphilis is transmitted efficiently during sexual intercourse. Sixty percent of partners acquire the infection through microscopic mucosal tears after a single encounter.

The manifestations of syphilis are wide-ranging, potentially affecting nearly every organ system. Pregnancy has little impact on the natural course of the

disease. With an intact immune system, some 60% remain in the latent phase (i.e. lack clinical manifestations). The maternal presentation (and risk) is dependent on whether the infection is primary (chancre, lasting 3–6 weeks with associated lymphadenopathy when untreated), secondary (characterized by dissemination – skin rash, condylomata lata, hepatitis, nephritis, CNS involvement: one-third of cases), or tertiary (granulomatous gummas of skin, bone and viscera, which is uncommon in women of reproductive age).

Fetal

Treponema pallidum crosses the placenta and infection may occur at any time,[193] though some believe the fetus is not at risk until immunocompetence develops (at approximately 18 weeks).[194] Manifestations include anemia, hydrops, growth deficiency, and systemic infection characterized by pneumonitis, myocarditis, nephrosis, osteochondritis, periosteitis, lymphadenopathy and death. Congenital infection approaches 90% with primary or secondary disease; 50% of fetuses are symptomatic while the remainder develop neonatal infection, or early latent syphilis (<1 year duration, 40%). These rates reflect the extent of maternal spirochaetemia. *Though the risk is lower, it should not be forgotten that congenital infection does occur with late latent infection (6–14%).*

Diagnosis

Maternal

The diagnosis can be difficult and is generally made on the basis of the history, physical examination and the result of dark-field microscopy, serology, CSF examination and/or chest x-ray. Dark-field microscopic imaging of the spirochaete in a specimen scraped from a primary or secondary lesion is accurate, rapid and inexpensive. However, a negative test does not preclude the possibility of infection.

Serological testing is the usual method to confirm infection but may not be positive until 3–5 weeks after inoculation (2 weeks after the chancre appears). They are either non-specific or specific for syphilis:[195]

Non-specific tests

Non-specific tests such as the Venereal Disease Research Laboratory (VDRL) or the rapid plasma reagin (RPR) tests are used for both screening and monitoring treatment, since the titer generally reflects the degree of infection. The titer is highest with secondary infection and lowest with latent infection. They

---

* Long-term for ampicillin: 4-6 g/day in four equal doses, i.v. for the first 2 days and 3 g per os for 14–21 days. Only 2 or 3 days for gentamycin (3 mg/kg/day).
** Chloramphenicol: caution with gray syndrome (cardiovascular collapse) in baby if mother treated at final stage of pregnancy.

are reactive in 75% of patients with primary disease and in virtually 100% of those with secondary syphilis. The major cause of a false-negative test is HIV infection.

The diagnosis should never be made on the basis of a non-specific test. The VRDL is negative in up to 50% of infected patients. A false-positive result (FPR) may occur because of (1) technical errors, (2) other treponemal infections (e.g. Yaws, a tropical treponemal disease) or (3) acute or chronic biological conditions. Acute conditions include postviral infections (measles, chicken pox, mumps, herpes simplex) or immunizations (typhoid, yellow fever) and can result in a false-positive result at a few weeks up to 6 months. Chronic conditions include autoimmune disease or more commonly intravenous drug abuse. A false-positive result can last for years and even a lifetime.[193] *Pregnancy is not an explanation for a false-positive result.*

Specific tests

Specific treponemal antigen serological tests include the fluorescent treponemal antibody (FTA) and the *Treponema pallidum* hemagglutination assay for antibodies (TPHA). These tests confirm a positive non-specific test and permit treponemal and non-treponemal disease to be distinguished. However, lifelong seropositivity despite adequate treatment means they cannot be used to monitor disease or differentiate between primary and recurrent infection.

The FTA is the first serological test to become positive (usually 3–4 weeks after infection). It is positive in 80–90% of cases of primary infection. The TPHA is the last to turn positive. Though almost 100% of patients with secondary syphilis are positive, only 60% of those with primary disease are positive. The CSF should be tested for cell count, total protein, TPHA, FTA and VDRL to exclude the diagnosis of neurosyphilis in a patient suspected of latent disease, or at follow-up in order to determine cure. The FTA and TPHA tests, if positive, do not necessarily mean active disease, but virtually rule out neurosyphilis if negative. In the UK, routine prenatal serological screening, with repeat testing at 28 weeks and at delivery in the high-risk population, has proven very effective.

Fetal

In general, infection during the first or second trimester places the fetus at significant risk. The detection of either hydramnios, placentomegaly hepatomegaly and/or hydrops fetalis in a woman with syphilis is presumptive evidence of fetal infection. Amniocentesis and cordocentesis are employed for confirmatory studies. Third-trimester fetal infection is generally symptomatic.

IgG-based testing is of no value. The presence of FTA IgM should be sought, though its absence does not exclude disease. More recently, an IgM antibody specific for *Treponema pallidum* wall antigen (anti-47-kDa) has been used.[196] Non-specific evidence of systemic disease would include thrombocytopenia, neutropenia and elevated liver enzymes.

Neonatal

Any neonate of a mother infected at some stage of pregnancy is suspect. Pertinent history or clinical findings include preterm delivery, systemic signs (hepatosplenomegaly, anemia, jaundice, skin rash, joint swellings, metaphyseal dystrophy), face and mouth abnormalities (e.g. rhagades, Hutchison's incisors). A long bone radiologic survey is made to search for osteochondritis or periosteitis. *Dark-field microscopy, serology VDRL and TPHA should be performed at birth and then repeated at 6 and 12 weeks to detect a rising titer.* Measurement of FTA IgM has been used to separate passive transfer from true congenital infection, but both false-positive and false-negative results occur. A CSF study is recommended. Untreated congenital syphilis may progress to a late phase characterized by Hutchinson teeth, mulberry molars, deafness, saddle nose, saber shins, mental retardation, hydrocephalus, general paresis and optic nerve atrophy.

Management Options

Maternal

The treatment of maternal syphilis is detailed in Chapter 51. Penicillin is the drug of choice – either procaine or, more pragmatically, benzathine.[197] The dose for early syphilis (primary, secondary or latent of less than 1 year's duration) during pregnancy is 2.4 million units benzathine penicillin G given intramuscularly at one session. For syphilis of more than 1 year's duration (latent disease, cardiovascular or late benign neurosyphilis), except neurosyphilis, 2.4 million units of benzathine penicillin G are adminstered weekly for 3 weeks (total 7.2 million units).

In the third trimester, penicillin is less effective treating fetal infection, and the neonate may still be infected. Non-penicillin regimes should be avoided whenever possible. Erythromycin does not cross the placenta well and tetracycline has untoward fetal effects *early* in gestation. Late in gestation, however, tetracycline may be an acceptable alternative. A Jarisch-Herxheimer reaction resulting from the release of prostanoids and beginning within 2–8 h of the injection is common with the treatment of primary (approaching 100%) and secondary (60%) syphilis. Fever is associ-

---

FETAL INFECTION
Summary of Management Options
(see also Chapters 29 and 30)

General approach

Presentation by abnormal ultrasound examination

(no maternal history of infection)

• See **Figure 1**

Presentation by maternal history of infection

• Document whether infection has genuinely occurred during pregnancy by serological testing (primary or reactivation)

• In cases of sexually transmitted diseases, arrange contact tracing

• When diagnosis confirmed, counsel about risks

• Consider whether maternal therapy is relevant or of proven benefit (after consideration of fetal diagnosis)

• Consider fetal diagnosis if appropriate for further management (e.g. maternal therapy, termination of pregnancy, novel fetal therapy)

• Careful pediatric assessment and investigation after birth

---

ated with decreased fetal movement, premature labor and fetal death.[198]

Fetal

Prenatal diagnostic evaluation depends upon presentation. Fetuses whose mothers are known to be infected and who present with hydramnios, placentomegaly and/or hydrops are presumptively infected. No further workup is necessary and prolonged, aggressive antibiotic treatment should be initiated. In contrast, if the presentation is hydrops and there is no maternal history, a full workup for hydrops including cordocentesis is indicated (see Chapter 45). The cause of syphilitic hydrops is not known, but may be myocarditis. The drug of choice is high-dose aqueous penicillin. Should hydrops be detected after 32 weeks, delivery with postnatal treatment is a consideration, but the mortality rate is high.

Neonatal

The drug of choice is penicillin. If the mother was treated appropriately before 20 weeks gestation, there is virtually no risk of congenital infection except by reinfection. Infant follow-up by examination and serology at 3 and 6 months for primary syphilis, and again at 12 months for secondary syphilis, is important.

REFERENCES

1   Remington JS, Desmonts G (1990) Toxoplasmosis. In Remington JS, Klein JO (eds), *Infectious Diseases of the Fetus and Newborn Infant*, pp. 89–195. London: W.B. Saunders.
2   Jeannel D, Niel G, Costagliola D *et al.* (1988) Epidemiology of toxoplasmosis among pregnant women in the Paris area. *International Journal of Epidemiology* **17**:595–602.

3 Editorial (1990) Antenatal screening for toxoplasmosis in the UK. *Lancet* **336**:346–348.

4 Desmonts G, Couvreur J (1974) Congenital toxoplasmosis: A prospective study of 378 pregnancies. *New England Journal of Medicine* **290**:1110–1116.

5 Wilson CB, Remington JS, Stagno S *et al.* (1980) Development of adverse sequelae in children born with subclinical congenital *Toxoplasma* infection. *Pediatrics* **66**:767–774.

6 Desmonts G, Couvreur J (1984) Toxoplasmose congenitale: Etude prospective de l'issue de la grossesse chez 542 femmes atteintes de toxoplasmose acquise en cours de grossesse. *Annales de Pédiatrie* **31**:805–809.

7 Couvreur J, Desmonts G, Aron-Rosa D 91985) Le pronostic oculaire de la toxoplsmose congenitale: Role du traitement. *Semaine des Hôpitaux de Paris* **61**:1734–1737.

8 Couvreur J, Desmonts G, Tournier G *et al.* (1985) Etude d'une serie homogene de 210 cas de toxoplasmose congenitale chez des nourrissons ages de 0 a 11 mois et depistes de facon prospective. *Semaine des Hôpitaux de Paris* **61**:3015–3019.

9 Daffos F, Forestier F, Capella-Pavlovsky M *et al.* (1988) Prenatal management of 746 pregnancies at risk for congenital toxoplasmosis. *New England Journal of Medicine* **318**:271–275.

10 Desmonts G, Couvreur J, Thulliez P (1990) Toxoplasmose congenitale: Cinq cas de transmission à l'enfant d'une infection maternelle anterieure à la grossesse. *Presse Médicale* **19**:1445–1449.

11 Koppe JG, Loewer-Sieger DH, DeRoever-Bonnet H (1986) Results of 20-year follow-up of congenital toxoplasmosis. *Lancet* **i**:254–256.

12 Desmonts G, Couvreur J, Thulliez P *et al.* (1985) Serodiagnostic de la toxoplasmose acquise: Des methodes simples pour des questions précises. *Le Concours Medical* **107**:227–234.

13 Dannemann BR, Vaughan WC, Thulliez P *et al.* (1990) Defferential agglutination test for diagnosis of recently acquired infection with *Toxoplasma gondii*. *Journal of Clinical Microbiology* **28**:1928–1933

14 Decoster A, Caron A, Darcy F *et al.* (1988) IgA antibodies against P30 as markers of congenital and acute toxoplasmosis. *Lancet* **2**:1104–1107.

15 Pinon JM, Poirriez J, Leroux B *et al.* (1986) Diagnostic precoce, surveillance et bilan therapeutique de la toxoplasmose congenitale. Indications des profils immunologiques compares ELIFA. *Revue Internationale de Pédiatrie* **157**:11–16.

16 Derouin F, Thulliez P, Candolfi E *et al.* (1988) Early prenatal diagnosis of congenital toxoplasmosis using amniotic fluid samples and tissue culture. *European Journal of Clinical Microbiology and Infectious Disease* **7**:423–425.

17 Grover CM, Thulliez P, Remington JS *et al* (1990) Rapid prenatal diagnosis of congenital toxoplasma infection by using Polymerase Chain Reaction and amniotic fluid. *Journal of Clinical Microbiology* **28**:2297–2301.

18 Cazenave J, Forestier F, Bessieres MH *et al.* (1992) Contribution of a new PCR assay to the prenatal diagnosis of congenital toxoplasmosis. *Prenatal Diagnosis* **12**:119–127.

19 Desmonts G, Daffos F, Forestier F *et al* (1985) Prenatal diagnosis of congenital toxoplasmosis. *Lancet* **i**:500–504.

20 Foulon W, Naessens A, De Catte L *et al.* (1990) Detection of congenital toxoplasmosis by chorionic villus sampling and early amniocentesis. *American Journal of Obstetrics and Gynecology* **163**:1511–1513.

21 Thulliez P, Marcon P, Daffos F *et al.* (1990) Results of prenatal diagnosis tests in 105 toxoplasma infected fetuses. In *Seventh ICOPA (International Congress of Parasitology)* Paris, August.

22 Hohlfeld P, Mac Aleese J, Capella-Pavlovsky M *et al.* (1991) Fetal toxoplasmosis: Ultrasonographic signs. *Ultrasound in Obstetrics and Gynecology* **1**:241–244.

23 Holliman RE, Johnson JD, Constantine G *et al.* (1991) Difficulties in the diagnosis of congenital toxoplasmosis by cordocentesis: Case report. *British Journal of Obstetrics and Gynaecology* **98**:832–834.

24 Desmonts G (1990) Preventing congenital toxoplasmosis. *Lancet* **336**:1017–1018.

25 Couvreur J, Thulliez P (1989) Devenir des toxoplasmoses congenitales. *Journal de Pediatrie et de Puericulture* **2**:80–88.

26 Hohlfeld P, Daffos F, Thulliez P *et al.* (1989) Fetal toxoplasmosis: Outcome of pregnancy and infant follow-up after *in utero* treatment. *Journal of Pediatrics* **115**:765–769.

27 Forestier F, Daffos F, Rainault M *et al.* (1987) Suivi therapeutique foeto-maternel de la spiramycine en cours de grossesse. *Archives Françaises de Pédiatrie* **44**:539–544.

28 Couvreur J (1987) traitement de la toxoplasmose congenitale. *Le Pediatre* **102**:5–16.

29 Marcon P, Thulliez P (1988) traitement de la toxoplasmose congenitale. *Journal de Pediatrie et de Puericulture* **4**:210–214.

30 Sibley LD, Boothroyd J (1992) Virulent strains of *Toxoplasma gondii* comprise a single clonal lineage. *Nature* **359**:82–85.

31 Capron A, Dessaint JP (1988) Vaccination against parasitic diseases: Some alternative concepts for the definition of protective antigens. *Annales de l'Institut Pasteur Immunologie* **139**:109–117.

32 Darcy F, Torpier G, Cesbron-Delauw MF *et al.* (1989) Antigenes de *Toxoplasma gondii* d'intérêt diagnostique et immunoprophylactique potentiel: Nouvelles strategies d'identification. *Annales de Biologie Clinique* **47**:457.

33 Stagno S (1990) Cytomegalovirus. In Remington JS, Klein JO (eds), *Infectious Diseases of the Fetus and Newborn Infant*, pp. 241–281. London: W.B. Saunders.

34 Merigan TC, Resta S (1990) Cytomegalovirus: Where have we been and where are we going? *Review of Infectious Diseases* **12**:S693–S700 (suppl.7).

35 Stagno S, Pass RF, Dworsky ME *et al.* (1982) Congenital cytomegalovirus infection: The relative importance of primary and recurent maternal infection *New England Journal of Medicine* **306**:945–949.

36 Stagno S, Pass RF, Dworsky ME *et al.* (1982) Maternal cytomegalovirus infection and perinatal transmission. *Clinical Obstetrics and Gynecology* **25**:563–576.

37 Peckham CS, Coleman JC, Hurley R *et al.* (1983) Cytomegalovirus infection in pregnancy: Preliminary findings from a propspective study. *Lancet* **1**:1352–1355.

38 Stagno S, Pass RF, Cloud G *et al.* (1986) Primary cytomegalovirus infection in pegnancy: Incidence, transmission to fetus, and clinical outcome. *Journal of the American Medical Association* **256**1904–1908.

39 Yow MD, Williamson DW, Leeds LJ *et al.* (1988) Epidemiologic characteristics of cytomegalovirus infection in mothers and their infants. *American Journal of Obstetrics and Gynecology* **158**:1189–1195.

40 Ho M (1990) Epidemiology of cytomegalovirus infections. *Review of Infectious Diseases* **12**:S701–S710 (suppl.7).

41 Ahlfors K, Ivarsson SA, Harris S *et al.* (1984) Congenital cytomegalovirus infection and disease in Sweden and the relative importance of primary and secondary maternal infections: Preliminary findings from a prospective study. *Scandinavian Journal of Infectious diseases* **16**:129–137.

42 Griffiths PD, Baboonian C, Rutter D *et al.* (1991) Congenital and maternal cytomegalovirus infections in a London population. *British Journal of Obstetrics and Gynaecology* **98**:135–140.

43 Handsfield HH, Chandler SH, Caine VA *et al.* (1985) Cytomegalovirus infection in sex partners: Evidence for sexual transmission. *Journal of Infectious Diseases* **151**:344–348.

44 Demmler GJ, O'Neil JH *et al.* (1986) Transmission of cytomegalovirus from husband to wife *Journal of Infectious Diseases* **154**:545–546.

45 Pass RF, Little EA, Stagno S *et al.* (1987) Young children as a probably source of maternal and congenital cytomegalovirus infection. *New England Journal of Medicine* **316**:1366–1370.

46 Adler SP (1988) Molecular epidemiology of cytomegalovirus: Viral transmission among children attending a day care center, their parents, and caretakers. *Journal of Pediatrics* **112**:366–372.

47 Yow MD (1989) Congenital cytomegalovirus disease: A now problem. *Journal of Infectious Diseases* **159**:163–167.

48 Pass RF, Hutto C, Ricks R *et al.* (1986) Increased rate of cytomegalovirus infection among parents of children attending day-care centers *New England Journal of Medicine* **314**:1414–1418.

49 Taber LH, Frank AL, Yow MD *et al.* (1985) Acquisition of cytomegaloviral infections in families with young children: A serological study *Journal of Infectious Diseases* **151**:948–952.

50 Adler SP (1986) Molecular epidemiology of cytomegalovirus: Evidence for viral transmission to parents from children infected at a day care center. *Pediatric Infectious Diseases* **5**:315–318.

51 Adler SP, (1989) Cytomegalovirus and child day care. Evidence for an increased infection among day-care workers *New England Journal of Medicine* **321**:1290–1296.

52 Pass RF, Hutto C, Lyon MD *et al.* (1990) Increased rate of cytomegalovirus infection among day care center workers *Pediatric Infectious Disease Journal* **9**:465–470.

53 Murph JR, Baron JC, Brown CK *et al.* (1991) The occupational risk of cytomegalovirus infection among daycare providers. **265**:603–608.

54 Wilfert CM, Huang ES, Stagno S (1982) Restriction endonuclease analysis of cytomegalovirus deoxyribonucleic acid as an epidemiologic tool. *Pediatrics* **70**:717–721.

55 Balfour CL, Balfour HH (1986) Cytomegalovirus is not an occupationsl risk for nurses in renal transplant and neonatal units: Results of a prospective surveillance study. *Journal of the American Medical Association* **256**:1909–1914.

56 Fowler KB, Stagno S, Pass RF *et al.* (1992) The outcome of congenital cytomegalovirus infection in relation to maternal antibody status. *New England Journal of Medicine* **326**:663–667.

57 Ramsay MEB, Miller E, Peckham CS (1991) Outcome of confirmed symptomatic congenital cytomegalovirus infection. *Archives of Diseases in Childhood* **66**:1068–1069.

58 Peckham CS (1989) Cytomegalovirus in the neonate. *Journal of Antimicrobial Chemotherapy* **23**:17–21 (suppl.E).

59 Alford CA, Stagno S, Pass RF *et al.* (1990) Congenital and perinatal cytomegalovirus infections. *Review of Infectious Diseases* **12**:S745–S810 (suppl.7).

60 Hayes K, Danks DM, Gibas H *et al.* (1972) Cytomegalovirus in human milk. *New England Journal of Medicine* **287**:177–178.

61 Stagno S, Reynolds DW, Pass RF *et al.* (1980) Breast milk and the risk of cytomegalovirus infection. *New England Journal of Medicine* **302**:1073–1076.

62 Sandler SG, Grumet FC (1982) Posttransfusion cytomegalovirus infections. *Pediatrics* **69**:650–653.

63 Spector SA, Rua JA, Spector DH *et al.* (1984) Detection of human cytomegalovirus in clinical specimens by DNA–DNA hybridization. *Journal of Infectious Diseases* **150**:121–126.

64 Demmler GJ, Six HR, Hurst SM *et al.* (1986) Enzyme-linked immunosorbent assay for the detection of IgM-class antibodies to cytomegalovirus. *Journal of Infectious Diseases* **153**:1152–1155.

65 Stirk PR, Griffiths PD (1987) Use of monoclonal antibodies for the diagnosis of cytomegalovirus infection by the detection of early antigen fluorescent foci (DEAFF) in cell culture. *Journal of Medical Virology* **21**:329–337.

66 Saltzman RL, Quirk MR, Jordan MC (1988) Disseminated cytonegalovirus infection: Molecular analysis of virus and leukocyte interactions in viremia. *Journal of Clinical Investiagation* **81**:75–81.

67 Griffiths PD (1989) Diagnosis of cytomegalovirus infection. *Journal of Antimicrobial Chemotherapy* **23**:11–16 (suppl.E).

68 Chou S (1990) Newer methods for diagnosis of cytomegalovirus infection. *Review of Infectious Diseases* **12**:S727–S736 (suppl.7)

69 Davis LE, Tweed GV, Chin TDY *et al.* (1971) Intrauterine diagnosis of cytomegalovirus infection: Viral recovery from amniocentesis fluid. *American Journal of Obstetrics and Gynecology* **109**:1217–1219.

70 Yambao TJ, Clark D, Weiner L *et al.* (1981) Isolation of cytomegalovirus from the amniotic fluid during the

third trimester. *American Journal of Obstetrics and Gynecology* **139**:937–938.

71 Huikeshoven FJM, Wallenburg HCS, Jahoda MGJ (1982) Diagnosis of severe fetal cytomegalovirus infection from amniotic fluid in the third trimester of pregnancy. *American Journal of Obstetrics and Gynecology* **142**:1053–1054.

72 Toma P, Magnano GM, Messano P *et al.* (1989) Cerebral ultrasound images in prenatal cytomegalovirus infection. *Neuroradiology* **31**:278–279.

73 Ghidini A, Sirtori M, Vergani P *et al.* (1989) Fetal intracranial calcifications. *American Journal of Obstetrics and Gynecology* **160**:663–664.

74 Meisel RL, Alvarez M, Lynch L *et al.* (1990) Fetal cytomegalovirus infection: A case report *American Journal of Obstetrics and Gynecology* **162**:663–664.

75 Grose C, Weiner CP (1990) Prenatal diagnosis of congenital cytomegalovirus infection: Two decades later. *American Journal of Obstetrics and Gynecology* **163**:447–450.

76 Weiner CP, Grose C (1990) Prenatal diagnosis of congenital cytomegalovirus infection by virus isolation from amniotic fluid. *American Journal of Obstetrics and Gynecology* **163**:1253–1255.

77 Drose JA, Dennis MA, Thickman D (1991) Infection *in utero*: US findings in 19 cases. *Radiology* **178**:369–374.

78 Lynch L, Daffos F, Emanuel D *et al.* (1991) Prenatal diagnosis of fetal cytomegalovirus infection *Obstetrics and Gynecology* **165**:714–718.

79 Hohfeld P, Vial Y, Maillard-Brignon C *et al.* (1991) Cytomegalovirus fetal infection: Prenatal diagnosis. *Obstetrics and Gynecology* **78**:615–618.

80 Pletcher BA, Williams MK, Mulivor RA *et al.* (1991) Intrauterine cytomegalovirus infection presenting as fetal meconium peritonitis. *Obstetrics and Gynecology* **78**:903–905.

81 Lamy ME, Mulongo KN, Gadisseux JF *et al.* (1992) Prenatal diagnosis of fetal cytomegalovirus infection. *American Journal of Obstetrics and Gynecology* **166**:91–94.

82 Brayman KL, Dafoe DC, Smythe WR *et al.* (1988) Prophylaxis of serious cytomegalovirus infection in renal transplant candidates using live khuman cytomegalovirus vaccine: Interim results of a randomized controlled trial. *Archives of Surgery* **123**:1502–1508.

83 Jeffries DJ (1989) The spectrum of cytomegalovirus infection and its management. *Journal of Antimicrobial Chemotherapy* **23**:1–10 (suppl.E).

84 Morris DJ (1990) Prevention of congenital cytomegalovirus disease *Journal of Infectious Diseases* **161**:149.

85 Porath A, McNutt RA, Smiley LM *et al.* (1990) Effectiveness and cost benefit of a proposed live cytomegalovirus vaccine in the prevention of congenital disease. *Review of Infectious Diseases* **12**:31–40.

86 Plotkin SA, Starr SE, Friedman HM *et al.* (1990) Vaccines for the prevention of human cytomegalovirus infection. *Review of Infectious Diseases* **12**:S827–S838 (suppl.7).

87 Balfour HH (1990) Management of cytomegalovirus disease with antiviral durgs. *Review of Infectious Diseases* **12**:S849–S860 (suppl.7).

88 Tookey P, Peckham CS (1991) Does cytomegalovirus

present an occupations risk? *Archives of Diseases in Childhood* **66**:1009–1010.

89 Meyers JD (1991) Prevention and treatment of cytomegalovirus infection. *Annual Reviews in Medicine* **42**:179–187.

90 Gregg NM (1941) Congenital cataract following German measles in the mother. *Transactions of the Ophthalmic Society of Australia* **3**:35–46.

91 Weller TH, Neva FA (1962) Propoagation in tissue culture of cytopathic agents from patients with rubella-like illness. *Proceedings of the Society for Experimental Biology and Medicine* **111**:215–225.

92 Parkman PD, Buescher EL, Artenstein MS (1962) Recovery of rubella virus from army recruits. *Proceedings of the Society for Experimental Biology and Medicine* **111**:225–230.

93 Plotkin JA, Farquhar JD, Katz M (1969) Attenuation of RA 27/3 rubella virus in WI-38 human diploid cells. *American Journal of Diseases of Children* **118**:178.

94 Sever JL (1967) The epidemiology of rubella. *Archives of Ophthalmology* **77**:427–429.

95 Lever AML, Ross MGR, Baboonian C *et al.* (1987) Immunity to rubella among women of child-bearing age. *British Journal of Obstetrics and Gynaecology* **94**:208–212.

96 Centers for Disease Control (1992) Congenital rubella syndrome among the Amish, Pennsylvania. 1991–1992. *Morbidity and Mortality Weekly Report* **41**:468–476.

97 Miller E (1990) Rubella reinfection. *Archives of Diseases in Childhood* **65**:820–821.

98 Green RH, Balsamo MR, Giles JP *et al.* (1965) Studies of the natural history and prevention of rubella. *American Journal of Diseases of Children* **110**:348–365.

99 Freij BJ, South MA, Sever JL (1988) Maternal rubella and the congenital rubella syndrome. *Clinics in Perinatology* **15**:247–257.

100 Best JM (1992) Rubella. In Greenough A, Osborne J, Sutherland S (eds), *Congenital, Perinatal and Neonatal Infections*, pp. 171–184. Edinburgh: Churchill Livingstone.

101 Sever JL, Nelson KB, Gilkeson MR (1965) Rubella epidemic, 1964. Effect on 6,000 pregnancies. *American Journal of Diseases of Children* **110**:395–407.

102 Horstmann DM, Banatvala JE, Riordan JT *et al.* (1965) Maternal rubella and the rubella syndrome in infants. *American Journal of Diseases of Children* **110**:408–415.

103 Bellanti JA, Artenstein MS, Olson LC *et al.* (1965) Congenital rubella. *American Journal of Diseases of Children* **110**:464–472.

104 South MA, Sever JL (1985) Teratogen update: The congenital rubella syndrome. *Teratology* **31**:297–307.

105 Miller E, Cradock-Watson JE, Pollock TM (1982) Consequences of confirmed maternal rubella at successive stages of pregnancy. *Lancet* **ii**:781–784.

106 Munro ND, Sheppard S, Smithells RW *et al.* (1987) Temporal relations between maternal rubella and congenital defects. *Lancet* **i**:201–204.

107 Enders G, Nickerl-Pacher U, Miller E *et al.* (1988) Outcome of confirmed periconceptional maternal rubella. *Lancet* **i**:1445–1447.

108 Mahony MJ, Fleming PJ, Roome APCH *et al.* (1985) Congenital rubella with fatal pneumonitis in two infants born to mothers reported as rubella immune. *Lancet* **i**:700–701.

109 Das BD, Kurz JB, Hunter N *et al.* (1990) Congenital rubella after previous maternal immunity. *Archives of Diseases in Childhood* **65**:545–546.

110 Morgan-Capner P, Thomas HIJ (1988) Serological distinction between primary rubella and reinfection. *Lancet* **i**:1397.

111 Best JM, Banatvala JE, Morgan-Capner P *et al.* (1989) Fetal infection after maternal reinfection with rubella: Criteria for defining reinfection. *British Medical Journal* **299**:773–775.

112 Huraux JM, Nicolas JC, Huraux-Rendu C (1981) Rubeole et grossesse. *Editions Merallino* :5–151.

113 Bricout F (1986) Interpretations des tests sérologiques de la rubeole *La Lettre de l'Infectiologue* **9**:243–245.

114 Grangeot-Keros L, Pillot J, Daffos F (1988) Prenatal and postnatal production of IgM and IgA antibodies to rubella virus studied by antibody capture immunoassay. *Journal of Infectious Diseases* **158**:138–143.

115 Ho-Terry L, Londesborough P, Rees KR *et al.* (1988) Diagnosis of fetal rubella infection by nucleic acid hybridization. *Journal of Medical Virology* **24**:175–182.

116 Daffos F, Forestier F, Grangeot-Keros L *et al.* (1984) Prenatal diagnosis of congenital rubella. *Lancet* **i**:1–3.

117 Enders G, Jonatha W (1987) Prenatal diagnosis of intrauterine rubella. *Infection* **15**:162–164.

118 Grose C, Itani O, Weiner CP (1989) Prenatal diagnosis of fetal infection: Advances from amniocentesis to cordocentesis – congenital toxoplasmosis, rubella, cytomegalovirus, varicella virus, parvovirus and human immunodeficiency virus. *Pediatric Infectious Disease Journal* **8**:459–468.

119 Daffos F, Forestier F, Grangeot-Keros L *et al.* (1984) Gradual appearance of total IgM in fetal serum during the second trimester of pregnancy: Application to the prenatal diagnosis of fetal infections. *Annales de Biologie Clinique* **42**:135.

120 Lebon P, Daffos F, Checoury A *et al.* (1985) Presence of an acid-labile alpha-interferon in sera from fetuses and children with congenital rubella. *Journal of Clinical Microbiology* **21**:755.

121 Preblud SR, Alford CA (1990) Rubella. In Remington JS, Klein JO (eds), *Infectious Diseases of the Fetus and Newborn Infant*, pp. 196–240. London:W.B. Saunders.

122 Morgan-Capner P, Hodgson J *et al.* (1985) Detection of rubella-specific IgM in subclinical rubella reinfection in pregnancy. *Lancet* **i**:244–246.

123 Enders G (1985) Rubella antibody titers in vaccinated and nonvaccinated women and results of vaccination during pregnancy. *Review of Infectious Diseases* **7**:S103 (suppl.1).

124 O-Shea S, Woodward S, Best JM *et al.* (1988) Rubella vaccination: Persistence of antibodies for 10–21 years. *lancet* **ii**:909.

125 Morgan-Capner P (1989) Diagnosing rubella. *British Medical Journal* **299**:338–339.

126 Forestier F, Daffos F, Lynch L (1991) Les foetopathies infectieuses: Prévention, diagnostic prénatal, attitude pratique. *Presse Medicale* **20**:1448–1454.

127 Cossart YE, Field AM, Cant B *et al.* (1975) Parvovirus-like particles in human sera. *Lancet* **i**:72–73.

128 Serjeant GR, Topley JM, Mason K *et al.* (1981) Outbreak of aplastic crises in sickle cell anaemia associated with parvovirus-like agent. *Lancet* **ii**:595–597.

129 Anderson LJ (1987) Role of parvovirus B19 in human disease. *Pediatric Infectious Disease Journal* **6**:711–718.

130 Thurn J (1988) Human parvovirus B19: Historical and clinical review. *Review of Infectious Diseases* **10**:1005–1011.

131 Carrington D, Gilmore DH,Whittle MJ *et al.* (1987) Maternal serum alpha-fetoprotein: A marker of fetal aplastic crisis during intrauterine human parvovirus infection. *Lancet* **i**:433–435.

132 Naides SJ, Weiner CP (1989) Antenatal diagnosis and palliative treatment of non-immune hydrops fetalis secondary to fetal parvovirus B19 infection. *Prenatal Diagnosis* **9**:105–114.

133 Young N, Harrison M, Moore J *et al.* (1984) Direct demonstration of the human parvovirus in erythroid progenitor cells infected *in vitro Journal of Clinical Investigation* **74**:2024–2032.

134 Centers for disease Control (1989) Risks asociated with human parvovirus B19 infection. *Morbidity and Mortality Weekly Report* **38**:81–97.

135 Public Health Laboratory Service Working Party on Fifth Disease (1990) Prospective study of human parvovirus (B19) infection in pregnancy. *British Medical Journal* **300**:1166–1170.

136 Young N (1988) Hematologic and hematopoietic consequences of B19 parvovirus infection. *Seminars in Hematology* **25**:159–172.

137 Kumar ML (1991) Human parvovirus B19 and its associated diseases. *Clinics in Perinatology* **18**:209–225.

138 Anand A, Gray ES, Brown T *et al.* (1987) Human parvovirus infection in pregnancy and hydrops fetalis. *New England Journal of Medicine* **316**:183–186.

139 Porter HJ, Quantrill AM, Fleming KA (1988) B19 parvovirus infection of myocardial cells. *Lancet* **i**:535–536.

140 Bloom MC, Rolland M, Bernard JD *et al.* (1990) Infection materno-foetale à parvovirus associée a une péritonite méconiale antenatale *Archives Françaises de Pediatrie* **47**:437–439.

141 Wright IMR, Williams ML, Cohen BJ (1991) Congenital parvovirus infection. *Archives of Diseases in Childhood* **66**:253–254.

142 Hartwig NG, Vermeij-Keers C, Van Elsacker-Niele AMW *et al.* (1989) Embryonic malformations in a case of intrauterine parvovirus B19 infection. *Teratology* **39**:295–302.

143 Shirley JA Revill S, Cohen BJ *et al.* (1987) serological study of rubella-like illnesses. *Journal of Medical Virology* **21**:369–379.

144 Schwarz TF, Roggendorf M, Deinhardt F (1988) Human parvovirus B19:ELISA and immunoblot assays. *Journal of Virological Methods* **20**:155–168.

145 Clewley JP, Cohen BJ, Field AM *et al.* (1987) Detec-

tion of parvovirus B19 DNA, Antigen and particles in the human fetus. *Journal of Medical Virology* 23:367–376.

146   Anderson MJ, Jones SE, Minson AC (1985) Diagnosis of human parvovirus infection by dot-blot hybridization using cloned viral DNA. *Journal of Medical Virology* 15:163–172.

147   Clewley JP (1985) Detection of human parvovirus using a molecularly cloned probe. *Journal of Medical Virology* 15:173–181.

148   Salimans MMM, Van de Rijke FM, Raap AK *et al.* (1989) Detection of parvovirus B19 DNA in fetal tissues by *in situ* hybridisation and polymerase chain reaction. *Journal of Clinical Pathology* 42:525–530.

149   Clewley JP (1989) Polymerase chain reaction assay of parvovirus B19 DNA in clinical specimens. *Journal of Clinical Microbiology* 27:2647–2651.

150   Koch WC, Adler SP (1990) Detection of human parvovirus B19 DNA by using the polymerase chain reaction. *Journal of Clinical Microbiology* 28:65–69.

151   Schwarz TF, Nerlich A, Hottenträger B *et al.* (1991) Parvovirus B19 infection of the fetus: Histology and *in situ* hybridization. *American Journal of Clinical Pathology* 96:121–126.

152   Burton PA (1986) Intranuclear inclusions in marrow of hydropic fetus due to parvovirus infection. *Lancet* ii:1155.

153   Francoisi RA, Tattersall P (1988) Fetal infection with human parvovirus B19. *Human Pathology* 19:489–491.

154   Gray ES, Davidson RJL, Anand A (1987) Human parvovirus and fetal anaemia. *Lancet* i:1144.

155   Woernle CH, Anderson LJ, Tattersall P *et al.* (1987) Human parvovirus B19 infection during pregnancy. *Journal of Infectious Diseases* 156:17–20.

156   Anderson LJ, Hurwitz ES (1988) Human parvovirus B19 and pregnancy. *Clinics in Perinatology* 15:273–286.

157   Maeda H, Shimokawa H, Satoh S *et al* (1988) Nonimmunologic hydrops fetalis resulting from intauterine human parvovirus B19 infection: Report of two cases. *Obstetrics and Gynecology* 72:482–485.

158   Rodis JF, Hovick TJ, Quinn DL *et al.* (1988) Human parvovirus infection in pregnancy. *Obstetrics and Gynecology* 72:733–738.

159   Samra JS, Obhrai MS, Constantine G (1989) Parvovirus infection in pregnancy. *Obstetrics and Gynecology* 73:832–834.

160   Brown KE (1989) What threat is human parvovirus B19 to the fetus? A review. *British Journal of Obstetrics and Gynaecology* 96:764–767.

161   Bernstein IM, Capeless EL (1989) Elevated maternal serum alpha-fetoprotein and hydrops fetalis in association with fetal parvovirus B19 infection. *Obstetrics and Gynecology* 74:456–457.

162   Peters MT, Nicolaides KH (1990) Cordocentesis for the diagnosis and treatment of human fetal parvovirus infection. *Obstetrics and Gynecology* 75:501–504.

163   Shmoys S, Kaplan C (1990) Parvovirus and pregnancy. *Clinical Obstetrics and Gynecology* 33:268–275.

164   Soothill P (1990) Intauterine blood transfusion for non-immune bydrops fetalis due to parvovirus B19 infection. *Lancet* ii:121–122.

165   Rodis JF, Quinn DL, Gary GW *et al.* (1990) Management and outcome of pregnancies complicated by human B_{19} infection: spontaneous reversal *in utero* and survival of a term infant. *American Journal of Obstetrics and Gynecology* 163:1168–1171.

166   Humphrey W, Magoon M, O'Shaughnessy R (1991) Severe nonimmune hydrops secondary to parvovirus B19 infection: Spontaneous reversal *in utero* and survival of a term infant. *Obstetrics and Gynecology* 78:900–902.

167   Sahakian V, Weiner CP, Naides SJ *et al.* (1991) Intauterine transfusion treatment of nonimmune hydrops fetalis secondary to human parvovirus B19 infection. *American Journal of Obstetrics and Gynecology* 164:1090–1091.

168   Pryde PG, Nugent CE, Pridjian G *et al.* (1992) Spontaneous resolution of nonimmune hydrops fetalis secondary to human parvovirus B19 infection. *Obstetrics and Gynecology* 79:859–861.

169   Kurtzman G, Frickhofen N, Kimball J *et al.* (1989) Pure red-cell aplasia of 10 years' duration due to persistent parvovirus B19 infection and its cure with immunoglobulin therapy. *New England Journal of Medicine.* 321:519–523.

170   Committee on Infectious Diseases (1990) Parvovirus, erythema infectiosum, and pregnancy. *Pediatrics* 85:131–133.

171   Kajigaya S, Fujita S, Ozawa K *et al.* (1988) A cell line that expresses B19 parvovirus structural proteins and produces empty capsids. *Blood* 72:44a (abstract 86).

172   Moss TR, Nathan PM (1988) (1988) General practitioners: prevention of HIV disease/AIDS. *Journal of the Royal College of General Practitioners* 38:427.

173   Tappin DM, Girwood RWA, Follett EAC *et al.* (1991) Prevalence of maternal infections in Scotland based on unlinked anonymous testing of newborn babies. *Lancet* 337:1565–1567.

174   Adies AE *et al.* (1991) Prevalence of maternal HIV-1 infection in Thames regions: Results from anonymous unlinked neonatal testing. *Lancet* 337:709–711.

175   McCarthy KH, Johnson MA, Studd JWW (1992) Antenatal HIV testing (Editorial). *British Journal of Obstetrics and Gynaecology* 99:867–868.

176   European Collaborative Study (1991) Children born to women with HIV-1 infection: Natural history and risk of transmission. *Lancet* 337:253–260.

177   Norman S, Studd J, Johnson M (1990) HIV infection in women. *British Medical Journal* 301:1231–1232.

178   Minkoff HL (1990) Serious infections during pregnancy among women with advanced human immunodeficiency virus infection. *American Journal of Obstetrics and Gynecology* 162:30–40.

179   Schoenbaum EE, Davenny K, Holbrook K (1992) The management of HIV disease in pregnancy. *Clinics in Obstetrics and Gynecology* 6:101–124.

180   Douglas GC, King BF (1992) Maternal–fetal transmission of human immunodeficiency virus: A review of possible routes and cellular mechanisms of infection. *Clin Infect Dis* 15:678–691.

181   Nanda D (1990) Human immunodeficiency virus

infection in pregnancy. *Obstetrics and Gynecology Clinics of North America* **17**:617–626.

182 Sperling RS (1992) A survey of Zidovudine use in pregnant women with human immunodeficiency virus infection. *New England Journal of Medicine* **326**:857–861.

183 Rogers MF *et al.* (1989) Use of the polymerase chain reaction for early detection of the proviral sequences of human immunodeficiency virus in infants born to seropositive mothers. *New England Journal of Medicine* **320**:1649.

184 Italian Multicentre Study (1988) Epidemiology, clinical features and prognostic factors of paediatric HIV infection. *Lancet* **ii**:1043–1045.

185 Van de Perre P, Simonson A, Msellati P *et al.* (1991) Postnatal transmission of human immunodeficiency virus type 1 from mother to infant. *New England Journal of Medicine* **325**:593–598.

186 Sison AV, Campos JM (1992) Laboratory methods for early detection of human immunodeficiency virus type 1 in newborns and infants. *Clin Microbiol Rev* **5**:238–247.

187 Centers for Disease Control (1989) Guidelines for prophylaxis against *Pneumocystis carinii* pneumonia for persons infected with human immunodeficiencey virus. *Morbidity and Mortality Weekly Report* **389**:1–9 (supp.).

188 Newton L, Hall SM, Pelerin M, McLauchlin J (1992) Listeriosis surveillance: 1991. *Communicable Disease Report* **2**:142–144.

189 McLauchlin J, Hall SM, Velani SK, Gilbert RJ (1991) Human listeriosis and paté: A possible association. *British Medical Journal* **303**:773–775.

190 Buchdahl R, Hird M, Gamsu H, Tapp A, Gibb D, Tzannatos C (1990) Listeriosis revisited: The role of the obstetrician. *British Journal of Obstetrics and Gynaecology* **97**:186–189.

191 Wilkinson P (1992) Uncommon infections: Listeriosis. *Prescribers' Journal* **32**:26–31.

192 Centers for Disease Control (1986) Congenital syphilis, United States, 1983–1985. *Morbidity and Mortality Weekly Report* **35**:625.

193 Adler MW (1984) ABC of sexually transmitted disease. *British Medical Journal* 46–48.

194 Silverstein AM (1962) congenital syphilis and the timing of immunogenesis in the human fetus. *Nature* **194**:196.

195 Larsen SA, Hunter EF, McGrew BE (1984) Syphilis. In Wentworth BB, Judson FN (eds), *Laboratory Methods for the Diagnosis of Sexually Transmitted Diseases*. Washington, DC: American Public Health Association.

196 Hallak M, Peipert JF, Ludomirsky A, Byers J (1992) Nonimmune hydrops fetalis and fetal congenital syphilis: A case report. *Journal of Reproductive Medicine* **37**:173–176.

197 Centers for Disease Control (1988) Guidelines for the prevention and control of congenital syphilis. *Morbidity and Mortality Weekly Report* **37**:1 (suppl.1).

198 Klein VR, Cox SM, Mitchell MD, Wendel GD Jr (1990) The Jarisch-Herxheimer reaction complicating syphilotherapy in pregnancy. *Obstetrics and Gynecology* **75**:375–380.

50

Craniospinal and Facial Defects

F.A. CHERVENAK, G. ISAACSON AND J. STRELTZOFF

INTRODUCTION

Craniospinal defects are of considerable importance since they often determine survival, physical appearance and function in society. A sonographic study of the craniospinal region necessarily focuses on morphologic abnormalities of the central nervous system, but at the same time includes facial defects, cervical and lymphatic dysgenesis. This regional approach is helpful, as abnormalities of varied embryological origins may have similar sonographic appearance.

SYSTEMATIC SCANNING OF THE CRANIOSPINAL REGION

It is important to have a systematic approach to the ultrasonic evaluation of the craniospinal region. A suggested order is:

HEAD

- lateral ventricles
- biparietal diameter view
- cerebellum
- base of skull
- sagittal and coronal views

FACE

- orbits and eyes
- ears
- lower face

NECK

- transverse

SPINE

- longitudinal

THE HEAD

Transverse planes are, for several reasons, preferred for prenatal ultrasound over the coronal and sagittal ones used by neonatal ultrasonographers and pathologists. First, the fetal head is most often in an occipito-transverse position. Second, the membranous bones of the fetal cranium do not reflect sound waves to the extent that they do in postnatal life, when they are more heavily calcified and rigid. Third, a transverse plane produces a large cross-section of the brain in which

multiple landmarks may be visualized at one time
(**Figure 1**).

The Lateral Ventricles

The lateral ventricles are identified as paired echo-
spared areas within the brain substance. The distal
ventricle (i.e. the one farthest from the ultrasound
transducer) is chosen for study, since reverberation
artifacts frequently obscure the anatomy of the proximal hemisphere. A prominent echogenic area which
represents the choroid plexus is usually seen within the
lateral ventricle.

As pregnancy advances, there is a decrease in the
proportion of the brain's cross-section occupied by the
lateral ventricles. Although the lateral-to-hemispheric
width ratio has been widely used to assess ventricular
volume (**Figure 2**),[1] the sonographic 'lateral wall' may
not be the true lateral wall. The authors prefer assessment of the atrium of the lateral ventricle which is well
defined and should always measure less than 1 cm^2
(**Figure 3**).[2]

The Biparietal Diameter

The most commonly studied transverse section of the
fetus is at the level of the biparietal diameter (BPD)

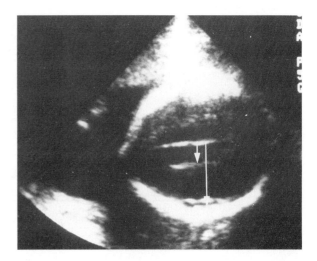

Figure 2. Transverse sonogram through bodies
of lateral ventricles. Arrows demonstrate distance
from midline echo to lateral wall of lateral ventricle
and distance from midline echo to inner skull table.[1]

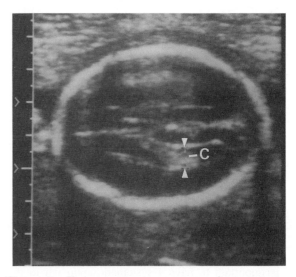

Figure 3. Transverse sonogram demonstrates
distal lateral ventricle with its atrial measurements
(arrows).

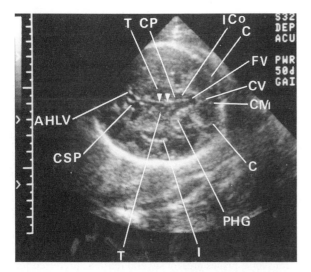

Figure 1. Transverse sonogram through fetal skull
at the level of BPD but angled posteriorly and
inferiorly, demonstrates cerebellum (C), cerebllar
vermis (CV), cisterna magna (CM), fourth ventricle
(FV), inferior colliculus (ICo), cerebellar peduncle
(CP), parahippocampal gyrus (PHG), insular cortex
(I), thalamus (T), third ventricle (arrowheads), cavum
septi pellucidi (CSP) and anterior horns of lateral
ventricles (AHLV).

(**Figure 4**). Several intracranial landmarks are located
within a plane 15° above the canthomeatal line and
parallel to the base of the skull. These are illustrated
in **Figure 4**.

In this plane, the BPD can be reproducibly measured as the distance from the proximal outer table
to the distal inner table of the skull. The head
perimeter/circumference can be determined by direct
measurement or calculated by summing the BPD and
occipitofrontal diameter measured from the midpoint
of frontal and occipital echo complexes and multiply-

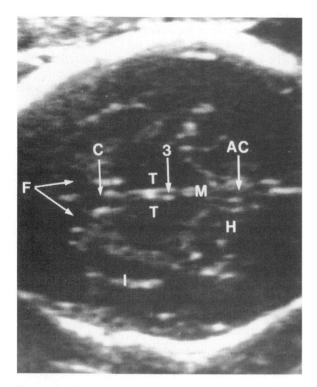

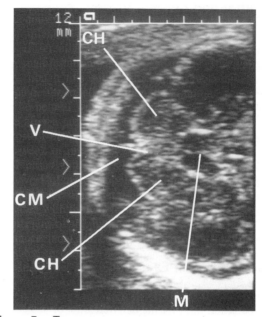

Figure 5. Transverse sonogram demonstrates cerebellar hemispheres (CH), vermis (V), midbrain (M) and cistern magna (CM).

Figure 4. Transverse sonogram at the level of the BPD demonstrates frontal horn of lateral ventricle (F), third ventricle (3), hippocampus (H), midbrain (M), great cerebral vein and ambient cistern (AC), insula (I) and thalamus (T). Reprinted with permission from Chervenak *et al.* [31]

ing by 1.62. The ratio of BPD to OFD defines the cephalic index (normal values 75–85). A high value determines brachycephaly and a low value dolichocephaly. With these variants of head shape, BPD may be an inaccurate determinant of gestational age and rarely there may be cranial pathology. Measurement of a head circumference eliminates this dating problem.

The Cerebellum

The cerebellum is visualized in a plane parallel to the BPD plane. Once located, the cerebellar structures are best studied by rotating the ultrasound transducer 15° farther from the canthomeatal line. In this plane, the cerebellum (with its brightly echogenic, centrally placed vermis, and two relatively non-echogenic hemispheres) can be viewed and measured [14] (**Figure 5**).

The Base of the Skull

The base of the skull level may be identified by an echogenic 'X' formed by the lesser wings of the sphe-

noid bone and the petrous pyramid. These bone ridges demark the anterior, middle and posterior fossae (**Figure 6**).

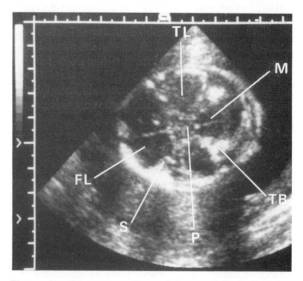

Figure 6. Sonogram through base of skull showing frontal lobe (FL), temporal lobe (TL), greater wing of sphenoid (S), temporal bone (TB), pituitary stalk (P) and medulla (M).

Sagittal and Coronal Views

Sagittal views of the fetal brain are sometimes helpful to delineate anatomy. The relationship of midline to cranial structures can be seen in **Figure 7**. Coronal views may also be of value (see Agenesis of the Corpus Callosum).

THE FACE

Unlike the cranium and its contents, which may be studied using an orderly progression of well-defined sonographic planes, characterization of the face requires both ingenuity and good luck on the part of the sonographer.

The Orbits and Eyes

Measurement of the distance between the bony orbits can be useful both for the determination of gestational age and the search for anomalies characterized by either hypotelorism or hypertelorism. Depending on the position of the fetal head, the inner and outer orbital distances can be measured in coronal or transverse planes and compared to nomograms. The outer orbital distance is the more valuable measurement because of greater normal variation across gestational age as compared with the inner orbital distance. The technique for obtaining these measurements and the charts are illustrated in **Figures 8a** and **b**.[3]

The lens of the fetal eye may be visualized as a circular area on the front of the globe. On occasion, the aqueous and vitreous humors, the extraocular muscles and the ophthalmic artery are seen.

The Ears

The pinna of the ear and the development of its cartilages have been observed sonographically. The pinna is initially smooth, but becomes increasingly ridged as gestation progresses. Occasionally, even the basal turn of the cochlea or superior semicircular canal may be visualized within the petrous of the temporal bone.

The Lower Face

The nares and the upper lip are visualized using an oblique transverse scan (**Figure 9**). This plane can be used in the search for cleft lip and cleft palate. The tongue may be observed and its motion in the act of swallowing studied. The fetal profile (i.e. the midline sagittal view) is useful for verifying the position of the nose, the contour of the chin and the shape of the facial midline.

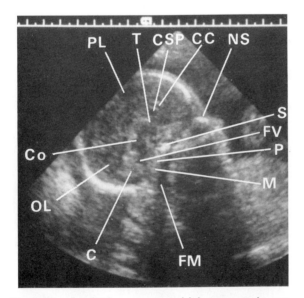

Figure 7. Sagittal sonogram which can supply supplemental information for midline cranial anatomy, including nasal septum (NS), body of sphenoid (S), thalamus (T), cavum septi pellucidi (CSP), corpus callosum (CC), parietal lobe (PL), occipital lobe (OL), colliculi (CO), cerebellum (C), fourth ventricle (FV), medulla (M), pons (P) and foramen magnum (FM).

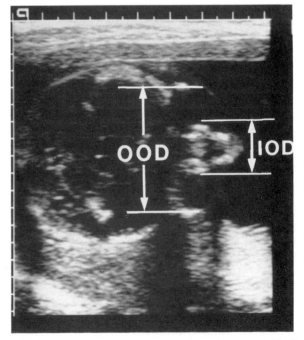

Figure 8a. Transverse sonogram with outer orbital distance (OOD) and inner orbital distance (IOD) indicated.

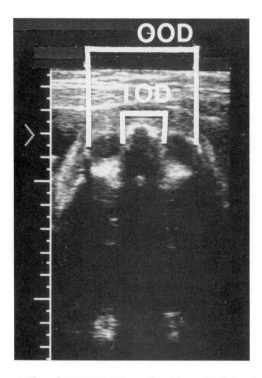

Figure 8b. Demonstration of orbits with fetus facing anteriorly. Reprinted with permission from Chervenak *et al.*[31]

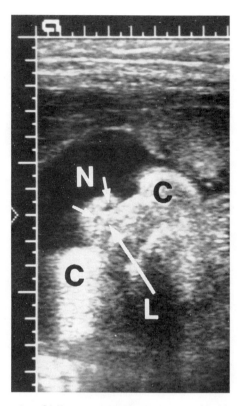

Figure 9. Oblique coronal sonogram looking up at fetal upper lip (L), cheeks (C) and nares (N). Reprinted with permission from Chervenak *et al.*[31]

THE NECK

The neck should be examined with particular attention to its surface contours as a variety of lesions may protrude from this area. The trachea and carotid bifurcation may be seen within the substance of the neck.

THE SPINE

An appreciation of the variability in the shapes of the vertebral bodies, and the changing sonographic appearance of the spine during gestation, is necessary to differentiate small defects in the spine from normal anatomic features. Their appearance at 18 weeks are shown in **Figures 10a–c**.

During the third trimester, more detail can be seen. The vertebral body, pedicles, transverse processes, posterior laminae and the spinous process, all may be identified as echogenic structures in transverse scans. In addition, the spinal canal and intervertebral foramina may be seen as non-echogenic areas (**Figure 11a**). In the sagittal plane, a line of vertebral bodies is still seen, but the posterior echoes are more complex with spinous processes seen jutting from the line of other elements (**Figure 11b**).

CRANIOSPINAL ANOMALIES: MANAGEMENT OPTIONS

Using the systematic approach to ultrasonic scanning described above, the common anomalies that might be identified are:

HEAD

lateral ventricles

BPD view

- anencephaly
- hydrocephaly
- cephalocele
- holoprosencephaly
- microcephaly
- choroid plexus cyst

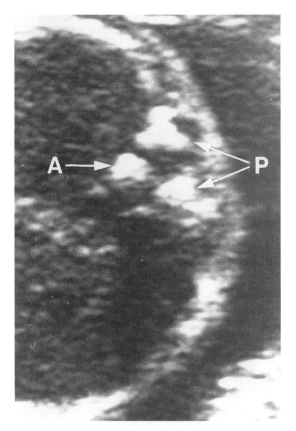

Figure 10a. Transverse sonogram of fetal spine at 18 weeks demonstrating one anterior (A) and two posterior (P) ossification centers. Reprinted with permission from Chervenak *et al.*[31]

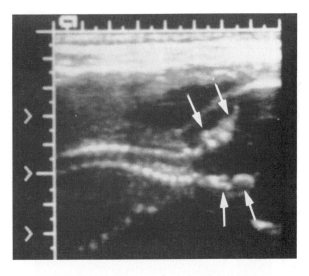

Figure 10c. Coronal sonogram of fetal spine demonstrates a cervical spine widening (arrows) toward the base of the skull.

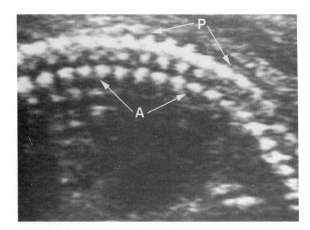

Figure 10b. Sagittal sonogram of fetus at 18 weeks gestation showing anterior (A) and posterior (P) perforation elements.

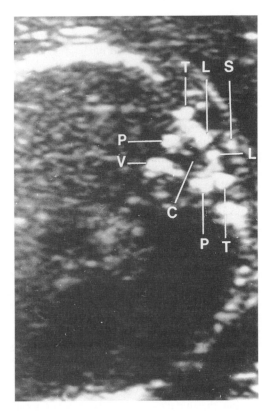

Figure 11a. Transverse sonogram of mature fetal spine shows vertebral body (V), pedicles (P), transverse processes (T), lamina (L), spinous process (S) and spine cord (C).

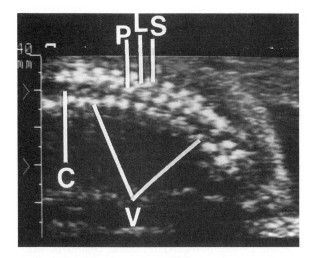

Figure 11b. Sagittal sonogram of mature lumbosacral spine shows vertebral bodies (V), spinal cord (C), pedicle (P), lamina (L) and spinous process (S). Note how the spinal cord moves posteriorly in the sacral region. Reprinted with permission from Chervenak et al.[31]

• hydranencephaly

Cerebellum

Base of skull

• Dandy-Walker malformation

Sagittal/Coronal

• agenesis of the corpus callosum

FACE

facial clefts

NECK

cystic hygroma

SPINE

• spina bifida

ANENCEPHALY

General

Anencephaly is a lethal anomaly in which much of the brain is absent and what remains is not covered by the vault of the skull. Remnants of forebrain may be present, and while the medulla is generally well-formed, the cerebral hemispheres and frequently the midbrain are completely absent.

The incidence of this disorder is highly variable, depending on geographic location, race and sex. Its incidence in the USA has been estimated at 1:1000 deliveries. Anencephaly is much more common in the UK, however, reaching a high of 6.7:1000 in Belfast. Anencephaly is more common in Whites than Blacks and Orientals, and approximately twice as common in female infants.

Anencephaly is thought to result from the failure of the rostral portion of the neural tube to close. This fusion normally begins in the region of the fourth somite and extends both rostrally and caudally. Closure in the region of the developing head is completed approximately 24 days after conception; in the region of the sacrum, closure occurs at about 26 days. This common embryologic origin may explain the concurrence of anencephaly with sacral spina bifida or complete non-closure of the neural tube.

In place of the cerebral hemispheres, a mass of thin-walled vascular channels known as the area cerebrovasculosa can be seen protruding from the base of the skull. This mass, which may be a derivative of the choroid plexus, is usually covered by a membrane contiguous with the scalp.

Diagnosis

The first suspicion of anencephaly may come from the finding of an elevated maternal serum alpha-fetoprotein (AFP) concentraftion before an ultrasound examination has been performed (see Chapter 37). The definitive diagnosis is made by ultrasound examination. *Amniocentesis to measure AFP and acetylcholinesterase are not justified when ultrasound is available.*

If routine screening with AFP and/or ultrasound is not available in the second trimester, the patient may present with hydramnios, presumably due to impaired swallowing. Anencephaly is easily diagnosed during the second and third trimesters. Caution, however, is necessary during the first trimester since the normal immature brain may be difficult at this early stage to differentiate from the area cerebrovasculosa.

The prenatal sonographic diagnosis of anencephaly is based on the absence of the calvaria, the dome-like portion of the cranial vault (**Figure 12**). After 14 weeks, it is abnormal not to see the bony structures of the skull above the orbits. Of course, the head must be accessible to the ultrasound (i.e. not hidden in the pelvis of the mother) for these structures to be adequately visualized. When the area cerebrovasculosa is prominent, an ill-defined mass of heterogeneous density may be seen by ultrasound.

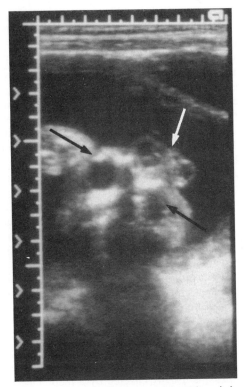

Figure 12. Coronal sonogram of fetal head demonstrating anencephaly. Black arrow points to orbits; white arrow points to area cerebrovasculosa.

While the diagnosis of anencephaly is usually straightforward, other diagnoses should be considered. In severe microcephaly, the bones of the skull may be difficult to locate, but are uniformly present. In the early amnion-rupture sequence, constricting bands may prevent the normal formation of the skull. However, the malformation is usually asymmetrical and brain tissue is present. An encephalocele might simulate anencephaly until a brain-filled sac is localized. Lastly, anencephaly is differentiated from acrania, as in the latter there is a normally formed brain absent skull.

Management Options

Anencephaly is a lethal anomaly. Most fetuses with anencephaly are stillborn or, if liveborn, die shortly after birth. A single report describes an infant with anencephaly that survived for $5\frac{1}{2}$ months.[4]

Prenatal

Anencephaly is diagnosable with a high degree of accuracy and is uniformly lethal. The authors believe that termination of pregnancy is an ethical option at any time in gestation.[5] If diagnosed during the third trimester and the parents elect termination, a number of methods are available which are discussed in Chapter 60. Laminaria placement and prostaglandin gel may facilitate induction of labor when the cervis in unripe.

Labor/delivery

Postmaturity is common in pregnancies complicated by anencephaly. Cesarean delivery is not recommended for fetal distress, but it may be necessary for maternal indications. If an anencephalic infant is liveborn, humane care should be provided until the time of its death. The use of anencephalic newborns as organ donors has been widely debated.[6,7]

Pathological examination of the fetus is important to confirm the diagnosis and to exclude conditions where the anencephaly is part of a genetic syndrome.

Postnatal/prepregnancy

The recurrence risk for any open neural tube defect including anencephaly may be as low as 1.7% in the USA. In populations where anencephaly is more common, the risk may be greater. The rate of recurrence is higher after the birth of two or more affected siblings and a 25% recurrence risk exists when anencephaly is part of the Meckel syndrome.

In future pregnancies, prenatal ultrasound should be performed in an attempt to make an anatomic diagnosis of an open neural tube defect and/or hydrocephalus. The use of periconceptual folate therapy is discussed later under 'spina bifida'.

HYDROCEPHALUS

General

Hydrocephalus (ventriculomegaly causing an enlarged head) is an abnormal increase in the volume of the cerebral ventricles compared with brain tissue. Hydrocephalus is almost always due to obstruction of cerebrospinal fluid (CSF) flow and the resulting increase in intracranial pressure. Rarely, hydrocephalus results from an increase in cerebrospinal fluid production or ventriculomegaly from a relative decrease in the amount of brain tissue. Hydrocephalus is said to be 'isolated' when the fetus is free from anomalies which are not the direct result of the ventricular enlargement and intracranial pressure. Meningomyelocele is the most common anomaly found in assocation with hydrocephalus.

The incidence of congenital hydrocephalus unassociated with neural tube defect is 5.8 per 10 000 total births in the USA and 3.1 per 10 000 total births in

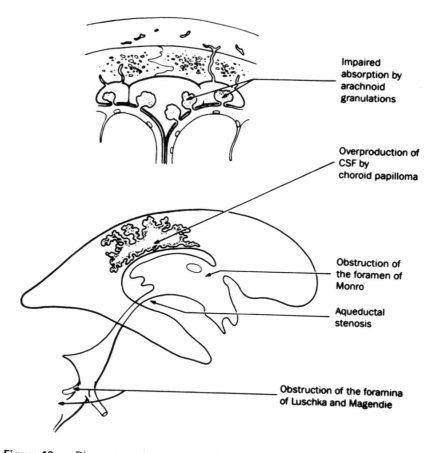

Impaired absorption by arachnoid granulations

Overproduction of CSF by choroid papilloma

Obstruction of the foramen of Monro

Aqueductal stenosis

Obstruction of the foramina of Luschka and Magendie

Figure 13a. Diagrammatic representation of mechanisms of ventriculomegaly.

England and Wales. How these neonatal data relate to the incidence of hydrocephalus *in utero* is uncertain, as spontaneous regression and antepartum death are possible.[8]

There are many and varied causes of hydrocephalus. It may result from abnormal formation of central nervous system structures. This category includes hydrocephalus inherited along a Mendelian pattern, or hydrocephalus associated with a malformation syndrome. Hydrocephalus may result from acquired defects *in utero*, as the result of infection with scarring or inflammation and CSF obstruction, from intraventricular hemorrhage, or intracranial tumors and mass lesions. Unfortunately, many cases of hydrocephalus cannot be assigned to one of these categories.

In general, there are four ways that the ventricles grow to an abnormal size (**Figure 13a**): (1) obstruction to outflow, usually at a point of narrowing in the system (frequently the aqueduct of Sylvius or the foramina of either Lushka or Magendie); (2) impaired resorption of CSF by the arachnoid granulations; (3) overproduction of CSF; and (4) underdevelopment or destruc-

tion of cortical tissue with a relative increase in the size of the ventricles. Our experience and that of others suggests that obstructive causes are the most common in both fetus and newborn.[8,9]

A variety of fetal anomalies have been described in association with fetal hydrocephalus. The most frequent coincident anomaly is spina bifida. This is probably due to the frequent association of spina bifida with the Arnold-Chiari malformation, where there is obstruction at the base of the fourth ventricle with a possible accompanying obstruction in the aqueduct (see later).

Diagnosis

A variety of techniques have been advocated for the diagnosis of hydrocephalus. The traditional method in the USA has been determination of the lateral ventricle to hemispheric width ratio (see **Figure 2**). This method has several advantages. Measurements are taken in the largest part of the ventricular system which can be identified quickly and consistently. Further, these measurements do not depend on identification of the medial wall of the lateral ventricle which was frequently difficult to visualize with earlier generation ultrasound machines and may still be a problem in difficult scanning situations. However, some have contended that the lateral ventricle to hemispheric width ratio is insensitive to early hydrocephalus as it ignores medial deviation of the medial wall of the lateral ventricle. Additional consideration of the lateral ventricular width may help to confirm normality during the second trimester when this measurement is less than 11 mm.[10] Further, several investigators have questioned whether the echo thought to represent the lateral wall of the lateral ventricle is truly derived from this structure. These authors have cast doubt on the value of *any* measurement of the body of the lateral ventricle.[2,11]

Cardoza *et al.* presented strong evidence that a single measurement of the lateral ventricular atrium accurately differentiates a normal ventricle system from one that is pathologically enlarged. In 100 normal fetuses, this measurement had a mean of 7.6 ± 0.6 mm (SD) in the range 14–38 weeks. All of 38 fetuses with hydrocephalus in this retrospective study had lateral ventricular atrial widths greater than or equal to 11 mm.[2]

In addition to the above methods, evaluation of the choroid plexus may be useful.[12] The choroid plexus usually fills the posterior portion of the lateral ventricles and appears symmetrical bilaterally, regardless of the orientation of the fetal head to gravity. In hydrocephalus, the choroid plexus assumes a dependent position in the enlarged ventricle. When the fetal head is transverse relative to the earth's surface, the choroid plexus of the two ventricles change asymmetrically relative to the middle echo. Attempts have been made to quantify this asymmetry be measuring a 'choroid angle' between the long axis of the choroid plexus in the dependent ventricle and the midline echo,[13] by measuring the distance between the choroid plexus and the medial wall of the lateral wall at the level of the atrium, or by evaluating changes in the shape of the frontal horn of the lateral ventricle.[12]

In cases of advanced hydrocephalus, any of these quantitative or qualitative assessements is bound to be accurate (**Figure 13b**). In cases of mild ventricular enlargement or when studying hydrocephalus in the early second trimester, it is the combination of these techniques in experienced hands which is most likely to lead to accurate diagnosis. The importance of serial examinations should be borne in mind when diagnosing or excluding fetal hydrocephalus.

Pitfalls in Diagnosis

Certain pitfalls in the detection of early fetal hydrocephalus should be considered to avoid false-positive

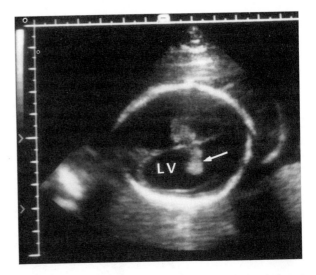

Figure 13b. Transverse sonogram of fetal head demonstrating hydrocephalus. LV, Dilated lateral ventricle; arrow points to dangling choroid plexus.

diagnoses. Because artifactual echoes often obscure accurate measurement on the proximal side of the head, hydrocephalus is best assessed in the distal hemisphere. Another potential source of confusion is a crescent-shaped, hypoechoic area, which is occasionally visualized in normal fetuses in the distal hemisphere. The differential diagnoses of large hydrocephalus (alobar holoprosencephaly, hydranencephaly, proencephaly and arachnoid cysts) are the other causes of large collections of intracranial fluid. They may be differentiated from hydrocephalus by the criteria listed later in this chapter. Another rare cause is an aneurysm of the vein of Galen. It is the only pathology in which flowing blood can be visualised by color flow Doppler ultrasound.

Management Options

Prior to the development of postnatal surgical shunting of the dilated ventricular system due to increased intracranial pressure, the outlook for the infant with hydrocephalus diagnosed after birth generally was poor. Although even unoperated obstructive hydrocephalus may progress slowly, or arrest spontaneously, massive head enlargement with blindness and mental retardation were far more common and still exist in the Third World.[15]

With the development of surgical shunting after birth, the prognosis for the infant with hydrocephalus has improved. For example, 200 consecutive infants with neonatal hydrocephalus at the Children's Memorial Hospital in Chicago underwent shunt procedures.[16] Of these, only five died. Intellectual development in the survivors was related to the type of hydrocephalus, age at initial shunt placement and shunt function, but not to the severity of the hydrocephalus or to the number of shunt revisions. For Caucasians with internal hydrocephalus, the mean IQ in this series was 84 ± 25.8. Infants with other forms of hydrocephalus such as those related to porencephaly or to Dandy-Walker cyst had significantly lower mean IQs.[16] Unfortunately, those infants with congenital hydrocephalus were not clearly differentiated from those who developed hydrocephalus during the neonatal period.

Others have corroborated the finding that well-treated infants without associated congenital malformations have a good chance to achieve normal intelligence, irrespective of the initial severity of their hydrocephalus.

Lorber followed 56 infants with severe congenital hydrocephalus (cortex 10 mm or less) over 8 years.[17] Of these, 46 infants survived, five of whom were of superior intelligence, 29 were of average to good intelligence, five were subnormal but educable, and six were profoundly retarded. Intellectual outcome was better when the shunting procedure was performed prior to 6 months of age. However, one cannot extrapolate from this data to neonates whose hydrocephalus is first diagnosed prenatally.

Several recent papers have focused on the outcome of hydrocephalus diagnosed during the fetal period. In each of these series, most of the fetuses (59–85%) had major structural anomalies in addition to hydrocephalus and most died during the perinatal period.[18,19] The much higher death rate observed in these fetal studies as compared to studies of children with hydrocephalus is at least partly attributable to the high frequency of associated anomalies and obstetrical trauma from cephalocentesis.

Prenatal

Once fetal hydrocephalus is identified, a careful sonographic search for associated anomalies including meningomyelocele is indicated. Fetal echocardiography should also be performed. The fetal karyotype should be determined, since 10% have a chromosomal aberration.[19]

The obstetric management of fetal hydrocephalus is dependent upon gestational age at the time of diagnosis, the association of other anomalies and the views of the parents. If the diagnosis is made prior to fetal viability, the initial options are either to terminate the pregnancy or to continue. If the decision is made to continue with the pregnancy, an attempt should be made to rule out an infectious etiology (see Chapter 49). Serial scans are performed to identify progressive

ventricular enlargement. A few cases have been documented which regressed in utero.

Further clinical investigation is necessary before the potential benefit and the potential harm of prenatal ventriculoamniotic shunt placement can be weighed, and the value of this procedure in the management of fetal hydrocephalus determined. Although experimental placement of these shunts in fetal rhesus monkeys yielded encouraging results, experience in human pregnancies has been disappointing. Of 44 fetuses in one large series, 34 survived. The death rate from the procedure was 10%, but only 12 of the liveborn infants are developing normally.[20]

Ventriculoamniotic shunt placement should be considered, if ever, only in those fetuses with progressive, isolated hydrocephalus who are too immature to be delivery for postnatal shunting. A multidisciplinary team composed of a perinatologist, sonographer, neurosurgeon, neonatologist, geneticist and social worker is important in order to provide integrated care. In addition, full disclosure to parents of currently known benefits and risks of the procedure is mandatory, so that parental consent is fully informed.[20,21] The principles of the technique for inserting a ventriculoamniotic shunt is the same as for inserting a vesicoamniotic shunt, which is described in detail in Chapter 51.

Where the decision has been taken to continue with the pregnancy, the next series of management decisions relate to the timing and method of delivery.

Labor/delivery

We recommend delivery of the fetus with hydrocephalus as soon as pulmonary maturity is demonstrated, so as to minimize the potential ill-effects of progressive ventricular enlargement. At the present time, there is no clear guideline for preterm delivery when hydrocephalus worsens prior to fetal lung maturity. The risks of respiratory distress syndrome with resultant delay in ventriculoperitoneal shunt placement must be balanced against potential ill-effects of progressive hydrocephalus. Serial sonography may be helpful if determining the management, arguing for early delivery if hydrocephalus is rapidly progressing. If delivery prior to fetal lung maturity is elected, than maternal corticosteroid adminstration is an option to reduce the risk and severity of respiratory distress syndrome in the neonate.

In cases of severe macrocephaly, fluid may be removed from the fetal ventricular system by a technique know as cephalocentesis. This method, which may avoid cesarean section, is performed by passing a 22-gauge needle transabdominally or transvaginally under ultrasound guidance and removing sufficient

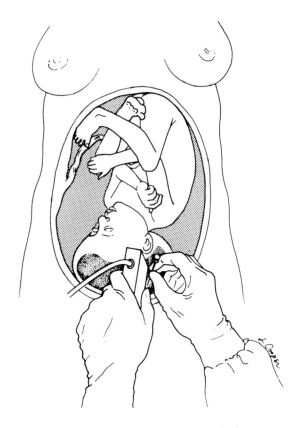

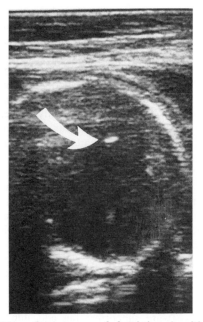

Figure 14b. Sonogram of fetal head with arrow pointing to tip of 18 gauge needle in dilated ventricle. Reprinted with permission from Chervenak *et al.*[19]

Figure 14a. Sonographic guidance of the needle during cephalocentesis.

CSF to permit vaginal delivery. The transabdominal technique is similar to that used for other invasive procedures (see Chapters 36, 40 and 41). The position of the needle tip should be followed throughout the procedure (see **Figures 14a,b**). After aspiration of CSF, overlapping of the cranial sutures can be observed with ultrasound.

Cephalocentesis is a potentially destructive procedure. In one series, perinatal death occurred following 91% of the cephalocenteses. The sonographic visualization of intracranial bleeding during cephalocentesis (see **Figure 15**), and the demonstration of this hemorrhage at autopsy, further emphasize the morbid nature of the procedure.

We believe that, in view of the potential for normal intelligence in those infants with hydrocephalus who are given optimum neonatal neurosurgical care, the parents of fetuses with apparent isolated hydrocephalus and macrocephaly should be encouraged to undergo cesarean section.[19] Because fetal cortical mantle thickness correlates poorly with subsequent intelligence, the authors do not advocate cephalocentesis in cases of severe isolated hydrocephalus. However, in those instances in which the parents decline cesarean section or the hydrocephalus is associated with anomalies that

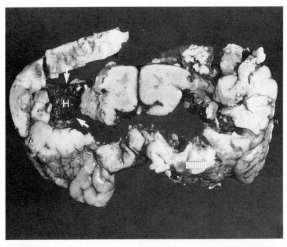

Figure 15. Coronal section of brain demonstrating a large subarachnoid hemorrhage (H) resulting from cephalocentesis. Modified from Isaacson.[32]

themselves carry a very poor prognosis (e.g. alobar holoprosencephaly or thanatophoric dysplasia with cloverleaf skull), cephalocentesis and subsequent vaginal delivery may be the most appropriate form of management. If there is no demonstrable cortex, hydranencephaly is most probably present. Since this condition has a dismal prognosis, cephalocentesis would be appropriate.[19]

The authors believe that cesarean delivery is not

necessary for all cases if there is a normal progression of labor. Attempted vaginal delivery may be appropriate when the fetus in a vertex presentation has a normal-sized head (head biometry < 2 SD above the mean for gestational age) or has mild macrocephaly (e.g. biparietal diameter of 98 mm at 38 weeks gestation). When fetal hydrocephalus is associated with a meningomyelocele, however, cesarean delivery may be less traumatic than vaginal delivery. This practice remains controversial.

Postnatal/prepregnancy

Hydrocephalus has diverse etiologies and the identification of its cause greatly aids in genetic counseling. A postmortem examination is essential. Several heritable patterns have been identified. Sex-linked recessive aqueductal stenosis carries a 1:4 risk of recurrence for future pregnancies and a 1:2 risk for male fetuses. Cerebellar agenesis with hydrocephalus is extremely rare but also may be sex-linked and thus have a similar recurrence risk.

Several syndromes which manifest dominant inheritance are associated with hydrocephalus (e.g. achondroplasia and osteogenesis imperfecta),[22] but the occurrence is irregular and the risk of hydrocephalus in future pregnancies cannot be accurately predicted. The Dandy-Walker syndrome has been reported in siblings and may sometimes follow an autosomal recessive pattern with a recurrence risk of 1:4 for future pregnancies. Several studies have suggested an increased risk of uncomplicated hydrocephalus in families with neural tube defects. Lorber and De studied uncomplicated congenital hydrocephalus and found an empiric risk of 4% for a central nervous system malformation and 2% for spina bifida or hydrocephalus in future pregnancies.[23]

Hydrocephalus may be associated with a variety of chromosomal abnormalities including triploidy, trisomy 13, trisomy 18, trisomy 21 and certain balanced translocations. The risk of recurrence is relatively low for sporadic chromosomal abnormalities, but may be much higher for balanced translocations.[22] Other causes of fetal hydrocephalus include prenatal infection, intracranial tumors and cysts, and vascular malformations. Such causes are unlikely to result in an increased risk of hydrocephalus in future pregnancies.[22]

CEPHALOCELE

General

A cephalocele is a protrusion of the meninges and, frequently, brain tissue through a defect in the cranium. The term includes both encephaloceles, which contain brain tissue, and cranial meningoceles, which do not. The incidence is approximately 1:2000 live births. In the West, 75% of these lesions are occipital but they may also be parietal, frontal or nasopharyngeal. The incidence of anterior lesions appears to be considerably greater in the Orient.

A cephalocele may arise from a failure of closure of the rostral end of the neural tube during the fourth week of fetal life. This fusion begins in the region of the fourth somite and extends both rostrally and caudally. It has been suggested that either a primary overgrowth of neaural tube tissue in the line of closure or a failure of induction by adjacent mesodermal tissues may interrupt this process. The majority of cephaloceles occur in the midline, and this mechanism may explain their genesis. If disruption of neural tube fusion occurs in the caudal region at the same time, then spina bifida and a cephalocele may be present simultaneously. This helps to explain the concurrence in 7–15% of cephaloceles.[24,25]

A cephalocele may also result from early disruption in the formation of the fetal skull. One clear example of this is the amnion rupture sequence. Rupture of the amnion early in gestation may produce bands of tissue capable of encircling any part of the fetus. Limb amputations, abdominal wall defects and malformations of the fetal skull are among the abnormalities that can result. In this disorder, cephaloceles do not have a single characteristic appearance or predictable location and often occur away from the midline. Other mechanisms may be responsible for the formation of a cephalocele, especially those in atypical locations.

Diagnosis

With cephaloceles, as with other open neural tube defects, alpha-fetoprotein (AFP) levels may be elevated in both amniotic fluid and maternal serum. Thus, potential cases of cephalocele may be referred to the sonologist as a result of AFP screening. If the lesion is covered with skin, however, both maternal and amniotic fluid AFP levels will be normal.

When scanned prenatally, a cephalocele appears as a sac-like protrusion from the head not covered by bone. The diagnosis can be made with certainty only if a bony defect in the skull is detected. When present, the position of the defect may be determined by using for orientation the bony structures of the face, the spine and (when possible) the midline echo of the brain. When the brain has herniated, the contents of the sac have a heterogeneous appearance. Large amounts of brain tissue are easily seen, but smaller amounts may be undetectable (**Figures 16, 17, 18**).

A diligent search for skull defects, using serial examinations if necessary, may help to improve diag-

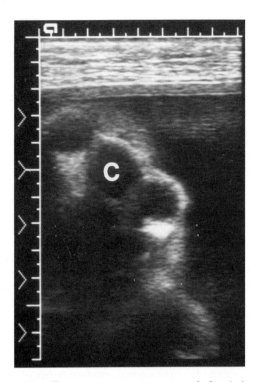

Figure 16. Transverse sonogram of fetal head demonstrating cephalocele (c) protruding between bony orbits resulting in hypertelorism. Reprinted with permission from Chervenak *et al.*[33]

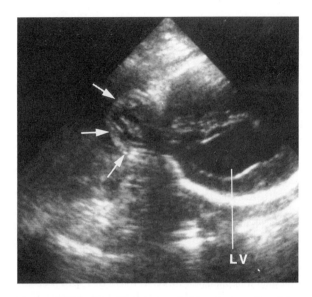

Figure 18a. Occipital encephalocele (outlined by arrows). LV, Dilated lateral ventricle.

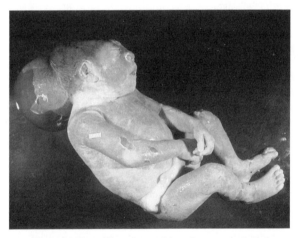

Figure 18b. Neonate with a large occipital enceptalocele.

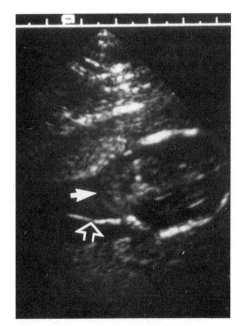

Figure 17. Sonogram demonstrating encephalocele (solid arrow) associated with amnion band (bottom arrow).

nostic accuracy. If a defect in the skull is still not found, the differential possibilities include cystic hygroma, teratoma and hemangioma, as well as cephalocele. It has been reported recently that fetal hair or a fetal ear can mimic the sonographic appearance of a cephalocele, emphasizing the importance of delineating a break in the skull.

Management Options

Once a cephalocele is diagnosed, the remainder of the fetal anatomy must be examined closely. Hydrocephalus is commonly seen. Since a second neural tube defect may be present, the spine should be examined in detail. In addition, cephaloceles may be present in association with a variety of genetic syndromes. Some features of these syndromes are currently detectable by ultrasound.

Several investigators have attempted to determine the prognosis of children with cephaloceles.[24,25] The larger series have focused on occipital lesions, but certain principles appear constant for all locations. The presence of brain in the protruding sac is the single most important discriminator.[24,25] Almost half of the infants with isolated cephaloceles have normal development after surgery. By contrast, the outlook is dismal for those children with microcephaly secondary to brain herniation. There are currently no good data regarding the significance of a small amount of brain in the sac. In the past, concurrent hydrocephalus was an adverse prognostic factor, but with modern shunt therapy it has less of an impact than the presence and amount of brain herniation. Frontal cephaloceles have a much better prognosis than those in other locations for several reasons. They tend to be smaller and so less brain herniates through, and the loss of frontal cortex produces fewer or less significant neurologic deficits. If a cephalocele is present concomitantly with other defects or as a part of certain severe genetic syndrome, the outlook is uniformly poor.

Labor/delivery

If a cephalocele is diagnosed before fetal viability, many parents will elect termination of pregnancy. After fetal viability has been reached, however, the mode of delivery at term becomes the critical issue. If a large amount of brain tissue is observed in the sac, and especially if one or more of the grave prognostic factors (i.e. microcephaly or associated anomalies) are also present, the parents should be counseled that the chance for a good outcome is remote, and cesarean section is avoided for fetal indication. In such cases, decompression of a large sac or associated hydrocephalus may be necessary to allow vaginal delivery.

There are, however, certain situations when cesarean delivery should be considered:

- a cephalocele sufficiently large and solid enough to cause dystocia;

- an isolated cephalocele is sonographically identified and the parents accept the risk of significant developmental defects. In such cases, cesarean delivery may theoretically minimize birth trauma and perhaps improve neonatal outcome. This approach is controversial.

Postnatal/prepregnancy

A cephalocele may develop as an isolated lesion or as a part of various syndromes, several with high recurrence risks. The most important of these is Meckel syndrome, which is characterized by polycystic kidneys, cephalocele and polydactyly, as well as a variety of other defects. Up to 5% of neural tube defects occur as part of the Meckel syndrome, which has an autosomal recessive pattern of inheritance. A cephalocele may also occur as a part of the Roberts, Chemke, Knoblock and cryptophthalmus syndromes and in dyssegmental dwarfism. These are all autosomal recessive disorders. In addition, cephaloceles have been reported with maternal warfarin ingestion.

The empiric risk for a cephalocele recurring in a subsequent pregnancy has been estimated as high as 5%. If, however, those cases appearing as a part of genetic syndromes – especially the Meckel syndrome – are excluded, the recurrence risk for cephaloceles may be as low as 1.7%.

HOLOPROSENCEPHALY

General

The term holoprosencephaly embraces a variety of cerebral abnormalities resulting from incomplete cleavage of the primitive prosencephalon, or forebrain (**Figure 19**). Various midline facial anomalies are closely

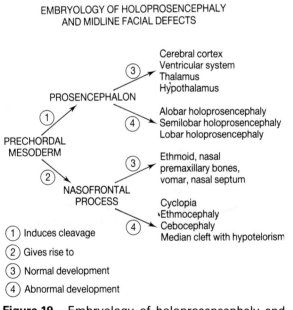

EMBRYOLOGY OF HOLOPROSENCEPHALY
AND MIDLINE FACIAL DEFECTS

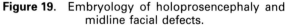

Figure 19. Embryology of holoprosencephaly and midline facial defects.

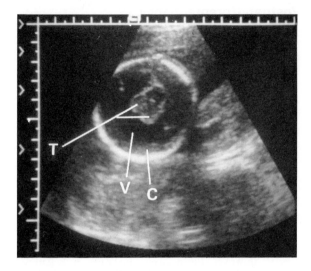

Figure 20a. Cranial sonogram demonstrating alobar holoprosencephaly V, Common ventricle; T, prominent fused thalamus; C, compressed cerebral cortex.

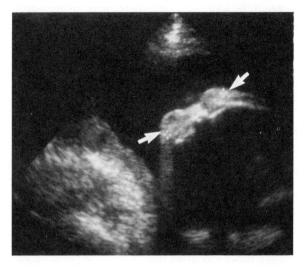

Figure 20b. Sonogram demonstrating hypotelorism (outlined by white arrows) in a fetus with a lobar holoprosencephaly.

associated with this entity. The incidence of holoprosencephaly has been reported to be between 1:5200 and 1:16 000 live births, but may affect as many as 0.4% of all conceptuses.

Holoprosencephaly is divided into alobar, semilobar and lobar categories, based on the degree of separation of the cerebral hemispheres. The alobar variety is the most severe, with no evidence of division of the cerebral cortex. The falx cerebri and interhemispheric fissure are absent. There is a common ventricle and only a rudimentary corpus callosum, if one is present at all. The semilobar and lobar varieties represent a higher degree of brain development, the semilobar having a partial separation of the hemispheres. There is much variability in the defects of the midline cerebral structures. Absent olfactory tracts and bulbs are usually associated with all of these conditions.

Diagnosis

Two intimately related abnormalities, namely hypotelorism and a single common ventricle, give rise to the sonographic markers of this abnormality: decreased intraorbital distance and absence of the midline echo (**Figures 20a, 20b**). In addition, the general appearance of the face, the position and configuration of the nose, and the integrity of the upper lip should be observed as they may define a specific facies of holoprosencephaly. It is not sufficient to see a central fluid collection in an abnormal brain, as it may also appear in hydranencephaly or a midline porencephalic cyst. Dif-

ferentiation of semilobar and lobar holoprosencephaly may not be possible before birth.

There are other anatomic aberrations related to holoprosencephaly that may be detected by prenatal ultrasound. These include hydrocephalus, midline facial cleft and polydactyly. Hydramnios may be a clinical feature.

Management Options

Prenatal

The prognosis for alobar holoprosencephaly is uniformly poor. Most infants die shortly after birth and the survivors have severe mental retardation.[26] Less is known about the prognosis in the lobar and semilobar varieties. A normal life-span has been reported for some, but many are severely mentally retarded.[26] It is possible that individuals with subtle forms of lobar holoprosencephaly with very little neurologic abnormality may exist without our knowledge.

Labor/delivery

The obstetric management of holoprosencephaly is dependent upon gestational age at the time of diagnosis. If this condition is detected prior to 24 weeks gestation, termination of pregnancy may be elected by the parents. In the third trimester, macrocephaly may prevent spontaneous vaginal delivery. To avoid cesarean delivery, cephalocentesis (see above) should be considered. The potentially destructive nature of this procedure must be explained to the parents.

Postnatal/prepregnancy

The diagnosis of holoprosencephaly signals the need for a careful postmortem and chromosomal determination to guide the management of future pregnancies. A chromosomal anomaly may predict either a recurrence risk of less than 1% (if a trisomy is demonstrated) or a much higher risk if the aneuploidy involves a translocation and one of the parents is a carrier of the translocation chromosomes.

In the absence of a chromosomal abnormality, an empiric recurrence risk of 6% has been calculated. However, some families may be faced with the 25% recurrence risk associated with autosomal recessive inheritance. It is usually impossible to identify these families, although co-sanguinity or a previously affected child may be suggestive. Rarely, autosomal dominant inheritance may be present, predicting a 50% recurrence rate. *Close examination of both parents of the proband for minor signs of midline facial anomaly (e.g. hypotelorism) is mandatory to rule out this possibility.* Finally, diabetes should be excluded as a cause (a 200–500 increase in the condition has been noted in such women).

MICROCEPHALY

General

Strictly translated, microcephaly means 'small head'. However, the clinical importance of the entity is its association with microencephaly (small brain) and mental retardation. At the present time, there is no universally accepted anthropometric definition of microcephaly. Some authors classify those infants with a head perimeter smaller than 2 SD below the mean as having microcephaly.[27] However, when this standard is used, the association with mental retardation is inconsistent. Three standard deviations below the mean for sex and age would appear to be a more reasonable criterion for the definition of microcephaly, since the correlation with mental retardation is stronger.[28]

Estimates of the incidence of microcephaly based on observations made at birth vary from 1:6250 to 1:8500 births. A much higher incidence, 1.6:1000 births was found in the US Collaborative Perinatal Project, when infants were observed through the first year of life.

Diagnosis

The way to determine that a head is small is to measure it. This simplistic remark belies the difficulty in accu-

rately determining when microcephaly is present and when it is clinically significant. Although the biparietal diameter (BPD) has been used in attempts to diagnose and exclude microcephaly, it carries a high false-positive rate. Thus, it is preferable to measure the head circumference. Serial examinations are especially important in suspected cases; measurable microcephaly may not be present during the second trimester.

Management Options

Prenatal

Since microcephaly can be a part of many malformation syndromes, a careful search using ultasound for other associated anomalies is warranted. Cortical mass may be decreased in microcephaly, leading to ventriculomegaly in the absence of obstructive hydrocephalus. In addition, a search for a cause should be made (teratogen exposure, family history, alcohol abuse, infections). The diagnosis of fetal infection may require both amniocentesis and cordocentesis.

It is difficult to make definitive statements concerning the prognosis of an entity with an unclear definition and multiple etiologies. Extreme caution should be used counseling parents. Several general remarks, however, can be made:

- The majority of microcephalic infants are mentally retarded, many severely.

- In general, the smaller the head, the worse the prognosis.

- If microcephaly occurs as part of certain genetic syndromes (e.g. Meckel syndrome), the outcome is uniformly poor.

- Despite very decreased head size, a child may be born with normal intelligence.

Labor/delivery

Uncomplicated vaginal delivery of a microcephalic child is to be expected. There exists, however, the possibility of shoulder dystocia due to incomplete dilatation of the cervix by a small fetal head.

Postnatal/prepregnancy

The risk of recurrence of microcephaly is dependent upon the underlying etiology. The search for an etiology should include a physical examination of the infant, maternal history of teratogenic exposure, careful family pedigree, chromosomal, microbiologic and serologic studies, and autopsy of stillborns and abortuses. It is increasingly recognized that alcohol is a common cause of mental retardation, often with microcephaly. If a chromosomal aberration of a defined genetic syndrome is identified, then that etiology defines the recurrence risk.

Several patterns of inheritance have been described within the subgroup of microcephaly without associated anomalies, i.e. 'true' microcephaly. These include autosomal recessive, autosomal dominant with incomplete penetrance, and sporadic.

Choroid Plexus Cyst

Small areas of cystic dilatation may be noted within the choroid plexus of the normal developing fetus (**Figure 21**). They are located in the choroid plexus of the lateral ventricles and generally resolve before the end of the second trimester without sequelae. A careful search for associated anomalies is indicated. An association with trisomy 18 and bilateral choroid plexus cysts has been described but not as yet confirmed. If no other abnormality is detected on ultrasound, then fetal karyotyping is not normally advised. However, careful counseling is required since there have been claims of aneuploidy in 1:200 cases. Further, a maternal serum AFP, hCG and estriol may prove useful (see Chapter 37).

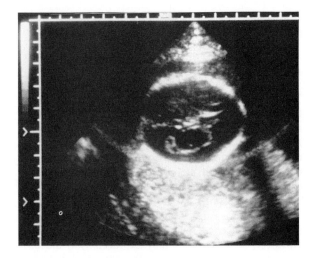

Figure 21b. Cranial sonogram demonstrating large choroid plexus cyst in a fetus with trisomy 18.

HYDRANENCEPHALY

General

Hydranencephaly is an intracranial anomaly characterized by replacement of the cerebral hemispheres with fluid covered by leptomeninges, dura mater, bone and skin. Only the basal ganglia and remnants of the mesencephalon remain within the normally formed skull above the tentorium cerebelli. The subtentorial structures are usually intact and the falx cerebri is frequently present.

Diagnosis

A ultrasound reveals a normal cranial vault filled with fluid. The cerebral cortex is absent, but a midline echo, the tentorium cerebelli and cerebellum may be visible. This disorder is differentiated from hydrocephalus, holoprosencephaly and porencephaly by the absence of cerebral cortex. In severe hydrocephalus, the thin cortical mantle may be hard to detect by ultrasound, and intrauterine computed tomography scanning or magnetic resonance imaging may be useful modalities to obtain a differential diagnosis (**Figure 22**).

Management Options

Most infants with hydranencephaly die within their first year. Severe retardation is uniformly present among survivors. Sporadic familial recurrences have been reported, but these are most exceptional and, in general, the recurrence risk should be considered negligible.

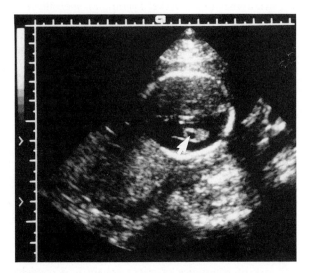

Figure 21a. Cranial sonogram demonstrating small choroid plexus cyst (arrow).

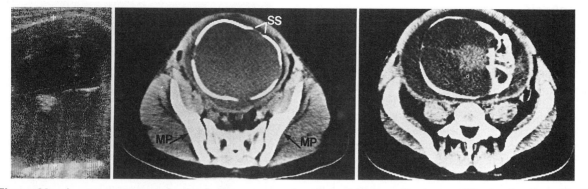

Figure 22. *In utero* computerized axial tomogram showing widening of sutures of fetal calvarium. Skull is filled by homogeneous low-density fluid with no evidence of cortex present. MP, Maternal pelvis; SS, separated suture. Reprinted with permission from Chervenak *et al.*[9]

DANDY-WALKER MALFORMATION

General

The neuropathology of the Dandy-Walker malformation is characterized by complete or partial absence of the cerebellar vermis and a posterior fossa cyst continuous with the fourth ventricle (**Figure 23**). Hydrocephalus is often present.

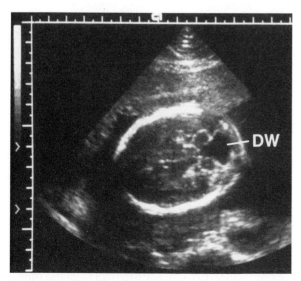

Figure 23. Cranial sonogram demonstrating Dandy-Walker cyst (DW) with defect in the cerebellar vermis.

Diagnosis

Dandy-Walker cysts appear on ultrasound as echo-spared areas in the posterior fossa. The cerebellar vermis, a bright echogenic midline structure caudal to the fourth ventricle, is absent or defective. Subsequently, the Dandy-Walker cyst can be seen in the posterior fossa to communicate with the fourth ventricle. Hydrocephalus involving all four cerebral ventricles is often observed in the fetus.

Management Options

While at one time the prognosis for all infants with the Dandy-Walker malformation was thought to be poor, a recent series of 40 infants showed greater than 80% survival with an IQ above 80 in almost all the survivors. For those cases diagnosed *in utero*, hydrocephalus and associated anomalies have been more common and the prognosis less favorable.

The Dandy-Walker malformation has been observed with increased frequency in families with a history of polycystic kidney disease and after the birth of a child with another central nervous system abnormality. Autosomal recessive inheritance has been suggested in some cases.

AGENESIS OF THE CORPUS CALLOSUM

General

The corpus callosum is the great commissural plate of nerve fibers interconnecting the cortical hemispheres. It lies at the depths of the interhemispheric fissure and curves in the midline just above to form the roof of the third ventricle.

Diagnosis

Agenesis of the corpus callosum is very difficult to diagnose *in utero* unless coronal or midline sagittal scans can be obtained to evaluate this structure. On midline sagittal scan, it appears as a hypoechoic structure below the pericallosal cistern where it forms the roof of the cavum septi pellucidi and cavum vergae. On coronal scan, it may be visualized as a hypoechoic structure above the lateral ventricles and beneath the pericallosal cistern. Failure to find it may suggest agenesis of the corpus callosum (**Figures 24 a–c**).

The corpus callosum itself cannot be seen on transverse scans, and it is necesary to search for associated anatomic abnormalities. These have included lateral displacement of the bodies of the lateral ventricle, enlargement of the atria and occipital horns and enlargement or upward displacement of the third ventricle in most reported cases (**Figures 25a, b**).

Management Options

Absence of the corpus callosum may occur as an isolated entity, or with other central nervous system lesions. The most consistent group of associated defects are those of the holoprosencephalic series.

The prognosis for a fetus with agenesis of the corpus callosum is highly variable and dependent upon associated defects. Management should be based on these underlying anomalies. Agenesis of the corpus callosum has been reported as an incidental autopsy finding in intellectually normal adults[29] and caution should be exercised in counseling patients when an isolated agenesis of the corpus callosum is suspected on ultrasound.

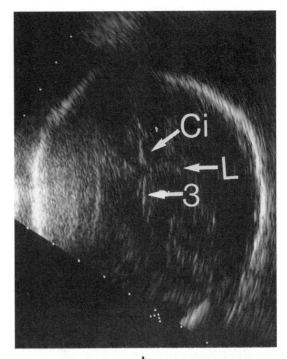

b

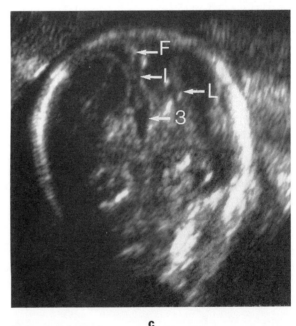

c

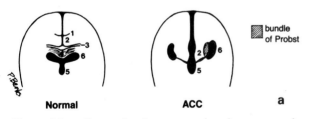

Figure 24a. Coronal diagrams showing normal anatomy and agenesis of the corpus callosum (1 = cingulate sulcus, 2 = cingulate gyrus, 3 = pericallosal cistern, 4 = corpus callosum, 5 = third ventricle, 6 = lateral ventricle.) Note that in ACC the third ventricle directly communicates with the interhemispheric fissure and that the lateral ventricle points upward instead of to the side. Reprinted with permission from Comstock.[34]

Figure 24b,c. Coronal scans of the fetal brain through the level of the third ventricle. (b) normal, (c) agenesis of the corpus callosum (3 = third ventricle, L = lateral ventricle, F = falx, I = interhemispheric fissure, CI = cingulate gyrus.) Note the rhomboid, instead of slit-shaped, third ventricle in ACC. Reprinted with permission from Comstock.[34]

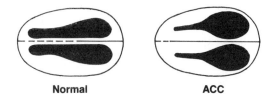

Figure 25a. Schematic representation of agenesis of the corpus callosum in transverse view.

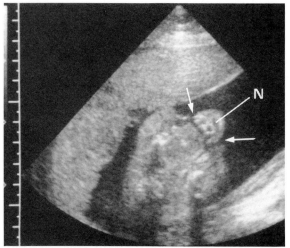

Figure 26. Sonogram along an oblique plane through lower part of fetal face demonstrating bilateral cleft lip (arrows). N, Nose.

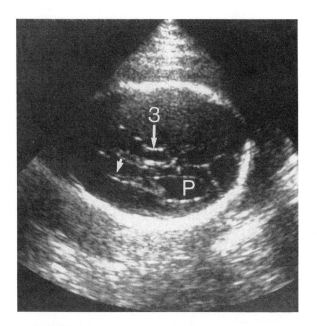

Figure 25b. Transverse sonogram of fetus with agenesis of the corpus callosum. The medial walls of the anterior horns are pushed away from the falx toward the lateral wall (arrow). The posterior horns are dilated (P) and the third ventricle is dilated and elevated (3). Reprinted with permission from Comstock.[34]

FACIAL CLEFTS

Diagnosis

In order to demonstrate a facial cleft before birth, the lower portion of the face must be anterior and clearly visualized (**Figure 26**). Both sagittal and oblique coronal planes of study may be useful. Undulating tongue movements, hypertrophied tissue at the edge of the cleft, and hypertelorism have all been described as useful adjuncts in the diagnosis of a facial cleft. An intact lip does not indicate an intact palate.

Management Options

After a facial cleft is identified, it is important to look carefully for ultrasonic evidence of other anomalies. Fetal karyotyping is recommended. The prognosis and management depends on the associated abnormality. If the clefting appears to be isolated, then the prognosis is excellent with plastic surgical correction being offered in early infancy. Difficulty with feeding may be experienced before such surgery occurs, but this is usually surmountable with the use of specially designed artificial palates for feeding.

CYSTIC HYGROMAS

General

Cystic hygromas are congenital malformations of the lymphatic system (**Figure 27a**), appearing as single or multiloculated fluid-filled cavities lined by true epithelium. In fetal life, they are associated with a generalized disorder of lymphatic formation. Cystic hygromas may occur as isolated defects or as a manifestation of a variety of genetic syndromes (**Figure 27b**). The incidence of this disorder has not been determined.

Diagnosis

Cystic hygromas may be diagnosed reliably by ultrasound. Their posterolateral position and cystic appearance are characteristic. Larger hygromas are frequently

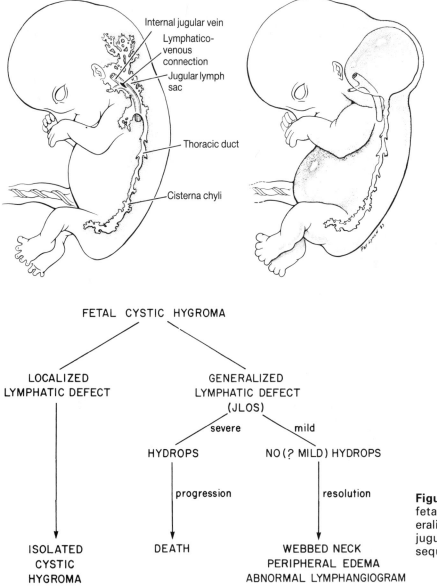

Figure 27a. Lymphatic system in a normal fetus (left) with a patent connection between the jugular lymph sac and the internal jugular vein and a cystic hygroma and hydrops from a failed lymphaticovenous connection (right). Reprinted with permission from Chervenak *et al.*[35]

Figure 27b. Natural history of fetal cystic hygroma. Generalized lymphatic results from jugular-lymphatic-obstruction sequence (JLOS). Reprinted with permission from Chervenak *et al.*[35]

divided by random, incomplete septa and they often have a dense midline septum extending from the fetal neck across the full width of the hygromas (**Figure 28a**). Fetal hydrops is often seen in association with cystic hygromas, as both may result from a defect in lymphatic formation (**Figure 28b**).

Sonographic features that differentiate cystic hygromas from other craniocervical masses (e.g. cephalocele or other neural tube defects, cystic teratoma, twin sac of a blighted ovum or nuchal edema) include the following: an intact skull and spinal column, and lack of a solid component to the mass, a constant position of the mass relative to the fetal head, and cysts separated by septa.

Management Options

Prenatal

Once a cystic hygroma is detected, a careful ultrasonic search is indicated for fetal skin edema, ascites, pleural and pericardial effusions, and cardiac or renal anomalies. The mother and fetus should be investigated as for non-immune fetal hydrops (see Chapter 45). This includes a fetal karyotype. The prognosis and management depend on the underlying cause and any associated abnormalities. If hydrops is present and no treatable cause is found, then the outlook is grave. Isolated

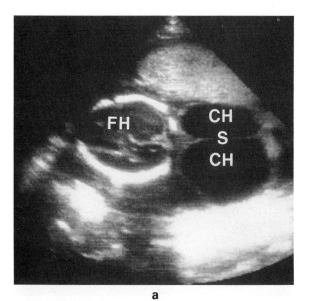

a

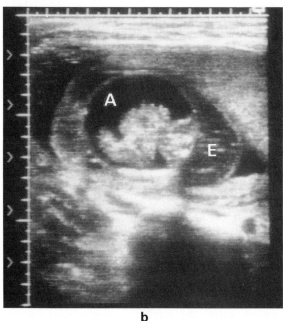

b

Figure 28 (a). Sonogram demonstrating nuchal cystic hygroma (CH), divided by midline septum (S). FH, Fetal head. **(b).** Transverse sonogram through fetal abdomen demonstrating fetal hydrops. E, Edema of abdominal wall; A, ascites.

cystic hygromas may be surgically corrected and have a good prognosis for survival.

It is possible that some cystic hygromas may regress *in utero*, leaving only a webbed neck. Such a mechanism has been postulated to account for neck webbing seen in patients with Turner's syndrome. If this is the case, some cystic hygromas must have a more favorable prognosis.

Labor/delivery

It is possible that termination of pregnancy will be chosen by the parents if the diagnosis is made before viability and especially if there is untreatable hydrops or an associated lethal malformation. When the decision has been taken to continue with pregnancy and the hygroma is so large that it potentially could interfere with delivery, there may be a role for transabdominal needle aspiration of cyst fluid. There is no evidence cesarean section *a priori* improves outcome.

Prenatal/prepregnancy

A careful postmortem is mandatory and tissue for cytogenic studies should be obtained where there is an aborted or stillborn fetus, from fetal membranes or from the newborn baby. Because these fetuses may have chromosomal mosaicism, several tissues should be studied. The counseling that is necessary following the pregnancy will depend on the underlying cause.

SPINA BIFIDA

General

Spina bifida refers to a defect in the spine resulting from a failure of both halves of the vertebral arch to fuse with each other. These lesions usually occur in the lumbo-sacral and cervical regions, but they may involve any segment of or all of the spine. If the meninges protrude through this defect, the lesion is designated a meningocele; if neural tissue is included, it is a meningomyelocele. The incidence of spina bifida varies greatly in different parts of the world, ranging from 0.3:1000 births in Japan to more than 4:1000 births in part of the UK. In the USA, there is an average incidnce of spina bifida of approximately 0.5:1000 births.

Spina bifida is also associated with the Arnold-Chiari malformation, wherein the cerebellar vermis, fourth ventricle and medulla are displaced caudally, obstructing CSF flow and resulting in hydrocephalus (90–95% of cases).

Diagnosis

Two important diagnostic tools are available to aid the search for neural tube defects: ultrasound and alpha-fetoprotein (AFP) determination (see Chapter 37). On ultrasound, spina bifida appears as a splaying of the posterior ossification centers of the spine, producing a

U-shaped vertebra (**Figures 29,30**). Normally, the spine progressively narrows as you scan caudally. The posterior ossification centers in a defective vertebra will be more widely spaced than those in vertebrae above and below the defect. Although spina bifida can be visualized on longitudinal scanning with loss of skin continuity in open defects, meticulous transverse examination of the entire vertebral column is necessary to detect smaller defects. In the third trimester, posterior vertebral elements, including the laminae and spinous processes, are normally visible sonographically. The absence of these structures further supports the diagnosis of spina bifida.

The Arnold-Chiari malformation can serve as an important marker for spina bifida. Two characteristic sonographic signs (the 'lemon' and the 'banana') of the Arnold-Chiari malformation have been described. (**Figure 31**). Scalloping of the frontal bones gives a lemon-like configuration to the skull of an affected fetus in axial section during the second trimester (**Figure 32**). The caudal displacement of the cranial contents within a pliable skull is thought to produce this effect. Similarly, as the cerebellar hemispheres are displaced into the cervical canal, they are flattened rostrocaudally and the cisterna magna is obliterated,

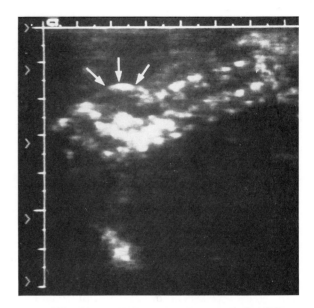

Figure 30. Longitudinal sonogram of fetal spine with arrows pointing to meningomyelocele.

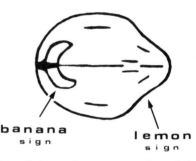

Figure 31. Schematic representation of the 'lemon' and 'banana' signs described by Nicolaides.[37]

thereby producing a flattened, centrally curved, banana-like sonographic appearance (**Figure 33**). In extreme cases, the cerebellar hemispheres may be absent from view during fetal head scanning.

It is currently controversial whether ultrasound alone is sufficient to evaluate an elevated maternal serum alpha-fetoprotein. The author agrees with others that amniocentesis is not routinely necessary to evaluate the elevated maternal serum alpha-fetoprotein provided the ultrasound examination is one of quality.[30]

Management Options

Prenatal

The prognosis in cases of spina bifida is dependent upon a number of factors. Most important are the pres-

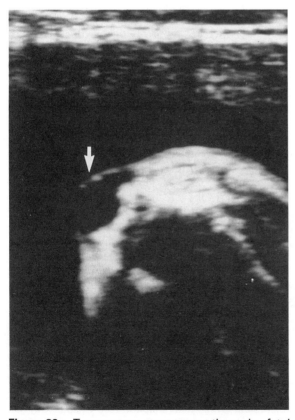

Figure 29. Transverse sonogram through fetal spine with arrow pointing to meningomyelocele.

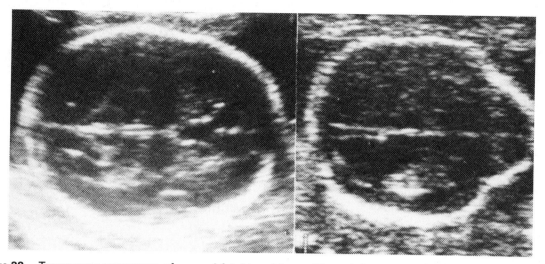

Figure 32. Transverse sonogram of normal fetal head in an 18 week fetus at level of cavum septi pellucidi (left). Transverse section of fetal head at level of cavum septi pellucidi in an 18 week fetus with open spina bifida showing 'lemon' sign (right). Reprinted with permission from Nicolaides *et al.*[36]

ence or absence of neural tissue in the meningeal sac and the spinal level and extent of the lesion. Lower extremity paralysis and incontinence of bowel and bladder are common and intelligence may be affected.

The outlook for spina bifida has changed. Over 90% of infants born with the condition survive long-term, and it is appreciated that many of these will grow to be productive adults with normal intelligence. Early closure of defects, ventriculo-peritoneal shunting of hydrocephalus, and management of urinary and fecal incontinence by surgery, dietary management and

biofeedback techniques, are in part responsible for these improvements. However, the obstetrician, faced with the diagnosis in pregnancy, is advised to be cautious and not present an over-optimistic outlook. The infants now born with the condition are a selected group; arguably, the more obvious and severe forms often end in termination at an early stage. Certainly the prognosis for those infants who are severely affected remains serious, with gross permanent multisystem defects. At present, it is impossible to predict in the first half of pregnancy, when the diagnosis is often

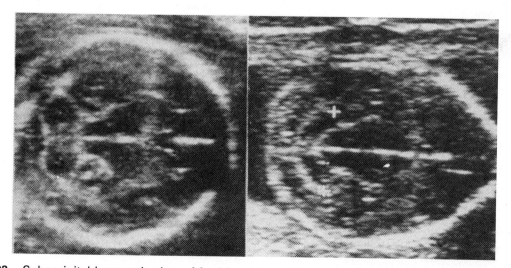

Figure 33. Suboccipital bregmatic view of fetal head in an 18 week fetus with normal cerebellum and cisterna magna (left). Suboccipital bregmatic view of fetal head in an 18 week fetus with open spina bifida demonstrating 'banana' sign (+) (right). Reprinted with permission from Nicolaides *et al.*[37]

CRANIOSPINAL AND FACIAL DEFECTS: HEAD
Summary of Management Options

HEAD

ANENCEPHALY

Prenatal

- Offer termination, induction of labor

Postnatal/prepregnancy

- Necroscopy
- Counseling
- Periconceptual folate

HYDROCEPHALY
Prenatal

- Search for other anomalies, karyotype
- Cautious counseling regarding prognosis if isolated
- Termination may be chosen by parents
- In continuing pregnancy:
  - serial scans for progressive dilatation
  - deliver fetus when risks of prematurity low
  - interdisciplinary care

Labor/delivery

- No evidence of which route is preferable
- Cephalocentesis is potentially destructive

Postnatal/prepregnancy

- Establish cause/type
- Counseling

CEPHALOCELE
Prenatal

- Consider termination
- Search for the defects, especially hydrocephalus

Labor/delivery

- Vaginal route

Postnatal/prepregnancy

- Necroscopy to establish whether isolated
- Counseling

HOLOPROSENCEPHALY
Prenatal

- Offer termination, induction of labor

Labor/delivery

- Vaginal delivery

Postnatal/pregnancy

- Necroscopy
- Karyotype
- Family history
- Screen for diabetes
- Counseling

MICROCEPHALY

Prenatal

- Careful search for other anomalies
- History of teratogens, alcohol, family, infection
- Caution with counseling

Labor/delivery

- Vaginal delivery
- Beware shoulder dystocia

Postnatal/prepregnancy

- Establish cause/type (teratogens, alcohol, family history, karyotype, infection serology, necroscopy)
- Counseling depending on cause

CHOROID PLEXUS CYST

Prenatal

- Careful search on ultrasound for other anomalies
- Karyotype if other anomalies found
- Careful counseling; usually benign if isolated findings (? 1:2000 risk of aneuploidy)

HYDRANENCEPHALY

Prenatal

- Offer termination, induction of labor

DANDY-WALKER SYNDROME

Prenatal

- Cautious counseling, prognosis difficult to predict

AGENESIS OF CORPUS CALLOSUM

Prenatal

- Careful search for other anomalies
- Counseling depends on other lesion: prognosis difficult to predict

---

CRANIOSPINAL AND FACIAL DEFECTS: FACE, NECK AND SPINE
Summary of Management Options

FACE

FACIAL DEFECTS

Prenatal

- Careful search for other anomalies

- Prognosis depends on cause (good if isolated)

NECK

CYSTIC HYGROMAS

Prenatal

- Investigate as for non-immune hydrops (Chapter 45)

- Prognosis and management depend on cause

- Termination may be chosen

Labor/delivery

- If pregnancy continues, aspiration of fluid may allow vaginal delivery; cesarean section is alternative

Postnatal/pregnancy

- Establish cause

- Counseling

SPINE

SPINA BIFIDA

Prenatal

- Prognosis difficult to predict

- Termination may be chosen by parents

- If pregnancy continues:
  - interdisciplinary approach
  - watch for development of hydrocephalus

Labor/delivery

- If pregnancy continues, optimal route of delivery is not known but cesarean delivery should be offered

- Care with delivery of back

Postnatal/prepregnancy

- Counseling

- Periconceptual folic acid

---

made, the prognosis for the baby. Most patients will opt for a termination of pregnancy.

If meningomyelocele is diagnosed in the third trimester, or if the option of pregnancy termination is declined when meningomyelocele is diagnosed earlier, a team approach – consisting of obstetrician, pediatric neurosurgeon, pediatric neurologist and neonatolo-gist – is advisable for optimum perinatal outcome. In addition, an actively involved perinatal social worker can provide invaluable support to the family both before and after birth.

Fetal surveillance consists of fetal heart rate monitoring and serial sonography to assess fetal growth, head size and severity of ventriculomegaly. Some obstetricians advise that unless an obstetric indication takes precedence, delivery should occur after documentation of fetal lung maturity.

Labor/delivery

There is no conclusive clinical information relating to the optimal route of delivery for the fetus with meningomyelocele. A randomized trial to study this question is unlikely. The best clinical study to date indicated that elective cesarean delivery before the onset of labor improved outcome in terms of functional level of spine defect. However, this study had flaws, not the least a biased control group. Subsequently, cesarean section should be offered to the parents only as a potentially beneficial procedure. If the lower uterine segment is well-developed, a low transverse incision is possible. After the head is delivered, the bisacromial diameter is positioned horizontally. Both fetal flanks are grasped, and gentle traction is applied in an outward direction away from the uterine wall near the meningomyelocele. The assistant retracts the edge of the uterine incision as the body of the infant is delivered.

After labor, there is no benefit to cesarean delivery. The recurrence risk after the birth of an affected child for any isolated open neural tube defect, including spina bifida, may be as low as 1.7% in the USA. In populations in which spina bifida is more prevalent, the recurrence risk may be higher. Where the neural tube defect is part of another syndrome, then the recurrence risk may be considerably higher (e.g. 25% for Meckel syndrome).

Postnatal/prepregnancy

The risk of recurrence in an isolated neural tube defect appears to be significantly reduced by periconceptual maternal folate therapy (5 mg orally three times a day). This should be offered to all women who have had a baby with anencephaly or spina bifida.

REFERENCES

1 Pretorius DH, Drose JA, Marco-Johnson ML (1986) Fetal lateral ventricular ratio determination during the second trimester. *Journal of Clinical Ultrasound* 5:121–124.

2 Cardoza JD, Goldstein RB, Filly RA (1988) Exclusion of fetal ventriculomegaly with a single measurement: The width of the lateral ventricular atrium. *Radiology* 169:711–714.

3 Jeanty P, Dramaix-Wilmet M, Delbeke D *et al.* (1982) Fetal ocular biometry by ultrasound. *Radiology* 143:513–516.

4 Brackbill Y (1971) The role of the cortex in orienting:

5 Chervenak FA, Farley MA, Walters LE et al. (1984) When is termination of pregnancy during the third trimester morally justifiable? *New England Journal of Medicine* 310:501–504.

6 Truog RD, Fletcher JC (1989) Anencephalic newborns. Can organs be transplanted before brain death? *New England Journal of Medicine* 321:388–390.

7 Medearis DN, Holmes LB. (1989) On the use of anencephalic infants as organ donors. *New England Journal of Medicine* 321:391–393.

8 Drugan A, Krause B, Canady A *et al.* (1989) The natural history of prenatally diagnosed cerebral ventriculomegaly. *Journal of the American Medical Association* 261:1785–1788.

9 Chervenak FA, Berkowitz RL, Romero R *et al.* (1983) The diagnosis of fetal hydrocephalus. *American Journal of Obstetrics and Gynecology* 147:703–716.

10 Pretorius DH, Drose JA, Manco-Johnson ML (1986) Fetal lateral ventricular ratio determination during the second trimester. *Journal of Ultrasound in Medicine* 5:121–124.

11 Hertzberg BS, Bowie JD, Burger PC *et al.* (1987) The three lines: Origin of sonographic landmarks in the fetal head. *American Journal of Radiography* 149:1009–1012.

12 Benacerraf BR, Birnholz JC (1987) The diagnosis of fetal hydrocephalus prior to 22 weeks. *Journal of Clinical Ultrasound* 15:531–536.

13 Cardoza JD, Filly RA, Podarsky AE (1988) The dangling choroid plexus: A sonographic observation of value in excluding ventriculomegaly. *American Journal of Radiography* 151:767–770.

14 Mahony BS, Nyberg DA, Hirsch JH *et al.* (1988) Mild idiopathic lateral cerebral ventricular dilatation in utero: Sonographic evaluation. *Radiology* 169:715–721.

15 Laurence KM, Coates S (1962) The natural history of hydrocephalus. *Archives of Diseases of Childhood* 37:345–362.

16 Raimondi AJ, Soare P (1974) Intellectual development in shunted hydrocephalic children. *American Journal of Diseases of Children* 127:664.

17 Lorber J (1968) The results of early treatment of extreme hydrocephalus. *Development Medicine and Child Neurology* (Suppl) 16:21–29.

18 Pretorius DH, David K, Manco-Johnson ML *et al.* (1985) Clinical course of fetal hydrocephalus: 40 cases. *American Journal of Radiology* 144:827–831.

19 Chervenak FA, Berkowitz RL, Tortora M *et al.* (1985) Management of fetal hydrocephalus. *American Journal of Obstetrics and Gynecology* 151:933–942.

20 Manning FA, Harrison MR, Rodeck C *et al.* (1986) Catheter shunts for fetal hydronephrosis and hydrocephalus. *New England Journal of Medicine* 315:336–340.

21 Glick PL, Harrison MR, Halks-Miller M *et al.* (1984) Correction of congenital hydrocephalus *in utero*. II. Efficacy of *in utero* shunting. *Journal of Pediatric Surgery* 19:870–871.

22 Smith DW (1982) *Recognizable Patterns of Human*

Orienting reflex in an anencephalic infant. *Development Psychology* 5:195–203.

Malformation 3rd edn. Philadelphia: W.B. Saunders, p. 617.

23 Lorber J, De NC (1970) Family history of congenital hydrocephalus. *Developmental Medicine and Child Neurology* (Suppl) **22**:94–100.

24 Mealey J, Ozenitis AJ, Hockley AA (1970) The prognosis of encephaloceles. *Journal of Neurosurgery* **32**:209–218.

25 Field B (1974) The child with an encephalocele. *Medical Journal of Australia* **1**:700–703.

26 Matsunaga E, Shiota K (1977) Holoprosencephaly in human embryos: Epidemiologic studies of 150 cases. *Teratology* **16**:261–272.

27 Avery GB, Menesses L, Lodge A (1972) The critical significance of "measurement microcephaly." *American Journal of Diseases of Children* **123**:214–217.

28 Bell WE (1977) Abnormalities in size and shape of the head. In *Diseases of the Newborn* 4th edn, pp. 717–719, Shaffer AJ, Avery ME (eds) Philadelphia: W.B. Saunders.

29 Babcock DS (1984) The normal, absent, and abnormal corpus callosum: Sonographic findings. *Radiology* **151**:449–453.

30 Nadel AS, Green JK, Holmes LB, *et al.* (1990) Absence of need for amniocentesis in patients with elevated levels of maternal serum alpha-fetoprotein and normal ultrasonographic examinations. *New England Journal of Medicine* **323**:557–567.

31 Chervenak FA, Isaacson G, Lorber J (1988) *Anomalies of the Fetal Head, Neck, and Spine: Ultrasound Diagnosis and Management* Philadelphia: W.B. Saunders. 1988.

32 Isaacson G (1984) Postmortem examination of infant brains. Techniques for removal, fixation, and sectioning. *Archives of Pathological and Laboratory Medicine* **108**:80–81.

33 Chervenak FA, Isaacson G, Rosenberg JC *et al.* (1986) Antenatal diagnosis of frontal cephalocele in a fetus with atelosteogenesis. *Journal of Ultrasound in Medicine* **5**:111–113.

34 Comstock C (1992). Agenesis of the corpus callosum in the fetus: Diagnosis and significance. *The Female Patient* **17**:40–45.

35 Chervenak FA, Isaacson G, Blakemore KJ *et al.* (1983) Fetal cystic hygroma. Cause and natural history. *New England Journal of Medicine* **309**:822–825.

36 Nicolaides KH, Campbell S, Gabbe SG, Guidetti R (1986) Ultrasound screening for spina bifida. Cranial and cerebellar signs. *Lancet* **2**:72–74.

51

Genitourinary Malformations

WOLFGANG HOLZGREVE, PETER MINY, MARK I. EVANS

INTRODUCTION

Anomalies of the fetal genitourinary tract are usually easily recognized by ultrasonography, since many have in common anomalous, fluid-filled spaces within the fetus. Frequently, functional renal impairment and/or outflow obstruction leads to oligo- or ahydramnios. In instances of fetal ovarian cysts or uterine anomalies, normal urinary tract and amniotic fluid volumes can be expected. The incidence of urinary tract malformations at birth, excluding hypospadias, is about 0.3%,[1] whereas in a prospective ultrasound study the incidence *in utero* was 0.65.[2] Large ovarian cysts are rare and comprise only about 1% of all tumors in childhood.[3]

Genitourinary malformations present in one of the following ways:

- chance finding on ultrasound examination

- oligohydramnios detected clinically

- family history of risk.

The conditions that will be considered in this section are:

- Renal agenesis/severe hypoplasia

- Urinary dilatation

  - ureteropelvic junction (UPJ or PUJ) obstruction

  - ureterovesical junction (UVJ or VUJ) obstruction

  - urethral obstruction (megacystis)

  - megaureter

  - reflux

- Renal cysts

  - autosomal recessive (infantile) polycystic kidney disease (Potter type I)

  - multicystic dysplastic kidney disease (Potter type II)

  - autosomal dominant (adult) polycystic kidney disease (Potter type III)

  - cystic renal dysplasia (Potter type IV)

  - syndromes associated with renal cysts

- Crossed renal ectopia and pelvic kidney

- Renal tumors

- Ambiguous genitalia

DIAGNOSIS

General Approach

If urinary tract abnormalities are sought or suspected, then the following checklist is helpful:

- Ultrasonic assessment of amniotic fluid volume. If oligohydramnios is found and there is no history of membrane rupture or evidence of growth deficiency, then urinary abnormalities should be strongly suspected.

- Ultrasonic examination for dilatation of the urinary tract. There is debate as to the definition of 'dilatation'. Some authors advocate pelvicalyceal dilatation of > 5 mm, whereas others recommend 10 mm as the threshold for diagnosis. Certainly if dilatation of 6–9 mm is identified, then careful evaluation as outlined in this checklist should be undertaken. If no other abnormal features are identified, it may be reasonable to repeat the scan after a 1–2 week interval before being certain about the significance of the observation. If dilatation is found, it is important to determine which portion of the system is dilated or if there has been decompression producing ascites or a urinoma.

- Ultrasonic examination for renal cysts.

- The size, shape and echogenicity of the kidneys should be assessed with ultrasound.

- The presence of the bladder should be determined with ultrasound.

- A general ultrasound examination of the fetus should be performed to look for other associated abnormalities suggestive of a syndrome and, if necessary, fetal karyotyping considered.

Prenatal Ultrasound and Laboratory Studies of Renal Function

Fetal urine is produced from 13 weeks gestation onward and consists of an ultrafiltrate of the fetal serum with subsequent selective tubular reabsorption of sodium and chloride. The levels of sodium and chloride normally fall progressively throughout gestation.[4] One retrospective study[5] suggested that urinary sodium levels above 100 mmol/l, chloride above 90 mmol/l and osmolarity above 210 mOsm generally were associated with insufficient tubular reabsorption capacity and irreversibly damaged kidneys at birth. It is unclear how biased these conclusions were by gestational age. Lenz *et al.*[6] found that high concentrations of neutral amino acids in the fetal urine reflected poor tubular capacity and are predictive of irreversibly destroyed kidneys.

Like others,[7,8] we have found that these parameters are not always able to select correctly those cases in which prenatal drainage of an obstructed urinary tract might be beneficial. In the postnatal as well as in the prenatal period, proteinuria is caused either by a pathologic process in the glomeruli and/or by damage in the tubular reabsorption capacity. The site and degree of the underlying lesions in kidneys with pathologic proteinuria can be identified by puncturing the dilated fetal bladder (**Figure 1a**) and separating the urinary proteins by polyacrylamide gel electrophoresis with sodium dodecyl sulfate as detergent (SDS-PAGE) (**Figure 1b**).[9] The color-coded Doppler sonography of the renal artery (**Figure 2**) may also be helpful in clarifying the prognosis of the fetal kidney by assessing the vascular peripheral resistance in the renal parenchyma, since presumably a damaged kidney will have higher resistance to flow than a normal kidney. Measurement of urinary output is largely a research tool at present.

Using the above general and specific approaches, it should be possible to define a differential diagnosis, though the precise diagnosis may not be possible until after delivery (see **Table 1**).

RISKS ASSOCIATED WITH GENITOURINARY MALFORMATIONS

Renal Agenesis

The incidence is approximately 1:3000 to 1:10000 births with a recurrence risk of 2–5%. It is presumed in most cases to be associated with a polygenic inheritance, though some cases inherited as X-linked recessive, autosomal recessive and autosomal dominant have been reported. Unilateral renal agenesis is probably much more common than bilateral agenesis, though because the diagnosis can be missed its true incidence is difficult to determine. Furthermore, provided the contralateral kidney is working normally, the prognosis for the fetus/baby is excellent without the need for any specific management.

Bilateral renal agenesis will result in the typical combination of pulmonary hypoplasia, limb deformities and Potter's facies. Oligohydramnios has been reported as early as 14 weeks. However, the kidneys do not become the major source of amniotic fluid until

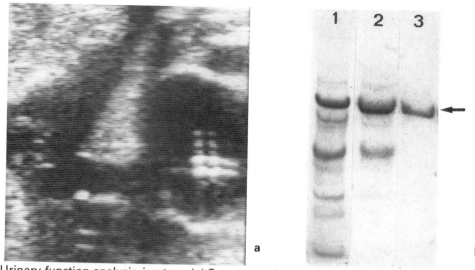

Figure 1. Urinary function analysis *in utero*. (a) Sonogram during puncture of 'key-hole' bladder. The tip of the needle can be recognized in the megacystis. (b) SDS-PAGE analysis of fetal urine samples obtained between 18 and 20 weeks gestation *in utero*. Protein bands are characterized by their mobility in relation to urine albumin (arrow). Severe tubular damage is expressed by the presence of at least six microproteins (molecular weight 10–40 kDa, lower half of the gel), exceeding the amount of macroproteins. Lane 1, fetus with irreversibly damaged kidney (Potter type IV dysplasia) due to urethral obstruction; lane 2, fetus with mild tubular damage who subsequently had successful *in utero* placement of vesicoamniotic shunt; lane 3, normal fetus for control.

14–16 weeks; thus the presence of apparently normal amniotic fluid volume between 10 and 14 weeks does not preclude the diagnosis. Approximately 15% of fetuses with bilateral renal agenesis have associated abnormalities. However, even without these, the outcome is fatal.

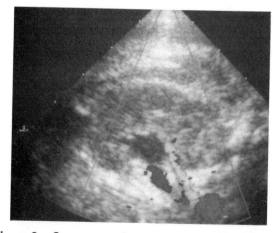

Figure 2. Sonogram of mild calyceal dilatation in a fetal kidney. The color-coded Doppler sonography allows easy identification of the renal artery and vein.

URINARY DILATATION

Ureteropelvic Junction (UPJ) Obstruction

This probably represents the most common cause of neonatal hydronephrosis and 20–50% of all urological disorders diagnosed before birth. It is more common in males. It is usually sporadic with a low risk of recurrence, though familial cases have been reported.

Unilateral UPJ obstruction may occur with contralateral renal agenesis or multicystic dysplasia, both of which can result in severe oligohydramnios if the UPJ obstruction is severe. In the extreme, a urinoma or urinary ascites may be seen. These are all poor prognostic features and there are limited prenatal therapeutic options in such circumstances.

Even in the absence of these urological abnormalities, associated anomalies have been reported in the gastrointestinal, skeletal, central nervous and adrenal systems. In such circumstances, the nature of these defects often determines the prognosis.

In contrast, if there is a normal amniotic fluid volume and no associated abnormality, the prognosis is generally good. There is probably no indication for prenatal therapeutic intervention. The advantage of identifying the abnormality before birth is that accurate

Table 1
Diagnosis of urinary tract abnormalities

Amniotic fluid	Dilated renal tract	Renal cysts	Kidneys	Bladder	Other anomaly
Renal agenesis/severe hypoplasia					
Absent > 14/weeks	No	No	Absent	Absent	Yes (15%)
Urinary dilatation					
UPJ obstruction					
Normal if no other lesion	Yes	Rarely multicystic	Normal if no other lesion	Normal if no other lesion	Yes
UVJ obstruction, megaureter, reflux					
Normal in most cases	Yes	Rarely cystic dysplastic	Rarely agenesis	Normal in most cases	Yes
Urethral obstruction, megacystis					
Absent usually	Yes	Cystic dysplastic	Hyperechogenic	Enlarged with dilated proximal urethra	Yes
Renal cysts					
Autosomal recessive (infantile) polycystic kidney disease (Potter type I)					
Absent if severe	No	Rarely visible	Enlarged, hyperechogenic	Absent if severe	Liver disease
Multicystic dysplastic kidney disease (Potter type II)					
Absent if bilateral	No	Variable in size	Type IIA = large; type IIB = normal	Absent if bilateral	Yes
Autosomal dominant (adult) polycystic kidney disease (Potter type III)					
Normal	No	Variably visible	Enlarged, hyperechogenic	Present	Cysts in other organs
Cystic renal dysplasia (Potter type IV)					
Absent if bilateral	Yes	Cortical size variable	Hyperechogenic	Dilated	Yes
Syndromes associated with renal cysts The renal tract appearances and associated anomalies depend upon the syndrome					
Crossed renal ectopia and pelvic kidney					
Normal usually	Rare	No	Abnormal size, shape location	Present	Yes
Renal/adrenal tumors					
Often excess fluid	No	No	Large mass in kidney or adrenal	Present	No

diagnosis, assessment of renal function and screening for urinary infection can be implemented in the newborn period. Spontaneous improvement in the condition can occur though surgery will be necessary at some stage in infancy in approximately 90%.

Megaureter, Reflux

A dilated ureter is more common in males and generally has a low risk of recurrence irrespective of the cause. However, familial cases of vesicoureteric reflux have been reported. While the ultrasonic diagnosis of ureteric dilatation is not difficult, prenatal differentiation of the various types/causes is less easy.

Other urological problems are more common with ureteric dilatation, including ectopic ureterocele, contralateral renal agenesis or dysplasia and duplicated collecting systems. Hirschsprung's disease has also been reported to be more common.

The prognosis in these cases is difficult to predict prenatally. Clearly, if there is bilateral hydronephrosis with oligohydramnios, the prognosis is poor. But even with normal amniotic fluid volume, the need for surgery during infancy can only be determined by postnatal pediatric assessment and surveillance. Prenatal invasive therapeutic procedures are probably not justified (see below).

Uretheral Obstruction, Megacystis

Bladder enlargement can be due to:

- posterior urethral valves

- urethral stricture

- urethral agenesis

- persistent cloaca with urethral agenesis/stenosis

- megacystis-microcolon-hypoperistalsis syndrome

Urethral valves are by far the most common cause and are found almost exclusively in males fetuses. They are generally sporadic and only rarely familial.

Irrespective of the cause, the *in utero* risks are due to the progressive effect of the obstruction, namely, bilateral hydronephrosis, cystic dysplasia and even rupture. The kidney damage can be asymmetrical. Renal hyperechogenicity is associated with a poor outlook. Oligohydramnios and subsequent pulmonary hypoplasia are the other effects which significantly influence prognosis. Other anomalies described in association with posterior urethral valves include cryptorchidism, hypospadias, patent ductus arteriosus, tracheal hypoplasia, cardiac defects and chromosomal abnormalities.

In general, the prognosis is related to the degree of oligohydramnios. The role of prenatal invasive therapeutic procedures is discussed below.

Renal Cysts

The four types of cystic kidney diseases according to Osathanondt and Potter[10-12] are summarized in **Table 2**.

Autosomal recessive (infantile) polycystic kidney disease (Potter type I)

Autosomal recessive polycystic kidney disease (ARPKD) has a variable presentation and expressivity depending on the degree of renal involvement. There is little to be done therapeutically to influence this prognosis. Also called 'infantile polycystic kidney disease' or 'microcystic kidney disease' (**Figure 3a**), ARPKD has an incidence of 1:50 000 births.[12] The sonographic picture of large fetal kidneys with hyperechogenic renal structure is easy to recognize (**Figure 3b**) and invariably bilateral. Though difficult to recognize prenatally, fetuses with Potter type I kidneys typically have associated portal and interlobular fibrosis of the liver accompanied by biliary duct hyperplasia and small distal venous branches. Perinatal, neonatal, infantile and juvenile types of ARPKD have been differentiated corresponding to differences in their manifestations and prognosis for survival.[11,13] Even though this subclassification is not universally accepted, the relatively high intrafamilial constancy may be helpful when counseling on the risk of recurrence after a prenatal diagnosis.

Most of the reported cases were diagnosed after the 24th week of pregnancy, but in our experience 9 out of 17 cases with ARPKD were identified before the 24th week. Pulsed Doppler examination of the renal artery may become useful based on the hypothesis that the cases with the worst prognosis are associated with impairment of the microcirculation and thus a higher resistance index. Once it is diagnosed, it is probably advisable to counsel about family studies for 'silent' disease.

Multicystic dysplastic kidney disease (Potter type II)

In this condition, the cysts are formed by dilated, collecting tubules. It can be unilateral, bilateral or segmental. It results possibly from atresia of the ureteric bud system during embryogenesis.

Potter type II kidney disease is characterized by a large variety of patho-anatomic and subsequently prenatal sonographic findings. Potter type IIA has enlarged or normal, often segmental multicystic kidneys (**Figure 4**). It is differentiated from type IIB which has rudimentary kidneys and a few or only small cysts.[11] The renal cysts may be large enough to compress the gastrointestinal organs or contralateral urinary tract. The prognosis depends on the involvement of the contralateral side. Even if one side is severely affected, the child will usually develop without renal insufficiency.

In bilateral multicystic dysplastic kidney disease, the prognosis is uniformly fatal. While in cystic dysplasia

Table 2
Synopsis of the different types of congenital cystic kidney disease according to Potter[10-12]

	Potter type 1	Pottery type II	Potter type III	Potter type IV
1. Patho-anatomic findings	Bilateral symmetrically enlarged kidneys; cysts up to 2 mm in diameter; congenital hepatic fibrosis	Great variety (hypoplastic and hyperplastic, 'multicystic'); frequently unilateral or asymmetric findings	Bilateral with considerable renal enlargement; different sized cysts up to several centimeters in diameter	Kidneys often slightly enlarged; ultimately cortical cysts due to urethral obstruction
2. Genetics	Autosomal recessive inheritance	Not hereditary isolated renal lesion; exclusion of a syndrome indispensable	Autosomal dominant inheritance; part of syndromes e.g. Meckel, or of tuberous sclerosis, etc.	Not hereditary; exclusion of syndromes indispensable
3. Clinical features	Renal insufficiency (childhood); portal hypertension (adolescence)	Clinically silent to 'renal non-function syndrome'; often some involvement of contralateral urinary tract	Onset usually in adulthood, but early manifestations possible	Depending on extent of involvement; megacystis, hydroureter, cortical renal cysts
4. Prenatal diagnosis	Bilateral enlargement with reniform configuration; increased echogenicity of renal parenchyma; in severe cases, oligohydramnios	Multicystic or hypoplastic kidney; in severe cases of bilateral involvement, hydramnios/oligohydramnios	Only a few documented cases; early diagnosis by DNA polymorphisms possible	Possible differentiation from type II by appearance of megacystis and peripheral renal cysts

(Potter type IV) there is the possibility of considering whether a bypass procedure will be of benefit, in multicystic dysplasia there is no such possibility.

Unilateral multicystic dysplasia has a good prognosis if the contralateral kidney is normal. Most pediatric surgeons practise close surveillance often with antibiotic prophylaxis and reserve nephrectomy for those with recurrent problems, especially infections.

Associated anomalies may be found in the cardiovascular, gastrointestinal and central nervous systems, together with diaphragmatic hernia and tracheoesophageal fistula. Chromosomal abnormalities can also be present.

Though maternal diabetes is said to be associated with the development of fetal Potter type II kidney disease,[14,15] in most cases no maternal risk factors are identified, and though Potter type II kidneys may be present in inherited syndromes such as Zellweger and Fryns syndrome, they are most often isolated and non-genetic.

Autosomal dominant (adult) polycystic kidney disease (Potter type III)

Although autosomal dominant polycystic kidney disease (ADPKD) most commonly manifests in adults between the third and fifth decade, early manifestations (**Figure 5**) have been reported.[16] The size and shape of the cysts prenatally are highly variable. In 1985, the mutation for ADPKD was localized[17] to the short arm of chromosome 16 after it had been demonstrated to be linked with the alpha-chain of human hemoglobin. Shortly afterwards, the first prenatal diagnosis in a 9 week fetus at risk for the disease was accomplished using a highly polymorphic DNA probe genetically linked to the locus of ADPKD.[18] The ethical justification for prenatal diagnosis of this frequent disease (1:1000) given by these authors was that 'ADPKD continues to impose a considerable burden on families and the community, accounting for approximately 10% of the total requirement for chronic replacement therapy.'

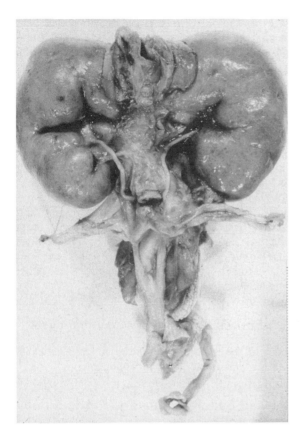

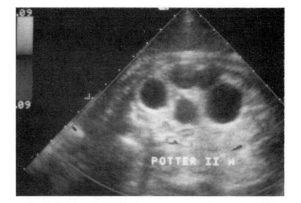

Figure 4. Potter type IIA unilateral multicystic kidney.

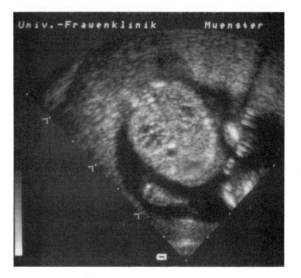

Figure 5. Transvaginal sonogram of a fetus with autosomal dominant polycystic kidney disease (positive family history).

Cystic lesions have also been reported in other organs, principally the liver but also the pancreas, spleen, lungs, testes and ovaries.

Cystic renal dysplasia (Potter type IV)

Urinary tract obstruction can produce increased intraluminal pressure during nephrogenesis and can lead to renal dysplasia. Controversy surrounds the theory that the type and severity of dysplasia probably depends on the time in fetal life that the obstruction develops. According to the Potter classification, type II multicystic dysplastic disease results from early obstruction (see above), whereas type IV cystic renal dysplasia results from an obstruction developing later in fetal life.

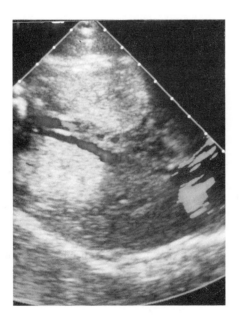

Figure 3. Potter type I autosomal recessive polycystic kidney disease (ARPKD). (a: upper) Situs post abortum (courtesy of Professor Rehder, University of Marburg, Germany). (b: lower) Sonogram showing that the enlarged kidneys reach the aorta.

Though Elizabeth Potter concluded that type IV kidney disease only occurs as a result of urethral occlusion (e.g. posterior urethral valves),[12] controversy continues among renal pathologists. In severe cases, the bladder is profoundly distended (**Figure 6a,b**), often with enlarged renal pelvises (**Figure 7a**) or cysts (**Figure 7b**). In fetuses with urethral obstruction (usually a male), the characteristic sonographic finding is dilatation of both the fetal urinary tract and the proximal urethra, producing a 'key-hole'-like appearance (**Figure 8a,b**).[19,20] Even in cases of urethral or bladder outlet obstruction where one might expect symmetric backup pressure with uniform degrees of hydronephrosis in both kidneys (**Figure 9**), there is often considerable asymmetry in the degree of hydronephrosis (**Figure 10a**). Although obstructive uropathies can sometimes be diagnosed in the early second trimester (**Figure 10b**), in one case Wladimiroff *et al.*[21] observed slight bilateral hydronephrosis as the first sign of an obstructive uropathy due to urethral valves where the diagnosis could not be established before 30 weeks gestation. Yet, postnatally, the child was anuric and bilateral ureterocutaneostomy had to be carried out. Cases of transient *in utero* hydronephrosis have also been reported,[22,23] some of which may be due to fetal vesicoureteral reflux resolving later in gestation.

Ureteropelvic junction (UPJ) obstruction is the most common cause of hydronephrosis in the neonate and child.[24] It can be differentiated prenatally since hydronephrosis is not associated with megacystis. In order to facilitate communication about the degree of hydronephrosis, a morphologic classification of *in utero* urinary tract dilatation has been proposed[25] based primarily on the degree of calyceal dilatation. The sonographic finding of cortical cysts has a sensitivity of 44% and specificity of 100% in the prediction of renal dysplasia, whereas increased echogenicity has a sensitivity of only 57% and a specificity of 89%.[26,27] Fetal kidneys that are obstructed severely enough to result in rupture of the collecting system and formation of a perinephric urinoma and urinary ascites (**Figures 11a,b**) are unlikely to have adequate residual renal function. It remains to be investigated systematically whether renal artery Doppler flow studies will be helpful for the prenatal assessment of kidney function.

Whatever the pathogenesis, extensive dysplasia indicates irreversible renal damage with significantly reduced renal function. Factors which influence the prognosis are whether the dysplasia is bilateral and what the residual renal function really is. These issues are discussed further below under 'Management Options'.

Syndromes associated with renal cysts

Some of the syndromes more commonly associated with renal cysts are given in **Table 3**.

Crossed Renal Ectopia and Pelvic Kidney

Crossed renal ectopia occurs in approximately 1:7000 births and may mimic unilateral renal agenesis. The ectopic kidney is abnormally large and bilobed in contrast to unilateral renal agenesis. The condition can cause obstructive uropathy, or reflux and can be found

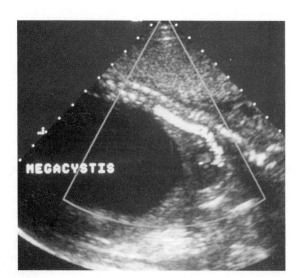
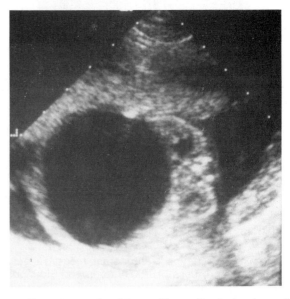

Figure 6.   (a: left, b: right) Urethral obstruction sequence: Sonogram of a fetus with urethral atresia and grossly distended bladder pushing the diaphragm upwards.

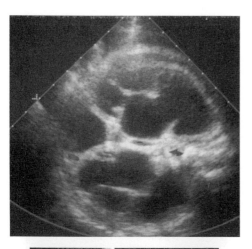

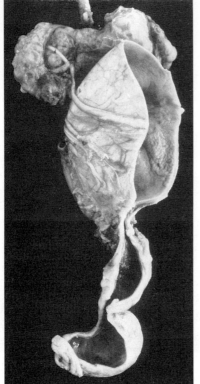

Figure 7. Potter type IV. (a: upper) Sonogram of bilateral severe hydronephrosis with parenchymal degeneration (shown by autopsy). (b: lower) Multicystic kidney degeneration in a fetus with urethral valves, megacystis and enlarged penis.

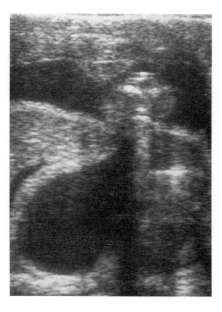

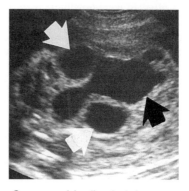

Figure 8. Sonographic 'keyhole'-appearance of a dilated bladder in cases of urethral obstructions. (a: upper) Male external genitalia; (b: lower) dilated ureters (white arrow) next to dilated bladder (black arrow).

with other cardiovascular or gastrointestinal anomalies. The prognosis is generally determined by these complications.

Pelvic kidney occurs in 1:1200 births and may also mimic unilateral renal agenesis. There is an association with other anomalies of the skeletal, cardiovascular, gastrointestinal and gynecological systems. Once again the prognosis is determined by these rather than the pelvic kidney *per se*.

Renal/Adrenal Tumors

These are rare in the fetus. Most are mesoblastic nephromas/hamartomas. Curative therapy consists of nephrectomy, though there have been reports of recurrences. Wilms' and other tumors are exceedingly rare in the fetus.

Focal renal dysplasia can produce an area of increased echogenicity which grows at a faster rate than the surrounding kidney and thus may mimic a tumor.

Adrenal neuroblastoma is the most common neonatal abdominal tumor. The incidence is between

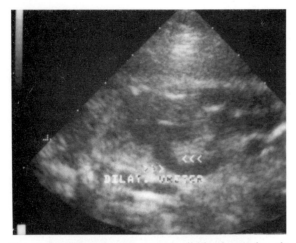

Figure 9. Dilated urether and mild hydronephrosis.

1:7000 and 1:100 000 births. While it is usually unilateral, 50% of affected newborns have metastases at the time of presentation. If the disease is disseminated *in utero*, it is possible for the increased circulating cathecholamines to produce maternal tachycardia and fetal hydrops.

Ambiguous Genitalia

While the identification of gender is part of a comprehensive ultrasonic evaluation of the fetus, a comparison with the results obtained from karyotype arguably yields the most useful information. This is especially true in the diagnosis of an intersex state such as testicular feminization or the adrenogenital syndrome. In multiple pregnancy, different gender documentation enables zygosity to be easily determined. Determining fetal sex is also of value in cases at risk of X-linked disorders.

Ovarian Cysts

Large cysts which are only rarely encountered clinically or by sonography[28] can be suspected prenatally if a cystic lesion is visualized next to a kidney in a female fetus (**Figure 12a**). Often, there is a characteristic sedimentation of cells with a sharp upper border in one part of the cyst (**Figure 12b**). Prenatally, these cysts are usually uncomplicated and typically disappear spontaneously postpartum. Rarely, surgery is necessary because of either their size or secondary complications. The risk of malignancy is exceedingly low.

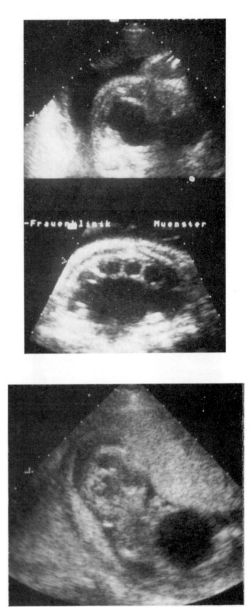

Figure 10. Urethral obstruction sequence. (a: upper) Different degrees of hydronephrosis in both kidneys of the same fetus. (b: lower) megacystis with oligohydramnios in a fetus early in the second trimester.

Management Options

In considering the management options for any case of a fetus with genitourinary malformations, there are some general guidelines which can be followed.

Counseling

Careful consideration must be given to counseling the parents when such an anomaly is recognized. The first

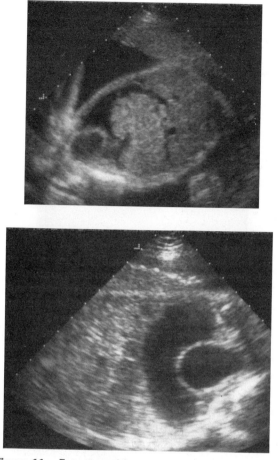

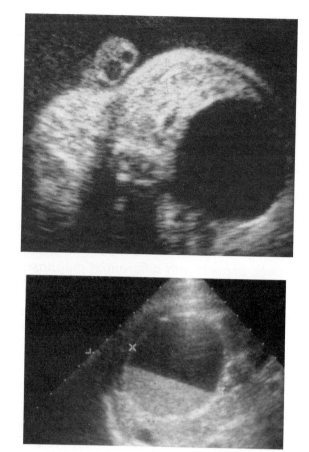

Figure 11. Fetuses with rupture of the collecting system resulting in urinary ascites.

Figure 12. Fetal ovarian cyst. (a: upper) Ovarian cyst next to normal kidney. Two-vessel cord can be recognized. (b: lower) Ovarian cyst with typical cell sedimentation on one side.

Table 3
Syndromes associated with renal cysts

Syndrome	Inheritance	Kidney involvement
Meckel-Gruber	AR	95%
Asphyxiating thoracic dystrophy	AR	Frequent
Zellweger	AR	Frequent
Various chromosomal	—	35%
VATER association	—	50%
Ehlers-Danlos	Different	Frequent
Prune belly	—	Frequent
Laurence-Moon-Biedl	AR	Frequent

prerequisite is that those counseling should try and establish the diagnosis as accurately as possible, if necessary with karyotyping. Despite this, it still may not be possible to be absolutely certain of the diagnosis and a differential diagnosis is the best that can be achi-

eved. In such circumstances, it is important not to 'over-prognosticate' about the outlook for the fetus. Some of the implications for specific conditions are considered above under 'Risks'.

Prognosis in children with prenatally recognized urinary tract abnormalities

Renal agenesis or a complete deficit of renal function is invariably lethal at birth usually because of pulmonary hypoplasia. While this could theoretically be prevented by the continuous infusion of fluid into the amniotic cavity, it is not currently feasible to transplant kidneys in the newborn period or to apply dialysis directly after birth preceding surgery. Although anencephalic donors have been used for kidney transplantation (and about 81 such cases are documented in the literature),[29] this potential source of organs is also very limited.

With all the current uncertainties about the prenatal

assessment of residual renal function, it is important to follow up all cases of prenatally diagnosed fetal genito-urinary anomalies in order to learn more about prognosis and to improve upon management protocols. In our experience, we have found that 20 of 89 (22.5%) children with prenatally recognized congenital uropathies developed arterial hypertension. Hypertension in children is a risk factor for progressive renal and cardiovascular disease, causing considerable morbidity and mortality if not recognized and treated early. The main risk factor for the development of arterial hypertension is pyelonephritis because of vesicorenal reflux, obstructive uropathy and fistulation of the renal pelvis. Each of these complications may follow successful surgery.

Genetic aspects and differential diagnosis of urinary tract abnormalities

Numerous syndromes are associated with cystic changes of fetal kidneys.[11] One of the more frequent is the autosomal recessive Meckel syndrome (1:40 000 births) characterized by neural tube defect, postaxial hexadactyly and polycystic kidneys similar to a Potter type III aspect. The identification of these major malformations can guide the search for minor malformations such as cleft lip or palate or genital malformations. Another autosomal recessive syndrome with renal involvement is Fraser syndrome, displaying the key symptoms of cryptophthalmos and syndactyly (**Figure 13a,b**).

The autosomal recessive Kaufman syndrome is characterized by hydrometrocolpos, polydactyly, congenital heart disease and secondary hydronephrosis due to pressure from the distended hydrometra on the ureters. We have also observed a syndrome with Potter sequence, persistent buccopharyngeal membrane type II, postaxial polydactyly, cleft palate, cardiac anomalies, intestinal non-fixation and intrauterine growth deficiency,[30] subsequently seen by others. In a survey of 80 cases with Potter sequence due to renal or urologic abnormalities, Curry *et al.*[31] found 15 patients with multiple congenital anomalies, four of which had autosomal recessive syndromes and three aneuploidies. Furlong *et al.*[32] also found a high rate of associated anomalies in fetuses with urinary tract abnormalities.

There is some confusion in the literature regarding the term 'prune belly' syndrome, which is defined as the triad of lax abdominal wall, cryptorchidism and urinary tract anomalies. The characteristic anterior wall defect can occur secondary to massive bladder dilatation and stretching of the abdominal walls.[33,34]

One common problem after ultrasonic detection of a fetal renal anomaly is distinguishing between megaureter and primary cysts of the kidney (**Figure 14a,b**). Avni *et al.* established a correct prenatal diagnosis in

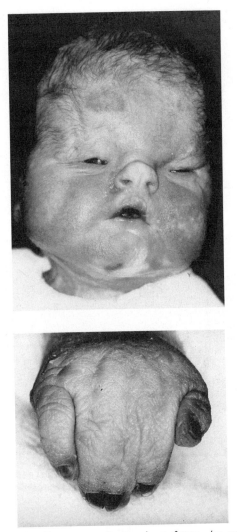

Figure 13. Fraser syndrome in a fetus. (a: upper) Bilateral cryptophthalmos; (b: lower) syndactyly and brachyphalangy of hand.

43 of 63 cases (70%).[35] Other problems include differentiating multicystic dysplastic kidneys from ureteropelvic junction obstruction owing to reflux or obstruction and nonvisualized, small, hypoplastic kidneys.

The prenatal ultrasound demonstration of bladder distention and/or hydronephrosis does not always signify true obstruction of the urinary tract, which is important to assess before contemplating a prenatal shunting procedure. Nor is it always possible to decide in cases with fetal renal pelvises of more than 10 mm between an obstructive lesion or exceptional extrarenal pelvises (**Figure 19**).[36] Greenblatt *et al.*[37] reported the first *in utero* diagnosis of crossed renal ectopia, and Vintzileos *et al.*[38] presented sonographic findings of the megacystis-intestinal hypoperistalsis syndrome which has an extremely bad prognosis. The prevalence

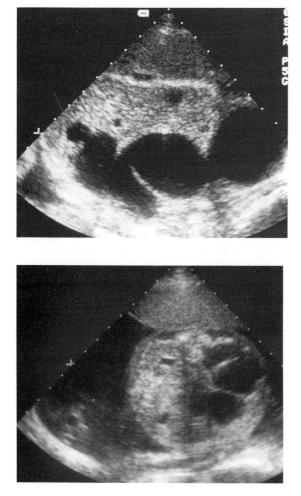

Figure 14. Dilated ureters. (a: upper) Longitudinal sonogram with slightly dilated renal pelvis in the left side of the picture. (b: lower) Transverse sonogram. The picture may be misinterpreted as a multicystic kidney.

of ureteral duplication is estimated to range from 0.7 to 1% of the general population and pathological manifestations such as vesicoureteral reflux occur in 20% of these cases.[39] Another important differential diagnosis for a simple urinary tract obstruction is the more complicated common cloaca sequence.[40] Cloaca malformation again has to be differentiated from a bladder diverticulum. We encountered an extreme case of a low bladder diverticulum in a fetus with urethral obstruction where the external aspect of the child *in utero* was similar to the one seen in cases with cystic sacrococcygeal teratoma (**Figure 15a–c**). In this situation, the condition could be classified prenatally as lethal, based on the pulmonary hypoplasia due to upward displacement of the diaphragm and on the result of urinary function studies.

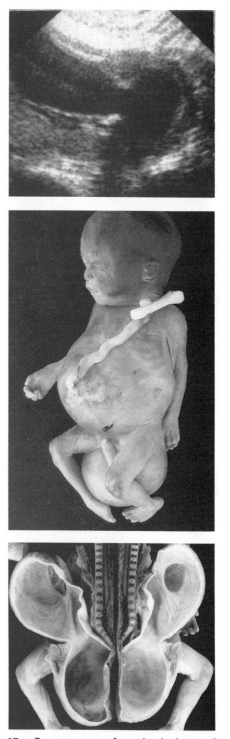

Figure 15. Severe case of urethral obstruction sequence. (a: upper) Sonogram showing megacystis and bladder diverticulum. (b: middle) Exterior aspect of the fetus resembling a sacrococcygeal teratoma. (c: lower) Autopsy preparation shows megacystis, bladder diverticulum and extremely dilated ureter ostia.

Termination of pregnancy

The possibility of a pregnancy termination should be discussed carefully and sensitively with the parents in those conditions diagnosed sufficiently early in pregnancy which have a poor prognosis.

Urinary diversion procedures with fetal urinary tract

Experimental[41] and clinical[42] evidence suggest that in some fetuses severe *in utero* urinary tract obstruction may ultimately lead to delivery of a neonate with advanced hydronephrosis and type IV cystic dysplasia incompatible with survival, and that the secondary oligohydramnios leads to pulmonary hypoplasia as well as to skeletal and facial deformities (Potter sequence). Therefore, several investigators have proposed that early *in utero* relief of the obstruction might allow both sufficient renal development to support postnatal life and 'catch-up growth' of the lungs. Two different approaches have been tried: placement of an indwelling suprapubic catheter *in utero*[42] and open fetal surgery with bilateral ureterostomies (**Figure 16a**).[27] The latter step was undertaken only after the early design catheters proved technically inadequate. Potential risks of open surgery, not only for the fetus but also for the

mother, include the need for repeated cesarean section. An improved *in utero* shunt device, originally introduced by Rodeck *et al.*[43] for pleuro-amniotic shunting, can now be placed from the inside of a trocar and has better material properties against clotting and dislocation (**Figure 16b**). The outcome of these treated fetuses has been maintained in an international registry. There is no apparent correlation between the gestational age at which the shunt is placed, the duration it functions, and the adequacy of renal function at birth.

Further, though many have adequate renal function at birth, long-term study suggests their disease is progressive. The ultimate need for dialysis and transplant remains high. Though the shunts prevent the development of the Potter sequence, it remains unclear whether they prevent renal disease. Thus at present these procedures should be considered novel therapy.

Bilateral renal agenesis is a uniformly lethal condition. Thus, reliable prenatal diagnosis is extremely important. Failure to identify a fetal bladder is an important diagnostic sign. The administration of furosemide to the mother has been suggested,[21] but its effect of inducing a fetal diuresis is doubtful. Oligohydramnios obscures sonographic visibility, hindering the diagnosis. Therefore, fluid can be infused into the amniotic cavity to enhance ultrasound imaging. It has also been shown recently that prophylactic

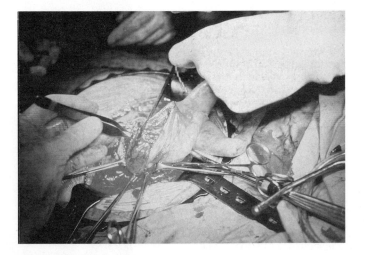

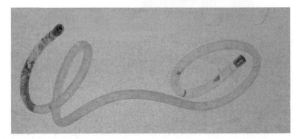

Figure 16. Urinary diversion procedures. (a: above) Open fetal surgery with ureterostomy because of prenatally recognized fetal obstruction. (b: left) Double pigtail indwelling catheter developed by Professor Charles Rodeck (London) which can be pushed through the inside of a needle.

amnioinfusion can improve the outcome of pregnancies complicated by thick meconium and oligohydramnios.[44] By adding some of Evans blue dye to the fluid, an unnoticed rupture of the membranes may become recognizable. For technical details, see Chapter 48. Color-coded sonography aids in delineating the blood flow in the umbilical cord from an open space (**Figure 17**). Tissue (blood, placenta or amniotic fluid cells) should always be obtained for a karyotype. In our experience, the most frequent aneuploidy associated with fetal renal anomalies or oligohydramnios is triploidy followed by trisomy 18.[45]

Place, timing and method of delivery

The decision to deliver in a tertiary referral center varies both with the normal practices of different institutions and also with the diagnosis. It is important that each unit develops its own guidelines on the basis of resources and geographical constraints.

Postnatal

Communication with pediatric colleagues during the pregnancy over cases with urogenital abnormality is mandatory. After birth, further evaluation of the genitourinary system will be undertaken and confirmation of diagnosis made. Once the diagnosis is made, subsequent management can be planned. There seems to be no consensus among pediatricians and/or pediatric surgeons about the use of prophylactic antibiotics in newborns with genitourinary malformations, though

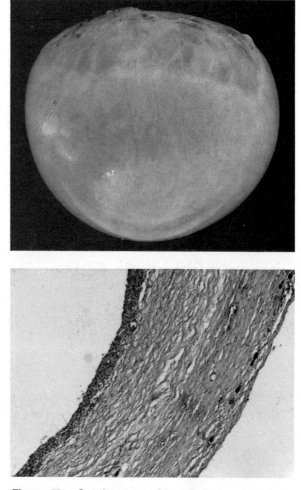

Figure 18. Ovarian cyst after surgical removal. (a: upper) The cyst has been removed microsurgically *in toto*. (b: lower) Nevertheless, primordial follicles can be recognized within the cyst wall.

it would appear that they are used more consistently where there is dilatation of the renal tract.

Naturally, postmortem examination should be requested if there is a lethal abnormality.

Conclusion

Although some congenital renal anomalies cannot be recognized prenatally (e.g. non-Finnish nephrotic syndrome without amniotic fluid AFP increase), most urogenital fetal anomalies can be detected by ultrasound. Prenatal recognition offers the chance to prevent postnatal complications (e.g. pyelonephritis from unrecognized hydronephrosis) and to make prognostic statements about the treatability of these conditions. The development of appropriate pre- and perinatal manage-

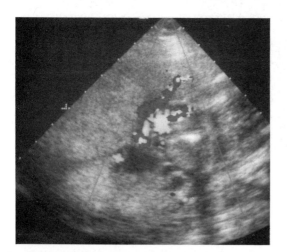

Figure 17. Color-coded Doppler sonogram of a case with severe oligohydramnios due to renal agenesis. The area which might be confused with an amniotic fluid pocket can easily be identified as an area with a coil of umbilical cord.

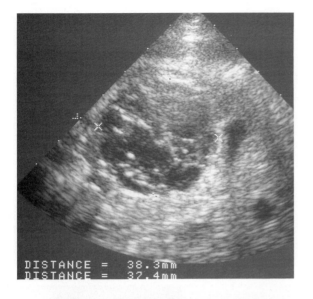

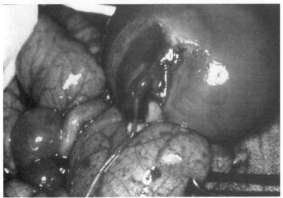

Figure 19. Torsion of a fetal ovarian cyst *in utero.* (a: upper) The irregular partly echogenic sono-graphic picture of the cyst is equivalent to the internal bleeding after torsion. (b: lower) Abdominal situs at the time of surgery right after birth confirming the intrauterine torsion of the fetal ovarian cyst.

ment protocols will require further studies, including careful postnatal follow-up investigations. It is suggested that these patients are referred to an appropriate consultant.

If ovarian cysts are taken out by laparotomy in the neonatal period, it is difficult even with microsurgery not to harm the small ovary which is often intimately integrated into the wall of the cyst (**Figure 18a,b**). It therefore seems prudent to either allow even large cysts to regress spontaneously or to puncture those requiring decompression due to secondary complications. In order to prevent torsion of the pedicle (**Figure 19a,b**) and subsequent necrosis or hemorrhage into the cyst, we recommend prenatal decompression, especially if the cyst is growing rapidly or a 'wandering mass'.

GENITOURINARY MALFORMATIONS
Summary of Management Options

Make diagnosis

Checklist

- Oligohydramnios?
- Dilatation of the urinary tract (or urinoma or urinary ascites)?
- Renal cysts?
- Size, shape and echogenicity of the kidneys?
- Bladder present?
- Associated abnormalities (including karyotype)?

Diagnostic guidelines

- See **Table 1**
- Establish whether family history of renal disease

Management options: general

- Counseling
- Consideration of invasive procedure
  - to clarify diagnosis
  - for possible therapeutic benefit
- Consideration of termination if appropriate
- Planning place, timing and method of delivery
- Pediatric involvement
  - prenatally for counseling
  - after birth for further evaluation, confirmation of diagnosis and planning subsequent management
- Postmortem examination if lethal abnormality

REFERENCES

1   Leck I, Record RG, McKeown T, Edwards JH (1968) The incidence of malformations in Birmingham, England, 1950–1959. *Teratology* **1**:263–280.

2   Livera LN, Brookfield DSK, Egginton JA, Hawnaur JN (1989) Antenatal ultrasonography to detect fetal renal abnormalities: A prospective screening programme. *British Medical Journal* **298**:1421–1423.

3   Costin ME, Kennedy RLJ (1972) Ovarian cysts in newborn. *American Journal of Roentgenology* **116**:664–672.

4   Nicolaides KH, Cheng HH, Snijders RJM, Moniz CF (1992) Fetal urine biochemistry in the assessment of obstructive uropathy. *American Journal of Obstetrics and Gynecology* **166**:932–937.

5   Appelman Z, Golbus MS (1986) The management of fetal urinary tract obstruction. *Clinics in Obstetrics and Gynecology* **29**:483–489.

6   Lenz S, Lund-Hansen T, Bang J *et al.* (1985) A possible prenatal evaluation of renal function by amino acid analysis on fetal urine. *Prenatal Diagnosis* **5**: 259–267.

7   Wilkins IA, Chitkara U, Lynch L *et al.* (1987) The nonpredictive value of fetal urinary electrolytes. Preliminary report of outcomes and correlations with pathologic diagnosis. *American Journal of Obstetrics and Gynecology* **157**:694–698.

8   Reuss A, Wladimiroff JW, Pijpers L *et al.* (1987) Fetal urinary electrolytes in bladder outlet obstruction. *Fetal Therapy* **2**:148–153.

9   Holzgreve W, Lison A, Bulla M (1989) SDS-PAGE as an additional test to determine fetal kidney function prior to intrauterine diversion of urinary tract obstruction. *Fetal Therapy* **4**:93–96.

10 Osathanondt V, Potter EL (1964) Pathogenesis of polycystic kidneys. *Archives of Pathology* **77**: 459–465.

11 Zerres K, Völpel MC, Weiß H (1984) Cystic kidneys. *Human Genetics* **68**:104–135.

12 Potter EL (1972) *Normal and Abnormal Development of the Kidney.* Chicago, IL: Year Book Medical Publishers.

13 Blyth H, Ockenden BG (1971) Polycystic disease of kidneys and liver presenting in childhood. *Journal of Medical Genetics* **8**:257–284.

14 Passarge E, Lenz W (1966) Syndrome of caudal regression in infants of diabetic mothers: Observations of further cases. *Pediatrics* **37**:672–675.

15 Grix A, Curry C, Hall BD (1982) Patterns of multiple malformations in infants of diabetic mothers. *Birth Defects* **18**:55–77.

16 Holzgreve W, Aydinli K, Evans M, Miny P. (1992) Prenatal diagnosis and management of fetal genitourinary tract abnormalities. In Kurjak A (ed.) *An Atlas of Ultrasonography in Obstetrics and Gynecology*, Carnforth: Parthenon pp. 61–79.

17 Reeders ST, Breuning MH, Davies KE *et al.* (1985) A highly polymorphic DNA marker linked to adult polycystic kidney disease on chromosome 16. *Nature* **317**: 542–544.

18 Reeders ST, Zerres K, Gal A (1986) Prenatal diagnosis of autosomal dominant polycystic kidney disease with a DNA probe. *Lancet* **ii**: 6–8.

19 Garrett WJ, Grunwald G, Robinson DE (1970) Prenatal diagnosis of fetal polycystic kidney by ultrasound. *Aus-tralia and New Zealand Journal of Obstetrics and Gynaecology* **10**: 7–9.

20 Harrison MR, Filly RA (1990) The fetus with obstructive uropathy: Pathophysiology, natural history, selection, and treatment. In Harrison MR *et al.* (eds) *The Unborn Patient*, pp. 328–398. Philadelphia, PA: W.B. Saunders.

21 Wladimiroff JW, Beemer FA, Scholtmeyer RJ *et al.* (1985) Failure to detect fetal obstructive uropathy by second trimester ultrasound. *Prenatal Diagnosis* **5**: 41–46.

22 Sanders R, Graham D (1982) Twelve cases of hydronephrosis *in utero* diagnosed by ultrasonography. *Journal of Ultrasound in Medicine* **1**: 341.

23 Baker ME, Rosenberg ER, Bowie JD *et al.* (1985) Transient *in utero* hydronephrosis. *Journal of Ultrasound in Medicine* **4**: 51–53.

24 Flake AW, Harrison MR, Sauer L *et al.* (1986) Ureteropelvic junction obstruction in the fetus. *Journal of Pediatric Surgery* **21**: 1058–1063.

25 Grignon A, Filion R, Filiatrault D *et al.* (1986) Urinary tract dilatation *in utero*: Classification and clinical applications. *Radiology* **160**: 645–647.

26 Mahony BS, Filly RA, Callen PW *et al.* (1984) Sonographic evaluation of renal dysplasia. *Radiology* **152**: 143.

27 Harrison MR, Golbus MS, Filly RA *et al.* (1982) Fetal surgery for congenital hydronephrosis. *New England Journal of Medicine* **306**: 591–593.

28 Holzgreve W, Beller FK, Buchholz B *et al.* (1987) Kidney transplantation from anencephalic donors. *New England Journal of Medicine* **316**: 1069–1070.

29 Kirkinen P, Jouppila P (1985) Perinatal aspects of pregnancy complicated by fetal ovarian cyst. *Journal of Perinatal Medicine* **13**: 245–251.

30 Holzgreve W, Wagner H, Rehder H (1984) Bilateral renal agenesis with Potter phenotype, cleft palate, anomalies of the cardiovascular system, skeletal anomalies including hexadactyly and bifid metacarpal: A new syndrome? *American Journal of Medical Genetics* **18**: 177–182.

31 Curry CJR, Jensen K, Holland J *et al.* (1984) The Potter sequence: A clinical analysis of 80 cases. *American Journal of Medical Genetics* **19**: 679–702.

32 Furlong LA, Williamson RA, Bonsib S *et al.* (1986) Pregnancy outcome following ultrasound diagnosis of fetal urinary tract anomalies and/or oligohydramnios. *Fetal Therapy* **1**: 134–145.

33 Bovicelli L, Rizzo N, Orsini LF *et al.* (1980) Prenatal diagnosis of the prune belly syndrome. *Clinics in Genetics* **18**: 79–82.

34 Burton BK, Dillard RG (1984) Prune belly syndrome: Observations supporting the hypothesis of abdominal overdistenson. *American Journal of Medicine and Genetics* **17**: 669–672.

35 Avni EF, Rodesch F, Schulman CC (1985) Fetal uropathies: Diagnostic pitfalls and management. *Journal of Urology* **134**: 921–925.

36 Arger PH, Coleman BG, Mintz MC (1985) Routine fetal genitourinary tract screening. *Radiology* **156**: 485–489.

37 Greenblatt AM, Beretsky I, Lankin DH *et al* (1985) *In utero* diagnosis of crossed renal ectopia using high-res-

olution real-time ultrasound. *Journal of Ultrasound in Medicine* **4**: 105–107.

38 Vintzileos, AM, Eisenfeld LI, Herson VC *et al.* (1986) Megacystis-microcolon-intestinal hypoperistalsis syndrome: Prenatal sonographic findings and review of the literature. *American Journal of Perinatology* **3**: 297–302.

39 Duval JM, Milon J, Coadou Y *et al.* (1986) Ultrasonographic anatomy and diagnosis of fetal uropathies affecting the upper urinary tract. *SRA* **8**: 131–145.

40 Holzgreve W (1985) Prenatal diagnosis of persistent common cloaca with prune belly and anencephaly in the second trimester. *American Journal of Medical Genetics* **20**: 729–732.

41 Adzick NS, Harrison MR, Gick PL *et al.* (1985) Fetal urinary tract obstruction: Experimental pathophysiology. *Seminars in Perinatology* **9**:79–90.

42 Golbus MS, Filly RA, Callen PW *et al.* (1985) Fetal urinary tract obstruction: Management and selection for treatment. *Seminars in Perinatology* **9**:91–97.

43 Rodeck CH, Fish NM, Fraser DI *et al.* (1988) Long-term *in utero* drainage of fetal hydrorthorax. *New England Journal of Medicine* **319**:1135–1138.

44 Macri CJ, Schrimmer DB, Leung A, Greenspoon JS, Paul RH (1992) Prophylactic amnioinfusion improves outcome of pregnancy complicated by thick meconium and oligohydramnios. *American Journal of Obstetrics and Gynecology* **167**:117–121.

45 Holzgreve W, Miny P (1989) Genetic aspects of fetal disease. *Seminars in Perinatology* **13**:260–277.

52

Gastrointestinal Malformations Including Diaphragmatic Hernia

PETER STONE

INTRODUCTION

Fetal gastrointestinal malformations are generally detected by chance during ultrasound examination in the second trimester performed either to check dating, exclude multiple pregnancy or examine for a structural abnormality. Abnormalities of fetal growth or amniotic fluid volume (usually hydramnios) or an abnormal maternal serum alpha-fetoprotein are other reasons for a targeted scan which may detect the abnormality. The most common gastrointestinal abnormalities detected prenatally by ultrasound are omphalocele, gastroschisis and diaphragmatic hernia. The other malformations to be discussed are both less common and less frequently diagnosed by ultrasound. Upon detection, the patient is managed in consultation with a multidisciplinary team which provides consistent advice and treatment. Team members often include an obstetrician with expertise in fetal medicine, a neonatal pediatrician, pediatric surgeon, clinical geneticist, midwife, a neonatal nurse and anesthetist. The patient may speak with these people individually or as a group depending on their needs.

OMPHALOCELE (EXOMPHALOS)

This defect is an extra-embryonic hernia due to failure of a portion of the abdominal wall to form normally (**Figure 1**). It is thought to be due to the arrest of ventral medial migration of the dermatomyotomes. 'Physiological' herniation of abdominal contents is common until 13 weeks gestation (**Figure 2**) and should be distinguished from an omphalocele.

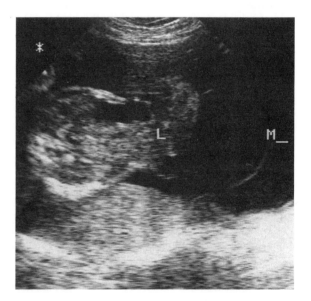

Figure 1. Characteristic ultrasound appearance of omphalocele. Note the membrane (M) surrounding the liver (L) and bowel.

Incidence

The incidence of this abnormality is variously quoted as 1:2500 to 1:5000 pregnancies. It is similar in incidence to gastroschisis, although recent publications and the author's experience suggest that the latter is slightly more common.[1]

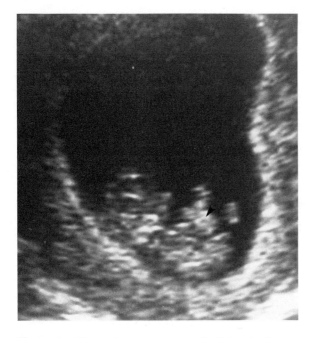

Figure 2. Normal appearance of abdominal contents outside the body cavity in the fetus at 11–12 weeks gestation illustrated by the arrow.

Presentation

Omphalocele usually presents as an abnormality detected on ultrasound (**Figure 1**). Detection occurs during careful scanning of the anterior abdominal wall, the cord insertion site and in performing abdominal circumference measurements. Omphalocele in particular may be associated with chromosomal abnormalities where fetal growth may also be abnormal.

Abdominal wall defects are commonly associated with increased amniotic fluid. In the situation with abnormal fetal growth associated with a chromosomal abnormality, oligohydramnios may be present. Small omphaloceles may be missed on ultrasound when the fluid volume is reduced, making it difficult to clearly delineate the anterior abdominal wall.

Abdominal wall defects produce very high maternal serum alpha-fetoprotein concentrations in the second trimester. However, the acetylcholinesterase bands associated with abdominal wall defects are faint and the pseudocholinesterase band dense – the reverse of the result in neural tube defects (see Chapter 37).[2]

Management Options

Prenatal

The first step is to exclude other abnormalities, which are present in 60–80% of cases. The ultrasound differ-

entiation between omphalocele and gastroschisis is important and is generally not difficult. The presence of a sac or membrane around the contents with the cord inserting upon it are important markers. Difficulties may arise when the sac has ruptured spontaneously *in utero*, or when the relationship of the herniated tissue to the umbilical cord insertion is unclear. Thickened loops of bowel in gastroschisis may give the appearance of a covering membrane. Distinguishing the membrane over an omphalocele with oligohydramnios may be difficult. **Table 1** lists associated abnormalities in omphalocele. Extracorporeal liver is very rare in gastroschisis, as opposed to omphalocele where the liver is in the sac in 40% of fetuses. Altogether, 30–70% of fetuses with omphalocele have other structural abnormalities.[3-5] An important part of the prenatal management therefore involves both obtaining a fetal karyotype and searching for other associated structural

Table 1
Associated anomalies in omphalocele

Pentalogy of Cantrell
   diaphragmatic hernia and pericardial defect
   distal sternal defect
   omphalocele
   cardiovascular malformations

Cloacal extrophy
   omphalocele
   bladder or cloacal extrophy
   other caudal abnormalities

Beckwith-Wiedemann syndrome
   omphalocele
   macroglossia
   generalized organomegaly (autosomal dominant)
   hypoglycemia

Trisomies
   13, 18, 21

Other aneuploidy
   Triploidy, Turner's syndrome

Other abnormalities
   Cardiac
      atrial septal defect
      ventricular septal defect
      patent ductus arteriosis
      pulmonary stenosis
   Gastrointestinal
      atresias
      Meckel's diverticulum
      imperforate anus
   Renal
   Neurological
      meningocele
      holoprosencephaly
      microphthalmos

abnormalities with a detailed ultrasound examination, including the heart.

The relationship between the omphalocele contents, associated abnormalities and prognosis has been examined. Fetuses with an omphalocele and intracorporeal liver are significantly more likely to have chromosomal abnormalities.[5] Advanced maternal age and other ultrasound abnormalities are also associated with an abnormal karyotype. However, there is probably little prognostic significance of the omphalocele contents if the karyotype is taken into account, though prognosis is worse in larger defects.

Having made the diagnosis, parental counseling involves discussing the need for a karyotype. Part of the counseling involves showing the parents illustrations of typical defects both pre- (**Figure 3**) and post-surgery. The counseling should emphasize a good prognosis. Even when the diagnosis is not made prenatally, the mortality rate for otherwise normal infants is low.[6] As the prognosis for surgery in neonates without chromosomal and other structural abnormalities is very good, termination of pregnancy before fetal viability is now rarely emphasized but remains an option. The main reasons for mortality in the otherwise normal infant relate to prematurity, sepsis or problems with short gut syndrome, which are more common in gastroschisis than in omphalocele. Survival is well in excess of 75–80%.

Labor/delivery

Delivery should occur in a center with a neonatal medical and surgical team in attendance to optimize the initial resuscitation and preoperative care of the neonate. A quasi-controversy at one time existed over the

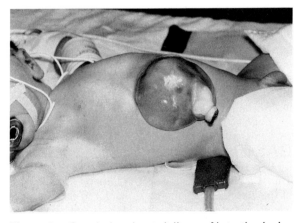

Figure 3. Omphalocele at delivery. Note the lesion is epigastric and the site of the umbilical cord insertion.

mode of delivery with omphalocele. Reviewed *in toto*, retrospective studies have been quite clear. There is no evidence to suggest that cesarean section confers *any* benefit to the fetus or neonate with omphalocele with or without a ruptured sac and irrespective of the contents of the sac.[7,8] The theoretical concerns about vaginal delivery – namely, visceral trauma, dystocia and infection – have not been supported by those that recommend cesarean delivery. In series where the diagnosis was either not suspected before birth or only known in a minority of cases, cesarean section made no difference to neonatal outcome.[1,9]

Neonatal morbidity in all recent series relates to associated anomalies and prematurity (isolated cases of late morbidity and mortality relate mostly to complications of bowel obstruction or short bowel syndrome in association with intestinal atresia).[10] Extracorporeal liver is relatively common in omphalocele, being found in nearly a quarter of cases. There seems to be no increase in survival with cesarean section in this group. Vaginal breech delivery with extracorporeal liver may present a special argument against vaginal delivery because of the mechanism of breech delivery, but this has not been examined in a controlled study and no specific recommendations can be made.

Postnatal

The principles of neonatal care apply in all cases of anterior abdominal wall defect. Steps are taken to ensure optimal initial management allowing stabilization of the baby while a definitive diagnosis of the type of abnormality is made and surgery planned. Prevention of heat and fluid loss and infection are the aims of initial post-delivery care.

Immediately after delivery, the neonate is lowered into a sterile bag containing warm electrolyte (no warmer than 37.5°C), plasma solution and antibiotics (Vi-Drape isolation bag, Becton Dickinson). In emergencies, any sterile bag with warmed normal saline or lactated Ringers solution and antibiotics will suffice. The solution in the bag consists of 1 liter of lactated Ringers solution, 500 ml stable plasma protein solution or similar solution and 1 million units of penicillin. The bag is tied at the level of the axillae and care is taken to avoid torsion of viscera (**Figure 4**). The temperature on arrival in the neonatal unit is critical to the success of resuscitation in general and these infants are at increased risk of hypothemia due to the large surface area of exposed viscera.

An alternative approach to the avoidance of heat and fluid loss is to place the baby in a sterile plastic bag up to the axillae without the fluid. A nasogastric tube is passed and when necessary ventilatory support is provided.

Neonates with major associated malformations or

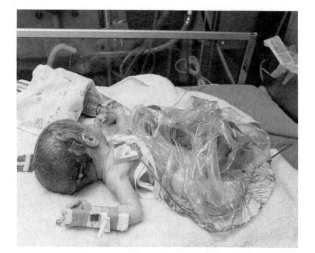

Figure 4. Neonate with an omphalocele showing bowel isolation bag tied above defect.

trisomy 13 or 18 are managed non-surgically. The options here are either to keep the neonate comfortable and provide supportive care only or, alternatively, to paint the unruptured omphalocele sac with 1% mercurochrome solution. Mercurochrome may be associated with renal failure. Neonates not treated generally die of dehydration or sepsis.

All other cases are managed surgically with operative repair within a few hours of delivery assuming the neonate's general condition is stable. It is not generally possible to predict prenatally whether primary surgical closure will be possible. Small omphaloceles with a defect less than 4 cm in diameter or without extracorporeal liver are almost always closed primarily. Large defects, or those containing liver, may not be closable during the first operation. Where primary closure is not possible, the defect and contents are covered with a silastic silo sutured to the edge of the defect. Over the following 7 days, the contents of the silo gradually enter the abdominal cavity under the influence of gravity coupled with daily compression of the silo. Care is taken to prevent the neonate developing respiratory or circulatory compromise during these maneuvers. Postoperative problems for both omphalocele and gastroschisis repair include respiratory embarrassment, pulmonary hypertension, small bowel perforation, bowel obstruction and malrotation. A period of parenteral nutrition is often necessary postoperatively for some days or weeks, while after a silo the average neonatal hospital stay ranges from 3 to 4 weeks. Up to 3 months has been necessary in some cases before satisfactory bowel function was achieved. Weakness of the anterior abdominal wall or poor cosmetic results at initial surgery may require a later plastic surgical revision.

The long-term prognosis for these infants is gener-

OMPHALOCELE
Summary of Management Options

Diagnosis

- Ultrasound after 13 weeks

- Elevated maternal serum alpha-fetoprotein

Management

- Exclude associated chromosomal or structural malformations (especially cardiac)

- Karyotype is advisable

Labor/delivery

- Delivery mode of a vertex presentation does not influence outcome

- Delivery is recommended in a tertiary unit with neonatal surgical facilities

- Place abdominal contents and/or baby in a sterile plastic bag with/without warm (37.5°C) isotonic solutions

---

ally very good and, in the absence of associated structural or chromosomal abnormalities, the risk of recurrence in a subsequent pregnancy is extremely low. The main recurrence risk is that for the associated abnormalities, though case reports of a familial recurrence have been recorded.[11]

GASTROSCHISIS

This is a paraumbilical defect usually on the right side of the anterior abdominal wall lateral to the umbilical vessels. Occasional left-sided defects are seen. Gastroschisis may be considered the result of an accident during development. Abnormal regression of (usually) the right umbilical vein has been proposed as a mechanism for the development of gastroschisis, but its etiology remains controversial.[12]

Iatrogenic abdominal wall defects with protrusion of viscera have been caused after bladder shunt procedures, e.g. vesico amniotic shunts for obstructive uropathy. Perhaps the main purpose of distinguishing the embryological development of gastroschisis from omphalocele is to emphasize the different incidence of associated abnormalities. The incidence with gastroschisis is <10%. The sonographic image is one of free-floating loops of bowel (**Figures 5, 6**).

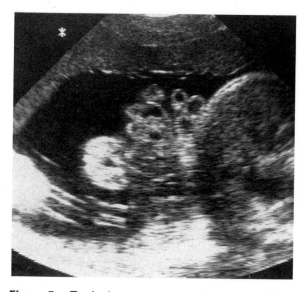

Figure 5. Typical appearance of gastroschisis: loops of bowel floating freely in the amniotic fluid (in this case, unusually, liver was also protruding through the defect).

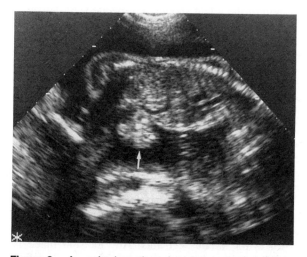

Figure 6. A sagittal section showing a gastroschisis. Note the absence of a membrane and the usual position, lower than omphalocele.

Incidence

The incidence of gastroschisis is approximately 1:2500–3000 live births with an equal sex ratio.[3]

Presentation

Prenatal detection is similar to that of omphalocele: ultrasound (**Figures 5, 6**), raised maternal serum alphafetoprotein or abnormal amniotic fluid volume beyond the mid second trimester when related to associated intestinal atresia.

Management Options

Prenatal

Though the risk of associated structural abnormalities is less than that for omphalocele, a search for these by detailed ultrasound is necessary. In one review, the incidence of anomalies was higher than the oft quoted 10%, but included isolated cases of ambiguous genitalia, undescended testes and hydrocele and dysmorphic faces. The risk of an abnormal karyotype is <1%. Hence many physicians do not consider a karyotype necessary. One review quoted only one case of trisomy 18.[8] The risk of an abnormal karyotype likely increases with the finding of other abnormalities. The most common abnormalities associated with gastroschisis are cardiac. The other abnormalities such as bowel stenosis or atresia are complications of the gastroschisis itself. Less frequently, cleft palate and diaphragmatic hernia have also been reported.[7] Other structures may, on rare occasions, be present within the gastroschisis: liver, uterus and undescended testes have all been noted.

Once the diagnosis is made, serial ultrasound examination has been suggested to assess fetal amniotic fluid volume and bowel appearance. However, accurate ultrasound measurements of fetal growth based on soft tissues may be difficult or impossible with large anterior abdominal wall defects. Long bone (femur) growth and head size can be assessed. Hydramnios may develop with associated small bowel atresia and reduced amniotic fluid volume may accompany poor uterine growth.

The appearance of the bowel and the diameter of the bowel loops is thought by some to have prognostic significance. The increased echogenicity and presumed thickening of the bowel wall in later pregnancy generally beyond 28 weeks may represent the fibrous coating or 'peel' that may cover and bind loops of bowel. The etiology of the peel is debated. While it has been suggested that amniotic fluid components cause a chemical peritonitis, an alternative explanation is that the thickening results from venous and lymphatic obstruction. The latter is supported by the observation that the intra-abdominal peritoneum, also exposed to amniotic fluid, does not always show a peel and that there is no evidence early delivery which would decrease exposure benefits outcome.[13] Though the presence of a peel can make the surgical closure more difficult, it otherwise has little correlation with outcome and resolves quickly after surgical closure of the abdominal wall as evidenced by findings at reoperation (K. Pringle, personal communication). Though increasing dilation of bowel loops may appear worrisome, it is not in itself an indication for delivery (**Figure 7**).[14]

Parental counseling, including the obstetrician and pediatric surgeon, should emphasize the high chance of a good outcome with over 80% survival (and primary closure in over 80%). Prolonged neonatal hospitalization with parenteral nutrition is sometimes necessary. In the absence of ultrasound abnormalities of growth, amniotic fluid volume or heart rate tracing abnormalities, the pregnancy may proceed to term. There is no evidence that early delivery generally improves outcome (**Figure 8**).

Close monitoring at term is suggested as unexplained death has been observed in a number of cases in the author's experience.

Labor/delivery

Similar to omphalocele, there is no objective evidence that cesarean section results in improved outcome. An international trial on delivery management of gastroschisis is currently in progress.

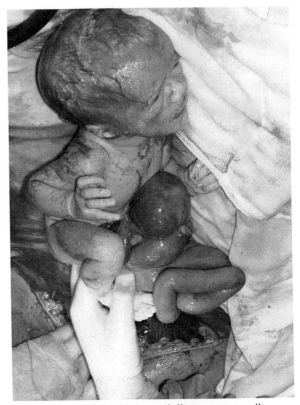

Figure 8. Gastroschisis at delivery, unusually containing the liver. Baby delivered by cesarean section, the indications being a footling breach presentation.

Postnatal

The immediate postnatal management is similar to omphalocele, but treatment may be more urgent as there is no protecting membrane over the components of the gastrochisis. The preoperative workup and stabilization of the infant should be expedited. At delivery, the neonate is placed in the isolation or Lehey bag or even a sterile plastic oven bag containing the warmed electrolyte and antibiotic solution as described for omphalocele (**Figure 4**). The bag is carefully tied at the axillary level so as not to kink or rotate the bowel. A nasogastric tube is passed and mechanical ventilation used if required. An average time of 7 h from delivery to surgery has been reported and has been associated with good results. Primary closure is achieved in 85% of cases.[6] Postoperative ventilation is generally required in all babies for about 72 h and total parenteral nutrition is often required until oral feeding can commence. The surgical approach favored by the author's unit is a transverse incision at the level of the defect if required. A careful examination of the bowel is made for atretic segments. Any incision made is closed transversely and the abdominal wall defect closed vertically with the umbilical cord left in place

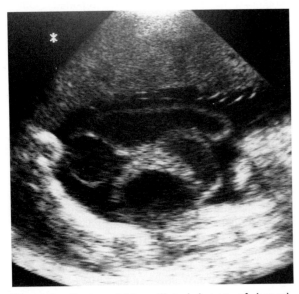

Figure 7. Gastroschisis: dilated loops of bowel. This fetus was delivered vaginally at term and primary abdominal wall closure was achieved.

to produce a 'normal' umbilicus (**Figure 9**). When primary closure is not possible, a silastic silo is employed (**Figures 10, 11**). Failure to pass stool by 28 days requires a further search for atresia which may occur in up to 5% of cases.[15]

The prognosis is generally good, but there is a mortality rate of approximately 10% associated with prematurity, intestinal ischemia or necrosis. Prolonged bowel dysfunction, especially motility disorders or malabsorption, occurs in a small number. There is only one investigation of very long-term follow-up of patients with gastrochisis.[16] Development beyond 5 years of age was normal in fetuses with isolated lesions, but those with bowel atresia or complications requiring bowel resection had a higher frequency of long-term bowel problems or non-specific abdominal complaints.

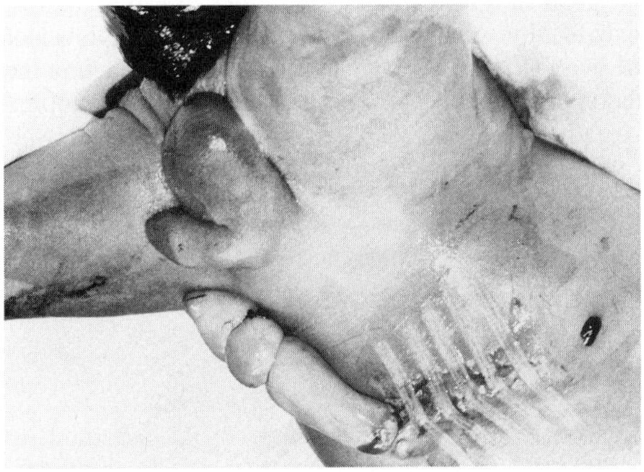

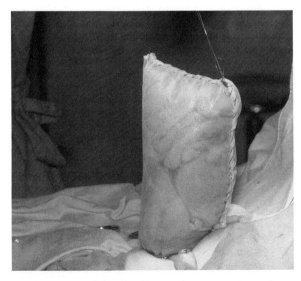

Figure 9. Abdominal wall closure in gastroschisis. Similar results are usually obtained with or without previous use of a silo.

Figure 10. Silastic silo used to cover bowel.

GASTROSCHISIS
Summary of Management Options

Diagnosis

- Ultrasound and/or raised serum alpha-fetoprotein

Prenatal

- Careful ultrasound examination of the fetal heart to exclude cardiac abnormality

- The indications for karyotype are unclear but the risk of an abnormal karyotype appears <1%.

- No indication to deliver prematurely, as the risk of this outweighs any possible advantages in terms of developing a peel or bowel dilation

Labor/delivery

- There is no evidence that delivery by cesarean section is beneficial

- Delivery in a center with neonatal surgical facilities

- Careful handling of the bowel

- Prevention of heat loss and early surgery

The risk of recurrence in subsequent pregnancies is very low. There have been isolated case reports suggesting a familial recurrence but the risk is very low.[17]

CONGENITAL DIAPHRAGMATIC HERNIA

Congenital diaphragmatic hernia may be considered an abdominal wall defect with some parallels to gas-

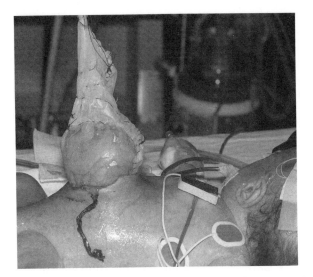

Figure 11. The silo is reduced in size over 7 days as its contents are returned to the abdomen.

troschisis and omphalocele. The associated pulmonary hypoplasia is often lethal.

Definition

Diaphragmatic hernia is a protrusion or herniation of abdominal contents into the thoracic cavity. Herniation can occur through a posterolateral defect in the pleuroperitoneal canal (the most common), defects in the sternocostal hiatus, the retrosternal or Morgagni hernia, a hiatus hernia, defects in the central tendon of the diaphragm and through complete eventration of the diaphragm.

Incidence

The incidence is 1:5000 live births, but higher if terminations, miscarriages and stillbirths are included. Left-sided hernias appear to be more common than right-sided ones. Over 15% of cases have associated abnormalities, and diaphragmatic hernia is associated with a number of syndromes, including Beckwith-Wiedeman syndrome, Pierre Robin syndrome, Fryns syndrome and chromosomal defects such as T13, T18 and deletion 9p-syndrome.

Presentation

The most common postnatal presentation is cyanosis soon after clamping the umbilical cord. Other signs

include a scaphoid abdomen (**Figure 12**), a barrel-shaped chest and dextrocardia. Diaphragmatic hernia is the most common cause of dextrocardia diagnosed in the delivery suite. With the widespread use of prenatal ultrasound, the diagnosis may be made prior to delivery. It is one of the differential diagnoses to be considered in the woman who presents in the late second or early third trimester with hydramnios.

The ultrasound diagnosis is not without difficulty. Small hernias may be missed and the diagnosis of right-sided diaphragmatic hernia is extremely difficult, since the liver and lung in early pregnancy have similar echogenicity. As pregnancy advances, the lungs tend to become more echogenic. The hyopechoic line seen on ultrasound separating the thoracic from the abdominal cavities may appear to be present, but is an unreliable sign in excluding diaphragmatic hernia. The most sensitive sign is an abnormal thoracic location of the heart (**Figure 13**).[18] Other signs are hydramnios, visualization of the bowel or stomach at the level of the heart (**Figure 13**) and absence of the stomach in the abdomen (**Figure 14**). The mechanism for developing hydramnios is unclear, but may involve impaired swallowing or obstruction of the upper gastrointestinal tract.

Management Options

Prenatal

Once diagnosed on ultrasound, it is important to exclude the presence of other structural abnormalities. The most common ones are cardiovascular, in particular VSD and tetralogy of Fallot, though gastrointestinal, skeletal and genitourinary abnormalities are also seen. A karyotype should be offered, as there is at least a 10–20% risk of aneuploidy.[19]

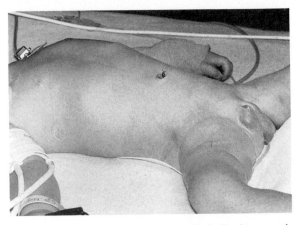

Figure 12. Neonate with congential diaphragmatic hernia showing scaphoid abdomen.

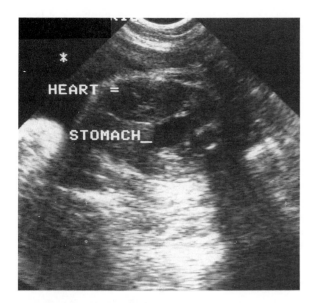

Figure 13. Prenatal ultrasound image of diaphragmatic hernia. Note the heart and stomach in the thorax and visualized together in the imaging plane.

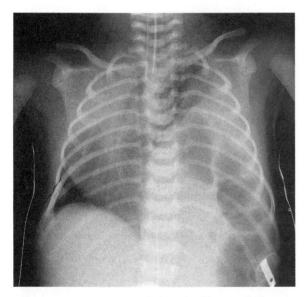

Figure 14. Diaphragmatic hernia. Neonatal chest x-ray showing the heart displaced to the right and abdominal contents in the left thorax.

In addition to excluding any other structural and chromosomal abnormalities, the differential diagnosis of intrathoracic ultrasound abnormalities or masses should be considered. These include cystic adenomatoid malformation of the lung and other cystic and solid masses within the mediastinum.

Where other abnormalities are detected in addition to diaphragmatic hernia, certainly prior to viability, termination of pregnancy needs to be discussed with the parents. The prognosis for isolated diaphragmatic hernia appears to be considerably higher than that previously reported. Studies examining the total population of an area (as opposed to mail surveys) document a 60% survival without the use of extracorporeal membrane oxygenation (ECMO) and with the repair being done in a variety of hospital levels.[20] Diaphragmatic hernia is generally fatal where there are other associated anomalies.

In the absence of other abnormalities, several investigations have attempted to predict outcome. If accurate, such predictions could help the parents decide whether to continue with the pregnancy or undergo termination. They might also guide immediate post-delivery management including the use of ECMO. Unfortunately, these schemes have not proven accurate enough to rely on. Factors considered influential in effecting prognosis are listed in **Table 2**.[21] While early diagnosis and the early development of hydramnios (i.e. before 28 weeks) are both associated with a poor prognosis, it is not invariable and the other proposed prognostic indicators require further study before being accepted as reliable.

The parents should meet with a member of the surgical team prior to delivery. Counseling involves an explanation of the fact that generally a period of preoperative stabilization after birth yields better results than that of immediate surgical repair. Poor ventilatory parameters that fail to improve with preoperative stabilization generally do not improve postoperatively and the prognosis is poor.

The wisdom of open fetal surgery for the treatment of isolated diaphragmatic hernia remains unclear. Several issues remain to be clarified – survival with postnatal surgery, appropriate fetal selection, ideal maternal techniques and quantification of the maternal risks. Despite protestation from some investigators, these issues must be resolved before any decision on an open fetal repair can be made.[22] Once the diagnosis is made, the pregnancy should be monitored closely for the development of hydramnios and any of its sequelae.

Table 2
Factors reported to affect prognosis in diaphragmatic hernia

Early diagnosis (<25 weeks gestation)
Hydramnios
Stomach in the chest
Liver in the chest
Lung to thoracic area ratio
Cardiac ventricular ratios

Labor/delivery

In the absence of associated abnormalities, labor and delivery are generally normal and there are no particular indications to deliver early or by cesarean section. However, these deliveries should be planned and affected in a center equipped for all likely complications.

Postnatal

After deliver, immediate intubation, ventilation and paralysis of the baby is necessary and the maintenance of good oxygenation from this time on is a good prognostic indicator. Typically, the neonatal chest x-ray will reveal a mediastinal shift with abdominal contents in the thorax (**Figure 14**).

In some centers, extracorporeal membrane oxygenation is available for those neonates not adequately oxygenated on conventional ventilatory support. The criteria for ECMO vary between centers, as do the data on what constitutes good response on ECMO. In a recent series of ECMO responders defined as a post-ductal pO_2 of greater than 100 mmHg, there was a 91% survival compared with only 7% in non-responders. In the same series, there was a similar high survival in those not requiring ECMO.[23] ECMO, however, is not without complications, including intracranial hemorrhage and vascular complications. Its place in the management of congenital diaphragmatic hernia, too, remains to be settled. Other postnatal treatments which may prove beneficial include artificial surfactant and pulmonary vasodilators. The comparative place of the new postnatal treatment *vs* prenatal surgery and its added maternal morbidity need to be fully assessed before clear guidelines for changes in the current management of diaphragmatic hernia can be given. A diaphragmatic hernia and its repair are illustrated in **Figures 15–18**.

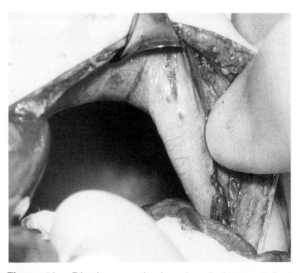

Figure 16. Diaphragmatic hernia. A large defect after the contents have been removed.

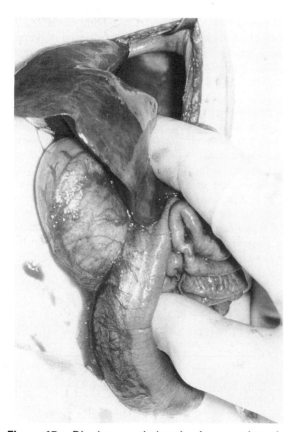

Figure 15. Diaphragmatic hernia. At operation, the contents of the hernia are being removed from the thorax. The defect is shown.

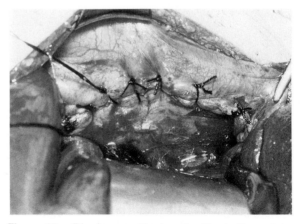

Figure 17. Diaphragmatic hernia illustrating closure of the defect.

CONGENITAL DIAPHRAGMATIC HERNIA
Summary of Management Options

Prenatal

- Diagnosis made by ultrasound

- Hydramnios is a common clinical finding

- Associated abnormalities should be sought by ultrasound and karyotype

- Prognosis is difficult to predict (**Table 2**)

- Termination is an option before viability

Labor/delivery

- Normal management but in tertiary center

Postnatal

- Immediate pediatric resuscitation with intubation and ventilation

- Preoperative stabilization with paralysis and ventilation may be necessary

- Early evidence suggests ECMO improves survival, though this technique is still experimental

- Recurrence risk is low

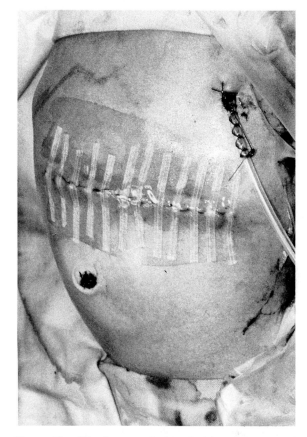

Figure 18. Diaphragmatic hernia showing wound closure and chest drain.

Prognosis

Survivors of postnatal repairs may suffer long-term morbidity, secondary bronchopulmonary dysplasia or other lung degenerative disorders such as emphysema.

However, these occur in the minority of cases. In general, the long-term prognosis is good if the neonate survives to surgery and especially beyond surgery.[24]

The recurrence risk is low, except where it is part of a genetic syndrome such as Fryns syndrome, which is an autosomal recessive trait including diaphragmatic hernia, dysmorphic facies and distal digital hypoplasia.

BODY STALK ANOMALY/LIMB BODY WALL COMPLEX

These are very rare abdominal wall defects.

Definition and Incidence

The etiology is variously due to maldevelopment of

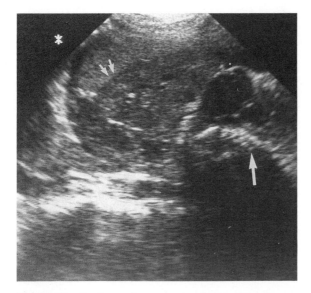

Figure 19. Body stalk anomaly. Illustration shows abnormal spine (arrow) and the appearance of the fetus being attached to the placenta and uterine wall (double arrows).

the body stalk or as part of the early amnion rupture sequence.[25] Its incidence is 1:14 000 births.

Presentation

Prenatal diagnosis is by ultrasound. Since this condition is incompatible with extrauterine life, the differentiation of a body stalk anomaly from other types of abdominal wall defects is important. There are multiple organ systems amomalies present in most cases. Sonographically, the viscera from the fetus appear to be attached to the placenta (**Figure 19**). Characteristically, there are associated neural tube defects, scoliosis and lower limb defects.[26] The fetal membranes may appear entangled with the eviscerated organs.

Management Options

Prenatal

Termination of pregnancy is offered to parents if the diagnosis is made within legal limits for your locale. Dystocia has not apparently been reported and vaginal delivery should be anticipated.

Prognosis

Lethal. This abnormality is thought to be sporadic and the recurrence risk is therefore extremely low.

BLADDER AND CLOACAL EXTROPHIES

While both are rare, bladder exstrophy is more common than cloacal exstrophy. The primary defect is failure of the caudal fold of the anterior abdominal wall to develop. The prenatal diagnosis of bladder exstrophy has been made and an omphalocele is seen in a high number.

Incidence

The incidence of this defect is approximately 1:200 000 live births. It constitutes less than 2% of anorectal malformations.[27]

Management Options

Prenatal

The prenatal diagnosis of cloacal exstrophy has rarely been suggested by ultrasound. Associated abnormalities include neural tube defect and omphalocele, and an elevated alpha-fetoprotein may occur if the fetus has these other abnormalities.

Bladder exstrophy has been diagnosed *in utero* by ultrasound. In view of the difficulties of surgical repair and the long-term problems of achieving continence and the associated genital abnormalities, termination of pregnancy is an option. Otherwise, management of the pregnancy is along standard lines with referral to the neonatal surgical team prior to delivery so that the parents are prepared as well as possible.

Labor/delivery

Standard obstetrical management is appropriate with delivery in a unit with neonatal extensive care and surgical facilities.

ESOPHAGEAL ATRESIA WITH OR WITHOUT TRACHEOSOPHAGEAL FISTULA

Definition and incidence

These abnormalities may occur together, the most common being esophageal atresia with a distal tracheoesophageal fistula in 87% of cases. They may also occur separately, isolated esophageal atresia and isolated tracheoesophageal fistulas occurring in 8 and 4% of the cases, respectively. The esophagus and trachea develop from a common diverticulum in the primitive pharynx with the upper respiratory and gastrointestinal tracts becoming separated between 3 and 5 weeks gestation.

Presentation

The most common prenatal presentations are preterm labor and hydramnios. Fetal swallowing is seen regularly from 16 weeks gestation and failure to visualize the stomach on scan after this is unusual. Failure to visualize the fetal stomach on serial scans after 20 weeks gestation should alert the ultrasonographer to the possibility.[28] The diagnosis should also be suspected in all cases of hydramnios (**Figure 20**) and careful scanning should also form part of the management of cases of preterm labor. The differential diagnosis of absence of stomach includes esophageal atresia, congenital diaphragmatic hernia and impaired fetal swallowing from 'neurological' causes. It may also simply be due to an empty stomach at the time of the scan. In the absence of other abnormalities, a repeat scan within a few days is warranted before further diagnoses are considered. Esophageal atresia with a tracheoesophageal fistula allowing passage of amniotic fluid into the stomach is not usually associated with either hydramnios or an absent stomach on ultrasound, and the diagnosis may not be made prenatally. A very small stomach in the presence of hydramnios suggests the diagnosis.

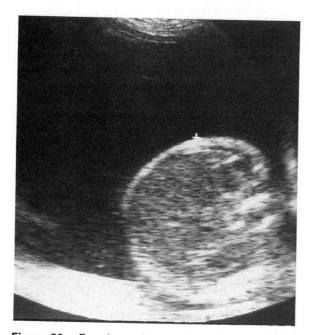

Figure 20. Esophageal atresia. Scan shows hydramnios and absent stomach in the imaging plane for the abdominal circumference measurement.

Occasionally, the proximal esophageal pouch in esophageal atresia can be seen on ultrasound when the stomach is absent. Failure to demonstrate the stomach necessitates a careful search for other abnormalities including the VATER or VACTERAL group of abnormalities. These abnormalities include vertebral, anal, cardiac (especially atrial and ventricular septal defects), renal and limb abnormalities, plus otocephaly, a major malformation of the mandible and temporal bones associated with abnormally placed ears.

Management Options

Prenatal

A karyotype should be obtained to rule out aneuploidy (particularly triploidy or trisomy 18). Esophageal atresia has also been recorded as part of the Di George sequence with deletion of chromosome 22.[29] In one recent series, nearly one-quarter of the patients had associated anomalies, the most common being the VATER syndrome, either in its complete or incomplete forms.[30] The other cluster of abnormalities sufficiently different from the VATER group to warrant distinction, is the CHARGE association (see **Table 3**). In the CHARGE association, most of the infants have some degree of mental retardation. In contrast, the majority of neonates with VATER have normal brain function (except those associated with either trisomy 18 or 13q- syndromes).

When the diagnosis is made before viability, parental counseling should include the influence of any associated abnormalities on neonatal outcome, the possible problems during the pregnancy (e.g. hydramnios) and the prognosis after neonatal surgery.

Table 3
Components of the CHARGE association

Colobomatous malformation
Heart defect
Atresia choanae
Retarded growth and/or CNS abnormalities
Genital abnormalities and/or hypogonadism
Ear anomalies and/or deafness

This association also includes:
  renal anomalies
  tracheoesophageal fistula
  facial palsy
  micrognathia
  cleft lip and palate
  omphalocele

Most have some degree of mental retardation

The latter has improved dramatically since the first recorded survival in 1939[31] due to both improvements in surgical techniques and neonatal intensive care.

The most common anomaly is esophageal atresia with a distal tracheoesophageal fistula. This is usually managed by thoractomy with division of the fistula and end-to-end esophageal anastomosis. In the absence of other abnormalities, survival rates of 100% have been reported.[31] After viability, the number of options may be reduced. In some centers, termination of pregnancy can still be offered, particularly for an abnormal karyotype or where a constellation of abnormalities suggests a poor prognosis. Karyotyping and careful ultrasound permit further management decisions to be made on the basis of results obtained.

If the decision is to continue the pregnancy, it is managed along standard obstetric lines. Hydramnios complicating esophageal atresia may prove to be difficult to manage and be associated with preterm labor. Medical management of hydramnios using indomethacin has helped in certain fetal abnormalities associated with increased fluid, but in the one published report did not do so in esophageal atresia.[32]

Labor/delivery

Labor and delivery are managed normally.

Postnatal

Awareness of the possiblity of esophageal atresia in all cases of hydramnios and in any newborn with excessive oral secretions, particularly if there are breathing difficulties or possibly cyanosis, should lead to the same management as that planned for the neonate where the diagnosis has been suspected prenatally. The secretions are aspirated and a polyethylene tube (e.g. a 10 French feeding tube) passed through the mouth or nose until resistance is felt. A chest x-ray should then be taken. Contrast media is not advisable at this stage, as there is considerable risk of aspiration. The absence of gas in the bowel does not exclude tracheoesophageal fistula, but where gas is present a communication between the esophageal atresia and a fistula exists. It is important to aspirate secretions from the mouth, pharynx and upper pouch of the esophagus frequently. Care should be taken with ventilation as a tracheoesophageal fistula may allow large volumes of air to enter the stomach causing the abdomen to become rapidly distended. Definitive surgery is offered once the infant's condition is stable.

Prognosis

The most important single determinant of outcome is the severity of associated anomalies. In most series, it is the Waterson C group[33] which has the lowest survival rate. Prematurity and low birthweight are generally associated with a good outcome, especially if the neonate weighs > 1500 g.[30] Immediate complications include anastomotic leaks, tracheal perforation and chest infection. Later complications are related to either esophageal stricture with obstruction to solids at

---

ESOPHAGEAL ATRESIA (WITH OR WITHOUT FISTULA)
Summary of Management Options

Prenatal

- Diagnosis by ultrasound in pregnancy is uncommon

- Hydramnios may be a clinical finding

- Associated abnormalities should be sought by ultrasound and karyotype

Labor/delivery

- Normal management but in tertiary center

Postnatal

- Excess secretions should be removed at birth and an esophageal tube passed and kept on continuous low-pressure suction

- Early chest x-ray

- Avoid feeding

- Check for other abnormalities

- Small risk of recurrence

the anastomosis site or respiratory complications including pneumonia, tracheomalacia and tracheal compression by the upper pouch. Only 10% of the series have respiratory complications beyond the first year and 8% have esophageal stricture.

The less common types of esophageal atresia with or without fisula (the types producing an airless abdomen either because of blind upper and lower pouches and no fistula or an atretic fistula) may require more complex surgery and the prognosis, especially in terms of morbidity, is poorer.[34] In this group, gastrostomy feeding and delayed anastomotic repair until the neonate grows are more frequently required.

Recurrence

Although this has been said to be a sporadic abnormality, there is a small recurrence risk and an increase in neural tube defects in subsequent offspring.[35] The familiar occurrence of esophageal atresia has also been reported.[36]

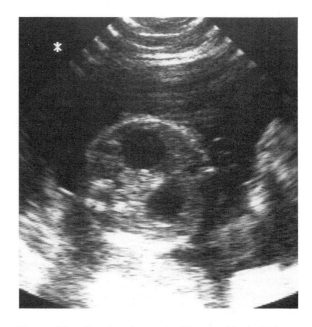

Figure 21. Duodenal atresia. The double bubble as seen on ultrasound.

ATRESIAS OF THE BOWEL: DUODENAL ATRESIA

Definition and Incidence

This is generally considered an early embryological insult to the duodenum most commonly either just proximal or distal to the ampulla of Vater with failure of canalization, which normally occurs around the 11 weeks gestation. Occasionally, vascular accidents or midgut strangulation associated with an omphalocele have been implicated as causes. The incidence of this defect has been reported as 1:10 000 live births.

Presentation

Hydramnios is a common feature in all upper intestinal atresias and is present in 50% of cases of duodenal atresia. The diagnosis may be made by the appearance of a 'double bubble' on ultrasound (**Figure 21**). Generally, this image occurs late in the second trimester but has been detected as early as 19 weeks.[37] It is important that a true transverse section of the abdomen is obtained and a connection between the two bubbles seen. This avoids confusion with an oblique scan of the stomach artificially producing a double bubble, or confusing the stomach and a choledochal cyst with a duodenal atresia. Increased peristaltic waves may be seen with real-time imaging.

Management Options

Prenatal

Other anomalies are present in over 50% of cases and should be sought. These include trisomy 21 in 30%, other gastrointestinal malformations in 25% and heart, tracheoesophagous, renal, hepatobiliary and pancreatic duct abnormalities in 48%. Other gastrointestinal abnormalities recorded include malrotation, esophageal atresia, imperforate anus, jejunal atresia, duplication of the duodenum and Meckel's diverticulum. Duodenal atresia may occur in association with multiple atresias of the bowel. Other chromosomal abnormalities associated with duodenal atresia include abnormalities of chromosome 9. About 50% of the infants have early onset growth deficiency.

This range of associated anomalies warrants both a detailed ultrasound search for structural abnormality and a karyotype. Knowledge of the karyotype is of value, even if termination is not considered. Fetuses with trisomy 21 have a high risk of cardiac abnormalities and may also have CTG abnormalities in labor which do not indicate hypoxia and do not require cesarean section. Indomethacin (or similar cycloxygenase inhibitors) may be given by mouth or by rectal suppository in an attempt to treat the hydramnios. Indomethacin given as 25 mg every 6 h has been effective in the treatment of symptomatic hydramnios.[32] No adverse effects on the fetus have been reliably documented when it is given for a short time prior to 32 weeks gestation. The main risk is constriction of the ductus arteriosus.

Labor/deliver

There is no *a priori* indication for cesarean section because of duodenal atresia. As the diagnosis of additional bowel atresias needs to be considered in any situation with hydramnios, delivery in a tertiary center is advised, both to manage the potential complications of the hydramnios and for access to neonatal surgical services. As with esophageal atresia where the cause for hydramnios may be in doubt, the passage of a nasogastric or orogastric tube at delivery and later x-rays of the neonate will help confirm the diagnosis. It is noted that a double bubble is not absolutely diagnostic of duodenal atresia and other possibilities must be excluded after delivery. These include an annular pancreas, peritoneal bands and duodenal stenosis.

Postnatal

After delivery, a tube is passed into the stomach and abdominal x-rays taken. The diagnosis can be confirmed at this stage by examination of the gas pattern. When the infant has been stabilized, the atretic area is excised (**Figure 22**) and the bowel closed with a primary end-to-end anastomosis.

DUODENAL ATRESIA
Summary of Management Options

Prenatal

- Diagnosis made by ultrasound

- Hydramnios is a common clinical finding

- Associated abnormalities should be sought by ultrasound and karyotype

Labor/delivery

- Normal management but in tertiary center

Postnatal

- A nasogastric tube is passed

- Diagnosis is made with x-ray

- At surgery, search for other abnormalities

Prognosis

The prognosis for this condition, if recognized and isolated, is good and the recurrence risk low.

Summary

This diagnosis is made by ultrasound or suggested by hydramnios. A careful search for multiple structural and chromosomal abnormalities is necessary.

ATRESIAS OF THE BOWEL: JEJUNAL ATRESIA

Definition and Incidence

This is the second most common form of atresia after the duodenum and the second most common site for

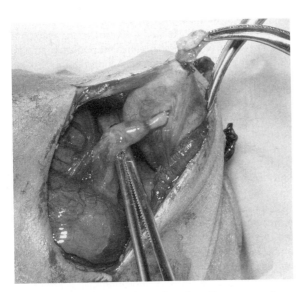

Figure 22. Duodenal atresia. Atretic segment as seen at neonatal surgery.

bowel obstruction in the neonate.[38] Jejuno-ileal atresias may occur throughout the small bowel. Its pathogenesis is thought to be due to vascular compromise of a bowel segment after organogenesis has been completed. Intestinal atresias are categorized according to the degree of occlusion or separation of the bowel on either side of the atretic segment. A special form of atresia called 'apple peel' deformity has a special significance both since it is an autosomal recessive trait and may have a poorer prognosis than the other forms of atresia.[39] Jejunal atresia has an incidence of approximately 1:5000 live births.

Presentation

Jejunal atresia manifests itself on ultrasound as multiple distended bowel loops. Hydramnios is more common with upper gastrointestinal obstruction (duodenal and jejunal) compared with lower obstructions. The development of ascites or an echogenic mass on scan is another sign of bowel perforation. Other features which may be useful in diagnosing bowel obstruction prenatally on ultrasound are increased peristalsis, failure to detect normal colon late in gestation and a disproportionately large abdominal circumference for dates.

Management Options

Prenatal

Jejunal and ileal atresias are usually isolated from other gastrointestinal lesions. It is important to exclude other causes of echolucent structures within the abdomen such as a urinary obstruction. It has been suggested that serial measurements of the diameter of the bowel loops may be of value in managing these patients and tables of bowel diameter are available.[40] However, these measurements do not correlate with either the diagnosis of bowel obstruction or prognosis. The appearance of the bowel is quite variable, particularly in the third trimester, and in our experience mild dilatation of the bowel has usually been associated with a normal outcome (**Figure 23**). However, it has been suggested that if the internal diameter of the small bowel is >7 mm,[41] there should be a high index of suspicion for bowel obstruction.

Labor/delivery

Fetuses believed to have a bowel obstruction should be delivered in a center with neonatal surgical facilities. Otherwise, obstetric management is unaltered by the

---

JEJUNAL ATRESIA
Summary of Management Options

Prenatal

- Diagnosis made by ultrasound

- Hydramnios may develop

- Serial ultrasound scans are advisable to recognize perforation (ascites, echogenic mass)

Labor/delivery

- Normal management but in tertiary center

Postnatal

- A nasogastric tube is passed

- Diagnosis is made by x-ray

- At surgery, search for other abnormalities

- Recurrence risk is low (except apple peel deformity with 1:4 risk)

---

presence of the abnormality. Hydramnios is not an *a priori* indication for a cesarean delivery.

Postnatal

After delivery, the neonate is evaluated to determine the site of obstruction and the presence of any associated congenital anomalies or meconium peritonitis. The prognosis is now very good for infants following repair with no losses in one series.[38] Even the group with apple peel deformity, early diagnosis and prolonged parenteral nutrition have seen a spectacular improvement in survival rates.[42]

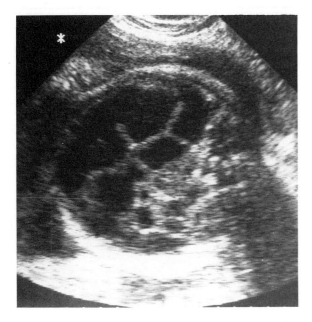

Figure 23. Dilated bowel on ultrasound. This fetus had a normal outcome.

Prognosis

The risk of recurrence for jejunal and ileal atresia is very small except in the group with apple peel syndrome, which would appear to be an autosomal recessive trait.[43]

ATRESIAS OF THE BOWEL: LARGE BOWEL OBSTRUCTION, ANAL ATRESIA AND IMPERFORATE ANUS

Colonic atresia is a rare condition largely confined to the right colon.[38] The distal colon becomes patent starting from the region of the descending colon. Anorectal malformations are complex and one way to classify them is by the level of the defect and its association with fistula formation.[44] Anal anomalies may also be part of multiple malformation syndromes, including the VATER complex. At least 25 such syndromes are recognized.[45] The incidence of imperforate anus is 1:2500 to 1:5000 live births.

Presentation

Prenatal

Large bowel abnormalities are rarely diagnosed on ultrasound, except perhaps as part of other multiple malformation syndromes. Apart from mechanical factors, other reasons for large bowel dilatation or increased echogenicity include meconium ileus and Hirschsprung's disease. Generally, the diagnoses of these conditions are made postnatally.

ATRESIAS OF THE BOWEL: MECONIUM ILLEUS/MECONIUM PERITONITIS

Definition and Incidence

Meconium ileus is an obstruction of the lower ileum by thick meconium. Perforation of the bowel may lead to meconium peritonitis and may occur after bowel obstruction secondary to any cause, including intestinal atresia, volvulus,[46] malrotation and meconium ileus. These conditions are rare. Most cases of meconium ileus are associated with cystic fibrosis; in contrast, most cases of meconium peritonitis are *not* associated with cystic fibrosis. However, this diagnosis should also be considered.

Presentation

Prenatal

Both meconium ileus and meconium peritonitis have been diagnosed in the second trimester.[47] Meconium ileus can present on ultrasound as a cluster of bright echoes or the bowel may appear both dilated and echogenic. Distinguishing it from normal, especially late in the third trimester, may be difficult (**Figure 24**).

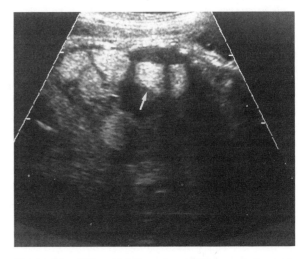

Figure 24. Ultrasound scan showing echogenic bowel (arrow) in the third trimester. This fetus had a normal outcome.

Fetal ascites and hydramnios are signs of perforation. A hyperechoic mass or diffuse hyperechoic deposits in the fetal abdomen indicate meconium peritonitis. The thorax may be compressed in the case of volvulus or other massive distention of the bowel.

Management Options

Prenatal

Suspected meconium ileus should lead to a search for cystic fibrosis. It is now possible to diagnose this condition on chorionic villous sampling, later placental biopsy or amniocentesis. Meconium peritonitis is a serious condition and the guidelines for management are suggested by the ultrasound appearances. A discrete lesion within the fetal abdomen which appears unchanging without ascites or hydramnios does not warrant intervention. The presence of ascites, increasing abdominal distention and hydramnios may warrant preterm delivery. In this situation and depending on gestation, antepartum corticosteriod administration could be considered to hasten pulmonary maturity. Drainage of the ascites, especially where there has been lung compression,[46] has been associated with a good outcome, but the result may not reflect cause and effect.

Labor/delivery

Meconium ileus in the absence of perforation is managed expectantly, though the neonatal intensive care team should be informed of the possible diagnoses. The management of meconium peritonitis in labor is determined by obstetric factors, e.g. the gestation and the ease of which labor can be induced. There is no objective information to suggest cesarean section is beneficial for meconium peritonitis.

Postnatal

Infants with meconium ileus usually become symptomatic within the first 24–48 h of life. Abdominal distention is noted and there is generally a delay in the passage of meconium. Vomiting is a relatively late sign. The overall prognosis for the neonate with meconium ileus is determined in part by the success of the gastrograffin enema or surgery in relieving the obstruction, but mainly by the severity of the cystic fibrosis if present. The prognosis for meconium peritonitis is not good, due in part to prematurity. The recurrence rate is low except where the condition is secondary to cystic fibrosis.

MECONIUM ILEUS/PERITONITIS
Summary of Management Options

Prenatal

- Diagnosis is made by ultrasound

- Consider diagnosis of cystic fibrosis (CF)

- Diagnosis of CF prior to viability allows termination as an option

- The development of ascites or hydramnios may be an indication for delivery

Labor/delivery

- Timing and mode based on:
  - obstetric factors
  - presence of perforation

- Delivery in tertiary center

Postnatal

- Outcome related to:
  - surgical feasibility of repair
  - associated abnormalities
  - perforation
  - gestation

MISCELLANEOUS INTRA-ABDOMINAL ULTRASOUND FINDINGS
ECHOLUCENT STRUCTURES WITHIN THE FETAL ABDOMEN

Echolucent or 'cystic' structures separate from normal bowel or the urinary tract may be identified on ultrasound. Possible diagnoses include cysts in the omentum, the mesentery, the ovary and liver in addition to choledochal cysts and duplication cysts of the bowel. Retroperitoneal cysts may also occur.

Management Options

Prenatal

The detection of intra-abdominal cysts is generally a chance finding on ultrasound. An attempt should be made to determine the origin of the structure and exclude other fetal abnormalities. Massive intra-abdominal cysts, especially those detected early in pregnancy, seem to have a poor prognosis, but in many cases remain unchanged or resolve.[48]

Hepatic cysts may be an isolated finding or be seen in association with adult type polycystic renal disease. Choledochal cysts (single or multiple) are seen in the right upper quadrant, below the liver, and intraperitoneal in location. As with most cystic lesions, their significance relates to postnatal management. Untreated, choledochal cysts may lead to biliary cirrhosis and portal hypertension.

The most common hypoechoic intra-abdominal lesion in the female fetus is an ovarian cyst. These are best observed postnatally, as most resolve over a period of weeks after delivery.

Labor/delivery

Obstetric care is unaltered by these abnormalities.

Postnatal

Awareness of the range of possible diagnoses is important. Ultrasound examination of the neonate soon after delivery is important. Duplications of the small and large bowel may rarely communicate with normal bowel lumen. In this instance the neonate may present with signs of bowel obstruction. Intestinal duplications in association with spinal cord and vertebral body anomalies have been reported.[49]

MISCELLANEOUS ECHOGENIC ('BRIGHT') LIVER

Echogenic liver (**Figure 25**) is an uncommon finding with a number of causes or associations, including liver tumors, congenital infection and vascular congestion. Hepatomegaly may occur in hemolytic disease or be part of a visceromegaly syndrome, e.g. Beckwith-Wiedemann syndrome.

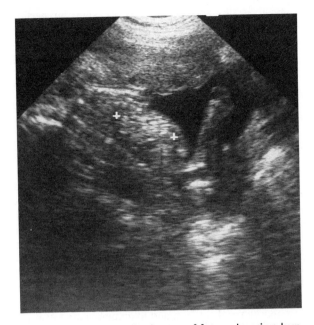

Figure 25. Longitudinal scan of fetus showing hyperechoic liver (crosses). This fetus had a normal outcome.

Management Options

Prenatal

Management is directed toward reaching a diagnosis. The association of hepatic calcification with congenital viral or toxoplasmosis infection is difficult to assess. Serologic screening of the mother is used to identify women at risk of giving birth to an affected child, but assumes one knows which infectious agent to screen for and that a maternal response has occurred. In a review of 49 at-risk cases of toxoplasmosis, fetal infection was diagnosed in five. The diagnosis of fetal infection was made on toxoplasmosis-specific IgM in fetal blood obtained by cordocentesis and isolation of the parasite from the blood. No abnormal fetal liver calcifications were recorded, but both hydrocephalus and intracranial calcifications were seen.[50]

Herpes virus, ECHO virus, varicella, coxsackie virus and adenovirus all have similar hepatic manifestations of infection. Hepatitis leading to ascites is not rare. The ultrasound appearances are non-specific and invasive tests are usually necessary for diagnosis (see Chapter 49). In the case of toxoplasmosis, the risk of fetal transmission where there has been proven maternal infection in the first trimester is thought to be low (~4%),[51] but invasive testing may provide reassurance with a negative result. Where proven infection is diagnosed before viability, termination is an option. Alternatively, treatment in the case of toxoplasmosis with spiramycin

3 g/day may be given until delivery. Four of the six neonatal survivors with toxoplasmosis in the study quoted were affected and two were asymptomatic at 6 months of age.[50]

Hepatic tumors including hepatoblastoma and hepatic adenoma[52] have been diagnosed *in utero*. Management involves observation until delivery, though as with any large tumor causing arteriovenous shunting, the fetus may develop congestive heart failure.

Labor/delivery

Standard obstetric management is generally appropriate.

Postnatal

This is determined by the likely diagnosis of the hepatic abnormality. Delivery in a center with pediatric surgical facilities as well as neonatal intensive care is advisable.

Acknowledgements

I would like to acknowledge the help of the following: Associate Professor Kevin Pringle, Pediatric Surgeon; Ms Louise Groossens, Medical Photographer; and Ms Jennie Flower, Ultrasonographer.

REFERENCES

1 Kirk EP, Wah RM (1983) Obstetric management of the fetus with omphalocele or gastroschisis: A review and report of one hundred twelve cases. *American Journal of Obstetrics and Gynecology* **146**:512–518.

2 Wald NJ, Cuckle HS (1983) Neural tube defects: Screening and biochemical diagnosis. In Rodeck CH, Nicolaides KH (eds), *Prenatal Diagnosis*, p. 234. Proceedings of the Eleventh Study Group of the Royal College of Obstetricians and Gynaecologists. London: RCOG.

3 Raine PAM (1991) Anterior abdominal wall defects. *Current Obstetrics and Gynaecology* **1**:147–153.

4 Nyberg DA, Fitzsimmons J, Mack LA, Hughes M, Pretorius DH, Hickok D, Shepard TH (1989) Chromosomal abnormalities in fetuses with omphalocele: Significance of omphalocele contents. *Journal of Ultrasound in Medicine* **8**:299–308.

5 Vanamo K, Sairanen H, Louhimo I (1991) The spectrum of Cantrell's syndrome. *Pediatric Surgery International* **6**:429–433.

6 Meller JL, Reyes HM, Loeff DS (1989) Gastroschisis and omphalocele. *Clinics in Perinatology* **16**:113–122.

7 Sermer M, Benzie RJ, Pitson L, Carr M, Skidmore M (1987) Prenatal diagnoses and management of congenital defects of the anterior abdominal wall. *American Journal of Obstetrics and Gynecology* **156**:308–312.

8 Sipes SL, Weiner CP, Spies DR, Grant SS, Williamson RA (1990) Gastroschisis and omphalocele: Does either antenatal diagnosis or route of delivery make a difference in perinatal outcome. *Obstetrics and Gynecology* **76**:195–199.

9 Moretti M, Khoury A, Rodriquez J, Lobe T, Shaver D, Sibai B (1990) The effect of mode of delivery on the perinatal outcome in fetuses with abdominal wall defects. *American Journal of Obstetrics and Gynecology* **163**:833–838.

10 Kohn MR, Shi ECP (1990) Gastroschisis and exomphalos: Recent trends and factors influencing survival. *Australia and New Zealand Journal of Surgery* **60**:199–202.

11 Baird PA, MacDonald EL (1981) An epidemiologic study of congenital malformations of the anterior abdominal wall in more than half a million consecutive live births. *American Journal of Human Genetics* **33**:470–478.

12 Glick PL, Harrison MR, Adzick NS, Filly RA, deLorimer AA, Callen PW (1985) The missing link in the pathogenesis of gastroschisis. *Journal of Pediatric Surgery* **20**:406–409.

13 Crabbe DCG, Thomas DFM, Beck JM, Spicer RD (1991) Prenatally diagnosed gastroschisis: A case for preterm delivery? *Pediatric Surgery International* **6**:108–110.

14 Sipes SL, Weiner CP, Williamson RA, Pringle KC, Kimura K (1990) Fetal gastroschisis complicated by bowel dilation: An indication for imminent delivery? *Fetal Diagnosis and Therapy* **5**:100–103.

15 Shah R, Woolley MM (1991) Gastroschisis and intestinal atresia. *Journal of Pediatric Surgery* **26**:788–790.

16 Swartz KR, Harrison MW, Campbell JR, Campbell TJ (1986) Long term follow-up of patients with gastroschisis. *American Journal of Surgery* **151**:546–549.

17 Lowry RB, Baird PA (1982) Familial gastroschisis and omphalocele. *American Journal of Human Genetics* **34**:517–518.

18 Romero R, Pilu G, Jeanty P, Ghidini A, Hobbins JC (1988) *Prenatal Diagnosis of Congenital Anomalies*, p. 215. Norwalk, CT: Appleton and Lange.

19 Benacerraf BR, Adzick NZ (1987) Fetal diaphragmatic hernia: Ultrasound diagnosis and clinical outcome in 19 cases. *American Journal of Obstetrics and Gynecology* **156**:573–576.

20 Wenstrom KD, Weiner CP, Hanson JW (1991) A five year state-wide experience with diaphragmatic hernia. *American Journal of Obstetrics and Gynecology* **165**:1302–1307.

21 Pringle KC (1990) Problems with selection of patients for antenatal repair of diaphragmatic hernia. *Clinical Consultations in Obstetrics and Gynecology* **2**:238–244.

22 Pringle KC (1991) Fetal surgery: Practical considerations and current status. Where do we go from here with Bochdalek diaphragmatic hernia? In Fallis JC,

Filler RM, Lemoine G (eds) *Pediatric Thoracic Surgery*, pp. 333–343. New York: Elsevier.

23 Wilson JM, Lund DP, Lillehei CW, Vacanti JP (1991) Congenital diaphragmatic hernia: Predictors of severity in the ECMO era. *Journal of Pediatric Surgery* **26**:1028–1034.

24 Molenaar JC, Bos P, Hazebroek FW, Tibboel D (1991) Congenital diaphragmatic hernia, what effect? *Journal of Pediatric Surgery* **26**:248–254.

25 Jones KL (1988) Early amnion rupture sequence. In *Smith's Recognizable Patterns of Human Malformation*, 4th edn, pp. 576–577. Philadelphia PA: W.B. Saunders.

26 Romero R, Pilu G, Jeanty P, Ghidini A, Hobbins JC (1988) *Prenatal Diagnosis of Congenital Anomalies*, pp. 226–227. Norwalk CT: Appleton and Lange.

27 Rintala R, Lindahl H, Louhimo I (1991) Anorectal malformations – results of treatment and longterm follow up in 208 patients. *Pediatric Surgery International* **6**:36–41.

28 Goldstein RB, Callen PW (1988) Ultrasound evaluation of the fetal thorax and abdomen. In Callen PW (ed.),*Ultrasonography in Obstetrics and Gynecology*, 2nd edn, p. 228. Philadephia, PA: W.B. Saunders.

29 Jones KL (1988) Di George Sequence *Smith's Recognizable Patterns of Human Malformation*, 4th edn, p. 556 Philadelphia, PA: W.B. Saunders.

30 Reys HM, Meller JL, Loeff DC (1989) Management of esophageal atresia and tracheosophageal fistula. *Clinics in Perinatology* **16**:79–84.

31 Myers NA (1991) Evolution of the management of oesophageal atresia from 1948 to 1988. *Pediatric Surgery International* **6**:407–411.

32 Kirshon B, Mari G, Morse K (1990) Indomethacin therapy in the treatment of symptomatic polyhydramnios. *Obstetrics and Gynecology* **75**:202–205.

33 Waterston DJ, Bonham-Carter RE, Aberdeen E (1962) Oesophageal atresia: Tracheo-oesophageal fistula. A study of survival in 218 infants. *Lancet*: **ii**:819–822.

34 Touloukian RJ (1981) Long term results following repair of esophageal atresia by end-to-side anastomosis and ligation of the tracheoesophageal fistula. *Journal of Pediatric Surgery* **16**:983–989.

35 McNay MB, Whittle MJ (1989) Gastrointestinal malformations. In Whittle MJ, Connor JM (eds), *Prenatal Diagnosis in Obstetric Practice*, p. 63. Oxford: Blackwell Scientific Publications.

36 Schimke RN, Leape LL, Holder TM (1972) Familial occurrence of esophageal atresia: A preliminary report. *Birth Defects: Original Article Series* **8**:22–23.

37 Romero R, Pilu G, Jeanty P, Ghidini A, Hobbins JC (1988) *Prenatal Diagnosis of Congenital Anomalies*, p. 237. Norwalk, CT: Appleton and Lange.

38 Reyes HM, Meller JL, Loeff D (1989) Neonatal intestinal obstruction. *Clinics in Perinatalogy* **16**:85–96.

39 Seashore JH, Collins FS, Markowitz RI, Seashore MR (1987) Familial apple peel jejunal atresia: Surgical, genetic and radiographic aspects. *Pediatrics* **80**:540–544.

40 Goldstein I, Lockwood C, Hobbins JC (1987) Ultrasound assessment of fetal intestinal development in the evaluation of gestational age. *Obstetrics and Gynecology* **70**:682–686.

41 Goldstein RB, Callen PW (1988) Ultrasound evaluation of the fetal thorax and abdomen. In Callen PW (ed.), *Ultrasonography in Obstetrics and Gynecology*, 2nd edn, p. 231. Philadelphia PA: W.B. Saunders.

42 Manning C, Strauss A, Gyepes MT (1989) Jejunal atresia with 'apple peel' deformity: A report of eight survivors. *Journal of Perinatology* **9**:281–286.

43 Smith MB, Smith L, Wells W, Shapira E, Hendrickson M, Moynihan PC (1991) Concurrent jejunal atresia with 'apple peel' deformity in premature twins. *Pediatric Surgery International* **6**:425–428.

44 Santulli TV, Kiesmetter WB, Bill AH Jr (1970) Anorectal anomalies: A suggested international classification. *Journal of Pediatric Surgery* **5**:281–287.

45 de Sa DJ (1991) The alimentary tract. In Wigglesworth JS, Singer DB (eds), *Textbook of Fetal and Perinatal Pathology*, pp. 968–969. Cambridge, MA: Blackwell Scientific Publications.

46 Suzumorik, Adachi R, Yagami Y, Togari H (1990) A fetal case of midgut volvulus. *Asia-Oceania Journal of Obstetrics and Gynaecology* **16**:13–16.

47 Romero R, Pilu G, Jeanty P, Ghidini A, Hobbins JC (1988) *Prenatal Diagnosis of Congenital Anomalies*, p. 240. Norwalk, CT: Appleton and Lange.

48 Zimmer EZ, Bronshtein M (1991) Fetal intra-abdominal cysts detected in the first and early second trimester by transvaginal sonography. *Journal of Clinical Ultrasound* **19**:564–567.

49 de Sa DJ (1991) The alimentary tract. In Wigglesworth JS, Singer DB (eds), *Textbook of Fetal and Perinatal Pathology*, p. 933. Cambridge, MA: Blackwell Scientific Publications.

50 Foulon W, Naessens A, Mahler T, de Waele M, de Catte L, de Meuter F (1990) Prenatal diagnosis of congenital toxoplasmosis. *Obstetrics and Gynecology* **76**:769–772.

51 Daffos F, Forestier F, Capella-Pavlovsky M *et al.* (1988) Prenatal management of 746 pregnancies at risk of congenital toxoplasmosis. *New England Journal of Medicine* **318**:271–275.

52 Marks F, Thomas P, Lustig I, Greco MA, Raghavendra BN, Wasserman R (1990) *In utero* sonographic description of a fetal liver adenoma. *Journal of Ultrasound in Medicine* **9**:119–122.

53

Fetal Cardiac Anomalies

LINDSEY D. ALLAN

INTRODUCTION

The majority of cardiac malformations are the result of fundamental abnormalities occurring during early fetal development. Although fetal heart motion has been identifiable by ultrasound for many years, it was not until the late 1970s that advances in image quality and development of 'real time' equipment allowed clear visualization of the cardiac structure. The cross-sectional appearance of the normal fetal heart was described by several authors almost simultaneously in 1980.[1-3] Since then, imaging systems have improved further such that a high degree of diagnostic accuracy in the detection of cardiac disease can be achieved from the midtrimester of pregnancy.[4] During the 1980s, the addition of pulsed and color Doppler to the echocardiographic study provided flow direction information to the cross-sectional images.

Congenital heart disease is now the most common congenital anomaly, present in about 8:1000 live births. Of these, 3 of 8 represent severe malformations. There are some forms of congenital heart disease which are associated with a high rate of spontaneous intrauterine loss. Despite enormous advances in pediatric cardiac surgery over the last 20 years, the outlook for children with many forms of heart disease remains poor, and though the short-term results of cardiac surgery for children are improving, the long-term results into early adult life remain uncertain. At the present time, there is little information about the late complications, quality of life and life-span in adults with major congenital heart disease which has been corrected in childhood.

Heart malformations are more common than many defects which are diligently sought for during routine scanning (e.g. neural tube defects). The most easily obtained view of the fetal heart is the four-chamber view (see **Figure 1**). Identifying the normality of this one section will either exclude many major defects or detect an abnormality in about 2:1000 pregnancies. The evaluation of the four-chamber view of the heart can be successfully performed during a routine ultrasound examination,[5] raising the possibility of screening pregnant women for major forms of fetal heart disease in countries where detailed ultrasound is offered in every case. At the present time, a cardiac scan which examines all cardiac structures is usually performed in specialized centers and limited to pregnancies at increased risk of congenital heart disease.

HIGH RISK PREGNANCIES

Certain groups of pregnancies are at increased risk of yielding a fetus with congenital heart disease (CHD). These patients should be referred to a specialized center for fetal echocardiography where the expertise of either a perinatal sonologist or a pediatric cardiologist with experience in prenatal diagnosis is available. The high risk pregnancies include:

- Women with a family history of CHD. If one previous child has CHD, the recurrence risk is 1–3% depending upon the defect. Where there have been two affected children, the risk increases to 10%.

If a parent is affected, the risk to the next generation is between 5 and 10%, probably greater if the mother is the affected parent and still higher yet if cyanotic.

- Maternal systemic disease, the most common example being diabetes, which doubles the risk of cardiac malformation. Euglycemic control prior to or during very early pregnancy diminishes this risk. Maternal phenylketonuria also increases the risk of fetal heart disease.

- Exposure to teratogens such as phenytoin and iso-retinoin, or to unconfirmed teratogens such as corticosteroids or lithium in early pregnancy.

- The detection of an extracardiac fetal anomaly on ultrasound should lead to a complete examination of the fetal heart, since many types of abnormalities, for example exomphalos, are associated with heart disease. Abnormalities in more than one organ system of the fetus increases the likelihood of a chromosome defect or a congenital syndrome.

- Though most fetal arrhythmias are not associated with structural heart disease, complete heart block producing a sustained bradycardia of less than 100 beats/min is often part of a complex abnormality.

- Non-immune fetal hydrops can be due to congenital heart disease and a fetal echocardiogram should be an essential part of the workup of these patients. Fetal hydrops will have a cardiac cause in up to 25% of cases.

- By far the most important high-risk group seen in our center are those 'normal' pregnancies whose obstetrician has noticed an abnormality of the four-chamber view on a routine scan. Over 80% of the anomalies now seen in our department are referred for this reason. Greater than 90% of pregnancies in the UK have a scan at some time during pregnancy. The timing and intensity of the routine scan varies, but in those units where a thorough 'anomaly' scan takes place at 18 weeks gestation or after, severe cardiac anomalies can be detected in up to 2:1000 studies.

ORGANIZATION OF FETAL ECHOCARDIOGRAPHY SERVICE

At-risk patients are seen at 18 and between 24 and 28 weeks gestation. Patients in whom an anomaly is suspected during an obstetric scan are seen as soon as they are referred. At 18 weeks, all the vascular connections are seen; later more minor defects are sought. Nearly 10 000 such patients have been evaluated in our department since early 1980. Over 800 anomalies have been detected with acceptable accuracy. In no patient has it proved impossible to visualize the atrioventricular connections and the two great arteries. Some minor defects such as small ventricular septal defects, secundum atrial septal defects, and valve stenosis have been overlooked. No major false-positive diagnoses have been made.

NORMAL FETAL CARDIAC ANATOMY

The practitioner must be familiar with the normal appearance of the fetal heart in its various projections or abnormalities will not be recognized. On the right side of the heart, the inferior and superior vena cavae drain to the right atrium, which connects through the tricuspid valve to the right ventricle. The pulmonary artery arises from the right ventricle. On the left side of the heart, the left atrium receives the pulmonary veins and connects via the mitral valve to the left ventricle from which the aorta arises.

Once the method to image all these connections is learned, major forms of heart disease can be excluded or diagnosed. Although many can be recognized prenatally, heart defects which do not involve a connection abnormality are usually relatively minor and associated with a good chance of successful correction.

The Four-chamber View

The four-chamber view demonstrates the pulmonary veins and atria, the atrioventricular connections and the two ventricles. In this one view alone, three of the connections are seen and clues to the normality of the great arteries can be identified. This view should be obtainable in every patient from 18 weeks gestation onward with generally available real-time equipment. *Failure to obtain a normal appearance of the four chambers of the heart necessitates referral for a specialized heart scan.*

The four chambers of the heart are seen in a horizontal section of the fetal thorax just above the level of the diaphragm (**Figure 1**). The heart lies mainly in the left chest with the apex pointing out of the left anterior chest wall. While the appearance of the four-chamber view varies according to the orientation of the fetus to the ultrasound beam, the normal position of the heart within the thorax and in relation to the spine should always be the same.

The same method of orientation should always be used in order to identify the cardiac chambers. The first

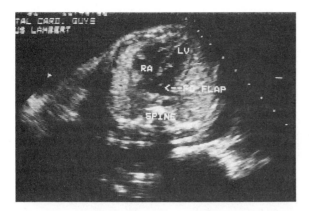

Figure 1. The four-chamber view of the fetal heart is obtained in a horizontal section of the thorax, just above the diaphragm. Here, the fetus is in an ideal position with the apex of the heart closest to the transducer. The ultrasound beam is almost parallel to the interventricular septum in this orientation. RA, Right atrium, LV, left ventricle; FO, foramen ovale.

step is to locate the spine. Opposite the spine is the anterior chest wall or sternum. Below the sternum is the right ventricle. Returning to the spine, the descending aorta is seen as a circle in the mediastinum lying anterior to the spine. Related to the aorta anteriorly is the left atrium. The remaining intracardiac chambers, the right atrium and left ventricle, can then be identified (**Figure 2**).

Figures 1 and **2** illustrate the images obtained when the apex of the heart is closest to the transducer. With the apex anterior, the beam is parallel to the intraventricular septum. **Figure 3** illustrates the view when the fetus lies with the right chest anterior and the beam is perpendicular to the septum. Compare **Figure 2** with **Figure 3**. When the fetus lies with either the left or right back anterior, the view will be less clear but sill recognizable (**Figure 4**). No matter how the fetus is lying, the following should always be seen if the heart is normal:

- the heart occupies about a third of the thorax

- there are two atria of approximately equal size

- there are two ventricles of approximately equal size, thickness and contraction in the moving image

- the atrial and ventricular septa meet the two atrioventricular valves at the crux of the heart in an offset cross

- two opening atrioventricular valves are seen in the moving image.

It should be noted that these rules are true for the fetal heart until about 32 weeks gestation, when the right ventricle may normally look slightly larger than the left. The septal leaflet of the tricuspid valve inserts

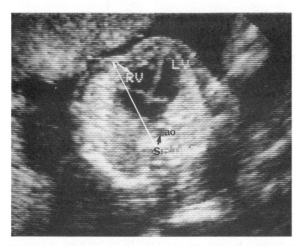

Figure 2. Whatever the fetal position the method of orientation is the same. The spine (S) is located first of all, the anterior chest wall lies opposite the spine with the right ventricle (RV) below it. The aorta (ao) is related to the spine anteriorly and the left atrium lies anterior to the aorta. Both ventricles lie in the left half of the chest. LV, left ventricle.

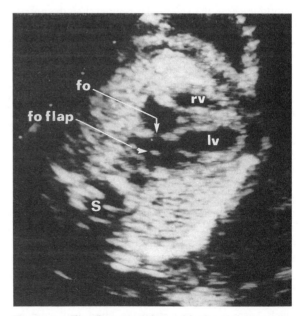

Figure 3. The fetus is lying with the right anterior thorax nearest the transducer such that the ultrasound beam is now perpendicular to the septum: lv, left ventricle; rv, right ventricle; fo, foramen ovale; S, spine.

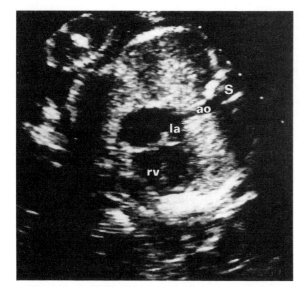

Figure 4. The right back of the fetus is lying anteriorly such that the fetal heart is at the opposite side of the chest from the transducer. The image quality when the fetus is in this position will be at its poorest, but the normal features are still recognizable. Note that when the beam is parallel to the septum as it is here, there is often dropout of the thin membranous portion of the septum just below the atrioventricular valves. This should not be mistaken for a ventricular septal defect. la, left atrium.

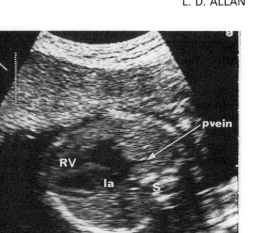

Figure 5. One pulmonary vein (p vein) can be seen entering the back of the left atrium.

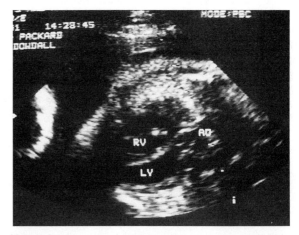

Figure 6. In a horizontal section above the four-chamber view, the origin of the aorta (AO) from the left ventricle (LV) can be seen.

slightly lower in the ventricular septum than the mitral valve. This means that the 'cross' at the crux of the heart is slightly offset. Scanning up and down in the four-chamber projection demonstrates the pulmonary veins entering the back of the left atrium (**Figure 5**).

Imaging the Great Arteries

The great arteries are imaged in a variety of projections in both horizontal and longitudinal sections of the fetus.[6] The horizontal views are usually the easiest views of the great arteries to find, although they may initially be difficult to understand. The longitudinal views are familiar to those used to postnatal cardiac imaging. Moving cranially from the four-chamber view and maintaining a horizontal projection, the aorta can be seen to arise in the center of the chest from the left ventricle (**Figure 6**). This artery sweeps out to the right of the thorax at its origin. The horizontal section cranial to this plane will visualize the pulmonary artery which arises anteriorly, close the chest wall, and is directed straight back toward the spine. The right ventricular outflow tract, the pulmonary valve, main and right pulmonary artery and the ductal junction with the descending aorta can be seen in this view (**Figure 7**).

The ascending aorta is seen in cross-section as a circle. Slightly further cranially, the crest of the arch of the aorta is seen in the inlet of the thorax (**Figure 8**). **Figure 9** illustrates the long axis of the left ventricle, which is achieved by tilting the transducer from the horizontal position to align the beam between the right shoulder and left hip. Transducer angulation in the other direction slightly to the right of a true longitudinal section permits the right heart connections to be seen (**Figure 10**). The aortic arch can also be imaged in a longitudinal section of the fetus (**Figure 11**).

The important features to note in these views are:

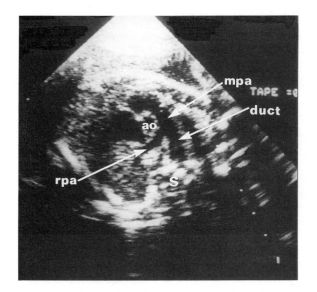

Figure 7. The main pulmonary artery (mpa) arises from close to the anterior chest wall and divides in front of the spine into the duct and right pulmonary artery (rpa).

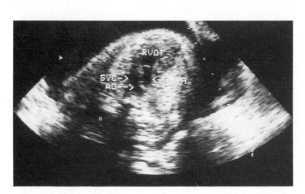

Figure 8. The crest of the arch of the aorta (AO) is seen just above the right ventricular outflow tract (RVOT) and main pulmonary artery (MPA) in the inlet of the thorax. SVC, Superior vena cava.

- two arterial valves can always be seen

- the aorta arises wholly from the left ventricle

- the pulmonary artery at the valve ring is slightly bigger than the aorta

- the pulmonary valve is anterior and cranial to the aortic valve

- at their origins the great arteries lie at right angles to, and cross over, each other

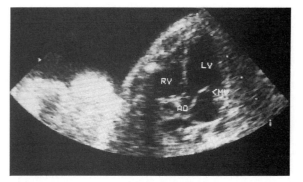

Figure 9. The long-axis view of the left ventricle is seen which illustrates all the left heart connections, the pulmonary vein to left atrium, the mitral valve (MV) between the left atrium and left ventricle and the aorta arising from the left ventricle.

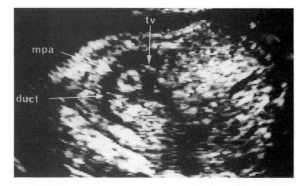

Figure 10. This section of the fetus demonstrates the right heart connections: the inferior vena cava entering the right atrium, the tricuspid valve (tv) between the right atrium and ventricle, the origin of the pulmonary artery from the right ventricle and its connection to the duct.

- the arch of the aorta is of a similar size to both the pulmonary artery and ductus, and is complete.

If all the normal features are seen, major anomalies of the great arteries can be excluded.

CARDIAC MALFORMATIONS

Risks and Management Options

When a fetal cardiac malformation is found, the management of the pregnancy will depend on:

- the nature of the cardiac malformation

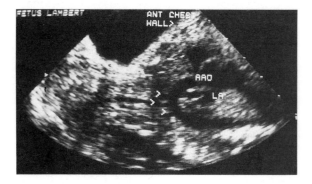

Figure 11. The arch of the aorta (AAO) is imaged. The aorta normally arises in the center of the thorax and forms a tight hook shape with the head and neck vessels (arrowed) arising from the crest of the arch.

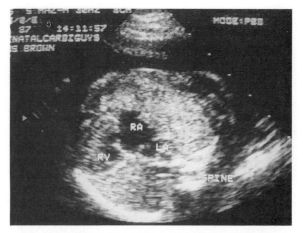

Figure 12. Only three chambers can be found in this heart as the left ventricle is absent.

- the association of extracardiac malformations

- the wishes of the parents

- the gestational age.

The Nature of the Cardiac Malformation

An exact diagnosis of the cardiac malformation is crucial if the parents are to be correctly counseled. A pediatric cardiologist should be consulted in the hope of providing the parents with a clear picture of the likely postnatal course, operability and outcome.

Aortic and mitral atresia (the hypoplastic left heart syndrome)

Aortic and mitral atresia is one of the most common anomalies recognized prenatally, since it is both common and associated with an abnormal four-chamber view. It is found in about 10% of infants with heart disease and up to 20% of fetuses in our experience. In typical cases, the aorta is tiny and the left ventricle small. Prenatally, the left ventricle can be impossible to find or the cavity small, thick-walled and echogenic (see **Figures 12** and **13**). The aorta is hypoplastic from its origin to the site of entry of the ductus where it becomes larger. Reversed blood in the ascending aorta can be seen on pulsed or color Doppler. It is rarely associated with extracardiac anomalies. Untreated neonates die in the first weeks of life. The Norwood operation or heart transplantation are recent options for treatment but the results are still disappointing. The experience with the Norwood operation has been dis-

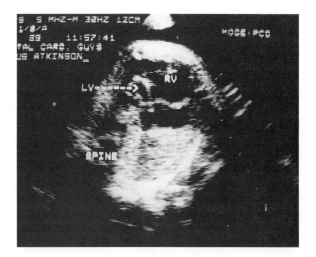

Figure 13. The left ventricle in this fetus is present but it is small, echogenic and poorly contracting on the moving image.

mal in the UK, although acceptable short-term results have been reported elsewhere.[7] There is a profound shortfall in donor material for transplantation and although the short-term results from some centers are reportedly good, the longer-term outcome is likely to be poor.[8–10]

Atrioventricular septal defect

A common atrioventricular valve results when there is a defect in both the atrial and ventricular septa at the crux of the heart where the two atrioventricular valves normally insert (**Figure 14**). The echocardiographic appearance is a single valve opening astride the crest of the ventricular septum. A common A-V valve is one of the most frequent types of heart disease seen pre-natally,[11] representing 17% of our series compared with the expected rate of 5% detected postnatally. This is because it is both frequently associated with extra-cardiac anomalies or fetal hydrops detected during obstetric ultrasound examination, and because it produces an abnormal four-chamber view. Atrioventricular valve regurgitation can be associated with the development of hydrops. The postnatal prognosis depends on the presence of other cardiac or extracardiac lesions which are common. Surgical repair usually takes place before the end of the first year of life. The mortality is between 20 and 30% depending on the associated lesions. It is often difficult to fashion two separate atrioventricular valve orifices from the common valve without leaving one valve regurgitant. This may mean a valve repair or even replacement at a later date.

Tricuspid atresia

In tricuspid atresia, there is no patent valve seen in the normal position between the right atrium and ventricle. It constitutes about 3–4% of both the neonatal and pre-natal series.[12] The right ventricular chamber is small or indiscernible as a consequence of no flow into the ventricle. There is a ventricular spetal defect of varying size. An example is shown in **Figure 15**. The great arteries can either be normally connected or trans-

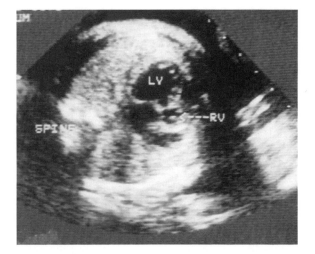

Figure 15. The right ventricle is much smaller than the left and there was no opening valve in the position of the tricuspid valve. This is tricuspid atresia.

posed. The arterial connection is important to identify as this will influence the management and prognosis. This form of heart disease is rarely associated with extracardiac anomalies. A Fontan procedure, which is the interposition of a conduit between the right atrium and main pulmonary artery, is the current repair of choice. While possible in the majority of cases, it is usually delayed until the fourth or fifth year of life. However, this palliative operation has many long-term complications which occur 10–20 years later.[13]

Mitral atresia

This is present when the mitral valve is not patent. It is seen more frequently prenatally than in postnatal series, constituting 5% in our experience. It can occur in combination with a normally connected but atretic aorta, as in the hypoplastic left heart syndrome, or with double outlet right ventricle. In the latter condition, there is no direct communication between the left atrium and ventricle, the floor of the left atrium being formed by muscular tissue. There is usually a ventricular septal defect as in the case illustrated in **Figure 16**. The great arteries arise from the right ventricle usually in abnormal parallel orientation. Surgical options for correction of this defect in the long-term are limited.

Double inlet connection

Double inlet connection is an uncommon defect where both atrioventricular valves drain to one ventricle. The sonographic appearance is of an absent interventricular

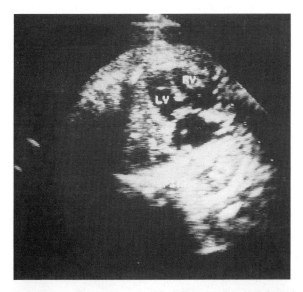

Figure 14. There is a large defect in the atrial and ventricular septum with a common atrioventricular valve seen closed in systole in this frame.

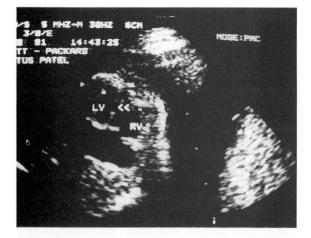

Figure 16. The mitral valve is atretic but the small left ventricle receives flow through a large trabecular ventricular septal defect (arrows).

septum (**Figure 17**). The origin of the geat arteries is variable. This condition has a poor prognosis for successful surgical repair.

Pulmonary atresia

In pulmonary atresia, the pulmonary root will either not be found in its usual position, or it will be very

tiny in relation to the aorta. It occurs in one of three settings:

- intact ventricular septum

- ventricular septal defect

- as part of complex congenital heart disease.

Pulmonary atresia with intact ventricular septum is the most common form seen postnatally and is characterized by a poorly contracting hypertrophied right ventricle with a small cavity (**Figure 18**). It represents 2% of CHD in both the prenatal and postnatal series. Pulmonary atresia is also commonly seen prenatally with a dilated right ventricle and severe tricuspid incompetence, (this form is described later under tricuspid dysplasia). In all forms of pulmonary atresia, the pulmonary blood flow needs to be increased by the creation of an aortic-to-pulmonary artery shunt. Definitive repair has poor results where the ventricular septum is intact. The outlook with a ventricular septal defect is usually better.

Transposition of the great arteries

The normal arrangement is lost in transposed great arteries. The aorta arises anterior and in parallel to the pulmonary artery instead of the normal appearance of being at right angles to the pulmonary artery at its ori-

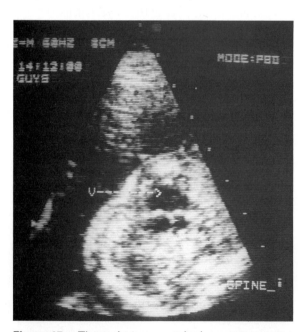

Figure 17. There is no ventricular septum seen dividing the single ventricular chamber (V). The two atrioventricular valves drain to this one ventricle.

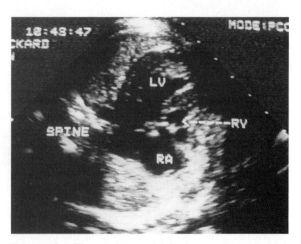

Figure 18. The right ventricle is small and thick-walled secondary to pulmonary atresia.

gin (**Figure 19**). Transposition represents around 10% of neonatal series, but is infrequent in prenatal series because the lesion is not detectable on the four-chamber view alone, and is rarely associated with extracardiac anomalies. It can be a difficult diagnosis to make unless the operator is experienced in the interpretation of both the horizontal and longitudinal views of the fetal heart.[6] However, prenatal diagnosis is important as transposition has a relatively good prognosis if early, corrective surgery takes place. The child will be cyanosed from birth and will either have an early balloon atrial septostomy and an atrial redirection procedure in the first 6 months of life, or will have an immediate arterial switch if the anatomy of the defect is suitable. The 20 year results of the first procedure are fairly good. Only 10 year results are available for the second, but these too are good.

Aortic override

In some forms of heart disease, the aorta is displaced anteriorly and arises astride the ventricular septum with a subaortic ventricular septal defect (**Figure 20**). This finding is seen in:

- Fallot's tetralogy

- pulmonary atresia with a ventricuar septal defect

- common arterial trunk

These conditions are differentiated by examination of the pulmonary outflow tract. The distinction is

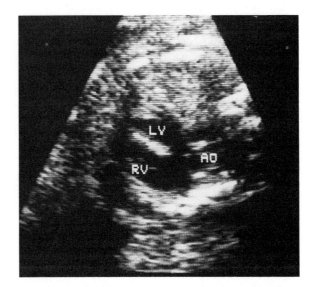

Figure 20. The aorta arises astride the ventricular septum. There is a large ventricular septal defect positioned below the aorta. Examination of the pulmonary outflow tract will differentiate between the three possible underlying diagnoses in this condition.

important since each carries a very different prognosis for corrective surgery. In the tetralogy, pulmonary outflow is obstructed but patent. In pulmonary atresia, it is completely obstructed and arises from the aorta as a common arterial trunk. The tetralogy of Fallot is by far the most common of three conditions. Tetralogy of Fallot is frequently (up to 50%) associated with extracardiac anomalies (particularly chromosomal). Corrective surgery in uncomplicated tetralogy carries a 5% mortality, but it will be much higher in pulmonary atresia. The surgery for a common arterial trunk is usually complicated by the dysplastic nature of the truncal valve, which must become the the aortic valve. Also, an artificial conduit is necessary between the right ventricle and main pulmonary artery. This conduit is subject to several common complications including obstruction. Further, repeated replacement is necessary to accommodate growth.

Double outlet right ventricle

In double outlet right ventricle, both great arteries arise from the right ventricle anterior to the ventricular septum. This anomaly is illustrated in **Figure 21**. Other lesions which can occur in association with double outlet right ventricle include:

- a ventricular septal defect

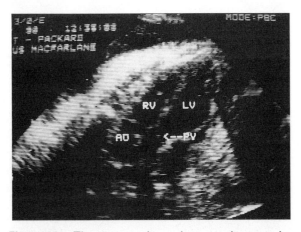

Figure 19. The aorta arises close to the anterior chest wall in parallel orientation to the pulmonary artery. The aorta connects to the right ventricle and the pulmonary artery to the left in this case of transposition of the great arteries.

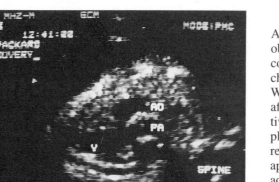

Figure 21. Both great arteries can be seen arising in parallel orientation from a single ventricular chamber. The aorta proved to be the anterior great artery.

- an atrioventricular septal defect

- mitral atresia

- pulmonary stenosis.

The position of the great arteries relative to each other can vary, but the normal 'crossing over' of the two is usually lost. Early palliation is often necessary. The long-term outlook for corrective surgery is reasonable, with a 20–30% mortality.

Additional abnormalities

Many other cardiac malformations can occur which do not involve abnormality of the connections of the heart. These tend to be less severe defects and more amenable to correction; some can, however, be recognized prenatally. They include:

- valve stenosis

- ventricular septal defect

- valvular dysplasia or displacement

- cardiac tumor

- aortic arch abnormalities

Valve stenosis

Any intracardiac valve can be stenosed or partially obstructed, but the aortic or pulmonary valve are most commonly affected. The respective ventricular chamber and the valve itself may appear thickened. When there is valvular obstruction prenatally, the affected artery is often disproportionately small relative to the other artery. Placement of the Doppler sample cursor in the sentosed artery may on occasion reveal increased flow velocity. The globular, echogenic appearance of the left ventricle characteristic of critical aortic stenosis is shown in **Figure 22**. On the moving image, diminished contraction of the left ventricle is evident. The high left ventricular diastolic pressure in this condition will often cause secondary left atrial hypertension with left to right shunting across the foramen ovale that can be demonstrated using Doppler color flow mapping. In critical aortic stenosis, the prognosis is very poor. When it is detected in the early fetus, the left ventricle fails to keep pace with normal growth and is hypoplastic by term. If it presents later in gestation, the outcome is still poor even if the obstruction is relieved immediately after delivery as the long-term damage to the ventricle appears irreversible. For this reason, prenatal balloon valvoplasty, accessing the left ventricle by transthoracic puncture, has been attempted with technical success but without survival.[14] In critical pulmonary stenosis, balloon valvoplasty soon after birth should be associated with a

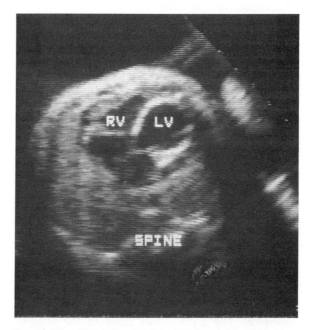

Figure 22. The left ventricle is echogenic, hypertrophied and globular in shape. In the moving image, the poor contraction could be appreciated. This was due to critical aortic stenosis.

good result. However, some cases will progress from stenosis to atresia during intrauterine life.

Ventricular septal defect

This is the most common heart malformation seen in childhood, constituting nearly 20% of cases.[15] However, ventricular septal defects (VSDs) are relatively uncommon in prenatal series. Ventricular septal defects vary in size and position and may be part of more complex anomalies. When found in the fetus, they tend to be large and/or be associated with extracardiac and chromosomal anomalies. These factors influence prognosis. The majority of isolated VSDs are small and close spontaneously postnatally, such as the one illustrated in **Figure 23**. A large inlet defect, which is unlikely to close, is shown in **Figure 24**. Less than 5% of VSDs require surgical correction.

Valvular dysplasia

Any cardiac valve can be dysplastic, but a dysplastic tricuspid valve is most commonly detected prenatally. This valve may also be displaced from its normal position into the body of the right ventricle producing Ebstein's anomaly. Both abnormalities result in incompetence of the tricuspid valve and right atrial dilatation. This can be very gross and associated with secondary

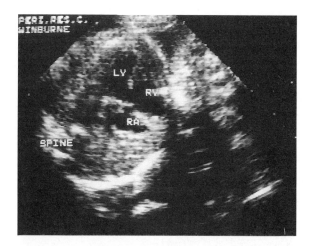

Figure 24. There is a large ventricular septal defect positioned in the inlet septum below the two atrioventricular valves.

lung compression and hypoplasia. An example of tricuspid dysplasia is illustrated in **Figure 25** and Ebstein's anomaly in **Figure 26**. These conditions are rare in pediatric practice but frequent in the prenatal series. The prognosis for a child with Ebstein's anomaly is variable, but the results of plication or replacement of the tricuspid valve if necessary are still unsatisfactory.

Tumor

Cardiac tumors are occasionally seen in prenatal life. They carry a high risk of blood flow obstruction with

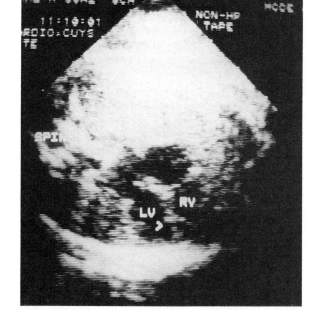

Figure 23. There is a small ventricular septal defect in the trabecular or muscular portion of the septum.

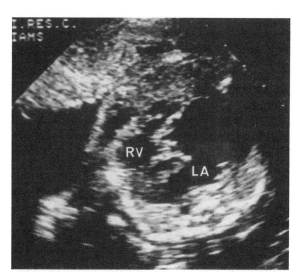

Figure 25. The right atrium is grossly enlarged due to severe tricuspid incompetence. The valve is dysplastic.

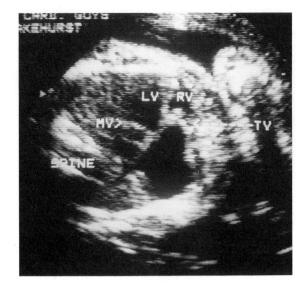

Figure 26. The right atrium is enlarged and the tricuspid valve is incompetent but also displaced into the right ventricle.

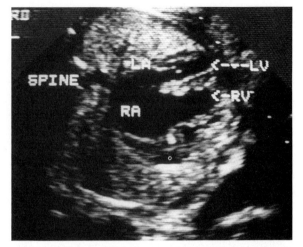

Figure 27. The right ventricle is dilated relative to the left in this case of coarctation of the aorta.

subsequent fetal hydrops and intrauterine death. The majority of tumors are histologically rhabdomyomas and associated with tuberous sclerosis.

Aortic arch anomalies

The aortic arch can be interrupted completely or partially obstructed as in coarctation, the latter being much more frequent. Coarctation can be a simple shelf region at the distal end of the arch, or be associated with severe arch hypoplasia. It is a common form of heart disease in infants, comprising about 10% of the total. Those cases recognized prenatally reflect the more severe end of the spectrum. Turner's phenotype, which includes cystic hygroma, fetal hydrops and coarctation, may be recognized in early fetal life. The clues to the diagnosis of arch anomalies in early pregnancy include recognition of an enlarged right ventricle and pulmonary artery relative to the left ventricle and aorta. An example of the four-chamber view in a fetus with coarctation is shown in **Figure 27**. A horizontal section of the arch of the aorta will show varying degrees of narrowing in coarctation and be incomplete in interruption. **Figure 28a** illustrates the appearance of the arch and duct imaged in the same section of a normal fetus. Severe aortic arch hypoplasia in associated with a coarctation lesion is shown in **Figure 28b**.

The presentation of this condition varies widely in children. The more severe cases become evident in the first days or weeks of life, whereas the milder cases manifest as asymptomatic hypertension in later life. Where the coarctation is discrete and there are no other anomalies, the prognosis for early corrective surgery

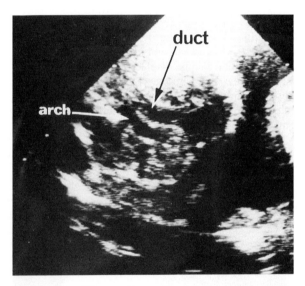

Figure 28a. The aortic arch and duct seen in the same section in a normal heart.

is good, although there is a re-coarctation rate of 20% in the cases surgically corrected during infancy. In neonates with complete interruption or severe arch hypoplasia, it can prove difficult or impossible to reconstruct the arch adequately and the mortality rate is high.

Artifacts

A common finding, that is not an abnormality, is illustrated in **Figure 29**. The bright mass within the cavity of the left ventricle is related to the papillary apparatus of the mitral valve. It probably represents fibrous deposition but has no pathological significance. It should

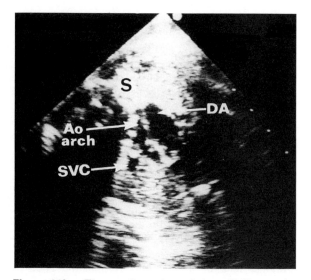

Figure 28b. The aortic arch and duct (DA) are visualized in the same plane in order to assess their relative size. The arch was severely hypoplastic in this case in association with coarctation.

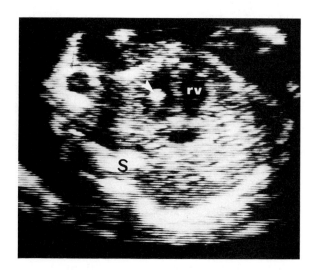

Figure 29. There is a densely echogenic lesion within the left ventricle. This is related to the free wall of the ventricle in the region of the papillary muscle of the mitral valve. It is not of pathological significance.

not be confused with the appearance of a tumor which can be at any site in the heart, is less echogenic, often larger or multiple and obstructive to blood flow.

In summary, the nature of a cardiac malformation can be accurately assessed prenatally and a prognosis offered based on the anatomical details and a knowledge of the prognosis for the condition as it occurs in children. Diagnosis and counseling should involve the

obstetric expert in fetal medicine and the pediatric cardiologist with expereince of fetal cardiology. However, there are some limitations of the fetal study which are important. First, some components of a cardiac defect are not detectable prior to 20 weeks gestation (for example, small or even moderate ventricular septal defects). Second, the degree of obstruction to flow, at either the valvar level or at a coarctation site, may increase as pregnancy advances. Third, the secondary effects of a cardiac lesion, such as the development of endocardial fibroelastosis in aortic stenosis or lung hypoplasia in tricuspid incompetence, may be the main determinant of outcome, although these findings may not be present when the case is seen initially. Fourth, some forms of fetal congenital heart disease are prone to the development of fetal hydrops, and spontaneous intrauterine death, which is difficult to predict. The potential for more complete diagnosis or for deterioration in the anatomical appearance of a defect must be taken into account when counseling the patient in the midtrimester.

The Association of Extracardiac Malformations

Nearly 20% of fetuses with congenital heart disease have a chromosomal abnormality.[16] A fetal karyotype should be performed either to help with a decision about terminating a pregnancy or to help in the management of prenatal care and delivery. A further 10% of fetuses have normal chromosomes but extracardiac anomalies. It is imperative to examine the whole fetus. There are some genetically inherited syndromes which have a heart malformation as a component, for example the Holt-Oram or Di George syndromes. The detection of such a syndrome within a family would influence the chance of a recurrence.

The Wishes of the Parents

When a fetal malformation is found, the wishes of the parents, once they have a clear understanding of the outlook, are paramount. Even if the lesion is operable, an affected child profoundly influences the lives of the parents and family. The author feels termination of pregnancy should be discussed in all cases if early enough in gestation. Many parents will have thought about their stance on termination prior to becoming pregnant. For some, the idea is discussed in the days between the detection of the possible anomaly and the specialist referral; for others, it occurs only after a major problem is described. Religious beliefs, social background and circumstances, education and previous experience are all important factors in making a decision concerning termination. The parents should be allowed freedom of choice, within the laws of the country or state, and supported whatever their decision. In many forms of congenital heart disease seen in prenatal life, the chances of the child reaching a healthy adult life are poor. Thus, the majority of parents in the UK at the present time – up to 75% in our series – will seek termination. A similar pattern is seen in the rest of Europe.

Where the pregnancy continues, the fetal heart should be examined sequentially in order to plan postnatal therapy. Changes in the findings should be sought and documented. The parents should be encouraged and supported throughout pregnancy and prepared for likely postnatal events. The site and method of delivery should be considered. In cases where there is no successful treatment, or alternatively where the neonate will not need early treatment, delivery may be local.

Where the neonate is likely to require treatment soon after birth, it is advisable to deliver within a center offering both obstetric and pediatric cardiac care. It is rarely necessary from the fetal cardiac point of view to deliver early or by cesarian section, though these options may need to be discussed in a small number of cases.

Gestational Age

The legal age limit for termination of pregnancy in the UK is 24 weeks gestation. However, in the presence of severe fetal anomaly, the age limit is unrestricted. In the USA and Europe, the time limit varies by state and country, respectively. In practice, the later the pregnancy, the more difficult it is to come to terms with the idea of termination. Termination after 24

CARDIAC MALFORMATIONS
Summary of Management Options

Prenatal – general

- Identification of high risk mothers

- Referral of high risk mothers to a specialist unit for a complete fetal echocardiogram

- Screening the normal obstetric population during routine scanning by four-chamber analysis

Prenatal – once fetal cardiac malformation identified

- Define/diagnose/characterize type of heart malformation

- Search for extracardiac, including chromosomal, anomalies

- Counseling offered by fetal cardiology specialist

- Termination of pregnancy offered if gestational age allows, prognosis poor and parents wish it

- Consider possible postnatal treatment depending on diagnosis

Labor/delivery

- Transfer care for delivery to center with appropriate obstetric and pediatric facilities

- Induce between 38 weeks and term at planned time

- Neonatal intensive care attendants at delivery for resuscitation

Postnatal

- Stabilization of neonate and cardiac investigation

- Interventional catheterization or surgery as indicated

weeks is usually reserved for those fetuses with lethal chromosome anomalies. Each case must be individually counseled and managed.

OUTCOME OF PRENATAL DIAGNOSIS OF CHD

Fetal echocardiography identifies cases of congenital heart disease (such as those associated with chromosome anomaly or atrial isomerism) which have a high rate of intrauterine loss, and which were not detected previously. Moreover, the spectrum of heart disease coming to the attention of the prenatal echocardiographer is different from that seen postnatally. Four-chamber view scanning identifies the more severe defects and the presence of fetal extracardiac anomalies leads to the detection of defects commonly associated with trisomies such as atrioventricular septal defects and tetralogy of Fallot. Fetal hydrops is a common presenting finding in cases of cystic hygroma, coarctation and Turner's syndrome. For these reasons, the epidemiology of congenital heart disease diagnosed prentally is quite different proportionally to that found in infants or children.

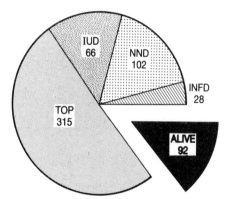

Figure 30. The outcome of 613 cases of congenital heart disease detected prenatally up to the end of 1989. TOP, Termination of pregnancy; IUD, intra-uterine death; NND, neonatal death; INFD, infant death; A, alive.

Figure 30 illustrates the outcome in 613 cases of congenital heart disease seen prenatally up to the end of 1991. There is a high mortality in the continuing pregnancies, with the majority of deaths occurring *in utero* or in the early postnatal period despite immediate

neonatal care. Only about half the survivors are leading a normal life as children.

REFERENCES

1 Lange LW, Sahn DJ, Allen HD, Goldberg SJ, Anderson C, Giles H (1980) Qualitative real-time cross-sectional echocardiographic imaging of the human fetus during the second half of pregnancy. *Circulation* **62**:799.

2 Kleinman CS, Hobbins JC, Jaffe CC *et al.* (1980) Echo-cardiographic studies of the human fetus: Prenatal diagnosis of congenital heart disease and cardiac dysrhythmias. *Pediatrics* **65**:1059.

3 Allan LD, Tynan MJ, Campbell S, Wilkinson J, Anderson RH (1980) Echocardiographic and anatomical correlates in the fetus. *British Heart Journal* **44**:444.

4 Allan LD, Crawford DC, Anderson RH, Tynan MJ (1984) Echocardiographic and anatomical correlates in fetal congenital heart disease. *British Heart Journal* **52**:542.

5 Allan LD, Crawford DC, Chita SK, and Tynan MJ (1986) Prenatal screening for congenital heart disease. *British Medical Journal* **292**:1717.

6 Allan LD (1986) *Manual of Fetal Echocardiography.* Lancaster: MTP Press.

7 Murdison KA, Baffa JM, Farrell PE, Chang AC, Barber G, Norwood WI, Murphy JD (1990) Hypoplastic left heart syndrome: Outcome after initial reconstruction and before modified Fontan procedure. *Circulation* **82**:199–207 (suppl. IV).

8 Stuart AG, Wren C, Hunter S, Sharples PN, Hey EN (1991) Neonatal transplantation for hypoplastic left heart syndrome: The shortage of suitable donors. *Lancet* **337**:957.

9 Boucek MM, Kanakriyeh MS, Trimm RF, Bailey LL (1990) Cardiac transplantation in infancy: Donor and recipients. *Journal of Pediatrics* **116**:171–176.

10 Pahl E, Fricker J, Armitage J, Griffith BP, Taylor S, Uretsky BF, Beerman LB, Zuberbuhler JR (1990) Coronary arteriosclerosis in pediatric heart transplant survivors: Limitation of long-term survival. *Journal of Pediatrics* **116**:177–183.

11 Machado MVL, Crawford DC, Anderson RH, Allan LD (1988) Atrioventricular septal defect in prenatal life. *British Heart Journal* **59**:352.

12 Anderson RH, Macartney FJ, Shinebourne EA, Tynan M (eds) (1987) *Paediatric Cardiology.* London: Churchill Livingstone.

13 Fontan F, Kirklin JW, Fernandez G, Costa F, Naftel DC, Tritto F, Blackstone EH (1990) Outcome after a 'perfect' Fontan operation. *Circulation* **81**:1520–1536.

14 Maxwell DJ, Allan LD, Tynan M (1991) Balloon aortic valvoplasty in the fetus: A report of two cases. *British Heart Journal* **65**: 256–258.

15 Fyler DC, Buckley LP, Hellenbrand WE, Cohn HE (1980) Report of the New England Regional Infant Cardiac Care Program. *Pediatrics* **65**:376 (suppl.).

16 Allan LD, Sharland GK, Chita SK, Lockhart S, Maxwell DJ (1991) Chromosomal anomalies in fetal congenital heart disease. *Ultrasound in Obstetrics and Gynecology* **1**:8–11.

54

Skeletal Abnormalities

DAVID R. GRIFFIN

INTRODUCTION

The pregnancy complicated by fetal limb or skeletal defect is one that may present the clinician with challenging diagnostic dilemmas and management options. Advances in real-time ultrasound image resolution have been such that fetal anatomy may be examined in great detail either from the conventional transabdominal route or transvaginally. In some instances the diagnosis of a lethal limb dysplasia may be readily apparent. In these cases discussion of pregnancy interruption would be appropriate. In others the diagnosis, prognosis and management options may be far less evident and require further biochemical, genetic or hematological investigation or karyotyping. The help of a geneticist with an interest in dysmorphology may be invaluable both in the initial diagnostic process and in counseling parents prior to final management discussions. A patient will present for prenatal diagnosis of a skeletal abnormality:

- because of a family history or genetic predisposition

- because a defect has been found during routine prenatal sonography which requires clarification

- because of adverse environmental influences.

CONDITIONS CONSIDERED

Heritable Defect in Family

In an increasing number of hereditable conditions mutant genes are being located so that prenatal diagnosis in high risk families may be achieved before skeletal manifestations are evident sonographically. In the remainder and in new presentations sonography remains the prime method for diagnosis.

This group of conditions will include dominant, recessive or sex-linked musculoskeletal disorders and chromosomal abnormality.

Dominant disorders (**Table 1**) carry a recurrence risk for the affected parent of 50% and are expressed in the heterozygous form. Some may show variable

Table 1
Dominant disorders

Achondroplasia
Cleidocranial dysostosis
Holt-Oram syndrome
Isolated polydactyly
Ectrodactyly
Ectrodactyly-ectodermal dysplasia-clefting syndrome
Spondylocostal dysplasia
Hypoglossia-hypodactyly syndrome
Distal dominant arthrogryposis
Dominant hypophosphatasia
Aase syndrome
Black fan diamond syndrome

expression such that the condition may be barely noticeable in an affected individual, e.g. ectrodactyly. Many dominant conditions are new mutations (sporadic). In these cases the risk of the condition recurring is very low (usually about 1%). Recurrence is thought to be due to gonadal mosaicism where some of the germ-line cells (but not somatic cells) of one parent carries the mutation. Recent evidence suggests that this is the mechanism of recurrence in osteogenesis imperfecta.

Recessive disorders (**Table 2**) are manifest in homozygous form. They occur in the offspring of unaffected heterozygous carriers. The risk of a heterozygous couple having an affected child is 25%, and 67% of unaffected children will be carriers. Close relatives in the same family are more likely to carry the gene than the general population so that in consanguineous marriages the likelihood of two carriers coupling is increased. Pregnancies from such consanguineous marriages should be considered at sufficiently increased risk of recessive disorders as to warrant detailed ultrasound examination of the fetus. Rapid progress has been made in the detection of gene loci for many of these conditions (see Chapter 2).

Table 2
Recessive disorders

Most of the osteochondrodystrophies
Roberts' syndrome
Jarcho-Levin syndrome
Fanconi pancytopenia syndrome
Thrombocytopenia-absent radius syndrome
Many polysyndactyly syndromes
Many multiple contracture syndromes

X linked disorders are very few in this group and thus they will not be discussed.

Chance Finding at Routine Ultrasound Examination

The ultrasonic abnormalities which may lead to the recognition of conditions with limb defects are listed in **Table 3**.

Unfavorable Intrauterine Environment

Examples of factors which can produce limb defects in this way are:

- diabetes mellitus

- adverse effect of drugs

- oligohydramnios

- maternal myasthenia gravis.

ULTRASOUND SCANNING FOR FETAL LIMB ABNORMALITIES

Limbs

It is assumed that the reader is familiar with the general fetal scanning techniques of locating and measuring long bones. The long bones should be measured as near to horizontal in the scanning plane as possible to avoid shadowing artifact (**Figure 1**). The strongest reflections occur from the most proximal bone interface so that a bone with thickened metaphyses may give an impression of being bowed. Hypomineralized long bones will reflect less ultrasound at the proximal interface and will show more even echogenicity across the diaphysis and a reduced acoustic shadow. Minor degrees of hypomineralization may be hard to detect.

Femur length measurements from some skeletal dysplasias encountered by the author are shown against a nomogram in **Figure 2**.

Full examination of a fetus at risk for a skeletal abnormality requires a detailed study of the remainder of the fetal general anatomy as this may give important clues to the diagnosis.

Head

Hypomineralization

Skull hypomineralization will reduce the reflection of ultrasound and increase transmission. The effect of this is to reduce both the echogenicity of the skull and the acoustic shadowing of tissues beyond it. The cranial contents are seen more clearly than in a normally calcified skull. In severe cases (osteogenesis imperfecta type 2a and c, achondrogenesis type 1) the cerebral hemispheres are anechoic lending the appearance of ventriculomegaly which is easily excluded by identifying the choroid plexus and the walls of the antrum of the lateral ventricle normally situated within the hemisphere (**Figure 6a**). The skull bones are soft and deform if subjected to pressure from the transducer. Hypomineralization is less obvious in milder cases such as hypophosphatasia or osteogenesis imperfecta type 2b and 3.

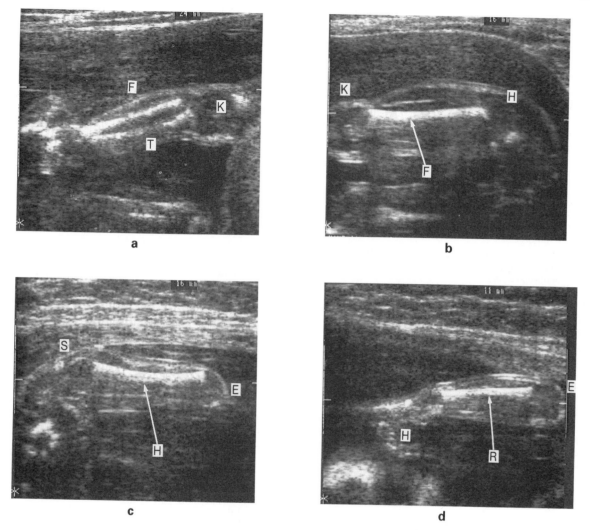

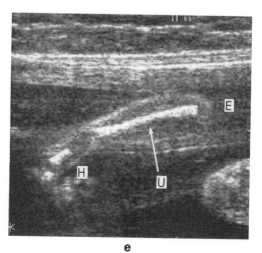

Figure 1. Normal long bones. The bones are measured as near as possible to horizontal in the scanning plane. The limb segment soft-tissue extremity is clearly visible beyond the end of the metaphyses. (**a**) T tibia, F, fibula, K, knee. (**b**) F femur, K knee, H hip. (**c**) H humerus, E elbow, S scapula. (**d**) R radius, E elbow, H hand. (**e**) U ulna, E elbow, H hand.

Table 3
Ultrasound abnormalities and skeletal defects

	Inheritance	Incidence	Prognosis
Short long bones – severe symmetrical			
Achondrogenesis (types 1 and 2)	AR	1:75 000	Lethal
Thanatophoric dysplasia	AD	1:30 000	Lethal
Campomelic dysplasia	AR	1:150 000	Mainly lethal
Osteogenesis imperfecta type 2	S	1:55 000	A + C: Lethal
			S: Often lethal
Hypophosphatasia (AR form)	AR or AD	1:110 000	AR: Lethal
			AD: Mild
Homozygous achondroplasia	AR	Very rare	Lethal
Schneckenbecken dysplasia[1]			
Atelosteogenesis[2]			
Grebe syndrome			
Short long bones – moderate symmetrical			
Hypochondrogenesis	5 (AR)	Very rare	Lethal
Jeune thoracic dystrophy	AR	Rare	70% Lethal
Short-rib polydactyly syndromes	AR	Very rare	Lethal
Ellis-van Creveld syndrome	AR	Very rare	33% Lethal
Diastrophic dysplasia	AR	Rare	Variable
Rhizomelic chondrodysplasia punctata	AR	Rare	Poor
Kniest dysplasia	AD/AR	Rare	Variable
Spondylo-epiphyseal dysplasia (severe form)	AD/AR	Very rare	Variable
Heterozygous achondroplasia	AD	1:66 000	Good
Noonan's syndrome	AD	Rare	Moderate
Down's syndrome			
Dyssegmental dysplasia[3]			
Metatrophic dysplasia[4,5]			
Mesomelic dysplasia			
Fibrochondrogenesis			
Short long bones: asymmetrical			
Isolated limb reductions			
Roberts' syndrome	AR	Rare	Poor
Femoral hypoplasia-unusual faces syndrome			
Femur-fibula-ulna syndrome			
Holt-Oram syndrome	AD	Rare	Variable
Thrombocytopenia-absent radius syndrome (TAR)	R	Very rare	Variable
Cleidocranial dysostosis (clavicles)	AD	Rare	Variable
Chromosomal abnormalities			
Phocomelias			
Congenital anemias[64] (e.g. Fanconi, Aase, Black Fan Diamond)			

AR: autosomal recessive; AD: autosomal dominant; S: sporadic   *continued*

Skull shape

The clover-leaf skull is characteristic of some cases of thanatophoric dysplasia. Measurement of orbital diameters[6,7] may reveal hypertelorism in some syndromes (e.g. Apert S.).

Face

Cleft lip and/or palate (see Chapter 50) is a feature of SRP type 2 (Majewski), fibrochondrogenesis, atelosteo-genesis, ectrodactyly-ectodermal dysplasia-clefting (EEC) syndrome and a number of other dysplasias. A facial profile in the sagittal plane may show frontal bossing, depressed nasal bridge or micrognathia. The mandible can be measured from the tempero-mandibular joint to the mental eminence[8,9] in the axial plane.

Thorax

The ribs may be short, thick, thin, beaded, flared or irregular in shape, arrangement or number. The thorax

Table 3
Continued

Bent femur/fractures
Campomelic dysplasia
Kyphomelic dysplasia
Osteogenesis imperfecta
Hypophosphatasia
Dyssegmental dysplasia
Thanatophoric dysplasia (some)

Missing bones/limbs
Phocomelias
Syrenomelia
Transverse reduction defects
Thrombocytopenia-absent radius syndrome
Syndactyly
Ectrodactyly
Fanconi pancytopenia syndrome
Apert's syndrome

Small thorax
Achondrogenesis syndromes
Thanatophoric dysplasia
Schneckenbecken dysplasia
Fibrochondrogenesis
Hypochondrogenesis
Short-rib polydactyly syndromes
Jeune thoracic dystrophy
Osteogenesis imperfecta type 2
Camptomelic dysplasia (some)

Hydrops
Hydramnios

Extra bones
Polydactyly
Short-rib polydactyly syndromes
Jeune thoracic dystrophy
Joubert's syndrome

Positional deformities
Diastrophic dysplasia
Rhizomelic chondrodysplasia punctata
Talipes
Rocker-bottom feet
Multiple joint contractures

Deformed spine
Isolated hemivertebrae
VACTERL association
Jarcho-Levine syndrome
Dyssegmental dysplasia
Spondylo-epiphyseal dysplasia
Fibrochondrogenesis
Atelosteogensis

Poor ossification
Achondrogenesis
Osteogenesis imperfecta type 2
Hypophosphatasia (severe form)

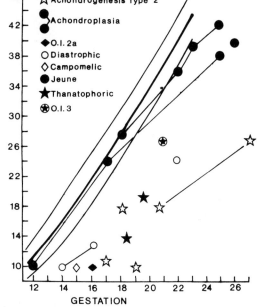

Figure 2. Diagram to show femur length measurements in many of the skeletal dysplasias described in the text set against a nomogram for femur length against postmenstrual age. Modified from Griffin 1990, 1992,[25,42] with permission.

may be normal, constricted, short or long. In cases with a constricted thorax the ratio of heart circumference to thoracic circumference (normally about 30%)[10] will be increased. Normal liver and abdominal circumference will cause abdominal wall protrusion in antero-posterior view. This is described as the 'champagne cork' appearance. Pulmonary hypoplasia resulting from restricted thorax is the major cause of death in neonates with this feature. Congenital heart abnormalities may be found in Ellis-van Creveld syndrome (50%), thanatophoric dysplasia, SRP type 2, camptomelic dysplasia, Holt-Oram syndrome, TAR syndrome, Noonan's syndrome, Carpenter's syndrome, trisomies and in pregnancies of diabetic mothers.

Kidneys

Renal dysplasia may be a feature of jeune thoracic dystrophy, thanatophoric dysplasia and caudal regression syndrome and the VACTERL association.

TERMINOLOGY

Table 4 contains a list of terms employed in the text.

Table 4
Terminology of limb defects

Acromelia – shortening predominantly of distal segments
(hands and feet)

Amelia – absence of a limb

Camptomelia – bent limbs

Diaphysis – central part of shaft of long bone

Epiphysis – bone ends with separate centres of ossification.
Many not apparent prenatally

Hemimelia – absence or hypoplasia of longitudinal segment
(e.g. radius)

Kyphoscoliosis – combination of lateral and convex
curvature

Kyphosis – dorsally convex curvature of spine (as thoracic)

Lordosis – dorsally concave curvature of the spine (as
lumbar)

Mesomelia – shortening predominantly in the intermediate
long bones (radius/ulna, tibia/fibula)

Metaphysis – more recently developed growing extremities
of shaft

Micromelia – severely shortened limb

Phocomelia (seal limb) – absence or hypoplasia of long
bones with hands or feet attached to trunk

Platyspondyly – flattening of the vertebral body

Rhizomelia – shortening predominantly in proximal long
bones (humerus, femur)

Scoliosis – lateral curvature of the spine

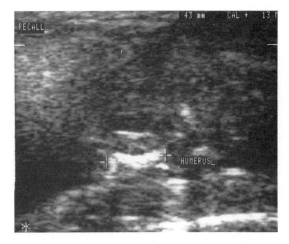

Figure 3a. Achondrogenesis. Short (13 mm)
humerus of a fetus with achondrogenesis type 2 at
18 weeks. Reproduced from Brock *et al.*, 1992,[29] with
permission.

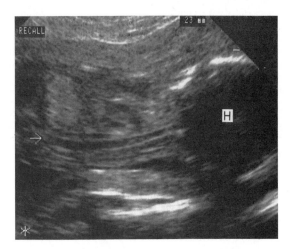

Figure 3b. Achondrogenesis. Sonogram of the
trunk and head (H) of the fetus in **Figure 3a**. The
spinal column is shown (arrowed) as an anechoic
cartilagenous column. The skull shows some
mineralization.

SHORT LONG BONES – SEVERE SYMMETRICAL

Skeletal dysplasias occur in about 1:5000 live births
and 1:550 still births.[11] No individual condition has a
frequency of greater than 1:10 000.

ACHONDROGENESIS

This group of conditions is characterised by severe
micromelia and hypomineralization. Fetal hydrops and
hydramnios may be evident in later pregnancy.

Diagnosis

Type 1 (Parenti-Fraccaro)

The long bones show extreme micromelia with very
poor modeling (e.g. femur length of 10 mm at 19
weeks.[12] The calvarium and vertebral column show
severe hypomineralization (**Figure 3b**).

Type 2 (Langer-Saldino)

The long bones are better modeled but still extremely
short, thick and straight (**Figure 3a**). The calvarium is
normally ossified in this variant but hypomineralization of the spine is variable but may be striking
(**Figure 3b, c, d**).

Risks and Management Options

Achondrogenesis is a lethal condition at or before
birth. Interruption of pregnancy should be offered. The

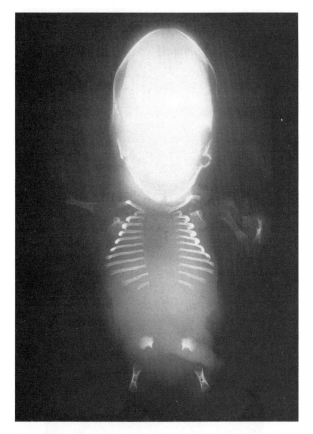

Figure 3c. Achondrogenesis. Radiograph of the fetus in **Figures 3a, b** showing total absence of ossification in all elements of the spinal column. The ribs are short and the thorax small. There is little mineralization of the skull. (Reproduced from Brock *et al.*, 1992,[29] with permission.

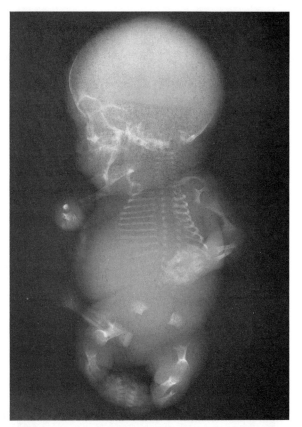

Figure 3d. Achondrogenesis. Postnatal radiograph of a different fetus with achondrogenesis type 2 at a similar gestation to that in **Figure 3c**. In this case only the vertebral bodies show lack of calcification. Other features are similar to those in **Figure 3c** with short, straight reasonably modeled long bones showing flared, cupped metaphyses. The ischial bones are unossified and the ilea small and halberd-shaped.

diagnosis is confirmed by postnatal radiography and expert pathology. The recurrence risk is 1:4.

THANATOPHORIC DYSPLASIA

Thanatophoric dysplasia is the most common skeletal dysplasia encountered in obstetric practice.

Diagnosis

Definitive diagnosis is possible by 18–20 weeks. Femur and other limb length measurements will be well below the third centile for postmenstrual age (**Figure 2**) and will show characteristic thickening of the metaphyses. Measurements from 14 mm to 21 mm at 18–20 weeks to 26 mm at 32 weeks have been

reported.[13–18] The femurs may appear bowed in some cases and straight in others (**Figure 4b**). The feet and hands are short. The short splayed fingers are described as 'trident hand'. The short stubby ribs produce a markedly small thorax (**Figure 4c**). The heart to thorax circumference is high (**Figure 4c**) and the characteristic champagne cork appearance will be evident on viewing the trunk in the sagittal plane (**Figure 4d**). Some cases show flattening of the vertebral bodies (platyspondyly) and a short spine. The skull is normally ossified and may be macrocephalic or brachycephalic. Some variants show the clover-leaf (**Figure 4a**) deformity produced by prominence of the parietal bones. This sign is more evident later in pregnancy. Lateral ventriculomegaly may occur. Sagittal view of the facial profile shows a depressed nasal bridge and frontal bossing. In later pregnancy soft tissue folds may

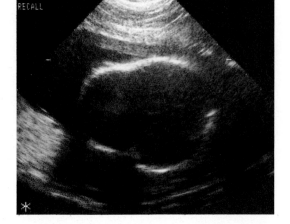

Figure 4a. Skull of a 20-week fetus with thanatophoric dysplasia showing the clover-leaf deformity.

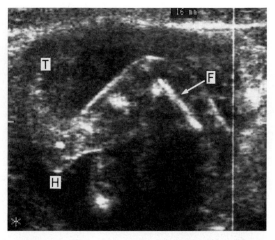

Figure 4b. Lower limb of a fetus of 18 weeks with thanatophoric dysplasia demonstrating short, short leg and femur (F) of 18 mm (H heel, T toes).

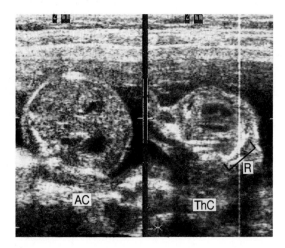

Figure 4c. Transverse sections of the trunk of fetus in **Figure 4b** at the level of the umbilical vein (AC) and the heart (ThC) showing marked reduction of the thoracic circumference and short ribs (R).

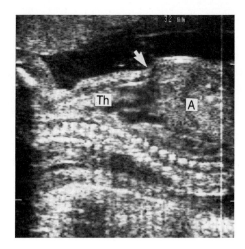

Figure 4d. Longitudinal antero-posterior sagittal scan of the trunk of fetus in **Figure 4b** showing the narrow thorax (Th) and abdomen (A) protruding anteriorly: the 'champagne cork' appearance. A normally mineralized spine is posterior.

be seen on the arms ('Michelin man' appearance). Cardiac and renal anomalies may be found. Hydramnios may be the presenting feature in later pregnancy.

Risks and Management Options

The condition is lethal and interruption of pregnancy should be offered. Confirmation of the diagnosis by radiography is essential. Parents should be advised that recurrence risks are low since this is a dominant sporadic condition.

CAMPTOMELIC DYSPLASIA

Diagnosis

Several cases of early diagnosis of this condition have been described.[19–25] The characteristic mid-shaft bowing of the femur should be recognized at a routine scan (**Figure 5**). The tibia is short and bowed and the fibula hypoplastic. Added to this, marked talipes causes the whole lower limb to be grossly bowed inward (camptomelia). The ribs may be short and the thorax

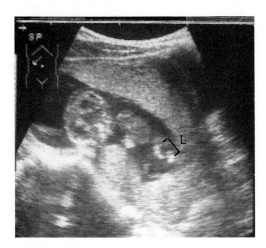

Figure 5. Campomelic dysplasia. Sonogram of a 15-week fetus with campomelic dysplasia. Note the short, bent leg (L). Micrognathia is evident in the facial profile. Reproduced with permission from Griffin (1990).[25]

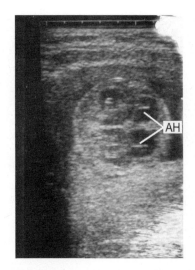

Figure 6a. Osteogenesis imperfecta type 2a (OI 2a). Skull of a 20-week fetus with OI 2a showing the features of severe hypomineralization of the skull. The skull bones are poorly echogenic and they cast no acoustic shadow. The cerebral hemispheres are anechoic, lending the appearance of cerebral ventriculomegaly (pseudohydrocephaly). However, the echoes from the anterior horns (AH) are normally placed. Reproduced with permission from Griffin 1990.[25]

constricted. Brachycephaly, micrognathia and short clavicle may also be recognized on careful skeletal survey. Associated soft tissue anomalies are found in one third of cases and include cardiac (ASD, VSD), hydronephrosis and ventriculomegaly. Hydramnios may complicate later pregnancy. Phenotypic sex reversal is common but would not be recognized prenatally unless karyotyping had been performed.

Risks and Management Options

Most cases result in a neonatal death from pulmonary hypoplasia and 95% die by 1 year.[26,27] The prognosis will depend upon the severity of associated malformations. Survivors fail to thrive and may show neurological impairment.

Interruption of pregnancy should be offered. Confirmation of the diagnosis by pathology and radiography is essential before counseling about the recurrence risk. Prenatal ultrasound diagnosis should be offered in subsequent pregnancies.

OSTEOGENESIS IMPERFECTA

Cases of osteogenesis imperfecta are characterized by poor bone mineralization. The condition is divided on a clinical and pathoradiologic basis into types 1–4. Types 1 and 4 are probably not open to early diagnosis by ultrasound in pregnancy. Types 2a, b, c and type 3

have been diagnosed in pregnancy. The overall incidence is 1:10 000 and that for type 2 is 1:55 000.

Type 2 is usually sporadic. Recent evidence using molecular methods has suggested that recurrences are probably due to gonadal mosaicism. Type 3 is possibly autosomal recessive in inheritance but again recurrences may be due to gonadal mosaicism. Both types 1 and 4 are autosomal dominant conditions.

Diagnosis

Osteogenesis imperfecta type 2a is the most commonly encountered variety of this condition. It is recognizable from very early pregnancy by the characteristic hypomineralization of the skull and long bones with severe micromelia and apparent bowing due to multiple fractures.[30–36] The appearance of the skull is such that the usual bright echo from the bones is lost and there is no acoustic shadow (**Figure 6a**). The orbits may be unusually prominent. The cerebral hemispheres take on a trans-sonic character suggestive of lateral ventriculomegaly which can be excluded on identifying the choroid plexus within normal ventricular walls and a normal posterior horn measurement. The head is brachycephalic. In later pregnancy the head will be easily deformed on pressure from the ultrasound transducer and details of cerebral structure will remain

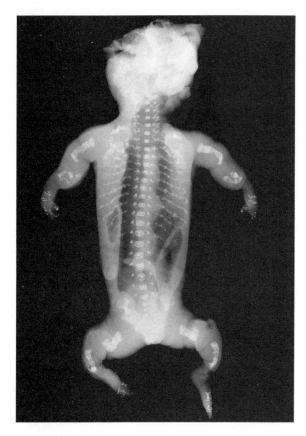

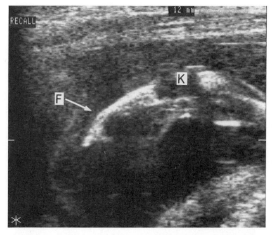

Figure 7. Osteogenesis imperfecta type 3 (OI 3). Femur (F) with mid-shaft bowing and poor mineralization. The cartilaginous epiphyses are evident at the knee (K).

Figure 6b. Osteogenesis imperfecta type 2a (OI 2a). Postnatal radiograph of fetus with OI 2a. The long bones are short bowed and crumpled by multiple intrauterine fractures. The lower limbs are held in a campomelic (bent) posture. The ribs are 'beaded' from fractures and hairline fractures are also evident in the vertebral bodies (the skull was lost in delivery). Reproduced with permission from Chamberlain 1990.[25]

prominent. The long bones are hypoechoic and irregularly bowed and crumpled due to multiple fractures and callous formation (**Figure 6b**). The limbs show marked fixed camptomelia and talipes. Further features such as beading of the ribs and small thorax may be recognized. Later pregnancy may be complicated by hydramnios or oligohydramnios. Munoz *et al.*[37] report reliable differentiation from other skeletal dysplasias on the basis of the three criteria: multiple fractures, hypoechoic skull and femoral length three or more standard deviations below the mean for gestational age.

Type 2b shows features intermediate between type 2a and type 3. Type 2c demonstrates skeletal features similar to type 2a. Poor cranial ossification is the worst in this type.

Type 3 may rarely demonstrate a poorly calcified skull. The femurs may show bowing (**Figure 7**) or

fracture with mild to moderate shortening but are generally well modelled. Typically the tibiae are bowed whereas the fibulae are straight.[34,38,39]

Type 1 has been diagnosed prenatally[20] but may not be reliably excluded before viability. The author has experience of an affected case scanned serially to 24 weeks with normal limb growth and morphology. Bowed femurs were apparent at birth and fractures occurred shortly afterwards. The clinical presentation and prognosis of types 1 and 4 are very variable and may show considerable overlap. Expert advice is recommended before counseling.

Risks and Management Options

Type 2a and c are lethal and while type 2b is often lethal, a child may survive to infancy. Type 3 may survive but with significant physical handicap due to multiple deforming fractures. Type 1 and type 4 show overlap and are not usually diagnosed in pregnancy.

For type 2, interruption of pregnancy should be offered. With type 3, interruption of pregnancy may be offered before viability. Abdominal delivery may reduce trauma or intracranial hemorrhage.

HYPOPHOSPHATASIA

This is another condition of bone hypomineralization due to a deficiency of alkaline phosphatase. It is a heterogeneous group varying from a severe lethal condition to milder forms only apparent in childhood. The appearance of the severe lethal form is similar to that of osteogenesis imperfecta type 2, although the bones are generally less 'crumpled'.

Diagnosis

Diagnosis of this condition may be biochemical, ultrasonic, molecular or a combination. There are surprisingly few reports of the prenatal diagnosis of this condition by ultrasound.[40–42] If cranial hypomineralization is marked, the skull will appear similar to osteogenesis imperfecta type 2 with anechoic calvarium, prominent intracranial structures and an easily deformed skull. The femora and humeri are short and may be markedly bowed in the mid-shaft such that full demonstration and measurement of the shaft may be difficult. Dislocations may be apparent at knees and elbows.[41] The ribs are thin and may show fractures. The spine may be markedly demineralized, particularly in the neural arch. Diagnosis of the milder form has been reported in which early femoral bowing was seen to resolve during pregnancy.[43]

Biochemical diagnosis by measuring alkaline phosphatase (ALP) in amniotic fluid[44] and cultured amniocytes has proven unreliable in the fourth to fifth month. Warren et al.[45] succeeded in diagnosing the condition in the first trimester in a high risk pregnancy by measuring cellular ALP in a chorion villous sample and further success with liver/bone/kidney (LBK) ALP has been reported by Brock and Barron.[46]

Risks and Management Options

The severe recessive form is lethal. In milder autosomal dominant forms, the osseous maldevelopment tends to improve with age.

Interruption of pregnancy should be offered in severe forms. The diagnosis must be confirmed by expert radiography and also by biochemical or genetic investigation of the parents. It is unclear whether milder forms should be delivered abdominally to avoid trauma.

HOMOZYGOUS ACHONDROPLASIA

This will only occur in the offspring of two heterozygous achondroplastic parents. Most fetuses probably perish in early pregnancy as the condition is rarely seen amongst achondroplastic couples.

Diagnosis

In a cased reported by Filly and Golbus[28] there was severe micromelia and a small thorax, similar to thanatophoric dysplasia.

Risks and Management Options

This is a lethal condition. Pregnancy termination should be offered.

SHORT LONG BONES – MODERATE SYMMETRICAL

Not all apparent mild shortening of bones is pathological. Symmetrical shortening of long bones may be seen as part of generalized growth deficiency.

HYPOCHONDROGENESIS

This condition is thought to represent the milder end of the spectrum of the achondrogenesis/spondyloepithelial dysplasia group of conditions.[47]

Diagnosis

The condition may be suspected if moderate long bone shortening (**Figure 8**) is found in association with a constricted thorax. The bones are straight and show some thickening of the metaphyses.[42]

Risks and Management Options

The condition is lethal due to pulmonary hypoplasia. Interruption of pregnancy may be offered if diagnosis is made before viability. Note that Jeune thoracic dystrophy and Ellis-van Creveld syndrome (both differential diagnoses) are not invariably fatal conditions and diagnostic distinction should be made if possible before undertaking counseling.

JEUNE THORACIC DYSTROPHY (ASPHYXIATING THORACIC DYSTROPHY)

The degree of limb shortening and the severity of this condition is very variable. Associated features include renal, hepatic, pancreatic and pulmonary dysplasia and occasionally postaxial polydactyly or facial clefts.

Diagnosis

Reports of the diagnosis of Jeune syndrome in the literature are based upon the finding of a small thorax in high risk families.[48,49] The chest will show reduced antero-posterior diameter and consequent protrusion of the anterior abdominal wall. Limb shortening may not be apparent, however until late (**Figure 8**).[49]

In *de novo* presentations the presence of polydactyly may make distinction between this condition and the short-rib polydactyly syndromes or Ellis-van Creveld syndrome difficult. Hydramnios is a common late pregnancy complication.

Risks and Management Options

The condition is about 70% lethal in the neonatal period due to respiratory failure. Survivors are of small stature and often succumb to respiratory, renal, hepatic or pancreatic complications in childhood. Intelligence is unimpaired. As mortality and morbidity are high interruption of pregnancy might be offered before viability.

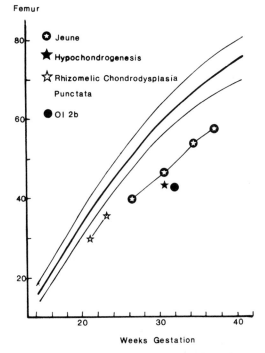

Figure 8. Diagram showing growth of the femur in a fetus with prenatal diagnosis (and postnatal confirmation) of Jeune thoracic dystrophy against nomogram of fetal growth against postmenstrual age. Single measurements are also shown for fetuses with hypochondrogenesis and OI type 2b.

SHORT-RIB POLYDACTYLY SYNDROMES (SRPS)

The main subdivisions of these conditions are:

- *Type 1 (Saldino-Noonan)* which shows severe micromelia and characteristic pointed ends to long bones

- *Type 2 (Majewski)* which is characterized by median cleft lip/palate and disproportionately short, ovoid tibiae.

Both syndromes may be associated with abnormalities of other organ systems. Fetal hydrops is a common finding and may be a consequence of cardiovascular anomaly. Phenotypic sex reversal (to apparent female) is a common finding.

Diagnosis

The basis of prenatal diagnosis is the identification of a small narrow thorax with short ribs, short limbs and postaxial polydactyly (**Figure 9**) and, if possible, the other minor distinguishing features.

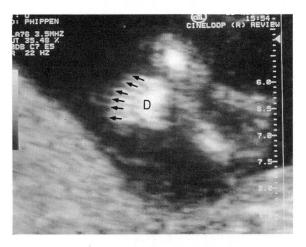

Figure 9. Short-rib polydactyly syndrome. Scan of the foot of a fetus with SRPS showing six digits (arrowed: D) (with thanks to Mr P. Smith).

Risks and Management Options

Because of respiratory failure, SRPSs are lethal and if diagnosed early enough, interruption of pregnancy should be considered.

ELLIS-VAN CREVELD SYNDROME (CHONDROECTODERMAL DYSPLASIA)

Diagnosis

Ultrasound diagnosis of polydactyly (hands more commonly than feet) should be possible.[50] Limb shortening is more pronounced in the forearm and lower leg (mesomelic). The diagnosis should be considered when the above findings are found with a small thorax.[51] In 50% there is congenital heart disease, typically ASD.

Risks and Management Options

One-third die during infancy. Survivors have normal intelligence but limited stature of about 3.5 to 5 feet.

Interruption of pregnancy may be offered before fetal viability but counseling should, as always, be cautious and sensitive to the views of the parents. In continuing pregnancy usual obstetric management procedures should be followed. Neonatal echocardiography is advisable.

DIASTROPHIC DYSPLASIA

This is a condition of variable presentation.

Diagnosis

Reports of prenatal diagnosis of diastrophic dysplasia have been based in severe cases on the combination of

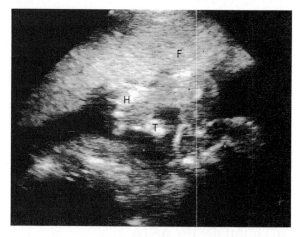

Figure 10. Diastrophic dysplasia. Scan of the hand (H) of a fetus with diastrophic dysplasia showing proximal displacement and abduction of the thumb (T) (the 'hitchhiker' thumb). Femur length measurement from this fetus at 22 weeks is shown in **Figure 2** (F: forearm).

rhisomelic limb shortening and bowing in association with the hitchhiker thumb (**Figure 10**).[52–54] Occasional associated features include micrognathia and cleft palate. Exclusion of the diagnosis before viability in high risk families may be difficult in milder cases as prenatal limb shortening may be minimal. Identification of normal thumbs may be helpful in excluding the diagnosis.

Risks and Management Options

A significant number of newborns die from respiratory failure and pneumonia. Survivors are of normal intellectual ability but have significant and progressive physical handicap coupled with limited mobility from kyphoscoliosis and arthropathy.

Interruption of pregnancy may be offered before viability. If the pregnancy continues, no specific measures are necessary before birth. Considerable mobility and physiotherapy support are likely to be needed in survivors. Limited surgical release of contractures may be possible.

RHIZOMELIC CHONDRODYSPLASIA PUNCTATA

This should be distinguished from the dominant and much milder form of chondrodysplasia punctata (Conradi-Hunerman syndrome).

Diagnosis

Individuals with rhizomelic chondrodysplasia punctata show rhizomelic shortening more pronounced in the humerus than the femur plus fixed flexion deformities of the limbs, again more pronounced in the arm. The characteristic feature on ultrasound is stippled epiphyses[42,55] (**Figure 11**).

Biochemically there is low dihydroxyacetone phosphate transferase activity (DHAP-TA) in cultured amniocytes and fibroblasts.[56]

Risks and Management Options

Many newborns die due to respiratory failure. Survivors exhibit failure to thrive, growth deficiency, microcephaly and severely retarded neurological development. Survival beyond the first year is unusual and the longest reported survival is 5 years.

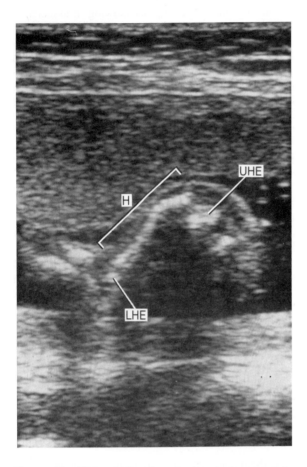

Figure 11. Rhizomelic chondrodysplasia punctata. Scan of the arm and shoulder of a 21-week fetus with rhizomelic chondrodysplasia punctata. The humerus (H) is short (25 mm) and bowed. At both the upper (UHE) and lower (LHE) humeral epiphyses there are echogenic accumulations representing disorganized calcification. Movement of the upper limb was limited during the examination.

Interruption of pregnancy should be discussed. Amniocentesis with measurement of DHAPT activity may be a helpful adjunct to ultrasonographic diagnosis.

KNIEST DYSPLASIA (METATROPIC DWARFISM: TYPE 2)

Diagnosis

Although limbs are noticeably short at birth, only one case of prenatal diagnosis has been reported[57] when features were not evident at 16 weeks but were at 31 weeks. This dysplasia is characterized by moderately short, dumb-bell shaped long bones with metaphyseal flaring, restricted joint mobility, platyspondyly with vertebral clefts and flat face with depressed nasal bridge.

Risks and Management Options

These children generally survive with normal intelligence but short stature (106–145 cm), limited mobility and severe orthopaedic disabilities. Ophthalmic complications and deafness may occur in childhood. An atypical, lethal Kniest dysplasia has been described in two sibs of one family.[58]

SPONDYLO-EPIPHYSEAL DYSPLASIA

Diagnosis

This condition has been observed prenatally. There was moderate shortening of the femur at 16+ weeks and more marked rhisomelic shortening at 27 weeks.[59] No other distinguishing features were evident. Definitive diagnosis was not achieved prenatally. There is deficient ossification of the spine, pubis, talus and calcaneum and delayed appearance of the lower femoral and upper tibial epiphyses. Vertebrae show marked platyspondyly with ovoid vertebral bodies, a narrow, bell-shaped thorax and moderate shortening of the long bones. Cleft palate may occur.

Risks and Management Options

This is a very heterogeneous group of disorders; some may be neonatally lethal whereas others may show prolonged survival. Myopia and retinal detachment are reported in about half of survivors. Hypotonic muscle weakness and restricted joint mobility inhibit mobilization and the spinal deformities cause progressive kyphoscoliosis.

HETEROZYGOUS ACHONDROPLASIA

'Achondroplasia' is a condition well recognized by the general population. Affected individuals, although markedly short in stature, are intelligent, productive members of society.

Diagnosis

The condition is characterized by predominantly acro-mesomelic limb shortening with stubby abducted fingers (trident hand). Typical facial features include a wide, prominent forehead (frontal bossing), depressed nasal bridge, hypertelorism and a wide mandible. Thoracic dimensions may be reduced but this is general insufficient to produce respiratory embarrassment. The spine is short and shows marked lumbar lordosis. Macrocrania and hydrocephalus may complicate the condition. Although the features are easily recognized in the neonate, it is well documented that the long bones may not show significant growth reduction until after the fifth to sixth month of gestation[40,60] (**Figure 2**).

Risks and Management Options

Life expectancy and intellectual performance are good. Hydrocephaly, probably resulting from partial obstruction at the restricted foramen magnum, is usually mild, non-progressive, and may be treated conservatively. Progressive neurological problems may result from spinal cord compression by progressive narrowing of the interpedicular distance, particularly in the lumbar spine as lordosis progresses. Corrective orthopaedic operations may be required to correct spinal deformities and bow-legs.

Affected mothers usually require elective cesarean section for reduced pelvic diameters. Cephalo-pelvic disproportion may also result during the delivery of an affected fetus to a normal mother if fetal macrocephaly is marked. Unaffected parents of an affected child should be given a low recurrence risk as this will represent a new mutation.

NOONAN'S SYNDROME

Previously known as male Turner's syndrome this condition is now recognized as a separate entity.

The diagnosis should be borne in mind on the ultrasonic finding of nuchal edema and short femur after the exclusion of Turner's syndrome or Down's syndrome by karyotyping. Congenital heart disease (pulmonary stenosis, VSD) is common. Intellectual impairment is common but not severe.

DOWN'S SYNDROME

Mild femoral shortening in Down's syndrome has been reported. Studies to date, however, have been retrospective and uncontrolled with differing conclusions.[61,62] On finding a significantly short femur

relative to other biometric parameters other markers should be sought and karyotyping discussed with the parents if no definitive diagnosis can be reached.

SHORT LONG BONES – ASYMMETRICAL

ISOLATED LIMB REDUCTIONS

This heterogeneous group of disorders comprises asymmetrical reductions of limbs or portions of limbs.

Risks and Management Options

The majority are non-genetic but they may occur as part of a genetic syndrome or chromosomal abnormality.[63] Because of these associations, it is essential to perform a detailed ultrasound examination of the whole fetus to exclude other markers and karyotyping should be considered. In the absence of associated physical or chromosomal abnormalities, the prognosis is generally good. Advances in prosthetics and orthopaedics have been such that much can be achieved to restore function and appearance of reduced limbs so that parents should be encouraged to discuss possibilities with appropriate professionals if they are worried about deformities or handicap. There are, however, some specific syndromes associated with isolated or asymmetric limb reductions.

ROBERTS' SYNDROME (PSEUDOTHALIDOMIDE)

Diagnosis

The marked reduction in all four limbs (tetraphocomelia) usually associated with this condition is similar to the teratogenic effects of thalidomide. Median facial clefting, microcephaly, joint flexion deformities, talipes, syndactyly and extremely short or missing fingers and toes are accompanying features. Other anomalies include hydrocephaly, encephalocoele and renal abnormalities including polycystic and horseshoe kidney. There is a similar condition of hypoglossia–hypodactyly syndrome in which there are similar reductions found in all limbs associated with micrognathia and microglossia. In this syndrome facial clefting is uncommon.

The two syndromes may be distinguished *in utero* by cytogenetic studies. In most cases of Roberts' syndrome, the premature separation of the centromeres produces a characteristic phenomenon of chromosome 'puffing'.

Risks and Management Options

Individuals with Roberts' syndrome have a high perinatal mortality (70–80%) and severe growth deficiency. Survivors are often severely mentally retarded. In contrast, survivors with hypoglossia–hypodactyly syndrome generally show satisfactory intellectual development.

FEMORAL HYPOPLASIA – UNUSUAL FACES SYNDROME

This condition appears to be more commonly encountered in children of diabetic mothers. Cleft palate and micrognathia are associated with varying degrees of hypoplasia/aplasia of the femur and fibula. There may be humeral reduction with flexion deformity at the elbow. Other abnormalities may include vertebral anomalies of the lower spine. Humeral reduction and cleft palate distinguish this syndrome from caudal regression. Most individuals have normal intelligence and are ambulatory.[64]

FEMUR–FIBULA–ULNA SYNDROME

Characterized by femoral and fibula hypoplasia/aplasia and varying degrees of paraxial ulna hemimelia this syndrome has been diagnosed prenatally.[65]

HOLT-ORAM SYNDROME

Diagnosis

The cardinal features of this condition are congenital heart disease (usually ASD or VSD) associated with various upper limb and limb girdle reductions. The limb reductions are described as being more severe in females and twice as common on the left as the right.[64,66,67]

Abnormalities in the hand and forearm include aplastic, hypoplastic or triphalangeal (finger-like) thumb, syndactyly and hypoplasia of the radius, ulna, humerus, clavicles, scapula or sternum. There is no consistent pattern and expression is variable.

Risks and Management Options

These will depend on the severity of the cardiac malformation and the skeletal deformities.

THROMBOCYTOPENIA ABSENT RADIUS (TAR) SYNDROME

The skeletal manifestations of TAR are variable bilateral radial aplasia or hypoplasia sometimes associated with humeral or ulna reductions. These are markers of underlying hemopoetic abnormality.

CLEIDOCRANIAL DYSOSTOSIS

Diagnosis

Hypoplastic clavicles (**Figure 12**) may be recognized on prenatal ultrasound scanning if plotted against published nomograms.[68] However, clavicles are not generally included in a routine prenatal survey of the fetus and may be shadowed by the chin, arms or scapulae. *De novo* presentations may therefore be missed. Mild femoral shortening and hypomineralized cranium with wide fontanelles may also be evident.

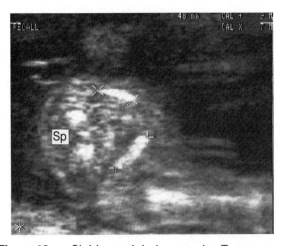

Figure 12a. Cleidocranial dysostosis. Transverse scan of the clavicles of the fetus of a mother with cleidocranial dysostosis. The clavicles are short, thick and straight. (Sp = spine)

Risks and Management Options

Individuals with this syndrome are generally of short stature. They may have respiratory difficulties in

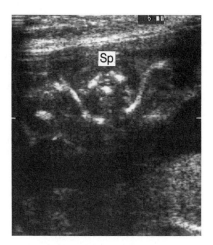

Figure 12b. Cleidocranial dysostosis. Similar PA scan of the clavicles of a normal 22-week fetus. Note the sigmoid form of the clavicles (Sp = spine).

.

infancy if the thorax is restricted. Dental and hearing problems may present in later childhood. Absent or hypoplastic clavicles do not cause significant handicap. Intelligence is unimpaired. Poor skull ossification tends to improve with age. The small pelvis may necessitate cesarean section in affected mothers.

CHROMOSOMAL ABNORMALITIES

Forearm reduction deformities may also occur in cases of chromosomal abnormalities including 13Q-, trisomies 8, 13 and 18, triploidy and others.[63]

POLYDACTYLY/SYNDACTYLY

These conditions frequently coexist.

Polydactyly can be either preaxial (on the radial side of the hand or medial side of the foot, including bifid thumb or great toe) or postaxial (on the ulnar side of the hand or lateral side of the foot). Isolated polydactyly may be inherited as an autosomal dominant trait with variable penetrance. The incidence of polydactyly is higher amongst some ethnic groups (Afro-Caribbean). Polydactyly is associated with numerous genetic and chromosomal syndromes listed in **Table 5**.

Syndactyly may be osseous (fusion of the bones) or cutaneous (fusion of the digits by soft tissues). Some syndromes featuring syndactyly are listed in **Table 6**. Many are common to those with polydactyly.

Table 5
Syndromes associated with polydactyly

Syndrome	Associated features
Ano-cerebro digital	CHD, renal agenesis, growth deficiency, anal atresia.
Bloom	Growth deficiency, syndactyly.
Carpenter	Craniosynostosis (acrocephaly).
C-trigonocephaly	Synostosis metopic suture, palate.
Egger	Cerebellar anomalies (see Joubert).
Ellis-van Creveld	Mesomelic dysplasia (see above).
Fanconi pancytopenia	Forearm reductions (see above).
Fitch (Oto-palato-digital type 2)	Cleft palate, micrognathia, joint contractures, camptodactyly.
Fuhrman	Polysyndactyly, fibula aplasia/hypoplasia, bowed femora.
Golabi-Rosen	Prenatal macrosomia, extra ribs.
Goltz	Syndactyly.
Grebe	Short limbs (see above).
Greig cephalopolysyndactyly	Macrocephaly.
Hydrolethalus	Hydrocephaly, micrognathia, CHD CL/CP (similar to Meckel S).
Jeune thoracic dystrophy	Short limbs, small thorax (see above).
Kaufman-McKusick	CHD, anal/vaginal atresia, urethral stenosis, intestinal malrotation.
Klippel-Trenaunay-Weber	Asymmetric limb hypertrophy, syndactyly, oligodactyly.
Meckel-Grubber	Encephalocoele, polycystic kidney or liver, microcephaly, CP.
Mohr (Oro-facial-digital type 2)	Median CL/CP.
(Oro-facial-digital type 1)	Median CL/CP, porencephalic cysts.
Robinow-Sorauf ACPS	Acrocephaly, bifid great toe.
Sakati-Nyhan ACPS	Acrocephaly, CHD, short limbs, dysplastic ears.
Tri 13, 3p-, dup(17q)	

Only those associated features which might be amenable to prenatal diagnosis have been included. For further details refer to Winter *et al.*[63] (Adapted from Winter *et al.*, 1988.)[63]

ECTRODACTYLY

Ectrodactyly (split hand) is a variant of syndactyly in which the hands resemble a 'lobster claw' (**Figure 13**). It may occur either as an isolated phenomenon or as part of a number of syndromes,[63] the chief of which is the EEC syndrome. Isolated ectrodactyly and EEC syndrome are both inherited as autosomal dominant traits.

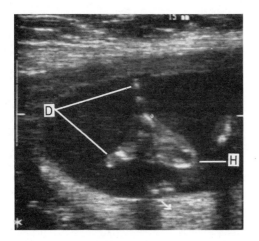

Figure 13. Ectrodactyly. Scan of a fetal foot showing ectrodactyly (H heel, D digits). Reproduced with permission from Griffin (1992).[42]

Diagnosis

Isolated ectrodactyly may affect one or more limbs and has extremely variable expression and penetrance so that the parent of an affected child may show only minimal changes in the skin creases.[69] In these mildly affected cases prenatal diagnosis may not be possible but a diagnosis should be achieved in more severe cases. In the EEC syndrome ectrodactyly is associated with cleft lip and/or palate and skin, hair and teeth dysplasia. Renal defects may be an accompanying feature.

Risks and Management Options

Individuals with EEC syndrome are of normal intelligence and generally manage to adapt to their deformities and lead normal lives. Facial clefting can be surgically corrected as can some of the orthopaedic deformities. Dentures and wigs may be required and attention to the lacrimal ducts is needed from an early stage to prevent corneal scarring.

Table 6
Syndromes associated with syndactyly

Syndrome	Associated features
Ablepharon-macrostomia (McCarthy)	Camptodactyly, cutaneous webs
Acrofacial dysostosis (Miller)	As Treacher Collins S, postaxial defects
Acrocephalo-syndactyly (Apert)	Coronal synostosis with brachycephaly, severe osseous syndactyly, CL/CP
(Pfeiffer)	2-3 Syndactyly, acrocephaly
Amniotic reduction	Oligohydramnios, CL/CP, limb reductions, abdominal wall defects (see text)
C-Trigonocephaly	As polydactyly
Carpenter	As polydactyly
Cenani-Lenz	Severe mesomelic limb hypoplasia. Complete syndactyly, radio-ulnar synostosis and severe hypoplasia
Cryptophthalmos	Renal agenesis, hypospadias
Ectrodactyly-ectodermal dysplasia-clefting	CL/CP, 'split' hands and feet (see below)
Fitch	As polydactyly
Fuhrmann	As polydactyly
Greig	As polydactyly
Goltz	As polydactyly
Golabi-Rosen	As polydactyly
Hypoglossia-hypodactyly	Limb reductions, micrognathia (see Roberts S.)
Klippel-Trenauny-Weber	As polydactyly
Lenz-Majewski	Growth retardation
Moebius	Micrognathia, CL/CP, radial
Nager	defects
Neu-Laxova	Microcephaly, flexion deformities, agenesis corpus callosum
Oculo-dental-digital	4-5 syndactyly
Oro-facio-digital (type 1)	Median CL, CP, polydactyly, asymmetrical syndactyly, porencephalic cysts
Oto-palato-digital	CP, 'tree frog' hands and feet (clynodactyly of peripheral digits)
Popliteal pterygium (severe, lethal AR form)	Popliteal webs, CL/CP, microcephaly
Poland sequence	Hypoplasia of fingers or hand
Roberts	As polydactyly
Robinow-Sorauf	As polydactyly
TAR	Radial aplasia (see above)
Triploidy	Growth retardation, large placenta, umbilical hernia, talipes, micrognathia, CHD, hydrocephaly, holoprosencephaly, renal dysplasia, hydronephrosis
Yunis-Varon	Cleidocranial dysostosis + micrognathia, absent thumbs distal aphalangia

POSITIONAL DEFORMITIES

Positional deformities may be found in several settings:

- in response to adverse intrauterine pressures (oligohydramnios, amniotic bands or tumors)

- diastrophic dysplasia

- rhizomelic chondrodysplasia punctata

- chromosomal disorders

- generalized neuromuscular deficiencies

- as specific isolated phenomena

The deformities are generally flexion but extension and bizarre combinations may be seen.

TALIPES

The commonest form of this condition is talipes equinovarus in which the foot is adducted and plantar inverted so that the sole of the foot points medially. In equinovalgus (calcaneovalgus) deformity the heel is elevated and the foot plantar everted. Talipes may occur as an isolated phenomenon with varying degrees of severity in about 1:1200 births or as a marker of chromosomal abnormalities or a number of genetic syndromes.

Diagnosis

Positional deformities of the feet can be recognized by employing sagittal and coronal scanning planes (**Figure 14**). When severe talipes equinovarus is present the plantar view of the foot will be seen in continuity with the leg in sagittal section (**Figure 15**). Because of the many associated syndromes a careful search for other abnormalities is mandatory prior to counseling. *The combination of talipes with polyhydramnios should raise the suspicion of myotonic dystrophy.*

Risks and Management Options

Isolated talipes is usually amenable to orthopedic correction. *An offer of karyotyping should be considered as talipes may be the only visible marker of chromosomal anomaly; it is advised if other structural abnormalities are found.* Management will depend upon the severity of associated defects and the results of karyotyping.

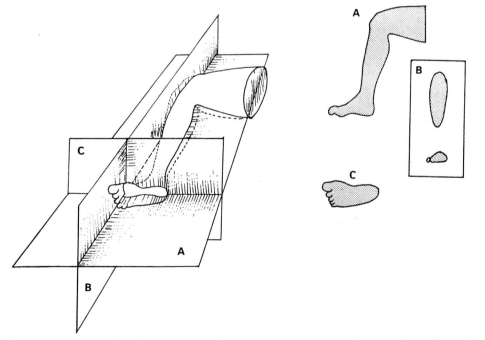

Figure 14. Diagram representing the scanning planes employed to visualize the foot. Plane A will show rocker-bottom feet; planes A and B will show talipes; planes B and C reveal polysyndactyly. Reproduced with permission from Griffin (1992).[42]

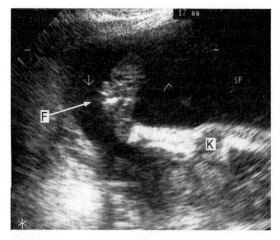

Figure 15. Positional deformities: Talipes. Longitudinal sonogram of the leg showing the lower end of the femur, knee (K), tibia/fibula and foot with talipes. The plantar view of the foot would not normally be seen in this plane.

ROCKER-BOTTOM FEET

The typical appearance of rocker-bottom feet, usually caused by a vertical talus, is a posteriorly prominent heel and convexity of the normally concave contour of the plantar arch (**Figure 16**). Rocker-bottom feet are strongly associated with trisomy 18, 18q syndrome, trisomy 13 and Pena-Shokeir type 2 syndrome. The finding of this deformity should lead to a diligent search for other abnormalities. A karotype is indicated.

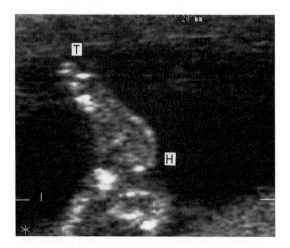

Figure 16. Rocker-bottom foot. Sagittal scan of the foot of a fetus with confirmed trisomy 18 showing prominent heel (H) and loss of the plantar arch (T toe).

MULTIPLE JOINT CONTRACTURES

This is a heterogeneous group of disorders characterized by multiple flexion deformities of the limbs, hands and feet resulting in fixed immobile limbs, sometimes with cutaneous webbing (pterygia) at joint flexures. The causes can be:

• CNS disease (55%)

• peripheral neuromuscular disorder (8%),

• connective tissue disease (11%)

• miscellaneous skeletal or other abnormality (19%).[70]

Table 7
Syndromes featuring positional deformities

Syndrome	Features
Aase-Smith-hydrocephalus-CP-joint contractures	CP, Dandy-Walker malformation (very variable presentation)
Amyoplasia	Multiple contractures with medial arm rotation (waiter's tip)
Bowed-Conradi	Like tri 18, rocker-bottom feet, micrognathia, camptodactyly
C-trigonocephaly	(see Polydactyly)
Cerebroarthrodigital	Digital hypoplasia, hydrocephalus microcephaly
Christian adducted thumbs	Craniosynostosis, micrognathia, CP adducted thumbs
Congenital myotonic dystrophy	More common with affected mother
Distal arthrogryposis	Camptodactyly of hands, talipes
Freeman-Sheldon	Ulnar deviation of hands, talipes
Marden-Walker	Camptodactyly, CHD, occ CP
Multiple pterygium (Lethal type)	Severe webbing, cystic hygroma, hydrops, pulmonary and cardiac hypoplasia, CP
Neu-Laxova	(see Syndactyly)
Pena-Shokeir type 1	Growth deficiency, pulmonary hypoplasia, camptodactyly, talipes
Syndesmoplastic dwarfism	No details
X linked arthrogryposis	

(Adapted from Winter *et al.*, 1988[63]).

Oligohydramnios may be present in 7%[70] and fetal hydrops has been reported in the second trimester.[25,71,72] Deficient swallowing and fetal breathing may be responsible for hydramnios and pulmonary hypoplasia in later pregnancy. Within this spectrum of disease, the more severe forms, commonly designated arthrogryposis multiplex congenita, a number of syndromes have been described including congenital muscular dystrophy, lethal multiple pterygium syndrome and Pena-Shokeir type 1 syndrome. These and other syndromes with varying degrees of contractures possibly amenable to prenatal diagnosis are listed in **Table 7**.

Risks and Management Options

The more severe of these syndromes associated with thoracic constriction, hydrops and multiple deformities including congenital muscular dystrophy, lethal multiple pterygium syndrome and Pena-Shokeir type 1 syndrome are lethal and pregnancy termination is an option. Definitive prenatal diagnosis of other syndromes may not be possible except in high risk families where detection or exclusion of relevant features might be possible. Discussion with geneticist prior to counseling is useful where any uncertainty exists. If the pregnancy continues, careful thought has to be given to the mode of delivery if the deformities are severe enough to produce dystocia or trauma with a vaginal delivery.

SPINAL DEFORMITIES

These may occur as a consequence of neural tube defects, hemivertebrae, dysplasia or agenesis of the vertebrae or asymmetrical muscle action (severe abdominal wall defects). Neural tube defects and abdominal wall defects are considered elsewhere in this volume (Chapters 50 and 52).

HEMIVERTEBRAE

A hemivertebra occurs when one of the pair of chondrification centers which fuse to form the vertebral body fails to appear. Only half of the vertebral body develops and produces a lateral angulation in the spine (scoliosis). Hemivertebrae may be isolated or found in association with cardiac, renal, radial or digital anomalies, tracheo-esophageal fistula and anal atresia in the VACTERL association or as a part of other genetic syndromes.

Diagnosis

A hemivertebra will be recognized by spinal scoliosis and asymmetry in vertebral echoes on ultrasound examination (**Figure 17**). A careful fetal survey for associated abnormalities is essential. Polyhydramnios may be the only clue to esophageal atresia. As a similar spectrum of deformities may be found in Trisomy 18 and 13Q syndromes, a karotype is indicated.

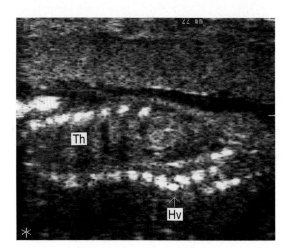

Figure 17. Hemivertebra. Longitudinal scan of the vertebral bodies of one of twin fetuses showing a mid-lumbar hemivertebra (HV). The spinal canal showed no evidence of narrowing on scan. Spinal deformity was minimal at birth (Th = thorax).

Risks and Management Options

These will depend upon the presence and severity of associated anomalies. Discussion with an orthopedic specialist regarding surgical correction of the spinal deformity may be helpful. Individuals with VACTERL association generally show normal intellectual potential.

JARCHO-LEVIN SYNDROME

This is an autosomal recessive most common in the Puerto-Rican population.

Diagnosis

The syndrome is characterized by a grossly disorganized axial skeleton and thorax (**Figure 18**). The spine may be missing or fused and hemivertebrae and ribs frequently reduced in number with posterior fusion

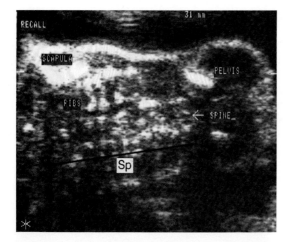

Figure 18. Jarcho-Levin syndrome. Longitudinal, coronal scan of the trunk of a fetus with Jarcho-Levin syndrome. The ribs are thick and irregular and the spinal components (Sp) grossly disorganized. Reproduced with permission from Griffin (1992).[42]

and anterior flaring (the 'crab chest' deformity).

Visceral and urogenital anomalies and diaphragmatic hernia have also been reported.[42,73,74]

Risks and Management Options

The majority of individuals with this condition die during the neonatal period or early infancy due to respiratory insufficiency. Termination of pregnancy should be discussed.

HYDROPS

Fetal hydrops may be a feature of the most severe forms of the following:

- chondrodysplasia (particularly achondrogenesis type 1 and 2
- thanatophoric dysplasia
- asphyxiating thoracic dystrophy
- SRP syndromes
- osteogenesis imperfecta type 2
- multiple contracture syndromes (including Pena-Shokeir syndrome type 1)
- Noonan's syndrome

- chromosomal abnormalities (Down's syndrome, trisomy 18)

A karotype is indicated.

HYDRAMNIOS

Many limb reduction deformities may be associated with hydramnios. These include:

- achondrogenesis
- asphyxiating thoracic dystrophy
- chondrodysplasia punctata
- dyssegmental dysplasia
- Roberts' syndrome

It may also be:

- esophageal atresia in the VACTERL association
- with fetal talipes in myotonic dystrophy.

Hydramnios generally presents late in pregnancy and may not be apparent at the time of a routine second trimester scan. As pregnancies complicated by diabetes mellitus may also develop hydramnios, spinal and lower limb deformities should also be sought.

UNFAVOURABLE INTRAUTERINE ENVIRONMENT

DIABETES MELLITUS

Patients with diabetes mellitus pre-dating pregnancy have an 8–12% risk of fetal malformation (see also Chapter 19). Skeletal malformations particularly associated with diabetes mellitus are the caudal regression syndrome and femoral hypoplasia-unusual faces syndrome (see above).

CAUDAL REGRESSION SYNDROME

This syndrome is highly variable in the severity and site of the malformation.

Diagnosis

The typical lesion is agenesis of the lower spine (**Figure 19**) which may be associated with lower limb reductions or deformities including fusion of the legs (sirenomelia) (**Figure 20**). Urogenital and anorectal organs of similar caudal origin are frequently evolved and may be malformed or atretic. Radial reduction and esophageal atresia may also occur in an association similar to VACTERL. Single umbilical artery is usual.

Risks and Management Options

Survival and prognosis will depend upon the severity of lesions. Minor degrees of sacral agenesis may be compatible with normal life whereas severe defects may cause considerable handicap or be incompatible with life if associated with renal agenesis. A careful assessment of lesions is essential and further discussions with relevant specialists may be appropriate before final counseling. Karyotyping is recommended as similar deformities may be associated with chromosomal abnormality. Pregnancy interruption should be discussed in severe cases before viability.

EARLY AMNION RUPTURE SEQUENCE

This bizarre and sporadic group of disorders (1:2000 births) consists of asymmetric anatomical disruptions associated in many cases with adherent bands or sheets of amnion. The consensus view seems to be that the deformities are secondary to early amnion rupture, the severity and site of the lesion being related to the stage of organogenesis at which rupture occurs.

Vascular occlusion during organogenesis may also be responsible for some of these anomalies. Abnormalities may not necessarily be associated with continued oligohydramnios and the diagnosis should be considered when transverse reduction defects or multiple asymmetrical disruptions are discovered even in the presence of normal amniotic fluid volume.

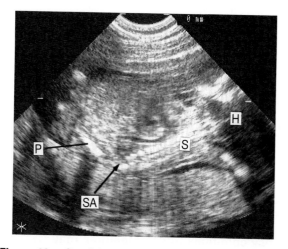

Figure 19. Caudal regression sequence. Longitudinal sagittal scan of the fetal trunk and spine of fetus with agenesis of the lumbo-sacral spine (SP). The spine terminates at the lower thoracic region (SA). The pelvis (P) is present (H head). Reproduced with permission from Griffin (1992).[42]

Diagnosis

Manifestations may include anencephaly, asymmetrical encephalocoele, facial clefts and disruptions, abdominal wall defects (usually gastroschisis) and limb deformities, constrictions or transverse reductions. Such malformations have also been reported following amniocentesis and, more recently, chorion villous sampling (CVS) before the tenth postmenstrual week.[75,76]

Amniotic bands may be seen attached to deformed structures. In known cases of early amnion rupture or continued 'bleeding' in the first trimester, such deformities should be excluded by detailed second trimester ultrasound examination. In the presence of oligohydramnios, visualization may be difficult if not impossible. Amnioinfusion may be performed to improve visualization.[77]

Karyotyping is appropriate as some chromosomal anomalies may present similar features.

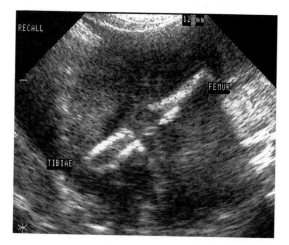

Figure 20. Sirenomelia. Sonogram of the lower 'limb' of an 18-week fetus diagnosed as sirenomelia. The single femur arose from the mid-pelvis and the broadened lower metaphysis articulated with two bones, presumed to be tibiae.

SKELETAL ABNORMALITIES
Summary of Management Options

Prepregnancy

- Ensure accuracy of diagnosis before counseling

- Counseling (possibly interdisciplinary)
  - recurrence risks
  - prenatal diagnostic options

Prenatal

- Careful ultrasound by experienced sonographer is vital, including general examination of fetus for other anomalies

- Consider a karyotype or other additional tests

- Interdisciplinary discussion before counseling parents (differential diagnosis rather than definitive diagnosis may be all that is possible)

- Ongoing review of ultrasonic findings if pregnancy continues (further features may develop allowing definitive diagnosis)

- Psychological support of parents

Labor/delivery

- Consider pregnancy termination with severe and/or lethal anomalies

- Psychological support of parents

- Cesarean section for obstetric indications

Postnatal

- If lethal, encourage postmortem (by experienced perinatal pathologist)

- Postnatal x-ray and review by specialist radiologist

- Tissue for karyotyping and other tests

- Ensure accuracy of diagnosis before counseling

- Counseling (possibly interdisciplinary)
  - recurrence risks
  - prenatal diagnostic options

It is important to recognize that amniotic band-like structures (synechiae) are commonly seen during routine examination. There is no evidence that these cause deformities if they are neither attached to the fetus nor restricting mobility.

Risks and Management Options

These will depend upon the severity of lesions. In cases of continuing severe oligohydramnios spontaneous miscarriage may ensue or pulmonary hypoplasia may threaten viability. Interruption of pregnancy should be discussed in non-viable or severely disrupted cases. Karyotyping should be considered when deformities are seen.

DRUGS IN EARLY PREGNANCY

Most drugs undergo extensive animal testing for teratogenicity before release for human consumption. A detailed fetal scan is recommended for any pregnant individual who has ingested significant medication during the first trimester. Some drugs specifically implicated in limb teratogenesis are thalidomide (withdrawn), warfarin, phenytoin, alcohol, cytotoxic drugs and lithium. A more comparative list of potentially teratogenic drugs has been produced by Koren et al.[78]

CONCLUSIONS

These can be extremely difficult malformations to diagnose sonographically. The ultrasonologist is rarely qualified to undertake parental counseling regarding exact diagnosis without expert assistance. In the initial stages of diagnosis, the complex fetal deformities should be discussed with a geneticist who has a specific interest in dysmorphology. Thereafter the diagnosis may be refined by further ultrasound examination, karyotyping (if not already performed) or other ancillary test.

Parents may find it useful to speak with other relevant specialists who have experience of these rare disorders before deciding on further management. All relevant professionals who may encounter the mother during her pregnancy and labour should be informed of the diagnostic findings and their significance (if known). Some parents may wish to continue pregnancy with a lethally malformed fetus; others may opt for a termination. Either option should always be respected and the parents treated with particular care and consideration by all carers.

If the condition is lethal the fetus or newborn should be photographed and x-rayed. Skin, blood, or placental samples should be obtained for karyotype/DNA analysis. When possible, the fetus should be examined by a pathologist specializing in perinatal pathology. Radiographs should be examined by a pediatric radiologist if there is any diagnostic doubt.

It is only when all information has been gathered that the final consultation with the parents is arranged with the obstetrician, geneticist or both. The parents can then be informed of recurrence risks in further pregnancies and offspring risks for their existing children or other family members. Management plans for prenatal diagnosis in a future pregnancy can then be discussed.

REFERENCES

1 Giedon A, Biedermann K, Briner J, Soler R, Spycher M (1991) Case report 693 (Schneckenbecken dysplasia). *Skeletal Radiology* **20**:534–538.

2 Chervenak FA, Isaacson G, Rosenberg JC, Kardon NB (1986) Antenatal diagnosis of frontal cephalocele in a fetus with atelosteogenesis. *Journal of Ultrasound in Medicine* **5**:111–113.

3 Kim HJ, Costales F, Bouzouki M, Wallach RC (1986) Prenatal diagnosis of dysegmental dwarfism. *Prenatal Diagnosis* **6**:143–150.

4 Nyberg DA, Mahony BS, Pretorius DH (1990) *Diagnostic Ultrasound of Fetal Anomalies: Text and Atlas*, pp. 196–197, 529. Chicago: Year Book Medical Publishers.

5 Smart LM, Muir BB, Lowles IE, Thomson AJ, Hardwick DJ (1994) Antenatal diagnosis of metatropic dysplasia by ultrasound: A case report. *Prenatal Diagnosis* (in press).

6 Mayden KL, Tortora M, Berkowitz RL, Bracken M. Hobbins JC (1982) Orbital diameters: a new parameter for prenatal diagnosis and dating. *American Journal of Obstetrics and Gynecology* **144**:289–297.

7 Jeanty P, Draimex-Wilmet M, Van Gansbeke D, Van Regemorter N, Rodesch F (1982) Fetal occular biometry by ultrasound. *Radiology* **143**:513–516.

8 Otto C, Platt LD (1991) The fetal mandible measurement: an objective determination of fetal jaw size. *Ultrasound in Obstetrics and Gynecology* **1**:12–17.

9 Chitty LS, Altman D, Campbell S (1993) Fetal mandible measurement: feasibility and development of centile charts. *Prenatal Diagnosis* (in press).

10 Allen LD, Tynan MJ, Campbell S, Anderson RH (1981) Normal fetal cardiac anatomy – a basis for the echocardiographic detection of abnormalities. *Prenatal Diagnosis* **1**:131–139.

11 Orioli IM, Castilla EE, Barbosa-Neto JG (1986) The birth prevalence rates for the skeletal dysplasias. *Journal of Medical Genetics* **23**:328–332.

12 Glenn LW, Teng SSK (1985) *In utero* sonographic diagnosis of achondrogenesis. *Journal of Clinical Ultrasound* **13**:195–198.

13 Chervenak FA, Blakemore KJ, Isaacson G, Mayden K, Hobbins JC (1983) Antenatal sonographic findings of thanatophoric dysplasia with cloverleaf skull. *American Journal of Obstetrics and Gynecology* **146**:984–985.

14 Beetham FGT, Reeves JS (1984) Early ultrasound diagnosis of thanatophoric dwarfism. *Journal of Clinical Ultrasound* 12:43–44.

15 Burrows PE, Stannard MW, Pearrow J, Sutterfield S, Baker ML (1984) Early antenatal sonographic recognition of thanatophoric dysplasia with cloverleaf skull deformity. *American Journal of Roentgenology* 143:841–843.

16 Camera G, Dodero D, De Pascale S (1984) Prenatal diagnosis of thanatoporic dysplasia at 24 weeks. *American Journal of Medical Genetics* 18:39–43.

17 Elejalde BR, de Elejalde MM (1985) Thanatophoric dysplasia: fetal manifestations and prenatal diagnosis. *American Journal of Medical Genetics* 22:669–683.

18 Weiner CP, Williamson RA, Bonsib SM (1986) Sonographic diagnosis of cloverleaf skull and thanatophoric dysplasia in the second trimester. *Journal of Clinical Ultrasound* 14:463–465.

19 Fryns JP, van den Berghe K, van Assche A, van den Berghe H (1981) Prenatal diagnosis of campomelic dwarfism. *Clinical Genetics* 19:199–201.

20 Hobbins JC, Bracken MB, Mahoney MJ (1982) Diagnosis of fetal dysplasias with ultrasound. *American Journal of Obstetrics and Gynecology* 142:306–312.

21 Redon JY, Le Grevellec JY, Marie F, Le Coq E, Le Guern H (1984) Un diagnostic antenatal de dysplasie campomelique. *Journal of Obstetrics Gynecology Biology and Reproduction* 13:437–441.

22 Winter R, Rosenkranz W, Hofmann H, Zierler H, Becker H, Borkenstein M (1985) Prenatal diagnosis of campomelic dysplasia by ultrasonography. *Prenatal Diagnosis* 5:1–8.

23 Gillerot Y, Vanheck C-A, Foulon M, Podevain A, Koulischer L (1989) Campomelic syndrome: manifestations in a 20-week fetus and case history of a five-year old child. *American Journal of Medical Genetics* 34:589–592.

24 Cordone M, Lituania M, Zampatti C, Passamonti U, Magnano GM, Toma P (1989) *In utero* ultrasonographic features of campomelic dysplasia. *Prenatal Diagnosis* 9:745–750.

25 Griffin DR (1990) Detection of congenital abnormalities of the limbs and face by ultrasound. In: Chamberlain G (ed.) *Modern Antenatal Care of the Fetus.* Oxford: Blackwell Scientific Publications, pp. 389–427.

26 Beluffy G, Fraccaro M (1982) Genetic and clinical aspects of campomelic dysplasia. In: Papadatos CJ, Bartsocas CS (eds) *Skeletal Dysplasias.* New York: Allan R. Liss, pp. 53–65.

27 Houston CS, Opitz JM, Spranger JW, Macpherson RI, Reed MA, Gilbert EF, Hermann J, Schinzel A (1983) The campomelic syndrome: review, report of 17 cases and follow-up on the currently 17-year old boy first reproted by Maroteaux *et al.* in 1971. *American Journal of Medical Genetics* 15:3–28.

28 Filly RA, Golbus MS (1982) Ultrasonography of the normal and pathologic fetal skeleton. *Radiologic Clinics of North America* 20:311–323.

29 Brock DJH, Rodeck, CH, Ferguson-Smith MA (eds) (1992) *Prenatal Diagnosis and Screening.* Edinburgh: Churchill Livingstone.

30 Dinno ND, Yacuob US, Kadlec JF, Garver KL (1982) Midtrimester diagnosis of osteogenesis imperfecta, type 11. *Birth Defects* 18:125–132.

31 Milsom I, Mattsson L-A, Dahlen-Nilsson I (1982) Antenatal diagnosis of osteogenesis imperfecta by real-time ultrasound: Two case reports. *British Journal of Radiology* 55:310–312.

32 Shapiro JE, Phillips JA, Byers PH, Sanders R, Holbrook KA, Levin LS, Dorst J, Barsh GS, Peterson KE, Goldstein P (1982) Prenatal diagnosis of lethal osteogenesis imperfecta (OI type II) *Journal of Paediatrics* 100:127–133.

33 Elejalde BR, de Elejalde MM (1983) Prenatal diagnosis of perinatally lethal osteogenesis imperfecta. *American Journal of Medical Genetics* 14:353–359.

34 Aylsworth AS, Seeds JW, Guilford WB, Burns CB, Washburn DB (1984) Prenatal diagnosis of a severe deforming type o osteogenesis imperfecta. *American Journal of Medical Genetics* 19:707–714.

35 Brons JTJ, van der Harten JJ, Wladimiroff JW, van Geijn HP, Dijkstra PF, Exalto NE, Reuss A, Niermeijer MF, Meijer CJLM, Th Arts NF (1988) Prenatal ultrasonographic diagnosis of osteogenesis imperfecta. *American Journal of Obstetrics and Gynecology* 159:176–181.

36 Constantine G, McCormack J, McHugo J, Fowlie A (1991) Prenatal diagnosis of severe osteogenesis imperfecta. *Prenatal Diagnosis* 11:103–110.

37 Munoz C, Filly R, Golbus MS (1990) Osteogenesis imperfecta type 11: prenatal sonographic diagnosis. *Radiology* 174:181–185.

38 Robinson LP, Worthen NJ, Lachman RS, Adomian GE, Rimoin DL (1987) Prenatal diagnosis of osteogenesis imperfecta type III. *Prenatal Diagnosis* 7:7–15.

39 Chitty LS, Griffin DR, Seller M, Maxwell M, Hall CN (1993) Prenatal diagnosis of osteogenesis imperfect type 3; report of two cases. *Ultrasound in Obstetrics and Gynecology* (in press).

40 Kurtz AB, Wapner RJ (1983) Ultrasonographic Diagnosis of second trimester skeletal dysplasias: a prospective analysis in a high risk population. *Journal of Ultrasound in Medicine* 2:99–106.

41 Wladimiroff JW, Niermeijer MF, Van der Harten JJ, Stewart FGA, Bloms W, Huijmans JGM (1985) Early prenatal diagnosis of congenital hypophosphatasia: case report. *Prenatal Diagnosis* 5:47–52.

42 Griffin DR (1992) Skeletal dysplasias. In: Brock DJH, Rodeck CH and Ferguson-Smith MA (eds) *Prenatal Diagnosis and Screening*, Edinburgh: Churchill Livingstone, pp. 257–313.

43 Walkinshaw SA, Burn J (1991) The diagnosis and management of pregnancies complicated by fetal abnormality. In Dunlop W, Calder AA (eds) *High Risk Pregnancy*, Guildford, Surrey: Butterworths.

44 Mulivor RA, Mennuti M, Zackai EH, Harris H (1978) Prenatal diagnosis of hypophosphatasia: Genetic, biochemical and clinical studies. *American Journal of Human Genetics* 30:271–282.

45 Warren RC, McKenzie CF, Rodeck CH, Moscoso G, Brock DJ, Barron L (1985) First trimester diagnosis of hypophosphatasia with a monoclonal antibody to the liver/bone/kidney isoenzyme of alkaline phosphatase. *Lancet* 2:856.

46 Brock JH, Barron L (1991) First trimester prenatal diag-
    nosis of hypophosphatasia: experience with 16 cases.
    Prenatal Diagnosis **11**:387–391.

47 Borochowitz Z, Ornoy A, Lachman R, Rimoin DL
    (1986) Achondrogenesis II – Hypochondrogenesis:
    variability versus heterogeneity. *American Journal of
    Medical Genetics* **24**:273–288.

48 Little D (1984) Prenatal diagnosis of skeletal dysplasias.
    In: Rodeck CH, Nicolaides KH (eds) *Prenatal Diag-
    nosis*. London: Royal College of Obstetricians &
    Gynaecologists, pp. 301–306.

49 Elejalde BR, de Elejalde MM, Pansch D (1985) Prenatal
    diagnosis of Jeune Syndrome. *American Journal of
    Medical Genetics* **21**:433–438.

50 Mahoney MJ, Hobbins JC (1977) Prenatal diagnosis of
    chondroectodermal dysplasia (Ellis-van Creveld
    syndrome) with fetoscopy and ultrasound. *New England
    Journal of Medicine* **297**:258–260.

51 Zimmer EZ, Weinraub Z, Raijman A, Perya A, Peretz
    BA (1984) Antenatal diagnosis of a fetus with an
    extremely narrow thorax and short-limbed dwarfism.
    Journal of Clinical Ultrasound **12**:112–114.

52 O'Brien GD, Rodeck C, Queenan JT (1980) Early pre-
    natal diagnosis of diastrophic dwarfism by ultrasound.
    British Medical Journal **280**:1300.

53 Mantagos S, Weiss RW, Mahoney M, Hobbins JC
    (1981) Prenatal diagnosis of diastrophic dwarfism.
    American Journal of Obstetrics and Gynecology
    139:111–113.

54 Gembruch U, Niesen M, Kehrberg H, Hansmann M
    (1988) Diastrophic dysplasia: A specific prenatal diag-
    nosis by ultrasound. *Prenatal Diagnosis* **8**:539–545.

55 Duff P, Harlass FE, Milligan DA (1990) Prenatal diag-
    nosis of chondrodysplasia punctata by sonography.
    Obstetrics and Gynecology **76**:497–500.

56 Hoefler S, Hoefler G, Moser AB, Watkins PA, Chen
    WW, Moser HW (1988) Prenatal diagnosis of rhi-
    zomelic chondrodysplasia punctata. *Prenatal Diagnosis*
    8:571–576.

57 Bromley B, Miller W, Foster SC, Benacerraf BR (1991)
    The prenatal sonographic freatures of Kneist syndrome.
    Journal of Ultrasound in Medicine **10**:705–707.

58 Sconyers SM, Rimoin DL, Lachman RS, Adomian GE,
    Crandall BF (1983) A distinct chondrodysplasia resem-
    bling Kniest dysplasia: Clinical, roentgenographic, his-
    tologic and ultrasound findings. *Paediatrics* **103**:898–
    904.

59 Kirk JS, Comstock CH (1990) Antenatal sonographic
    appearance of spondyloepithelial dysplasia congenita.
    Journal of Ultrasound in Medicine **9**:173–175.

60 Filly RA, Golbus MS, Cary JC, Hall JG (1981) Short
    limbed dwarfism: ultrasonographic diagnosis by men-
    suration of fetal femoral length. *Radiology* **138**:653–
    656.

61 Benacerraf B, Gelman R, Frigoletto FD Jr (1987) Sono-
    graphic identification of second-trimester fetuses with
    Down's syndrome. *New England Journal of Medicine*
    317:1371–1376.

62 LaFollette L, Filly RA, Anderson R, Golbus MS (1989)
    Fetal femur length to detect trisomy 21: A reappraisal.
    Journal of Ultrasound in Medicine **8**:657–660.

63 Winter RM, Knowles SAS, Bieber FR, Baraitser M

(1988) *The Malformed Fetus and Stillbirth: A Diagnos-
    tic Approach*. Chichester: John Wiley and Sons,
    pp. 166–182.

64 Smith DW (1982) *Recognizable Patterns of Human
    Malformations: Genetic, Embryologic and Clinical
    Aspects*. Philadelphia: W. B. Saunders.

65 Hirose K, Koyanagi T, Hara K, Inoue M, Nakano H
    (1988) Antenatal ultrasound diagnosis of the femur-fib-
    ula-ulna syndrome. *Journal of Clinical Ultrasound*
    16:199–203.

66 Muller LM, de Jong G, van Heerden KMM (1985) The
    antenatal ultrasonographic detection of the Holt-Oram
    syndrome. *South African Medical Journal* **68**:313–315.

67 Brons JTJ, Van Geijn HP, Wladimiroff JW, Van Der
    Harten JJ, Kwee ML, Sobotka-Plojhar M, Th.Arts NF
    (1988) Prenatal ultrasound diagnosis of the Holt-Oram
    Syndrome. *Prenatal Diagnosis* **8**:175–181.

68 Yarkoni S, Schmidt W, Jeanty P, Reece EA, Hobbins
    JC (1985) Clavicular measurement: a new biometric
    parameter for fetal evaluation. *Journal of Ultrasound in
    Medicine* **4**:467–470.

69 Penchaszadeh VB, Negrotti TC (1976) Ectrodactyly-
    ectodermal dysplasia-clefting (EEC) syndrome: domi-
    nant inheritance and variable expression. *Journal of
    Medical Genetics* **13**:281–284.

70 Hageman G, Ippel EPF, Beemer FA, de Pater JM, Lind-
    hout D, Willemse J (1988) The diagnostic management
    of newborns with congenital contractures: A nosologic
    study of 75 cases. *American Journal of Medical Gen-
    etics* **30**:883–904.

71 Shenker L, Reed K, Anderson C, Hauck L, Spark R
    (1985) Syndrome of camptodactyly, ankyloses, facial
    anomalies and pulmonary hypoplasia. (Pena-Shokeir
    syndrome): Obstetric and ultrasound aspects. *American
    Journal of Obstetrics and Gynecology* **152**:303–307.

72 Kirkinen P, Herva R, Leisti J (1987) Early prenatal
    diagnosis of a lethal syndrome of multiple congenital
    contractures. *Prenatal Diagnosis* **7**:189–196.

73 Tolmie JT, Whittle MJ, McNay MB, Gibson AAM,
    Connor JM (1987) Second trimester prenatal diagnosis
    of the Jarcho-Levin syndrome. *Prenatal Diagnosis*
    7:129–134.

74 Romero R, Ghidini A, Eswara MS, Seashore MR, Hob-
    bins JC (1988) Prenatal findings in a case of spon-
    dylocostal dysplasia type I (Jarco-Levin syndrome).
    Obstetrics and Gynecology **71**:988–991.

75 Firth HV, Boyd PA, Chamberlain P, MacKenzie IZ,
    Huson SM (1991) Severe limb abnormalities after chor-
    ion villous sampling at 56–66 days gestation. *Lancet*
    337:762–763.

76 Burton BK, Schultz CJ, Burd LI (1992) Limb abnor-
    malities associated with chorionic villous sampling.
    Obstetrics and Gynecology **79**:726–730.

77 Gembruch U, Hansmann M (1988) Artificial instillation
    of amniotic fluid as a new technique for the diagnostic
    evaluation of cases of oligohydramnios. *Prenatal Diag-
    nosis* **8**:33–45.

78 Koren G, Edwards MB, Miskin M (1987) Antenatal
    sonography of fetal malformations associated with
    drugs and chemicals: A guide. *American Journal of
    Obstetrics and Gynecology* **176**:79–85.

55

Miscellaneous Fetal Disorders: Tumors, Hyperthyroidism, Hypothyroidism, Congenital Adrenal Hyperplasia, Pathologies Specific to Twins

MARY PILLAI

FETAL TUMORS

Fetal neoplasms are a rare and heterogeneous group of disorders whose etiology is poorly understood. The most common true neoplasm of the fetus is a teratoma, composed of multiple tissues foreign to the part in which they arise. Sacrococcygeal teratomas comprise over 50% of teratomas found at birth.[1] Other locations include the intracranium, palate, cervical spine, mediastinum, retroperitoneal space and gonads. For convenience, the fetal tumors have been grouped according to the region affected – the cranium, oronasopharyngeal region, neck, thorax, abdomen and pelvis, placenta and cord, other vascular tumors, and fetal tumors of maternal origin.

INTRACRANIAL TUMORS

Congenital brain tumors account for approximately 0.3% of neonatal deaths at less than 28 days.[2] They are usually teratomas which can be either benign or malignant. However, in this location, even benign lesions tend to have devastating consequences. Other tumors reported in this location include glioblastoma,[3] meningeal sarcoma,[4] lipoma of the corpus callosum[5] and oligodendroglioma.[6] In general, these are limited to isolated case reports. Although craniopharyngiomas account for 5–10% of all childhood intracranial tumors, they are seldom detected prior to the age of 2 years, and there has been only one case reported in a fetus.[7]

INTRACRANIAL TUMORS: TERATOMA

Presentation

A number of fetal intracranial teratomas have been reported, most often presenting with a sudden increase in uterine size with hydramnios.[6,8–12] The ultrasound appearance is a bizarre array of cystic and solid regions. Growth of the tumor may result in hydrocephalus, destruction of the intracranial contents and erosion of the cranial vault.

Risks and Management Options

In contrast to teratomas in other locations, intracranial teratomas carry a particularly poor prognosis – most children are either stillborn or die in the neonatal period. The tumor mass itself may greatly expand the calvara, or this may occur secondary to hydrocephalus. Cephalocentesis is an option when there is severe hydrocephalus or a large cystic component to the tumor. However, some cases will need to be delivered by cesarean section because vaginal delivery is likely to be impossible even after cephalocentesis.

Treatment consists of postnatal surgical excision. Though long-term survival has been achieved in a minority of cases, the risk of neurologic impairment is high.[13,14] Two inoperable newborns were treated by shunting; each died within 3 months due to shunt obstruction secondary to the high protein content of the cerebrospinal fluid (CSF).[10]

INTRACRANIAL TUMORS: CHOROID PLEXUS PAPILLOMA

Presentation

These benign tumors of variable size are attached to a normal choroid plexus. Most are unilateral and located in the atrial portion of the lateral ventricle. They are most often diagnosed following recognition of hydrocephalus. The image of an echogenic mass in the atrium of one lateral ventricle is highly suggestive of a choroid plexus papilloma.

Risks and Management Options

Postnatal surgery is the preferred treatment. Delivery should be at term, or if the associated hydrocephalus is rapidly increasing, as soon as pulmonary maturity has been demonstrated. The mode of delivery depends on the head size. Cesarean section is preferred if disproportion is likely. Cephalocentesis to avoid cesarean section is not desirable since a normal outcome is possible with surgery.

ORONASOPHARYNGEAL TUMORS

Presentation

Teratomas are the most common tumors of this region. An epignathus is a nasopharyngeal teratoma arising from the fetal facial bones, especially the palate or ethmoid. Prenatal diagnosis is based on the appearance of a solid and cystic mass arising from the mouth or face.[15–17] An elevated maternal serum alpha-fetoprotein and hydramnios are likely to occur, the latter when they are large enough to obstruct fetal swallowing.[15]

Risks and Management Options

When the tumor involves the neck or oral cavity, a pediatric surgeon should be present at delivery and prepared to perform a tracheostomy if necessary. These tumors are generally benign, and complete surgical extirpation offers the best chance of cure. However, the tumor site may preclude complete excision and death may occur secondary to asphyxia or meningitis if the base of the skull is involved. With large tumors,

staged procedures and flap reconstruction may be necessary.

NECK

The differential diagnosis of sonographically detected tumors in the fetal cervical region includes occipital encephalocele, cervical meningomyelocele, hygromas (lymphangiomas), teratoma, hemangioma, sarcoma, and congenital goiter. An occipital encephalocele appears as a complex mass in the midline dorsal region with a bony defect in the skull on cross section. The intracranial image is usually abnormal and the head measurements smaller than expected. Cervical meningomyelocoeles are also located in the midline dorsal region with a bony defect in the cervical spine.

NECK: CYSTIC HYGROMA

Risks and Management Options

Cystic hygroma is undoubtedly the most common of all fetal tumors. The position and prognosis of these tumors are very different to cystic hygroma in infancy; prognosis is governed by the appearance of the tumor and gestational age of the fetus.

In the first and second trimesters there is a strong association between fetal nuchal cystic hygromas or nuchal edema and chromosomal anomalies.[18,19] The risk of chromosome anomaly increases with the thickness of the nuchal swelling. In chromosomally normal fetuses the natural history is disappearance of the nuchal swelling by 18–20 weeks gestation.[18,19] In second trimester fetuses with pathological accumulation of fluid in the nuchal region, there is a difference between cystic hygromas and edema both in terms of pathogenesis and in terms of their association with chromosomal defects. Hygromas which are bilateral and septated are strongly associated with Turner's syndrome and are thought to represent overdistension of the jugular lymphatic sacs which have failed to communicate with the internal jugular vein.[20] In contrast, nuchal edema is due to subcutaneous accumulation.

NECK: CERVICAL TERATOMA

Risks and Management Options

Cervical teratomas account for 3–4% of childhood teratomas and are usually evident as a large mass at birth. Their size and location may prevent swallowing, cause hydramnios, and be responsible for the relatively high mortality; 17% of affected fetuses are stillborn, and 35% die before surgery.[21] The vast majority of cervical teratomas are benign with only 4 of 118 cases reported in the literature metastasizing.[22] Fetal and placental hydrops may occur with large tumors and delivery by cesarean section is indicated if dimensions of the tumor are such that it may obstruct labour. A pediatrician should attend the delivery and be prepared for a difficult intubation secondary to compression of the trachea by tumor. Definitive treatment is by surgical excision.

NECK: GOITRE

Risks and Management Options

A large goiter in a fetus is a rare but potentially serious consequence of maternal ingestion of excessive quantities of goitrogens (typically iodides), stimulation of the fetal thyroid by maternal thyroid stimulating antibodies in maternal Grave's disease, or fetal hypothyroidism secondary to therapy of maternal Grave's disease with antithyroid drugs. A large goiter may cause hyperextension of the fetal neck resulting in malpresentation with obstructed labour. In the neonate it may obstruct the trachea.

Diagnosis and management of this is discussed below under Fetal Thyrotoxicosis.

THORAX

Tumors involving the thoracic region originate from the lungs, the heart and the mediastinum. A differential of space-occupying lesions found in the fetal chest is given in **Table 1**.

Table 1
Lesions found in the fetal chest

Solid lesions
Type III cystic adenomatoid malformation
Pulmonary sequestration (lobar or extralobar)
Mediastinal teratoma
Rhabdomyoma

Cystic lesions
Types I and II cystic adenomatoid malformation
Diaphragmatic hernia
Bronchogenic cyst
Gastric cyst

THORAX: LUNGS

Risks and Management Options

There are no true tumors originating from the fetal lungs, but malformations which may appear as a mass include congenital cystic adenomatoid malformation (CAM), bronchogenic cysts and extralobar pulmonary sequestration. Although these lesions are not true tumors, CAM and pulmonary sequestration can give the echogenic appearance of a solid or mixed solid-cystic tumor (**Figure 1**) and so have been included.

Pulmonary sequestration

Pulmonary sequestration is a forgut malformation in which a segment of lung parenchyma is isolated from

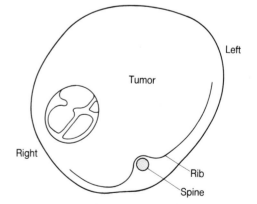
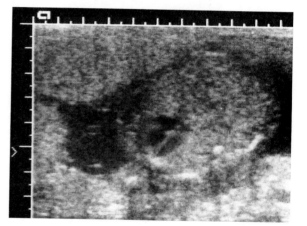

Figure 1. a (upper): Ultrasound transverse section of thorax of a 20 week fetus with type 111 cystic adenomatoid malformation. The lungs are replaced by a solid mass and there is extreme dextroposition of the heart on the right due to extrinsic compression by the tumor. Hydrops and fetal death supervened at 22 weeks. **b** (lower): Diagrammatic interpretation.

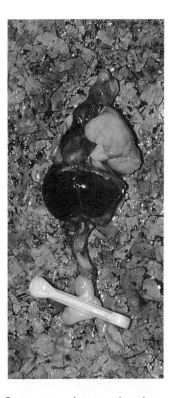

Figure 1c. Gross specimen showing umbilical cord, liver, diaphragm and thoracic contents. The white mass is the 'tumor' and the heart is seen on the right of the chest.

eral, but occasionally they may appear to completely replace the normal lung tissue (**Figure 1**). The presence of an isolated CAM does not carry an increased risk of abnormal karyotype. According to the size of cysts, CAM have been classified into three subtypes:

- type I have large cysts (**Figure 2**)

- type II have multiple cysts <1.2 cm

- type III are microcystic <5 mm diameter and have a solid appearance (**Figure 1**).

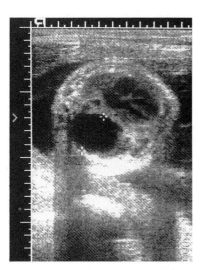

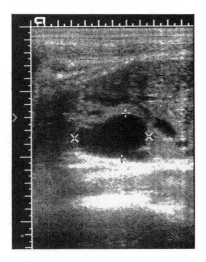

Figure 2. Type 1 cystic adenomatoid malformation. A 3 × 5 cm cystic mass occupies the left thorax and the heart occupies the right thorax. **a** (upper): Transverse view of thorax. **b** (lower): Longitudinal view of thorax.

normal lung tissue. In most cases, the sequestration has no trachobronchial connection, and is supplied by an aberrant systemic artery arising from the aorta rather than a pulmonary vessel. Drainage may be to pulmonary or systemic veins. In some cases the abnormal mass of lung may be replaced by cysts. A recent review of the literature described only 17 published reports, with antenatal diagnosis being relatively uncommon.[23–25] The prognosis depends on the development of pleural effusions which may lead in turn to hydrops.

Placement of pleuroamniotic shunts in the fetus with hydrops may relieve the obstruction to cardiac return and cure the hydrops.

Congenital cystic adenomatoid malformation (CAM)

This is thought to result from failure of the endodermal bronchiolar epithelium to induce the formation of bronchopulmonary segments by the surrounding mesenchyme. The resulting hamartoma tissue can cause mediastinal shift, pulmonary, esophageal and vena caval compression which decreases cardiac return leading to hydramnios and hydrops. Most CAMs are unilat-

Type I tends to have the best prognosis; however the natural history of CAM is variable, and there have been several reports of spontaneous diminution in size of fetal chest masses.[26-28] Survival rates are most closely linked to the presence or absence of non-immune hydrops.[29]

Because of this, a number of investigators have undertaken repetitive thoracentesis[30] or placement of thoracoamniotic shunts.[31,32] The aspiration of a cystic lesion generally provides only short-term benefit because fluid rapidly reaccumulates. Placement of a catheter may be complicated by malfunction after relatively short periods of time, and will not provide adequate drainage of multilocular cysts.

Kuller et al.[28] described 18 patients who elected to continue their pregnancy after the diagnosis was made. In nine cases fetal hydrops did not develop, and all these infants survived after delivery at 32–42 weeks. In four of these nine cases the neonate underwent resection of the CAM. In the other nine cases non-immune hydrops developed between 20 and 27 weeks. In one case the infant delivered at 33 weeks and died of respiratory distress at 1 h of life. In six cases, fetal surgery (hysterotomy and resection of the CAM) was performed at 21–27 weeks. Four survived and are apparently well.

This initial report suggests that fetal surgery may have a place in the management of CAM complicated by hydrops. However, the bias of case ascertainment is clear. The results of randomized controlled studies must be awaited before a conclusion can be reached.

CARDIAC

Cardiac tumors are very rare in early life. When they occur, they may represent the earliest manifestation of several genetic disorders including tuberous sclerosis, Gorlin's syndrome (nevoid basal cell carcinoma syndrome), neurofibromatosis and familial myxomas.[33] In the neonate and infant the most common primary cardiac tumor is a rhabdomyoma (a non-malignant smooth muscle hamartoma), associated with concomitant tuberous sclerosis in most cases.[34,35] Groves et al. recently reported a series of 11 fetal cardiac tumors out of 794 congenital cardiac malformations seen over 11 years at a tertiary referral center for fetal cardiac problems; 10 cases were rhabdomyomas and one was a pericardial teratoma.[35] Myxomas are not seen in infants and have not been reported in the fetus.

Rhabdomyomas are solid in appearance occurring within the myocardium. They usually arise from the ventricular wall or interventricular septum (**Figure 3**). If large, they can compress the ventricular cavity, and produce fetal hydrops by limiting cardiac output.[36] Arrhythmias also occur, possibly due to disruption of

the conducting tissue by tumor within the interventricular septum.

Development of rhabdomyomas has been reported during the course of gestation,[35,37] so they cannot be excluded by a single normal examination. Though there is no evidence that these tumors regress during perinatal life, they do regress postnatally.[35,38,39] Rhabdomyomas have been associated with tuberous sclerosis in 50–78% of cases. Since other features of tuberous sclerosis are often absent in the fetus and early postnatal life, it is possible that nearly all cases would develop the disease if they survived long enough. The finding of a cardiac rhabdomyoma is currently the most likely means of diagnosing tuberous sclerosis prenatally as the prevalence of tumors in young infants with the disease is considerably above 50%.[40] How-

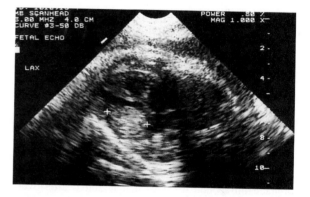

Figure 3a. A single large cardiac rhabdomyoma arising within the left ventricular wall. Courtesy of Dr Christopher Harman, Winnipeg.

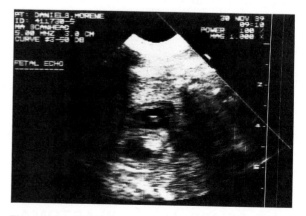

Figure 3b. Multiple cardiac rhabdomyomas. The diagnosis of tuberous sclerosis was confirmed in infancy. Courtesy of Dr Christopher Harman, Winnipeg.

ever, the absence of a cardiac tumor in a fetus at risk for tuberous sclerosis does not exclude the diagnosis.

Management Options

If no fetal complications occur, delivery is at term and the route determined by obstetrical indications. The chances of tumor regression in infancy and again in adolescence are high and this has led some to suggest conservative postnatal management.[38,40] Others have suggested that the risk of sudden death is in the order of 23% and that the optimum management is either complete surgical resection of the tumor, or partial resection and consideration of transplantation for large unresectable tumors.[41] The development of fetal hydrops, unless associated with a rhythm disturbance, is an indication for delivery and consideration of surgery. However, the prognosis is very poor.

TUMORS OF THE ABDOMEN AND PELVIS: THE LIVER

Risks and Management Options

Malignant and benign primary liver tumors are rare in children and those diagnosed antenatally are confined to a few case reports. The embryonic origin of the liver is both mesenchymal and endodermal. Therefore, the differential diagnosis on finding a liver 'tumor' on a prenatal ultrasound includes hemangioma, arteriovenous malformation, hamartoma, teratoma, hepatoblastoma and polycystic disease affecting the liver or liver and kidneys. Arteriovenous malformations usually present in the newborn with congestive cardiac failure, thrombocytopenia and/or a huge abdominal mass.[42] Large tumors are likely to be visible on prenatal ultrasound and pulsed colour Doppler sonography can be extremely useful in determining their vascularity (**Figure 4**).

Mesenchymal hamartomas may be congenital and their prenatal diagnosis has been reported. In one case there were several large transonic intrahepatic masses, oligohydramnios and a thickened placenta.[43] The fetus was stillborn at 34 weeks.

A single case of hepatic teratoma has been reported in an anencephalic fetus.[44]

TUMORS OF THE ABDOMEN AND PELVIS: NEUROBLASTOMA

Neuroblastoma is the most common solid tumor in infancy and prenatal diagnosis by ultrasound has been

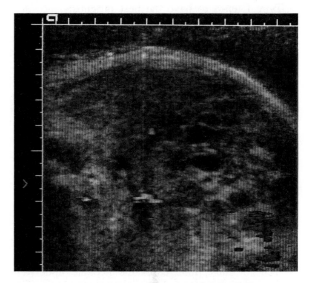

Figure 4a. Hemangioepithelioma of the fetal liver. Multiple fluid filled spaces are evident within the tumor – only one third of these showed flow on colour Doppler sonography.

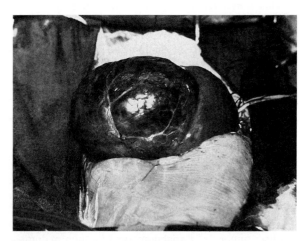

Figure 4b. Neonatal surgical excision of this hepatic tumor.

reported.[45,46] It is an embryonal tumor of neural crest origin that may arise at any site in the sympathetic nervous system, the most common site being the adrenal gland. In the fetus, neuroblastoma may appear as an echogenic abdominal mass displacing the kidney caudally (**Figure 5**). Though the primary tumor is often small, 50% of cases have metastases at birth and liver metastases are a common mode of presentation in the newborn.

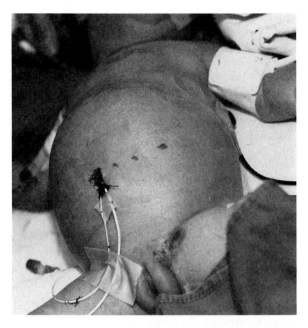

Figure 5a. Newborn infant with abdominal swelling due to a retroperitoneal neuroblastoma. Courtesy of Dr Christopher Harman, Winnipeg.

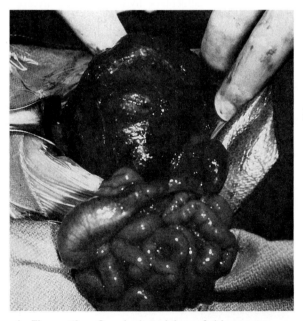

Figure 5b. Surgical excision of this tumor.

Risks and Management Options

Children under 1 year of age have a better prognosis than older children, but there are insufficient data on fetal neuroblastoma. Retroperitoneal tumors do worse than neuroblastoma in other sites.[47] Treatment is based on the extent of the disease according to staging criteria. For localized disease (stages I and II), surgical resection is most often the only treatment required. For advanced metastatic disease (stages III and IV) the therapy is aggressive and includes combined treatment with multiagent chemotherapy, total body irradiation, and transplantation with autologous marrow purged of tumor cells with monoclonal antibodies.[47]

TUMORS OF THE ABDOMEN AND PELVIS: THE KIDNEY

Fetal renal tumors are extremely rare. Wilms' tumor accounts for most renal tumors diagnosed in children, but the author found no documented fetal cases. The most common renal tumor reported in the fetus and newborn is mesoblastic nephroma (fetal renal hamartoma). This appears on ultrasound as a solid tumor with low level echoes replacing the kidney.[48–50] Hydramnios is common as with most other fetal tumors.

Risks and Management Options

Most mesoblastic nephromas are unilateral and are benign. A policy of delivery at term in the absence of any other problem would therefore seem appropriate. Postnatally, the management is surgical, most often unilateral nephrectomy without irradiation or chemotherapy.

TUMORS OF THE ABDOMEN AND PELVIS: FETAL OVARIAN CYSTS

An incidence of ovarian cysts in female fetuses of 1 in 2625 pregnancies has been reported.[51]

Diagnosis usually follows the coincidental finding of a lower abdominal cyst off midline on ultrasound. The diagnosis is supported by confirmation of female genitalia, identification of normal urinary tract anatomy and normal gastrointestinal structures (stomach, small and large bowel). Anomalies mistakenly reported as ovarian cysts include mesenteric and urachal cysts, mesonephric cysts, GI duplication cysts and hematometra with vaginal agenesis. No particular association with other congenital anomalies has been established.

Risks and Management Options

Management should be based on knowledge of the natural history. Sakala *et al.* recently reviewed 66 cases.[52] Of these, 95% were unilateral and all cases were diagnosed in the third trimester. The size of most cysts remained unchanged from diagnosis to delivery while two cases resolved *in utero*. Hydramnios was present in 18% and was associated with larger ovarian cysts (mean size 6.7 × 9.0 cm compared with 4.7 × 5.5 cm without hydramnios). It has been suggested that this reflects a partial bowel obstruction secondary to compression by the larger cysts. Intrauterine torsion was suspected in 12 of 66 cases based on a change in cyst appearance on serial sonograms (a simple cyst becoming echodense with septa formation, development of a fluid-debris level or finding of a retracting clot). These findings were not associated with any evidence of deterioration in fetal condition. These 12 patients were managed conservatively and the neonatal outcome was good.

After delivery, 41 of 64 neonates with a persisting cyst (those with the largest persisting cysts) underwent operative management: two cases resolved *in utero* and 23 were initially managed conservatively with serial sonography postnatally. Of these, 16 (64%) underwent spontaneous involution, and 90% did so within 3 months. Seven of the 23 (30%) underwent torsion. The main predictor of torsion was not size but rather the length of the pedicle (cysts with long pedicles were often noted to 'change side' on examination). These infants presented with vomiting, anemia and an acute surgical abdomen. These cases underwent surgery and the outcome was good. Of the 48 operated infants, 43 (90%) underwent oophorectomy with the remaining 5 having cystectomy. All histologically examined fetal ovarian cysts were benign.

In summary most fetal ovarian cysts are functional in origin, histologically benign and do not pose a risk to the fetus. Delivery at term is appropriate. There is a strong case for conservative postnatal observation as many will regress spontaneously and in those complicated by torsion or increase in size, the outcome of surgery is good. Surgery carries the risk of adhesion formation and removal of significant amounts of functional ovarian tissue which could impact negatively on future fertility. When it is necessary, an attempt should be made to conserve any normal ovarian tissue.

TUMORS OF THE ABDOMEN AND PELVIS: SACROCOCCYGEAL TERATOMAS

Teratomas arising in the presacral and coccygeal regions are the most common true congenital neoplasm in the fetus and newborn, with a female predominance and an estimated incidence of 1 in 40 000 births. There is an increased incidence of associated congenital anomalies, most of which are musculoskeletal.[53]

Sacrococcygeal teratomas appear as a mass arising from the sacral area and extending around to the perineum (**Figure 6**). They may grow to an enormous size, and be associated with hydramnios and hydrops, presumably secondary to high blood flow through the tumor.[54] The sonographic appearance of the tumor may be solid, cystic or mixed. Cystic cases may be difficult to differentiate from meningomyelocele, however there is characteristic bulging of the latter when the infant's fontanelle is compressed. Further, the spine should be intact with sacrococcygeal teratoma. Serum and amniotic fluid alpha-fetoprotein may be elevated if the teratoma contains neural tissue.

While intracranial teratomas carry a poor prognosis, sacrococcygeal tumors have a relatively good prognosis, provided any associated abnormalities have been excluded.[55,56] Shanbhogue *et al.* reported 43 patients of whom 36 (84%) survived long-term, and there were no deaths since 1982.[56]

Management Options

Prenatal

Serial sonograms coupled with weekly visits should detect the development of hydramnios and hydrops. The size of the tumor towards term should be taken into account when determining the mode of delivery. *These tumors are very fragile and their hemorrhage lethal.* Cesarean delivery is usually indicated via a vertical uterine incision. In the absence of other complications, delivery is performed after documentation of fetal lung maturity or after 36 weeks. The development of hydrops is usually associated with tumors of large size and rapid growth, and is an indication for immediate delivery. Hydrops with a fetal tumor carries a grave prognosis, although survival has been reported.[54]

The main causes of death with sacrococcygeal teratoma have been death prior to transfer or intraoperative

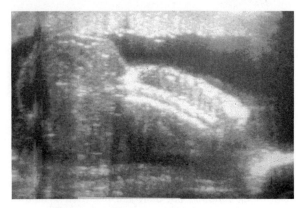

Figure 6. Sacrococcygeal teratoma.
Courtesy of Dr Peter Twining, Nottingham.

death related to heavy blood loss, or malignant change related to delayed treatment or incomplete excision.[56] Ideally, delivery should occur in a centre with neonatal surgical facilities. Blood should be available in case hemorrhage into the teratoma occurs at delivery.

Postnatal

Early surgery is recommended because of the malignant potential of some sacrococcygeal teratomas. The risk of malignancy is less than 10% before the age of 2 months but rises to 65–90% if the diagnosis and surgical excision are delayed beyond 4 months. At birth, pulmonary insufficiency may be severe where there is associated hydrops but can respond dramatically to removal of the tumor,[54] possibly because elimination of excess blood tumor blood volume results in improvement of the ventilation-perfusion ratio. Alternatively, the tumor may be a source of vasoactive substances or extremely desaturated blood that leads to pulmonary hypertension and right-to-left shunting.

Bladder outlet obstruction may develop in association with intrapelvic extension of the tumor and postoperative urological complications are relatively common.[57] They probably result from surgical injury to sacral nerves. Urinary and anorectal dysfunction or lower extremity weakness were present in 41% of 27 patients reviewed at a mean of 5 years after excision of a sacrococcygeal teratoma, and 67% of those with intrapelvic primary tumors. A high incidence of bladder dysfunction persists to adult life.[57] Repositioning the anteriorly displaced anus and preserving as much of the overstretched levator ani as possible for a normal anatomical pelvic floor reconstruction are important factors in preserving continence.[56]

Prevention of tumor recurrence and malignancy depend on complete excision and long-term follow-up. A delay in presentation may occur with intrapelvic tumors which were not diagnosed prenatally. The most common presenting symptoms in this group are constipation or urinary dribbling because of bladder and rectal outlet compression by the large tumor. Rectal examination of the newborn will detect these. Rectal examination, serial ultrasound and serum alpha-fetoprotein can be used to detect a recurrence,[58] the treatment of which is chemotherapy.

VASCULAR TUMORS

Risks and Management Options

'Tumors' of the extremities are nearly always vascular abnormalities. Vascular hamartosis (angioma) is a rare proliferation of new vessels which might be considered neoplastic. In a case described at 24 weeks gestation, the affected fetus was deformed with large subcutaneous masses.[59] A further case seen by the author was diagnosed at 18 weeks as huge subcutaneous masses with solid and cystic components distributed over the thorax and upper limbs (**Figures 7a and b**). Termination was declined and the size of the tumors increased with fetal growth. At 32 weeks the fetus became hydropic and a much extended classical uterine incision was necessary to extract the fetus (**Figures 7c and d**). The infant was ventilated from birth. Unfortunately, the tumors did not respond to chemotherapy.

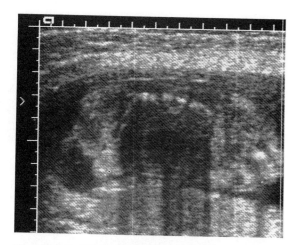
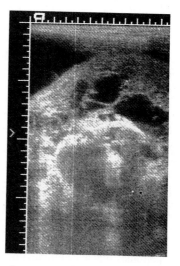

Figure 7a (left) and b (right). Ultrasound views of fetal thorax showing a massive subcutaneous angiomatous tumor with solid and cystic components.

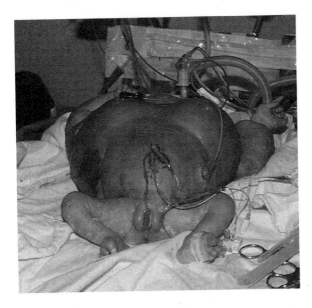

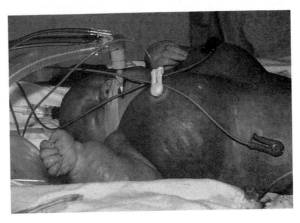

Figure 7c (left) and d (above). Hydropic neonate with massive angiomas.

There is no evidence that fetal therapy has any place in these cases.

TUMORS OF THE UMBILICAL CORD AND PLACENTA

Umbilical cord tumors are very infrequent. They can be divided into angiomyxomas or hemangiomas derived from embryonic vessels, teratomas, and vestigial cysts derived from remnants of the allantois or omphalomesenteric duct. Conditions which may mimic one of these on ultrasound include cord hematoma and a true knot. The ultrasound appearance is a mass of mixed echogenicity adjacent to the cord or placenta. Colour Doppler can be useful in establishing the vascular nature of the mass.

Cord hemangiomas have been associated with extremely high alpha-fetoprotein levels,[60] and the development of hydrops.[61] Fetal hemorrhage has been reported as a further life-threatening complication of a hemangioma.[62]

TUMORS OF THE UMBILICAL CORD AND PLACENTA: PLACENTAL CHORANGIOMA

Hemangiomas (chorioangiomas) occur in about 1% of placentae.[63] Most are small, single, discrete and indistinguishable from fresh infarcts on macroscopic examination of the placenta. Large hemangiomas (>5 cm

diameter) are comparatively rare, but will be visible on ultrasound (**Figure 8**) and may be associated with very high maternal serum alpha-fetoprotein values. They may lie on the maternal surface within the membranes, or they may be attached to the placenta by a vascular pedicle.

Risks and Management Options

Colour Doppler can be useful in delineating the vascularity of the tumor. The absence of blood flow in the

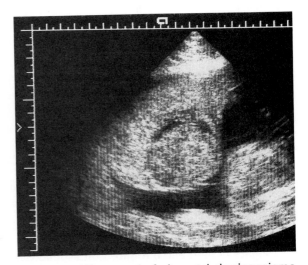

Figure 8a. Ultrasound of placental chorioangioma. Courtesy of Dr Christopher Harman, Winnipeg.

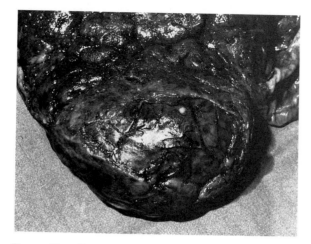

Figure 8b. Gross specimen at delivery. Courtesy of Dr Christopher Harman, Winnipeg.

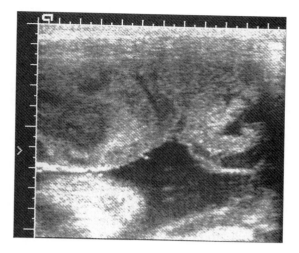

Figure 9. Ultrasound of placental Brues mole.

tumor may result from spontaneous infarction in which case the risks to the fetus are minimal. Large or multiple hemangiomas with high blood flow can produce the same fetal problems associated with any large arteriovenous anastomoses: hydramnios, cardiomegaly, cardiac failure, hydrops, anemia and thrombocytopenia. In pregnancies where a large vascular chorangioma is identified, the fetus requires close surveillance for signs of these complications and delivery if they occur. Steroids may be appropriate for promoting lung maturity, but it not known whether they may have a direct effect on the hemangioma to reduce complications.

TUMORS OF THE UMBILICAL CORD AND PLACENTA: BRUES MOLE

Risks and Management Options

A Brues mole is not a true tumor but is a massive subchorial collection of blood dissecting the membranes off the fetal surface of the placental disc. On histologic section, the collection of blood is a thrombus of maternal origin which is seen to be dissecting the chorionic plate from underlying villi and sometimes extending into the placenta. It is not always associated with fetal death.[64] Sonographically, a Brues mole appears as a mass with large cystic spaces (**Figure 9**) which may be so extensive that they dominate the appearance of the placenta. Swirling of clotted blood may be seen within these hypoechoic subchorionic areas.

DISSEMINATED CARCINOMA (see also Chapter 32)

Cancer in pregnancy is not uncommon and the main risk to the fetus is the need for preterm delivery either because of deterioration in maternal condition or the need to institute maternal therapies incompatible with pregnancy. Congenital malignant neoplasms very rarely arise in this way, with malignant melanoma the only tumor with a propensity to metastasize to the placenta and involve the fetus.[65-67]

Fetal Risks and Management Options with Maternal Malignant Melanoma

In all the reported cases of fetal metastases, the mother had advanced disease. The actual number of cases is small. Rapid progression can occur, and infant death within the first year of life approaches 100%.[67] Mothers with advanced or recurrent disease should undergo ultrasound examinations during pregnancy to look for any obvious fetal tumor mass.

Attention should be directed towards placental thickness, fetal liver size and spleen size. These infants should be followed up for a further one year, when prenatal sonogram is negative and there is no obvious involvement of the infant at birth. Cord blood should be examined for malignant cells, and the placenta subjected to thorough histological examination. Fetal involvement may appear as an unusual tumor mass involving any area of the body – an external mass or an enlargement of internal organs. If the neural tube is involved, then hydrocephalus may develop.[67]

In the above instance prompt delivery[67] has been recommended, although this decision will be influ-

---

FETAL TUMORS
Summary of Management Options

Prenatal

- Diagnosis by ultrasound generally including color flow imaging

- Biopsy should not be necessary with most, and could be dangerous

- Definitive diagnosis may not be possible

- Counsel parents

- Liaison with pediatricians and pediatric surgeons

Labor/delivery

- Mode of delivery depends on
  - prognosis
  - tumor size/anatomical considerations

Postnatal

- Pediatric assessment and management

---

enced by whether a viable gestational age has been reached.

FETAL THYROID DISEASE
(see also Chapter 21)

FETAL HYPERTHYROIDISM

Although rare, fetal/neonatal thyrotoxicosis carries a significant risk of morbidity and mortality for an affected baby. Most cases are associated with maternal Grave's disease, and cause problems which resolve within a few weeks of birth.

Grave's disease is common among young women, and it has been estimated that as many as 0.2% of pregnant women have hyperthyroidism and 2% of their infants have congenital thyrotoxicosis due to this disease.[68] It is an autoimmune disorder in which thyroid stimulating IgG autoantibodies (TSI) directed against thyroid receptors for TSH produce hyperthyroidism. The fetal thyroid is known to function by the 12th week of pregnancy,[69] however extrapolating from other alloimmune fetal diseases, significant levels of thyroid stimulating IgG are unlikely to reach the fetus before 18–20 weeks gestation.

Risks

Consequences of uncontrolled thyrotoxicosis for the fetus and newborn can be very serious; a high incidence of growth deficiency is reported, particularly if the mother has been thyrotoxic for 30 weeks or more of pregnancy,[70,71] has a TSI level above 30% at the time of delivery, had onset of disease before the age of 20 or duration of disease greater than 10 years.[72] These fetuses/neonates are also at risk of thrombocytopenia, postnatal craniosynostosis, neurodevelopmental abnormalities, and high-output cardiac failure secondary to tachycardia.[73–75] Stillbirth due to fetal hyperthyroidism has been reported without associated tachycardia or growth deficiency antemortem.[76] *A neonatal death rate of 16%[77] and a perinatal death rate of 50% have been reported in affected fetuses.[78]* Conversely, adverse effects resulting from maternal therapy are infrequent. For this reason, aggressive maternal therapy has been advocated, especially when the pregnancy is advanced.[79]

Maternal treatment outside pregnancy is usually in the form of antithyroid drugs or ablation of the thyroid with surgery or radioactive iodine followed by thyroxine replacement therapy. While ablative and replacement therapy renders the patient clinically euthyroid, the persistence of TSI places their pregnancies at risk.

Management Options

Prenatal

Pregnancy is one of the few conditions where measurement of TSI is clinically helpful, indicating the need for fetal and neonatal surveillance. *All women with a history of Grave's disease should be tested for the production of TSI at the outset of pregnancy. Those with positive tests should be referred to a fetal therapy unit.*

By mid gestation, the intact fetal thyroid is responsive to TSI and fetal thyrotoxicosis may result.

Therapeutic goals for the management of Grave's disease during pregnancy are to maintain the mother in a euthyroid or slightly hyperthyroid state and to keep the fetus in a euthyroid state.[71,73,80]

The choice of treatment for the hyperthyroid pregnant women lies between antithyroid drugs and surgery. Radioactive-iodine is contraindicated in pregnancy. Surgery is rarely necessary in pregnancy and even then the disease must first be controlled with medical therapy.

In addition to TSI, antithyroid drugs are also readily transferred across the placenta.[81,82] Medical treatment is predominantly with thioamides, most often propylthiouracil (PTU) because it passes through the placenta less easily than methimazole or carbimazole.[83] These drugs may cause side-effects, the most serious of which is an allergic agranulocytosis. Chemical hepatitis is fairly common.

Patients must be warned of these risks and a white-cell count should be determined if they develop a sore throat or fever during treatment. Drug therapy also poses the risk of fetal hypothyroidism although in practice problems are rarely encountered except when high doses are used in pregnancy (for example 800–1200 mg of PTU daily). For this reason the patient should be maintained on the lowest dose that keeps values for thyroid function in the upper normal range for non-pregnant women once the disease is controlled. Goiter has been reported both in fetuses with hyperthyroidism and in those with thyroid suppression from maternal PTU.[84,85]

No ultrasound findings characteristic of fetal hyper or hypothyroidism have been described. Hyperthyroidism is associated with intrauterine growth deficiency, tachycardia and other signs of fetal stress; however these are not specific and may result from many conditions. In rare cases, a fetal goiter may be visualized as a bilobed symmetrical mass in the anterior portion of the fetal neck.[86] Yet no assumption can be made about the fetal thyroid status since fetal goiter may occur with a fetus in a hypo or hyperthyroid state.

It is an important principle to realize that the fetal endocrine status may be entirely different from the maternal endocrine status and cannot be definitively ascertained by indirect methods. Amniotic fluid thyroid hormone levels do not reliably predict fetal thyroid status,[87,88] although TSH concentrations in normal fetuses have been reported in the range <0.15 to 1.7 μU/ml, and significantly higher amniotic fluid levels of TSH were found in a hypothyroid fetus.[89] The only reliable means of determining fetal thyroid status is by cordiocentesis. Data from cordocentesis in unaffected pregnancies has confirmed that there is no relation between fetal and maternal values. Free serum

TSH levels are higher and T_4 and T_3 levels are lower than adult values. Total and free T_4 levels reach adult levels by 36 weeks.[90]

Thioamides block the synthesis but not the release of thyroid hormone, so an effect may not be seen for several days. Where rapid control of symptoms is desired, it can be achieved with the addition of beta-blocking agents and iodide. Long-term iodide carries a significant risk of producing a large, obstructive fetal goiter. Its use should be limited to initial disease control or treatment of thyroid storm (life-threatening exacerbation of signs and symptoms of hyperthyroidism). The administration of propranolol in pregnancy has been associated with fetal growth deficiency, impaired fetal response to anoxic stress, and neonatal bradycardia and hypoglycemia. However, there is sufficient data to suggest pregnant women may safely be treated with beta-blockers if these are indicated for maintaining a clinically euthyroid state.

Postnatal

Lactation

Small amounts of thioamides appear to be transferred in breast milk.[91,92] The amount of PTU transferred is less than that of methimazole and would be unlikely to affect neonatal thyroid function markedly.[92] There is the small theoretical risk of drug reactions, though none so far have been reported. If a mother taking thioamides wishes to breast feed, she should be given an explanation of possible adverse effects and neonatal thyroid function monitored.

The neonate

In the fetus, signs of thyrotoxicosis can include tachycardia, growth deficiency and rarely goiter. In the newborn, it may present with jaundice, irritability, tremulousness, diarrhea, fever, failure to gain weight, tachycardia, cardiac failure, hepatosplenomegaly, goiter, and prominent eyes.[75] It occurs in around 1 in 70 infants born to mothers with Grave's disease with both male and female infants equally affected. The risk relates more closely to maternal TSI levels than maternal thyroid hormone levels.[72] When the mother has been on PTU, the signs may not occur in the first few days because of the continued effects of transplacental PTU.[82] The diagnosis is confirmed by elevated T_4 and low TSH in the newborn. However, umbilical cord levels may be normal after maternal treatment with antithyroid drugs and should be repeated after 5–10 days. The morbidity and mortality of neonatal thyrotoxicosis is significant and the first aim of treatment is control of cardiac symptoms usually with propranolol (1–2 mg/kg/day in three divided doses). Sup-

FETAL HYPERTHYROIDISM AND HYPOTHYROIDISM
Summary of Management Options

HYPERTHYROIDISM
(see also Chapter 21)

Prenatal

- Fetal risk in mothers with thyrotoxicosis is indicated by the production of TSI antibodies

- Maternal therapy is aimed at keeping her euthyroid or slightly hyperthyroid (propylthiouracil rather than carbimazole)

- Monitor fetus for
  - tachycardia
  - hydrops
  - growth deficiency
  - goiter

- Cordocentesis justified if fetal hyperthyroidism suspected

- Maternal administration of beta-blockers if fetal hyperthyroidism

Postnatal

- Pediatric assessment and management

HYPOTHYROIDISM

Prenatal

- Fetal goitrous hypothyroidism confirmed by cordocentesis

- Treatment by intra-amniotic injection of thyroxine

pression of hypersecretion is with a saturated solution of potassium iodide (10% solution, one drop every 8 h) and PTU 5–10 mg/kg/day in three divided doses. Carbimazole can be used as an alternative to PTU. T4 levels should be kept in the middle of the normal range. If the thyroid is over-suppressed, the infant may temporarily require L-thyroxine 5–15 µg/kg/day at the same time as the antithyroid regime is continued. Neonatal Grave's disease is transient and will regress as the maternal TSI is cleared from the infants circulation, usually within 2–6 months.

FETAL HYPOTHYROIDISM

Risks and Management Options

Where fetal hypothyroidism is confirmed, prenatal treatment requires the direct administration of thyroid hormones to the fetus, because the placenta is relatively impermeable to thyroxine and triiodothyronine.[93,94] The most convenient route of administration is by intraamniotic injection. It is easy to do, has a low complication rate and allows a long interval between injections. In the last few weeks of pregnancy, goitrous hypothyroidism has been successfully treated with 500 µg at 10–14 day intervals[95] and with 250 µg at weekly intervals.[85,96]

CONGENITAL ADRENAL HYPERPLASIA

Risks

Most cases of congenital adrenal hyperplasia (CAH) are caused by 21-hydroxylase deficiency, where the impaired metabolism of cholesterol to cortisol results in an excess of 17-hydroxyprogesterone. This is metabolized to androstenedione and testosterone. As a consequence genetic females are exposed to excess androgens and virilized. The abnormal differentiation can vary from clitoral hypertrophy to complete formation of a phallus and fusion of the labia which has resulted in erroneous assignment of gender. When female sex is correctly assigned, the genitalia may require multi-stage surgical correction. In male infants, the genitalia may give no clue to the diagnosis at birth and they are at risk of adrenocortical insufficiency with severe salt losing crisis.

Unfortunately, a first affected child remains unsuspected until after birth as carriers of the autosomal recessive gene are completely normal. Subsequent offspring have a 1:4 likelihood of the disease with a 1:8 chance of a virilized female.

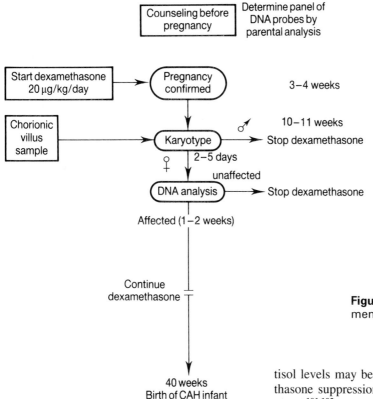

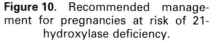

Figure 10. Recommended management for pregnancies at risk of 21-hydroxylase deficiency.

Management Options

Prenatal diagnosis of 21-hydroxylase deficiency was originally made by finding elevated levels of 17-hydroxyprogesterone in midtrimester amniotic fluid.[97] It now relies on DNA analysis for linked HLA or C4 genes, or direct detection of mutant 21-hydroxylase alleles by molecular genetic techniques. The most recent clinical advance is a program of combined prenatal diagnosis with karyotyping and suppression of fetal androgen production in females by steroid administration to the mother.[98,99]

Pharmacological suppression of the fetal adrenal gland by maternal administration of dexamethasone 0.25–1.5 mg daily has been used to prevent masculinization of fetuses, and studies suggest that this should be started by 7 weeks menstrual age.

Maternal administration of dexamethasone from the first trimester to birth is associated with excessive weight gain, cushingoid facies, severe striae, and development of hyperglycemia.[100] Other symptoms include hypertension, gastrointestinal intolerance, and extreme irritability.

First and second trimester amniotic fluid 17-hydroxyprogesterone androstenedione and testosterone may be elevated on this treatment regardless of genital outcome. The measurement of maternal estriol and cor-

tisol levels may be preferable for monitoring dexamethasone suppression of the maternal and fetal adrenal gland.[101,102] *Because of the high incidence of side-effects, the dose should be lowered during the second half of gestation.*

The duration of unnecessary prenatal dexamethasone treatment for an unaffected fetus is substantially reduced if first trimester chorionic villus sampling (CVS) is employed for diagnosis.[98]

The current recommended management for pregnancies known to be at risk of 21-hydroxylase deficiency is outlined in **Figure 10**. It consists of pre-pregnancy investigation of known carrier parents to determine the appropriate DNA probes; commencement of dexamethasone 20 μg/kg/day as soon as the pregnancy is confirmed and before 7 weeks gestation, and CVS at around 11 weeks. If this reveals a male karyotype or an unaffected female, the dexamethazone is discontinued. If DNA analysis reveals an affected female the dexamethasone is continued for the remainder of the pregnancy, but the dose can be reduced after 20 weeks. Obviously, affected infants of both sexes will require postnatal treatment.

Experience to date indicates that starting dexamethasone as early as possible in the first trimester, proper dosage and non-interruption of therapy all contribute to the likelihood of a favourable outcome.[98] Prior to the era of prenatal dexamethasone therapy, the birth of a female with classical 21-hydroxylase deficiency with completely normal genitalia had not been reported.

CONGENITAL ADRENAL
HYPERPLASIA
**Summary of Management
Options**

Prenatal (see Figure 10)

PATHOLOGIES SPECIFIC TO TWINNING (see also Chapter 10)

MONOAMNIOTIC TWINS

Only 1% of all twin pregnancies are monoamniotic 3–5 per 1000 pregnancies.[103] A predominance of female sex has been reported among monoamniotic twins.[104–106]

Risks

The high mortality of this unusual form of twinning is thought to result predominantly from cord entanglement with resultant cord occlusion and fetal asphyxia. Vaginal delivery poses further risk of fetal interlocking and cord entanglement.

Pseudomonoamniotic twinning occurs when the membrane separating twins becomes disrupted. It carries the same potential for cord and twin entanglement as monoamniotic twinning and can occur whether the membrane is mono- or dichorionic. It has been reported following both amniocentesis and cordocentesis,[107] though it may occur spontaneously.[108] Because of the risk of this complication traversing the membrane of twin sacs at these procedures should be avoided where possible.

Diagnosis

While visualization of a membrane separating twin fetuses allows confident diagnosis of a diamniotic gestation, in most cases the apparent absence of a membrane is not diagnostic of monoamniotic pregnancy. Townsend *et al.* reported 10 cases in which no membrane could be found on careful evaluation, and of

whom only three were in fact monoamniotic.[109] The appearance of one twin 'stuck' to the uterine wall/placenta without visualization of a membrane allows presumptive diagnosis of diamniotic twins, and is due to severe oligohydramnios in one sac. In about 50% of cases, the 'stuck twin' appearance represents twin–twin transfusion in a monochorionic diamniotic gestation (see below). Congenital infection may produce the same findings. The same appearance without hydramnios may occur in dizygous pregnancies where fetal anomaly or severe early growth deficiency results in severe oligohydramnios in one of the sacs.

In cases where there is uncertainty of amnionicity, injection of dye into the sac under ultrasound guidance may be conclusive. Indigo carmine or Evans blue are currently the dyes of choice because (unlike methylene blue) no fetal morbidity has been reported with these two agents.[110] An alternative method described includes intra-amniotic injection of either aerated dye or renografin followed by a single-slice computed tomographic scan at the level of the umbilicus.[111,112] The latter must be viewed as excessive.

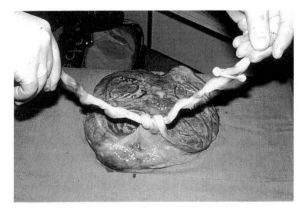

Figure 11.   Monoamniotic twin placenta with cord entanglement.

Management Options

The timing and mode of delivery have been areas of controversy. Because of the risk of cord entanglement, some obstetricians advocate intensive antenatal surveillance and prophylactic early delivery by cesarean section.[113] Others have suggested a more conservative approach with a trial of labour at term.[114] Because of the high mortality, if one aims not to intervene until a mature gestation is reached, a program of close surveillance would seem appropriate. Hospital admission either once viability has been reached or after cord entanglement has been demonstrated have each been recommended. With colour flow Doppler, it is now possible to identify cord entanglement by following the two cords to an area of suspected entanglement, where there may be apparent 'branching' of the umbilical vessels.[115] With pulsed Doppler it may be possible to demonstrate two different heart rates within the entwined area. Entanglement should also be suspected when there are antepartum decelerations on a non-stress test. Entanglement *per se* does not necessarily imply fetal compromise or the need for immediate delivery[116] but rather the need for intensive surveillance. Surveillance advocated includes twice or thrice daily fetal heart rate monitoring and biweekly biophysical profiles.[115] However, there is no evidence presently that this improves outcome.

With the increases in fetal size relative to total intrauterine volume in later pregnancy, it is likely that changing position relative to one another, and hence episodes of cord entanglement, would decrease in the last trimester. Two recent reports support this; Carr *et al.* found that the greatest risk of intrauterine death occurs before 30 weeks' gestation,[117] and Tessen and Zlatnik retrospectively reviewed 20 pairs of monoamniotic twins after 20 weeks gestation and found that no fetal death occurred after 32 weeks.[114] Labor and vaginal delivery were also not associated with an increased risk of death. These findings challenge the concept of prophylactic preterm cesarean section to avoid fetal demise.

In the 20 cases reported by Tessen and Zlatnik, the majority were delivered vaginally; no fetal death occurred in labor and only one case of fetal distress required emergency cesarean section.[114]

These two relatively large series challenge the widely stated edict that early prenatal diagnosis is important to ensure optimal perinatal care. Indeed it has been the author's experience that the obstetrician and patient anxiety generated by this diagnosis is likely to result in iatrogenic prematurity.

TWIN–TWIN TRANSFUSION SYNDROME

Two-thirds of monozygotic twins are monochorionic and susceptible to a variety of developmental abnormalities which may lead to discordant fetal size and amniotic fluid volume.[118] Twin–twin transfusion syndrome is one such complication and is seen almost exclusively in monochorionic gestations. The sonographic description of a 'stuck twin' refers to a lack of amniotic fluid around one twin transfixing the fetus against either the uterine or placental walls, and normal to increased amniotic fluid volume around the co-twin. It is usually associated with discordant fetal size.

Though many practitioners equate the finding of a stuck twin with twin–twin transfusion,[119] the differential diagnosis for stuck twin includes uteroplacental dysfunction, discordant aneuploidy or structural malformations, and congenital infection.

Definition

The diagnosis of twin–twin transfusion has traditionally been made postnatally when both the neonatal weights and hemoglobin concentrations were divergent. The scientific basis for this tradition is weak. Rausen reported that 19 of 130 monochorionic twins pairs had a hemoglobin concentration which differed by ≥ 5 g/dl while none of 43 dichorionic pairs had a similar difference.[120] They proposed that the presence of vascular anastomoses and a 5 g/dl difference was indicative of twin–twin transfusion. However, virtually all monochorionic twin pregnancies have anastomoses[121] and other pregnancy complications can cause fetal polycythemia. Danskin and associates found that the incidence of discordant hemoglobin was similar for dichorionic and monochorionic twin gestations.[122]

Tan and coworkers reported that hemoglobin concentrations were discordant only when the neonatal weights differed by $\geq 15\%$.[123] Unfortunately, discordant hemoglobin was their sole criterion for the diagnosis; chorionicity was not considered. Danskin found that the distribution of discordant birthweight between monochorionic and dichorionic gestations was similar.[122]

The application of the postnatal criteria for twin–twin transfusion also fails to consider the timing of transfusion – either chronic, or acute at delivery. Wenstrom observed that only 18% of monochorionic twin gestations were discordant for both weight and hemoglobin.[124] However, the smaller twin was polycythemic in one-third of such cases, a finding more consistent with uteroplacental dysfunction than twin–twin transfusion syndrome. Thus, only 12% of monochorionic twin pairs had postnatal findings classic for twin–twin transfusion. About a third of the twin pairs studied were concordant for weight, but discordant for hemoglobin. Unusually, the second twin had the higher hematocrit. This is consistent with either acute twin–twin transfusion or uteroplacental dysfunction.

Differentiating between acute and chronic twin to twin transfusion is important. Though neonates with acute twin–twin transfusion may have problems in the immediate neonatal period associated with hyperviscosity or hypotension, pulmonary hypertension and the cardiomyopathy secondary to chronic volume overload are not typically seen. It is the chronic twin–twin transfusion syndrome with its associated acute and massive second trimester hydramnios, hydrops fetalis and preterm delivery which without therapy carries the extremely high perinatal morbidity and mortality (<90%) rates. Thus, it is this syndrome we focus on.

Postnatal Diagnosis

This may not be as straightforward as once thought. The studies of Danskin and Wenstrom demonstrate that contrary to common practice, the diagnosis of chronic twin–twin transfusion syndrome cannot be made with any certainty postnatally. Clearly, chronic twin–twin transfusion syndrome exists, but how to make the diagnosis? It is relevant to ask whether the symptoms of twin–twin transfusion syndrome are the result of volume transfer? If so, can a stuck twin be the result of twin–twin transfusion syndrome if there is no difference in hematocrit or if the smaller twin is polycythemic?

Prenatal Diagnosis

Practitioners have employed a variety of non-invasive and invasive techniques for the prenatal diagnosis of twin–twin transfusion syndrome. All techniques utilize ultrasonography in one manner or another.

A full medical and obstetric history should be taken. Determine if the growth of the uterine fundus has been consistent with acute hydramnios and whether there has been any suggestion of maternal infection. A complete ultrasound examination of the uterine contents performed by an individual with expertise in obstetric anomaly scanning is essential. Because of the rarity of this entity, a referral to a tertiary care unit, and preferably a Fetal Diagnosis and Treatment Unit, is recommended.

Differentiating between acute and chronic hydramnios is important. The initial separation is based on the patient's oral history and the referring physician's records. Objective measurement of the fundus or the abdominal girth should reveal an increase of many centimeters per week.

Therapeutic amniocentesis

The first diagnostic step is a therapeutic amniocentesis (in the fundus to minimize the risk of rupturing membranes) to reduce the amniotic fluid pressure into normal range and the uterine cavity down to a workable size. If more than 1500 ml must be removed, stop there and repeat the amniocentesis 8–12 h later.

Therapeutic amniocentesis has several benefits. First, it enhances maternal comfort during the rest of the examination. Second, it facilitates the sonographic examination permitting the use of a higher frequency ultrasound transducer than would have otherwise been

possible. Third, it often facilitates cordocentesis which may be part of the diagnostic work-up prior to 25 weeks gestation. Fourth, therapeutic amniocentesis appears to decrease the risk of both preterm labor and premature rupture of the membranes compared with historic controls.[119,125–127] And finally, and perhaps most importantly, it allows the physician to estimate the rate of fluid accumulation. No or little reaccumulation is inconsistent acute hydramnios secondary to chronic twin–twin transfusion syndrome.

Sonography

2-D ultrasound

The goals of the initial sonographic examination are to document monochorionicity, fetal biometric discordance, and to seek evidence of discordant fetal anomalies or infection. Monochorionic twins are the same sex and have one placental mass with a paper thin dividing membrane.[128] Because the dividing membrane is so thin, it is often difficult to identify and the pregnancies misidentified as monoamniotic. Visualization is facilitated by searching over the fetal chin or away from the fetal body and around the limbs. A dichorionic placenta essentially eliminates the diagnosis of TTTS. The likelihood of a chromosome abnormality is increased greatly in the presence of a structural malformation.

The absence of acute hydramnios, a stuck twin, size discordance, structural malformations and monochorionic placentation does not necessarily exclude twin–twin transfusion syndrome. However, the lack of these minimal findings suggests that any existing shunt is small and not likely to account for a size discordance at a previable stage (<25 weeks).

There should be near anhydramnios in the sac of the growth deficient twin and hydramnios in the sac of the other. The bladder of the small twin may not be seen at all. The larger twin has a full bladder which rarely completely empties. If twin–twin transfusion syndrome is detected early, the difference in fetal size may be small. On occasion, the portion of the placenta supplying the recipient appears echodense. This is an early sign of hydrops.

The heart of the recipient twin is structurally normal, but the ventricular walls hypertrophied and the cardiothoracic ratio increased. Prior to the development of hydrops, ventricular contractility is diminished and on M-mode, A-V valve regurgitation is present.

Doppler ultrasound

There have been multiple attempts to apply Doppler velocimetry to the antenatal diagnosis of chronic twin–twin transfusion syndrome.[129–134] It had been suggested that a 0.4 difference in the umbilical artery S/D ratios of the co-twins was consistent with the diagnosis[130-131] (the higher one identifying the donor). Unfortunately, the diagnosis of twin–twin transfusion syndrome was based on postnatal criteria. Inequitable division of the placental mass at the time of twinning could yield the same Doppler findings. Not surprisingly, others have failed to find a consistent difference in the umbilical artery Doppler resistance index of monochorionic twin gestations with discordant sizes.[132-134]

Cordocentesis

The diagnosis of chronic twin–twin transfusion syndrome is greatly facilitated by cordocentesis. However, cordocentesis is not indicated in all patients suspected of twin–twin transfusion syndrome. Pregnancies which present after 25 weeks with acute hydramnios and a stuck twin have a much lower perinatal mortality rate. It is difficult to justify the risk of the procedure when there is no effective therapy to offer (see below). Cordocentesis is indicated when the syndrome manifests prior to 25 weeks or if one twin has hydrops and delivery is felt to be undesirable. In this instance, the loss rate far outweighs the risks of the diagnostic procedures. *Both* fetuses should be sampled. The hematocrit is measured and evidence of fetal infection sought.[135] If the shunt is large and sustained enough to produce acute hydramnios and discordant size, at least one fetus should have a hematocrit above or below the norm for gestation.[136] The possibility of a fetal infection as an explanation for the pathology should always be suspected (approximately 15% of those twin pregnancies referred for evaluation of possible twin–twin transfusion syndrome). Parvovirus and cytomegalovirus have each been reported. When the small or stuck twin is found to have polycythemia, uteroplacental dysfunction is the most common cause.

There are few biochemical markers for chronic twin–twin transfusion syndrome. It is, however, one of the only pathologic fetal states consistently alters the total serum protein and albumen concentrations. The recipient twin has hyperproteinemia while the donor tends to have hypoproteinemia.[137]

The passage of a marker from the donor twin to the recipient supports the diagnosis. Its absence all but precludes the diagnosis. Adult red blood cells provide an excellent marker. Infuse 15–20 ml of 70% hematocrit O-negative blood into the presumed donor if the initial hematocrit measurements are consistent with chronic twin–twin transfusion syndrome and then check for the presence of adult red blood cells (RBCs) in the presumed recipient twin 12–24 hours later.

Even after completing a full antenatal evaluation, one can only say that the findings are consistent with the diagnosis.

Management Options

While the diagnosis can now be made antenatally with some accuracy, therapy for chronic twin–twin transfusion presenting prior to 25 weeks gestation or for hydrops after 25 weeks remains an elusive problem. Any interpretation of past experience must be colored by the lack of a firm diagnosis. A variety of therapeutic techniques have been advocated (**Table 2**). No technique has yet been shown to stabilize or reverse the flow of blood.

Table 2
Management options in twin–twin transfusion syndrome presenting <25 weeks

| Conservative observation: >90% mortality |
| maternal morbidity |

| Interventional management |
| Therapeutic termination |
| Therapeutic serial amniocentesis |
| Indomethacin alone |
| Indomethacin with serial amniocentesis |
| Selective feticide |
| Laser ablation of placental vascular anastomoses |
| Phlebotomy/transfusion |

Therapeutic amniocentesis

Therapeutic amniocentesis is the only treatment that should be offered to a woman who presents after 25 weeks in the absence of hydrops. First, the evaluation has risks and the fetuses are already potentially viable. Second, the likelihood of chronic twin–twin transfusion syndrome presenting after 25 weeks is low. Third, there is no treatment that is both safe and effective at this time. Though there have been no randomized trials testing serial therapeutic amnioscenteses for either the prolongation of pregnancies complicated by acute hydramnios or the stabilization of a shunt in pregnancies complicated by chronic twin–twin transfusion syndrome, and all prior reports, by their selection criteria, included pregnancies with a heterogeneous set of problems, a few conclusions can be drawn.

First, the major complications of severe hydramnios of any cause are preterm labor and/or premature rupture of membranes leading to delivery. Therapeutic amniocentesis appears to prolong pregnancy compared with historical controls. For this reason alone, therapeutic amniocentesis is of value.

Second, amniocentesis has been associated with the reappearance of fluid in the sac of the stuck twin. From the standpoint of minimizing the risk of postural deformation and pulmonary hypoplasia in a pregnancy prior to 25 weeks gestation, this is beneficial. It has been suggested that the reappearance of fluid means that the amniocentesis, perhaps by decreasing hydrostatic pressure on the placenta altered the size of the shunt. In chronic twin–twin transfusion syndrome, this assumption is probably incorrect for several reasons. First, though most patients with a stuck twin have an elevated amniotic fluid pressure, a significant percentage do not. Second, hydramnios in a singleton gestation is rarely associated with growth deficiency in the absence of a chromosome abnormality or congenital infection. Third, there was no evidence in the patients with chronic twin–twin transfusion syndrome diagnosed using invasive techniques that the shunt either stabilized or reversed despite multiple therapeutic amniocenteses. And fourth, induction of massive hydramnios in the gravid ewe has no detectable effect on either placental function or fetal blood gases.[138] Frequently, when fluid reappears in the sac of the growth deficient twin, its bladder remains small or undetectable. This suggests a fluid source other than urination. Rather than altering the shunt, it may be that the dividing membrane, while pressed against the uterine wall was inadvertently punctured and fluid from the other sac leaked in. A patient treated at the University of Iowa Fetal Diagnosis and Treatment Unit illustrates this point well. She presented at 23 weeks gestation with a fundal height of 40 cm, a history of rapid uterine growth, and a stuck twin. Sonographic examination revealed discordant fetal size, like sex and presumed monochorionic placentation. However, both twins had similar and normal hematocrits. Daily therapeutic amniocenteses were required to keep the fundal height at a reasonable level. The large twin became hydropic 5 days after admission. A repeat cordocentesis of the large twin revealed that the hematocrit was unchanged and the umbilical venous pressure (UVP) normal. The normal UVP eliminated a cardiac explanation for the hydrops. However, the fetal liver enzymes were massively elevated. The following morning after another therapeutic amniocentesis, fluid was noted around the small twin. The amount gradually increased over the next 10 days. Though the small twin's stomach became visible, its bladder was not seen. After birth, the neonate remained oliguric for days. Subsequently, copious B-19 parvovirus viral particles were identified in the fetal blood by electron microscopy.

Pregnancy termination

While it might seem radical to offer a termination, it should be viewed in the reality that interventional management is invasive, frequently unsuccessful and even with intervention the prognosis may be no better than in many fetal diseases for which termination is readily considered. Notwithstanding this, termination is always likely to be less acceptable when the fetuses are not anomalous.

Indomethacin

Clague et al. retrospectively reviewed 20 cases to determine the impact of intervention with indomethacin and amniocentesis on the 'stuck twin' syndrome.[139] They concluded that indomethacin alone prolonged the pregnancy and reduced perinatal mortality for the larger but not the smaller twin. Combing indomethaacin with amniocentesis may further prolong pregnancy and improve the outcome for both twins. Clearly, there is little information available on the effect of indomethacin on the renal function of the smaller twin.

Partial exchange transfusion

The UVP is elevated when A-V valve regurgitation is present; hydrops usually develops shortly thereafter. In the recipient, hydrops means heart failure from hyperviscosity. Decreasing viscosity by reducing the hematocrit with a partial exchange transfusion effectively reduces preload and the UVP declines.

Though there have been several attempts to phlebotomize the recipient or transfuse the donor in an attempt to salvage both previable fetuses, none have been successful. The magnitude of the shunt in pregnancies presenting prior to 25 weeks appears to be huge, with the hematocrits returning to their pretreatment differences within 24–72 h.

Laser ablation

DeLia et al. reported the presumed successful treatment of twin–twin transfusion syndrome using in utero laser ablation of fetal vessels seen to traverse the dividing membrane.[140] If further research supports the initial results, laser ablation will be a fine solution to the problem. There is, however, reason for caution at this stage. First, in none of the pregnancies treated was chronic twin–twin transfusion syndrome objectively documented prior to the intervention. At delivery, sometimes shortly after the procedure, the smaller twin was often polycythemic rather than normal or anemic. Second, the patient may be required to undergo both general anesthesia and laparotomy. Third, the placenta must be posterior. Each of these limit the number of potential candidates. Fourth, it may well be that the hemodynamically significant shunts exist within the substance of the placenta, hidden from the laser.

Selective feticide

The spontaneous death of one twin has historically been associated with either the loss of the other soon thereafter, or resolution of the hydramnios.[141,142] This observation led some to conclude that a controlled death of one fetus might allow the survival of the other. But how to produce death without endangering the other twin? No noxious substance which could endanger the co-twin may be injected while there is still cardiac activity. Wittman reported the selective killing of a twin at 25 weeks in a pregnancy complicated by presumed chronic twin–twin transfusion syndrome.[143] Death of the presumed donor was brought about by the creation of a fetal pericardial effusion. The donor twin was selected because it had not grown in many weeks. The pregnancy continued until 37 weeks when labor was induced.

Clearly, causing the death of one previable fetus in hopes of preserving the other is a less than desirable approach. Yet, it remains an option for chronic twin–twin transfusion syndrome presenting prior to 25 weeks.

The donor twin is selected for two reasons. First, it is easily accessible. And second, the donor by definition supplies the net high pressure portion of the shunt. Death of the recipient might create a parasitic twin. Ventricular action can reliably be stopped for 20–30 seconds by injecting sterile water or lactated Ringer's solution into the right fetal ventricle. During asystole, 1 ml of KCl is injected into the ventricle to prevent repolarization. After death of one twin, hydramnios stabilizes. However, if there are A:V anastomoses in the opposite direction, shunt reversal with exsanguination of the recipient into the now dead donor may occur.

Other

Two other 'therapeutic' procedures for the treatment of chronic twin–twin transfusion syndrome have been reported. In one report, maternally administered digoxin reversed hydrops.[144] However, the diagnosis of chronic twin–twin transfusion syndrome was not confirmed and the presentation was atypical. Further, there are several reasons why such therapy could not be effective which have previously been addressed.[145] The second option is the surgical removal of one twin.[146] This approach seems rather extreme compared with selective feticide.

TWIN REVERSED ARTERIAL PERFUSION SEQUENCE

Twin reversed arterial perfusion (TRAP sequence, acardiac monster or chorioangiopagus parasiticus) occurs in one in 35 000 births.[147] These are usually monochorionic and often monoamnionic gestations, although it has been reported in a set of dizygotic twins with a fused placenta. The TRAP sequence is thought to result from direct artery-to-artery anastomoses early in the first trimester which allows competition between the two circulations. When the arterial pressure in one twin exceeds that of the other, blood flow is reversed in the 'perfused' twin. A spectrum of gross reduction anomalies is found and is thought to result from perfusion of deoxygenated blood from the donor or pump twin (**Figure 12**). Blood gas analysis has shown severe hypoxemia in acardiac fetuses.[148]

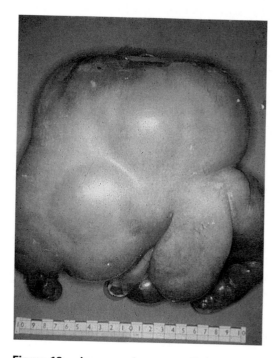

Figure 12. An amorphous acardiac monster.

Risks

The absence of an identifiable heart and multiple reduction anomalies in one twin is diagnostic. However, there may be difficulty distinguishing a fetal heart from large, pulsating mediastinal vessels.[149] The sonographic diagnosis has been made as early as 10 weeks.[150] Though the anatomy of the 'pump' twin is usually normal, it is at risk because of the extra cardiac work-load. Hydramnios is common; high cardiac output in the pump twin also increases the risk of decompensation during labor if not before then. In one series of five pump twins who died and had autopsies all had cardiomegaly, hepatomegaly, ascites and growth failure.[151] They had no evidence of malformations or embolic phenomenon. The mortality is obviously 100% for the acardiac twin and approximately 50% in the 'pump' twin. Death usually results from heart failure and extreme prematurity. Long-term developmental data were available in only one of the live born twins and were normal.[151]

Management Options

Close surveillance of the pump twin is indicated. Control of amniotic fluid volume may usefully prolong the pregnancy. This can be accomplished with either serial amniocentesis or pharmacologically with indomethacin.[152] Midtrimester hysterotomy with removal of the acardiac twin has been reported resulting in the delivery of a healthy infant at 37 weeks.[153] This strikes the authors as being fairly radical. Another approach would be the insertion of a helical metal coil in the umbilical artery of the acardiac twin to induce thrombosis or ligation of the cord using spontaneous techniques.[154]

The mode and timing of delivery depends on evidence of compromise in the pump twin. Consideration must also be given to the size of the parasitic acardiac twin which may grow to several times the size of its co-twin and obstruct labour.[155]

SINGLE FETAL DEATH IN TWINS

The incidence of single fetal death in a multiple pregnancy appears to be in the order of 2–6%.[108,156–158]

Maternal risks

There is the risk of maternal disseminated intravascular coagulation, but in practice its occurrence with one dead and one live intrauterine twin is very rare.[159] It has been reversed by the administration of heparin at a dose of 5000–12 000 U s.c. twice daily.[160] The incidence of pre-eclampsia may also be increased. However in cases where pre-eclampsia has predated the fetal death, an improvement in maternal condition has sometimes been observed.[161]

Psychological trauma may be considerable and will be enhanced by concerns about the health of the surviving fetus.

Fetal Risks

Early single fetal demise

The death of one twin in the first half of pregnancy is relatively common, but until recent years went largely undetected since the placenta of the survivor appears as a normal singleton placenta. With the advent of routine ultrasound, it is now a relatively common diagnosis. In the first trimester, it may only be evident as a cyst on the fetal surface of the surviving placenta, while in the early second trimester fetal skeletal remnants or papyraceus are evident within the placenta. It has been reported that this early reduction in fetal number has little effect on the surviving fetus who has a good prognosis,[162] however a recent report of 47 such cases found that 38% of the remaining fetuses died in utero, usually within 2 weeks of the demise of the first twin.[163]

It is currently unknown whether there is an excess of early twinning failures in infants with neurological pathology, yet this issue is of great importance if selective termination is offered as a therapeutic solution for multiple gestation where one twin is affected by a genetic disorder.

Late single fetal demise

Certainly the death of one twin after the first 20 weeks carries an increased risk for the surviving twin and this risk is much greater with monozygous twinning.

Management Options

Prenatal

Women who have lost a twin require extensive time for counseling and support with close surveillance for the remainder of the pregnancy. The risk of coagulopathy is low (see above), however, it is reasonable to check the maternal platelet count and fibrinogen concentration on a regular basis to exclude this diagnosis.

Three major factors which influence the management from the fetal viewpoint are:

- gestational age at death

- cause of death

- chorionicity of the twins

With dichorionic fetuses, provided the cause of death is intrinsic to that fetus (for example congenital anomaly), complications are rare for the surviving twin. In this circumstance the pregnancy should be allowed to continue to maturity with surveillance of the mother for evidence of coagulopathy. More often the cause of death is not known and close surveillance of the well-being of the remaining fetus is necessary, particularly in the immediate future, lest the insult which was lethal to one twin was sublethal to the other but may continue to present a risk. If the gestational age is 37 weeks or more, then the documented increased risk to the survivor justifies immediate delivery. If the gestational age is between 34 and 37 weeks then there is a case for assessment of lung maturity – and delivery if there is evidence of maturity. If the gestational age is 34 weeks or less and tests of fetal well-being are satisfactory, then a period of close surveillance while awaiting further maturity would seem most appropriate since there is no evidence that delivery improves the outcome even for monochorionic twin gestations. The prognosis for the surviving, monozygous twin appears poor. In one published review, of 53 reported infants, 15 (28%) died and only 11 (29%) of the survivors were known to be developmentally normal.[164]

The problems described in a monozygous co-twin following single fetal death include microcephaly, hydrocephaly, porencephaly, cerebral atrophy, cerebral palsy, limb reduction, intestinal atresia, renal necrosis, and pulmonary, hepatic and splenic infarction.[164] The high frequency of neurological damage in the surviving twin has been attributed to degenerated products from the blood of the dead co-twin entering the circulation of the survivor. However, there is no evidence for the existence of these products. Although the spectrum of pathology is consistent with single or repeated vascular events, the precise mechanism is unknown. It is equally possible that vascular shunting from the survivor to the dying fetus associated with falling blood pressure of the dying twin may induce acute hypovolemia and hypoxic ischemic damage. This leaves the therapeutic dilemma that the damage may already have occurred when a dead co-twin is diagnosed, and prompt delivery may only serve to add prematurity to the survivors problems. The evidence of vascular damage to the brain and other organs may take several days or weeks to evolve following the causative insult. Equally the possibility exists that prompt delivery following the diagnosis may protect the surviving co-twin from continuing vascular injury. In surviving co-twins who subsequently died in the neonatal period, Szymonowicz et al. describe evidence of an ongoing process with multiple infarcts ranging in age from a few days to 8 weeks.[164] However, evidence from the literature does not conclusively support one or other method of management. In practice therefore, if pulmonary maturity can be anticipated or demonstrated, or there is evidence of acute compromise in the survivor then prompt delivery can be advocated. If delivery is likely to result in

pathology from immaturity and the survivor appears well, then awaiting maturity with close surveillance is appropriate. Currently used methods of fetal assessment such as the non-stress test, Doppler studies and the biophysical profile will give no indication of brain damage unless there is brain stem involvement. Antenatal diagnosis of intracranial hemorrhage, or encephaloclastic lesions may be detected by high resolution ultrasound, but are only prognostic and cannot be reversed. If several weeks have elapsed with no apparent ill-effect on the survivor (for example where death was diagnosed at 22 or 24 weeks) then continuing conservative management to 37 weeks seems appropriate.

Postnatal

Because of the high incidence of morbidity, when a surviving monozygous twin is delivered the infant should be monitored for seizures and other neurological dysfunction. It may be helpful to look for evidence of cerebral, renal or hepatic infarcts with ultrasound, as a guide to prognosis and follow-up. Following delivery, consideration and support must be given to the mother and her family. They need to grieve for their perinatal loss.

CONGENITAL ANOMALY IN ONE TWIN

Risks

Technical difficulties and the risks attached to invasive procedures may be increased and the possibility that one twin will be sampled twice exists. Though a fetal loss rate of 8.1% prior to 28 weeks and 6.1% prior to 20 weeks has been reported after genetic amniocentesis in viable twin pregnancies,[165] it seems excessive.

Management Options

When ultrasound or genetic studies reveal that the twins are discordant for major disease, the parents are faced with a serious dilemma. Their choices are: continuation of the pregnancy on behalf of the normal twin, termination of pregnancy in spite of the normal twin, or consideration of selective feticide in the hope of allowing continuation only of the normal twin.

Health and survival of the normal twin, except in a few instances, will best be served by the first option. Acceptance of this option will obviously depend on the severity of disease and life expectance/quality in the co-twin.

PATHOLOGIES SPECIFIC TO TWINNING
Summary of Management Options (See also Chapter 10)

MONOAMNIOTIC TWINS

Prenatal

- Surveillance of fetal health until term (see Chapters 39 and 43)

- Delivery at term or sooner if evidence of fetal compromise (with maternal steroid administration)

Labor/delivery

- Vaginal delivery is not contraindicated provided continuous fetal heart rate monitoring of both twins and facilities for immediate cesarean section

TWIN–TWIN TRANSFUSION SYNDROME

Prenatal

See **Table 1**

TWIN REVERSED ARTERIAL PERFUSION SEQUENCE

Prenatal

- Control hydramnios with serial amniocenteses

- Fetal surveillance of 'pump' twin (see Chapters 39 and 43) intervention prematurely if compromise

- Role of umbilical occlusion not yet established

Labor/delivery

- Mode of delivery depends on factors such as presentation and fetal health

SINGLE FETAL DEATH

Prenatal

- Counseling and support for mother and family

- Screening for maternal coagulopathy

- Fetal surveillance in surviving twin (see Chapters 39 and 43) though this may not accurately predict neurodevelopmental prognosis

- Role of high resolution ultrasound of fetal brain is uncertain

Labor/delivery

- Timing is controversial but most would delay until 37 weeks if fetal surveillance is normal

Postnatal

- Counseling and support for mother and family

- Paediatric assessment and follow-up and appropriate management depending on problems

CONGENITAL ANOMALY IN ONE TWIN

Prenatal

- Options
  - continuation of pregnancy (? commonest chosen option)
  - termination of pregnancy
  - selective termination (see Chapter 57)

The option to terminate the pregnancy again involves consideration of severity of disease and parental desire for birth of the normal twin.

Selective termination is undoubtedly the most difficult and potentially dangerous option[166] and the issues relating to this option are discussed in Chapter 57.

REFERENCES

1 Barson AJ (1978) Congenital neoplasia: The society's experience. *Archives of Diseases in Childhood* **53**:436.

2 Fraumeni JR, Miller RW (1969) Cancer deaths in the newborn. *American Journal of Diseases of Children* **117**:186.

3 Riboni G, DeSimoni M, Leopardi O, Molla R (1985) Ultrasound appearance of a glioblastoma in a 33 week fetus *in utero. Journal of Clinical Ultrasound* **13**:345.

4 Van Vliet MAT, Bravenboer B, Kock MCLV, Teepen JLJM (1983) Congenital meningeal sarcoma: A case report. *Journal of Perinatal Medicine* **11**:249.

5 Christensen RA, Pinckney LE, Higgins S, Miller KE (1987) Sonographic diagnosis of lipoma of the corpus callosum. *Journal of Ultrasound in Medicine* **6**:449–450.

6 Wienk MAThP, van Geijn HP, Copray FJA, Brons JTJ (1990) Prenatal diagnosis of fetal tumors by ultrasonography. *Obstetrical Gynecological Survey* **45**:639–653.

7 Snijder JR, Lustig Gillman I, Milio L *et al.* (1986) Antenatal ultrasound diagnosis of an intracranial neoplasm (craniopharyngioma). *Journal Clinical Ultrasound* **14**:304–306.

8 Hoff NR, MacKary LM (1980) Prenatal ultrasound diagnosis of intracranial teratoma. *Journal of Clinical Ultrasound* **8**:247–248.

9 Crade M (1982) Ultrasound demonstration *in utero* of intracranial teratoma. *Journal of the American Medical Association* **247**:1173.

10 Lipman SP, Pretorious DH, Rumack CM, Manco-Johnson ML (1985) Fetal intracranial teratoma: Ultrasound diagnosis of three cases and a review of the literature. *Radiology* **157**:491–494.

11 Chervenak FA, Isaacson G, Touloukian R, Tortora M, Berkowitz RL, Hobbins JC (1985) Diagnosis and management of fetal teratomas. *Obstetrics and Gynecology* **66**:666–671.

12 Sherer DM, Abramowicz JS, Eggers PC, Metlay LA, Sinkin RA, Woods JR (1993) Prenatal ultrasonographic diagnosis of intracranial teratoma and massive craniomegaly with associated high-output cardiac failure. *American Journal of Obstetrics and Gynecology* **168**:97–99.

13 Whittle JR, Simpson DA (1981) Surgical treatment of neonatal intracranial teratomas. *Surgery and Neurology* **15**:268–272.

14 Ventureyra ECG, Herder S (1983) Neonatal intracranial teratomas. *Journal of Neurology and Surgery* **59**:879–883.

15 Anderson RL, Simpson GF, Sherman S, Dedo HH, Golbus MS (1984) Fetal pharyngeal teratoma – another cause of elevated amniotic fluid alpha-fetoprotein. *American Journal of Obstetrics and Gynecology* **150**:432–433.

16 Chervenak FA, Tortora M, Moya FR *et al.* (1984) Antenatal sonographic diagnosis of epignathus. *Journal of Ultrasound in Medicine* **3**:235.

17 Kang KW, Hissong SL, Langer A (1978) Prenatal ultrasonic diagnosis of epignathus. *Journal of Clinical Ultrasound* **6**:330.

18 Nicolaides KH, Azar G, Byrne D *et al.* (1992) Fetal nuchal translucency: ultrasound screening for chromosomal defects in first trimester of pregnancy. *British Medical Journal* **304**:867–869.

19 Johnson MP, Johnson A, Holzgreve W *et al.* (1993) First-trimester simple hygroma: Cause and outcome. *American Journal of Obstetrics and Gynecology* **168**:156–161.

20 Van der Putte SCJ (1977) Lymphatic malformation in human fetuses. *Virchows Archives A* **376**:233–246.

21 Rosenfeld CR, Coln CD, Duenholter JH (1979) Fetal cervical teratoma as a cause of polyhydramnios. *Pediatrics* **64**:176–179.

22 Baumann FR, Nerlich A (1993) Metastasizing cervical teratoma of the fetus. *Pediatric Pathology* **13**:21–27.

23 Dolkart LA, Reimers FT, Helmuth WV, Porte MA, Eisinger G (1992) Antenatal diagnosis of pulmonary sequestration: A review. *Obstetrics and Gynecology* **47**:515–520.

24 Weiner C, Varner M, Pringle K *et al.* (1986) Antenatal diagnosis and palliative treatment of nonimmune hydrops fetalis secondary to pulmonary extralobar sequestration. *Obstetrics and Gynecology* **68**:275–280.

25 Meizner I, Carmi R, Mares AJ, Katz M (1990) Spontaneous resolution of isolated fetal ascites associated with extralobar lung sequestration. *Journal of Clinical Ultrasound* **18**:57–60.

26 Saltzman DN, Adzick NS, Benacerraf BR (1988) Fetal cystic adenomatoid malformation of the lung: apparent improvement *in utero. Obstetrics and Gynecology* **71**:1000–2.

27 Kuller JA, Laifer SA, Tagge EP, Nakayama DK, Hill LM (1922) Diminution in size of a fetal intrathorciac mass: caution against aggressive *in utero* management. *American Journal of Perinatology* **9**:223–224.

28 Kuller JA, Yankowitz J, Goldberg JD *et al.* (1992) Outcome of antenatally diagnosed cystic adenomatoid malformations. *American Journal of Obstetrics and Gynecology* **167**:1038.

29 Adzick NS, Harrison MR, Glick PL (1985) Fetal cystic adenomatoid malformation: prenatal diagnosis and natural history. *Journal of Pediatric Surgery* **20**:483–488.

30 Nugent CE, Hayashi RH, Rubin J (1989) Prenatal treatment of type I congenital cystic adenomatoid malformation by intrauterine fetal thoracentesis. *Journal of Clinical Ultrasound* **17**:675–677.

31 Clark SL, Vitale DJ, Minton SD, Stoddard RA, Sabey PL (1987) Successful fetal therapy for cystic adenomatoid malformation associated with second-trimester hydrops. *American Journal of Obstetrics and Gynecology* **157**:294–295.

32 Nicolaides KH, Blott M, Greenough A (1987) Chronic drainage of fetal pulmonary cyst. *Lancet* **1**:618.

33 Vidaillet HJ Jr (1988) Cardiac tumors associated with hereditary syndromes. *American Journal of Cardiology* **61**:1355.

34 Fenoglio JJ, McAllister HA, Ferrans VJ (1976) Cardiac rhabdomyoma: A clinicopathologic and electron microscopic study. *American Journal of Cardiology* **38**:241–250.

35 Groves AM, Fagg NL, Cook AC, Allen LD (1992) Cardiac tumors in intrauterine life. *Archives of Diseases in Childhood* **67**:1189–1192.

36 DeVore GR, Hakim S, Kleinman CS, Hobbins JC (1982) The *in utero* diagnosis of an interventricular septal cardiac rhabdomyoma by means of real-time directed M-mode echocardiography. *American Journal of Obstetrics and Gynecology* **143**:967–968.

37 Gava G, Buoso G, Beltrame GL, Memo L, Visentin S, Cavarzerani A (1990) Cardiac rhabdomyoma as a marker for the prenatal detection of tuberous sclerosis. *British Journal of Obstetrics and Gynaecology* **97**:1154–1157.

38 Farooki ZQ, Ross RD, Paridon SE, Humes R, Karpawich PP, Pinsky WW (1989) Spontaneous regression of cardiac rhabdomyomas. *American Journal of Cardiology* **64** (Abstracts):416.

39 Smythe JF, Dyck JD, Smallhorn JF, Freedom RM (1990) Natural history of cardiac rhabdomyoma in infancy and childhood. *American Journal of Cardiology* **66**:1247–1249.

40 Smith HC, Watson GH, Patel RG, Super M (1989) Cardiac rhabdomyomata in tuberous sclerosis: their course and diagnostic value. *Archives of Diseases in Childhood* **64**:196–200.

41 Parmley LF, Salley RK, Williams JP, Head GB (1988) The clinical spectrum of cardiac fibroma with diagnostic and surgical considerations. Non-invasive imaging enhances management. *Annals of Thoracic Surgery* **45**:455–465.

42 Davidson PM, Waters KD, Brown TCK, Auldist AW (1988) Liver tumors in children. *Pediatric Surgery International* **3**:377–381.

43 Fourcar E, Williamson RA, Yiu-Chiu V, Varner MW, Kay BR (1983) Mesenchymal hamartoma of the liver identified by fetal sonography. *American Journal of Radiology* **140**:970–972.

44 Robinson RA, Nelson L (1986) Hepatic teratoma in an anencephalic fetus. *Archives of Pathology and Laboratory Medicine* **110**:655–657.

45 Janetchek G, Weitzel D, Stein W *et al* (1984) Prenatal diagnosis of neuroblastoma by sonography. *Urology* **24**:397.

46 Fowlie F, Giacomantonio M, McKenzie E *et al* (1986) Antenatal sonographic diagnosis of adrenal neuroblastoma. *Journal of the Canadian Association of Radiologists* **37**:50.

47 Grosfeld JL (1990) Neuroblastoma: a 1990 overview. *Pediatric Surgery* **6**:9–13.

48 Apuzzio JJ, Unwin W, Adhate A, Nicols R (1986) Prenatal diagnosis of fetal renal mesoblastic nephroma. *American Journal of Obstetrics and Gynecology* **154**:636–637.

49 Giulian B (1984) Prenatal ultrasonographic diagnosis of fetal renal tumors. *Radiology* **152**:69–70.

50 Hartman DS, Lesar MSL, Madewell JE (1981) Mesoblastic nephroma: radiologic-pathologic correlation of 20 cases. *American Journal of Radiology* **136**:96–100.

51 Kirkinen P, Jouppila P (1985) Perinatal aspects of pregnancy complicated by fetal ovarian cyst. *Journal of Perinatal Medicine* **13**:245.

52 Sakala EP, Leon ZA, Rouse GA (1991) Management of antenatally diagnosed fetal ovarian cysts. *Obstetrics and Gynecology Survey* **46**:407–414.

53 Birch JM, Marsden HB, Swindell R (1982) Pre-natal factors in the origin of germ cell tumors of childhood. *Carcinogenesis* **3**:75–80.

54 Nakayama DK, Killian A, Hill LM, Miller JP, Hannakan C, Lloyd DA, Rowe MI (1991) The newborn with hydrops and sacrococcygeal teratoma. *Journal of Pediatric Surgery* **26**:1435–1438.

55 Engelskirden R, Holschneider AM, Rhein R, Hecker WCh, Hopner F (1987) Sacrococcygeal teratomas in children. An analysis of long-term results in 87 children. *Zeitschift Fur Kinderchirurgie* **42**:358–361.

56 Shanbhogue LRK, Bianchi A, Doig CM, Gough DCS (1990) Management of benign sacrococcygeal teratoma: reducing mortality and morbidity. *Pediatric Surgery International* **5**:41–44.

57 Lahdenne P, Wikstrom S, Heikinheimo M, Simes MA (1992) Late urological sequelae after surgery for congenital sacrococcygeal teratoma. *Pediatric Surgery* **7**:195–198.

58 Billmire DF, Grosfield JL (1986) Teratomas in childhood: analysis of 142 cases. *Journal of Pediatric Surgery* **21**:548–551.

59 Arienzo R, Ricco CS, Romeo F (1987) A very rare malformation: The cutaneous widespread vascular hamartomatosis. *American Journal of Obstetrics and Gynecology* **157**:1162–1163.

60 Resta RG, Luthy DA, Mahony BS (1988) Umbilical cord hemangioma associated with extremely high alpha-fetoprotein levels. *Obstetrics and Gynecology* **72**:488–490.

61 Seifer DB, Ferguson JE, Behrens CM, Zemel S, Stevenson DK, Ross JC (1985) Nonimmune hydrops fetalis in association with hemangioma of the umbilical cord. *Obstetrics and Gynecology* **66**:283–286.

62 Dombrowski MP, Budev H, Wolfe HM, Sokol RJ, Perrin E (1987) Fetal hemorrhage from umbilical cord hemangioma. *Obstetrics and Gynecology* **70**:439–442.

63 Fox H (1966) Haemangiomata of the placenta. *Journal of Clinical Pathology* **19**:133–137.

64 Shanklin DR, Scott JS (1975) Massive subchorial thrombohaematoma (Brues' mole). *British Journal of Obstetrics and Gynaecology* **82**:476–487.

65 Holland E (1949) A case of transplacental metastasis of malignant melanoma from mother to fetus. *Journal of Obstetrics and Gynaecology of the British Empire* **56**:529.

66 Smythe AR, Underwood PB, Kreutner A (1976) Metastatic placental tumors. Report of three cases. *American Journal of Obstetrics and Gynecology* **125**:1146–1151.

67 Campbell WA, Storlazzi E, Vintzileos AM, Wu A, Schneiderman H, Nochimson DJ (1987) Fetal malignant

melanoma: ultrasound presentation and review of the literature. *Obstetrics and Gynecology* **70**:434–439.

68 Burrow GN (1988) Thyroid diseases. In: Burrow GN, Ferris TF (eds) *Medical Complications During Pregnancy* 3rd edn. Philadelphia: W.B. Saunders, pp. 224–253.

69 Evans TC, Kretzschmar RM, Hodges RE *et al.* (1967) Radioiodine uptake studies of the human fetal thyroid. *Journal of Nuclear Medicine* **8**:157.

70 Sugrue D, Drury MI (1980) Hyperthyroidism complicating pregnancy: Results of treatment by antithyroid drugs in 77 pregnancies. *British Journal of Obstetrics and Gynaecology* **87**:970–975.

71 Stice RC, Grant CS, Gharib H, Heerden JA (1984) The management of Graves disease during pregnancy. *Surgery Obstetrics and Gynecology* **158**:157–160.

72 Mitsuda N, Tamaki H, Amino N, Hosono T, Miyai K, Tanizawa O (1992) Risk factors for developmental disorders in infants born to women with Graves disease. *Obstetrics and Gynecology* **80**:359–364.

73 Hollingsworth DR (1983) Graves disease. *Clinical Obstetrics and Gynecology* **26**:615–634.

74 Wenstrom KD, Weiner CP, Williamson RA, Grant SS (1990) Prenatal diagnosis of fetal hyperthyroidism using funipuncture. *Obstetrics and Gynecology* **76**:513–517.

75 Daneman D, Howard NJ (1980) Neonatal thyrotoxicosis: Intellectual impairment and craniosynostosis in later years. *Journal of Pediatrics* **97**:257–259.

76 Page DV, Brady K, Mitchell J, Pehrson J, Wade G (1988) The pathology of intrauterine thyrotoxicosis: Two case reports. *Obstetrics and Gynecology* **72**:479–481.

77 Hollingsworth DR, Mabry CC (1976) Congenital Graves' disease: four familial cases with long-term follow-up and perspective. *American Journal of Diseases of Childhood* **130**:148–155.

78 Pekonen F, Teramo K, Makinen T, Ikonen E, Osterlund K, Lamberg BA (1984) Prenatal diagnosis and treatment of fetal thyrotoxicosis. *American Journal of Obstetrics and Gynecology* **150**:893–894.

79 Davis LE, Lucas MJ, Hankins GDV, Roark ML, Cunningham FG (1989) Thyrotoxicosis complicating pregnancy. *American Journal of Obstetrics and Gynecology* **160**:63–70.

80 Burrow GN (1985) The management of thyrotoxicosis in pregnancy. *New England Journal of Medicine* **31**:562–565.

81 Tamaki H, Amino N, Aozasa M (1988) Universal predictive criteria for neonatal overt thyrotoxicosis requiring treatment. *American Journal of Perinatology* **5**:152–158.

82 Tamaki H, Amino N, Takeoka K *et al.* (1989) Prediction of later development of thyrotoxicosis or central hypothyroidism from the cord serum thyroid-stimulating hormone level in neonates born to mothers with Graves disease. *Journal of Pediatrics* **115**:318–321.

83 Marchant B, Brownlie BEW, Hart DM, Horton PW, Alexander WD (1977) The placental transfer of propylthiouracil, methimazole and carbimazole. *Journal of Clinical Endocrinology and Metabolism* **45**:1187–1193.

84 Cheron RG, Kaplan MM, Larsen PR, Selenkow HA, Crigler JF Jr (1981) Neonatal thyroid function after propylthiouracil therapy for maternal Graves disease. *New England Journal of Medicine* **304**:525–528.

85 Davidson KM, Richards DS, Schatz DA, Fisher D (1991) Successful *in utero* treatment of fetal goitre and hypothyroidism. *New England Journal of Medicine* **324**:543–546.

86 Bromley B, Frigoletto FD, Cramer D, Osathanondh R, Benacerraf BR (1992) The fetal thyroid: normal and abnormal sonographic measurements. *Journal of Ultrasound in Medicine* **11**:25–28.

87 Hollingsworth DR, Alexander NM (1983) Amniotic fluid concentrations of iodothyronines and thyrotropin do not reliably predict fetal thyroid status in pregnancies complicated by maternal thyroid disorders or anencephaly. *Journal of Clinical Endocrinology and Metabolism* **57**:349–355.

88 Sack J, Fisher DA, Hobel CJ, Lam R (1975) Thyroxine in human amniotic fluid. *Journal of Pediatrics* **87**:364–368.

89 Kourides IA, Berkowitz RL, Pang S, Van Natta FC, Barone CM, Ginsberg-Fellner F (1984) Antepartum diagnosis of Goitrous hypothyroidism by fetal ultrasonography and amniotic fluid thyrotropin concentration. *Journal of Clinical Endocrinology and Metabolism* **59**:1016–1018.

90 Thorpe-Beeston JG, Nicolaides KH, Felton CV, Butler J, McGregor AM (1991) Maturation of the secretion of thyroid hormone and thyroid stimulating hormone in the fetus. *New England Journal of Medicine* **324**:532–536.

91 Low LCK, Lang J, Alexander WD (1979) Excretion of carbimazole and propylthiouracil in breast milk. *Lancet* **i**:1011.

92 Cooper DS, Bode HH, Nath B, Saxe V, Maloof F, Ridgeway EC (1984) Methimazole pharmacology in man: studies using a newly developed radioimmunoassay for methimazole. *Journal of Clinical Endocrinology and Metabolism* **58**:473–479.

93 Roti E, Gnudi A, Braverman LE (1983) The placental transport, synthesis and metabolism of hormones and drugs that affect thyroid function. *Endocrine Review* **4**:131–149.

94 Vulsma T, Gons MH, de Vijlder JJM (1989) Maternal–fetal transfer of thyroxine in congenital hypothyroidism due to total organification defect or thyroid agenesis. *New England Journal of Medicine* **321**:13–16.

95 Perelman AH, Johnson RL, Clemons RD, Finberg HJ, Clewell WH, Trujillo L (1990) Intrauterine diagnosis and treatment of fetal goitrous hypothyroidism. *Journal of Clinical Endocrinology and Metabolism* **71**:618–621.

96 Weiner S, Scharf JI, Bolognese RJ, Librizzi RJ (1980) *Journal of Reproductive Medicine* **24**:39–42.

97 Frasier SD, Thorneycroft IH, Weiss BA, Horton R (1975) Elevated amniotic fluid concentration of 17-hydroxyprogesterone in congenital adrenal hyperplasia. *Journal of Pediatrics* **86**:310–312.

98 Speiser PW, Laforgia N, Kato K (1990) First trimester prenatal treatment and molecular genetic diagnosis of congenital adrenal hyperplasia (21-hydroxylase deficiency). *Journal of Endocrinology and Metabolism* **70**:838–848.

99 Karaviti LP, Mercado AB, Mercado MB *et al.* (1992) Prenatal diagnosis/treatment in families at risk for infants with steroid 21-hydroxylase deficiency (congenital adrenal hyperplasia). *Journal of Steroid Biochemistry and Molecular Biology* **41**:445–451.

100 Pang S, Clark AT, Freeman LC *et al.* (1992) Maternal side effects of prenatal dexamethasone therapy for fetal congenital adrenal hyperplasia. *Journal of Clinical Endocrinology and Metabolism* **75**:249–253.

101 David M, Forest MG (1984) Prenatal treatment of congenital adrenal hyperplasia resulting from 21-hydroxylase deficiency. *Journal of Pediatrics* **105**:799–803.

102 Pang S, Pollack MS, Marshall RN, Immken L (1990) Prenatal treatment of congenital adrenal hyperplasia due to 21-hydroxylase deficiency. *New England Journal of Medicine* **322**:111–115.

103 Benirschke K (1961) Accurate recording of twin placentation: A plea to the obstetrician. *Obstetrics and Gynecology* **18**:334–347.

104 James WH (1980) Sex ratio and placentation in twins. *Annals of Human Biology* **7**:273–276.

105 Derom C, Vlietinck R, Derom R, Berghe H Van Den, Thiery M (1988) Population based study of sex proportion in monoamniotic twins. *New England Journal of Medicine* **319**:119–120.

106 James WH (1991) A further note on the sex ratio of monoamniotic twins. *Annals of Human Biology* **18**:471–474.

107 Megory E, Weiner E, Shalev E, Ohel G (1991) Pseudomonoamniotic twins with cord entanglement following genetic funipuncture. *Obstetrics and Gynecology* **78**:915–917.

108 D'Alton ME, Newton ER, Cetrulo CL (1984) Intrauterine fetal demise in multiple gestation. *Acta Geniticae Medicae et Gemollogiae (Roma)* **33**:43–49.

109 Townsend RR, Simpson GF, Filly RA (1988) Membrane thickness in ultrasound prediction of chorionicity of twin gestations. *Journal of Ultrasound in Medicine* **7**:327–332.

110 McFadyen I (1992) The dangers of intraamniotic methylene blue. *British Journal of Obstetrics and Gynaecology* **99**:89–90.

111 Tabsh K (1990) Genetic amniocentesis in multiple gestation: A new technique to diagnose monoamniotic twins. *Obstetrics and Gynecology* **75**:296–298.

112 Carlan SJ, Angel JL, Sawai SK, Vaughn V (1990) Late diagnosis of non-conjoined monoamniotic twins using computed tomographic imaging. *Obstetrics and Gynecology* **76**:504–506.

113 Rodis JF, Vintzileos AM, Campbell DJ (1987) Antenatal diagnosis and management of monoamniotic twins. *American Journal of Obstetrics and Gynecology* **157**:1255–1257.

114 Tessen JA, Zlatnik FJ (1991) Monoamniotic twins: a retrospective controlled study. *Obstetrics and Gynecology* **77**:832–834.

115 Belfort MA, Moise KJ, Kirshon B, Saade G (1993) The use of color flow Doppler ultrasonography to diagnose umbilical cord entanglement in monoamniotic twin gestations. *American Journal of Obstetrics and Gynecology* **168**:601–604.

116 Annan B, Hutson RC (1990) Double survival despite cord entwinement. Case report. *British Journal of Obstetrics and Gynecology* **97**:950–951.

117 Carr SR, Aronson MP, Coustan DR (1990) Survival rates of monoamniotic twins do not decrease after 30 weeks' gestation. *American Journal of Obstetrics and Gynecology* **163**:719–722.

118 Weir PE, Ratten GJ, Beischer NA (1979) Acute polyhydramnios – a complication of monozygous twin pregnancy. *British Journal of Obstetrics and Gynaecology* **86**:849–853.

119 Elliott JP, Urig MA, Clewell WH (1991) Aggressive therapeutic amniocentesis for treatment of twin–twin transfusion syndrome. *Obstetrics and Gynecology* **77**:537–540.

120 Rausen AR, Seki M, Strauss L (1965) Twin transfusion syndrome. A review of 19 cases studied at one institution. *Journal of Pediatrics* **66**:613–628.

121 Robertson EG, Neer KJ (1983) Placental injection studies in twin gestation. *American Journal of Obstetrics and Gynecology* **147**:170–174.

122 Danskin FH, Neilson JP (1989) Twin-to-twin transfusion syndrome: what are appropriate diagnostic criteria? *American Journal of Obstetrics and Gynecology* **161**:365–369.

123 Tan KL, Tan R, Tan SH, Tan AM (1979) The twin transfusion syndrome. Clinical observations on 35 affected pairs. *Clinical Pediatrics* **18**:111–114.

124 Wenstrom KD, Tessen JA, Zlatnik FJ (1992) Frequency, distribution, and theoretic mechanisms for hematology and weight discordance in monochorionic twins. *Obstetrics and Gynecology* **80**:257–261.

125 Feingold M, Cetrulo CL, Newton ER, Weiss J, Shakr C, Shmoys S (1986) Serial amniocentesis in the treatment of twin to twin transfusion complicated with acute polyhydramnios. *Acta Geniticae Medicae et Gemollogiae (Roma)* **35**:107–113.

126 Saunders NJ, Snijders RJM, Nicolaides KH (1992) Therapeutic amniocentesis in twin–twin transfusion syndrome appearing in the second trimester of pregnancy. *American Journal of Obstetrics and Gynecology* **166**:820–824.

127 Mahoney BS, Petty CN, Nyberg DA, Luthy DA, Hickok DE, Hirsch JH (1990) The stuck twin phenomenon: Ultrasonographic findings, pregnancy outcome, and management with serial amniocenteses. *American Journal of Obstetrics and Gynecology* **163**:1513–1522.

128 Barss VA, Benacerraf BR, Frigoletto FD (1985) Ultrasonographic determination of chorion type in twin gestation. *Obstetrics and Gynecology* **66**:779–783.

129 Yamada A, Kasugai M, Ohno Y, Ishizuka T, Mizutani S, Tomoda Y (1991) Antenatal diagnosis of twin–twin transfusion syndrome by Doppler ultrasound. *Obstetrics and Gynecology* **78**:1058–1061.

130 Pretorius DH, Manchester D, Barkin S, Parker S, Nelson TR (1988) Doppler ultrasound of twin transfusion syndrome. *Journal of Ultrasound in Medicine* **7**:117–124.

131 Farmakides G, Schulman H, Saldana LR, Bracero LA, Fleischer A, Rochelson B (1985) Surveillance of twin pregnancy with umbilical arterial velocimetry. *Amer-*

ican Journal of Obstetrics and Gynecology **153**:789–792.

132 Giles WB, Trudinger BJ, Cook CM, Connelly AJ (1990) Doppler umbilical artery studies in the twin–twin transfusion syndrome. *Obstetrics and Gynecology* **76**:1097–1099.

133 Gaziano EP, Knox GE, Bendel RP, Calvin S, Brandt D (1991) Is pulsed Doppler velocimetry useful in the management of multiple-gestation pregnancies? *American Journal of Obstetrics and Gynecology* **164**:1426–1431.

134 Neilson JP, Danskin F, Hastie SJ (1989) Monozygotic twin pregnancy: diagnostic and Doppler ultrasound. *British Journal of Obstetrics and Gynaecology* **96**:1413–1418.

135 Weiner CP, Grose CF, Naides SJ (1993) Diagnosis of fetal infection in the patient with an abnormal ultrasound examination and without a positive clinical history. *American Journal of Obstetrics and Gynecology* **168**:6–11.

136 Weiner CP, Williamson RA, Wenstrom KD, Sipes SL, Grant SS, Widness JA (1991) Management of fetal hemolytic disease by cordocentesis: I. Prediction of fetal anemia. *American Journal of Obstetrics and Gynecology* **165**:546–553.

137 Weiner CP, Ludomirsky A (1992) Diagnosis and treatment of twin to twin transfusion syndrome (TTTs). *Proceedings, Society of Perinatal Obstetricians.*

138 Fisk NM, Giussani DA, Parkes MJ, Moore PJ, Hanson MA (1991) Amnioinfusion increases amniotic pressure in pregnant sheep but does not alter fetal acid-base status. *American Journal of Obstetrics and Gynecology* **165**:1459–1463.

139 Clague N, Connors G, Hopkins C, Lange I (1992) The impact of intervention with indomethacin and amniocentesis on twin–twin transfusion syndrome. *Abstract-Society of Obstetricians and Gynecologists of Canada, Vancouver,* p. 59.

140 DeLia JE, Cruickshank DP, Keye WR (1990) Fetoscopic neodymium YAG laser occlusion of placental vessels in severe twin–twin transfusion syndrome. *Obstetrics and Gynecology* **75**:1046–1053.

141 Shiroshita K, Kimura J, Kato Y, Sudo S, Tsujii H (1988) A live birth in twin transfusion syndrome complicated with intrauterine death of one fetus: a case report. *Acta Obstetrica et Gynaecologica Japonica* **40**:1559–1562.

142 Kirshon B, Moise KJ, Mari G, Rothchild S, Wasserstrum N (1990) *In utero* resolution of hydrops fetalis following the death of one twin in twin–twin transfusion. *American Journal of Perinatology* **7**:107–109.

143 Wittmann BK, Farquharson DF, Thomas WD, Baldwin VJ, Wadsworth LD (1986) The role of feticide in the management of severe twin transfusion syndrome. *American Journal of Obstetrics and Gynecology* **155**:1023–1026.

144 DeLia JE, Emergy MG, Sheafor SA, Jennison TA (1985) Twin transfusion syndrome: successful in utero treatment with digoxin. *International Journal of Gynaecology and Obstetrics* **23**:197–201.

145 Weiner CP (1990) Use of digoxin in pregnancy. *Amer-*

ican Journal of Obstetrics and Gynecology **162**:607–608.

146 Urig MA, Simpson GF, Elliott JP, Clewell WH (1988) Twin–twin transfusion syndrome: the surgical removal of one twin as a treatment option. *Fetal Diagnosis and Therapy* **3**:185–188.

147 Napolitani FD, Schreiber I (1960) The acardiac monster. *American Journal of Obstetrics and Gynecology* **80**:582–589.

148 Ko TM, Tzeng SJ, Hsieh FJ, Chu JS (1991) Acardius anceps: report of 3 cases. *Asia Oceania Journal of Obstetrics and Gynecology* **17**:49–56.

149 Fusi L, Fisk N, Talcert D, Gau G, Rodeck C. When does death occur in an acardiac twin? Ultrasound diagnostic difficulties. *Journal of Perinatal Medicine* **18**:223–227.

150 Shalev E, Zalel Y, Ben-Ami M, Weiner E (1992) First trimester ultrasonic diagnosis of twin reversed arterial perfusion sequence. *Prenatal Diagnosis* **12**:219–222.

151 Van Allen MI, Smith DW, Shepard TH (1983) Twin reversed arterial perfusion (TRAP) sequence: a study of 14 twin pregnancies with acardius. *Seminars in Perinatology* **7**:285–293.

152 Ash K, Harman CR, Gritter H (1990) TRAP sequence-successful outcome with indomethacin. *Obstetrics and Gynecology* **76**:960–962.

153 Ginsberg NA, Applebaum M, Rabin SA *et al.* (1992) Term birth after midtrimester hysterotomy and selective delivery of an acardiac twin. *American Journal of Obstetrics and Gynecology* **167**:33–37.

154 Porreco RP, Barton SM, Haverkamp AD (1991) Occlusion of the umbilical artery in acardiac, acephalic twin. *Lancet* **337**:326–327.

155 Imai A, Hirose R, Kawabata I, Tamaya T (1991) Acardiac acephalic monster extremely larger than its co-twin. A case report. *Gynecological and Obstetrical Investigations* **32**:62–64.

156 Litschgi M, Stucki D (1980) Course of twin pregnancies after fetal death *in utero*. *Z Geburtshilfe Perinatology* **184**:227.

157 Melnick M (1977) Brain damage in survivor after *in utero* death in monozygous co-twin. *Lancet* **2**:128.

158 Enbom JA (1985) Twin pregnancy with intrauterine death of one twin. *American Journal of Obstetrics and Gynecology* **152**:424–429.

159 Landy HJ, Weingold AB (1989) Review of the management of multiple gestation complicated by antepartum fetal demise. *Obstetrics and Gynecology Survey* **44**:171.

160 Romero R, Duffy TP, Berkowitz RL, Chang E, Hobbins JC (1984) Prolongation of a preterm pregnancy complicated by death of a single twin *in utero* and disseminated intravascular coagulation. *New England Journal of Medicine* **310**:772–774.

161 Fusi L, Gordon H (1990) Twin pregnancy complicated by single intrauterine death. Problems and outcome with conservative management. *British Journal of Obstetrics and Gynaecology* **97**:511–516.

162 Landy HJ, Weiner S, Corson SL, Batzer FR, Bolognese RJ (1986) The "vanishing twin": Ultrasonographic assessment of fetal disappearance in the first

trimester. *American Journal of Obstetrics and Gynecology* **155**:14–19.

163 Shackley D, Daw E (1992) Effect on the survivor of the early demise of its twin. *Journal of Obstetrics and Gynecology* **12**:373–374.

164 Szymonowicz W, Preston H, Yu VYH (1986) The surviving monozygotic twin. *Archives of Diseases of Childhood* **61**:454–458.

165 Pruggmayer M, Baumann P, Schutte H, Osmers R, Bartels I, Jovanovich V, Rauskolb R (1991) Incidence of abortion after genetic amniocentesis in twin pregnancies. *Prenatal Diagnosis* **11**:637–640.

166 Toth Z, Bolodar A, Torok O, Ccsecsei K, Papp Z (1991) Selective termination of the development of the defective fetus in discordant twin pregnancies. *Orv Hetil* **132**:2617–2621.

56

Fetal Tissue Biopsies

MARK I. EVANS, MARK PAUL JOHNSON, ERIC P. HOFFMAN, WOLFGANG HOLZGREVE

INTRODUCTION

The development of prenatal diagnostic techniques has centered in two major areas, the first of which has been visualization of fetal structure and function. These techniques have included x-ray, amniography, direct visualization by fetoscopy and ultrasound.[1] The second major approach to prenatal diagnosis has been through laboratory study of fetal tissue. The first and predominant technique has been amniocentesis (see Chapter 40). Chorionic villus sampling (CVS) and cordocentesis are two additional techniques for obtaining fetal material (see Chapters 36 and 41). The combination of cytogenetic, biochemical and, more recently, molecular analyses in conjunction with highly detailed ultrasound examination has enabled the prenatal diagnosis of multiple fetal diseases and anatomic defects.

There has been a movement over the last 5 years away from needing specific tissue material for diagnosis. However, in some cases, the availability of DNA diagnoses has increased both the possibilities for diagnosis and the need for fetal tissue-specific biopsies. The major advantage of molecular diagnosis is that it allows, in general, for the use of any fetal tissue to look at DNA structure and expected function rather than at enzymatic reactions which are tissue-limited to their actual site of action.[2]

In this chapter, we will divide the discussion of fetal tissue biopsies into the different tissues involved. The majority of data available concern fetal skin, liver and, more recently, fetal muscle biopsies.

FETAL SKIN BIOPSY

Only a few of the serious dermatologic disorders are associated with chromosomal abnormalities or enzyme defects that can be detected in amniotic fluid or chorionic villi.[3] Furthermore, in the majority of serious cutaneous abnormalities, ultrasonic visualization is useless. Actual visualization of the skin and histology are the only ways to make such diagnoses. Examples of conditions for which prenatal diagnosis requires study of the fetal skin include:

- harlequin ichythyosis

- Sjogren-Larsson syndrome

- epidermolytic hyperkeratosis

- epidermolysis bullosa dystrophica

- epidermolysis bullosa lethalis

- oculocutaneous albinism

- congenital ichthyosiform erytheraderma

- congenital bullous epidermolysis[3-8]

Clinical Procedures

*Fetal skin biopsies have been obtained in one of two ways: either under direct visualization via fetoscopy or under ultrasound guidance (**Figures 1, 2**).[9]*

Fetoscopy

For fetoscopy, the site of entry of the fetoscope is chosen to allow easy access to biopsy sites such as the back, thighs or scalp.[10-12] Traditionally, fetal skin biopsies have been obtained by fetoscopic methods which carry a 2–5% risk of miscarriage. The skin is prepared as for any invasive fetal procedure. Lidocaine 1% is injected subcutaneously into the maternal skin for anesthesia. A no. 15 scalpel blade is used to nick the skin and, if the patient is thin, down to the fascia. Then, under ultrasound guidance, the trocar of the fetoscope – which can be as simple as a 16 or 18 gauge needle – is inserted into the amniotic sac. If the procedure is being performed under direct visualization, the fetoscope is directed to the biopsy site. A significant advantage of direct visualization is that the specimen can be obtained at the site of obvious pathology. Though ultrasound-guided 'blind' biopsy has gained popularity because the quality of fiber optics has been so poor, recent advances of fiber optiscopes may change the equation back in favor of direct visualization.

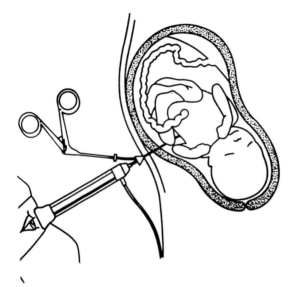

Figure 1. Schematic of fetal skin biopsy under fetoscopic visualization.

Ultrasound-guided biopsies

Recently, a modified approach to obtaining percutaneous ultrasound-guided fetal skin biopsies has been developed using a fine needle system.[13] The maternal skin is anesthetized with 1% zylocaine. A good site is the occipital area midway between the vault and base of the fetal head. An 18 gauge, 16 cm long needle with trocar is inserted into the abdominal wall through the uterine cavity. Then, the sharp point of the trocar is withdrawn to avoid trauma. The tip of the needle is guided until it is about 1 cm away from the biopsy site. A 20 cm long, 20 gauge biopsy forceps is inserted until it touches the fetal scalp, and a biopsy is obtained. The biopsy may be repeated up to three times to ensure that adequate material is obtained.

One potential concern applicable to all skin biopsies is scarring from the procedure. However, recent evidence, predominantly secondary to fetal surgical experience, suggests that fetal skin heals by a different mechanism than it does postnatally. The process of regeneration is to reorganize properly, and fetal incisions therefore tend to heal without scar.[14]

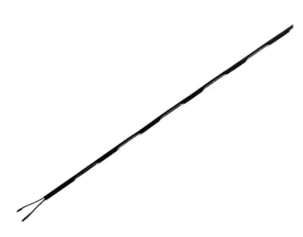

Figure 2. Biopsy forceps for skin biopsy.

Laboratory Procedures

Methods of diagnosis include histology and biochemical studies. For example, in harlequin ichythyosis, there is premature hyperkeratosis, most marked around the hair follicles and sweat ducts. (**Figures 3, 4**).[10] Sjogren-Larsson syndrome is diagnosed by finding of hyperkeratosis and increased keratohyaline.[15] In epidermolysis bullosa dystrophica, a cleavage plane below the basal lamina, and focal collagenolysis of the upper dermis, appears below the dermal/epidermal junction in unseparated regions.[16]

Significant advances in the biochemical examination of pathological fetal skin have been made over the past 5 years concurrent with our understanding of the ontogeny of structural proteins of normal fetal skin.[8,17] Biochemical studies have the advantage of allowing diagnoses earlier in gestation before direct visualization would be possible. The biochemical analyses of skin may also be applicable for genetic diagnosis using amniocytes and amniotic fluid. For example, prenatal diagnosis of several ichthyoses and other genetic disorders of which ichythyosis is a component, has been performed using amniotic fluid obtained between 14 and 16 weeks gestation.

Such studies have concluded, for example, that harlequin ichythysis is not one disorder, but a genetically heterogeneous group of disorders with altered glomerular granules, intercellular lipids, and variation in expression and/or processing of structural protein markers of normal epidermal keratinization.

FETAL LIVER BIOPSY

The liver has hundreds of metabolic functions. For a large number of these enzymatic reactions, enzyme activity can be documented in many different tissues including amniotic fluid and chorionic villi.[18] While it was necessary to learn that there were different normal activity values in different tissues,[19,20] the diagnoses of conditions such as the mucopolysaccharidoses and Tay Sachs disease (among countless others) have been routine for a number of years. Unfortunately, enzyme activity is strictly limited to the liver for certain disorders.

Fetal liver biopsies have been used successfully for the prenatal diagnosis of:

- ornithine transcarbamylase deficiency[21–25]

- Von Gierke's disease

- carbamyl phosphate synthetase deficiency

- primary hyperoxaluria type 1

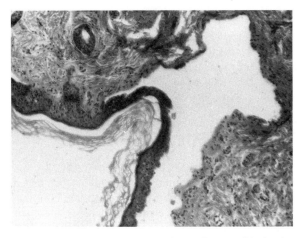

Figure 3. Histology of skin from fetus with harlequin ichythyosis.

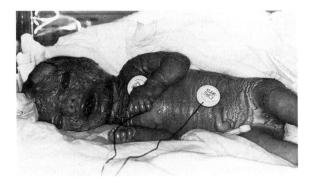

Figure 4. Baby with harlequin ichythyosis.

Clinical Procedures

*The technique for fetal liver biopsy is similar to that for skin except that a needle or coring biopsy instrument is inserted into the upper right quadrant of the fetal abdomen. (**Figures 5–7**) If a needle is used, a syringe is attached to create suction and the needle removed taking a core of specimen with it.[22] It is important for all of these biopsy techniques to have a dissecting microscope readily available to ensure that an adequate specimen has been obtained (**Figure 8**).*

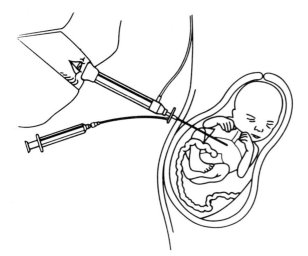

Figure 5. Schematic depiction of fetal liver biopsy with fetoscope.

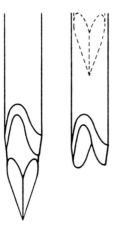

Figure 6. Cutting needle with aspiration trocar.

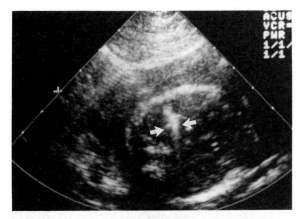

Figure 7. Ultrasound showing needle in liver (arrows).

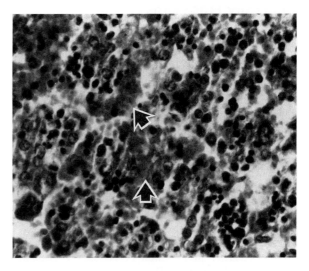

Figure 8. Histologic picture of fetal liver biopsy at 18 weeks; besides hepatic tissue, blood (arrows) can be seen.

Laboratory Procedures

Multiple enzymes, in addition to the one of interest, must be tested to eliminate the possibility that a low level of activity is a function of a poor specimen rather than disease. Otherwise, the enzymatic procedures are similar to those well known for pediatric specimens.

FETAL MUSCLE BIOPSY

After nearly three decades of research in the USA and millions of dollars in funding from highly publicized charitable campaigns, the gene for the muscle protein dystrophin, whose absence causes Duchenne muscular dystrophy (DMD), was finally isolated in 1987.[26] This gene encompasses more that two and a half million base pairs on the X chromosome and is by far the largest gene ever described.[27] Analyses of children with DMD have revealed that multiple molecular defects can produce the clinical picture of DMD.[28]

Many of the children with DMD have sizable deletions of the gene. In about 45% of patients, however, no deletion is detectable. Attempts to diagnose DMD prenatally had been futile for nearly 20 years. It was hoped, for example, that muscle proteins could be demonstrable in fetal blood, as it is known that elevated levels of creatine phosphokinase (CPK) are often elevated in carriers of DMD as well as significantly elevated in patients with DMD. Unfortunately, these levels do not begin to rise until at least the very end of pregnancy, making it impractical for prenatal diagnosis.

With the isolation of the DMD gene, the majority of fetal cases could be diagnosed by the molecular analysis of the gene either through detection of deletion mutations or by linkage analysis. Thus, the majority of cases of DMD are currently diagnosed from tissue specimens obtained via chorionic villus sampling. However, there are a number of situations where a deletion mutation is not found and DNA molecular diagnosis will not work. These can be divided into four different categories:

- Where there is only one prior family member affected and it cannot be determined whether the single affected family member inherited an abnormal X chromosome from his mother, or was a spontaneous mutation himself.

- Where analysis of polymorphisms proves uninformative (i.e. fails to reveal any differences between two maternal X chromosomes).

- Where there has been a crossover in meiosis between maternal X chromosomes such that it cannot be determined whether or not the DMD gene mutation was inherited.[29]

- Where there is an X-autosomal translocation in a male or even female fetus. Such female DMD cases are possible because an X-autosomal translocation break can be in the DMD region,[30] and these translocations will usually not be inactivated because Barr bodies are intact X chromosomes.

For example, a 41-year-old, gravida 3, para 2, woman came for prenatal diagnosis at 11 weeks gestation by chorionic villus sampling for advanced maternal age. On family history, however, it was first revealed that she had a 19-year-old son from a previous marriage, who had classic Duchenne muscular dystrophy. No other family members were affected. Chorionic villus sampling was obtained demonstrating a normal male karyotype. DNA analysis was performed on the fetus, the mother and the son with DMD which showed that the fetus had inherited the same X chromosome as his affected half-brother. Using Bayesian analysis, it was determined that the chance that the fetus was affected was the same risk as that the mother was a carrier, which was felt to be about 30% in this case. Typically, patients in this circumstance have been advised to consider termination of pregnancy followed by postmortem analysis for dystrophin. If dystrophin was absent, then the fetus was affected by DMD and the mother was a carrier. Therefore, future fetuses would be at risk. If dystrophin were present, it could be concluded that the deceased brother was affected

with DMD due to a spontaneous mutation, and that there was little risk to future pregnancies. Because of this patient's age, she did not wish to terminate and wait for another pregnancy. The presence of dystrophin was documented both by Western blotting and by immunofluorescence of muscle tissue.[31] The pregnancy continued successfully, and the child was born without symptoms or scarring.

Clinical Procedure

*Under ultrasound guidance, a site of entry for a KlearCut® kidney biopsy gun (Perry group, St Louis; **Figure 9**) is chosen, the maternal abdomen anesthetized, and a small nick made in the skin to ease entry. The gun is inserted into the uterine cavity and into the fetal buttock in a downward and outward direction. The coring guide is extended and then the trigger pulled, creating a core biopsy (**Figure 10**).*

Complications of the procedure include ruptured membranes, infection and damage to the fetus from the biopsy (both nerve and vascular abnormalities). In principle, there is no reason why the fine-cut tissue biopsy technique cannot be used for skin or liver biopsy.

Laboratory Procedures

The dystrophin protein is present only in muscle. Assays for the dystrophin protein are immunoblotting

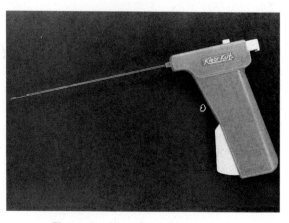

Figure 9. KlearCut® biopsy gun.

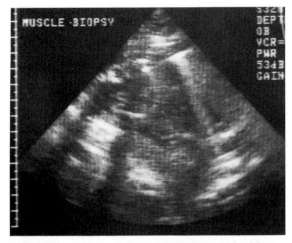

Figure 10. Ultrasound of gluteal muscle biopsy. Arrow shows biopsy gun entering fetal buttock.

and immunofluorescence (**Figures 11, 12**), though the former requires a relatively large amount of muscle tissue (50 μg). Immunofluorescence is accurate with as few as a half dozen muscle cells.[30] It is important to use multiple antibodies directed against different regions of the very large dystrophin protein, and to include control antibodies which demonstrate the presence of fetal muscle cells in the biopsy, which is usually predominantly epidermal tissue. Additional tissue controls of known normal and known affected fetal muscle should be carried out in parallel. Our initial experience with five pregnancies suggests that the incubation of serial cryostat sections with anti-dystrophin antibodies 60 kD (amnio-terminal region) and d10 (carboxyl-terminal region), and a myosin heavy chain antibody (F59), allows the accurate differentiation of Duchenne dystrophy from normal.

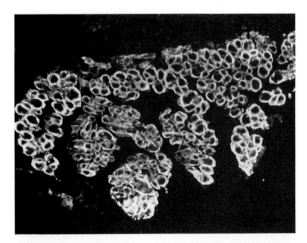

Figure 11. Immunofluorescent muscle tissue positive for dystrophin, and therefore normal.

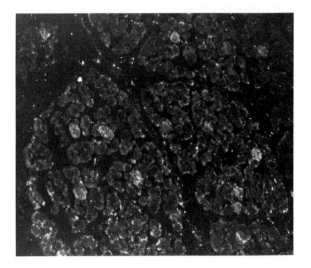

Figure 12. Muscle tissue not immunofluorescent for dystrophin, and therefore abnormal for Duchenne muscular dystrophy.

The high incidence of DMD and the frequent difficulties encountered in arriving at unambiguous molecular genetic predictions suggest that fetal muscle biopsy will become a standard procedure for the *in utero* diagnosis of DMD. As progress is made in the molecular pathology of other neuromuscular conditions, it is conceivable that this methodology could be extended to the diagnosis of other muscle diseases.

OTHER ORGANS

It is easy to imagine the desirability of having a fetal tissue biopsy of a tumor or mediastinal mass.[9] Kidney biopsies may be useful to document the degree and type of renal dysplasia associated with an obstructive uropathy. At the current time, however, most of these other indications would not seem strong enough to outweigh the risk of obtaining the fetal tissue.

A major risk in biopysing a tumor or a mediastinal mass would be uncontrollable bleeding. As visualization techniques and instrumentation improve, however, the balance of the equation might certainly change, and one should be very hesitant to be dogmatic about the desirability of any particular procedure.

CONCLUSIONS

Though most prenatal diagnoses can be made either by visualization or the obtaining of either amniotic fluid or blood, other rare disorders require a specific tissue such as skin, liver or muscle. Fetal tissue biopsy may

---

FETAL TISSUE BIOPSIES
Summary of Management Options

Indications

- Possible/potentially lethal or severely handicapping conditions in the fetus affecting:
  - skin
  - liver
  - muscle

- Occasionally for diagnosis of fetal tumors (see Chapter 55)

Procedure

- Prior counseling

- Options
  - fetoscopic directed biopsy
  - ultrasound-guided aspiration
  - ultrasound-guided 'tru-cut' technique

- Immediate/bedside microscopic confirmation of correct tissue biopsied

---

be performed either fetoscopically or under sonographic guidance. The risks of pregnancy wastage are relatively high. Thus, these biopsies should be performed only when the yield exceeds that risk. Because of their rarity and the complexity involved in the analyses of the specimens, these procedures should be performed only in specialized referral units.

REFERENCES

1 Charrow J, Nadler HL, Evans MI (1991) Prenatal diagnosis. In Emery AEH, Rimoin DL (eds), *Principles and Practice of Medical Genetics* 2nd edn, pp. 1959–1994. New York: Churchill Livingstone.

2 Caskey CT, Rossiter BJF (1992) Molecular genetics. In Evans MI (ed.) *Reproductive Risks and Prenatal Diagnosis*, pp. 265–277. Norwalk, CT: Appleton and Lange.

3 Epstein E (1984) Diagnosis of metabolic diseases that affect the skin using cultured amniotic fluid cells. *Seminars in Dermatology* 3:167–171.

4 Nazzaro V (1989) Sviluppo normale della cute umana fetale. *Giornale Italiano di Dermatologia E Venereologia* 124:421–427.

5 Dale BA, Holbrook KA, Fleckman P, Kimball JR, Brumbaugh S, Sybert VP (1990) Heterogeneity in harlequin ichthyosis, an inborn error of epidermal keratinization: Variable morphology and structural protein expression and a defect in lamellar granules. *Journal of Investigative Dermatology* 94:618.

6 Holbrook KA, Dale BA, Williams ML, Perry TB, Hoff MS, Hamilton EF, Fisher C, Senikas V (1988) The expression of congenital ichthyosiform erythroderma in second trimester fetuses of the same family: Morphologic and biochemical studies. *Journal of Investigative Dermatology* 91:521–531.

7 Nazzaro V, Nicolini U, DeLuca L, Berti E, Caputo R (1990) Prenatal diagnosis of junctional epidermolysis bullosa associated with pyloric atresia. *Journal of Medical Genetics* 27:244–248.

8 Dale BA, Perry TB, Holbrook KA, Hamilton EF, Senikas V (1986) Biochemical examination of fetal skin biopsy specimens obtained by fetoscopy: Use of the method for analysis of keratins and filaggrin. *Prenatal Diagnosis* 6:37–44.

9 Rodeck CH, Nicolaides KH (1986) Fetal tissue biopsy: Techniques and indications. *Fetal Therapy* 1:46–58.

10 Elias J, Mazur M, Sabbagha R, Esterly J, Simpson JL (1980) Prenatal diagnosis of harlequin ichthyosis. *Clin Genet* 17:275–279.

11 Hobbins JC, Mahoney MJ (1974) *In utero* diagnosis of hemoglobinopathies: Technique for obtaining fetal blood. *New England Journal of Medicine* 290:1065–1067.

12 Bang J (1985) Intrauterine needle diagnosis. In Holm K (ed.), *Interventional Ultrasound*, pp. 122–128. Copenhagen: Munksgaard.

13 Buckshee K, Parveen S, Mittal S, Verma K, Singh M (1991) Percutaneous ultrasound-guided fetal skin biopsy: A new approach. *International Journal of Gynecology and Obstetrics* 34:267–270.

14 Adzick NS, Longaker MT (1992) *Fetal Wound Healing*, pp. 53–70. New York: Elsevier.

15 Kusseff BG, Matsouka LY, Stenn KS, Hobbins JC, Mahoney MJ, Hashimoto K (1982) Prenatal diagnosis of Sjogren-Larsson syndrome. *Journal of Pediatrics* 101:998–1001.

16 Ant N, Lambrect L, Jovanovic V et al. (1981) Prenatal diagnosis of epidermolysis bullosa dystrophica hallopean siemens with electron microscopy of fetal skin. *Lancet* 2:1677–1679.

17 Moll R, Moll I, Wiest W (1983) Changes in the pattern of cytokeratin polypeptides epidermis and hair follicles during skin development in human fetuses. *Differentiation* 23:170–178.

18 Ben-Yoseph Y (1992) Biochemical genetics. In Evans MI (ed.), *Reproductive Risks and Prenatal Diagnosis*, pp. 251–265. Norwalk, CT: Appleton and Lange.

19 Evans MI, Moore C, Kolodny E, Schulman JD, Landsberger EJ, Karson EM, Dorfmann AD, Larsen

JW, Barranger JA (1986) Lysosomal enzymes in chorionic villi, cultured amniocytes, and cultured skin fibroblasts. *Clinica Chemica Acta* **157**:109–113.

20 Ben-Yoseph Y, Evans MI, Bottoms SF, Pack BA, Mitchell DA, Koppitch FC, Nadler HL (1986) Lysosomal enzyme activities in fresh and frozen chorionic villi and in cultured trophoblasts. *Clinica Chemica Acta* **161**:307–313.

21 Rodeck CH, Patrick AD, Pemberg ME, Tzanatos C, Whitfield AE (1982) Fetal liver biopsy for prenatal diagnosis of ornithine carbamyl transferase deficiency. *Lancet* **1**:297–299.

22 Holzgreve W, Golbus MS (1984) Prenatal diagnosis of ornithine transcarbamylase deficiency utilizing fetal liver biopsy. *American Journal of Human Genetics* **36**:320–328.

23 Danpure CJ, Jennings PR, Penketh RJ, Wise PJ, Cooper PJ, Rodeck CH (1989) Fetal liver alanine: Glyoxylate aminotransferase and the prenatal diagnosis of primary hyperoxaluria type I. *Prenatal Diagnosis* **9**:271–291.

24 Golbus MS, Simpson TJ, Koresawa M, Appelman Z, Alpers C (1988) The prenatal determination of glucose-6-phosphatase activity by fetal liver biopsy. *Prenatal Diagnosis* **8**:401–404.

25 Piceni Sereni L, Bachmann C, Pfister U, Buscaglia M, Nicolini U (1988) Prenatal diagnosis of carbamoyl-phosphate synthetase deficiency by fetal liver biopsy. *Prenatal Diagnosis* **8**:307–309.

26 Hoffman EP, Brown RH, Kunkel LM (1987) Dystrophin: The protein product of the Duchenne muscular dystrophy locus. *Cell* **51**:919–928.

27 Hoffman EP, Fishbeck KH, Brown RH et al. (1988) Dystrophin characterization in muscle biopsies from Duchenne and Becker muscular dystrophy patients. *New England Journal of Medicine* **318**:1363–1368.

28 Hoffman EP (1993) Genotype/phenotype correlations in Duchenne/Becker muscular dystrophy. In Partridge TA (ed.), *Molecular and Cell Biology of Muscular Dystrophy*, pp. 57–63. London: Chapman and Hall.

29 Evans MI, Greb A, Kunkel LM, Sacks AJ, Johnson MP, Boehm C, Kazazian HH Jr, Hoffman EP (1991) *In utero* fetal muscle biopsy for the diagnosis of Duchenne muscular dystrophy. *American Journal of Obstetrics and Gynecology* **165**:728–732.

30 Evans MI, Farrell SA, Greb A, Ray P, Johnson MP, Hoffman EP (1993) *In utero* fetal muscle biopsy for the diagnosis of Duchenne muscular dystrophy in a female fetus 'suddenly at risk'. *American Journal of Medical Genetics* **46**:309–312.

31 Kuller JA, Hoffman EP, Fries MJ, Golbus MS (1992) Prenatal diagnosis of Duchenne muscular dystrophy by fetal muscle biopsy. *Human Genetics* **90**:34–40.

57

Multifetal Pregnancy Reduction and Selective Termination

MARK I. EVANS, LINDA LITTMANN, NELSON B. ISADA, MARK P. JOHNSON

THE PROBLEM AND THE OPTIONS

Fertility drugs such as human menopausal gonadotrophin (Perganol® or Metrodin®) have helped thousands of couples each year to conceive their own children. However, these drugs with or without associated reproductive technologies such as *in vitro* fertilization (IVF) or gamete in the fallopian tube (GIFT), have created one of the most bitter ironies in medicine. Women previously infertile suddenly bear more fetuses than they can either carry to viability, or at least are at significant increased risk for perinatal mortality or morbidity.[1,2]

Although advances in both prenatal and neonatal care have reduced the mortality, and to a lesser extent the morbidity of prematurity,[3-6] the obstetric outcome for triplets or higher numbers of fetuses is significantly worse than for singleton or even twin pregnancies.[1,3-6] The ability to carry four or more fetuses is, by any reasonable definition, significantly compromised, and in the case of six or more fetuses, it has hardly ever been seen. While recent reports have certainly shown markedly diminished mortality, particularly with triplets, there is still great concern about long-term morbidity.[3,4]

When caught in such a dilemma, couples are faced with three unpleasant options (**Table 1**). The first option is termination of the entire pregnancy. This choice, especially for infertility patients, has generally been very unpalatable. The second option is to continue with all of the fetuses. In cases of quadruplets or

Table 1
Options in multifetal gestation

Abortion
Attempt to carry
Multifetal pregnancy reduction

even quintuplets, survival of some or all is certainly realistic but problematic, and there is a significant risk of long-term morbidity. With six or more fetuses, the chance of survival is extremely low.

A third option is consideration of multifetal reduction (MFR) (alternatively called selective termination), which has become a realistic option in the face of perinatal tragedy from multiple fetuses.[7-13] Those in the field have generally adopted the convention of calling first trimester procedures for fetal number MFR, and second trimester procedures provided for fetal abnormalities selective termination (ST).

MULTIFETAL REDUCTION (MFR)

Techniques

The number of cases performed has significantly risen as awareness of MFR has spread. Three different technical procedures have been reported (**Table 2**).[9-13]

Table 2
Techniques of multifetal
pregnancy reduction

Transcervical
Transvaginal
Transabdominal

Procedure: Multifetal Reduction

Transcervical suction

Originally, Dumez and Oury reported a technique involving transcervical, low-pressure suction to remove embryos at 8–11 weeks.[9] Under ultrasound guidance, a mini suction curettage was performed. Technical success was achieved in the majority of cases, but with loss of the entire pregnancy in about 50%.[1] This technique has largely been abandoned, but has now reemerged in a few centres.

Transvaginal aspiration

Transvaginal aspiration of the early embryo at about 6–7 weeks has been tried successfully. This technique is analogous in many respects to oocyte aspiration for in vitro fertilization and may be useful particularly when the attempt is very early in gestation.
A speculum is inserted into the vagina which is then cleaved with Betadine®. A long, sharp needle is passed through the vaginal wall into the uterine cavity. The needle is maneuvered into a chosen sac and moved up against the embryo. Suction is applied, and the embryo is aspirated or disrupted. The amniotic fluid is left in utero. The same needle is partially withdrawn and then repositioned for additional embryos as needed.

Transabdominal KCl

The technique many believe to be most feasible involves the transabdominal insertion of a spinal needle (usually a 22 gauge) under ultrasound guidance. The abdomen is prepared as for an amniocentesis procedure. The insertion site is carefully chosen for each embryo to attempt a direct, vertical, downward

*approach, since it is usually less painful for the patient to go straight down as opposed to maneuvering through the abdomen at a significant angle from vertical. When the position over the fetal heart is confirmed (**Figures 1 and 2**), the needle is thrust into the thorax (**Figure 3**). If too gentle, the embryo will bounce away and the needle repositioned. It is rarely necessary to remove the needle completely. Proper placement of the needle is important. While one aims for the heart,*

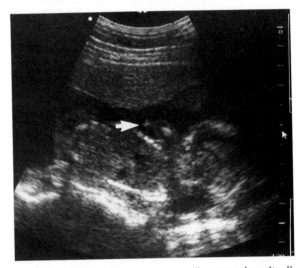

Figure 1. Tip of 22 gauge needle seen longitudinally positioned above fetal thorax just before needle insertion.

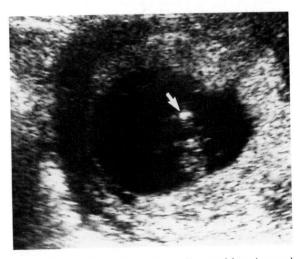

Figure 2. Confirmation of needle position (arrow) in transverse plane prior to insertion.

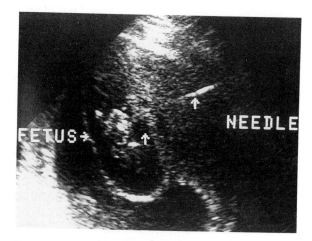

Figure 3. Intrathoracic position of needle ready for KCl injection.

anywhere within the fetal thorax is acceptable in the first trimester. Placement below the diaphragm will lead to failure.

Once the needle is properly positioned, the inner stylet is removed, a 3 cc syringe attached, and the plunger is pulled back gently. There should be negative pressure on a small amount of blood from the heart. There should not be any amniotic fluid.

Once the operator is certain of the position, a small dose of KCl (about 0.5 ml) is injected. Cardiac standstill occurs within 1–2 min of the injection. A pleural or car-

*diac effusion can often be appreciated (**Figure 4**). On occasion, cardiac motion continues for a longer period, but is associated with a definite slowing which appears 'preterminal'. Ultimately, the sac is resorbed.*

Selection

Embryo selection

It is not uncommon for an embryo to appear abnormal at 9–12 weeks. Thus, the decision of which embryo to choose is usually based on which embryos are easiest to reach.[4] Anecdotal experience suggests that is is better not to choose the embryo closest to the cervix as persistent vaginal bleeding is likely. Also, there is concern about removal of amniotic fluid as a sudden decrease in uterine size might induce contractions. With six or more embryos, performing the procedure at two separate times about a week apart may be technically easier, allowing the remaining embryos to grow and become easier to reach. With experience, it is possible to reduce octuplets to twins at one time without problem, so this decision should be individualized.

Timing

Most of the transabdominal cases reported to date have been performed at 9–12 weeks of pregnancy. Although the data are limited, it seems that transabdominal attempts prior to 8 weeks are technically more difficult. The transvaginal approach will probably be better at very early gestational ages. However, the chance of a spontaneous loss of remaining embryos 'naturally' is still a considerable possibility, and therefore adds to the risk of losing the remaining embryo(s).[14,15] Beyond 13 weeks, the chance of spontaneous loss is minimal, but there are theoretic risks of infectious necrosis from the tissue mass left and disseminated intravascular coagulation. However, there are no reliable data and no known cases to date.

Number

In the author's personal experience, the decisions of both the patient and physician have almost always been to leave twins. We feel that by leaving twins there will still be some 'margin for error'. Although the obstetric outcome for twins is not quite as good as that for singleton pregnancies, it is considerably better than for triplets or more. Triplets have been left[7,8] and the outcome can be satisfactory. However, the risks of prema-

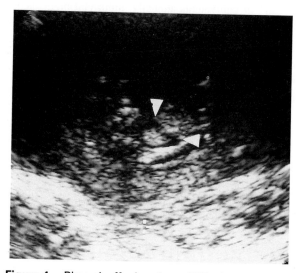

Figure 4. Pleural effusion from KCl after injection (arrows).

turity and morbidity are certainly increased above those with twins. Such risks are justifiable if the couple understands the likelihood of alterations of lifestyle during the pregnancy, despite which there may still be an unsatisfactory outcome.

While pooled collaborative data suggest longer gestations and slightly lower morbidity with a singleton, we do not believe leaving one is generally the best medical decision, since the pregnancy will be lost if there is a problem with the remaining embryo. Especially for an infertility couple, taking home one baby is very different than none. Exceptions to the aforementioned would include a woman with diethyl-stilbestrol-induced uterine malformations, cervical incompetence, or very significant medical disease such as cardiac failure for which the added burden of a multiple gestation might be the difference between a viable pregnancy or not. For the first few years of our experience, we insisted on reducing to two fetuses. With increased experience and documented safety, we believe the factors of patient autonomy and a small decrease in the risk of morbidity for a singleton makes the issue more complex.

Outcome of MFR

An essentially 100% technical success rate is possible. Composite data from those centers with the most experience suggest success (defined as the live birth of an infant) to be approximately 75–80%, which must be viewed against the background risks of multifetal pregnancies which we believe to be about 10% for twins. Complications are primarily a function of the initial starting number of fetuses (**Table 3**).[16] It is not surprising that a three to two reduction would be less risky than a six to two reduction. Overall results from 463 completed cases show reduction to twins being the

safest in terms of fetal loss rate and lowest rate of early premature deliveries.[16]

Management of Pregnancies after MFR

There is concern for the possibility of midtrimester pregnancy loss, since a large proportion of late losses have had confounding factors involved and it is not possible to delineate exact components of risk. The available natural history data on the early and midtrimester of multifetal pregnancies are poor and hinder evaluation of selective termination assessment. The risks of congenital malformations should be no different, and invasive studies such as amniocentesis should be considered as otherwise indicated. CVS would seem less desirable as excessive manipulation of the uterine contents around the time of the procedure might increase the risks of fetal loss. Once past the midtrimester, there is no reason to believe that late pregnancy management should be any different than that for any other twins.

Treatment of Infertility and Multiple Pregnancy

Nearly all quadruplets or higher are iatrogenic. Many result from suboptimal Pergonal® use or *in vitro* fertilization and embryo transfer of large numbers of embryos. With the development of cryopreservation, the incidence of IVF multiple gestations has been decreasing.[17]

In response to malpractice litigation initiated by patients who had poorly controlled Pergonal® cycles, such cases may diminish further. However, it is clear that with about 20 000 patients in the USA receiving Pergonal® or equivalents annually, multifetal pregnancies

Table 3
Results of multifetal pregnancy reduction

Finishing no.	Starting no.				Total
	2	3	4	5+	
Singletons					
Losses	3	6	3	2	14
Total	18	26	10	3	57
Percentage	16.7%	23.0%	30.0%	66.7%	24.6%
Twins					
Losses		10	26	18	54
Total		149	170	61	380
Percentage		6.7%	15.3%	29.5%	13.7%
Triplets					
Losses			2	5	7
Total			13	13	26
Percentage			15.4%	38.5%	26.9%

can and will happen occasionally to excellent physicians using the best of equipment, skill and intent. Furthermore, there are some patients for whom there is a very narrow margin of Pergonal® use between no response and hyperstimulation. The availability of MFR allows the physician to take 'calculated' risks for patients who otherwise would probably not become pregnant.

SELECTIVE TERMINATION

In contrast to the above in which the problem is fetal number *per se*, selective termination of an abnormal twin has been practised for a decade as a means of dealing with a known fetal problem. In 1978, Aberg reported cardiac puncture of a twin fetus with Hurler Syndrome.[18] In 1981, Kerenyi and Chitkara reported a twin pregnancy.[19] One fetus had Down's syndrome. They selectively terminated the abnormal twin when the mother threatened to abort the pregnancy. MFR and ST differ in that both fertile and post-fertile couples will face the dilemma. Further, these abnormalities are discovered in the second trimester, not the first.

Procedure: Selective Termination

*The technique for ST also differs from MFR in some aspects. First, the injection of KCl must be done directly into the cardiac chamber in order to achieve cardiac standstill (**Figure 5**). Pleural injection will not suffice. The dose required increases with gestational age. We have found that 3 ml is more than adequate up to 20 weeks gestation. Another method is to use air embolization. While effective, the air clouds the ultrasound image, making assessment of cardiac status difficult and enhancing the difficulty of making a repeat injection if necessary.*

Selection

Case selection is critical. Two major factors need to be considered. First, one must make sure which is the abnormal twin. While obvious in many instances, discrimination can in some instances be difficult. Second, if the placenta is shared, then the demise of one twin potentially puts the other at significantly increased risk. Occasionally, even if the circulation does not appear to be joined based on the sonographic image, there may be vascular consequences.

Outcome and Dilemma

Though the combined experience is relatively small, ST is associated with term delivery of a healthy neonate. The management of resulting problems associated with fetal death are discussed in Chapter 58.

Just as there are difficulties in the appropriate indications for MFR, the same is true for ST. Ethical reasoning[7,13] gives concern to the risk imposed upon a normal twin by killing the other. In MFR, the issues center on fetal number as well as associated morbidity and mortality. In ST, the morbidity of the abnormal co-twin can usually be predicted, along with the morbidity of prematurity for the normal one. When ST was a new procedure with undefined risks, some authors attempted to define which abnormalities were significant enough and which were not. As experience has been gained and the safety of ST has emerged, indications for the procedure would seem to most people to be more liberalized. Different conditions may be perceived in widely divergent fashions by different people, though its use for sex selection is widely condemned.

CONCLUSION

Advanced reproductive technologies have created a bitter irony. Previously infertile women suddenly bear more fetuses than they are likely to carry successfully. The obstetric outcome for triplets or higher preg-

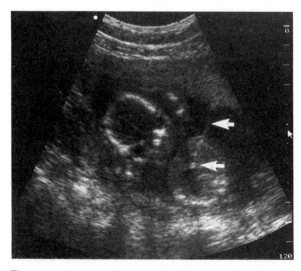

Figure 5. Intracardiac needle placement in 15 week fetus with unbalanced translocation.

SELECTIVE REDUCTION OF PREGNANCY
Summary of Management Options

Multifetal reductions

- Careful prior discussion and counseling

- Ideally at 9–12 weeks

- Avoid fetuses over cervix

- ? Reduce to 2 fetuses

- Technical options:
  - transabdominal KCl
  - (transcervical suction)
  - (transvaginal aspiration)

- Outcome – see **Table 3**

- If viable survivors, subsequent management as for twin pregnancy (see Chapter 10)

Selective termination of abnormal twin

- Careful prior discussion and counseling
- Second trimester

- Careful identification of abnormal twin

- Mono-amniotic twins are a contraindication

- Technique = intracardiac KCl

- If other twin survives:
  - monitor maternal platelets and clotting
  - monitor fetal growth and health

---

nancies is significantly worse than that of the singleton. These women have only three options: end the pregnancy, carry knowing the likelihood of a complete success is low, or reduce the number of fetuses. Multifetal reduction (MFR) has become a realistic option. It is performed in the late first trimester. Fetal selection is based on the ease of approach. The most common technique involves the intrathoracic injection of potassium chloride. The technical success rate approaches 100% in experienced hands. The procedure-related pregnancy loss rates depend upon the number of fetuses killed and ranges from 6 to 12%.

In contrast to MFR, selective termination (ST) applies to the killing of a maldeveloped fetus after the completion of the first trimester. The most common technique involves the intracardiac injection of potassium chloride. However, this method is contraindicated if the pregnancy is of monozygotic origin. The indications for the procedure will vary among societies. However, the use of either MFR or ST for sex selection is widely condemned. Both MFR and ST should be performed only by experienced operators.

REFERENCES

1 Bronsteen RA, Evans MI (1989) Multiple gestation. In Evans MI, Fletcher JC, Dixler AO, Schulman JD (eds), *Fetal Diagnosis and Therapy: Science, Ethics and the Law*, pp. 242–265. Philadelphia, PA: J.B. Lippincott.

2 Lunenfeld B, Lunenfeld E (1992) Ovulation induction: HMG. In Seibel MM (ed.), *Infertility: A Comprehensive Text*, pp. 311–323. Norwalk, CT: Appleton and Lange.

3 MacLennan AH (1984) Multiple gestations. In Creasy RK, Resnik R (eds), *Maternal Fetal Medicine: Principles and Practice*, pp. 527–538. Philadelphia, PA: W.B. Saunders.

4 Newman RB, Hamer C, Miller C (1989) Outpatient triplet management: A contemporary revue. *American Journal of Obstetrics and Gynecology* 161:547–555.

5 Collins MS, Bleyl JA (1990) Seventy one quadruplet pregnancies: Management and outcome. *American Journal of Obstetrics and Gynecology* 162:1384–1392.

6 Petrokovsky B, Vintzileos A (1989) Management and outcome of multiple pregnancies of higher fetal order: Literature review. *Obstetrical and Gynecological Survey* 44:578.

7 Evans MI, Fletcher JC, Zador IE, Newton BW, Quigg MH, Struyk CD (1988) Selective first trimester termination in octuplet and quadruplet pregnancies: Clinical and ethical issues. *Obstetrics and Gynecology* 71:289–296.

8 Berkowitz RL, Lynch L, Chitkara U *et al.* (1988) Selective reduction of multifetal pregnancies in the first trimester. *New England Journal of Medicine* 318:1043.

9 Dumez Y, Oury JF (1986) Method for first trimester selective abortion in multiple pregnancy. *Contributions to Gynecology and Obstetrics* 15:50.

10 Kanhai HH, VanRijssel EJC, Meerman RJ *et al.* (1986) Selective termination in quintuplet pregnancy during first trimester *Lancet* **ii**:1447.

11 Lynch L, Berkowitz RL, Chitakara U *et al.* (1990) First trimester transabdominal multiple pregnancy reduction: A report of 85 cases. *Obstetrics and Gynecology* **75**:735.

12 Tabsh KM (1990) Transabdominal multifetal pregnancy reduction: Report of 40 cases. *Obstetrics and Gynecology* **75**:739.

13 Evans MI, May M, Drugan A *et al.* (1990) Selective termination: Clinical experience and residual risks. *American Journal of Obstetrics and Gynecology* **162**:1568–1575.

14 Varma TR (1979) Ultrasound evidence of early pregnancy failure in patients with multiple conceptions. *British Journal of Obstetrics and Gynaecology* **86**:290.

15 Gindoft PR, Yeh MN, Jewelewicz R (1986) The van-ishing sac syndrome. *Journal of Reproductive Medicine* **31**:322.

16 Evans MI, Dommergues M, Wagner RJ *et al.* (1993) Efficacy of transabdominal multifetal pregnancy reduction: Collaborative experience of the world's largest centers. *Obstetrics and Gynecology* **82**:61–66.

17 Cohen J, DeVane GW, Elsner CW, Fehilly CB, Kort HI, Massey JB, Turner Jr TG (1988) Cryopreservation of zygotes and early cleaved human embryos. *Fertility and Sterility* **49**:283–289.

18 Aberg A, Miterian F, Cantz M, Geliler J (1978) Cardiac puncture of fetus with Hurler's disease avoiding abortion of unaffected co-twin. *Lancet* **2**:990–991.

19 Kerenyi T, Chitkara U (1981) Selective birth in twin pregnancy with discordancy for Down's syndrome. *New England Journal of Medicine* **304**:1525–1527.

58

Fetal Death

CARL P. WEINER

INTRODUCTION

There is usually great sadness when a fetus dies. The known threat of an embryonic miscarriage has past, and both patient and caregiver have become optimistic about the future. But whether the death has occurred in a singleton or multiple gestation, it triggers a change in management and the patient's psychosocial needs.

Management Options

Evaluation

An evaluation of a fetal death involves both the fetus and mother. It is essential that the cause of death be determined whenever possible. Only then can the likelihood of a recurrence and the possibility of prevention be ascertained. Further, knowledge of the actual cause of death often aids the parental grieving process, since it usually eliminates the natural tendency for self-recrimination. A thorough maternal past and current medical history should again be obtained and the physical examination repeated in search of an unsuspected pre-existing or acquired systemic illness. A targeted ultrasound examination of the uterus and its contents is performed to search for fetal or placental malformations and evidence of fetal growth deficiency. The more common causes of fetal death are listed in **Table 1**.

Unless the history and examination pinpoint the cause, a basic group of laboratory tests should be per-

Table 1
Causes of fetal death

Maternal

Systemic illness
  diabetes mellitus
  hypertension: includes prepregnancy- and pregnancy-
    associated connective tissue disorders
  any causing septicemia with associated hypoperfusion

Fetal
  malformations: structural and chromosomal
  infection-bacterial, viral, protozoan
  fetal immune hemolytic disease
  cord accident: includes prolapse, thrombosis,
    strangulation by bands or knots, and torsion (all
    likely to be greatly overdiagnosed)
  metabolic disorders

Placental
  dysfunction causing hypoxemia and includes those
    associated with fetal growth deficiency and
    'postmaturity'
  abruption causing hypoxemia
  previa or infarction
  twin to twin transfusion
  fetal to maternal hemorrhage

formed prior to delivery. These are listed in **Table 2**. If delivery is not likely to occur in the near future, an amniocentesis both to search for fetal infection (see Chapter 49) and to obtain a karyotype is recommended. A chromosome abnormality is seen in 15% of second

Table 2
Routine laboratory evaluation and follow-up of fetal death

On detection

Maternal
fasting blood glucose or glycosylated hemoglobin
platelet count
fibrinogen
indirect Coombs
specific serologic screening targeted for common
infections
stain of a peripheral smear for fetal red blood cells
(Kleihauer test)
anticardiolipins
antinuclear antibodies
lupus anticoagulant

Fetal
karyotype
aminiotic fluid culture for cytomegalovirus, anaerobic
and aerobic bacteria

Subsequent

Maternal
weekly fibrinogen measurements and platelet counts if
fetal death more than 4 weeks duration until delivery

Fetal (at delivery)
repeat infection workup (see Chapter 49)
karyotype (if not done prenatally) (placenta may be
more likely to yield a successful culture)
fetogram (total body X-ray)
postmortem examination

---

trimester stillbirths. The karyotype should be determined in most fetuses even in the apparent absence of structural malformations, since the usual dysmorphic features may be obscured by postmortem changes. In contrast to fetal fascia or subcutaneous tissue, amniocytes can be successfully cultured weeks after a demise has occurred. The placenta is an alternative site for obtaining material for karyotype.

After delivery, photographs of the child are made for both the medical record and the parents, a fetogram obtained and permission sought for a postmortem examination. The fetal organ cavities should be cultured for both bacteria and virus even if an infectious workup had been initiated prenatally.

Pregnancy management

The approach to the pregnancy after the fetus has died depends upon the gestational age and whether it is a single or multiple gestation (**Table 3**).

Singleton gestation

Prior to 15 weeks, a dilation and evacuation should be performed. This option remains until 24 weeks, though it has been suggested that the risk of maternal hemorrhage may be increased with a demise.[1] Caution is indicated. The second, and more common alternative, is an induction of labor (see Chapter 60).

The management of a fetal demise after 15 weeks gestation has changed with the introduction of prostaglandin analogs for the induction of labor. Prior to their availability, management was guided by a number of pragmatic realities. First, 90% or more of women with an intrauterine demise spontaneously labored within 3 weeks of its detection.[2,3] Second, oxytocin was frequently ineffective in bringing about labor, most likely because of the early gestation. As a result, prolonged labor was the rule. And though the intra-amniotic instillation of hypertonic saline or glucose was said to hasten induction, they were also associated with several maternal deaths. Thus, despite the considerable social pressure for delivery, observation was the best medical approach.

The disadvantage to observation is that some 25% of women with a demise after 20 weeks gestation who retain their dead fetus for 4 or more weeks, develop a chronic consumptive coagulopathy characterized by varying degrees of decreased fibrinogen, plasminogen, antithrombin III and platelets, and increased fibrin degradation products.[4-7] The etiology of the coagulopathy has never been conclusively determined. Using sensitive coagulation tests, pathologic activation of the clotting cascade can be demonstrated within 48 h of the demise. The incidence of the coagulopathy increases with the duration of the delay, but <2% of these women experience a hemorrhagic complication. Fortunately, this chronic, low-grade intravascular coag-

Table 3
Management options for delivery following fetal death of singleton (see also Chapter 60)

≤15 weeks
Dilation and evacuation
Prostaglandins (12–15 weeks)

15–28 weeks
Prostaglandins
(some centers use dilatation and morcellation up to 20
weeks)

>28 weeks
If cervix favorable: oxytocin and amniotomy
If cervic unfavorable:
laminaria
prostaglandins

ulopathy can be reversed by the administration of a low-dose heparin.[8-10] Traditionally, labor was induced after treatment of the coagulopathy even if the cervix was unfavorable. If left to a natural course, the coagulopathy resolves within 48 h of delivery.

The development of the prostaglandin E and F series for the induction of labor has eliminated the need to wait. The efficacy of these agents for the induction of labor exceeds 90%.[11] Delivery shortly after detection of the demise has several advantages. First, it brings an end to an emotionally painful event and allows the psychological healing process to begin. Second, any postmortem examination is more likely to yield useful information if done prior to the development of severe autolysis. The various prostaglandin preparations may be administered either vaginally, intracervically, extraovularly or intramuscularly depending upon regional availability. In the USA , prostaglandin E_2 (PGE$_2$) vaginal suppositories are not yet approved by the Food and Drug Administration (FDA) for the termination of pregnancy after an intrauterine demise beyond 28 weeks. However, clinical experience supports both their reliability and safety.[11] Common complications include nausea and vomiting, fever and tachycardia. Their frequency is generally route of administration and dose dependent, and greatly reduced by premedication.[12]

Multiple gestation

The optimal management of the multiple gestation with a singleton demise remains unclear. The incidence of this complication is low (<1% of all twin gestations), but the prematurity and neonatal death rates among the survivors high.[13,14] Several factors must be considered. First is the cause of death. Could the same stimulus, such as congenital infection or a maternal systemic illness, cause a sublethal insult yielding a damaged survivor? If so, will continuation of the pregnancy worsen the outcome by prolonging the exposure? Clearly, an informed decision requires knowledge of the cause and is a matter for individualization.

The second item to consider is whether the dead twin's very presence poses a risk to the surviving twin. A syndrome has been reported in survivors of monochorionic gestations with one demise which can include bilateral renal cortical necrosis, multicystic encephalomalacia, gastrointestinal structural malformations and even a disseminated intravascular coagulopathy.[15-20] These varied disorders could share a vascular etiology and it has been suggested that they result from feto–feto transfer of necrotic, thromboplastic emboli through placental anastomoses. If true, delivery of the surviving twin as soon as reasonable would seem prudent. However, there has been no prenatal documentation of a fetal coagulopathy and the evidence for necrotic emboli (as opposed to thrombotic

phenomena) weak. Further, the syndrome has been reported in neonates born of monochorionic gestations uncomplicated by a demise. There are other potential etiologies which could result in either thrombosis or hypoperfusion. The most likely is an abrupt hypotensive event at the time of the co-twin's death, which might occur with extensive vascular anastomoses.[21,22] If this is the mechanism underlying the development of the syndrome, preterm delivery would come too late to prevent it and only add the complications of prematurity to the neonatal course. If the gestation appears to be monochorionic, it would seen prudent to observe the surviving co-twin very closely, perhaps continuously during the 7 day interval following the demise. Since the risk of death to the surviving co-twin in a dizygotic gestation is less than 5%,[13] the author does not favor iatrogenic delivery prior to 36 weeks solely for the indication of a dead co-twin.

The third and final concern is the development of a maternal coagulopathy should the pregnancy be continued. Hypofibrinogenemia and thrombocytopenia should be tested for weekly after 4 weeks delay (**Table 4**). Though the incidence is likely to be as high as that for a retained singleton gestation, the same treatment is effective. Low-dose heparin, between 10 and 30 000 units given in divided doses subcutaneously, is usually adequate to reverse the hypofibrinogenemia.[23,24] There is no need to prolong the partial thromboplastin time. However, the amount of heparin necessary to reverse the hypofibrinogenemia may be quite high, possibly reflecting the low antithrombin III concentration. Of significance, the need for heparin is temporary. It can usually be discontinued 6–8 weeks later without recurrence of the hypofibrinogenemia.[24,25]

Parental psychosocial care

Many hospitals have a grieving support counselor or a psychologist as part of the perinatal team. In addition, there are frequently support groups in the locale consisting of women who have also experienced an intra-

Table 4
Summary of management options for a multiple gestation with a singleton demise (see also Chapter 55)

Ascertain chorionicity by ultrasound
Seek etiology and confirm the survivor is unaffected
Serial maternal fibrinogen measurements and platelet counts
Consider low-dose heparin (10 000–30 000 IU/day in divided doses adjusted individually)
Delivery for evidence of fetal compromise or after 36–37 weeks gestation

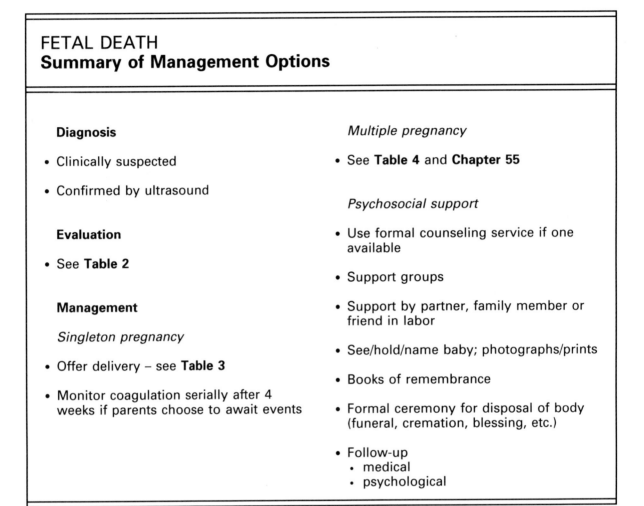

FETAL DEATH
Summary of Management Options

Diagnosis

- Clinically suspected

- Confirmed by ultrasound

Evaluation

- See **Table 2**

Management

Singleton pregnancy

- Offer delivery – see **Table 3**

- Monitor coagulation serially after 4 weeks if parents choose to await events

Multiple pregnancy

- See **Table 4** and **Chapter 55**

Psychosocial support

- Use formal counseling service if one available

- Support groups

- Support by partner, family member or friend in labor

- See/hold/name baby; photographs/prints

- Books of remembrance

- Formal ceremony for disposal of body (funeral, cremation, blessing, etc.)

- Follow-up
  - medical
  - psychological

---

uterine demise. It is very helpful if a representative of one of these groups meets with the patient shortly after the diagnosis is made. Where appropriate, pastoral care may also be helpful. During labor and after delivery, her partner is encouraged to stay and provide support. When far enough along in gestation, the patient should be encouraged to view and hold the newborn. Too often patients incorrectly assume they have conceived a monstrosity. They should also be informed that bruising and facial marks may well be present even if the child looks otherwise normal. Neonatal footprints and handprints are made, and the parents encouraged to name the child. Photographs are helpful. If the patient does not immediately want any of these remembrance items, they should be stored. Many women change their mind and later write to request them.

Upon discharge from the hospital, the patient is given an appointment for a return visit. The timing of this visit varies. Many centers see the couple for an initial counseling visit within 1–2 weeks when the result of the postmortem is known. While the results

of all the investigations may not be available, there may be psychological benefit in such an early preliminary discussion. A comprehensive discussion should take place within 3–6 months. The results of all studies performed are reviewed and the parents given an opportunity to voice any questions they may have. If the cause of death was ascertained, its implications (if any) to subsequent pregnancies should be discussed. It is important to reinforce to both the patient and her partner that these events are not usually under their control.

REFERENCES

1   Gerl D, Noschel H (1968) Course of delivery in intrauterine fetal death with special reference to blood loss. *Zentralbl Gynakol* **90**:1463–1466.

2   Dippel AL (1934) Death of foetus *in utero*. *Johns Hopkins Medical Journal* **54**:24–34.

3   Tricomi V, Kohl SG (1957) Fetal death *in utero*. *Amer-*

ican Journal of Obstetrics and Gynecology 1957; **74**:1092–1098.

4   Weiner AE, Reid DE, Roby CC, Diamond LK (1950) Coagulation defects with intrauterine death from Rh isoimmunization. *American Journal of Obstetrics and Gynecology* **60**:1015–1018.

5   Pritchard JA (1959) Fetal death *in utero*. *Obstetrics and Gynecology* **14**:573–580.

6   Pritchard JA, Ratnoff OD (1955) Studies of fibrinogen and other hemostatic factors in women with intrauterine death and delayed delivery. *Surgery Gynecology and Obstetrics* **101**:467–473.

7   Goldstein DP, Reid DE (1963) Circulating fibrinolytic activity: A precursor of hypofibrinogenemia following fetal death *in utero*. *Obstetrics and Gynecology* **22**:174–181.

8   Lerner R, Margolin M, Slate WG *et al.* (1967) Heparin in the treatment of hypofibrinogenemia complicating fetal death *in utero*. *American Journal of Obstetrics and Gynecology* **97**:373–381.

9   Jimenez JM, Prichard JA (1968) Pathogenesis and treatment of coagulation defects resulting from fetal death. *Obstetrics and Gynecology* **32**:449–445.

10 Waxman B, Gambrill R (1972) Use of heparin in disseminated intravascular coagulation. *American Journal of Obstetrics and Gynecology* **112**:434–439.

11 Kochenour NK (1987) Management of fetal demise. *Clinics in Obstetrics and Gynecology* **30**:322–330.

12 Lauersen NH, Cederqvist LL, Wilson KH (1980) Management of intrauterine fetal death with prostaglandin E₂ vaginal suppositories. *American Journal of Obstetrics and Gynecology* **137**:753–764.

13 Hagay ZJ, Mazor M, Leiberman JR, Biale Y (1986) Management and outcome of multiple pregnancies complicated by the antenatal death of one fetus. *Journal of Reproductive Medicine* **31**:717–720.

14 Litschgi M, Stucki D (1980) Course of twin pregnancies after fetal death *in utero*. *Z Geburtshife Perinatol* **184**:227–239.

15 Reisman LE, Pathak A (1966) Bilateral renal necrosis in the newborn. *American Journal of Diseases of Children* **111**:541–555.

16 Moore CM, McAdams AJ, Sutherland J (1969) Intrauterine disseminated coagulation: A syndrome with multiple pregnancy with a dead twin fetus. *Journal of Pediatrics* **74**:523–528.

17 Melnick M (1977) Brain damage in a survivor after *in utero* death of monozygous co-twin. *Lancet* **ii**:1287–1289.

18 Yoshioka H, Kadomoto Y, Mino M *et al.* (1979) Multicystic encephalomalacia in liveborn twin with a stillborn macerated co-twin. *Journal of Pediatrics* **95**:798–804.

19 Fusi L, Gordon H (1990) Twin pregnancy complicated by single intrauterine death: Problems and outcome with conservative management. *British Journal of Obstetrics and Gynaecology* **97**:511–516.

20 Anderson RL, Golbus MS, Curry CJ, Callen PW, Hastrup WH (1990) Central nervous system damage and other anomalies in surviving fetus following second trimester antenatal death of co-twin: Report of four cases and a review of the literature. *Prenatal Diagnosis* **10**:513–518.

21 Fusi L, McParland P, Fisk N, Nicolini U, Wigglesworth J (1991) Acute twin–twin transfusion: A possible mechanism for brain-damaged survivors after intrauterine death of a monochorionic twin. *Obstetrics and Gynecology* **78**:517–520.

22 Bejar R, Vigliocco G, Gramajo H *et al.* (1990) Antenatal origin of neurologic damage in newborn infants. II. Multiple gestations. *American Journal of Obstetrics and Gynecology* **162**:1230–1236.

23 Skelly H, Marivate M, Norman R, Kenoyer G, Martin R (1982) Consumptive coagulopathy following fetal death in a triplet pregnancy. *American Journal of Obstetrics and Gynecology* **142**:595–601.

24 Romero R, Duffy TP, Berkowitz RL *et al.* (1984) Prolongation of a preterm pregnancy complicated by death of a single twin *in utero* and disseminated intravascular coagulation. *New England Journal of Medicine* **310**:772–774.

25 Levine W, Rosengart M, Siegler A (1962) Spontaneous correction of hypofibrinogenemia with fetal death *in utero*. *Obstetrics and Gynecology* **19**:551–555.

59

Labor: An Overview

PHILIP J. STEER

THE PURPOSE OF INTRAPARTUM CARE

When asked this question, contributors to this section gave an interesting variety of answers. One considered that it was to ensure the delivery of the fetus in optimal condition for gestation while minimizing the potential hazards of childbirth and any underlying pathology to the mother; a very medical approach. Another also put this aspect first, but went on to mention easing the physical and emotional burden on the parturient and her husband, and the creation of a healthy family. A third said it was the reassurance and guidance of the woman and her partner, and put identification of abnormalities in labor second. When considering the place of birth, the first said hospital predominantly, the second said home intrapartum care and delivery was discouraged, while the third said that 40% of births in his area took place at home, and that 60% of births were supervised by midwives and family doctors.

These answers illustrate the current tension between the medical and midwifery models of care. The former declares that labor is only ever normal in retrospect (i.e. all labors should be considered a complication waiting to happen until proved otherwise), whereas the latter says that most labors are normal and should be treated as such, lest negative thoughts impair the natural process. Doctors tend to intervene surgically in labor because they are trained to do so, because they are afraid of litigation, because they have a heavy workload with conflicting demands, and because they have a perverse financial incentive to do so[1] – obstetricians are often paid more for surgical intervention than for normal delivery, and even if they are not, an operative delivery taking at the most an hour is much more cost-effective for the physician (although not for the patient or hospital) than the often protracted process of natural birth taking up to a day. Midwives, on the other hand, sometimes miss abnormalities in their ardent desire that things will be normal, are sometimes reluctant to recommend intervention because they will lose control of the case, and are less likely to be able to provide continuity of care because they commonly work in large teams (often because of their own family commitments).

Perhaps the only sensible compromise in this situation is to expect a positive outcome to labor, while retaining an awareness that the negative can sometimes happen ('accentuate the positive, but do not eliminate the negative', with apologies to Cole Porter). A positive, reassuring but vigilant attitude is surely even more important in maternity care than in any other branch of medicine.

THE PATTERN OF INTRAPARTUM CARE

There is currently no evidence to suggest that any particular pattern of care is associated with a better perinatal outcome than any other. The first contributor quoted above works in a country which spends much more on maternity care than the third, but which has substantially higher perinatal mortality rates. In particular, there is no documented evidence that home birth in low-risk cases (probably at least 70% of the population in most developed countries) is associated with higher perinatal mortality rates; indeed, some have argued that morbidity is lower with home birth because of lower rates of surgical intervention and cross-infection. What therefore must take priority is delivering care which is appropriate to the individual mother. Even in the USA, probably home to the archetypal medical model, demand for birthing centers with all the comforts of home has grown substantially over the last 15 years, and the practice of midwifery is also increasing. In Holland, the midwifery model is still pre-eminent, although there has been a gradual shift to more hospital births over the last 20 years. In the UK, midwifery reached a low point in the mid-1970s, when medical intervention peaked (e.g. with a national induction rate of 45%), but with the widespread introduction of midwifery teams with improved continuity, and a named caseload with full responsibility for total care in normal cases, has developed renewed confidence. Perhaps most important has been the consumer revolution, with women wanting and demanding a greater participation in decisions affecting their care. This has been facilitated by increasing moves to patient held records, which is now official government policy for maternity records in the UK. It is spreading to include a parent held pediatric record, and may become universal with the patient held electronic patient record being developed by the National Health Service Management Executive.

Another current issue is cost-effectiveness; the employment of expensively trained medical staff to perform normal deliveries is hard to defend and even harder to pay for. While this may be a common pattern in a free market system, there are increasing moves to 'managed competition', in which audit and cost considerations play an important part. The widespread publication of birth statistics, including cesarean section rates, will result in a better informed and increasingly vocal public.

THE NEED FOR WOMEN TO HAVE CHOICE

The first aim in intrapartum care should therefore be to select women without obvious risk factors, and offer them choice. They should be able to choose their birth attendant, the place of birth and their mode of birth. There can be no justification for arbitrary rules, and if normal women wish to deliver on a bean bag on the floor surrounded by their family, or in a birthing pool with their partner, they should be allowed to do so. There is no evidence that they are exposing themselves or their baby to undue risk, and there is some evidence that a supportive emotional atmosphere is beneficial to the progress in labor. In the past, many women have been subjected to demeaning procedures such as pubic shaving and routine enemas, without a shred of evidence that they were beneficial; such practices have fortunately been discontinued in most institutions.

On the other hand, many women wish to avail themselves of effective pain relief. In the UK over the last 10 years, a remarkably consistent 30% of women in their first labors have elected to have epidural anesthesia. The provision of a safe service requires a hospital setting with full staffing and equipment for maternal resuscitation, in case of a rare complication. For this reason alone, hospital maternity units are likely to remain popular. Even apparently normal nulliparas who choose to have their babies at home have a 25% chance of needing transfer to hospital for specialized help, and therefore adequately trained paramedical staff need to be available for such emergencies (and for high-risk women who have some sudden complication at home).

ELECTRONIC FETAL MONITORING: YES OR NO? (see Chapter 62)

Electronic fetal monitoring (EFM) remains a conundrum. Despite its many advocates, it has proved impossible to demonstrate its effectiveness conclusively. In addition, the contribution of perinatal events to long-term handicap is now believed to be much less than was at one time thought. There is some optimism that this might help to reduce the tide of litigation which is engulfing obstetric practice in many Western countries, but it also reduces the apparent need for detailed and continuous monitoring in low-risk cases. Again, it is important that the parents be involved in the decision about the way their baby will be monitored in labor. Many obstetricians will have experienced the trauma of parents who decline EFM and who then have an unexpected stillbirth. On the other hand, there can be little doubt that EFM is responsible for many unnecessary cesarean sections, especially in those units where fetal blood sampling and pH estimation is not routinely practiced. The indications for EFM are clearly spelled out in the chapter on fetal distress (Chapter 62); if there are no such indications, the woman's choice must be paramount. For the professionals' sake, however, clear records of her choice, and the reasons for it, should be kept. If the woman has risk factors but declines monitoring, explanation of the need for EFM should be clearly given and its use firmly advised. However, her choice must be respected, and there is no place for compromising other aspects of her care if she refuses advice on any particular issue.

Choice should also be extended to women with complications. As explained in the chapter on breech delivery (Chapter 13), there is no scientific proof that cesarean section for a preterm infant in breech presentation results in a better outcome for the child, although most obstetricians practise operative delivery in this situation. It may be difficult to share this uncertainty with a couple at a time of great stress; but not to do so removes from them the option of choosing a vaginal birth should they prefer it. This is particularly important at 24–26 weeks gestation, when the prognosis for the child is very poor and the morbidity from a vertical incision in the uterus very considerable. The physician's first duty is to his or her patient, not to his or her self-esteem.

ACTIVE OR EXPECTANT MANAGEMENT OF LABOR (see Chapter 61)

The active management of labor, like EFM, has its passionate devotees. However, like EFM, the scientific evidence for its superiority is lacking. While there is little doubt that use of oxytocin in labors progressing more slowly than average shortens labor, the evidence that the mode of delivery is affected is conflicting. Certainly, the risks of inadvertent uterine hyperstimulation are considerable, and inappropriate use of oxytocics is the single most common cause of litigation in obstetrics. A study from my own unit[1] showed that even if the cervix was dilating at less than 1 cm every 2 h, 50% of women still achieved a vaginal delivery without the use of oxytocics. An editorial in the *Lancet* in 1988[2] commented: 'since 50% of the untreated control group achieved a vaginal delivery, the conservative approach remains a valid clinical option. At present, low dose oxytocin infusion with careful assessment of uterine activity is the best policy in most cases.' The need for cautious, low-dose oxytocin infusion was reinforced by the American College of Obstetricians and Gynecologists in 1987.[3] Certainly, women should not be sold active management on the basis that it has proven medical benefit for themselves if the real reason for using it is to speed labor and thus economize on staff time. On the other hand, many women in desultory labor, or with spontaneous prelabor rupture of the membranes, wish to 'get on with it', and there is no reason why their views should not be the deciding factor.

INDUCTION OF LABOR (see Chapter 60)

The major factors influencing the outcome of induced labor are parity and the state of the cervix. Failed induction should be a rarity in parous women, and is uncommon in nulliparas provided the cervix is favorable (a Bishop score of 6 or more). In such women, induction of labor can be undertaken with confidence if there are medical indications (which probably do not exist in more than about 5% of pregnancies), or if the woman requests it for social reasons. Following an era in which so-called medical indications were said to exist in more than half of all pregnancies in some institutions, it would seem perverse if the expertise in induction of labor thus gained should be denied to women who wish to take advantage of it for reasons that to them are compelling. In nulliparous women with an unfavorable cervix, two (small) doses of vaginal prostaglandin E_2 24 h apart can be tried; if they do not precipitate labor or improve the ripeness of the cervix, the indications for induction should be critically reviewed.

OPERATIVE DELIVERY (see Chapters 65, 66 and 67)

The competition between the vacuum extractor and forceps continues; the former causes less maternal trauma but the latter is more often successful at achieving delivery. Perhaps the priority is that the operator should know thoroughly the indications for, and the hazards of, the procedure used ('it's not what you do, it's the way that you do it', with apologies again to Cole Porter). Cesarean section has become ubiquitous; in some South American countries, the incidence is said to have reached 80%.[4] Rates above 20% seem hard to defend; above 30% impossible. A return to rates below 10% seems unlikely, given the remarkable safety of the modern procedure, medicolegal pressures, and the reluctance of most women to put up with prolonged labor. However, it should not be forgotten that delivery by emergency cesarean section increases maternal morbidity and mortality four- or five-fold – and for the unfortunate few this is not only a statistical concept.

Therefore, if cesarean sections are to be performed, safety must remain the top priority. For this reason, regional blockade should be used for anesthesia whenever possible (in at least 80% of cases). The evidence that they minimize mortality and morbidity is overwhelming; they also provide a much more satisfactory birth experience for most parents. Routine prophylactic antibiotics are also of proven benefit. There is also an increasing awarenenss of the importance of prophylactic subcutaneous heparin, particularly in the obese patient.

REFERENCES

1 Bidgood KA, Steer PJ (1987) A randomized control study of oxytocin augmentation of labour. 1. Obstetric

outcome. *British Journal of Obstetrics and Gynaecology* **94**:512–517.

2 Editorial (1988) How actively should dystocia be treated?. *Lancet* **i**:160–160.

3 American College of Obstetricians and Gynecologists (1987) Technical Bulletin No. 110, Washington, DC, November.

4 King JE (1993) Obstetric intervention and the financial imperative. *British Journal of Obstetrics and Gynaecology* **100**:303–304.

60

Labor Induction Including Pregnancy Termination for Fetal Anomaly

IAN Z. MACKENZIE

DEFINITIONS

Labor Induction

Labor induction is the initiation of uterine contractions prior to their spontaneous onset, leading to cervical dilatation and effacement and delivery of the baby. The term generally refers to the third trimester and, occasionally, to the last 3 weeks of the second trimester, when fetal survival is an anticipated outcome.

Termination of Pregnancy

This is the removal of a pregnancy, generally before 24 weeks gestation, when sustained fetal survival is not considered a possibility either because of extreme fetal immaturity or a congenital anomaly not compatible with sustained extrauterine life.

INDUCTION OF LABOR: INDICATIONS

Labor is induced when delivery of the pregnancy will be of benefit to the health of the fetus or mother or both. Induction of labor or abortion excludes those situations where it is considered more expedient to maternal and/or fetal safety and well-being to deliver the pregnancy by cesarean section or hysterotomy.

Some general categories and specific indications are illustrated in **Table 1**.

The specific definitions and relative importance of these indications, as well as obstetricians' attitudes, vary considerably: for example, 'post-term' may be defined as a gestation of any length beyond 40 weeks; cephalopelvic disproportion may be managed by early induction at 38 weeks gestation or ignored in the belief that spontaneous labor, even post-term, is to be preferred and results in a more favorable outcome. Some obstetricians consider that cervical state determines the timing of induction, while others acknowledge that there is often little relationship between cervical favorability and either maternal health and fetal health or gestational age. The indications for terminating pregnancy are based on legal constraints and, at the more advanced gestations, are largely confined to those cases with abnormalities that would result in an inability to maintain sustained extrauterine life.

The decision about which method(s) to use for inducing labor or terminating pregnancy is influenced by a variety of factors, including pregnancy gestation, maternal health and parity, indication for induction or termination, any primary or secondary pregnancy complications, significant previous labor or delivery complications, fetal health, lie and presentation, cervical condition, maternal preference and obstetric unit facilities.

METHODS OF INDUCING LABOR

Cervical condition, including form, consistency and dilatation, appears to exert the most significant influ-

Table 1
Indications for inducing labor

Maternal reasons		Fetal reasons		Social reasons
Evident	Theoretical	Evident	Theoretical	
Deteriorating health	Hypertension	Macrosomia	Prolonged pregnancy	Maternal care provision,
renal	Ruptured membranes	Growth deficiency	Growth deficiency	e.g. blood cross-
hypertension	Fetopelvic disproportion	Diabetes	Diabetes	matching
autoimmune	Maternal height	Hydramnios	Breech	Fetal care provision,
malignancy	Fetal death	Red cell	Isoimmunization	e.g. fetal surgery
psychological	Previous cesarean	isoimmunization	Multiple pregnancy	Staff availability,
	section	Unstable lie	Antepartum hemorrhage	e.g. anesthesia
Diabetic instability		Antepartum	Ruptured membranes	Domestic provision,
Intrauterine infection		hemorrhage	Previous obstetric	e.g. husband at home
Coagulopathy		Infection	history	
Abruptio placentae				
Discomfort (multiples)				
Hydramnios				

ence upon induced labor outcome and in consequence the most appropriate method to use. The methods presently used include those that rely upon mechanical stimulation to provoke cervical effacement, dilatation and uterine contractility, those that employ pharmacological agents to modify cervical form, those that stimulate uterine contractions to establish labor, and those that employ a combination of methods. As a general principle, the simplest inductions, those which probably precede the spontaneous onset of labor by a few hours to a day or two, rely upon mechanical techniques alone, while the most difficult inductions are often managed with pharmacological agents, frequently involving more than one drug and combined with a mechanical stimulus. **Table 2** gives an outline of the various methods used.

As a prelude to induction, a final check should be made to ensure that the indication to induce still pertains and any specific labor management that may be required as a consequence of the indication should be reaffirmed. Immediately prior to the induction, whichever method is used, palpation of the abdomen should confirm the anticipated fetal lie and presentation: an induction should not proceed if the fetal lie is not longitudinal without prior agreed arrangements (see Chapter 14). The fetal heart rate should be checked, if preferred by electronic equipment, to confirm that the fetus is in a satisfactory condition.

Cervical condition is probably the most important consideration when deciding which induction method should be used. Bishop's pelvic scoring system[1] provides the basis for cervical assessment for induction and other systems have been described which detail minor variations upon his assessment.[2–4] **Table 3** illustrates the components of the Bishop pelvic scoring system.

Induction When the Cervix is Very Unfavorable (Bishop score <5)

This can present a major problem, especially in nulliparas; rarely is it a problem for multiparas, except occasionally for those women previously delivered by cesarean section.

During the last 15 years, the concept of cervical ripening or priming has gained momentum and involves treatment to render the cervix more favorable followed by a formal induction method. The distinction between ripening and labor induction is artificial, making a subdivision between the latent prelabor phase and active acceleratory phase. Such a subdivision may encourage the idea of abandoning the attempt to induce labor if cervical ripening is not easily achieved; such an approach to management must question the initial indication to induce labor.

Ripening may be achieved either medically or mechanically. Three principles of management have been explored using pharmacological agents in this situation: those that primarily stimulate uterine contractions (oxytocin), those that modify the cervix and stimulate uterine contractions (prostaglandins), and those that influence cervical form and consistency, by modifying the cervical ground-substance without seemingly provoking any change in myometrial contractility (estrogens, antiprogestins, relaxin, DHEAS). All three groups of substances may be used in isolation, or in combination with other modalities of treatment.

Prostaglandins

Powerful oxytocics at all stages of gestation, both prostaglandin E_2 (PGE$_2$) and $F_{2\alpha}$ (PGF$_{2\alpha}$), have been used,

Table 2
An outline of methods which are used and have been explored for the induction of labor

Cervical state	Induction methods			
Unfavorable cervix (nulliparas score < 5)	Medical	Myometrial stimulants	Prostaglandins Oxytocin	Followed by amniotomy and further oxytocic
		Cervical modifying drugs	Prostaglandins (?) Estrogens Relaxin DHEAS Antiprogestins	Followed by amniotomy and/or oxytocic
	Mechanical	Bougies Hygroscopic tents Catheters and balloons		Followed by oxytocic and/or amniotomy
Moderately favorable cervix (all multiparas and nulliparas score 5–8)	Mechanical	Amniotomy	Followed by oxytocic immediately or after a variable delay	
	Medical	Oxytocin (i.v.)	Followed by amniotomy immediately or after a variable delay – usually < 6 h	
		Prostaglandin (oral or vaginal)	Followed by amniotomy after 3 h and i.v. oxytocin after a further 3 h	
			Or repeated prostaglandins and amniotomy or i.v. oxytocin if necessary	
Favorable cervix (scores > 8)	Mechanical	Sweep and stretch	Followed by amniotomy and/or i.v. oxytocin or oral prostaglandins	
		Amniotomy (high or low)	Followed after 4–6 h by i.v. oxytocin or oral prostaglandins	

Table 3
Bishop's pelvic scoring system for the assessment of induced labor outcome

Score	0	1	2	3
Station of presenting part	−3	−2	−1, 0	+1
Cervical dilatation (cm)	closed	1–2	3–4	5+
Cervical effacement (%)	0–39	40–59	60–79	80+
Cervical consistency	firm	medium	soft	
Cervical position in pelvis	posterior	mid-position	anterior	
			Total score =	

Total score is the summation of the scores of the five criteria.

although there are fewer studies reported using $PGF_{2\alpha}$. Various synthetic prostaglandin analogs have been explored for pregnancy termination and in cases of fetal death, but have been avoided for labor induction with a viable fetus, due to uncertainty over effects upon the fetus and neonate. When the cervix is unripe, local administration routes are most applicable, as illustrated in **Figure 1**. Oral and intravenous administration (see later) can be used, but side-effects are frequent with the doses required to achieve clinical benefit.

Extra-amniotic infusion or instillation

With prior vulval and vaginal toilet, and using aseptic techniques, a self-retained 14 or 16 gauge Foley's catheter

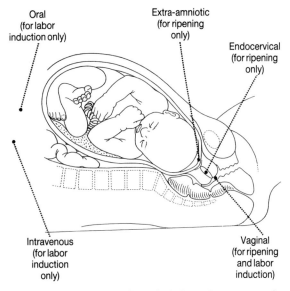

Figure 1. Prostaglandin administration routes for cervical ripening before labor and for labor induction.

is guided either by the vaginal examining fingers or under direct vision using a Cusco's bivalve speculum and swan-necked forceps, through the cervical canal. Once in place, and with the balloon distended with 20–50 ml sterile isotonic saline, the catheter is connected to an infusion pump. PGE_2 solution is infused into the extra-amniotic space at 20–150 μg/h, with 10 μg/h incremental increases at 15 min intervals as necessary using a concentration of 1.5–5 μg/ml.[5,6] The infusion is maintained until the catheter is expelled into the vagina, at which point labor is usually establishing. Amniotomy may be performed then or delayed until later. Oxytocin augmentation (see later) may be started 3 h or more after discontinuing the prostaglandin infusion. Inadvertent perforation of the fetal membranes is a disadvantage and disturbance of a previously unsuspected placenta previa may provoke excessive hemorrhage, requiring immediate cesarean section.

An alternative approach is single bolus instillation of prostaglandins using a disposable polyethylene catheter (e.g. Nelaton) introduced into the extra-amniotic space as described above. PGE_2 240–500 μg in 7–10 ml viscous gel is injected and the catheter withdrawn.[7,8] Subsequent management is as described for the infusion technique.

$PGF_{2\alpha}$ 3–10 μg/min infusion or 5 mg in viscous gel by single instillation has been described, but there is relatively little experience reported with this compound.

Endocervical instillation

An introducing catheter is passed into the cervical os and PGE_2 500–1000 μg in 2–4 ml in viscous gel is discharged into the endocervical canal.[9,10] Subsequent management is as described for the extra-amniotic instillation approach. There must be considerable doubt about the precise location of the gel after initial injection, with some probably reaching the extra-amniotic space and some leaking into the vagina. Attempts have been made to confine the drug to the cervical canal using a system of balloons, but the benefits of the system have yet to be demonstrated.[11] The disadvantages of the extra-amniotic approach should be avoided using endocervical instillation, but otherwise the results are virtually the same.

Vaginal instillation

Many different vehicles including dry tablets,[12] wax pessaries,[13] viscous gels,[14] non-biodegradable hydrogel polymers,[15] and water'soluble polymers,[16] incorporating many different doses, have been tried. There is no single most appropriate protocol to advocate. Published results suggest that PGE_2 2–5 mg in biodegradable pessaries and gels and PGE_2 5–10 mg in the non-biodegradable formulations as a single instillation are appropriate, that the lower dose is probably as effective as the higher dose, and that a latent period of 12 h is necessary in many cases to achieve the desired clinical effect upon the cervix to improve the outcome of labor before formal induction is performed if required.[17] Some protocols use repeated prostaglandin treatments at 6 h intervals for three or more doses; others describe amniotomy and oxytocin titration 15 h after a single prostaglandin treatment unless labor has already supervened.

Repeated small doses of PGE_2 0.5 mg at 2–3 h intervals have been used,[18,19] but have not been widely adopted. It appears that tachyphylaxis may occur in those women with a resistant cervix and this approach does not improve outcome. Personal experience using a second prostaglandin treatment 15 h after the initial dose, compared with immediate intravenous oxytocin titration and amniotomy if possible, indicates that no benefit accrues from repeated prostaglandin treatments, but results in a delay in delivery.[20,21]

Prostaglandin $F_{2\alpha}$ 25–50 mg in viscous gel has also been studied, but the objective evidence available suggests that it is less efficient that PGE_2 although it has demonstrable benefits over placebo.[22,23]

Oxytocin

Oxytocin may be given by intravenous infusion as described later (see p. 1046) or as buccal tablets of 50 units of demoxytocin[24] or oxytocin citrate 100 units increasing to 400 units[25] at 30 min intervals. Intramuscular injections and nasal sprays have been used but have now been abandoned. Controlled studies have indicated that oxytocin is not very effective when the cervix is unfavorable when compared with local prostaglandins.[24,26] Prior to the introduction of prostaglandins, inductions were managed by infusions or buccal courses over an 8–15 h period with a break overnight and repeated the next day and as often as necessary until labor was induced, or the attempt at induction abandoned.

Estrogens

Estradiol 150–300 mg in viscous gel extra-amniotically[27–29] or endocervically or vaginally[30] or estradiol 10 mg intramuscularly[31] and estriol 15–25 mg in viscous gel extra-amniotically,[32,33] can provide improvement in cervical scores with minimal myometrial stimulation. When formal induction is performed 12–24 h later, there appears to be little improvement in the outcome of labor. However, since estradiol has a tenfold higher estrogenic potency than estriol and there was a considerable dosage range in these studies, the true value of estrogens for cervical ripening remains uncertain.

Dehydroepiandrosterone sulfate

Intravenous dehydroepiandrosterone sulfate (DHEAS), which is transformed into estrogens in the fetoplacental unit, has been explored as a possible cervical ripening agent, achieving effacement without inducing uterine contractions. The results were not encouraging when DHEAS 100 mg injected intravenously twice a week from 38 weeks gestation was compared with placebo[34] and the concept has received little further attention.

Relaxin

Like DHEAS, this has been studied in the human, using purified porcine relaxin 1–4 mg in viscous gel vaginally[35] or endocervically[36] in the hope that it has the same properties as exhibited in certain animal species. To date, there have been no well-conducted trials to determine its value for ripening the unfavorable cervix and enhancing the outcome of induced labor without stimulating uterine activity, and more studies enabling a critical scientific assessment to be made are required before considering it to be of any clinical value.

Antiprogestins

The antiprogestional agent mifepristone (RU486), 200 mg orally, has been given daily for 2 days prior to surgical induction and has been shown to produce significant cervical ripening and frequently to induce labor when compared with placebo.[37] Experience using this drug to date is extremely limited and there must be some uncertainty about the overall safety for the fetus and neonate. However, the prospects of this drug revolutionizing labor induction in the future are considerable.

Catheters and balloons

Dilatation, and to a lesser extent effacement, can be produced by the introduction through the cervical canal of a catheter with an inflatable balloon. Using aseptic precautions, the catheter is introduced most easily using the lithotomy position. The catheter is held in swan-necked forceps and guided into the cervical os either along the two vaginal examining fingers, or under direct vision using a Cusco's speculum. The catheter only needs to be introduced just above the level of the internal cervical os and the balloon distended with 30–50 ml sterile isotonic saline. It should be spigotted and may either be left free or connected to a 'weight' to provide traction to the catheter and hold the distended balloon against the internal cervical os to enhance effacement and dilatation.[38,39] Once adequate dilatation has been achieved, the catheter will pass through the cervix and the balloon will present at the vulva. Thereafter, the induction can be advanced either by low amniotomy or administration of an oxytocic (see later). Intrauterine infection is a theoretical risk, which probably increases with prolonged retention of the catheter. A careful watch should be kept on maternal pulse and temperature. There seems little place for this method if prostaglandins are available, although when successful the improvement in cervical condition has generally occurred without significant uterine activity, which would reduce the chances of fetal distress being provoked in the at-risk case.

Bougies

Rubber bougies 7 × 30 mm passed through the cervix into the extra-amnotic space have been used and can produce improvements in cervical condition and may occasionally induce labor[40] This does not appear to be an efficient method and infection is a potential hazard, since 18–24 h are frequently necessary before any physiological benefit accrues.

Hygroscopic tents

Compared with their use for therapeutic abortion, they have been used relatively little for term labor induction. Insertion of the tent is best achieved using the lithotomy position and the cervix exposed with a Cusco's speculum. Aseptic procedures should be followed and the tent introduced into the cervical canal using swan-necked forceps or sponge-holders; one or more tents may be inserted as considered appropriate according to cervical state. A period of 12 h is generally needed to provide the required improvement in cervical condition. If labor does not start, amniotomy and/or oxytocin administration can be used to establish labor. Both natural inert laminaria tents[41] and compressed synthetic polyvinyl alcohol polymer sponges impregnated with 450 mg magnesium sulfate[42] have been tried, the latter apparently inducing their effect in fewer hours than the former. Compared with the pharmacological approaches, there has been relatively little work exploring the value of these newer tents and so firm conclusions are impossible. However, infection remains a concern if the attempt to induce is prolonged.

Induction When the Cervix is Moderately Favourable (Bishop score 5–8)

Oxytocin

Buccal

Buccal oxytocin citrate 100–400 units every 30 min,[25] or demoxytocin 50 units at 30 min intervals[24] as tablets held under the tongue to allow the oxytocin to be absorbed across the buccal mucous membrane, is not widely used because of fears of unpredictable absorption and uterine response and has thus largely been abandoned.

Intravenous infusion

Present-day intravenous infusions of oxytocin have largely been based on the work of Turnbull and Anderson.[43] Although originally given at a constant low-dose infusion at less than 10 mU/min, this has been replaced by titrated doses, determined by the intensity and frequency of the uterine contraction pattern. The rate is then commonly determined using basic clinical observations of contraction rate, duration and intensity assessed by clinical staff who alter the infusion rate using a crude compression switch or a mechanical and latterly electronic drip counter or infusion pump. Automatic infusion pumps governed by intrauterine contraction pressure have also been explored (**Figure 2**).

• *Clinically determined infusion rates*

Mechanically controlled peristaltic drip counters are almost certainly safer than gravity-feed drip counters, which are influenced by changes in pressure at the venous access point; an alternative is the mechanical syringe pump.[44] Infusion solutions vary between oxytocin 5–20 units/1000 ml saline, N/5 dextrose-saline, or 5% dextrose solution. Infusion rates normally start at 1–4 mU/min and increase variably,[45] arithmetically[46] or logarithmically[47] at 15–30 min intervals often to a maximum of around 32 mU/min or until satisfactory labor has been established, which on occasions may be much higher.[47] Most workers consider that the rate required to establish labor should be maintained into the second stage, and increased once the third stage of labor is reached, and maintained for approximately 1 h following delivery of the placenta and membranes. A modification was suggested, to reduce the chances of unnecessarily overdosing the patient, by giving 1 min infusions every 10 min;[48] this approach has not been widely adopted.

• *Automatically controlled infusion rates*

To eliminate the vagaries of human assessment of uterine contractions by repeated fundal palpation, an automatic open-loop infusion system was devised, which controls the infusion rate by a continuous objective measure of intrauterine pressure using a transcervical intrauterine pressure catheter.[49] Once contractions are adequate, the rate is controlled manually. Subsequent modifications have been introduced.[50,51] The more recent modification incorporates a closed-loop feedback system which allows a decrease in infusion rate which the earlier systems did not permit; it was anticipated that overall doses of oxytocin administered would be reduced, and avoidance of overdosage could more easily be guaranteed. Dosage rates with these systems are essentially similar to those using manual control. In a prospective randomized study, Steer et al.[52] demonstrated a marked reduction in total and mean maximum oxytocin infused with the automated system compared with the non-automated peristaltic pump, while Gibb et al.[53] concluded no difference existed in a non-randomized trial. Despite the apparent enhanced safety features, the automated systems have not found wide acceptance, probably due at least in part to patient resistance. More work is required to assess the possible advantages of these systems.

The place of amniotomy in inductions using intravenous oxytocin varies. Most obstetricians combine the two, with low amniotomy followed immediately (or within 1 h) by intravenous oxytocin titration, while some advocate a delay of 4–6 h. The titrated infusion of oxytocin can be started and amniotomy delayed until contractility is established in cases where the pre-

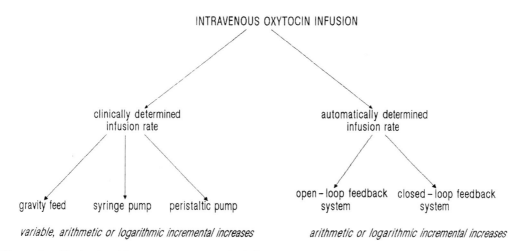

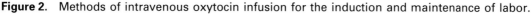

Figure 2. Methods of intravenous oxytocin infusion for the induction and maintenance of labor.

senting part is very mobile at or above the pelvic brim; such a method should reduce the chances of cord prolapse or malpresentation occurring at amniotomy.

Prostaglandins

Oral administration

This is most appropriate with a favorable cervical score. PGE_2 0.5 mg tablets taken hourly with an incremental increase of 0.5 mg every 2 h to a maximum of 2.0 mg/h should establish labor in most cases; some advocate half-hourly medication.[54] Treatment may be continued for a maximum of 6 h or maintained as long as necessary to establish labor. Amniotomy may be performed before prostaglandin treatment, when cervical dilatation starts to occur, when labor begins to establish, or after 6 h. Some clinicians favor leaving the membranes intact unless rupturing them is indicated for other reasons. $PGF_{2\alpha}$ is not used orally for labor induction.

Intravenous infusions

These are not widely used because of the gastrointestinal side-effects and local erythema at the infusion site associated with their use. Infusions usually start at PGE_2 0.1–0.5 μg/min or $PGF_{2\alpha}$ 3–5 μg/min remaining constant or increasing arithmetically or logarithmically at 30 min intervals as necessary to a maximum of PGE_2 2–4 μg/min or $PGF_{2\alpha}$ 18–30 μg/min.[55,56] As with oxytocin, the infusion rate may be adjusted using routine clinical criteria, and a peristaltic drip counter, or an automatic feedback loop system. The place of amniotomy when using intravenous prostaglandins is similar to that described for oxytocin.

Vaginally

A single PGE_2 1–3 mg dose administered into the posterior vaginal fornix as a dry tablet, viscous gel or wax pessary, followed by low amniotomy after 3 h will induce labor in approximately 60% of primiparas and 80% of multiparas.[12,13,57] Augmentation can be given with intravenous oxytocin, or repeated prostaglandin treatments at 6 h intervals. Timing of the amniotomy and further oxytocic augmentation is debatable, but most consider that oxytocin should not be administered for at least 3 h after prostaglandin treatment.

Induction When the Cervix is Favorable (Bishop score >8)

Membrane sweep and cervical stretch

This is performed by a simple vaginal examination using a sterile glove, introducing one or two fingers through the cervix and stretching the os. In addition, one of the fingers is swept around the internal surface of the effaced cervix, dislodging the membranes from the cervical surface. This commonly causes no more discomfort than that associated with a vaginal examination in late pregnancy, but occasionally some dysmenorrhea-like pains are provoked which are short-lived. Following this procedure, uterine contractions are frequently stimulated, probably due to the release of endogenous prostaglandins, which either lead immediately to established labor, or provoke labor after a latent period of a few hours. When performed daily for 3 days, labor is induced in 69% of cases, depending upon the degree of cervical favorability at the time of the initial examination.[58] A 'show' and mild short-lived blood-staining frequently occurs during the first few hours following the procedure, whether labor is established or not. If labor does not start, formal amniotomy may be performed.

Low or forewater amniotomy

Abdominal palpation must confirm that the presenting part, head or breech, is either engaged or apparently securely sited in the pelvic brim. Usually performed in the labor suite with the facilities allowing 'sterile' procedures to be performed, the maternal bladder should be emptied by spontaneous voiding immediately before the procedure and ideally the rectum should be empty, if necessary following the prior administration of a rectal suppository or enema. However, the use of suppositories or enemas can be omitted if the patient considers them objectionable. The dorsal or lithotomy position with some mild degree of left lateral tilt is used to reduce the chances of supine hypotension decreasing placental bed blood flow. The decision to use the dorsal or lithotomy position is predominantly dependent upon the skill and experience of the accoucheur and the favorability of the cervix – the latter position generally aids the completion of the amniotomy but causes more distress to the patient. Vulval toilet is performed and vulval drapes may be applied; the use of full gowning procedures and hats and masks has been abandoned by some without apparent compromise to mother or baby.

An initial vaginal examination is performed assessing the condition of the cervix, noting the features described in the Biship's scoring system (**Table 2**), at which time the forewaters are confirmed to be intact. The size and shape of the mid-cavity and outlet of the pelvis is noted. Following a sweep and stretch as described above, if the cervical dilation allows it, the presentation and position of the presenting part are determined, excluding any evidence of low-lying placenta or umbilical cord. The membranes over the presenting part are then ruptured using a pair of toothed forceps, or a purpose-designed instrument such as an amniotomy hook. With tearing of the membranes, amniotic fluid is released, more being released by controlled elevation of the presenting part. A further check is made to ensure the presentation is unchanged, the cord is not palpable, and the position and station of the presenting part are maintained. Finally, the condition of the amniotic fluid is noted and the fetal heart rate checked to ensure there is no evidence of distress. If continuous electronic monitoring is to be used, the preferred electrode can be attached to the most appropriate area of the presenting part before completing the procedure. Labor is then awaited.

The interval between amniotomy and any necessary pharmacological augmentation is variable, ranging from a few minutes to a delay of up to 24 h. Approximately 88% of women with a favorable Bishop score will labor after amniotomy alone.[59] Amniotomy with early intravenous oxytocin infusion, however, produces a significant reduction in women undelivered after 24 h compared with those managed by amniotomy alone.[60–62]

Hindwater amniotomy

This method of inducing labor is now rarely used. The mechanism by which the technique stimulates labor is almost certainly the same as that associated with low amniotomy. It is usually reserved for inductions when the presenting part is high in relation to the pelvic cavity and for cases of hydramnios, aiming to achieve a controlled release of amniotic fluid from a puncture in the membranes above the level of the presenting part to reduce the chances of malpresentation and placental abruption (see Chapter 14 on unstable lie).

Nipple stimulation

Uterine contractions can be induced by mechanical stimulation of the nipples, even to the extent of causing uterine hypertonus.[63,64] Although probably effective, especially in those women with a favorable cervix, and on the point of spontaneous labor, it is difficult to define a quantitative controlled level of stimulation.

Induction in Complicated Circumstances

Intrauterine fetal death

When fetal death occurs, spontaneous labor will usually occur within a few days in the majority of cases. Once the diagnosis of fetal demise has been confirmed, delivery of the baby can be arranged at the request of the woman to relieve emotional distress. There are also medical indications for terminating the pregnancy. If the fetal membranes have ruptured, prolonged retention may result in intrauterine infection, and if the dead fetus is retained for longer than 4 weeks, a consumptive coagulopathy may develop.[65] The methods of achieving evacuation are either mechanical or pharmacological.

Mechanical evacuation

Up to 16 weeks gestational size, evacuation by cervical dilatation and aspiration or morcellation under general or local anesthetic is probably the most expedient management. Some advocate the method at more advanced gestations, but there is little reported in the literature of this approach in cases of fetal death and it will not be considered further.

Prostaglandins

The prostaglandins have revolutionized the management of these cases. The administration routes appropriate in this situation are illustrated in **Figure 3** and include intravenous, extra-amniotic, intramuscular and vaginal, and some protocols described are illustrated in **Table 4**.[68–73] The oral route is not appropriate with the natural or analogous prostaglandins available, since the doses required cause very high rates of side-effects. The intra-amniotic route has been used[66] but may be unwise for two reasons: (1) puncturing the fetal membranes by amniocentesis may enhance the possibility of amniotic fluid embolism, a hazard thought to be more common in cases of fetal death *in utero*,[67] and (2) the risk of intrauterine infection may be increased. The few reports of this method for managing such cases have not, however, observed these problems.

Management is essentially the same whichever protocol is used. A check of the clotting status should be made if fetal death is thought to have occurred at least 3 weeks previously, and appropriate investigations initiated to assist in determining the etiology for those cases where death was unexpected. Progress, once treatment has started, is assessed by vaginal examinations as indicated and adequate analgesia provided according to needs. Delivery of the dead fetus and placenta is similar to that when the fetus is liveborn, although attempts are made to avoid perineal damage if possible. Ergometrine or intramuscular prostaglandin analog should be given to enhance uterine contractility following delivery to reduce the chances of excessive hemorrhage.

Other methods

Prior to the introduction of the prostaglandins, these cases were managed conservatively, or given repeated high doses of estrogens,[74] intra-amniotic injections of hypertonic solutions[75] or, more frequently, repeated high-dose infusions of oxytocin.[76–78] With the advent of the prostaglandins, it now seems inappropriate to consider using any of these other techniques.

Fetal breech presentation

Some obstetricians are of the opinion that when the breech presents, labor should not be induced, and that labor should always be allowed to occur spontaneously; the logic for this philosophy is not clear. If labor is to be induced, the approach to the induction is the same as that when the head presents. There are advocates for radiological pelvimetry, but results of retrospective analyses do not demonstrate any convincing evidence of benefit. There is a view that delaying membrane rupture until labor is well advanced, and the breech well into the pelvis, reduces the chances of cord prolapse. This has not been substantiated. Protocols that use prostaglandins as outlined for general labor induction may offer some advantage in this respect, but this is also speculative.

Previous cesarean section

As with fetal breech presentation, opinions vary over the wisdom of inducing labor in women previously delivered by lower segment cesarean section; the majority appear to consider a previous classical section and previous repeated lower segment sections should usually be considered contraindications to attempting labor. For those who favor an attempt at labor and induction is indicated, the most appropriate method is debated. Some believe it only appropriate to induce labor by low amniotomy, others to limit the oxytocic to low doses of oxytocin, while there are those who do not restrict the method to be used and are prepared to use whichever method seems most suitable from those outlined earlier.

There is widespread agreement that fetopelvic disproportion should not usually be anticipated in a woman entering labor who has been delivered previously by cesarean section, unless there is specific

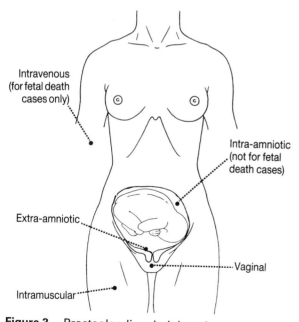

Intravenous (for fetal death cases only)

Intra-amniotic (not for fetal death cases)

Extra-amniotic

Vaginal

Intramuscular

Figure 3. Prostaglandin administration routes used for the induction of labor and abortion in cases of fetal death *in utero* and for pregnancy termination because of fetal abnormality.

Table 4
Examples of prostaglandin administration protocols for evacuation of missed abortion and late fetal death *in utero*

Drug administration protocol	Vomiting	Diarrhea	Expulsion time (h)	Reference
Vaginal PGE$_2$ 20 mg every 3–6 h	87%	70%	14.6	**68**
Vaginal PGE$_2$ 25 mg single instillation + i.v. oxytocin after 15–20 h	31%	8%	14.4	**69**
Vaginal 16, 16-dimethyl-PGE$_1$ 1 mg every 3 h × 3 + i.v. oxytocin after 15–20 h	15%	10%	14.2	**69**
Extra-amniotic PGE$_2$ 1–4 µg/min infusion	29%	0%	10.0±	**70**
Intramuscular 16-phenoxy-PGE$_2$ 500 µg every 4–6 h	48%	48%	12.4	**71**
Intramuscular 15-methyl-PGF$_{2\alpha}$ 125–500 µg every 2 h	52%	59%	8.6	**72**
Intravenous 16-phenoxy-PGE$_2$ 1 µg/min infusion	19%	2%		**73**
Intravenous 16-phenoxy-PGE$_2$ 3 µg/min infusion	38%	14%		**73**

evidence such as a known contracted pelvis secondary to trauma (most commonly associated with horse-riding or road traffic accidents). Prelabor radiological pelvimetry is of unproven value, although frequently used. Management of the induction is either little different from other 'uncomplicated' inductions or conducted with greater caution and monitoring. Continuous electronic monitoring of the fetal heart rate is advocated by many, and continuous intrauterine pressure recording by a smaller number.[79–81] Although logical as a way of anticipating or avoiding scar rupture, the major concern in this situation, experience has not confirmed the benefits of such monitoring.

The pharmaceutical company marketing PGE$_2$ in the UK states that previous cesarean sections are a contraindication to the use of prostaglandins for the induction of labor. However, a recent survey of consultant obstetric units in the UK found that 78% used prostaglandins to induce labor following a previous cesarean section.[81] It has been argued that PGE$_2$ might have advantages in patients with a scarred uterus, since the characteristic contractions provoked by prostaglandins are of low amplitude and theoretically less likely to compromise the scar.[82] More recent work has substantiated that view, comparing pressures generated by prostaglandins and oxytocin in both spontaneous labor and following labor induction.[45]

Scar rupture appears to occur as frequently following spontaneous onset of labor as after prostaglandin and oxytocin-induced labors.[82–84] The combination of prostaglandins and oxytocin possibly increases the risk of rupture.[85]

Multiple pregnancy

When multiple pregnancies are considered in texts or monographs, little attention is paid to the place or method of inducing labor. In a series of 391 twin pregnancies managed in Oxford, labor started spontaneously in 50%, was induced in 37% and elective cesarean section performed in 13% (I.Z. MacKenzie, unpublished data).

The methods previously described for labor induction are equally applicable to twin pregnancies. As with other complicated pregnancy situations, continuous electronic fetal monitoring of both babies is considered by some to be essential. Since postpartum hemorrhage due to uterine hyptonia is a recognized added risk of labor for twin pregnancies, it has been suggested[86] that the prostaglandins might be particularly appropriate.

Complications of Induction of Labor

There are a number of potential hazards for both mother and fetus/neonate from induction of labor, either as a result of initiating labor before spontaneous onset, or as a consequence of the method of induction used. Among the hazards are the following.

Hyponatremia

Hyponatremia may occur as a consequence of intravenous oxytocin infusions and is most likely to occur with prolonged infusions of relatively high doses of oxytocin in dextrose or dilute solutions of saline. This can result in maternal fluid retention, electrolyte derangement, coma and death.[87] Similar derangements to neonatal biochemistry leading to neonatal seizures can occur in severely disturbed cases.[88]

'Failed' induction

There is no universally accepted definition of 'failed induction'. It should perhaps be reserved for those cases where the cervix does not dilate beyond 3 cm despite adequate and appropriate oxytocic stimulation over a reasonable period of time, perhaps 8 h in a nullipara and 4 h in a multipara; there should be no fetopelvic disproportion. It is most likely to occur in nulliparas with an unfavorable cervix at the time of induction. It is a rare complication in multiparas except those whose only previous delivery was by cesarean section. In the high-risk group of nulliparas with an unfavorable cervix, failed inductions probably occur in 15–35% of cases induced with intravenous oxytocin, and 3–5% induced with local prostaglandins.

Uterine hyperstimulation

Hypersystole and hypertonia occur during both spontaneous and induced labors. The true incidences are unclear, but hypertonus occurs in about 1:500 labors, whether induced or spontaneous. The prostaglandins classicially provoke low-amplitude contractions at 1–2 min intervals which are often subclinical and generally do not cause fetal or maternal disturbance.

If hypertonus occurs, it can be counteracted by tocolytic administration. Intravenous injections and aerosol inhalation have been used,[89] although the latter route is of uncertain benefit.[90] This management strategy can either be used to treat the acute episode and allow labor to continue if the fetus is not distressed and normal uterine contractility is restored, or as a first aid measure while preparing for emergency cesarean section.

Fetal distress

Fetal distress should be expected to occur more frequently during induced than spontaneous labor, since some induction indications, such as those for intrauterine growth deficiency, predispose to fetal distress. When diagnosed, management will depend upon circumstances at the time and the identified cause of the distress – such as abruptio placenta, cord prolapse, hyperstimulation, previously suspected placental insufficiency – and tocolytic therapy may be given prior to emergency cesarean section.[89]

Cord prolapse

This occurs most commonly with low amniotomy. It is especially likely to occur when there is a flexed breech presentation, or in cases induced with a high presenting part managed with an oxytocic to stimulate contrac-

tions in which the membranes spontaneously rupture during the stimulation. An urgent operative vaginal delivery may be appropriate if the cervix is fully dilated. However, delivery is usually by emergency cesarean section, with mechanical measures taken to prevent pressure on the cord at the pelvic brim by use of the knee–chest position, or a vaginal examination exerting counter-pressure against the presenting part.

Abruptio placentae

This may occur at any stage of labor, but is most likely to occur when the membranes rupture either spontaneously or at amniotomy, especially in cases of hydramnios. There has been a suggestion that prostaglandins may predispose to this complication when used for labor induction.[91] Only one report has appeared suggesting the relationship, and at present the evidence for such an association is unconfirmed.

Uterine rupture

Extremely uncommon in nulliparas, this complication may occur in any labor whether induced or spontaneous. It is a particular risk in multiparas of high parity and those previously delivered by cesarean section.

Inadvertent preterm delivery

This is a risk with any induction, whichever method is used. With the widespread use of ultrasound examinations in early pregnancy, there is a belief that the incidence has declined. Cases still occur when gestation has been inappropriately assigned by ultrasound measurements.

Hyperbilirubinemia

The incidence of neonatal hyperbilirubinemia is increased following induction with intravenous oxytocin compared with prostaglandin inductions and spontaneous labor.[92,93] Prostaglandins are not associated with increased rates of hyperbilirubinemia, possibly because of their apparent steroidogenic properties.[94]

Hypotonic uterine postpartum hemorrhage

Postpartum hemorrhage is more commonly encountered following induced labor than spontaneous labor.[95] The rate is possibly lower following prostaglandin –

than oxytocin-induced labors; this is yet to be established for certain.

TERMINATION FOR FETAL ABNORMALITY

As with labor induction, evacuation of the uterus can be achieved using pharmacological agents singularly, in combination, or with a mechanical method. The decision over which method to use is made according to pregnancy gestation, as well as unit facilities, and operators' preferences and experience. The techniques described refer to pregnancy termination before 24 weeks gestation.

Unlike labor induction, there are few factors which influence the method of termination to be used. Pre-existing maternal health may be important, expecially if it is important that a general anesthetic be avoided. Patients with a history of hysterotomy or cesarean section often cause anxiety, but in fact such a history has little bearing upon management. The major concern is whether or not postmortem structural examination of the fetus is desirable to establish the cause of death; this is often important in relation to counseling for future pregnancies. The surgical termination method outlined below will not allow the post-abortion confirmation or elucidation of the prenatal diagnosis of any structural abnormalities.

Methods

Dilatation and evacuation

This method, which is widely favored in the USA, may be performed as a day-case under local anesthesia with a cervical block,[96] or under general anesthesia as a single-stage procedure,[97] or a two-stage procedure, the second operation performed to complete the abortion which was initiated the previous day.[98]

The technique used varies from mechanical cervical dilatation up to Hegar 10 followed by compression of the fetal parts with ring forceps and removal with a 10 mm suction curette,[96] to cervical dilatation up to Hegar 22 preceded by multiple insertions of cervical tents for 48 h preoperatively, and morcellation and retrieval of fetal parts using crushing forceps.[99] The procedure is one requiring considerable expertise to ensure cervical damage is reduced to a minimum, uterine wall perforation and bowel damage is not caused, and the entire contents of the uterus have been removed at the initial operation, unless a second operation is planned.

Prostaglandins

This approach is more favored in the UK than dilatation and evacuation with 66% performed using prostaglandins in a nationwide survey in 1982.[100] Four basic administration routes have evolved over the past 15 years: extra-amniotic, intra-amniotic, vaginal and intramuscular (**Figure 3**). The place for each differs marginally, and is essentially determined by gestation and availability of the appropriate prostaglandin analog as well as the physician's preference. Although intravenous prostaglandin administration has been used, the side-effects provoked are severe and the method has largely been abandoned.

Extra-amniotic administration

This route is applicable at any gestation during the second trimester, but is most appropriate up to 18 weeks. PGE_2, $PGF_{2\alpha}$ or an analog may be used with the dosages outlined in **Table 5**. For repeated injections at 2 h intervals or continuous infusions, a self-retained Foley's catheter is passed through the cervix under sterile conditions as described for labor induction and left *in situ* until spontaneously expelled once sufficient cervical dilatation has occurred. With each regime, the concomitant intravenous infusion of oxytocin at 100 mU/min will shorten induction-to-abortion intervals.

Intra-amniotic protocols

As a general principle, the intra-amniotic route has been employed for terminations beyond 15 weeks gestation. Many protocols have been developed over the past 20 years and involve either single instillation of prostaglandins at amniocentesis, or repeated injections through an indwelling transabdominal intra-amniotic catheter inserted through a Tuohy needle at the time of amniocentesis. **Table 5** illustrates some of the protocols developed. By combining a single dose of prostaglandins with 100–200 ml of a hypertonic solution, having removed a similar volume of amniotic fluid, abortion can be reliably induced within 24 h in more than 90% cases. This is particularly useful at the more advanced gestations, since fetal death occurs before expulsion from the uterus, reducing the distress for the patient and the attending staff. However, use of hypertonic saline has been associated with severe maternal side-effects if the solution accidentally enters a maternal vein. Use of hypertonic solutions of urea largely avoided this problem and for a while was widely used in the UK, but appropriate preparations of urea were withdrawn from the market in the UK in the late 1980s. Fetal demise before delivery can be produced by air embolization of the fetal circulation by cord puncture under ultrasound guidance immediately prior to the intra-amniotic injection of prostaglandins, using

Table 5
Examples of prostaglandin administration protocols for the induction of midtrimester abortion

Drug administration protocol	Vomiting	Diarrhea	Abortion time (n)	Reference
Extra-amniotic 15-methyl-PGF$_{2\alpha}$ 1 mg single injection	36%	34%	15.0±	**103**
Extra-amniotic PGE$_2$ 1.5–2.5 mg single injection + i.v. oxytocin after 6 h	45%	17%	14.8	**104**
Extra-amniotic PGE$_2$ 46–333 μg/min infusion	41%	2%	20.5	**101**
Extra-amniotic PGF$_{2\alpha}$ 750 μg/h infusion	25%	—	24.9	**102**
Intra-amniotic PGF$_{2\alpha}$ 10 mg + hypertonic urea	70%	1%	16.3	**106**
Intra-amniotic PGE$_2$ 5–10 mg + i.v. oxytocin at 6 h	39%	5%	14.8	**104**
Intra-amniotic PGF$_{2\alpha}$ 25 + 25 mg every 6 h	53%	15%	19.7	**105**
Intra-amniotic 15-methyl-PGF$_{2\alpha}$ 2.5 mg single injection	42%	24%	20.0±	**103**
Vaginal 12-methyl-PGF$_{2\alpha}$ 1.5 mg every 3 h	67%	70%	14.2	**107**
Vaginal 15-methyl-PGF$_{2\alpha}$ 3 mg single pessary	72%	77%	14.7	**108**
Vaginal 16, 16-dimethyl-PGE$_1$ 1 mg every 3 h × 5	14%	20%	19.3	**109**
Vaginal 16, 16-dimethyl-PGE$_1$ 1 mg every 3 h × 3 + i.v. oxytocin at 6 h	30%	27%	19.5	**110**
Intramuscular 16-phenoxy-PGE$_2$ 1 mg every 8 h	50%	25%	14.8	**111**
Intramuscular 15-methyl-PGF$_{2\alpha}$ 250 μg every 2 h 12 h after laminaria insertion	64%	65%	23.2[a]	**112**
Intramuscular 16-phenoxy-PGE$_2$ 500 μg every 2 h 12 h after laminaria insertion	41%	17%	22.8[a]	**112**

[a] Includes 12 h pretreatment with laminaria tents.

one of the protocols outlined in **Table 5**. However, this is a more difficult technique and correspondingly is not widely used except in centers specializing in the diagnosis of fetal anomaly.

Vaginal administration

Repeated administration of vaginal pessaries of prostaglandins, as shown in **Table 5**, offers a relatively non-invasive method, which can be enhanced by the concomitant intravenous infusion of oxytocin at 100 mU/min. Gastrointestinal side-effects vary with the protocol used. The vaginal route is probably most appropriate up to 18 weeks gestation.

Intramuscular prostaglandins

Repeated intramuscular injections of a prostaglandin analog offer the least invasive approach. This method is most appropriate up to 18 weeks gestation, and the results are similar to those for other routes of administration, although gastrointestinal side-effects are more common (**see Table 5**). Laminaria tents inserted in the cervix 12 h before the start of prostaglandin treatment have been used but do not appear to improve the results.

Prostaglandins and an antiprogestin

The oral administration of the antiprogestational agent, epostane, a 3β-hydroxy steroid dehydrogenase inhibitor or mifepristone (RU 486), the progesterone receptor blocker 600 mg, 24–72 h prior to prostaglandin treatment reduces the induction-to-abortion interval by 40–60% and thus can lower the dose of prostaglandins required with consequent decreased gastro-intestinal side-effects and need for analgesia.[113–115] A product licence in the UK for the use of mifepristone in the second trimester is awaited.

Complications of Late Pregnancy Termination

The incidence of complications occurring after pregnancy termination is low, although it tends to increase with advancing gestation. To some extent, the complications are related to the method of termination used, with some being more common after certain procedures.

INDUCTION OF LABOR AND TERMINATION FOR FETAL ABNORMALITY
Summary of Management Options

Induction of labor

Indications

- See **Table 1**

Methods

- See **Table 2**

Complications

- Hyponatremia (mother and fetus)

- 'Failure'

- Hyperstimulation

- 'Fetal distress'

- Cord prolapse

- Placental abruption

- Uterine rupture

- Preterm delivery (unexpected)

- Neonatal hyperbilirubinemia

- Hypotonic uterine postpartum hemorrhage

Termination for fetal abnormality

Methods

- Dilatation and evacuation

- Prostaglandins:
  - extra-amniotic
  - intra-amniotic
  - vaginal
  - intramuscular

- Prostaglandins and antiprogestin

Complications

- Incomplete abortion

- Excess hemorrhage

- Cervical damage

- Uterine damage

- Coagulopathy

- Infection

Incomplete abortion

Incomplete abortion following medically induced late abortion is influenced by gestation, with 60% being incomplete at 12 weeks, falling to 20% by 19 weeks gestation.[104] Following expulsion of the fetus, the placenta is usually expelled within 2 h. The longer the delay before surgical removal, the greater the rate of excessive bleeding.[116]

Excess hemorrhage

The incidence of excessive hemorrhage (>500 ml) at the time of abortion, whether surgically or medically managed, is in the region of 1%, with 0.5% requiring transfusion. The administration of an oxytocic such as ergometrine 0.5 mg intramuscularly at the time of abortion is believed to reduce the chances of excess blood loss.

Cervical damage

Cervical lacerations may occur with all methods of termination, while cervico-vaginal fistulas or buckethandle lacerations of the cervix requiring surgical repair may occur in cases managed medically, especially with intra-amniotic injections of prostaglandins if given in combination with a hypertonic solution. Post-abortion vaginal examination should be performed to exclude this complication and appropriate repair surgery organized when indicated.

Uterine body damage

Perforation may occur with the surgical approach and rupture of the body with the medical methods: damage is more common with dilatation and evacuation, occurring in 0.2–1.0%.

Coagulopathy

This is provoked by the use of hypertonic solutions but not by the use of prostaglandins alone.[117–119] It has also been described with dilatation and evacuation.[98,120]

Infection

This may occur with both the surgical and medical methods of managing abortion. It is more common if there is a long induction-to-abortion interval with medically induced abortion.

CONCLUSIONS

There is a large variety of methods of inducing labor. The most important factor to influence which method to use is the state of the cervix. The prostaglandins have been shown to improve the outcome of labor induction significantly if the cervix is unfavorable, but are probably of little benefit if the cervix is very favorable. Oxytocin is best given by intravenous infusion, preferably using a mechanical peristaltic pump, and the rate controlled by the quality of uterine contractions. Contractions can be assessed clinically or by use of an intrauterine catheter. For complicated pregnancies, there is insufficient information to recommend a particular method.

Late pregnancy termination is best achieved using prostaglandins locally, combined with oxytocin, or by cervical dilatation and uterine evacuation. Other pharmacological agents have been tried and some could well have a major impact upon both late pregnancy termination and labor induction in the near future.

REFERENCES

1 Bishop EH (1964) Pelvic scoring for elective induction. *Obstetrics and Gynecology* **24**:266–268.

2 Friedman EA, Niswander KR, Bayonet-Rivera NP, Sachtleben MR (1966) Relation of prelabor evaluation to inducibility and the course of labor. *Obstetrics and Gynecology* **28**:495–501.

3 Calder AA, Embrey MP, Hillier K (1974) Extra-amniotic prostaglandin E₂ for the induction of labour at term. *Journal of Obstetrics and Gynaecology of the British Commonwealth* **81**:39–46.

4 Lange AP, Secher NJ, Westergaard JG, Slovgard I (1982) Prelabor evaluation of inducibility. *Obstetrics and Gynecology* **60**:137–147.

5 Calder AA, Embrey MP, Hillier K (1974) Extra-amniotic prostaglandin E₂ for induction of labour at term. *British Journal of Obstetrics and Gynaecology* **81**:39–46.

6 Miller AWF, Mack DS (1974) Induction by extra-amniotic prostaglandins. *Journal of Obstetrics and Gynaecology of the British Commonwealth* **81**:706–708.

7 Calder AA, Embrey MP, Tait T (1977) Ripening of the cervix with extra-amniotic prostaglandin E₂ in viscous gel before induction of labour. *British Journal of Obstetrics and Gynaecology* **84**:264–268.

8 Sims CD, Mellows JH, Spencer PJ, Craft I (1979) Routine induction of labour with extraamniotic prostaglandin E₂ in a viscous gel. *British Journal of Obstetrics and Gynaecology* **86**:329–332.

9 Wingerup L, Andersson K-E, Ulmsten U (1979) Ripening of the cervix and induction of labour in patients at term by single intracervical application of prostaglandin E₂ in viscous gel. *Acta Obstetricia et Gynecologica Scandinavica* **84**:11–14 (suppl.).

10 Ulmsten U, Wingerup L, Belfrage P, Ekman G, Wiqvist N (1982) Intracervical application of prostaglandin gel for induction of term labor. *Obstetrics and Gynecology* **59**:336–339.

11 Atad J, Bornstein J, Petrikovsky B, Calderon I, Sorokin Y, Abramovici H (1990) A non-pharmaceutical ripening of the unfavourable cervix and induction of labor by a novel double balloon device. *Obstetrics and Gynecology* **77**:146–152.

12 Kennedy JH, Stewart P, Barlow DH, Hillan E, Calder AA (1982) Induction of labour: A comparison of a single prostaglandin E₂ vaginal tablet with amniotomy and intravenous oxytocin. *British Journal of Obstetrics and Gynaecology* **89**:704–707.

13 Shepherd JH, Bennett M, Laurence D, Moore F, Sims CD (1981) Prostaglandin vaginal suppositories: A simple and safe approach to the induction of labour. *Obstetrics and Gynecology* **58**:596–600.

14 MacKenzie IZ, Embrey MP (1977) Cervical ripening with intravaginal prostaglandin E₂ gel. *British Medical Journal* **2**:1381–1384.

15 Embrey MP, Graham NB, McNeill ME (1980) Induction of labour with a sustained release prostaglandin E₂ vaginal pessary. *British Medical Journal* **281**:901–902.

16 Arulkumaran S, Adaikan PG, Anandakumar C, Viegas OAC (1989) Comparative study of a two dose schedule of PGE₂ 3 mg pessary and 1700 μg film for

induction of labour in nulliparae with poor cervical score. *Prostaglandins, Leukotrienes and Essential Fatty Acids* **38**:37–41.

17 Walker E, Gordon AJ (1983) Lengths of exposure to prostaglandin E₂ and cervical ripening in primigravidae. *Journal of Obstetrics and Gynecology* **4**:88–89.

18 Liggins GC (1979) Controlled trial of induction of labour by vaginal suppositories containing prostaglandin E₂. *Prostaglandins* **18**:167–172.

19 Hunter IWE, Cato E, Ritchie J (1984) Induction of labor using high dose or low dose prostaglandin vaginal pessaries. *Obstetrics and Gynecology* **63**:418–420.

20 MacKenzie IZ (1981) Clinical studies on cervical ripening. In Ellwood, DA, Anderson ABM (eds), *The Cervix in Pregnancy and Labour*, pp. 161–186. London: Churchill Livingstone.

21 Taylor AVG, Boland J, MacKenzie IZ (1991) A randomised trial to assess the benefits of repeated vaginal prostaglandin treatment for cervical ripening in primiparae with an unfavourable cervix. Unpublished data.

22 MacKenzie IZ, Embrey MP (1979) A comparison of PGE₂ and PGF₂α vaginal gel for ripening the cervix before induction of labour. *British Journal of Obstetrics and Gynaecology* **85**:657–661.

23 Neilson DR, Prins RP, Bolton RN, Mark C, Watson P (1983) A comparison of prostaglandin E₂ gel and prostaglandin F₂α gel for pre-induction cervical ripening. *American Journal of Obstetrics and Gynecology* **146**:526–530.

24 Sorensen SS, Brocks V, Lenstrup C (1985) Induction of labor and cervical ripening by intracervical prostaglandin E₂. *Obstetrics and Gynecology* **65**:110–114.

25 Pentecost AF (1973) The effect of buccal 'Pitocin' on the unripe cervix. *Current Medical Research Opinions* **1**:482–484.

26 Roberts WE, North DH, Speed JE, Martin JN, Palmer SM, Morrison JC (1986) Comparative study of prostaglandin, laminaria, and minidose oxytocin for ripening of the unfavourable cervix prior to induction of labor. *Journal of Perinatalogy* **6**:16–19.

27 Gordon AJ, Calder AA (1977) Oestradiol applied locally to ripen the unfavourable cervix. *Lancet* **ii**:1319–1321.

28 Craft I, Yovich J (1978) Oestradiol and induction of labour. *Lancet* **ii**:208.

29 Tromans PM, Beazley JM, Shenouda PI (1981) Comparative study of oestradiol and prostaglandin E₂ vaginal gel for ripening the unfavourable cervix before induction of labour. *British Medical Journal* **282**:679–681.

30 Magnani M, Cabrol D (1986) Declenchement artificiel du travail par la prostaglandine E₂ après maturation du col par l'estradiol. *Inserm* **151**:109–118.

31 Luther ER, Roux J, Popat R, Gardner A, Gray J, Soubiran E, Korcaz Y (1980) The effect of estrogen priming on induction of labor with prostaglandins. *American Journal of Obstetrics and Gynecology* **137**:351–357.

32 Thiery M, De Grezelle H, Van Kets H, Voorhoof L, Verheugen C, Smis B, Gervis J, Derom R, Martens G (1979) The effect of locally administered estrogen on

the human cervix. *Zeitschrift für Geburtshilfe und Perinatologie* **183**:448–445.

33 Quinn MA, Murphy AJ, Juhn RJP, Robinson HP, Brown JB (1981) A double blind trial of extra-amniotic oestriol and prostaglandin F₂α gel in cervical ripening. *British Journal of Obstetrics and Gynaecology* **88**:644–649.

34 Sasaki K, Nakano R, Kadoya Y, Iwao M, Shima K, Sowa M (1982) Cervical ripening with dehydroepiandrosterone sulphate. *British Journal of Obstetrics and Gynaecology* **89**:195–198.

35 MacLennan AH, Green RC, Bryant-Greenwood GD, Greenwood FC, Seamark RF (1980) Ripening of the human cervix and induction of labor with purified porcine relaxin. *Lancet* **i**:220–223.

36 Evans MI, Dougan MB, Moawad AH, Evans WJ, Bryant-Greenwood GD, Greenwood FC (1983) Ripening of the human cervix with porcine ovarian relaxin. *American Journal of Obstetrics and Gynecololgy* **147**:410–414.

37 Frydman R, Baton C, Lelaidier C, Vial M, Bourget P, Fernandez H (1991) Mifepristone for induction of labour. *Lancet* **337**:488–489.

38 Embrey MP, Mollison BG (1967) The unfavourable cervix and induction of labour using a cervical balloon. *Journal of Obstetrics and Gynaecology of the British Commonwealth* **74**:44–48.

39 Lewis GJ (1983) Cervical ripening before induction of labour with prostaglandin E₂ pessaries or a Foley's catheter. *Journal of Obstetrics and Gynaecology* **3**:173–176.

40 Manabe Y, Manabe A, Sagawa N (1982) Stretch-induced cervical softening and initiation of labor at term: A possible correlation with prostaglandins. *Acta Obstetrica et Gynecologica Scandinavica* **61**:279–280.

41 Lackritz R, Gibson M, Frigoletto FD (1979) Preinduction use of laminaria for the unripe cervix. *American Journal of Obstetrics and Gynecology* **134**:349–350.

42 MacPherson M (1984) Comparison of Lamicel with prostaglandin E₂ gel as a cervical ripening agent before the induction of labour. *Journal of Obstetrics and Gynaecology* **4**:205–206.

43 Turnbull A, Anderson A (1968) Induction of labour. Part III: Results with amniotomy and oxytocin 'titration'. *Journal of Obstetrics and Gynaecology of the British Commonwealth* **75**:32–41.

44 O'Brien WF, Cefalo R (1986) Labour and delivery. In Gabbe SG, Niebyl JR, Simpson JL (eds), *Obstetrics: Normal and Problem Pregnancies*, pp. 351–378. New York: Churchill Livingstone.

45 Lamont RF, Neave S, Baker AC, Steer PJ (1991) Intrauterine pressures in labours induced by amniotomy and oxytocin or vaginal prostaglandin gel compared with spontaneous labour. *British Journal of Obstetrics and Gynaecology* **98**:441–447.

46 Kurup A, Chua S, Arulkumaran S, Tham KF, Tay D, Ratnam SS (1991) Induction of labour in nulliparae with poor cervical score: Oxytocin or prostaglandin vaginal pessaries. *Australia and New Zealand Journal of Obstetrics and Gynaecology* **31**:223–226.

47 Toaff ME, Hezrom J, Toaff R (1978) Induction of labour by pharmacological and physiological doses of

intravenous oxytocin. *British Journal of Obstetrics and Gynaecology* **85**:101–108.

48 Pavlou C, Barker GH, Roberts A, Chamberlain GVP (1978) Pulsed oxytocin infusion in the induction of labour. *British Journal of Obstetrics and Gynaecology* **85**:96–100.

49 Francis JG, Turnbull AC, Thomas FF (1970) Automatic oxytocin infusion equipment for induction of labour. *Journal of Obstetrics and Gynaecology of the British Commonwealth* **77**:594–602.

50 Butterworth MJ (1974) Automated incremental oxytocin infusion in the induction of labor. *Obstetrics and Gynecology* **44**:238–245.

51 Carter MC, Steer PJ (1980) An automatic infusion system for the measurement and control of uterine activity. *Medical Instruments* **14**:169–173.

52 Steer PJ, Carter MC, Choong K, Hanson M, Gordon AJ, Pradhan P (1985) A multicentre prospective randomised trial of induction of labour with an automatic closed-loop feedback controlled oxytocin infusion system. *British Journal of Obstetrics and Gynaecology* **92**:1127–1133.

53 Gibb DMF, Arulkumaran S, Ratnam SS (1985) A comparative study of methods of oxytocin administration for induction of labour. *British Journal of Obstetrics and Gynaecology* **92**:688–692.

54 Miller JF, Welpy GA, Elstein M (1975) Prostaglandin E$_2$ tablets compared with intravenous oxytocin in induction of labour. *British Medical Journal* i:14–16.

55 Calder AA, Embrey MP (1975) Comparison of intravenous oxytocin and prostaglandin E$_2$ for induction of labour using automated and non-automated infusion techniques. *British Journal of Obstetrics and Gynaecology* **82**:728–733.

56 Thiery M, Vroman S, De Hemptinne D, Yo Le Sian S, Vanderheyden K, Van Kets H, Martens G, Derom R, Rolly G (1977) Elective induction of labor conducted under epidural block. *European Journal of Obstetrics and Gynecology and Reproductive Biology* **7**:181–200.

57 MacKenzie IZ, Bradley S, Embrey MP (1981) A simpler approach to labour induction using a lipid-based prostaglandin E$_2$ vaginal suppository. *American Journal of Obstetrics and Gynecology* **141**:158–162.

58 Swann RO (1958) Induction of labour by stripping membranes. *Obstetrics and Gynecology* **11**:74–78.

59 Booth JH, Kurdizak VB (1970) Elective induction of labor: a controlled study. *Canadian Medical Association Journal* **103**:245–248.

60 Patterson WM (1971) Amniotomy with or without simultaneous oxytocin infusion. *Journal of Obstetrics and Gynaecology of the British Commonwealth* **78**:310–316.

61 Saleh YZ (1975) Surgical induction of labour with and without oxytocin infusion: A prospective study. *Australia and New Zealand Journal of Obstetrics and Gynaecology* **15**:80–83.

62 Drew-Smythe JH (1931) Indications for the induction of premature labour. *British Medical Journal* 1:1018–1020.

63 Elliott JP, Flaherty JF (1983) The use of breast stimulation to ripen the cervix in term pregnancies. *American Journal of Obstetrics and Gynecology* **145**:553–556.

64 Viegas OAC, Arulkumaran S, Ratnam SS (1984) Nipple stimulation in late pregnancy causing uterine hyperstimulation and profound bradycardia. *British Journal of Obstetrics and Gynaecology* **91**:364–366.

65 Pritchard JA (1959) Fetal death *in utero*. *Obstetrics and Gynecology* **14**:593–580.

66 Sher G (1976) Intra-amniotic use of urea and prostaglandin F$_{2\alpha}$ to induce labour in pregnancies complicated by death of the fetus. *South African Medical Journal* **50**:510–512.

67 Peterson EP, Taylor HB (1970) Amniotic fluid embolism: An analysis of 40 cases. *Obstetrics and Gynecology* **35**:787–793.

68 El-Demarawy H, El-Sahwi S, Toppozada M (1977) Management of missed abortion and fetal death *in utero*. *Prostaglandins* **14**:583–590.

69 Hill NCW, Selinger M, Ferguson J, MacKenzie IZ (1991) Management of intra-uterine fetal death with vaginal administration of gemeprost or prostaglandin E$_2$: A random allocation controlled trial. *Journal of Obstetrics and Gynaecology* **11**:422–426.

70 Calder AA, MacKenzie IZ, Embrey MP (1976) Intrauterine (extra-amniotic) prostaglandins in the management of unsuccessful pregnancy. *Journal of Reproductive Medicine* **16**:271–275.

71 Toppozada M, Warda A, Ramadan M (1979) Intramuscular 15 phenoxy PGE$_2$ ester for pregnancy termination. *Prostaglandins* **17**:461–467.

72 Wallenburg HCS, Keirse MJNC, Freie HMP, Blacquiere JF (1980) Intramuscular administration of 15(s)-15-methyl prostaglandin F$_{2\alpha}$ for induction of labour in patients with fetal death. *British Journal of Obstetrics and Gynaecology* **87**:203–209.

73 Kanhai HHH, Keirse MJNC (1989) Induction of labour after fetal death: A randomised controlled trial of two prostaglandin regimens. *British Journal of Obstetrics and Gynaecology* **96**:1400–1404.

74 Martin RH, Menzies DN (1955) Oestrogen therapy in missed abortion and labour. *Journal of Obstetrics and Gynaecology of the British Empire* **62**:256–258.

75 Courtney LD, Boxall RR, Child P (1971) Permeability of membranes of dead fetus. *British Medical Journal* i:492–493.

76 Loudon JDO (1959) The use of high concentration oxytocin intravenous drips in the management of missed abortion. *Journal of Obstetrics and Gynaecology of the British Empire* **66**:277–281.

77 Liggins GC (1962) The treatment of missed abortion by high dosage Syntocinon intravenous infusion. *Journal of Obstetrics and Gynaecology* **69**:227–281.

78 Ursell W (1972) Induction of labour following fetal death. *Journal of Obstetrics and Gynaecology of the British Commonwealth* **79**:260–264.

79 Flamm BL, Dunnett C, Fischermann E, Quilligan EJ (1984) Vaginal delivery following cesarean section: Use of oxytocin augmentation and epidural anaesthesia with internal tocodynamic and internal fetal monitoring. *American Journal of Obstetrics and Gynecology* **148**:759–763.

80 Hibbard LT (1986) Cesarean section and other surgical

procedures. In Gabbe SG, Niebyl JR, Simpson JL (eds), *Obstetrics: Normal and Problem Pregnancies*, pp. 517–546. New York: Churchill Livingstone.

81 MacKenzie IZ, Boland J (1993) Current therapeutic uses of prostaglandins in obstetrics in the United Kingdom. *Contemporary Reviews in Obstetrics and Gynaecology* **5**:9–14.

82 MacKenzie IZ, Bradley S, Embrey MP (1984) Vaginal prostaglandins and labour induction for patients previously delivered by caesarean section. *British Journal of Obstetrics and Gynaecology* **91**:7–10.

83 Molloy BG, Sheil O, Duignan NM (1987) Delivery after caesarean section: Review of 2176 consecutive cases. *British Medical Journal* **294**:1645–1647.

84 Phelan JP, Clark SL, Diaz F, Paul RH (1987) Vaginal birth after caesarean section. *American Journal of Obstetrics and Gynecology* **157**:1510–1515.

85 MacKenzie IZ (1991) Prostaglandin induction and the scarred uterus. In Keirse MJNC, Elder MG (eds), *Induction of Labour: Special Issues*, pp. 29–39. Amsterdam: Excerpta Medica.

86 MacKenzie IZS (1990) The therapeutic roles of prostaglandins in obstetrics. In Studd J (ed.), *Progress in Obstetrics, Vol. 8*, pp. 149–174. Edinburgh: Churchill Livingstone.

87 Hatch MC (1969) Maternal deaths associated with induction of labor. *New York State Journal of Medicine* **69**:599–602.

88 Schwartz RH, Jones RWA (1978) Transplacental hyponatraemia due to oxytocin. *British Medical Journal* **i**:152–153.

89 Ingemarsson I, Arulkamaran S, Ratnam SS (1985) Single injection of terbutaline in term labor. I. Effect on fetal pH in cases with prolonged bradycardia. *American Journal of Obstetrics and Gynecology* **153**:859–865.

90 Kurup A, Arulkumaran S, Tay D, Ingemarsson I, Ratnam SS (1991) Can terbutaline be used as a nebuliser instead of intravenous injection for inhibition of uterine activity? *Gynecological and Obstetric Investigation* **32**:84–87.

91 Leung A, Kwok P, Chang A (1987) Association between prostaglandin E_2 and placental abruption. *British Journal of Obstetrics and Gynaecology* **94**:1001–1002.

92 Beazley JM, Weekes ARL (1976) Neonatal hyper-bilirubinaemia following the use of prostaglandin E_2 in labour. *British Journal of Obstetrics and Gynaecology* **83**:62–67.

93 Conway DI, Read MD, Baver C, Martin RH (1976) Neonatal jaundice: A comparison between intravenous oxytocin and oral prostaglandin E_2. *Journal of International Medical Research* **4**:241–246.

94 Saruta T, Kaplan NM, (1972) Adrenocortical steroidogenesis: The effects of prostaglandins. *Journal of Clinical Investigation* **51**:2246–2251.

95 Brinsden PRS, Clark AD (1978) Postpartum haemorrhage after induced and spontaneous labour. *British Medical Journal* **ii**:855–856.

96 Beekhuizen W, Van Schie KJ, Van Lith DAF, Du Plessis M, Keirse MJNC (1982) Aspirotomy for outpatient termination of pregnancy in the second trimes-

ter. In Keirse MJNC, Bennebroek Gravenhorst J, Van Lith DAF, Embrey MP (eds), *Second Trimester Pregnancy Termination*, pp. 52–64. The Hague: Leiden University Press.

97 Hodari AA, Peralta J, Quiroga PJ, Gerbi EB (1977) Dilatation and curettage for second-trimester abortion. *American Journal of Obstetrics and Gynecoogy* **127**:850–854.

98 Davis G (1972) Midtrimester abortion. *Lancet* **ii**:1026–1027.

99 Herr WM (1984) Serial multiple laminaria and adjunctive urea in late outpatient dilatation and evacuation abortion. *Obstetrics and Gynecology* **63**:543–549.

100 Stanwell-Smith R (1984) Procedures used for legal abortion. In Alberman I, Denis KJ (eds), *Late Abortions of England and Wales: Report of a National Confidential Study*, pp. 45–67. London: Royal College of Obstetricians and Gynaecologists.

101 Midwinter A, Bowen M, Shepherd A (1972) Continuous intrauterine infusion of prostaglandin E_2 for termination of pregnancy. *Journal of Obstetrics and Gynaecology of the British Commonwealth* **79**:807–809.

102 Embrey MP, Hillier K, Mahendran P (1973) Termination of pregnancy by extraamniotic prostaglandins and the synergistic action of oxytocin. *Advances in Biosciences* **9**:507–513.

103 Tejuja SS, Choudhury SS, Manchanda PK (1978) Use of intra- and extra-amniotic prostaglandins for the termination of pregnancies: Report of multicentric trials in India. *Contraception* **18**:641–652.

104 Hill NCW, MacKenzie IZ (1989) 2308 second trimester terminations using extraamniotic or intraamniotic prostaglandin E_2: An analysis of efficacy and complications. *British Journal of Obstetrics and Gynaecology* **96**:1424–1431.

105 World Health Organization (1976) Comparison of intra-amniotic prostaglandin $F_{2\alpha}$ and hypertonic saline for second trimester abortion. *British Medical Journal* **i**:1373–1376.

106 Burkman RT, Atienza MF, King TM, Burnett LS (1976) Intra-amniotic urea and prostaglandin $F_{2\alpha}$ for midtrimester abortion: A modified regimen. *American Journal of Obstetrics and Gynecology* **126**:328–333.

107 World Health Organization Task Force (1977) Repeated vaginal administration of 15-methyl $PGF_{2\alpha}$ for termination of pregnancy in the 13th to 20th week of gestation. *Contraception* **16**:175–181.

108 Tejuja SS, Choudhury SD, Manchanda PK, Malhotra U (1979) Indian experience with a single long-acting vaginal suppository for the termination of pregnancy. *Contraception* **19**:191–196.

109 Cameron IT, Michie AF, Baird DT (1987) Prostaglandin induced pregnancy termination: Further studies using gemeprost (16,16-dimethyl-trans-Δ2-PGE$_1$ methyl ester) vaginal pessaries in the early second trimester. *Prostaglandins* **34**:111–117.

110 Hill NCW, Selinger M, Ferguson J, MacKenzie IZ (1991) Midtrimester termination of pregnancy with 16,16-dimethyl-trans-Δ2-prostaglandin E_1 vaginal pessaries: A comparison with intra- and extra-amniotic

prostaglandin E$_2$ administration. *International Journal of Gynaecology and Obstetrics* **35**:337–340.

111 World Health Organization Task Force (1982) Termination of second trimester pregnancy by intra-muscular injection of 16-phenoxy-ω-17,18,19,20-tetranor-PGE$_2$ methyl sulfonylamide. *International Journal of Gynaecology and Obstetrics* **20**:383–386.

112 World Health Organization Task Force (1988) Termination of second trimester pregnancy with laminaria and intramuscular 15-methyl-PGF$_{2\alpha}$ or 16-phenoxy-ω-17,18,19,20-tetranor-PGE$_2$ methyl sulfonylmide: A randomised multicentre study. *International Journal of Gynaecology and Obstetrics* **26**:129–135.

113 Selinger M, MacKenzie IZ, Gillmer MDG, Phipps SL, Ferguson J (1987) Progesterone inhibition in midtrimester termination of pregnancy: Physiological and clinical effects. *British Journal of Obstetrics and Gynaecology* **94**:1218–1222.

114 Hill NCW, Selinger M, Ferguson J, Lopez Bernal A, MacKenzie IZ (1990) The physiological and clinical effects of progesterone inhibition with RU 38,486 (mifepristone) in the second trimester. *British Journal of Obstetrics and Gynaecology* **97**:487–492.

115 Rodger MW, Baird DT (1990) Pretreatment with mifepristone (RU 486) reduces interval between prostaglandin administration and expulsion in second trimester abortion. *British Journal of Obstetrics and Gynaecology* **97**:41–45.

116 Brenner WE, Hendricks CH, Fishbourne JI, Braaksma JT, Staurovsky LG, Harrell LC (1973) Induction of therapeutic abortion with intraamniotically administered prostaglandin F$_{2\alpha}$: A comparison of three repeated injection dose schedules. *American Journal of Obstetrics and Gynecology* **116**:923–930.

117 Stander RW, Flessa HC, Gueck HI, Kisker CT (1971) Changes in maternal coagulation factors after intraamniotic injection of hypertonic saline. *Obstetrics and Gynecology* **37**:660–665.

118 MacKenzie IZ, Sayers L, Bonnar J, Hillier K (1975) Coagulation changes during midtrimester abortion induced with intra-amniotic prostaglandin E$_2$ and hypertonic solutions. *Lancet* **ii**:1066–1069.

119 Burkman RT, Bell WR, Atienza MF, King TM (1977) Coagulopathy with mid-trimester induced abortion: Association with hyperosmolar urea administration. *American Journal of Obstetrics and Gynecology* **127**:553–556.

120 Stubblefield PG (1986) Surgical techniques of uterine evacuation in first and second trimester abortion. In Laferla JJ (ed.), *Clinics in Obstetrics and Gynaecology: Termination of Pregnancy*, pp. 53–70. London: W.B. Saunders.

61

Poor Progress in Labor Including Augmentation, Malpositions and Malpresentations

SABARATNAM ARULKUMARAN

INTRODUCTION

The management of spontaneous labor has become an important issue both in the developing and the developed world. In the developing world, prolonged labor associated with high levels of morbidity and mortality is still common because of a lack of adequate health care, in particular antibiotics and the surgical facilities necessary for cesarean section. The causes of death and morbidity include obstructed labor, sepsis, rupture of the uterus and postpartum hemorrhage.[1] The World Health Organization has embarked on clinical trials of the use of partograms as a simple managerial tool for the early detection and appropriate management of prolonged labor and its sequelae.[2] In the developed world, the increasing cesarean section (CS) rate for dystocia or difficult labor contributes at least a third to the overall CS rate, and repeat CS following primary CS contributes up to another third.[3] CS leads to increased maternal morbidity as well as mortality, especially when it is performed as an emergency procedure.[4] Maternal and fetal morbidity and mortality due to prolonged labor and the CS rate for dystocia can be reduced by proper management of poor progress in labor.

NORMAL LABOR

Normal labor is difficult to define precisely but the archetype can be described as spontaneous painful uterine contractions associated with effacement and dilatation of the cervix and descent of the head in a vertex presentation. The process culminates in the birth of a healthy fetus followed by expulsion of the placenta. In most cases, the outcome can be predicted prospectively by observing the progress of cervical dilatation. The basis for the scientific study of the progress of labor was developed by Friedman,[5] who described it graphically by plotting the rate of cervical dilatation against time. The resulting graph of cervical dilatation forms the basis of the modern partogram, which now incorporates many additional aspects of labor, and in most cases is capable of standing alone as a sufficient record.

The Partogram

The modern partogram contains many relevant parameters related to labor, mother and the fetus in relation to each other chronologically on one page. These parameters include cervical effacement and dilatation, descent of presenting part (in fifths of the head palpable and station in centimeters above or below the ischial spines), fetal heart rate (FHR), frequency and duration of uterine contractions, color and quantity of amniotic fluid passed per vaginam, maternal parameters such as temperature, pulse and blood pressure, and drugs used (**Figure 1**). The pictorial documentation of labor facilitates early recognition of poor progress. Plotting of cervical dilatation also enables prediction of the time of onset of the second stage of labor. The partogram helps in easy recognition of omissions and highlights inefficient clinical practice.

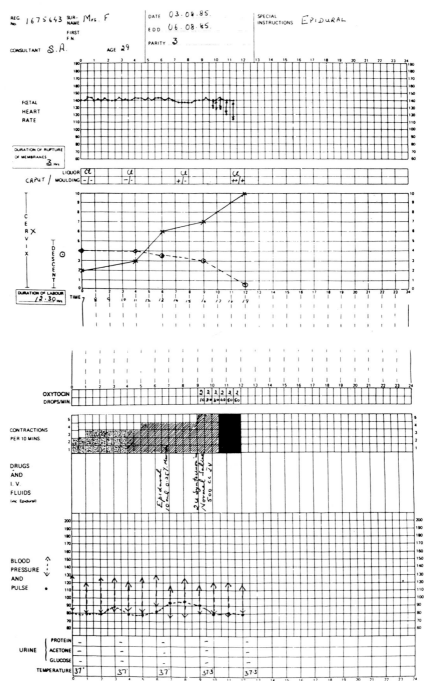

Figure 1. Partogram showing parameters of cervical effacement and dilatation, descent of the head in fifths, fetal heart rate, frequency and duration of contractions, color of amniotic fluid, maternal parameters and drugs used in relation to each other chronologically on one page.

Because it enables the recording of nearly all relevant data on one page, it reduces the bulk of documentation, facilitates the 'handing over' of patients, and improves the efficiency of the labor ward.

Nomograms of cervical dilatation

The rate of cervical dilatation in labor has been studied in various ethnic groups.[6-9] Based on the observed pattern of cervical dilatation in parturients not requiring augmentation and achieving a spontaneous vaginal delivery of neonates in good condition, centiles of cervical dilatation pattern have been constructed. The nomograms derived show similar rates of cervical dilatation in different ethnic groups and comparative studies have confirmed that differences in ethnicity have little influence on the rate of cervical dilatation[10] or uterine activity in spontaneous normal labor.[11] Observations during the first stage of labor (defined as from the time of admission to the labor ward to full dilatation of the cervix) show that the rate of cervical dilatation has two phases: a slow 'latent phase' of labor during which the cervical canal shortens from about 3 cm long to less than 0.5 cm long (effacement), and dilates to 3 cm open; and a faster 'active phase', when the cervix dilates from 3 cm to full dilatation (taken by convention to be 10 cm, although in reality it will of course depend on the size of the presenting part). In order to identify parturients at risk of prolonged labor, a line of acceptable progress is drawn on the partogram. If the rate of cervical dilatation in any particular case crosses to the right of the line, progress is deemed unsatisfactory. The line of acceptable progress can be based on the mean, median or slowest 10th percentile rate of cervical dilatation, or it can be a line parallel and 1–4 h to the right of these. Accordingly, the proportion of labors deemed to have unsatisfactory progress can vary from 5 to 50%. In the presence of good contractions, the latent phase may last for up to 8 h in nulliparas and up to 6 h in multiparas. During the peak of the active phase of labor, the cervix dilates at an average rate of approximately 1 cm/h in both nulliparas and multiparas. Multiparas appear to dilate faster because they have shorter labors overall; not only do they have a shorter latent phase resulting in a more advanced cervical dilatation on admission, they have an increased rate of progress approaching full dilatation.[10] Construction of nomograms of expected progress, with the addition of alert lines, prevents prolongation of labor being overlooked and is of considerable diagnostic and educational value.

DIAGNOSIS OF POOR PROGRESS OF LABOR

The term dystocia or difficult labor refers to poor progress of labor and is diagnosed when the rate of cervical dilatation in the active phase is slower than the mean, median or slowest 10th centile, according to the policy of the obstetrician. When a woman is admitted in the active phase of labor with regular painful contractions, her cervical dilatation can be plotted on the partogram and an expected progress line or alert line can be constructed. Another line, the action line, can be constructed 1–4 h parallel and to the right of the alert line (**Figure 2**). Alternatively, an action line can be added by the use of a stencil,[12] in which an individualized alert line is contructed from the cervical dilatation on admission. If the progress of labor is to the right of the action line, it is considered to be poor needing augmentation. The outcome of such labors has been studied and various abnormal labor patterns have been described.[12–14] The latent phase is usually considered prolonged if it is greater than 8h in a nullipara and 6 h in a multipara, although to some extent this will depend on the Bishop score on admission (the slowest 20% of labors will dilate at less than one Bishop score point per hour in the latent phase of induced labor).[15] If the progress of labor is slow in the active phase of labor and is to the right of the nomogram, it is termed 'primary dysfunctional labor' (**Figure 3**(c)). If labor progresses normally in the early active phase but subsequently fails to dilate or dilates slowly, prior to full dilatation of the cervix, it is termed 'secondary arrest' of labor (**Figure 3**(b)). The same patient may exhibit both a prolonged latent phase and primary dysfunctional labor.

The use of a partogram with the expected progress line constructed for an individual patient allows easy recognition of an unsatisfactory rate of cervical dilatation. The descent of the presenting part is also plotted at each vaginal examination and a poor rate of descent also indicates a potentially problematic labor. Poor progress may be related to inadequate uterine contractions and/or to an increased resistance of the birth canal to passage of the fetus. This latter can be due to disproportion between the presenting part and the birth canal, or to an unfavorable cervix. Poor progress in labor does not identify the specific cause (i.e. a fault with the powers, passage or passenger). Secondary arrest of labor need not indicate cephalopelvic disproportion, as sometimes in these patients inadequate uterine contractions can be corrected by oxytocin, resulting in spontaneous vaginal delivery.[16] When there is failure to progress, obvious problems in the passenger (e.g. hydrocephalus, brow presentation, undiagnosed shoulder presentation, large/macrosomic baby) and passage (e.g. congenitally small pelvis, deformed pelvis due to accident or disease or masses in the pelvis) should be excluded. Commonly, there is no recognizable compromise in the cephalopelvic relationship. Unfavorable pelvic diameters may result in cephalopelvic disproportion. However, the fetus is more commonly the cause of relative disproportion due to malposition or deflexion attitudes. In such cases, dystocia may be overcome by further flexion, rotation and molding of the head to the occipito-anterior position, or by efficient uterine contractions. Inefficient uterine contractions have been recognized as the most common cause for poor progress of labor.[17,18] In these cases, the appropriate use of oxytocin will usually

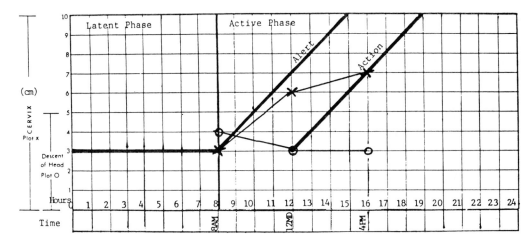

Figure 2. The partogram used in the WHO trials showing an 'alert line' in the active phase progressing at 1 cm/h from 3 cm. Note the 'action line' at the end of 8 h for the latent phase and 4 h parallel and to the right of the 'alert line' in the active phase.

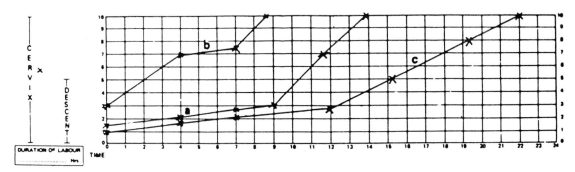

Figure 3. Abnormal labor patterns. (a) Prolonged latent phase of labor; (b) secondary arrest of labor; (c) prolonged latent phase and primary dysfunctional labor.

produce efficient contractions and bring about vaginal delivery.[17,18]

Management Options for Poor Progress of Labor (First Stage)

Augmentation

The case for augmentation

Prolonged labor may culminate in obstructed labor, and is associated with maternal infection, uterine rupture and postpartum hemorrhage. It is a significant cause of maternal death. It has been a common axiom 'not to allow the sun to set twice on a laboring woman', in order to prevent such tragic events. Philpott in Africa[6] O'Driscoll in Dublin[7] and Studd in the UK[8] advocated

and popularized the concept of augmentation to reduce the incidence of prolonged labor. The Dublin school promulgated the concept of active management of labor to diagnose and correct poor progress of labor.[7,8] The main components of 'the active management of labor' are regular assessment to enable early diagnosis of slow cervical dilatation rates, prompt administration of oxytocin (to correct 'inefficient uterine action', although the regime does not include direct intrauterine pressure measurement), reassurance provided by one-to-one support by a nurse or a medical student, pain relief (although not usually using epidural anesthesia, which they claim is rarely necessary with their regime), and hydration. Initially, the presence of the husband or partner was discouraged, although this aspect has now been changed. The use of active management as practised in the National Maternity Hospital, Dublin, has been associated with much lower overall intervention rates (in particular, instrumental and operative delivery) than in most other Western settings.[18,19] The word 'augmentation' is more appropriate than acceleration of labor, as the latter might denote accelerating a labor with normal progress.

When to augment labor

The 'efficiency' of uterine contractions should be defined in terms of the work done, i.e. the progress of cervical dilatation and descent of the head, and not in relation to the magnitude of uterine contractions, because normal progress of labor is observed with a wide range of uterine activity in nulliparas and multiparas.[20,21,22] The more rapid the rate of progress for a given level of uterine activity, the more 'efficient' the contractions. It is also important to recognize the difference between the concept of inefficient uterine activity and that of 'incoordinate' uterine contractions. Inefficiency is the failure of the uterus to work in such a way that labor progresses satisfactorily. It can be demonstrated only when the end-point of such activity has been observed to be deficient. This clinical situation is one of poor cervimetric progress in the absence of cephalopelvic disproportion or malposition (although both of these may co-exist with inefficient uterine action). Incoordinate uterine action is a descriptive term for a tocographic tracing. Most records of uterine contractions show some degree of irregularity. Quantification of irregularity is difficult, but there appears to be an instrinsic pattern of uterine contractile rhythm, which each individual patient assumes once labor is established. This pattern does not change substantially during active labor. Irregular uterine contractions are often associated with normal progress of labor. **Figures 4, 5,** and **6** illustrate incoordinate contraction patterns seen in labor progressing normally. While incoordinate patterns may also be inefficient, this can only be concluded once vaginal examination has confirmed that labor has failed to progress. Therefore, the decision to augment labor should be governed primarily by the rate of cervical dilatation after exclusion of gross disproportion or malpresentation. The issue of whether oxytocin augmentation is appropriate in the presence of slow progress but apparently normal contractions as demonstrated by intrauterine pressure measurement is discussed further in the overview of labor (see Chapter 59).

Practical aspects of labor management

A variety of techniques are used for the detection of slow progress in labor. However, it is universally agreed that the diagnosis of active labor depends fundamentally on a careful assessment of cervical state

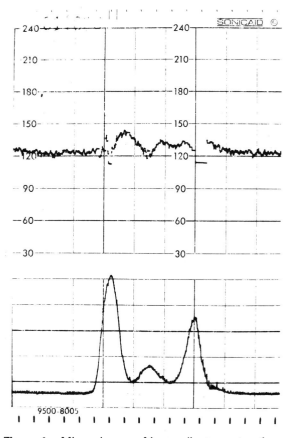

Figure 4. Minor degree of incoordinate contractions.

(dilatation, effacement, consistency, position, descent of the head) and not on soft indicators such as regular painful contractions, a show, or even rupture of the amniotic membranes. On admission, the cervical dilatation should be plotted on a partogram. In our unit, an alert line is drawn at 1 cm/h once the active phase of labor is reached and an action line is drawn parallel to it and 2 h to the right. Alternatively, a labor stencil, such as that described by Studd,[8] can be used. If the observed progress is slow and is to the right of the action line, augmentation should be considered. There is no consensus as to the placement of the action line – whether it should be 1, 2, 3 or 4 h to the right of the alert line. Various centers use different intervals. Modifying factors include the level of nursing and medical care available for supervision of labor (because oxytocin is likely to be used once the cervical dilatation rate crosses the action line), the risk of complications associated with prolonged labor (which is likely to be higher in disadvantaged communities) and the social milieu of the clients (in many Western settings there is consumer demand for 'natural childbirth', which basically means avoiding intervention unless this become inescapable). The fact that there is a line drawn

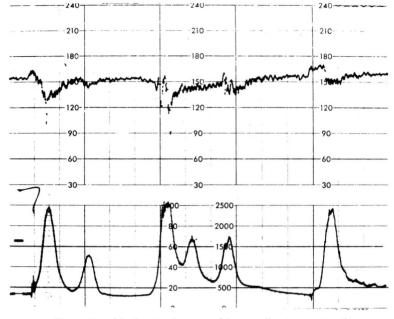

Figure 5. Moderate degree of incoordinate contractions.

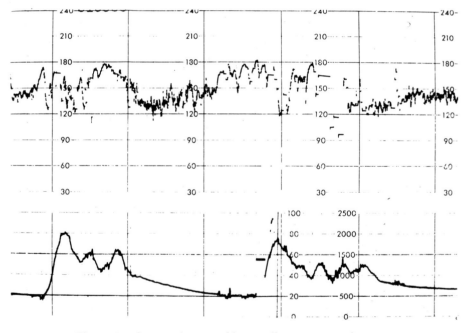

Figure 6. Severe degree of incoordinate contractions.

to indicate that action is necessary at some point is more important than the time interval between the alert and action lines. When action is needed, amniotomy alone may be adequate to correct slow progress, although oxytocin will be needed in most cases.

Augmentation in the latent phase of labor

The duration of the latent phase of labor varies widely and makes the diagnosis of labor more difficult. An appreciable proportion of women have painful contractions for long periods in the latent phase of labor with little cervical change. These contractions may subside and the labor may not become established. Due to the variation in the duration of the latent phase and the uncertainty regarding the establishment of labor, management of the latent phase should usually be conservative. This involves reassurance, hydration, nutrition and ambulation. The decision to augment labor in the latent phase should be based on medical or obstetric indications. In women with 'spurious labor' who have been managed conservatively, there is a slightly higher risk of fetal distress in subsequent labor.[23] Hence it may be useful to confirm fetal well-being by cardiotocography before managing the latent phase conservatively. Augmentation of labor in the latent phase with a poor cervical score may be associated with a higher risk of cesarean section and as such a clear indication is a prerequisite for intervention. There is limited literature available in relation to the prolonged latent phase. The results of a large WHO multicenter study using a partogram with a cut-off at 8 h in the latent phase (**Figure 2**) may shed some light regarding the management of the prolonged latent phase (B. Kwast, WHO personal communication).

Augmentation in the active phase of labor

When women are admitted in the active phase of labor (cervical dilatation > 3 cm), the 'alert line' can be constructed using a stencil[12] or a line drawn at a rate of 1 cm/h from the initial assessment.[2,24] O'Driscoll et al[7,19] advocate augmentation of labor when the progress of labor is less than 1 cm/h, whereas others are less stringent and advocate augmentation when the progress has deviated to the right of the 'action line' drawn 2, 3, or 4 h parallel to the alert line. By allowing a 2 h 'period of grace', fewer patients will be augmented: 55% of nulliparas with no period of grace[7] compared to 19% with a 2 h period of grace.[16] Both methods of management yield comparable results, although prompt intervention does decrease duration of labor and therefore may be most appropriate when labor ward staffing is very limited. Alternatively, if clients are more in favor of 'natural childbirth', preference should be given to a protocol with lower intervention rates if obstetric outcomes are not very different. The WHO has conducted a study with the action line drawn 4 h to the right of the alert line in the active phase (**Figure 2**) to reduce the number of patients needing oxytocin. The results of this trial are awaited with interest.

Oxytocin dosage and time increment schedules

The uterus of a patient in labor is sensitive to oxytocin and may be hypersensitive even to small doses.[25] The drug is best titrated in an arithmetic or geometric manner starting from a low dose. Oxytocin is often administered by gravity-fed drips which are not reliable. Overdosage may lead to fetal distress, while a suboptimal dose may lead to failure to progress resulting in unnecessary intervention. The dangers to the fetus[26–28] and the mother[29] of uncontrolled infusion are well documented. Ideally, for precise control, a peristaltic infusion pump should be utilized.

Published protocols variously recommend a starting dose of 2–6 mU/min of oxytocin and geometric increases every 15–30 min for induction of labor.[30–32] They have been adapted for augmentation of labor in many centers. The recommendations were based on earlier in vitro pharmacological studies in which the half-life of oxytocin was thought to be 3–4 min.[33,34] However, recent in vivo studies [35] have suggested that the half-life of oxytocin is in fact 10–15 min. Continuous intravenous infusion of oxytocin has also shown first-order kinetics, with a progressive stepwise increase. With every increase in infusion rate, a steady plasma concentration is reached 40–60 min after the alteration of an infusion.[35] A shorter increment interval results in the dose being increased before maximum plasma levels are reached. These findings, along with a number of litigation cases due to the misuse of oxytocin,[36] have prompted a closer look at intervals between dose increments. Seitchik et al.[35] recommend an incremental interval of 30 min as a reasonable compromise to avoid overdosage and danger of uterine hyperstimulation leading to fetal distress on the one hand, and undue delay in delivery on the other. Retrospective[37] and prospective[38,39] studies on induced labor have confirmed that the optimal interval between dose increments is 30 min. Recent radioimmunoassays in vivo and retrospective studies on contraction patterns in augmented labor[40] are in favor of 30 min incremental intervals (also the recommendation of the American College of Obstetricians and Gynecologists[41]).

Achievement of optimal uterine activity

The literature is limited regarding the level of uterine activity that should be produced by oxytocin titration to effect good obstetric outcome. It has been suggested that the use of pre- and post-augmentation uterine activity measurements from the use of an intrauterine catheter may identify those who are likely to need cesarean section for failure to progress.[42] It is known that active contraction area measurements using an intrauterine catheter correlate better with the rate of cervical dilatation than the individual variables of frequency or amplitude of contractions.[43] Hence if there is no progress with optimal uterine activity, it may suggest disproportion. Despite this possible theoretical advantage, measurement of uterine activity using an intrauterine catheter or oxytocin titration to achieve preset active contraction area profiles has not been shown to produce better obstetric outcome in augmented labor compared with oxytocin titration to achieve a present frequency of contractions.[44]

If oxytocin titration to achieve a preset frequency gives a good obstetric outcome, what should this frequency be? In a prospective study, two-thirds of women who showed failure to progress despite no evidence of cephalopelvic disproportion had two or fewer contractions in 10 min, while one-third had an 'optimal' contraction frequency of one in 3 min over a period of 4 h. In the latter group, oxytocin titration to achieve a contraction frequency of 4 in 10 min with each contraction duration lasting >40s was associated with vaginal delivery of babies in good condition in 96% (24/25) of these women.[18] It may therefore be that three contractions in 10 min should be the target uterine activity with oxytocin titration, but if there is no progress with that frequency of contractions, the oxytocin dose should be increased to achieve a contraction frequency of four in 10 min (always providing that the FHR pattern is normal).

How should uterine contractions be measured – external or internal tocography?

The frequency of contractions can be assessed by either external or internal tocography. Some centers use intrauterine catheters when oxytocin is used because they consider that hyperstimulation of the uterus can be identified early and oxytocin infusion rates adjusted accordingly, resulting in a reduction in fetal hypoxic episodes and a better neonatal outcome. In most instances, prior to hyperstimulation there is an increase in frequency followed by an increase in amplitude of contractions, which precedes elevation of the baseline tone. However, excessively frequent contractions can also be identified by external tocography. A prospective randomized study did not show better obstetric outcome when an intrauterine catheter was used, compared with the use of external tocography, in augmented labor.[45] In a busy clinical practice, it may be easier, less invasive and cheaper to assess uterine contractions using external tocography. On the other hand, in high-risk cases (such as pregnancies complicated by intrauterine fetal growth deficiency, or in practices where medicolegal concerns are important), there are theoretical advantages to the use of intrauterine pressure measurement. In addition, the use of intrauterine catheters may be of value in restless or obese parturients where external tocography does not give a good recording. There are circumstances where the contraction frequency is three or four in 10 min with each contraction lasting >40 s but with poor progress of labor. In these situations and in cases where high doses of oxytocin (>15 mU/min) are used, quantification of

uterine activity by the use of an intrauterine catheter may prevent hyperstimulation with consequent fetal hypoxia. The use of intrauterine pressure measurement has also been recommended in patients with previous cesarean scar who are augmented with oxytocin as a sudden decline in uterine activity may be the first and only sign of scar dehiscence in a proportion of cases.[46,47]

Duration of augmentation

There is a general agreement that the use of partograms and oxytocic augmentation for the management of poor progress of labor is valuable. There is, however, debate as to how long one should augment labor prior to deciding on cesarean section for failure to progress. A prospective study of 2803 patients admitted in spontaneous labor evaluated the mode of delivery and neonatal outcome when augmentation was continued in those who had unsatisfactory progress (<1 cm/h) in the first 4 h of augmentation.[15] Of the 19.0% of nulliparas and 7.3% of multiparas who had poor progress, 65.5% of nulliparas and 83.8% of multiparas showed good response to oxytocic augmentation and dilated at a rate >1 cm/h in the first 4 h. In those who showed such good progress, only 1.4% of nulliparas and 1.2% of multiparas needed cesarean section and these were for reasons other than poor progress. In those who had poor progress in the first 4 h (35.5% of nulliparas and 16.2% of multiparas), a further 4 h of augmentation was allowed. In this group, 62.5% of nulliparas and 50% of multiparas needed cesarean section. The neonatal outcome was uniformly good. These data suggest that augmentation of slow labors (<1 cm in 3 h) benefits both nulliparas and multiparas. A period of 8 h of augmentation with adequate monitoring in the absence of gross disproportion should result in the majority of nulliparas and multiparas delivering vaginally with little risk of intrauterine or birth asphyxia or injury. It is doubtful whether more than 8 h of augmentation in the presence of poor progress will result in a significantly greater number of patients delivering vaginally without compromise to the fetus.

Augmentation: Special circumstances

• Multiparas

Caution has to be exercised in augmenting multiparas, especially grand multiparas, where the cause of the poor progress may be unrecognized disproportion. Augmentation in such situations might lead to rupture of the uterus. In these women, if there is no progress despite adequate spontaneous uterine contractions, it may be better to observe them for a few hours than to use oxytocin. One has also to be careful when augmentation is undertaken for failure to progress in the late first stage of labor (>7 cm cervical dilatation). A prolonged period of augmentation should be avoided. Failure to progress despite augmentation may be due to disproportion and an early decision should be made as to the mode of delivery.

- ## Previous cesarean section

Opinion regarding augmentation if there is poor progress in cases of previous cesarean section or breech presentation varies widely. When there is failure to progress in cases of previous cesarean section, and major disproportion seems unlikely (there is no history of pelvic injury, clinical pelvimetry is normal and the head is no more than three-fifths palpable per adbomen), if contractions are not optimal (frequency less than three in 10 min and active pressure less than 40 mmHg) it may be justified to augment labor. The role of intrauterine pressure measurement in this situation is disputed. There are no prospective studies which show an overall increase in scar rupture rate with oxytocin augmentation and yet some clinicians refuse to sanction use of oxytocin in trial of scar for fear that rupture will occur. On purely logical grounds, it would seem reasonable to augment contractions at least to the average level for spontaneous labor. In practice, augmentation may lead to higher levels of uterine activity than spontaneous normal labor.[48,49] In addition, a substantial proportion of those who fail to make adequate progress in the first 4 h of augmentation need operative delivery,[16] and they are also more susceptible to scar rupture.[46,47] Thus the period of augmentation should probably be limited to 4 h unless adequate cervical dilatation rates resume. Those who show satisfactory progress can be allowed a further period of augmentation.

- ## Breech

Dysfunctional labor in breech presentation is more common than in cephalic presentation.[50] If augmentation is carried out in the presence of breech presentation, it should be performed cautiously. It is probably wise to estimate fetal weight by ultrasound before augmentation, as fetal weights greater than 3.8 kg are associated with a significantly higher rate of obstructed labor. X-ray pelvimetry can be used to exclude gross disproportion,[51] although it is becoming increasingly appreciated that pelvimetry is a poor indicator of likely mode of delivery and that a normal pelvimetry is not associated with a reduced scar rupture rate.[52] Knowledge of the adequacy of uterine activity may also be useful before a decision is made about augmentation.[53] Good results have been reported provided there is ready resort to cesarean section if there is no progress in the first 4 h of augmentation.[53,54]

Genuine cephalopelvic disproportion and disproportion due to malposition

If the progress of labor is unsatisfactory despite adequate augmentation mechanical factors that might contribute to disproportion have to be considered. Disproportion may be diagnosed when two-fifths or more of the head are palpable abdominally. Vaginal examination may reveal a loosely applied presenting part, an edematous cervix, gross molding and caput. Furthermore, deflexion or malposition of the head may be identified with the maximal diameter of the head still high in the pelvis. A cardiotocographic tracing may show either early or variable decelerations suggestive of head compression. Meconium-stained amniotic fluid sometimes appears. These signs indicate an absolute cephalopelvic disproportion if the occiput is anterior with a well-flexed vertex presentation, and relative disproportion due to malposition if the head is deflexed with the occiput felt laterally or posteriorly.

In relative cephalopelvic disproportion due to malposition, the degree of flexion is unsatisfactory and a larger anteroposterior occipitofrontal (11 cm) diameter is presented instead of the smaller suboccipito bregmatic (9.5 cm) diameter in a well-flexed occipitoanterior position. The subtle distinction between 'absolute' cephalopelvic disproportion and 'relative' cephalopelvic disproportion due to malposition may be useful in deciding on trial of labor or a repeat elective cesarean section in the next pregnancy. A patient who has a cesarean section for disproportion due to malposition and deflexed head in her first pregnancy may well have a normal delivery in her subsequent labor if the head flexes and presents in an occipito-anterior position with a smaller diameter. Thus two-thirds of patients allowed a trial of labor despite a previous cesarean section for failure to progress due to 'disproportion', deliver vaginally in their subsequent pregnancy without a significant increase in maternal or fetal morbidity.[55–57]

X-ray pelvimetry

In the majority of patients who fail to progress in labor, the relative contribution by the passenger and the passage is difficult to evaluate. The dynamic nature of labor continuously alters the dimensions of the pelvis, and of the presenting part by flexion, rotation and molding. Static measurements are probably of little value in such situations. Prospective studies of prenatal and intrapartum x-ray pelvimetry have been shown not to alter planned management policies.[58–60] In a woman with a cephalic presentation, unless there is evidence of gross disproportion, a well-conducted trial of labor is the best test for the adequacy of the pelvis.

POOR PROGRESS IN THE SECOND STAGE OF LABOR

The second stage of labor is defined as the period from full cervical dilatation to delivery of the fetus. Traditional teaching advocates instrumental vaginal delivery if this stage is more than 1 h. This practice stems from the fear of fetal distress when the second stage is prolonged. There are problems associated with such a regimen.

The stage of full dilatation of the cervix is a continuum in the process of labor and not a static phase. Oscillatory changes of cervical dilatation with contractions have been well documented.[61] Full dilatation is usually identified either on routine vaginal examination or when the patient expresses a desire to bear down. The sensation of bearing down and full cervical dilatation are not functionally related and do not always occur synchronously.

The second stage of labor has a pelvic and perineal phase. In the pelvic phase the cervix may be fully dilated, but since the presenting part is high, it does not give rise to the sensation of bearing down. In the perineal phase the patient feels the sensation of bearing down because the presenting part is deep in the pelvis and exerts pressure on the rectum. In the pelvic phase it is not advisable to request a patient to bear down or to carry out a difficult instrumental vaginal delivery after an arbitrary 1 h.

In the presence of malposition the second stage of labor is often prolonged, and if the head is high it is not necessary to adhere strictly to a time limitation provided that fetal condition remains satisfactory and the mother is happy to continue. Uterine activity may also be augmented if necessary. Care should be taken that this does not induce hypoxia in a previously well fetus, as this can compromise the safety of instrumental delivery. In addition, there is a risk of uterine rupture in grand multiparas, and in women with a scarred uterus.

Instrumental vaginal deliveries for failure to progress in the second stage are not without danger. A prolonged first stage (especially a protracted late first stage) followed by prolonged second stage sets the scene for the possibility of difficult instrumental vaginal delivery and shoulder dystocia. A loosely hanging rim of cervix or part of it which is not well applied to the head in the late first stage is also a warning sign of possible disproportion. Prior to attempting an instrumental vaginal delivery, an abdominal palpation should be performed to confirm that no more than one-fifth of the head is palpable. Vaginally there should be no sign of excessive caput or molding, the head should descend with uterine contractions and bearing down effort and a fetal ear should be palpable. If these conditions are not fulfilled, instrumental vaginal delivery is probably not advisable. When a trial of forceps is undertaken, it should be in the operating theater with full preparations for cesarean section having been made. There should be no hesitation in abandoning the forceps delivery if difficulty is encountered with the application of the blades or locking of the handles. Such difficulty signifies a possible malposition and a wrong application of the forceps, one on the face and the other over the occipital bone. Forcible locking and traction might result in fracture of the skull and tentorial tearing in addition to injury to the eyes. If a rotational forceps delivery is attempted, failure of rotation is also an indication for cesarean section. With any forceps or vacuum delivery, if the presenting part shows no descent with bearing down efforts and traction over three contractions, consideration should be given to abandoning the procedure and proceeding to cesarean section.

Prolongation of the second stage is common with the use of epidural anesthesia.[20,62] This has been attributed to reduced uterine acitivity due to absence of the normal surge of oxytocin secretion seen in the second stage[63] secondary to the abolition of the Ferguson reflex (stretching of the cervix and upper vagina).[64] Correction of the deficiency by administering oxytocin and, in addition, allowing more time and coordinating the mother's bearing down efforts with uterine contractions, can reduce the number of instrumental vaginal deliveries.[65] Care must be taken not to overstimulate the uterus and produce fetal hypoxia, as this will then contraindicate any further attempt at rotational vaginal delivery. Extra care should be exercised when dealing with grand multiparas because of the risk of uterine rupture.

Malpresentation

Presentation is defined as the lowermost part of the fetus which presents to the pelvis and the lower uterine segment. It is more precisely determined by vaginal examination than by abdominal palpation. More than 95% of fetuses at term present in labor by the vertex, and any other presentation is called malpresentation. About 3% of fetuses at term present by the breech. Face (incidence 1:500) and brow (incidence 1:1500) presentation are malpresentations, not being vertex although cephalic.[66] The other rare malpresentation is a shoulder with an incidence of 3:10 000. When the cord presents at the cervical os with intact membranes it is termed a cord presentation. The incidence, etiology and management of breech presentation is discussed in Chapter 13.

Brow presentation is due to a deflexed head. On vaginal examination, the forehead is the leading part felt through the cervix but is termed brow presentation because the brow is the most definable portion of the head beyond the forehead. Because of extension of the head, the presenting anteroposterior diameter is 'mentovertical' and is about 13 cm at term. The mid-pelvis of the female is circular and the average anteroposterior and lateral diameters are equal (12 × 12 cm). Thus a brow presentation at term will generally not negotiate the mid-pelvis. The head in a brow presentation can flex and become a vertex presentation or extend and become a face presentation (submento bregmatic diameter of 9.5 cm).[67] Progress in labor can then resume and vaginal delivery occur. Hence if a brow presentation is diagnosed at term in the prenatal period, the patient can be managed conservatively. If diagnosed in early labor, time (2–3 h) may be allowed without oxytocic augmentation to see whether spontaneous flexion or extension will take place to a favorable presentation. If there is no progress over a few hours and the presentation remains as a brow, it is safer to deliver the fetus by cesarean section. There are others who prefer to augment with oxytocin for 1 h (with caution in a multipara and not at all in a grand multipara) to see whether the increased contractions will bring about flexion to a vertex or extension to a face presentation in addition to promoting cervical dilatation. If there is no change in presentation, or poor progress, delivery by cesarean section is necessary.[68] Although there is no etiological factor identified for most cases of brow presentation, thyroid goitre (or other tumors in the neck of the fetus) and anencephaly have occasionally been implicated. Where facilities exist, these possibilities are best excluded by an ultrasound examination. In the case of a preterm fetus, the anteroposterior diameter even with a brow presentation may be small and the patient may deliver vaginally without difficulty. Cesarean section should be considered if progress is poor even in a preterm fetus to avoid possible cervical cord and intracranial injuries.

Anecdotal reports exist of vacuum delivery of a brow presentation by direct traction or progressive reapplication toward the occiput to flex the head followed by traction.[68] This is an exercise only for the very experienced obstetrician. It is safe and acceptable to deliver a brow presentation identified at full dilatation by cesarean section when there is no progress.

Face presentation is diagnosed by palpation of the chin, mouth, nose and the orbital ridges. Presenting diameters are the transverse 'biparietal' (9.5 cm) and the anteroposterior 'submento bregmatic' (9.5 cm). Mentoanterior positions are reasonably likely to deliver vaginally either spontaneously or with assistance. Because of the favorable diamaters (9.5 × 9.5 cm), a trial of labor is allowed with face presentation. The use of oxytocic augmentation in cases associated with poor progress is controversial, and some opt for a cesarean section and refrain from using oxytocin for fear of cervical cord and intracranial injuries. Should oxytocin be used, labor may be continued if there is satisfactory progress, but a cesarean section is advisable if there is

no progress in 1–2 h. Face presentation in a preterm fetus may not pose a problem because of the relatively small size of the fetal head but cesarean section is advisable if progress is poor. In a case of intrauterine death, the fetus no longer needs to be considered, and augmentation can be carried out to achieve vaginal delivery.

Delay in the second stage can be managed by a forceps delivery if the presenting part is low and is in the mentoanterior position. If it is presenting in the mentoposterior position, rotation of the head to the mentoanterior position is desirable, as the diameter of the head negotiating the retropubic area and the subpubic arch is adequate. This may not be easy if the presenting part is high. Cesarean section is preferable to a difficult rotation forceps delivery.

Malposition

Position is defined as the relationship of the denominator of the presenting part of the fetus to fixed points of the maternal pelvis. The denominator is usually the most definable peripheral point of the presenting part. The occiput is the denominator for vertex presentations, the sacrum for breech presentations and the mentum (chin) for face presentations. The fixed points of the maternal pelvis are the symphysis pubis anteriorly, the ileopectineal eminences anterolaterally, the sacroiliac joints posterolaterally and the sacrum posteriorly. If the occiput is pointing to the sacrum it is termed a direct occipitoposterior position, and if it points to the right sacroiliac joint it is termed a right occipitoposterior position.

Most fetuses with a cephalic presentation have the vertex presenting to the cervix because of the shape and curvature of the pelvis and direction of the pelvic floor which promotes flexion at the atlanto-occipital joint. In labor, about 90% of vertex presentations have the occiput in the anterior half of the pelvis (occipitoanterior position).[69] Of the remainder, half turn to occipitoanterior with the advance of labor and deliver vaginally. The other half remain in an occipitoposterior or occipitolateral position. Delivery can occur spontaneously but assistance is commonly required. When the vertex is in the occipitolateral or occipitoposterior position, it is termed a malposition. Although face and breech presentations have denominators and positions can be defined, the term malposition is not applicable when there is malpresentation. Malposition indicates the possibility of poor progress in labor because of the larger anteroposterior ('occipitofrontal') diameter of 11 cm associated with the deflexed head.

The etiology of malposition is difficult to identify. Postulated mechanisms are increased tonus of the extensor muscles of the fetus which prevent flexion, and suboptimal shapes of the birth canal such as and-

---

POOR PROGRESS IN LABOR
Summary of Management Options

First stage

Diagnosis

With partogram

Management

- Poor progress in latent phase:
  - conservative approach in most cases
  - check CTG intermittently
  - trials of augmentation awaited

- Poor progress in active phase:
  - augmentation (some set 8 h limit; some argue for stopping if no progress after 4 h)

Second stage

Diagnosis

- No spontaneous delivery with a second stage of 1 h (arbitrary; some set shorter limit with parous women)

Management

- Augmentation if poor uterine activity
- Assisted vaginal delivery otherwise

Vigilance for

Malposition

- Occipitolateral or occipitoposterior; augmentation (with 4–8 h limit) is acceptable for poor progress in first stage
- Assisted delivery for second stage delivery (ventouse, rotational forceps, cesarean section are the options)

Malpresentation

- Breech – see Chapter 13
- Cord
  - options are prompt assisted vaginal delivery or cesarean section
- Brow
  - if diagnosed early in first stage, conservative approach can be followed (will it convert to flexed vertex?)
  - if no change or diagnosed in late labor for cesarean section, augmentation used with caution
- Face
  - if mento-anterior vaginal delivery possible.
  - mentoposterior will mostly have to be delivered by cesarean section;
  - use of augmentation is controversial

Disproportion

Delivery by cesarean section

---

roid, anthropoid and platypelloid.[70,71] However, the fact that a reasonable number of patients with malposition and poor progress of labor respond to oxytocin augmentation and deliver vaginally points to the fact that inadequate force of uterine contractions may also be an important factor.

Malposition in labor can cause poor progress in the first stage of labor due to a larger presenting diameter and the poor fit of the presenting part to the cervix and lower segment. Oxytocin augmentation may produce flexion and rotation of the head with consequent spontaneous or assisted vaginal delivery. If despite augmentation for 6–8 h the progress of labor remains poor, cesarean section is probably advisable.

CONCLUSIONS

Labor is a natural phenomenon leading to childbirth. Many women have the rewarding experience of a safe vaginal delivery, while a small proportion die of the consequences of prolonged labor and its sequelae. In an attempt to reduce adverse events, obstetric interventions have become popular. However, public suspicions about unnecessary interventions have often threatened to bring the medical profession into disrepute (Sir Anthony Carlisle first voiced these concerns in the British Parliament as long ago as 1834 when speaking to the Select Committee on Medical Education, concerns echoed in the most recent report on childbirth produced by the Select Committee on Health in 1992). These concerns, widely expressed by the general public in recent years, are perfectly valid and will increase if practice is not continually scrutinized and subjected to appropriate clinical trials whenever possible. Interventions in labor should not only be made in good faith but should be based on sound knowledge of normal labor and its variations. Perhaps in obstetrics more than in other fields of medicine, opinions differ as to management policies especially when an intervention is needed. The physician is in a dilemma when he intervenes because, on the one hand, if complications ensue the decision to intervene may be questioned and, on the other, if fetal or maternal morbidity or mortality follow non-intervention the consequences may be even more difficult to face. During the last four decades, research concerning the management of labor has been directed to formulating guidelines based on scientific data. Further research is needed to improve current practice. Some areas of current interest related to poor progress of labor concern the usefulness of prostaglandins[72] and the use of catheter-mounted transducers to quantify intrauterine pressure and head-to-cervix force.[73]

REFERENCES

1 Rao B (1992) Obstructed labor. In Ratnam SS, Rao B, Arulkumaran S (eds), *Obstetrics and Gynaecology for Postgraduates*, Vol. 1, pp. 127–133. Madras:Longman.

2 World Health Organization (1988) *The Partograph*, Sections I, II, III and IV. WHO/MCH/88.4. Geneva: WHO/Maternal and Child Health Unit, Division of Family Health.

3 Editorial (1981) Cesarean child birth: Summary of a National Instiues of Health Consensus statement. *British Medical Journal* **282**:1600–1604.

4 Hall MH (1990) Confidential enquiry into maternal death. *British Journal of Obstetrics and Gynaecology* **97**:752–753.

5 Friedman EA (1954) The graphic analysis of labour. *American Journal of Obstetrics and Gynecology* **68**:1568–1571.

6 Philpott RH (1972) Graphic records in labour. *British Medical Journal* **iv**:163–165.

7 O'Driscoll K, Stronge JM, Minogue M (1973) Active management of labour. *British Medical Journal* **iii**:135–138.

8 Studd JWW (1973) Partograms and nomograms in the management of primigravid labour. *British Medical Journal* **iv**:451–455.

9 Illancheran A, Lim SM, Ratnam SS (1977) Nomograms of cervical dilatation in labour. *Singapore Journal of Obstetrics and Gynaecology* **8**:69–73.

10 Duignan NM, Studd JWW, Hughes AO (1975) Characteristics of labour in different racial groups. *British Journal of Obstetrics and Gynaecology* **82**:593–601.

11 Arulkumaran S, Gibb DMF, Chua S, Piara Singh, Ratnam SS (1989) Ethnic influences on uterine activity in spontaneous normal labour. *British Journal of Obstetrics and Gynaecology* **96**:1203–1206.

12 Studd J, Clegg DR, Saunders RR, Hughes AO (1975) Identification of high risk labours by labour nomogram. *British Medical Journal* **ii**:545–547.

13 Cardozo LD, Gibb DMF, Studd JWW, Vasant RV, Cooper DJ (1982) Predictive value of cervimetric labour patterns in primigravidae. *British Journal of Obstetrics and Gynaecology* **89**:33–38.

14 Gibb DMF, Cardozo LD, Studd JWW, Magos AL, Cooper DJ (1982) Outcome of spontaneous labour in multigravidae. *British Journal of Obstetrics and Gynaecology* **89**:708–711.

15 Beazley JM, Alderman S (1976) The 'inductograph', a graph describing the limits of the latent phase of induced labour in low risk situations. *British Journal of Obstetrics and Gynaecology* **83**:513–517.

16 Arulkumaran S, Koh CH, Ingemarsson I, Ratnam SS (1987) Augmentation of labour: Mode of delivery related to cervimetric progress. *Australia and New Zealand Journal of Obstetrics and Gynaecology* **27**:304–308.

17 Steer PJ, Carter MC, Beard RW (1985) The effect of oxytocin infusion on uterine activity levels in slow labour. *British Journal of Obstetrics and Gynaecology* **92**:1120–1126.

18 Arulkumaran S, Chua S, Chua TM, Yang M, Piara S, Ratnam SS (1991) Uterine activity in dysfunctional labour and target uterine activity to be aimed at with oxytocin titration. *Asia and Oceania Journal of Obstetrics and Gynaecology* **17**:101–106.

19 O'Driscoll K, Jackson RJA, Gallagher JT (1970) Active management of labour and cephalopelvic disproportion. *Journal of Obstetrics and Gynaecology of the British Commonwealth* **77**:385–389.

20 O'Driscoll K, Meagher D (1980) *Active Management of Labour: Clinics in Obstetrics and Gynaecology*, pp. 3–17. Philadelphia, PA: W:B: Saunders.

21 Gibb DMF, Arulkumaran S, Lun KC, Heng SH, Ratnam SS (1984) Characteristics of uterine activity in nullipar-

ous labour. *British Journal of Obstetrics and Gynaecology* **91**:220–227.

22 Arulkumaran S, Gibb DMF, Lun KC, Heng SH, Ratnam SS (1984) The effect of parity on uterine activity in labour. *British Journal of Obstetrics and Gynaecology* **91**:843–848.

23 Arulkumaran S, Michelson J, Ingemarsson I, Ratnam SS (1987) Obstetric outcome of patients with a previous epidode of spurious labor. *American Journal of Obstetrics and Gynecology* **157**:17–20.

24 Arulkumaran S, Ingemarsson I (1985) New concepts in the management of spontaneous labour. *Singapore Journal of Obstetrics and Gynaecology* **16**:163–172.

25 Sica Blanco Y, Sala NL (1961) *Oxytocin: Proceedings of an International Symposium*, pp. 127–134. Oxford: Pergamon Press.

26 Kubli F, Ruttgers H (1961) Iatrogenic fetal hypoxia. In Gevers RH, Ruys JH (eds), *Physiology and Pathology in the Perinatal Periods*, pp. 55–75. Leiden: Leiden University Press.

27 Liston WA, Campbell AJ (1974) Dangers of oxytocin induced labour to the fetus. *British Medical Journal* **3**:606–607.

28 Gibb DMF, Arulkumaran S (1982) Oxytocin: A reappraisal. *Singapore Journal of Obstetrics and Gynaecology* **13**:152–158.

29 Daw E (1973) Oxytocin induced rupture of the primigravid uterus. *Journal of Obstetrics and Gynaecology of the British Commonwealth* **80**:374–375.

30 Turnbull AC, Anderson AB (1968) Induction of labour. *Journal of Obstetrics and Gynaecology of the British Commonwealth* **75**:32–41.

31 Steer PJ, Carter MC, Choong K *et al.* (1985) A multicentre prospective randomized controlled trial of induction of labour with an automatic closed-loop feedback controlled oxytocin infusion system. *British Journal of Obstetrics and Gynaecology* **92**:1127–1133.

32 Knutzen VK, Tanneberger U, Davey DA (1977) Complications and outcome of induced labour. *South African Medical Journal* **52**:482–485.

33 Fuchs AR, Fuchs F (1984) Endocrinology of human parturition: A review. *British Journal of Obstetrics and Gynaecology* **91**:948:967.

34 Saameli K (1963) an indirect method for the estimation of oxytocin blood concentration and half-life in pregnant women near term. *American Journal of Obstetrics and Gynecology* **85**:186–192.

35 Seitchik J, Amico J, Robinson AG *et al.* (1984) Oxytocin augmentation of dysfunctional labour. iv. Oxytocin pharmacokinetics. *American Journal of Obstetrics and Gynecology* **150**:225–232.

36 Fuchs F (1985) Caution on using oxytocin for inductions. *Contemporary Obstetrics and Gynecology* **25**:13–16.

37 Foster TCS, Jacobson JD, Valenzuela GJ (1988) Oxytocin augmentation of labour: A comparison of 15 and 30 minute dose increment intervals. *Obstetrics and Gynecology* **71**:147–149.

38 Blakemore KJ, Qin NG, Petrie RH, Paine LL (1990) A prospective comparison of hourly and quarter hourly oxytocin dose increase intervals for the induction of labour at term. *Obstetrics and Gynecology* **75**:757–761.

39 Chua S, Arulkumaran S, Kurup A, Tay D, Ratnam SS (1991) Oxytocin titration for induction of labour: A prospective randomized study of 15 versus 30 minute dose increment schedules. *Australia and New Zealand Journal of Obstetrics and Gynaecology* **31**:134–137.

40 Brindley BA, Sokol RJ (1988) Induction and augmentation of labour: Basis and methods for current practice. *Obstetrics and Gynecological Survey* **43**:730–743.

41 American College of Obstetricians and Gynecologists (1987) *Induction and Augmentation of Labour*, Technical Bulletin No. 110, November.

42 Reddi K, Kambaran SR, Philpott PA (1988) Intrauterine pressure studies in multigravid patients in spontaneous labour. Effect of oxytocin augmentation in delayed first stage. *British Journal of Obstetrics and Gynaecology* **95**:771–777.

43 Steer PJ (1977) The measurement and control of uterine contractions. In Beard RW, Campbell S (eds), *The Current Status of Fetal Heart Rate Monitoring and Ultrasound in Obstetrics*, pp. 48–70. London: Royal College of Obstetricians and Gynaecologists.

44 Arulkumaran S, Yang M, Ingemarsson I, Piara S, Ratnam SS (1989) Augmentation of labour: Does oxytocin titration to achieve preset active contraction area values produce better obstetric outcome? *Asia and Oceania Journal of Obstetrics and Gynaecology* **15**:333–337.

45 Chua S, Kurup A, Arulkumaran S, Ratnam SS (1990) Augmentation of labor: Does internal tocography result in better obstetric outcome than external tocography? *Obstetrics and Gynecology* **76**:164–167.

46 Beckley S, Gee H, Newton JR (1991) Scar rupture in labour after previous lower segment caesarean section: The role of uterine activity measurement. *British Journal of Obstetrics and Gynaecology* **98**:265–269.

47 Arulkumaran S, Chua S, Ratnam SS (1992) Symptoms and signs with scar rupture: Value of uterine activity measurements. *Australia and New Zealand Journal of Obstetrics and Gynaecology* **32**:208–212.

48 Arulkumaran S, Gibb DMF, Ingemarsson I, Kitchener CH, Ratnam SS (1989) Uterine activity during spontaneous normal labour after previous caesarean section. *British Journal of Obstetrics and Gynaecology* **96**:933–938.

49 Arulkumaran S, Ingemarsson I, Ratnam SS (1989) Oxytocin augmentation in dysfunctional labour after previous caesarean section. *British Journal of Obstetrics and Gynaecology* **96**:939–941.

50 Borten M (1983) Breech presentation. In Friedman EA, Cohen WR (eds), *Management of Labor*, pp. 253–256. Baltimore, MD: University Park Press.

51 Arulkumaran S, Tariq K, Ingemarsson I (1988) Management of the term breech presentation in labour. *Singapore Journal of Obstetrics and gynaecology* **19**:44–52.

52 Krishnamurthy S, Fairlie F, Cameron AD, Walker JJ, MacKenzie JR (1991) The role of postnatal pelvimetry after caesarean section in the management of subsequent delivery. *British Journal of Obstetrics and Gynaecology* **98**:716–718.

53 Arulkumaran S, Ingemarsson I, Gibb DMF, Ratnam SS (1988) Uterine activity in spontaneous labour with

breech presentation. *Australia and New Zealand Journal of Obstetrics and Gynaecology* **28**:275–278.

54 Ingemarsson I, Arulkumaran S, Westgren M (1989) Breech delivery: Management and long term outcome. In Tejani N (ed.), *Obstetrical events and developmental sequelae* pp. 143–159. Boca Raton, FL: CRC Press.

55 Clark SL, Eglinton GS, Beall M, Phelan JP (1984) Effect of the indication for previous caesarean section on subsequent delivery outcome in patients undergoing a trial of labour. *Journal of Reproductive Medicine* **29**:22–25.

56 Phelan JP, Clark SL, Diaz F, Paul RH (1987) Vaginal birth after caesarean. *American Journal of Obstetrics and Gynecology* **157**:1510–1515.

57 Chua S, Arulkumaran S, Piara S, Ratnam SS (1989) Trial of labour after previous caesarean section: Obstetric outcome. *Australia and New Zealand Journal of Obstetrics and Gynaecology* **29**:12–17.

58 Hanna WJ (1965) X-ray pelvimetry: Critical appraisal. *American Journal of Obstetrics and Gynecology* **91**:333–341.

59 Laube WD, Varner MW, Cruikshank DP (1981) A prospective evaluation of x-ray pelvimetry. *Journal of the American Medical Association* **246**:2187–2190.

60 Jagani N, Schulman H, Chandra P, Gonzalez P, Fleischer A (1981) The predictability of labor outcome from a comparison of birth weight and X-ray pelvimetry. *American Journal of Obstetrics and Gynecology* **139**:501–511.

61 Richardson JA, Sutherland IA, Allen DW (1978) A cervimeter for continuous measurement of cervical dilatation in labour: Preliminary results. *British Journal of Obstetrics and Gynaecology* **85**:178–184.

62 Paintin DB, Vincent F (1980) Forceps delivery: Obstetric outcome. In Beard RW, Paintin DB (eds), *Outcome of Obstetric Intervention in Britain*, pp. 17–32.

London: Royal College of Obstetricians and Gynaecologists.

63 Vascika A, Kumaresan P, Han GS, Kumaresan M (1978) Plasma oxytocin in initiation in labour. *American Journal of Obstetrics and Gynecology* **130**:263–273.

64 Ferguson JKW, (1941) A study of the motility of the intact uterus at term. *Surgery, Gynecology and Obstetrics* **73**:359–366.

65 Goodfellow CF, Studd C (1979) the reduction of forceps in primigravidae with epidural analgesia: A controlled trial. *British Journal of Clinical Practice* **33**:287–288.

66 Cruikshank DP, Cruikshank JE (1981) Face and brow presentation: A review. *Clinical Obstetrics and Gynecology* **24**:33–351.

67 Clinch J (1989) Abnormal fetal presentations and positions. In Turnbull A, Chamberlain G (eds), *Obstetrics*, pp. 793–812. London: Churchill Livingstone.

68 Seeds JW, Cefalo RC (1982) Malpresentations. *Clinical Obstetrics and Gynecology* **25**:145–156.

69 Myerscough P (1989) Cephalopelvic disproportion. In Turnbull A, Chamberlain G (eds), *Obstetrics*, pp. 813–821. London: Churchill Livingstone.

70 Holmberg NG, Lilieqvist B, Magnusson S, Segerbrand E (1977) The influence of the bony pelvis in persistent occiput posterior position. *Acta Obstetrica et Gynecologica Scandinavica* **66**:49–54 (Suppl.).

71 Stewart DB (1984) The pelvis as a passageway. II. The modern human pelvis. *British Journal of Obstetrics and Gynaecology* **91**:618–623.

72 Keirse MJNC (1989) Augmentation of labour. In Chalmers I, Enkin M, Keirse MJNC (eds), *Effective Care in Pregnancy and Childbirth*, pp. 951–968. Oxford: Oxford University Press.

73 Gough GW, Randall NJ, Genevier ES, Sutherland IA, Steer PJ (1990) Head to cervix forces and their relationship to the outcome of labour. *Obstetrics and Gynecology* **75**:613–618.

62

Fetal Distress in Labor

PHILIP J. STEER, P.J. DANIELIAN

INTRODUCTION

What Is Fetal Distress, And Can It Be Measured?

'Fetal distress' is a widely used but poorly defined term.[1,2] It is commonly used to signify a fetal indication for a cesarean section or instrumental delivery. However, such an indication might be hypoxia and acidosis, or intrauterine infection causing fetal tachycardia, or the passage of meconium in association with prolonged labor. To equate such differing pathophysiologies is akin to saying that a non-pregnant patient needs a laparotomy 'because she is ill'. Some have suggested that 'fetal distress' should be used to indicate the likely occurrence of 'birth asphyxia', but this expression is no easier to define[3] and recently some authors have suggested that it should be abandoned.[4]

Strictly speaking, fetal distress applies only to the condition of the fetus *in utero*, although the ultimate concern of the clinician is that the diagnosis of fetal distress implies the danger of a poor neonatal outcome, usually termed 'birth asphyxia'. The original form of this expression was 'asphyxia neonatorum', subdivided into 'asphyxia livida' (asphyxia with cyanosis) and 'asphyxia pallida' (asphyxia with shock, and thus a vasoconstricted periphery). It was used to indicate failure of the newly born baby to breathe, for whatever reason, be this drugs given to the mother (such as anesthetics), trauma, infection, congenital abnormality or hypoxia.[5] Gradually, however, the assumption crept

in that it was usually due to hypoxia, and in 1976 it was defined by Towell[6] as 'depletion of oxygen and accumulation of carbon dioxide, leading to a state of acidosis, which during intrauterine life is due to interference with placental gaseous exchange'. This assumption was fuelled by surveys such as the National Birthday Trust Survey of perinatal mortality in the UK in 1958, which recorded an overall perinatal mortality rate of 31 per 1000 births; the toll attributed to 'trauma and/or hypoxia' in labor amounted to approximately 1:100 normally formed babies weighing 1 kg or more, about a third of the total.[7] However, the diagnosis that these deaths were primarily caused by hypoxia could not at that time be validated scientifically. The diagnosis of fetal condition was essentially limited to auscultating the fetal heart rate (FHR) and examining the amniotic fluid for meconium (see later for a full description of the significance of meconium in the amniotic fluid). Intermittent auscultation of the FHR, performed according to standard practice at the time – noting the fetal heart rate, rhythm and intensity every 2 h during the first stage (of labor) while the membranes were intact, and every 30 min after they had ruptured[5] – had manifestly failed to prevent these deaths. It was in an attempt to diagnose 'fetal distress' in labor and hence this toll of stillbirth, that fetal blood sampling (FBS) and pH estimation were introduced into clinical practice by Erich Saling in 1962.[8] His original major indications for sampling were: passage of meconium found at amnioscopy or after rupture of membranes (accounting for 42% of samplings), and/or alteration of the fetal heart rate with a rise above 150 beats/min (known then as 'acceleration' and accounting for 40% of samplings) or a fall below 120 beats/min (11% of samplings).[8] By 1967, the study of 306 fetuses born in a vigorous condition had established the mean pH of a fetal blood sample as 7.33 with a range (± 2 SDs) of 7.2 – 7.5;[9] 7.2 rapidly became the accepted lower limit of normal. However, it was soon noted that despite the assumption that most cases of poor neonatal condition at birth were associated with biochemical asphyxia and therefore should be preceded by acidosis detectable with fetal blood sampling and pH estimation, there was in a 'certain number of cases' a discrepancy between the condition of the neonate predicted from the measured pH and its actual condition.[10] For example, in 1967, Beard et al.[10] reported that 15 of 116 fetuses with a FBS pH of >7.205 in the late first stage of labor were unexpectedly born with a 1 min Apgar score of <7, whereas 25 of 126 neonates with a 1 min Apgar score >7 had a FBS pH ≤ 7.205. Estimation of base deficit did not provide a more accurate prediction of which babies would be depressed at birth, and the authors concluded that 'the Apgar score does not differentiate between asphyxial and non-asphyxial depression of the newborn'. In this comment, the authors were limiting the use of the expression 'asphyxia' to indicate acid–base disturbance, rather than using it in the previous global sense of 'failure to breathe after birth'.

One of the early problems of using FBS was that known risk factors gave insufficient indication of which fetuses should have FBS performed. Beard[11] further reported in 1968 that 'despite the availability of fetal blood sampling a number of intrapartum stillbirths caused by intrauterine asphyxia during labour still occur each year. Characteristically the fetal heart rate of these babies often remains within the normal range right up to the moment of death.' In the 1969 study of Coltart et al.,[12] no cases of acidosis were discovered in 69 fetuses sampled because of obstetric risk factors but in whom the FHR (assessed by intermittent auscultation) remained normal and there was no meconium staining of the amniotic fluid. On the other hand, there was one intrapartum stillbirth in which FBS had not been carried out because there were no clinical signs of distress during labor.

The introduction of continuous electronic fetal heart rate monitoring (EFM) in the late 1960s might have been expected to boost the use of fetal blood sampling, by revealing FHR abnormalities undetectable using the Pinard stethoscope (for example, shallow late decelerations). Unfortunately, the relative ease of performing EFM compared with FBS had the opposite effect, and the use of EFM became widespread whereas the use of FBS did not. For example, in a survey of UK practice carried out by Gillmer and Combe in 1978,[13] only 1 of 244 maternity units responding did not possess an electronic fetal heart rate monitor. However, only 98 supplemented the use of

EFM with FBS. This was despite the work of Beard et al., which showed that the majority of abnormal FHR patterns were not associated with an abnormally low pH.[14] Beard et al. concluded that 'if continuous monitoring of FHR is used on its own in clinical practice a number of false positive diagnoses of fetal asphyxia are likely to be made. In practical terms an abnormal FHR trace should be regarded as a warning sign indicating the need to check the fetal pH.' Their warning was confirmed when five randomized controlled trials of EFM vs intermittent auscultation carried out during the next 10 years failed to show any improvement in neonatal outcome, but did show an overall 2.4-fold increase in the cesarean section rate, associated with the use of EFM without FBS.[15–19] In the single largest prospective randomized controlled trial of EFM vs auscultation, in which FBS was used (often referred to as the 'Dublin Trial,' after the city in which it was performed), no such increase in the cesarean section rate was observed.[20]

The reason for the increase in intervention with EFM is that in only about 60% of labors does the FHR remain unequivocally normal throughout labor[21] (a normal FHR tracing indicates less than a 2% chance of finding a pH <7.20 on a FBS[14] and a less than 1% chance of the 5 min Apgar score being less than 7, provided that the amniotic fluid is not meconium-stained[21]). This means that up to 40% of fetuses show variations in the FHR, which can be interpreted as 'suspicious' or 'abnormal'. Unfortunately, 80% of abnormalities are only suspicious, and 80% of these will not be associated either with fetal acidosis or depression at birth.[14] Even with the most abnormal pattern, a baseline tachycardia with late decelerations, only 50% of fetuses will be found to be acidotic on FBS.[14] Thus routine intervention on the basis of an abnormal FHR, without the additional information of a FBS pH, will prove to be unnecessary in a majority of cases.

Moreover, recent studies have shown that there is only a weak relationship between biochemical disturbance of the fetus (measured as hypoxia, hypercarbia and acidosis) and indicators of neonatal condition such as the Apgar score. Sykes et al.,[22] in a study in Oxford, UK, showed that only 1:5 babies with either a 1 or 5 min Apgar score <7 had a severe acidosis (umbilical artery pH <7.1 and a base deficit ≥ 13 mmol/l). Similarly, only 1:4 babies with a severe acidosis had a 1 min Apgar score ≤7 and only 1:7 a 5 min Apgar score ≤7. Lissauer and Steer[23] found that almost 60% of babies born at 32 weeks gestation or later and needing resuscitation by intubation and positive pressure ventilation had no evidence of biochemical disturbance; they had either entirely normal FHR patterns throughout labor and/or normal values for umbilical cord blood pH measurement. Steer et al.[21] subsequently reported that variation in umbilical artery pH accounted for only 7.5% of the variation in the 1 min

Apgar score and only 1.8% of the variation in the 5 min Apgar score. Hall[24] has commented that the concept, of birth asphyxia as a state of perinatal hypoxia and acidosis, which had developed since the 1960s, was no longer tenable. He considered that: 'Asphyxia is hard to define and measure; hypoxic-ischaemic encephalopathy is the most reliable indicator of asphyxia; neither traditional clinical signs nor electronic monitoring allow reliable recognition of asphyxia.' Thorp[25] suggested that birth asphyxia be redefined to include not only acidemia (pH ≥ 2 SDs below the mean, e.g. <7.10), but also neonatal depression and evidence of hypoxic end-organ damage such as early neonatal seizures, renal or cardiac dysfunction. Subsequently, the Oxford group widened their definition of birth asphyxia even more, to include a variable combination (at least two) of umbilical artery or capillary blood pH at birth <7.20, an Apgar score < 7 at 1 min, the need for intermittent positive pressure ventilation, signs of cerebral irritability – cycling, fisting, staring – clinical convulsions treated with anticonvulsant drugs, and meconium aspiration syndrome.[26] Perhaps one solution to the problem of defining birth asphyxia would be to revert to its original definition of failure to breathe at birth, and simply to list the associated features, such as acidosis or convulsions.

As well as making clear the weak relationship between fetal acid-base status and condition at birth, recent studies have suggested that acidosis *per se* has little value in the prediction of long-term problems. Ruth and Raivio followed for 1 year a cohort of 964 infants having had umbilical artery blood acid–base measurements.[27] They found that a pH <7.11 only had a sensitivity of 21% and a specificity of 89% in the prediction of abnormal development. Dennis et al.[28] failed to find a statistically significant association between acidosis at birth and developmental outcome in 203 infants followed up to age 4.5 years. Low et al.[29] found no difference in the Brazelton newborn assessment score between 51 newborns with an umbilical buffer base <34 mmol/l and a non-acidotic matched control group and concluded that 'many newborns who have undergone an intrapartum asphyxial insult will not have evidence of central nervous system injury'. Winkler et al.[30] reported that none of 335 infants born with an umbilical artery pH <7.2 but >7.0 had any neonatal complications, and only 2 of 23 born with a pH <7.0 had any complications attributable to asphyxia (one had convulsions and the other ischemic necrosis of the tricuspid papillary muscle). Goodwin et al.[31] reviewed 129 term normally formed singleton infants born with an umbilical artery pH <7.0. In total, 78% were entirely normal at follow-up; only 8% had a major neurological defect (4% died, 4% were suspect and 6% were lost to follow-up).

Does this mean therefore that FBS and pH measurement during labor are of no value? The Dublin Trial did show one significant benefit associated with EFM, a neonatal seizure rate which was significantly lower (1.4 per 1000) than when intermittent auscultation was used (3.8 per 1000). It is possible, indeed likely, that this was associated with fewer cases of hypoxia and acidosis in the EFM group. In support of this hypothesis is the fact that in a subgroup of 1075 babies who had routine umbilical venous blood pH measurement, there were fewer with a pH < 7.1 in the EFM group (5/540, 1%) than in the intermittent auscultation (IA) group (11/535, 2.1%)(P=0.1, Fisher's exact test, one-tailed). This was associated not only with a higher rate of FBS in the EFM group (4.4%) than in the IA group (3.5%) but, more importantly, a higher pick-up of low FBS pHs <7.20: 29 in the EFM group compared with only 16 in the IA group (P=0.036, Fisher's exact test, one-tailed). In the EFM group, 173 FBSs were performed for abnormalities in the FHR compared with only 49 for this indication in the IA group. In contrast, fewer FBSs were performed in the EFM group solely because of labor being prolonged for more than 8 h (77 vs 139), presumably because a normal FHR tracing gave sufficient reassurance about fetal well-being.

It is perhaps surprising that the higher incidence of neonatal seizures in the IA group in the Dublin study was not associated with a higher rate of perinatal mortality, as other studies have emphasized the adverse prognostic significance of seizures[32] and there was a higher incidence of neonatal neurological abnormalities persisting for at least 1 week (20 vs 12). However, even the Dublin study was too small to detect clinically significant differences in perinatal mortality rate. The overall perinatal mortality rate (PNMR) was so low (2.16 per 1000) that the 95% confidence interval of the difference between the PNMR in the EFM compared with the IA group ranged from −1.59 to +1.6 per 1000. This means that, statistically, the result of the trial was compatible with a true halving of the PNMR associated with the use of EFM and FBS.

Another assumption which has recently been questioned is the relationship between any event in labor, even when unrelated to acidosis, and long-term neurological or intellectual handicap. Illingworth[33] was among the first to question the assumption that brain damage, cerebral palsy and mental subnormality were often related to difficulties in labor. Paneth and Stark[34] pointed out that 50% of cases of cerebral palsy had no demonstrable depression at birth and estimated that no more than 15% of severe mental retardation could be attributed to perinatal events; they considered that mental retardation without cerebral palsy was not due to birth asphyxia. In 1985, the National Institutes of Health in the USA[35] reported that 'the causes of severe mental retardation are primarily genetic, biochemical, viral and developmental, and not related to birth events. Associated factors include maternal life-styles such as poor nutrition, cigarette smoking, and alcohol and drug abuse.' Hensleigh and Fainstat[36] reported that the causes of perinatal mortality correlated poorly with the occurrence of cerebral palsy. Even more recently, concern has been expressed that despite improvements in perinatal mortality in the developed world, cerebral palsy rates are not declining,[37] which is further evidence that birth asphyxia is not a major cause of cerebral palsy.

Does all this mean that routine EFM in labor, even with FBS, cannot be justified? In an editorial in the *British Medical Journal*, Neilsen[38] opined in 1993 that 'the available evidence does not support routine continuous fetal heart rate monitoring in all labours. In a normal labour intermittent auscultation with a Pinard stethoscope could not be regarded as an inadequate or negligent form of assessment.' However, he overlooked the fact that there is no scientific evidence that monitoring the FHR with the Pinard stethoscope has any value; no randomized controlled trials have been performed to demonstrate the superiority of auscultation to expectant management without knowledge of the FHR. Neither is there any consensus as to how auscultation should be performed; in the main UK midwifery text book,[39] it states simply that the FHR should be auscultated 'at intervals'. It may also be that it is not cardiotocography in principle which is not efficacious, but the way it is used. For example, an important audit of the antecedents of birth asphyxia was carred out in Oxford, UK, over a 17 month period.[40] The diagnosis of birth asphyxia was a clinical one, made by the pediatrician who admitted the infant to the special care baby unit. It relied on the presence of a variable number (at least two) of the following indicators: umbilical artery or capillary blood pH at birth <7.20; Apgar score < 7 at 1 min; the need for intermittent positive pressure ventilation; signs of cerebral irritability (cycling, fisting, staring); clinical convulsions treated with anticonvulsant drugs; and meconium aspiration syndrome. It was found that the cardiotocogram (CTG) had been severely abnormal in 61% of 38 babies with birth asphyxia, compared with only 9% of 120 controls. The criteria for the diagnosis of a severe CTG abnormality was that at least two of three expert reviewers thought that a FBS or immediate delivery should have been performed (inter-observer agreement on the diagnosis of severe CTG abnormality was approximately 90%). The mean cord arterial pH at birth was 7.01 for cases (n=34) and 7.23 for controls (n=62). Despite this high rate of severely abnormal CTG in the asphyxia group, FBS was performed in only 15% of cases (5/34) compared with 8% (5/62) of controls (P=0.25, one-tailed). This suggests that a primary problem was failure to recognize and react to the abnormal CTG; indeed, the mean time taken by staff before they reacted in any recorded way to the CTG abnormality was 99 min, with one case remaining unremarked upon for 475 min (almost 8 h). Medico-

legal experience suggests a similar conclusion, that in many cases the failure of CTG and FBS monitoring to prevent adverse events has more to do with human error than with the technology itself. Ennis[41] has shown that the majority of errors leading to litigation stem from the assumption of responsibility by inadequately trained and overconfident junior staff.

Conclusion

In summary, there is no conclusive evidence of the value of fetal monitoring in labor. It seems unlikely that it can play a major part in preventing long-term handicap; its most likely role is in the prevention of intrapartum death. Monitoring FHR with the Pinard stethoscope is probably acceptable in low-risk cases; EFM is appropriate in more complicated labors, such as those that are prolonged, augmented or induced, multiple pregnancies, those with thick meconium staining of the amniotic fluid, and those where there is a known or suspected growth-deficient or preterm fetus (See **Table 1**).[38]

FETAL HEART RATE MONITORING

Intermittent Auscultation

In 1963, Sir Andrew Claye wrote:

> 'The fetal heart rate, rhythm and intensity should be noted every two hours during the first stage (of labour) provided the membranes are intact – after the membranes have ruptured, it should be done every half an hour. Auscultation should be done as long after a contraction as possible, to allow the heart which has slowed to return to its normal rate.[5]

If the EFM has taught us anything, it is that this advice is no longer acceptable. Although there is no published standard for the technique of auscultation, the consensus view of the contributors to the labor section of this book is that the heart rate should be counted over at least 15 s (and preferably over 1 min), at least every 30 min (and preferably ever 15 min), during the first stage of labor. Auscultation should be performed just after a contraction, to detect persisting deceleration of the FHR. If the baseline rate is above 150 beats/min, or below 110 beats/min (FIGO guidelines[42]), or slows noticeably after a contraction, EFM should be employed to elucidate the pattern of the FHR. The frequency of auscultation should be increased in the second stage of labor, preferably taking place after every contraction. Decelerations are probably acceptable in the second stage of labor, provided prompt

Table 1
Indications for continuous electronic fetal monitoring

Labor abnormalities
Induced labor
Augmented labor
Prolonged labor
Prolonged membrane rupture
Regional analgesia
Previous cesarean section
Abnormal uterine activity

Suspected fetal distress in labor
Meconium staining of amniotic fluid
Suspicious fetal heart rate on auscultation
Abnormal FHR on admission CTG
Vaginal bleeding in labor
Intrauterine infection

Fetal problems
Multiple pregnancies (all fetuses)
Small fetus
Preterm fetus
Breech presentation
Oligohydramnios
Post-term pregnancy
Rhesus isoimmunization

Maternal medical disease
Hypertension
Diabetes
Cardiac disease (especially cyanotic)
Hemoglobinopathy
Severe anemia
Hyperthyroidism
Collagen disease
Renal disease

recovery (within 30 s) takes place to a normal baseline. If the fetal heart is difficult to hear, then a portable ultrasound fetal heart detector should be used. These are particularly useful if the mother is active, making application of the Pinard stethoscope difficult. Waterproof versions are available for use during pool deliveries. Intermittent auscultation of the FHR is not easy to perform properly. It is very time-consuming to carry out with the recommended frequency. If may inadvertently be omitted when procedures such as the insertion of epidural anesthetics are being performed; the midwife or obstetric nurse is busy helping the anesthetist. This may have serious consequences if there is maternal hypotension or some other complication and the FHR is discovered to be abnormal after the procedure; the birth attendants are not able to know whether the abnormality is transient or has been present for some time. Recordings may also become unacceptably infrequent during the second stage, when the midwife or obstetrician is busy conducting the delivery

and is scrubbed up with sterile gloves on. If there is no second midwife or nurse in attendance, and the baby does not emerge as quickly as expected, the deadly combination of prolongation of the second stage and inadequate FHR recording can easily occur. Second, the FHR normally varies considerably from one minute to another (normal baseline variability is from 5 to 15 beats/min) and this is very difficult to assess using a counting technique (it can be done,[43] but requires considerable patience). Third, intermittent auscultation cannot detect unusual FHR abnormalities such as a fixed rate with loss of baseline variability, or shallow late decelerations. Fourth, adherence to a strict regime of 15 min auscultation is very demanding on the birth attendant. Allowing for placing the mother in a suitable position, siting the Pinard stethoscope correctly, counting the rate and then recording it on the partogram, means that at least 5 min in every 15 min is taken up with this task. It seems unlikely that in routine practice such high levels of surveillance are achieved.

Electronic Fetal Monitoring

Because of the problems associated with intermittent auscultation, and despite the lack of proven superiority of EFM, the use of EFM has become widespread in the Western world. A cardiotocograph machine is used to produce a continuous recording of FHR and uterine contractions, known as a cardiotocogram (CTG). It produces information about aspects of FHR such as baseline variability which cannot be measured using intermittent auscultation. It also produces recordings of FHR decelerations in relation to contractions which are easier to detect and analyze, and there is automatically a paper record for archival purposes (in the future other media, such as optical discs or cards, are likely to take over, on the grounds of storage convenience). This record is available for subsequent independent review, which is very valuable for audit and teaching, although it may be a mixed blessing in medicolegal terms if it reveals abnormalities previously overlooked.

Electronic fetal monitors can measure the FHR and uterine contractions via external transducers using Doppler ultrasound and a tocodynamometer (strain gauge attached to a belt) or via internal sensors such as a fetal electrode and an intrauterine catheter. Despite the fact that the latter methods are more reliable and accurate, and probably more comfortable for the average woman in labor than the belts necessary to attach the external transducers, they are more 'invasive' and thus most EFM is performed using the external devices. This mode of EFM has a number of problems.

First, systems produced prior to 1982 often had poor ultrasound processing circuits with the result that the true FHR record was obscured by considerable artefactual jitter.[44] Traces produced using such systems were commonly misinterpreted as showing normal FHR variability when in fact variability was reduced and the observer was being misled by artefact. Equally unfortunately, many obsolete machines using such inadequate ultrasound systems are still in use because of financial constraints on their replacement. Although to the experienced eye pathologically reduced variability is still evident using these old systems, the average junior doctor, midwife or nurse often finds such ultrasound recordings confusing when compared with the electrode-derived trace. Modern machines generally use a form of autocorrelation or cross-correlation analysis[45] and are much better at producing a clear FHR trace, but the systems are now so sensitive that if the fetus is dead they sometimes produce a recording of the maternal rate which can be mistaken for that of the fetus.[46,47] This is particularly likely if the mother is anxious and has a tachycardia, so that her heart rate is similar to that expected of her fetus, and can even lead to the erroneous emergency delivery of a dead fetus.[48]

Second, good recording of the FHR is very dependent on correct placement of the transducers on the abdomen. This is not always achieved, and constant readjustment is often necessary if the mother is very active. Unfortunately, it is often the mothers who wish to have an active birth and who are very mobile who decline the use of internal monitoring. This commonly results in loss of adequate signal and FHR information at a most critical time in the labor, the second stage.

Third, the information which can be obtained about uterine contractions using an external transducer is essentially limited to timing them. The tocodynamometer gives only a relative indication of contraction strength, and the recording is attenuated if, for example, the mother is obese or the transducer is poorly placed. This may mislead the birth attendant into underestimating the strength of contractions, particularly in a stoical woman, and thus lead to overdosage with uterine stimulants such as oxytocin.

By comparison, the recordings obtained from a directly applied fetal electrode and an intrauterine catheter are much more accurate and less susceptible to recording failure. Nonetheless, there remains a small number of babies in whom the fetal ECG signal is weak (for reasons as yet obscure, which do not appear in most cases to be pathological) and mothers who cannot tolerate the insertion of an intrauterine catheter. In these cases, there is no substitute for either continuous ultrasound or assiduous intermittent FHR monitoring and clinical assessment of contractions.

In the USA more EFM is performed using the internal methods, while in the UK a larger proportion is performed using external methods. This may be due to the fact that in the USA the monitoring is generally applied by physicians who will not be present throughout the labor, and who therefore place a premium on continuity and reliability of the recording. One factor

that is beginning to militate against the use of scalp electrodes is the increasing prevalence of the HIV virus. In the UK, the Royal College of Obstetricians' advice is that women who carry the HIV virus should not have their fetuses monitored using an electrode which breaches the skin, for fear of increasing the risk of transmission of the virus to the fetus. Work is currently in progress to develop contact electrodes which do not breach the skin, so that FHR monitoring using the fetal ECG as a trigger will still be possible in these women.

Interpretation of FHR Recordings

The key to reliable and consistent interpretation of FHR tracings from CTG machines is a systematic approach. Four main aspects of the FHR should be assessed:

- the baseline rate

- the baseline variability

- the presence or absence of accelerations

- the presence and classification of decelerations (slowings of the FHR, or 'dips').

Many errors of interpretation occur because of an excessive concern with decelerations, and a consequent failure to appreciate the significance of the other three aspects of the FHR. One suggested approach to the assessment of the FHR in labor using cardiotocography is given in **Table 2**. These guidelines are taken from a more detailed account supplied in the Appendix to this book (p. 1259).

A normal CTG pattern is highly reassuring that the fetus is not acidotic; only about 2% of babies with a normal pattern will have a pH on a fetal blood sample (FBS) taken in labor <7.25.[14] The significance of an abnormal pattern is much more difficult to judge. In general, the more of the four basic aspects of the FHR (baseline rate, baseline variability, accelerations, decelerations) which are abnormal, the more likely the fetus is to be acidotic.

Management Options with FHR Abnormality

In general, the management options advocated with FHR are (see **Table 2**):

Table 2
Interpretation of fetal heart rate pattern (cardiotocograph, CTG) (see also Appendix, p. 1259)

Admission test
Normal/reassuring/reactive
  2 or more accelerations (> 15 beats/min for > 15 s) in
    20 min
  baseline FHR 110–150 beats/min
  baseline variability 5–25 beats/min
  absence of decelerations
  moderate tachycardia/bradycardia and accelerations
Interpretation/action: Risk of fetal hypoxia in next 2–3 h
in spontaneous labor is low other than following acute
events

Suspicious/equivocal/non-reactive
  absence of accelerations, reduced baseline variability
    (5–10 beats/min), or silent pattern (5 beats/min), for
    > 40 min, although baseline rate normal (110–
    150 beats/min)
  baseline FHR < 110 beats/min or > 150 beats/min
  variable decelerations (depth < 60 beats/min, duration
    < 60 s)
Interpretation/action: Continue CTG, consider
vibroacoustic stimulation/amniotomy/fetal scalp pH
estimation if CTG not normal in 1 h
Pathological/ominous
  silent pattern and baseline FHR > 150 beats/min or
    < 110 beats/min with no accelerations
  repetitive late decelerations and/or complicated variable
    decelerations
  baseline FHR < 100 beats/min or prolonged bradycardia
    (> 10 min)
Interpretation/action: Exclude cord prolapse, placental
abruption and scar dehiscence. If small fetus, or thick
meconium, or previously abnormal trace, consider
immediate delivery. In other situations, consider fetal scalp
pH estimation (and, for example, tocolysis if uterine
hyperstimulation, i.v. fluids if related to epidural 'top-up')

First stage intrapartum CTG
Normal/reassuring/reactive
  2 or more accelerations (> 15 beats/min for > 15 s) in
    20 min
  baseline FHR 110–150 beats/min
  baseline variability 5–25 beats/min
  early decelerations (in late first stage)

Suspicious/equivocal/non-reactive
  absence of accelerations for > 40 min
  baseline FHR 150–170 beats/min or 100–110 beats/min
    (normal baseline variability, no decelerations)
  silent pattern > 40 min (normal baseline rate, no
    decelerations)
  baseline variability > 25 beats/min in the absence of
    accelerations
  variable decelerations (depth < 60 beats/min, duration
    < 60 s)
  occasional transient prolonged bradycardia (FHR drops
    to < 80 beats/min for > 2 min or < 100 beats/min
    for > 3 min)
Interpretation/action: Continue CTG, vibroacoustic
stimulation or fetal scalp pH estimaion if CTG not normal
in 1 h

Pathological/ominous
  baseline FHR > 150 beats/min and silent pattern and/or
    repetitive late or variable decelerations
  silent pattern for > 90 min
  complicated variable decelerations (depth > 60
    beats/min, duration > 60 s) and changes in shape
    (overshoot, decreased or increased baseline heart rate
    following the deceleration, absence of baseline
    variability slow recovery)
  combined/biphasic decelerations (variable followed by
    late)
  prolonged bradycardia (FHR drops to < 80 beats/min
    for > 2 min or < 100 beats/min for > 3 min) in a
    suspicious trace
  prolonged bradycardia (FHR drops to < 80 beats/min
    for > 2 min or < 100 beats/min for > 3 min)
  > 10 min
  repetitive late decelerations
  pronounced loss of baseline variability
  sinusoidal pattern with no accelerations
Interpretation/action: Consider fetal scalp pH
  estimation

Second stage intrapartum CTG
Normal/reassuring/reactive
  normal baseline heart rate, normal baseline variability
    and no decelerations. Frequent accelerations, both
    periodic and scattered
  baseline heart rate 110–150 beats/min and baseline
    variability 5–25 beats/min or > 25 beats/min, with or
    without early and/or variable decelerations

Suspicious/equivocal/non-reactive
  basline heart rate > 150 beats/min, persisting or
    compensatory following each deceleration
  reduced baseline variability or silent pattern
  decelerations of > 60 s duration
  mild bradycardia, heart rate catches up between
    contractions and may reach above 100 beats/min,
    especially when baseline variability is normal
Interpretation/action: Observe trace for increasing baseline
heart rate or bradycardia

Pathological/ominous
  baseline heart rate < 100 beats/min of different patterns
  a. progressive bradycardia: baseline heart rate gradually
     decreases between contractions; absence of baseline
     variability can be seen especially when heart rate is
     < 80 beats/min
  b. persisting bradycardia, baseline < 80 beats/min. The
     additional absence of baseline variability represents
     a more ominous feature
  baseline tachycardia (> 150 beats/min) with reduced
    variability and severe variable and late decelerations
Interpretation/action: Expedite delivery if not imminent

The authors are grateful to Hewlett Packard Asia-Pacific Medical Products Group for allowing us to reproduce the guidelines
for interpretation of antepartum and intrapartum cardiotocography, which they published in 1992. The authors are also grateful
to the writers of the guidelines: S. Arulkumaran, I. Ingemarsson, S. Montan, D.M.F. Gibb, R. Paul, B. Schifrin, J.A.D. Spencer
and P.J. Steer.

In the first stage

- Suspicious/equivocal/non-reactive: continue CTG, vibroacoustic stimulation or fetal scalp pH estimation if CTG not normal in 1 h

- Pathological/ominous: consider fetal scalp pH estimation

In the second stage

- Suspicious/equivocal/non-reactive: observe trace for increasing baseline heart rate or bradycardia

- Pathological/ominous: expedite delivery if not imminent

However, a number of other factors should modulate the response to such a pattern. These are listed below.

Time

The fetus does not become acidotic as soon as the FHR becomes abnormal. Fleischer et al.[49] have shown that a well-grown fetus can cope with a hypoxic stress for as long as 90 min before the pH of fetal blood starts to fall. Thus, a normal fetal scalp blood pH 60 min after the CTG has become abnormal does not indicate that the abnormality is a 'false-positive'. The pH of the fetus may begin to fall at any subsequent time; accordingly, the only safe plan is to repeat the fetal blood sampling at hourly intervals (more often if the pattern is severely abnormal), or deliver the baby.

In contrast, a low pH may be an acute response to temporary interference with maternal placental blood flow and gas exchange. This can occur, for example, after an epidural top-up (with or without maternal hypotension) or because of uterine hyperstimulation with oxytocics.[50] Action should be taken to correct the problem. This can include turning the mother to the left lateral position to correct supine hypotension, stopping any infusions of oxytocic drugs, and giving the mother oxygen by face mask; persisting hypotension from epidural anesthesia can usually be corrected by intravenous injection of a vasoconstrictor such as ephedrine, and excessive uterine activity may be corrected by an infusion of a tocolytic drug such as ritodrine or salbutamol. If the FHR pattern rapidly returns to nor-

mal, then a low pH is often rapidly corrected and immediate delivery of the fetus would be inappropriate. Therefore, it is probably unnecessary to take a FBS in response to an acute FHR abnormality unless the resuscitative measures described above fail to correct the abnormality of the FHR within 15–20 min.

Small for gestational age fetuses

The expression 'small for gestational age' (SGA) refers to the size of a fetus or neonate in relation to its peers of the same gestational age ('size' suggests that the dimensions measured are crown heel length or head and abdomen circumference; in fact, it is weight which is usually assessed and SGA should therefore probably by renamed 'weight for gestational age'). Because the distribution of birthweight is not Gaussian, the relative size of the baby is described in terms of its centile position, rather than in terms of standard deviations (which by contrast are usually used in ultrasound charts, a discrepancy which is a common cause of confusion). Weight below the 10th centile is commonly taken to indicate that the baby is growth-deficient, however, this is often not true. Many babies are simply genetically small and are otherwise functionally normal (see Chapter 42).[51] For example, most babies between the 5th and 10th centiles perform as well as their larger peers in labor.[52] True growth deficiency can only be demonstrated by detecting a fall-off in the normal rate of growth,[53] or signs in the neonate such as a reduced skinfold thickness or a low Ponderal Index (birthweight in g $\times$ 100 divided by crown heel length in cm^3), or assessed by functional measures such as neonatal hypoglycemia.[54]

Despite these caveats, babies below the 5th centile do exhibit a doubled incidence of dysfunction in labor, as measured by FHR abnormalities, low FBS pHs and low Apgar scores.[52,55,56] Thus any baby thought to be seriously SGA on prenatal assessment, or with intrauterine growth deficiency demonstrated on serial ultrasound scanning, should be treated as particularly at risk during labor. The significance of an abnormal FHR pattern is enhanced, FBSs should be taken promptly and more often than with well-grown babies, and the threshold for operative delivery should be reduced.

Early gestational age

Preterm babies are more susceptible to the effects of intrauterine hypoxia than term babies; in particular, hypoxia has a damaging effect on the type 2 pneumocytes that produce surfactant in the lungs, increasing the incidence and severity of the neonatal respiratory distress syndrome (hyaline membrane disease).[57] However, the incidence of hypoxia and acidosis in fetuses in preterm labor is not increased compared with fetuses in term labor.[58–60] Preterm babies are more likely to have low Apgar scores than term babies, but this is due to functional immaturity and not to the effects of hypoxia.[61,62] A baby born at 28 weeks gestation is likely to have poor respiratory effort, to have reduced tone and to have less reflex irritability, and thus a lower Apgar score than its term counterpart; however, given a normal FHR pattern, it is no more likely to be hypoxic or acidotic.[58–62]

The interpretation of the FHR pattern of the preterm fetus in labor is similar to that of its term counterpart.[63] However, there are some subtle differences which may be seen in the FHR pattern. Short-term baseline variability is often rather less, and FHR accelerations less frequent and less marked (the differentiation between quiet and active sleep patterns sometimes does not develop until 32 weeks gestation). Small, brief (<20 s) decelerations are often seen and are insignificant (cause unknown).

Presentation of the fetus

The second stage of labor is more stressful for the fetus in breech presentation than for the fetus in cephalic presentation, and some authors have reported a 20-fold increase in perinatal mortality for babies delivered vaginally by the breech compared with their counterparts in cephalic presentation,[64] although their conclusions have been disputed. However, it is probably wise not to embark on a vaginal breech delivery if there is any suggestion of fetal compromise at the onset of the second stage. Thus, if the FHR pattern is entirely normal, vaginal delivery can proceed, but if the FHR is abnormal, fetal condition should be checked by a FBS pH measurement. This can readily be taken from the buttock and guidelines for interpretation of pH values are the same as for babies in cephalic presentation.[65] If the FBS pH is normal, then the delivery can be allowed to proceed, but if the FHR abnormality persists, the FBS should probably be repeated if delivery has not occurred within 30 min. The passage of meconium is common with a breech presentation and unless it occurs very early in labor is not a useful monitoring variable.

Instrumental delivery

'Fetal distress' is commonly cited as an indication for urgent instrumental vaginal delivery. However, great caution should be applied if the fetal head needs to be rotated. Hypoxia and acidosis can cause cerebral edema and an edematous brain is stiffer and less flexible than normal. Twisting forces applied in this situation may cause tentorial tears which would otherwise

not occur. Thus, rotational deliveries where the FHR pattern is abnormal should probably only be undertaken after a FBS pH has been measured and found to be normal.[66] What represents normality in this situation has not been defined by prospective trials, but in 1968 Beard[11] proposed that pHs of 7.30 or above should be considered normal, pHs from 7.25 to 7.29 equivocal and below 7.25 abnormal, and this classification has since become widely adopted in the UK. Some European workers have suggested that values for the lower limit of normal should be related to the stage of labor; for example, Saling[8] and Rooth et al.[67] suggested that the lower limit of normal could be as low as 7.20 in the first stage of labor and 7.15 in the late second stage.

Maternal preferences/risk factors

As explained in the introduction to this chapter, a scientific basis for deciding when labor should be terminated operatively for fetal indications remains elusive. Such decisions cannot therefore be taken in isolation from the social context, and the wishes and anxieties of the parents should always be taken into account. Some parents have particular anxieties about labor; for example, they may have a sibling with residual damage attributed to birth asphyxia or trauma. In such cases, they may request delivery by cesarean section if there is any sign of fetal dysfunction, or delay in labor. In view of the very low mortality and morbidity associated with cesarean section in modern practice,[68] especially in the absence of any acute emergency, it is probably wise to accede to such requests unless delivery is imminent and the obstetrician very confident of a successful outcome.

Twin or higher order pregnancy

Until the development of ultrasound as a means of monitoring fetal heart rate, the second twin was largely ignored in labor. This was because its heart beat was often difficult to detect with the Pinard stethoscope, especially if the first twin was overlying it. In addition, it is not usually possible to rupture the membranes of the second twin to determine whether the amniotic fluid is meconium-stained. Now, however, the use of ultrasound allows the heart rate of the second twin to be recorded accurately, and in view of the higher mortality of the second twin, such monitoring is recommended.[69] The second twin may develop heart rate changes suggestive of hypoxia, while that of the first twin remains normal.[69] In this case, since fetal blood sampling is impossible until the first twin has delivered, cesarean section is probably appropriate.

Use of intravenous fluids during labor and their effect on fetal acid-base balance

Women in labor are commonly advised not to eat, because of the risk of Mendelson's syndrome (aspiration of stomach contents), should they unexpectedly need general anesthesia. As a result, they often develop ketonemia.[70] For this reason, it is common practice to give parenteral fluid containing glucose and electrolytes, particularly if labor lasts more than a few hours. However, in 1975, Ames et al. reported that infusion of glucose-containing solutions could give rise to maternal lactic acidosis.[71] This is because the rise in maternal blood glucose concentration increases the production rate of lactate, according to Michaelis-Menton kinetics. Subsequently, it was confirmed[72] that maternal infusion of glucose at 100 g/h (1 liter of 10% glucose over 1 h) produced a significant fall in average pH and rise in lactate in fetal as well as maternal blood. These results were subsequently confirmed during a study of the infusion of 1 liter of 5% dextrose over 30 min as part of a policy of preloading for epidural anesthesia.[73] However, it has since been shown that lactic acidosis does not occur if the glucose infusion rate is restricted to 30 g/h.[74] These studies indicate that, in labor, as at other times, care must be taken to monitor the volume and content of intravenous infusions to ensure they are compatible with the maintenance of normal physiology.

There remains a controversy as to whether low-risk women in labor should be allowed unrestricted oral intake. The argument for feeding women in labor is that oral intake reduces both psychological stress[75,76] and physiological stress. It has recently been suggested in the midwifery press that if parturients take a light diet in labor, they become less distressed, require fewer analgesic drugs and are more likely to progress normally in labor, although these claims remain anecdotal. It is certainly true that in units where epidural analgesia is used for high-risk labors and cesarean sections, general anesthesia is seldom needed. The importance of keeping the mother with an effective epidural block nil by mouth therefore decreases. It is currently common practice in the UK for women to be given clear fluids in labor in many units; such fluids may contain glucose, for example in the form of honey. It is likely that women laboring at home eat freely if they feel hungry, and the case for insisting on starvation in low-risk labors seems weak. There is, however, a stronger case for keeping the stomach empty if women are likely to be subjected to general anesthesia in labor, as aspiration of gastric contents is a known cause of maternal death, and it is most likely to occur in combination with general anesthesia. In one reported series, almost 90% of women delivered by emergency cesarean section had earlier indications that abdominal delivery was likely,[77] and therefore in most units the risk of a woman needing a cesarean section unexpectedly will only be 1–2%. It has been shown that feeding women 2–3 h before elective cesarean section increases the volume of gastric contents,[78] but that there is little benefit to fasting for longer than 4 h. There seems little justification, therefore, for starving women for 12 h or more in obstetric units with efficient epidural services, if the woman has no obvious risk factors and is prepared to have a regional block if, unexpectedly, she needs a cesarean section.

Iatrogenic causes of fetal distress

Excessive oxytocin augmentation of labor

Every uterine contraction above 4–6 kPa causes a cessation of maternal intervillous placental blood flow.[79] This produces a period of relative hypoxia for the fetus, such that the fetal pO_2 falls by about 0.5–0.75 kPa during each contraction, reaching its lowest level at the end of the contraction, following which the flow is restored and the pO_2 recovers.[80,81] Because it takes some time for the oxygen-depleted maternal pool of blood to be replaced, recovery takes about 60–90 s. The total period of reduced oxygenation is therefore 120–150 s, emphasizing the importance of an adequate inter-contraction interval to ensure fetal oxygenation. Poorly controlled oxytocin infusions, which produce excessively frequent contractions, can therefore result in iatrogenic fetal hypoxia and acidosis.[82] There is some evidence that this hypoxia can result in an increase in neonatal convulsions.[83,84] Since oxytocin infusion rates greater than 8–12 mU/min are associated with 30–40% hyperstimulation rates,[85–89] great caution should be used before such doses are administered. Uterine activity should probably be measured using an intrauterine catheter if there is no apparent clinical response to lower doses.[90] According to the data sheet currently supplied with Syntocinon®, the manufacturers recommend that it should never be administered if there is any evidence of fetal distress, and in practical terms this means if there is any abnormality of the FHR. If such an abnormality occurs during Syntocinon® infusion, then the infusion should be stopped immediately.

Epidural anesthesia

Before preloading of the circulation with colloid came into practice, abnormalities of the FHR occurred in approximately one-third of cases following insertion of an epidural anesthetic.[91] With preloading, this can be reduced by two-thirds (see Chapter 63).

Epidural anesthetics may also cause a fetal tachycardia by inducing hyperthermia in the mother (and hence in the fetus).[92,93] This can occur in up to 25% of women after 16 h of labor.[50] The tachycardia is not likely to be associated with significant fetal hypoxia, and fetal pH is not affected, but it can give rise to an erroneous diagnosis of fetal distress. The correct response is to cool the mother with tepid sponging.

Drugs

Drugs given to the mother may cross the placenta and affect the fetus. Beta-blockers such as propranolol, and alpha- and beta-blockers such as labetalol may interfere with the reflex responsiveness of the fetal circulation, and impair its response to hypoxia.[94] Other hypotensives such as hydrallazine may cause hypoxia by producing maternal hypotension.[95] Sedatives such as pethidine and valium may depress the fetal central nervous system, producing reduced variability of the FHR and neonatal depression.[96] Care must be taken to give the minimum of any necessary drug in labor, and the effects on the fetus must always be considered.

Non-hypoxic causes of fetal distress

Intrapartum trauma

Intrapartum trauma can cause cephalhematoma, cerebral injury, facial nerve palsy, Erb's palsy, and fractured bones. Trauma has been reported to complicate up to 2% of all labors, even when breech delivery is excluded.[97] Cerebral trauma can also occur due to excessive molding in cases of cephalopelvic disproportion.[98] Careful note must be taken at all vaginal examinations of the degree of molding of the fetal skull, and if there is ++ or more (overlapping of the fetal skull bones), consideration should be given as to whether it is safe to allow the labor to proceed.

Intrapartum infection

Intrapartum chorioamnionitis, commonly with beta-hemolytic streptococcus, poses a major threat to the fetus. In Hauth and co-workers' study of 103 acute cases, one baby died in labor and 43 had serious neonatal problems related to sepsis.[99] Despite this high level of morbidity, only 24 had a cord artery pH <7.20, a proportion which is not different from that found in the general population.[22] It is likely that in many cases a fall in pH is a relatively late event in sepsis, and the decision regarding the timing and mode of delivery has to be made on the basis of a clinical assessment of the severity and duration of the infection.

Procedure: Performance of Fetal Blood Sampling

First, the woman needs to be placed in a suitable position for sampling. The use of the lithotomy position should be avoided because of the risk of supine hypotension.[50] This can produce iatrogenic hypoxia and acidosis in the fetus and therefore lead to unnecessary operative delivery. The sampling is most comfortably performed with the woman in the left (or right) lateral position. An amnioscope is passed up the vagina to rest on the presenting part of the fetus. Sufficient pressure must be used to exclude amniotic fluid, which will otherwise contaminate the sample. The fetal skin is then dried with a dental swab in a holder, and sprayed with ethyl chloride. The evaporation of the ethyl chloride cools the skin, and as it warms up again, a reactive hyperemia is produced which aids bleeding. The skin is smeared with a water-repellent gel (often silicone), so that when the skin is stabbed with a guarded 2 mm blade a droplet of blood forms. This droplet is allowed to flow into a pre-heparinized thin glass tube by capillary action (it helps to tilt the tube slightly downward at the operator's end). Mouth-operated suction should not be used because of the risk of the operator ingesting potentially infected blood. The sample is then transferred to a blood gas analyzer for measurement. It is preferable to measure pO_2 with pCO_2, pH, and calculate the base deficit. If the values are normal, but the FHR pattern remains abnormal, it will usually be necessary to repeat the sampling within 15–30 min.

CORD PROLAPSE

General

Prolapse of the umbilical cord in labor is an uncommon event, occurring in less than 1:200 labors; three recent series reported incidences of 1:385,[100] 1:703[101] and 1:277 births.[102] The occurrence of cord prolapse is most commonly associated with breech and other mal-presentations, a high head at the onset of labor, multiple gestation, grand multiparity, abnormal placentation, preterm labor, hydramnios, and obstetric manipulations such as forceps delivery.[100] In one series of 117 cases, the presentation was breech in just over half the cases (16% complete breech, 21% footling breech and 18% a foot presentation).[101] The diagnosis is commonly made during a vaginal examination, the examiner feeling a soft, usually pulsatile structure. In one series,[101] in 4% the cord was presenting, in 11% it was alongside the presenting part, in 45% it was in the vagina and in 39% it appeared at the introitus. The latter is more likely to occur following artificial, or sudden sponaneous, rupture of the forewaters than in association with a hindwater leak. Occasionally, the diagnosis may be suggested by the sudden appearance of large variable decelerations on the cardiotocogram.

Management Options

The mode of delivery remains controversial. As neonatal care has improved, so there has been a steady decline in the perinatal mortality associated with cord prolapse, irrespective of the mode of delivery. For example, in one series reported in 1977, the perinatal mortality rate was 430 per 1000 births,[103] in 1985 162 per 1000 births[101] and in 1988 55 per 1000 births.[104] Some studies have emphasized the danger of a prolonged prolapse-to-delivery interval[101] and have urged prompt cesarean section[104] unless the cervix is fully dilated and the presenting part at or below the ischial spines so that the fetus is immediately deliverable by forceps (which is the case in about 20–30%).[100,104] While the woman is being prepared for the operation, it is usually recommended that she be nursed in the tranditional knee–chest position facing downwards, or alternatively (and often more practically) in the steep Trendelenberg position. It may be necessary for a birth attendant to keep a gloved hand in the vagina to elevate the presenting part and relieve pressure on the cord. One technique first suggested by Vago[105] and since commended by others[104] is to fill the urinary bladder with 500–700 ml of saline, elevating the presenting part and thus relieving pressure on the cord. However, more recently, one paper has championed manual replacement of the cord (termed funic reduction), describing a successful vaginal delivery in 7 of 8 cases so treated (one was too far advanced in labor for this to be feasible and a cesarean section was performed).[102] The interval between replacement of the cord and vaginal delivery ranged from 14 to 512 min (8.5 h!).

MECONIUM STAINING OF AMNIOTIC FLUID

Aspiration of meconium by the fetus remains a common cause of perinatal mortality and morbidity for which at present there are no effective preventative measures available. The fetus passes meconium into the amniotic fluid in approximately 10% of all pregnancies; in 5% of these (i.e. in 1:200 of all pregnancies) the meconium is aspirated and can then lead to meconium aspiration syndrome (MAS). MAS causes, or contributes to neonatal death in approximately 0.5% (i.e. 1:2000) of all pregnancies.[106–108] Extrapolating these figures for England and Wales, it can be estimated that of the approximately 600 000 labors annually, 60 000 are complicated by meconium-stained amniotic fluid, 3000 by aspiration of meconium and 300 deaths occur in the neonatal period from, or in association with, MAS. A third of all cases in which aspiration occurs are likely to have long-term mild respiratory compromise.[109–112] The overall incidence of meconium staining of the amniotic fluid (MSAF) may be increasing. In 1991, Dysart et al, reported an increasing trend over a 6 year period with a peak incidence of 26.5% of all deliveries.[113] In our own unit, the incidence has increased from 17.5% to over 20% in 3 years.

It seems likely that the causes of meconium *passage* by the fetus are not necessarily the same as those which cause *aspiration*, and so in the account which follows, the two aspects will be addressed separately.

Meconium passage *in utero*

Mechanism

Meconium is passed into the amniotic fluid by peristalsis of the fetal gut accompanied by relaxation of the internal and external anal sphincters. In the adult, this process is a complex interaction of hormonal, myogenic and neurogenic factors. Peristalsis is principally controlled by local reflexes acting via the neural complexes in the gut wall, but is modified by extrinsic innervation. Sympathetic activity inhibits rectal activity and causes constriction of the internal anal sphincter, while parasympathetic activity has the reverse effects. In the resting state, the internal and external sphincters are constricted. In the human adult, involuntary defecation can occur in response to emotional stress, mediated centrally by the hypothalamus (and possibly the amygdala) which in turn causes stimulation of the visceral parasympathetics.[114,115] In contrast, physiological stresses such as pain, heat, cold, injury, exercise and non-intestinal infections, all produce gut stasis and constipation.[114] Although it is attractive to suggest that the fetus may exhibit a similar response to the 'emotional' stress of labor, there is no way to ascertain its emotions *in utero* and the concept is likely to remain an untestable theory. The fetus in labor can be stressed physiologically by hypoxia, pyrexia or compression, which by extrapolation from known adult physiology would be as likely to produce gut stasis as increased motility. However, fetal physiology differs in many important ways from that of the adult, and our knowledge of the mechanisms of bowel motility and hence meconium passage in the fetus remains very slight.

The effect of fetal maturity on its passage of meconium

Meconium has been found in the fetal gut from 10 weeks gestation,[116] but passage of meconium into the amniotic fluid is rare before 34 weeks gestation.[117] The incidence of meconium passage increases with gestational age and reaches approximately 30% at 40 weeks gestation and 50% at 42 weeks.[117-119] It has therefore been suggested that the presence of meconium in the amniotic fluid may simply be a physiological reflection of fetal gastrointestinal maturity.[120] Studies have confirmed that fetal gut transit time decreases with gestational age, from an average of 9 h at 32 weeks to 4.5 h at term, and gastrointestinal motility also increases with gestational age.[121] The lower motility in the preterm fetus has been attributed to a relative lack of gut musculature, but this explanation is unlikely because peristalsis begins before 12 weeks gestation and muscle development must have occurred before this.[122] It is more likely that there is immaturity of the innervation of the fetal gut, with preterm infants having more unmyelinated axons and fewer ganglion cells in the colon than term infants. Nonetheless, meconium passage by the preterm fetus can still occur if it becomes infected.[123] The organisms implicated (*Listeria monocytogenes, Ureaplasma urealyticum*, rotaviruses) produce a fetal enteritis and hence passage of meconium. The musculature and intramural plexuses of the fetal gut must therefore be sufficiently developed for peristalsis to occur and meconium to be passed even in the preterm fetus.

Hormonal control of meconium passage

The intestinal hormone motilin has also been implicated in the passage of meconium *in utero* by the fetus; it acts on the smooth muscle of the gastrointestinal tract, causing it to contract. Motilin levels in the umbilical vein are significantly higher in term as opposed to preterm infants, and if they reflect levels in the bowel, could be a factor in explaining the increased

tendency of the mature fetus to pass meconium.[124] Cord motilin levels are also higher in infants that have passed meconium prenatally,[124,125] and one report found higher levels if there had been a fetal heart rate abnormality in labor.[124] This latter finding was not confirmed in a more recent paper,[125] but different definitions of heart rate abnormality were used in the two studies. It is possible that stress on the fetus could cause release of motilin and thus passage of meconium, but this remains conjectural. The hormonal and other factors which control and interact with motilin are still largely unkown even in the adult. An increasing response of the fetal gut to exogenous drugs with increasing maturity has been noted,[126] but whether this acts through the agency of motilin is unknown.

Risks of Meconium Staining of Amniotic Fluid

Fetal hypoxia

An association between passage of meconium *in utero* and poor condition of the neonate has been suggested for many years. The name meconium is derived from the Greek for opium poppy juice, and Aristotle reported opium-like effects in neonates born through meconium-stained amniotic fluid. There have been references to meconium in association with perinatal death from as early as 1676 (quoted in Schulze).[127] Although subsequently many authors have suggested that fetal hypoxia causes intestinal peristalsis, relaxation of the anal sphincter and thus passage of meconium, this has largely been an assumption, with little or no direct evidence being reported to support such a hypothesis. Stander[128] claimed that meconium was a sign of impending fetal 'asphyxia' due to 'relaxation of the sphincter and muscle induced by faulty aeration of the blood' and proposed prompt delivery whenever meconium was seen. Desmond *et al.*[129] stated that meconium staining of the amniotic fluid was a marker of fetal hypoxia, but performed no measurements of fetal or neonatal blood oxygen or pH, the diagnosis of hypoxia being made on clinical grounds alone.

These observations were made despite the report of Schulze,[127] who had concluded from the study of a series of more than 5500 births in California, that passage of meconium during labor 'is in the large majority of cases independent of fetal asphyxia' and that the presence of old meconium in the amniotic fluid was of no prognostic significance for the later development of asphyxia (asphyxia here was not defined but appears to mean lack of respiratory effort at birth). She also observed that in cases associated with asphyxia, there were always changes of the fetal heart rate during labor, and that these changes should be the sole guide as to the necessity for delivery. However, in a later study, meconium passage was found to be associated with low umbilical vein oxygen saturation, and thick meconium to be associated with lower levels of pO_2 than thin meconium.[130] This remained the principal experimental evidence linking fetal hypoxia with meconium passage and was widely quoted, often as the sole evidence, for at least the subsequent 20 years.

Fenton and Steer[131] made one of the first attempts to separate meconium passage from other markers of fetal compromise such as abnormality of heart rate, but again had only presumptive evidence of hypoxia in the fetus. They did, however, state that there were other, benign causes of meconium passage, and suggested that the passage of meconium was not significant if the fetal heart rate was greater than 110 beats/min. Fujikura and Klionsky[132] conceded that the stimulus to pass meconium before birth was 'by tradition' fetal anoxia or hypoxia, but produced no evidence to support this assertion. The introduction of fetal blood sampling began to clarify the situation. Miller et al.[133] found no difference in scalp blood pH, umbilical cord artery and vein pH and neonatal arterial pH up to 64 min of life, between meconium and non-meconium groups, if the fetal heart rate during labor had been normal. They concluded that the presence of meconium in the absence of other signs was not an indication of 'fetal distress' (defined as late decelerations on the CTG and umbilical artery acidosis). A dissenting opinion was expressed by Starks,[134] who found that thick meconium was associated with lower fetal scalp blood pH than thin or absent meconium and concluded that thick meconium usually indicates fetal hypoxia or acidosis regardless of fetal heart rate. However, more recent studies have confirmed that infants who have normal fetal heart rate patterns have similar outcomes whether or not meconium is present.[135–138]

If the fetal heart rate pattern is abnormal, however, the presence of meconium is associated with a higher chance of a baby being acidotic, born in poor condition and needing resuscitation at birth.[117,133] For example, in the data presented by Steer et al,[117] 140 babies had an abnormal CTG pattern in the first stage of labor. In the 108 with clear amniotic fluid, the mean cord artery blood pH was 7.22 (SD=0.10) compared with 7.17 (SD=0.12) in the 32 cases where the amniotic fluid was meconium-stained (t=2.37, P=0.0096). The incidence of 1 min Apgar scores <7 was 19% (3% at 5 min) if the amniotic fluid was clear, compared with 56% (9% at 5 min) if the amniotic fluid was meconium-stained – the difference is significant at 1 min (P=0.196; Fisher's exact test, one-tailed). However, they commented that the reduction in the 1 min Apgar score may have been due at least in part to the use of pharyngeal suction and/or endotracheal intubation by the attending pediatrician, which tends to suppress spontaneous respiratory effort and thus iatrogenically reduce the Apgar score.

Despite the lack of a clear relationship between meconium staining of the amniotic fluid and fetal acidosis in the absence of fetal heart rate changes, we cannot conclude that the presence of meconium in the amniotic fluid is not a threat to the fetus/neonate even if the FHR is normal. Yeomans et al.[139] studied 323 pregnancies with meconium-stained amniotic fluid at 36–42 weeks gestation. Although there was a significantly higher incidence of meconium below the vocal cords if an umbilical artery pH was <7.20 [31/89 (34%) compared with 74/323 (23%) when the umbilical artery pH was >7.2; P=0.0174, Fisher's exact test, one-tailed], there was no significant difference in the incidence of clinical meconium aspiration syndrome according to pH. Moreover, 51 of 74 (69%) babies born with meconium below the cords had a cord arterial pH of ≥7.2. Thus, the finding of a normal pH does not rule out the possibility of meconium aspiration, and the majority of babies suffering meconium aspiration will not have an acidosis. These data do not support the hypothesis that fetal hypoxia is a major cause of meconium passage in labor, and indeed Naeye et al.[140] reported that meconium staining of the amniotic fluid was not more common even in cases where the neonate was known to be hypoxic.

In fact, evidence that hypoxia *per se* does not lead to passage of meconium has been available for many years. Becker et al.[120] showed *reduced* peristalsis in the fetal guinea-pig after induction of maternal hypoxemia, and a similar result has been demonstrated in the monkey fetus. Saling[141] proposed that meconium passage was due to redistribution of intestinal blood flow in the hypoxemic fetus, but this remains supposition. If meconium passage does occur in response to reduced intestinal blood flow, it must be an early event for the neurogenic reflexes still to be present. Meconium passage may occur as a result of vagal stimulation, which could account for any co-existing reduction in the fetal heart rate.[131] The parasympathetic stimulation may be due to cord compression.[142] This is supported by meconium passage being more common with increasing gestational age. However, Emmanouilides et al.[143] found that in the sheep fetus, if one umbilical artery was ligated, passage of meconium only occurred as a very late phenomenon, after chronic fetal wasting had developed. In an otherwise authoritative review article, Katz and Bowes[144] stated that fetal hypoxia led to meconium passage in laboratory animals. However, both the studies cited were concerned with the investigation of fetal breathing movements,[145,146] and do not in fact state that meconium was passed in response to hypoxia.

Meconium aspiration

The passage of meconium is not of itself a risk to the fetus, but aspiration of the meconium into the fetal or neonatal lung is associated with clinical disease ranging from mild transitory respiratory distress to severe respiratory compromise, and occurs in up to one-third of cases. Meconium aspiration is commonly defined as the presence of meconium below the vocal cords,[146] and occurs in up to 35% of live births with meconium-stained amniotic fluid,[107,147] with a range of 21–58%.[148,149]

Aspiration of meconium was originally thought to occur at delivery as the newborn infant took its first breath.[133,149,150,151] Oropharyngeal suction, and endotracheal intubation of the infant before the first breath, were widely promoted in order to prevent meconium aspiration. However, it now seems likely that aspiration of meconium most commonly occurs *in utero*. This change of view has occurred because of reports that severe meconium aspiration syndrome still occurs despite adequate suction at delivery.[107,139,147,148,152–155] The current view is that meconium aspiration occurs due to fetal breathing movements, causing inhalation of amniotic fluid, with meconium if present. The breathing movements that cause inhalation of amniotic fluid are of two types: gasping and deep breathing. Gasping is a normal response to hypoxemia and can be induced experimentally by occluding the umbilical cord, or by occluding the maternal aorta.[145,146,156] The fetus may also inhale meconium by deep irregular breathing *in utero*, not initiated by hypoxia. These breaths become more frequent as gestation advances, and comprise 10% of all fetal breathing movements.[145] The passage of amniotic fluid deep into the lung has been demonstrated by radio-labeling experiments. The human fetus inhales up to 200 ml/kg/24 h of amniotic fluid.[157] Fetal hypercapnia and acidemia also increase these breathing movements, but they still occur in most, if not all, normal fetuses.[145,158] Although there are infants with meconium aspiration who are already severely compromised at birth, two studies have found little or no difference in umbilical cord acid–base status between infants with meconium below the cords and those without.[139,148] Meconium aspiration is more common if the meconium is thick rather than thin.[107] This may be a reflection of the fact that oligohydramnios (and therefore thick undiluted meconium) is more likely to lead to fetal hypoxia due to cord compression, and consequently increased fetal breathing.

Meconium aspiration syndrome

General

Meconium aspiration syndrome (MAS) represents a wide spectrum of disease ranging from transient respiratory distress with little therapy required, to severe respiratory compromise requiring prolonged mechanical ventilation and high levels of oxygen administration. Neonatal death occurs in up to 40% of cases.[152]

Severe MAS is associated with profound hypoxia, which is secondary to right-to-left shunting, a persistent fetal circulation, resistant pulmonary hypertension, pulmonary hemorrhage, necrosis of the pulmonary vessels and muscularization of the distal pulmonary arterioles.[107,108,118,147,148,159–161] These changes may be due to intrauterine hypoxia, rather than to the meconium itself, although the inhalation of meconium exacerbates the problem in several ways in the neonatal period.

Meconium inhaled in an infant which has not been subjected to hypoxia usually causes mild disease only, and is asymptomatic in 90% of cases.[107,147,148] Exposure to intrauterine hypoxia causes pulmonary vasoreactivity which persists after birth. Large increases in pulmonary artery pressure in response to very small falls in oxygen tension then result. The severity of this pulmonary vasospasm seems to be dependent on the severity of the fetal hypoxia, and may be fixed (completely unresponsive) in the most severe cases. These changes have been demonstrated experimentally, and observed clinically.[162–164] A vicious circle of hypoxia, pulmonary vasospasm, shunting and therefore worsening hypoxia can develop.

Jovanovic and Nguyen[165] have demonstrated in the guinea-pig that meconium or amniotic fluid aspiration in the absence of hypoxia caused minimal damage, whereas there was severe lung damage (necrosis of alveoli and diffuse hemorrhage) in the hypoxic cases, whether the amniotic fluid contained meconium or not. The degree of lung destruction seems to be primarily dependent on the length and degree of hypoxia, and not simply on the aspiration of meconium. Hypoxic damage also reduces the clearance of aspirated meconium or amniotic fluid.[166,167] Meconium does, however, exacerbate the problems faced by the neonate.[168] It displaces surfactant, causing atelectasis and hyaline membrane formation[169–171] and causes a chemical pneumonitis possibly due to cytotoxicity to the type II pneumocytes caused by bile-salt induced accumulation of calcium.[172] In addition, it enhances bacterial growth and is associated with intrauterine infections. Aspiration may therefore lead to an infectious pneumonitis.

Some bacterial toxins cause pulmonary vascular spasm, exacerbating the effects of hypoxia.[123,173–175] Recently, meconium has been demonstrated to cause vascular necrosis and vasoconstriction in the umbilical cord; by analogy it may also cause similar damage in the lung.[176] The umbilical vasoconstriction may cause hypoxia *in utero* leading to aspiration. The factor in meconium responsible for this effect has not been identified, but is is heat-labile and therefore may be a protein or prostaglandin. Inhaled thick meconium may cause a physical obstruction to the airways, leading to distal lung collapse, with hyperinflation in other areas. In total, 95% of severe cases of MAS occur when the meconium is thick, and this is more common in postterm pregnancies when a relative oligohydramnios develops.[107,118] Oligohydramnios may also be due to hypoxia causing reduced fetal urine output,[177] or may be a sign of uteroplacental insufficiency.[178]

Methods of preventing MAS

During the 1950s and 1960s, it was thought that meconium-stained amniotic fluid was a marker of fetal compromise, and therefore efforts were made to detect the meconium in late pregnancy, and to deliver the fetus before, or as soon as, meconium appeared. Saling[141] introduced amnioscopy for pregnancies more than 10 days past the expected date of confinement. It was stated that meconium indicated 'impending danger' and that, if detected, immediate amniotomy and fetal blood sampling should be performed; the ensuing uterine contractions were thought to be therapeutic for the fetus. This study was not controlled in any way, and gestational age was estimated from menstrual dates only. However, a three-fold reduction in perinatal mortality was claimed. Other workers have been unable to reproduce these results.[179,180] Saldana et al.[181] showed no benefit from amnioscopy and delivery. Tchabo[182] has recently claimed that amnioscopy reduced the incidence of meconium aspiration, but this too was an uncontrolled study. The method, which has yet to be shown to be beneficial, is uncomfortable for the mother, may result in accidental rupture of the membranes or induce labor, can cause infection and has to be repeated at arbitrary intervals until delivery of the infant.

Benacerraf et al.[183] reported the detection of thick meconium by ultrasonography, but further studies have shown that vernix can produce an ultrasonically indistinguishable image in the absence of meconium.[184,185]

Because meconium passage is more common with advanced gestational age, many studies have investigated the effect of inducing labor at an earlier gestation. Cole et al.[186] in a controlled trial, significantly reduced the incidence of meconium-stained amniotic fluid by inducing labor at 39–40 weeks gestation, but no effect on perinatal mortality or respiratory disease was demonstrated. Dyson et al.[187] did find significantly less meconium aspiration in the induced group, but perinatal mortality, and morbidity as assessed by 5 min Apgar score and length of infant stay, were not significantly different. Other studies of induction of labor have failed to show any decrease in meconium aspiration, even if the incidence of meconium staining of the amniotic fluid was reduced.[188–192] There is thus no evident benefit from induction of labor before meconium appears, or in the routine use of amnioscopy, and disadvantages to both procedures exist.

In the 1970s, it was widely belived that meconium aspiration developed by inhalation of meconium at delivery. To prevent this, aggressive policies of oropharyngeal suction, endotracheal intubation and splinting of the thorax to prevent inspiration were proposed (see also Chapter 71).[149–151] Despite these interventions, cases of meconium aspiration still occurred, and further studies have shown little or no reduction in meconium aspiration syndrome.[106,107,147,154,160] A decline in the mortality from meconium aspiration has probably been due to advances in perinatal medicine, rather than to the introduction of suction protocols. Indeed, suction and intubation are not free of risk. Cordero and Hon[193] reported apnea and bradycardias in infants having nasopharyngeal suction, and Linder et al.[194] found no benefit from the intubation at birth of meconium-stained but otherwise normal infants. All cases of meconium aspiration in this study occurred in the intubated group, as did two cases of laryngeal stridor which required repeated hospitalization, with residual hoarseness at 6 months of age. Cunninham et al.[155] supported this approach and recommended routine oropharyngeal suction but not intubation. There is now widespread acceptance that routine suctioning and intubation of neonates that have passed meconium has little if any effect on aspiration, and may have deleterious side-effects.

Amnioinfusion, the instillation of normal saline into the uterus during labor, has been proposed as a method to reduce meconium concentration and therefore the effects of aspiration. It may also reduce cord compression in cases of oligohydramnios, and therefore possibly fetal gasping. Three small studies have suggested that this technique may be useful. Sadovsky et al.[195] showed a reduction in meconium below the cords and an improvement in cord arterial pH in a group managed with amnioinfusion compared with controls managed conventionally, but there were no cases of meconium aspiration syndrome in either group. Wenstrom and Parsons[196] did demonstrate a significant reduction in both meconium aspiration and MAS. More recently, a report has suggested that amnioinfusion in labor reduces the incidence of meconium passage, as well as reducing the incidence of aspiration.[197] A larger randomized trial with 85 women in each group confirmed these findings with a significant reduction in CTG abnormalities (3 vs 19), meconium aspiration (4 vs 33) and meconium aspiration syndrome (0 vs 5).[198]

Attempts have been made to classify meconium in labor according to its concentration, because thick meconium has been associated with increased incidence and severity of the aspiration syndrome.[107,118,134,153] However, any grading system remains subjective because amniotic fluid draining during labor may not be representative of the fluid in utero, and no fluid may drain at all in cases of oligohydramnios, masking the presence of meconium. Quantifying the meconium concentration by centrifuging samples of amniotic fluid and measuring the amount of solid matter in the sample has been attempted,[199,200] but the same problems of obtaining amniotic fluid representative of the intrauterine milieu exist. In addition, neither of these two studies addressed the problem of vernix, and solid matter other than meconium in the fluid, producing false-positive or falsely elevated results.

There have been two reports that suggest that social support during labor reduces the incidence of meconium staining,[201,202] but in both cases more oxytocin was used in the group with no support, which could have led to unphysiological contractions and therefore fetal hypoxia.

Katz and Bowes[144] suggest that the data linking fetal distress and meconium should be viewed with caution because the events during labor and delivery do not represent the intrauterine environment at the time of meconium passage. In addition, it is unlikely that prevention of meconium passage or aspiration will be successful until there is some elucidation of the underlying causes. In our unit, we have designed an intrauterine probe which measures meconium concentration in the amniotic fluid continuously during labor, using a light reflectance method.[203] This enables observation of events at the time of meconium passage and may lead to further information on some of the antecedents of meconium passage during labor. In addition, meconium not visible to the birth attendants can be detected, and the efficacy of amnioinfusion to reduce meconium concentration can be monitored. Preliminary results have revealed three cases in which there were sudden increases in meconium concentration synchronous with the development of fetal heart rate abnormalities shortly after top-up of epidural analgesia. Meconium has also been detected in three cases where its presence was unknown to the attendants, one of which developed meconium aspiration syndrome. If the presence of meconium is not detected, the labor may be managed suboptimally: fetal heart rate abnormalities may not be acted upon appropriately, and the attendance of a pediatrician for the birth of a possibly hypoxic infant may be delayed.

Conclusions: risks of meconium

Meconium aspiration syndrome remains a significant cause of perinatal mortality and morbidity. Little is know about the cause of meconium passage, but it is strongly associated with increasing gestational age, presumably as a result of maturation of the neuromuscular system of the fetal intestine. There is no evidence that passage of meconium is commonly related to hypoxia. Meconium aspiration is predominantly a intrauterine event, but is probably not usually a serious problem unless caused by, or associated with, severe hypoxia. Meconium, especially if thick, can seriously exacerbate the respiratory disease caused by hypoxia.

Prevention of meconium aspiration syndrome remains problematical; there is usually lack of knowledge of the timing of meconium passage in utero, even in labor, and therefore it is impossible to correlate this event with data which may have been available at the time. Previously reported lack of correlation between data collected at birth and presence of meconium that may have been passed several hours earlier may therefore not be surprising. Investigation of the pathophysiology of meconium passage during labor may help to identify some of the causes of meconium passage, and enable preventative measures to be taken. In addition, better directed management of the labor complicated by meconium staining of the amniotic fluid may be possible.

Management Options with Meconium Staining of Amniotic Fluid

When amniotic fluid is seen to drain, it should always be inspected carefully for the presence of meconium. If meconium is detected, continuous electronic fetal heart rate monitoring is recommended. If the FHR pattern remains normal, no specific action need be taken except to avoid actions which might precipitate acute fetal hypoxia (notably supine hypotension, epidural hypotension and uterine hyperstimulation with oxytocics). In particular, there is no indication for routine fetal blood sampling and pH estimation so long as the FHR pattern remains normal. At delivery, a pediatrician should be present. If the baby is vigorous and cries promptly, there is probably no need for further action. Although there is no proof of efficacy, some pediatricians prefer to suction the pharynx as soon as possible after delivery of the head, and this is probably acceptable so long as care is taken not to traumatize the pharynx or larynx, as this may of itself precipitate meconium aspiration (see Chapter 71).

If the FHR pattern becomes abnormal during labor, the likelihood of acidosis is substantially increased. Consideration should be given to immediate delivery, if necessary, by cesarean section. If rapid progress in cervical dilatation is occurring, it may be appropriate to perform a fetal blood sample and allow the labor to continue if the pH is above 7.20, but this decision must take into account other factors such as the wishes of the mother, and whether there are other risk factors such as suspected intrauterine growth deficiency. Amnioinfusion should be considered if it is decided to allow the labor to continue. Amnioinfusion can also be considered even if the FHR pattern is normal, as a preventative measure, although the technique remains experimental.

FETAL DISTRESS IN LABOR
Summary of Management Options

FETAL HEART RATE

Methods

- Low risk – regular auscultation of FHR during labour:
  - every 15 min during first stage
  - after every contraction in second stage
  - count for 1 min as contraction is abating

- High risk – continuous electronic FHR monitoring:
  - facilities for fetal blood sampling and pH estimation should be available
  - see **Table 1** for indications

Interpretation and management options

- General approach
  - turn patient on to left side
  - oxygen by face mask
  - stop oxytocic
  - i.v. fluids if epidural
  - consider tocolysis if hyperstimulation

- Special circumstances
  - small fetus
  - preterm fetus
  - prolonged labor
  - intrapartum infection and pyrexia

- drugs administered to mother
- trauma during birth

- Specific options
  - see **Table 2**

Cord prolapse

- Cesarean section while relieving pressure on cord until delivery

- Forceps if in second stage, presenting part below ischial spines and easy and prompt vaginal delivery anticipated

- Role of fundic reduction not clear

Meconium staining of amniotic fluid

- Continuous FHR recording with guidelines for management as above except perhaps an earlier recourse to cesarean section if FHR becomes abnormal

- Avoid events which may precipitate hypoxia

- Role of amnioinfusion has not been established

- Pediatrician for delivery (see Chapter 71)

REFERENCES

1 Steer PJ (1982) Has the expression 'fetal distress' outlived its usefulness? *British Journal of Obstetrics and Gynaecology* **89**:690–693.
2 Parer JT (1990) What is fetal distress? *American Journal of Obstetrics and Gynecology* **162**:1421–1427.
3 Hall DB (1989) Birth asphyxia and cerebral palsy. *British Medical Journal* **299**:279–282.
4 Clark RB, Quirk JG (1990) What is birth asphyxia? *American Journal of Obstetrics and Gynecology* **163**:1367–1368.
5 Claye Sir A (1963) Management of labour. In Claye A,

Bourne A (eds), *British Obstetric and Gynaecological Practice*, pp. 184–204. London: Heinemann Medical.
6 Towell M (1976) Fetal acid base physiology and intrauterine asphyxia. In Goodwin JW, Godden JO, Chance GW (eds), *Perinatal Medicine: The Basic Science Underlying Clinical Practice*, pp. 187–208. Baltimore, MD: Williams and Wilkins.
7 Butler NR, Bonham DG (1963) *Perinatal Mortality*. Edinburgh: Churchill Livingstone.
8 Saling E (1962) Neues Vorgehen zur Untersuchung des Kindes unter der Geburt – Ein Fuhrung, Technick und Grundlagen. *Archiv für Gynakologie* **197**:108–122.
9 Bretscher J, Saling E (1967) pH values in the human

fetus during labour. *American Journal of Obstetrics and Gynecology* **97**:906–911.

10 Beard RW, Morris ED, Clayton SG (1967) pH of foetal capillary blood as an indicator of the condition of the fetus. *Journal of Obstetrics and Gynaecology of the British Commonwealth* **74**:812–822.

11 Beard RW (1968) The effect of fetal blood sampling on Caesarean section for fetal distress. *Journal of Obstetrics and Gynaecology of the British Commonwealth* **75**:1291–1295.

12 Coltart TM, Trickey NRA, Beard RW (1969) Foetal blood sampling: Practical approach to management of foetal distress. *British Medical Journal* **i**:342–346.

13 Gillmer MDG, Combe D (1979) Intrapartum fetal monitoring practice in the United Kingdom. *British Journal of Obstetrics and Gynaecology* **86**:753–760.

14 Beard RW, Filshie GM, Knight CA, Roberts GM (1971) The significance of the changes in the continuous fetal heart rate in the first stage of labour. *Journal of Obstetrics and Gynaecology of the British Commonwealth* **78**:865–880.

15 Haverkamp AD, Orleans M, Langendoerfer S, McFee J, Murphy J, Thompson HEA (1979) A controlled trial of the differential effects of intrapartum fetal monitoring. *American Journal of Obstetrics and Gynecology* **134**:399–412.

16 Renou P, Chang A, Anderson I, Wood C (1976) Controlled trial of fetal intensive care. *American Journal of Obstetrics and Gynecology* **126**:470–476.

17 Kelso IM, Parsons RJ, Lawrence GF, Arora SS, Edmonds DK, Cooke ID (1978) An assessment of continuous fetal heart rate monitoring in labour. *American Journal of Obstetrics and Gynecology* **131**:526–532.

18 Haverkamp AD, Thompson HE, Mcfee JG, Cetrulo C (1976) The evaluation of continuous fetal heart rate monitoring in high risk pregnancy. *American Journal of Obstetrics and Gynecology* **125**:310–320.

19 Wood C, Renou P, Oats J, Farrell E, Beischer N, Anderson I (1981) A controlled trial of fetal heart rate monitoring in a low risk obstetric population. *American Journal of Obstetrics and Gynecology* **141**:527–534.

20 MacDonald D, Grant A, Sheridan-Pereira M, Boylan P, Chalmers I (1985) The Dublin randomized controlled trial of intrapartum fetal heart rate monitoring. *American Journal of Obstetrics and Gynecology* **152**:524–539.

21 Steer PJ, Eigbe FE, Lissauer TJ, Beard RW (1989) Interrelationships among abnormal cardiotocograms in labor, meconium staining of the amniotic fluid, arterial cord blood pH, and Apgar scores. *Obstetrics and Gynecology* **74**:715–721.

22 Sykes G, Molloy PM, Johnson P, Gu W, Ashworth F, Stirrat GM, Turnbull AC (1982) Do Apgar scores indicate asphyxia? *Lancet* **i**:494–495.

23 Lissauer TJ, Steer PJ (1986) The relation between the need for intubation at birth, abnormal cardiotocograms in labour and cord artery blood gas and pH values. *British Journal of Obstetrics and Gynaecology* **93**:1060–1066.

24 Hall DB (1989) Birth asphyxia and cerebral palsy. *British Medical Journal* **299**:279–282.

25 Thorp JA (1990) What is birth asphyxia: Reply. *American Journal of Obstetrics and Gynecology* **163**:1368.

26 Murphy KW, Johnson P, Moorcraft J, Pattinson R, Russell V, Turnbull A (1990) Birth asphyxia and the intrapartum cardiotocograph. *British Journal of Obstetrics and Gynaecology* **97**:470–479.

27 Ruth VJ, Raivio KO (1988) Perinatal brain damage: Predictive value of metabolic acidosis and the Apgar score. *British Medical Journal* **297**:24–247.

28 Dennis J, Johnson A, Mutch, L, Yudkin P, Johnson P (1989) Acid–base status at birth and neuro-developmental outcome at four and one half years. *American Journal of Obstetrics and Gynecology* **161**:213–220.

29 Low JA, Muir D, Pater EA, Karchmar EJ (1990) The association of intrapartum asphyxia in the mature fetus with newborn behaviour. *American Journal of Obstetrics and Gynecology* **163**:1131–1135.

30 Winkler CL, Hauth JC, Tucker JM, Owen J, Brumfield CG (1991) Neonatal complications at term as related to the degree of umbilical artery acidemia. *American Journal of Obstetrics and Gynecology* **164**:637–641.

31 Goodwin TM, Belai I, Hernandez P, Durand M, Paul RH (1992) Asphyxial complications in the term newborn with severe umbilical acidemia. *American Journal of Obstetrics and Gynecology* **167**:1506–1512.

32 Dennis J, Chalmers I (1982) Very early neonatal seizure rate: A possible epidemiological indicator of the quality of perinatal care. *British Journal of Obstetrics and Gynaecology* **89**:418–427.

33 Illingworth R (1979) Why blame the obstetrician? A review. *British Medical Journal* **1**:797–801.

34 Paneth N, Stark RI (1983) Cerebral palsy and mental retardation in relation to indicators of perinatal asphyxia. *American Journal of Obstetrics and Gynecology* **147**:960–966.

35 National Institutes of Health (1985) Causes of Mental Retardation and Cerebral Palsy. Report of the Task Force on Joint Assessment of Prenatal and Perinatal Factors Associated with Brain Disorders. *Pediatrics* **76**:745–748.

36 Hensleigh PA, Fainstat T, Spencer R (1986) Perinatal events and cerebral palsy. *American Journal of Obstetrics and Gynecology* **154**:978–981.

37 Stanley FJ, Watson L (1992) Trends in perinatal mortality and cerebral palsy in Western Australia, 1967 to 1985. *British Medical Journal* **304**:1658–1662.

38 Neilsen JP (1993) Cardiotocography during labour. *British Medical Journal* **306**:347–348.

39 Bennett V, Brown LK (eds) (1989) *Myles Textbook for Midwives*. Edinburgh: Churchill Livingstone.

40 Murphy KW, Johnson P, Moorcraft J, Pattinson R, Russell V, Turnbull A (1990) Birth asphyxia and the intrapartum cardiotocograph. *British Journal of Obstetrics and Gynaecology* **97**:470–479.

41 Ennis M, Vincent CA (1990) Obstetric accidents: A review of 64 cases. *British Medical Journal* **300**:1365–1367.

42 FIGO (1987) Guidelines for the use of fetal monitoring. *International Journal of Gynaecology and Obstetrics* **25**:159–167.

43 Steer PJ, Beard RW (1970) Continuous record of fetal

heart rate obtained by serial counts. *British Journal of Obstetrics and Gynaecology* **77**:908–914.

44   Steer PJ (1982) Technical aspects of fetal and intrauterine pressure monitoring. In Beard RW, Nathanielscz P (eds), *Fetal Physiology and Medicine*. pp. 679–711. New York: Marcel Dekker.

45   Carter MC, Steer PJ (1988) Technology and fetal monitoring. *Hosptial Update* **14**:1820–1827.

46   Amato JC (1983) Fetal heart rate monitoring. *American Journal of Obstetrics and Gynecology* **147**:967–969.

47   Divon MY, Torres FP, Yeh S, Paul RH (1985) Autocorrelation techniques in fetal monitoring. *American Journal of Obstetrics and Gynecology* **151**:2–6.

48   Steer PJ, Carter MC, Pentecost AF (1986) Fetal monitoring in labour. *British Medical Journal* **292**:827–827.

49   Fleischer A, Schulman H, Jagani N, Mitchell J, Randolph G (1982) The development of fetal acidosis in the presence of an abnormal fetal heart rate tracing. *American Journal of Obstetrics and Gynecology* **144**:55–60.

50   Steer PJ (1985) Fetal distress. In Crawford J (ed.), *Risks of Labour*, pp. 11–31. Chichester: John Wiley.

51   Teberg AJ, Walther FJ, Pena IC (1988) Mortality, morbidity and outcome of the small for gestational age infant. *Seminars in Perinatology* **12**:84–94.

52   Steer PJ (1989) Intrapartum monitoring in IUGR. In Sharp F, Milner RDG, Fraser RB (eds), *Fetal Growth*, pp. 381–387. London: Royal College of Obstetricians and Gynaecologists.

53   Danielian PJ, Allman ACJ, Steer PJ (1992) Is obstetric and neonatal outcome worse in fetuses who fail to reach their own growth potential? *British Journal of Obstetrics and Gynaecology* **99**:452–454.

54   Chard T, Costeloe K, Leaf A (1992) Evidence of growth retardation in neonates of apparently normal weight. *European Journal of Obstetrics and Gynecology and Reproductive Biology* **45**:59–62.

55   Low JA, Pancham SR, Worthington D (1976) Fetal heart deceleration patterns in relation to asphyxia and weight–gestational age percentile of the fetus. *Obstetrics and Gynecology* **47**:14–20.

56   Low JA, Karchmar J, Broekhoven L, Leonard T, McGrath MJ, Pancham SR, Piercy WN (1981) The probability of fetal metabolic acidosis during labour in a population at risk as determined by clinical factors. *American Journal of Obstetrics and Gynecology* **141**:941–951.

57   Hobel CJ, Hyvarinen MA, Oh W (1972) Abnormal fetal heart rate patterns and fetal acid–base balance in low birth weight infants in relation to the respiratory distress syndrome. *Obstetrics and Gynecology* **39**:83–88.

58   Perkins RP, Papile L-A (1985) The very low birthweight infant: Incidence and significance of low Apgar scores, 'asphyxia', and morbidity. *American Journal of Perinatology* **2**:108–113.

59   Ramin SM, Gilstrap LC, Leveno KJ, Burris J, Little BB (1989) Umbilical artery acid–base status in the preterm infant. *Obstetrics and Gynecology* **74**:256–258.

60   Dickinson JE, Eriksen NL, Meyer BA, Parisi VM (1992) The effect of preterm birth on umbilical cord blood gases. *Obstetrics and Gynecology* **79**:575–578.

61   Catlin EA, Carpenter MW, Brann BS, Mayfield SR, Shaul PW, Goldstein M, Oh W (1986) The Apgar score revisited: Influence of gestational age. *Journal of Pediatrics* **109**:865–868.

62   Marlow N (1992) Do we need an Apgar score? *Archives of Diseases of Children* **67**:765–767.

63   Zanini B, Paul RH, Huey JR (1980) Intrapartum fetal heart rate: Correlation with scalp pH in the preterm fetus. *American Journal of Obstetrics and Gynecology* **136**:43–47.

64   Thorpe-Beeston JG, Banfield PJ, Saunders N StG (1992) Outcome of breech delivery at term. *British Medical Journal* **305**:746–747.

65   Eliot BW, Hill JG (1972) Method of breech management incorporating use of fetal blood sampling. *British Medical Journal* **4**:703–706.

66   Paintin DB (1982) Midcavity forceps delivery. *British Journal of Obstetrics and Gynaecology* **89**:495–500.

67   Rooth G, Jacobsen L, Heinrich J, Seidenschnur G (1972) The acidbase status of the fetus during normal labour. Testing a model of maternal–fetal acid base exchange on two different series of patients. In Longo LD, Bartels H (eds), *Respiratory Gas Exchange and Blood Flow in the Placenta*, pp. 477–480. Bethesda, MD: US Department of Health Education and Welfare.

68   Sachs BP, Yeh J, Acker D, Driscoll S, Brown DAJ, Jewett JF (1988) Cesarean section related maternal mortality in Massachusetts, 1954–1985. *Obstetrics and Gynecology* **71**:385–388.

69   Steer PJ, Beard RW (1973) Two cases of continuous fetal heart rate monitoring in twins. *British Medical Journal* **3**:263–265.

70   Dumoulin JG, Foulkes JEB (1984) Ketonuria during labour. *British Journal of Obstetrics and Gynaecology* **91**:97–98.

71   Ames AC, Cobbold S, Maddock J (1975) Lactic acidosis complicating treatment of ketosis of labour. *British Medical Journal* **4**:611–613.

72   Lawrence GF, Brown VA, Parsons RJ, Cooke ID (1982) Fetomaternal consequences of high-dose glucose infusion during labour. *British Journal of Obstetrics and Gynaecology* **89**:27–32.

73   Philipson EH, Kalhan SC, Riha MM, Pimentel R (1987) Effects of maternal glucose infusion on fetal acid-base status in human pregnancy. *American Journal of Obstetrics and Gynecology* **157**:866–873.

74   Piquard F, Hsiung R, Haberey P, Dellenbach P (1989) Does fetal acidosis develop with maternal glucose infusions during normal labor? *Obstetrics and Gynecology* **74**:909–914.

75   Simkin P (1986) Stress, pain and catecholamines in labour. Stress associated with childbirth events: A pilot survey of new mothers. *Birth* **13**:234–240.

76   Broach J, Newtown N (1988) Food and beverages in labor: The effects of cessation of oral intake during labor. *Birth* **15**:88–92.

77   Morgan BM, Magni V, Goroszenuik T (1990) Anaesthesia for emergency caesarean section. *British Journal of Obstetrics and Gynaecology* **97**:420–424.

78   Lewis M, Crawford JS (1987) Can one risk fasting the

obstetric patient for less than 4 hours? *British Journal of Anaesthesia* **59**:312–314.

79 Brotanek V, Hendricks CH, Yoshida T (1969) Changes in uterine blood flow during uterine contractions. *American Journal of Obstetrics and Gynecology* **103**:1108–1116.

80 Huch R, Huch A (1977) Continuous measurement of fetal pH and pO$_2$. In Beard RW, Campbell S (eds), *The Current Status of Fetal Heart Rate Monitoring and Ultrasound in Obstetrics*, pp. 71–100. London: Royal College of Obstetricians and Gynaecologists.

81 Schneider H, Strang F, Huch R, Huch A (1980) Suppression of uterine contractions with fenoterol and its effect on fetal tcPO$_2$ in human term labour. *British Journal of Obstetrics and Gynaecology* **87**:657–665.

82 Kubli F, Ruttgers H (1971) Iatrongenic fetal hypoxia. In Gevers RH, Ruys JH (eds), *Physiology and Pathology of the Perinatal Period*, pp. 57–75. Leiden: Leiden University Press.

83 Goodlin RC (1985) Is oxytocin the culprit? *American Journal of Obstetrics and Gynecology* **153**:928–929.

84 MacDonald D, Sheridan-Pereira M, Boylan P, Grant A, Chalmers I (1985) Is oxytocin the culprit? Reply. *American Journal of Obstetrics and Gynecology* **153**:929–929.

85 Caldeyro-Barcia R, Sica-Blanco Y, Poseiro JJ, Gonzalez-Panniza V, Mendez-Bauer C, Fielitz C, Alvarez H, Pose SV, Hendricks CH (1957) A quantitative study of the action of synthetic oxytocin on the pregnant human uterus. *Journal of Pharmacology* **121**:18–31.

86 Seitchik J, Castillo M (1982) Oxytocin augmentation of dysfunctional labour. *American Journal of Obstetrics and Gynecology* **144**:899–905.

87 Arulkumaran S, Ingemarsson I, Ratnam SS (1987) Oxytocin titration to achieve preset active contraction area values does not improve the outcome of induced labour. *British Journal of Obstetrics and Gynaecology* **94**:242–248.

88 Bidgood KA, Steer PJ (1987) A randomised control study of oxytocin augmentation of labour. 1. Obstetric outcome. *British Journal of Obstetrics and Gynaecology* **94**:512–517.

89 Mercer B, Pilgrim P, Sibai B (1991) Labor induction with continuous low dose oxytocin infusion: A randomized trial. *Obstetrics and Gynecology* **77**:659–663.

90 Leading Article (1988) How actively should dystocia be treated?/*Lancet* **i**:160.

91 Collins KM, Bevan DR, Beard RW (1978) Fluid loading to reduce abnormalities of fetal heart rate and maternal hhypotension during epidural analgesia in labour. *British Medical Journal* **2**:1460–1461.

93 Fusi L, Steer PJ, Maresh MJA, Beard RW (1989) Maternal pyrexia associated with the use of epidural analgesia in labour. *Lancet* **i**:1250–1252.

93 Macauley JH, Randall N, Bond K, Steer PJ (1992) Continuous monitoring of fetal temperature by non-invasive probe and its relationship to maternal temperature, fetal heart rate and cord arterial oxygen and pH. *Obstetrics and Gynecology* **79**:469–474.

94 Redmond GP (1982) Propranolol and fetal growth retardation. *Seminars in Perinatology* **6**:142–147.

95 Berkowitz J (1980) Antihypertensive drugs in the preg-nant patient. *Obstetrical and Gynecological Survey* **35**:191–204.

96 Cree JE, Meyer J, Hailey DM (1973) Diazepam in labour: Its metabolism and effect on the clinical condition and thermogenesis of the newborn. *British Medical Journal* **4**:251–255.

97 Dunn P (1976) Breech delivery, perinatal morbidity and mortality. In Rooth G, Bratteby LE (eds), *Perinatal Medicine: Proceedings of the 5th European Congress of Perinatal Medicine*. Stockholm: Almquist and Wiksell.

98 Stewart KS, Philpott RH (1981) Fetal response to cephalo-pelvic disproportion. *British Journal of Obstetrics and Gynaecology* **87**:641–649.

99 Hauth JC, Gilstrap LC, Hankins GDV, O'Connor KD (1985) Term maternal and neonatal complications of acute chorioamnionitis. *Obstetrics and Gynecology* **66**:59–62.

100 Levy H, Meier PR, Makowski EL (1984) Umbilical cord prolapse. *Obstetrics and Gynecology* **64**:499–502.

101 Yla-Outinen A, Heinonen PK, Tuimala R (1985) Predisposing and risk factors of umbilical cord prolapse. *Acta Obstetrica Gynecologica Scandinavica* **64**:567–569.

102 Barrett JM (1991) Funic reduction for the management of umbilical cord prolapse. *American Journal of Obstetrics and Gynecology* **165**:654–657.

103 Migliorini GD, Pepperell RJ (1977) Prolapse of the umbilical cord. Medical Journal of Australia **:**522–527.

104 Katz Z, Shoham Z, Lancet M, Blickstein I, Mogilner BM, Zalel Y (1988) Management of labor with umbilical cord prolapse – a five year study. *Obstetrics and Gynecology* **72**:278–281.

105 Vago T (1970) Prolapse of the umbilical cord: A method of management. *American Journal of Obstetrics and Gynecology* **107**:967–969.

106 Coltart TM, Byrne DL, Bates SA (1989) Meconium aspiration syndrome: A 6-year retrospective study. *British Journal of Obstetrics and Gynaecology* **96**:411–414.

107 Rossi EM, Philipson EH, Williams TG, Kalhan SC (1989) Meconium aspiration syndrome: Intrapartum and neonatal attributes. *American Journal of Obstetrics and Gynecology* **161**:1106–1110.

108 Wiswell TE, Tuggle JM, Turner BS (1990) Meconium aspiration syndrome: Have we made a difference. *Pediatrics* **85**:715–721.

109 Macfarlane PI, Heaf DP (1988) Pulmonary function in children after neonatal meconium aspiration syndrome. *Archives of Diseases of Children* **63**:368–372.

110 Leading Article. (1988) Lung function in children after neonatal meconium aspiration. *Lancet* **i**:317–318.

111 Swaminathan S, Quinn J, Stabile MW, Bader D, Platzker ACG, Keens TG (1989) Long-term pulmonary sequelae of meconium aspiration syndrome. *Journal of Pediatrics* **114**:356–361.

112 Gupta AK, Anand NK (1991) Wheezy baby syndrome – a possible sequelae of neonatal meconium aspiration syndrome. *Indian Journal of Pediatrics* **58**:525–527.

113 Dysart M, Graves BW, Shapr ES, ζotsonis G (1991) The incidence of meconium-stained amniotic fluid

from 1980 through 1986, by year and gestational age. *Journal of Perinatology* **11**:245–248.

114 Thomas JE (1964) Organ systems in adaptation: The digestive system. In Dill DB, Adolp EF, Wilber CG (eds), *Handbook of Physiology, Section 4: Adaptation to the Environment*, pp. 207–214. Washington DC: American Physiological Society.

115 Guyton AC (1991) Behavioural and motivational mechanisms of the brain – the limbic system and the hypothalamus. In *Textbook of Physiology*, 8th edn, pp. 651–656. Philadelphia, PA: W.B. Saunders.

116 Smith CA (1976) In *The Physiology of the Newborn Infant*. Springfield, IL: Charles C. Thomas.

117 Steer PJ, Eigbe F, Lissauer TJ, Beard RW (1989) Inter-relationships among abnormal cardiotocograms in labor, meconium staining of the amniotic fluid, arterial cord blood pH and Apgar scores. *Obstetrics and Gynecology* **74**:715–721.

118 Meis PJ, Hall M, Marshall JR, Hobel CJ (1978) Meconium passage: A new classification for risk assessment during labor. *American Journal of Obstetrics and Gynecology* **131**:509–513.

119 Miller FC, Read JA (1981) Intrapartum assessment of the postdate fetus. *American Journal of Obstetrics and Gynecology* **141**:516–520.

120 Becker RF, Windle WF, Barth EE, Schulz MD (1940) Fetal swallowing, gastro-intestinal activity and defecation in amnio. *Surgery Gynecology Obstetrics* **70**:603–614.

121 McLain CR (1963) Amniography studies of the gastro-intestinal motility of the human fetus. *American Journal of Obstetrics and Gynecology* **86**:1079–1087.

122 Woods JR, Dolkart LA (1989) Significance of amniotic fluid meconium. In Creasy RK, Resnik R (eds), *Maternal–Fetal Medicine: Principles and Practice*, 2nd edn, pp. 404–413. Philadelphia, PA: W.B. Saunders.

123 Romero R, Hanaoka S, Mazor M, Athanassiadis AP, Callahan R, Chiung Hsu Y, Avila C, Nores J, Jimenez C (1991) Meconium-stained amniotic fluid: A risk factor for microbial invasion of the amniotic cavity. *American Journal of Obstetrics and Gynecology* **164**:859–862.

124 Lucas A, Christofides ND, Adrian TE, Bloom SR, Aynsley-Green A (1979) Fetal distress, meconium, and motilin. *Lancet* **i**:718.

125 Mahmoud EL, Benirschke K, Vaucher YE, Poitras P (1988) Motilin levels in term neonates who have passed meconium prior to birth. *Journal of Pediatric Gastroenterology and Nutrition* **7**:95–99.

126 Grand RJ, Waykins JB, Torti FM (1976) Development of the human gastrointestinal tract. *Gastroenterology* **70**:790–810.

127 Schulze M (1925) The significance of the passage of meconium during labor. *American Journal of Obstetrics and Gynecology* **10**:83–88.

128 Stander HJ (1941) Prolapse of the cord-asphyxia. In *Williams' Obstetrics*, 8th edn, p. 1104. New York: Appleton-Century.

129 Desmond MM, Moore J, Lindley JE, Brown CA (1957) Meconium staining of the amniotic fluid. *Obstetrics and Gynecoloogy* **9**:91–103.

130 Walker J (1954) Foetal anoxia. *Journal of Obstetrics and Gynaecology of the British Empire* **61**:162–180.

131 Fenton AN, Steer CM (1962) Fetal distress. *American Journal of Obstetrics and Gynecology* **83**:354–362.

132 Fujikura T, Klionsky B (1975) The significance of meconium staining. *American Journal of Obstetrics and Gynecology* **121**:45–49.

133 Miller FC, Sacks DA, Yeh S-Y, Paul RH, Schifrin BS, Martin CB, Hon EH (1975) Significance of meconium during labor. *American Journal of Obstetrics and Gynecology* **122**:573–580.

134 Starks GC (1980) Correlation of meconium-stained amniotic fluid, early intrapartum fetal pH, and Apgar scores as predictors of perinatal outcome. *Obstetrics and Gynecology* **56**:604–609.

135 Wong WS, Wong KS, Chang A (1985) Epidemiology of meconium staining of amniotic fluid in Hong Kong. *Australia and New Zealand Journal of Obstetrics and Gynaecology* **25**:90–93.

136 Bochner CJ, Medearis AL, Ross MG, Oakes GK, Jones P, Hobel CJ, Wade ME (1987) The role of antepartum testing in the management of postterm pregnancies with heavy meconium in early labor. *Obstetrics and Gynecology* **69**:903–907.

137 Shaw K, Clark SL (1988) Reliability of intrapartum fetal heart rate monitoring of the postterm fetus with meconium passage. *Obstetrics and Gynecology* **72**:886–889.

138 Baker N, Kilby MD, Murray H (1992) An assessment of the use of meconium alone as an indication for fetal blood sampling. *Obstetrics and Gynecology* **80**:792–796.

139 Yeomans ER, Gilstrap LC, Leveno KJ, Burris JS (1989) Meconium in the amniotic fluid and fetal acid–base status. *Obstetrics and Gynecology* **73**:175–178.

140 Naeye RL, Peters EC, Bartholomew M, Landis JR (1989) Origins of cerebral palsy. *American Journal of Diseases of Children* **143**:1154–1161.

141 Saling E (1966) *Amnioscopy. Clinics in Obstetrics and Gynecology* **9**:472–490.

142 Hon EH (1963) The foetal heart rate. In Carey HM (ed), *Modern Trends in Human Reproductive Physiology*, pp. 245–256. London: Butterworths.

143 Emmanoulides GC, Townsend DE, Bauer RA (1968) Effects of single umbilical artery ligation in the lamb fetus. *Pediatrics* **42**:919.

144 Katz VL, Bowes WA (1992) Meconium aspiration syndrome: Reflections on a murky subject. *American Journal of Obstetrics and Gynecology* **166**:171–183.

145 Dawes GS, Fox HE, Leduc BM, Liggins GC, Richards RT (1972) Respiratory movements and rapid eye movement sleep in the foetal lamb. *Journal of Physiology* **220**:119–143.

146 Duenhoelter JH, Pritchard JA (1977) Fetal respiration: A review *American Journal of Obstetrics and Gynecology* **129**:326–338.

147 Falciglia HS (1988) Failure to prevent meconium aspiration syndrome. *Obstetrics and Gynecology* **71**:349–353.

148 Dooley SL, Pesavento DJ, Depp R, Socol ML, Tamura RK, Wiringa KS (1985) Meconium below the vocal cords at delivery: Correlation with intrapartum events.

American Journal of Obstetrics and Gynecology **153**:767–770.

149 Gregory GA, Gooding CA, Phibbs RH, Tooley WH (1974) Meconium aspiration in infants – a prospective study. *Journal of Pediatrics* **85**:848–852.

150 Ting P, Brady JP (1975) Tracheal suction in meconium aspiration. *American Journal of Obstetrics and Gynecology* **122**:767–771.

151 Carson BS, Losey RW, Bowes WA, Simmons MA (1976) Combined obstetric and pediatric approach to prevent meconium aspiration syndrome. *American Journal of Obstetrics and Gynecology* **126**:712–715.

152 Davis RO, Philips JB, Harris BA, Wilson ER, Huddleston JF (1985) Fetal meconium aspiration syndrome occurring despite airway management considered appropriate. *American Journal of Obstetrics and Gynecology* **151**:731–736.

153 Mitchell J, Schulman H, Fleischer A, Farmakides G, Nadeau D (1985) Meconium aspiration and fetal acidosis. *Obstetrics and Gynecology* **65**:352–355.

154 Sepkowitz S (1987) Influence of the legal imperative and medical guidelines on the incidence and management of the meconium-stained newborn. *American Journal of Diseases of Children* **141**:1124–1127.

155 Cunningham AS, Lawson EE, Martin RJ, Pildes RS (1990) Tracheal suction and meconium: A proposed standard of care. *Journal of Pediatrics* **116**:153–154.

156 Block MF, Kallenberger DA, Kern JD, Nepveux RD (1981) *In utero* meconium aspiration by the baboon fetus. *Obstetrics and Gynecology* **57**:37–40.

157 Duenholter JH, Pritchard JA (1976) Fetal respiration: Quantitative measurements of amniotic fluid inspired near term by human and rhesus fetuses. *American Journal of Obstetrics and Gynecology* **125**:306–309.

158 Harding R (1984) Fetal breathing. In Beard RW, Nathanielsz PW (eds), *Fetal Physiology and Medicine*, 2nd edn, pp. 255–286. New York: Marcel Dekker.

159 Murphy JD, Vawter GF, Reid LM (1984) Pulmonary vascular disease in fatal meconium aspiration. *Journal of Pediatrics* **104**:758–762.

160 Hageman JR, Conley M, Francis K, Stenske J, Wolf I, Santi V, Farrell EE (1988) Delivery room management of meconium staining of the amniotic fluid and the development of meconium aspiration syndrome. *Journal of Perinatology* **8**:127–131.

161 Brown BL, Gleicher N (1981) Intrauterine meconium aspiration. *Obstetrics and Gynecology* **57**:26–29.

162 Gersony WM (1984) Neonatal pulmonary hypertension: Pathophysiology, classification, and etiology, *Clinics in Perinatology* **ii**:517–524.

163 Drummond WH, Peckham GJ, Fox WW (1977) The clinical profile of the newborn with persistent pulmonary hypertension. *Clinics in Pediatrics* **16**:335–341.

164 Fox WW, Gewitz MH, Dinwiddie R, Drummond WH, Peckham CJ (1977) Pulmonary hypertension in the perinatal aspiration syndromes. *Pediatrics* **59**:205–211.

165 Jovanovic R, Nguyen HT (1989) Experimental meconium aspiration in guinea pigs. *Obstetrics and Gynecology* **73**:652–656.

166 Hutchinson AA, Russell G (1976) Effective pulmonary capillary blood flow in infants with birth asphyxia. *Acta Paediatrica Scandinavica* **65**:669–672.

167 Tyler DC, Murphy J, Cheney FW (1978) Mechanical and chemical damage to lung tissue caused by meconium aspiration. *Pediatrics* **62**:454–459.

168 Thibeault DW, Hall FK, Sheehan MB, Hall RT (1984) Postasphyxial lung disease in newborn infants with severe perinatal acidosis. *American Journal of Obstetrics and Gynecology* **150**:393–399.

169 Clark DA, Neiman GF, Thompson JE, Paskanik AM, Rokhar BA, Bredenberg CE (1987) Surfactant displacement by meconium free fatty acids: An alternative explanation for atelectasis in meconium aspiration syndrome. *Journal of Pediatrics* **110**:765–770.

170 Auten RL, Notter RH, Kendig JW, Davis JM, Shapiro DL (1991) Surfactant treatment of full-term newborns with respiratory failure. *Pediatrics* **87**:101–107.

171 Moses D, Holm BA, Spitale P, Liu M, Enhorning G (1991) Inhibition of pulmonary surfactant function by meconium. *American Journal of Obstetrics and Gynecology* **164**:477–481.

172 Oelberg DG, Downey SA, Flynn MM (1990) Bile salt-induced intracellular Ca^{++} accumulation in type II pneumocytes. *Lung* **168**:297–308.

173 Hammerman C, Komar K, Abu-Khudair H (1988) Hypoxic *vs* septic pulmonary hypertension. *American Journal of Diseases of Children* **142**:319–325.

174 Florman AL, Teubner D (1969) Enhancement of bacterial growth in amniotic fluid by meconium. *Journal of Pediatrics* **74**:111–114.

175 Hoskins IA, Hemming VG, Johnson TRB, Winkel CA (1987) Effects of alterations of zinc-to-phosphorus ratios and meconium content on Group B *Streptococcus* growth in human amniotic fluid *in vitro*. *American Journal of Obstetrics and Gynecology* **157**:770–773.

176 Altshuler G, Arizawa M, Molnar-Nadasy G (1992) Meconium-induced umbilical cord vascular necrosis and ulceration: A potential link between the placenta and poor pregnancy outcome. *Obstetrics and Gynecology* **79**:760–766.

177 Drummond WH, Bissonnette JM (1978) Persistent pulmonary hypertension in the neonate: Development of an animal model. *American Journal of Obstetrics and Gynecology* **131**:761–763.

178 Cucco C, Osborne MA, Cibils LA (1989) Maternal–fetal outcomes in prolonged pregnancy. *American Journal of Obstetrics and Gynecology* **161**:916–920.

179 Huntingford PJ, Brunello LP, Dunstan M *et al.* (1968) The technique and significance of amnioscopy. *Journal of Obstetrics and Gynaecology of the British Commonwealth* **75**:610–615.

180 Browne ADH, Bernan RK (1968) The application, value, and limitations of amnioscopy *Journal of Obstetrics and Gynaecology of the British Commonwealth* **75**:616.

181 Saldana LR, Schulman H, Chin-Chu Lin (1976) Routine amnioscopy at term. *Obstetrics and Gynecology* **47**:521–524.

182 Tchabo J-G (1989) The effect of hysteroscopy on the incidence of meconium aspiration in high risk obstetric patient. *Journal of International Surgery* **74**:188–190.

183 Benacerraf BR, Gatter MA, Ginsburgh F (1984) Ultrasound diagnosis of meconium-stained amniotic fluid.

American Journal of Obstetrics and Gynecology **149**:570–572.

184 Sepulveda WH, Quiroz VH (1989) Sonographic detection of echogenic amniotic fluid and its clinical significance. *Journal of Perinatal Medicine* **17**:333–335.

185 Sherer DM, Abramowicz JS, Smith SA, Woods JR (1991) Sonographically homogeneous echogenic amniotic fluid in detecting meconium-stained amniotic fluid. *Obstetrics and Gynecology* **78**:819–822.

186 Cole RA, Howie PW, Macnaughton MC (1975) Elective induction of labour: A randomised prospective trial. *Lancet* **ii**:767–770.

187 Dyson DC, Miller PD, Armstrong MA (1987) Management of prolonged pregnancy: Induction of labor versus antepartum fetal testing. *American Journal of Obstetrics and Gynecology* **156**:928–934.

188 Martin DH, Thompson W, Pinkerton JHM, Watson JD (1978) A randomized controlled trial of selective planned delivery. *British Journal of Obstetrics and Gynaecology* **85**:109–113.

189 Knox GE, Huddleston JF, Flowers CE (1979) Management of prolonged pregnancy: Results of a prospective randomised trial. *American Journal of Obstetrics and Gynecology* **134**:376–384.

190 Cardozo L, Fysh J, Pearce JM (1986) Prlonged pregnancy: The management debate. *British Medical Journal* **293**:1059–1063.

191 Augensen K, Bergsjo P, Eikeland T, Askvik K, Carlsen J (1987) Randomised comparison of early versus late induction of labour in post-term pregnancy. *British Medical Journal* **294**:1192–1195.

192 Witter FR, Weitz CM (1987) A randomized trial of induction at 42 weeks gestation versus expectant management for postdates pregnancies. *American Journal of Perinatology* **4**:206–211.

193 Cordero L, Hon EH (1971) Neonatal bradycardia following nasopharyngeal suction. *Journal of Pediatrics* **78**:441–447.

194 Linder N, Aranda JV, Tsur M, Matoth I, Yatsiv I, Mandelberg H, Rottem M, Feigenbaum D, Ezra Y, Tamir I (1988) Need for endotracheal intubation and suction in meconium-stained neonates. *Journal of Pediatrics* **112**:613–615.

195 Sadovsky Y, Amon E, Bade ME, Petrie RH (1989) Prophylactic amnioinfusion during labour complicated by meconium: A preliminary report. *American Journal of Obstetrics and Gynecology* **161**:613–617.

196 Wenstrom KD, Parsons MT (1989) The prevention of meconium aspiration in labor using amnionfusion. *Obstetrics and Gynecology* **73**:647–651.

197 Strong TH, Hetzler G, Sarno AP, Paul RH (1990) Prophylactic intrapartum amnioinfusion: A randomized clinical trial. *American Journal of Obstetrics and Gynecology* **162**:1370–1375.

198 Macri CJ, Schrimmer DB, Leung A, Greenspoon JS, Paul RH (1992) Prophylactic amnioinfusion improves outcome of pregnancy complicated by thick meconium and oligohydramnios. *American Journal of Obstetrics and Gynecology* **167**:117–121.

199 Weitzner JS, Strassner HT, Rawlins RG, Mack SR, Anderson RA (1990) Objective assessment of meconium content of amniotic fluid. *Obstetrics and Gynecology* **76**:1143–1144.

200 Trimmer KJ, Gilstrap LC (1991) 'Meconiumcrit' and birth asphyxia. *American Journal of Obstetrics and Gynecology* **165**:1010–1013.

201 Sosa R, Kennell J, Klaus M, Robertson S, Urrutia J (1980) The effect of a supportive companion on perinatal problems, length of labor, and mother–infant interaction. *New England Journal of Medicine* **303**:597–600.

202 Klaus MH, Kennell JH, Robertson SS, Sosa R (1986) Effects of social support during parturition on maternal and infant morbidity. *British Medical Journal* **293**:585–587.

203 Genevier ES, Danielian PJ, Randall NJ, Smith R, Steer PJ (1993) A method for continuous monitoring of meconium in the amniotic fluid during labour. *Journal of Biochemical Engineering* **15**:229–234.

63

Maternal Anesthesia and Analgesia in Labor

BARBARA MORGAN

INTRODUCTION

The function of pain is probably to provide a warning that tissue is being, or may be about to be, damaged. The functional value of pain due to dilatation of the cervix is not known for certain but it can be conjectured that it is a signal to the mother that the important event of birth is about to take place. Unexpected delivery in an unsuitable environment is a hazard even under the optimum conditions of modern civilized society. Thus the pain of labor can be imagined as a signal to the expectant mother to find a suitable safe haven (secure, warm and draft-free) before the birth of the child occurs.

If the function of pain in labor is to provide a warning, and this warning is heeded, then one may hypothesize that there is no need for the pain to continue. If this hypothesis is true, then pain may be relieved without any inevitable adverse effect on the mother, fetus, or progress of labor. Not only humanitarian but also physiological considerations suggest the need for safe efficient pain relief in obstetric as well as surgical patients, particularly in complicated labors and for surgical delivery, whether that be abdominal or vaginal. For women with pregnancy-related pathology, analgesia and anesthesia may be essential to ensure maternal safety. Effective analgesia in labor can also benefit the fetus by relieving maternal distress leading to disordered physiology and can thus also enhance the probability of delivering a neonate in good condition.

In normal labor, pain relief must not deprive the mother of the emotional rewards of her experience of childbirth. Although this experience has for many years been seen in almost wholly negative terms by a male-dominated society, it is now being viewed by many women as valuable and worth having even if only during part of the labor. Complete loss of sensation or even unconsciousness during childbirth is often not the woman's aim. The major function of pain relief in normal (as opposed to abnormal) labor is to improve the mother's experience if her emotional support is insufficient or if she is unwilling to negotiate unmedicated labor.

ASSESSMENT OF PAIN RELIEF

The study of pain and its relief has many pitfalls. There are no objective measurements. Three methods of measurement of successful analgesia are frequently used in pain studies, but all of them are subject to criticism. First, quantal measurements or the number of women who declared themselves pain-free after the treatment is often used but is obviously inadequate if the aim of the analgesia is reduction rather than elimination of pain. Second, the visual linear analog scale can be used, such as a 10 cm line ranging from 'no pain' at one end to 'unbearable pain' at the other, and marked by the mother at a point she considers representative of her state or experience. The distance of this mark from either end is then measured, giving an index of the degree of pain. This technique sufers from the subjective nature of the measurement and the mother's occasional inability to understand the method. Third, rank scoring or rating the pain before and after treatment on a 3- or 5-point scale of severity or a descriptive scale of mild, moderate or severe, can also be used. This produces only discrete values which must be analysed by non-parametric tests (such as the Fisher's exact or chi-squared tests), unlike the linear analog method which produces a measurement on a continuous scale which can therefore be analyzed by parametric techniques (such as Student's t-test).

Melzack[1] has compiled a scoring system in which not only the quantity of pain but also the quality of pain can be estimated by using a series of adjectives and having the mother select those that best describe the pain that she is experiencing. These adjectives describe the sensory quality of pain by the use of words such as 'cramping' or 'pulling', the affective quality with words like 'exhausting' or 'terrifying' and evaluative words to describe the overall pain experience.

The only absolute certainty about pain, its measurement and its relief is that only the woman herself can say whether she is in pain, how severe it is and how effective the treatment has been. The opinion of the midwife, the obstetrician, the anesthetist, a companion or the husband is relatively worthless.

The measurement of pain in labor is further bedevilled by the unpredictable rate of progress of each labor and thus the rate at which pain increases. Comparison of the effects of an analgesic drug between patients or using the patient as her own control is therefore unreliable.

The round-the-clock nature of obstetric care frequently results in mothers being questioned postpartum about their pain relief, commonly 24–48 h after delivery. The mother's perception of pain changes after the birth, and therefore the time at which enquiry is made should always be taken into account when her responses are evaluated. Pain during labor is exaggerated by fear that is of course not present after the event.

THE NATURE OF PAIN IN LABOR

There is some evidence that pain in the first stage of labor is visceral and caused by the dilatation of the cervix. Both paravertebral block at T11–T12 and paracervical block will eliminate first-stage pain. Women who completed a visual linear analog of pain every 30 min during normal labor revealed that pain increases with increasing cervical dilation. **Figure 1** shows the mean and upper limit of the range of analog pain scores of 45 nulliparas as related to the cervical dilatation. These women all had minimal analgesia with psychoprophylaxis, transcutaneous electrical stimulation (TENS) or Entonox®, and spontaneous vaginal deliveries. There is a wide inter-patient variability, as has been shown previously.[2] It is common knowledge that low pain scores are a sign of normal labor and that severe pain very early in labor is an adverse prognostic sign

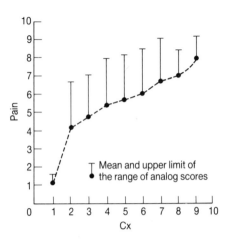

Figure 1. Pain scores hourly in labor related to cervical dilatation: 45 nulliparas with minimal analgesia.

for both labor and delivery. However, the wide range of pain scores and the inaccuracy of the pain measurement prevent this from being a clinically useful diagnostic test for abnormal labor. Bundsen[3] found that the most consistent influence on the woman's assessment of the success of systemic analgesia was the patient's cervical dilatation on admission.

There is wide variation in the degree of pain recorded in the various reported studies. At one extreme, in a study by Melzack[4] of 87 mothers in normal labor, pain was described as intolerable by almost 30% of the women. Over 80% of all women in this study elected to have epidural analgesia. This may be a reflection of cultural attitude, as Melzack reported. More American women expect labor to be very painful than comparable Dutch women and, for example, three times as many American as Dutch women expected analgesia in labor.[5] It is therefore inappropriate to extrapolate levels of pain reported by women in one culture to women in other cultures.

Pain in the second stage of labor is different from first-stage pain. It is possibly not visceral but somatic and caused by vaginal and perineal tissue trauma; in support of this hypothesis, it can easily be eliminated by pudendal block.

MANAGEMENT OPTIONS FOR PAIN RELIEF IN LABOUR

General

Even where epidural analgesia is freely available on maternal request, it is not used by the majority of mothers. Rates of epidural analgesia for vaginal delivery range between 20 and 50% in most obstetric units in the UK where the technique has been offered routinely for at least 20 years. The reason why this startlingly successful analgesic does not have an even higher take-up rate is unclear, although as previously suggested, it may relate to women's desire to 'experience' labor fully. The familiarity of mothers, midwives obstetricians and anesthetists with epidural analgesia and its lack of serious complications have not greatly increased its popularity.

The profile of analgesia selected by women who achieve a vaginal delivery at our hospital is shown in **Figure 2**. One noticeable trend over recent years is the considerable increase in the numbers of women using minimal analgesia, including non-pharmacological methods of analgesia and Entonox® (50% nitrous oxide premixed with oxygen). The use of opiate analgesia in labor has fallen to less than 10% over the period shown. Thus although conduction anesthesia has provided a real improvement in the effectiveness of methods available for the relief of pain in labor, it has been paralleled by the need for an understanding of psychoprophylactic techniques.

Non-Pharmacological Analgesia

The Gate Control theory of pain[6] suggests that the pain impulses or messages can be modified at several stations along the route. This can be achieved because both excitatory and inhibitory impulses affect the conscious preception of pain. Many of the psychoprophylactic techniques rely on this theory to provide an explanation for their mode of action. The pain impulses can be inhibited in the dorsal horn where touch and pressure impulses as well as pain impulses synapse; for example, allowing a reduction in the patient's perception of pain with massaging.

Inhibitory effects also come from fibers descending from the brainstem and cerebral cortex, which decrease the excitability of the pain neurons in the dorsal horn. Pain sensation is commonly known to be suppressed by more demanding, threatening or exciting events that absorb cortical activity. Hypnotic states may be an example of this mechanism. Central nervous system sedation is, in contrast to excitation, a means of enhancing the perception of pain.[7]

Education of the mother prenatally so that she understands the birthing process helps her to accept the accompanying pain as a necessary part of childbirth, and 'part of a task willingly undertaken'.[8] This is particularly the case in societies where women are in control of their own fertility and childbearing is a choice.

Psychoprophylaxis is generally considered a technique for minimizing but not eliminating pain. Having the mother actively involved with her own pain-reducing techniques helps her to feel in control of herself during labor.[9] Women are encouraged to manage their pain relief during the early part of labour even if they progress to epidural analgesia later. The success of psychoprophylaxis depends on (1) the mother's willingness to attempt it, (2) her determination to succeed and (3) the labor being normal – these techniques are usually ineffective in obstructed labor.

Transcutaneous electrical stimulation is a method of exciting sensory receptors in the skin and, by bombarding the dorsal column with innocuous stimuli, inhibiting pain. It has been used in labor[10–13] with a success rate that is measured as a reduction in the amounts and frequency of use of other analgesic drugs and techniques. It has been found to be of some value in eary labor, but is of little benefit after 6 cm dilatation. Nevertheless, it is fashionable and popular with mothers. Harrison *et al.*[14] reported that only 18% of women in their study completed their labor using TENS alone, but this rose to 48% of women if Entonox® analgesia in the second stage was the only additional analgesic used. Despite these not very impressive results, 96% of mothers reported partial pain relief with TENS and a high consumer satisfaction at 24 h postpartum.

Entonox® (Nitrous Oxide in 50% Oxygen)

Nitrous oxide in a 50/50 mixture with oxygen in premixed cylinders has been shown to be a more effective analgesic in labor than pethidine,[14,15] with no adverse effect on the neonatal condition.[16] Its effectiveness can be enhanced by supplementing intermittent self-administered Entonox® with continuous nasal supplement.[17] It is similar in efficacy to other inhalational agents[18] but shorter-acting. The fear of aspiration of gastric contents is held to be a possible problem but there is no evidence that women ever become unconscious with self-administered Entonox®. It is popular with mothers, as it allows them the feeling of being in control of their analgesia. It is the most rapidly acting analgesic available.

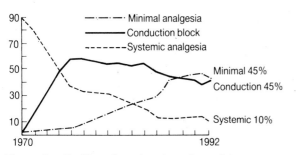

Figure 2. Profile of analgesia selected by women who achieve vaginal delivery at Queen Charlotte's and Chelsea Hospital.

Systemic Analgesics

Since its introduction in 1939, pethidine has become the most commonly used analgesic in obstetric units throughout the world; in some units, it is even used on a routine basis. However, randomized double-blind studies to assess its effectiveness as an intramuscular analgesic in labor are lacking, as are such trials to assess its effectiveness in the control of any severe pain. Two placebo-controlled studies using intramuscular pethidine have, however, been described.[19] Both report some analgesic effect but neither is convincing. One of the studies[20] suggested that intramuscular pethidine is twice as good as a placebo, and slightly better than a phenothiazine, at 30 min following administration, but at 1, 2 and 3 h methotrimeprazine (phenothiazine) gave better analgesia than did pethidine (although pethidine was still better than placebo). As the phenothiazines are not known to be analgesics, these results suggest that the action of pethidine in labor is not analgesic but possibly sedative, as is the phenothiazine. The obstetricians were more impressed by the adequacy of pain relief than were the mothers.

A larger study by Cullhed and Lofstrom compared five different treatments: intramuscular pethidine 50 mg, pethidine 50 mg with scopolamine 0.2 mg, scopolamine 0.2 mg, placebo and a non-injection group.[21] All the women in the study had free access to pure nitrous oxide delivered intermittently, or trilene 0.5% in air. In total, 34% of the pethidine and scopolamine groups, 48% of the placebo group and 56% of the non-injection group used inhalational analgesia. In the three injection groups, 31% of mothers claimed inadequate analgesia compared with 40% in the placebo group; however, only 28% of the non-injection group felt that their analgesia was inadequate when questioned during labor (they had free access to the inhalational drugs). This perhaps indicates that mothers relying on intramuscular analgesia are less likely to have adequate analgesia than those using inhalational drugs. Other studies[15,20–28] performed over a 20 year period have recorded that between 20 and 75% of mothers report poor to no pain relief with varying intramuscular doses of pethidine, pentazocine or meptazinol with or without additional drugs. When assessed by the visual analog scale with no pain set at 0 and maximum pain set at 100, studies using different doses of pethidine intramuscularly have reported pain scores of between 65 and 72, with the maximum being 100.[29–33] Intravenous, rather than intramuscular, administration of pethidine in doses ranging between 50 and 100 mg has been shown to be more effective at 30 min after administration, with 30–60% of women reporting substantial pain relief.[34–36] Studies which report the highest rates of successful analgesia, between 65 and 72%, have usually reported the analgesic effectiveness as assessed by the midwife or the obstetrician and not by the mother.[37,38] Even when patient-controlled intravenous or intramuscular analgesia was used, disappointingly high pain scores were reported.[39–43] These studies also reported a wide range of drug dosage selected by the mothers, indicating that a standard dose of opiate is an inadequate way of achieving the desired therapeutic effect.

The results of the trials reported are in the main not readily comparable because the obstetric situation is often not precisely defined. Normal and abnormal labors are compared and even parity is often overlooked, as well as the cervical dilatation when the drug is given, the state of the membranes, the time from administration to delivery and the mode of delivery. Further doses of pethidine or additional local blocks are often not clearly specified, additional drugs given with the pethidine are ignored and the initial dose of pethidine varied from 50 to 200 mg with usually no relationship to maternal bodyweight. Measures of successful pain relief are varied, usually taken postpartum, and at different times.

The therapeutic aim of systemic opiates as well as non-pharmacological techniques is merely the reduction, not the elimination, of pain, and this must be explained to the mother before labor if disappointment is to be avoided. In maternity services with no regional anesthesia available and where no attempt is made to educate the mother prenatally about the birth process or, teach her psychoprophylaxis or provide her with effective emotional support, the only way she can achieve some degree of analgesia is with intramuscular opiates or inhalational agents.

Maternal side-effects of systemic analgesics

The increased likelihood of reflux in pregnancy that results in over 70% of women at term having heartburn[44] is aggravated by opiates and several other anesthetic drugs.[45] Narcotics have also been shown to delay gastric emptying when used during labor,[46] and thus increase the risk of there being substantial gastric contents if an emergency general anesthetic is necessary. The presence of substantial gastric contents is thought to be one factor leading to an increased risk of aspiration (Mendelson's syndrome) in association with general anesthesia for emergency cesarean section. This dangerous side-effect of pethidine and other narcotics has been highlighted in the *Report on Confidential Enquiries into Maternal Deaths 1982–84*,[47] which suggests that 'their omission would be a contribution to maternal safety', and again in the 1985–87 report where it is suggested that women who have received pethidine should have a naso- or oro-gastric tube passed before general anesthesia to empty the stomach.[48] Increasing numbers of obstetric units are giving ranitidine 50 mg i.m. 6 hourly to all women who have recieved a dose of pethidine in labor to ensure that the gastric contents are less acid and are diminished in volume despite the gastric stasis which still occurs.

One reason for the poor analgesic efficacy of pethidine in labor is the small doses that are used to avoid producing maternal and neonatal respiratory depression. Respiratory depression is an unavoidable side-effect of all opiates. A decrease in respiratory rate and a shift of the carbon dioxide response curve to the right is also produced. During labor, the repeated pain of contractions produces hyperventilation which helps to counteract this effect to some extent, but oxygen desaturation still occurs.[49] Maternal respiratory depression may be enhanced by the combination of pethidine and epidural block, because the latter removes pain and thus reduces hyperventilatory drive. Orthostatic hypotension may also occur following the administration of pethidine, thus confining the woman to her bed.

Nausea and vomiting is a commonly encountered side-effect more serious in some patients than others. Antiemetic drugs are not required by all women and therefore should be given only when needed rather than routinely.

Fetal side-effects of systemic analgesics

The depressant effects of opiates can also be observed in the fetus. Altered electroencelophalogram and electrocardiogram patterns have been recorded.[50] A decrease in baseline variability of the fetal heart rate pattern is often observed when the fetus is monitored by cardiotocography. Despite these changes, fetal oxygenation *in utero* appears unaffected by the drug.[51]

Neonatal effects of systemic analgesics

All drugs that affect the mother's central nervous system and that cross the placenta must necessarily produce central nervous depression in the neonate. The neonate who has received drugs transplacentally may well have a reduced Apgar score, although this is not likely to have an adverse effect on the child's long-term outcome provided it is resuscitated and not subsequently allowed to become hypoxic due to respiratory depression. A reduction in both the 1 min and 5 min Apgar scores may be caused either by depressant drugs and/or intrauterine hypoxia. The history of the mother's analgesic and anesthetic drug intake in labor must be known if conclusions are to be drawn from the Apgar scores.

The respiratory depression seen in the neonate following pethidine is evidenced by prolonged time to sustained respiration, lower oxygen saturation[52] and respiratory acidosis.[53] The severity of these side-effects can be minimized by reducing the dose of pethidine,

avoiding where possible any additional drugs, and keeping the administration to delivery time to a minimum, as fewer infants have low Apgar scores if delivered within 1 h of an intramuscular dose. The reason for this may well be related to the speed of the distribution of pethidine through the maternal and fetal tissues. The initial level of drug in the umbilical vein is higher than that of the umbilical artery, reflecting the fetal tissue uptake of the drug. If delivery occurs within 1 h of the drug administration the umbilical vein drug concentration is greater than the arterial because of fetal tissue uptake. In those with a longer interval the drug concentration of umbilical vein and artery are equal indicating saturation of fetal tissues with whatever dose of pethidine has been given. The neonatal respiratory depressant effect is greatest if the delivery occurs 2–3 h after the drug is given.[54] The longer the interval between administration and delivery, the more pronounced the effect on the neurobehavioral scores rather than on respiration. This may indicate the effect of norpethidine. This active metabolite occurs in very high concentrations in the fetus if the administration to delivery time is longer than 4 h[55].

Even if the neonate shows no respiratory depression following analgesic drugs, neurobehavioral changes have been demonstrated. There are several tests of neurobehavior which concentrate on different aspects of neonatal condition. The Brazelton neonatal behavioral assessment scale has been simplified to reflect a cluster of altered responses and thus allows easier comparison between infants.[56]

The early neonatal neurobehavioral scale (ENNS)[57] and the neurologic adaptive capacity score (NACS)[58] were designed to assess the effects of anesthetic and analgesic drugs. The tests concentrate on reflexes, muscle tone, response to stimulation, states of consciousness and general behavioral status, and have been used to investigate the effects of analgesic and anesthetic drugs on the neonate.[59] Pethidine has been reported to be associated with decreased alertness,[60,61] abnormal reflexes and decreased social responsiveness and self-quieting.[55] These studies suggest that the effects of pethidine last for at least 24 h. This suggests the involvement of an active metabolite, possibly norpethidine.

Regional (Epidural) Analgesia

The epidural space can be approached via the lumbar or caudal routes. The caudal approach has largely been abandoned in obstetric practice as it is more painful. In addition, the anatomy of the sacral hiatus is variable and the bony landmarks are often obscured by fatty tissue, making it a more difficult technique. Although it makes the possibility of dural puncture less likely, it is not avoided altogether. Epidural injections through the sacral hiatus require much larger volumes of local anesthetic solution to produce effective anesthesia than via the lumbar route. Perineal anesthesia is produced readily with the caudal approach, and this may be an advantage in advanced labor. However, perhaps the major disadvantage is the risk of accidental injection of local anesthetic into the fetal head,[62] making its use in the second stage inadvisable.

The neural blockade that results from the injection of local anesthetic drugs into the epidural space is described by Bromage[63] as 'not a single entity but a range of blocks from the barely perceptible sensory block to a block of most of the nerve fibers'. This allows the block to be used both for pain relief in labor and for cesarean section. It offers startlingly good analgesia in labor, drawing clear attention to the inadequate analgesia offered by all other methods.

It is, however, an expensive method of analgesia both in demands on staff time and expertise. It is not suitable for use in obstetric units where a skilled anesthetist is not immediately available throughout the entire period of the neural blockade or where the staff on the labor ward are not fully conversant with cardiopulmonary resuscitation of the pregnant woman. It requires anesthetic expertise for the insertion of the epidural catheter as well as for maintaining and monitoring the resulting neural blockade. In countries where trained midwives give epidural top-ups, the anesthetist still retains responsibility for the patient and her anesthesia. It also requires expertise in the conduct of the labor and delivery, as the second stage in particular is affected by the blockade. It is an essential tool in the management of high-risk labors, as there are therapeutic indications for epidural analgesia in labor that have become a necessary feature of modern obstetric practice. Fetal indications may include vaginal delivery where the fetus is presenting by the breech[64] although this remains controversial. The ability of the mother to cooperate with the maneuvers necessary in many cases to secure a safe assisted vaginal breech delivery is greatly increased, although her ability to bear down and assist the delivery process is often impaired.

Vaginal or abdominal delivery of twins is a less controversial indication for conduction anesthesia. The major risk with twin delivery is to the second twin, and this often relates to malpresentation. Correction of an abnormal lie, for example by internal podalic version, can only be carried out safely and without causing undue distress to the mother or fetus if the mother has adequate anesthesia, preferably from regional block. Given good analgesia, the condition of the second twin can consistently be safeguarded.[65,66]

The preterm and low-birthweight neonate is particularly sensitive to systemic analgesic drugs, and neonatal mortality is reduced in low-birthweight infants delivered with analgesia provided by epidural analgesia rather than narcotics.[67]

The use of epidural anesthesia is appropriate in women with pre-eclampsia, whether vaginal or abdominal delivery is planned.[68,69] Judicious use can limit the progressive rise in blood pressure which can occur due to the stress of progressive labor without adequate analgesia, and in particular the sudden intense rise of blood pressure which commonly occurs during endotracheal intubation.[69] In addition, the effective analgesia of an epidural allows the obstetrican to avoid the use of systemic sedative and analgesic drugs in patients likely to be receiving other potent drugs such as hypotensive agents and anticonvulsants. An important advantage of epidurals in pre-eclampsia can be an improvement in placental perfusion,[70] which can in turn improve the condition of an hypoxic fetus. Patients with fulminating pre-eclampsia or eclampsia may be unsuitable for epidural anesthesia if they are already convulsing, have a coagulopathy[71] or have a very low plasma protein concentration with incipient preoperative pulmonary edema. These seriously ill women require careful monitoring and meticulous attention to management whatever analgesia and anesthesia are used. In addition, if epidural anesthesia is used in women with the constricted vascular system of severe pre-eclampsia, extra care must be taken to avoid hypotension from excessively rapid or large top-ups, and the supine posture (caval compression syndrome). Acute vascular changes can be limited by use of weak solutions of local anesthetic, e.g. 0.25% Marcaine® rather than 0.5%.

Analgesia for labor in women with medical disorders is usually best provided by epidural analgesia. Cardiac disease, with the relative exception of aortic stenosis, pulmonary hypertension or right-to-left shunt, is an indication for epidural analgesia for both labor and cesarean section, because it provides the best analgesia and therefore limits the cardiac demand imposed by the stress of a painful labor. Respiratory diseases where central sedation must be avoided is also an indiction for epidural analgesia. However, serious medical disorders combined with pregnancy and delivery place the mother at high risk and she requires detailed monitoring; access to intensive care expertise and facilities should always be available. Delivery should only be planned in obstetric units that are properly equipped to deal with the seriously ill patient.

Epidural opioids

Epidural opioids do not provide satisfactory analgesia in labor[72] and as with intramuscular opioids they are associated with various side-effects:[73] nausea, sedation, respiratory depression and also, unlike the intramuscular route, pruritis. There have been no definitive studies on the neonatal effects or the delay in gastric emptying seen with their intramuscular use. They do, however, have a considerable advantage when mixed with local anesthetics by allowing lower concentrations of local anesthetics to be used, giving satisfactory analgesia with less motor blockade[74] and possibly improving the mother's psyche. Fentanyl and pethidine are commonly used; how they should be given, whether by an initial bolus dose or by addition to epidural infusion solutions or with top-ups, is not yet clear.[75]

Side-effects and complications of epidural analgesia

Hypotension

The chemical sympathectomy that constitutes epidural blockade can cause hypotension, especially if the mother is relatively hypovolemic with a growth-deficient fetus, or with pre-eclampsia. However, this is less of a problem when using epidural block for analgesia in labor rather than for cesarean section, as the dose – both volume and concentration – of bupivacaine is much lower. It is common practice for a preload of 500–1000 ml Ringer-Lactate solution to be given before regional analgesia is commenced, to limit the fall in blood pressure when the vascular compartment expands in response to sympathetic blockade. Ephedrine can be used to treat or avoid hypotension, as it has been shown to be the one vasoconstrictor that does not reduce placental perfusion.[76] Once the block has been established, no further hypotension should occur unless caval occlusion develops.[77] Fetal acidosis can occur with prolonged hypotension and a fall in maternal cardiac output,[78] but hypotension should be avoidable or treatable in the great majority of cases, leaving neonatal condition unimpaired.[79] Usually, the biochemical condition of the fetus is improved when epidural anesthesia is used during labor.[80,81]

Effect on labor

Epidural analgesia has been shown not to prolong the duration of the first stage of labor, but it does prolong the second stage.[82] This effect is particularly evident in nulliparas, and is associated with a high rate of instrumental delivery, although the association has never conclusively been shown to be causal. Some studies have shown little or no association between the use of epidural anesthesia and an increase in forceps delivery rate; but they have suffered from design faults related to the selection of patients for the block, the nature of the epidural analgesia and the change in obstetric practice, required for the effective use of epidural anesthesia.[83–86] A similar number of studies show an increase in instrumental delivery, but again most of these studies are not conclusive for similar reasons.[74,87–89]

Prospective randomized studies of epidural *vs* other forms of analgesia are difficult to perform, as expectant mothers are generally not willing to enter such a study as they frequently have strong views about the analgesia they wish to use in labor. The two published studies[29,32] both suffer from design flaws, which mean that neither are convincing. The first study[29] had dissimilar groups with 56% of the epidural group having labor induced *vs* 19% in the pethidine group. Only 36% of patients used solely the analgesia allotted. The higher instrumental delivery rate observed in the epidural group (51 *vs* 27%) of nulliparas may thus have been caused by obstetric factors. In the second study[32] epidural analgesia was stopped at 8 cm cervical dilatation, thus eliminating analgesia for the second stage. As a result, only 41% of the epidural and 39% of the pethidine groups had a painless delivery, and 85% of all patients received a pudendal block. There was a 25% forceps or ventouse rate in both groups. Thus, although any increase in instrumental delivery rate appeared to have been avoided, this was at the expense of a loss of the analgesic effect, which is the whole point of epidural anesthesia.

If epidural block does indeed cause an increase in instrumental delivery, it is important to elucidate what aspect of the blockade does so and how this can be diminished. Suggestions that it is perineal analgesia in the second stage, motor block, the duration of the second stage or the lack of oxytocin increase in the second stage, have all been investigated.

There is evidence that analgesia throughout the second stage is associated with a doubling of the instrumental delivery rate (52 *vs* 27%)[90] and that inadequate analgesia at this stage is not associated with higher instrumental delivery rates.[91,92] However, the option to allow the analgesia to wear off would seem only to be applicable to epidural infusions allowing rapid return of perineal sensation. It is not merely the return of pain anywhere,[93] but the return of pain and sensation in the perineum (which promotes the urge to push) that may make the difference to the mode of delivery.

Motor block appears to be related to instrumental delivery rates only as much as it is a sign of the density and analgesic efficacy of the block.[94] A reduction of motor block while maintaining analgesia with low doses of local anesthetic mixed with opiates has not been shown to reduce forceps rates in some studies[95] but has in others.[96]

Another feature in the management of labor with epidural analgesia that may be manipulated to reduce forceps rate is the duration of the second stage. Allowing longer for the descent of the presenting part is widely promoted but has not been shown significantly to reduce the instrumental delivery rate[97,98] Problems associated with a prolonged second stage are the possible neuropraxis of the perineum (associated with both duration of second stage and birthweight), which may result in an increased incidence of incontinence in old age.[99,100]

The instrumental delivery rate has been shown to be diminished by the use of Syntocinon® augmentation in the second stage.[100] Uterine contractions normally increase in the second stage of labor; this is attributed to the Ferguson reflex in which stretching of the perineum is said to cause an increase in oxytocin secretion from the posterior pituitary.[101] This increase is not seen in labors managed with epidural analgesia in the second stage.[102] Oxytocin levels increase in the normal way during the second stage when systemic analgesia is used, but not when epidural anesthesia is used.[103] This can be corrected by judicious oxytocin infusion, which in several studies has been shown to limit the increase in instrumental delivery rate.[104,105] It should be borne in mind, however, that the second stage is a time of particular stress for the fetus, and each labor must be carefully assessed to exclude as far as possible by careful clinical examination the presence of outlet disproportion before oxytocin augmentation is commenced. Uterine hyperstimulation can interfere with oxygenation of the fetus, producing hypoxia and acidosis. If it then proves impossible to complete the delivery vaginally, whether spontaneously or instrumentally, cesarean section will be required. The delay before this procedure can be performed, with continuing hypoxia, and the difficulty of extracting a very molded fetal head wedged deep in the pelvis, may result in damage to the fetus and/or mother.

Fetal heart rate abnormalities

Epidural analgesia in labor can cause changes in the fetal heart rate which will appear as abnormalities of the cardiotocogram. Fetal bradycardia[106] may be evidence of maternal hypotension and aortocaval compression. This results from a fall in cardiac output in a patient vasodilated and unable to increase her peripheral resistance. The treatment or avoidance of this danger requires that the mother be nursed in the (left) lateral position (or the uterus displaced to the left if the mother must be placed supine) and ephedrine can also be administered if necessary. The supine position during labor can produce up to a 50% fall in fetal pO_2[107] and pH.[108] Conduction anesthesia is not associated with reduced placental perfusion provided hypotension and aortocaval compression are avoided or treated.[109] Several studies indicate an improvement in intervillous blood flow with epidural analgesia especially in pre-eclamptic mothers.[110–112] This increase in placental perfusion may be the result of preload, reduction in maternal pain and catecholamines and reduced intensity of uterine contractions.

Neonatal effects of local anesthetics

Studies on neonatal condition after bupivacaine, lignocaine or chloroprocaine epidural analgesia have shown no adverse effects compared with infants of mothers who received no drugs at all for labor[113,114] or who were delivered by elective cesarean section.[115,116] However, using various neurobehavioral tests, some alteration of infant behavior has been measured.[117,118] Kuhnert suggests that since such sophisticated tests are required to find the effects, they are probably not clinically meaningful.[119]

Backache

Backache following immediately after recovery from the epidural block is usually due to bruising. However, very severe or worsening bachache indicates a need for a full neurological examination, as it is the first symptom of an epidural hematoma or abscess. Long-term backache after epidural vaginal delivery is almost twice as common as after vaginal delivery with other analgesia;[120] this is likely to be the result of poor posture during labor, as it does not occur following epidural for elective cesarean section.

Unexpectedly extensive conduction blocks

The epidural catheter may lie either completely in the subarachnoid space, or partially subarachnoid and partially in the epidural space, or wholly in the epidural space with a rent in the dura after a known or unknown dural tap. This can result in a more extensive block than expected and a potentially fatal total spinal block can occur with the first dose, or even more dangerously with a subsequent top-up dose.[121] This is one reason why a person capable of cardiopulmonary resuscitation of the pregnant woman must always be available when epidurals are in use. Epdiural catheters can also be placed in the subdural space and the result of a local anesthetic injection here would be an extensive but patchy block.[122]

Headache

Postdural tap headache results from loss of cerebrospinal fluid and dragging on the pain-sensitive structures in the brain. The characteristics of dural tap headaches are posture-related pain in the occipital or frontal areas, pain and stiffness in the neck, photophobia, nausea and vomiting; one or all of these symptoms may be present. Symptoms improve on lying flat but return within a short time on standing or sitting. There have been numerous case reports of intracranial subdural hematoma following dural puncture with an epidural or subarachnoid needle.[123–125] Symptomatic treatment is achieved by maintaining the supine position. An epidural blood patch of 10–20 ml of the patient's blood usually cures the problem. The sooner this is done after the puncture, the more likely it is to fail and one must speculate that this may be the dilutional effect of the cerebrospinal fluid on the blood injected. A second patch may be required in some patients.

Neurological sequelae

Direct damage to nerve roots with the epidural or spinal needle is unlikely to occur as the awake patient is unable to tolerate the severe pain that even touching the nerve roots causes. Bromage has reviewed the cases in which permanent damage has been reported.[126] He draws attention to the fact that the unprotected cord and nerve roots in the subarachnoid space are more sensitive to damage by chemical contaminants, than they are in the epidural space. Cases that he reports to uphold this view are damage following the injection of benzyl alcohol,[127] detergent[128] and chloroprocaine[129–131] into the subarachnoid space.

Cases have been reported of accidental thiopentone and potassium chloride injection in the epidural space with no long-term consequences, but there are reports of devastating sequelae as a result of possible contaminants[132] in the injected fluid.

Neurological lesions related to obstetric events are frequently attributed to epidural or spinal anesthesia. The most common of these is compression of the lumbosacral trunk by the fetal head as it passes through the pelvis, or trauma to the femoral nerve or lateral cutaneous nerve of the thigh due to the parturient being in lithotomy stirrups for a prolonged period. These injuries usually recover in 12–16 weeks. They are characterized by mixed motor and sensory loss, in particular foot drop and loss of sensation over the outer thigh, calf and foot.

Other neurological complications may result from diabetes, porphyria, multiple sclerosis and AIDS; epidurals are often seen as the obvious culprit, mostly without any possible justification.

Toxicity of local anesthetics

The main toxic reactions to local anesthetic drugs involve the central nervous and the cardiovascular systems. These reactions usually follow accidental intravascular injection, or use of excessive doses. Signs and symptoms of central nervous system (CNS) toxicity include light-headedness, numbness of the tongue, visual disturbances, unconsciousness and convulsions. Bupivacaine is toxic at lower plasma concentrations than lignocaine[133] and its toxicity is increased in pregnancy.[134] The slower the rate of intravenous injection of the local anesthetic, the higher the plasma levels that can be tolerated before CNS toxicity occurs.[135]

Cardiac toxicity of local anesthetics is particularly important given the case reports of cardiac arrest following administration of bupivacaine.[136] Lignocaine increases the conduction time of electrical impulses in the heart and high doses will depress spontaneous pacemaker activity with resulting sinus bradycardia and sinus arrest.[137] Bupivacaine, however, causes ventricular arrhythmias not observed with lignocaine.[138,139] Lignocaine/bupivacaine mixtures may be protective to the heart by delaying or suppressing cardiac arrhythmias.[140]

Space-occupying lesions

Hematoma formation in the epidural space with consequent cord compression and permanent neurological damage can occur from accidental venous puncture in anticoagulated patients.[141–143] Perhaps, more surprisingly, it can also occur spontaneously.[144] Nonetheless, large series of epidural anesthetics performed on anticoagulated patients have been reported in whom no ill-effects were observed.[145,146]

Low-dose heparin prophylaxis is no longer considered a contraindication to regional block, but anticoagulation screening should be performed before inserting the epidural catheter, to exclude inadvertent excessive anticoagulation.[147] There should be no change in a clotting screen,[148] as low-dose heparin prevents spontaneous thrombus formation but not clot formation in response to injury; any change is a contraindication to proceeding with the epidural. Aspirin has been implicated as a speculative cause of epidural hematoma,[149] but doubt has been cast on this idea.[150] The bleeding time has been discredited as a test of clotting competence with aspirin.[151]

Patients with disseminated intravascular coagulopathy are not considered suitable for regional anesthesia in many units if they have a prolonged clotting time and a platelet count of below 100×10^9 l. However, patients with idiopathic thrombocytopenia and normal clotting are not regarded as having a contraindication to regional anesthesia.

Whenever patients are considered at possible risk of epidural hematoma, it is mandatory to maintain a close review of their neurological state after the local anesthetic block has recovered. The signs and symptoms of epidural hematoma are severe and include persistent backache, headache, neck stiffness and local tenderness. Subsequent neurological signs of bilateral numbness or weakness with decreased reflexes demand instant diagnostic imaging and decompression of the cord if necessary.

An epidural abscess can form after epidural injection,[152,153] although they can also occur spontaneously. Its symptoms are similar to those described for epidural hematoma, except that the patient is usually also systemically unwell and usually has a fever.

MANAGEMENT OPTIONS FOR ANESTHESIA FOR CESAREAN SECTION

Advantages of Neural Blockade

Epidural and spinal anesthesia has become the method of choice for both elective and emergency cesarean section. Anesthesia for cesarean section at Queen Charlotte's Hospital is detailed in **Table 1**. The reasons for the decline in popularity of general anesthesia for the obstetric patient are the maternal fetal and neonatal disadvantages that are inherent in the technique. The maternal disadvantages include the risk of failed intubation, which may be followed by aspiration of stomach contents, the lack of maternal awareness of the birth itself, and the effects of the anesthetic agents on the fetus and neonate, particularly in relation to the establishment of spontaneous ventilation in the newborn. The maternal advantages of regional anesthesia for cesarean section are the virtual elimination of the two major causes of anesthetic maternal death, failed endotracheal intubation and aspiration of gastric contents. In addition, maternal postoperative morbidity is decreased;[154,155] in particular, blood loss is almost half that in cases where general anesthesia is used.[156] It is possible that the decline in postoperative deep vein thrombosis seen in orthopedic patients[157] will also occur in obstetric cases. There has been only one case report of fatal pulmonary embolism following epidural cesarean section.[158] The psychological advantages for the mother include increased involvement in the birth process[159,160] and the improvement in maternal–infant

bonding which occurs when the mother is conscious during childbirth.[161,162]

The fetal and neonatal advantages result from improved placental perfusion[163,164] and better fetal perfusion of its own tissues,[165,166] greater sympathoadrenal activity in the neonate[167] and less central nervous depression.[168,169] These advantages are reflected in the improved condition of the neonate following cesarean section for fetal distress using regional blockade for maternal anesthesia as compared to general anesthesia,[170,171] and the improved condition of growth-deficient neonates.[67] Even in urgent cases, when there is already a working epidural *in situ*, it is usually possible to top-up the anesthesia to be suitable for cesarean section by the time the surgeons are ready to start. In less urgent cases, an experienced anesthetist will be able to institute a block within 15–20 min, or even quicker if a spinal anesthetic is used. The combined approach of spinal plus epidural is increasingly finding favor due to a combination of speed of onset, density of block, and ability for topping up for procedures which are longer than planned, or for postoperative pain relief. On rare occasions, however, it may be necessary to use the speed of general anesthesia (for example, if there is severe pain and shock, together with acute fetal hypoxia, from sudden rupture of a uterine scar). In such cases, it may be inappropriate for the woman to be awake. In emergency cases, it is particularly important that the anesthetist is experienced with epidural anesthesia, in order to avoid complications (particularly hypotension, which may compromise maternal and/or fetal condition) or treat those that arise and have the knowledge and ability to assess the extent and density of the anesthetic block before surgery commences.

Indications for General Anesthesia in Obstetric Practice

General anesthesia retains a role in obstetrics, albeit a small one. In elective cesarean section, the mother's wish to be unconscious for the delivery should be respected unless there is a specific contraindication to general anesthesia. Known or suspected placenta accreta or percreta is considered in many units a relative indication for general anesthesia, as these patients require invasive cardiac monitoring and preparation for replacement of massive blood loss. Emergency cesarean sections may require general anesthesia when severe antepartum hemorrhage has occured and/or where coagulopathy and disseminated intravascular coagulopathy are known or suspected. Sudden unexpected severe fetal bradycardia may be a relative indication for general anesthesia, but this is a rare event occuring in less than 1% of a reported obstetric population and 10% of emergency cesarean sections.[172] Severe pre-

Table 1
Anesthesia for cesarean section at Queen Charlotte's Hospital, 1991

Epidural	Elective		Emergency	
	n	%	*n*	%
Block inserted for CS	51	17.8	23	
Block *in situ* for labor extended for CS	—		242	74.4
Spinal				
Single dose combined spinal/epidural	219	76.8	12 56	16.2
General anesthesia	15	5.2	28	
Epidural + GA	—		5	9.2
Total	285		356	
Overall conduction anesthesia (%)		95.0		91.0

CS, Cesarean section.

eclampsia and eclampsia with coagulopathy and a seriously ill mother requires general anesthesia with invasive cardiovascular monitoring. Certain congenital heart conditions may require intensive monitoring and general anesthesia. Patients with cardiac disease considered suitable for conduction anesthesia should have epidural rather than spinal anesthesia, and the epidural block should be of a slow onset and extension so that hemodynamic changes can be compensated for.

All sick women require intensive monitoring during and after anesthesia. General anesthesia for manual removal of the placenta is usually unnecessary. It is sometimes suggested that high doses of a volatile anesthetic agent such as halothane are necessary so as to cause uterine relaxation and aid the obstetrician in his exploration of the uterus. However, other means of causing uterine relaxation, such as intravenous salbutamol, are more effective than agents such as halothane, and are shorter acting, so limiting postpartum hemorrhage. Severe hemorrhage and any suggestion of a coagulopathy are, however, once again contraindications to epidural anesthesia.

ANESTHETIC MATERNAL MORTALITY

From 1967 to 1987, the reports on confidential enquiries into maternal deaths in England and Wales[48,173] discuss 195 direct anesthetic deaths and a further 40 deaths where anesthesia was indirectly the cause. Only 10 of these deaths occurred as a result of regional anesthesia. Two of these women had general anesthesia as well and one excessive sedation; these three died from complications related to these additional agents. Three further mothers died of inadvertent total spinal blocks, another two from an asthmatic response to dextran and ergometrine, and two

from the cardiovascular consequences of regional block.

Anesthesia was among the top three causes of maternal death between 1967 and 1984.[48,173] However, it has now fallen to being the sixth most common cause. **Table 2** shows the numbers of women who died from direct and indirect anesthetic causes as well as the precentage of these women who had general anesthesia, those who were in labor at the time and the percentage who died of failed intubation or gastric aspiration.

Deaths from aspiration of gastric contents can be reduced by preparing the gastric contents to lessen the danger. This involves preoperative doses of ranitidine to reduce acid secretion and volume of contents, metoclopramide to increase gastric emptying, the avoidance of pethidine or other opiates that delay gastric emptying, and the administration of sodium citrate before induction of anesthesia. The avoidance whenever possible of general anesthesia, especially during labor by early epidural blockade in women at risk, is also an important prophylactic measure. When general anesthetic is necessary, rapid sequence induction with cricoid presure applied by a skilled assistant is essential, especially in the laboring woman. A planned sequence of action for failed intubation is necessary as this is reported to occur in 1:300 cases.[174]

The avoidance of anesthetic death from regional block makes it imperative that equipment and the ability to resuscitate the mother is always available and no epidural anesthetic should be embarked upon or continued without immediate access to anesthetic facilities.

Midwives should be aware of all the possible complications of epidural anesthesia and be encouraged to call the anesthetist for any untoward event, preferably before anoxic cardiac arrest has occurred. The anesthetist retains responsibility for the patient during the entire

Table 2
Anesthetic maternal deaths 1967–87[a]

	Direct + indirect deaths (n)	Deaths in labor (%)	Deaths from aspiration and failed intubation (%)	Deaths having general anesthesia
1967–69	50	70	70	100
1970–72	37	68	52	97
1973–75	31 + 6	62	65	94
1976–78	30 + 10	67	77	87
1979–81	22 + 7	78	73	96
1982–84	19 + 1	58	79	100
1985–87	6 + 16	84	84	84

Data from Department of Health.[46,173]

MATERNAL ANESTHESIA AND ANALGESIA IN LABOR
Summary of Management Options

Pain relief in labor

General

- Flexibility and choice are important

Non-pharmacological methods

- Education, preparation classes, etc.

- Psychoprophylaxis

- TENS

Entonox®

- Rapid effect

- Limited to use in late labor

Systemic analgesics

- (timing and dosage vary; units are encouraged to have written guidelines)

- Pethidine (50–150 mg)

- Pentazocine (45–60 mg)

- Meptazinol (75–100 mg)
  NOTE: Beware respiratory depression in mother and/or neonate; naloxone should be available

Regional (epidural)

- Anesthetic and trained support staff should be available constantly

- Preferred method with:
  - vaginal breech delivery
  - multiple pregnancy
  - preterm/low-birthweight baby
  - hypertension/pre-eclampsia
  - many medical problems (see below for exceptions)
  - prolonged labor

- Contraindications:
  - maternal wishes
  - clotting disorder
  - certain cardiac problems:
    — aortic stenosis
    — pulmonary hypertension
    — right-to-left shunt

Anesthesia for cesarean section

- Neural blockade probably the preferred method for most

- General anesthesia indicated with:
  - maternal wishes
  - speed
  - clotting abnormality
  - certain medical contraindications to regional block (see above)

---

duration of epidural analgesia and must not abandon the patient solely to the care of the midwife.

There is rarely any justification for neglecting the preoperative assessment of the obstetric patient on the spurious grounds of emergency. The anesthetist should be called to assess the patient when there is 'anything more than just a possibility of abdominal delivery'.[48] There is no longer any defence for the flying squad approach to anesthesia for obstetric patients; rather, anesthetists – even those with other hospital duties – must be involved in treating high-risk cases on the labor ward as one would in a high dependency unit.

There is little if any need for an anesthetist to be involved with normal women in normal labor with normal infants, as the presence of a sympathetic midwife is more important than analgesia.[175]

CONCLUSIONS

- Opiates have doubtful value as analgesics in labor; their action is more probably via sedation. They are becoming less popular. Their most serious complication is gastric aspiration in the mother and respiratory depression of the newborn.

- Pain in labor has an important psychological component, and is therefore susceptible to amelioration by a variety of psychological methods.

- Epidural anesthesia is indicated for pain relief in labor at maternal request; it is particularly indicated in prolonged labor, twin delivery and possibly breech delivery.

- Epidural anesthesia probably prolongs the second stage of labor and doubles the instrumental delivery rate by obtunding the Ferguson reflex.

- There are few fetal or maternal contraindications for epidural anesthesia; the main contraindications are coagulopathy, severe hemorrhage and the need for extreme speed.

- Hypotension is an important complication of epidural anesthesia; it can be minimized by using low concentrations of local anesthetic, avoiding the supine position, and preloading the circulation with crystalloid fluids.

REFERENCES

1 Melzack R (1975) The McGill pain questionnaire: Major properties and scoring methods. *Pain* 1:277–299.

2 Hardy JD, Javert CT (1949) Studies on pain: Measurements of pain intensity in childbirth. *Journal of Clinical Investigation* 28:153–162.

3 Bundsen P, Peterson L, Selstam U (1982) Pain relief during delivery. *Acta Obstetrica et Gynecologica Scandinavica* 61:289–297.

4 Melzack R (1984) The myth of painless childbirth. *Pain* 19:321–337.

5 Senden IPM, Wetering MD, Eskes AB, Bierkens PB, Laube DW, Pitkin RM (1988) Labor pain: A comparison of parturients in a Dutch and an American Teaching Hospital. *Obstetrics and Gynecology* 71:541–543.

6 Melzack R, Wall PD (1965) Pain mechanism: A new theory. *Science* 150:971–979.

7 Dundee JW (1960) Alterations in response to somatic pain associated with anaesthesia: II. The effect of Thiopentone and Pentobarbitone. *British Journal of Anaesthesia* 32:407–414.

8 Kitzinger S (1980) *The Complete Book of Pregnancy and Birth*. New York: A.A. Knopf.

9 Humenick JS (1981) Mastery: The key to childbirth satisfaction. A review. *Birth* 6:79–83.

10 Augustinsson L, Bohlin P, Bundsen P, Carlson CA, Forssman L, Sjoberg P, Tyremen NO (1977) Pain relief during delivery by transcutaneous electrical nerve stimulation. *Pain* 4:59–65.

11 Harrison RF, Woods T, Shaw M, Mathews G, Unwin A (1986) Pain relief in labour using transcutaneous electrical nerve stimulation (TENS): A TENS placebo controlled study, in two parity groups. *British Journal of Obstetrics and Gynaecology* 93:739–746.

12 Nesheim BI (1981) The use of transcutaneous nerve stimulation for pain relief during labour. *Acta Obstetrica et Gynecologica Scandinavica* 60:13–16.

13 Miller Jones CMH (1980) Transcutaneous nerve stimulation in labour. *Anaesthesia* 35:372–375.

14 Harrison RF, Shore M, Woods T, Matthews G, Gardiner J, Unwin A (1987) A comparative study of transcutaneous electrical nerve stimulation (TENS) entonox, pethidine and promazine and lumbar epidural for pain relief in labor. *Acta Obstetrica et Gynecologica Scandinavica* 66:9–14.

15 Holdcroft A, Morgan M (1974) An assessment of the analgesic effect in labour of pethidine and 50% nitrous oxide in oxygen (Entonox). *Journal of Obstetrics and Gynaecology of the British Commonwealth* 81:603–607.

16 Stefani SJ, Hughes SC, Shnider SM *et al.* (1982) Neonatal neurobehavioral effects of inhalation analgesia for vaginal delivery. *Anesthesiology* 56:351–355.

17 Arthurs GJ, Rosen M (1981) Acceptability of continuous nasal nitrous oxide during labour – a field trial of six maternity hospitals. *Anaesthesia* 36:384–388.

18 Rosen M, Mushin WW, Jones PL *et al.* (1969) Field trial of methoxyflurane, nitrous oxide and trichlorethylene as obstetric analgesic. *British Medical Journal* 3:263–267.

19 Dickersin K (1989) Pharmacological control of pain during labour. In Chalmers I, Enkin M, Keirse MJNC (eds), *Effective Care in Pregnancy and Childbirth, Vol. 2: Childbirth*, pp. 917–920. Oxford: Oxford University Press.

20 De Kornfield TJ, Pearson JW, Lasagna L (1964) Methotrimeprazine in the treatment of labour pain. *New England Journal of Medicine* 270:391–394.

21 Cullhed S, Lofstrom B (1961) Obstetric analgesia with pethidine and scopolamine. *Lancet* 1:75–77.

22 Duncan SB, Ginsburg J, Morris NF (1965) Comparison of pentazocine and pethidine in normal labor. *American Journal of Obstetrics and Gynecology* 105:197–202.

23 Nicholas ADG, Robson PJ (1982) Double-blind comparison of meptazinol and pethidine in labour. *British Journal of Obstetrics and Gynaecology* 89:318–322.

24 Osler M (1987) A double-blind study comparing meptazinol and pethidine for pain relief in labour. *European Journal of Obstetrics and Gynecology and Reproductive Biology* 26:15–18.

25 Jensen F, Quist I, Brock V, Secher V, Westergaard LG (1984) Submucous paracervical blockade compared with intramuscular meperidine as analgesia during labor: A double blind study. *Obstetrics and Gynecology* **64**:724–727.

26 Grant AM, Holt EM, Noble AD (1970) A comparison between pethidine and phenazocine for relief of pain in labour. *Journal of Obstetrics and Gynaecology of the British Commonwealth* **77**:824–829.

27 Moore J, Carson RM, Hunter RJ (1970) A comparison of the effects of pentazocine and pethidine administered during labour. *Journal of Obstetrics and Gynaecology of the British Commonwealth* **77**:860–863.

28 Jackson MBA, Robson PJ (1980) Preliminary experience of the use of meptazinol as obstetric analgesic. *British Journal of Obstetrics and Gynaecology* **87**:296–301.

29 Robinson JO, Rosen M, Evans JM, Revill SI, David H, Rees GAD (1980) Maternal opinion about analgesia in labour: A controlled trial between epidural block and intramuscular pethidine combined with inhalation. *Anaesthesia* **35**:1173–1181.

30 Robinson JO, Rosen M, Evan JM, Revill SI, David H, Reese GAD (1980) Self administered intravenous and intramuscular pethidine. *Anaesthesia* **35**:763–770.

31 Deckhart R, Fembacher P), Scheider K, Graeff H (1987) Maternal arterial oxygen saturation during labor and delivery. *Obstetrics and Gynecology* **70**:21–25.

32 Philipsen T, Jensen NH (1989) Epidural block or parental pethidine as analgesia in labour: A randomized study concerning progress in labour and instrumental deliveries. *European Journal of Obstetrics and Gynecology and Reproductive Biology* **30**:27–33.

33 Philipsen T, Jensen NH (1990) Maternal opinion about analgesia in labour and delivery: A comparison of epidural blockade and intramuscular pethidine. *European Journal of Obstetrics and Gynecology and Reproductive Biology* **34**:205–210.

34 Moore J, Ball HB (1974) A sequential study of IV analgesic treatment during labour. *British Journal of Anaesthesia* **46**:365–372.

35 Girvan CB, Moore J, Dundee JW (1976) Pethidine compared with pethidine–nalaxone administered during labour. *British Journal of Anaesthesia* **48**:563–569.

36 Rayburn W, Smith CV, Parriott JE, Woods RE (1989) Randomised comparison of meperidine and fentanyl during labor. *Obstetrics and Gynecology* **74**:604–606.

37 McQuitty FM (1967) Relief of pain in labour: A controlled double-blind trial comparing pethidine and various phenothiazine derivatives. *Journal of Obstetrics and Gynaecology of the British Commonwealth* **74**:925–928.

38 Levy DL (1971) Obstetric analgesia: pentazocine and meperidine in normal primiparous labor. *Obstetrics and Gynecology* **38**:907–911.

39 Harper NJN, Thompson J, Brayshaw SA (1983) Experience with self-administered pethidine with special reference to the general practitioner's obstetric unit. *Anaesthesia* **38**:52–55.

40 Rayburn W, Leuschen P, Earl R, Woods M, Lorkovic M, Gaston-Johansson F (1989) Intravenous meperidine during labor: A randomised comparison between nurs-

ing and patient controlled administration. *Obstetrics and Gynecology* **74**:702–706.

41 Frank M, McAteer EJ, Cattermole R, Loughnan B, Stafford LB, Hitchcock AM (1987) Nalbuphine for obstetric analgesia: A comparison of nalbuphine with pethidine administered by patient controlled analgesia. *Anaesthesia* **42**:697–703.

42 Li DFH, Rees GAD, Rosen M (1988) Feasibility of self-administration analgesia by intramuscular route in labour. *European Journal of Obstetrics and Gynecology and Reproductive Biology* **27**:99–104.

43 Scott JS (1970) Obstetric analgesia. *American Journal of Obstetrics and Gynecology* **106**:959–978.

44 Lind JF, Smith AM, McIver DK, Coopland AT, Crispin JS (1968) Heartburn in pregnancy – a manometric study. *Canadian Medical Association Journal* **98**:571–574.

45 Cotton BR, Smith G (1984) The lower oesophageal sphincter and anaesthesia. *British Journal of Anaesthesia* **56**:37–45.

46 Nimmo WS, Wilson J, Prescott LF (1975) Narcotic analgesics and delayed gastric emptying during labour. *Lancet* **i**:890–893.

47 Department of Health (1989) *Report on Confidential Enquiries into Maternal Deaths in England and Wales 1982–84*. London: HMSO.

48 Department of Health (1991) *Report on Confidential Enquiries into Maternal Deaths in the United Kingdom 1985–87*. London: HMSO.

49 Huch A, Huch R (1974) Maternal hypoxaemia after pethidine. *Journal of Obstetrics and Gynaecology of the British Commonwealth* **81**:608–614.

50 Rosen MG, Scibetta JJ, Hochberg CJ (1970) Human fetal electroencephalogram. III. Pattern changes in presence of fetal heart rate alterations and after use of maternal medications. *Obstetrics and Gynecology* **36**:132–140.

51 Jenkins VRII, Dilts PV Jr (1971) Some effects of meperidine hydrochloride on maternal and fetal sheep. *American Journal of Obstetrics and Gynecology* **109**:1005–1010.

52 Shnider SM, Moya F (1984) Effects of meperidine on the newborn infant. *American Journal of Obstetrics and Gynecology* **89**:1009–1015.

53 Koch G, Wandel H (1968) Effect of pethidine on the postnatal adjustment of respiration and acid–base balance. *Acta Obstetrica et Gynecologica Scandinavica* **47**:27–37.

54 Kuhnert BR, Linn PL, Kuhnert PM (1985) Obstetric medication and neonatal behaviour: Symposium on developmental and behavioural issues in perinatology. *Clinics in Perinatology* **12**:423–440.

55 Kiuhnert BR, Liun PL, Kennard MJ, Kuhnert PM (1985) Effects of low doses of meperidine on neonatal behavior. *Anesthesia and Analgesia* **64**:335–342.

56 Lester BM, Als H, Brazelton TB (1982) Regional obstetric anesthesia and newborn behavior. *Child Development* **53**:687–692.

57 Scanlon JW (1981) Effects of obstetric anesthesia and analgesia on the newborn: A select annotated bibliography for the clinician. *Clinics in Obstetrics and Gynecology* **24**:649–670.

58 Amiel-Tison C, Barrier G, Shnider SM *et al.* (1988) A new neurologic and adaptive capacity scoring system for evaluating obstetric medication in full-term newborns. *Anesthesiology* **56**:340–350.

59 Dailey PA, Baysinger CL, Levinson G *et al* (1982) Neurobehavioral testing of the newborn infant: Effects of obstetric anesthesia. *Clinics in Perinatology* **9**:191–214.

60 Hodgkinson R, Husain FJ (1982) The duration of effect of maternally administered meperidine on neonatal neurobehavior. *Anesthesiology* **56**:51–52.

61 Belsey EM, Rosenblatt DB, Lieberman BA *et al.* (1981) The influence of maternal analgesia on neonatal behavior. I. Pethidine. *British Journal of Obstetrics and Gynaecology* **88**:398–406.

62 Sinclair JC, Fox HA, Leatz JF (1965) Intoxication of the fetus by a local anaesthetic: A newly recognised complication of maternal caudal anesthesia. *New England Journal of Medicine* **273**:1173–1177.

63 Bromage PR (1978) *Epidural Analgesia.* Philadelphia, PA: W.B. Saunders.

64 Crawford JS (1974) An appraisal of lumbar epidural blockade in patients with singleton fetus presenting by the breech. *Journal of Obstetrics and Gynaecology of the British Commonwealth* **81**:867–872.

65 Crawford JS (1987) A prospective study of 200 consecutive twin deliveries. *Anaesthesia* **31**:1054–1059.

66 Jarvis GJ, Whitfield HF (1981) Epidural analgesia and the delivery of twins. *Journal of Obstetrics and Gynaecology* **2**:90–92.

67 David H, Rosen M (1976) Perinatal mortality after epidural analgesia. *Anaesthesia* **31**:1054–1059.

68 Abboud T, Artal R, Sarkis F, Henriksen EH, Kammula RK (1982) Sympathoadrenal activity, maternal, fetal and neonatal responses after epidural anesthesia in the preeclamptic patient. *American Journal of Obstetrics and Gynecology* **144**:915–918.

69 Hodgkinson R, Husain FJ, Hayashi RH (1980) Systemic and pulmonary blood pressure during caesarean section in parturients with gestational hypertension. *Canadian Anaesthestists' Society Journal* **27**:389–394.

70 Joupilla P, Joupilla R, Hollmen A, Korvula A (1982) Lumbar epidural analgesia to improve intervillous blood flow during labor in severe preeclampsia. *Obstetrics and Gynecology* **59**:158–161.

71 Leduc L, Wheeler JM, Kirshon B, Mitchell P, Cotton DB (1992) Coagulation profile in severe pre-eclampsia. *Obstetrics and Gynecology* **79**:14–18.

72 Husemeyer RP, O'Connor MC, Davenport HT (1980) Failure of epidural morphine to relieve pain in labour. *Anaesthesia* **35**:161–163.

73 Husemeyer RP, Davenport HT, Cummings AJ, Rosankiewicz JR (1981) Comparison of epidural and intramuscular pethidine for analgesia in labour. *British Journal of Obstetrics and Gynaecology* **88**:711–717.

74 Kaminski HM, Stafl A, Aiman J (1987) The effect of epidural analgesia on the frequency of instrumental obstetric delivery. *Obstetrics and Gynecology* **69**:770–773.

75 Skjoldebrand A, Garle M, Gustafsson LL, Johansson H, Lunell NO, Rane A (1982) Extradural pethidine with and without adrenaline during labour: A wide variation in effect. *British Journal of Anaesthesia* **54**:415–420.

76 Ralston DH, Shnider SM, de Lorimier AA (1974) Effects of equipotent ephedrine, metaraminol, mephentermine and methoxamine on uterine blood flow in the pregnant ewe. *Anesthesiology* **40**:354–370.

77 Kerr MG, Scott DB, Samuel E (1964) Studies of the inferior vena cava in late pregnancy. *British Medical Journal* **1**:532–533.

78 Antoine C, Young BK (1982) Fetal lactic acidosis with epidural anesthesia. *American Journal of Obstetrics and Gynecology* **142**:55–59.

79 Brizgys RV, Dailey PA, Shnider SM, Kotelko DM, Levinson G (1987) The incidence and neonatal effects of maternal hypotension during epidural anesthesia for cesarean section. *Anesthesiology* **67**:782–786.

80 Thalme B, Belfrage P, Roabe U (1974) Lumbar epidural analgesia in labour. 1. Acid–base balance and clinical condition of mother, fetus and newborn child. *Acta Obstetrica et Gynecologica Scandinavica* **53**:27–53.

81 Pearson JF, Davies P (1974) The effect of continuous lumbar epidural analgesia upon fetal aid–base status during the first stage of labour. *British Journal of Obstetrics and Gynaecology* **81**:971–974.

82 Studd JWW, Crawford JS, Duignan NM *et al.* (1980) The effect of lumbar epidural analgesia on the rate of cervical dilatation and the outcome of labour of spontaneous onset. *British Journal of Obstetrics and Gynaecology* **87**:1015–1021.

83 Bailey PW, Howard FA (1983) Epidural analgesia and forceps delivery: Laying a bogey. *Anaesthesia* **35**:282–285.

84 Potter N, MacDonald RD (1971) Obstetric consequences of epidural analgesia in nulliparous patients. *Lancet* **1**:1031–1034.

85 Matouskova A, Dottori O, Forssman L, Victorin L (1979) An improved method of epidural analgesia with reduced instrumental delivery rate. *Acta Obstetrica et Gynecologica Scandinavica* **83**:9–13.

86 Maltau JM, Andersen HT (1975) Continuous epidural anaesthesia with a low frequency of instrumental deliveries. *Acta Obstetrica et Gynecologica Scandinavica* **54**:401–406.

87 Crawford JS (1972) The second thousand epidural blocks in an obstetric hospital practice. *British Journal of Anaesthesia* **44**:1277–1287.

88 Hoult IJ, MacLennon AH, Carrie LES (1977) Lumbar epidural analgesia in labour: Relation to fetal malposition and instrumental delivery. *British Medical Journal* **1**:14–16.

89 Studd JWW, Crawford JS, Duignan NW, Rowbotham CJF, Hughes AO (1980) The effect of lumbar epidural analgesia on the rate of cervical dilatation and the outcome of labour of spontaneous onset. *British Journal of Obstetrics and Gynaecology* **87**:1015–1021.

90 Chestnut DH, Vanderwalker GE, Owen CZ, Bates JM, Choi WW (1987) The influence of continuous epidural bupivacaine analgesia on the second stage of labor and method of delivery in nulliparous women. *Anesthesiology* **66**:774–780.

91 Chestnut DH, Bates JN, Choi WW (1987) Continuous infusion epidural analgesia with lidocaine: Efficacy

and influence during the second stage of labour. *Obstetrics and Gynecology* **69**:323–327.

92 Chestnut DH, Laszewski LJ, Pollack KL, Bates JN, Manago NK, Choi WW (1990) Continuous epidural infusion of 0.0625% bupivacaine and 0.0002% fentanyl during the second stage of labor. *Anesthesiology* **72**:613–618.

93 Phillips KC, Thomas TA (1982) Second stage of labour with or without extradural analgesia. *Anaesthesia* **38**:972–976.

94 Thorburn J, Moir DD (1981) Extradural analgesia: The concentration of bupivacaine on the mode of delivery, analgesia efficacy and motor blockade. *British Journal of Anaesthesia* **53**:933–939.

95 Chestnut DH, Owen CL, Bates JN *et al.* (1988) Continuous infusion epidural analgesia during labor: A randomized double blind comparison of 0.0625% bupivacaine/0.0002% fentanyl versus 0.125% bupivacaine. *Anesthesiology* **68**:754–759.

96 Vertommen JD, Vandermeulen E, Van Aken H *et al.* (1991) The effects of the addition of sufentanil to 0.125% bupivacaine on the quality of analgesia during labor and on the incidence of instrumental deliveries. *Anesthesiology* **74**:809–814.

97 McQueen J, Mylrea L (1977) Lumbar epidural analgesia in labour. *British Medical Journal* **i**:640–641.

98 Maresh M, Choong KH, Beard RW (1983) Delayed pushing with lumbar epidural analgesia in labour. *British Journal of Obstetrics and Gynaecology* **90**:623–627.

99 Snooks SJ, Swash M, Setchell M, Henry MM (1984) Injury to innervation of pelvic floor musculature in childbirth. *Lancet* **i**:546–550.

100 Allen RE, Hosker GL, Smith ARB, Warrell DW (1990) Pelvic floor damage and childbirth: A neurophysiological study. *British Journal of Obstetrics and Gynaecology* **97**:770–779.

101 Saunders NJ, Spiby H, Gilbert L *et al.* (1989) Oxytocin infusion during second stage of labour in primiparous women using epidural analgesia: A randomised double blind placebo controlled trial. *British Medical Journal* **299**:1423–1426.

102 Bates RG, Helm CW, Duncan A, Edmonds DK (1985) Uterine activity in the second stage of labour and the effect of epidural analgesia. *British Journal of Obstetrics and Gynaecology* **92**:1246–1250.

103 Goodfellow CF, Hull MGR, Swaab DK *et al.* (1983) Oxytocin deficiency at delivery with epidural analgesia. *British Journal of Obstetrics and Gynaecology* **90**:214–219.

104 Goodfellow CF, Studd C (1979) The reduction of forceps in primigravidae with epidural analgesia: A controlled trial. *British Journal of Clinical Practice* **33**:287–288.

105 Turner MJ, Silk JM, Alagesan K, Egan DM, Gordon H (1986) Epidural bupivacaine concentration and forceps delivery in primiparae. *British Journal of Obstetrics and Gynaecology* **9**:122–125.

106 Schifin BS (1972) Fetal heart rate patterns following epidural anaesthesia and oxytocin infusion during labour. *Journal of Obstetrics and Gynaecology of the British Commonwealth* **79**:332–334.

107 Huch A, Huch R (1976) Transcutaneous noninvasive monitoring of pO$_2$. *Hospital Practice* **11**:43–52.

108 Humphrey MD, Chang A, Wood EC *et al.* (1974) A decrease in fetal pH during the second stage of labour when conducted in the dorsal position. *Journal of Obstetrics and Gynaecology of the British Commonwealth* **81**:600–602.

109 Shnider SM, de Lorimier AA, Hall JW *et al* (1986) Vasopressors in obstetrics. 1. Correction of fetal acidosis with ephedrine during spinal hypotension. *American Journal of Obstetrics and Gynecology* **102**:911–919.

110 Hollmen A, Joupilla R, Joupilla P *et al.* (1982) Effect of extradural analgesia using bupivacaine and 2-chloroprocaine on intervillous blood flow during normal labour. *British Journal of Anaesthesia* **54**:837–842.

111 Joupilla P, Joupilla R, Hollmen *et al.* (1982) Lumbar epidural analgesia to improve intervillous blood flow during labor in severe pre-eclampsia. *Obstetrics and Gynecology* **59**:158–161.

112 Datta S, Alper MH, Ostheimer GW (1982) Method of ephedrine administration and nausea and hypotension during spinal anesthesia for cesarean section. *Anesthesiology* **56**:68–70.

113 Abboud TK, Khoo SS, Miller F *et al* (1982) Maternal, fetal and neonatal responses after epidural anesthesia with bupivacaine, 2-chloroprocaine or lidocaine. *Anesthesia and Analgesia* **61**:638–641.

114 Abboud TK, Sarkis F, Blikian *et al.* (1983) Lack of adverse neonatal neuro-behavioural effects of lidocaine. *Anesthesia and Analgesia* **62**:473–475.

115 Abboud TK, Kim KC, Noueihed R *et al* (1983) Epidural bupivacaine, chloroprocaine or lidocaine for cesarean section – maternal and neonatal effects. *Anesthesia and Analgesia* **62**:L914–919.

116 Kileff ME, James FM, Dewan DM (1984) Neonatal neurobehavioral responses after epidural anesthesia for cesarean section using lidocaine and bupivacaine. *Anesthesia and Analgesia* **63**:413–417.

117 Kuhnert BR, Harrison MJ, Linn PL (1984) Effects of maternal epidural anesthesia on neonatal behavior. *Anesthesia and Analgesia* **63**:301–308.

118 Murray AD, Dolby RM, Nation RL *et al.* (1981) Effects of epidural anesthesia on newborns and their mothers. *Child Development* **52**:71–82.

119 Kuhnert BR, Linn PL, Kuhnert PM (1985) Obstetric medication and neonatal behavior: Current controversies. *Clinics in Perinatology* **12**:423–440.

120 MacArthur C, Lewis M, Knox EG, Crawford JS (1990) Epidural anaesthesia and long term backache after childbirth. *British Medical Journal* **301**:9–12.

121 Morgan BM (1990) Unexpectedly extensive conduction blocks in obstetric epidural analgesia. *Anaesthesia* **45**:148–152.

122 Reynolds F, Speedy HM (1990) The subdural space: The third place to go astray. *Anaesthesia* **45**:120–123.

123 Edelman JD, Wingard DW (1980) Subdural hematomas after lumbar dural puncture. *Anesthesiology* **52**:166–167.

124 Jack TM (1979) Postpartum intracranial subdural hematoma. *Anaesthesia* **34**:176–180.

125 Mantia AM (1981) Clinical report of an intracerebral

hemorrhage following post-lumbar puncture headache. *Anesthesiology* **55**:684–685.

126 Bromage PR (1987) Neurologic complications of regional anesthesia. In Shnider SM, Levinson G (eds), *Anesthesia for Obstetrics*, pp. 321–323. Baltimore, MD: Williams and Wilkins.

127 Craig DB, Habib GG (1977) Flaccid paraparesis following obstetrical epidural anesthesia: Possible role of benzyl alcohol. *Anesthesia and Analgesia* **56**:219–221.

128 Winkelman NW (1952) Symptoms following accidental intraspinal detergent injection. *Neurology* **2**:284–285.

129 Covino BG, Marx GF, Finster M, Zsigmund EK (1980) Prolonged sensory/motor deficits following inadvertent spinal anesthesia. *Anesthesia and Analgesia* **59**:399–400.

130 Usubiaga JE (1975) Neurological complications following epidural analgesia. *International Anesthesiology Clinics* **13**:19–50.

131 Reisner LS, Hockman BN, Plumer MH (1982) Persistant neurologic deficit and adhesive arachnoiditis following intrathecal 2-chloroprocaine injection. *Anesthesia and Analgesia* **59**:452–454.

132 Brahams D (1982) Record award for personal injuries sustained as a result of negligent administration of epidural anaesthetic. *Lancet* **1**:159.

133 Liu PL, Feldman HS, Giasi R, Patterson MK, Covino GH (1983) Comparative CNS toxicity of lidocaine, etidocaine, bupivacaine and tetracaine in awake dogs following rapid IV administration. *Anesthesia and Analgesia* **62**:375–379.

134 Morishima HO, Pedersen H, Finster M *et al.* (1985) Bupivacaine toxicity in pregnant and non-pregnant ewes. *Anesthesiology* **63**:134–139.

135 Scott DB (1975) Evaluation of clinical tolerance of local anesthetic agents. *British Journal of Anaesthesia* **47**:328–331.

136 Albright GA (1979) Cardiac arrest following regional anesthesia with etidocaine or bupivacaine. *Anesthesiology* **51**:285–287.

137 Lieberman NA, Harris RS, Katz RI *et al.* (1968) The effects of lidocaine on the electrical and mechanical activity of the heart. *American Journal of Cardiology* **22**:375–378.

138 de Jong RH, Ronfeld RA, De Rosa RA (1982) Cardiovascular effects of convulsant and supraconvulsant doses of amide local anesthetics. *Anesthesia and Analgesia* **61**:3–9.

139 Kotelko DM, Shnider SM, Dailey PA *et al.* (1984) Bupivacaine induced cardiac arrhythmias in sheep. *Anesthesiology* **60**:10–18.

140 de Jong RH, Bonin JD (1974) Mixtures of local anesthetics are no more toxic than the parent drug. *Anesthesiology* **54**:177–181.

141 Harik SI, Raichle ME, Reis DJ (1971) Spontaneously remitting spinal epidural hematoma in a patient on anticoagulants. *New England Journal of Medicine* **284**:1355–1357.

142 Varkey GP, Bridle GF (1974) Peridural anaesthesia and anticoagulant therpay. *Canadian Anaesthetists' Society Journal* **21**:106–109.

143 De Angelis J (1972) Hazards of subdural and epidural anesthesia during anticoagulant therapy: A case report and review. *Anesthesia and Analgesia* **51**:676–679.

144 Scott DB, Quisling RG, Miller CA (1976) Spinal epidural hematoma. *Journal of the American Medical Association* **235**:513–517.

145 Rao TKL, El-Etr AA (1981) Anticoagulation following placement of epidural and subarachnoid catheters: An evaluation of neurologic sequelae. *Anesthesiology* **55**:618–20.

146 Odoom JA, Sih IL (1983) Epidural analgesia and anticoagulant therapy: Experience with one thousand cases of continuous epidurals. *Anaesthesia* **38**:254–259.

147 Cooke ED (1976) Monitoring during low dose heparin prophylaxis. *New England Journal of Medicine* **264**:1066–1067.

148 Heglund PO, Blomback M (1979) The effect of prophylaxis with low dose heparin on blood coagulation parameters. *Thrombosis and Haemostasis* **41**:337–339.

149 Locke GE, Giorgio AJ, Biggers SL (1976) Acute spinal epidural hematoma secondary to aspirin-induced prolonged bleeding. *Surgical Neurology* **5**:292–294.

150 Benzon HJ, Brunner EA, Vaisrub N (1984) Bleeding time and nerve blocks after aspirin. *Regional Anesthesia* **9**:86–87.

151 Channing Rodgers RP, Levin J (1990) A critical reappraisal of the bleeding time. *Seminar in Thrombosis and Hemostasis* **16**:1–20.

152 Baker AS, Ojemann RG, Swartz MN, Richardson EP (1975) Spinal epidural abscess. *New England Journal of Medicine* **293**:463–466.

153 Ferguson JF, Kirsch WM (1974) Epidural empyema following thoracic extradural block. *Journal of Neurosurgery* **41**:762–764.

154 Morgan BM, Aulakh JM, Baler JP, Reginald PW, Gorosszenuik T, Trojanowski A (1984) Anaesthetic morbidity following caesarean section under epidural or general anaesthesia. *Lancet* **i**:328–330.

155 Kehlet H (1984) Influence of regional anaesthesia on postoperative morbidity. *Annales Chirugiae et Gynaecologica* **73**:171–176.

156 Moir DD (1970) Anaesthesia for caesarean section: An evaluation of a method using low concentrations of halothane and 50% oxygen. *British Journal of Anaesthesia* **42**:136–139.

157 Poikeleninen E, Hendolin H (1983) Effects of lumbar epidural analgesia and general anaesthesia on flow velocity in the femoral vein and postoperative deep vein thrombosis. *Acta Chirurgica Scandinavica* **149**:361–364.

158 McHale SP, Tilak MDV, Robinson PN (1992) Fatal pulmonary embolism following spinal anaesthesia for Caesarean section. *Anaesthesia* **47**:128–130.

159 Hardwick M (1983) Caesarean section under epidural: A personal account. *British Medical Journal* **287**:35–36.

160 Marut J, Mercer R (1979) Comparison of primiparas' perception of vaginal and caesarean births. *Nursing Research* **28**:260–266.

161 McClennan M, Cabiaca W (1980) Effects of early mother–infant contact following caesarean birth. *Obstetrics and Gynecology* **56**:52–55.

162 Trowell J (1982) Possible effects of emergency caesarean section on the mother–child relationship. *Early Human Development* **7**:41–51.

163 Joupilla R, Joupilla P, Kinika J *et al.* (1978) Placental blood flow during caesarean section under lumber extradural analgesia. *British Journal of Anaesthesia* **50**:275–279.

164 Giles WB, Lah FX, Trudinger BJ (1987) The effect of epidural anaesthesia for caesarean section on maternal uterine and fetal umbilical artery blood flow velocity wave forms. *British Journal of Obstetrics and Gynaecology* **94**:55–59.

165 Lindblad A, Bernow J, Marsal K (1987) Obstetric analgesia and fetal aortic blood flow during labour. *British Journal of Obstetrics and Gynaecology* **94**:306–311.

166 Lindblad A, Bernow J, Vernersson E, Marsal K (1987) Effects of extradural anaesthesia on human blood flow *in utero*: Comparison of three local anaesthetic solutions. *British Journal of Anaesthesia* **59**:1265–1272.

167 Irestedt L, Lagtercrantz H, Hjemdahl P, Hagnevik K, Belfrage P (1982) Fetal and maternal plasma catecholamine levels at elective cesarean section under general and epidural anaesthesia versus vaginal delivery. *American Journal of Obstetrics and Gynecology* **142**:1004–1010.

168 Fox GS, Smith GB, Namba Y, Johnson RC (1979) Anesthesia for cesarean section: Further studies. *American Journal of Obstetrics and Gynecology* **133**:15–18.

169 Crawford JS, Davies P (1982) Status of neonates delivered by elective caesarean section. *British Journal of Anaesthesia* **54**:1015–1017.

170 Marx GF, Luyx WM, Cohen S (1984) Fetal–neonatal status following caesarean section for fetal distress. *British Journal of Anaesthesia* **56**:1009–1012.

171 Ramanathan J, Ricca DM, Sibai BM, Angel JJ (1988) Epidural *vs* general anesthesia in fetal distress with various abnormal fetal heart rate patterns. Anesth. Analg. **67**:180 (suppl.).

172 Morgan BM, Magni V, Goroszenuik T (1990) Anaesthesia for emergency caesarean section. *British Journal of Obstetrics and Gynaecology* **97**:420–424.

173 Department of Health (1972, 1975, 1979, 1982, 1986, 1989) *Reports on Confidential Enquiries into Maternal Deaths in England and Wales 1967–69, 1970–72, 1973–75, 1976–78, 1979–81, 1982–84*. London: HMSO.

174 Lyons G (1985) Failed intubation: Six years' experience in a teaching maternity unit. *Anaesthesia* **40**:759–762.

175 Morgan BM, Bulpitt CJ, Clifton P, Lewis PJ (1984) The consumer's attitude to obstetric care. *British Journal of Obstetrics and Gynaecology* **90**:624–628.

64

Maternal Distress in Labor

BARBARA MORGAN

INTRODUCTION

Labor almost always causes at least a degree of maternal distress. This is because childbirth is commonly accompanied by severe pain, physical exhaustion, an awareness in the mother of danger for herself and her baby, and anxiety or even fear about the outcome. Often sleep deprivation, hunger, nausea and the demands of physical and mental exertion combine to cause considerable and at times extreme stress. Diminishing maternal distress in labor requires a broad approach rather than just the administration of drugs. Prenatal preparation, the mother's surroundings in labor, her mental and physical well-being, as well as effective treatment for pain, must be addressed.

Risks

Distress within tolerable limits, in normal labor with a healthy mother and fetus, is not disadvantageous. This is not the case when the distress is great or the mother or fetus are not in optimum condition. It is well known that stress affects pregnancy. High levels of maternal stress have been associated with low birthweight,[1-3] prematurity,[4-5] and other prenatal complications including pre-eclampsia.[6,7] During labor, maternal fear and anxiety have been associated with fetal distress, postpartum hemorrhage, prolonged labor and an increased incidence of interventions such as forceps delivery and manual removal of the placenta.[8-13] On the other hand, reducing maternal distress in labor by the simple expedient of providing her with a sympath-

etic companion has been shown to decrease complications in labor, especially fetal distress and failure to progress.[14-16]

Both mental and physical stress such as occur in labor cause a stimulation of the sympathetic nervous system with release of the neurotransmitters noradrenaline and adrenaline. Together, these catecholamines mediate the increased activity that allows the 'fright, fight or flight' response to stress. Changes required to face the dangers for which this extensive mechanism has evolved are an increase in heart rate, a rise in blood pressure, a shift of blood flow from the splanchnic bed (including the uterus) to the skeletal muscles, a rise in blood glucose, and dilatation of the pupils and bronchioles. Sympathetic stimulation of the beta-2 receptors in the uterus by adrenaline also relaxes the pregnant uterus. This property of beta-2 stimulation is of therapeutic value in premature labor; sympathomimetic drugs such as salbutamol and ritodrine are used to suppress unwanted uterine activity.

The consequence of the sympathetic outpouring of adrenergic transmitters resulting from maternal distress is therefore a decrease in uterine contractility,[17] a decrease in uterine blood flow[18] and an increase in maternal heart rate and blood pressure.[19] Catecholamines administered to the mother have been shown to cause uterine artery vasoconstriction.[18,20,21,22]

In animal studies, maternal stress caused by pain or fear has been shown to result in a reduction in fetal arterial oxygenation,[20,23] which can have a profound effect on the fetus. This is especially prolonged and severe when the fetus is already hypoxic.[24]

The cardiovascular effects of the stress of labor are

particularly important in women with hypertension or cardiac disease. During labor, there is a progressive increase in cardiac output[25] until almost the maximum output of 12 l/min is achieved by the time the cervix is fully dilated. One cause of this increased output is the autotransfusion that occurs with each uterine contraction; another is the increasing stress, fear and pain of labor. Although blood flow is shifted from the splanchnic bed, the usual response of the cardiovascular system to sympathetic nervous stimulation is altered in pregnancy. Part of the usual response is arteriolar vasoconstriction and an increase in peripheral resistance, but in pregnancy there is also an active vasodilatation of several vascular compartments, especially in the placental bed, skin and kidneys. In addition, there is a relative refractoriness to the increase in catecholamines, angiotensin and serotonin, so that the normal mother has relatively little hypertensive response to the increase in cardiac output and peripheral resistance remains low. The main exception to this difference is in pre-eclampsia, where the increase in peripheral resistance and in arterial reactivity to catecholamines is similar to the non-pregnant woman. This means that there are greater rises in blood pressure during labor and especially during stress, such as during the induction of general anesthesia, in pre-eclampsia than in normal pregnancies.[26]

Management Options (see also Chapter 63)

General measures

Women's consumer groups have long argued that laboring women should not be made to feel that they are about to undergo a dangerous surgical procedure but encouraged to feel that childbirth is a normal, natural event. By such encouragement, it is believed that maternal distress is lessened. Apprehension and fear can also be lessened to the benefit of mother and baby by simple techniques such as allowing women to wear their own clothes, avoiding enemas and pubic shaves, and having partners, relatives or other support persons with them during labor. The demand of some women for home deliveries centers on the idea that in secure and familiar surroundings, maternal stress and fear are reduced and thereby labor is made easier, with a reduced requirement for analgesia and fewer complications.[27]

Encouraging the mother to feel at ease in the hospital environment decreases her sense of alienation. At the present time, clinical institutional surroundings are being widely discarded for more domestic interiors with curtains, pictures on the walls, subdued lighting and concealment of medical equipment.

Women able to have coping-related thoughts are less distressed in early labor (before 3 cm of cervical dilatation) and more likely to have shorter labors with less pain, fewer fetal heart rate abnormalities, and less need for instrumental deliveries or pediatric assistance to the neonate at birth.[28] This emphasizes the importance of prenatal training and psychoprophylactic techniques that attempt to teach mothers coping techniques in labor.[29] It may be that those women who can achieve a less stressful early phase of labor benefit irrespective of whether analgesia is used later during the active phase or not. There is, however, no consistent view as to how women should be trained for childbirth. Classes should at least convey information regarding the birth process and an explanation of possible medical interventions and what these entail.[30]

Psychoprophylaxis is a method of focusing the attention on something other than pain, such as specific breathing patterns or other distractions. Women are often very highly motivated to learn these techniques, as they believe that coping better with the stress of labor will result in a more satisfactory experience of childbirth,[31] although there is evidence that pain is not greatly reduced by psychoprophylaxis.[32] However, acceptance of the pain is one means of coping with it, helping to reduce distress and improve the mother's sense of satisfaction.[33] High levels of maternal anxiety in the prenatal period have been reported as being related to higher levels of pain experienced in labor,[34] although whether this is cause and effect or merely the result of a generally lower pain threshold is difficult to establish.

Fear prior to interventions such as artificial rupture of membranes, internal fetal monitoring and epidural analgesia, has been shown to increase maternal catecholamine levels.[35] Explanation and reassurance is essential if these fears are to be calmed.[36] When parents are informed of options, and given explanations for specific practices, they are more likely to have a positive childbirth experience and be less distressed.[37]

Studies suggest that levels of pain are relatively similar for all women in labor regardless of attitudes.[32,38] However, the experience of childbirth (of which pain is only a component) varies greatly with maternal attitudes. Women who desire and are given the opportunity of taking an active part in childbirth have a more satisfying experience.[38,39]

An important feature in decreasing maternal distress is giving the mother the freedom to conduct labor in the way she feels will best suit her. The feeling of control she experiences decreases stress – not being in control is a well-known cause of stress-related conditions in the non-obstetric patient.

Some women wish to experience natural unmedicated childbirth in the hope of a normal vaginal delivery without medical intervention. These women wish to take responsibility for their own actions and for the progress and outcome of the birth. Being in control of their circumstances allows them to feel less stress and anxiety than they would if they were being controlled by others.[39] However, if medical intervention is required, these women may become particularly distressed. In contrast, if women are very anxious, painless labor with regional blockade can allow them to feel in control of themselves in a way which would be impossible if their experience was dominated by pain.[40] For these women, an active unmedicated normal childbirth may be a harrowing experience, adding considerably to maternal distress in labor.[41]

Mothers who feel a sense of self-reliance, independence and self-control often wish to remain physically active in labor. Walking about, changing positions and adopting the most comfortable birthing position can be a means of reducing maternal distress. In some studies, these positions have been reported to be associated with a higher rate of normal deliveries than the traditional recumbent position,[42,43] whereas others have not been able to demonstrate any such advantage.[44,45] Possibly the most important conclusion to be drawn from these studies is that there is no reason why the mother's wishes should not be respected. This means supporting the mother who wishes to be physically active in labor to be so, but not forcing those who would prefer a more passive experience into a prescribed active routine.

Companionship during labor is clearly important in decreasing maternal fear and stress. Continuous uninterrupted physical and emotional support, with close proximity, frequent touching and talking by 'doulas' or sympathetic lay women has been shown in some settings to decrease labor complications[15] and to have a positive impact on perinatal outcome,[46] mother–infant interactions[14] and the mother's view of how she coped with labor.[47] Whether the presence of a professional member of staff such as a midwife is helpful in a similar way is not known, but it has been reported that mothers regard the presence of a sympathetic midwife throughout labor as more important than analgesia.[48]

Although the presence of the father during labor and delivery has become almost routine, there is no evidence to suggest that this has a direct impact on the outcome of labor, although it is usually reassuring for both mother and father.[49]

Pharmacological methods

The most important means of decreasing maternal stress is effective pain relief. Pain in labor inadequately treated with intramuscular opiates has been shown to be associated with increased levels of maternal catecholamines,[50] and may result in an increase in the incidence of fetal and neonatal acidosis.[51,52]

Biochemical and metabolic changes are known to be associated with pain and surgical stress, and have been shown to occur in labor.[53–56] Whether these metabolic changes have an adverse effect on the labor, the fetus and the mother is a matter of dispute. However, it seems likely that adverse effects are only likely to be observed in the sick mother, in excessively long labors, or where the fetus is already small or ill or has poor placental function. The fetus, and not just the mother, is the beneficiary of effective analgesia in such labors.

The use of sedative drugs in labor to reduce maternal distress has a long history, from the use of scopolamine in combination with morphine as twilight sleep at the turn of the century to the more modern benzodiazepines. Sedatives have not proved as useful in women in labor as they have in other patients in whom sleep and anxiolysis is desirable. The reasons for this are that sedative drugs have anti-analgesic properties[57] and enhance the perception of pain, sometimes causing the mother to be disorientated and more difficult to manage. The effect on the neonate limits the dose that can be given and therefore the maternal therapeutic effect.

The phenothiazine group of drugs has retained some place in obstetric use because of their anxiolytic and antiemetic effects. However, they have a very long duration of action. Their effects on the neurobehavioral responses of the neonate remain largely unknown. Double-blind studies have shown no advantages in the use of these drugs as judged by the mother,[58] although others have claimed considerable analgesic and sedative advantages.[59]

Benzodiazepines have been used in obstetrics especially as anticonvulsants, particularly diazepam. It is a very long-acting drug with a half-life of about 90 h in the mother and persists for about 1 week in the neonate.[61] It has been used in small doses as anxiolytic in women having cesarean section and in combination with narcotics[61–63] to improve analgesia. Because of its prolonged action in both the mother and neonate, it is not favored for obstetric use. Midazolam, which is much shorter-acting, has been used in small doses as a premedication for those mothers who are very anxious prior to cesarean section, as reducing maternal stress may be more advantageous for the neonate than the neonatal disadvantages of the drug. In addition, the benzodiazepine antagonist flumazenil is now available to reverse the neonatal effects. Midazolam has little effect on the maternal cardiovascular system and is anxiolytic in doses that are not sedative. Its major disadvantage is the anterograde amnesic effect. Amnesia is not considered desirable by the mother who does not wish to be deprived of the important experience of childbirth.

Drugs, however useful in pathological states in labor, should not be used to overcome maternal distress in normal labor. The mother is more likely to have a positive experience of childbirth with psychological and social support and a greater understanding of her needs. Women believe that a satisfying experience of childbirth is related subsequently to positive mental health, confidence and greater self-esteem.[64] An unsatisfactory experience leads to increased rates of depression, which can have a profound effect on the entire family.[65,66]

Anesthesia

Regional blockade has been shown to reduce maternal distress and the associated high catecholamine levels.[53,55,67] This benefit is especially important in the pre-eclamptic mother with poor placental perfusion.[68,69] Numerous reports have measured the improvements in the fetal environment that follow elimination of pain. A reduction in maternal noradrenaline levels[50,54] occurs following epidural analgesia with complete pain relief. A reduction in maternal hyperventilation and consequently oxygen consumption can benefit the hypoxic fetus,[70,71] and result in an improvement in maternal and fetal acid–base balance.[72] Incoordinate uterine action is an important complication of first labors and may in part be a result of maternal distress. Various reports have suggested the value of regional blockade in its management,[73] as well as the more familiar syntocinon augmentation of labor.[74]

General anesthesia for operative delivery, either abdominal or vaginal, is associated with a considerable stress response leading to a rise in blood pressure, heart rate, plasma cortisol, insulin, catecholamines and glucose.[75] These well-known stress responses during surgery under general anesthesia can only be prevented by deep anesthesia[76] or very large doses of intravenous opiates.[77] These anesthetics are not suitable for most obstetric patients. The rapid sequence induction with endotracheal intubation at a light plane of anesthesia causes marked cardiovascular responses[78] and leads to considerable hypertension which is of special concern in the pre-eclamptic patient. The evidence that large doses of alfentanil[79] can block this response has persuaded many obstetric anesthetists that this is the technique of choice in the pre-eclamptic patient who is unsuitable for regional anesthesia.[80] The effects of opiates are less serious for the neonate than extreme hypertension for the mother.

General anesthesia has for many situations become obsolete in obstetric practice. Maternal distress as an indication for general anesthesia and delivery by cesarean section is now almost never seen in obstetric units where regional blockade is available. The combination of the stress response to general anesthesia and the increased risk of failed endotracheal intubation and aspiration of gastric contents means that general, rather than regional, anesthesia has been implicated in over 80% of the maternal deaths associated with anesthesia in England and Wales since 1972.[81] The increased maternal risk, the possibility of awareness under anesthesia and the psychological disability caused by

unconsciousness at birth,[82] all discourage the use of this form of anesthesia for most obstetric patients.

The fact that there is a readily available alternative anesthetic for vaginal or abdominal operative delivery, namely spinal or epidural regional blockade, has been the most important factor in the decreased use of general anesthesia. Less maternal surgical stress occurs with regional blockade and this may have advantages for the fetus. Epidural anesthesia prevents the rise in blood glucose levels[83] secondary to surgery that can result in subsequent neonatal hypoglycemia. Circulating catecholamines are actually reduced with spinal[84] and epidural[85] anesthesia in non-obstetric patients. A well-conducted regional block results in less cardiovascular response than a well-conducted obstetric general anesthetic. This is especially important in preeclampsia, where the hypertensive response to endotracheal intubation can be dramatic.[86]

The response to a particular anesthetic technique of the fetus suffering chronic or acute hypoxia has not been well studied. There is little evidence that a healthy term infant is adversely affected by either general or regional anesthesia. However, some reports suggest that with acute intrapartum fetal distress requiring delivery by cesarean section, the use of regional block is associated with better neonatal condition than if general anesthesia is used.[87]

Food and fluids

Maternal distress may be aggravated by hunger and the rationale for feeding low-risk women in labor is that oral intake reduces both psychological stress[88,89] and physiological stress, as once glycogen stores are depleted the demands for glucose must be met by metabolism of body fat. This leads to the release of increased ketones into the blood, resulting in acidosis and ketonuria. Women at term have what has been described as accelerated starvation,[90] which is aggravated during labor.[91] This leads to early hypoglycemia and ketonuria. This has long been regarded as an indication for intervention in labor, usually with intravenous fluids. Ketoacidosis has been regarded as causing maternal distress and preventing efficient uterine contractions. However, treating ketonuria during labor with infusions of 10% dextrose in water, or excessive volumes of 5% dextrose, has been shown to be dangerous, causing hyponatremia in the mother[92] and causing rebound hypoglycemia[93] and hyponatremia[94] in the neonate. In addition, Ames et al. reported in 1975 that such treatment could give rise to maternal lactic acidosis.[95] This was attributed to the rise in maternal blood glucose concentrations increasing the production rate of lactate, which is an acid produced as part of the metabolism of glucose. Subsequently, Lawrence et al.[96] showed that maternal infusion of glucose at 100

MATERNAL DISTRESS IN LABOR
Summary of Management Options

General

- Avoid enemas and pubic shaves

- Familiarity with surroundings (arrange visits to labor suite during pregnancy)

- Prenatal training/classes

- Psychoprophylaxis exercises

- Explanation and reassurance from care givers

- Flexibility of approach to position/ambulation, etc., provided safety maintained

- Companionship and support during labor

Pharmacological methods

- See Chapter 63

- Experience and discussion with mother about choice and timing

Anesthesia

- Regional analgesia
  - see Chapter 63
  - ensure adequate fluid preloading

- General anesthesia
  - should not be necessary except in very exceptional circumstances

Food and fluids

- Food and fluids probably can be consumed in the early/latent phase

- Oral clear fluids probably can be drunk in limited amounts in the late/active phase of normal labor

- Any case of possible/potential cesarean section should avoid any oral intake during labor (? have an epidural electively in place in anticipation)

- If i.v. fluids necessary to correct ketosis, saline or Hartman's should be used in preference to dextrose solutions

g/h (1 liter of 10% glucose over 1 h) produced a significant fall in pH and rise in lactate in fetal as well as maternal blood. In 1987, Philipson et al.[97] confirmed these results when they studied the infusion of 1 liter of 5% dextrose over 30 min as part of a policy of preloading for epidural anesthesia. However, in 1989, Piquard et al.[98] subsequently showed that these adverse events did not occur if the glucose infusion rate was restricted to 30 g/h. These studies indicate that in labor, as at other times, care must be taken to monitor the volume and content of intravenous infusions to ensure they are compatible with the maintenance of normal physiology. In general, intravenous infusions used during labor should consist only of electrolyte-containing solutions[99] to avoid hyponatremia and hyperglycemia. If it is felt that glucose administration is needed, for example in prolonged labor, the amount should be physiological (normally no more than 6 g/h) and care must be taken to ensure that disturbance of electrolyte concentrations or fluid overloads do not occur.

Maternal distress in labor may be influenced by a lack of oral nutrition and the need for intravenous infusion. This subject remains a constant source of disagreement between anesthetists, midwives and mothers. Midwives and mothers believe that if allowed a light diet in labor, mothers become less distressed, require fewer analgesic drugs and less intervention, and they suggest that this is another benefit of home delivery as mothers are allowed to eat and drink at will. In units where epidural analgesia is used for high-risk labors and cesarean sections, general anesthesia is seldom needed. The importance of keeping the mother with an effective epidural block nil by mouth therefore decreases. Certainly, it is currently common practice for women to be given clear fluids in labor in many units; such fluids may contain glucose, for example in the form of honey. However, keeping the stomach empty is essential if women are likely to be subjected to general anesthesia in labor. In these circumstances, the use of pethidine is contraindicated as one of its side-effects is to delay gastric emptying,[100,101] leading to the accumulation of large volumes of gastric secretions. The anesthetic case for an empty stomach prior to general anesthesia is powerful, as aspiration of gastric contents is a known cause of maternal death, and it is most likely to occur in combination with general anesthesia. It has been shown that feeding women 2–3 h before elective cesarean section increases the volume of gastric contents,[102] but that there is little benefit to fasting for longer than 4 h.[103] There seems little justification for starvation of 12 h or more in obstetric units with access to efficient epidural services. In one reported series, almost 90% of women delivered by emergency cesarean section had earlier indications that abdominal delivery was likely.[60] Some of the women unexpectedly needing cesarean section will have arrived in the labor ward from home, not starved. Women admitted in labor in whom problems are anticipated ought to have early epidural blockade to avoid a hurried emergency general anesthetic.

CONCLUSIONS

- Maternal distress is associated with low birthweight, preterm delivery, fetal hypoxia in labor, prolonged labor, an increased intervention rate and neonatal dysfunction.

- Maternal distress can be ameliorated by careful prenatal preparation and appropriate emotional support during labor.

- Maternal distress as an indication for general anesthesia and/or cesarean section can be almost completely abolished by the use of regional block.

- Routine treatment of ketosis in labor is not necessary; intravenous infusions should preferably be crystalloid; and dextrose infusions should be limited to a physiological rate of not more than 6 g/h.

- Healthy women in normal labor should be allowed clear fluid intake as desired; women in whom cesarean section seems likely should be considered candidates for regional anesthesia.

The relief of maternal distress in labor should be limited to those cases where the women requests it or there is a clearly demonstrated advantage of intervention to the mother and fetus. Appropriate management of maternal distress (which may include doing nothing, or simply providing emotional or psychological support, as well as providing analgesia and physiological support) leads not only to the short-term reduction of complications in labor, but also to the long-term advantage of the family.

REFERENCES

1 Newton RW, Hunt LP (1984) Psychosocial stress in pregnancy and its relation to low birth weight. British Medical Journal 288:1191–1194.
2 Wilson-Evered E, Stanley G (1986) Stress and arousal during pregnancy and childbirth. British Journal of Medical Psychology 59:57–60.
3 Magann EF, Nolan TE (1991) Pregnancy outcome in an active-duty population. Obstetrics and Gynecology 78:391–393.
4 Newton RW, Webster PA, Binu PS, Maskrey N, Phillips AB (1979) Psychosocial stress in pregnancy and

its relation to the onset of premature labour. *British Medical Journal* 2:411–413.

5   Norbeck JS, Tilden VP (1983) Life stress, social support, and emotional disequilibrium in complications of pregnancy: A prospective multivariate study. *Journal of Health and Social Behaviour* 1:30–46.

6   Nuckolls KB, Cassels J, Kaplan BH (1972) Psychosocial assets, life crisis and the prognosis of pregnancy. *American Journal of Epidemiology* 95:431–434.

7   Rizzardo R, Magni G, Andreoli C *et al.* (1985) Psychosocial aspects during pregnancy and obstetrical complications. *Journal of Pschosomatic Obstetrics and Gynecology* 4:11–22.

8   Kartchner FD (1950) A study of emotional reactions during labor. *American Journal of Obstetrics and Gynecology* 60:19–29.

9   Lederman RP, Lederman E, Work BA, McCann DS (1978) The relationship of maternal anxiety, plasma catecholamines and plasma cortisol to progress in labor. *American Journal of Obstetrics and Gynecology* 132:495–500.

10 Beck NC, Siegel LJ, Davidson NP *et al.* (1980) The prediction of pregnancy outcome: Maternal preparation, anxiety and attitudinal sets. *Journal of Psychosomatic Research* 24:343–351.

11 Burns JK (1976) Relation between blood levels of cortisol and duration of human labour. *Journal of Physiology* 254:12.

12 Burns JK (1992) Parameters of catecholamine metabolism in pregnancy presage the duration of labor. *Journal of Psychosomatic Obstetrics and Gynecology* 13:37–49.

13 Crandon AJ (1979) Maternal anxiety and obstetric complications. *Journal of Psychosomatic Research* 23:109–111.

14 Sosa R, Kennell J, Klaus M, Robertson S, Urrutia J (1980) The effect of a supportive companion on perinatal problems, length of labor and mother–infant interaction. *New England Journal of Medicine* 303:597–600.

15 Klaus MH, Kennell JH, Robertson SS, Sosa R (1986) Effects of social support on maternal and infant morbidity. *British Medical Journal* 293:585–587.

16 Kennell J, Klaus M, McGrath S, Robertson S, Hinkley C (1988) Medical intervention: The effect of social support during labor. *Pediatric Research* 23:211 (abstract).

17 Zauspan FP, Cibils LA, Pose SV (1962) Myometrial and cardiovascular responses to alterations in plasma epinephrine and norepinephrine. *American Journal of Obstetrics and Gynecology* 84:841–851.

18 Greiss FC, Gabble LL (1987) Effect of sympathetic nerve stimulation on the uterine vascular bed. *American Journal of Obstetrics and Gynecology* 97:962–967.

19 Schnider SM, Wright RG, Levinson G, Roizen M, Wallis KL, Rolbin SH, Craft JB (1979) Uterine blood flow and plasma norepinephrine changes during maternal stress in the pregnant ewe. *Anesthesiology* 50:524–527.

20 Myers RE (1975) Maternal psychological stress and fetal asphyxia: A study in the monkey. *American Journal of Obstetrics and Gynecology* 122:47–53.

21 Rosenfeld CR, Barton MD, Meschia G (1976) Effects of epinephrine on distribution of blood flow in the pregnant ewe. *Amercian Journal of Obstetrics and Gynecology* 124:156–163.

22 Rosenfeld CR, West J (1977) Circulatory response to systemic infusion of norepinephrine in the pregnant ewe. *American Journal of Obstetrics and Gynecology* 127:376–383.

23 Adamson SK, Mueller-Heubach E, Myers RE (1971) Reproduction of fetal asphyxia in the rhesus monkey by administration of catecholamines to the mother. *American Journal of Obstetrics and Gynecology* 109:248–262.

24 Morishima HO, Pederson H, Finster M (1978) The influence of maternal psychological stress on the fetus. *American Journal of Obstetrics and Gynecology* 131:286–290.

25 Robson SC, Dunlop W, Boys RJ, Hunter S (1987) Cardiac output during labour. *British Medical Journal* 295:1169–1172.

26 Hodgkinson R, Hussain FJ, Hayashi RH (1980) Systemic and pulmonary blood pressure during caesarean section in parturients with gestational hypertension. *Can Anaes Soc J* 27:385–394.

27 Van Alten D, Eskes M, Treffers PE (1989) Midwifery in the Netherlands. The Wormerveer Study: Selection, mode of delivery, perinatal mortality and infant morbidity. *British Journal of Obstetrics and Gynaecology* 96:656–662.

28 Wuitchik M, Bakal D, Lipshitz J (1989) The clinical significance of pain and cognitive activity in latent labor. *Obstetrics and Gynecology* 73:35–42.

29 Beck NC, Siegel LJ (1980) Preparation for childbirth and contemporary research on pain, anxiety and stress reduction: A review and critique. *Psychosomatic Medicine* 42:429–447.

30 Crowe K, Von Baeyer C (1989) Predictors of a positive childbirth experience. *Birth* 16:59–63.

31 Simkin P, Enkin M (1989) Antenatal classes. In Chalmers I, Enkin M, Keirse M (eds), *Effective Care in Pregnancy and Childbirth*, Vol.1, pp. 318–334. Oxford: Oxford University Press.

32 Melzack R, Taenzer P, Feldman P, Kinch RA (1981) Labour is still painful after prepared childbirth training. *Canadian Medical Association Journal* 125:357–363.

33 Huttle FA, Mitchell Fisher MZ, Meyer AE (1972) A quantitative evaluation of psychoprophylaxis in childbirth. *Journal of Psychosomatic Research* 16:81–85.

34 Klusman LE (1975) Reducing pain in childbirth by the alleviation of anxiety in pregnancy. *J Consult Clinic Psycho* 43:162–165.

35 Buchan PC (1980) Emotional stress in childbirth and its modification by variations in obstetric management. *Acta Obstetrica et Gynecologica Scandinavica* 59:319–321.

36 Hayward J, Chalmers B (1990) Obstetricians' and mothers' perceptions of obstetric events. *Journal of Psychosomatic Obstetrics and Gynecology* 11:57–71.

37 Morcos FH, Snart FD, Harley DD (1989) Comparison

of parents expectations and importance rating for specific aspects of childbirth. *Canadian Medical Association Journal* **141**:909–915.

38 Davenport-Slack B, Boylan C (1974) Psychological correlates of childbirth pain. *Psychosomatic Medicine* **36**:215–223.

39 Humenick JS (1981) Mastery: The key to childbirth satisfaction. A review. *Birth* **6**:79–83.

40 Kitzinger S (1987) *Some Women's Experience of Epidurals: A Descriptive Study*. London: National Childbirth Trust.

41 Poore M, Cameron Foster J (1989) Epidural and no epidural anaesthesia: Differences between mothers and their experience of birth. *Birth* **12**:205–213.

42 Stewart P, Spiby H (1989) Posture in labour. *British Journal of Obstetrics and Gynaecology* **66**:1258–1260.

43 Flynn N, Kelly J, Hollins G, Lynch PF (1978) Ambulation in labour. *British Medical Journal* **2**:591–593.

44 McManus TJ, Calder AA (1978) Upright posture and the efficiency of labour. *Lancet* **1**:72–74.

45 Gardosi J, Sylvester S, Lynch CB (1989) Alternative positions in the second stage of labour: A randomised controlled trial. *British Journal of Obstetrics and Gynaecology* **66**:1290–1296.

46 Kennell JH, Klaus M, McGrath S, Robertson S, Hinkley C (1989) Labor support: What's good for the mother is good for baby. *Pediatric Research* **25**:15A.

47 Hofmeyr GJ, Nikodem VC, Wolman W, Chalmers BE, Kramer T (1991) Companionship to modify the clinical birth environment: Effects on progress and perceptions of labour and breast feeding. *British Journal of Obstetrics and Gynaecology* **98**:756–764.

48 Morgan BM, Bulpitt CJ, Clifton P, Lewis PJ (1984) The consumer's attitude to obstetric care. *British Journal of Obstetrics and Gynaecology* **91**:624–628.

49 Bertsch TD, Nagashima, Whalen L, Dykeman S, Kennell JH, McGrath S (1990) Labor support by first time fathers: Direct observations with a comparison to experienced doulas. *Journal of Psychosomatic Obstetrics and Gynecology* **11**:251–260.

50 Thornton CA, Carrie LES, Sayers L, Anderson ABM, Turnbull AC (1976) A comparison of the effect of extradural and parenteral analgesia on maternal plasma cortisol concentrations during labour and the puerperium. *British Journal of Obstetrics and Gynaecology* **83**:631–635.

51 Deckhardt R, Fembacher PM, Schneider KTM, Graeff H (1987) Maternal arterial oxygen saturation during labour and delivery: Pain-dependent alterations and effects on the newborn. *Obstetrics and Gynecology* **70**:21–25.

52 Pearson JF, Davies P (1974) The effect of continuous lumbar epidural analgesia upon fetal acid–base status during the second stage of labour. *Journal of Obstetrics and Gynaecology of the British Commonwealth* **84**:975–979.

53 Lederman RP, McCann DS, Work B, Huber MJ (1977) Endogenous plasma epinephrine and norepinephrine in last trimester pregnancy and labor. *American Journal of Obstetrics and Gynecology* **129**:5–8.

54 Falconer AD, Powles AB (1982) Plasma noradrenaline levels during labour: Influence of elective lumbar epidural blockade. *Anaesthesia* **37**:416–420.

55 Abboud TK, Sarkis F, Hung TT et al. (1983) Effects of epidural anesthesia during labor on maternal plasma beta-endorphine levels. *Anesthesiology* **59**:1–5.

56 Thomas TH, Fletcher JE, Hill RG (1982) Influence of medication pain and progress in labour on plasma beta-endorphine-like immunoreactivity. *British Journal of Anaesthesia* **54**:401–408.

57 Dundee JW (1960) Alterations in response to somatic pain associated with anaesthesia: The effect of thiopentone and pentobarbitone. *British Journal of Anaesthesia* **32**:407–414.

58 Matthews AEB (1963) Double blind trials of promazine in labour. *British Medical Journal* **2**:423–427.

59 de Kornfeld TJ, Pearson JW, Lasagna L (1964) Methotrimeprazine in the treatment of labour pain. *New England Journal of Medicine* **270**:391–394.

60 Morgan BM, Magni V, Goroszenuik T (1990) Anaesthesia for emergency caesarean section. *British Journal of Obstetrics and Gynaecology* **97**:420–424.

61 Cree IE, Meyer J, Hailey DM (1973) Diazepam in labour: its metabolism and effect on the clinical condition and thermogenesis of the newborn. *British Medical Journal* **4**:251–255.

62 Friedman EA, Niswander KR, Sachtleben MR (1969) Effect of diazepam on labour. *Obstetrics and Gynecology* **34**:82–86.

63 Flowers CE, Rudolph AJ, Desmona MM (1969) Diazepam (Valium) as an adjunct in obstetric analgesia. *Obstetrics and Gynecology* **34**:68–81.

64 Oakley A (1989) Can social support influence pregnancy outcome? *British Journal of Gynecology* **96**:260–262.

65 Plotsky H, Sherenshefsky P (1973) Psychological meaning of labour delivery experience. In Yarrow L, Sherenshefsky P (eds), *Psychological Aspects of a First Pregnancy and Early Postnatal Adaptation*. New York: Raven Press.

66 Lee MC, Gotlib IH (1989) Maternal depression and child adjustment: A longitudinal analysis. *Journal of Abnormal Psychology* **98**:78–85.

67 Jouppila R, Puolakka J, Kauppila A, Vuori J (1984) Maternal and umbilical cord plasma noradrenaline concentrations during labour with and without segmental extradural analgesia and during caesarean section. *British Journal of Anaesthesia* **56**:251–254.

68 Jouppila P, Jouppila R, Hollmen A, Koivula A (1982) Lumbar epidural analgesia to improve intervillous blood flow during labor in severe pre-eclampsia. *Obstetrics and Gynecology* **59**:158–161.

69 Jouppila R, Jouppila P, Hollmen A, Koivula A (1979) Epidural analgesia and placental blood flow during labour in pregnancies complicated by hypertension. *British Journal of Obstetrics and Gynaecology* **86**:969–972.

70 Hagerdal M, Morgan C, Sumner AE, Gutsche B (1983) Minute ventilation and oxygen consumption during labour with epidural analgesia. *Anesthesiology* **59**:425–427.

71 Sangoul F, Fox GS, Houle GL (1975) Effect of regional analgesia on maternal oxygen consumption

during first stage of labour. *American Journal of Obstetrics and Gynecology* 121:1080–1083.

72 Reynolds F (1989) Epidural analgesia in obstetrics: Pros and cons for mother and baby (Editorial). *British Medical Journal* 299:751–752.

73 Moir DD, Willocks J (1966) Continuous epidural analgesia in inco-ordinate uterine action. *Acta Anaesthetica Scandinavica* 23:144–148.

74 O'Driscoll K, Foley M, MacDonald D (1984) Active management of labor as an alternative to cesarean section for dystocia. *Obstetrics and Gynecology* 63:485–490.

75 Loughran PG, Moore J, Dundee JW (1986) Maternal stress response associated with caesarean delivery under general and epidural anaesthesia. *British Journal of Obstetrics and Gynaecology* 93:943–949.

76 Roizen MF, Holligan RW, Frazer BM (1981) Anaesthetic doses blocking adrenergic (stress) and cardiovascular responses to incision. *Anesthesiology* 54:390–398.

77 Blunnie WP, McIlroy PAA, Merrett JD, Dundee JW (1983) Cardiovascular and biochemical evidence of stress during major surgery associated with different techniques of anaesthesia. *British Journal of Anaesthesia* 55:611–618.

78 Russell WJ, Morris RG, Frewin DB, Drew SE (1981) Changes in plasma catecholamine concentrations during endotracheal intubation. *British Journal of Anaesthesia* 53:837–839.

79 Stanley TH, Bermahl Green O, Robertson D (1980) Plasma catecholamine and cortisol responses for fentanyl-oxygen anesthesia for coronary artery operation. *Anesthesiology* 53:250–253.

80 Dann WL, Hutchinson A, Cartwright DP (1987) Maternal and neonatal responses to alfentanil administration before induction of general anaesthesia for caesarean section. *British Journal of Anaesthesia* 59:1392–1396.

81 Department of Health (1991) *Report on Confidential Enquiries into Maternal Deaths in the United Kingdom 1985–87.* London: HMSO.

82 Lynch MA, Roberts J (1977) Predicting child abuse: Signs of bonding failure in maternity hospitals. *British Medical Journal* 1:624–626.

83 Brandt M, Kehlet H, Binder C, Hagen C, McNeilly AS (1976) Effect of epidural analgesia on the glycoregulatory endocrine response to surgery. *Clinical Endocrinology* 5:107–114.

84 Pflug AE, Hatter JB (1981) Effect of spinal anesthesia on adrenergic tone and the neuro-endocrine response to surgical stress in humans. *Anesthesiology* 55:120–126.

85 Hall GM (1985) The anaesthetic modification of the endocrine and metabolic response to surgery. *Annals of the Royal College of Surgeons* 67:25–29.

86 Fox EJ, Skar GJ, Hill CH, Villanueva R, King BP (1977) Complications related to pressor response. *Anesthesiology* 47:524–525.

87 Marx GF, Luykx WM, Cohen S (1984) Fetal–neonatal status following caesarean section for fetal distress. *British Journal of Anaesthesia* 56:1009–1012.

88 Broach J, Newton N (1988) Food and beverages in labor: The effects of cessation of oral intake during labor. *Birth* 15:88–92.

89 Simkin P (1986) Stress pain and catecholamines in labour. Stress associated with childbirth events: A pilot survey of new mothers. *Birth* 13:234–240.

90 Metzger BE, Ravnikar V, Vileisis RA, Freinkel N (1982) Accelerated starvation and the skipped breakfast in late normal pregnancy. *Lancet* 1:588–592.

91 Dumoulin JG, Foulkes JE (1984) Ketonuria during labour (Editorial). *British Journal of Obstetrics and Gynaecology* 91:97–98.

92 Evans SE, Crawford JS, Stevens ID, Durbin GM, Daya H (1986) Fluid therapy for induced labour under epidural analgesia: Biochemical consequences for mother and infant. *British Journal of Obstetrics and Gynaecology* 93:329–333.

93 Kenepp NB, Kumar S, Shelley WC, Stanley CA, Gabbe SG, Gutsche BB (1982) Fetal and neonatal hazards of maternal hydration with 5% dextrose before caesarean section. *Lancet* 1:1150–1152.

94 Tarnow-Mordi WO, Shaw JC, Liu D, Gardner DA, Flynn FV (1981) Iatrogenic hyponatremia of the newborn due to maternal fluid overload: A prospective study. *British Medical Journal* 283:639–642.

95 Ames AC, Cobbold S, Maddock J (1975) Lactic acidosis complicating treatment of ketosis of labour. *British Medical Journal* 4:611–613.

96 Lawrence GF, Brown VA, Parsons RJ, Cooke ID (1982) Fetomaternal consequences of high-dose glucose infusion during labour. *British Journal of Obstetrics and Gynaecology* 89:27–32.

97 Philipson EH, Kalhan SC, Riha MM, Pimentel R (1987) Effects of maternal glucose infusion on fetal acid–base status in human pregnancy. *American Journal of Obstetrics and Gynecology* 157:866–873.

98 Piquard F, Hsiung R, Haberey P, Dellenbach P (1989) Does fetal acidosis develop with maternal glucose infusions during normal labor? *Obstetrics and Gynecology* 74:909–914.

99 Lind T (1983) Fluid balance during labour: A review. *Journal of the Royal Society of Medicine* 76:870–875.

100 Nimmo W, Wilson J, Prescott FF (1975) Narcotic analgesics and delayed gastric emptying during labour. *Lancet.* 1:890–893.

101 Holdsworth JD (1978) Relationship between stomach contents and analgesia in labour. *British Journal of Anaesthesia* 50:1145–1148.

102 Lewis M, Crawford JS (1987) Can one risk fasting the obstetric patient for less than 4 hours? *British Journal of Anaesthesia* 59:312–314.

103 Thomas EA (1987) Preoperative fasting: A question of routine? *Nursing Times* 83:46–47.

65

Forceps Delivery

PHILIP C. DENNEN

INTRODUCTION

Forceps delivery, as an extricating maneuver, has the potential safely to remove the infant, mother and obstetrician from a difficult or even hazardous situation. For several centuries, obstetrical forceps have been the subject of controversy and wide swings in popularity both inside and outside the profession. Currently, the use of forceps is widely taught.[1,2] However, reviewing hospital statistics reveals that there is considerable variation in the percentage of deliveries in which forceps are used. In the USA, the range can be from near zero to 20%. In the UK and Ireland, most institutions report the use of forceps in 10–15% of deliveries. In some maternity units, figures for instrumental delivery include the use of the ventouse (vacuum extractor). On the European continent, the ventouse is often more popular than forceps but use of the latter is still reported in significant numbers. In underdeveloped areas of the world, where large sections of the population have inadequate access to medical care and maternal and perinatal mortality rates are high, the use of forceps is much less common.

INDICATIONS

Maternal indications are most commonly those of maternal distress, maternal exhaustion, or simply undue prolongation of the second stage of labor. Less common but arguably more medically significant indications include cardiopulmonary or vascular conditions in which the stresses of the second stage of labor

should be minimized. The increased forceps rate following epidural anesthesia has been well documented.[3,4] Prolongation of the second stage of labor is a relative indication. Many have argued that specific time limits are not needed if monitoring of the fetus shows no evidence of distress and progress is not obviously arrested. However, in practice, it is probably more realistic to propose intervention in cases without regional anesthesia if the second stage is prolonged beyond 2 h in the nullipara or 1 h in the multipara. An additional hour should probably be added in the presence of regional anesthesia.[5]

A further indication for the use of forceps is failure of delivery using the vacuum extractor. Some authors have suggested that if use of the vacuum extractor has failed to deliver the infant but the fetal vertex has been brought down sufficiently, a safe low or outlet forceps procedure may be attempted.[6]

Maternal bleeding can be a valid indication for terminating labor. This may overlap with bleeding in relation to which there is also a fetal indication, for example placental abruption.

In relation to *fetal indications*, malposition with relative dystocia is the most frequent indication for forceps intervention. The commonly encountered occiput posterior and occiput transverse positions occur more frequently with regional anesthesia.[4,7,8] This may result from disturbing the tone of the musculature of the pelvic floor and impeding spontaneous rotation to the optimal occiput anterior position. Similarly, maternal expulsive forces may be compromised.

Early in the twentieth century, Dr Joseph DeLee proposed the use of prophylactic forceps to protect the fetal skull and its contents from the trauma of delivery. Although the concept became quite popular, particularly in relation to delivery of the preterm infant, conclusive scientific proof of the validity of this idea has never been established. Indeed, in the infant weighing less than 1500 g, routine forceps delivery (in cases where there is no specific indication) offers no advantage[9] and may in fact be deleterious,[10] due to an increased incidence of intracranial bleeding. Spontaneous delivery with a generous episiotomy and manual control of the head appear preferable. Some have argued that if operative delivery is necessary in this weight range, delivery by cesarean section is indicated.[10]

However, there is no general agreement on this point. In low-birth weight infants, between 1500 and 2500 g, forceps delivery has been more widely accepted, although care should be taken not to use excessive traction.[11,12]

'Fetal distress' is a commonly cited indication for forceps delivery. 'Presumed fetal jeopardy' may be preferable to the term fetal distress, as the latter term is subject to various interpretations.[13] For example, a common reason for making the diagnosis of 'fetal distress' is an abnormality of the cardiotocogram, and yet most babies born following such an indication are healthy. For the purposes of accuracy and subsequent review, the medical record should contain as precise a description of the situation as possible to validate the indication,[5] rather than vague and ill-defined comments such as 'fetal distress'.

Vaginal delivery of the breech is considered by some to be an indication for forceps to the 'aftercoming head'.[14–16] The procedure becomes mandatory if the body has delivered and the Mauriceau-Smellie-Veit maneuver has failed. A putative advantage of the use of forceps is the avoidance of traction on the trunk and cervical spine, together with automatic control of the flexion of the fetal head, which may decrease the chance of hyperextension and cervical plexus injury.[16,17]

In cases of shoulder dystocia, should the usual management such as McRobert, Wood and other maneuvers not be effective, the use of forceps is a possible option. Parallel forceps such as those of Shute or Kielland may be applied beneath the head to the anterior and posterior aspects of the chest. Subsequent rotation of the chest should result in the shoulders moving to an oblique diameter of the inlet with resolution of the impaction.

CONTRAINDICATIONS

There are many relative contraindications to the use of obstetric forceps, although few are so absolute that no-one has suggested a technique to overcome them. Lack of engagement of the fetal head suggests inlet dystocia and is usually quoted as an absolute contraindication for forceps delivery, although some forceps have been designed specifically for this situation.[18] In some conditions, vaginal delivery *per se* is contraindicated, such as known pelvic abnormality or fetal anomalies, if obstructive or subject to damage from vaginal delivery. The rarely encountered Bandl's retraction ring of the uterus is an indication for abdominal delivery rather than forceps. Fetal malpositions such as a brow with occiput anterior or face presentation with chin posterior are not suitable for forceps delivery, nor is the dead fetus with postmortem changes. An inability to diagnose the position of the fetal head or an inability to apply the instrument are absolute contraindications.

Contraindications include a presenting part above the level of the ischial spines – the higher it is, the stronger the contraindication. Similarly, an increased risk of shoulder dystocia following mid-cavity delivery has been reported if the fetus is macrosomic.[19] Lack of training or experience on the part of the operator must also be considered a relative contraindication.

DEFINITIONS

Significant comparative statistics have always been difficult to collect due to differences in the classifications of forceps deliveries. The American College of Obstetricians and Gynecologists has proposed a more specific classification,[1,5] which has shown itself to be of clinical value.[20,21] The classification is given in **Table 1**. It applies equally to vacuum extraction procedures.[5] To the classification of low forceps, a significant clinical addition would be that on examination the head must fill the hollow of the sacrum. The inclusion of an occiput posterior position in the outlet category is questionable due to the fact that the biparietal diameter is higher in relation to the leading bony point than with an occiput anterior position. Also, greater force is required for delivery with an occiput posterior position because the presenting diameters are less favorable than with an occiput anterior position.[15] Station is measured in centimeters of distance between the leading bony point of the skull and the ischial spines, negative distances meaning that the leading point is above the spines, and positive distances below.

Fetal results comparable with those of spontaneous delivery can be expected with forceps procedures categorized as outlet or low forceps with rotation less than 45°.[20,22–26] Mid-forceps and rotational procedures are generally associated with a higher rate of morbidity than spontaneous delivery. However, when contrasted more properly with appropriate alternatives of management, namely manual rotation followed by forceps extraction or delivery by cesarean section, mid-forceps

Table 1
Classification of forceps deliveries according to
station and rotation

Type of procedure	Classification
Outlet forceps	Scalp is visible at the introitus without separating labia
	Fetal skull has reached pelvic floor
	Sagittal suture is in anteroposterior diameter or right or left occiput anterior or posterior position
	Fetal head is at or on perineum
	Rotation does not exceed 45°
Low forceps	Leading point of fetal skull is at station ≥ + 2 cm, and not on the pelvic floor
	Rotation ≤ 45° (left or right occiput anterior to occiput anterior, or left or right occiput posterior to occiput posterior)
	Rotation > 45°
Mid-forceps	Station above +2 cm but head engaged
High	Not included in classification

Reproduced from American College of Obstetricians and Gynecologists.[5]

results are the same.[27–31] Studies have been reported from both protagonists[12,27,31] and antagonists[9,23,32] of mid-forceps to support their own preferred management. The controversy continues; appropriate selection of cases and skill in execution of the maneuver remain the unmeasurable variables which often determine the results of trials.

'Failed forceps' is a term with a pejorative implication. Historically associated with high morbidity and mortality, it carries the implication of poor judgement, poor obstetrics, and perhaps negligence, in that disproportion was unrecognized.[33] A trial of forceps, on the other hand, connotes a cautious attempt at vaginal delivery with the option to alter management if unusual difficulty is met.[16] The procedure deserves greater utilization.[28] A gentle negative trial of forceps (perhaps a better term psychologically than 'failed forceps') should not alter outcome.[8,28]

PREREQUISITES

In the management of a forceps delivery, certain prerequisites must be met.[5,16] The head should be engaged as defined by the biparietal diameter, having passed through the plane of the inlet of the pelvis (see **Figure 2**).

Generally, this will have occurred when the leading bony point has reached the ischial spines, and thus estimation of the station is a prerequisite for any attempt at instrumental delivery. However, it must be remembered that certain conditions lead to a higher than anticipated level of the biparietal diameter. A common example is molding of the fetal head, particularly if the fetus is macrosomic. Asynclitism and occiput posterior positions are also associated with a higher level of the widest diameter for a given station as is any extension of the fetal vertex away from a well-flexed position.

The bladder should be emptied for procedures other than outlet forceps. The amniotic membranes must be ruptured and the cervix should be fully dilated and retracted. Forceps application under even a small rim of cervix is difficult and may result in fetal or maternal trauma. With any form of delivery the cervix may be lacerated, while with a rotational delivery direct posterior application of the blade of Kiellands' forceps can result in perforation of the posterior fornix. Even if application of the blades is accomplished, marked obstruction to rotation or descent of the head may occur. There is probably no place in modern obstetrics for manual or mechanical dilatation of the cervix or for cervical incisions to facilitate a forceps procedure.[16]

The position of the head must be established so that an accurate biparietal bimalar application of the forceps blades can be made. The design of the instrument is such that the forces required to move the head are transmitted symmetrically to non-vital areas of the skull only when the application is correct. An incorrect application, such as a brow mastoid application, produces asymmetrical forces and these may cause damage to intracranial structures. Should the operator be unable to diagnose position from fontanelles and suture lines, feeling for the location of an ear can be of assistance. This may entail an unfortunate loss of station and backward rotation of the head due to the displacement of the vertex which is necessary during this maneuver.

Careful consideration of factors such as maternal overweight or diabetes (which predispose to macrosomia) and the pattern of cervical dilatation can give the obstetrician a warning that malposition or dystocia may develop. Clinical evaluation of the pelvis for adequacy of the fetopelvic relationship is important, particularly if an arrest pattern develops. Additional radio-graphic pelvimetry is not usually necessary.

Appropriate anesthesia is needed for any forceps delivery. On occasion, outlet and some low forceps procedures may be performed with a local perineal infiltration. For minimal anesthesia, a pudendal block is usually required. For any rotational or mid-forceps procedure, a regional block – epidural or saddle – is necessary. In rare circumstances, a quick general anesthesia may be used.

Although the simplest forceps operations may be undertaken in an informal birthing room environment,

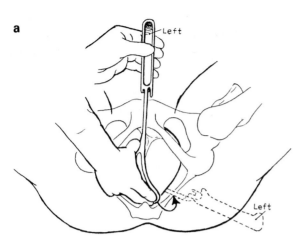

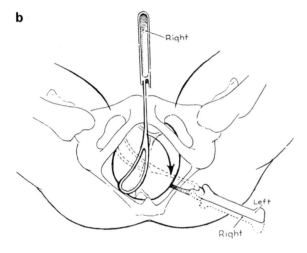

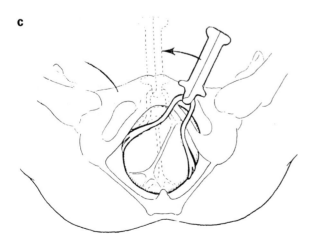

Figure 1. Forceps application LOA.

most procedures deserve a delivery room/operating theater setting. Facilities, equipment and personnel should be adequate for support of patient, infant and operator in case any adverse unforseen situations develop. A negative trial of forceps should be capable of moving swiftly to an abdominal approach.

Forceps complications tend to increase in inverse ratio to the technical skill and experience of the operator. The operator must know his or her limitations and be prepared to abandon the procedure in case of difficulty. The use of greater force is the worst of the available options.

INSTRUMENTS AND CHOICE

Obstetrical forceps in current use may be loosely grouped in two major categories – classical and special. Classical instruments are related to those devised by Sir James Y. Simpson (1848) and by George T. Elliot (1858). Both the Simpson and Elliot forceps are still widely used. The Simpson-type forceps are characterized by a spread shank and somewhat longer cephalic curve. Examples of the type are the long and short Simpsons', Simpson-Braun, Luikart-Simpson, DeLee, Hawks-Dennen, Barnes, Wrigley, as well as the DeWees and many obsolescent axis traction instruments. They are preferred by many for their superior traction ability. The Elliot-type forceps are characterized by overlapping shanks and a shorter cephalic curve. Examples of the type include the Elliot, Tucker-MacLane and its Luikart modification, Bailey-Williamson and others.

Special instruments include the Piper forceps designed for the 'aftercoming head' in breech delivery, the Kielland forceps for rotational delivery at any station, the Barton forceps for transverse arrest in the flat pelvis, the divergent forceps of Laufe and Zeppelin, the Moolgaoker, the Shute, and other cleverly designed instruments.

The choice of instrument is often influenced by regional as well as personal preferences. For example, the Wrigley and Barnes instruments commonly used in the UK and Canada are almost unknown in the USA. Some operators prefer to approach most clinical situations with the same instrument, thereby losing the unique clinical advantages of the various available forceps. The larger, more molded head is more accurately contacted by the blade with the longer tapering cephalic curve of a Simpson type. The unmolded head is better accommodated by a short. full cephalic curve of an Elliot type.[34]

With the occiput in an anterior quadrant, any classical instrument with the appropriate cephalic curve may be chosen. Most commonly used for outlet forceps are the Wrigley, the Simpson (short or long) or an Elliot type of instrument. For low forceps with rotation less than 45°, one of the previously listed longer Simpson-type or Elliot-type forceps are usually chosen. For low forceps with rotation greater than 45°, several alternatives are available. Most operators prefer a special instrument for rotation, such as the Kielland or the Moolgaoker, Shute, etc. Either an Elliot or Simpson type of classical forceps may also be used. At the mid-forceps level, the same choices apply, but the need for axis traction principles must also be considered. For forceps to the 'aftercoming head', Piper forceps are generally preferred, although the Kielland forceps and even classical forceps have been used effectively.

Procedure: Forceps Delivery

Position

Definitive texts are available which outline many of the specifics of procedure for forceps delivery. Certain principles given here have universal pertinence to the use of forceps regardless of the type of instrument chosen. In some areas, the least complicated procedures may be performed with the patient in the Sims lateral recumbent position. For clarity, the use of the lithotomy position is assumed in the following discussion. Once the prerequisites for forceps delivery have been observed, the aspects of application and traction must be considered.

Application (see **Figure 1**)

Application is extremely important to the safe control of the head when force is transmitted from operator to fetal skull via the instrument. A correct application allows the operator to know the exact attitude of the head. To minimize the amount of force required and the potential of trauma, descent of the long axis of the head must be accomplished in the axis of the pelvis. If the landmarks are obscured and fetal position is unknown, the operator should not use forceps.

In an oblique anterior position of the occiput, the blade going to the posterior segment of the pelvis should be inserted first. Some operators believe that the left

blade of any classical instrument should always be inserted first. This avoids having to cross the handles to engage the lock. If the occiput is to the right side, this minor advantage is counterbalanced by the tendency to rotate the head backwards to a much less favorable transverse position during the wandering to apply the anterior blade. This does not happen if a posterior blade is in place splinting the head. Therefore, in a right-sided position of the occiput, the right blade should probably be inserted first. In a left-sided position of the occiput, the left blade is the posterior blade and should be inserted first.

With application of the classical instrument, the left blade is held in the left hand, is applied to the left side of the mother's pelvis and to the left side of the fetal skull. The laterality is preversed for the right blade. Exceptions include application to an occiput posterior (OP) or to an aftercoming head, when the left blade goes to the right side of the head. The dictum may also not apply with certain special instruments or maneuvers such as the Scanzoni rotation.

To commence insertion, the posterior blade is held perpendicular to the long axis of the patient. The cephalic curve of the instrument is approximated to the curve of the fetal skull, guided by the fingers of the opposite hand. The handle is gently moved in an arc away from the midline toward the thigh, then down, then back toward the midline. The toe of the blade is moved high in the pelvis to seat over the malar eminence. This is repeated with the anterior blade. The amount of downward component in the arc traversed by the handles is the same for each blade in the case of an occiput anterior (OA) position. Increasing rotation of the occiput away from OA decreases the downward component of the arc of the posterior blade insertion while increasing the downward arc of the anterior blade insertion. The anterior blade is often more subject to temporary obstruction as it is wandered into the anterior segment of the pelvis. The blades are locked and the application is checked.

Checks for accurate application are as follows: the sagittal suture should be perpendicular to the plane of the shanks of the forceps. Any other situation is an asymmetrical application with increased risk of fetal injury. Second, the posterior fontanelle should be midway between the blades and one finger's breadth above the plane of the shanks. A greater distance above the plane of the shanks indicates an extended head, whereas a lesser distance indicates an overflexed attitude. In either case, a longer, less favorable diameter is presented to the pelvic axis and relative resistance to descent results. This applies to all vertex presentations. Last, with fenestrated blades, a small but equal fenestration should be felt. The presence of a large amount of palpable fenestration suggests a short application of the blades on the head, rather than correct application below the malar eminences. The risk of facial nerve injury and slipping of the blades is increased if the application is short.

When the checks indicate improper application, readjustment is necessary. Should the sagittal suture be oblique to the plane of the shanks rather than perpendicular, a brow mastoid application is present. The blades must be unlocked, then separately wandered to the correct position. This is accomplished with slight movement of the handle away from the midline to move the toe away from the head. Pressure is then exerted on the heel of the blade with pressure in the opposite direction on the handle to shift the blade to the correct position. The other blade is similarly adjusted. The blades are relocked and rechecked. Correction of the flexion attitude is readily accomplished by unlocking and adjusting the blades. They are shifted separately to bring the plane of the shanks to one finger's breadth below the posterior fontanelle. The presence of more than a fingertip of fenestration is an indication to unlock the blades and separately adjust them higher in the pelvis. These readjustments are all done without removal of the forceps. If proper application cannot be accomplished, removal of the forceps, re-evaluation of the situation, and then re-application are indicated.

Traction

The ultimate and dominant function of the obstetrical forceps is traction to accomplish descent of the head in the birth canal following application. The pelvic curve, so carefully designed into the instrument, is mechanically effective with the occiput in the anterior position. Increasing rotation of the occiput away from OA decreases the pelvic curve until it is non-existent in occipito-transverse (OT). Thus, a correctional rotation to OA should be accomplished either before or with the onset of traction. The head should be rotated along its long axis, since an 'off-center' rotation increases resistance. The instrumental rotation should be performed with the toes describing as small an arc as possible in the upper pelvis. This maintains the direction of the long axis of the head. The handles are directed in a wide arc ending with the occiput at OA. Rotation of the instrument along its own axis would result in a wide arc of the toes due to the pelvic curve.

Compression of the fetal head with the forceps is an undesirable effect and should be minimized by the use of the fingerguards rather than squeezing the handles during traction. Force applied at the fingerguards is so close to the fulcrum at the adjacent lock that negligible compressive force is applied to the head. The natural compression supplied by the pelvic walls and intervening soft tissues serves to maintain the position of the instrument on the head.

Assuming the clinical situation permits, traction should be timed to coincide with uterine contractions and voluntary expulsive effort by the mother. The operator may be seated or standing, well balanced, using principally shoulder and arm muscles. Traction force should be increased gradually rather than rapidly. Jerking the instrument increases the risk of injury to fetus and mother. A steady pull should be maintained and then gradually released as the contraction wears off. The number of tractions and the force required will vary with the case, but usually delivery should be effected by traction with no more than three contractions and employing no more than moderate force. There are two components of traction, both of which must be considered: direction and amount.

The direction of traction must be in the axis of the pelvic curve. This direction alters with the different obstetrical planes of the pelvis (see **Figure 2**). The critical head diameter which must be moved is the biparietal diameter. The application of tractive force in the correct direction can be done manually with the Pajot-Saxtorph maneuver with traction outwards on the fingerguards and downwards on the shanks of the instrument. The resultant vector of force is ideally perpendicular to the plane of the biparietal diameter at its level in the pelvis (**Figure 3**). This vector must be estimated by the operator and is more difficult with the biparietal diameter

at higher station. The axis traction principle is more easily accomplished instrumentally with an attachment such as the Bill handle, which will fit any classical forceps, or with a forceps specially designed for axis traction.

As the biparietal diameter descends, the direction of traction rises and the level of the handles is elevated (see **Figure 4**). The long axis of the head tends to be held in the axis of the pelvis by pressure from maternal structures. With traction and elevation of the handles, observation of the edge of the instrument in relation to the adjacent scalp will show the operator the proper direction of pull. If the instrument is elevated too soon, the scalp appears to sink in relation to the upper

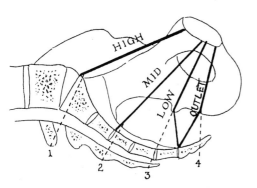

Figure 2. The obstetrical planes of the pelvis and forceps classification. 1, Plane of inlet; 2, plane of greatest pelvic dimension; 3, plane of least pelvic dimension; 4, plane of outlet. Reproduced with permission from Dennen.[16]

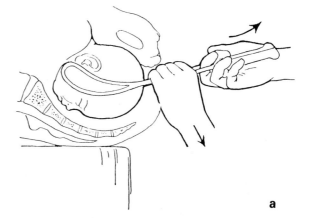

a

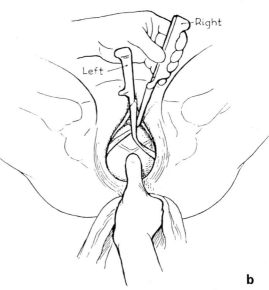

b

Figure 3. Line of axis traction (perpendicular to the plane of the pelvis at which the head is stationed) at different planes of the pelvis. 1, High; 2, mid; 3, low; 4, outlet. Reproduced with permission from Dennen.[16]

Figure 4. **a** Traction. **b** Removal of forceps; Ritgen head control.

edge of the blade. Conversely, late elevation of the instrument results in the scalp rising as the head is forced to extend. As the occiput passes under the symphysis pubis, the handle elevation may reach 45° above the horizontal. A higher elevation of the handles increases the risk of sulcus laceration.

The amount of tractive force should always be the least possible to accomplish reasonable descent. The maximum permissible safe force is 45 lb (20 kg) in the nullipara or 30 lb (13 kg) in the multipara.[16] Most deliveries are accomplished with considerably less force. The amount of vectored force may be difficult to estimate when using manual axis traction. With a traction attachment, the vectored force is equal to the entire pull.

Episiotomy, quite popular in North America, is less so in other parts of the world. Regardless of the controversy over routine use of the procedure, episiotomy results in the need for less tractive force. There is continuing controversy about whether the episiotomy should be mediolateral or midline; this author prefers the median approach as it heals up more quickly and is less painful in the puerperium. However, although data from controlled trials are lacking, it seems likely that the median episiotomy is associated with a higher rate of third-degree tears than the mediolateral[35] and thus either approach remains valid at the present time.

During extension of the head over the perineum, the forceps may be removed and a Ritgen maneuver performed for completion of delivery of the head. The fetus should be monitored between contractions throughout the procedure.

Should reasonable effort not produce descent of the head, the initial move should be to direct tractive force to a lower plane, rather than using more force. If this is not helpful, the blades should be removed and the situation re-evaluated for cervical dilatation, fetal position and pelvic abnormality. The same or another instrument may be carefully reapplied. Although high failure rates are quoted for ventouse use after negative forceps trials, it is an available option with cesarian section as the ultimate alternative.

MANAGEMENT OF SPECIAL SITUATIONS

Occiput Transverse

Should delivery become necessary with a persistent occiput transverse (OT) position, several options are available. Fetal results with all of the options should be equivalent.[36]

Procedure: Occiput Transverse Position

Manual rotation (see Figure 5)

Manual rotation is a method used successfully by some operators. Used alone and followed by spontaneous delivery, there is a significant decrease in the danger of sulcus and vaginal tears.[37] Assuming the need for subsequent forceps use, the hand used for rotation depends upon the location of the occiput. The left hand would be used to guide the toe of the right forceps blade after rotation from a right occipit transverse (ROT) to OA. Thus the left hand is used to rotate a ROT. The fingers are introduced into the vagina behind the posterior parietal bone with the palm upward and the thumb over the anterior parietal bone. The head is then flexed, if possible, and rotated toward OA. Fundal pressure fixes the head and the posterior blade of the forceps is applied as the fingers splint the head in its new position. Rotation is usually easiest with the biparietal diameter at the plane of greatest pelvic dimension.

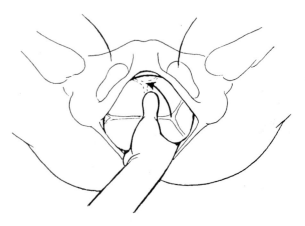

Figure 5.   Manual rotation of the head.

Higher displacement of the head, even disengagement, is considered potentially hazardous. However, some operators feel that resorting to this alternative is an acceptable risk, with fundal pressure reengaging the rotated head in OA, provided that immediate recourse to abdominal delivery is available.

Classical forceps

Forceps rotation with a classical instrument is also commonly used, although accurate application of the forceps to the head in OT is more difficult to accomplish than in anterior positions. More points of obstruction may be met in wandering the anterior blade. Mid-forceps rotations are particularly difficult, since the pelvic curve of the instrument is not available to aid application when the fetal head is in the transverse position and the perineum may obstruct adequate depression of the handle of the anterior blade. The Simpson-type instrument may be used, but the Elliot-type overlapping shanks offer less resistance to rotation and application may be slightly easier.[34]

Initial application of the anterior blade has been advocated.[38] The author prefers application of the posterior blade first. The blade (the left blade in a LOT) is introduced directly posterior to the head following the plane of least resistance until the handle is below the horizontal. The handle is lower with increasing height of the head. To compensate for the pelvic curve of the instrument, the handle must deviate laterally away from the midline during insertion so that the toe stays in the midline. The anterior blade (the right blade in the case of a LOT) is introduced as high as possible under the pubic ramus with the handle initially almost vertical. The handle descends through an arc of nearly 180°. The heel of the blade is simultaneously wandered upward with pressure from the fingers of the vaginal hand. The blades are locked with the shanks as close as possible to one finger's breadth medial to the posterior fontanelle. Standard checks of application apply. Rotation is then accomplished with rotation of the handles through a wide arc consistent with the pelvic curve of the instrument. If obstruction is met the head may require slight upward displacement so that

rotation may be facilitated close to the plane of greatest pelvic dimension. The application is rechecked and readjusted, if required, prior for traction for delivery.

Kielland's forceps (see **Figure 6**)

The Kielland's forceps is the most popular instrument worldwide for transverse positions of the occiput. The construction of the instrument offers a single accurate application for easy rotation and extraction, correction of asynclitism, and a semi-axis traction pull. Use of the instrument should result in fetal results equivalent to those of cesarean section for the same clinical situation.[28,29,31,39]

The instrument should not be used in a flat pelvis or when short anteroposterior diameters are present, as in such cases rotation is associated with an increased risk of maternal injury. The lack of pelvic curve may also increase the risk of injury during extension of the head at delivery. Due to the special characteristics of this instrument, the operator must not use the same approach as with conventional forceps.

Prior to application, the bladder should always be emptied and the patient positioned with the buttocks overhanging the edge of the delivery table. The instrument is held in a position of use so that the knobs, or buttons, on the shanks can be oriented toward the occiput. The anterior blade is usually inserted first. Four application methods are possible. With a very low station, the blade may be applied directly from below upward. In Kielland's original inversion application, the blade is inserted in an inverted manner, concavity of the cephalic curve upward, beneath the symphysis and anterior to the head. The toe is carried into the uterus until the 'elbow' of the leading edge of the shank is close to the pubis. At this point, the blade can be rotated 180° on its own axis. The forcep will then drop onto the head with the cephalic curve applied to the anterior parietal bone. If difficulty is encountered, the anterior blade is removed in favor of a wondering application. It may be wandered over the occiput in case of a flexed head or over the face in case of an extended head. Some operators fear the inversion application (sometimes called the classical application) and rou-

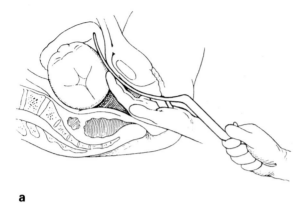

a

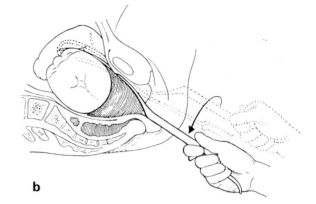

b

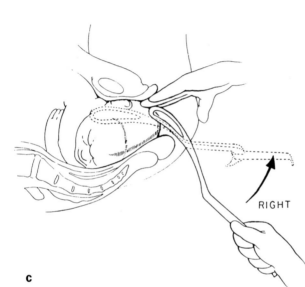

c

RIGHT

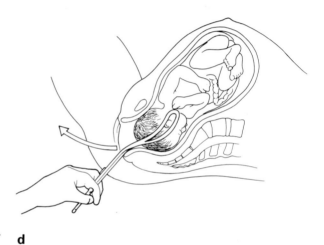

d

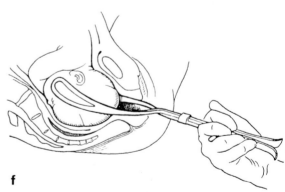

e

f

Figure 6. The use of Kielland's forceps. LOT **a**, **b** Classical (inversion) method of application of anterior blade. **c** Direct application of anterior blade to low head. **d** Wandering application of anterior blade. **e** Direct application of posterior blade (anterior blade in place). **f** Traction after rotation to OA.

tinely use the wandering method. The chance of meeting obstruction is greater with wandering.

With the anterior blade in place, the posterior blade is introduced posterior to the head, with the cephalic curve upward, following the plane of least resistance. Obstruction is frequently met at the sacral promontory. This is overcome with a lateral shift to avoid the obstruction. When in place, the instrument's sliding lock is engaged with the handles at approximately 45° below the horizontal in a midforceps procedure. The level of the handles depends upon the level of the biparietal diameter, being higher with a lower head. Any asynclitism is corrected by equalizing the level of the fingerguards. Correction of inadequate flexion is facilitated if the blades are unlocked and separately wandered to one finger's breadth medial to the posterior fontanelle. They are then relocked and moved back toward the midline. Rotation toward OA is accomplished, usually with remarkably little effort, by rotating the instrument along its axis. If resistance is met, lowering the plane of the handles should be tried. Continued resistance may be due to a relative obstruction at that level. The head should first be drawn downward in transverse position for 1 cm and rotation attempted. If unsuccessful, displacement of the head to above the original station for rotation at a better level should then be performed.

Following rotation to OA, application should be rechecked. Extraction may be performed with the Kielland forceps. The operator must remember that the nearly straight instrument must be pulled in a lower plane below the horizontal and should not be raised above the horizontal at delivery. Some change to another instrument for better traction. In the experience of the author, such a change is usually unnecessary.

Other forceps

The Barton forceps, with its hinged anterior blade, is another alternative for managing transverse arrest. Its main indication is the rare contraindications for the Kielland's, the short or flat maternal pelvis.[35,38] In a woman with short anteroposterior pelvic dimensions, the head is brought down in the transverse position. It is then rotated to OA as it traverses the plane of the outlet. The need for this instrument is so infrequent that the reader is referred to standard texts for its use.[16,38]

In the USA and Canada, specialty instruments (Mann, Laufe, Shute and other forceps) have been devised for rotation from OT or from OP. These instruments have regional advocates. Similarly, the Moolgaoker[18], has attracted followers in the UK and on the European continent. The ventouse and, of course, cesarean section are also alternative management options.

Occiput Posterior

Many occiput posterior (OP) positions will eventually rotate spontaneously to OA and deliver. Similar options to those for the OT are available when delivery is required from an OP position. Before any procedure is carried out, the operator must know in which direction to rotate the head, if it is not in an oblique posterior position. Position earlier in labor, palpation of the fetal back, or even ultrasound location of the back should resolve the question.

Procedure: Occiput Posterior Position

Manual rotation

Manual rotation either with or without subsequent forceps extraction is an option. The technique is similar to that for an OT with rotation being carried up to 180° rather than 90°.

Classical forceps

A classical instrument rotation from OP is usually performed with the modified Scanzoni maneuver, a double application method. A single upside-down application from below followed by a 180° rotation has been described, but is not popular.[37] In the Scanzoni technique, an Elliot-type instrument is preferred. It is applied to the OP as if it were in an OA position. In a ROP position, the blades would be applied as if the position were LOA. The shanks should be just above the posterior fontanelle on checking application. The rotation to OA is accomplished with rotation of the handles through a wide arc, ending with the handles pointing downward. The blades are now upside-down with toes pointing posteriorly. One blade should be left as a splint against backward rotation, while the other is removed downward, then inverted and reinserted between the splinting blade and the head. The splinting blade is then removed downward prior to reapplication in standard manner to the OA vertex. An ordinary forceps technique is then used for delivery. Some operators prefer to substitute a better tractor at the reapplication. The use of a solid blade or indented fenestration instrument for rotation prevents insertion of one blade through a fenestration in the other blade inside the vagina.

Kielland's forceps

Kielland's forceps is probably the most popular method of rotation of an OP. The previous comments on the instrument (see OT management) apply. Application to a posterior occiput differs in that the blades, with buttons toward the occiput, are applied directly from below the thighs to the appropriate position on the head. The inversion method of application is not used if the occiput is from 5 to 7 o'clock in position. Other aspects of technique are not different from those discussed in rotation from OT. Similarly, special rotational instruments as previously noted are very effective for rotation of the posterior occiput.

Delivery as OP

Delivery as a posterior is an option which is advocated by those who fear that rotational procedures may be traumatic. An indication for delivery without rotation can exist in an anthropoid pelvis with dangerously narrow transverse dimensions. Also, with a funnel pelvis, usually android, with the head molded into the outlet under a narrow arch, delivery in OP is indicated. An OP delivery is relatively traumatic, as unfavorable diameters must be brought through the pelvis. The biparietal diameter is usually higher than

anticipated. More force is required and the direction of the force is critical. More perineal space is required. An axis traction instrument or at least a Simpson-type instrument should be employed. Applied as in the first step of a Scanzoni, the shanks are depressed against the perineum to get close to the posterior fontanelle. The blades are then locked and the application is checked. With traction, after the anterior fontanelle clears the symphysis, the head is delivered by flexion rather than by extension.

Procedure: The 'Aftercoming Head' of a Breech

Following delivery of the arms and body of the infant, the body is wrapped in a towel, care of which is placed in the hands of the assistant. The presence of an assistant is mandatory. The assistant is admonished to avoid elevating the body of the child above the horizontal. Thus the extremities are removed from the field but the risk of cervical hyperextension injury due to elevation of the body is avoided. In the controlled breech delivery, the back is upwards and the head enters the pelvis within a few degrees of mentum posterior. Position is determined manually. The Piper forceps are applied upward from a kneeling position. The left blade is applied first, guided by two fingers of the right hand. The handle is started beneath the patient's right thigh, then swept downward and medially as the toe passes upward to the right parietal area of the infant. The handle then rests 45°–50° below the horizontal. The right blade is similarly applied upwards from beneath the left thigh and the lock is engaged. Application is checked by palpation of the chin between the shanks of the instrument. The infant is then allowed to straddle the instrument and traction is applied to the fingerguards in a direction similar to routine forceps use. Vectoring is not necessary, since the reverse pelvic *curve gives the required axis traction. The head is routinely delivered with the forceps in place.*

Procedure at Cesarean Section

The use of forceps to deliver the head from the uterine incision at cesarean section[37] can sometimes decrease traumatic extension of the incision. Wrigley or short Simpson forceps are usually employed. A single vectis blade, to turn and elevate the occiput through the uterine incision, can have the same effect. The Murless instrument, with a single, hinged, locking blade, is more popular in England. It is introduced unlocked, laterally, and swept beneath the head. When locked in position, it acts as a vectis and elevator to deliver the head.[37] The ventouse has also been advocated for this purpose, and is a reasonable alternative.

COMPLICATIONS

The complications of forceps operations may be maternal or fetal. Most of the complications have also been reported following spontaneous vaginal and even abdominal delivery, but the incidence is greater with forceps delivery. Since operative vaginal delivery is so often accompanied by other fetal and labor factors which are associated with birth injury, assessment of causation is frequently problematic. It is obviously difficult for the operator to disclaim responsibility for an injury found following a delivery in which forceps were used.

Maternal complications are usually those of soft tissue trauma. They can include uterine, cervical or vaginal injury, laceration or hematoma. Bladder or urethral injury may occur, including postpartum urinary retention and late fistula formation. Rectal laceration, with or without episiotomy, and subsequent fistula may occur. Increased blood loss is not uncommon with more difficult procedures.

Fetal complications include transient facial forceps marks, bruising, abrasion, laceration, cephalhematoma, subgaleal hematoma and intracranial hemorrhage. Cephalhematoma may be associated with an underlying skull fracture.[40] Brachial plexus palsy related to shoulder dystocia is more common with operative vaginal delivery. Facial nerve palsies are slightly more common than in spontaneous deliveries.[41] The questions of related long-term neurologic damage is inconclusive and is under continued investigation.[12] Some studies show a relationship between cerebral palsy and difficult forceps procedures, whereas others have failed to confirm such a relationship.[27] It is generally believed that most neurologic deficit problems are unrelated to incidents occurring at delivery or to substandard obstetrical care.[42]

CONCLUSIONS

The thinking related to forceps delivery should include several significant points:

- Injury is the result of force applied to tissues which resist that force. Such resistance can be felt and should be obvious. The operator who does not apply force of injurious magnitude does not injure.

- More important than the leading bony point of the head is the biparietal diameter – the widest and most critical diameter, which must be moved. It contains the pivot point of the head.

- The location and movement of the blade and toes of the forceps are the critical factors in safe application and should be the primary consideration in movement of the handle.

- The forceps should be checked prior to use. Rogue instruments from different manufacturers differ in dimensions and a mismatch of blades can apply asymmetrical force to the head.[43]

- All forceps procedures should be considered a trial, to be performed with care and with adequate facilities for timely abdominal delivery in the case of a negative trial.

- Protection is afforded to the operator by recording of the cognitive processes of decision for and execution of the forceps operation. A specific detailed documentation in the patient's record is always indicated.

FORCEPS DELIVERY
Summary of Management Options

Indications

Maternal

- Distress/exhaustion

- Certain maternal medical disorders

Fetal

- Presumed fetal jeopardy

- ? Breech delivery

Process

- Malposition (OP/OT)

Contraindications

- Unengaged head

- Malposition (face/brow)

- Inability to define position

- ? Head above level of ischial spines

- Macrosomic fetus (>4.0 or 4.5 kg estimated weight, especially if diabetes)

- Inexperience/lack of training

Prerequisites

- Engaged head

- ? At or below level of spines

- Fully dilated

- Known presentation and position

- Empty bladder (? not for outlet forceps)

- Adequate analgesia

- Experienced operator and adequate support facilities

Procedure

Normal (OA)

- Usually lithotomy position

- Clean, gown and catheterize (see above)

- Left blade first (unless ROA oblique)

- Recheck application placing both blades

- Traction of appropriate amount and direction with contractions (not usually more than three)

- Episiotomy (some consider this optional)

- If no descent, recheck application, dilatation, position, pelvic capacity/pathology

- Cesarean section (rather than ventouse) if no descent on second attempt

- Make adequate written record after

OT/OP

- Options are manual rotation/ventouse/rotational forceps; selection is based on personal preference or experience rather than scientific guidelines

Breech

- Options are forceps/manual for head

- No guidelines exist for best method

Complications

Maternal

- Trauma (bladder, urethra, uterus, cervix vagina)

- Hemorrhage

- Thromboembolic disease

Fetal

- Trauma

- Neurological

REFERENCES

1   American College of Ostetricians and Gynecologists (1989) *Obstetric Forceps*. ACOG Committee Opinion No. 71, August, Washington, DC.

2   Healy DL, Laufe LE (1985) Survey of obstetric forceps training in North America in 1981. *American Journal of Obstetrics and Gynecology* 151:54.

3   Kaminski HM, Stafl A, Aiman J (1987) The effect of epidural analgesia on the frequency of instrumental obstetric delivery. *Obstetrics and Gynecology* 69:770.

4   Hoult IJ, MacLennan AH, Carrie LES (1977) Lumbar epidural analgesia in labour: Relation to fetal malposition and instrumental delivery. *British Medical Journal* 1:14.

5   American College of Obstetricians and Gynecologists (1991) *Operative Vaginal Delivery*. ACOG Technical Bulletin No.152, Wasington, DC.

6   Williams MC, Knuppel RA, O'Brien WF, Weiss A, Kanarek KS (1991) A randomized comparison of assisted vaginal delivery by obstetric forceps and polyethylene vacuum cup. *Obstetrics and Gynecology* 78:789.

7   Perkins RP (1987) Fetal dystocia. *Clinics in Obstetrics and Gynecology* 30:56.

8   Boyd ME, Usher RH, McLean FH, Norman BE (1986) Failed forceps. *Obstetrics and Gynecology* 68:779.

9   Fairweather DVI (1981) Obstetric management and follow-up of the very low birth-weight infant. *Journal of Reproductive Medicine* 26:387.

10 O'Driscoll K, Meagher D, MacDonald D, Goeghegan F (1981) Tramatic intracranial hemorrhage in firstborn infants and delivery with obstetric forceps. *British Journal of Obstetrics and Gynaecology* 88:577.

11 Schwartz DB, Miodovnik M, Lavin JP (1983) Neonatal outcome among low birth weight infants delivered spontaneously or by low forceps. *Obstetrics and Gynecology* 62:283.

12 Laube DW (1986) *Clinics in Obstetrics and Gynecology* Forceps delivery. 29:286.

13 Steer, PJ. (1982) Has the expression 'fetal distress' outlived its usefulness? *British Journal of Obstetrics and Gynaecology* 89:690–693.

14 Milner RDG (1975) Neonatal mortality of breech deliveries with and without forceps to the aftercoming head. *British Journal of Obstetrics and Gynaecology* 82:783.

15 Myers SA, Gleicher N (1987) Breech delivery: Why the dilemma? *American Journal of Obstetrics and Gynecology* 156:6.

16 Dennen PC (1988) *Forceps Deliveries*, 3rd edn. Philadelphia, PA: F.A. Davies.

17 Tan KL (1973) Brachial palsy. *Journal of Obstetrics and Gynaecology of the British Empire* 117:51.

18 Moolgaoker A (1962) A new design of obstetric forceps. *Journal of Obstetrics and Gynaecology of the British Commonwealth* 69:450.

19 Benedetti TJ, Gabbe SG (1978) Shoulder dystocia: A complication of fetal macrosomia and prolonged second stage of labor with midpelvic delivery. *Obstetrics and Gynecology* 52:526.

20 Hagadorn-Freathy AS, Yoemans ER, Hankins GDV (1991) Validation of the 1988 ACOG forceps classification system. *Obstetrics and Gynecology* 77:356.

21 Robertson PA, Laros RK, Zhao RL (1990) Neonatal and maternal outcome in low-pelvic and midpelvic operative deliveries. *American Journal of Obstetrics and Gynecology* 162:1436.

22 Niswander KR, Gordon M (1973) Safety of the low forcep operation. *American Journal of Obstetrics and Gynecology* 117:619.

23 Friedman EA, Sachtleben-Murray MS, Dahrouge D, Neff RK (1984) Long term effects of labor and delivery on offspring: A matched pair analysis. *American Journal of Obstetrics and Gynecology* 150:941.

24 Gilstrap LC, Hauth JC, Schiano S, Connor KD (1984) Neonatal acidosis and method of delivery. *Obstetrics and Gynecology* 63:681.

25 Seidman DS, Laor A, Gale R, Stevenson DK, Mashiach S, Danon YL (1991) Long-term effects of vacuum and forceps deliveries. *Lancet* 337:1583.

26 Yancey MK, Herpolsheimer A, Jordan GD, Benson WL, Brady K (1991) Maternal and neonatal effects of outlet forceps delivery compared with spontaneous vaginal delivery in term pregnancies. *Obstetrics and Gynecology* 78:646.

27 Richardson DA, Evans MI, Cibils LA (1983) Midforceps delivery: A critical review. *American Journal of Obstetrics and Gynecology* 145:621.

28 Lowe B (1987) Fear of failure: A place for the trial of instrumental delivery. *British Journal of Obstetrics and Gynaecology* 94:60.

29 Dierker LJ, Rosen MG, Thompson K, Lynn P (1986) Midforceps deliveries: Long-term outcome of infants. *American Journal of Obstetrics and Gynecology* 154:764.

30 Bashore RA, Phillips WH, Brinkman CR (1990) A comparison of the morbidity of midforceps and cesarean delivery. *American Journal of Obstetrics and Gynecology* 162:1428.

31 Dierker LJ, Rosen MG, Thompson K, Debanne S, Linn P (1985) The midforceps: Maternal and neonatal outcomes. *American Journal of Obstetrics and Gynecology* 152:176.

32 Hughey MJ, McElin TW, Lusskey R (1978) Forceps operations in perspective, I. Mid-forcep rotation operations. *Journal of Reproductive Medicine* 20:253.

33 Hughey, MJ, McElin TW (1978) Forceps operations in perspective. II. Failed operations. *Journal of Reproductive Medicine* 21:177.

34 Dennen EH (1959) Choice of forceps. *Clinics in Obstetrics and Gynecology* 2:367.

35 Buekens P, Lagasse R, Dramaix M, Wollast E (1985) Episiotomy and third degree tears. *British Journal of Obstetrics and Gynaecology* 92:820–823.

36 Healy DL, Quinn MA, Pepperell RJ (1982) Rotational delivery of the fetus: Kielland's forceps and two other methods compared. *British Journal of Obstetrics and Gynaecology* 89:501.

37 Douglas-Stromme (1988) *Operative Obstetrics*, 5th edn. Norwalk, CT: Appleton and Lange.

38 O'Grody JP (1988) *Modern Instrumental Delivery*. Baltimore, MD: Williams and Wilkins.

39 Traub AI, Morrow RJ, Ritchie JWK, Dornan KJ (1984) A continuing use for Kielland's forceps? *British Journal of Obstetrics and Gynaecology* 91:894–898.

40 Zelson C, Lee SJ, Pearl M (1974) The incidence of skull fractures underlying cephalhematomas in newborn infants. *Journal of Pediatrics* **85**:371.

41 Levine MG, Holroyde J, Woods JR, Siddiqi TA, Scott M, Miodovnik M (1984) Birth trauma: Incidence and predisposing factors. *Obstetrics and Gynecology* **63**:792.

42 Niswander K, Henson G, Elborne D *et al.* (1984) Adverse outcome of pregnancy and the quality of obstetric care. *Lancet* **2**:827.

43 Hibbard BM, McKenna DM (1990) The obstetric forceps – are we using the appropriate tools? *British Journal of Obstetrics and Gynaecology* **97**:374.

66

Ventouse Delivery

ROBERT H. HAYASHI

INTRODUCTION

Ventouse delivery is an operative vaginal delivery using a vacuum extractor instrument. Early descriptions of attempts at using vacuum extraction for delivery were published in Europe by Youngs (1706) and Simpson (1849), but it was not until Malstrom introduced his metal cup in 1952 that the technique came into general use.[1] Today, the vacuum extractor has nearly replaced forceps use in some parts of the world; however, for reasons which are not clear, there has been some reluctance to use it in English speaking countries.

INSTRUMENTATION

The principal idea of the vacuum extractor is to use a cup device attached by tubing to a pump to create enough negative pressure to allow traction on the cup. In this way, traction is transferred to the fetal head (scalp) which is thereby pulled along the birth canal axis. Traction is applied during a uterine contraction, resulting in descent of the fetal head by a push–pull effect. Positioning of the cup on the fetal head and the development of a caput succedaneum are important considerations.

Malstrom devised a metal cup with rounded edges and an outside diameter of 60 mm, with the vacuum tubing and traction chain coming off the center of the back of the cup dome. By gradual increments of negative pressure, the fetal scalp is sucked into the hollow of the shallow cup to create a caput succedeaneum called a 'chignon'. Placement of the chignon is very important and a major determinant of outcome. If properly placed at the 'flexing point' of the fetal head, a point located on the sagittal suture 3 cm in front of the posterior fontanelle, traction will result in maximal flexion of a synclitic head.[2,3] Deviations of the placement may result in deflexed and asynclitic fetal head attitudes and consequent failure of the vacuum extractor technique (see **Figure 1**). Assuming that the length of the sagittal suture is approximately 9 cm at term, when the cup is properly placed on the 'flexion point', the leading edge of the cup will be about 3 cm away from the anterior fontanelle.[3] Proper cup positioning is crucial to move the fetal head from a mid-pelvic level to the plane of the outlet of the birth canal and thus positioning should always be a primary concern when performing a ventouse delivery.

An important modification to the Malstrom vacuum extractor was designed by Bird.[2] He moved the vacuum hose and traction chain attachment from the dome to the lateral wall or rim of the cup. This modified cup was to be used specifically for posterior and lateral positions of the occiput. This alteration allowed easier placement of the cup over the flexing point and its utility has been supported by an observational study in Portsmouth.[4]

Traction force studies have suggested that 22.7 kg (50 lb) of traction force may be the upper limit of fetal safety for assisted deliveries.[5–7] Duchon noted that with a vacuum cup having a diameter of 60 mm, a vacuum of 550–600 mmHg (0.8 kg/cm^2) will allow 22 kg of traction force before detachment or 'pop off' occurs.[8] This should be considered the end-point of safety and

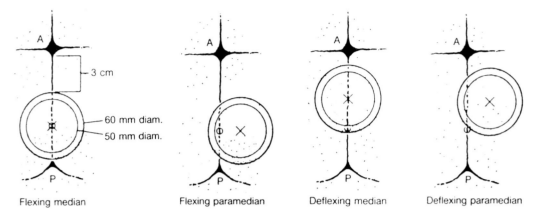

Figure 1. Applications of a 50 mm vacuum cup: the 'flexing median' application should be used in order to avoid deflexion and/or asynclitism. Reproduced with permission from Chalmers I, Enkin M, Keirse MJNC (eds) (1989). *Effective Care in Pregnancy and Childbirth.* Oxford: Oxford University Press.

inappropriate increases in vacuum should be avoided to minimize fetal morbidity. Repeated detachments of the cup are often associated with scalp injury.

In 1973, Koboyashi introduced a single unit pliable Silastic cup with a stainless steel valve on the stem that allows for relief of a significant amount of the suction force to the scalp between contractions without loss of application of the cup to the fetal head.[9] The Silastic cup diameter is 65 mm and it fits over the fetal occiput like a skull cap. The advantage of this design over the metal cup is that there is less scalp trauma because the cup has no rigid edge and can shape to the fetal head. Also, there is no need to take time to develop a chignon so that traction can be applied shortly after proper application. The disadvantage is that placement of the cup center over the flexing point of the fetal head is not easily done on a non-flexed head in the mid-pelvic area. Two randomized comparisons of the soft cups with rigid cups have been reported.[10,11] Both found a higher failure rate with the Silastic cup, especially with occiput posterior positions. On this basis, Silastic cup use should be restricted to easy or to outlet procedures. Nevertheless, because of the perceived increased safety and convenience of the soft cup, this device has nearly replaced the metal cup for use in vacuum extractor deliveries in the USA.

In 1973, a three-component plastic system vacuum extractor composed of a disposable plastic replica of the Malstrom cup with a flexible handle stem that can be attached to disposable plastic tubing and reusable hand pump was described by Paul *et al.*[12] from the University of Southern California. They reported favorably on their experience with the device. The cup was 50 mm in diameter and required the development of a chignon as with the rigid cup. The advantage over the rigid cup was the simplicity of assembly because

there were fewer parts to fit together. Also, defective tubing and rough edges on the cup were avoided. In later years, the cup was modified to remove the necessity of forming a chignon before traction. The cup diameter was increased to 60 mm and the cup shaped like a tea-cup (i.e. the dome was deepened). This device is called a Mityvac.

Since maintained vacuum or negative pressure is crucial for effective use of the vacuum extractor and 'pop offs' can result in fetal scalp trauma, properly maintained equipment to provide an airtight seal within the pump and tubing is essential. The equipment should be regularly serviced and defective parts (including smooth rimmed cups) replaced. The operators should test run the system for air leakage immediately before applying the cup to the fetal head.

INDICATIONS

The indications are essentially the same as for forceps delivery (see Chapter 65). The vacuum extractor should be used to assist the gravida by the push–pull effect in the second stage of labor if there is a demonstrated lack of progress in descent despite adequate uterine contractility. This may occur due to maternal exhaustion or lack of maternal effort secondary to conduction anesthesia or be secondary to a malposition of the fetal head.

The vacuum extractor can be used electively to shorten the second stage, particularly in gravidas with heart disease or other maternal complications requiring the avoidance of stress. Finally, the vacuum extractor can be used if fetal distress in the second stage indicates the need for a rapid delivery. Some have advocated use of the vacuum extractor for delivery of the vertex presenting second twin.

CONTRAINDICATIONS

The contraindications are essentially the same as for forceps delivery (see Chapter 65). The vacuum extractor should not be used in situations where dystocia is thought to be due to cephalopelvic disproportion or where fetal position cannot be confidently determined. It should not be applied to an unengaged fetal head or used to deliver a premature fetus, since the incidence of serious fetal injury is probably increased in such cases. Caution should be used if a vacuum extractor is used on a fetus who has had fetal scalp blood samplings performed earlier in labor, since there has been one report of exsanguination of an infant when ventouse delivery followed fetal blood sampling.[13]

PREREQUISITES

Use of the vacuum extractor should be confined to the second stage of labor, even though some have advocated its use at 9–10 cm cervical dilatation. The operator should be experienced in its use (or if learning, should have an experienced operator physically present to advise) and be willing to abandon the technique if progressive descent does not occur. The majority of ventouse deliveries occur in 3–5 pulls.[3,14]

Procedure: Ventouse Delivery

After determining that there is a clear indication for a ventouse delivery, the operator should discuss the following issues with the patient and/or her partner: the options at this juncture of her care, the advantages and disadvantages of the vacuum extractor, the expected outcome and any complications (both minor and serious). These issues should be recorded at some time close to the procedure.

Ideally, the operator should have a choice of vacuum extractor types depending on the situation. A Silastic or plastic cup can be used for a flexed, relatively synclitic fetal head at the pelvic outlet, whereas for a deflexed, asynclitic fetal head, use of the Malstrom cup carries a higher chance of successful delivery. If fetal head malposition such as occiput posterior or transverse causes dystocia, then use of the Bird cup (or similar device) would be a good choice. An improperly chosen instrument lessens the chance of a successful outcome. Prior to application

of the cup to the fetal head, the operator must check the pump, hose and cup, fully assembled, for proper and maintained negative pressure when the cup is applied to the palm of a gloved hand.

After the patient has been washed with antiseptic solution and draped in the dorsal lithotomy position for delivery, the operator should empty the urinary bladder and then check the fetal head position and station. Analgesia should preferably be by regional block, placed previously. However, an alternative for deliveries expected to be straightforward is a pudendal block with perineal infiltration of local anesthetic.

The application technique of the cup will differ depending on whether the cup is metal or soft.

Malstrom metal cup

For the Malstrom metal cup, betadine or an antiseptic soap solution is applied to the rim of the cup and the cup slipped carefully into the vagina. The cup is then positioned over the flexing point of the fetal head with the rim nearest to the anterior fontanelle positioned 3 cm from it (see **Figure 1**). *The negative pressure of the system is increased to 0.2 kg/cm² and the perimeter of the cup is checked for entrapped cervical or vaginal tissue. Negative pressure is increased by 0.2 kg/cm² every 2 min to a maximum pressure of 0.8 kg/cm² in order to build the chignon. At this point, traction in the axis of the birth canal can be applied during uterine contractions.*

By placing a hand in the vagina with the thumb on the cup and index finger on the fetal scalp, traction force can be monitored in the following manner. Gradually increase the traction force until the cup begins to slip away from the fetal scalp, diminish the traction somewhat and hold for the remainder of the uterine contraction. Release traction between uterine contractions. The expectation is that the presenting part should descend with each push–pull event and the head be delivered within 3–5 pulls. The fetal heart rate is monitored throughout the procedure with an external fetal heart rate monitor. Once the head is delivered, the suction is disconnected and the cup removed.

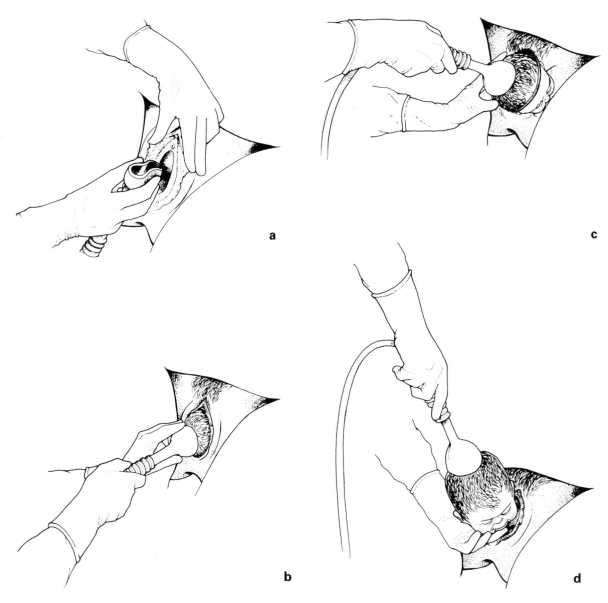

Figure 2. Delivery with ventouse.

Soft Cup (see **Figure 2**)

For application of the soft cup, a flexed synclitic fetal head position is presumed. After application of betadine or antiseptic soap solution to the cup rim, the edges of the cup are carefully folded in to diminish its diameter and it is then inserted into the vagina. Because of the larger overall size of the Silastic cup, periurethral and labial lacerations can occur easily unless extra care is taken. Once on the fetal head, the operator should palpate around the edges of the cup to clear any trapped tissues, move the stem of the cup as close to the flexing point near the occiput as possible and pump the negative pressure to 0.2 kg/cm². A further check should be made for any tissue under the cup rim, then a uterine contraction should be awaited. With the onset of a uterine contraction, the negative pressure is increased to 0.8

VENTOUSE DELIVERY
Summary of Management Options

Indications

Maternal

- Distress/exhaustion
- Certain maternal medical disorders

Fetal

- Presumed fetal jeopardy
- ? Breech delivery

Process

- Malposition (OP/OT)

Contraindications

- Unengaged head
- Malposition (face/brow)
- Inability to define position
- ? Head above level of ischial spines
- Macrosomic fetus (>4.0 or 4.5 kg estimated weight; especially if diabetes)
- Inexperience/lack of training
- ? Repeated scalp pH estimations

Prerequisites

- Engaged head
- ? At or below level of spines
- ? Fully dilated (some argue for 9+ cm)
- Known presentation and position
- Empty bladder (? not for outlet delivery)
- Adequate analgesia
- Experienced operator and adequate support facilities

Procedure

- Lithotomy, clean, gown and catheterize
- Choose cup of appropriate size and orientation
- Ensure correct position of application
- Recheck position after initial 0.2 kg/cm^2
- Increase to 0.8 kg/cm^2
- Appropriate traction with contractions in correct direction
- Episiotomy (some consider this optional)
- If no descent, recheck application, dilatation, position, pelvic capacity/pathology
- Options if no descent on second attempt are forceps or cesarean section
- Make adequate written record after

Complications

Maternal

- Trauma (bladder, urethra, uterus, cervix vagina)
- Hemorrhage
- Thromboembolic disease

Fetal

- Trauma
- Alopecia in infancy
- Neurological

*kg/cm² and traction exerted, placing the intravaginal hand and fingers as above to monitor the traction force (**Figure 2b**). After the contraction, the partial release valve mechanism is triggered to drop the negative pressure to 0.2 kg/cm² between contractions. Expectations for progress are the same as above. The operator using a vacuum extractor must be willing to abandon the technique if obvious progress of descent is not evident within 3–5 push–pull events or after several 'pop offs'.*

COMPLICATIONS

Maternal injury using the vacuum extractor is usually reported to be less common than with forceps delivery,[4,15,16] although not invariably so.[17] Entrapment of the cervix or vaginal wall between the cup edge and fetal head can cause laceration but should rarely occur with careful use. Placement of the cup intravaginally can result in periurethral and vaginal lacerations if done carelessly or forcefully. Neonatal morbidity is higher overall when using vacuum extractor over forceps; cephalohematoma, bruising and superficial lacerations are a particular risk with the rigid cup. However, even the soft cup has been associated with serious sequelae. Both subgaleal hematomas and tentorial tears with intracranial hemorrhage have been reported but the overall incidence is unknown at this time. Subgaleal hematomas are thought to be due to disruption of the diploic vessels in the loose subaponeurotic scalp tissue that allows a large volume of bleeding to occur over time.[18] The entire scalp can be elevated. Tentorial tears have been associated with mechanical injury to the fetal cranium and are thought to be related to the shearing forces on the tentorium resulting in rupture of the deep venous system or laceration of the inferior surface of the cerebellum.[19] Although the pathophysiology is not clearly understood, the vacuum extractor may produce stress on the fetal cranium in the occipital frontal diameter, with tension on the tentorium. The tentorium may then rupture, causing intracranial hemorrhage. Because of these uncommon, but serious sequelae in infants following a ventouse delivery, all such infants should be carefully observed for a reasonable period of time for any neurologic signs of irritability, drowsiness, tachypnea, seizure activity or an enlarging head size.[16] All such signs should be carefully investigated. Fortunately, most reported series of vacuum extractions have not recorded these complications.

Several long-term studies of term infants delivered by vacuum extractor have shown no increase in mental retardation or cerebral palsy, nor any differences from infants delivered by forceps.[20–23]

REFERENCES

1 Malstrom T (1961) The vacuum extractor. I. Indications and results. *Acta Obstetrica et Gynecologica Scandinavica* **43**:5–52.

2 Bird GC (1976) The importance of flexion in vacuum extractor delivery. *British Journal of Obstetrics and Gynaecology* **83**:194–200.

3 Vacca A (1990) The place of the vacuum extractor in modern obstetric practice. *Fetal Medicine Review* **2**:103–122.

4 Vacca A, Grant A, Wyatt G, Chalmers I (1983) Portsmouth operative delivery trial: A comparison of vacuum extraction and forcep delivery. *British Journal of Obstetrics and Gynaecology* **90**:1107–1112.

5 Wylie B (1935) Traction in forceps deliveries *American Journal of Obstetrics and Gynecology* **29**:425.

6 Moolgaoker A, Ahamed O, Payne P (1979) A comparison of different methods of instrumental delivery based on electronic measurements of compression and traction. *Obstetrics and Gynecology* **54**:299–309.

7 Laufe LE (1971) Divergent and crossed obstetric forceps: Comparative study of compression and traction forces. *Obstetrics and Gynecology* **38**:885–887.

8 Duchon M, DeMund M, Brown R (1988) Laboratory comparison of modern vacuum extractors. *Obstetrics and Gynecology* **71**:155–158.

9 Maryniak G, Frank J (1984) Clinical assessment of the Kobayashi vacuum extractor. *Obstetrics and Gynecology* **64**:431–435.

10 Hammarstrom M, Csemiczky G, Belfrage P (1986) Comparison between the conventional Malstrom extractor and a new extractor with Silastic cup. *Acta Obstetrica et Gynecologica Scandinavica* **65**:791–792.

11 Dohn M, Barclay C, Fraser R, Zaklama M, Johanson R, Anderson D, Walker C (1989) A multicentre randomized trial comparing delivery with a silicone rubber cup and rigid metal vacuum extractor cups. *British Journal of Obstetrics and Gynaecology* **96**:545–551.

12 Paul R, Staisch K, Pine S (1973) The 'new' vacuum extractor. *Obstetrics and Gynecology* **41**:800–802.

13 Ott WJ (1975) Vacuum extraction. *Obstetrics and Gynecological Survey* **30**:643–649.

14 Lasbrey A, Orchard C, Critchton D (1964) A study of the relative merits and scope for vacuum extraction as opposed to forceps delivery. *South African Journal of Obstetrics and Gynecology* **2**:1–3.

15 Johanson R, Pusey J, Livera N, Jones P (1989) North Staffordshire/Wigan assisted delivery trial. *British Journal of Obstetrics and Gynecology* **96**:537–544.

16 Chalmers JA, Chalmers I (1989) The obstetric vacuum extractor is the instrument of first choice for operative

vaginal delivery. *British Journal of Obstetrics and Gynaecology* **96**:505–509.

17 Punnonen R, Aro P, Kuukankorpi A, Pystynen P (1986) Fetal and maternal effects of forceps and vacuum extraction. *British Journal of Obstetrics and Gynaecology* **93**:1132–1135.

18 Boo N (1990) Subaponeurotic haemorrhage in Malaysian neonates. *Singapore Medical Journal* **31**:207–210.

19 Hannigan W, Morgan A, Kokinski L, Stahlberg M, Hiller J (1990) Tentorial hemorrhage associated with vacuum extraction. *Pediatrics* **85**:534–539.

20 Byre I, Dahlia K (1974) The long term development of children delivered by vacuum extraction. *Dev Med Child Neurol* **16**:378–381.

21 Plena G, Svenningsen M, Gustafson B, Sunder B, Cronquist S (1977) Neonatal and prospective follow up study of infants delivered by vacuum extraction. *Acta Obstetrica et Gynaecologica Scandinavica* **56**:189–194.

22 Carmody F, Grant, A Mutch M, Vacca A, Chalmers I (1986) Follow up of babies delivered in a randomized comparison of vacuum extraction and forceps delivery. *Acta Obstetrica et Gynecology Scandinavica* **65**:763–766.

23 Ngan H, Miu P, Ko L, Ma H (1990) Long term neurological sequelae following vacuum extractor delivery. *Australia and New Zealand Journal of Obstetrics and Gynaecology* **30**:111–114.

67

Cesarean Section

JAN E. DICKINSON

INTRODUCTION

Cesarean birth has been reported sporadically throughout medical history, but has been technically refined and rendered safe for both mother and fetus only in this century. Today, cesarean birth is performed in 15–25% of all deliveries in most developed countries, with an associated maternal mortality of less than 1 : 1000. The safety of the lower uterine segment technique, the development of skilled anesthesia (both general and regional), the availability of blood products and antibiotics, the broadening of indications for the operation, the recognition of the fetus as a patient, the feasibility of vaginal delivery following cesarean section and the acceptance of this procedure by women have characterized this operation in the twentieth century. These factors have all contributed to the rapid rise in the incidence of cesarean birth over the past 50 years.

The lower uterine segment operation, pioneered by Munro Kerr in the early twentieth century, is now performed in over 90% of cesarean operations.[1] This operative procedure is now enabling many women safely to achieve a vaginal delivery in a subsequent pregnancy. It is, however, sobering to remember that a cesarean section is a major surgical procedure and that perioperative complications remain a cause of maternal mortality and morbidity.

INDICATIONS FOR CESAREAN SECTION

During the past decade, the cesarean delivery rate has risen progressively throughout the world, though more dramatically in some countries than in others. In 1984, cesarean delivery became the number one in-hospital operative procedure in the USA[2] and accounted for 21% of all live births. In 1987, this figure climbed to 25%,[3] and is projected to reach 30% in this decade. This increasing rate has been attributed to the performance of elective repeat cesareans and primary cesareans for fetal distress and breech presentation.[4] In Europe and the UK, the increase in the cesarean section rate has been less dramatic, with reported operative rates half those of their trans-Atlantic neighbor.

There are four major indications for cesarean section in the USA: previous cesarean section (35%), dystocia (29%), malpresentation (10%) and fetal distress (8%) (**Table 1**).[3] The percentages for previous cesarean section are lower in the UK and for the other indications

Table 1
Indications for cesarean section

Dystocia	35%
Elective repeat cesarean section	29%
Malpresentation	10%
Fetal distress	8%
Others	18%
multifetal gestations	
placental abruption	
placenta previa	
fetal disease	
gynecologic cancer	
obstruction	

Data from Taffel *et al.*[3]

correspondingly higher. There is, however, no single indication for a cesarean delivery; this procedure is necessary whenever vaginal delivery cannot be safely accomplished without risk to the mother or fetus.

The contemporary obstetric literature is replete with articles on methods to decrease the cesarean birth rate. Despite the multitude of such articles, there is little evidence to suggest that a reduction in the number of abdominal deliveries will occur and the need for all obstetricians to be adept at this surgical procedure remains.

OPERATIVE TECHNIQUE OF CESAREAN SECTION

Observation and participation in surgical procedures during training will assist each individual to evolve his or her own personal operative method and style. In this time-honored way, all surgeons develop their individual variations of operative procedures. The cesarean section is no exception to this adage, and each surgeon stamps the operation with his or her personal style and technique.

Cesarean section is the most frequent major surgical procedure performed in obstetrics and gynecology.[5] The majority of women undergoing cesarean section are young and frequently in their first pregnancy. There is therefore a need to balance a cosmetic skin incision with adequate exposure to safely deliver the infant and complete the surgical procedure. The size of the abdominal incision is a critical factor in the degree of difficulty of delivery. In a prospective study, a significant negative correlation between perceived delivery difficulty and incision size was reported.[6] An abdominal incision size of 15 cm or greater was associated with significantly less difficulty in cesarean delivery. It is of no benefit to anyone to substitute a technically difficult cesarean section for a difficult vaginal delivery.

The Abdominal Incision for Cesarean Birth

As with any surgical procedure, preoperative positioning of the patient and preparation of the surgical area is important. Left lateral tilt will minimize maternal inferior vena caval compression. A urinary catheter usually remains *in situ* perioperatively, draining continuously to a closed system. The removal of pubic and abdominal hair down to the upper level of the labia majora is followed by application of antiseptic solution to the skin, usually povidone iodine. It is important to perform shaving as short a time before the procedure as possible, as shaving several hours before (or, even worse, the previous day) encourages skin infections in the nicks and grazes which are unavoidable during the procedure and increases the incidence of wound infections subsequently. Plastic adhesive drapes are no more effective than linen drapes in preventing wound infections and may adversely affect healing.[7]

The choice of the abdominal incision and its closure should be individualized to the characteristics of the patient and the circumstances demanding operative intervention. The massively obese gravida will require a different operative technique than used on the unscarred abdomen of a thin nulligravida. The ideal incision provides prompt surgical access, adequate exposure and a secure wound closure.

Two basic types of skin incisions are used:

- suprapubic (Pfannenstiel) transverse

- midline vertical

Each has its advantages under particular surgical and obstetric circumstances. The transverse skin incision has the advantage of improved cosmesis, less postoperative pulmonary dysfunction (being performed in the skin lines it is less painful for the mother to breathe deeply postoperatively) and superior wound strength. Mowat and Bonnar[8] reported that abdominal wound dehiscence after cesarean delivery was eight times more common with vertical compared with transverse incisions, although this differential has probably been reduced by the use of the mass closure technique using a continuous nylon suture. However, the transverse incision is more difficult to enlarge quickly (it is necessary to use diathermy to cut the rectus muscles) and postoperative wound collections are not infrequent, particularly in patients who are obese or have bleeding disorders. The vertical incision allows rapid surgical access to the abdomen, superior visualization of the intra-abdominal contents and can be enlarged without difficulty. In 1976, Haeri[9] reported no significant difference between the two incisions in terms of operating time (53 *vs* 45 min, transverse *vs* vertical incision, respectively), postoperative febrile morbidity (30/100 *vs* 48/100) and post-cesarean hemoglobin <10 g/dl (28/100 *vs* 36/100).

Procedure: Abdominal Incision

The Pfannenstiel incision

The excellent cosmetic appearance and low incidence of wound dehiscence and hernia formation have made this incision extremely popular among obstetricians and patients. The disadvantages stated in the previous paragraph render it unsuitable for complicated surgical cases such as the exploratory laparotomy for hemorrhage. In a series of 48 cases, Ayers et al.[6] noted that 75% of cesarean sections with a Pfannenstiel incision less than 13 cm in diameter were associated with a perceived increase in difficulty of fetal delivery.

The skin and subcutaneous tissue are incised using a transverse, slightly curvilinear incision made at the level of the pubic hairline and extending beyond the lateral borders of the rectus muscles. The subcutaneous tissue and underlying fascia are separated, and the latter is then transversely incised along the central 1–2 cm. Scissors then cut the fascia bilaterally. Both subcutaneous tissue and fascia can alternatively be divided by traction in opposite lateral directions by the surgeon and assistant, the so-called 'rip' technique. The fascial sheath is separated from the underlying rectus muscles superiorly and inferiorly by blunt dissection. The perforating blood vessels may bleed during this maneuver and care with hemostasis is necessary. Separation is performed cephalad to permit an adequate longitudinal incision of the peritoneum. The rectus muscles are separated from each other and the underlying transversalis fascia and peritoneum. The latter are then incised to expose the peritoneal cavity and the uterus.

Closure is performed in anatomic layers. Evidence is accumulating against routine closure of the peritoneum.[10–13] Many surgeons place drains in the subfascial space to reduce hematoma formation. Drains should be used when there is preoperative infection or when a large moist potential space is left. A continuous running synthetic suture to close the rectus fascia is used in patients with clean wounds. Fascia should not be closed with chromic catgut, which has a low relative strength and high tissue reactivity. The high strength and low tissue reactivity of polyglycolic acid (Dexon®), polyglactin (Vicryl®) or one of the sutures with delayed absorption such as monofilament polyglyconate or polydioxanone, make these sutures ideal for fascial closure. Interlocking continuous sutures may slow the healing process by decreasing vascularization. A Smead-Jones internal retention suture using monofilament polypropylene has been suggested for obese patients or patients with altered healing mechanisms who are at higher risk for dehiscence and incisional hernias.[14–16] A closed drainage system may be required anterior to the fascia (e.g. in the obese patient, or with unsatisfactory hemostasis). Subcutaneous sutures are usually unnecessary, although a few interrupted plain catgut sutures may be needed to eliminate dead space and reduce skin tension. The skin can be closed with staples or a subcuticular suture. Occasionally, a case of peritoneal contamination occurs (presence of frank pus or enterotomy) and delayed closure with open packing for 5–7 days is advisable.[14]

The Cohen incision

This incision[17] permits quick and bloodless entry to the peritoneal cavity. A straight transverse incision is made between two points 2 cm inferior and medial to the anterior superior iliac spines. The subcutaneous tissue is divided in the relatively bloodless midline for 3 cm and the central rectus sheath is then similarly incised. By blunt dissection and traction vertically and laterally, the subfascial space is opened. The peritoneum is opened transversely, high above the bladder.

The Cherney incision

The modified Cherney incision may be used when the low transverse abdominal incision is not adequate to deliver the fetus safely or is too small to obtain adequate exposure to deal with intraoperative complications. The incision is about 25% longer than a midline incision from the umbilicus to the symphysis[18] and pelvic sidewall exposure is provided. Prior to incising the rectus abdominus muscles, the inferior epigastric vessels are located by developing the space of Retzius in the midline with blunt dissection. The recti are sharply dissected from their pubic insertion and the peritoneal incision can then be extended laterally 1–2 cm above the bladder. Following closure of the uterus, the rectus tendons are sutured to the lower segment of the rectus sheath. The remainder of the closure is routine, although drainage of the subfascial space may be necessary.

The Maylard incision

The Maylard transverse muscle-cutting incision provides good pelvic exposure but the delivery time is significantly longer when compared with the Pfannenstiel incision.[6] This renders the incision unsuitable for most routine cesarean deliveries.[19] The incision can be used for exploration for postpartum bleeding and in pregnant patients with adnexal masses, although it provides only limited upper abdominal exposure. Reapproximation of the recti is best achieved by suturing to the overlying fascia. Fascial closure will then result in reapproximation of the muscles.

The infraumbilical vertical incision

The vertical skin incision has been the traditional approach to enter the peritoneal cavity, although it now has been usurped by the more cosmetic low transverse incision. The main indications are a previous midline vertical incision, obesity or if the operative diagnosis is uncertain, for example in trauma to the pregnant abdomen or an intra-abdominal tumor mass.

The lower midline incision is made from the umbilicus to the symphysis pubis. It may be extended around the umbilicus toward the xiphisternum for additional exposure, although this is infrequently required with the abdominal distension of pregnancy. Sharp dissection is performed to the level of the anterior rectus sheath, which is freed of subcutaneous fat to expose a strip of fascia in the midline about 2 cm wide. Physiologic separation of the rectus abdominus muscles is usually present. The rectus sheath may be incised with the scalpel or, after an initial small opening, be completed with the scissors. This latter approach is probably more common, due to a putative reduction in bleeding and accidental damage to the underlying structures. Midline separation of the rectus and the pyramidalis muscles exposes the transversalis fascia and peritoneum. Using two hemostats, the peritoneum is elevated at the cephalad end of the incision to create a fold. This maneuver permits inspection and palpation of the underlying peritoneal contents. The peritoneum is incised superiorly and then inferiorly to the vesical peritoneal reflection.

In the massively obese patient, a vertical skin incision with avoidance of the subpanniculus fold is indicated. The higher wound infection rates in this subpopulation[20] requires modification of perioperative procedures. Gallup et al.[14] reduced the wound infection rate from 42 to 3% by careful perioperative techniques. If a transverse incision is chosen for the obese patient, it should be away from the subpanniculus fold.

Closure of midline incisions should be effected with a running continuous suture of polyglycolic acid, large-bore monofilament polypropylene or similar delayed absorbable suture.[21–24] A Smead-Jones internal retention suture closure with monofilament polypropylene is recommended in the massively obese patient to reduce dehiscence and incisional hernia rates.[25] The continuous running closure is rapid, cost-efficient, minimizes foreign material in the wound and distributes tension equally. Fagniez et al.[25] reported no difference in dehiscence rates in a randomized prospective trial of 3135 patients when assessing the use of running vs polyglycolic acid sutures in midline incisions. A closed drainage system, located anterior to the rectus sheath, may be required. Subcutaneous sutures may be used and the skin closed with surgical staples or subcuticular suture.

The paramedian incision

In the upper abdomen, paramedian incisions have been recommended due to their wound strength. Secondary to the *termination of the posterior rectus sheath at the level of the arcuate line, this advantage is not present in the lower abdomen. In a prospective study, Guillou et al.[26] found the incidence of hernia occurrence in midline and paramedian incisions to be essentially the same. Suspected appendicitis remains a possible indication for a right paramedian incision in pregnancy.*

The Uterine Incision for Cesarean Birth

The clinical situation prompting the need for abdominal delivery determines the uterine incision to deliver the fetus (**Figure 1**). The low transverse uterine incision is used in over 90% of cesarean deliveries.[1] This high prevalence is due to its ease of repair, reduced adhesion formation, lower blood loss and low incidence of dehiscence or rupture in subsequent pregnancies.[1] A previous low transverse uterine incision renders most women eligible for a trial of labor in a subsequent pregnancy. The disadvantages of the low transverse incision are primarily restricted to situations in which the lower uterine segment is undeveloped. In this circumstance, there is a greater chance of lateral extension into the major uterine vessels, resulting in maternal morbidity from hemorrhage. If the initial incision is inadequate to deliver the fetus, extension of the uterine incision to a 'J' or a 'U' or an inverted 'T' incision will be required, creating a more vulnerable scar.

The low vertical incision,[27] also a lower segment incision, may be used in situations where the transverse incision is inappropriate, predominantly in patients with an underdeveloped lower uterine segment. When used in these circumstances, there is a lower risk of lateral extension into the uterine vessels. The incision may be extended upward into the body of the uterus if more room is needed. An upper uterine segment extension renderes closure more difficult and precludes a subsequent trial of labor. More extensive dissection of the bladder is necessary to keep the vertical incision within the lower uterine segment. If the incision extends downward, it may tear through the cervix into the vagina and possibly the bladder. The low vertical incision may be used if a contraction ring needs to be cut in order to deliver the infant. If the vertical incision is confined to the lower uterine segment, there is a low probability of dehiscence and/or rupture in a subsequent pregnancy,[1] and such patients may be eligible for a subsequent trial of labor.

Infrequently performed in modern obstetrics, the classical uterine incision is a vertical incision into the upper uterine segment. It is required in circumstances where exposure of the lower uterine segment is inadequate, in elective cesarean hysterectomy, or in cases of a non-correctable back-down transverse lie. The incision permits rapid delivery and reduces the risk of bladder injury as the bladder is not dissected. When an anterior placenta previa is present, an upper segment incision may be used to avoid incising the placenta. However, dissection around the placenta following a lower segment incision will eliminate the need for a classical uterine incision. The many disadvantages of the classical uterine incision result in its limited use in obstetrics today. The incision is more complicated and time-consuming to repair, the incidence of infection is higher and adhesion formation is common. There may be a greater risk of incision rupture during subsequent pregnancies[1,28] and, if rupture occurs, the resultant bleeding is much greater than with the relatively avascular lower segment. The fetus is also more likely to be completely expelled from the uterus into the peritoneal cavity. For these reasons, most obstetricians consider a vertical upper uterine incision to be a contraindication to a trial of vaginal delivery, committing women to elective repeat cesarean deliveries.

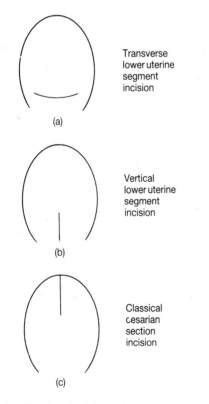

(a) Transverse lower uterine segment incision

(b) Vertical lower uterine segment incision

(c) Classical cesarian section incision

Figure 1. Uterine incisions for cesarean section.

Procedure: Uterine Incision

Low transverse uterine incision

The uterus is palpated to identify the size and the presenting part of the fetus and to determine the direction and degree of rotation of the uterus. Moistened laparotomy packs may be placed in the paracolic gutters to absorb uterine contents; however, this is probably unnecessary.

A Balfour retractor blade is inserted inferiorly and the loose reflection of vesicouterine serosa overlying the uterus held in the midline with forceps, cut with scissors and opened transversely just above the upper margin of the bladder. The inferior visceral peritoneum is then grasped with forceps and the bladder is reflected from the underlying lower uterine segment with sharp or blunt dissection. The developed bladder flap is held beneath the symphysis pubis with the bladder retractor.

A 1–2 cm transverse uterine incision is made in the lower uterine segment above the detached bladder through the myometrium. Suction is useful during this maneuver to assist visualization and avoid inadvertent fetal laceration. The incision is then extended laterally with scissors. A lateral wall retractor can aid visualization as the incision is extended. Lateral and upward pressure with each index finger is useful to complete the uterine incision. Some surgeons prefer to split the myometrium digitally after the initial incision; this is a quicker technique but it does not protect the uterine vessels as well, the incision is more ragged and it increases the risk of downward extension of the uterine angles. The uterine incision should be adequate to deliver the fetus without extension into the broad ligament and trauma to the uterine vessels. Curving the incision upward bilaterally, avoiding the lateral uterine vessels, will provide additional room if required. Conversion of the incision to a 'J', a 'U', inverted 'T' or anchor incision by upward midline extension into the upper uterine segment may be necessary if these steps are insufficient, usually secondary to inadequate assessment of the uterus prior to commencement. Although preferable to a traumatic delivery through an inadequate incision, these latter circumstances will contraindicate a subsequent trial of labor because of the greater risk of uterine rupture.[1,28] Conversion to a Cherney incision will permit improved exposure if the abdominal incision is inadequate.

The bladder retractor is removed and if the fetal presentation is cephalic, the membranes are ruptured (if still intact) and the fetal head delivered by elevation through the uterine incision manually or with forceps.

Fundal pressure assists the delivery of the fetal head. Short-handle forceps (Wrigley's or short Simpson's) are useful if the fetal head is high. Some surgeons advocate the use of the vacuum extractor in place of forceps, although the application and delivery time is longer with this instrument. In situations of fetal malpresentation, the infant is manually extracted as appropriate to the individual case. If the placenta is in the incision line, it should be detached, rather than incised, as the latter is associated with fetal hemorrhage. If the head is wedged in the maternal pelvis, disimpaction by the upward pressure of an assistant per vaginam may be required.

Commonly, the nose and oropharynx of the baby are suctioned before the body is delivered. The body is then delivered using gentle traction and fundal pressure. The infant is maintained at the level of the maternal abdomen, the umbilical cord is clamped and cut, and the infant handed to the neonatal staff after parental visualization of the infant if appropriate.

Once the fetus is delivered, oxytocin is administered to aid uterine contraction and placental separation. Regimens differ markedly from country to country. In the UK, 5 IU oxytocin is administered intravenously to the mother and a dilute intravenous solution of oxytocin commenced. In North America, the bolus injection is not given and the oxytocin infusion (20 units/liter, titrated to produce adequate uterine contraction) alone is administered. In Australia, the infusion is omitted in routine cases and parenteral oxytocics alone are used. Maternal antibiotics are administered prophylactically in most centers, though sometimes this is on a reflective rather than comprehensive basis (e.g. in cases of non-elective cesarean section with prior rupture of the membranes) to decrease the incidence of postoperative endomyometritis (see below). Umbilical cord blood samples are then obtained from the placental end of the cord.

The placenta is delivered manually or with cord traction and inspected for completeness. The uterus may be exteriorized for repair. This procedure is not necessary but does assist visualization and technically facilitates repair of the uterine incision, especially if there have been lateral extensions. The relaxing uterus can be promptly recognized and massage applied, potentially decreasing intraoperative blood loss. Hershey and Quilligan[29] reported lower blood loss in women undergoing exteriorization repair (mean reduction in hematocrit 6.2 ± 0.35 vs 7.0 ± 0.43, exteriorization vs intraperitoneal, respectively; $P < 0.01$). No increase in febrile morbidity has been reported with uterine exteriorization.[29] The main adverse effect is pain and vagal-induced vomiting with traction when the woman is awake and the cesarean is being performed under regional anesthesia. The uterine cavity is examined and wiped with a moist laparotomy sponge to remove any remaining debris. Some surgeons probe for cervical patency with a ring forceps to ensure lochia drainage in non-labored cases.

The placement of a ring or Green-Armytage forceps at each uterine angle and the inferior incision edge improves visualization and reduces blood loss during incision repair. On occasion, the thinned lower uterine incision edge may be missed and the bulging posterior wall inadvertently incorporated into the closure; care should be taken to avoid this error. The uterine incision can be closed with one or two layers. The initial stitch should be positioned just beyond the angle of the incision. If closing in two layers, then a continuous locking stitch of absorbable suture through the myometrium can be used in the first layer. Interrupted sutures may also be used. Once inserted, the needle should not be withdrawn to minimize bleeding from myometrial vessels perforated and then not enclosed in the suture. The running-lock suture is continued just beyond the opposite angle of the incision. Traditionally, chromic catgut was used to close the uterine incision. The current trend is toward use of the less reactive and stronger synthetic absorbable sutures, although there is no convincing evidence of their advantage and they sometimes have a tendency to cut through the muscle tissue with a 'cheesewire' type of effect. Early reports expressed concern at the incorporation of decidua in the incision line resulting in scar endometriosis and weakening of the scar.[30,31] This now appears to be a rare complication[32] and the avoidance of decidual incorporation is probably an unnecessary prolongation of operating time. If the lower uterine segment is thin or reapproximation with one layer has been achieved with adequate hemostasis, a two-layer closure is unnecessary.[33] If a second layer is used, an inverting suture is used with a continuous vertical or horizontal Lembert's stitch. Once repaired, the incision is assessed for hemostasis and figure-of-eight sutures used to control any bleeding.

The pelvic organs are inspected and necessary adnexal procedures, such as tubal ligation, performed. The uterus is then returned to the peritoneal cavity. Recent reports indicate the closure of peritoneal surfaces to be unnecessary[10] and, indeed, detrimental with higher adhesion formation rates.[11-13] If the individual surgeon deems closure necessary, the vesicouterine serosa may be reapproximated with a running suture of 00 chromic or polyglycolic acid. The lower edge of the peritoneum and the attached bladder should not be carried above the line of the uterine incision, as urinary frequency and discomfort during later pregnancies[34] and difficult dissection of adherent peritoneum with subsequent cesarean section or hysterectomy may result.

The incision site is reinspected for evidence of bleeding, blood and amniotic fluid are suctioned from the paracolic gutters and cul de sac, and with a correct needle and sponge count the abdominal wall is closed as previously described.

Low vertical incision

The low vertical incision is most useful where there is a malpresentation, in multifetal pregnancies, or where there is delivery of a very immature fetus through *a non-labored uterus. This uterine incision requires more extensive bladder mobilization than the low transverse incision. The incision is commenced as low as possible in the exposed lower segment and is extended superiorly for a distance to enable safe delivery of the fetus. Encroachment into the active upper segment may occur.*

In closure of the low vertical uterine incision, the initial stitch is positioned beyond the inferior edge of the incision and a running or running-lock stitch of absorbable suture used to close the incision. One or two layers of myometrial suture may be used, depending upon the individual surgeon's preference. Following completion of the uterine closure, the operative procedure is completed as outlined in the previous section.

Classical cesarean section

There are few remaining indications for performing a classical cesarean section in contemporary obstetrics. Inadequate exposure or development of the lower uterine segment, transverse fetal lie at or near term and some cases of anterior placenta previa form the major indications for the procedure. Most obstetric surgeons rarely perform this procedure.

The classical cesarean incision extends anteriorly from just above the bladder to the upper uterine fundus. There is no dissection of the bladder. The initial scalpel incision is usually extended with bandage scissors to the uterine fundus. Continuous or interrupted layers of absorbable suture are used to close the uterine incision. A three-layer surgical closure is usually required, secondary to the myometrial thickness of the active segment. Potter and Elton[35] have suggested that interrupted sutures placed in the outer third of the uterus only may be adequate for uterine closure. The final layer is inverted to eliminate any raw surface areas and help reduce adhesion formation. The upper segment uterine incision is a well-known contraindication for a subsequent trial of labor.[1,28]

Extraperitoneal cesarean section

Prior to the advent of effective antibiotics, extraperitoneal cesarean section was rec-ommended in cases of infection as an alternative to cesarean hysterectomy.[36,37] Although there remain a few advocates of this procedure today,[38] it is generally considered obsolete and the increased operative morbidity has essentially relegated it to the history books.

COMPLICATIONS OF CESAREAN SECTION

Cesarean section is a major abdominal surgical procedure and is thus subject to the well-known complications – medical, anesthetic and surgical – that are associated with any laparotomy (**Table 2**). It is beyond the scope of this chapter to deal with all the potential complications that may surround a cesarean section. However, it is important to remember that the maternal morbidity and mortality associated with cesarean section are often related to the administration of anesthesia.[39,40] An emergency cesarean performed on an unprepared patient, who may also have other medical disorders, is not a procedure for an anesthesiologist inexperienced in obstetric anesethesia. Identification of potential high-risk surgical patients and preliminary anesthetic assessment before delivery is vital.

Table 2
Complications of cesarean section

Anesthesia-related
    aspiration syndrome
    hypotension
    spinal headache

Hemorrhage
    uterine atony
    placenta previa/accreta
    lacerations

Urinary tract and gastrointestinal injuries

General postoperative complications
    respiratory: atelectasis/pneumonia
    gastrointestinal: ileus
    urinary tract infections
    thromboembolism

Endomyometritis

Wound infection

Hemorrhage

Hemorrhage at the time of cesarean section may be related to the operative procedure, such as damage to the uterine vessels, or be incidental, such as due to uterine atony or placenta previa/accreta. The origin of the excess blood loss is generally apparent at the time of surgery. Hemorrhage secondary to uterine atony is initially dealt with by conservative measures such as bimanual pressure, infusion of oxytocin, administration of methergine and/or 15 methyl PGF$_{2\alpha}$. If there is inadequate response to these measures, uterine artery ligation and/or hypogastric artery ligation may be proceeded to, with hysterectomy if these procedures fail. Severe post-cesarean atony is associated with the use of magnesium sulfate, oxytocin augmentation of labor, preoparative chorioamnionitis, fetal macrosomia, and cesarean delivery for dystocia.[41]

The incidence of placenta accreta appears to be increasing[42] and is now second only to uterine atony as an indication for emergency hysterectomy for obstetric hemorrhage.[41] There is an association of placenta accreta with placenta previa and previous cesarean delivery, both of which have been increased by the recent trend toward more liberal indications for cesarean delivery. Clark *et al.* reported that 25% of patients undergoing cesarean section for placenta previa in the presence of one or more uterine scars subsequently underwent cesarean hysterectomy for placenta accreta.[42] This risk appears to increase directly with the number of previous uterine incisions. Effective management almost always requires total abdominal hysterectomy.[41,42] The uterus, vagina or broad ligament may be lacerated during a cesarean delivery. Traumatic deliveries or poor delivery technique are associated with an increased frequency of operative lacerations. Lacerations involving uterine tissue are usually sutured without difficulty. Vertical lacerations into the vagina or lateral extensions into the broad ligament may be associated with significant blood loss and the potential for ureteric damage during their repair. Prior to commencement of the repair of lacerations into the broad ligament, identification of the ureter is frequently necessary. The initial suture must be inserted just distal to the apex of the laceration.

Urinary Tract Injuries

Injuries to the urinary bladder occur with variable incidence during the course of cesarean delivery.[43,44] The Pfannenstiel incision with lower entry into the peritoneal cavity increases the risk of inadvertent cystotomy, especially after prolonged labor where the bladder is pulled cephalad. Scarring and secondary obliteration of the vesicouterine space following previous cesarean section increase the incidence of trauma secondary to attempts at dissection. The bladder may also be damaged secondary to a uterine laceration, particularly in association with a low vertical uterine incision.

Various techniques are employed to reduce the incidence of intraoperative bladder injury. Preoperative catheterization of the bladder and peritoneal entry as far cephalad as possible are important. Injuries to the base of the bladder are most frequent during a repeat procedure where clear tissue planes do not always exist. Careful sharp rather than blunt dissection of the bladder will reduce the occurrence of inadvertent cystotomy as well as reducing blood loss. If there is concern as to possible bladder injury, the abdomen must not be closed until the issue is resolved by transurethral instillation of methylene blue-colored saline with leakage of fluid identifying the cystotomy site.

Full thickness bladder lacerations should be repaired with a two-layer closure with continuous or interrupted 2-0 or 3-0 chromic catgut. The site of the bladder laceration is important as a laceration of the bladder dome and its subsequent repair are usually straightforward. The bladder base appears to heal more slowly, is thinner, receives less blood flow and occlusion of the ureteric orifice is a possibility. Fistula formation is usually not a problem if accidental cystotomy is promptly recognized and repaired.

Ureteral injury is one of the most dreaded complications of any pelvic operation. It is, however, an uncommon occurrence at cesarean section. Eisenkop *et al.*[45] reported seven ureteral injuries in 7527 patients undergoing cesarean delivery. In five, the ureteric injury occurred during an attempt to control hemorrhage from an extension of the uterine incision. When controlling hemorrhage, it is useful to apply direct pressure while identifying the course of the ureter to permit accurate suture placement and reduce the potential for ureteral injury.

Postoperative Complications

As with any surgical procedure, various complications may occur following cesarean section. Medical personnel caring for the woman recovering from a cesarean delivery need to be aware of the major postoperative complications and to act promptly to provide effective therapy when required.

Basic supportive care to provide adequate analgesia, fluids and nutrition, early ambulation and respiratory therapy to minimize postoperative atelectasis are mandatory. The postoperative observation of cardiovascular and respiratory status, in addition to uterine consistency, vaginal blood loss and incision care, are axiomatic. Respiratory complications remain a primary cause of postoperative morbidity following major surgical procedures. Deep breathing exercises, incentive spirometry, chest percussion and postural drainage all have merit, depending on the clinical circumstance.

Gastrointestinal dysfunction is not common after a cesarean delivery and is usually restricted to a transient ileus. Urinary tract infections occur with a reported frequency of 2–16%.[46]

Thromboembolic disease during pregnancy is an uncommon event but remains a major cause of maternal morbidity and mortality. The greatest incidence in the puerperium is among cesarean patients. The risk of a deep venous thrombosis after cesarean delivery is 3–5 times greater than after vaginal delivery.[47] In the management of the cesarean patient, the physician must consider the risks associated with the hypercoagulable state of pregnancy.

Endomyometritis

In the absence of prophylactic antibiotics, post-cesarean endomyometritis occurs with an incidence of 35–40%.[48] Postoperative infections may be reduced by 50–60% with the use of prophylactic antibiotics at the time of cesarean delivery.[49,50] In approximately 10% of cases, concurrent bacteremia will accompany post-cesarean endomyometritis.[48,49] Uncommonly, post-cesarean endomyometritis may be complicated by pelvic abscess, septic shock and septic pelvic thrombophlebitis. The major risk factors for the development of post-cesarean infection are young age, low socioeconomic status, prolonged labor, prolonged ruptured membranes and multiple vaginal examinations.

Post-cesarean section endomyometritis is a polymicrobial infection secondary to bacteria normally present in the lower genital tract – aerobic streptococci (group B and D streptococci), anaerobic Gram-positive cocci (peptococcus and peptostreptococcus), aerobic (E. coli, Klebsiella pneumoniae, Proteus spp.) and anaerobic Gram-negative bacilli (Bacteroides spp. and Gardnerella vaginalis).[48] The symptoms and signs of endomyometritis usually develop 24–48 h post-surgery. The main clinical manifestations are fever, tachycardia, lower abdominal pain, uterine and adnexal tenderness, and peritoneal irritation. Following appropriate laboratory investigation, including complete blood count, aerobic and anaerobic blood cultures and aerobic and anaerobic endometrial cultures, antibiotic therapy is instituted. There are several effective regimens available: clindamycin plus an aminoglycoside or aztreonam; penicillin plus aminoglycoside and metronidazole; or one of the extended spectrum penicillins such as ticarcillin–clavulinic acid or ampicillin–sulbactam. If a cephalosporin has been administered for prophylaxis, a penicillin should be used due to the possibility of enterococcus infection.

Most patients show a clear response to treatment within 72 h. The two most common causes of apparent treatment failure are concurrent wound infection and resistant microorganisms. If a wound infection develops, incision and drainage is indicated, but a change in antibiotics is not usually necessary. The principal microorganisms likely to be resistant to initial treatment regimes are aerobic Gram-negative bacilli, enterococci and Bacteroides spp. If a resistant organism is thought to be present, antibiotic therapy should be modified. Parenteral therapy should be continued for a minimum of 24 h after the patient becomes afebrile and asymptomatic. At this point, therapy may be discontinued. Patients do not need to be maintained on oral antibiotics after discharge from hospital. Extended therapy of this nature is expensive and increases the risk of side-effects without providing any measurable therapeutic benefit.

In patients who fail to improve after a change in antibiotic therapy, another detailed examination should be performed to detect a wound infection or pelvic abscess. Other possible causes of poor treatment response include viral syndrome, venous thrombophlebitis and drug fever.

Wound Infection

Adverse outcomes associated with abdominal wounds in obstetric patients occur more frequently in the presence of anemia, premature rupture of the membranes, prolapsed cord and meconium staining. Reported wound infection rates associated with cesarean section range from 2.5 to 16.1%.[51]

Nielson[52] found rates of 4.7% for elective cases and 24.2% for emergency cases. A mixture of anaerobic and aerobic bacteria (Staphylococcus aureus, E. coli, Proteus mirabilis, Bacteroides spp., beta-hemolytic streptococci) are isolated from post-cesarean wound infections, similar to those of postpartum endomyometritis.[53] Early diagnosis is important, and frequent inspection of the cesarean wound is paramount.

The prevention of wound infections involves careful preoperative preparation. Preoperative hexachlorophene showers,[54] clipping of the abdominal hair rather than shaving,[54,55] liberal application of skin antiseptic agents in the operating room and use of wound drapes are simple but effective measures to decrease the incidence of wound infection. Sterile technique, attention to hemostasis, obliteration of tissue dead space and removal of devitalized tissues are important surgical factors that promote appropriate wound healing and prevent wound infection. The use of closed drainage systems are preferable to Penrose-type drains, as the former remain sterile as long as flow continues.

As with any infective process, prompt recognition and treatment are essential. An infected wound is usually characterized by local pain, tenderness, erythema and purulent discharge. Systemic evidence may also be present with fever and leukocytosis. Initial treatment

---

CESAREAN SECTION
Summary of Management Options

Indications

- See **Table 1**

Operative technique

Skin incision options

- Pfannenstiel/suprapubic transverse

- Vertical subumbilical midline

Uterine incision options

- Transverse lower segment (commonest)

- Lower vertical
  - malpresentation
  - poorly formed lower segment

- 'Classical' (rarely performed) disputed/rarely accepted indications include:
  - malpresentation with little amniotic fluid
  - poorly formed lower segment
  - anterior placenta previa

Delivery of the fetus

- Head either manually or with forceps and fundal pressure

- Body with traction and fundal pressure

Oxytocic agent

- Practice varies (drug, dose and timing)

- Delivery of placenta

Prophylactic antibiotics

- Practice varies

Other techniques

- Probing cervix is not uniformly practised

- Uterine closure after inspection (± swabbing uterine cavity) with one or two layers of interrupted or continuous sutures

- 'Figure-of-eight' sutures for bleeding points

- Inspect adnexal structures

- Not all agree closure of peritoneum necessary

Complications

- See **Table 2**

---

involves opening the wound along the affected area to the fascia and culturing the exudate (anaerobic and aerobic). Incision and drainage with debridement of necrotic tissue is vital. Applications of hydrogen peroxide to chemically debride the area should follow initial local surgical efforts. As antiseptic solutions are cytotoxic, saline lavage must follow their application with the application of wet-to-dry dressings. When all necrotic tissue is removed and granulation tissue forms,

cessation of debriding agents is important and the use of wet-to-wet dressings instituted. The wound may be reapproximated once granulation tissue appears or be left to close by secondary intention. Drainage is usually sufficient and systemic antibiotics are not indicated for simple wound infections. A serious complication of wound infection is necrotizing fasciitis, a synergistic infection that destroys subcutaneous tissues. Repeated, aggressive debridement is vital in association with broad-spectrum antibiotics and hyperbaric oxygen therapy to achieve cure.

CONCLUSION

With the cesarean birth rate showing no evidence of declining, it is paramount for the obstetrician to be adept at the procedure and knowledgeable in the management of associated perioperative complications, which constitute a major portion of maternal mortality and morbidity statistics.

REFERENCES

1 Tahilramaney MP, Boucher M, Eglinton GS et al. (1984) Previous cesarean section and trial of labor: Factors related to uterine dehiscence. Journal of Reproductive Medicine 29:17–21.

2 Rutkow IM (1986) Obstetric and gynecologic operations in the United States, 1979 to 1984. Obstetrics and Gynecology 67:755–759.

3 Taffel SM, Placek PJ, Liss T (1985) Trends in the United States cesarean section rate and reasons for the 1980–85 rise. American Journal of Public Health 77:955–959.

4 Shiono PH, McNellis D, Rhoads GG (1987) Reasons for the rising cesarean delivery rates. Obstetrics and Gynecology 69:696–700.

5 Bottoms SF, Rosen MG, Sokol RJ (1980) The increase in cesarean birthrate. New England Journal of Medicine 302:559–563.

6 Ayers JWT, Morley GW (1987) Surgical incision for cesarean section. Obstetrics and Gynecology 70:706–708.

7 Alexander JW, Aerni S, Plettner JP (1985) Development of a safe and effective one-minute preoperative skin preparation. Archives of Surgery 120:1357–1361.

8 Mowat J, Bonnar J (1971) Abdominal wound dehiscence after cesarean seciton. British Medical Journal 2:256–257.

9 Haeri AD (1976) Comparison of transverse and vertical skin incisions for caesarean section. South African Medical Journal 52:33–34.

10 Hull DB, Varner MW (1991) A randomized study of closure of the peritoneum at cesarean delivery. Obstetrics and Gynecology 77:818–821.

11 Ellis H (1962) The aetiology of post operative abdominal adhesions: An experimental study. British Journal of Surgery 50:10–16.

12 Elkins TE, Stovall TG, Warren J et al. (1987) A histologic evaluation of peritoneal injury and repair: Implications for adhesion formation. Obstetrics and Gynecology 70:225–228.

13 Tulandi T, Hum HS, Gelfand MM (1988) Closure of laparotomy incisions with or without peritoneal suturing and second look laparoscopy. American Journal of Obstetrics and Gynecology 158:536–537.

14 Gallup DG (1984) Modification of celiotomy techniques to decrease morbidity in obese gynecologic patient. American Journal of Obstetrics and Gynecology 150:171–178.

15 Wallace D, Hernandez W, Schlaerth JB et al. (1980) Prevention of abdominal wound disruption using the Smead-Jones closure technique. Obstetrics and Gynecology 56:226–230.

16 Morrow CP, Hernandez WL, Townsend DE et al. (1977) Pelvic celiotomy in the obese patient. American Journal of Obstetrics and Gynecology 127:335–339.

17 Cohen SJ (1972) Abdominal and Vaginal Hysterectomy, pp. 19–30. Oxford: Allen and Mowbray.

18 Cherney LS (1941) Modified transverse incision for low abdominal operations. Surgery Gynecology Obstetrics 72:92.

19 Maylard AE (1907) Direction of abdominal incision. British Medical Journal 2:895.

20 Pitkin RM (1976) Abdominal hysterectomy in obese women. Surgery Gynecology Obstetrics 142:532–536.

21 Knight CD, Griffen FD (1983) Abdominal wound closure with a continuous monofilament polypropylene suture: Experience with 1,000 consecutive cases. Archives of Surgery 118:1305–1308.

22 Archie JP, Feldtman RW (1981) Primary abdominal wound closure with permanent, continuous running monofilament sutures. Surgery Gynecology Obstetrics 153:721–722.

23 Kratzer FL (1978) Intestinal anastomosis and abdominal wound closure using monofilament prolene polypropylene suture: report of fifty cases. Diseases of the Colon and Rectum 21:342–345.

24 Shepherd JH, Cavanagh D, Riggs D et al. (1983) Abdominal wound closures using a nonabsorbable single layer technique. Obtetrics and Gynecology 61:248–252.

25 Fagniez PL, Hay JM, Lacaine F et al. (1985) Abdominal midline incision closure. Archives of Surgery 120:1351.

26 Guillou PJ, Hall TJ, Donaldson DR et al. (1980) Vertical abdominal incisions – a choice? British Journal of Surgery 67:395–399.

27 Kronig B (1912) Transperitonealer Cervikaler Kaiser-Schnitt. In Doderlein A, Kronig B (eds), Operative Gynakologie, p. 879. Berlin.

28 Pedowitz P, Schwartz RM (1957) The true incidence of silent rupture of cesarean section scars: A prospective analysis of 403 cases. American Journal of Obstetrics and Gynecology 74:1071–1081.

29 Hershey DW, Quilligan EJ (1972) Extraabdominal uterine exteriorization at cesarean section. Obstetrics and Gyencology 52:189–192.

30 Sortor RF, Brines OA (1957) Endometriosis involving cesarean section abdominal scar: Report of a case. Obstetrics and Gynecology 10:425.

31 Kale S, Shuster M, Shangold J (1971) Endometrioma in a cesarean section scar: Case report and review of the literature. American Journal of Obstetrics and Gynecology 111:596–597.

32 Chatterjee SK (1980) Scar endometriosis: A clinicopathologic study of 17 cases. Obstetrics and Gynecology 56:81–84.

33 Hibbard LT (1986) Cesarean section and other surgical procedures. In Gabbe SG, Niebyl JR, Simpson JL (eds),

Obstetrics: Normal and Problem Pregnancies, pp. 517–546. New York: Churchill Livingstone.

34 Cunningham FG, MacDonald PC, Gant NF (eds) (1989) *Williams' Obstetrics*, 18th edn, pp. 441–459. Norwalk, CT: Appleton and Lange.

35 Potter MG, Elton NW (1942) An improved method of closure in high classical cesarean section. *American Journal of Obstetrics and Gynecology* **43**:303–308.

36 Frank F (1907) Suprasymphysial delivery and its relation to other operations in the presence of contacted pelvis. *Arch. Gynaekol.* **81**:46–94.

37 Latzko W (1909) Ueber den extraperitonealen Kaiserschnitt. *Zentralblatt für Gynaekologie* **33**:275.

38 Perkins RP (1977) Extraperitoneal section: A viable alternative. *Contemporary Obstetrics and Gynecology* **9**:55–59.

39 Shaw DB, Wheeler AS (1984) Anesthesia for obstetric emergencies. *Clinics in Obstetrics and Gynecology* **27**:112–124.

40 Rubin G, Peterson HB, Rochat RW *et al.* (1981) Maternal death after cesarean section in Georgia. *American Journal of Obstetrics and Gynecology* **139**:681–685.

41 Clark SL, Yeh S-Y, Phelan JP *et al.* (1984) Emergency hysterectomy for obstetric hemorrhage. *Obstetrics and Gynecology* **64**:376–380.

42 Clark SL, Koonings PP, Phelan JP (1985) Placenta previa/accreta and previous cesarean section. *Obstetrics and Gynecology* **66**:89–92.

43 Nielson TF, Hokegard K-H (1984) Cesarean section and intraoperative surgical complciations. *Acta Obstetrica et Gynecologica Scandinavica* **63**:103–108.

44 Mattingly RF, Borkowf HI (1978) Acute operative injury to the lower urinary tract. *Clinics in Obstetrics and Gynecology* **5**:123–149.

45 Eisenkop SM, Richman R, Platt LD *et al.* (1982) Urinary tract injury during cesarean section. *Obstetrics and Gynecology* **60**:591–596.

46 Farrell SJ, Anderson HF, Work BA (1980) Cesarean section: Indications and postoperative morbidity. *Obstetrics and Gynecology* **56**:696–700.

47 Hirsh J, Cade JF, Gallus AS (1972) Anticoagulants in pregnancy: A review of indications and complications. *American Heart Journal* **83**:301–305.

48 Duff P (1986) Pathophysiology and management of postcesarean endomyometritis. *Obstetrics and Gynecology* **67**:269–276.

49 Swartz WH, Grolle K (1981) The use of prophylactic antibiotics in cesarean section: A review of the literature. *Journal of Reproductive Medicine* **26**:595–609.

50 Cartwright PS, Pittaway DE, Jones HW *et al.* (1984) The use of prophylactic antibiotics in obstetrics and gynecology: A review. *Obstetrical and Gynecological Survey* **39**:537–554.

51 Mead PB (1979) Managing infected abdominal wounds. *Contemporary Obstetrics and Gynecology* **14**:69–75.

52 Nielsen TF, Hokegard K-H (1983) Postoperative cesarean section morbidity: A prospective study. *American Journal of Obstetrics and Gynecology* **146**:911–916.

53 Sweet RL, Yonekura ML, Hill G *et al.* (1983) Appropriate use of antibiotics in serious obstetric and gynecologic infections. *American Journal of Obstetrics and Gynecology* **136**:719–739.

54 Cruse PJE, Foord R (1973) A five-year prospective study of 23,649 surgical wounds. *Archives of Surgery* **107**:206–210.

55 Alexander JW, Fischer JE, Boyajian M *et al.* (1983) The influence of hair removal methods on wound infections. *Archives of Surgery* **118**:347–352.

68

Postpartum Hemorrhage and Other Problems of the Third Stage

DOUGLAS KEITH STILL

PRIMARY POSTPARTUM HEMORRHAGE

Postpartum hemorrhage is still a major contributor to maternal morbidity and mortality. The incidence in developed countries is 4–6% of pregnancies with 0.5% resulting in hemorrhage severe enough to cause hypotension and shock. Postpartum hemorrhage is the most common cause of excessive blood loss in pregnancy and occupies third place in the leading causes of maternal mortality in North America.[1] Hemorrhage is the fourth most common cause of maternal mortality in the UK;[2] two-thirds of hemorrhages are postpartum (the remaining fatalities being due to placental abruption). The morbidity of postpartum hemorrhage is due not only to the consequences of anemia and shock, but also to the complications of treatment such as infections with cytomegalovirus, human immunodeficiency virus and hepatitis C virus, and transfusion reactions. Acute renal failure and postpartum panhypopituitarism (Sheehan's syndrome) can also occur after severe hemorrhage.

Definition

Postpartum hemorrhage is the loss of greater than 500 ml of blood in the first 24 h postpartum. This is termed 'primary' or 'acute'. Hemorrhage occurring after the first 24 h is termed 'secondary' or 'late' postpartum hemorrhage. The clinical estimation of blood loss is notoriously inaccurate. The normal healthy gravida may not show a fall in blood pressure or a rise in pulse until 10–15% of blood volume is lost. More subtle is the slow but constant loss that goes unnoticed or ignored until vascular collapse occurs.

Because mortality and morbidity from postpartum hemorrhage is largely preventable, prompt assessment and treatment is mandatory. Because 1 g of blood is approximately equal to 1 ml, the practice of weighing linen or tampons is of value.

Postpartum collapse is evidenced by the sudden onset of fainting, dizziness and distress following delivery. Serious cases have a dramatic onset with the manifestations of circulatory collapse such as pallor, sweating and unconsciousness. The most common reason for postpartum collapse is postpartum hemorrhage, but the differential diagnosis includes dehydration, diabetic ketoacidosis and septicemia. Uterine inversion, amniotic fluid embolism, thromboembolic phenomena, and other catastrophes such as ruptured aneurysms (of the hepatic or splenic artery or cerebral berry aneurysms), or rupture of the liver or spleen may also occur. Myocardial infarction, while extremely uncommon, can also occur in the postpartum period.[2]

Etiology

The most common cause of postpartum hemorrhage is uterine atony. Other causes include trauma to the genital tract (which for the purposes of this chapter will include uterine inversion and rupture), placenta accreta and coagulation disorders. Uterine atony accounts for 75–90% of postpartum hemorrhage, while trauma and retained placenta account for most of the remainder.

About 3% of postpartum hemorrhages result from coagulation disorders.[3,4]

The predisposing factors that contribute to uterine atony are listed in **Table 1**. Many patients who experience postpartum hemorrhage due to uterine atony have multiple predisposing factors.[5] A history of previous postpartum hemorrhage is associated with a 20–25% recurrence rate.[6,7]

Trauma, the second most important cause of postpartum hemorrhage, may be due to episiotomy, lacerations or extension of the uterine incision laterally at the time of cesarean section. Placenta accreta, uterine inversion and rupture of the uterus are also causes. Coagulation disorders include congenital conditions such as von Willibrand's disease and acquired problems such as liver failure, hepatitis or anticoagulant therapy. Acute coagulopathies may develop with placenta previa, abruption, pre-eclampsia or amniotic fluid embolism. The diagnosis and treatment of the acute coagulopathies are discussed in Chapter 23. The rare appearance of acquired Factor VIII inhibitors may occur near term, to produce a condition similar to von Willibrand's syndrome. These inhibitors may lead to life-threatening hemorrhage. Treatment is by administration of cryoprecipitate and other measures to support the circulation.[8]

Patients with von Willibrand's disease seldom present a problem unless there is a significant reduction in Factor VIII C. The increasing level of clotting factors in pregnancy including Factor VIII complex may result in an improved bleeding time as pregnancy progresses.[9] It is important to evaluate these patients, preferably prior to the onset of pregnancy.

Options for Prevention and Management of the Third Stage

The management of primary postpartum hemorrhage (secondary hemorrhages will be discussed in Chapter 69) is best described in terms of anticipation and pre-

Table 1
Factors predisposing to uterine atony

Previous postpartum hemorrhage
Uterine overdistension (e.g. with twins)
High parity
Antepartum hemorrhage
Precipitate labor
Prolonged labor
Chorioamnionitis
Retained placental products
Uterine anomalies or fibroids
Uterine trauma (rupture or inversion)
Operative delivery
General anesthesia

vention. This includes identification of the women at risk for uterine atony or with a history of previous third-stage hemorrhage (from any cause), the active management of the third stage of labor and the routine use of oxytocics in the third stage. The patient with a history of previous postpartum hemorrhage requires adequate predelivery counseling regarding place of delivery and a full explanation of the preventive measures that should be used. This includes cross-matched blood held in reserve, establishing access to the circulation after the onset of labor by siting an intravenous cannula, and the preventive use of oxytocics.

The 'active management' of the third stage of labor means prophylactic use of oxytocic drugs, early clamping of the umbilical cord and controlled cord traction (Brandt-Andrews method) for the delivery of the placenta.[10,11] However, some recent authors have questioned the routine use of all the components (as defined above) of an 'active' approach to the third stage of labor.[12–15] Their arguments to date have applied more heat than light to this issue, as they range from those who promote the policy of routine manual removal/exploration of the uterus to the employment of a totally passive approach with intervention only if excessive bleeding occurs.

A comprehensive review of this issue has recently been published.[16] The conclusion of these authors was that 'the evidence from controlled trials supports the routine use of oxytocic drugs in the third stage of labour because of a reduced risk of postpartum hemorrhage. The reduction in risk is likely in the order of 30–40%. This advantage must be weighed against the somewhat small risk of hypertension and the disadvantages attending the routine use of injections'. These same authors go on to conclude that the routine use of ergonovine (ergometrine in the UK) should be stopped, because of the unpleasant side-effects of nausea and hypertension. Oxytocin is as effective as either ergonovine or the prostaglandin preparations in reducing postpartum hemorrhage and has fewer side-effects when given routinely in the third stage of labor. This does not mean that these drugs (ergonovine or prostaglandins) should never be used. They are extremely valuable in the treatment of postpartum hemorrhage as described below.

While the recommended timing of administration of oxytocics has varied from crowning until after the placenta has been delivered, there is no evidence to support any particular advantage of one method over another. My personal bias is to give an oxytocic (oxytocin 5 units) i.v. or i.m. after the placenta has been delivered, to avoid the increase in placental retention which may occur if oxytocics are given earlier.[17]

Early cord clamping reduces the length of the third stage of labor but does not have any effect on postpartum hemorrhage. In Rhesus-negative women, early clamping increases the risk of feto-maternal transfusion.

An aggressive approach to delivery of the placenta remains controversial. Brandt[11] did not originally describe this procedure as including cord traction. His technique probably evolved gradually into the technique described by Spenser[18] and commonly called the Brandt-Andrews maneuver.

Procedure: Brandt-Andrews Method (Figure 1)[19]

This method is applied after the signs of placental separation (show, lengthening of the cord, change of uterine shape), by which time the placenta is usually lying in the cervix or upper vagina. The cord is clamped close to the vulva and the clamp held with one hand. The other hand is placed on the woman's abdomen, between the symphysis pubis and the uterine fundus. As the cord is held taut, this hand is pushed upward against the uterus. There will be little resistance if the placenta has separated, and it will emerge from the uterus. If tension on the cord develops, and the bleeding is not excessive, nothing further should be done for several minutes. After this, the process is repeated until the placenta is delivered. This process rarely takes more than 5–10 min. The use of Crede's maneuver (forceful squeezing of the fundus) lacks specific advantage in prophylaxis against postpartum hemorrhage and is painful. Cord traction in one study resulted in the rupture of the umbilical cord in 3% of women managed this way.[20]

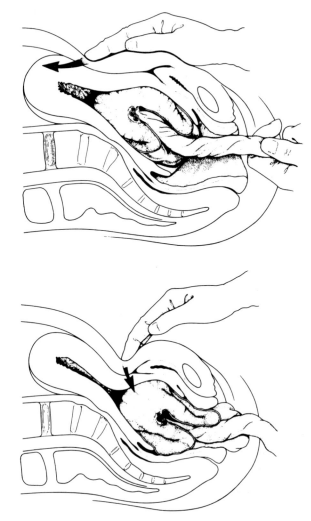

Figure 1. Brandt method of expression of placenta. (a, upper) Fundus is elevated by external pressure combined with gentle traction on cord. (b, lower) Placenta is expelled from vagina by external pressure directed into the pelvis. Reproduced with permission from Zuspan and Quilligan.[19]

In summary, the prophylactic use of oxytocics will reduce the incidence of postpartum hemorrhage. Other components of the 'active management' of the third stage have yet to be proved. There is then a place for those who would follow a kinder, gentler (less interventionist) approach to the management of the third stage. It is important to osberve the postpartum mother carefully for the first few hours following childbirth. The uterus should be checked gently to confirm that it has contracted, and any clots which have accumulated in the vagina should be removed. A full bladder should be emptied. As Ian Donald has said, 'Beware therefore of inertia – not only of the uterus but also of the attendant'.[21]

Diagnosis of Postpartum Hemorrhage

While some bleeding is inevitable during the third stage of labor because of separation of the placenta, sudden massive bleeding makes the diagnosis of postpartum hemorrhage obvious. However, excessive bleeding may also be intermittent or protracted.

Management Options

General

When the bleeding is excessive, a logical sequence of actions is:

- accurately to identify and correct the cause of bleeding;

- implement resuscitation measures (see Chapter 73).

Initial measures

Given these important underlying principles, the initial steps that should be taken are:

- to 'rub up' a contraction by massaging the fundus of the uterus and giving an extra dose of oxytocin (5–10 units), preferably i.v. since atony is the the most likely cause;

- to ensure i.v. access and dispatch blood for cross-match of at least 4 units.

Uterine atony

Uterine atony is the most common cause of excessive bleeding and initial attention should be given to this. A boggy, soft uterus with the placenta in place requires removal of the placenta; preferably by the Brandt technique. If this does not result in the delivery of the placenta, and the bleeding is excessive, manual removal may be required. This procedure (**Figure 2**) should be done under adequate anesthesia or analgesia but, in rare circumstances and in order to save life, it may have to be done without. The first step is to site a large

bore (16–18 gauge) cannula in a large vein. Blood should be sent for hemoglobin estimation and cross-matching (4 units/2 liters minimum). It is best not to proceed with the manual removal until the blood is available on the delivery suite. Once the cannula is *in situ* and the blood samples sent off, a crystalloid solution can be infused. The bladder should always be catheterized. The procedure should not be commenced until the anesthesiologist has prepared the patient appropriately.

Procedure: Manual Removal

*An aseptic technique is very important. The fundus of the uterus is grasped with one hand while the other hand is inserted into the vagina and through the cervix. The palm of this hand is introduced between the uterine wall and the placenta using the fingers in a side-to-side motion. After separation of the placenta is complete, the entire placenta is grasped and removed. It is important to re-explore the hopefully emptied uterus to confirm that no placental fragments remain. Once the uterus is confirmed empty, an intravenous infusion containing 20–40 units of oxytocin in 1 liter of crystalloid should be commenced. If bleeding is persistent, massage and manual compression can be effective (**Figure 3**).*

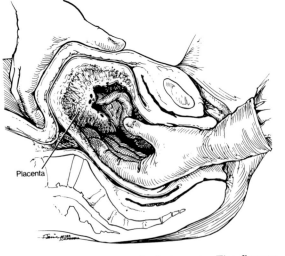

Figure 2. Manual removal of placenta. The fingers are moved from side to side until the placenta is completely detached. Reproduced with permission from Cunningham *et al.*[22]

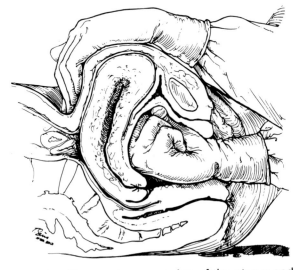

Figure 3. Bimanual compression of the uterus and massage with the abdominal hand usually will effectively control hemorrhage from uterine atony. Reproduced with permission from Cunningham *et al.*[22]

Should excessive bleeding continue and there is the possibility of retained placental fragments, curettage should be performed under general anesthesia. The postpartum uterus can easily be perforated and so great caution should be employed. This is not a maneuver to delegate to an inexperienced practitioner.

Pharmacological methods

If the uterus remains boggy and soft, ergometrine 0.25–0.5 mg may be given i.m. or i.v. The side-effects of this drug include hypertension, nausea and vomiting, especially if it is given intravenously. The main benefit of ergometrine is sustained action. Syntometrine® (5 units oxytocin and 0.5 mg ergometrine) combines the rapid onset of oxytocin with the prolonged effect of ergometrine. This drug is routinely used in some centers for prophylaxis. If the uterus remains hypotonic, a repeat injection of ergometrine is worthwhile. Great caution regarding the use of ergot derivatives should be employed in patients with pre-eclampsia, as severe hypertension may be provoked by the use of these drugs.

Prostaglandin E_2, $F_{2\alpha}$ and an analog of $F_{2\alpha}$ (the 15-methyl derivative) have been used successfully by direct injection into the uterine muscle either through the abdominal wall or into the uterine muscle at the time of laparotomy.[23,24] Injection at laparotomy is safer as it can be administered under direct vision into the myometrium. Administration through the intact abdominal wall increases the risk of inadvertent injection into a vein, with consequent collapse of the patient due to the vasodilatory effects of prostaglandin. PGE_2 can also be administered intravaginally or rectally as suppositories, or even instilled directly into the uterine cavity and held there by bimanual compression. Alternative dosage regimes for the prostaglandins are:

- $PGF_{2\alpha}$ 0.25–1.0 mg injected into the myometrium.

- 15-methyl-$PGF_{2\alpha}$ 0.25 mg i.m., or directly into the myometrium every 15–90 min;

- PGE_2 (dinoprostone), one rectal suppository every 4–6 h.

15-Methyl-$PGF_{2\alpha}$ (carboprost trimethamine) has been given intravenously (0.25 mg in 500 ml 5% glucose solution).[25] While 15-methyl-$PGF_{2\alpha}$ is the most effec-tive of the prostaglandins with the least side-effects, the original investigators found it to be ineffective if chorioamnionitis or uterine sepsis was present. Uterine tone was maintained after one injection (86%) and the remainder (except those with chorioamnionitis) responded to a second injection.[24] Side-effects reported were gastrointestinal upset and mild pyrexia. Severe hypotension has been reported with the intramuscular injection of 1 mg PGE_2 at the time of laparotomy.[26] Hogdall[27] recently concluded that the use of prostaglandins for the control of severe postpartum hemorrhage due to uterine atony resulted in the avoidance of surgical intervention in at least 60% of cases.

If bleeding persists despite these efforts, careful inspection of the vulva, vagina and cervix should be made to rule out an undiagnosed or an incompletely repaired laceration. Placenta accreta, inversion, rupture or perforation of the uterus must also be considered. In thin patients, aortic compression may be attempted. The uterus is lifted out of the pelvis, with the lower hand grasping the lower part of the uterus and the upper hand pressing the fundus firmly toward the patient's spine. In theory, this should compress the aorta while attenuating the flow in the uterine vessels.

Hot uterine douching together with uterine packing is a historical technique that predates the use of transfusion and oxytocics. Both techniques have recently been reviewed.[28–30] Uterine packing is one of the most controversial methods in the management of postpartum hemorrhage. It must be done meticulously and methodically if it is to be successful. Uterine packing should only be considered when the previously described methods have failed, and all other possible causes for bleeding have been ruled out. Huff is likely to be correct when he says 'Improper use of a poorly placed pack probably has contributed to the low esteem of this form of therapy'.[31]

Procedure: Uterine Packing

*Packing should be done under adequate analgesia or anesthetic (**Figure 4**). With an oxytocic solution running, 15–20 m of dry sterile gauze is used (some suggest gauze moistened with saline may be easier to use). Ring forceps are placed on the anterior and posterior lips of the cervix, which is thereby steadied by an assistant. The gauze is 'fed' into the uterus over the operator's fingers which should lie along the posterior wall of the vagina. It is imperative that the fundus is packed firmly in a layered fashion working down toward the cervix and packing the vagina as well. The patient should be*

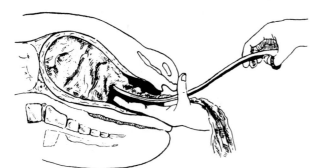

Figure 4. Packing the uterus. The left hand serves as a cervical speculum, while the uterus is tightly packed with gauze with the aid of packing forceps. Reproduced with permission from Cavanagh et al.[32]

commenced on a broad-spectrum antibiotic and an indwelling catheter inserted into the bladder. The pack, if successful in controlling the bleeding, should be left in place for 24–36 h and then removed in circumstances where immediate surgery can be undertaken. Packing may be indicated when other methods to control hemorrhage have failed, and the patient is being prepared for transport to a tertiary care unit. It is unfortunate that packs are often placed in a panic and the patient arrives at the receiving hospital with little more than an absorbent cork in place. When packing becomes a consideration, it may be wiser to proceed to laparotomy, since most practitioners have had little experience with the technique and its effectiveness has not been proved.

The use of a Foley catheter with a large bulb has been reported as a successful method to control postpartum hemorrhage where there has been a low-lying placenta.[33] The tip of the catheter is inserted inside the cervix and the bulb is inflated to its maximum. Traction is then applied to the catheter, causing the bulb to exert a downward pressure against the cervix, thereby creating a tamponade.

Surgical management

When medical management fails to control postpartum hemorrhage, surgical therapy is indicated. Hysterectomy is the definitive treatment for hemorrhage from uterine atony unresponsive to other measures. In one review of 70 hysterectomies done for postpartum

hemorrhage, the predisposing cause was uterine atony in 43%.[34] Of the remainder requiring hysterectomy, 30% had placenta previa and 13% had experienced a ruptured uterus. Hysterectomy may be avoided by using other methods such as uterine artery ligation, and bilateral hypogastric artery ligation, alone or with bilateral ovarian artery ligation.

Uterine artery ligation will only control bleeding from the uterus, and not from the vagina, which is supplied by the vaginal branch of the internal iliac artery (internal iliac artery ligation will control bleeding from both sites). Despite this limitation, uterine artery ligation has not been given enough attention according to O'Leary.[35] The advocates of this procedure point out that 90% of flow to the uterus is via the uterine arteries and they are readily accessible.

Procedure: Uterine Artery Ligation

*The operator preferably stands on the left side of the patient (**Figure 5**). The ligation of the left uterine artery is accomplished by elevating the uterus and placing a large atraumatic needle including a suitable suture (the type is not important) from front to back 2–3 cm medial to the uterine artery (including the myometrium in this bite). The needle is then brought forward through an avascular area in the*

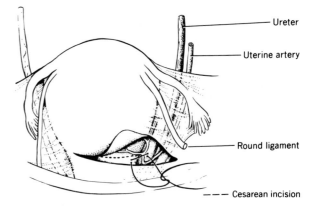

Figure 5. Operative technique for uterine artery ligation. The vesicouterine fold of peritoneum has been incised transversely and the bladder mobilized inferiorly. A number 1 chromic catgut suture on a large smooth needle has been placed through the avascular space of the broad ligament and through the uterus. The suture includes the uterine vessels and several centimeters of myometrium. Reproduced with permission from Pauerstein.[36]

broad ligament. Ligation of the right uterine artery is accomplished in a similar manner. The ligation is best done at a level equal to or just below the site where the transverse incision for cesarean section is performed. The procedure is effective, safe and technically easier than internal iliac artery ligation. There are few associated complications, but the usual caution regarding inadvertent ligation of a ureter should be exercised.[37]

Internal iliac ligation

Internal iliac artery ligation is performed as follows (**Figure 6**). The common iliac artery bifurcates into the external and internal iliac arteries at the pelvic brim (at the level of the sacral promontory). The ureter crosses the common iliac artery at the level of its bifurcation. An 8–10 cm incision is made in the peritoneum lateral and parallel to the ureter. The peritoneal flap is retracted medially with the ureter still attached. The internal iliac artery is dissected free for approximately 5 cm to avoid ligation above the posterior branch. If the flow to the posterior branch is interrupted, it can result in compromised flow to the gluteal muscles and buttocks.

The anterior branch of the internal iliac artery is identified and the adventitia carefully removed. This allows the artery to bulge away from the internal iliac vein. A right-angled clamp is then used to place two sutures around the artery. The suture of choice is usually said to be silk but others describe equal success with mersilene or chromic 1-0 catgut. Complications include injury to the iliac vein, external iliac artery ligation with subsequent ischemic damage to the pelvis, or failure of the procedure to achieve its objective. It has recently been stated that the procedure succeeds in approximately 40% of cases.[38,39] While internal iliac artery ligation is often described, and is reasonably

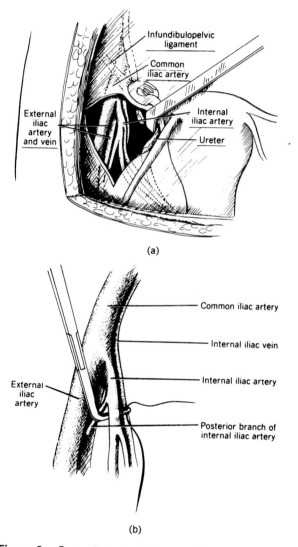

Figure 6. Operative technique of internal iliac artery ligation. (a) The retroperitoneal space over the right internal and external iliac vessels has been opened and the ureter retracted medially. (b) A right-angled clamp is passed between the iliac artery and vein to receive a ligature of number 0 silk. The vessel should be doubly ligated. Reproduced with permission from Pauerstein.[36]

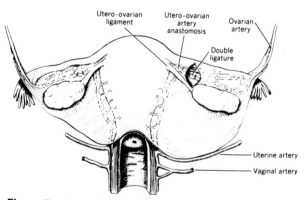

Figure 7. Area for ovarian artery ligation. Two free ties of 2-0 silk suture are used to ligate the ovarian artery bilaterally near its anastomosis with the uterine artery. An avascular area of mesovarium near the junction of the utero-ovarian ligament with the ovary is the site chosen. Reproduced with permission from Pauerstein.[36]

easy to do, it is usually undertaken with reluctance because of the circumstances in which it is indicated. The patient is often compromised, and there may be edema and hematoma complicating the anatomy. If an operator is not familiar with the retroperitoneal pelvic anatomy, it may be more prudent to proceed with hysterectomy, unless assistance from a more experienced operator is available. Ovarian artery ligation can be used as an adjunct to uterine artery ligation or internal iliac artery ligation (**Figure 7**).[40]

POSTPARTUM HEMORRHAGE
Summary of Management Options

Prevention

Options for women at risk (see **Figure 1**)

- Intravenous access

- Save serum for rapid cross-match if needed or actually cross-match two units

Active management of third stage

- Oxytocic agent

- Controlled cord traction

- Clamp and cut cord

Management

Initial emergency measures

- Rub-up contraction

- Intravenous oxytocin (10 units) (ergometrine 0.5 mg i.m. is an alternative but should be avoided in hypertensive patients)

- Establish i.v. access

- Cross-match blood

- See Chapter 73 for general management of major obstetric hemorrhage

Specific measures

- Examine uterus to confirm atony is cause

- Confirm placenta appears intact (manual removal or uterine exploration and removal of placental fragments if suspicion of incomplete third stage)

- Commence i.v. oxytocin infusion

- Give further i.v. bolus of oxytocin

- Rule out trauma to vagina, cervix or uterus

- Bimanual compression

- Prostaglandin options:
  - $PGF_{2\alpha}$ (0.5–1.0 mg) into uterine muscle
  - 15-methyl-$PGF_{2\alpha}$ (0.25 mg) i.m. or into uterine muscle

- Bilateral uterine artery ligation

- Bilateral internal iliac artery ligation

- Hysterectomy

Hysterectomy

Should these procedures fail, or if preservation of future child-bearing is not an issue, hysterectomy is indicated. In any event, hysterectomy may be life-saving and further measures to temporize may only lead to further deterioration in the patient's cardiovascular and hemodynamic status. The choice of total *vs* subtotal hysterectomy will depend on the current situation, the experience of the operator, the condition of the patient and difficulty of the procedure. The amount of bleeding during hysterectomy will not be reduced by performing internal iliac artery ligation beforehand.

Other methods

Finally, arterial embolization under angiographic control and the infusion of vasopressin into the internal iliac artery has been used to control massive postpartum hemorrhage.[41,42] Vasopressin was infused via catheters directly into the internal iliac arteries, using a solution of 0.2 units/min, continued over 24 h. Embolization using absorbable gelatin and sponge has also been described. In situations where there is unavoidable delay in organizing surgical intervention, the use of MAST (military antishock trousers) may be a lifesaving measure.[43]

PLACENTA ACCRETA

Definition

Immediate postpartum hemorrhage seldom results from retained small placental fragments. Usually, the fragment is large, such as a succenturiate lobe, the remaining portion of a bifid placenta or morbid adherence (placenta accreta). Placenta accreta is 'an abnormal adherence, either in whole or in part, of the afterbirth to the underlying uterine wall'.[44–46] The incidence of an abnormally adherent placenta in North America is approximately 1 : 7000 deliveries. Three types are described:

- *Placenta accreta*: pathological adherence due to the paucity of underlying decidua.

- *Placenta increta*: the placenta invades the uterine wall.

- *Placenta percreta*: the invasion reaches the uterine serosa and may even lead to rupture of the uterus.

Placenta accreta is commonly associated with placenta previa (in over 50% of cases), probably because of a deficiency of decidua in the lower uterine segment. Any condition resulting in reduction of decidua can lead to either partial or complete abnormal adherence; this includes multiparity, previous infection, uterine scar or previous traumatic curettage.

Management Options

The management of the condition begins with prompt recognition, especially in any patient where placental separation is delayed (>30 min), or when manual removal of the placenta has been required and is difficult. It should be noted that a fundally implanted adherent placenta may lead to uterine inversion in the attempt to remove it. In any situation where the placenta is unduly adherent, further attempts at removal should abandoned. If not already done, access to the patient's circulation should be obtained with a large-bore needle and an intravenous infusion of crystalloid commenced. Preparation for surgery should then be made.

In remote areas, the patient is better off being transferred with the placenta *in situ* rather than undergoing repeated attempts to remove it. At the time of surgery, curettage with manual removal is the next step. Uterine atony is treated with oxytocics as previously described.

Placenta accreta is associated with significant maternal mortality; but the lowest mortality in one study occurred when immediate hysterectomy was performed. In this study, maternal mortality was four times greater when conservative management was used.[47] The more aggressive approach is supported in another recent study.[48]

In summary, the preferred treatment for a pathological adherent placenta is hysterectomy. Conservative treatment should be reserved for the young patient who wishes to retain fertility at all costs. There is no place in management for allowing chronic retention, and the inherent difficulties related to infection and hemorrhage that will occur later.

UTERINE INVERSION

Definition

Uterine inversion is a rare but serious complication. Its incidence is approximately 1 : 10 000 deliveries. Uterine inversion may be complete, where the fundus has passed completely through the cervix, or incomplete, where the fundus is still above the cervix. Hemorrhagic shock is common.[49] The etiology of uterine inversion is not completely understood, and while 'mismanagement' of the third stage (undue tugging on the umbilical cord) has often been quoted as a cause for uterine inversion, this is not proved. Other reported causes are the use of the Crede maneuver and too rapid withdrawal of the placenta from the uterus during manual removal. Other causes include a sudden rise in intra-abdominal pressure (such as, for example, with coughing or vomiting) in the presence of a relaxed uterus, and a short umbilical cord with fundal insertion of the placenta.

Management Options

Treatment must be immediate and direct. Assistance including an anesthetist should be sought. Antishock measures begin when the condition is recognized. A freshly inverted uterus with the placenta separated can often be replaced immediately (**Figure 8**).[50] If immediate replacement fails or if the placenta remains adherent, no further attempts should be made to replace it until the patient is hemodynamically stable. Part of the 'shock' seen with this condition is probably neurogenic due to traction on the uterine supports. A general anesthetic that relaxes the uterus (such as Halothane) is of assistance in replacing the inverted uterus. Further relaxation may be achieved by using betamimetic agents such as terbutaline and ritodrine.[51]

After the placenta has been removed, the palm of the hand is placed on the fundus of the uterus with the fingers extended to identify the margins of the cervix. Upward pressure is applied to force the fundus through the cervix. Oxytocin is then (and not before) infused to maintain uterine tone, using 40 units in 1000 ml crystalloid.

If these measures fail to restore the uterus to its proper position, the O'Sullivan method of hydrostatic replacement can be tried. A warm antiseptic douche solution is forced into the vagina with one hand sealing the labia. Ballooning of the vaginal fornices with hydrostatic pressure will force open the constricting cervix and restore the uterus to its original position.[52]

Procedure: Laparotomy

*Laparotomy may be necessary in the event that the uterus cannot be replaced by these methods. At laparotomy, the inverted uterus resembles a 'funnel' (**Figure 9**). Traction is placed on the round ligaments with ring forceps or Allis forceps, and an assistant pushes from below. If necessary, a vertical incision in the posterior cervix may be used (the Haultain technique; **Figure 10**) to effect the restoration of the uterus.*

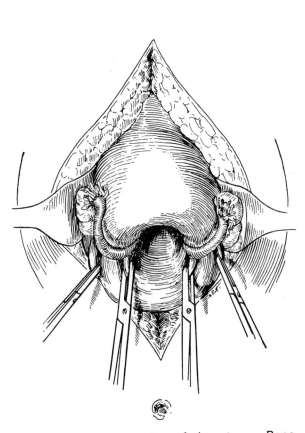

Figure 9. Acute inversion of the uterus. Repositioning partially completed. Reproduced with permission from Zuspan and Quilligan.[19]

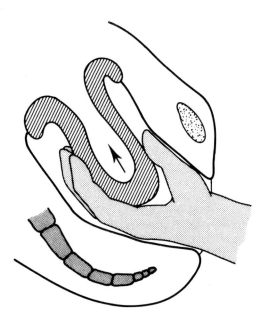

Figure 8. Manual replacement of uterine inversion. Reproduced with permission from Baskett.[50]

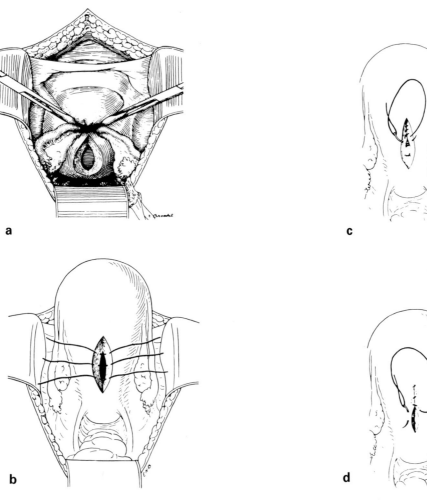

Figure 10. Haultain operation for correction of inversion of the uterus. (a) An incision is made in the posterior uterine wall through the ring. The uterus has already been partially replaced by traction on the round ligaments, while an assistant exerts pressure on the fundus below. (b) The inversion has been completely corrected. The incision in the uterus is repaired with interrupted 2-0 chromic catgut sutures. (c) Further closure with a continuous 2-0 chromic catgut suture. (d) The serosa is approximated with a 3-0 chromic catgut Lembert stitch. Reproduced with permission from Zuspan and Quilligan.[19]

UTERINE RUPTURE

Definition

The incidence of uterine rupture does not appear to be falling in North America as it has done in the UK.[53,54] The reported rate varies from 1 : 1000 to 1 : 1500 deliveries.

The definition of uterine rupture is described by Plauche[55] 'as those cases of complete separation of the wall of the pregnant uterus with or without expulsion of the fetus that endanger the life of the mother and/or the fetus'. The rupture may be incomplete (not including the peritoneum) or complete (when it includes the visceral peritoneum). Asymptomatic dehiscences are not included in this definition.

Risks

The significance of uterine rupture lies in the risk it carries for the mother and for her infant. It has been a significant factor in the causation of maternal mortality in England and Wales,[56] but its incidence has recently fallen sharply.[54]

Diagnosis

The most common antecedent cause for uterine rupture is a previous uterine scar, especially a cesarean section scar. A vertical incision ('classical scar') predisposes to a rupture rate of 3–4%, compared with 0.25% for a lower segment scar. Other predisposing factors are previous uterine surgery (e.g. myomectomy), manipulations during pregnancy or delivery such as version or the use of forceps. Spontaneous rupture may occur during labor, especially in patients with high parity (who are more sensitive to oxytocin as well).[57] Rupture of the unscarred uterus is sudden and dramatic with a high fetal and maternal mortality.[58] There is a higher perinatal mortality rate associated with rupture of a classical uterine scar than rupture of a low transverse scar.[59]

The most common clinical indication that uterine rupture has occurred is fetal distress,[60] followed by vaginal bleeding, abdominal pain and alterations in uterine contractility.[63] The diagnosis of uterine rupture is made by exploring the uterus and identifying the rent.

Management Options

Treatment is surgical, either hysterectomy or repair. Hysterectomy is the best option, especially if the patient does not desire further child-bearing, is of high parity or in poor condition. Repair of the rupture is a reasonable option in the younger woman who is in a stable clinical condition with an uncomplicated rupture (**Figure 10**). Subsequent pregnancy in these patients carries a risk of recurrence of 4–10%.[64,65] One author advises repeat cesarean section at 36 weeks or when fetal lung maturity has been attained in those patients where a rupture has been repaired.[66]

In summary, uterine rupture is a sudden and generally unforeseen, uncommon event, which carries a significant maternal and perinatal mortality. Prompt diagnosis and surgical treatment are lifesaving. Repair of the rupture is a reasonable option given favorable circumstances.

AMNIOTIC FLUID EMBOLISM

While amniotic fluid embolism is rare (1 : 80 000 deliveries), it is associated with a mortality rate greater than 80%.[67,68] This incidence has remained the same in England and Wales over the past decade.[54]

The underlying etiology is related to the passage of amniotic fluid and particulate debris (e.g. fetal squames) into the maternal circulation causing an anaphylactic-like reaction.[69] The onset is dramatic with the clinical manifestation of respiratory distress, cyanosis, cardiovascular collapse, hemorrhage and coma.

The use of triple lumen catheters has been useful in providing information regarding the pathophysiology.[70] It has shown that the initial onset of severe pulmonary hypertension and profound hypoxia is followed by left heart failure. If the patient survives this initial phase, there is a 40% probability that disseminated intravascular coagulation will develop.

High parity, maternal age more than 35 years, overdistension of the uterus, complete or partial uterine rupture, large babies and/or hypertonic labor, particularly associated with the excessive use of oxytocics, are features commonly found when amniotic fluid embolism occurs.[2] However, they are not specific and most women who have these features do not develop amniotic fluid embolism.

Diagnosis

In the past, the definitive diagnosis of amniotic fluid embolism was made by the pathologist. More recently, examination of blood from the central circulation has led to the diagnosis, and sometimes successful treatment.[61,62] The differential diagnosis must include septic or anaphylactic shock, aspiration pneumonitis, pulmonary embolism or myocardial infarction.

Management Options

The treatment of amniotic fluid embolism is not specific, but uses the general principles of treatment for shock. This includes oxygen administration and the maintenance of cardiac output (in the hypotensive patient, infusion of a dopamine drip 2–20 µg/kg/min). Insertion of a pulmonary artery catheter is necessary to maintain surveillance of the circulation. If necessary, administration of digoxin (0.5–1.0 mg in divided doses) may be beneficial. Treatment of the severe but usually transient coagulopathy is accomplished by the use of blood and blood products including fresh frozen plasma and cryoprecipitate.

OTHER PROBLEMS OF THE THIRD STAGE
Summary of Management Options

Placenta accreta

- Recognition of problem is difficult

- Intravenous access and resuscitation

- Options for treatment:
  - curettage
  - manual removal
  - hysterectomy

- Treat any associated uterine atony as described under 'Primary Postpartum Hemorrhage'

Uterine inversion

- Prompt recognition and treatment are keys to successful outcome

- Intravenous access and resuscitation

- Options for treatment:
  - manual replacement (with/without a general anesthetic such as Halothane or tocolytics)
  - hydrostatic replacement
  - laparotomy and correction 'from above'

Uterine rupture

- Diagnosis confirmed by EUA or laparotomy

- Surgical options:
  - hysterectomy
  - repair

- In subsequent pregnancies, elective cesarean section is advocated by most

Amniotic fluid embolism

- If diagnosed before death, management is largely directed toward general, resuscitative and supportive measures:
  - oxygen
  - maintain circulation (e.g. dopamine, digoxin)
  - intensive care unit
  - treat any DIC (see Chapter 73)

REFERENCES

1 Kaunitz AM, Hughes JM, Grimes DA, Smith JC, Rochat RW, Kafrissen ME (1984) Causes of maternal mortality in the United States. *Obstetrics and Gynecology* **65**:605–612.

2 Department of Health (1991) *Report of Confidential Enquiries into Maternal Deaths in the United Kingdom 1985–1987*. London: HMSO.

3 Gibb DMF (1991) *Common Obstetric Emergencies*. Oxford: Butterworth-Heineman.

4 Hayashi R (1983) Postpartum haemorrhage. In Queenan JT (ed.), *Managing OB/GYN Emergencies*, 2nd edn, p. 156. New Jersey: Medical Economic Books.

5 Doran JR, O'Brien SA, Randall JA (1955) Repeated post-partum haemorrhage. *Obstetrics and Gynecology* **5**:186–192.

6 Hayashi RH, Castillo MS, Noah ML (1981) Management of severe postpartum haemorrhage due to uterine atony using an analogue of prostaglandin F2 alpha. *Obstetrics and Gynecology* **58**:426–429.

7 Baskett TF (1985) Complications of the third stage of labor. In Baskett TF, *Essential Management of Obstetric Emergencies*, pp. 159–161. Chichester: John Wiley.

8 Reece EA, Romero R, Hobbins J (1984) Coagulopathy associated with Factor VIII inhibitor: A literature review. *Journal of Reproductive Medicine* **29**:53–58.

9 Kasper CK, Hoag MS, Aggeler PM, Stone S (1964) Blood clotting factors in pregnancy: Factor VIII concentrations in normal and AHF-deficient women. *Obstetrics and Gynecology* **24**:242–247.

10 Garcia J, Garforth S, Ayers S (1987) The policy and practise of midwifery study: Introduction and methods. *Midwifery* **3**:2–9.

11 Brandt ML (1933) The mechanism and management of the third stage of labor. *American Journal of Obstetrics and Gynecology* **25**:662–667.

12 Chamberlain GVP (1985) Discussion. In Chamberlain GVP, Orr CJB, Sharp F (eds), *Litigation and Obstetrics and Gynaecology*, pp. 272–278. London: Royal College of Obstetricians and Gynaecologists.

13 Milton PSD (1985) Natural childbirth and home deliveries – clinical aspects. London: Royal College of Obstetricians and Gynaecologists, pp. 279–299.

14 Dunn PM (1988) Management of childbirth in normal women: The third stage of fetal adaptation. In *Perinatal Medicine, Report of the IXth European Congress on Perinatal Medicine*. Lancaster: MTP Press.

15 Inch S (1985) Management of the third stage of labor: Another cascade of intervention. *Midwifery* **1**: 114–122.

16 Prendiville W, Elbourne D (1989) Care during the third stage of labor. In Chalmers I, Enkin M, Keirse MJNC (eds), *Effective Care in Pregnancy and Childbirth*, Vol. 2, pp. 1145–1170. Oxford: Oxford University Press.

17 Sorbe B (1978) Active pharmacologic management of the third stage of labor: A comparison of oxytocin and ergometrine. *Obstetrics and Gynecology* **52**:694–697.

18 Spencer PM (1962) Controlled cord traction in management of the third stage of labor. *British Medical Journal* **1**:1728–1732.

19 Zuspan FP, Quilligan EJ (1988) *Douglas-Stromme Operative Obstetrics*, 5th edn. Norwalk, CT: Appleton and Lange.

20 Kemp J (1971) A review of cord traction in the third stage of labor from 1963 to 1969. *Medical Journal of Australia* **1**:899–903.

21 Donald I (1979) *Practical Obstetric Problems*, 5th edn. London: Lloyd-Luke, p. 764.

22 Cunningham FG, MacDonald PC, Gant NF (1989) *Williams' Obstetrics*, 18th edn. Norwalk, CT: Appleton and Lange.

23 Buttino L, Garite TJ (1986) The use of 15 Methyl F2 alpha prostaglandin (prostin 15M) for the control of postpartum haemorrhage. *American Journal of Perinatology* **3**:241–243.

24 Hayashi RH, Castillo MS, Noah ML (1984) Management of severe postpartum haemorrhage with a prostaglandin F2 alpha analogue. *Obstetrics and Gynecology* **63**:806–808.

25 Granstrom L, Ekman G, Ulmsten U (1989) Intravenous infusion of 15 Methyl-prostaglandin F2 alpha (Prostinfenem) in women with heavy postpartum haemorrhage. *Acta Obstetrica et Gynecologica Scandinavica* **68**:365–367.

26 Kilpatrick AW, Thorburn J (1990) Severe hypotension due to intramyometrial injection of prostaglandin E2. *Anaesthesia* **45**:848–849.

27 Hogdall CK, Hogdall E (1989) Treatment of severe postpartum atony with prostaglandin. *Uqueskr-Laeger* **151**:2410–2413.

28 Fribourg SRC, Rothman LA, Rovinsky JJ (1973) Intrauterine lavage for control of uterine atony. *Obstetrics and Gynecology* **41**:876–883.

29 Hester JD (1975) Postpartum haemorrhage and re-evaluation of uterine packing. *Obstetrics and Gynecology* **45**:501–504.

30 Drucker M, Wallach RC (1979) Uterine packing: A reappraisal. *Mount Sinai Journal of Medicine* **46**:191–194.

31 Huff RW (1987) Postpartum haemorrhage. In Pauerstein CJ (ed.), *Clinical Obstetrics*, p. 931. New York: John Wiley.

32 Cavanagh D, Woods RE, O'Conner TCF, Knuppel RA (1982) *Obstetrics Emergencies*, 3rd edn. Philadelphia, PA: Harper and Row.

33 Bowen LW, Beeson JH (1985) Use of a large Foley catheter balloon to control postpartum haemorrhage resulting from a low placental implantation. *Journal of Reproductive Medicine* **30**:623–625.

34 Clark SL, Yeks Y, Phelan JP, Bruce S, Paul RH (1984) Emergency hysterectomy for obstetric haemorrhage. *Obstetrics and Gynecology* **64**:376–380.

35 O'Leary JA (1988) Postpartum haemorrhage. In Charles D, Glover Douglas D (eds), *Current Therapy in Obstetrics*, pp. 216–222. Toronto: B. C. Decker.

36 Pauerstein C (1987) *Clinical Obstetrics*. New York: John Wiley.

37 O'Leary JL and O'Leary JA (1966) Uterine artery ligation in the control of intractable postpartum haemorrhage. *American Journal of Obstetrics and Gynecology* **94**:920–924.

38 Evans S, McShane P (1985) The efficacy of internal iliac artery ligation in obstetric haemorrhage. *Surgery, Gynecology and Obstetrics* **160**:250–253.

39 Clark SL, Phelan JP, Yesh S, Bruce SR, Paul RH (1985) Hypogastric artery ligation for obstetric haemorrhage. *Obstetrics and Gynecology* **66**:353–356.

40 Cruickshank SH, Stoelk EM (1983) Surgical control of pelvic haemorrhage; Method of bilateral ovarian artery ligation. *American Journal of Obstetrics and Gynecology* **147**:724–725.

41 Greenwood LH, Glickman MG, Schwartz PE, Morse SS, Denny DF (1987) Obstetric and nonmalignant gynecologic bleeding: Treatment with angiographic embolization. *Radiology* **164**:155–159.

42 Sacks BA, Palestrand AM, Cohen WR (1982) Internal iliac artery vasopressin infusion for postpartum haemorrhage. *American Journal of Obstetrics and Gynecology* **143**:601–603.

43 Pearse CS, Magrina JF, Finley BE (1984) Use of MAST suit in obstetrics and gynaecology. *Obstetrical and Gynecological Survey* **39**:416–422.

44 Irving FC, Hertig AT (1937) A study of placenta accreta. *Surgery, Gynecology and Obstetrics* **64**:178–200.

45 Breen JL, Neubecher R, Gregori CA, Franklin JE (1977) Placenta accreta, increta, and percreta: A survey of 40 cases. *Obstetrics and Gynecology* **49**:43–47.

46 Hutton L, Yang SS, Bernstein J (1983) Placenta accreta: A 26 year clinicopathologic review (1956–1981). *New York State Journal of Medicine* **83**:857–866.

47 Fox H (1972) Placenta accreta, 1945–1949. *Obstetrical and Gynecological Survey* **27**:475–490.

48 Read JA, Corron DB, Miller FC (1980) Placenta accreta: Changing clinical aspects and outcome. *Obstetrics and Gynecology* **56**:31–34.

49 Platt LD, Druzin ML (1981) Acute puerperal inversion of the uterus. *American Journal of Obstetrics and Gynecology* **141**:187–190.

50 Baskett TF (1985) *Essential Management of Obstetric Emergencies*. Chichester: John Wiley.

51 Catanzarite VA, Moffit KD, Baker ML, Awadalla SG, Argubright KF, Pechins RP (1986) New approaches to the management of acute puerperal uterine inversion. *Obstetrics and Gynecology* **68**:7–10 (suppl.).

52 O'Sullivan JV (1945) Acute inversion of the uterus. *British Medical Journal* **2**:282–284.

53 Eaden RD, Parker RT, Gall SA (1986) Rupture of the pregnant uterus: A 53 year review. *Obstetrics and Gynecology* **68**:671–674.

54 Department of Health (1989) *Report on Confidential Enquiries into Maternal Deaths in England and Wales 1982–1984*. London: HMSO.

55 Plauche WC, Von Almen W, Muller R (1984) Catastrophic uterine rupture. *Obstetrics and Gynecology* **64**:792–797.

56 Department of Health and Social Security (1982) *Report on Confidential Enquiries into Maternal Deaths in England and Wales 1976–1978*. London: HMSO.

57 Fuchs K, Peretz BA, Marcovici R, Paldi E, Timor-Trish I (1985) The 'grand multipara': Is it a problem? A review of 5785 cases. *International Journal of Gynecology and Obstetrics* **23**:321–326.

58 Shrinsky DC, Benson RC (1978) Rupture of the pregnant uterus. A review. *Obstetrical and Gynecological Survey* **33**:217–232.

59 Sufrin-Disler C (1990) Vaginal birth after caesarean. *ICEA Review* **14**:1–12.

60 Rodriquez MH, Masaki DI, Phelan JP, Diaz FG (1989) Uterine rupture: Are intrauterine pressure catheters useful in the diagnosis? *American Journal of Obstetrics and Gynecology* **161**:666–669.

61 Resnik R, Swartz WH, Plumer MH, Benirschke K, Stratthaus ME (1976) Amniotic fluid embolism with survival. *Obstetrics and Gynecology* **47**:295–298.

62 Duff P, Engelsgjerd B, Zingery LW, Huff RW, Monteil M (1983) Hemodynamic observations in a patient with intrapartum amniotic fluid embolism. *American Journal of Obstetrics and Gynecology* **146**:112–115.

63 Fedorkow DM, Nimrod CA, Taylor PJ (1987) Ruptured uterus in pregnancy: A Canadian hospital's experience. *Canadian Medical Association Journal* **137**:27–29.

64 Sheth SS (1988) Results of treatment of rupture of the uterus by suturing. *Journal of Obstetrics and Gynaecology of the British Commonwealth* **75**:55–58.

65 Aguero O, Kizer S (1968) Obstetric prognosis of the repair of uterine rupture. *Surgery, Gynecology and Obstetrics* **127**:528–530.

66 Ritchie EH (1971) Pregnancy after rupture of the pregnant uterus. *Journal of Obstetrics and Gynaecology of the British Commonwealth* **78**:642–648.

67 Morgan M (1979) Amniotic fluid embolism. *Anaesthesia* **34**:20–32.

68 Mulder JI (1985) Amniotic fluid embolism: An overview and case report. *American Journal of Obstetrics and Gynecology* **152**:430–435.

69 Azegami M, Mori N (1986) Amniotic fluid embolism and leukotrines. *American Journal of Obstetrics and Gynecology* **155**:1119–1124.

70 Clark SL, Colton DB, Gonik B, Greenspoon J, Phelan JP (1988) Central dynamic alteration in amniotic fluid embolism. *American Journal of Obstetrics and Gynecology* **158**:1124–1126.

69

Puerperal Problems

DOUGLAS KEITH STILL

INTRODUCTION

The puerperium may seem uneventful compared with the rapid and dramatic events that occur with delivery. However, major physiological changes occur following childbirth, and these can lead to problems which arise without warning, and are often difficult to predict.

PUERPERAL HEMATOMAS

Hematomas do not necessarily result from lacerations or because of episiotomy. In fact, they usually result from damage to a vessel wall without laceration of overlying tissues. This trauma may be the result of pressure during the normal course of labor, the application of forceps, or the result of the infiltration of a local anesthetic for paracervical or pudendal anesthesia. Massive hematomas may occur at the apex of an episiotomy and this area should be checked immediately after repair. The patient who complains of increasing perineal discomfort or pain after delivery should be examined for the presence of a hematoma.

Management Options

The management of a hematoma in the vulva or vagina is immediate surgical drainage and establishment of hemostasis. Reflex retention of urine is common and a self-retaining catheter should be inserted for at least 24 h.

A retroperitoneal hematoma should be suspected in the presence of increasing pelvic pain and a falling hemoglobin. These large hematomas may develop insidiously, and present as an abdominal mass, or result in hypovolemic shock. The source of the hematoma is usually an unrecognized cervical laceration, but it may develop spontaneously because of injury to the uterine artery or vein.

The management of a large progressive retroperitoneal hematoma is laparotomy and evacuation. If a specific bleeding point cannot be found, bilateral hypogastric artery ligation should be performed. Conservative management is an option if the hematoma is non-progressive and the patient is hemodynamically stable.

SECONDARY POSTPARTUM HEMORRHAGE

Secondary postpartum hemorrhage (an equivalent term is 'late postpartum hemorrhage') is abnormal bleeding between 24 h and 6 weeks postpartum. Most hemorrhages occur between 5 and 10 days after delivery. Secondary postpartum hemorrhage occurs following about 1% of births.

Retained placental fragments have traditionally been implicated in the causation of secondary postpartum hemorrhage in about one-third of cases.[1] However, recent studies using ultrasound in which retained placental fragments were demonstrated in only 5% of cases of postpartum hemorrhage, suggest that the presence of retained placental material is less common than was at one time thought.[2] From a practical point of view, it is advisable to tell patients with retained fragments of placenta following a vaginal birth and controlled cord traction for management of the third stage that 'not all the placenta has come out as it should', rather than 'some placenta has been left behind', as this tends to suggest that someone has been negligent by failing to remove all the placenta.

Subinvolution (arrest of involution) frequently accompanies retained placental or membrane fragments. Subinvolution can also occur because of local infection. In either case, the result is prolongation of lochia or profuse hemorrhage. When examined, the uterus is soft, bulky and can be tender. The cervix will usually remain open and patulous. Ultrasound examination of the uterus can be performed as an aid to the diagnosis of retained placental products; however, it should always be remembered that organized clot can present appearances similar to placental tissue on ultrasound. Inexperienced ultrasonographers commonly report 'retained products of conception' even following cesarean sections when all the placenta has been removed manually and there can be no doubt that the uterus is empty, at least of placenta and membranes. In the end, management must always be based on sound clinical judgment.

Management Options

The traditional management of secondary postpartum hemorrhage is curettage, but curettage may aggravate the problem by removing fibrin and clot, and inflict further trauma upon the underlying endometrium. The increase in bleeding that frequently happens after curettage is often unresponsive to oxytocics. Other methods of management include suction curettage,[3] which may sometimes be of value for removing necrotic decidua even where there is no actual placental tissue retained, and the use of a vasopressin-soaked pack with operative hysteroscopy.[4] Because endometritis and pelvic infection is a common concomitant of secondary postpartum hemorrhage (and may even be causal in many cases), the value of conservative management with bed rest, antibiotics (intravenously if necessary) and blood transfusion should not be forgotten.

Thus the challenge in the management of secondary postpartum hemorrhage arises in the selection of those patients who have retained placental or membrane material and who require uterine evacuation from those who have not and do not. Because retained placental products are found in a minority of patients, the initial management should probably be the combined use of oxytocics (oxytocin, ergotamine, prostaglandin $F_{2\alpha}$ or E_2), with broad spectrum antibiotics. If the bleeding persists or is initially severe, exploration of the uterus should be performed. Immediate exploration is also appropriate if there are strong clinical grounds for suspecting retained placental material, for example if the

placenta was reported to be incomplete after delivery. Whenever dilatation and curettage are performed under these circumstances, it is important to inform the patient that hysterectomy may be necessary. Conventional or preferably suction curettage should then be done under general anesthesia (the only real drawback with suction evacuation is that if perforation occurs, as it can more easily in the rather soggy infected postpartum uterus, damage to the bowel and other intra-abdominal structures is likely to be more severe than with a simple curette). When bleeding cannot be controlled by these methods, a uterine pack, or laparotomy with internal iliac artery ligation, may be considered. Packing or internal iliac ligation should be reserved for the situation where the patient has requested that every possible attempt be made to maintain fertility, otherwise a hysterectomy is usually the better management decision (see also Chapter 68).

PUERPERAL INFECTION

Puerperal infection is infection of the genital tract after delivery. Infection is a significant factor in maternal mortality, forming part of a lethal triad with hemorrhage and hypertension. Infection is becoming a less common cause of maternal mortality in North America, England and Wales.[5,6]

Fever is the main sign of infection and is generally the basis for commencing antibiotic therapy and assessing its effectiveness. The definition of postpartum febrile morbidity is a temperature of 38°C (100.4°F) or higher in any two of the first 10 days postpartum except in the first 24 h. Remember that fever and infection are not synonymous; but any patient experiencing fever in the puerperium should be investigated for a source of infection. Conversely, not all patients with clinical endometritis will have fever meeting the definition of postpartum febrile morbidity.[7]

While most puerperal infections involve the uterus, other sites to examine are the chest, bladder and breasts, and the presence of thrombophlebitis must be considered. Other possibilities include appendicitis or cholecystitis.

Antepartum factors reported to predispose to puerperal infection are anemia, poor nutrition, intercourse and premature rupture of the membranes. Apart from premature rupture of the membranes, there is no conclusive evidence to incriminate these factors in the causation of postpartum infection.

Intrapartum factors of considerable importance in the etiology of postpartum infection are contamination from frequent vaginal examinations (four or more), trauma and hemorrhage. Cesarean section is now the most important factor in the etiology of puerperal infection.[8]

Management Options

Precise identification of the bacteria responsible for puerperal infection in the genital tract is difficult because one or more potential pathogens will usually be found in routine cultures taken from the uterine cavity in clinically healthy puerperal women.[9] Cultures taken from the uterine fundus are more likely to identify the pathogen responsible when uterine infection is present. **Table 1** lists the most commonly isolated bacteria thought to be responsible for puerperal infections.

Infections of the lower genital tract (perineum, vagina, cervix) are surprisingly uncommon. These sites represent less than 1% of puerperal infections.[7] Most common is infection of an episiotomy, although even this is unusual (and should be distinguished from breakdown of a suture repair due to poor primary healing). If infection can be demonstrated (a tense, tender swelling surrounded by erythema), all remaining sutures should be removed and drainage of the infection site ensured, if necessary by a surgical incision. A broad-spectrum antibiotic should be prescribed. Although urinary retention is uncommon with infections of the lower genital tract, it may occasionally be necessary to catheterize the patient for 24–48 h. Usually, healing by secondary intention occurs without incident. Once the swelling subsides and any purulent discharge settles, it is sometimes helpful to suture the perineal skin with interrupted non-absorbable sutures, leaving the vaginal aspect open to drain. This helps to stabilize the perineal surfaces and reduce discomfort, and by bringing the healing surfaces closer together

Table 1
Bacteria commonly responsible for female genital infections

Aerobes
Group A, B and D streptococci
Enterococcus
Gram-negative bacteria
   Escherichia coli, *Klebsiella* and *Proteus* spp.
Staphylococcus aureus

Anaerobes
Peptococcus spp.
Peptostreptococcus spp.
Bacteroides bivius, B. fragilis, B. disiens
Clostridium spp.
Fusobacterium spp.

Other
Mycoplasma hominis
Chlamydia trachomatis

From the American College of Obstetricians and Gynecologists.[10]

(although not sealing them) can shorten the time before union occurs. The sutures must be removed after the perineal skin has healed firmly.

Necrotizing infection is an uncommon but serious complication of lower genital tract infections, and may occur in an abdominal incision. The mortality is significant (20–50%), but can be reduced if recognized and treated early. 'Necrotizing cellulitis' refers to infection involving the skin and subcutaneous tissue. If the fascia and underlying tissues become involved, the term 'necrotizing fasciitis' applies. These two conditions are differentiated as either 'clostridial' or 'non-clostridial', depending on the causative organism.

The management of clostridial infections requires large doses of penicillin and immediate surgical debridement. Alternative antibiotics that are equally effective are tetracycline and cloramphenicol. Clostridial myonecrosis usually follows cesarean section in which spores have contaminated the wound. It should be remembered that *Clostridium perfringens* is normal flora in approximately 8% of the population. Transfer of the patient to a center with hyperbaric oxygen equipment is recommended.[11,12]

Necrotizing infections of the 'non-clostridial' variety are caused by a mixed group of aerobic and anaerobic organisms. Immediate surgical debridement and wide antibiotic coverage with penicillin, and aminoglycoside and clindamycin or metronidazole should be used.

Infection of the postpartum uterus is the most common site of puerperal sepsis. The infection usually involves the decidua and myometrium and can extend to the perimetrial tissue via the lymphatics. The most common predisposing factor is cesarean section (which will have been undertaken in about 50% of cases), and other factors, such as prolonged labor and multiple vaginal examinations, will be found in a further 40%.[13] Untreated infection (now rarely seen) can extend to the abdominal cavity via the lymphatics and cause peritonitis. Adnexal structures involved in puerperal infections are usually only superficially affected and rarely result in tubal occlusion or sterility.

Uncommonly, and usually following cesarean section, a pelvic abscess may form. Toxic shock syndrome has also been reported to occur in the puerperium.[14]

The management of postpartum uterine infection includes general supportive measures such as administration of intravenous fluids, analgesics, antipyretics, and use of other methods to reduce fever. Appropriate culture material should be taken from the uterine fundus. Initially, a single agent antibiotic is the preferred treatment and is generally effective in the uncomplicated case. Surgical drainage is required if an abscess is present.

Prophylactic measures have received much attention and study in recent years. While not all agree upon the indications for prophylaxis, or what antimicrobial agent to use, the consensus view is that antibiotic prophylaxis is justified for all non-elective cesarean sections. Usually, one of the first-line cephalosporins, or ampicillin, in one to three doses is given, starting immediately before or during surgery and continuing for the first 12 h following delivery. Beyond this there is no increase in effectiveness.[15] Peritoneal lavage is a less effective method for antibiotic adminstration than the intravenous route.[16]

Septic thrombophlebitis

Septic pelvic vein thrombophlebitis is an uncommon complication of pregnancy. In total, 1–2% of patients with puerperal infection will be affected, and cesarean section is the most significant predisposing event. The bacterial invasion probably begins at the placental site with thrombosis eventually involving the ovarian veins with extension to the renal veins. The diagnosis, based on exclusion or the clinical suspicion that septic thrombophlebitis is present, is often made when antibiotic treatment seems ineffective or failing. Computed tomography or magnetic resonance imaging is often helpful to show the presence of thrombus. The effectiveness of the 'heparin challenge test', promoted both as a diagnostic and therapeutic tool, has been questioned.[17] However, management involves the appropriate use of both heparin and antimicrobials. While life-threatening pulmonary embolism is rare, recurrent septic thrombi during convalescence may require vena cava ligation or the insertion of a filter.

Urinary tract infection

During the puerperium, the bladder may contain residual urine for several reasons. These include overdistension during labor as the result of intravenous infusion, epidural or general anesthesia, and trauma from delivery. The incidence of postpartum urinary tract infection is 2–4% of deliveries.

If it is suspected that the bladder is overdistended, catheterization should be performed. If more than 200 ml of urine is measured, the catheter should be left in place. Appropriate cultures should be taken and treatment prescribed if indicated. After 24 h, the catheter should be removed and, after the first voiding if it is suspected that the bladder is not completely empty, the residual urine should be measured.

The combination of residual urine and incomplete emptying frequently leads to cystitis. Pyelonephritis may occur in the puerperium, but is not usually present until several days after delivery unless there was pre-existing cystitis. The treatment of these infections is with the appropriate antimicrobials; *Escherichia coli* is the most common pathogen.

THROMBOEMBOLIC DISEASE

Thromboembolic disease is covered in Chapter 33, but must be underlined as a major contributor to maternal mortality and morbidity in the puerperium. A recent report now ranks pulmonary embolism as the major cause of maternal mortality in England and Wales.[6] The incidence of deep vein thrombosis (DVT) associated with pregnancy in North America is probably 1–2 per 1000 deliveries.[18] Since the 1950s, there has been a reduction in the incidence of DVT in the puerperium coincidental with the practice of early postdelivery ambulation. However, the risk of thromboembolic disease still increases as pregnancy advances and is greatest in the puerperium.[19] Most patients who develop pulmonary embolism during or following pregnancy have no prior history of DVT or other medical problems. The two most common predisposing factors are a previous history of thrombosis and operative delivery.[20] All patients who experience thromboembolic disease must be investigated for a coagulation defect such as antithrombin III deficiency, protein C deficiency, protein S deficiency, or the presence of lupus anticoagulant.

Management Options

The diagnosis and management of thromboembolic disease in the puerperium are similar to that in the antepartum period. Warfarin may be used for long-term therapy instead of heparin, but heparin should be continued for 5 days after the therapeutic prothrombin time is reached.[21] Breast-feeding is safe with either drug; heparin is not absorbed via the gastrointestinal tract, and though warfarin appears in the breast milk, the amounts are too small to pose any threat to the neonate.[22]

DISORDERS OF THE BREASTS
AND PROBLEMS WITH
LACTATION
SUPPRESSION OF LACTATION

When breast-feeding is stopped, the main reasons given are: nipple trauma, breast engorgement, mastitis and insufficient milk. These problems have been extensively studied, and it has been concluded that 'the majority of these problems can be prevented by unrestricted breast feeding by a baby who has been well positioned from the first feed on'.[23] This advice should be enhanced by appropriate practical and emotional support. Unfortunately, there is no good evidence to suggest that there are any drugs that will improve milk production where the natural supply is inadequate.

Management Options

For those women who choose not to breast-feed their babies, there are a variety of approaches to hasten lactation suppression and reduce the associated symptoms. The non-pharmacologic approaches include the use of breast binding, a good supporting brassiere and fluid restriction. Symptomatic relief is provided by analgesics. Pumping or manual expression of milk may be necessary. Ice packs also may provide relief from the pain of engorgment. The pharmacologic methods available range from the use of sex hormones (Stilbestrol® (diethystilbestrol), Estrovis® (quinestrol)) to bromocriptine. The use of sex hormones is not recommended because of the risk of thromboembolism.[24] Bromocriptine, a commonly emplyed dopamine antagonist, is effective when 2.5 mg is given daily for 14 days: 25% of those who choose this treatment still have rebound engorgement after therapy is completed.[25]

In summary, the available evidence suggests that fluid restriction and other non-pharmacologic methods of lactation suppression such as firm breast support (binding, brassiere) are more effective in the long term (i.e. less rebound); but there is more pain experienced during the process.

MASTITIS

Puerperal fever from breast engorgement is not an uncommon event. In one study, and confirmed by others, the incidence is 18% of otherwise healthy mothers.[26,27] The temperature can range from 37.8°C to 39°C. While puerperal fever can be entirely due to breast engorgement, 2.5% of postpartum women will develop infectious mastitis.[28] Approximately 5% of these patients will develop an abscess in the infected breast.

Mastitis is a non-specific term and there is some confusion over the terminology employed to describe puerperal breast infection. Sporadic puerperal mastitis, often called 'non-epidemic mastitis', is more often caused by *Staphylococcus aureus* and usually occurs sometime remote from hospital discharge.[29] The infection involves the interlobular connective tissue and presents as mammary cellulitis. Milk stasis, nipple trauma and poor nursing technique are implicated in its etiology. Pathogenic bacteria enter via the traumatized nipple and set the stage for the evolution of cellutitis. While *Staphylococcus aureus* is frequently the causative organism, several other organisms have been implicated. These include *Staph. epidermidis* beta-hemolytic streptococci of Lancefield groups B, F and A, *Escherichia coli*, *Haemophilus influenza* and others.[28,30]

Management Options

Cellulitis

The symptoms of mastitis are sudden in onset with a dramatic febrile response, general malaise and flu-like symptoms. The initial management is the prompt administration of a penicillinase-resistant form of penicillin or erythromycin, with acetaminophen or aspirin to control fever. Breast-feeding should continue or milk should be expressed manually or by pumping.

Epidemic mastitis refers to infection acquired in hospital. This infection involves the ductal system and peripheral lymphatics of the breast. Nipple fissure with associated pain is less of a feature compared with the sporadic (non-epidemic) form. Both *Staph. aureus* and *Staph. epidermis* may be encountered. The onset of the disease is usually 2–3 weeks postpartum. The management is similar to that described for the non-epidemic form of mastitis.

Abscess

Both forms of mastitis may result in abscess formation. A major factor in the prevention of an abscess is to decrease milk stasis with the continuation and encouragement of breast-feeding.[31,32] Most authorities suggest that breast-feeding should be stopped when pus is discharging from the nipple or when an abscess develops. The management of abscess formation is surgical drainage plus administration of antibiotics.[33]

An abscess in the breast is drained under general anesthesia. After appropriate preliminary preparation, a radial or circumferential incision is made over the site where the abscess is pointing. The index finger is inserted into the cavity, breaking down any or all adhesions (**Figure 1**). Hemostasis may be helped by packing the wound.[34] Usually, no attempt is made to

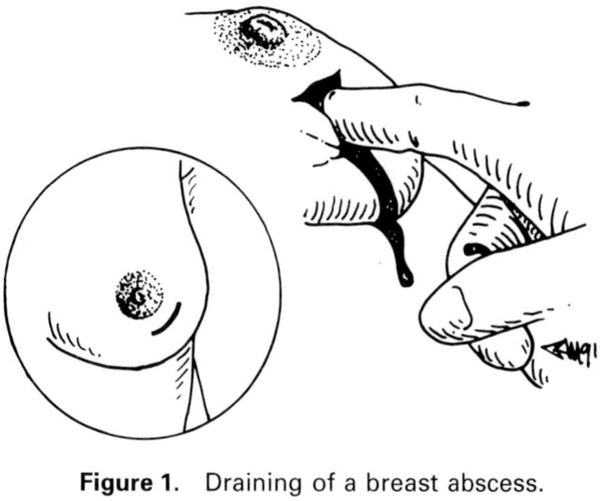

Figure 1. Draining of a breast abscess.

close the skin and the wound is allowed to heal by secondary intention. An alternative method is to close the wound using deep mattress sutures, without formal drainage. It is claimed that this technique results in more rapid healing, but it requires more meticulous follow-up, with mandatory antibiotic coverage.[33] The specimen obtained at the time of the surgery must be sent for bacteriological culture as well as histological examination to rule out an underlying carcinoma.

There is also some controversy regarding the type of incision which should be made. **Figure 1** shows a circumferential incision, and while this incision probably produces a better cosmetic result, a deep incision of this type may damage other lactiferous ducts. Thus the incision should be tailored to the situation. If the abscess is deeply situated, then a radial incision would probably be the best choice.

OTHER MEDICAL DISORDERS OF THE PUERPERIUM

Medical conditions unique to the puerperium were covered in the appropriate sections on that system. Two examples of this are postpartum cardiomyopathy (Chapter 20) and postpartum hypothyroidism (Chapter 21).

INJURIES TO THE PELVIC GIRDLE

Rupture of the symphysis pubis is an uncommon occurrence that can be partial or complete. It can occur spontaneously or as the result of a difficult instrumental delivery. The pain is severe and localized to the symphysis with radiation down the thighs. Generally, analgesics and bedrest result in relief of the pain, but infiltration of a local anesthetic may be necessary on occasion. Healing is nearly always spontaneous, but occasionally orthopedic surgery is necessary.

Separation of the symphysis pubis and sacroiliac joints is a common complication of the third trimester and the puerperium. The onset of the pain is generally gradual and is specific to the joint or joints. Movement will aggravate the pain. Often the pain will be felt when rolling from one side to the other. Occasionally, an orthopedic belt that encircles the trochanters will be necessary for symptomatic relief. There are seldom any sequelae.

Frequently, the coccyx is pushed backward during delivery. If the sacrococcygeal joint is fixed, it can fracture. The loud 'snap' this produces can sometimes be heard during delivery. Sitting can be very painful, and infiltration with a local anesthetic may be necessary to relieve it. Analgesics, heat therapy and rest are usually sufficient. A ring cushion can be very comforting for these patients.

MATERNAL OBSTETRICAL PARALYSIS

This condition is an uncommon lower limb paralysis that manifests itself as 'foot drop' during or after labor. The underlying pathophysiology is not clear and has been the subject of much debate. Whether the damage occurs at the origin of the lumbosacral trunk or to the perineal nerve peripherally is not resolved.

The presentation can range from a 'shooting pain' down the affected leg to an inability of the patient to support their weight on that side. Most patients will show a limp and a gait in which the toe drags on the affected side. The muscle groups involved are the dorsiflexors of the foot and perineal muscles. There is frequently an associated sensory loss. Occasionally, weakness in the quadriceps will be found. Management is aimed at resting the affected limb with the anticipation of gradual recovery. A splint to prevent plantar flexor deformity may be necessary. When the pain allows, physiotherapy should be initiated; progressing from massage to nerve stimulation, and then from passive to active movements. If the cause is a disc protrusion, then surgical intervention may be necessary.

POSTPARTUM DEPRESSION

There has been general acceptance that 'postpartum depression' is an illness and therefore a medical subject.[35] This 'illness' is divided into three categories that have at times indistinct clinical separation. These are 'postpartum blues' occurring in 50–70% of postpartum patients, 'postpartum depression' occurring in 10–15% and 'postpartum psychosis' occurring in 0.15–0.25%.

Clinical Types and Risks

'Postpartum blues' describes the frequently observed and transient experience of weepiness, mood instability, anxiety and irritability observed in the first few days following childbirth. It is usually self-limiting, but should it persist beyond 10–14 days the risk of psychosis is increased.[36] Marital conflict is presently the only definable link between 'postpartum blues' and progression to the more serious affective disorder of postpartum depression. In one study, 12% of women developed clinically relevant depressive disorders by 6 weeks postpartum, but in 90% of these pre-existing situational and longstanding conditions existed.[37] A previous history of psychosis indicates a significant risk that postpartum depression will develop.[38]

Postpartum depression may be difficult to differentiate clinically from 'postpartum blues'. Besides the previously described symptoms, the woman experiences a profound sense of incapacity to love her family, and a feeling of ambivalence toward her infant. Suicidal thoughts should be taken seriously, but actual suicide is exceedingly rare in a patient who does not have a psychiatric history.[6]

Postpartum psychosis is a major affective disorder with manifestations of mania (40%) that can rapidly fluctuate to symptoms of severe depression, clouding of consciousness, confusion, restlessness, irritability and visual hallucinations.[39,40] Often delusional ideas will be incorporated into the patient's memory of the childbirth experience.

Management Options

The diagnosis of postpartum depression even in its mildest forms must not overlook the possibility of a co-existing, underlying medical abnormality. Abnormal thyroid function, toxic effects from drugs, systemic lupus erythematosis, or intracranial events such as hemorrhage or tumor should be considered in the broad perspective. While the true medical nature of postpartum depression has been challenged,[40] the management and treatment remain clinical.[41]

Postpartum blues are so common, a biological cause rather than a psychological cause has been proposed. So far, no specific endocrine, biochemical or hormonal abnormality has been found. The management includes empathy, understanding, affirmation (this is real), also freedom to allow the emotions to be expressed. Reassurance about its transience should be given.

Postpartum depression requires more intense therapy, usually including the assistance of a psychiatrist and the adminstration of tricyclic antidepressants. Sex steroid therapy has been proposed but its effectiveness remains unproven.[42] In addition, relief from child care responsibilities and access to other mothers with babies in a formal or informal setting is helpful.

Postpartum psychosis is usually treated in hospital but successful management in an out-patient setting or in combination with hospitalization has been reported.[43] If possible, the mother should not be separated from her infant. Sometimes if facilities are available, admission of the father as well may be beneficial.[44] Psychiatric supervision of antidepressants and neuroleptics is essential. Failure of medication may indicate the need for electroconvulsive therapy. Immediate contraception is important as unstable moods may lead to unprotected intercourse.

PERINATAL GRIEVING (see also Chapter 58)

While the outcome of an obstetric event is usually happy and positive, the loss of a baby either *in utero*

Table 2
Checklist of guidelines for management of a couple who have lost a baby

1.	Keep the mother informed, be honest and forthright
2.	Recognize and facilitate anticipatory grieving
3.	Encourage the presence of the mother's major support person throughout labor and delivery
4.	Support and encourage the couple in seeing or touching the infant
5.	Describe the infant in detail, for those who choose not to see. Take a photograph, but in a tasteful setting, i.e. wrapped in a blanket with the face showing
6.	Show the infant as often in the postpartum period as requested. Those who choose not to see it initially may change their minds
7.	Encourage the mother to make as many choices regarding her care as possible
8.	Offer genetic counseling
9.	Encourage autopsy, help deal with the paperwork related to death certificates and disposal of the body
10.	Discuss funeral, memorial, or 'naming' services
11.	Help the couple deal with informing other siblings and family members
12.	Avoid sedation
13.	Discuss future pregnancies
14.	Schedule an office visit(s) before the patient leaves hospital to discuss the loss, the autopsy and the implications for the future

or in the postpartum period is a particularly tragic event. Often the woman will experience and express feelings of personal failure or defeat. Grieving is a natural consequence of her loss. A similar sense of grief can also be seen in the loss of an 'ideal', such as occurs when a handicapped child is born.

While ready support for those who are grieving must be found in all those in attendance (physician, nurse, social worker and pastoral care), this is not a highly complex endeavor requiring sophisticated training or skill. Simple acquaintance with the symptoms and signs of grieving combined with understanding and a willingness to listen and respond to questions are important. A helpful list of guidelines previously published is modified for this chapter[45] and is given in **Table 2**.

PUERPERAL PROBLEMS
Summary of Management Options

Hematomata

- Drainage ± resuture

- Secure hemostasis

- Conservative approach is rarely adopted

Secondary postpartum hemorrhage

- Oxytoxics

- Antibiotics

- EUA if severe/continuing ± curettage

- Send tissue for histology

- If severe despite these options (see Chapter 68):
  - packing
  - internal iliac ligation
  - hysterectomy

Infection

General

- Appropriate bacterial culture (see **Table 1**)

- Antibiotics (i.v. initially)

- Intravenous fluids and supportive/general measures

Specific

- Wound infection
  - remove sutures and drain

- Septic thrombophlebitis
  - radiological diagnosis important
  - treat with antibiotics and anticoagulation

- Urinary infection
  - fluids (i.v. if not tolerating oral)
  - catherization may be necessary
  - i.v. antibiotics (change to oral after 24–48 h)

Thromboembolic disease

- See also Chapter 33

- Prophylactic heparin to those at very high risk (e.g. lupus, previous DVT)

- Radiological diagnosis if suspected clinically

- Anticoagulation (i.v. heparin changing to warfarin)

Breast

Suppression of lactation – options

- Analgesia and support

- Bromocriptine

'Mastitis'

- Cellulitis
  - penicillinase-resistant penicillin or erythromycin
  - anti-inflammatory agents
  - continue breast-feeding or express milk on affected side

- Abscess
  - surgical drainage
  - antibiotics
  - most advocate cessation of breast-feeding on affected side

Postnatal psychiatric problems

General

- Consider other medical problems (e.g. thyroid disease, drug effects, lupus, intracranial pathology)

'Blues'

- Reassure

- Psychological support

Depression

- Psychiatric referral

- Psychotherapy

- Tricyclic antidepressants

- Rarely need hospitalization in mother and baby psychiatric unit

Psychosis

- Hospitalization in mother and baby psychiatric unit

- Extensive psychiatric input

Perinatal grieving for loss of a baby

- See also Chapter 58

- See **Table 2**

REFERENCES

1 Dewhurst CJ (1966) Secondary postpartum hemorrhage. *Journal of Obstetrics and Gynaecology of the British Commonwealth* **73**:53–58.

2 Lee CY, Madrazo B, Drukker BH (1981) Ultrasonic evaluation of the postpartum uterus in the management of postpartum bleeding. *Obstetrics and Gynecology* **58**:227–232.

3 King PA, Duthie SJ, Dong ZG, Ma HK (1989) Secondary postpartum haemorrhage. *Australia and New Zealand Journal of Obstetrics and Gynaecology* **29**:394–398.

4 Townsend DE, Barbis SD, Mathews RD (1991) Vasopressin and operative hysteroscopy in the management of delayed postabortion and postpartum bleeding. *Journal of Obstetrics and Gynecology* **165**:616–618.

5 Rockat RW, Koonin LM, Atrash HK, Jewett JF (1988) Maternal mortality in the United States: Report from the Maternal Mortality Collaborative. *Obstetrics and Gynecology* **72**:91–97.

6 Department of Health (1989) *Report on Confidential Enquiries into Maternal Deaths in England and Wales 1982–1984*. London: HMSO.

7 Sweet RL, Ledger WJ (1973) Puerperal infectious morbidity: A two year review. *American Journal of Obstetrics and Gynecology* **117**:1093–1100.

8 Apuzzio JJ, Reyelt C, Pelosi M, Sen P, Louria DB (1982) Prophylactic antibiotics for cesarean section: Comparison of high and low risk patients for endomyometritis. *Obstetrics and Gynecology* **59**:693–698.

9 Gibbs RS, O'Dell TN, MacGregor RR, Schwartz RH, Morton H (1975) Puerperal endometritis: A prospective microbiologic study. *American Journal of Obstetrics and Gynecology* **121**:919–925.

10 American College of Obstetricians and Gynecologists (1988) *Antimicrobial Therapy for Obstetric Patients*. Technical Bulletin No. 117, June. Washington DC: ACOG.

11 Pearse CS, Magrina JF, Finley BE (1984) Use of MAST suit in obstetrics and gynecology. *Obstetrics and Gynecological Survey* **39**:416–422.

12 Riseman JA, Zamboni WA, Curtis A, Graham DR, Konrad HR, Ross DS (1990) Hyperbaric oxygen therapy for necrotizing fasciitis reduces mortality and the need for debridements. *Surgery* **108**:847–850.

13 Depalma RT, Cunningham FG, Leveno KJ, Roark ML (1982) Continuing investigation of women at high risk for infection following cesarean delivery: Three dose perioperative antimicrobial therapy. *Obstetrics and Gynecology* **60**:53–59.

14 Wager GP (1983) Toxic shock syndrome: A review. *American Journal of Obstetrics and Gynecology* **146**:93–102.

15 Stiver HG, Forward KR, Livingstone RA, Fugere P, Lemay M, Verschelden G, Hunter JD, Carson GD, Beresford P, Tyrell DL (1983) Multicenter comparison of cefoxaltin *vs* cefazolin for prevention of infectious morbidity after non-elective cesarean section. *American Journal of Obstetrics and Gynecology* **145**:158–163.

16 Conover WB, Moore TR (1984) Comparison of irrigation and intravenous antibiotic prophylaxis at cesarean section. *Obstetrics and Gynecology* **63**:787–791.

17 Brown CE, Lowe TW, Cunningham FG, Weinreb JC (1986) Puerperal pelvic thrombophlebitis: Impact on diagnosis and treatment using x-ray computed tomography and magnetic resonance imaging. *Obstetrics and Gynecology* **68**:789–794.

18 Weiner CP (1985) Diagnosis and management of thromboembolic disease during pregnancy. *Clinics in Obstetrics and Gynecology* **28**:107–118.

19 Aaro LA, Jeurgens JL (1971) Thrombophlebitis associated with pregnancy. *American Journal of Obstetrics and Gynecology* **109**:1128–1136.

20 Tengborn L, Bergquist D, Matzsch T, Bergquist A, Hedner U (1989) Recurrent thromboembolism in pregnancy and puerperium: Is there a need for thromboprophylaxis? *American Journal of Obstetrics and Gynecology* **160**:90–94.

21 Moser KM (1990) State of the art: Venous thromboembolism. *American Review of Respiratory Diseases* **141**:235–249.

22 Orme ML, Lewis PJ, de Swiet M, Serlin MJ, Sibeon R, Baty JD, Breckenridge AM (1977) May mothers given warfarin breast-feed their infants? *British Medical Journal* **1**:1564–1565.

23 Inch S, Renfrew MJ (1989) Common breastfeeding problems. In Iain Chalmers I, Enkin M, Keirse MJNC (eds), *Effective Care in Pregnancy and Childbirth*, Vol. 2, pp. 1375–1389. Oxford: Oxford University Press.

24 Turnbull AC, (1968) Puerperal thromboembolism and suppression of lactation. *Journal of Obstetrics and Gynaecology of the British Commonwealth* **75**:1321–1323.

25 Blakemore K (1986) Lactation suppression is a matter of choice. *Contemporary Obstetrics and Gynecology* **28**:39.

26 Roser DM (1966) Breast engorgement and postpartum fever. *Obstetrics and Gynecology* **27**:73–77.

27 Almeida OD, Kitay DZ (1986) Lactation suppression and puerperal fever. *American Journal of Obstetrics and Gynecology* **154**:940–941.

28 Marshall BR, Hepper JK, Zirbel CC (1975) Sporadic puerperal mastitis: An infection that need not interrupt lactation. *Journal of the American Medical Association* **233**:1377–1379.

29 Gibberd GF (1953) Sporadic and epidemic puerperal breast infections: A contrast in morbid anatomy and clinical signs. *American Journal of Obstetrics and Gynecology* **65**:1038–1041.

30 Niebyl J, Spence M, Parmley T (1978) Sporadic (nonepidemic) puerperal mastitis. *Journal of Reproductive Medicine* **20**:97–100.

31 Thomsen AC, Hansen KB, Moller BR (1984) Leukocyte counts and microbiologic cultivation in the diagnosis of puerperal mastitis. *American Journal of Obstetrics and Gynecology* **146**:938–941.

32 Thomsen AC, Espersen T, Maigaard S (1984) Course and treatment of milk stasis, noninfectious inflammation of the breast and infectious mastitis in nursing women. *American Journal of Obstetrics and Gynecology* **149**:492–495.

33 Benson EA (1989) Management of breast abscesses. *World Journal of Surgery* **13**:753–756.

34 Zuspan FP, Quilligan EJ (1988) *Douglas-Stromme*

Operative Obstetrics. Norwalk, CT: Appleton and Lange.

35 Day S (1982) Is obstetric technology depressing? *Radical Science Journal* **12**:17–45.

36 Robinson GE, Stewart DE (1986) Postpartum psychiatric disorders. *Canadian Medical Association Journal* **134**:31–37.

37 Watson JP, Elliott SA, Rugg AJ, Brough DI (1984) Psychiatric disorders in pregnancy and the first postnatal year. *British Journal of Psychiatry* **144**:453–462.

38 Vendenbergh RL (1980) Postpartum depression. *Clinics in Obstetrics and Gynecology* **23**:1105–1111.

39 Hall RC, Popkin MK, Stickney SK, Gardner ER (1979) Presentation of the steroid psychosis. *Journal of Nevous and Mental Diseases* **167**:229–236.

40 Weiner A (1982) Childbirth related psychiatric illness. *Comprehensive Psychiatry* **23**:143–154.

41 Romito P (1989) Unhappiness after childbirth. In Chalmers I, Enkin M, Keirse MJNC (eds), *Effective Care in Pregnancy and Childbirth*, Vol. 2, pp. 1433–1446. Oxford: Oxford University Press.

42 Kane FJ (1968) Psychiatric reactions to oral contraceptives *American Journal of Obstetrics and Gynecology* **102**:105–133.

43 Nurnberg HG, Prudic J (1984) Guidelines for treatment of psychosis during pregnancy. *Hospital and Community Psychiatry* **35**:67–71.

44 Luepker E (1972) Joint admissions and evaluation of postpartum psychiatric patients and their infants. *Hospital and Community Psychiatry* **23**:284–286.

45 Kowalski K (1980) Managing perinatal loss. *Clinics in Obstetrics and Gynecology* **23**:1113–1123.

70

Postnatal Contraception and Sterilization

JOHN HUTTON

CONTRACEPTION

When Does Contraception Become Necessary?

The time of first intercourse after a pregnancy depends on the mother's physical and psychological response to the birth and attitude to parenting, as well as cultural factors.

It has been generally advised that intercourse should not occur until at least 6 weeks after birth, when involution is said to be complete. However, it is perhaps more logical to suggest that intercourse should not begin after birth until:

- the perineum is not tender to touch (indicating that any damage by a tear or episiotomy has healed)

- the lochia has ceased (indicating that the endometrium has healed and there is thus little risk of ascending infection).

Libido after birth is reduced, particularly in women who are breast-feeding when the interval until first coitus is prolonged. The reasons for this are uncertain, but one reason may be tiredness.

Partner attitudes to sex do not appear to be affected by breast-feeding. This delay in first coitus with breast-feeding in comparison with bottle-feeding mothers may also somehow be related to ovarian dysfunction, with the consequent low production of estrogens causing atrophic vaginitis and superficial dyspareunia. If this is considered a factor, an estrogen cream inserted weekly into the vagina by an applictor or as a pessary relieves symptoms and has no apparent effect on lactation but, if used, it must be stressed that it has no contraceptive benefit.

Contraceptive Effect of Breast-Feeding

Breast-feeding in the puerperium causes amenorrhea. Women of all cultures generally shun contraceptive use until the first menses again prompts fertility awareness. In most cultures, over 90% of breast-feeding women will be anovulatory, and thus do not need contraception, provided:

- the infant is not taking supplemental feeds of >150 ml (6 oz) of milk per day

- frequency of feeding is at least 4 hourly including twice during the night

- the infant is not more than 5 months of age.

Indeed, breast-feeding under these circumstances is probably more effective than all forms of contraception as the factor most likely to delay the pregnancy interval after a birth.

Couples should, however, not rely on breast-feeding as a contraceptive, and thus use contraception after birth when:

- a fully breast-fed infant is aged >5 months

- a younger infant (<5 months) is having solids, or >150 ml per day of other milk feeds, or is sleeping through the night (i.e. interval between feeds is >6 h)

- when menses recur.

Choice of Contraceptive Method

The factors affecting the choice of contraceptive method include whether the mother is breast-feeding and when in the postnatal period the contraceptive is being initiated.

The reversible methods (i.e. not permanent contraception in the form of sterilization) are:

- male barrier methods (condom)

- female barrier methods (e.g. diaphragm, cervical cap, vaginal sheath)

- intrauterine devices

- combined oral estrogen and progestagen preparations

- oral progestagen preparations

- injectable hormones (usually progestagens)

- progestagenic implants and vaginal rings

- spermicidal agents

- natural family planning.

Other methods are under study and include the use of a luteinizing hormone agonist. While its effectiveness is encouraging, further research and development is required before it will be an acceptable method of postnatal contraception.

Contraceptive Methods

Male barrier (condom)

This is the most widely used postnatal contraceptive method. Condoms do not need to be used with other methods such as spermicides or creams in breast-feeding mothers, although this should be encouraged in other mothers.

The use of condoms should be initiated at the onset of postnatal coitus and not be delayed until the infant is no longer dependent on breast-feeding. This use of condoms at the outset allows the contraceptive effect of breast-feeding to act as a 'second line of defence' and is especially valuable in a couple who have not used this technique before. The introduction of condoms with first coitus in breast-feeding mothers also avoids the need for the additional spermicide which is often recommended during the initial learning phase, when condoms are being introduced in other situations as the contraceptive of choice.

Female barrier methods

The diaphragm is used much more commonly than the cervical cap for female contraception. If the woman has used a diaphragm previously, it must be checked, as initially a larger size is usually needed. A diaphragm fitting should not occur until 4–6 weeks after birth, often at the postnatal check.

The fitting occurs in the standard way with an estimate of the likely size being made at the time of checking the completeness of involution. With the index finger in the posterior fornix, the point on the finger where the posterior rim of the symphysis pubis lies is noted; the distance to the tip of the finger is the size of the first fitting ring that should be tested. As the interval after birth lengthens in breast-feeding mothers, so the function of the ovaries increases – the associated estrogenization of the vagina thus means that a further check on the diaphragm size is advisable once menses recur.

The choice of coiled or flat spring rim is entirely arbitrary and really depends on patient comfort. Unlike the use of condoms in breast-feeding women, a spermicide should always be used with every application of a diaphragm.

If the woman has used a cervical cap previously, it is unlikely that the same size will be suitable because of the changes to the cervix during birth. The fitting of the cervical cap should occur at the 6 week check and the comments above that relate to the diaphragm also apply to the cervical cap.

Intrauterine contraceptive devices

There are three general types of intrauterine contraceptive devices (IUCDs): non-medicated, medicated with copper and medicated with progestagen. There are various designs, especially of the copper IUCDs (see **Table 1**). These can be inserted immediately after the placenta is delivered (post-placental insertion) or, preferably, at the 6 week check when involution is complete.

Table 1
Types of intrauterine devices available for contraceptive use in the puerperium

Types	Example
Non-medicated	Lippes loop (usually size D)
Medicated	
copper	TCu 200
	TCu 220
	Multiload Cu 375
	Multiload Cu 250
	Nova T pp
	Dimelys R
progestagen	IPCs – 52 mg

An IUCD is a particularly useful method of contraception for parous women who do not wish sterilization. The string on the end of the device that projects through the cervical os to allow a check on placement or retrieval of the device also facilitates the transfer of organisms into the upper genital tract, and thus predisposes to infection and ectopic pregnancies. Therefore, the device cannot be advised in promiscuous women or women with a history of, or at risk of, a sexually transmitted disease.

The insertion of the IUCD is best done at the 6 week check ('internal insertion') when fundal application can best be ensured. While the placement of an IUCD can be attained with post-placental insertion, the device may slip during involution and thus the contraceptive effectiveness of IUCD may be compromised.

Some researchers believe the expulsion rate of postpartum IUCDs with either a post-placental insertion or insertion at the postnatal check is more dependent on the insertion technique than the design of the device. Thus those undertaking procedures should first become experienced in the use of one device used at one particular time before using other devices at other times.

Procedure: Insertion of IUCD (see Figure 1)

Interval insertion

Fully informed consent must first be obtained.

1. Check the size of the uterus for completeness of involution (and the possibility of pregnancy)

2. Determine the position of the uterus (anteverted vs retroverted), noting especially whether the uterus is acutely anteflexed.

3. Position the patient in the most favored position for examination of the cervix. If there is any difficulty in visualizing the cervix with the patient in the dorsal position, the patient should be placed in the left lateral or lithotomy position.

4. Insert a warmed and sparsely lubricated bivalve (Cusco's) speculum and open the blades to visualize the complete cervix and os.

5. Take a cervical smear for cytology if indicated.

6. Swab the cervix with a cotton gauze held in sponge forceps and soaked in an antiseptic such as chlorhexidine (**Figure 1a**). (The concomitant use of an oral antibiotic or devices that also have an antiseptic does not appear to affect the infection rate after insertion.)

7. Attach a single toothed tenaculum to the anterior lip of the cervix to steady the cervix and straighten the angle at the internal os of the uterine cavity with the cervical canal.

8. Measure the length of the uterine cavity with a sound remembering to angle the sound anteriorly or posteriorly depending on the position of the uterus (**Figure 1b**). The length should normally be 7–8 cm.

9. Fix the stop on the device applicator to the appropriate length to ensure the IUCD is placed at the fundus and not lower in the uterine cavity where it is less effective, and expulsion more likely (**Figure 1c**).

10. Insert the IUCD (**Figure 1d**). The actual method of insertion depends on the design of the device but withdrawal methods are preferable to devices that require a plunger action. The 'Multiload' with its free 'arms' requires simple inser-

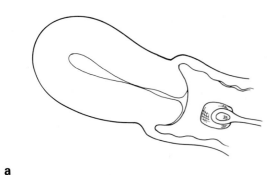

a

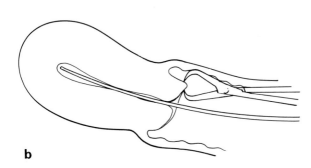

b

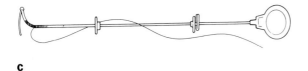

c

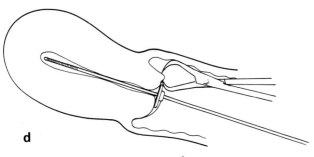

d

Figure 1a–d.

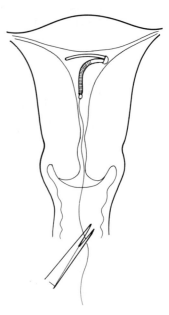

Figure 1e.

tion to the fundus, a slight twist to engage the arms on the endometrial walls, and then withdrawal of the applicator.

11. Cut the strings so that 2–3 cm only are visible (**Figure 1e**). It is important not to apply any traction to the string to avoid displacement of the device or getting retraction of the string into the uterus after trimming.

Complications

Caution is necessary if the woman has had a cesarean section and the uterus is retroverted as the sound or device applicator can pass easily through the soft uterine scar. Conversely, it is easy to perforate the uterus posteriorly if the uterus is acutely anteverted. Fortunately, the appropriate use of the tenaculum avoids this problem by straightening out the angle of the cervical canal with the uterine cavity.

The procedure usually causes no or little discomfort to the woman. If the woman develops pain during or shortly after the insertion, perforation should be suspected and the device should be immediately withdrawn after reintroducing the speculum and pulling on the threads. Asking the woman to push down may be helpful. If the woman becomes faint with a slow pulse, vagal shock from partial expulsion should be expected and immediate removal rather than atropine is then advisable.

Postplacental insertion

Insertion of an intrauterine device within 10 min of delivery of the placenta is advisable if there is a strong possibility of the woman not returning for an interval insertion. *Thus, the usual reasons for choosing post-placental insertion of an IUCD are patient unreliability or health personnel problems.*

Surprisingly, the copper IUCDs are as effective at this time as the larger Lippes loops (size D), and have no higher expulsion or failure rates. However, the safety and effectiveness of these post-placental insertions are significantly lower than interval insertions. Nevertheless, postplacental insertion is not associated with increased puerperal bleeding problems.

Method

Post-placental insertion does require good sterile technique and fundal insertion must be ensured either by placement of the device by hand or by using an inserter or applicator. The insertion of an IUCD at the time of cesarean section has, surprisingly, lower expulsion rates than with immediate postpartum vaginal insertion; indeed, continuation rates are almost comparable to interval insertions, perhaps because fundal placement can be ensured visually.

Progestagenic intrauterine devices

Earlier progestagenic devices fell into disrepute because of a possible increased risk of ectopic pregnancy. However, this is not a common problem with the newer devices which contain levonorgestrel. A major benefit of these devices is reduced menstruation, which is likely to be a major health benefit especially in developing nations. The higher expulsion rate with post-placental insertion with this device in comparison with the copper devices probably relates to user unfamiliarity rather than the device itself.

Combined oral contraceptive hormones

This method is generally contraindicated in the early puerperium in the breast-feeding woman because of an inhibitory effect on the initiation of lactation. There are also concerns about latent effects on the infant of ingestion of the estrogen and progestagen that is secreted in the breast milk.

The combined oral contraceptive can, however, be initiated in women who are not breast-feeding. It is

doubtful if there is any significant thromboembolic risk with the initiation of the oral contraceptive in this situation, and it can be effectively begun within the first 7 days of birth. This contraceptive does not appear to affect involution. Nevertheless, it is not a common choice for women in the immediate postnatal period, despite its obvious health benefits and safety. It does not appear to have any effect on the development of choriocarcinoma.

Progestagen-only pill (POP or mini-pill)

This is the common hormonal contraceptive postnatally. Because it has no effect on lactation, it is especially favored for breast-feeding women. There are also no effects on the infant because the amount of circulating progestagen absorbed is small in comparison to other progestagenic methods such as injections, implants or vaginal rings.

A major problem with the mini-pill is irregular or intermenstrual bleeding. The effectiveness of the mini-pill largely depends on the reliability of the woman in taking the pill at the same time each day.

Injectable progestagens

The most effective contraceptive postnatally is a depot injection of medroxyprogesterone acetate (DMPA) or northisterone enanthate ('Norgest'). However, when irregular bleeding occurs, it is difficult to differentiate this progestagenic effect from retained products of conception or an endometritis. Irregular bleeding that is associated with the progestagenic injection usually resolves with the second injection at an interval of 12 or 13 weeks, (the timing depending on the preparation used).

The progestagen is secreted in the breast milk and levels in the fetus tend to parallel those in the mother. The biological significance of the absorbed progestagen in the neonate is uncertain.

Progestagenic implants and vaginal rings

These newer methods of delivering progestagens such as levonorgestrel have the advantage over injections of reversibility should there be complications that are potentially attributable to the progestagen, such as irregular bleeding. Because of a relatively high expulsion with vaginal rings in the early postnatal period, their use should not be advocated until involution is complete at about 6 weeks after birth.

Studies with 'Norplant', the levonorgestrel implant, have shown very good effectiveness and safety but, unfortunately, its use is lactating women is not promoted because of the absorption from breat milk. It is unlikely that there is an adverse effect from this progestagen, and it certainly does not affect the amount of gonadotrophin or gonadal steroid secreted in infants.

Spermicides

Spermicides are usually used coincidentally with a barrier method such as a diaphragm or cervical cap. The usual spermicide is nonoxynol. The effectiveness of

gossypol is still being studied. There is no evidence that the use of these spermicides in the puerperium, even in douche or foam form, is associated with an increased risk of genital tract infection.

Natural family planning

The detection of estrogenic mucus in the postnatal period is possible if women have had prior experience of the technique. However, this mucus may be present for some days without ovulation occurring, and this consequently affects the reliability of this method until regular menses again become established. There are difficulties in the reliability of this technique when infants are not fully breast-fed and younger than 5 months.

PUERPERAL CONTRACEPTION
Summary of Management Options

- Until the infant is 5 months old, and provided it is fully breast-fed (i.e. <150 ml supplement) including at night, lactation is probably an effective contraceptive

- Contraception is advisable if the infant is more than 5 months old or, if less than 5 months old, is not fully breast-fed and therefore requiring solid or supplementary bottle feeds

- The most popular puerperal contraceptive method is condoms

- Diaphragms or cervical caps should be fitted at the 6 week visit and checked once menses recur

- IUCDs are more reliable if inserted at the postnatal check rather than post-placentally

- Progestagen-only preparations are available as tablets, injections, vaginal rings and implants, and all can cause irregular bleeding – the infant's absorption of the progestagen does not seem to produce any adverse effects

- Natural family planning may be a difficult method to use in the puerperium

---

STERILIZATION

Sterilization is now the most common form of contraception in the world. The incidence of puerperal sterilization is, however, falling in the Western world in preference to 'interval' sterilization.

Benefits

The major benefit of sterilization after delivery is convenience, either for the woman or the doctor. The most convenient puerperal sterilization is at the time of an elective cesarean section.

Risks

The major disadvantage of puerperal sterilization is psychological with dissatisfaction of the procedure resulting in an increased demand for reversal (rates up to 10%), especially in younger women aged < 25 years. The second major risk is that associated with the general anesthesia, especially if undertaken shortly after prolonged labor or difficult delivery. The use of H2-antagonists prophylactically and probably during labor may reduce the risk of the acid-aspiration syndrome. Thromboembolism is a further risk and if puerperal sterilization is indicated at a time of increased thrombogenic activity, specific prophylaxis by thromboembolic stockings is also indicated.

Prenatal Care

Couples should be counseled about puerperal sterilization during the prenatal period. If appropriate, the procedure can then be agreed and consent signed. Preconditions may be agreed such as the infant being normal and not requiring resuscitation. Discussion about the knowledge of the sex of the child at birth may reveal uncertainty about the decision for permanent contraception, in which case the procedure should not be agreed.

Indications

At cesarean section:

- completed family

- age >30 years (relative indication)

- elective rather than emergency cesarean section that is necessary because of previous cesarean sections

- decision made and confirmed during second or early third trimester

- no anticipated neonatal risk

Puerperal sterilization:

- completed family

- age >30 years

- parity 4+

- unable to return for interval laparoscopic sterilization

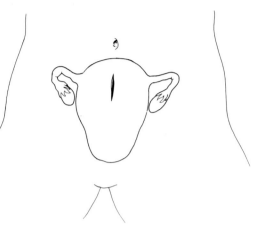

Figure 2a.

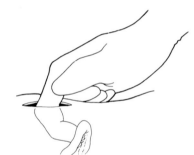

Figure 2b.

Procedure: Sterilization (Figure 2)

Pomeroy tubal ligation is the preferred method. Other techniques such as the Irving technique or Hulka clips have been used but do not appear to be of greater benefit.

1. Incision: for puerperal sterilization: 3 cm mid-line incision, 2–3 cm below fundus (Figure 2a).

2. The middle portion of the tube is drawn out through the incision with the index finger (Figure 2b). The fimbrial end is then identified visibly to ensure that it

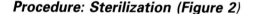

Figure 2c.

is the tube and not the round or ovarian ligament that is being ligated.

3. The tube is then clamped with small artery forceps (Figure 2c).

4. The mesenteric vessels are identified and a T10 chromic catgut suture brought through the mesentery about 2 cm below the forceps grasping the tube – this is then tied around either the medial or lateral segment of the tube (**Figure 2d**).

5. The other portion is then tied with the same catgut.

6. Using the end of the catgut, a 1 cm ischemic segment is created by drawing a suture around the tubes 1 cm below the first transfixed suture (**Figure 2e**).

7. The 3–4 cm segment of the tube is removed about 0.5 cm distal to the first suture and the stump checked hemostatically prior to cutting the second suture (**Figure 2f**).

8. The tubal segment is sent for histology.

9. The procedure is repeated on the other tube.

10. The abdomen is then closed in three layers. The procedure for Pomeroy tubal ligation at cesarean section is similar.

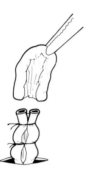

Figure 2f.

Complications

There are few complications of the procedure. Women should be warned that there is approximately a 1:200 failure rate, and this should be noted in the consent form. An ileus is a rare complication and usually suggests hemorrhage or infection.

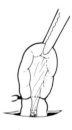

Figure 2d.

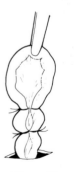

Figure 2e.

PUERPERAL STERILIZATION
Summary of Management Options

- Puerperal sterilization is better performed as an interval procedure using the laparoscope

- If immediate puerperal sterilization is required, a mini-laparotomy using the Pomeroy technique is simpler, quicker, safer and probably more reliable than any laparoscopic technique

- The Pomeroy technique is the most common surgical technique of early puerperal sterilization

FURTHER READING

Puerperal Contraception

1   Knodel J, Kamnuansilpa P, Chamratrithirong A (1985) Infant feeding practices, postpartum amenorrhea, and contraceptive use in Thailand. *Studies in Family Planning* 302–311.

2   Laukaran VH, Winikoff B (1985) Contraceptive use, amenorrhea, and breastfeeding in postpartum women. *Studies in Family Planning* 293–301.

3   Hatherley LI (1985) Lactation and postpartum infertility: The use-effectiveness of natural family planning (NFP) after term pregnancy. *Clin Reprod Fertil* 3:319–334.

4   Abdulla KA, Elwan SI, Salem HS, Shaaban MM (1985) Effect of early postpartum use of the contraceptive implants, NORPLANT, on the serum levels of immunoglobulins of the mothers and thier breastfed infants. *Contraception* 32:261–266.

5   Chi IO, Wilkens L, Rogers S (1985) Expulsions in immediate postpartum insertions of Lippes Loop D and Cooper T IUDs and their counterpart Delta devices: An epidemiological analysis. *Contraception* 32:119–134.

6   Chick PH, Frances M, Paterson PJ (1985) A comprehensive review of female sterilisation: Tubal occlusion methods. *Clin Reprod Fertil* 81–97.

7   Thiery M, Van Kets H, Van der Pas H (1985) Immediate post-placental IUD insertion: The expulsion problem. *Contraception* 31:331–349.

8   Ellis DJ, Hewat RJ (1985) Mothers' postpartum perceptions of spousal relationships. *J Obstet Gynecol Neonatal Nurs* 14:140–146.

9   Shaaban MM, Salen HT, Abdullah KA (1985) Influence of levonorgestrel contraceptive implants, NORPLANT, initiated early postpartum upon lactation and infant growth. *Contraception* 32:623–635.

10 Diaz S, Jackanicz TM, Herreros C, Juez G, Peralta O, Miranda P, Casado ME, Schiapacasse V, Salvatierra AM, Brandelis A *et al.* (1985) Fertility regulation in nursing women: VIII. Progesterone plasma levels and contraceptive efficacy of a progesterone-releasing vaginal ring. *Contraception* 32:603–622.

11 Sivin I (1985) Insertion technique, not design, affects expulsion rates of postpartum intrauterine devices. *Contraception* 31:553–555.

12 Zacharias S, Aguilera E, Assenzo JR, Zanartu J (1986) Effects of hormonal and nonhormonal contraceptives on lactation and incidence of pregnancy. *Contraception* 33:203–213.

13 Shikary ZK, Betrabet SS, Patel ZM, Patel S, Joshi JV, Toddywala VS, Toddywala SP, Patel DM, Jhaveri K, Saxena BN (1987) ICMR task force study on hormonal contraception: Transfer of levonorgestrel (LNG) administered through different drug delivery systems from the maternal circulation into the newborn infant's circulation via breast milk. *Contraception* 35:477–486.

14 Pedron N, Mondragon H, Marcushamer B, Gallegos AJ (1987) The effect of post-partum IUD insertion on postpartum bleeding. *Contraception* 35:245–251.

15 Chi IC, Farr G (1989) Postpartum IUD contraception: A review of an international experience. *Advances in Contraception* 5:127–146.

16 Fraser HM, Dewart PJ, Smith SK, Cowen GM, Sandow J, McNeilly AS (1989) Luteinizing hormone releasing hormone agonist for contraception in breast feeding women. *Journal of Clinical Endocrinology and Metabolism* 69:996–1002.

17 Chick PH, Frances M, Paterson PJ (1985) A comprehensive review of female sterilisation: Tubal occlusion methods. *Clin Reprod Fertil* 3:81–97.

18 Elder MG, Lawson JP, Elstein M, Nuttall ID (1991) The efficacy and acceptability of a low-dose levonorgestrel intravaginal ring for contraception in a UK cohort. *Contraception* 43:129–137.

19 Lahteenmaki PL, Diaz S, Miranda P, Croxatto H, Lahteenmaki P (1990) Milk and plasma concentrations of the progestin ST-1435 in women treated parenterally with ST-1435. *Contraception* 42:555–562.

20 Diaz S, Miranda P, Brandeis A, Cardenas H, Croxatto HB (1991) Mechanism of action of progesterone as contraceptive for lactating women. *Annals of the New York Academy of Science* 626:11–21.

21 Kennedy KI, Rivera R, McNeilla AS (1989) Consensus Statement on the Use of Breastfeeding as a Family Planning Method. *Contraception* 39:477–495.

Puerperal Sterilization

1   De Villiers VP (1986) Postpartum sterilization by mini-incision at Paarl, CP: A multicentre international comparison. *South African Medical Journal* 70:540–541.

2   Klaerke M, Brunn Nielsen JE, Vilsgaard K (1986) Laparoscopic sterilization with the Falope-ring technique in the puerperium. *Acta Obstetrica et Gynecologica Scandinavica* 65:99–101.

3   de Villiers VP (1987) Postpartum sterilisation with the Filshie titanium silicone-rubber clip and subsequent pregnancy. *South African Medical Journal* 71:498–499.

4   Griffin WT, Mandsager NT (1987) Spring clip sterilisation: Long-term follow-up. *Southern Medical Journal* 80:301–304.

5   Chick PH, Frances M, Paterson PJ (1985) A comprehensive review of female sterilisation: Tubal occlusion methods. *Clin Reprod Fertil* 3:81–97.

71

Resuscitation and Immediate Care of the Newborn

DAVID JAMES

INTRODUCTION

The percentage of newborn infants requiring 'active resuscitation' in the form of assisted ventilation is probably less than 5%. However, approximately one-third of babies requiring such resuscitation are delivered after an apparently normal labor with no evidence of fetal compromise either before or during the labor and delivery. Thus, wherever babies are delivered, someone should be available at all times capable of commencing expert resuscitation of the newborn. While in many cases this individual will be a pediatrician, this is not so for every delivery. Thus it is imperative that obstetricians understand the principles of neonatal resuscitation and, furthermore, can institute appropriate and effective resuscitation either by intubation or by bag and mask.

In summary, the obstetrician has two responsibilities relating to neonatal resuscitation:

- To ensure that the provision of facilities for resuscitation are adequate.

- To ensure that he/she understands the principles and can initiate resuscitation of the newborn.

PREREQUISITES FOR A NEONATAL RESUSCITATION SERVICE

Normally, the responsibility for ensuring adequate neonatal resuscitation facilities are available lies with pediatricians. However, in units or settings where no pediatric support is available, that responsibility lies with the obstetrician. The prerequisites are:

- Provision of adequate training (including the preparation of appropriate protocols) in neonatal resuscitation for all medical professionals likely to be involved in providing care in labor, including obstetricians, nurses, midwives, anesthetists as well as pediatricians. In practice, the degree of training varies considerably.

- Posting of a roster of trained staff immediately available for neonatal resuscitation in the delivery suite, telephone exchange and the pediatric department.

- Summoning trained assistance in good time whenever a resuscitation problem is anticipated. The deliveries where a pediatrician or someone trained in resuscitation of the newborn should be present are summarized in **Table 1**.

- Ensuring that resuscitation equipment is available and working (**Table 2**).

- Ensuring that the delivery rooms are draught-free with a temperature of at least 24°C.

NEONATAL RESUSCITATION AND IMMEDIATE CARE BY THE OBSTETRICIAN

When potential resuscitation problems are anticipated before delivery, then the normal practice should be to have a pediatrician present at the delivery (see **Table 1**). The practical skills in neonatal resuscitation required by the obstetrician, therefore, are to be able to initiate resuscitation and maintain it:

- in such cases until the pediatrician arrives

- in cases where the baby is delivered and requires resuscitation which has not been anticipated. When this occurs, pediatric support should be mobilized urgently.

Table 1
Deliveries at which pediatric staff or those trained in neonatal resuscitation should be present

Factors related to labor/delivery

Cesarean section
Breech delivery or other malpresentation
Forceps/ventouse delivery (except simple 'lift outs')
Delivery after significant antepartum hemorrhage
Prolapsed cord

Maternal factors

Mother with severe pregnancy-induced hypertension
Mother with other medical disorders which can affect the fetus
Mother with a history of current drug or alcohol abuse
Delivery under heavy sedation or general anesthesia
Fever

Fetal factors

Multiple pregnancy (one pediatrician for each baby)
Preterm delivery (< 37 weeks) (two pediatricians are advisable if the baby is < 32 weeks or if the anticipated weight is < 1500 g)
Prolonged membrane rupture (> 24 h) or suspected chorioamnionitis
Hydramnios
Fetal distress (meconium staining of amniotic fluid, fetal heart rate abnormality, abnormal fetal scalp pH)
Fetal abnormality or disease, either known or suspected
Isoimmuinization

Preparation

If not already known to the parents, the obstetrician should introduce him/herself to the parents and briefly

Table 2
Neonatal resuscitation equipment (checked daily and after use)

Immediately available in every delivery room

Resuscitation trolley with overhead heater, lighting, stop-clock with a sweep second hand
Oxygen and air supply (with reducing valve, flow-meter, pressure blow-off device set at 30 cm H_2O and pressure manometer)
Connecting tubes to supply air/oxygen to bag and mask and ETT
Face masks of appropriate size range (00, 0 and 1) (see **Figure 1**)
Resuscitation bag (volume 250–500 ml) (see **Figure 2**) with fitting for face mask and ETT adaptor and blow-off valve
Two laryngoscopes, with preterm and term sized straight blades, respectively, and spare bulbs and batteries
Endotracheal tubes (see text for sizes) and connectors and fixation devices
ETT introducer (nylon or metal)
Oropharyngeal airways (range of sizes)
Suction device (maximum suction setting = 200 mmHg; normal setting = 100 mmHg) and suction catheters (sizes 8 and 10)
Sterile towel, scissors and cord clamps
Antiseptic cleaning solution
Silver swaddler and warmed dry towels
Intravenous cannulas, three-way taps, connecting tubing
Sterile syringes (2, 5 and 10 ml) and needles (21 and 23 g)
Nasogastric tubes (F.G. 6 and 8)
Oral mucus extractors
Adhesive tape and safety pins
Sterile containers and specimen bottles for samples
Drugs (naloxone, 20 μg/ml; vitamin K)
Capillary glucose test strips
Stethoscope with infant endpiece
Alcohol swabs

Available at all times within the delivery suite (not in every room)

Equipment for umbilical catheterization
Pneumothorax drains and valves
10% glucose solution for infusion (500 ml)
Pediatric i.v. giving sets
Intravenous infusion pumps
Fresh frozen plasma
Fresh blood (group O, Rh-negative)
Drugs
    glucose 25% (25 ml ampoules)
    adrenaline/epinephrine (1:10 000 solution)
    calcium gluconate 10%
    0.9% sodium chloride for injection
    sterile water for injection

Facilities that are assumed to be present on the Neonatal Intensive Care Unit

EKG electrodes and monitor
Blood pressure monitor
Transcutaneous O_2 and CO_2 monitors
Blood gas analyzers
Oxygen saturation monitors

A list of already calculated emergency drug doses for a range of baby sizes/gestations is advisable.

explain that he/she is going to be involved in the resuscitation of the baby.

As full a history as possible should be obtained as quickly as possible from the mother, medical professionals involved in the delivery and the maternal notes. In particular, it is important to establish:

- the gestational age

- whether any drugs have been given to the mother

- whether there has been any evidence of fetal distress (heart rate abnormality or meconium)

- whether there has been any vaginal bleeding

- the duration of membrane rupture

- the maternal health in labor

- any obstetric or medical history with potential effects on the fetus.

The resuscitation equipment should be checked and prepared:

- check that the equipment is available and in working order (especially the clock, the oxygen supply, the suction equipment, the laryngoscopes and lights, the resuscitation bag, a range of face masks and endotracheal tubes)

- turn on the overhead heater

- ensure that dry warm towels are available

- if the mother has had a narcotic analgesic during labor, ensure that an antagonist (e.g. naloxone) is readily available.

Management at Birth (see **Figure 3**)

Basic care for all newborns

Timing of birth

The time that the baby is born should be noted so that the timing of any subsequent interventions can be accurately documented.

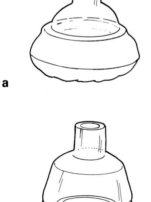

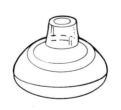

Figure 1. Neonatal face masks.
a Ambu. **b** Laerdal. **c**. Bennet.

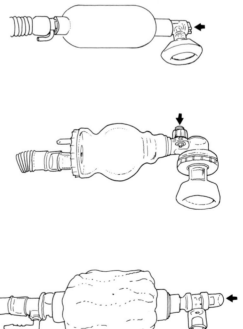

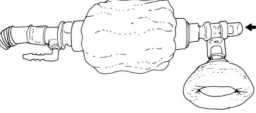

Figure 2. Self-inflating resuscitation bags.
a Cardiff. **b** Laerdal. **c** Ambu.
(Arrows indicate position of blow-off valve.)

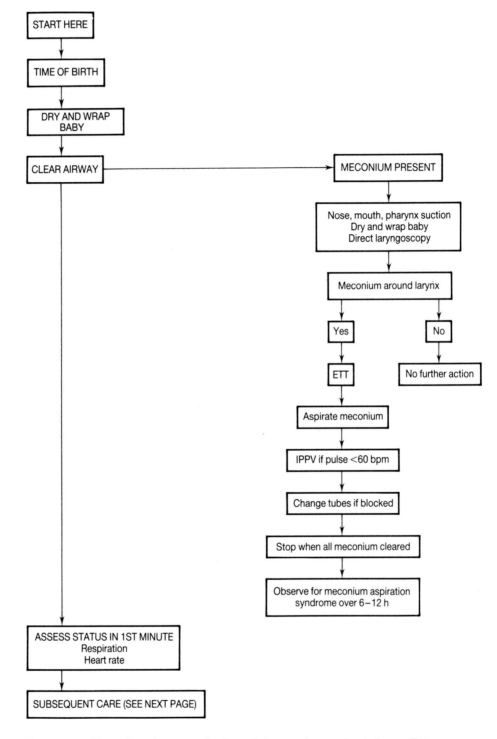

Figure 3a. Flow chart for resuscitation of the newborn – basic immediate care.

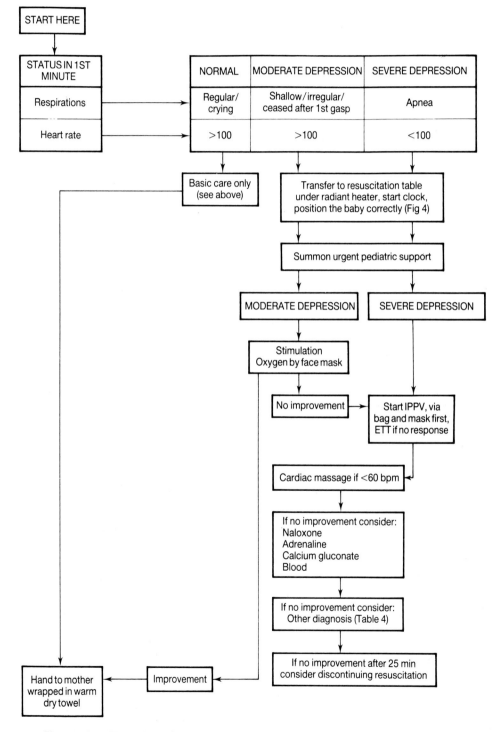

Figure 3b. Flow chart for resuscitation of the newborn – subsequent care.

Thermal care

Even healthy infants have difficulty maintaining body temperature soon after delivery. The risk of cold stress is even greater in growth-deficient, preterm, ill or sedated babies. Oxygen requirements will rise if the baby's temperature is allowed to drop below normal. Heat loss is minimized by immediately drying the infant, removing wet linen and wrapping the infant in a warm towel. If resuscitation has to occur, this should take place with the wrapped infant under an overhead heater. An incubator or a silver foil swaddler may be needed for transfer of babies at great risk of hypothermia. Silver foil should not be used under a radiant heater, as it reflects radiant heat and reduces the effectiveness of the heater. A clothed infant may lose up to 85% of its total heat loss through its head; therefore, using a bonnet is advisable to reduce heat loss during prolonged resuscitations.

Care of the airway

The majority of babies do not require aspiration of the upper airway with a mucus suction catheter. Direct mouth suction is no longer used because of the potential risk of HIV infection. The alternatives are oral suction using a system with a double mucus trap or artificial suction. It is usually sufficient to wipe the lips and nose during the process of drying the baby. Suction should normally be confined to aspiration of the anterior nose or mouth. The tip of the catheter should not be inserted into the pharynx unless there is clear evidence of obstruction (inspiratory retraction of the chest wall and poor/absent air entry), in which case it should be done under direct vision with the use of a laryngoscope. There is a danger of reflex bradycardia, apnea and hypotension with overvigorous probing around the larynx.

When the upper airway is obstructed, the blockage is usually located in the nose and is due to either debris or choanal atresia or stenosis. The patency of the nasal passages can be tested by listening to each nostril in turn with the stethoscope while temporarily occluding the opposite nostril. If the diagnosis is made and aspiration fails to remove any debris and the problem persists, insertion of an airway of appropriate size will encourage breathing through the infant's mouth and, if necessary, allow intermittent positive pressure ventilation (IPPV), by face mask using the same route and may be lifesaving.

When meconium has been passed *in utero* (approximately 10% of all deliveries), inhalation of that meconium may lead to severe respiratory distress. The pathogenesis of this condition includes chemical pneumonitis, partial airway obstruction with patchy atelectasis, overinflation and pneumothoraces, and a persistent fetal circulation. Meconium aspiration syndrome is largely preventable by correct delivery room management. This comprises:

Procedure: Management After Delivery Where Meconium is Present

1. Once the face is delivered on the perineum, meconium is cleared from the nose, mouth and pharynx using an oral mucus extractor.

2. After delivery, the infant should be transferred to the resuscitation table.

3. The infant should be quickly dried and wrapped by an assistant.

4. The mouth, pharynx and nose are gently sucked out using a laryngoscope to visualize the vocal cords; the posterior pharynx and larynx are sucked out under direct vision.

5. If meconium is seen in the posterior pharynx and larynx, the infant should be intubated. Gentle suction should be applied to the endotracheal tube (ETT) until no more meconium is obtained. The aim is to delay the application of positive pressure to the airway until there is no more meconium below the vocal cords. However, if there is a bradycardia and the baby's condition deteriorates, the baby should then be resuscitated by IPPV using the ETT with the lowest pressure and inspiratory time compatible with good chest expansion and oxygenation.

6. If the catheter or ETT blocks, then it should be removed and replaced.

7. Where meconium has been found below the vocal cords, close observation is advisable over the first 6–12 h of life to watch for the development of meconium aspiration syndrome.

Note: *This process of checking and clearing the airways of meconium should be completed as quickly as possible, since a delay in providing adequate oxygenation by resuscitation may be counterproductive, especially if the fetus has suffered intrapartum asphyxia as a cause for the passage of meconium. In such cases, aspiration of the meconium may have already occurred* in utero.

Assessment of clinical status

The status of the infant at birth may be assessed using the Apgar score (**Table 3**). While this is conventionally only recorded at 1, 5 and, perhaps, 10 min, if resuscitation continues it is worth recording the score every 5 min after that. The Apgar score was originally introduced to quantitate the initial status of the baby and to determine appropriate resuscitation measures. In this respect, it is as valuable as ever, although its usefulness in predicting long-term outcome, especially neurodevelopmental, is less certain. In practice, the baby's heart rate and respirations are the most useful guides to management.

Table 3
The Apgar score

Sign	Score = 0	Score = 1	Score = 2
Heart rate	Absent	< 100 beats/min	> 100 beats/min
Respiration	Absent	Gasping/weak	Regular/crying
Muscle tone	Flaccid	Some flexion of extremities	Well flexed, active
Reflex/ irritability	No response	Grimace	Cough, sneeze, cry
Color	White/blue	Body pink, extremities blue	Completely pink

Subsequent care: when the infant requires resuscitation

The infant that will require resuscitation should be recognized promptly *within the first minute* by one of the following criteria:

- no regular respiration

- heart rate which remains below 100 beats/min

- Apgar score which remains below 7

In addition, it is probably wise to anticipate resuscitation problems in infants that are less than 37 weeks and/or less than 2500 g.

1. Such babies should be transferred promptly to the resuscitation table at the same time taking measures to avoid hypothermia (see above).

2. If it has not already been done, pediatric assistance should be mobilized urgently.

3. If resuscitation problems are anticipated, the clock on the resuscitation tables should be started when the baby leaves the mother's body (not when the cord is clamped). In other circumstances, the clock will be started when the baby is brought to the resuscitation table and an estimate of the intervening delay made.

4. The infant should be placed either in the horizontal position or with a slight head-down tilt. The shoulders should be supported and the neck neither excessively extended nor excessively flexed so that the larynx is visible (see **Figure 4**).

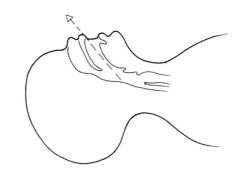

a

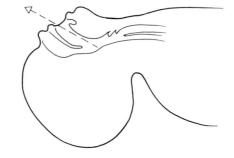

b

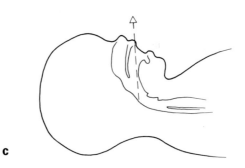

c

Figure 4. Positioning the head for resuscitation.
a Correct. **b** Incorrect. **c** Incorrect.

5. If the baby has a heart rate over 100 beats/min (usually with an Apgar score of 4–6), then the infant is only moderately depressed and simple stimulation either by drying the baby with a towel, by gently clearing the nose with a mucus catheter or by gently flicking the feet may be sufficient to stimulate respiration. Administration of 100% oxygen by face mask is often performed at the same time.

6. If the baby shows no response to simple stimulation, or if the heart rate is less than 100 beats/min, or if the Apgar score is less than 4, then IPPV should be instituted. Oxygen (100%) at pressures of up to a maximum of 30 cm H_2O should be administered to the airway at a rate of 30–60 puffs/min using either a bag and mask, or through an ETT. The purpose of the former method is to provoke the onset of respiration by reflex stimulation of pressure receptors in the lower airway rather than to inflate the lungs mechanically. Occasionally, with large babies or infants with severe underlying lung disease, higher pressures (up to 40 cm H_2O) may be necessary.

- *Using bag and mask*: it is mandatory that all medical, midwifery and nursing staff involved in labor care should know how to use the bag and mask. It is a simple method and is non-invasive. It is the technique of choice if the infant is moderately depressed (Apgar score 4–6) because intubation in such babies is sometimes difficult and, furthermore, intubation may produce reflex apnea. It is important to ensure that the upper airway is clear (see above) and an airway should be inserted if there is any doubt over nasal patency. There should be a tight seal where the mask is applied to the baby's face and overforceful compression of the bag should be avoided. There should be synchronous movement of the chest wall with compression and relaxation of the bag. If this fails to occur, then the baby's head should be repositioned to ensure that the airway is adequately extended and the seal of the face mask checked.

- *Using endotracheal intubation*: this is the preferred method for infants not responding within 1 min to bag and mask IPPV (rise in heart rate, improved color, onset of respiration) and for those with more severe asphyxia (Apgar score less than 4). It is a technique which should be learnt ideally with pediatric supervision and advice using a model before it is first used in a clinical setting.

Procedure: Neonatal Endotracheal Intubation (see Figure 5)

Endotracheal tube sizes

ETT size	Baby weight (g)	Gestation (weeks)
2.0	< 750	< 26
2.5	750–1000	26–29
3.0	1000–2000	30–34
3.0 or 3.5	2000–3000	30–34
3.5	> 3500	> 34

Technique

1. Ensure the head and neck are in line with the rest of the body and the neck is slightly extended (see **Figure 4**).

2. Insert the laryngoscope blade over the tongue in the midline to the back of the larynx. The uvula and then the epiglottis will come into view.

3. Lift the epiglottis forward by exerting traction parallel to the handle of the laryngoscope (not by tilting the blade upwards).

4. The vocal cords should then be visualized. Brief suction may be needed to clear secretions. Gentle cricoid pressure with the fifth finger of the left hand or by an assistant may help visualization.

5. Keeping the trachea central, with the right hand insert the appropriate size ETT with adaptor attached through the vocal cords until the shoulder or mark on the tube (about 2 cm from the tip) is at the vocal cords.

6. Once the ETT is in the correct position, gently stabilize this for ventilation by holding the ETT with the thumb and forefinger of the right hand while maintaining the fixed position with the other three fingers placed against the side of the baby's face and jaw.

7. Carefully remove the laryngoscope

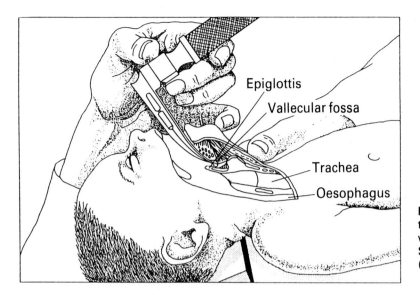

Figure 5. The technique for endotracheal intubation. Reproduced with permission from Fleming PJ, Speidel BD, Marlow N, Dunn PM (1991) *A Neonatal Vade-Mecum.* London: Edward Arnold.

(and introducer from the ETT if one has been used).

8. Request an assistant to connect tubing from the oxygen source to the adaptor of the ETT.

9. Commence IPPV – starting at 30 cm H₂O blow-off valve setting, 2–3 l/min flow rate and 30 breaths/min (the method of applying IPPV will depend on the ETT and adaptor design).

10. Observe equal movement of both sides of the chest and auscultate the chest for heart rate and breath sounds. Check for equal air entry on both sides; if there is unilateral air entry, the ETT is probably in one main bronchus and should be withdrawn slightly.

If the first attempt is unsuccessful, then bag and mask resuscitation should be recommenced for another 30–60 s before a further attempt at intubation. There is a great danger of the baby becoming cold and/or hypoxic as a result of prolonged or many unsuccessful attempts at resuscitation. If the baby does not respond to IPPV within 30 s, then the tube should be rechecked to ensure that it is not dislodged or blocked. With either bag and mask or endotracheal IPPV, the air/oxygen supply should normally have the blow-off set at 30 cm H₂O (lower pressures should be used if possible with babies < 1500 g) and the flow rates should not exceed 2–3 l/min. Higher pressures (up to 40 cm H₂O) and

flow rates (4–6 l/min) can be considered if there is no response with large babies. Higher pressures and rates of ventilation also can be used with the baby that still does not improve despite the above measures. Once the baby is pink and breathing spontaneously, the tube should be removed. An open ETT should not be left in place as this will impair oxygenation by increasing the dead space.

7. If the heart beat is undetectable or remains below 50–60 beats/min despite IPPV, then cardiac massage should be commenced.

Procedure: Cardiac Massage

1. Place the fingers of one or both hands behind the baby's chest with one or both thumbs on the lower sternum.

2. The sternum is then depressed by about 2 cm and at a rate of 100/min (i.e. effectively 'squeezing' the heart at that rate). This compression should not be vigorous in order to avoid damage to the chest wall, heart or liver.

3. During cardiac massage, assisted ventilation should continue. It is advisable for the senior person at the resuscitation to coordinate the two activities by repeatedly calling out '1-2-3-breath' until the rhythm of massage and ventilation is established at rates of about 100/min and 30/min, respectively.

8. If the baby shows no response and the mother has received an opiate such as pethidine, morphine or heroin within the previous 8 h, administration of naloxone (10 μg/kg) by intramuscular or subcutaneous injection into the thigh is advisable. Attempting to inject this drug intravenously may result in unacceptable delay. This specific antagonist given intramuscularly usually produces a response within 2 min. The dose may be repeated after 30–60 min. However, the first priority is always to establish and maintain cardiorespiratory support.

9. If there is a persisting bradycardia/asystole despite adequate ventilation and cardiac massage, then the following therapeutic options are available:

- administration of 1 : 10 000 adrenaline/epinephrine 0.1 ml/kg dilution either i.v. (umbilical vein) or via the ETT

- calcium gluconate 10% solution 1 ml/kg

- if there is no response to these two approaches, then intracardiac adrenaline and calcium gluconate in the same doses can be given.

10. If there is a possibility from the maternal history that there may have been placental blood loss and the baby is white/pale, apneic and hypotensive with a weak

Table 4
Causes for difficulty at resuscitation

Respiratory
Extreme prematurity/severe RDS
Meconium aspiration syndrome
Diaphragmatic hernia
Pneumothorax/pneumomediastinum
Pleural/pericardial effusion
Congenital pneumonia
Pulmonary edema/hemorrhage
Pulmonary hypoplasia
Malformation of the respiratory tract

Cardiovascular
Congenital heart disease
Persistent fetal circulation
Hypovolemia due to blood loss

Neurological
Cerebrospinal trauma/hypoxia/malformation
Cerebral depression from drugs
Neuromuscular disorders

Other
Severe metabolic disturbance

RESUSCITATION AND IMMEDIATE CARE OF THE NEWBORN BY THE OBSTETRICIAN
Summary of Management Options

Wherever babies are delivered, someone should always be available capable of commencing expert resuscitation of the newborn. Because pediatricians are not immediately available for every delivery, obstetricians must be able to institute effective neonatal resuscitation.

Prerequisites for a neonatal resuscitation service

- Adequate training of medical professionals involved in deliveries
- Preparation of appropriate protocols
- Posting of a roster of trained staff on-call for resuscitation
- Anticipating resuscitation problems (**Table 1**)
- Ensuring that resuscitation requipment is available and working
- Delivery room temperature at least 24°C and no draughts

Neonatal resuscitation and immediate care by the obstetrician

Preparation

- If possible, introduce yourself to the parents
- Obtain a relevant history as quickly as possible
- Check and prepare the resuscitation equipment (**Table 2**); switch on heater

Management at birth

- See Flow Chart for Resuscitation of the Newborn (**Figure 3**)

pulse that may be either slow or rapid from the moment of birth, then the baby may be hypovolemic. If the baby in such circumstances fails to respond to IPPV, then a rapid transfusion of 10–20 ml/kg of blood via the umbilical vein over 5–10 min should be considered using either uncross-matched O rhesus-negative blood or blood taken from the mother. Close observation of the response should be made.

11. If these resuscitation measures fail or are inadequate, it is worth rechecking that there is no fault in the resuscitation procedure (misplaced, blocked or too small ETT; too low blow-off valve setting; disconnected oxygen). If there is still no response, then a number of differential diagnoses are possible (see **Table 4**). However, by this stage, pediatric help should be present, since the obstetrician should have summoned assistance at an earlier stage (see above). Thus the ongoing resuscitation will no longer be the responsibility of the obstetrician.

12. In rare circumstances, the obstetrician will be faced with a baby who fails to respond to resuscitation despite implementation of all the above measures and no pediatric support has arrived. The obstetrician is faced with a difficult ethical decision in such circumstances. However, it is probably wise to consider ceasing resuscitation after 25 min with no response. This decision should be discussed with the parents wherever possible.

13. The use of intravenous alkali or the use of inotropic agents during resuscitation are controversial and are probably best avoided by obstetricians. Intravenous alkali given as a bolus to a poorly ventilated asphyxiated acidotic infant, may exacerbate hypercarbia and intracellular acidosis while lowering blood pressure via its vasodilator and negative inotropic actions.

CONCLUSION

In most hospitals, a pediatrician will be available at all times to perform neonatal resuscitation. As far as possible, deliveries where such skills might be necessary should be identified in advance and the pediatric staff alerted in good time in advance of the delivery. However, deliveries will occur where such skilled assistance is not immediately available. Thus it is mandatory that all obstetricians should receive training in and feel confident to carry out effective neonatal resuscitation.

Acknowledgement

I am grateful to Dr Neil Marlow for his advice and comments on the text.

FURTHER READING

1 Fleming PJ, Speidel BD, Marlow N, Dunn PM (1991) *A Neonatal Vade-Mecum*, 2nd edn. London: Edward Arnold.

2 Roberton NRC (1986) *Textbook of Neonatology*. Edinburgh: Churchill Livingstone.

3 Taeusch HW, Ballard Ra, Avery ME (1991) *Diseases of the Newborn*. Philadelphia, PA: W. B. Saunders.

4 Working Party on Neonatal Resuscitation (1991) *Resuscitation of the Newborn. Part 1. Basic Resuscitation and Resuscitation of the Newborn. Part 2. Advanced Resuscitation*. London: Royal College of Obstetricians and Gynaecologists.

72

Counseling About Pediatric Problems

DAVID JAMES

THE PRACTICE OF COUNSELING

In most developed countries, counseling about pediatric problems is normally and appropriately undertaken by pediatricians. However, on occasions, the obstetrician has to provide some counseling. These circumstances include:

- When a patient is referred for prepregnancy counseling and unanticipated questions arise about neonatal problems.

- When the patient books for delivery in a pregnancy following a previous neonatal problem, the obstetrician should be able to assess the relevance of the more common problems to the current pregnancy.

- When a potential neonatal problem is identified during pregnancy, the ideal approach is an interdisciplinary one with the relevant nursing and medical staff and other professionals being involved in counseling the mother and her family. Nevertheless, when the problem is initially recognized and during ongoing prenatal care, the obstetrician must be prepared to give a limited amount of counseling.

- After the delivery of a baby with a problem, while the majority of any counseling of parents will be undertaken by the pediatrician, it is not uncommon for the obstetrician to be asked questions about the problem by the parents.

COUNSELING BY OBSTETRICIANS: CONDITIONS

Neonatal conditions where the obstetrician may feel able to provide some support counseling to that offered by the pediatrician are listed in **Table 1**. The degree of confidence that an obstetrician has in providing that counseling will depend on the problem and his/her training and experience in neonatal medicine. Many units have weekly meetings with their pediatric colleagues where they discuss both potential (undelivered)

Table 1
Neonatal conditions where the obstetrician
may provide counseling

The small-for-dates baby
The large-for-dates baby
The preterm baby
Birth trauma
Congenital abnormalities
Respiratory problems
Cardiac problems
Neurological disorders
Gastrointestinal problems
Metabolic problems
Hematological problems
Perinatal infection
Jaundice
Neonatal surgical problems

pediatric problems and also current neonatal (delivered) problems. This practice is to be commended. Not only does it encourage communication about problems, but it is also educational – for both obstetricians and pediatricians! As a result, obstetricians feel more able to provide complementary counseling about neonatal problems in addition to that provided by pediatricians.

However, one important warning is necessary when obstetricians do provide such counseling. It is imperative that nothing is said which is at variance with what the pediatrician has said so that confusion in the patient's mind is avoided. If there is ever doubt, it is best for the obstetric and pediatric staff to communicate and agree upon the substance of what is to be said.

The Small-For-Dates (SFD) Baby

The incidence of this problem depends on the population studied and the definitions used (see also Chapter 42). However, the morphologically normal baby that is undergrown is an risk from the complications summarized in **Table 2**.

The Large-For-Dates (LFD) Baby

The definitions used the LFD baby also vary, e.g. babies weighing >90th, >95th or >97th centiles. While many such babies are merely constitutionally of large size (a feature which is often familial), the ones which have neonatal problems are the LFD infants of diabetic mothers (IDM; see also Chapter 19). The latter group manifest complications mainly as a result of excessive insulin production both before and after birth. How-

ever, all LFD babies should be managed as IDM because not all women with gestational diabetes are identified during pregnancy. Problems that the IDM may manifest are summarized in **Table 3**.

The Preterm Baby

Approximately 4–5% of newborns are delivered before 37 weeks; however, it is the smaller number that are delivered before 34 or even 32 weeks which give rise to most problems. These problems are summarized in **Table 4**.

Birth Trauma

All signs of birth injury, even minor ones, should be shown to and discussed with the parents with appropriate explanation and reassurance. The more common injuries and their implications are summarized in **Table 5**.

Congenital Abnormalities

The incidence varies between different areas and populations, but approximately 5% of all newborns have a congenital anomaly ('a morphological defect present at birth'). Of these, 3% are malformations ('a primary error of morphogenesis arising in embryogenesis or prenatal life') and 2% are deformations ('a secondary alteration in the morphology of a previously normally formed part of the body arising during the fetal period'). Counseling implications for many congenital

Table 2
Complications of the small-for-dates baby

Complication	Comments
Hypoglycemia	Due to low glycogen and fat stores
Birth asphyxia	The baby is less able to tolerate intrapartum anoxia as a result of depleted glycogen (especially cardiac) and fat stores. Prognosis for this problem depends on severity; if a baby does not manifest an encephalopathy by the end of first week, prognosis is generally good
Meconium aspiration syndrome	Intrapartum anoxia is more common, hence passage of meconium and its aspiration *in utero* are more likely. Management at birth is discussed in Chapter 71. See below for neonatal management/outlook
Cold stress	More likely because of reduced fat stores. If it occurs, it makes other problems (e.g. hypoglycemia, asphyxia and respiratory distress) worse. To prevent this, SFD babies are nursed with extra blankets and even an electric blanket. If these measures are unsuccessful at maintaining the temperature, nursing in an incubator may be necessary
Polycythemia	May result in hyperviscosity (which in turn may exacerbate hypoglycemia and respiratory problems) and/or jaundice

Table 3
Complications of the large-for-dates baby (especially IDM)

Complication	Comments
Birth injury	Because of the large size
Hypoglycemia	Develops during the first 1–2 h and lasts for 24–48 h. Early feeding and frequent early blood glucose monitoring are part of standard care
Respiratory distress	Either due to transient tachypnea of the newborn in association with a higher cesarean section rate or respiratory distress syndrome primarily in those babies that are electively delivered preterm
Jaundice	See specific section
Hypocalcemia	See specific section
Polycythemia	This may exacerbate respiratory problems and hypoglycemia
Immaturity of sucking and swallowing reflexes	May require orogastric feeding
Cardiomyopathy	Can lead to congestive cardiac failure and even ventricular outflow obstruction; treated by propranolol rather than digoxin. For most babies, the condition resolves over a few weeks
Congenital malformations	Up to 13% of IDM have congenital malformations, especially musculoskeletal (e.g. neural tube, sacral agenesis) and cardiac defects (e.g. ventricular septal defects, transposition of the great vessels)
Risk of diabetes in later life	Up to 5% risk

Table 4
Complications of the preterm infant

Complication	Comments
Cold stress	Can be minimized by monitoring core and peripheral temperature and ensuring measures are taken both at birth and afterwards to prevent hypothermia. The peripheral temperature must be maintained in the range 35–36°C. The neutral thermal environment is the ambient temperature range which leads to minimum oxygen consumption. Charts give the values for the neutral thermal ranges for infants of different birthweights and ages
Respiratory problems	Due to respiratory distress syndrome, apnea or aspiration pneumonia
Neurological problems	Related to the immaturity of sucking, swallowing and respiratory control and also periventricular/intraventricular hemorrhage
Gastrointestinal problems	Abdominal distension with feeding and compromised respiration, poor absorption of fat and necrotizing enterocolitis
Jaundice	Due to hepatic immaturity
Hemorrhage	Due to low levels of vitamin K leading to defective blood clotting
Renal problems	Low glomerular filtration rates and poor tubular function lead to inability to excrete large water or solute load and a poor ability to conserve water or sodium
Metabolic problems	Including hypoglycemia and hypocalcemia
Infection	Especially group B streptococci, *Escherichia coli*, *Staphylococcus epidermidis* and *Pseudomonas aeruginosa*
Patent ductus arteriosus	Can lead to cardiac failure treated with antifailure therapy (oxygen, fluid restriction and diuretics) and may require indomethacin or even surgical closure
Social	Related to the enforced separation of mother and baby

Table 5
Birth injuries and their implications

Injury	Implications
Caput succedaneum	Quickly subsides; no action necessary
'Chignon'	Caused by vacuum extractor; local toilet necessary; scarring and alopecia rare
Subaponeurotic hemorrhage	If hemorrhagic shock/anemia/jaundice (very rare), treat as acute hemorrhage
Cephalhematoma	Anemia and jaundice can occur; resolve spontaneously; no action necessary
Scalp lacerations	Local toilet required, sepsis rare; rarely require suturing
Facial cyanosis	Commonly seen after delivery; pink body excludes heart disease; reassure
Superficial injuries	Subconjunctival hemorrhages, petechiae and bruising spontaneously resolve
Scalpel incisions	(Occur during cesarean section); consult with plastic surgeon; take photographs
Facial palsy	Can follow spontaneous delivery; usually unilateral; artificial tears for open eye; spontaneous recovery for the majority
Brachial plexus injuries	(After should dystocia or breech); x-rays to exclude fractures; physiotherapy is treatment; complete recovery in two-thirds
Fractures	
skull	Rare; consult with neurosurgeon
clavicle	Gentle handling; heal (sometimes with figure-of-eight bandage) in 2–3 weeks
cervical spine	Rare; often follows breech extraction; flaccid quadriplegia and urinary retention common; prognosis poor
limb long bones	Often after breech delivery; light splinting produces healing in 3 weeks
Intra-abdominal trauma	Rare (after breech delivery); delayed shock common; treat as acute hemorrhage; vitamin K mandatory; surgery in extreme
Genital bruising	10% of male breech deliveries; minimal handling; follow-up for infertility (rare)
Severe bruising	Beware shock, anemia, jaundice, oliguria

malformations are discussed the relevant chapters in the Fetal Medicine Section and Chapter 2. Information relevant to other more common malformations not covered in those chapters (especially skin and face) and the more common deformations are summarized in **Tables 6** and **7**.

Respiratory Problems

Many neonatal cardiac and respiratory disorders present with the same clinical signs of tachypnea, grunting, chest retraction and cyanosis. Although the supportive care for each is much the same, it is essential to make a definitive diagnosis so that specific treatment can be given. The more common respiratory disorders leading to distress are summarized in **Table 8**. It is usually possible to distinguish easily between the different conditions on the basis of the history, clinical examination and chest x-ray appearances. The basic supportive therapy that all babies with respiratory distress receive includes nursing in a thermoneutral environment, minimal handling, screeing for infection and monitoring blood pressure. The form and degree of ventilatory support is determined by the diagnosis and serial blood gas and pH measurements. The type of respiratory support can vary from an increased ambient oxygen concentration, through continuous positive airways pressure (CPAP) to intermittent positive pressure ventilation (IPPV). Additional measures that may be necessary with IPPV include paralysis to prevent the baby 'fighting' against the ventilator and alpha-blockade to overcome pulmonary hypertension.

Cardiac Problems

Congenital heart disease is found in approximately 7:1000 live births. It may occur as an isolated defect, but is often found in association with other malformations. In general, cardiac problems can present in the newborn as cyanosis, heart failure, as an asymptomatic heart murmur or as an arrhythmia. Some of the more important causes are summarized in **Table 9**, but are also discussed in Chapters 47 and 53.

Table 6
Congenital malformations of skin and face

Malformation	Implications
'Stork mark'	(Midline upper lip, forehead, upper nose, nape of neck); tend to fade in first months; no treatment required
Port wine stain	Capillary nevus which may persist and be cosmetically unacceptable; plastic surgery can be considered; when over ophthalmic division of trigeminal nerve, there can be underlying intracranial hemangioma ('Sturge-Weber syndrome')
Cavernous hemangioma	Present at birth or appear in 1–2 weeks; 'strawberry nevus'; can enlarge and then resolve spontaneously; usually disappears within a few years; medical (prednisolone) or surgical treatment if fail to resolve or occlude eye or cause thrombocytopenia
Pigmented naevus	If small, requires no treatment; large hairy 'bathing trunk' types may need plastic surgery (risk of later malignancy)
Dermal sinuses	Often sacral ('pilonidal') or nuchal ('brachial') or preauricular; consider excision if recurrent infection
Cystic hygroma	Lymphangiomata of neck or axilla; treatment is surgical; can be underlying chromosomal problem
Cleft lip/palate	1:700 births; 1:7 other abnormalities; can be familial (1:20 recurrence); approach is interdisciplinary; special feeding techniques needed before surgery; early problems are middle ear and pulmonary infections; late problems are hearing, speech and orthodontic
Congenital teeth	Usually lower incisors present from birth; 1:200 births; remove if supernumerary or loose to prevent inhalation
Craniostenosis	1:5000 births; premature closure of cranial sutures; can be isolated or with other anomalies; growth arrested in direction perpendicular to suture; surgery may be necessary to prevent compression
Choanal atresia	1:10 000 births; present with airway obstruction and cyanosis; cured by opening mouth with oral airway before surgery

Table 7
Congenital deformations

Deformation	Implications
Sternomastoid torticollis	1:300 births; may not appear for 2 weeks; treatment is by passive gentle stretching of the damaged muscle from 6 weeks; rarely tenotomy and neck collar required
Congenital dislocation of the hip	1:75 births (10% dislocated, 90% dislocatable); early and regular examination necessary to detect; treatment is by use of various splints; more common in girls ($\times 4$) and breech presentations ($\times 10$)
Talipes	1:250 babies; such deformities if mild can be treated with regular gentle manipulation to the overcorrected position; more severe cases may need strapping or even surgery
Neurapraxias	Temporary lower motor neurone paralyses due to pressure on peripheral nerve before birth; facial, radial, sciatic and obturator nerves are the most commonly affected; muscle weakness resolves within days or weeks; physiotherapy for more severe cases

Table 8
Respiratory problems

Condition	Comments
Respiratory distress syndromes (RDS)	Due to surfactant deficiency; onset of distress within 1 h of birth; signs persist beyond 24 h but improvement often starts by 96 h; chest x-ray shows typical reticulogranular pattern with air bronchogram; air leaks (pneumothorax, interstitial emphysema, pneumomediastinum) and pneumonia are common complications; prognosis dramatically improved with the advent of ventilatory support and more recently exogenous surfactant therapy
Transient tachypnea of new born (TTN)	Usually a term infant with mature lungs but distress due to delayed clearance of lung fluid; often follows CS; onset within 2–3 h of birth; chest x-ray shows coarse streaking and fluid in fissures; requires only 30–40% oxygen; resolves in 3–4 days
Meconium aspiration syndrome	Usually a term baby often beyond 40 weeks; can be prevented by care at birth; early-onset respiratory distress; can be severe; chest x-ray shows hyperinflation and patchy consolidation; treated with antibiotics and ventilatory support
Congenital pneumonia	More common with prolonged membrane rupture; onset often within 2–3 h of birth but can be delayed for 1–2 days; chest x-ray can show patchy consolidation but may mimic RDS; treatment is intensive ventilatory support and antibiotics (usually penicillin and an amninoglycoside)
Pulmonary hypoplasia	Associated with oligohydramnios of any cause; presents as severe respiratory failure unresponsive to ventilation
Diaphragmatic hernia	Respiratory distress varies in severity and onset
Persistent fetal circulation	Persistent pulmonary hypertension with right-to-left shunting can complicate any of the above respiratory problems and polycythemia; alpha-blockade may improve the condition
Chronic lung disease	Long-term oxygen dependency may follow any of these conditions or long-term IPPV

Table 9
Cardiac problems

Problem	Causes/comments
Cyanosis	Cardiac anomalies (transposition of great arteries, pulmonary atresia, tetralogy of Fallot, Ebstein's malformation, total anomalous pulmonary venous connection) Persistent fetal circulation Severe lung disease

Heart failure	Congenital heart defects
	    left heart obstructive lesions (e.g. hypoplastic left heart, coarctation)
	    left-to-right shunts (e.g. patent ductus, ventricular septal defect, truncus arteriosus)
	    primary myocardial failure (e.g. myocarditis, endocardial fibro-elastosis, ischemia secondary to birth asphyxia, hypertrophic cardiomyopathy especially in IDM)
	    arrhythmias (e.g. supraventricular tachycardia, congenital heart block)
	Anemia
	Polycythemia
	Severe sepsis
	Severe metabolic abnormality (hypoglycemia, hypocalcemia)
	Thyroid disease (hypo- or hyper-)
	Fluid overload

Asymptomatic heart murmur	Common in the newborn period; often innocent; the murmur of a patent ductus is often present in first 24 h but thereafter disappears with closure of duct; all babies with murmurs persisting beyond 36–48 h should be investigated and followed up

Table 10
Neurological problems

Problem	Causes/comments
Convulsions	Should be promptly investigated and treated; 90% have definable etiology: Metabolic (e.g. hypoglycemia, hypocalcemia, hypomagnesemia, inborn errors of metabolism) Hemorrhagic/ischemia encephalopathy (see below) Infections (e.g. septicemia, meningitis, severe systemic infection, encephalitis) Drugs/toxins (e.g. drug withdrawal, hyperbilirubinemia causing kernicterus) Vascular (e.g. cerebral venous thrombosis, cerebral vascular malformation)
Hemorrhagic and ischemic brain lesions	With the advent of ultrasound visualization of the neonatal brain, a whole spectrum of lesions have been recognized; many may result in long-term neurodevelopmental disability. *Causes*: Perinatal asphyxia Prenatal asphyxia Subarachnoid hemorrhage Tentorial tear Subdural hemorrhage Periventricular hemorrhage in preterms Cerebral contusion The prognosis for these lesions varies with cause, timing, severity and coincidental pathologies. In general, it is very difficult to predict outcome
Neurological sequelae of perinatal asphyxia	Perinatal asphyxia remains an important cause of neurological disability. Management includes fluid restriction, and close monitoring of blood gases, blood glucose and renal function and implementation of appropriate support therapy if these parameters deteriorate; prognosis may be estimated by the degree of *encephalopathy*: *mild*: 'hyperalert', restless, jittery, poor feeding, resolution within 7 days *moderate*: 'lethargic', hypotonic, poor suck, decreased responsiveness, if fits they are easy to control, mainly resolved by 7 days, usually no long-term sequelae *severe*: 'stuporose', profound hypotonia, unresponsive, absent/decreased reflexes, fits common (control difficult), high mortality, disability common

Neurological Disorders

A variety of pathologies can present with neurological dysfunction. Long-term neurological integrity is arguably the most important factor in determining the quality of life for the child and parents. The common problems and their causes and implications are summarized in **Table 10**.

Gastrointestinal Problems

Necrotizing enterocolitis is arguably the most important gastrointestinal problem in the newborn. Although most common in low-birthweight babies, the frequency varies widely between centers. It is rare among those babies that have not been fed. Risk factors include low birthweight, apshyxia, artificial feeds, intrauterine growth deficiency, polycythemia and vascular catheterization. The cause is multifactorial and a number of pathogenic processes have been suggested to be important, including decreased vascular perfusion of the bowel secondary to asphyxia or hypoperfusion and anaerobic colonization of the bowel. The babies classically present with abdominal distension, bile-stained aspirates and bloody diarrhea. Management comprises withholding oral feeds, antibiotic therapy and supportive therapy for systemic disturbance. Recovery occurs in most cases within 7–10 days; however, occasionally, surgery and bowel resection may be necessary. Other causes of diarrhea in the newborn are summarized in **Table 11**.

Table 11
Causes of diarrhea in the newborn

Gastroenteritis (viral and bacterial)
Systemic infection
Necrotizing enterocolitis
Metabolic disorders (e.g. adrenal deficiency)
Surgical problems (e.g. Hirschsprung's disease)
Lactose intolerance
Opiate withdrawal
Phototherapy for jaundice
Prostaglandin therapy (for patent ductus arteriosus)

Metabolic Problems

Hypoglycemia, hypocalcemia and hypomagnesemia are the most common metabolic problems found in the newborn. Their features are summarized in **Table 12**.

Hematological Problems

The main hematological problems affecting the newborn are summarized in **Table 13**.

Perinatal Infection

The newborn infant is especially susceptible to infection because of reduced defence mechanisms and is rapidly colonized by organisms in the environment. Even 'weak' pathogens can cause severe infection. Humoral immunity is mainly conferred by transplacental IgG only. Leucocytes have decreased chemotaxis, phagocytosis and bactericidal properties and opsonization is defective. These features are more pronounced in the preterm infant. The clinical signs of sepsis in the newborn are non-specific and overlap with

the clinical features of many other disorders. The general approach to neonatal sepsis is summarized in **Table 14**. The implications of more specific infections in the newborn, especially those acquired *in utero*, are discussed in Chapters 29, 30 and 49.

Jaundice

'Physiological' jaundice can result from the changeover from fetal to neonatal bilirubin metabolism. Circulating bilirubin levels reach a maximum at the third or fourth day (with a mean of approximately 120 µmuol/l) and fall over the next 4–5 days. Bilirubin levels above 150 µmol/l in the first 48 h or above 220 µmol/l at any time should be regarded as potentially pathological. The causes of pathological jaundice and their management are summarized in **Table 15**.

Neonatal Surgical Problems

Many surgically treated abnormalities are identified prenatally and are considered and discussed in the appropriate chapters of the Fetal Medicine Section.

Table 12
Metabolic problems

Problem	Causes/risk groups	Management

Hypoglycemia	Small-for-dates
	Preterm
	Maternal steroid or beta-mimetic therapy
	Inborn errors of metabolism
	Congenital heart disease
	Infection
	Hypothermia
	Hypoxia
	Polycythemia
	Diabetic mother
		Prevention
		Avoid risk factors
		Check capillary glucose every 3 h
		Early feeding if at risk (or i.v. dextrose)
		
		Treatment
		If asymptomatic:
		  correct hypothermia
		  correct hypoxia
		  feed baby (or i.v. dextrose if feeding
		    contraindicated)
		If symptomatic:
		  i.v. dextrose (bolus and infusion)
		  investigate for cause

Hypocalcemia
  a. Early
	Preterm
	Diabetic mother
	Exchange transfusion
		Calcium supplementation (form and route
		  depends on whether symptomatic)
		Investigate for cause

b. Late	Hypomagnesemia Hypoparathyroidism Renal failure Maternal hypercalcemia or hyperparathyroidism	
Hypomagnesemia	Idiopathic (often with hypocalcemia) Exchange transfusion Malabsorption	Magnesium sulfate supplementation Investigate for cause

Table 13
Hematological problems

Problem	Comments
Hemorrhagic disease of newborn	Vitamin K stores are low at birth and rapidly depleted. Breast milk contains very little vitamin K and breast-fed infants may develop bleeding from depletion of Factors II, VII, IX and X. Phenytoin and/or phenobarbitone therapy in the mother may interfere with vitamin K metabolism and further deplete these factors and produce bleeding at birth. *Prevention* is by giving all newborn infants vitamin K *Treatment* is by administration of fresh whole blood or packed cells, platelets and fresh frozen plasma

Thrombocytopenia	This presents with petechiae, bruising, cephalhematoma or more rarely major hemorrhage.
	Causes include:
	    Maternal autoimmune disease (throbocytopenia, lupus)
	    Maternal drugs (quinine, hydralazine)
	    Severe pre-eclampsia or IUGR
	    Alloimmune thrombocytopenia
	    Severe bacterial sepsis
	    TORCH agents
	    Trisomies 13 and 18

Anemia
    a. Early
	Causes include:
	    Hemorrhage
	        fetomaternal
	        twin-to-twin
	        placental
	        trauma
	        neonatal (from many causes)
	    Hemolysis
	        rhesus or other antibodies
	        hemoglobinopathies
	        infection

b. Late	Causes include:
	    Hemorrhage
	        hemorrhagic disease
	        excessive venesection
	        intraventricular
	        gastrointestinal
	    Hemolysis
	        as above
	        red cell defects
	    Decreased production
	        iron/folate
	        deficiency
	        infection
	        drugs

Table 14
General approach to sepsis in the newborn

Signs suggestive of neonatal infection
   Non-specific (poor color, lethargy, poor feeding,
     unstable temperature)
   vomiting
   loose stools
   distended abdomen, hepatosplenomegaly
   jaundice
   thrombocytopenia
   irritability, convulsions
   apnea, cyanotic attacks
   tachycardia
   hypo- or hyperglycemia

Investigation of infant with suspected sepsis (sepsis screen)
   Gram-stain and culture (bacterial and viral) nose, throat,
     stools and any skin lesions
   Gram-stain and bacterial culture of urine
   blood culture (aerobic and anaerobic)
   hemoglobin, platelets, white cell count and differential,
     film
   blood gases, glucose, urea, electrolytes
   cerebrospinal fluid for microscopy, culture (viral and
     bacterial), protein and glucose
   chest x-ray (abdominal x-ray if necrotizing enterocolitis
     suspected)

General management of septic infant
   general supportive measures
   respiratory support if apnea or abnormal gases
   correct hypotension
   transfuse if anemic
   correct glucose, fluid or electrolyte imbalance
   immediate antibiotics after cultures taken and review
     when sensitivities known

Table 15
Pathological jaundice in the newborn

Causes

Unconjugated hyperbilirubinemia
   Acute hemolysis
     rhesus/other antibodies
     red cell abnormalities
     infection
   Polycythemia
   Sequestered blood
     swallowed blood
     bruising
     hemorrhage
   Decreased conjugation
     infection
     congenital enzyme defects

Increased enterohepatic circulation
   breast milk jaundice
   delayed meconium
   intestinal obstruction
Conjugated hyperbilirubinemia:
   Impaired liver function
     infection
     metabolic disorders
     severe hemolysis
   Biliary obstruction
     choledochal cyst
     biliary atresia

Management

General
   Measures employed depend gestational age and size,
     postnatal age and degree of hyperbilirubinemia. The
     aim is to avoid bilirubin encephalopathy
     ('kernicterus'). The range of options includes:
   observation and monitoring only
   phototherapy
   exchange transfusion

Specific
   Investigation and treatment of cause if indicated in
     addition to general measures when the jaundice is
     severe, early in onset or prolonged

COUNSELING ABOUT PEDIATRIC PROBLEMS
Summary of Management Options

General

- Communicate with pediatrician if there is any doubt about information to be conveyed

- Do not confuse the issue for parents

- Do not provide information if uncertain

Specific

- The small-for-dates baby – see **Table 2**

- The large-for-dates baby – see **Table 3**

- The preterm baby – see **Table 4**

- Birth trauma – see **Table 5**

- Congenital malformations – see specific chapters and **Table 6**

- Congenital deformations – see **Table 7**

- Respiratory problems – see **Table 8**

- Cardiac problems – see Chapters 47 and 53 and **Table 9**

- Neurological disorders – see **Table 10**

- Gastrointestinal problems – see **Table 11**

- Metabolic problems – see **Table 12**

- Hematological problems – see **Table 13**

- Perinatal infection – see **Table 14** and Chapters 29, 30 and 49

- Jaundice – see **Table 15**

- Neonatal surgical problems – see appropriate chapters in Fetal Medicine Section

---

CONCLUSION

There are several 'musts' for obstetricians with regard to pediatric problems:

- They must understand the more common problems and their management.

- They must communicate with pediatricians about any potential pediatric problems in undelivered patients.

- They must learn of the outcome of babies after delivery both where problems were anticipated and where they were never suspected.

- They must only counsel parents about pediatric problems when they are sure of their facts and that what they say is in keeping with what the pediatrician is saying.

FURTHER READING

1 Fleming PJ, Speidel BD, Marlow N, Dunn PM (1991) *A Neonatal Vade Mecum*, 2nd edn. London: Edward Arnold.
2 Roberton NRC (1986) *Textbook of Neonatology*. Edinburgh: Churchill Livingstone.
3 Taeusch HW, Ballard RA, Avery ME (1991) *Diseases of the Newborn*. Philadelphia, PA: W.B. Saunders.

73

High Dependency Care of the Obstetric Patient

MICHAEL MARESH, KATE NEALES

SEVERE HYPERTENSION IN PREGNANCY (see also Chapter 18)

Definition

There is widespread agreement that a diastolic blood pressure of ≥110 mmHg diastolic on more than one occasion should be classified as severe hypertension. The 4th Korotkov sound has been used for this. This definition is in agreement with the International Society for the Study of Hypertension in Pregnancy.[1] Systolic levels are less easily agreed upon, but ≥160 mmHg is often used. The presence of significant proteinuria is not needed for the definition, but will alter management.

Incidence

Estimates vary between 0.5 and 5.0%. This variation is no doubt due in part to some authors including intrapartum rises in blood pressure.

Maternal Risks

Some risks relate more to the degree of hypertension:

- cerebrovascular hemorrhage
- cardiac failure

Other risks relate more to the usual association of the problem with the pre-eclampsia syndrome, which is a multi-system disorder. Risks to the mother from this may be unavoidable or may be minimized through appropriate therapy. Such risks include:

- eclamptic convulsions and cerebral edema
- liver dysfunction (rarely acute fatty liver)
- disseminated intravascular coagulopathy (DIC)
- hemorrhage
- acute renal failure
- adult respiratory distress syndrome.

In addition, there are iatrogenic risks such as:

- fluid overload
- toxic effects of drugs (e.g. magnesium sulfate, phenytoin)
- inhalation of gastric contents secondary to profound sedation.

Finally, if delivery is by cesarean section, this has its own morbidity.

Estimation of these risks is difficult. Eclampsia has been estimated to occur currently in about 0.5 per 1000 pregnancies.[2] Deaths from eclampsia are reported as 5 per million maternities.[3] Thus currently perhaps 1% of cases of eclampsia are associated with maternal death. The 1985–87 UK confidential enquiry also reported 6 per million deaths associated with hypertensive disorders when eclampsia was not present. The immediate cause of death was classified for all cases as being almost evenly divided between intracerebral hemorrhage or pulmonary complications, with half the cases having DIC.

Fetal/Neonatal Risks

True pre-eclampsia (significant proteinuria and hypertension) is usually accompanied by intrauterine growth deficiency secondary to poor spiral artery development. Accordingly, the fetus is at particular risk of intrauterine asphyxia and, once delivered, the neonate is at risk of all the problems associated with growth deficiency (e.g. hypothermia, hypoglycemia, polycythemia, hypocalcemia).

Apart from the hypoxial stress of labor on a growth-deficient fetus, hypoxial stress may also occur secondary to hypotension associated with:

- placental abruption secondary to hypertension

- rapid dropping of blood pressure secondary to hydralazine or a poorly managed epidural

The other major risk to the fetus and neonate is that since the maternal condition almost always has to be treated by termination of the pregnancy, the fetus is often delivered prematurely with all its attendant neonatal risks. Of relevance prior to delivery is the increased risk of a malpresentation which may influence mode of delivery or cause unexpected problems with a planned vaginal delivery.

Management Options

Prepregnancy

There is nothing which can be done prior to pregnancy to reduce the risk of severe hypertensive disorders occurring. All that can be done is to explore whether the woman is at significant increased risk. Risk prediction is unsatisfactory (see below) and it is unlikely to deter a woman from pregnancy.

Prenatal

Discussion on severe hypertensive disorders in the prenatal period centers around four areas:

- prediction

- prevention

- early detection

- management

Prediction

The prediction of women who are at risk of severe hypertensive disorders is worthwhile, since there may be ways of preventing it or reducing its severity (see below). Women with essential hypertension have always been regarded as being at increased risk of proteinuric hypertension, with a five-fold increase commonly being quoted,[4] although current consensus views would suggest it is not as high.

Women who had the condition in a previous pregnancy are also at increased risk, although the condition is rarely as severe.[5] There does appear to be an inherited susceptibility to the condition,[6] but the exact genetic basis is controversial and the concept of the single gene model[7] has been challenged.[8]

Whatever the actual risks are for women who fit into these categories, since they do only constitute a small percentage of a typical prenatal population, it would be prudent to provide closer prenatal surveillance for them.

Prevention

There is some evidence from a number of small studies[9,10,11] that pre-eclampsia is associated with an imbalance in thromboxane A_2 and prostacyclin and that treatment with low-dose aspirin may alter this and prevent or reduce the severity of pre-eclampsia (see Chapter 18). This is currently being investigated in a large randomized controlled trial (CLASP).

It has also been claimed that treatment of pregnancy associated hypertension may reduce the chance of subsequent superimposed proteinuria.

Early detection

When one attempts to analyze the purpose of many aspects of routine prenatal clinical assessments, one finds them to be of dubious significance, with little impact on subsequent outcome. However, an assessment regime with regular checks for hypertension and proteinuria would appear justifiable in the primigravid woman, especially after 34 weeks gestation,[12] but the multiparous woman will not need such close monitoring. Clearly, blood pressure measurement does not need a doctor and neither does the estimation of proteinuria, which can be assessed by the woman herself. This has been incorporated into prenatal programmes.[13]

In view of the multisystem nature of the condition, a number of other markers have been investigated to see if these can provide an early warning of the condition. Those that appear to be of use include serum uric acid concentrations[14] and platelet concentrations.[15] Since the condition is associated with poor placental perfusion, Steel et al.[16] investigated the Doppler blood flow velocity profiles in the uterine arcuate arteries and suggested this could be a useful screening test. More simply, the prenatal detection of growth deficiency should also alert one to the increased possibility of a subsequent hypertensive disorder.

Management (see also Chapter 18)

Mild hypertension (no proteinuria, diastolic blood pressure 90–99 mmHg) is usually managed on an outpatient basis with additional domiciliary assessments to predict a worsening of the condition.

Moderate hypertension (proteinuria with mild hypertension, or moderate hypertension alone – diastolic 100–109 mmHg) is usually managed in hospital. Antihypertensive therapy is usually commenced in women with persistent moderately elevated blood pressure (e.g. methyl dopa or beta-blockers or nifedipine).[17] Since early delivery may be required in this group, consideration should be given to the use of maternal steroid therapy to enhance fetal lung maturation if the fetus is likely to be very preterm. Although this view has been challenged by Redman,[18] studies have suggested no adverse effects on the mother and there are fetal benefits.[19]

Severe hypertension (diastolic blood pressure persistently more than 110 mmHg) requires complex management, which is ideally carried out in a high-dependency care environment and decisions about terminating the pregnancy need to be at the forefront. Accordingly, this is discussed below under labor and delivery management.

Labour/Delivery

General

Women with severe hypertension (diastolic >110 mmHg) are best transferred to a high-dependency care environment and senior staff should be informed. Most units prefer to manage these cases in their own delivery units rather than moving them to an adult intensive care unit. However, post-delivery, when the problems frequently still persist or even deteriorate and management may be further complicated by the postoperative state, transfer to an intensive care unit is more frequent (e.g. 1–2 per 1000 deliveries). Nursing such cases on a delivery unit entails having midwives or nurses with training and experience in intensive care techniques and experienced anesthetic involvement. If these conditions are not met, then transfer to an intensive care unit is necessary. All maternity units in the UK are expected to have written protocols for these cases and these should be followed. Departure from them should only be done by a consultant. One of the key areas of such a protocol should be that it states who is to be responsible for the various aspects of care. The management is best broken down into specific areas.

Management of hypertension

A sustained diastolic blood pressure >110 mmHg requires hypotensive medication to be instituted. However, there is rarely a need to lower the blood pressure rapidly over minutes and such a rapid drop may be associated with a diminution of cardiac output to the uterus and possible fetal hypoxia. Continuous fetal heart rate monitoring should be performed during initial therapy to detect such effects and thus allow early remedial action. The objective of therapy should be a gradual reduction in blood pressure to levels about 140/90 mmHg. Three acceptable options are currently used:

- *Hydrallazine (Apresoline®)*

This is a vasodilator and although available as an oral form is usually given parenterally. It can be given in slow intravenous boluses of 10 mg, but this can have dramatic hypotensive effects and a slow intravenous infusion is preferable. It is best given via a syringe pump, as this allows easier control of fluid balance, rather than added to an intravenous infusion bag. The infusion should run at 2–20 mg/h, the rate being determined by titration against the blood pressure response. The typical side-effects of vasodilators such as headaches, palpitations and tachycardia may occur. There is no doubt about its efficacy in acute hypertension in pregnancy, but side-effects appear to be more common than with labetalol.[20]

- *Nifedipine (Adalat®)*

This is a calcium channel blocker and is rapidly effective orally in acute hypertensive episodes in pregnancy.[21] Normally, effects become apparent 30 min after an oral dose of 10–20 mg. More rapid adminstration can be obtained by breaking up the capsule and adminstering it sublingually. Again marked hypotension can occur with this drug and other side-effects include headaches and palpitations. If nifedipine treatment is achieving a satisfactory effect, then the dosage will need to be repeated every 8 h. Nifedipine has been used to try to suppress labor through blocking calcium channels, so theoretically it should not be given in a case where induction of labor is proposed.

- *Labetalol (Trandate®) and other beta-blockers*

With its popularity for managing acute hypertension outside pregnancy, labetalol has become one of the most popular drugs used in the UK for managing severe hypertension.[17] Labetalol is a combined alpha-beta-blocker and is contraindicated in asthmatic patients. It may be useful if the other agents cause unacceptable tachycardias. While it can be given orally, the majority use the parenteral approach. If using the latter approach, it is preferable to use a syringe pump. A bolus dose should be given and the infusion run at 1–2 mg/min (maximum 160 mg/h). Once control is achieved, consideration may be given to an oral preparation of labetalol or one of the alternatives such as atenolol or oxprenolol. Alternatively, these may be considered initially if the hypertension is not so severe and parenteral therapy is not felt necessary.

Blood pressure is usually assessed every 5–15 min initially, prefereably using an automatic monitor. Once the blood pressure is stabilized, the interval can be lengthened to 30 min.

Prevention of eclamptic convulsions

This is discussed in detail in the section on eclampsia. The presence of severe hypertension, proteinuria and other symptoms such as epigastric discomfort coupled with hyperreflexia alert one to the possibility of an eclamptic fit. Accordingly, many clinicians use drug regimes to try to prevent eclampsia.[17] This approach remains controversial and others regard the management to be purely early recourse to delivery and control of hypertension. The likelihood of carrying out a randomized trial of prophylactic drug treatment *vs* placebo remains remote, as the study would need to be extremely large. For instance, in our unit, where prophylactic treatment is used, in over 100 consecutive patients treated over the last 6 years, no fits occurred. Eclamptic fits are estimated to occur in about 1:2000 pregnancies[2] and were surveyed in 1992 throughout the UK.

Assessment of renal function and fluid balance

Acute renal failure is a very rare but serious complication of severe hypertension in pregnancy. In fact, there is frequently excessive concern about oliguria with resulting fluid overload causing serious iatrogenic problems.

Severe hypertension of pregnancy is associated with a decrease in plasma volume and increasing vascular resistance. However, catheterization of the right side of the heart has suggested that these women have normal or hyperdynamic left ventricular function.[22] The classic renal lesion results in leakage of protein into the urine and accumulation of waste products such as urea, uric acid and creatinine. The loss of plasma proteins such as albumin results in a decrease in plasma oncotic pressure and fluid leakage into the extracellular compartment – the nephrotic syndrome. Accordingly, a number of urgent baseline assessments should be performed once intensive care is required.

- *Urinary assessment*

A strict fluid balance chart should be commenced and an indwelling urinary catheter inserted. A device with a measuring chamber allows easier, regular measurement, which is best done hourly. Protein estimations can be done on these samples using dipsticks. It is essential to obtain a clean urine sample for microscopy and culture. A urinary tract infection will increase the estimated magnitude of the proteinuria and thus may exaggerate the severity of the condition and cause possible unnecessary invasive procedures. Microscopy is also helpful by looking for granular casts which suggest renal disease. It is prudent to save all the urine, since if delivery is not performed early, then total protein excretion and creatinine clearance may subsequently be determined. Most feel that urine output should be maintained at about 0.5 ml/kg body weight/h. Thus for a woman of normal weight (60 kg) this will be in the order of 30 ml/h, which is half the rate some have previously used (1 ml/kg/min).

- *Blood tests*

An intravenous cannula should be inserted for initial venous access and a blood sample taken for a number of investigations. With regard to the monitoring of renal function and fluid balance, the following should be performed: sodium, potassium, urea, creatinine, albumin, hemoglobin and packed cell volume. The frequency of repeating these tests will vary, but it is likely that they should be repeated at least daily and, apart from plasma albumin concentrations, usually twice a day during the most acute phase of the condtion.

- ● *Central pressure monitoring*

Althougth central venous pressure monitoring has its critics, it is our view that on balance it should be used. Some regard it as an unnecessary invasive procedure, but in the presence of a severe hypertensive disorder and reduced urine output, additional information is mandatory for safe management. Others criticize it as it does not correlate that well with pulmonary capillary wedge pressure. Cotton *et al.* have shown in a large series of initially untreated severe cases of hypertension that pulmonary capillary wedge pressure was normal to high in most cases, while central venous pressure was rarely elevated.[22] However, there is no reason why a healthy myocardium could not generate higher intracardiac pressures with severe systemic hypertension and accordingly the filling pressures for the left and right side of the heart could be different. Accordingly, central venous pressure monitoring might reflect intravascular volume better than capillary wedge pressure. However, the assessment of whether the left side of the heart is handling any major therapeutic volume expansion can only be assessed by pulmonary capillary wedge pressure measurement.

As a simple guide, the presence of oliguria should be managed with central venous pressure monitoring. The presence of persistent oliguria or pulmonary edema may best be managed by the addition of pulmonary capillary wedge pressure measurement, which is likely to entail managing the patient on an intensive care unit.

All patients in whom a central venous pressure catheter is inserted should have a chest x-ray performed to check on correct placement. In addition, this can serve as a baseline for lung field markings if there is a need for subsequent assessment of pulmonary edema.

- ● *Intravenous fluid therapy*

The safest principle is to keep the patient as 'dry' as possible. Since the patient is likely to be hypovolemic and protein-depleted, a number of further principles can be applied. The use of intravenous water (e.g. 5% dextrose) has no place. Drug infusions such as hydralazine or oxytocin should be given via a syringe pump using normal saline as the medium. The 1 ml/kg body weight/h regime is a useful starting rate for total fluid input. There are different opinions on which fluid to use. Hartmann's, however, is widely used as first choice. Since these women are usually hypoalbuminemic (<30 mg/1), human albumin solution is often given (e.g. 200–400ml over a 12 h period).

In the presence of oliguria and reduced central venous pressure (<5 mmHg), 200 ml albumin is often given as a fluid challenge. If central venous pressure is normal, then the normal basal rate of Hartmann's should be continued and urine output measured every 30 min along with central venous pressure. When central venous pressure is raised (>10 mmHg) and there is oliguria, then a diuretic such as 40 mg frusemide is advisable.

It is impossible to be proscriptive when these fluid regimes fail. However, there is one simple rule and that is that a consultant with experience in the subject, such as an obstetric anesthetist or a renal physician, must be involved directly with care. The hazards for the woman (e.g. pulmonary edema) are too great in this type of case to be managed by an obstetrician who sees one or two cases a year.

Clotting abnormality (see also section on DIC)

As mentioned above, severe proteinuric hypertension is usually associated with some disturbance of clotting function. Some degree of thrombocytopenia will occur and platelet numbers should be assessed every 12 h. If less than 50×10^9/liter, 6 units of platelets should be available to cover delivery. In addition to thrombocytopenia, there may be some disturbance of clotting and so the prothrombin time, fibrinogen and fibrin degradation products should be measured. If abnormal, they should be repeated at least 12 hourly. Fresh frozen plasma should be given to cover the delivery. If there is clinical evidence of a coagulopathy occurring, fresh fresh frozen plasma and platelets should be given and a consultant hematologist should be actively involved. The latter usually facilitates obtaining the appropriate blood products.

Pulmonary function

Pulmonary function may be impaired through early pulmonary edema coupled with respiratory depression if opiate analgesia has been used for labor. The simple measurement of respiratory rate should be done at the same frequency as pulse and blood pressure recordings (e.g. every 30 min). Ideally, a pulse oximeter should be used on all these patients to record continuous oxygen saturation pressure. If this falls to 95 mmHg or less, careful clinical and x-ray assessment of the chest is necessary for early signs of pulmonary edema. Oxygen therapy should be commenced early and titrated against the pulse oximeter readings.

Fetal assessment

As mentioned above, the fetus is at particular risk under these circumstances, as it is likely to be growth-deficient and is now subjected to further potential problems such as: variations in blood supply secondary to maternal hypertension and its treatment; placental separation secondary to maternal hypertension or a coagulopathy; and risk of hypoxia secondary to reduced maternal pulmonary function. For initial fetal assessment, ultrasound assessment is preferable to assess fetal size, look for evidence of growth deficiency, assess amniotic fluid volume, determine presentation and examine fetal activity. Umbilical artery Doppler blood flow velocity profiles, if available, may be helpful. They are likely to be abnormal, but if grossly so, such as reversed end-diastolic flow, this might influence the decision about mode of delivery, as reversed flow is associated with an increased risk of abnormal cardiotocographs in labor with an associated increased chance of cesarean section.

Intermittent non-stress testing should be performed at regular intervals (e.g. every 4 h) for as long as necessary to obtain a normal reactive recording. If not obtained, a decision will have to be taken with regard to urgent delivery.

Corticosteroids should be administered to aid lung maturation (e.g. betamethasone 12 mg i.m., two doses, 12 h apart.)[19] Thyrotropin-releasing hormone (TRH) has also been shown to be of value when given predelivery in reducing the incidence of chronic lung disease in infants born prematurely who were also given betamethasone.[23] The regime used in this study was 400 μg TRH given intravenously in 50 ml normal saline during a 20 min infusion, every 8 h for a total of four doses.

Timing of delivery

There is little debate when the pregnancy is near to term, but the severe problems frequently occur when immediate delivery of the neonate may put it at high risk of morbidity or mortality. Once it is clear that the condition is severe and progressive, the only real considerations to be undertaken are:

- Whether it is safe for the mother for the pregnancy to continue for 48 h post-steroid adminstration so that neonatal benefit may be obtained.

- Delivering at an appropriate time for the neonatologists and, if necessary and safe for the mother, transferring her to a unit which can provide skilled neonatal care. If transferred, the mother must be accompanied by an experienced doctor.

Delaying delivery for more than 48 h becomes increasingly fraught with risks for the mother and fetus. There is increasing risk of any of the above complications occurring and there are the iatrogenic risks associated with central pressure monitoring and drug therapy. The uteroplacental circulation will be impaired so that chronic fetal acidemia may occur insidiously, which may lead to fetal demise *in utero* or subsequent morbidity. Accordingly, the likely benefit for the fetus of a significant delay is probably non-existent.

If significant complications such as liver involvement, non-responsive oliguria, eclampsia, pulmonary edema or coagulopathy occur, then delivery should not be delayed and a decision made about mode of delivery.

Mode of delivery

There is disagreement about what is the best mode of delivery under these circumstances. This is mainly due to lack of information.

- *Fetal considerations*

If the fetus is viable and the decision is made that cesarean section is justifiable for fetal reasons, then there may still be a case for a trial of labor with continuous fetal monitoring and recourse to cesarean if a persistent abnormality persists. Similarly, just because it may be a breech presentation does not necessarily dictate a cesarean, as the data currently published do not support routine cesarean section for the preterm breech (see Chapter 13). However, since the fetus is likely to be growth-deficient, the combination of a premature, growth-deficient fetus suffering the hypoxia of a breech delivery results in many obstetricians performing a cesarean section under these circumstances. This is not without the risk of head entrapment in a poorly formed lower uterine segment when not delivered by a very experienced operator.

- *Maternal considerations*

Cesarean section undoubtedly puts the mother at increased risk of morbidity and mortality. There are well-recognized anesthetic problems (see below) and in the presence of a coagulopathy further problems may arise. Having had one cesarean will increase the chance of future deliveries also being done by this method. In addition, some operators use a classical vertical uterine incision under these circumstances. This is usually unnecessary provided a large 'smile' or U-shaped incision is performed in the lower part of the uterus. If a vertical incision is performed, then a subsequent cesarean is usually considered mandatory.

Balanced against these risks are those of continuing to provide high-dependency care during labor and the increasing risks of maternal complications occurring with time. Accordingly, if the mother is stable, the fetus does not appear to be suffering from hypoxia, and there are staff and support facilities continuing to be available, an attempt to deliver vaginally has much to be commended.

Labor management

Intensive maternal monitoring must continue as outlined above. In view of the increased likelihood of a worsening maternal condition with time, labor progress needs to be assessed regularly, and cesarean performed early if progress slows. In practice, this is uncommon provided labor can be induced. Induction may be with either vaginal prostaglandins or intravenous oxytocin. In order to keep a closer control on fluid balance, it is preferable to give the oxytocin using a syringe driver, since this will reduce the fluid input, a factor of particular relevance because of the anti-diuretic properties of oxytocin.

Continuous electronic fetal monitoring should be performed because of the major fetal risks under these circumstances. If satisfactory monitoring cannot be obtained using an abdominal ultrasound transducer, then a scalp clip should be used even in the preterm infant. Fetal scalp blood samples can be taken from a preterm fetus, although most prefer to perform a cesarean section if there is a persistently abnormal cardiotocograph.

Traditionally, the bearing down effort by the mother is limited because of the possible increase in hypertension associated with this effort. However, if the fetal and maternal condition is satisfactory, maternal expulsive efforts should continue in an attempt to achieve a spontaneous delivery. The second stage and delivery must be managed by someone experienced with preterm deliveries.

Oxytocin rather than preparations containing ergometrine should be used for the active management of the third stage of labor, in view of possible effects of the latter on maternal blood pressure.

There is debate about the choice of analgesia for labor. Nitrous oxide analgesia, if sufficient, has the advantage of no significant side-effects and the additional benefit of oxygen therapy, as it is administered as a 50:50 mixture of N_2O and O_2. Epidural analgesia has a number of advantages because it is usually highly effective, may prevent major fluctuations in blood pressure and allows more control in the second stage, preventing a precipitous delivery if the fetus is very small. However, epidural analgesia is contraindicated in the presence of any blood coagulation changes, as an epidural hematoma could occur, causing serious neurological morbidity through compression. Accordingly, if the platelets are less than 80×10^9/liter or there are any disturbances in any of the other clotting tests, an epidural anesthetic should not be inserted.

If an epidural is indicated, then intravenous preloading should be performed with care. If central venous pressure is being measured, then the initial response to a small preload (e.g. 200 ml) intravenous Hartmann's solution can be assessed. If the central venous pressure does not return to its previous level, then no more fluid should be given; if it does, then the full preload of 500 ml should be administered. Continuous fetal monitoring needs to be performed during the procedure and subsequently, because of the possible effects of reduced blood flow to the fetus and direct toxic effects of the drugs on the fetal myocardium.[24]

If an epidural cannot be used, than a traditional opiate analgesia (e.g. pethidine) will need to be employed if any pain relief is required. Effects on the fetus are not of major concern prior to delivery and can be reversed postdelivery. However, maternal respiratory depression can occur and coupled with any minor degree of pulmonary edema can cause a reduction in maternal and fetal oxygenation. Accordingly, the respiratory rate must be measured regularly, preferably by transcutaneous oxygen saturation using a pulse oximeter.

Assuming that there is no clotting disturbance (see above), epidural regional anesthesia may be preferable to general anesthesia for a cesarean section for the following reasons:

- intubation may be difficult due to laryngeal edema;

- intubation is sometimes associated with dramatic reflex hypertension;

- post-delivery pulmonary complications may be worse after general anesthesia;

- immediately post-delivery may be the only opportunity the mother will have of seeing her baby alive if extremely preterm.

Postnatal

Early management

- *General*

Intensive monitoring (as outlined above) should be continued. The patient's condition should now begin to recover. The following points relate mainly to the gradual reduction of intensive management as this occurs.

SEVERE HYPERTENSION
Summary of Management Options

Prepregnancy

- Counsel those women at risk

Prenatal

Prediction

- Increased risk with pre-existing hypertension, renal disease, connective tissue disorders, diabetes mellitus, previous pre-eclampsia

Prevention

- ? Fish liver oil

- ? Low-dose aspirin

Early detection

- ? Uric acid

- ? Platelets

- ? Uterine artery Doppler velocimetry

- ? Fetal growth

Management

- General: high-dependency care with appropriately trained staff and support

- Reduce BP (options = hydralazine, nifedipine, labetalol)

- Prevent convulsions (controversial, see eclampsia section)

- Assess/monitor renal function and fluid balance

- ? Central pressure monitoring (? CVP, ? pulmonary wedge pressure)

- Intravenous fluids but avoid overload

- Assess clotting status

- Fetal assessment

- Give steroids if preterm (? and TRH)

- Timing of delivery dependent on: e.g. gestation, steroid administration, fetal status, maternal complications

- Mode of delivery depends on maternal and fetal factors/considerations

Labor/delivery

- If labor undertaken, close monitoring of progress, maternal condition and fetal heart rate (continuous)

- Avoid fluid overload

- Epidural may be of benefit (if no coagulopathy) – caution with preloading

- Assisted second stage more likely

- Oxytocin for third stage

Postnatal

- Early: confirm resolution, monitoring: BP, fluid balance/renal function, pulmonary function, neurological and coagulation status

- Late: investigate for underlying cause

- *Fluid balance and renal function*

Once a maintained diuresis is occurring, then central venous pressure monitoring can be discontinued. Urinary measurements can be lengthened from an hourly basis and the urinary catheter taken out as soon as convenient from the patient's viewpoint. Renal function tests can be discontinued once they have returned to normal. Edema may not immediately improve but no specific action is required.

- *Pulmonary function*

The respiratory rate should continue to be monitored and preferably oxygen saturation using a pulse oximeter. Clinical examination of the chest should be performed regularly. If there is any suggestion of pulmonary edema then this should be treated with diuretics, and if there are signs of infection physiotherapy and antibiotics should be used. If oxygen has been required, then this should be reduced gradually with monitoring of the oxygen saturation by a pulse oximeter.

- *Blood pressure*

Oral antihypertensive drugs (for example a beta-blocker) should be started so that no intravenous agents are necessary.

- *Eclamptic convulsions*

These can still occur post-delivery. Prophylactic anticonvulsants are not routinely given unless the patient shows any suggestion of cerebral irritability, such as marked hyperreflexia (see section on Eclampsia).

- *Coagulopathy*

If the clotting tests have been abnormal, these should be repeated approximately every 12 h (or sooner if clinically indicated) to ensure that they are returning to normal; once they are, they need not be repeated. Any abnormalities should be managed as outlined in the section on coagulopathies.

- *Long-term follow-up*

These women are likely to have problems either in a subsequent pregnancy or in the long term. Accordingly, it is necessary to investigate them fully after the puerperium. As a minimum, there should be a 24 h urine collection to determine creatinine clearance and total protein excretion, and measurements of blood urea and creatinine concentrations. If hypertension persists, then other causes such as renal pathology or a pheochromocytoma should be sought by renal ultrasound and the measurement of catecholamines (by whichever test is performed by the local laboratory).

If there is any suggestion of an underlying renal disorder, then the patient should be referred to a renal team to help in reaching a diagnosis and the institution of long-term follow-up. How common this is is uncertain. In one series, detailed renal investigation suggested 65% of women had underlying renal pathology.[25] However, the outcome in the subsequent pregnancies in this series has not yet been reported. If there is no evidence of persistent renal pathology, then the woman can be reassured that a subsequent pregnancy is unlikely to have such severe problems. It is possible when current trials are reported, that low-dose aspirin may be beneficial for such women in future pregnancies.

MAJOR OBSTETRIC HEMORRHAGE

Definition

Major obstetric hemorrhage is an imprecise term, but it has been defined as estimated blood loss of more than 1500 ml from the genital tract in association with pregnancy, and this is generally accepted by clinicians. It has also been defined as a loss of greater than 30% of blood volume, or a sustained fall in systolic blood pressure to less than 80 mmHg. All these definitions have problems in clinical application as blood loss is notoriously underestimated and the degree of hypotension produced is not always related to the amount of blood loss.

The term usually refers to a major peripartum bleeding episode in a pregnancy of viable gestation and includes the puerperium. Bleeding can be revealed, or concealed into the uterine cavity, broad ligament or peritoneal cavity.

Incidence

This is difficult to estimate as the definition includes all severe episodes of antepartum, intrapartum, primary and secondary postpartum hemorrhage, and these figures are not recorded collectively or statutorily. The incidence is likely to be about 0.5%, with the largest number of cases being due to primary postpartum hemorrhage.

Maternal Risks

Death

The *Report on Confidential Enquiries into Maternal Deaths in the United Kingdom* shows that hemorrhage is the fourth most common cause of direct maternal death and accounted for 7.2% of cases in 1985–87.[3] Bleeding was also a contributory factor in a further 8% of cases. This incidence has halved in the last 15 years and the death rate from hemorrhage per million maternities now stands at 4.5. The risk of death from hemorrhage increases with parity and maternal age to 20 per million maternities in the 35 year and over age group.[26] Postpartum hemorrhage, often in association with cesarean section and coagulation failure, remains the most common cause of death.

In the developing world, postpartum hemorrhage accounted for 28% of maternal mortalities in 11 different countries studied, and is one of the most feared complications of labor and delivery.[27]

Major morbidity

Although death due to hemorrhage is rare in developed countries, major episodes of bleeding causing significant morbidity are not uncommon, and often require intensive management and heroic resuscitation to avoid disaster. Hypovolemic shock, disseminated intravascular coagulation and renal failure are the major complications encountered. The incidence of these problems is extremely difficult to estimate and there may be other confounding factors present, such as pregnancy-induced hypertension. Whether renal failure develops depends much on the management and adequacy of resuscitation. Adult respiratory distress syndrome and hepatic failure are late sequelae and are particularly likely to occur if initial replacement of blood volume was inadequate.

Iatrogenic morbidity

The management of patients with major obstetric hemorrhage involves fluid and blood replacement to treat hypovolemia, intensive monitoring and often surgical intervention. Complications arising from treatment include fluid overload and left ventricular failure, and adverse reactions to blood or blood products. Failure to transfuse fresh frozen plasma or platelets, or to consider vitamin K and other clotting agents when large quantities of blood are given, may worsen any coagulopathy present. Pneumothorax and other complications may result from the insertion of central venous and arterial lines. Surgical procedures to repair genital tract trauma or to stop hemorrhage by vessel ligation or hysterectomy may result in damage to the bladder, ureters or other pelvic structures.

The most common medical error, however, is to underestimate the degree of blood loss and give inadequate replacement in the initial stages. Any delayed decision to proceed to delivery, or to surgery in an attempt to obtain hemostasis, will also increase morbidity.

Anemia

The patient is at risk of both iron deficiency and folic acid deficiency after delivery and supplementation should be given. Transfused blood has a relatively shorter half-life and a period of increased marrow activity and reticulocytosis will occur in the recovery phase, when iron stores are already depleted.

Sheehan's syndrome

Severe postpartum hemorrhage (less commonly antepartum) can cause permanent hypopituitarism by avascular necrosis of the pituitary gland. The anterior pituitary is particularly vulnerable due to its two- to three-fold increase in size in late pregnancy. There is failure of lactation, amenorrhea, and features of hypothyroidism and adrenocortical insufficiency. Several hundred cases have been reported and any patient with a history of severe hemorrhage and impaired lactation should be followed for 12 months to check endocrinological status.[28]

Reduced fertility

Future pregnancy rates in women who have suffered a major antepartum or postpartum hemorrhage are reduced. A hysterectomy may have been necessary or there may have been extensive genital tract damage requiring other surgical procedures. Uterine adhesions may have formed and secondary infection is relatively common, leading to tubal occlusion. Because of their traumatic experience, many of these patients feel unable to contemplate another pregnancy, even when antepartum hemorrhage has resulted in a perinatal death.

Fetal/Neonatal Risks

There are risks for the fetus secondary to prenatal and intrapartum hemorrhage and these are greater when the bleeding is caused by placental abruption rather than placenta previa. With modern care, the total perinatal mortality rate for abruption is about 300 per 1000 cases, with half of the deaths occurring prior to admission.[29,30] Surviving infants have higher rates of respiratory distress, low Apgar scores, patent ductus arteriosis and anemia.[30] The perinatal mortality rate for placenta previa is approximately 50 per 1000 cases and surviving infants generally have normal long-term development.[31] Most neonatal deaths occur as a consequence of prematurity.

Death due to asphyxia

The fetus may be stillborn following severe placental abruption and placental separation, or die from intrauterine hypoxia secondary to maternal blood loss and shock.

Cerebral hypoxia

Antepartum or intrapartum hypoxia may result in an infant in poor condition at delivery, with subsequent development of convulsions, intracerebral edema and hemorrhage. This may lead to conditions such as periventricular leucomalacia and porencephalic cysts, and long-term neurological handicap. Pulmonary hemorrhage and necrotizing enterocolitis may also occur after an hypoxic episode.

Complications associated with prematurity

These account for most of the cases of neonatal death if the infant has survived the initial insult, and include respiratory distress syndrome and persistent fetal circulation with patent ductus arteriosis. Complications associated with prolonged neonatal intensive care such as sepsis and bronchopulmonary dysplasia are relatively common.[30]

Management Options (see also Chapters 7, 9 and 68)

Prenatal

Identification of 'at-risk' patients

Massive blood loss cannot always be anticipated or prevented. The prediction of such an event in the general obstetric population is poor and as the incidence is less than 0.5%, no specific preventative measures can be provided. If a woman is anemic when coming into labor, or refuses blood products on religious grounds, she is at increased risk of morbidity from blood loss and should be booked in a large unit with appropriate staff and facilities. Some high-risk patients and situations can be identified, such as a placenta previa occurring after cesarean section.

Patients who have had a previous hemorrhage in pregnancy are at risk of recurrence and should be counseled about such risk and delivered in larger obstetric units with full resuscitative measures available. They should be aware of the procedures for urgent admission to the unit and the need to attend with any degree of bleeding. Iron prophylaxis is advisable in this group (although the risk of major hemorrhage is not generally seen as an indication for routine iron therapy).

Risk of placenta previa

Advancing age and parity are associated with the development of placenta previa, although the relative importance of these two factors is disputed.[31,32] Uterine scars, previous miscarriages, terminations and dilatation and curettage are reported as predisposing factors, possibly due to endometrial damage.[33,34] Placenta previa is more common in multiple pregnancy, due to increased placental size.[33] Maternal age is the most important factor in recurrent placenta previa and the risk of recurrence is quoted as between 10 and 15%.[35]

There is an association between cesarean section scars and the subsequent development of placenta previa, which is reported as between 3 and 10%, and increases with the number of prvious cesarean sections.[32,36] This group of patients is also at risk of placenta accreta, which is stated at between 10 and 67%, increasing again with the number of previous cesarean sections.[32] Any patient with a placenta previa and previous cesarean section should be informed of the possible necessity of a hysterectomy. The repeat cesarean section should be booked in an appropriate unit and performed by a senior obstetrician with blood crossmatched and immediately available.

However, the overall incidence of placenta previa is between 0.3 and 1%, and only 15–20% of cases of placenta previa have major bleeding episodes.[37,38] It should be stressed to the woman with a placenta previa that she is much more likely not to have a severe hemorrhage than she is to have one, especially as ultrasound diagnosis has led to increased detection of asymptomatic placenta previa that may prove to be of little clinical significance.

Vasa previa and velamentous insertion of the cord are associated with placenta previa, and neonatal anemia of varying degrees is relatively common.[39] Although bleeding with a placenta previa is assumed to be of maternal origin, it has been suggested that a proportion of the blood loss may be fetal in origin.[31] A denaturation test to detect the presence of fetal cells should be carried out in the presence of hemorrhage if delivery is not planned.[37]

Risk of placental abruption

The causative factors are known in only a minority of cases of placental abruption but an association with increasing parity, smoking, low socioeconomic status and pre-existing intrauterine growth deficiency is reported.[29,40–42] The role of pregnancy-induced hypertension in the etiology of abruption is controversial. The two conditions do co-exist, but no increase in hypertension was found in the prenatal period prior to the abruption in the two reported series.[29,40] Some cases of abruption will be due to trauma or sudden reduction in uterine volume, typically seen at membrane rupture in the presence of hydramnios.[42]

The importance of maternal factors is shown by the recurrence rate of 6–16% after one placental abruption and 20–25% after two previous placental abruptions.[29,42] The women should be told that maintenance of a normal blood pressure and cessation of smoking may reduce the risk, although this has not been proved in controlled trials. There is some evidence that stress may precipitate a placental abruption, but discussions on this subject must be conducted tactfully, as a woman will look for a factor to account for a previous abruption and may well blame herself. Folic acid supplementation has not been shown to reduce the risk of recurrent abruption. Low-dose aspirin is increasingly given to women who have had a previous placental abruption, and the results of controlled trials are now awaited.[43]

Risk of postpartum hemorrhage

Any woman having a baby is at some risk of postpartum hemorrhage, estimated at 3–5% of deliveries, and women contemplating a home delivery should be informed of this, as most cases occur unexpectedly. If there has been a previous postpartum hemorrhage, the risks of recurrence are increased to approximately 8–10%.[44] Women with a history of retained placenta and those with multiple pregnancy are also at risk. Appropriate management of labor and delivery, with timely use of oxytocic drugs at delivery, should reduce the risk of recurrent postpartum hemorrhage. Abnormalities of labor and delivery predispose to postpartum hemorrhage of different causes and this will be discussed when management is considered.

Management of major hemorrhage: general measures

The essential management of major bleeding episodes is the same whatever the underlying cause of hemorrhage and involves:

- identifying the cause and treating it to stop blood loss

- replacing the ciruclating blood volume and other blood constituents.

Every obstetric unit should have its own protocol for management of massive hemorrhage available on the delivery unit for all nursing and medical staff. This enables the appropriate clinical and laboratory staff to be summoned early and a clear management strategy to be adopted.

An example of a general management protocol for major hemorrhage is given in **Table 1**, and should be followed without delay as soon as a major bleeding episode is recognized. This protocol clearly outlines the necessary steps to be taken and similar guidelines could be drawn up for any obstetric unit.

There are specific consideration relating to the underlying cause of hemorrhage. In addition to the initial regimen for resuscitation with intravenous fluids outlined above, and which is the same for all episodes of hemorrhage whatever the underlying cause, there is a need to monitor fluid balance and renal function. A central venous line should be inserted as soon as practicable and the management of fluid replacement ideally performed by the senior anesthetist. Failure to appreciate the degree of blood loss or to resuscitate adequately in the initial phases remains the most common critisism in the 1985–87 Maternal Mortality Report.[3] Up to 2 liters of crystalloid and 1.5 liters of colloid can be given while arranging for urgent blood supplies. The hematologist must be kept informed at all times for the continuing need for blood and blood products. Massive hemorrhage will invariably lead to the depletion of labile coagulation factors and platelets and 1 unit of fresh frozen plasma (FFP) should be given for every 4–6 units of blood transfused routinely. Platelets and further FFP are transfused if coagulation screening tests indicate the need.[45]

The renal output should be monitored throughout via an indwelling catheter and once control of hemorrhage has been obtained careful stock must be taken of hourly urine output and CVP readings. If the urine output remains below 30–40 ml per hour after adequate replacement of blood volume, intravenous mannitol (0.2 g/kg) or dopamine infusion (2 μg/kg/min) may be given to avoid acute renal failure.

Ideally, the patient should be managed in a high-dependency unit in association with the labor/delivery suite.[26] Arterial lines and determination of pulmonary pressures should only be necessary if there is cardiac or lung disease, or if fluid overload has occurred and there is failure to respond to the above measures. In these cases, there is a high likelihood of significant morbidity and mortality with prolonged intensive care and organ failure.

Major antepartum hemorrhage due to placental abruption (see also Chapter 9)

In severe abruption, the woman is usually in severe pain and may be shocked due to hypovolemia. There may be heavy vaginal bleeding or evidence of increas-

Table 1
Major hemorrhage protocol

___

Organization

1. Switchboard operator sends for:
   a. Obstetric registrar and SHO if not present
   b. Duty obstetric anesthetist
   c. Obstetric nursing officer to arrange extra staff
   d. Blood bank technician
   e. Porter to maternity unit

2. Consultant hematologist and obstetrician informed of the clinical situation

3. One nurse to be solely assigned to record-keeping:
   a. Patient vital signs, CVP and urine output
   b. Amount and type of all fluids the patient receives
   c. Dosage and types of drugs given

4. Prepare for theater as soon as possible – most diagnoses require surgical intervention

Clinical management

1. Insert two large-bore (preferably 14 gauge) cannulas. Take 20 ml of blood for cross-matching and order at least 6 units of blood

2. Place the patient in a head-down position and give oxygen via face mask

3. Commence fluid replacement quickly:
   a. Initially crystalloid and colloid. Hartmann's solution to a maximum of 1.5–2 liters, Haemaccell®, Hespan® 1.5–2 liters
   b. Uncrossed blood. Rh-negative, matched with the patient's ABO group should be given next if cross-matched blood not ready
   c. Cross-matched blood as soon as possible
   d. O-negative blood only if none of the above available (but it may be life-saving)
   All fluids and blood should be given through a warming device

4. Insert central venous line and urinary catheter

5. Stop the bleeding
   a. If antepartum, deliver the fetus (see text)
   b. If postpartum, deliver the placenta if still *in utero*, commence bimanual compression of the uterus and give ergometrine 0.5 mg i.v. Commence syntocinon infusion of 40 units of Syntocinon® in 500 ml of Hartmann's solution to run over 4 h
   c. If bleeding because of genital tract trauma or retained products, take the patient to theater promptly to explore the uterine cavity and repair damage
   d. If bleeding continues, consider coagulation failure. Temporary direct aortic compression may give valuable time. Uterine packing can be considered in women of low parity where every effort is made to conserve the uterus
   e. Other surgical measures:
   f. Direct intramyometrial injection of prostaglandin E_2 0.5 mg, or $F_{2\alpha}$ 0.25 mg
   g. Ligation of uterine arteries on both sides
   h. Ligation of internal iliac arteries
   i. Hysterectomy

ing girth if the abruption is concealed. A coagulation defect with severe hypofibrinogenemia may already be evident, with absence of clotting in the vaginal loss, or hematuria and bleeding from puncture sites. Coagulopathy occurs in some 38% of cases where the fetus is dead, but is comparatively rare with a live fetus.[37] Labor occurs spontaneously in approximately 50% of patients.[46]

Maternal resuscitation is the immediate priority and has been outlined above. Adequate analgesia should be given if required, usually by intravenous narcotics supplemented by nitrous oxide/oxygen mixtures self-administered by mask. Epidural analgesia is contraindicated because peripheral blood pooling may cause further hypotension in an already compromised patient, and there may be a developing coagulopathy even in the presence of acceptable blood clotting studies.

The only treatment for severe placental abruption is to terminate the pregnancy as soon as feasible. If the fetus is dead, then normal management is to aim for a vaginal delivery, except where there is an obvious obstetric indication for cesarean section such as transverse lie. There will be rare situations where uterine contractions cannot be stimulated or maternal shock is uncorrectable. Cesarean section may have to be undertaken in such cases, although the maternal risk is considerable, as coagulopathy is common in this group.[47] If there is no response to Syntocinon®, prostaglandins may be administered with appropriate surveillance in an attempt to stimulate uterine contractions. There is an increased risk of uterine rupture with a large abruption, particularly if blood has infiltrated the myometrium to produce a Couvelaire uterus.[42]

Determining if the fetus is alive may be difficult because of a tender, hypertonic uterus and interference with transmission of heart sounds if there is a retroplacental clot and anterior placenta. Accordingly, visualizing the heart using ultrasound is usually the quickest method if a machine is available. If not, it may be necessary to rupture the membranes and attach a fetal ECG electrode. Exclusion of placenta previa may be difficult on clinical grounds if the presenting part cannot be palpated, and the two conditions may co-exist. Ideally, location of the placental site is checked by ultrasound before any vaginal examination.

If the fetus is alive, then consideration should be given to early delivery by cesarean section for fetal reasons.[37,48] This will depend on the fetal gestation, as it is extremely improbable that a fetus under 26 weeks gestation will survive such an asphyxial episode. The mode of delivery will also depend on the fetal condition as judged by cardiotocography. If the fetal heart rate pattern is totally normal (which is unlikely), induction of labor with continuous monitoring can be considered. If the cardiotocograph is grossly abnormal (e.g. severe bradycardia of 80 or less), then the place of immediate cesarean is debatable. If one leaves the fetus *in utero* while active maternal resuscitation takes place, then it will either die or improve. A fetus with such severe antepartum hypoxia that does not respond to improved maternal oxygenation is unlikely to do well in the neonatal period.

Current clinical practice seems to favor cesarean section if the fetus is judged viable, but one study has suggested that the rate could be reduced by up to 50% without affecting fetal outcome by aiming for vaginal delivery in selected patients, and avoidance of surgery is certainly in the best interests of the mother.[31] The specific problem of disseminated intravascular coagulation will be considered later.

Major antepartum hemorrhage due to placenta previa (see also Chapter 9)

Placenta previa may cause bleeding from 16 weeks gestation onwards, but in 80% of cases the bleeding occurs after 32 weeks gestation.[49] Outcome is reported to worsen as the degree of placenta previa increases, and an early initial bleeding episode seems to have a worse prognosis, although the evidence is conflicting.[38,49] Only 2% of cases of significant placenta previa will not bleed before the onset of labor.[38]

Placenta previa will be suspected if there is painless vaginal bleeding in the absence of labor. The fetal heart is usually still present and additionally there may be evidence of uterine contractions (20%) or premature rupture of membranes (10%). Massive hemorrhage will follow smaller 'warning' bleeds in the majority of cases, and the placental site will often already be known.[37,38]

Initial management involves maternal resuscitation as previously described. A patient with such a severe hemorrhage due to placenta previa will usually require delivery by cesarean section whatever the gestation, and the decision is not dependent on whether the fetus is dead or alive. The cesarean section may need to be performed as resuscitative efforts are underway if the mother's condition cannot be stabilized. Occasionally, vaginal delivery may be contemplated if the fetus is dead or extremely premature,[50] but the general consensus is that cesarean section is safer because of the risk of precipitating catastrophic uncontrolled hemorrhage. A digital examination is absolutely contraindicated where there is any possibility of placenta previa, except in theater after the decision has been made to deliver and the diagnosis of placenta previa is in doubt.[50]

Cesarean section for placenta previa is often a difficult procedure associated with fetal malpresentation, a poorly developed lower uterine segment, and excessive blood loss that further compromises the condition of the patient. The operation should be performed by a senior obstetrician with extra blood immediately available. Postpartum hemorrhage is also more common because of the inability of the lower uterine segment

to contract efficiently and should be anticipated and prophylactic measures taken.

Placenta previa/accreta may be encountered in 5% of cases with no previous scar in the uterus, and in up to 67% of cases with multiple cesarean sections, as stated previously.[32] Early recourse to hysterectomy may be necessary but conservative management has been attempted, using curettage, uterine packing and oversewing of the placental bed.[32,50]

Major primary postpartum hemorrhage (see also Chapter 68)

Most cases of massive postpartum hemorrhage are primary and occur within the first hour after delivery. It is relatively uncommon for secondary hemorrhage to present with blood loss of greater than 1000 ml.[46,51,52] Initial management and resuscitation is outlined in **Table 1**. It is imperative that early steps are taken to identify the cause of the bleeding, which may include retained products, uterine atony, trauma or coagulation defects, and that the appropriate definitive action is taken to stop further blood loss. More than one etiological factor may be present and this possibility should always be considered.

- #### *Retained products of conception*

If the whole placenta or a large part of it is still *in utero*, the likely cause for the hemorrhage is obvious and the placenta should be delivered immediately by whatever means necessary (often manual removal under general anesthetic). Even a small piece of membrane may stop the uterus from contracting properly, leading to bleeding from the placental bed. The placenta may be retained due to failure of separation, or because of misuse of oxytocin causing constriction above the level of the cervix when delivery by controlled cord traction may still be possible.[46] Difficulty arises if the retained portion is a small cotyledon or succenturiate lobe, and the diagnosis may not be made on inspection of the placenta and membranes. This procedure should never be relied upon to exclude retained products and an early examination under anesthesia is required.

Occasionally, the placenta may be morbidly adherent to the uterus and no plane of cleavage found (placenta accreta). The etiological features of this have already been discussed and surgical intervention with uterine packing, intenal iliac ligation, or often hysterectomy is required. Rupture of the uterus may occur in an attempt to remove a placenta accreta, and also is more common during curettage for secondary postpartum hemorrhage with retained products in association with infection.[51]

- *Uterine atony*

The main factors involved in achieving hemostasis after delivery are vascular constriction and thrombosis. Constriction of the vascular bed occurs because of vessel wall contraction and external pressure from intermittent and sustained myometrial contractions which squeeze bleeding vessels from the placental bed and obstruct blood flow.

Before the routine use of oxytocic agents, uterine atony as a cause of postpartum hemorrhage was more common. The incidence is markedly reduced with all oxytocic drugs, even though the type of agent used and timing and route of delivery are disputed.[54,55] Nevertheless, it still remains the most common cause of postpartum hemorrhage. Conditions such as prolonged labor, high parity, sepsis and overdistension may predispose to uterine atony, but uterine atony is most commonly seen with either retained products or uterine trauma and these conditions must be excluded. In some cases, the oxytocic has been inadvertently omitted, administered incorrectly, or not been available if the delivery was outside hospital.

Initial management involves the administration of further oxytocic agents. Commonly, ergometrine 0.5 mg is given intravenously followed by a Syntocinon® infusion. Bimanual compression of the uterus will temporarily contract the uterus and reduce the bleeding, thus giving valuable time to organize resuscitation and identify the cause of bleeding.

If there has been no response to conventional agents, prostaglandins should be given. Both $PGF_{2\alpha}$ and PGE_2 analogs have been used and these can be given intramuscularly, by vaginal pessary, or as a direct myometrial injection, especially at cesarean section or laparotomy.[55–57] If these measures fail to cause uterine contraction and hemostasis, then there should be early recourse to other surgical measures, such as internal iliac ligation or hysterectomy. Uterine packing has been employed in certain cases with success.[58]

- *Genital tract trauma*

Any trauma to the birth canal may cause excessive blood loss due to the marked increase in vascularity during pregnancy. Tears of the upper vagina and uterus are more likely to cause massive hemorrhage because of the larger vessels that may be damaged, difficulty in access to control bleeding, and difficulty in diagnosis, especially if the bleeding is concealed into the broad ligament. In the 1985–87 Maternal Mortality Report, all six cases of deaths due to postpartum hemorrhage were due to trauma to the uterus and cervix.[3]

Although uterine rupture often occurs before or at the time of delivery, it has been considered in relation to postpartum hemorrhage, as the diagnosis may not be made until after delivery. The clinical picture differs depending on whether there is rupture of the lower segment at the site of an old cesarean scar or rupture that arises *de novo* or occurs in the upper segment, and it is usually the latter group that cause massive hemorrhage. Uterine rupture is much more common in multiparas, regardless of the cause.[46] Predisposing factors include a previous hysterotomy or upper cesarean section scar (or much less commonly a previous myomectomy or uteroplasty). Obstructed labor with or without the use of oxytocic drugs may lead to rupture, as may operative trauma including ventouse delivery through an incompletely dilated cervix, mid-cavity forceps (especially rotational) and other intrapartum manipulations. Cervical laceration extending to the lower uterine segment may follow a precipitate delivery, especially if bearing down occurred before full dilatation. Rupture of the upper segment is usually a dramatic event, with sudden onset of severe pain, bright vaginal bleeding, collapse and loss of the fetal heart. There may be early warning signs of fetal distress, alteration in maternal observations, lack of progress and a small amount of vaginal bleeding. Management of uterine rupture involves resuscitation as outlined before, laparotomy and often hysterectomy. If the woman is anxious to have further children, repair may be undertaken in certain cases, but there should be early recourse to hysterectomy if hemorrhage cannot be controlled.

Vaginal and cervical lacerations typically occur following delivery, and bleeding can be profuse due to the vascularity of the vagina and cervix. If the laceration is confined to this region, bleeding will continue despite a well-contracted uterus.[52] Maternal resuscitation should commence and repair of the laceration should be performed under anesthesia as soon as possible. The repair should not be attempted under inadequate local anesthesia, as careful exploration of the uterine cavity and vaginal fornices must be carried out. Bimanual compression of the cervix can be employed while the patient is taken to theater. If there is any suggestion of the laceration extending upward into the uterus or broad ligament, then laparotomy should be undertaken. Careful examination to exclude hematoma formation must be carried out, as these can result from tearing of the vessels beneath the surface as well as an obvious laceration. Concealed blood loss above the levator ani and into the broad ligament can be massive, and is suspected when a pelvic mass can be felt beside the uterus.

Major secondary postpartum hemorrhage

Massive blood loss occurring after the first 24 h post-delivery is less common than primary postpartum hemorrhage and is usually due to sub-involution of the uterus caused by retained pieces of placenta or membrane and superimposed infection. In one reported series, seven of 505 patients with secondary postpartum

MAJOR OBSTETRIC HEMORRHAGE
Summary of Management Options
(see also Chapters 7, 9 and 68)

Prenatal

Identification of the patient at risk

- Previous APH or PPH
- Patients with proven placenta previa
- Patients with anemia at the onset of labor
- Previous cesarean section (increased risk of placenta previa)
- Women of higher age and parity

Such women should be booked in larger obstetric units with full facilities (resuscitation; cesarean section)

Correct anemia; prophylactic iron/folate if high risk

? Low-dose aspirin in patients with previous abruption

Management of major hemorrhage

Principles of management are the same whatever the cause

- Stop blood loss
- Replace circulating blood volume

*A management protocol for major hemorrhage should be available on every labor ward (see **Table 1** for example)*

Placental abruption (see also Chapter 9)

- Check for and treat coagulopathy
- Analgesia (probably not epidural)

- Route and mode of delivery depends on:
  - condition of mother and fetus
  - gestation
  - presentation
- Vigilance for PPH

Placenta previa (see also Chapter 9)

- Delivery is usually by cesarean section
- Vigilance for PPH

Primary PPH (see also Chapter 68)

- Management depends on cause (more than one might exist in same patient):
  - atony
    - —complete third stage
    - —extra i.v. oxytocin
    - —? packing uterus
    - —prostaglandins
    - —surgery (ligation, hysterectomy)
  - repair trauma
  - treat coagulopathy

Secondary PPH (see also Chapter 68)

- Oxytocics
- IV antibiotics
- ? EUA and curettage if continued bleeding
- ? Then packing and surgical options

Postnatal

- Transfer to high-dependency or intensive care unit for continuation of monitoring and support
- Intravenous broad-spectrum antibiotics
- Oral iron and folate supplementation

hemorrhage required hysterectomy to control bleeding.[46] Management involves maternal resuscitation and blood transfusion as outlined in **Table 1**. Bimanual compression and ergometrine is adminstered and intravenous antibiotics commenced. If the bleeding continues, the patient must be taken to theater for examination and careful curettage, although risk of perforation is considerable. If bleeding continues, then hysterectomy or uterine artery ligation may be necessary. Uterine packing has been successfully employed and is more successful in secondary postpartum hemorrhage than primary postpartum hemorrhage.[58]

Postnatal

After prolonged or massive hemorrhage, all patients will require continuous close monitoring of pulse rate, blood pressure, oxygenation, central venous pressure and urine output. Acid–base status, biochemical parameters and hematology should be checked regularly.

After delivery, transfer back to the high-dependency or intensive care unit is advisable where appropriately trained nursing and medical staff are immediately available. There is a place for short-term ventilation for 24–48 h to prevent adult respiratory distress syndrome and to assist recovery if there has been a degree of fluid overload and pulmonary edema.

Intravenous broad-spectrum antibiotics should be commenced because of prolonged or repeated surgical procedures and vaginal examinations in a compromised patient. Iron and folic acid supplementation should be started after the acute phase and continued for 3 months.

Healthy women generally respond to treatment for massive hemorrhage remarkably well and their recovery can be very rapid if long-term sequelae and organ failure have been avoided by prompt and effective management.

ECLAMPSIA (see also Chapters 18 and 26)

Definition

Fits can occur at any stage during the pregnancy and the puerperium. Eclamptic convulsions are considered to occur in a more narrow time-frame between 20 weeks gestation and 10 days postpartum. A fit which does not appear to be of epileptic origin, nor appears to be caused through metabolic or other known causes, should be classified as an eclamptic convulsion. Convulsions should only be classified as such if they have the features of grand mal convulsions such as auror, clonic and tonic movements, involuntary activity and

a post-ictal state. Eclampsia is normally regarded as the occurrence of convulsions superimposed on pre-eclampsia.

Incidence

The incidence of epileptic fits in pregnancy is uncertain. Epilepsy is thought to be present in about 0.5% of pregnant women. Epileptic fits are more likely to occur in pregnancy than outside for a number of reasons, including non-compliance with drugs because of concern about fetal effects, plasma expansion and alterations in drug metabolism (see also Chapter 26).

Eclamptic convulsions have been estimated as occurring in 1:2000 pregnancies.[2] This may well be an underestimate and one objective of the 1992 UK survey of eclampsia is to try to establish the true incidence. The majority of eclamptic convulsions occur post-delivery.

Maternal Risks

Maternal death in association with eclamptic convulsions has been estimated at 5 per million maternities.[3] This would suggest a mortality rate of about 1% for the condition. Epileptic convulsions are unlikely to be associated with maternal death.

Major maternal morbidity associated with eclampsia relates to the underlying intracranial pathologies which have caused the fits, namely:

- cerebral edema
- cerebral petechial hemorrhages
- major cerebral hemorrhage.

Other significant morbidity relates to eclampsia being just one manifestation of a multisystem disorder, usually associated with severe hypertension, which may result in the following pathologies:

- liver dysfunction
- disseminated intravascular coagulopathy (DIC)
- hemorrhage
- acute renal failure
- adult respiratory distress syndrome.

In addition, there are significant iatrogenic risks to the mother, such as:

- fluid overload

- side-effects from drugs (e.g. magnesium sulfate, phenytoin)

- inhalation of gastric contents secondary to profound sedation.

Delivery may need to be performed by cesarean, which has specific additional risks:

- difficulties with intubation during general anesthesia leading to hypoxia

- severe hypertension associated with induction of general anesthesia

- general morbidity associated with cesarean section.

Fetal/Neonatal Risks

Epileptic fits are likely to be associated with transient fetal hypoxia, but there is no evidence to suggest that these cause significant morbidity.

Eclamptic convulsions that occur prior to delivery cause major risks to the fetus. As fetal growth deficiency is more likely to be present as part of the multisystem disorder of pre-eclampsia/eclampsia, the fetus is more likely to be affected by the hypoxia associated with the eclamptic convulsion. This may result in fetal death or hypoxic brain damage. This damage may cause an ischemic encephalopathy with cerebral edema and convulsions and long-term structural brain damage such as porencephalic cysts. The infant may thus be handicapped to varying degrees with cerebral palsy.

Since eclamptic fits may occur at any time during pregnancy, and as part of their management require delivery, the neonate may be delivered prematurely. Accordingly, the baby is exposed to the risks of prematurity, such as respiratory distress syndrome and chronic lung disease, periventricular hemorrhage with subsequent chronic neurodevelopmental compromise, and necrotizing enterocolitis. All of these complications and others are potentially fatal.

Management Options

Only the management of eclamptic convulsions will be considered in this chapter. The management of epilepsy and convulsions from other causes is covered in Chapter 26.

Prepregancy

Nothing can be done prepregnancy to prevent eclampsia other than advising women not to conceive. This cannot be justified even in a woman who has had eclampsia in her first pregnancy, as the risk of recurrence is low. Occasionally, the experience may have been such a severe physical and emotional experience that the woman is not prepared to conceive again.

Prenatal

Prenatal management of eclamptic convulsions centers on three main areas:

- prediction

- prevention

- management.

Prediction

Eclampsia usually occurs in primiparous women, but since they constitute about 40% of a prenatal population, this is of minimal help. Since eclampsia is a complication of pre-eclampsia, then the factors which one can use for predicting this condition, such as essential hypertension, current pre-eclampsia and previous eclampsia, could be used. However, eclampsia is such a rare condition and may present in apparently atypical ways, that prediction does not have a significant impact on clinical practice.

Prevention

Any measures which reduce the incidence of hypertensive disorders in pregnancy may reduce the incidence of eclampsia. Accordingly, low-dose aspirin therapy may well have a major role here in reducing the incidence of hypertensive disorders (see above).

Similarly, the early detection of hypertension allows antihypertensive management to be instituted. Such effective control of the blood pressure in itself may prevent eclampsia from occurring.[2] Hypertension should be treated if the diastolic blood pressure is >110 mmHg and many institute treatment when it is persistently >100 mmHg.[17] When it is considered that the blood pressure needs to be rapidly lowered, the drugs commonly used are parenteral hydrallazine, parenteral labetalol and oral nifedipine. Milder hypertension (e.g. diastolic 100–110 mmHg) is more usually managed with oral methyl dopa, beta-blockers or nifedipine. The use of all these has been detailed in the section on hypertension (see above).

The early detection of proteinuria through routine prenatal urine dipstick testing remains a simple and cheap method for the early detection of pre-eclampsia/eclampsia. This can be performed by the woman herself. Other markers which have been proposed are major increases in the serum urate concentrations[14] and decreasing platelet concentrations.[15]

Classic symptoms may be associated with impending eclampsia. With increasing technology in obstetrics, these are sometimes ignored with potentially disastrous results. They are simple to ask about, and their significance can usually be confirmed by examination so that management can be instituted. Epigastric pain arises from the liver capsule suggesting intrahepatic pathology such as edema or hemorrhage. Tenderness in the right hypogastrium should be regarded as confirmation of this and urgent action instituted. Headache and visual symptoms, while common, may be indicative of underlying cerebral edema or petechial hemorrhages. Fundoscopy must be part of the routine assessment in all cases. In the absence of any signs suggestive of intracerebral pathology, simple analgesia may be given as a therapeutic trial for headache.

It is controversial whether 'prophylactic' anticonvulsants should be given to women with severe hypertensive disorders but without any features of imminent eclampsia. Since the underlying pathology from the hypertension alone is cerebral hemorrhage either of a petechial or of a larger nature, then anticonvulsants cannot modify the process. Accordingly, it is argued that treatment should be aimed at control of hypertension and delivery at an appropriate time reserving the use of anticonvulsants to those women with features of imminent eclampsia. The contrasting view is that the additional risks of a fit such as maternal and fetal hypoxia and/or the possibility of inhalation of gastric contents, outweigh any minor side-effects from anticonvulsant drugs and that such drugs should be used. The efficacy of such 'prophylactic' anti-convulsant treatment for this condition has not been proven. Trials comparing treatment with no treatment, or comparing different drugs, are difficult to mount because of the rarity of the condition. In addition, the majority of doctors are unhappy about placebo-controlled studies for this condition.[17]

The current consensus view in the UK is that 'prophylactic' convulsants should be used with severe pre-eclampsia. Hutton *et al.*[17] reported that 84% of obstetricians advised such therapy. If one is going to use 'prophylactic' anticonvulsants, what are the acceptable conditions? One such protocol is only to use 'prophylactic' anticonvulsants in the presence of severe hypertension (diastolic >110), proteinuria >2+ and signs such as epigastric discomfort and hyperreflexia or severe headache. It would appear logical to give the drugs parenterally to ensure that adequate concentrations are achieved quickly and are maintained. The same drugs are used prophylactically as are used for actual treatment and these are discussed in the next section.

Management

A number of the aspects of care have already been discussed in detail in the section on hypertensive disorders (see above). Accordingly, these will only be mentioned again briefly in this section.

• *Immediate action*

The first action is to obtain resuscitation equipment and protect the airway against inhalation. An oral airway should be inserted and the patient placed in the semi-prone position. A facial oxygen mask should be attached to reduce the degree of hypoxia. An intravenous anticonvulsant should be given, the most commonly used one in the UK being diazepam.[17] A dose of 10 mg should be given by slow intravenous injection over 1–2 min. Additional obstetric and anesthetic help should be mobilized and the woman moved to the delivery unit where high-dependency nursing care should be available. The senior obstetrician and senior anesthetist should be notified.

• *Prevention of further convulsions*

Four drugs are currently widely used, one (magnesium sulfate) in North America and three (diazepam, phenytoin and chlormethaziole) elsewhere.

• *Diazepam*

Diazepam is the most widely used drug in the UK.[17] Its main disadvantages are profound sedation in the mother and therefore care is needed with regard to the airway and monitoring respiration. In addition, transplacental transport to the fetus results in loss of variability of the fetal heart rate, making this less useful as a test of fetal well-being. Chronic maternal administration of diazepam will have neonatal effects due to the long half-life of diazepam and its active metab-olites. These include delayed onset of respiration, apnea, hypotonia, poor temperature control and poor sucking, and some of these effects can be prolonged for up to 10 days. However, the advantages of diazepam are that it is readily available, used in this formulation for other purposes, and is familiar, cheap and easy to administer. Recurrence of convulsions after initiation of treatment was found in 26% of women in a recent controlled study.[59] However, other studies have reported a figure as high as 46% (L. Duley, 1991 – personal communication).

The recommended regime is 40 mg diazepam in 500 ml 5% dextrose or 0.9% saline. The infusion rate should be titrated against the patient's level of sedation to keep her drowsy but rousable. The regime should continue for 24 h after the last convulsion and then be reduced to half the concentration for the next 24 h. Further convulsions should be managed with an additional intravenous injection of 5–10 mg over 1–2 min. The woman should be nursed in the recovery position to reduce the risks of inhalation.

- *Chlormethiazole*

Chlormethiazole is also quite widely used.[60] Like diazepam, it produces profound sedation of the mother and respiratory depression is a risk. Its only apparent advantage over diazepam is that while it does cross the placenta, it is rapidly excreted from the fetus/neonate and therefore the adverse effects reported with diazepam should be less common. However, respiratory depression, sedation and hypotonia have all been reported. Another disadvantage is that it not so widely used in other areas of medicine and therefore less familiar to medical staff.

It is administered as 0.8% solution at a rate to produce sedation. This preparation may result in large volumes of crystalloid fluid being given and so careful attention to fluid balance is essential.

- *Phenytoin*

Phenytoin was proposed as a drug for consideration in the management of eclampsia, as it avoided the severe sedation and respiratory depression which occur with diazepam and chlormethiazole.[61] Hypotension can occur, but this depends on the rate of infusion rather than total dosage, so should be avoidable. Cardiac conduction defects have been reported in association with phenytoin therapy in the non-pregnant patient, but this appears to be more likely when there is pre-existing cardiac disease. Phenytoin has membrane-stabilizing properties but ECG abnormalities are very rare.[61] Breast-feeding is not contraindicated in view of the low neonatal concentrations being reported in mothers with phenytoin concentrations in the therapeutic range. The disadvantages are that it is not commonly used intravenously and the regime is slightly more complicated than diazepam or chlormethaziole. Routine ECG monitoring does not appear necessary.

Large studies on the use of phenytoin are not yet available. In the only controlled study, 4 of the 11 women treated with phenytoin had further convulsions while being actively treated, although the phenytoin concentrations were at the lower end of the therapeutic range.[62] In an uncontrolled study, two out of eight patients had further convulsions.[64]

The recommended total dosage of Slater *et al.*[63] was based on maternal weight: 750 mg for 40–50 kg, 1000 mg for 51–70 kg and 1250 mg for >70 kg. Phenytoin 250 mg was made up in 250 ml normal saline. The infusion rate was for the initial 250 mg phenytoin to be given rapidly (over 15, 12 and 10 min, respectively, by weight group) and for the rest to be given more slowly (at 2 mg/min). A further dose is given after 12 h.

- *Magnesium sulfate*

Magnesium sulfate has been used extensively in North America.[64] Its mode of action is uncertain as it does not cross the blood-brain barrier and does not effect the EEG abnormalities found in eclampsia.

Hypotension may occur initially with treatment. Cardiorespiratory arrest is the most worrying side-effect of magnesium therapy. This is associated with magnesium intoxication and great care must be taken with the regime. In Crowther's series,[59] 1 of 29 women had a cardiac arrest immediately after the loading dose of magnesium was given, probably because of too rapid an infusion. There was one maternal death in the large American series of 245 cases associated with overdosage[64] and there were other cases of severe respiratory depression associated with magnesium intoxication. Accordingly, any unit introducing this protocol must do so with great care.

The recurrence rate of convulsions has been estimated from published data to be 24% (L. Duley, 1991 – personal communication). Magnesium has relaxant effects on uterine smooth muscle. This may cause increased blood loss at delivery and postpartum. In addition, this uterine tocolytic effect could interfere with attempts to achieve a vaginal delivery. An increase in cesarean section rate was demonstrated in the magnesium-treated arms of the two published controlled trials,[59,62] although the increase was not statistically significant.

The advantages of magnesium therapy are that it does not cause sedation and although it crosses the placenta no significant neonatal effects have been demonstrated. While not used in other areas of medicine, it is a cheap preparation.

If magnesium is to be used for the initial management of convulsions, the regime recommended by Pritchard and Pritchard[65] is 4 g magnesium sulfate (8 ml 50% magnesium sulfate solution diluted with 12 ml of sterile water) given intravenously over 3–5 min. In view of the toxicity of magnesium, a larger volume of fluid (e.g. 50–200 ml) and a longer time for injection (e.g. 10–20 min) may be preferable, especially for units not experienced in use of the drug. This is followed immediately by 10 ml 50% magnesium sulfate solution (5 g) intramuscularly deep into each buttock (total dose 20 ml, 10 g). Recurrent convulsions are managed by 2–4 g magnesium intravenously over 4–8 min. Maintenance therapy is 5 g every 4 h intramuscularly (alternating the buttocks) for 24 h after the last fit, provided that the signs of toxicity (respiratory rate <16/min, knee jerks absent and urine output <25 ml/h) are not present. The antidote to magnesium sulfate is 1 g calcium gluconate given intravenously.

An alternative to the intramuscular maintenance therapy is to adminster the drug intravenously at 2 g/h (e.g. 16 ml 50% magnesium sulfate solution in 200 ml N-saline at 50 ml/h) for 24 h. In such circumstances, magnesium levels should be estimated after 60 min and then every 6 h to maintain them in the therapeutic range of 2–3 mmol/l/

The four drug regimes have not been compared adequately in controlled trials. All of them appear efficacious, but have significant side-effects. The best method will only come out of such studies and a large international trial is currently underway. Until that time, units should follow only one of these protocols, which should be agreed by all concerned, well documented and readily available. Where possible, regions should aim to use one or at the most two regimes which makes it easier for junior medical staff, who routinely rotate through a number of hospitals.

- *Treatment of hypertension (see also previous section)*

The majority of women will have associated hypertension which requires specific treatment. A diastolic of 110 mmHg is commonly regarded as an indication for urgent treatment in eclampsia. In view of the concern about intracranial hemorrhage in these cases, a lower threshold such as 100 mmHg would appear justified. Intravenous hydrallazine is the agent most commonly used in the UK.[17] While it can be given in slow intravenous 10 mg boluses, an infusion is preferable. The infusion is best given using a syringe pump, as this allows more control over fluid balance when compared with a standard infusion bag. The infusion should be given at 2–20 mg/h, the rate being determined by the blood pressure response. Typically, one should be aiming for readings in the order of 140/90. Too large a

hypotensive effect may result in the prenatal case in a reduction in *uteroplacental* blood supply and fetal hypoxia. Pritchard *et al.*[64] found hydrallazine to be efficacious without any additional antihypertensive drugs and had no cases of suspected intracranial hemorrhage.

Continuation of the use of intravenous therapy should be for 24 h after convulsions have ceased. Often little therapy is needed after this time. If the blood pressure does remain elevated, oral agents are usually commenced. The options regarding which agents should be used are discussed in Chapter 18.

- *Assessment of renal function and fluid balance*

This is critical in the patient with eclampsia and has been discussed in detail in the section on the management of severe hypertension (see above).

- *Clotting abnormality*

Eclampsia is frequently associated with clotting disturbances. Accordingly, a full clotting screen should be performed and repeated regularly (e.g. every 12 h) during the acute phase. If the platelets are less than 50 ×10⁹/liter, 6 units of platelets should be available to cover delivery. If other clotting tests are abnormal, then fresh frozen plasma should be given to cover the delivery. The management of clotting abnormalities is discussed in detail below.

- *Assessment of pulmonary function*

Pulmonary function is likely to be impaired if respiratory depressants such as diazepam and chlormethiazole are used as anticonvulsants. In addition, magnesium sulfate cause respiratory depression if too much is administered. If the woman needs analagesia either in labor or post-cesarean section, then opiate analgesia is likely to be given which may depress respiration further. Also, excessive intravenous fluids may cause pulmonary edema, thus exacerbating the problem.

Accordingly, respiratory rate should be assessed at the same frequency as pulse and blood pressure recordings (e.g. every 15–30 min. Ideally, a pulse oximeter should be used on all these patients to record oxygen saturation pressure continuously. If this falls to <95 mmHg, then careful clinical and x-ray assessment of the chest is necessary. Oxygen therapy should be commenced early and titrated against the pulse oximeter readings. Intravenous diuretics should be used if pulmonary edema develops.

- *Fetal assessment*

Prenatal eclamptic fits are one of the few obstetric situations where the fetal condition automatically takes second place to that of the mother. Once the immediate urgent management has been instituted and the mother is stabilized in a high-dependency or intensive care environment, it is necessary to determine whether the fetus has survived the eclamptic fit. If he/she has survived, then it is helpful to know whether he/she is showing any signs suggestive of asphyxia, resulting from one of the following:

- he/she may be growth-deficient, since eclampsia is usually a sequela of pre-eclampsia with its associated spiral artery disease and poor uteroplacental blood supply

- the eclamptic fit will have been associated with maternal and subsequently fetal hypoxia

- hypotensive agents may have significantly reduced uteroplacental blood supply.

The most readily available method for determining whether any degree of asphyxia may be present is by means of continuous cardiotocography. Interpretation of this may be difficult as baseline variability is usually reduced if drugs such as diazepam and chlormethiazole have been given. In addition interpretation may be difficult if the fetus is very preterm. If the tracing is considered to be significantly abnormal (e.g. late decelerations and a tachycardia), then a decision has to be taken as to whether it is feasible with regard to maternal safety, and reasonable with regard to fetal viability, to contemplate a cesarean as opposed to a vaginal delivery (see below). There is usually little time to consider further investigations (such as a biophysical profile score), nor is it easy when a patient is receiving intensive care.

Labor/delivery

Timing and mode of delivery

Eclamptic fits can continue to occur until delivery has occurred and shortly after. The only way of curing the condition is through delivery. Accordingly, for those who have fits prenatally, part of the management must be planning delivery as soon as practical. This is not the occasion for considering delaying for possible beneficial fetal effects of steroid therapy. Once the patient is stabilized, she should either be induced or prepared for a cesarean section.

There is no consensus view as to the mode of delivery. In a large American series, Pritchard et al.[64] showed that attempts to achieve a vaginal delivery can result in an overall high success rate (67%), without high neonatal morbidity and mortality. Of the 27 cesareans, only five were for fetal distress, the majority being for failed induction of labor. In Crowther's series of 51 cases of antepartum eclampsia, the policy was to plan for vaginal delivery if delivery was considered likely within 8 h.[59] If this was not anticipated a cesarean section was carried out immediately. This policy resulted in a 73% cesarean rate.

Accordingly, it would seem appropriate to attempt a vaginal delivery with continuous fetal heart rate monitoring. This is essential because the fetus is likely to be growth-deficient. Other complications such as prematurity and abnormal presentation may also need to be taken into consideration, but do not necessarily dictate that a cesarean is mandatory.

There are maternal risks associated with cesarean delivery. These include performing surgery if there is a coagulopathy and anesthetic problems (see below). It will also increase the likelihood of future cesareans. Balanced against this is the risk of further convulsions (approximately 25%), although when occurring in intensive care surroundings, these should not result in major morbidity. However, with time the risk of other medical problems increases and so a definite time limit should be set for how long to persevere for a vaginal delivery.

Labor management

This is similar to that discussed in the section on hypertensive disorders (see above). In summary, it should be:

- induction with prostaglandins or oxytocin (using a syringe pump preferably to minimize fluid input)

- continuous electronic fetal heart rate monitoring

- assisted instrumental delivery to minimize bearing down

- oxytocin rather than Syntometrine® in the third stage

- recourse to cesarean if failed induction or delay in labor.

Analgesia for labor

If a coagulopathy is present, epidural anesthesia cannot be used because of the risk of an epidural hematoma occurring and causing compression. Entenox® analgesia (50% N_2O: 50% O_2) is safe, giving additional oxygen with no maternal respiratory depression. If not sufficient, then opiate analgesia must be given. Effects on the fetus are not a major concern and can be reversed after delivery. More worrying are potential maternal respiratory depression effects. Accordingly, respiratory rate must be accurately recorded and should be >16/min. It is preferable to monitor oxygen saturation continuously using a pulse oximeter.

Anesthesia for cesarean

General anesthesia is more commonly employed for reasons of speed and potential or real coagulopathy. Particular problems associated with general anesthesia under these circumstances are:

- difficult intubation due to laryngeal edema

- reflex hypertension associated with induction of anesthesia.

After delivery, anesthesia is often continued with elective ventilation for some hours in an intensive care environment as this should minimize the risks of hypoxia, pulmonary edema, further convulsions and inhalation.

Postnatal

Those who have eclamptic fits post-delivery should be managed in exactly the same way as those who fit prior to delivery. Management is clearly simplified by there being no fetal considerations. Fits occurring immediately post-delivery may not be eclamptic fits, but be caused through intracerebral bleeding secondary to a cerebral vascular anomaly. Despite this possibility, the management must follow the standard eclampsia protocol to ensure maternal risks are minimized.

Intensive maternal monitoring is typically required for 24–48 h post-delivery. Management should continue as outlined above under Labor Management. Specific points are discussed below.

Convulsions

After 48 h free of convulsions, anticonvulsant therapy is usually stopped. Oral anticonvulsants are not used routinely.

Blood pressure

The patient usually requires oral antihypertensive agents and these should be commenced when the patient's condition is improving and her blood pressure is stable on intravenous therapy. Oral medication may need to be continued after discharge from hospital. The

options regarding which antihypertensive agents should be used are discussed in Chapter 18.

Fluid balance – renal function

Central venous pressure monitoring can be discontinued once a diuresis has occurred. The frequency of urinary measurements can be reduced and the catheter removed once the patient is mobile. Renal function should continue to be assessed on a daily basis until returning to normal or the patient's overall condition is improved. Peripheral lines may be removed once there is no further need.

Coagulopathy

Evaluation of coagulation is best repeated approximately every 12 h until it is returning to normal.

Pulmonary function

Respiratory rate and prefereably oxygen saturation measurements must continue while there is any evidence of respiratory depression. Oxygen therapy should continue until oxygen saturation can be maintained at over 95 mmHg. Regular clinical chest examination should continue and be supplemented by x-ray examination if there is any suggestion of pulmonary edema or aspiration. Once the patient is alert and able to begin to mobilize, then these routine observations can be discontinued.

Any woman who has gone through an eclamptic episode is likely to have found it a frightening event and will be very anxious about the future. Accordingly, she should be counseled that she will be investigated postnatally for any underlying medical problems (see below). In the likely event that nothing is detected, she should be told that the chance of recurrence is extremely low and that it should be perfectly safe for her to consider a further pregnancy. She should be advised that aspirin therapy in a future pregnancy may be beneficial and appears to have no adverse effects.

Long-term follow-up

There is a strong case for the patient who had convulsions atypical of eclampsia, or who had further fits despite adequate anticonvulsive therapy, to have neurological follow-up. Ideally, this should include computed tomography to exclude intracerebral vascular malformations. Blood pressure should be monitored at home and treatment reduced and stopped when appropriate. The timing for this cannot be predicted.

Just as for women with sever hypertensive disorders, a hospital review after 4–6 weeks is ideal to review renal function, and if proteinuria persists on routine stick testing then formal 24 h quantification is prefer-

ECLAMPSIA
Summary of Management Options

Prepregnancy

- Discuss relatively low recurrence risk
- Counsel regarding prevention (see below)

Prenatal

Prediction

- Vigilance with pre-eclampsia, previous eclampsia, hypertension

Prevention

- ? Low-dose aspirin, etc. (see Hypertension section and Chapter 18)
- Antihypertensive therapy
- Prompt action with warning clinical features
- ? Prophylactic anticonvulsants (debated)

Management

- General: resuscitation, maintain airway, nurse, semi-prone, oxygen
- Give i.v. anticonvulsant (diazepam or magnesium sulfate – see text for doses)
- Transfer to high-dependency area
- Anticonvulsant to prevent recurrence (diazepam, chlormethiazole, phenytoin, magnesium sulfate – see text for doses)
- Control BP (see previous section and Chapter 18)
- Assess renal function and fluid balance; avoid fluid overload

- Assess clotting status
- Assess pulmonary function
- Assess fetal health
- Deliver when stable

Labour/delivery

- Mode of delivery will depend on maternal status and fetal viability
- If labor:
  - continuous FHR monitoring
  - assisted second stage
  - oxytocin for third stage
  - avoid prolonged labor
- Regional analgesia for labor and delivery contraindicated with clotting abnormality

Postnatal

- Maintain high-dependency care for 24–48 h
- Stop anticonvulsants after 48 h fit-free
- Intravenous antihypertensives or oral after 24 h
- Reduce intensive monitoring when recovery noted
- Counseling about risks of recurrence
- Long-term follow-up – consider neurological assessment if atypical fits (see Chapter 26); monitor BP and proteinuria and consider investigation if remain abnormal

able. This will also give the opportunity to measure creatinine clearance. Any derangements of renal function at this point should be managed by transfer to the appropriate renal medicine follow-up program.

DISSEMINATED INTRAVASCULAR COAGULATION

Definition

The combination of massive hemorrhage and coagulation failure is one of the most feared complications that can arise in pregnancy, but disseminated intravascular coagulation (DIC) is associated with a wide variety of clinical situations in obstetrics. It is always a secondary phenomenon following a 'trigger' of generalized coagulation activity. Consumption of clotting factors, fibrin and platelets occurs, setting up a vicious cycle that results in continued disastrous bleeding and coagulation failure. The clinical manifestations can vary from mild coagulation disorders detected on laboratory tests only, to massive uncontrollable hemorrhage with very low fibrinogen and platelet levels. A failure to anticipate or detect the early stages of DIC is cited as a major deficiency in the care of women who die from obstetric hemorrhage,[3,66] and despite advances in obstetric care and hematological services, hemorrhage with associated DIC remains a major cause of maternal mortality and morbidity.

Incidence

Due to the wide range of obstetric complications that may be associated with DIC and the variation in degree of severity, it is impossible to quote an overall incidence for the condition, but the incidence of severe DIC with uncontrollable hemorrhage has been estimated at 0.1% of pregnancies. There are no population-based or controlled trials looking at coagulation failure in pregnancy because of the small numbers seen in any one unit.

Mechanisms

Disseminated intravascular coagulation is triggered by various mechanisms that include the release of thromboplastic agents into the circulation, endothelial damage to small vessels, and pro-coagulant phospholipids produced in response to intravascular hemolysis (**Table 2**). With obstetric complications associated with coagulation failure, there may be interaction of several mechanisms, and blood loss itself with trans-

Table 2
Mechanism of DIC occurring during pregnancy

Injury to vascular endothelium	Pre-eclampsia Hypovolemic shock Septicemic shock
Release of thromboplastic tissue factors	Placental abruption Amniotic fluid embolism Retained dead fetus Chorioamnionitis Hydatidiform mole Placenta accreta Hypertonic saline used to induce abortion
Production of procoagulant phospholipids	Feto-maternal hemorrhage Incompatible blood transfusion Septicemia Intravascular hemolysis

In many obstetric complications, there may be interaction between several mechanisms and more than one trigger factor present

fusion and volume replacement can precipitate or exacerbate DIC.

Once DIC has occurred, a vicious cycle ensues, with further consumption of clotting factors and platelets and bleeding continues until the underlying cause is corrected (**Figure 1**). The spectrum of severity of the condition is extremely wide and has been classified by

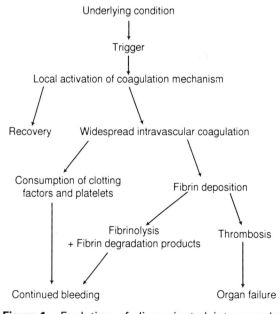

Figure 1. Evolution of disseminated intravascular coagulation

Letsky (**Table 3**). The incidence of DIC reported in association with specific complications varies widely because of differences in the criteria on which the diagnosis was made.

Risks

The risks to both the mother and the fetus from coagulation failure in terms of mortality and morbidity are the same as those discussed under major obstetric hemorrhage in this chapter. The specific situations where DIC and coagulation failure may occur and the risks of each underlying condition will now be considered.

Placental abruption

This remains the most common cause of coagulation failure in obstetrics and is related to the degree of placental separation and hypovolemic shock. In severe placental abruption with a dead fetus, profound hypofibrinogenemia (Stage 3 DIC) was reported in 35–38% of cases but is much less common if the fetus is alive.[37,47] Earlier stages of DIC are common with mild to moderate abruption but can usually be corrected early if delivery is not delayed.[48] The initial mechanism is due to the release of thromboplastic substances, but in severe abruption hypovolemic shock, large volume transfusion and high levels of FDPs that act as anticoagulants themselves will exacerbate the situation.

Table 3
Classification of severity of DIC

Severity of DIC		*In vitro* findings
Stage 1	Low-grade compensated	Elevated fibrin degradation products (FDPS) Increased soluble fibrin complexes
Stage 2	Uncompensated, but no hemostatic failure	Findings as above, but also: Decreased platelet count Decreased fibrinogen levels Reduced factor V and VIII
Stage 3	Rampant DIC, with hemostatic failure	Very low platelet count Gross depletion of coagulation factors, especially fibrinogen Very high levels of FDPS

Stage 3 is most common after severe placental abruption, amniotic fluid embolism or severe pre-eclampsia, but there may be rapid progression in other conditions if early manifestations of DIC are not recognized and corrected

After Letsky.[83]

Amniotic fluid embolism

This obstetric disaster classically occurs during a relatively rapid labor with intact membranes and can also occur at cesarean section. It is thought that amniotic fluid enters the circulation through lacerations in the placenta and or lower uterine segment, causing platelet thrombi in the pulmonary vessels and severe cardiorespiratory failure. There is a high mortality at this stage, but if the patient survives the initial insult she will develop massive DIC with almost undetectable levels of clotting factors. The diagnosis is confirmed at postmortem by the detection of amniotic fluid and fetal squames within the maternal lungs, and therefore the incidence of successfully treated cases is difficult to determine as the diagnosis is only suggestive and cannot be proven.[67,68] The incidence of death from amniotic fluid embolism between 1970 and 1987 in England and Wales was 7.1 per million maternities. Possible risk factors include maternal age over 35 years, parity of more than 3, and use of oxytocic drugs for augmentation with excessively strong contractions, but no specific etiology was identified in the maternal mortality report.[3] In most cases, the maternal death was unpredictable and unavoidable, and as obstetric care improves, amniotic fluid embolism has been responsible for an increasing proportion of maternal deaths, and is now the fifth most common cause.[3]

Retention of a dead fetus

A gradual reduction in clotting factors occurs following intrauterine fetal death, but these changes are not detectable on laboratory testing for 3–4 weeks. Approximately 80% of patients with a retained dead fetus will go into spontaneous labor within 3 weeks, but 30% of patients who remain undelivered for more than 4 weeks will develop DIC, usually of a mild degree.[69,70] Release of thromboplastic substances from the dead fetus into the maternal circulation is thought to be the trigger mechanism. The condition is much less common today, as ultrasound scanning confirms the diagnosis of fetal death, coagulation screening is routinely performed and induction of labor is carried out much earlier, usually before 3–4 weeks have elapsed.

Pre-eclampsia

Although the etiology and pathogenesis of this condition has not been defined, the development of the syndrome known as pre-eclampsia appears to result from generalized endothelial injury caused by circulatory factors released from the placenta.[71] The stimulus for the release of these factors is uteroplacental insufficiency and placental ischemia, and widespread endothelial injury explains the multiple organ systems involved, including the clotting system.[72]

Early disturbances can be detected by a falling platelet count in an otherwise asymptomatic patient, due to endothelial injury and consumption of maternal platelets. This trigger mechanism can lead to full DIC, and severe clotting abnormalities in pre-eclampsia are particularly associated with liver pathology, as in the HELLP syndrome.[73] Interactions between platelets and the damaged endothelium at the early stage may explain why low-dose aspirin can prevent the development of the maternal syndrome of pre-eclampsia.[43]

Sepsis

Endotoxic shock can be associated with chorioamnionitis, septic abortion or postpartum intrauterine infection. Gram-negative organisms are the most common isolated, although *Clostridium welchi* and *Bacteroides* sp. may be encountered, particularly in septic abortion. The bacterial endotoxin produces severe endothelial damage leading to fibrin deposition and DIC. Secondary intravascular hemolysis, which produces hematuria and oliguria characteristic of the condition, then occurs, and microangiopathic hemolysis can also cause purpuric skin lesions. Hypotension and coagulation failure are poor prognostic features in the presence of sepsis.[74,75]

Other risk factors

Other rarer conditions of pregnancy that have been associated with DIC and coagulation failure include induced abortion with hypertonic saline,[76] acute fatty liver of pregnancy and other hepatic disorders.[77] Hydatidiform mole and placenta accreta are associated with DIC because of loss of the intact decidua basalis, and passage of amniotic fluid and other thromboplastic substances into the maternal circulation is more likely.[78,79] Incompatible blood transfusions, large fetomaternal hemorrhage, and other causes of intravascular hemolysis including drug reactions and the use of other replacement fluids can also precipitate or exacerbate existing DIC.[45]

Management Options

General

The management of the bleeding obstetric patient is essentially the same whether or not coagulation failure is present and a planned protocol should be available on every delivery unit, as discussed in the previous section. The mainstay of treatment is to locate and deal with the source of bleeding and to instigate adequate resuscitation and fluid replacement. Prolonged hypovolemic shock may trigger DIC not initially present and lead to hemostatic failure. If an effective circulation is restored without too much delay in the presence of DIC, renal shutdown can be avoided and fibrin degradation products can be cleared from the circulation by the liver, thus aiding the restoration of normal hemostasis.

Laboratory investigation of suspected DIC

As soon as there is concern about bleeding from any source, 10–20 ml of blood should be taken and sent for cross-matching and appropriate laboratory tests before commencing intravenous resuscitation (**Table 4**).

The thrombin time, which provides a rapid estimation of clottable fibrinogen in a blood sample, is the most useful rapid test of hemostatic competence, as the thrombin time will be prolonged when there is depleted fibrinogen and also where FDPs are raised. Blood should be taken for FDP estimation, as elevated levels in the acute situation will confirm the diagnosis of DIC, but the assay should be delayed until after the emergency is over as the result does not assist in the acute management of the patient. Blood can be observed for evidence of clotting, but there is little point in performing whole blood clotting tests at the bedside as they are unreliable and time-consuming.[80]

Screening tests should be repeated at regular intervals throughout resuscitation and treatment to assess the need for other component replacement therapy such as platelets.

Table 4
Laboratory investigations

1. Full blood count including platelet estimation
   (2.5 ml in EDTA bottle)

2. Coagulation screen:
   Prothrombin time — extrinsic system
   Partial thromboplastin time — intrinsic system
   Thrombin time
   Fibrinogen titer
   (4.5 ml with 0.5 ml citrate anticoagulant)

3. Fibrin degradation products
   (2.0 ml in special bottle with antifibrinolytic agent)

4. Cross-matching, at least 6 units
   (10 ml in plain tube)

Ideally, 20 ml of blood should be sent, but 10 ml is sufficient for essential tests. The sample should be collected as atraumatically and quickly as possible, and any heparinized i.v. lines avoided

Fluid replacement in coagulation failure

The urgent necessity in the initial stages is to maintain circulatory volume and tissue perfusion, and resuscitation with crystalloid and colloid solutions should be undertaken as soon as possible, as outlined in the previous section. Dextran solutions should not be used as they interfere with platelet function and can aggravate bleeding and DIC, as well as invalidating the laboratory investigations. Prompt and adequate fluid replacement will also prevent renal shutdown and help in the clearance of elevated levels of FDPs from the circulation via the liver, aiding the restoration of normal hemostasis.[70]

Initial fluid replacement is only a temporary stop-gap measure, and blood products should be given as soon as available. Fresh frozen plasma (FFP) and stored red cells provide all the necessary components in fresh whole blood apart from platelets, and the clotting factors in FFP are well preserved for at least 12 months provided the sample is stored correctly. The use of fresh whole blood should not be encouraged, as it cannot be screened for possible infections. It is rarely necessary to give extra fibrinogen in the form of cryoprecipitate, as sufficient amounts are provided in FFP, which also contains Factors V, VIII and anti-thrombin III in higher concentrations. Platelets are not found in FFP, and their functional activity rapidly deteriorates in stored blood. The platelet count reflects both the degree of DIC and the amount of transfused blood given. If there is persistent bleeding and the platelet count is very low (less than 60×10^9/liter), the patient may be given concentrated platelets, but these are not usually necessary to gain hemostasis.[45,81]

As stated previously, there is a wide spectrum in the manifestation of the process of DIC, but the aims of treatment are:

- to remove the initiating stimulus

- to maintain circulating blood volume

- to replace clotting factors and red blood cells.

In many cases, such as placental abruption, amniotic fluid embolism, pre-eclampsia, fetal death *in utero* and antepartum sepsis, this will mean delivery as soon as practicable. A spontaneous recovery from the coagulopathy can be expected once the uterus is contracted and empty, providing that circulating blood volume has been maintained by adequate fluid replacement.

The importance of locating and dealing with the source of bleeding cannot be overstated, and every attempt must be made to limit blood loss during resuscitation. Measures should be taken to maintain a

---

DISSEMINATED INTRAVASCULAR COAGULATION
Summary of Management Options

Diagnosis

- Vigilance in high-risk pregnancies:
  - placental abruption
  - amniotic fluid embolism
  - pre-eclampsia
  - retained and prolonged fetal death
  - APH or PPH
  - septicemic shock

- Investigate such high-risk cases for possible diagnosis (see **Table 4**)

- Diagnosis should be possible in such cases before clinically suspected allowing prompt treatment

Treatment

- Involve hematologist and support sevices (blood transfusion, etc.) early

- Treat/remove cause (e.g. empty uterus, antibiotics for sepsis)

- Hematological priorities are to replace blood constituents and coagulation factors

- Heparin and antithrombolytic therapy have both been used in DIC to break the cycle of consumptive coagulopathy. Neither has been subjected to controlled trials and their use is considered inappropriate by most authorities

---

firm contracted uterus and limit bleeding from the placental site. FDPs can have a direct inhibitory effect on myometrial contractility, which can further exacerbate the problem.[82]

Other treatment options in DIC

Once coagulation failure has developed, a vicious cycle is established, as seen in **Figure 1**, and there is a theoretical risk at least that transfusion with fibrinogen, FFP and platelets may 'fuel the fire' and encourage further DIC. The main thrust of treatment is therefore directed at removing the underlying stimulus for the DIC, and in most cases hemostasis will be restored after this, providing the circulatory volume has been maintained. Many other therapies have been tried in an attempt to break the cycle of DIC, but in no case has a controlled trial been performed, as the number of cases encountered by any one researcher is too small to be statistically significant.

Heparin therapy has been used to treat DIC of many different underlying causes, but there is no definite evidence to suggest that its use confers any benefit over supportive therapy. Most authorities suggest that heparin is contraindicated if the circulation is not intact and this would include placental abruption.[75,80,83] There may be a place for the use of heparin therapy in the management of conditions such as amniotic fluid embolism and sepsis, and the successful management of small numbers of patients has been reported in several small uncontrolled trials.[68,82] Antifibrinolytic drugs have also been used, but there is the risk that their use would prevent the removal of microvascular thrombi from organs such as kidney or brain as the DIC resolves, leading to long-term sequelae.[83,84] The cornerstone of treatment remains supportive, with restoration of circulating volume, replacement of blood and clotting factors, and correction of the underlying cause of the coagulation failure the vital measures.

REFERENCES

1 Davey DA, MacGillivray I (1988) The classification and definition of the hypertensive disorders of pregnancy. *American Journal of Obstetrics and Gynecology* **158**:892–898.

2 Redman C (1988) Eclampsia still kills. *British Medical Journal* **296**:1209–1210.

3 Department of Health. (1991) *Report on Confidential Enquiries into Maternal Deaths in the United Kingdom, 1985–87*. London: HMSO.

4 Butler NR, Bonham DG (1963) *Toxaemia in Pregnancy: Perinatal Mortality*, pp. 87–100. Edinburgh: E. and S. Livingstone.

5 Campbell DM, MacGillivray I, Carr-Hill R (1985) Pre-eclampsia in a second pregnancy. *British Journal of Obstetrics and Gynaecology* **92**:131–140.

6 Chesley LC, Annitto JE, Cosgrove RA (1968) The familial factor in toxaemia of pregnancy. *Obstetrics and Gynecology* **32**:303–311.

7 Chesley LC, Cooper DW (1986) Genetics of hypertension in pregnancy: Possible single gene control of pre-eclampsia and eclampsia in the descendants of eclamptic women. *British Journal of Obstetrics and Gynaecology* **98**:898–908.

8 Thornton JG, Onwude JL (1991) Pre-eclampsia: Discordance among identical twins. *British Medical Journal* **303**:1241–1242.

9 Beaufils M, Uzan S, Donsimoni R, Colau JA (1985) Prevention of pre-eclampsia by early antiplatelet therapy. *Lancet* **ii**:840–842.

10 Schiff E, Peleg E, Goldenburg M, Rosenthal T, Ruppin E, Tamarkin M, Barkai G, Ben-Baruch G, Yahal I, Blankstein K, Goldman B, Mashiach S (1989) The use of aspirin to prevent pregnancy-induced hypertension and lower the ratio of thromboxane A_2 to prostacyclin in relatively high risk pregnancies. *New England Journal of Medicine* **321**:351–356.

11 Wallenburg HCS, Dekker GA, Makovitz JW, Rotmans P (1986) Low-dose aspirin prevents pregnancy-induced hypertension and pre-eclampsia in angiotensin-sensitive primigravidae. *Lancet* **i**:1–3.

12 Hall HM, Chang PK, MacGillivray I (1980) Is routine antenatal care worthwhile? *Lancet* **ii**:78–80.

13 Mathews DD (1977) A randomised controlled trial of bed rest and sedation or normal activity and non-sedation in the management of non-albuminuric hypertension in late pregnancy. *British Journal of Obstetrics and Gynaecology* **84**:108–114.

14 Redman CWG, Beilin LJ, Bonnar J, Wilkinson RH (1976) Plasma urate measurements in predicting fetal death in hypertensive pregnancy. *Lancet* **ii**:1370–1373.

15 Redman CWG, Bonnar J, Beilin LJ (1978) Early platelet consumption in pre-eclampsia. *British Medical Journal* **1**:467–469.

16 Steel SA, Pearce JM, McParland P, Chamberlain GVP (1990) Early Doppler ultrasound screening in prediction of hypertensive disorders of pregnancy. *Lancet* **335**:1548–1551.

17 Hutton JD, James DK, Stirrat GM, Douglas KA, Redman CWG (1992) Management of severe pre-eclampsia and eclampsia by UK Consultants. *British Journal of Obstetrics and Gynaecology* **99**:554–556.

18 Redman CWG (1989) Hypertension in pregnancy. In de Swiet M (ed.), *Medical Disorders in Obstetric Practice*, 2nd edn, pp. 249–305. Oxford: Blackwell Scientific Publications.

19 Crowley P (1989) Promoting pulmonary maturity. In: Chalmers I, Enkin M, Keirse MJNC (eds), pp. 746–764. *Effective Care in Pregnancy and Childbirth*. Oxford: Oxford University Press.

20 Mabie WC, Gonzalez AR, Sibai BM, Amou E (1987) A comparative trial of labetalol and hydrallazine in the acute management of severe hypertension complicating pregnancy. *Obstetrics and Gynecology* **70**:328–333.

21 Walters BNJ, Redman CWG (1984) Treatment of severe pregnancy associated hypertension with the calcium antagonist nifedipine. *British Journal of Obstetrics and Gynaecology* **91**:330–336.

22 Cotton DB, Lee W, Huhta J, Dorman K (1988) Hemodynamic profile of severe pregnancy-induced hypertension. *American Journal of Obstetrics and Gynecology* **158**:523–529.

23 Ballard RA, Ballard PL, Creasy RK, Padbury J, Polk DH, Bracken M, Moya FR, Gross I (1992) Respiratory disease in very low birth weight infants after prenatal thyrotropin-releasing hormone and glucocorticoid. *Lancet* **339**:510–515.

24 Abboud TK, Khoo SS, Miller F, Doan T, Henriksen EH (1982) Maternal, fetal and neonatal responses after epidural anesthesia with bupivicaine, 2-chloroprocaine or lidocaine. *Anesthesia and Analgesia* **62**:638–644.

25 Ihle BU, Long P, Oats J (1987) Early onset preeclampsia: Recognition of underlying renal disease. *British Medical Journal* **294**:79–81.

26 Royal College of Obstetricians and Gynaecologists (1992) *Maternal Mortality: The Way Forward*. London: Chameleon Press.

27 Maine D *et al.* (1987) *Prevention of Maternal Deaths in Developing Countries*. New York: Centre for Population of Family Health, University of Columbia.

28 Grimes H, Brooks M (1980) Pregnancy in Sheehann's syndrome: Report of a case and review. *Obstetrical and Gynecological Survey* **35**:481–488.

29 Paterson ME (1979) The aetiology and outcome of abruptio placentae. *Acta Obstetrica et Gynaecologica Scandinavica* **58**:31–35.

30 Hurd WH, Miodovnik M, Hertzberg V, Lavin JP (1983) Selective management of abruptio placentae: A prospective study. *Obstetrics and Gynecology* **27**:155–167.

31 Naeye RL (1978) Placenta praevia: Predisposing factors and effects on the fetus and surviving infants. *Obstetrics and Gynecology* **52**:521–525.

32 Clark SL, Koonings PP, Phelan JP (1985) Placenta praevia/accreta and prior cesarean section. *Obstetrics and Gynecology* **66**:89–92.

33 Brenner WE, Edelman DA, Hendricks CH (1978) Characteristics of patients with placenta praevia and results of expectant management. *American Journal of Obstetrics and Gynecology* **132**:180–184.

34 Rose GL, Chapman MG (1985) Aetiological factors in placenta praevia – a case controlled study. *British Journal of Obstetrics and Gynaecology* **93**:585–588.

35 Gorodeski IG, Bahari CM, Schachter A, Neri A (1981) Recurrent placenta praevia. *European Journal of Obstetrics and Gynecology and Reproductive Biology* **12**:7–11.

36 Singh PM, Rodrigues C, Gupta AN (1981) Placenta praevia and previous cesarean section. *Acta Obstetrica et Gynaecologica Scandinavica* **292**:371–372.

37 Green-Thompson RW (1982) Antepartum haemorrhage. *Clinics in Obstetrics and Gynecology* **9**:479–503.

38 Cotton DB, Read JA, Paul RH, Quilligan EJ (1980) The conservative aggressive management of placenta praevia. *American Journal of Obstetrics and Gynecology* **137**:687–695.

39 Carp HJ, Mashiach S, Serr DM (1979) Vasa praevia: A major complication and its management. *Obstetrics and Gynecology* **53**:273–275.

40 Naeye RL, Harkness WL, Utts J (1977) Abruptio placentae and perinatal death: A prospective study. *American Journal of Obstetrics and Gynecology* **128**:701–704.

41 Naeye RL (1980) Abruptio placentae and placenta praevia. Frequency, perinatal mortality and cigarette smoking. *Obstetrics and Gynecology* **55**:700–703.

42 Hibbard BM, Jeffcoate TNA (1966) Abruptio placentae. *Obstetrics and Gynecology* **27**:155–167.

43 Sibai BM, Mirro R, Chesley M, Leffler C (1989) Low dose aspirin in pregnancy. *Obstetrics and Gynecology* **74**:551–557.

44 Kelly JV (1976) Post-partum haemorrhage. *Clinics in Obstetrics and Gynecology* **19**:595–606.

45 Hewitt PE, Machin SJ (1990) Massive blood transfusion. *British Medical Journal* **300**:107–109.

46 Beischer NA, McKay EV (1986) *Obstetrics and the Newborn*. London: Baillière Tindall.

47 Pritchard JA, Brekken AL (1967) Clinical and laboratory studies on severe abruptio placentae. *American Journal of Obstetrics and Gynecology* **97**:681–695.

48 Knab DR (1978) Abruptio placentae: An assessment of the time and method of delivery. *Obstetrics and Gynaecology* **52**:625–629.

49 Silver R *et al.* (1984) Placenta praevia: Aggressive expectant management. *American Journal of Obstetrics and Gynecology* **150**:15–22.

50 Myersclough PR (1982) *Munro Kerr's Operative Obstetrics*, 10th edn. London: Baillière Tindall.

51 Gilbert L, Porter W, Brown V (1987) Post-partum haemorrhage: A continuing problem. *British Journal of Obstetrics and Gynaecology* **94**:67–71.

52 Lucas WE (1980) Post-partum haemorrhage. *Clinics in Obstetrics and Gynecology* **23**:637–646.

53 Whitfield CR (1981) Complications of the third stage of labour. In Dewhurst J (ed.), *Integrated Obstetrics and Gynaecology for Postgraduates*, p. 437. Oxford: Blackwell Scientific Publications.

54 Prendeville WJ, Elbourne DR, Chalmers I (1988) The effects of routine oxytocic adminstration in the management of the third stage of labour: An overview of clinical trials. *British Journal of Obstetrics and Gynaecology* **95**:3–16.

55 Toppozada M, El-Bossati M, El Rahman HA (1981) Control of intractable atonic post-partum haemorrhage by 15-methyl prostaglandin $F2_{2\alpha}$. *Obstetrics and Gynecology* **58**:327–330.

56 Jacobs MM, Arias F (1979) Intramyometrial prostaglandin $F2_{2\alpha}$ in the treatment of severe post-partum haemorrhage. *Obstetrics and Gynecology* **55**:665–666.

57 Hertz RH, Sokal RJ, Dieker LJ (1980) Treatment of postpartum uterine atony with prostaglandin E_2 vaginal suppositories. *Obstetrics and Gynecology* **56**:120–130.

58 Hester JD (1975) Post-partum haemorrhage and re-evaluation of uterine packing. *Obstetrics and Gynecology* **45**:501.

59 Crowther C (1990) Magnesium sulphate versus diazepam in the management of eclampsia: A randomized controlled trial. *British Journal of Obstetrics and Gynaecology* **97**:110–117.

60 Duffus GM, Tunstall ME, MacGillivray I (1968) Intravenous chlormethiazole in pre-eclamptic toxaemia in labour. *Lancet*. **i**:335–337.

61 Slater RM, Smith WD, Patrick J, Mawer GE, Wilcox FL, Donnai P, Richardson T, D'Souza S (1987) Pheny-

toin infusion in severe pre-eclampsia. *Lancet* **i**:1417–1420.

62 Dommisse J (1990) Phenytoin sodium and magnesium sulphate in the management of eclampsia. *British Journal of Obstetrics and Gynaecology* **97**:104–109.

63 Slater M, Wilcox FL, Smith WD, Maresh MJA (1989) Phenytoin in pre-eclampsia. *Lancet* **ii**:1224.

64 Pritchard JA, Cunningham G, Pritchard SA (1984) The Parkland Memorial Hospital protocol for treatment of eclampsia: Evaluation of 245 cases. *American Journal of Obstetrics and Gynecology* **148**:951–960.

65 Pritchard JA, Pritchard SA (1975) Standardized treatment of 154 cases of eclampsia. *American Journal of Obstetrics and Gynecology* **123**:543–552.

66 Department of Health (1989) *Report on Confidential Enquiries into Maternal Deaths in England and Wales, 1982–1984*. London: HMSO.

67 Morgan M (1979) Amniotic fluid embolism. *Anaesthesia* **34**: 20–34.

68 Chung AF, Merkatz IR (1973) Survival following amniotic fluid embolism with early heparinisation. *Obstetrics and Gynecology* **42**:809–814.

69 Pritchard JA (1959) Fetal death *in utero*. *Obstetrics and Gynecology* **14**:573–580.

70 Pritchard JA (1973) Haematological problems associated with delivery, placental abruption, retained dead fetus and amniotic fluid embolism. *Clinics in Hematology* **2**:563–586.

71 Roberts JM, Taylor RN *et al.* (1989) Pre-eclampsia, an endothelial cell disorder. *American Journal of Obstetrics and Gynecology* **161**:1200–1204.

72 Redman CWG (1991) The placenta and pre-eclampsia. *Placenta* **12**:301–308.

73 Weinstein L (1982) Syndrome of haemolysis, elevated liver enzymes and low platelet count: A severe consequence of hypertension of pregnancy. *American Journal of Obstetrics and Gynecology* **142**:159–167.

74 Hawkins DF, Sevitt LH, Fairbrother PF, Totill AU (1975) Management of chemical septic abortion with renal failure: Use of a conservative regimen. *New England Journal of Medicine* **292**:722–725.

75 Beller FK, Uszynski M (1974) Disseminated intravascular coagulation in pregnancy. *Clinics in Obstetrics and Gynaecology* **17**:264–278.

76 Stander RW, Flessa HC, Glueck HC *et al.* (1971) Changes in maternal coagulation factors after intra-amniotic injection of hypertonic saline. *Obstetrics and Gynecology* **37**:660–666.

77 Harpey J, Charpentier C (1983) Acute fatty liver of pregnancy. *Lancet* **i**:586–587.

78 Read JA, Cotton DB, Miller FC (1980) Placenta accreta: Changing clinical aspects and outcome. *Obstetrics and Gynecology* **56**:31–34.

79 Breen JL, Neubecker R, Gregori CA, Franklin JE (1977) Placenta accreta, increta and percreta: A survey of 40 cases. *Obstetrics and Gynecology* **49**:43–47.

80 Letsky EA (1992) In Royal College of Obstetricians and Gynaecologists (ed.), *Maternal Mortality: The Way Forward*, pp. 63–71. London: Chameleon Press.

81 Letsky EA (1991) Mechanism of coagulation and changes induced by pregnancy. *Current Obstetrics and Gynaecology* **1**:203–209.

82 Basu HK (1969) Fibrinolysis and abruptio placentae. *Journal of Obstetrics and Gynaecology of the British Commonwealth* **76**:481–496.

83 Letsky EA (1985) *Coagulation Problems During Pregnancy*. Edinburgh: Churchill Livingstone.

84 Bonnar J (1981) Haemostasis and coagulation disorders in pregnancy. In Bloom AL, Thomas DP (eds), *Haemostasis and Thrombosis*, Ch. 6. pp. Edinburgh: Churchill Livingstone.

Appendix of Normal Values

MARGARET RAMSAY

MATERNAL PARAMETERS

WEIGHT GAIN

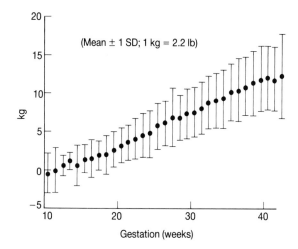

(Mean ± 1 SD; 1 kg = 2.2 lb)

Figure 1. Maternal weight gain in 988 normal women who had uneventful pregnancies; they were all booked at < 20 weeks and delivered between 37 and 41 weeks. (Longitudinal study.) *Data source*: ref. **1**, with permission.

PLACENTAL BIOCHEMISTRY

Serum Alpha-fetoprotein (SAFP)

	First tri-mester	Second tri-mester	Third tri-mester	Labour at term	First post-partum day
	(n = 22)	(n = 10)	(n = 18)	(n = 10)	(n = 10)
serum alpha-feto-protein (ng/ml)	37 30–54	178 151–258	292 270–418	143 153–250	104 65–275

(Median and IQ range)

Figure 2. Cross-sectional study, although samples from women in labor and on the first postpartum day were paired. SAFP measured by radioimmunoassay. *Data source*: ref. **2**, with permission.

Comment: In the second trimester, SAFP rises by approximately 15% per week.[3] Reference ranges for SAFP in the second trimester are established by individual screening laboratories for their own population. Twin pregnancies are associated with SAFP levels approximately twice as high as those of singleton pregnancies.[3] Maternal weight is inversely related to SAFP levels, probably due to the dilutional effect of a larger vascular compartment.[3]

Human Chorionic Gonadotrophin (HCG)

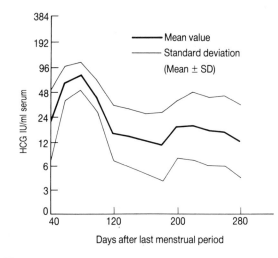

Figure 3. Longitudinal study of 20 healthy women. The first samples were drawn as early in pregnancy as possible, with subsequent samples every 3–4 weeks; the last sample was taken during labor. Samples were classified into groups with a class interval of 30 days. HCG was determined by a radioimmunoassay; the international HCG standard was used as a reference. *Data source*: ref. **4**, with permission.

Comment: Women with male fetuses have significantly lower HCG levels than do those with female fetuses.[4]

Human Placental Lactogen (HPL)

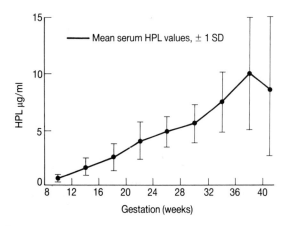

Figure 4. Cross-sectional study of 151 normal women with singleton pregnancies attending the prenatal clinic. HPL was measured by radioimmunoassay. *Data source*: ref. **5**, with permission.

Comment: HPL levels in women with multiple pregnancies are outside these ranges; however, if values are corrected for predicted placental weight then they are appropriate for ges-

tational age.[5] Plasma HPL is virtually undetectable 4 h after delivery of the placenta; the half-life of HPL in the plasma is 21–23 min.[6]

Estriol (E₃)

Table 1
Cross-sectional study in women with uncomplicated pregnancies. Plasma estriol was measured by a fluorometric method

Gestation (weeks)	No. of samples	Plasma estriol (μg/dl) Mean	SD	Range
20–23	29	5.6	4.0	2.1–21.7
24–27	34	6.2	2.4	3.0–10.6
28–31	50	9.4	5.6	3.6–33.7
32–33	29	12.8	7.7	4.1–33.0
34–35	40	15.6	7.6	4.1–36.0
36–37	44	17.8	7.3	5.7–34.0
38–39	44	21.5	8.0	10.5–36.5
40	37	24.8	9.7	12.5–58.0

Data source: ref. **7**, with permission.

HEMATOLOGY

Hemoglobin and Red Cell Indices

Table 2
Longitudinal study (mean and SD) of women recruited at 12 weeks who delivered after 37 weeks (n = 24). No iron/folate supplements given. 'Non-pregnant' samples were taken 4–6 months postdelivery. Samples were analyzed in a Coulter Counter

Investigation	Non-pregnant (SD)	12 weeks (SD)	36 weeks (SD)	Post-partum (SD)
Red blood cell count (× 10¹²/l)	4.688 (0.309)	4.008 (0.247)	3.880 (0.304)	4.493 (0.338)
Hemoglobin concentration (g/dl)	13.30 (0.77)	12.03 (0.70)	11.07 (0.84)	12.69 (0.92)
Hematocrit (l/l)	0.3936 (0.0233)	0.3515 (0.0226)	0.3311 (0.0232)	0.3787 (0.0289)
Mean cell volume (fl)	83.7 (3.1)	86.2 (3.6)	85.0 (5.3)	84.1 (3.8)
Mean cell hemoglobin (pg)	28.39 (1.06)	30.07 (1.16)	28.65 (2.00)	28.23 (1.45)
Mean cell hemoglobin concentration (g/dl)	33.75 (0.68)	34.23 (1.13)	33.46 (0.82)	33.47 (0.93)

Table 3

Longitudinal study (mean and SD) of women recruited at 12 weeks who delivered after 37 weeks (*n* = 21). *Given iron/folate supplements from 12 weeks.* 'Non-pregnant' samples were taken 4–6 months postdelivery. Samples were analyzed in a Coulter Counter

Investigation	Non-pregnant (SD)	12 weeks (SD)	36 weeks (SD)	Post-partum (SD)
Red blood cell count ($\times 10^{12}$/l)	4.621 (0.238)	4.109 (0.227)	4.119 (0.246)	4.370 (0.169)
Hemoglobin concentration (g/dl)	13.42 (0.66)	12.06 (0.57)	12.66 (0.81)	13.03 (0.45)
Hematocrit (l/l)	0.3971 (0.0190)	0.3539 (0.020)	0.3666 (0.020)	0.3880 (0.0123)
Mean cell volume (fl)	85.7 (2.2)	86.0 (3.3)	88.8 (2.9)	88.4 (3.3)
Mean cell hemoglobin (pg)	29.00 (0.77)	29.43 (1.03)	30.76 (1.24)	29.86 (1.20)
Mean cell hemoglobin concentration (g/dl)	33.63 (0.69)	34.05 (1.08)	34.50 (0.82)	33.59 (0.66)

Data source: ref. **8**, with permission.

Comment: Hemoglobin concentration falls in the first trimester, whether or not iron and folate supplements are given. Pregnancy-induced hematological changes are still present 6–8 weeks postpartum.

White Cell Count (Total and Differential)

	Non-pregnant	12 weeks	36 weeks	6–8 weeks postpartum
Total white cell count ($\times 10^9$/l)	5.64 (1.01)	6.89 (1.71)	10.24 (3.39)	7.27 (2.38)

Figure 5. Longitudinal study (mean and SD) of 24 women recruited at 12 weeks, who delivered after 37 weeks. 'Non-pregnant' samples were taken 4–6 months postdelivery. Samples were analyzed in a Coulter Counter. *Data source*: ref. **8**, with permission.

Comment: Supplementation with iron and folate does not affect total white cell count (WBC) during or after pregnancy. Pregnancy related changes in WBC are still present 6–8 weeks postdelivery. Another (cross-sectional) study found no change in numbers of circulating lymphocytes and monocytes, but decreased eosinophils in the third trimester.[8] Immature granulocytes (myelocytes and metamyelocytes) are found frequently in peripheral blood smears during pregnancy.[9,10]

Platelet Count and Indices

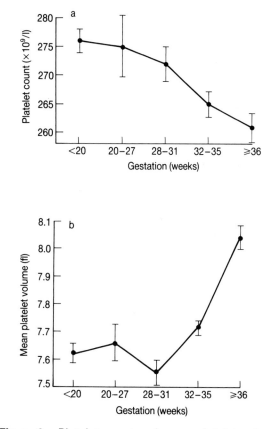

Figure 6. Platelet count and mean platelet volume (mean ± SEM) during pregnancy. Study was largely cross-sectional in design (2881 samples from 2114 women). Samples were analyzed in a Coulter Counter. At the end of the study, any patients who had developed hypertension were excluded. *Data source*: ref. **11**, with permission.

Comment: It has been suggested that there is hyperdestruction of platelets in pregnancy, with a consequent decrease in platelet life span. Young platelets are known to be larger than old platelets. Another study[12] of longitudinal design, but with much smaller numbers (*n* = 44) did not find evidence of significant change in the platelet count with gestational age.

Serum Iron, Transferrin (Iron Binding Capacity), Ferritin

Serum and Red Cell Folate

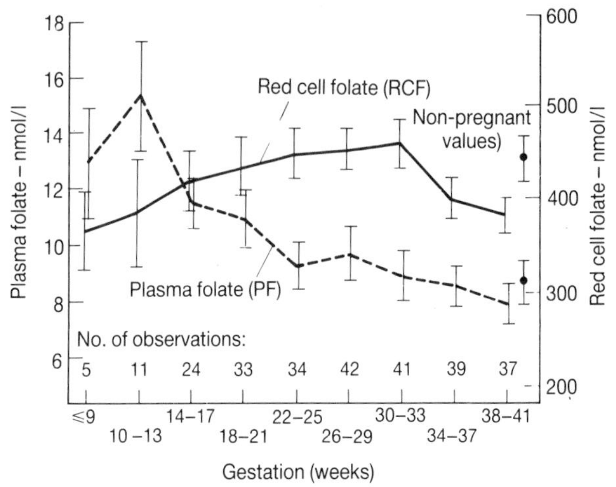

Patients	Hb (g/dl)	Serum iron (μmol/l)	Trans-ferrin/TIBC sat$^{n.}$ (%)	Serum ferritin (μg/l)
Not treated ($n = 30$)				
First trimester	12.9	23	36	96
Term	12.0	14	13	13
Given FeSO$_4$ ($n = 82$)				
First trimester	12.5	22	33	67
Term	12.5	25	27	41

Figure 7a. Longitudinal study (mean values) of women recruited in the first trimester. At the start, 72 were randomized to the 'no treatment' group, but any whose Hb fell below 11 g/dl were prescribed ferrous sulfate 60 mg tds; thus only 30 progressed through pregnancy without iron supplements. In all subjects studied, serum ferritin rose rapidly postpartum, reaching similar values to those found in early pregnancy by 5–8 weeks after delivery (NB no iron supplements were given following delivery.) *Data source*: ref. **13**, with permission.

Figure 8. Serial study (mean ± SEM) of plasma and red cell folate levels during singleton pregnancy; all women were taking iron supplements from approximately 12 weeks gestation, but none took folate supplements ($n = 43$). Samples were taken after overnight fasting, with patients seated. Non-pregnant reference samples were from 50 healthy women (non-lactating) aged 19–37 years, taken 3–5 h following their last meal. None of the women developed anemia during pregnancy (Hb and MCV values remained stable). *Data source*: ref. **14**, with permission.

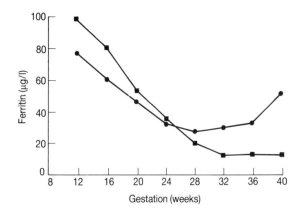

Figure 7b. Mean serum ferritin levels during pregnancy in: (●) women given oral iron supplements and (■) untreated women.

Comment: Iron stores (as indicated by serum ferritin) become depleted during pregnancy, whether or not iron supplements are given.

Comment: In other studies, red cell folate has been shown to have a slight downward trend with advancing gestation and those patients with low red cell folate at the beginning of pregnancy develop megaloblastic anemia in the third trimester.[15] These differences may relate to dietary folate intake. Plasma and red cell folate values are similar in pregnant women at term, regardless of their parity.[14] In the 6 weeks following delivery, plasma and red cell folate return towards non-pregnant values, although lactation (which constitutes an added folate stress) may delay recovery.[16]

Vitamin B$_{12}$

		Serum vitamin B$_{12}$ (pg/ml)	
Stage of pregnancy (weeks)	No. of cases	Mean (SEM)	(Range)
First visit (≤ 24)	154	239 (12)	(50–950)
32	152	164 (6)	(40–480)
36	134	162 (7)	(50–475)
40	133	165 (7)	(20–510)
3 months postdelivery	53	338 (21)	(not stated)
Non-pregnant reference group	36	454 (31)	(205–1025)

Figure 9. Serum vitamin B$_{12}$ levels measured longitudinally in pregnancy; only 53 of the original group had levels measured postpartum. Non-pregnant reference values were from 36 different women in the child-bearing years. *Data source*: ref. **17**, with permission.

Comment: Serum vitamin B$_{12}$ levels fall in the first trimester.[17] They tend to be lower in smokers. Muscle and red cell vitamin B$_{12}$ concentrations also fall during pregnancy; however, vitamin B$_{12}$ absorption does not change.[16]

Coagulation Factors

Table 4

Longitudinal study in 72 women (healthy primigravidae, or multigravidae whose previous pregnancies had been uncomplicated), aged 19–42 years. Postdelivery samples were taken between 6 h and 4 days following delivery (mean 52 h); postnatal samples were taken after 6 weeks. The postnatal samples yielded similar values to those from an age-matched non-pregnant group of women ($n = 66$)

No. examples examined		41	48	47	66	62	48	61	61
Weeks		11–15	16–20	21–25	26–30	31–35	36–40	Postdelivery	Postnatal
Factor VII	Mean	111	129	150	158	162	171	134	94
	Range	60–206	68–244	80–280	75–332	84–312	87–336	70–255	52–171
Fibrinogen (g/l)	Mean	3.63	3.65	3.65	3.78	4.17	4.23	4.61	2.65
	Range	2.64–5.00	2.55–5.22	2.53–5.26	2.67–5.35	2.90–6.00	2.90–6.15	2.98–7.14	1.71–4.11
Factor X	Mean	103	111	115	126	123	127	117	90
	Range	62–169	74–166	74–177	78–203	78–194	72–208	72–191	54–149
Factor V	Mean	93	84	82	82	82	85	91	81
	Range	46–188	46–155	36–185	32–214	34–195	39–184	36–233	42–155
Factor II	Mean	125	128	125	124	115	115	112	106
	Range	70–224	75–218	73–214	79–193	74–179	68–194	74–170	68–165
Factor VIII:C	Mean	122	150	141	188	185	212	206	95
	Range	53–283	53–419	44–453	67–528	69–499	79–570	74–569	46–193
Factor VIII R: Ag	Mean	133	156	167	203	262	376	421	89
	Range	56–318	55–439	66–427	84–492	95–718	133–1064	169–1042	29–272
Factor VIIIR: Ag/VIII: C ratio	Mean	1.09	1.04	1.18	1.08	1.42	1.77	2.05	0.95
	Range	0.43–2.74	0.40–2.72	0.43–3.27	0.41–2.81	0.48–4.21	0.62–5.09	0.71–5.92	0.36–2.52

(Means and 95% ranges. Where no units are stated, values are expressed as % of standard.) *Data source*: ref. **18**, with permission.

Comment: Normal pregnancy is a hypercoagulable state associated with increased levels of Factors VII, VIII and X, also a very marked increase in fibrinogen levels due to increased synthesis. Factor IX levels rise and Factor XI levels fall.[16]

Naturally Occurring Anticoagulants and Fibrinolytic Factors

Table 5
Longitudinal study in 72 women (healthy primigravidae, or multigravidae whose previous pregnancies had been uncomplicated), aged 19–42 years

No. examples examined		41	48	47	66	62	48	61	61
Weeks		11–15	16–20	21–25	26–30	31–35	36–40	Postdelivery	Postnatal
FDPs. μg/ml	Mean	1.07 —	1.06 —	1.09 —	1.13 —	1.28 —	1.32 —	1.66 —	1.04 —
Fibrinolytic activity	Mean	7.6	7.4	7.3	5.5	4.5	5.6	14.8	17.4
Lysis time in hours	Mean	13.25	13.5	13.75	18.25	22.25	17.8	6.75	5.75
Antithrombin III: C	Mean	85	90	87	94	87	86	87	92
	Range	49–120	46–133	42–132	47–141	42–132	40–132	48–127	38–147
Antithrombin III: Ag	Mean	93	94	93	97	96	93	95	100
	Range	60–126	56–131	56–130	56–138	59–132	50–136	58–133	64–134
Alpha$_1$-antitrypsin	Mean	124	136	125	146	149	154	172	77
	Range	66–234	86–214	53–295	85–249	89–250	91–260	84–352	44–135
Alpha$_2$-macroglobulin	Mean	176	178	170	160	157	153	146	142
	Range	100–309	98–323	92–312	88–294	85–292	85–277	81–265	82–245

(Means and 95% ranges, except for fibrinolytic activity where full ranges. Where no units are stated, values are expressed as % of standard.
Patients were those described in **Table 4**. *Data source*: ref. **18**, with permission.

	Protein C: Ag units/dl	Protein S: Ag units/dl
Booking visit (7–17 weeks)	111.1 (20.8)	97.9 (13.8)
Second visit (28–32 weeks)	121.6 (26.4)	84.9 (19.7)
Third visit (36–40 weeks)	113.3 (25.0)	81.1 (16.4)
Delivery	117.6 (28.8)	79.8 (12.8)
Reference ranges for the laboratory	75–140	70–130

Figure 10.   Longitudinal study (mean and SD) in 14 healthy women aged 24–38 years. *Data source*: ref. **19**, with permission.

Comment: Free protein S levels fall progressively during pregnancy but remain within the normal reference ranges; protein C levels change little. Antithrombin III levels are stable during pregnancy, fall in labor and then rise 1 week postpartum.[16] Fibrinolysis is depressed during pregnancy; both fibrinogen and plasminogen levels are elevated, but there are decreased levels of circulating plasminogen activator.[20]

CARDIOVASCULAR FUNCTION

Blood Pressure

Table 6
Study (mean and SD) of 226 primigravidae

Period of pregnancy	Weight (kg)	No. of patients	Blood pressure (mmHg)	
			Diastolic sitting	Systolic sitting
Initial visit	57.5 (7.9)	226	56.3 (9.7)	102.9 (10.7)
< 16 weeks	56.1 (7.1)	114	54.4 (7.7)	102.8 (9.8)
16–20 weeks	58.5 (8.0)	182	53.7 (8.6)	101.7 (9.5)
21–28 weeks	61.9 (8.3)	221	56.2 (8.6)	103.1 (9.6)
29–34 weeks	64.8 (8.5)	220	60.2 (9.5)	104.5 (10.1)
35–38 weeks	66.9 (8.7)	226	65.7 (10.5)	107.9 (10.6)
39–40 weeks	68.0 (8.5)	150	67.4 (11.2)	108.9 (11.1)
> 40 weeks	67.9 (8.2)	38	68.8 (9.4)	109.2 (12.2)
6 weeks postpartum	59.4 (8.3)	144	70.3 (11.2)	110.4 (12.4)

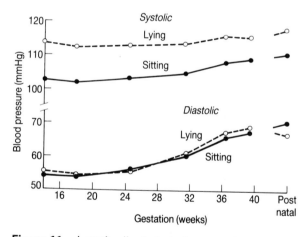

Figure 11. Longitudinal study (mean values) of 226 primigravidae whose first attendance at the antenatal clinic was before 20 weeks of pregnancy. Their mean age was 24.3 (SD 4.9) years. Blood pressure measurements were taken with the London School of Hygiene sphygmomanometer to avoid terminal digit preference and observer bias; diastolic pressures were recorded at the point of muffling (phase 4). *Data source*: ref. **21**, with permission.

Comment: Systolic pressure changes little during pregnancy, but diastolic pressure falls markedly towards mid-pregnancy, then rises to near non-pregnant levels by term. Thus there is a widening of the pulse pressure for most of the pregnancy.

Pulse Rate

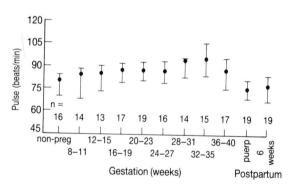

Figure 12. Longitudinal study (median ± IQ ranges) of 20 healthy women recruited in early pregnancy and studied every 2 weeks thereafter; 'non-pregnant' measurements were made 8–12 months after delivery. All women finished the study but not all participated in every visit. *Data source*: ref. **22, with permission.**

Comment: The typical increase in heart rate during pregnancy is approximately 15 beats/min, present from as early as 4 weeks after the last menstrual period.[23]

Blood Gases

Arterial oxygen pressure (P_{O_2}), carbon dioxide pressure (P_{CO_2}) and standard bicarbonate

Transcutaneous Oxygen Pressure (tcP_{O_2}), Carbon Dioxide Pressure (tcP_{CO_2})

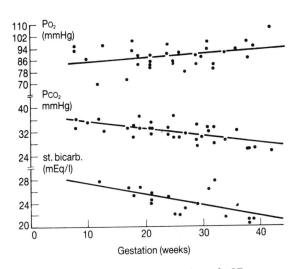

Figure 13. Cross-sectional study of 37 women between 8 and 42 weeks of pregnancy (individual values, with regression lines shown). Blood sampling was done from a cannula inserted into the brachial artery under local anesthesia, after 30 min rest in a quiet, darkened room. *Data source*: ref. **24**, with permission.

Comment: Arterial pH was found to be constant (7.47) during pregnancy in this study. P_{CO_2} and standard bicarbonate showed significant decrease with advancing gestation, but P_{O_2} levels did not alter significantly.

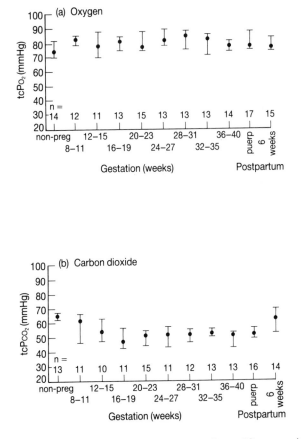

Figure 14. Longitudinal study (median ± IQ ranges) of 20 healthy women recruited in early pregnancy and studied every 2 weeks thereafter; 'non-pregnant' measurements were made 8–12 months after delivery. All women finished the study but not all participated in every visit. *Data source*: ref. **22**, with permission.

Comment: Transcutaneous P_{CO_2} is higher than arterial P_{CO_2} due to temperature differences between the skin surface and blood, as well as addition of CO_2 by skin metabolism (conversion factor approx 1.4).[22] Transcutaneous P_{O_2} values in adults are 10–20% lower than arterial P_{O_2} values. In this study the rise in tcP_{O_2} and fall in tcP_{CO_2} during pregnancy were both significant.

PULMONARY FUNCTION

Respiration Rate

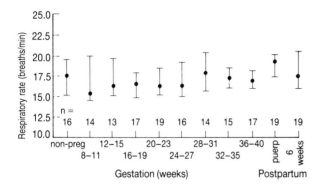

Figure 15. Longitudinal study (median and IQ ranges) of 20 healthy women recruited in early pregnancy and studied every 2 weeks thereafter; 'non-pregnant' measurements were made 8–12 months after delivery. All women finished the study but not all participated in every visit. *Data source*: ref. **22**, with permission.

Comment: Respiration rate is similar in pregnant and non-pregnant women.

Tidal Volume

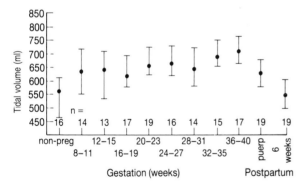

Figure 16. Longitudinal study (median and IQ ranges) of 20 healthy women recruited in early pregnancy and studied every 2 weeks thereafter; 'non-pregnant' measurements were made 8–12 months after delivery. All women finished the study but not all participated in every visit. *Data source*: ref. **22**, with permission.

Comment: Tidal volume increases early in pregnancy and continues to rise until term; overall, there is a 30–40% rise. By 6–8 weeks postpartum, tidal volumes have returned to non-pregnant values. Minute ventilation rises in parallel with tidal volume; typical values are 7.5 l/min for a non-pregnant woman, and 10.5 l/min in late pregnancy.[25]

Respiratory Function Tests

	During ← pregnancy →			After delivery
	10 weeks	24 weeks	36 weeks	10 weeks postpartum
Vital capacity (l)	3.8	3.9	4.1	3.8
Inspiratory capacity (l)	2.6	2.7	2.9	2.5
Expiratory reserve volume (l)	1.2	1.2	1.2	1.3
Residual volume (l)	1.2	1.1	1.0	1.2

Figure 17. Longitudinal study (mean values) of eight healthy women, aged 18–29 years, studied through pregnancy and then again 10 weeks postpartum. All tests were done in the sitting position. *Data source*: ref. **25**, with permission.

Comment: Some women increase their vital capacity (by 100–200 ml) during pregnancy, but the converse has been demonstrated in obese women.[26] Anatomical changes (flaring of the lower ribs, a rise in the diaphragm and increase in transverse diameter of the chest) are responsible for the alterations in lung volume subdivisions.[26] Forced expiratory volume in one second (FEV_1) and peak expiratory flow rate (PFR) are unaffected by normal pregnancy.[25] Gas transfer factor (i.e. pulmonary diffusing capacity with carbon monoxide) decreases in pregnancy.[25] This has been attributed to altered mucopolysaccharides in the alveolar capillary walls, as well as lower circulating hemoglobin.

CARBOHYDRATE METABOLISM

Fasting Plasma Glucose

Gestation (weeks)	Plasma glucose (mmol/l)	
10	4.2	(0.5)
20	4.0	(0.4)
30	4.1	(0.4)
38	3.8	(0.4)
10–12 weeks after delivery	4.4	(0.3)

Figure 18. Longitudinal study (mean and SD; 1 mmol/l = 18 mg/dl) of plasma glucose levels following an overnight fast (of at least 10 hours duration) in 19 healthy women, none of whom was obese or had a family history of diabetes mellitus. *Data source*: ref. **27**, with permission.

Comment: Plasma glucose levels fall with advancing gestation. In most women, the fall has taken place by the end of the first trimester.[27] Plasma insulin levels rise in the third trimester.[27]

75 g Glucose Tolerance Test (GTT)

		Plasma glucose (mmol/l) before and after a 75 g glucose load		
		0 h	1 h	2 h
Second trimester (14–20 weeks)	$n=43$	4.19 (3.59–4.88)	5.02 (2.87–8.78)	4.91 (3.20–7.53)
Third trimester (28–37 weeks)	$n=168$	4.07 (3.40–4.85)	6.71 (4.11–10.98)	6.11 (3.89–9.59)

Figure 19. Cross-sectional (median, 2.5 and 97.5 centiles) study of healthy women under the age of 35 years, weighing less than 85.0 kg, with singleton pregnancies. None had a personal or family history of diabetes mellitus. *Data source*: ref. **28**, with permission.

Comment: The plasma glucose concentrations 1 and 2 h following an oral glucose load differ substantially between mid and late pregnancy. When judged by the World Health Organisation's criteria for a 75 g GTT outside pregnancy (fasting plasma glucose < 6 mmol/l, 2-h value < 7.7 mmol/l), women in the third trimester have decreased glucose tolerance. An alternative view is that the upper limit of normal for plasma glucose 2 h after a 75 g glucose load is higher in late pregnancy.

Serum Fructosamine, Glycosylated Hemoglobin

Table 7
Cross-sectional study (median, 5th and 95th centiles) of 1200 pregnant women at different gestational ages, compared with 1650 non-pregnant woman, aged between 15 and 40 years. Women with known diabetes or previous gestational diabetes were excluded from the study

		Serum fructosamine		
	No. of observations	Median (mmol/l)	5th Percentile (mmol/l)	95th Percentile (mmol/l)
Non-pregnant women	1650	2.46	2.02	2.82
Pregnant women (weeks' gestation)				
4–8	90	2.46	2.21	2.67
8–12	254	2.47	2.23	2.68
12–16	167	2.46	2.19	2.70
16–20	138	2.43	2.19	2.62
20–24	130	2.39	2.14	2.61
24–28	189	2.35	2.15	2.55
28–32	215	2.36	2.15	2.61
32–36	152	2.31	2.11	2.58
36–40	232	2.31	2.11	2.58

Comment: Serum fructosamine concentrations are significantly lower in the second and third trimester than in the first trimester or non-pregnant state. Falling total protein and albumin concentrations in pregnancy may contribute to this reduction in serum fructosamine levels.[29] Values for glycosylated hemoglobin (Hb A_{1c}) during pregnancy in healthy women are similar to those found in non-pregnant women.[30,31]

THYROID FUNCTION

Total Thyroxine (T₄) and Tri-iodothyronine (T₃), T₃-Uptake T₃U, Thyroid Binding Globulin (TBG)

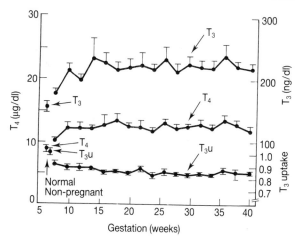

Figure 20. Mostly cross-sectional study (mean ± SEM) of 339 women at various stages of pregnancy; 10–45 were sampled in each 2-week period from 6 to 40 weeks gestation. The controls were 40 non-pregnant women of similar age. *Data source*: ref. **32**, with permission.

Comment: Serum total T₄ and T₃ concentrations are significantly elevated in pregnancy. The T₃ uptake test is low in pregnancy, indicating unsaturation of thyroid binding globulin. Thyroid binding globulin (TBG) concentrations are doubled by the end of the first trimester, remain elevated throughout pregnancy, and fall slowly in the 6 weeks following delivery.[33]

Conversion: T₄: 1 μg/dl ≈ 13 nmol/l
T₃: 1 ng/dl ≈ 0.015 nmol/l

Free Thyroxine (Free T₄), Free Tri-iodothyronine (Free T₃), Thyroid Stimulating Hormone (TSH)

Table 8
Cross-sectional study of 159 women attending antenatal clinics; all were free from metabolic illness. The control samples were from 109 patients (male and female), taken from the routine workload of the laboratory (excluding those with thyroid disease, diabetes, cardiac disease, carcinoma, or patients in a postoperative state)

Subject group	FT₃ (pmol/l)			FT₄ (pmol/l)		
	Mean	SD	Mean ± 2 SD	Mean	SD	Mean ± 2 SD
Adult reference population (n = 109/143)	6.34	1.06	4.2–8.5	16.92	2.97	11.0–22.9
1st trimester pregnancy (n = 54)	6.34	1.03	4.3–8.4	16.65	2.60	11.4–21.8
2nd trimester pregnancy (n = 45)	5.27	0.69	3.9–6.6	14.97	2.21	10.5–19.4
3rd trimester pregnancy (n = 49(FT₃)/60(FT₄))	3.87	0.54	2.8–4.9	11.29	2.01	7.3–15.3

Data source: ref. **34**, with permission.
Conversion: FT₃: 1 pmol/l ≈ 65.1 pg/100 ml
FT₄: 1 pmol/l ≈ 77.7 pg/100 ml

Comment: Free T₄ and T₃ concentrations in pregnancy, measured directly (rather than derived from resin uptake measurements) lie within normal non-pregnant ranges, generally.[35] However, a number of different assay methods are available; some yield lower values in late pregnancy.[34] TSH levels, measured by radioimmunoassay, are unchanged in normal pregnancy, although some studies have found low levels towards the end of the first trimester in association with the highest circulating concentrations of HCG.[32]

ADRENAL HORMONES

Catecholamines: Adrenaline, Noradrenaline

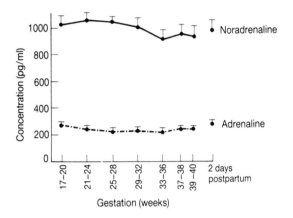

Figure 21. Longitudinal study (mean ± SEM) of 52 women, mean age 28 years, who remained normotensive throughout pregnancy; 39 were primigravidae. Samples were taken by venepuncture after 20 min rest in the left lateral position; a radioenzymic method was used for the assays. *Data source*: ref. **36**, with permission.

Comment: This study showed a decline in plasma levels of both adrenaline and noradrenaline as pregnancy progressed. Other studies (in which blood samples were taken from indwelling intravenous cannulae) have shown steady levels through pregnancy, with no difference between values during pregnancy and those in the early puerperium.[37] In healthy pregnant women, plasma noradrenaline and adrenaline show a diurnal pattern, with lowest levels during the night.[38] Urinary vanillomandelic acid (VMA) excretion has not been studied in healthy pregnancies, but is likely to be within the normal adult range.

Glucocorticoids: Adrenocorticotrophic Hormone (ACTH), Cortisol, Cortisol Binding Globulin (CBG)

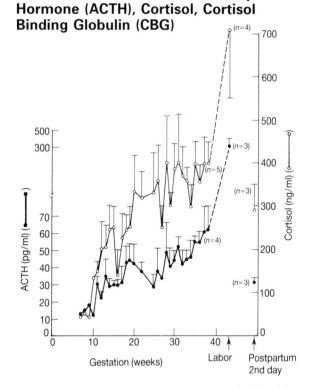

Figure 22. Longitudinal study (mean ± SEM) of five healthy pregnant women, aged 17–28 years. Blood samples were taken weekly at 0800 to 0900 h after an overnight fast, from early pregnancy until delivery. Samples for ACTH measurement were collected improperly from one woman and had to be discarded. Samples were also taken from three of these subjects during labor and on the second postpartum day. *Data source*: ref. **39**, with permission.

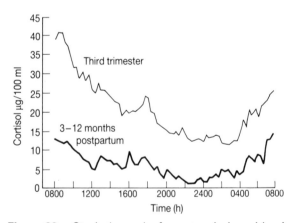

Figure 23. Study (mean) of seven primigravidae in the third trimester and three non-pregnant women, two of whom had been studied during pregnancy. The non-pregnant women were at least 3 months after delivery and none was breast-feeding or using oral contraceptives (20 min samples). *Data source*: ref. **40**, with permission.

| | Plasma cortisol (μg/dl) | | | Free cortisol index | |
| | minimum | mean | maximum | minimum | maximum |
	(in	24-h	period)	(in 24-h period)	
Pregnant Third trimester ($n = 7$)	7.1 (0.9)	20.9 (1.0)	43.4 (3.4)	2.2 (0.3)	15.7 (1.7)
Non-pregnant ($n = 3$)	0.8 (0.2)	6.3 (0.9)	16.2 (1.2)	0.22 (0.05)	5.7 (0.9)

Mean ± 1 SD

Figure 23. Continued.

Comment: Total plasma cortisol, free plasma cortisol and free cortisol index are increased in pregnancy compared with the non-pregnant state. ACTH levels during pregnancy are variously reported as remaining within the normal range for non-pregnant subjects, increasing, or decreasing,[39,41] but there is agreement that levels rise with advancing gestation. The rise in ACTH during pregnancy is attributed to placental production of the peptide.[41] Normal diurnal patterns of cortisol (despite overall elevated levels) are found during pregnancy (i.e. lowest values at 2400 h, highest values at 0800 h[40]). Cortisol binding globulin (CBG) concentrations rise steadily during pregnancy, reaching twice normal values by mid-gestation.[42] Cortisol production rate during pregnancy has been described as being depressed[43] or elevated.[40] Urinary free cortisol more than doubles during pregnancy.[44] Plasma cortisol levels measured at 0800 h following 1 mg of dexamethasone given orally at 2300 h the previous evening suppress to < 5 μg/dl (a normal response);[45] however, urinary cortisol levels do not suppress as much in pregnant as in non-pregnant subjects.[41]

PROLACTIN

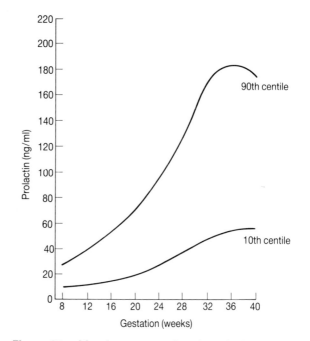

Figure 24. Mostly cross-sectional study (10th and 90th centiles) of 839 women with uncomplicated singleton pregnancies, between 8 and 40 weeks gestation; a total of 980 blood samples were taken. All samples were collected between 0900 and 1100 h. Any woman who developed a pregnancy complication was rejected from the normal series. *Data source*: ref. **46**, with permission.

Comment: Prolactin concentrations increase 10–20 fold during the course of pregnancy. There is a normal circadian rhythm, with a nocturnal rise.[47] In labour, there is an acute fall in levels, then a postpartum surge during the first 2 h following delivery.[48] these changes are not seen in women undergoing elective cesarean deliveries. Prolactin levels approach the normal range 2–3 weeks after delivery in non-lactating women, but remain elevated in those who breast-feed their infants.[49]

TOTAL AND IONIZED CALCIUM, MAGNESIUM, ALBUMIN, PARATHYROID HORMONE (PTH), CALCITONIN (CT)

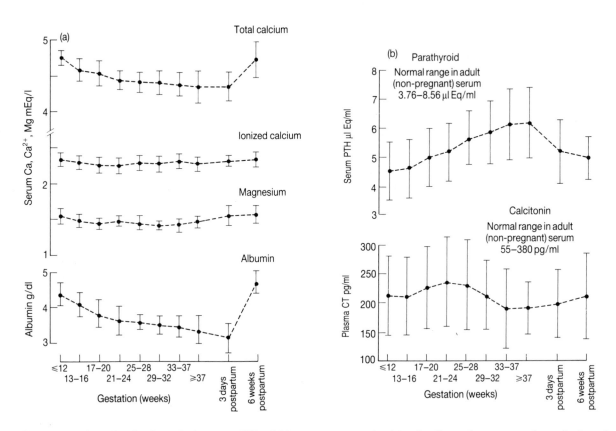

Figure 25. Longitudinal study (mean ±SD) of 30 women, recruited in the first trimester and studied at 4-week intervals. Samples were also taken on the third postpartum day and during the sixth postpartum week. The subjects ranged in age from 19 to 33 years, 20 were primigravidae. Samples were collected by venepuncture after an overnight fast. *Data source*: ref. **50**, with permission.

Comment: Total serum calcium declines during pregnancy, in association with the fall in serum albumin; however, ionized calcium levels remain constant. PTH levels are lower in early gestation than in the puerperium; they rise progressively through pregnancy. A menstrual cyclicity in PTH has also been noted, with higher values corresponding to times of increased estrogen secretion.[50]

Conversion: Serum Ca, Ca²⁺, Mg: 1mEq/l = 0.5 mmol/l.

RENAL FUNCTION

Serum Electrolytes, Urea, Creatinine, Osmolality

Table 9

Longitudinal study (mean and SD) of 83 healthy pregnant women (77 of whom were primigravidae), recruited at 12 weeks gestation. Samples were collected every 4 weeks during pregnancy, 7 days postpartum, then at 6 and 26 weeks postpartum

Gestation (weeks)	No. of estimations	Total osmolality (mOsm/kg)		Sodium (mEq/l)		Potassium (mEq/l)		Chloride (mEq/l)		Blood urea (mg/100 ml)	
		Mean	SD	Mean	SD	Mean	SD	Mean	SD	Mean	SD
12	82	280.2	2.86	139.8	3.64	4.27	0.28	105.1	2.91	21.0	4.48
16	83	279.8	4.23	139.5	3.29	4.25	0.39	104.9	2.76	20.2	4.43
20	83	280.1	3.23	139.6	3.87	4.19	0.31	105.1	2.47	19.5	4.38
26	83	280.0	3.29	138.7	3.78	4.24	0.30	105.2	2.52	19.7	4.48
28	80	280.5	3.63	138.5	3.65	4.18	0.35	105.1	2.56	19.5	4.22
30	83	280.4	3.58	139.0	3.41	4.17	0.31	105.3	2.47	19.3	4.03
32	83	280.2	3.18	139.2	3.02	4.20	0.32	105.1	2.34	18.6	4.12
34	83	280.8	3.48	139.4	2.90	4.18	0.28	104.7	2.58	18.9	4.44
36	83	280.7	3.85	139.0	3.34	4.22	0.32	105.0	2.37	18.9	4.52
38	79	280.0	3.36	138.8	3.36	4.25	0.30	105.2	2.79	18.7	4.62
7 days postpartum	82	287.0	4.74	138.3	3.77	4.37	0.28	104.0	2.98	24.3	4.72
6 weeks postpartum	83	289.5	4.52	139.4	3.57	4.30	0.31	104.5	2.73	25.9	5.56
26 weeks postpartum	73	289.3	4.06	140.6	3.27	4.29	0.32	104.7	3.37	23.5	5.13

Data source: ref. **51**, with permission.

Comment: Total osmolality falls by the end of the first trimester to a nadir 8–10 mOsm/1 below non-pregnant values. The major serum electrolytes (sodium, potassium, chloride) have almost unchanged concentrations during pregnancy. Bicarbonate and phosphate concentrations decline during pregnancy.[52] Both plasma urea and creatinine fall during pregnancy; typical mean (SD) values for plasma creatinine are 60 (8), 54 (10) and 64 (9) μmol/l in first, second and third trimesters respectively, rising to 73 (10) μmol/l by 6 weeks postpartum.[53,54]

Conversion: Sodium, potassium, chloride: 1mEq/l = 1mmol/l
Urea: 1mg/100 ml ≈ 0.17 mmol/l.

Serum Urate

Gestation (weeks)		Serum urate (μmol/l)
Non-pregnant	$n = 33$	246 (59)
4	$n = 16$	240 (44)
8	$n = 32$	190 (70)
12	$n = 32$	173 (47)
16	$n = 35$	189 (48)
24	$n = 35$	196 (40)
32	$n = 36$	216 (53)
36	$n = 32$	232 (56)
38	$n = 32$	269 (56)
12 weeks postpartum	$n = 35$	275 (57)

Figure 26. Longitudinal study (mean and SD) of 31 healthy women, aged 23–37 years, five of whom were studied during two pregnancies. They were studied preconceptually, at least 3 months after stopping oral contraceptives (if used), in the luteal phase of their menstrual cycle, then monthly during pregnancy and again 12 weeks postpartum. All samples were taken between 0900 and 0930 h, after overnight fasting. *Data source*: ref. **55**, with permission.

Comment: Serum urate levels decrease during the first trimester, probably due to altered renal handling of uric acid.[55] During late pregnancy, serum urate rises to reach levels higher than non-pregnant values at term; these may remain elevated for 12 weeks after delivery.[55]

Creatinine Clearance

Early pregnancy

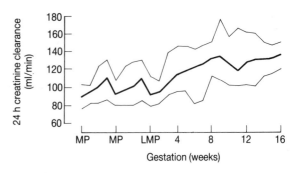

Figure 27. Longitudinal study (mean + range) of nine healthy women, recruited prior to pregnancy. Measurements of 24-h creatinine clearance were made weekly, through the different phases of the menstrual cycle and up to 16 weeks gestation. No diet, fluid or exercise restrictions were imposed. *Data source*: ref. **56**, with permission.

Second/third trimester

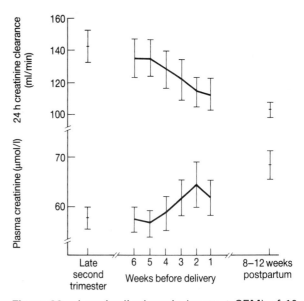

Figure 28. Longitudinal study (mean ± SEM) of 10 healthy pregnant women. Creatinine clearance measurements were made once between 25 and 28 weeks gestation, then weekly from 32 weeks until delivery and finally once between 8 and 12 weeks postpartum. *Data source*: ref. **57**, with permission.

Comment: Glomerular filtration rate (GFR) and effective renal plasma flow increase in early pregnancy to levels approximately 50% above non-pregnant values; in the third trimester, GFR declines by about 15%.[57] 24-h creatinine clearance measurements mirror these changes. During the menstrual cycle, there is a 20% mean increase in creatinine clearance between the week of menstruation and the late luteal phase.[56]

Urine Composition

Glucose, amino acids, protein

Glycosuria is common in pregnancy in individuals whose plasma glucose concentrations and glucose tolerance tests are normal. It is thought to arise because of increased glomerular filtration plus decreased tubular resorption of glucose.[58] Aminoaciduria has also been demonstrated during pregnancy[59] and there is an increase in urinary albumin excretion.[60]

HEPATIC FUNCTION

Serum Proteins

Total serum protein and albumin

Table 10
Longitudinal study (mean and SD) of 83 healthy pregnant women (77 of whom were primigravidae), recruited at 12 weeks gestation. Samples were collected every 4 weeks during pregnancy, 7 days postpartum, then at 6 and 26 weeks postpartum

Gestation (weeks)	Total protein g/dl mean	Total protein g/dl SD	Albumin g/dl mean	Albumin g/dl SD
12	6.47	0.43	3.22	0.40
16	6.36	0.40	3.04	0.30
20	6.29	0.40	2.93	0.37
26	6.22	0.38	2.81	0.26
28	6.30	0.37	2.85	0.36
30	6.24	0.42	2.80	0.29
32	6.22	0.31	2.82	0.26
34	6.20	0.35	2.75	0.28
36	6.18	0.36	2.75	0.30
38	6.24	0.39	2.76	0.30
7 days postpartum	6.21	0.46	2.69	0.34
6 weeks postpartum	7.04	0.48	3.39	0.35
26 weeks postpartum	6.98	0.38	3.42	0.36

Data source: ref. **51**, with permission.

Comment: Decreased total serum protein and albumin concentrations in pregnancy are associated with a decrease in colloid osmotic pressure.[51] Serum immunoglobulin levels do not change significantly in pregnancy.[61]

Lipids

Cholesterol, triglyceride

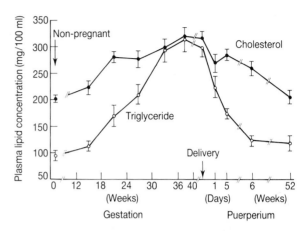

Figure 29. Longitudinal study (mean ± SEM) of 43 women aged 20–41 years. Samples were taken following an overnight fast and 10 min supine rest at 4–6 weekly intervals through pregnancy, during labor and the puerperium; also 12 months after delivery in 14 of the subjects. The non-pregnant reference samples were from 15 subjects of comparable age. No dietary restrictions were imposed. *Data source*: ref. **62**, with permission.

Comment: Plasma cholesterol doubles and there is a threefold increase in plasma triglyceride concentration during pregnancy. The lipid content of the low density lipoproteins increases in pregnancy, as does high density lipoprotein triglyceride content.[63]. Serum lipid levels fall rapidly after delivery, but both cholesterol and triglyceride concentrations remain elevated at 6–7 weeks postpartum. Lactation does not influence lipid levels.[61]

Liver Enzymes, Bilirubin

Table 11
Cross-sectional study (mean ± SEM) of 108 normal women attending a hospital prenatal clinic in Nigeria; the non-pregnant controls of similar age were patients attending the gynecological clinic. No patients were clinically anemic and all were normotensive

Patient group	No. of subjects	Total plasma Alkaline phosphatase (IU/l)
Non-pregnant controls	118	61.6 (2.8)
First trimester	40	60.2 (2.1)
Second trimester	38	74.2 (3.5)
Third trimester	30	139.3 (6.3)

Data source: ref. **63**, with permission.

Comment: Total plasma alkaline phosphatase (AP) levels are approximately doubled by late pregnancy. Almost half of the total plasma AP in pregnancy is placental AP isoenzyme, but bone AP isoenzyme levels are also markedly increased; liver AP isoenzyme levels do not change significantly in pregnancy.[63] Serum gammaglutamyl transpeptidase (GGT) and transaminase levels do not change significantly during pregnancy, labour or the puerperium.[64] Bilirubin levels remain within normal levels during pregnancy.[65]

IMMUNOLOGY
Complement System, Immune Complexes

	C3 (g/l)	C4 (g/l)
Non-pregnant controls	0.81 (0.12)	0.33 (0.06)
Weeks gestation		
17–20	0.96 (0.16)	0.39 (0.10)
21–24	1.00 (0.17)	0.39 (0.09)
25–28	1.02 (0.16)	0.43 (0.12)
29–32	1.05 (0.22)	0.41 (0.11)
33–36	1.14 (0.18)	0.44 (0.13)
37–40	1.10 (0.19)	0.42 (0.11)

Figure 30. Longitudinal study (mean and 1 SD) of 147 healthy women, who remained normotensive throughout pregnancy. The control population was 32 normal non-pregnant women, aged 15–41 years, 11 of whom were taking oral contraceptives. *Data source*: ref. **66**, with permission.

Comment: Levels of C3 and C4 are significantly elevated during the second and third trimesters of pregnancy. Another cross-sectional study[67] showed elevated levels of C4, but not C3, during the 1st trimester. Circulating immune complexes are low during pregnancy.[67] There is some disagreement as to whether C3 degradation products are elevated[67] or normal;[68] no longitudinal studies have been done.

Markers of Inflammation: Erythrocyte Sedimentation Rate (ESR), C-Reactive Protein (CRP)

Values of ESR are high in pregnancy (typically > 30 mm in the first hour) due to elevated plasma globulins and fibrinogen.[69] Thus, ESR cannot be used as a marker for inflammation. Levels of C-reactive protein are undetectable in healthy pregnant women; elevations are due to intercurrent disease.

FETAL PARAMETERS

EARLY EMBRYONIC STRUCTURES: YOLK SAC, FETAL POLE, HEART BEAT, AMNIOTIC MEMBRANE, MIDGUT HERNIA

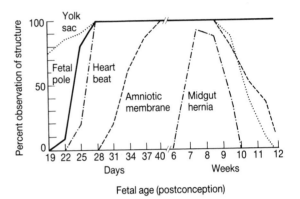

Figure 31. Longitudinal study of 39 women with known dates of ovulation; most were patients from an assisted conception unit. They were scanned using a vaginal probe weekly, once pregnancy had been confirmed, starting as early as 18 days postconception. Five subjects had twin pregnancies. *Data source*: ref. **70**, with permission.

Comment: Transvaginal ultrasound scanning yields better images in the first trimester than does transabdominal scanning. By 28 days postconception, fetal viability may be confirmed by visualization of a heart beat. The fetal heart rate increases from 90 bpm to 145 bpm by 7 weeks postconception.[70]

FETAL BIOMETRY

Crown-Rump Length (CRL)

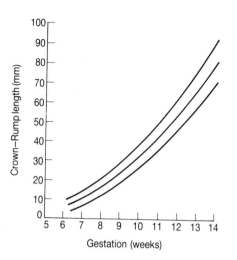

Figure 32. Cross-sectional study (mean ± 2 SD) of 334 women who were certain of the date of their last menstrual periods (LMP) and had normal regular menstrual cycles. The study covered the time period from 6 to 14 weeks post-LMP. A transabdominal ultrasound technique was used and the longest length of fetal echoes was found and measured. *Data source*: ref. **71**, with permission.

Comment: CRL measurements can only be used effectively in the first trimester. Other studies have found very similar values for CRL; measurements are not influenced by maternal age, height or parity.[72] In a smaller, longitudinal study CRL was found to be significantly smaller in female than male fetuses.[72] No differences have been found in CRL measurements between Asian and European patients.[73]

Biparietal Diameter (BPD)

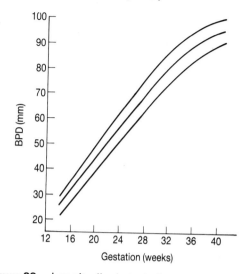

Figure 33. Longitudinal study (mean ± 2 SD) of 41 women with regular menstruation and a known last menstrual period (LMP). They were scanned every 2–4 weeks, beginning 13–14 weeks post-LMP; in total 493 scans were performed. *Data source*: ref. **74**, with permission.

Comment: Other studies have found similar values for BPD.[73,75] No differences in BPD measurements have been found between Asian and European patients living in the same city.[73]

Head Circumference (HC)

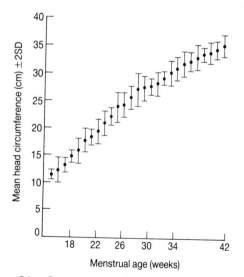

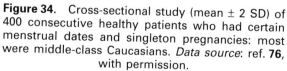

Figure 34. Cross-sectional study (mean ± 2 SD) of 400 consecutive healthy patients who had certain menstrual dates and singleton pregnancies: most were middle-class Caucasians. *Data source*: ref. **76**, with permission.

Comment: HC measurements are particularly useful in the assessment of gestational age when there is an abnormality of fetal head shape, e.g. dolicocephaly.

Abdominal Circumference (AC)

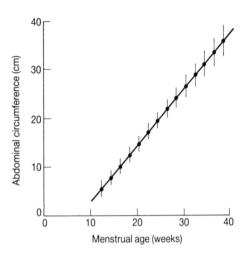

Figure 35. Longitudinal study (mean ± 1 SD) of 20 women with certain last menstrual periods (LMP); most were patients in an Infertility Program. They were scanned every 3 weeks, beginning 14–16 weeks post-LMP. *Data source*: ref. **77**, with permission.

Comment: Another study of fetal AC measurements suggests that there is a flattening off of growth towards term.[78] Some of the discrepancies between studies are due to different mathematical curve-fitting techniques applied to the experimental data, as well as to differences in the design of studies and numbers of subjects involved.[77,79]

Femur Length (FL)

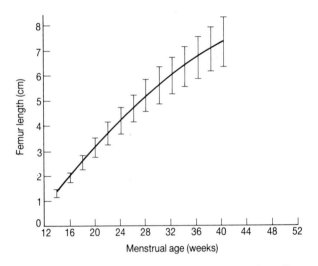

Figure 36. Cross-sectional study (regression line and 95% confidence intervals) of 254 women between 13 and 39 weeks gestation; all were certain of the dates of their last menstrual periods and had regular cycles. Ultrasound scans were performed transabdominally using a 2.4 or 3.5 MHz transducer. The longest image of the femur was measured in a straight line with the transducer along the long axis of the femur (to avoid foreshortening). *Data source*: ref. **80**, with permission.

Comment: The rate of growth of the femur decreases with advancing gestational age, but the variability increases.[80] Another study from a different geographical location found very similar values for FL in pregnancy.[81]

Limb-Bone Lengths (Tibia, Fibula, Humerus, Radius, Ulna)

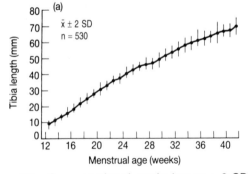

Figure 37. Cross-sectional study (mean ± 2 SD) of 530 healthy women between 13 and 42 weeks gestation. Menstrual age was confirmed in each case by an early ultrasound scan to measure CRL. Lengths of the tibia, humerus and radius were measured in every case, but those of the fibula and ulna in 339 cases. *Data source*: ref. **82**, with permission.

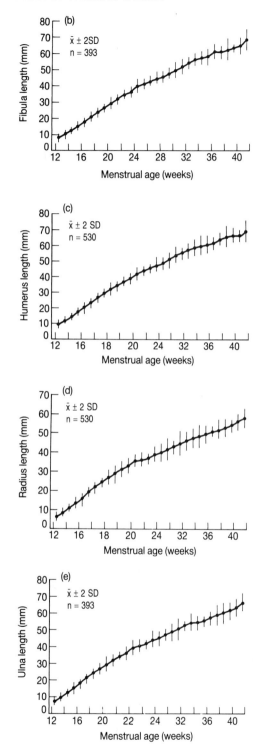

Figure 37. Continued.

Comment: All limb bones show linear growth from 13–25 weeks; thereafter the growth is non-linear. Good agreement has been found between ultrasound and x-ray measurements of limb bones.

Foot

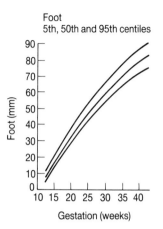

Figure 38. Cross-sectional study (5th, 50th, 95th centiles) of 669 healthy women with singleton pregnancies; any who subsequently delivered an infant with a significant malformation, abnormal karyotype, or other disease was excluded from the analysis. All women had a known last menstrual period and there was agreement between menstrual age and ultrasound dating (at the time of the initial scan). Approximately 20 measurements were obtained for each variable for each week of pregnancy from 12 until 42 weeks gestation. *Data source:* ref. **75**, with permission.

Kidney

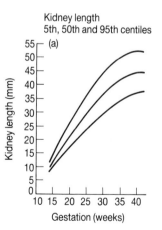

Figure 39. Cross-sectional study (5th, 50th and 95th centiles) of 669 healthy women with singleton pregnancies; all had a known last menstrual period and there was agreement between menstrual age and ultrasound dating (at the time of the initial scan). Approximately 20 measurements were obtained for each variable for each week of pregnancy from 12 until 42 weeks gestation. (Figure 39 is continued on page 1280.)*Data source:* ref. **75**, with permission.

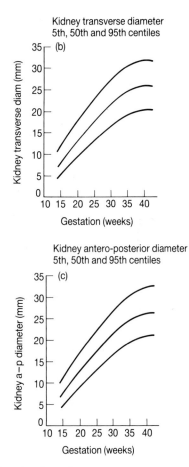

Figure 39. Continued.

Comment: The ratio of the transverse renal circumference to the abdominal circumference (in a section at the level of the umbilical vein) is a simple way of assessing normal kidney size; values are 0.27–0.30 from 17 weeks until term.[83]

Orbital Diameters

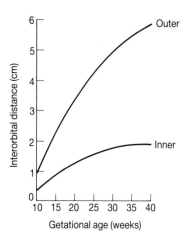

Figure 40. Cross-sectional (mean) study of 180 healthy women from 22 to 40 weeks gestation. A scan plane was obtained which transected the occiput, orbits and nasal processes. *Data source*: ref. **84**, with permission.

Comment: Outer-orbital diameter (IOD) is closely related to biparietal diameter (BPD). It is a useful measurement when the fetal position precludes accurate measurement of BPD.

Cerebral Ventricles

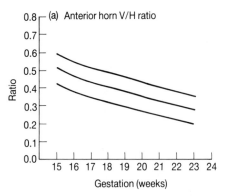

Figure 41. Cross-sectional study (mean ± SD) of 101 women in the second trimester. The ratio of the distance from the lateral border of the frontal horn of the lateral cerebral ventricle to the midline echo compared with the hemispheric width at the same axial scan plane was computed as the anterior V/H ratio. Similarly, the posterior V/H ratio was calculated from measurements of the temporal horn of the lateral ventricle. *Data source*: Personal communication, S. Campbell (Data from the Ultrasound Department, King's College Hospital, London, UK).

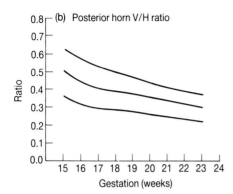

Figure 41. Continued.

Comment: The most reliable measurements of the ventricular system are made using the frontal horns of the lateral cerebral ventricles as they are the easiest to identify.

Cerebellum

Table 12

Cross-sectional study (10th, 50th, 90th centiles) of 371 normal pregnant women of gestational age 13–40 weeks. In all women, gestational age was confirmed by ultrasonography before 14 weeks. The transverse cerebellar diameter was measured in an axial scan plane through the posterior fossa

Gestational age (weeks)	Cerebellum (mm)		
	Centiles		
	10th	50th	90th
15	10	14	16
16	14	16	17
17	16	17	18
18	17	18	19
19	18	19	22
20	18	20	22
21	19	22	24
22	21	23	24
23	22	24	26
24	22	25	28
25	23	28	29
26	25	29	32
27	26	30	32
28	27	31	34
29	29	34	38
30	31	35	40
31	32	38	43
32	33	38	42
33	32	40	44
34	33	40	44
35	31	41	47
36	36	43	55
37	37	45	55
38	40	49	55
39	52	52	55

Data source: ref. **85**, with permission.

Comment: The cerebellum may be visualized as early as 10–11 weeks gestation.

Fetal Weight

Birth weight

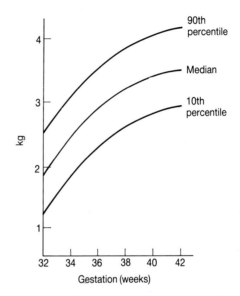

Figure 42. Analysis of 46703 singleton births in Aberdeen, Scotland, during 1948–1964. Most of the mothers were of Caucasian origin and were themselves born in Scotland. *Data source*: ref. **86**, with permission.

Comment: Birth weight ranges by gestational age need to be established for different populations, as they are influenced by ethnic, socioeconomic and geographic factors etc.[87] Different ranges apply to infants from multiple pregnancies.

Weight estimated from ultrasound measurements

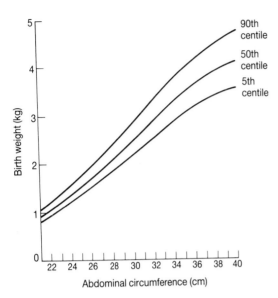

Figure 43. Study of 138 women who had an ultrasound examination within 48 hours of delivery for the measurement of fetal AC. The actual birth weights were compared with the AC measurements and a polynomial equation derived to describe the relationship. *Data source*: ref. **88**, with permission.

Comment: Equations have also been derived for estimating fetal weight from various combinations of ultrasonic measurements (AC, BPD, HC, FL)[88,89,90] which are claimed to be more accurate than those based on AC measurements alone.

AMNIOTIC FLUID

Volume

Total volume

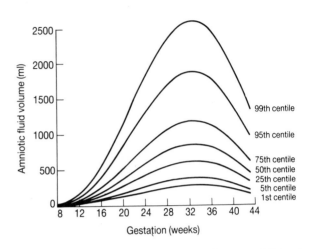

Figure 44. Composite analysis of 12 published reports of amniotic fluid volume in human pregnancy, totalling 705 measurements. Amniotic fluid volumes were either measured directly at the time of hysterotomy or indirectly using an indicator dilution technique. Only healthy pregnancies were included; any complicated by fetal death or anomaly, or by maternal disease were excluded. *Data source*: ref. **91**, with permission.

Amniotic fluid index (AFI)

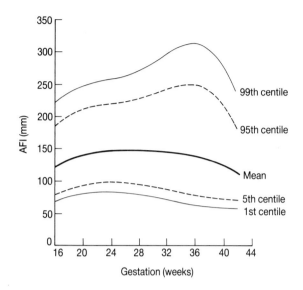

Figure 45. Prospective study of 791 patients. Any who did not have a normal pregnancy outcome (i.e. infant born at term, between 10th and 90th centile for birthweight, with 5-min Apgar score above 6, and without congenital anomaly) were subsequently excluded. Ultrasound imaging was performed and the uterus divided into four quadrants along the sagittal midline and midway up the fundus. Amniotic fluid index was calculated as the sum of the deepest vertical dimension (in millimetres) of the amniotic fluid pocket in each quadrant of the uterus. *Data source*: ref. **92**, with permission.

Comment: Amniotic fluid volume rises to a plateau between 22 and 39 weeks gestation of 700–850 ml. This corresponds to an AFI of 140–150 mm. After term, there is a significant decline in amniotic fluid volume.

Pressure

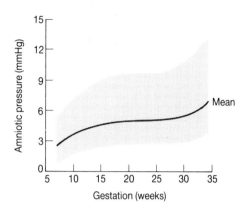

Figure 46. Cross-sectional study (mean and 95th CI) of 171 singleton pregnancies, subsequently shown to have normal karyotype, in whom amniotic fluid volume was subjectively assessed as normal on ultrasonic appearances. All patients were scheduled to undergo a transamniotic invasive procedure for diagnostic reasons or else were to undergo therapeutic termination of pregnancy. Amniotic fluid pressure was measured using a manometry technique referenced to the top of the maternal abdomen. *Data source*: ref. **93**, with permission.

Comment: Amniotic fluid pressure rises with gestation, although there is a mid-trimester plateau of 4–5 mmHg. Pressure was not influenced by parity or maternal age and was similar in twin and singleton pregnancies.[93]

Osmolality

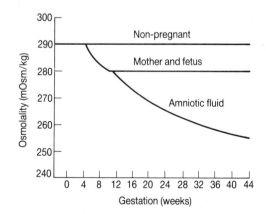

Figure 47. Composite analysis (mean) of six published reports of amniotic fluid osmolality. *Data source*: ref. **94**, with permission.

Comment: In early pregnancy the composition of amniotic fluid is consistent with a transudate of maternal or fetal plasma.[95] The fetal skin becomes keratinized by mid-pregnancy and the amniotic fluid solute concentrations decrease as fetal urine becomes more dilute.[95] Thus there is an osmotic gradient between amniotic fluid and both maternal and fetal plasma.

Umbilical Artery

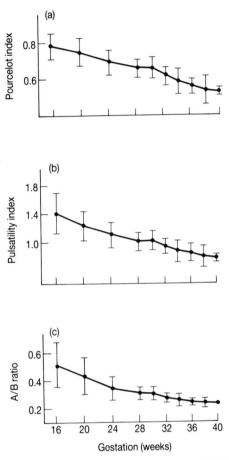

DOPPLER INDICES

Uteroplacental Vessels

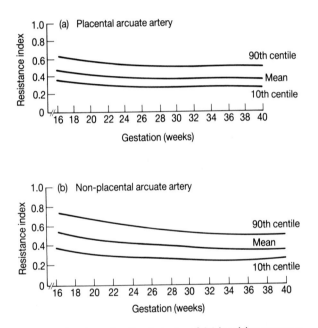

Figure 48.   Longitudinal study of 34 healthy women recruited at 16–18 weeks gestation and studied every 4 weeks until delivery. All remained free from pregnancy complications. Doppler-shift waveforms were obtained from vessels within the myometrium running towards the placenta using a duplex pulsed Doppler system. Resistance Index (i.e. [systolic − diastolic frequency] ÷ systolic frequency) was calculated from three recorded waveforms. *Data source:* ref. **96**, with permission.

Figure 49.   Longitudinal study (mean ± 2 SD) of 15 normal pregnancies scanned every 2 weeks from 24–28 weeks gestation until delivery; eight of these patients had been recruited at 16 weeks and also scanned every 4 weeks through the second trimester. In all subjects gestational age had been confirmed by ultrasound scanning at 16 weeks gestation. A range-gated pulsed Doppler beam was guided from the ultrasound image to insonate the umbilical artery. Pulsatility Index ([A–B] ÷ M), Resistance Index ([A–B] ÷ A) and A/B Ratio (A ÷ B) were calculated (where A = maximum systolic frequency, B = maximum diastolic frequency, M = mean frequency as measured from the Doppler-shift waveforms). *Data source:* ref. **97**, with permission.

Comment: There is a fall in Resistance Index values from uteroplacental Doppler-shift waveforms with gestational age due to increasing end-diastolic frequencies. This is interpreted as being due to decreasing resistance in the placental circulation as pregnancy advances.

Comment: After 16 weeks gestation there is forward flow in umbilical arteries throughout the cardiac cycle, as evidenced by positive Doppler-shift frequencies even at the end of diastole. Declining values of Pulsatility Index, Resistance Index and A/B Ratio with gestation are interpreted as indicating decreasing resistance in the placental circulation.

HEMATOLOGY

Red Cell Count (RBC), White Cell Count (WBC), Platelets (PLT), Hemoglobin (HB), Hematocrit (HCT), Mean Cell Volume (MCV)

Table 13
Cross-sectional study (mean ± 1 SD) of 1233 normal fetuses between 18 and 36 weeks gestation. These were pregnancies referred for fetal blood sampling for prenatal diagnosis (mostly toxoplasmosis), but the fetuses were normal and subsequently shown to be healthy at birth. Fetal blood samples were taken by ultrasound-guided cordocentesis

Gestational age (weeks)	WBCC (10^9/l)	PLT (10^9/l)	RBC (10^{12}/l)	Hb (g/dl)	Ht (%)	MCV (fl)
18–23 ($n = 771$)	4.41 ± 1.2	241 ± 45	2.87 ± 0.28	11.7 ± 0.8	37.4 ± 3.18	131.2 ± 7.3
24–29 ($n = 407$)	4.6 ± 1.3	267 ± 49	3.38 ± 0.32	12.8 ± 1.1	40.4 ± 3.4	119.1 ± 5.6
30–35 ($n = 55$)	5.8 ± 1.6	265 ± 59	3.86 ± 0.43	14.1 ± 1.4	44.3 ± 4.4	114.3 ± 7

Data source: ref. **98**, with permission.

Comment: Fetal red cell count increases with gestation, but white cell count and platelet count do not change. Lymphocytes form the main population of white cells in the fetus; erythroblast numbers decrease with advancing gestation. Fetal hemoglobin (HbF) decreases with advancing gestation, from over 80% of total hemoglobin in mid-pregnancy to approximately 70% by term.[99]

Coagulation Factors

Table 14
Blood samples obtained by cordocentesis from 103 fetuses of 19–27 weeks gestational age, subsequently shown to be healthy (percentage of normal adult values; mean ± 1 SD)

Coagulation factors	%	Inhibitors	%
VIIIC	40 ± 12	Fibronectin	40 ± 10
VIIIRAg	60 ± 13	Protein C	11 ± 3
VII	28 ± 5	Alpha$_2$-macroglobulin	18 ± 4
IX	9 ± 3	Alpha$_1$-antitrypsin	40 ± 4
V	47 ± 10	AT III	30 ± 3
II	12 ± 3	Alpha$_2$-antiplasmin	61 ± 6
XII	22 ± 3		
Prekallikrein	19 ± 2		
Fibrin-stabilizing factor	30 ± 5		
Fibrinogen	40 ± 15		
Plasminogen	24 ± 15		

Data source: ref. **98**, with permission.

Comment: No changes in levels or activity of the various coagulation factors and their inhibitors were observed through the 8 weeks of gestation studied.

BIOCHEMISTRY

Table 15
Blood samples obtained by cordocentesis from 78 fetuses of gestational age 20–26 weeks; all fetuses were subsequently shown to be healthy at birth

	Mean ± SD
Glucose (mmol/l)	4.3 ± 0.6
Cholesterol (g/l)	0.59 ± 0.11
Uric acid (μmol/l)	179 ± 39
Triglycerides (g/l)	0.4 ± 0.1
Total bilirubin (μmol/l)	26.3 ± 5.8
Alkaline phosphatase (IU/l)	260 ± 65
Gamma GT (IU/l)	60 ± 34
Aspartate aminotransferase (IU/l)	17 ± 6.5
Creatinine (μmol/l)	1.8 ± 0.3
Calcium (mmol/l)	2.3 ± 0.2

Data source: ref. **98**, with permission.

BLOOD GASES

P_{O_2}, P_{CO_2}, pH

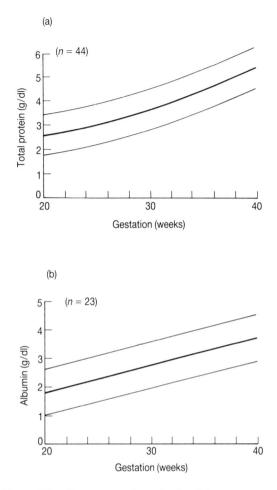

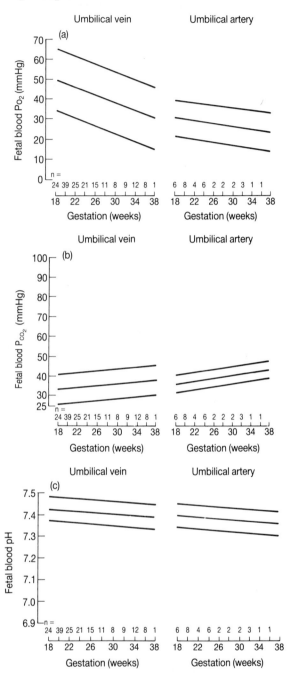

Figure 50. Blood samples obtained by cordocentesis from 45 fetuses, subsequently shown to be normal at birth (regression curve and 95% confidence range). *Data source*: ref. **99**, with permission.

Comment: Plasma total protein and albumin concentrations increase significantly with gestational age.[99] Little information is available regarding other biochemical variables; over the 6-week time period studied,[98] triglyceride levels fell but other parameters remained stable. Fetal concentrations of bilirubin are higher, and those of triglyceride and cholesterol lower, than in maternal serum.[98]

Figure 51. Blood samples obtained by cordocentesis from 208 appropriately-grown-for-gestational-age fetuses between the gestational ages of 18 and 38 weeks (mean and 95% confidence intervals). Fetal blood sampling was performed for karyotyping or prenatal diagnosis of inherited genetic disease or infections; all these fetuses were normal. *Data source*: ref. **100**, with permission.

Comment: Umbilical arterial and venous P_{O_2} and pH decrease, and P_{CO_2} increases with gestational age. Concentrations of lactate do not change with gestation; mean (SD) values are 0.99 (0.32) mmol/l for umbilical vein and 0.92 (0.21) mmol/l for umbilical artery.[100] Intervillous blood has a higher P_{O_2} and lower P_{CO_2}, but similar pH and lactate concentrations as umbilical venous blood.[101] The decrease in P_{O_2} in umbilical venous blood with advancing gestation is offset by increasing fetal hemoglobin concentration, such that blood oxygen content remains constant; mean umbilical venous oxygen content is 6.7 (SD 0.6) mmol/l.[101]

URINARY BIOCHEMISTRY

Phosphate, Creatinine

	16 weeks	33 weeks
Phosphate (mmol/l)	0.91	0.10
Creatinine (μmol/l)	99.9	172.9

(mean values)

Potassium, Calcium, Urea

	Mean value	95% Confidence intervals
Potassium (mmol/l)	3.0	0–6.1
Calcium (mmol/l)	0.21	0.04–1.2
Urea (μmol/l)	7.9	2.6–13.1

Sodium

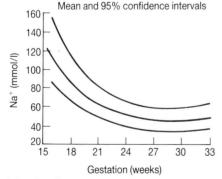

Figure 52. Study (mean and 95% confidence intervals) of 26 women between 16 and 33 weeks gestation, with normal amniotic fluid volume and normal fetal anatomy. Seventeen of the women had pregnancies complicated by rhesus alloimmunization; in these the fetal bladder was emptied prior to intraperitoneal blood transfusion. The other women had aspiration of the fetal bladder prior to therapeutic termination of pregnancy. *Data source:* ref. **102**, with permission.

Comment: Fetal urinary biochemistry has previously only been studied indirectly from examination of the amniotic fluid.[95] This direct study found that urinary sodium and phosphate levels decreased significantly with gestational age over the period studied (16–33 weeks); creatinine levels increased. Urinary potassium, calcium and urea did not show gestational changes. The pattern of electrolyte changes suggests parallel maturation of both glomerular and tubular function with advancing gestation.

ENDOCRINE FUNCTION

Thyroid Function: TSH, TBG, Total T_4, Free T_4, Total T_3, Free T_3

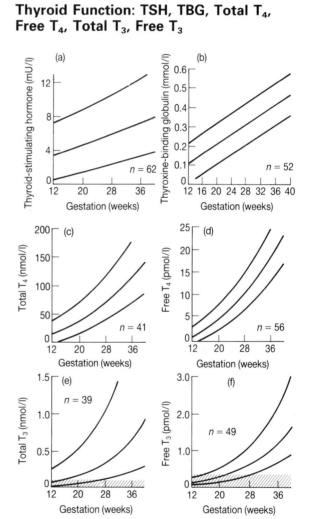

Figure 53. Study of 62 women (mean, 5th, 95th centiles) who underwent cordocentesis or cardiocentesis for prenatal diagnosis, and whose fetuses were subsequently shown to be normal. Cross-hatched area is lower limit of sensitivity of assay. *Data source:* ref. **103**, with permission.

Comment: No significant associations have been found between fetal and maternal thyroid hormones and TSH concentrations, suggesting that the fetal pituitary-thyroid axis is independent of that of its mother.[103] Fetal TSH levels are always higher than those in the mother. Free and total T_4 levels and those of TBG rise through pregnancy and reach adult levels by 36 weeks gestation; however free and total T_3 levels are always substantially less than adult levels. The increase in fetal blood levels of TSH, thyroid hormones and TBG during pregnancy indicates independent and autonomous maturation of the pituitary, thyroid and liver respectively.[103] There does not appear to be feedback control of pituitary secretion of TSH by circulating thyroid hormones *in utero*.

AMNIOTIC FLUID BILIRUBIN (ΔOD_{450})

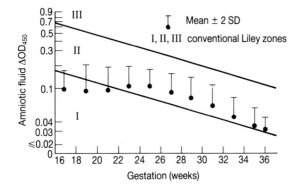

Figure 54. A total of 475 samples of amniotic fluid obtained from pregnancies between 16 and 36 weeks gestation not complicated by fetal haemolysis. Amniotic fluid samples taken at the time of fetoscopy or by amniocentesis were placed in darkened containers to protect against photodecomposition and centrifuged to remove vernix and cellular debris. The liquor bilirubin concentration was measured spectrophotometrically by the deviation in optical density of the amniotic fluid at a wavelength of 450 nm. *Data source*: ref. **104**, with permission.

Comment: The normal range of liquor ΔOD_{450} falls through the third trimester and the values are widely scattered. There is clearly a discrepancy with what has been taken as the 'gold standard' in the past – the Liley zones (I = mild disease or unaffected, II = moderate disease, III = severe disease).

FETAL HEART RATE (FHR)

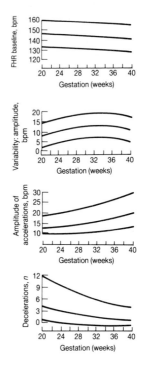

Figure 55. Cross-sectional (mean and 95th CI) study of 119 pregnancies between 20 and 39 weeks gestation who had been referred for prenatal diagnosis by cordocentesis. In all these cases, fetal blood gases, hemoglobin and karyotype were subsequently shown to be normal; none had hydops fetalis or any cardiac defect. Fetal heart rate monitoring was performed immediately before cordocentesis for a period of 30 minutes. The traces were examined for FHR baseline, variability, accelerations and decelerations. *Data source*: ref. **105**, with permission.

Antepartum Cardiotocogram (Non-stress test, NST)

- At least two accelerations (> 15 beats for > 15 s) in 20 min, baseline heart rate 110–150 bpm, baseline variability 5–25 bpm, absence of decelerations.

- Sporadic decelerations amplitude < 40 bpm are acceptable if duration < 15 s, or < 30 s following an acceleration.

- When there is moderate tachycardia (150–170 bpm) or bradycardia (100–110 bpm) a reactive trace is reassuring of good health.

Figure 56. Antepartum cardiotocogram (non-stress test). *Data source*: ref. **106**, with permission.

Comment: Baseline FHR decreases with gestation, but the variability of the baseline increases. The number and amplitude of accelerations increase with gestation. Spontaneous decelerations are commonly found in the second trimester and early third trimester, but rarely in healthy fetuses approaching term. During labor, criteria for the interpretation of FHR traces alter (see Chapter 62). Early decelerations (i.e. synchronous with contractions) are common towards the end of the first stage of labor; during the second stage of labor both early and variable decelerations are normal findings.

PROGRESS OF LABOR

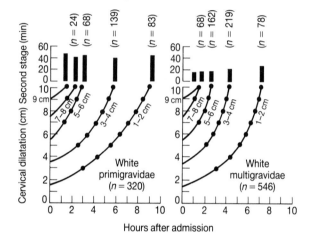

Figure 57. Study (mean) of 3217 consecutive women in labor, from which a group of 1306 who had normal labor were identified (i.e. women with a cephalically presenting fetus, who did not have epidural block, receive oxytocic drugs, or require instrumental delivery). The progress of labor was followed by vaginal examination to establish cervical dilatation; the first examination being performed soon after admission to the labor suite. The onset of second stage was confirmed when full cervical dilatation was found at the time of routine examination, or when the patient was beginning to bear down. *Data source*: ref. **107**, with permission.

Comment: This study found that mean cervimetric progress from 1 to 7 cm was faster in Caucasian multiparae than primiparae, but thereafter progress in the two groups was similar. No significant differences in the cervimetric progress of labor between women from different racial groups has been found.[107] The mean duration of the second stage of labor is approximately 42 min in primiparae and 17 min in multiparae,[107] although it is recognized that the precise onset of full cervical dilatation is difficult to establish.

REFERENCES

1   Dawes MG, Grudzinkas JG (1991) Patterns of maternal weight gain in pregnancy. *British Journal of Obstetrics and Gynaecology* **98**:195–201.

2   Seppala M, Ruoslahti E (1972) Radioimmunoassay of maternal alpha fetoprotein during pregnancy and delivery. *American Journal of Obstetrics and Gynecology* **112**:208–212.

3   Haddow JE, Palomaki GE (1992) Maternal protein enzyme analyses. In Reece EA, Hobbins JC, Mahoney MJ, Petrie RH (eds) *Medicine of the Fetus and Mother*, pp. 653–667. Philadelphia: J.B. Lippincott.

4   Brody S, Carlstrom G (1965) Human chorionic gonadotrophin pattern in serum and its relation to the sex of the fetus. *Journal of Clinical Endocrinology* **25**:792–797.

5   Josimovich JB, Kosor B, Boccella L, Mintz DH, Hutchinson DL (1970) Placental lactogen in maternal serum as an index of fetal health. *Obstetrics and Gynecology* **36**:244–250.

6   Beck P, Parker ML, Daughaday WH (1965) Radioimmunologic measurement of human placental lactogen in plasma by a double antibody method during normal and diabetic pregnancies. *Journal of Clinical Endocrinology* **25**:1457–1462.

7   Mathur RS, Leaming AB, Williamson HO (1972) A simplified method for estimation of estriol in pregnancy plasma. *American Journal of Obstetrics and Gynecology* **113**:1120–1129.

8   Taylor DJ, Lind T (1979) Red cell mass during and after normal pregnancy. *British Journal of Obstetrics and Gynaecology* **86**:364–370.

9   Efrati P, Presentey B, Margalith M, Rozenszajn L (1964) Leukocytes of normal pregnant women. *Obstetrics and Gynecology* **23**:429–432.

10 Kuvin SF, Brecher G (1962) Differential neutrophil counts in pregnancy. *New England Journal of Medicine* **266**:877–878.

11 Fay RA, Hughes AO, Farron NT (1983) Platelets in pregnancy: hyperdestruction in pregnancy. *Obstetrics and Gynecology* **61**:238–240.

12 Fenton V, Saunders K, Cavill I (1977) The platelet count in pregnancy. *Journal of Clinical Pathology* **30**:68–69.

13 Fenton V, Cavill I, Fisher J (1977) Iron stores in pregnancy. *British Journal of Haematology* **37**:145–149.

14 Ek J, Magnus M (1981) Plasma and red blood cell folate during normal pregnancies. *Acta Obstetrica et Gynecologica Scandinavica* **60**:247–251.

15 Chanarin I, Rothman D, Ward A, Perry J (1968) Folate status and requirement in pregnancy. *British Journal of Medicine* **2**:390–394.

16 Letsky E (1991) The haematological system. In Hytten F, Chamberlain G (eds) *Clinical Physiology in Obstetrics* 2nd edn, pp. 39–82. Oxford: Blackwell Scientific Publications.

17 Temperley IJ, Meehan MJM, Gatenby PBB (1968) Serum vitamin B12 levels in pregnant women. *Journal of Obstetrics and Gynaecology of the British Commonwealth* **75**:511–516.

18 Stirling Y, Woolf L, North WRS, Seghatchian MJ,

Meade TW (1984) Haemostasis in normal pregnancy. *Thrombosis Haemostasis* **52**:176–182.

19   Warwick R, Hutton RA, Goff L, Letsky E, Heard M (1989) Changes in protein C and free protein S during pregnancy and following hysterectomy. *Journal of the Royal Society of Medicine* **82**:591–594.

20   Bonnar J, McNicol GP, Douglas AS (1969) Fibrinolytic enzyme system and pregnancy. *British Medical Journal* **iii**:387–389.

21   MacGillivray I, Rose GA, Rowe B (1969) Blood pressure survey in pregnancy. *Clinical Science* **37**:395–407.

22   Spatling L, Fallenstein F, Huch A, Huch R, Rooth G (1992) The variability of cardiopulmonary adaptation to pregnancy at rest and during exercise. *British Journal of Obstetrics and Gynaecology* **99** (Suppl 8).

23   Clapp JF III (1985) Maternal heart rate in pregnancy. *American Journal of Obstetrics and Gynecology* 659–660.

24   Lucius H, Gahlenbeck H, Kleine H-O, Fabel H, Bartels H (1970) Respiratory functions, buffer system, and electrolyte concentrations of blood during human pregnancy. *Respiratory Physiology* **9**:311–317.

25   Gazioglu K, Kaltreider NL, Rosen M, Yu PN (1970) Pulmonary function during pregnancy in normal women and in patients with cardiopulmonary disease. *Thorax* **25**:445–450.

26   De Swiet M (1991) The respiratory system. In Hytten F, Chamberlain G (eds) *Clinical Physiology in Obstetrics* 2nd edn pp. 83–100. Oxford: Blackwell Scientific Publications.

27   Lind T, Billewicz WZ, Brown G (1973) A serial study of changes occurring in the oral glucose tolerance test during pregnancy. *Journal of Obstetrics and Gynaecology British Commonwealth* **80**:1033–1039.

28   Hatem M, Anthony F, Hogston P, Rowe DJF, Dennis KJ (1988) Reference values for 75 g oral glucose tolerance test in pregnancy. *British Medical Journal* **296**:676–678.

29   Roberts AB, Baker JR (1986) Serum fructosamine: a screening test for diabetes in pregnancy. *American Journal of Obstetrics and Gynecology* **154**:1027–1030.

30   Shah BD, Cohen AW, May C, Gabbe SG (1982) Comparison of glycohemoglobin determination and the one-hour oral glucose screen in the identification of gestational diabetes. *American Journal of Obstetrics and Gynecology* **144**:7744–777.

31   Ylinen K, Hekalir R, Teramo K (1981) Haemoglobin A_{1c} during pregnancy of insulin-dependent diabetic and healthy control. *British Journal of Obstetrics and Gynaecology* **1**:223–228.

32   Harada A, Hershman JM, Reed AW *et al.* (1979) Comparison of thyroid stimulators and thyroid hormone concentrations in the sera of pregnant women. *Journal of Clinical Endocrinology and Metabolism* **48**:793–797.

33   Man EB, Reid WA, Hellegers AE, Jones WS (1969) Thyroid function in human pregnancy. *American Journal of Obstetrics and Gynecology* **103**:338–347.

34   Parker JH (1985) Amerlex free triiodothyronine and free thyroxine levels in normal pregnancy. *British Journal of Obstetrics and Gynaecology* **92**:1234–1238.

35   Osathanondh R, Tulchinsky D, Chopra IJ (1976) Total and free thyroxine and triiodothyronine in normal and complicated pregnancy. *Journal of Clinical Endocrinology and Metabolism* **42**:98–102.

36   Natrajan PG, McGarrigle HHG, Lawrence DM, Lachelin GCL (1982) Plasma noradrenaline and adrenaline levels in normal pregnancy and in pregnancy-induced hypertension. *British Journal of Obstetrics and Gynaecology* **89**:1041–1045.

37   Rubin PC, Butters L, McCabe R, Reid JL (1986) Plasma catecholamines in pregnancy-induced hypertension. *Clinical Science* **71**:111–115.

38   Beilin LJ, Deacon J, Michael CA *et al.* (1983) Diurnal rhythms of blood pressure, plasma renin activity, angiotensin II and catecholamines in normotensive and hypertensive pregnancies. *Clinical and Experimental Hypertension – Hypertension in Pregnancy* **B2** (2):271–293.

39   Carr BR, Parker CR, Madden JD, MacDonald PC, Porter JC (1981) Maternal plasma adrenocorticotrophin and cortisol relationships throughout human pregnancy. *American Journal of Obstetrics and Gynecology* **139**:416–422.

40   Nolten WE, Lindheimer MD, Rueckert PA, Oparil S, Ehrlich EN (1980) Diurnal patterns and regulation of cortisol secretion in pregnancy. *Journal of Clinical Endocrinology and Metabolism* **51**:466–472.

41   Rees LH, Burke CW, Chard T, Evans SW, Letchworth AT (1975) Possible placental origin of ACTH in normal human pregnancy. *Nature* **254**:620–622.

42   Doe RP, Fernandez R, Seal US (1964) Measurement of corticosteroid-binding globulin in man. *Journal of Clinical Endocrinology* **24**:1029–1039.

43   Migeon CJ, Kenny FM, Taylor FH (1968) Cortisol production rate VIII. Pregnancy. *Journal of Clinical Endocrinology* **28**:661–666.

44   Pearson Murphy BE, Okouneff LM, Klein GP, Ngo SH (1981) Lack of specificity of cortisol determinations in human urine. *Journal of Clinical Endocrinology and Metabolism* **53**:91–99.

45   Nolten WE, Lindheimer MD, Oparil S, Ehrlich EN (1978) Desoxycorticosterone in normal pregnancy. I. Sequential studies of the secretory patterns of desoxycorticosterone, aldosterone, and cortisol. *American Journal of Obstetrics and Gynecology* **132**:414–420.

46   Biswas S, Rodek CH (1976) Plasma prolactin levels during pregnancy. *British Journal of Obstetrics and Gynaecology* **83**:683–687.

47   Boyer RM, Finkelstein JW, Kapen S, Hellman L (1975) Twenty-four hour prolactin (Prl) secretory patterns during pregnancy. *Journal of Clinical Endocrinology and Metabolism* **40**:1117–1120.

48   Rigg LA, Yen SSC (1977) Multiphasic prolactin secretion during parturition in human subjects. *American Journal of Obstetrics and Gynecology* **128**:215–218.

49   Jacobs HS (1991) The hypothalamus and pituitary gland. In Hytten F, Chamberlain G (eds) *Clinical Physiology in Obstetrics* 2nd edn, pp. 345–356. Oxford: Blackwell Scientific Publications.

50   Pitkin RM, Reynolds WA, Williams GA, Hargis GK (1979) Calcium metabolism in normal pregnancy: a longitudinal study. *American Journal of Obstetrics and Gynecology* **133**:781–787.

51   Robertson EG, Cheyne GA (1972) Plasma biochemistry

in relation to the oedema of pregnancy. *Journal of Obstetrics and Gynaecology of the British Commonwealth* **79**:769–776.

52 Newman RL (1957) Serum electrolytes in pregnancy, parturition, and puerperium. *Obstetrics and Gynecology* **10**:51–55.

53 Kuhlback B, Widholm O (1966) Plasma creatinine in normal pregnancy. *Scandinavian Journal of Laboratory and Clinical Investigations* **18**:654–656.

54 Davison J (1989) Renal disease. In de Swiet M (ed) *Medical Disorders in Obstetric Practice* 2nd edn, pp. 306–407. Oxford: Blackwell Scientific Publications.

55 Lind T, Godfrey KA, Otun H (1984) Changes in serum uric acid concentrations during normal pregnancy. *British Journal of Obstetrics and Gynaecology* **91**:128–132.

56 Davison JM, Noble MCB (1981) Serial changes in 24 hour creatinine clearance during normal menstrual cycles and the first trimester of pregnancy. *British Journal of Obstetrics and Gynaecology* **88**:10–17.

57 Davison JM, Dunlop W, Ezimokhai M (1980) 24-hour creatinine clearance during the third trimester of normal pregnancy. *British Journal of Obstetrics and Gynaecology* **87**:106–109.

58 Davison JM, Dunlop W (1980) Renal haemodynamics and tubular function in normal human pregnancy. *Kidney International* **18**:152–161.

59 Hytten FE, Cheyne GA (1972) The aminoaciduria of pregnancy. *Journal of Obstetrics and Gynaecology of the British Commonwealth* **79**:424–432.

60 Lopez-Espinola I, Dhar H, Humphreys S, Redman CWG (1986) Urinary albumin excretion in pregnancy. *British Journal of Obstetrics and Gynaecology* **93**:176–181.

61 Mendenhall HW (1970) Serum protein concentrations in pregnancy. *American Journal of Obstetrics and Gynecology* **106**:388–399.

62 Potter JM, Nestel PJ (1979) The hyperlipidaemia of pregnancy in normal and complicated pregnancies. *American Journal of Obstetrics and Gynecology* **133**:165–170.

63 Adeniyi FA, Olatunbosun DA (1984) Origins and significance of the increased plasma alkaline phosphatase during normal pregnancy and pre-eclampsia. *British Journal of Obstetrics and Gynaecology* **91**:857–862.

64 Walker FB, Hoblit DL, Cunningham FG, Combes B (1974) Gamma glutamyl transpeptidase in normal pregnancy. *Obstetrics and Gynecology* **43**:745–749.

65 McNair RD, Jaynes RV (1960) Alterations in liver function during normal pregnancy. *American Journal of Obstetrics and Gynecology* **80**:500–505.

66 Gallery ED, Raftos J, Gyory AZ, Wells JV (1981) A prospective study of serum complement (C3 and C4) levels during normal human pregnancy: effect of the development of pregnancy-associated hypertension. *Australian and New Zealand Journal of Medicine* **11**:243–245.

67 Schena FP, Manno C, Selvaggi L, Loverro G, Bettocchi S, Bonomo L (1982) Behaviour of immune complexes and the complement system in normal pregnancy and pre-eclampsia. *Journal of Clinical and Laboratory Immunology* **7**:21–26.

68 Jenkins JS, Powell RJ (1987) C3 degradation products (C3d) in normal pregnancy. *Journal of Clinical Pathology* **40**:1362–1363.

69 Hytten FE, Lind T (1973) Volume and composition of the blood. In *Diagnostic Indices in Pregnancy*, pp. 36–54. Basle, Switzerland: Documenta Geigy.

70 Mills MS (1992) Ultrasonography of early embryonic growth and fetal development. MD Thesis, University of Bristol.

71 Robinson HP, Fleming JEE (1975) A critical evaluation of sonar "crown-rump length" measurements. *British Journal of Obstetrics and Gynaecology* **82**:702–710.

72 Pedersen JF (1982) Fetal crown-rump length measurement by ultrasound in normal pregnancy. *British Journal of Obstetrics and Gynaecology* **89**:926–930.

73 Parker AJ, Davies P, Newton JR (1982) Assessment of gestational age of the Asian fetus by the sonar measurement of crown-rump length and biparietal diameter. *British Journal of Obstetrics and Gynaecology* **89**:836–838.

74 Erikson PS, Secher NJ, Weis-Bentzon M (1985) Normal growth of the fetal biparietal diameter and the abdominal diameter in a longitudinal study. *Acta Obstetrica et Gynecologica Scandinavica* **64**:65–70.

75 Chitty LS, Altman DG (1993) Charts of fetal size. In Dewbury K, Meire H, Cosgrove D (eds) *Ultrasound in Obstetrics and Gynaecology*, pp. 513–595. Edinburgh: Churchill Livingstone.

76 Hadlock FP, Deter RL, Harrist RB, Park SK (1982) Fetal head circumference: relation to menstrual age. *American Journal of Roentgenology* **138**:647–653.

77 Deter RL, Harrist RB, Hadlock FP, Poindexter AN (1982) Longitudinal studies of fetal growth with the use of dynamic image ultrasonography. *American Journal of Obstetrics and Gynecology* **143**:545–554.

78 Hadlock FP, Deter RL, Harrist RB, Park SK (1982) Fetal abdominal circumference as a predictor of menstrual age. *American Journal of Roentgenology* **139**:367–370.

79 Deter RL, Harrist RB, Hadlock FP, Carpenter RJ (1982) Fetal head and abdominal circumferences: II A critical re-evaluation of the relationship to menstrual age. *Journal of Clinical Ultrasound* **10**:365–372.

80 Warda AH, Deter RL, Rossavik IK, Carpenter RJ, Hadlock FP (1985) Fetal femur length: a critical reevaluation of the relationship to menstrual age. *Obstetrics and Gynecology* **66**:69–75.

81 Shalev E, Feldman E, Weiner E, Zuckerman H (1985) Assessment of gestational age by ultrasonic measurement of the femur length. *Acta Obstetrica et Gynecologica Scandinavica* **64**:71–74.

82 Merz E, Kim-Kern M-S, Pehl S (1987) Ultrasonic mensuration of fetal limb bones in the second and third trimesters. *Journal of Clinical Ultrasound* **15**:175–183.

83 Grannum P, Bracken M, Silverman R, Hobbins JC (1980) Assessment of fetal kidney size in normal gestation by comparison of ratio of kidney circumference to abdominal circumference. *American Journal of Obstetrics and Gynecology* **249**–254.

84 Mayden KL, Tortora M, Berkowitz RL, Bracken M, Hobbins JC (1982) Orbital diameters: a new parameter for prenatal diagnosis and dating. *American Journal of Obstetrics and Gynecology* **144**:289–297.

85 Goldstein I, Reece EA, Pilu G, Bovicelli L, Hobbins JC (1987) Cerebellar measurements with ultrasonography in the evaluation of fetal growth and development. *American Journal of Obstetrics and Gynecology* **156**:1065–1069.

86 Thompson AM, Billewicz WZ, Hytten FE (1968) The assessment of fetal growth. *Journal of Obstetrics and Gynaecology British Commonwealth* **75**:903–916.

87 Williams RL, Creasy RK, Cunningham GC, Hawes WE, Norris FD, Tashiro M (1982) Fetal growth and perinatal viability in California. *Obstetrics and Gynecology* **59**:624–632.

88 Campbell S, Wilkin D (1975) Ultrasonic measurement of fetal abdomen circumference in the estimation of fetal weight. *British Journal of Obstetrics and Gynaecology* **82**:689–697.

89 Shepard MJ, Richards VA, Berkowitz RL, Warsof SL, Hobbins JC (1982) An evaluation of two equations for predicting fetal weight by ultrasound. *American Journal of Obstetrics and Gynecology* **142**:47–54.

90 Hadlock FP, Harrist, RB, Carpenter RJ, Deter RL, Park SK (1984) Sonographic estimation of fetal weight. *Radiology* **150**:535–540.

91 Brace RA, Wolf EJ (1989) Normal amniotic fluid volume changes throughout pregnancy. *American Journal of Obstetrics and Gynecology* **161**:382–388.

92 Moore TR, Cayle JE (1990) The amniotic fluid index in normal human pregnancy. *American Journal of Obstetrics and Gynecology* **162**:1168–1173.

93 Fisk NM, Ronderos-Dumit D, Tannirandorn Y, Nicolini U, Talbert D (1992) Normal amniotic pressure throughout gestation. *British Journal of Obstetrics and Gynaecology* **99**:18–22.

94 Gilbert WM, Moore TR, Brace RA (1991) Amniotic fluid volume dynamics. *Fetal Medicine Review* **3**:89–104.

95 Lind T, Parkin FM, Cheyne GA (1969) Biochemical and cytological changes in liquor amnii with advancing gestation. *Journal of Obstetrics and Gynaecology British Commonwealth* **76**:673–683.

96 Pearce JM, Campbell S, Cohen-Overbeek T, Hackett G, Hernandez J, Royston JP (1988) Reference ranges and sources of variation for indices of pulsed Doppler flow velocity waveforms from the uteroplacental and fetal circulation. *British Journal of Obstetrics and Gynaecology* **95**:248–256.

97 Erskine RLA, Ritchie JWK (1985) Umbilical artery blood flow characteristics in normal and growth-retarded fetuses. *British Journal of Obstetrics and Gynaecology* **92**:605–610.

98 Forestier F (1987) Some aspects of fetal biology. *Fetal Therapy* **2**:181–187.

99 Takagi K, Tanaka H, Nishijima S *et al.* (1989) Fetal blood values by percutaneous umbilical blood sampling. *Fetal Therapy* **4**:152–160.

100 Nicolaides KH, Economides DL, Soothill PW (1989) Blood gases, pH, and lactate in appropriate- and small-for-gestational-age fetuses. *American Journal of Obstetrics and Gynecology* **161**:996–1001.

101 Soothill PW, Nicolaides KH, Rodeck CH, Campbell S (1986) Effect of gestational age on fetal and intervillous blood gas and acid-base values in human pregnancy. *Fetal Therapy* **1**:168–175.

102 Nicolini U, Fisk NM, Rodeck CH, Beacham J (1992) Fetal urine biochemistry: an index of renal maturation and dysfunction. *British Journal of Obstetrics and Gynaecology* **99**:46–50.

103 Thorpe-Beeston JG, Nicolaides KH, Felton CV, Butler J, McGregor AM (1991) Maturation of the secretion of thyroid hormone and thyroid stimulating hormone in the fetus. *New England Journal of Medicine* 1991; **324**:532–536.

104 Nicolaides KH, Rodeck CH, Mibashan RS, Kemp JR (1986) Have Liley charts outlived their usefulness? *American Journal of Obstetrics and Gynecology* **155**:90–94.

105 Sadovsky G, Nicolaides KH (1989) Reference ranges for fetal heart rate patterns in normoxaemic nonanaemic fetuses. *Fetal Therapy* **4**:61–68.

106 Arulkumaran S, Ingemarsson I, Montan S *et al.* (1992) *Guidelines for Interpretation of Antepartum and Intrapartum Cardiotocography.* Hewlett Packard.

107 Duignan NM, Studd JWW, Hughes AO (1975) Characteristics of normal labour in different racial groups. *British Journal of Obstetrics and Gynaecology* **82**:593–601.

Index